# The Glaucoma Book

Paul N. Schacknow • John R. Samples
Editors

# The Glaucoma Book

A Practical, Evidence-Based Approach
to Patient Care

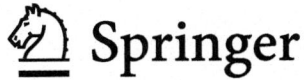

Editors
Dr. Paul N. Schacknow
Visual Health Center
2889 10th Avenue, N.
Palm Springs, FL 33461
USA

Dr. John R. Samples
Oregon Health & Sciences University
Casey Eye Institute
Department of Ophthalmology
3375 SW, Terwilliger Blvd.
Portland OR 97201-4197
USA

ISBN 978-0-387-76699-7        e-ISBN 978-0-387-76700-0
DOI 10.1007/978-0-387-76700-0
Springer New York Dordrecht Heidelberg London

Library of Congress Control Number: 2010921595

© Springer Science+Business Media, LLC 2010
All rights reserved. This work may not be translated or copied in whole or in part without the written permission of the publisher (Springer Science+Business Media, LLC, 233 Spring Street, New York, NY 10013, USA), except for brief excerpts in connection with reviews or scholarly analysis. Use in connection with any form of information storage and retrieval, electronic adaptation, computer software, or by similar or dissimilar methodology now known or hereafter developed is forbidden.
The use in this publication of trade names, trademarks, service marks, and similar terms, even if they are not identified as such, is not to be taken as an expression of opinion as to whether or not they are subject to proprietary rights.
While the advice and information in this book are believed to be true and accurate at the date of going to press, neither the authors nor the editors nor the publisher can accept any legal responsibility for any errors or omissions that may be made. The publisher makes no warranty, express or implied, with respect to the material contained herein.

Custom illustrations by Alice Y. Chen, aliceychen.com

Printed on acid-free paper

Springer is part of Springer Science+Business Media (www.springer.com)

The gestational period for *The Glaucoma Book* has exceeded that of the African elephant (Loxodonta africana) whose pregnancy lasts an average of 660 days. The 2-year period from its conception to parturition has been filled with both pain and joy, similar to the human birth process. When two friends and colleagues decide to create a major textbook on glaucoma, it places a great strain not only upon them, but upon the ones that they love. Our wives, Sharma Schacknow and Griffen Samples, and our children Wesley Samples, Laura Samples, and Jeffrey Schacknow have shared with us our ups and downs, our late night phone calls, our unavailability for normal social functions, our thousands of e-mails to parts unknown and our happiness that this project has finally come to a wonderfully successful conclusion. No marriages were lost, no children abandoned. We dedicate this book with love to all of these family members who helped us maintain our mental equilibrium. We are back more fully in your lives. Hopefully, the copy of *The Glaucoma Book* that each family will have on the living room coffee table, will daily serve to remind each family that Paul and John have worked very hard to better the lives of our patients for whom they took an oath to serve and cure.

Paul Schacknow and John Samples

# Foreword

Putting together a comprehensive, multiauthored text is a daunting task. However, the benefits may justify the effort. Such is the case with regards to the present *Glaucoma Book*. It is not likely that many ophthalmologists (or others) will decide, at the end of a busy day, to pour themselves a cocktail, and settle into a comfortable chair with this large tome in hand, with the intent of reading it from start to finish. A pity. It would make several enjoyable and profitable days of good reading.

The text starts with comments by an individual who is strongly grounded in the fundamentals of being a good physician. Ivan Goldberg has used his brilliance, his wide international experiences and knowledge, and his commitment to assuring that physicians know their craft, to provide a penetrating perspective on ophthalmology today and tomorrow. *The Glaucoma Book* ends with commentaries by the editors, John Samples, a true physician/scientist, and Paul Schacknow, an experienced community-based clinician. Samples' essay "What Really Causes Glaucoma?" nicely describes the leading theories underlying the cell biology of glaucoma. In "What Do We Know Now, What Do We Need to Know About Glaucoma?," Schacknow offers an essay on some of the controversial ideas raised within the book and speculates on future research. The stage is set for comments by the world's leading experts in the field of glaucoma, and their trainees, to deal with the issues raised by Goldberg: the final curtain closes with the difficult but valid idea that while we know a lot, and are knowing more, there is no substitute for observing clearly and pondering thoughtfully.

It is disturbing that half (or more) of the world's people who have glaucoma never even get diagnosed; it is tragic that glaucoma is the leading cause of irreversible blindness in the world, when the overwhelming bulk of that misery could have been prevented by proper diagnosis and treatment. We are not clearly doing our job well; there is clearly much to learn and lots to do.

While it is not the traditional way physicians use large texts, ophthalmologists would do well to spend several hours by the fire with *The Glaucoma Book*. The people who would really benefit would be patients.

George L. Spaeth<br>
Esposito Research Professor<br>
Wills Eye Institute<br>
Philadelphia, PA<br>
USA

# Preface

Do we really need another book about glaucoma diagnosis and management? There are probably several classic, fairly up-to-date, texts about glaucoma sitting on your bookshelf. Who would have the audacity to write a new text entitled *"The" Glaucoma Book*, as though it would be the one you would turn to first for definitive, pragmatic answers to questions about diagnosis and management of your patients? Not just a comprehensive academic work with evidence-based science and exhaustive bibliographies, but also an everyday, pragmatic guide for comprehensive ophthalmologists, optometrists, and resident physicians, who would look to it for answers to clinical questions while patients are being examined in their offices.

*The Glaucoma Book* has been written by physicians. Many of them are members of the American Glaucoma Society; all are either fellowship-trained glaucoma specialists, their current glaucoma fellows, and exceptional residents, optometric physicians, or experts on some special topics. These colleagues have large clinical practices and years of experience dealing with the everyday issues that confront eye physicians who manage glaucoma patients.

Our goal was to create both a clinically based book and an academic reference that would serve to bring the explosion of new glaucoma diagnostic techniques and therapeutic interventions to those doctors in the trenches who see the great majority of glaucoma patients. We invited not only "the usual suspects" from well-known academic institutions, whose names you are familiar with from the literature and international scientific congresses, but also community-based, real world ophthalmologists, who both know the latest science and also how to see 50 patients in a day while still delivering state-of-the-art care.

This book is nontraditional in several ways. We do not include a great deal of discussion on eye anatomy. We do have sidebar essays, inside of major chapters, that discuss important subtopics in greater detail. We have allowed the style to vary among manuscripts, some are more formal, with a large number of references, and some are more informal with a reflective or philosophical bent and few or no references. Photos, illustrations, and tables are sprinkled liberally throughout the book where most appropriate. The topic choices range from the conventional (e.g., open angle glaucoma, pigmentary dispersion syndrome) to those that have not previously appeared in a glaucoma textbook (e.g., medical-legal aspects of glaucoma care, doing community-based glaucoma research). *The Glaucoma Book* is intentionally idiosyncratic in its design.

We have allowed each author the space needed to discuss their assigned topic, so some chapters are longer than others. There is considerable overlap and redundancy in this multiauthored text. This repetition of ideas and facts, from different perspectives, adds strength to the volume. While some topics may be explored to different depths within different chapters, each chapter stands on its own and may be read without having a need to build upon a previous chapter. Cross-referencing of similar topics between chapters and sidebars is done within chapters.

*The Glaucoma Book* is divided into six sections, containing 92 chapters and 38 sidebar essays. Topics are presented in what seemed like a logical order. The book can be read from front to back or sampled intermittently as interesting patients present themselves in your practice. We did not censor our authors from expressing unconventional scientific ideas, as long as they could present convincing arguments for their opinions. This book is not meant for glaucoma subspecialists who are surely familiar with most of the information it contains. (Of course, we hope that a few of them too will buy a copy!) Rather, the editors feel that we have created an informative, useful tool for the working ophthalmologists and the ophthalmologists in training on current thinking in glaucoma circles. This should ultimately benefit our glaucoma patients who place their trust in us for proper diagnosis and treatment.

Lake Worth, FL  Paul Schacknow
Portland, OR  John Samples

# Contents

**Part I  The Basics**

1. Glaucoma in the Twenty-First Century .................................................. 3
   Ridia Lim and Ivan Goldberg

2. An Evidence-Based Approach to Glaucoma Care ................................... 23
   Louis R. Pasquale

3. Glaucoma Risk Factors: Intraocular Pressure ....................................... 35
   Nils A. Loewen and Angelo P. Tanna

4. Glaucoma Risk Factors: Fluctuations in Intraocular Pressure ................ 51
   Felipe A. Medeiros

5. Glaucoma is a 24/7 Disease ................................................................. 55
   Amish B. Doshi, John H.K. Liu, and Robert N. Weinreb

6. Continuous Monitoring of Intraocular Pressure .................................... 59
   Ron E.P. Frenkel, Max P.C. Frenkel, and Shamim A. Haji

7. Aqueous Veins and Open Angle Glaucoma .......................................... 65
   Murray Johnstone, Annisa Jamil, and Elizabeth Martin

8. Glaucoma Risk Factors: The Cornea .................................................... 79
   Lionel Marzette and Leon Herndon

9. Glaucoma Risk Factors: Family History – The Genetics of Glaucoma ..... 91
   John R. Samples

10. Glaucoma Risk Factors: Ethnicity and Glaucoma ................................ 101
    M. Roy Wilson and Mark Gallardo

11. Glaucoma Risk Factors: Ocular Blood Flow ....................................... 111
    Brent Siesky, Alon Harris, Rita Ehrlich, Nisha Kheradiya,
    and Carlos Rospigliosi Lopez

12. Glaucoma Risk Factors: Sleep Apnea and Glaucoma ......................... 135
    Rick E. Bendel and Janet A. Betchkal

13. Evaluating Ophthalmic Literature ..................................................... 139
    Dan Eisenberg and Paul N. Schacknow

| 14 | Indications for Therapy | 155 |

George L. Spaeth

## Part II  The Examination

| 15 | Clinical Examination of the Optic Nerve | 169 |

Scott J. Fudemberg, Yuanjun Zhao, Jonathan S. Myers, and L. Jay Katz

| 16 | Clinical Cupping: Laminar and Prelaminar Components | 185 |

Claude F. Burgoyne, Hongli Yang, and J. Crawford Downs

| 17 | Disc Hemorrhages and Glaucoma | 195 |

David J. Palmer

| 18 | Some Lessons from the Disc Appearance in the Open Angle Glaucomas | 199 |

Stephen M. Drance

| 19 | Evaluating the Optic Nerve for Glaucomatous Progression | 203 |

Felipe A. Medeiros

| 20 | Digital Imaging of the Optic Nerve | 209 |

Shan Lin and George Tanaka

| 21 | Clinical Utility of Computerized Optic Nerve Analysis | 219 |

Neil T. Choplin

| 22 | Photography of the Optic Nerve | 223 |

Roy Whitaker Jr. and Von Best Whitaker

| 23 | Detecting Functional Changes in the Patient's Vision: Visual Field Analysis | 229 |

Chris A. Johnson

| 24 | Using Electroretinography for Glaucoma Diagnosis | 265 |

Kevin C. Leonard and Cindy M. L. Hutnik

| 25 | Glaucomatous Versus Nonglaucomatous Visual Loss: The Neuro-Ophthalmic Perspective | 269 |

Matthew D. Kay, Mark L. Moster, and Paul N. Schacknow

| 26 | Gonioscopy | 283 |

Reid Longmuir

| 27 | Beyond Gonioscopy: Digital Imaging of the Anterior Segment | 293 |

Robert J. Noecker

| 28 | Office Examination of the Glaucoma Patient | 301 |

Paul N. Schacknow

| 29 | Glaucoma and Driving | 339 |

Odette Callender

| 30 | Electronic Medical Records in the Glaucoma Practice | 343 |

Mildred M.G. Olivier and Linda Hay

| | | |
|---|---|---|
| 31 | **Advanced Glaucoma and Low Vision: Evaluation and Treatment**.................... | 351 |
| | Scott Robison | |
| 32 | **Glaucoma and Medical Insurance: Billing and Coding Issues**....................... | 383 |
| | Cynthia Mattox | |
| 33 | **Medical Legal Considerations When Treating Glaucoma Patients**.................. | 391 |
| | J. Wesley Samples and John R. Samples | |

**Part III    The Glaucomas**

| | | |
|---|---|---|
| 34 | **Primary Open Angle Glaucoma**....................................................... | 399 |
| | Matthew G. McMenemy | |
| 35 | **Normal Pressure Glaucoma**............................................................ | 421 |
| | Bruce E. Prum | |
| 36 | **Primary and Secondary Angle-Closure Glaucomas**................................. | 461 |
| | Marshall N. Cyrlin | |
| 37 | **Malignant Glaucoma (Posterior Aqueous Diversion Syndrome)**................... | 489 |
| | Marshall N. Cyrlin | |
| 38 | **Pigmentary Dispersion Syndrome and Glaucoma**................................... | 499 |
| | Celso Tello, Nathan Radcliffe, and Robert Ritch | |
| 39 | **Exfoliation Syndrome and Glaucoma**................................................. | 507 |
| | Anastasios G. P. Konstas, Gábor Holló, and Robert Ritch | |
| 40 | **Neovascular Glaucoma**................................................................. | 517 |
| | Donald Minckler | |
| 41 | **Inflammatory Disease and Glaucoma**................................................. | 527 |
| | Sunita Radhakrishnan, Emmett T. Cunningham Jr, and Andrew Iwach | |
| 42 | **Posner–Schlossman Syndrome**........................................................ | 537 |
| | Raghu C. Mudumbai and Sarwat Salim | |
| 43 | **Fuchs' Uveitis Syndrome and Glaucoma**............................................. | 539 |
| | Edney R. Moura Filho and Thomas J. Liesegang | |
| 44 | **Herpes Simplex Related Glaucoma**................................................... | 545 |
| | Edney R. Moura Filho and Thomas J. Liesegang | |
| 45 | **Herpes Zoster Related Glaucoma**.................................................... | 549 |
| | Edney R. Moura Filho and Thomas J. Liesegang | |
| 46 | **Iridocorneal Endothelial Syndrome and Glaucoma**................................. | 553 |
| | Sarwat Salim and Peter A. Netland | |
| 47 | **Ghost Cell Glaucoma**................................................................... | 555 |
| | Dinorah P. Engel Castro and Cynthia Mattox | |
| 48 | **Fuchs' Endothelial Dystrophy and Glaucoma**....................................... | 557 |
| | Blair Boehmer and Clark Springs | |

## 49 Ocular Trauma and Glaucoma ... 561
Helen Tseng and Kenneth Mitchell

## 50 Infantile, Childhood, and Juvenile Glaucomas ... 567
David S. Walton

## Part IV  The Medical Treatment

## 51 Medications Used to Treat Glaucoma ... 583
Paul N. Schacknow and John R. Samples

## 52 Choosing Adjunctive Glaucoma Therapy ... 629
Jess T. Whitson

## 53 Monocular Drug Trials for Glaucoma Therapy in the Community Setting ... 643
Tony Realini

## 54 Neuroprotection of Retinal Ganglion Cells ... 647
Alvaro P.C. Lupinacci, Howard Barnebey, and Peter A. Netland

## 55 Compliance and Adherence: Lifelong Therapy for Glaucoma ... 651
Alan Robin, Betsy Sleath, and David Covert

## 56 Alternative and Non-traditional Treatments of Glaucoma ... 657
Joseph R. Zelefsky and Robert Ritch

## 57 Intravitreal Steroids and Glaucoma ... 671
Yousuf Khalifa and Sandra M. Johnson

## 58 Pregnancy and Glaucoma ... 673
Jeff Martow

## 59 Systemic Side Effects of Glaucoma Medications ... 677
Paul Lama

## 60 Systemic Diseases and Glaucoma ... 689
Paul Lama

## Part V  The Surgical Treatment

## 61 Laser Therapies: Iridotomy, Iridoplasty, and Trabeculoplasty ... 713
Douglas Gaasterland

## 62 Laser Iridoplasty Techniques for Narrow Angles and Plateau Iris Syndrome ... 741
Baseer U. Khan

## 63 Laser Therapies: Cyclodestructive Procedures ... 749
Christopher J. Russo and Malik Y. Kahook

## 64 Laser Therapies: Newer Technologies ... 753
Michael S. Berlin and Kevin Taliaferro

## 65 Incisional Therapies: Trabeculectomy Surgery ... 765
Shlomo Melamed and Daniel Cotlear

| 66 | **Incisional Therapies: Trabeculotomy Surgery in Adults** | 789 |
|---|---|---|
| | Ronald L. Fellman | |
| 67 | **Incisional Therapies: Canaloplasty and New Implant Devices** | 795 |
| | Diamond Y. Tam and Iqbal "Ike" K. Ahmed | |
| 68 | **Incisional Therapies: Shunts and Valved Implants** | 813 |
| | John W. Boyle IV and Peter A. Netland | |
| 69 | **Incisional Therapies: What's on the Horizon?** | 831 |
| | Richard A. Hill and Don S. Minckler | |
| 70 | **Incisional Therapies: Complications of Glaucoma Surgery** | 841 |
| | Marlene R. Moster and Augusto Azuara-Blanco | |
| 71 | **Amniotic Membrane Grafts for Glaucoma Surgery** | 861 |
| | Hosam Sheha, Lingyi Liang, and Scheffer C.G. Tseng | |
| 72 | **Treating Choroidal Effusions After Glaucoma Surgery** | 867 |
| | Jody Piltz-Seymour | |
| 73 | **Cyclodialysis Clefts: Surgical and Traumatic** | 871 |
| | George R. Reiss | |
| 74 | **Epithelial Downgrowth** | 877 |
| | Matthew C. Willett, Sami Al-Shahwan, and Deepak P. Edward | |
| 75 | **Penetrating Keratoplasty and Glaucoma** | 883 |
| | Michele L. Scott and Peter A. Netland | |
| 76 | **Descemet's Stripping Endothelial Keratoplasty (DSEK) and Glaucoma** | 885 |
| | Theodoros Filippopoulos, Kathryn A. Colby, and Cynthia L. Grosskreutz | |
| 77 | **Cataract and Glaucoma Surgery** | 889 |
| | Joseph R. Zelefsky and Stephen A. Obstbaum | |
| 78 | **Cataract Extraction as Treatment for Acute and Chronic Angle Closure Glaucomas** | 905 |
| | Baseer U. Khan | |
| 79 | **Refractive Surgery and Glaucoma** | 913 |
| | Sarwat Salim and Peter A. Netland | |
| 80 | **Glaucoma after Retinal Surgery** | 917 |
| | Annisa L. Jamil, Scott D. Lawrence, David A. Saperstein, Elliott M. Kanner, Richard P. Mills, and Peter A. Netland | |

**Part VI   The Future**

| 81 | **Immunology and Glaucoma** | 925 |
|---|---|---|
| | Michal Schwartz and Anat London | |
| 82 | **How the Revolution in Cell Biology Will Affect Glaucoma: Biomarkers** | 933 |
| | Paul A. Knepper, Michael J. Nolan, and Beatrice Y. J. T. Yue | |

| 83 | **CD44 and Primary Open Angle Glaucoma** | 939 |

Paul A. Knepper, Michael J. Nolan, and Beatrice Y.J.T. Yue

| 84 | **Stem Cells and Glaucoma** | 953 |

Shan Lin, Mary Kelley, and John Samples

| 85 | **Cytoskeletal Active Agents for Glaucoma Therapy** | 955 |

Jennifer A. Faralli, Marie K. Schwinn, Donna M. Peters, and Paul L. Kaufman

| 86 | **The Drug Discovery Process: How Do New Glaucoma Medications Come to Market?** | 961 |

Michael Bergamini

| 87 | **Glaucoma Clinical Research in the Community Setting** | 977 |

Harvey DuBiner, Helen DuBiner, and Paul N. Schacknow

| 88 | **Future Glaucoma Medical Therapies: What's in the Pipeline?** | 983 |

Abbot F. Clark

| 89 | **Anecortave Acetate: A New Approach for the Medical Treatment of Glaucoma** | 989 |

Amy Lewis Hennessy and Alan L. Robin

| 90 | **Future Glaucoma Instrumentation: Diagnostic and Therapeutic** | 995 |

Kelly A. Townsend, Gadi Wollstein, and Joel S. Schuman

| 91 | **What Really Causes Glaucoma?** | 1011 |

John R. Samples

| 92 | **The Glaucoma Book: What Do We Know Now, What Do We Need to Know About Glaucoma?** | 1015 |

Paul N. Schacknow

**Index** .................................................................................................. 1023

# Sidebars

Sidebar 4.1 Rapid Oscillations in Intraocular Pressure
*W. Daniel Stamer and Renata F. Ramos*

Sidebar 8.1 Pachymeters for Measuring Central Corneal Thickness
*Odette Callender*

Sidebar 10.1 Glaucoma in Latinos
*Elizabeth Salinas-Van Orman*

Sidebar 11.1 Ocular Perfusion Pressure and Glaucoma: Another View
*Edney R. Moura Filho and Arthur J. Sit*

Sidebar 15.1 Alpha-beta Peripapillary Atrophy
*S. Fabian Lerner*

Sidebar 15.2 Relative Afferent Pupillary Defects in Glaucoma Patients
*Edney R. Moura Filho and Rajesh K. Shetty*

Sidebar 23.1 Lens Induced Artifacts During Visual Field Testing
*Andrew C. S. Crichton*

Sidebar 23.2 Another Perspective on the Need for Goldmann Visual Fields in the Era of Automated Visual Fields
*Andrew C. S. Crichton*

Sidebar 31.1 Contact Lenses and the Glaucoma Patient
*Jane Bachman Groth*

Sidebar 34.1 Glaucoma Suspects - When to Treat, When to Observe
*Sophio Liao and Alan Robin*

Sidebar 34.2. Proteoglycan Biosynthesis and Degradation: What Really Causes Glaucoma?
*Ted Acott, Kate Keller, Mary Kelley, and John Samples*

Sidebar 36.1 Topiramate, Uveal Effusion and Secondary Angle Closure Glaucoma
*Theodoros Filippopoulos and Cynthia L. Grosskreutz*

Sidebar 40.1 Open Angle Glaucoma and Central Retinal Vein Occlusion
*Meena Beri*

Sidebar 40.2 Central Retinal Vein Occlusion and Monitoring Risk of Neovascular Glaucoma
*John Hyatt, Sarwat Salim, and Peter A. Netland*

Sidebar 41.1 Laboratory Testing for Uveitis in the Glaucoma Patient
*Omar Chaudhary and Sandra M. Johnson*

Sidebar 51.1 Circadian Variation of Aqueous Humor Dynamics: Implications for Glaucoma Therapy
*Arthur J. Sit*

Sidebar 51.2 How to Use Eye Drops to Treat Glaucoma
*Odette Callender*

Sidebar 51.3 Preservatives and Glaucoma Medications
*Clark L. Springs*

Sidebar 51.4 Carbonic Anhydrase Inhibitors
*Sophio Liao and Alan Robin*

Sidebar 51.5 Hyperosmotic Agents for the Acute Management of Glaucoma
*Kayoung Yi and Teresa C. Chen*

Sidebar 52.1 Combination Medical Therapy for Glaucoma
*Todd D. Severin*

Sidebar 60.1 Antihypertensive Medications and Glaucoma
*Kevin C. Leonard and Cindy M. L. Hutnik*

Sidebar 60.2 Glaucoma, Diet, Exercise, and Life Style
*Janet Betchkal and Rick Bendel*

Sidebar 60.3 Statin Medications and Glaucoma
*Kevin C. Leonard and Cindy M. L. Hutnik*

Sidebar 61.1 Comparing Laser Instruments
*Yara Catoira-Boyle*

Sidebar 61.2 New Forms of Trabeculoplasty
*Giorgio Dorin and John Samples*

Sidebar 61.3 Corneal Edema Following Angle Closure - How to Perform Laser Iridotomy
*Peter T. Chang*

Sidebar 65.1 Incisional Glaucoma Surgery—Making the Decision to Operate
*Claudia U. Richter*

Sidebar 65.2 Anticoagulants and Glaucoma Surgery
*Siva S. Radhakrishnan Iyer, Sarwat Salim, and Peter A. Netland*

Sidebar 65.3 Fornix Versus Limbal Based Flaps
*Kenneth B. Mitchell*

Sidebar 65.4 Antimetabolites and Glaucoma Surgery
*Claudia U. Richter*

Sidebar 68.1 Trabeculectomy or Tube Shunt Surgery – Which to Perform?
*Daniel A. Jewelewicz*

Sidebar 68.2 Encapsulated Filtering Blebs after Glaucoma Shunt Surgery
*Sandra M. Johnson*

Sidebar 70.1 Postoperative Flat Anterior Chamber
*Janet Betchkal and Rick Bendel*

Sidebar 70.2 Hypotony Maculopathy After Glaucoma Surgery
*Raghu C. Mudumbai and Sarwat Salim*

Sidebar 70.3 Fibrin Glue and Glaucoma Surgery
*Andrew M. Hendrick and Malik Y. Kahook*

Sidebar 77.1 Flomax: Implications for Glaucoma and Cataract Surgery
*Maria Basile and John Danias*

Sidebar 77.2 Anterior Chamber Intraocular Lenses, Pupillary Block and Peripheral Iridectomy
*Christopher C. Shen, Sarwat Salim, and Peter A. Netland*

# Contributors

**Ted S. Acott, PhD**
Professor, Department of Ophthalmology, Casey Eye Institute, Oregon Health and Science University, Portland, OR, USA

**Iqbal "Ike" K. Ahmed, MD, FRCSC**
Department of Ophthalmology, Credit Valley Eye Care, Mississauga, ON, Canada

**Sami Al-Shahwan, MD**
Senior Academic Consultant, Department of Glaucoma Services, King Khaled Eye Specialist Hospital, Riyadh, Kingdom of Saudi Arabia

**Augusto Azuara-Blanco, MD, PhD, FRCS(Ed)**
Consultant Ophthalmologist and Honorary Senior Lecturer, Department of Ophthalmology, Aberdeen Royal Infirmary, The Eye Clinic, University of Aberdeen, Foresterhill, Aberdeen, Scotland, UK

**Howard Barnebey, MD**
Glaucoma Director, Specialty Eyecare Centre, Bellevue, WA, USA

**Maria Basile, MD**
Assistant Professor, Department of Ophthalmology, New York Eye and Ear Infirmary, Beth Israel Hospital, New York, NY, USA

**Rick E. Bendel, MD**
Assistant Professor of Ophthalmology, Mayo Clinic Jacksonville, Mayo School of Medicine, Consultant, Department of Ophthalmology, Jacksonville, FL, USA

**Michael V. W. Bergamini, BS, PhD**
Adjunct Professor, Department of Pharmacology and Neuroscience, University of North Texas Health Services Center, Fort Worth, TX, USA

**Meena Beri, MD**
Beri Eye Care Associates, Portland, OR, USA

**Michael S. Berlin, MS, MD**
Director, Glaucoma Institute of Beverly Hills, Los Angeles, CA, USA

**Janet Betchkal, MD**
Chairman, Department of Ophthalmology, St. Vincent's Medical Center, Jacksonville, FL, USA

**Blair Boehmer, MD**
Department of Ophthalmology, Indiana University School of Medicine, Indianapolis, IN, USA

**John W. Boyle IV, MD**
Instructor of Ophthalmology, Hamilton Eye Institute, University of Tennessee Health Science Center, Memphis, TN, USA

**Claude F. Burgoyne, MD**
Senior Scientist and Van Buskirk Chair for Ophthalmic Research, Research Director, Optic Nerve Head Research Laboratory, Discoveries in Sight Research Laboratories, Devers Eye Institute, Legacy Health System, Portland, OR, USA

**Odette V. Callender, MD**
Chief of Ophthalmology, Wilmington VA Medical Center, Wilmington, DE, USA

**Dinorah P. Engel Castro, MD**
New England Eye Center, Department of Ophthalmology/Glaucoma Service, Tufts Medical Center, Boston, MA, USA

**Yara Paula Catoira-Boyle, MD**
Assistant Professor of Clinical Ophthalmology, Department of Ophthalmology, Indiana University School of Medicine, Indianapolis, IN, USA

**Peter T. Chang, MD**
Assistant Professor of Ophthalmology, Department of Ophthalmology, Baylor College of Medicine, Houston, TX, USA

**Omar Chaudhary, MD**
Resident, Department of Ophthalmology and Visual Science, Yale University School of Medicine, New Haven, CT, USA

**Teresa C. Chen, MD**
Assistant Professor of Ophthalmology, Department of Ophthalmology, Glaucoma Service, Massachusetts Eye and Ear Infirmary, Harvard Medical School, Boston, MA, USA

**Neil T. Choplin, MD**
Eye Care of San Diego, San Diego, CA, USA

**Abbot F. Clark, PhD**
Professor, Department of Cell Biology & Genetics, Director, The North Texas Eye Research Institute, University of North Texas Health Sciences Center, Fort Worth, TX, USA

**Kathryn Colby, MD, PhD**
Department of Ophthalmology, Cornea Service, Massachusetts Eye and Ear Infirmary, Harvard Medical School, Boston, MA, USA

**Anastasios P. Costarides, MD, PhD**
Firman Professor of Ophthalmology, Department of Emory Eye Center, Emory University School of Medicine, Atlanta, GA, USA

**Daniel Cotlear, MD**
Director, the Glaucoma Service-Barzilai Medical Center, Ashkelon, Tel – Hashomer, Israel
Consultant, the Sam Rothberg Glaucoma Center, Sheba Medical Center, Tel – Hashomer, Israel
Department of Ophthalmology, Goldschleger Eye Institute, Ashkelon, Tel – Hashomer, Israel

**David W. Covert, MBA**
Associate Director, Department of Health Economics, Alcon Research Limited, Fort Worth, TX, USA

**Andrew C. S. Crichton, MD, FRCS**
Clinical Professor of Surgery, Department of Ophthalmology, University of Calgary, Calgary, AB, Canada

**Emmett T. Cunningham Jr., MD, PhD, MPH**
Adjunct Clinical Professor, Stanford University School of Medicine, Stanford, CA, USA
Director, Department of Ophthalmology, The Uveitis Service, California Pacific Medical Center, San Francisco, CA, USA

**Marshall N. Cyrlin, MD**
Clinical Professor of Ophthalmology, Oakland University William Beaumont
School of Medicine, Rochester, MI, USA
Emeritus Director, Glaucoma Services, William Beaumont Eye Institute, Royal Oak, MI, USA
Associated Vision Consultants, Southfield, MI, USA

**John Danias, MD, PhD**
Associate Professor, Department of Ophthalmology, Mount Sinai Medical Center,
New York, NY, USA

**Giorgio Dorin**
Nuclear Electronics Engineer, Director, Clinical Applications Development,
IRIDEX Corporation Inc., Mountain View, CA, USA

**Amish B. Doshi, MD**
Director of Glaucoma Service, Kaiser Permanente, Department of Ophthalmology,
Antioch, CA, USA

**J. Crawford Downs, PhD**
Associate Scientist and Director, Ocular Biomechanics Laboratory, Discoveries in Sight
Research Laboratories, Devers Eye Institute, Legacy Health System, Portland, OR, USA

**Stephen M. Drance OC, MD**
Department of Ophthalmology, University of British Columbia, Vancouver, BC, Canada

**Harvey DuBiner, MD**
Glaucoma Director, Clayton Eye Center, Morrow, GA, USA

**Helen DuBiner, PharmD**
Clayton Eye Center, Clinical Study Coordinator, Morrow, GA, USA

**Deepak P. Edward, MD, FACS**
Professor, Chair, Program Director, Department of Ophthalmology, Northeastern Ohio
Universities College of Medicine, Summa Health Systems, Akron, OH, USA

**Rita Ehrlich, MD**
Department of Ophthalmology, Indiana University School of Medicine,
Indianapolis, IN, USA

**Dan Eisenberg, MD**
The Shepherd Eye Center, Las Vegas, NV, USA

**Jennifer A. Faralli, PhD**
Research Associate, Department of Pathology, University of Wisconsin,
Madison, WI, USA

**Ronald L. Fellman, MD**
Associate Clinical Professor of Ophthalmology, University of Texas Southwestern
Medical Center, Dallas, TX, USA
Glaucoma Associates of Texas, Dallas, TX, USA

**Edney de Resende Moura Filho, MD**
Fellow, Mayo Clinic, Jacksonville, FL, USA

**Theodoros Filippopoulos, MD**
Glaucoma Fellow, Assistant in Ophthalmology, Department of Ophthalmology,
Massachusetts Eye & Ear Infirmary, Harvard Medical School, Boston, MA, USA
Athens Vision Eye Institute, Kallithea, Athens, Greece

**Max P. C. Frenkel**
Department of Ophthalmology, Eye Research Foundation, Stuart, FL, USA

**Ronald E. P. Frenkel, MD, FACS, FICS**
Voluntary Associate Professor, Department of Ophthalmology, University of Miami, Bascom Palmer Eye Institute, Miami, FL

**Scott J. Fudemberg, MD**
Instructor, Glaucoma Department, Wills Eye Institute, Jefferson Medical College, Philadelphia, PA, USA

**Douglas E. Gaasterland, MD**
Clinical Professor, Eye Doctors of Washington, Department of Ophthalmology, Georgetown University & George Washington University, Chevy Chase, MD, USA

**Mark Gallardo, MD**
Assistant Professor/Director of Ophthalmology Services, Department of Ophthalmology, Texas Tech Health Sciences Center – El Paso, El Paso, TX, USA

**Ivan Goldberg, MBBS, FRANZCO, FRACS**
Clinical Associate Professor, Department of Ophthalmology, Eye Associates, Sydney Eye Hospital, University of Sydney, Floor 4, Sydney, NSW, Australia

**Cynthia L. Grosskreutz, MD, PhD**
Associate Professor of Ophthalmology, Co-Director, Glaucoma Service, Department of Ophthalmology, Massachusetts Eye & Ear Infirmary, Harvard Medical School, Boston, MA, USA

**Jane A. Bachman Groth, OD**
Attending Clinical Faculty, Department of Ophthalmology, Medical College of Wisconsin, Milwaukee, WI, USA

**Shamin A. Haji, MD**
Eye Research Foundation, East Florida Eye Institute, Stuart, FL, USA

**Alon Harris, PhD**
Lois Letzter Professor of Ophthalmology, Professor of Cellular and Integrative Physiology, Department of Ophthalmology, Indiana University School of Medicine, Indianapolis, IN, USA

**Linda J. Hay, JD**
Alholm, Monahan, Klauke, Hay & Oldenburg, LLC, Chicago, IL, USA

**Andrew M. Hendrick, MD**
Resident Physician, Department of Ophthalmology, University of Colorado, Denver, CO, USA

**Amy Lewis Hennessy, MD, MPH**
Glaucoma Specialist, Associate, International Health, Johns Hopkins Bloomberg School of Public Health, Baltimore, MD, USA
Glaucoma Specialists, PA, Department of Ophthalmology/Glaucoma, Greater Baltimore Medical Center, Baltimore, MA, USA

**Leon W. Herndon Jr, MD**
Associate Professor of Ophthalmology, Department of Glaucoma, Duke University Eye Center, Durham, NC, USA

**Richard A. Hill, MD**
Professor Emeritus, Founder Orange County Glaucoma and Glaukous Corporation, Department of Ophthalmology, Santa Ana, CA, USA

**Gábor Holló, MD, PhD**
1st Department of Ophthalmology, Semmelweis University School of Medicine, Budapest, Hungary

**Cindy M. L. Hutnik, MD, PhD**
Associate Professor, Departments of Ophthalmology and Pathology, Ivey Eye Institute,
St. Joseph's Health Care, University of Western Ontario, London, ON, Canada

**John D. Hyatt, MD**
Resident, Hamilton Eye Institute, University of Tennessee Health Science Center,
Memphis, TN, USA

**Andrew Iwach, MD**
Department of Ophthalmology, Glaucoma Center of San Francisco,
University of California – San Francisco, San Francisco, CA, USA

**Annisa L. Jamil, MD**
Glaucoma Consultants Northwest, Swedish Medical Center, Seattle, WA, USA

**Daniel A. Jewelewicz, MD**
Delray Eye Associates, Delray Beach, FL, USA

**Chris A. Johnson, Ph.D**
Professor, Department of Ophthalmology and Visual Sciences, University of Iowa Hospitals
and Clinics, Iowa City, IA, USA

**Sandra M. Johnson**
Associate Professor of Ophthalmology, Glaucoma Service, University of Virginia
School of Medicine, Charlottesville, VA, USA

**Murray Johnstone, MD**
Consultant in Glaucoma, Department of Ophthalmology, Swedish Medical Center,
Seattle, WA, USA

**Malik Kahook, MD**
Associate Professor, Department of Ophthalmology, University of Colorado, Denver, CO, USA

**Elliott M. Kanner, MD, PhD**
Assistant Professor, Hamilton Eye Institute, University of Tennessee Health Science Center,
Memphis, TN, USA

**L. Jay Katz, MD**
Professor, Jefferson Medical College, Director of Glaucoma Service, Wills Eye Institute,
Philadelphia, PA, USA

**Paul L. Kaufman, MD**
Professor and Chair, Department of Ophthalmology and Visual Sciences,
School of Medicine and Public Health, Madison, WI, USA

**Matthew D. Kay, MD**
Neuro-ophthalmologist, Private Practice, West Palm Beach, FL, USA

**Kate E. Keller, PhD**
Assistant Professor, Department of Ophthalmology, Casey Eye Institute,
Oregon Health and Science University, Portland, OR, USA

**Mary J. Kelley, PhD**
Assistant Professor, Department of Ophthalmology, Casey Eye Institute,
Oregon Health and Science University, Portland, OR, USA

**Yusuf Khalifa, MD**
Cornea Fellow, Moran Eye Institute, University of Utah, Salt Lake City, UT, USA

**Baseer U. Khan, MD, FRCS(C)**
Lecturer, Department of Ophthalmology, University of Toronto, Toronto, ON, Canada

**Nisha Kheradiya, BS**
Department of Ophthalmology, Indiana University School of Medicine, Indianapolis, IN, USA

**Paul A. Knepper, MD, PhD**
Research Scientist, Department of Ophthalmology and Visual Science,
University of Illinois, Chicago, IL, USA

**Anastasios G. P. Konstas, MD, PhD**
Associate Professor in Ophthalmology, Head Glaucoma Unit, 1st University Department
of Ophthalmology, Ahepa Hospital, Thessaloniki, Greece

**Paul J. Lama, MD**
Associate Clinical Professor of Ophthalmology, Columbia University, New York, NY, USA
Director, Glaucoma Division, Department of Ophthalmology, Saint Barnabas
Health Care System, Hackensack, NJ, USA

**Scott D. Lawrence, MD**
Instructor, Department of Ophthalmology, The Hamilton Eye Institute,
University of Tennessee, Memphis, TN, USA

**Kevin C. Leonard, MSC, MD**
Resident, Departments of Ophthalmology and Pathology, Ivey Eye Institute,
St. Joseph's Health Care, University of Western Ontario, London, ON, Canada

**S. Fabian Lerner, MD**
Director, Glaucoma Section, Postgraduate Department, University Favaloro,
Buenos Aires, Argentina

**Lingyi Liang, MD, PhD**
Fellow, Ocular Surface Center, Miami, FL, USA

**Sophie D. Liao, MD**
House Staff, Wilmer Eye Institute, Johns Hopkins University, Baltimore, MD, USA

**Thomas J. Liesegang, MD**
Professor, Department of Ophthalmology, Mayo Clinic, Jacksonville, FL, USA

**Ridia Lim, MB BS, MPH, FRANZCO**
Doctor, Glaucoma Department, Sydney Eye Hospital, Sydney, NSW, Australia

**Shan Lin, MD**
Associate Professor, Department of Ophthalmology, University of California San Francisco,
School of Medicine, San Francisco, CA, USA

**John H. K. Liu, PhD**
Professor, Department of Ophthalmology, University of California, San Diego,
La Jolla, CA, USA

**Nils A. Loewen, MD**
Northwestern University, Department of Ophthalmology, Feinberg School of Medicine,
Chicago, IL, USA

**Anat London**
Department of Neurobiology, Weizmann Institute of Science, Rehovot, Israel

**Reid Longmuir, MD**
Assistant Professor, Department of Ophthalmology, University of Iowa
Hospitals and Clinics, Iowa City, IA, USA

**Carlos Rospigliosi Lopez, MD**
Department of Ophthalmology, Indiana University School of Medicine, Indianapolis, IN, USA

**Alvaro P.C. Lupinacci, MD**
Glaucoma Fellow, Hamilton Eye Institute, University of Tennessee Health Science Center, Memphis, TN, USA

**Elizabeth Martin, BA**
Medical student, University of Washington, School of Medicine, Seattle, WA, USA

**Jeff Martow, MDCM, FRCS(C)**
Clinical Instructor, Department of Ophthalmology, St. Michael's Hospital, University of Toronto, ON, Canada

**Lionel Marzette, MD**
Research Associate, Department of Ophthalmology, Duke University Eye Center, Durham, NC, USA

**Cynthia Mattox, MD**
Director of Glaucoma and Cataract Service, Department of Ophthalmology, New England Eye Center, Tufts University School of Medicine, Boston, MA, USA

**Matthew G. McMenemy, MD**
Department of Ophthalmology, Lone Star Eye Care, PA, Sugar Land, TX, USA

**Felipe A. Medeiros, MD, PhD**
Associate Professor, Department of Ophthalmology, University of California San Diego, La Jolla, CA, USA

**Shlomo Melamed**
Professor of Ophthalmology, Director, The Sam Rothberg Glaucoma Center, Goldschleger Eye Institute, Sheba Medical Center, Tel Aviv University Medical School, Hashomer, Israel

**Richard P. Mills, MD, MPH**
Glaucoma Consultants Northwest, Seattle, WA, USA

**Don S. Minckler, MD, MS**
Professor of Ophthalmology and Pathology, Department of Ophthalmology & Pathology, University of California, Irvine, CA, USA

**Kenneth B. Mitchell, MD**
Associate Professor, Department of Ophthalmology, West Virginia University School of Medicine, Morgantown, WV, USA

**Mark L. Moster MD**
Chairman, Neuro-Ophthalmology, Albert Einstein Medical Center, Professor of Neurology, Jefferson Medical College, Neuro-Ophthalmology Service, Wills Eye Institute, Elkins Park, PA, USA

**Marlene R. Moster, MD**
Professor of Ophthalmology, Department of Ophthalmology, Thomas Jefferson University Hospital, Philadelphia, PA, USA

**Raghu Chary Mudumbai, MD**
Residency Program Director, Associate Professor, Department of Ophthalmology, University of Washington Medical Center, Seattle, WA, USA

**Jonathan S. Myers, MD**
Spaeth/Katz/Myers, P.C., Wills Eye Institute, Philadelphia, PA, USA

**Peter A. Netland, MD, PhD**
Professor and Chair, Department of Ophthalmology, University of Virginia School of Medicine, Charlottesville, VA, USA

**Robert J. Noecker, MD, MBA**
Vice Chair Clinical Affairs, Director Glaucoma Service, Associate Professor,
Department of Ophthalmology, UPMC Eye Center, University of Pittsburgh
School of Medicine Pittsburgh, PA, USA

**Michael J. Nolan, BS, MA**
Research Coordinator, Department of Ophthalmology and Visual Science,
University of Illinois, Chicago, IL, USA

**Stephen A. Obstbaum, MD**
Professor of Ophthalmology, NYU School of Medicine, New York, NY, USA
Chairman, Department of Ophthalmology, Lenox Hill Hospital, New York, NY, USA

**Mildred M. G. Olivier, MD**
Associate Clinical Professor, Department of Ophthalmology, Midwestern University,
Rosalsind Franklin University of Medicine and Science, Hoffman Estates, IL, USA

**David J. Palmer, MD**
Clinical Assistant Professor, Department of Ophthalmology, Northwestern University
Feinberg School of Medicine, Chicago, IL, USA

**Louis R. Pasquale, MD**
Co-Director, Glaucoma Service, Department of Ophthalmology, Massachusetts
Eye and Ear Infirmary, Boston, MA, USA

**Donna Peters, PhD**
Professor, Departments of Pathology and Laboratory Medicine and Ophthalmology
and Visual Sciences, University of Wisconsin School of Medicine and Public Health,
Madison, WI, USA

**Jody Piltz-Seymour, MD**
Director, Glaucoma Care Center PC, Century Eye Care LLC, Bristol, PA, USA

**Bruce E. Prum, Jr., MD**
Associate Professor of Ophthalmology, Department of Ophthalmology,
University of Virginia, Charlottesville, VA, USA

**Nathan Radcliffe, MD**
Assistant Professor, New York Presbyterian Hospital, Weill Cornell Medical College,
New York, NY, USA

**Sunita Radhakrishnan, MD**
Glaucoma Center of San Francisco & Glaucoma Research and Education Group,
San Francisco, CA, USA

**Siva S. Radhakrishnan Iyer, MD**
Resident, Department of Ophthalmology, University of Tennessee Health Science Center,
Memphis, TN, USA

**Renata Fortuna Ramos, PhD**
Postdoctoral Fellow, Department of Bioengineering, Rice University, Houston, TX, USA

**Tony Realini, MD**
Associate Professor of Ophthalmology, Department of Ophthalmology,
West Virginia University, Morgantown, WV, USA

**George R. Reiss, MS, MD**
Instructor, Department of Ophthalmology, Maricopa Medical Center, Glendale, AZ, USA

**Claudia U. Richter, MD**
Clinical Instructor, Department of Ophthalmology, Harvard Medical School, Boston, MA, USA

**Robert Ritch, MD**
Shelley and Steven Einhorn Distinguished Chair in Ophthalmology, Chief, Glaucoma Service, Surgeon Director, Department of Ophthalmology, The New York Eye and Ear Infirmary, New York, NY, USA
Professor of Clinical Ophthalmology, Department of Ophthalmology,
The New York Medical College, Valhalla, NY, USA

**Alan L. Robin, MD**
Associate Professor, International Health, Bloomberg School of Public Health,
Wilmer Institute, Johns Hopkins School of Medicine, Baltimore, MD, USA

**Scott Robison, OD**
Adjunct Assistant Professor, Department of Ophthalmology, Medical College of Wisconsin, Milwaukee, WI, USA

**Christopher J. Russo, MD**
Department of Ophthalmology, Rocky Mountain Lions Eye Institute, University of Colorado Denver, Aurora, CO, USA

**Sarwat Salim, MD**
Assistant Professor, Department of Ophthalmology, Hamilton Eye Institute,
University of Tennessee Health Science Center, Memphis, TN, USA

**John R. Samples, MD**
Clinical Professor, Oregon Health and Sciences University, Portland, OR, USA
Clinical Professor, Rocky Vista University, Parker, CO, USA
Director, Western Glaucoma Foundation
Executive Secretary, Pacific Coast Oto-Ophthalmology Society
Specialty Eye Care, Parker CO

**John Wesley Samples, BS, BA**
.D. Candidate, Case Western Reserve University School of Law, Class of 2011Submissions Editor, Case Western Reserve Journal of Law, Technology & theInternet

**David A. Saperstein, MD**
Vitreoretinal Associates, Glaucoma Consultants Northwest, Seattle, WA, USA

**Paul N. Schacknow, MD, PhD**
Clinical Associate Professor, Division of Ophthalmology,
Nova Southeastern University, Fort Lauderdale, FL, USA
Chief of Glaucoma Services, Visual Health Center, Palm Springs, FL USA

**Joel S. Schuman, MD, FACS**
Eye and Ear Foundation Professor and Chairman, University of Pittsburgh
School of Medicine, Pittsburgh, PA, USA
Director, UPMC Eye Center, Pittsburgh, PA, USA
Professor of Bioengineering, Swanson School of Engineering, University of Pittsburgh, Pittsburgh, PA, USA
Professor, Center for the Neural Basis of Cognition, Carnegie Mellon
University and University of Pittsburgh, Pittsburgh, PA, USA

**Michal Schwartz, PhD**
Professor of Neuroimmunology, Department of Neurobiology,
The Weizmann Institute of Science, Rehovot, Israel

**Marie K. Schwinn, PhD**
Postdoctoral Fellow, Department of Pathology and Laboratory Medicine,
University of Wisconsin-Madison, Madison, WI, USA

**Michele L. Scott, MD**
Instructor, Hamilton Eye Institute, University of Tennessee Health Science Center,
Memphis, TN, USA

**Todd Severin, MD**
Director, Glaucoma Services, East Bay Eye and Glaucoma Diagnostic Centers,
San Ramon, CA, USA

**Hosam Sheha, MD, PhD**
Director of Medical Education and Clinical Studies, Ocular Surface Center,
Miami, FL, USA

**Christopher C. Shen, MD**
Resident, Department of Ophthalmology, University of Tennessee Health Science Center,
Memphis, TN, USA

**Rajesh K. Shetty, MD**
Assistant Professor, Department of Ophthalmology, Mayo Clinic, Jacksonville, FL, USA

**Brent Siesky, PhD**
Research Associate, Department of Ophthalmology, Indiana University School of Medicine,
Indianapolis, IN, USA

**Craig Simms, COMT, ROUB, CDOS**
Clinical Instructor, Program Director, Calgary Ophthalmic Medical Technology Program,
Rockyview Hospital Eye Clinic, Calgary, AB, Canada

**Arthur J. Sit, SM, MD**
Assistant Professor, Department of Ophthalmology, Mayo Clinic College of Medicine,
Rochester, MN, USA

**Betsy Lynn Sleath, PhD**
Professor of Pharmaceutical Outcomes and Policy, University of North Carolina,
School of Pharmacy, Chapel Hill, NC, USA

**George L. Spaeth, BS, MD**
Esposito Research Professor, Department of Ophthalmology, Wills Eye Institute,
Jefferson Medical College, Philadelphia, PA, USA

**Clark Springs, MD**
Assistant Professor, Department of Ophthalmology, Indiana University,
Indianapolis, IN, USA

**W. Daniel Stamer, PhD**
Professor, Department of Ophthalmology and Vision Science,
University of Arizona, Tucson, AZ, USA

**Kevin Taliaferro, BA**
Glaucoma Institute of Beverly Hills, Los Angeles, CA, USA

**Diamond Y. Tam, MD**
Glaucoma and Advanced Anterior Segment Surgery Fellow, Department of Ophthalmology
and Vision Sciences, Credit Valley Eye Care, University of Toronto, Mississauga, ON,
Canada

**H. George Tanaka, BSE, MD**
Clinical Instructor, Department of Ophthalmology, California Pacific Medical Center,
San Francisco, CA, USA

**Angelo P. Tanna, MD**
Assistant Professor, Department of Ophthalmology, Northwestern University,
Feinberg School of Medicine, Chicago, IL, USA

**Celso Tello, MD**
Associate Professor of Ophthalmology, Director, Glaucoma Clinic,
Department of Ophthalmology, New York Eye and Ear Infirmary, New York, NY, USA

**Kelly A. Townsend, BS**
Research Specialist, Biomedical Engineer, UPMC Eye Center, Eye and Ear Institute,
University of Pittsburgh School of Medicine, Pittsburgh, PA, USA
Department of Ophthalmology, Ophthalmology and Visual Science Research Center,
University of Pittsburgh School of Medicine, Pittsburgh, PA, USA

**Helen Tseng, MD**
Clinical Instructor, Department of Ophthalmology, University of California,
Irvine, CA, USA

**Scheffer C. G. Tseng, MD, PhD**
Director, Ocular Surface Center, Miami, FL, USA

**Elizabeth Salinas Van Orman, MD**
Director of the Research Department, Specialty Eye Care, Parker, CO, USA

**David S. Walton, MD**
Clinical Professor of Ophthalmology, Department of Ophthalmology, Harvard Medical
School, Boston, MA, USA

**Robert N. Weinreb, MD**
Distinguished Professor of Ophthalmology, Department of Ophthalmology,
University of California, La Jolla, San Diego, CA, USA

**Roy Whitaker Jr., MD**
Medical Director, Eye Consultants of Greensboro, Greensboro, NC, USA

**Von Best Whitaker, RN, MS, MA, PhD**
Research Associate Professor, North Carolina Agricultural and Technical State University,
School of Nursing, Greensboro, NC, USA

**Jess T. Whitson, MD**
Professor, Department of Ophthalmology, UT Southwestern Medical Center at Dallas,
5323 Harry Hines Boulevard, Dallas, TX, USA

**Matthew C. Willett, MD**
Department of Ophthalmology, Summa Health Systems, Akron, OH, USA

**M. Roy Wilson, MD, MS**
Chancellor and Professor, Department of Ophthalmology, University of Colorado Denver,
Denver, CO, USA

**Gadi Wollstein, MD**
Assistant Professor of Ophthalmology, UPMC Eye Center, Eye and Ear Institute,
University of Pittsburgh School of Medicine, Pittsburgh, PA, USA
Ophthalmology and Visual Science Research Center, Department of Ophthalmology,
University of Pittsburgh School of Medicine, Pittsburgh, PA, USA

**Hongli Yang, MS**
Graduate Research Assistant, Department of Biomedical Engineering,
Tulane University, New Orleans, LA, USA

**Kayoung Yi, MD, PhD**
Associate Professor, Department of Ophthalmology, Kangnam Sacred Heart Hospital, Hallym University, Seoul, South Korea

**Beatrice Y. J. T. Yue, PhD**
Thanis A. Field Professor of Ophthalmology, Department of Ophthalmology and Visual Sciences, University of Illinois, Chicago, IL, USA

**Joseph R. Zelefsky, MD**
Clinical Instructor in Ophthalmology, Department of Ophthalmology, New York University, New York, NY, USA

**Yuanjun Zhao**
Wills Eye Institute, Philadelphia, PA, USA

# Part I
# The Basics

# Chapter 1
# Glaucoma in the Twenty-First Century

Ridia Lim and Ivan Goldberg

## 1.1 What is Glaucoma for the Twenty-First Century?

Our concepts of the glaucomas evolve as our understanding of disease processes increases, technology advances, and our treatment strategies become more sophisticated. Technology has always corralled our definitions and our understanding of the glaucomas; the challenge of this new century is to focus our progress for the direct benefit of our patients.

To understand and to modify where we are heading, we must know where we are now, and how we arrived here.

Since the time of Hippocrates, the glaucomas have mystified physicians. In the mid-nineteenth century, the truth began to emerge.[1] The link with disc cupping followed Hermann von Helmholtz's 1860s invention of the ophthalmoscope and Albrecht von Graefe's observations. Thus, there arose the structural nerve head-based definitions: Glaucoma was considered a neurological disease. The association with raised intraocular pressure (IOP) occurred over several centuries but was boosted by improvements in tonometers between 1880 and 1910 (Table 1.1). Improved functional assessment established the mid-twentieth century triad definition: raised IOP with characteristic optic disc and visual field changes. As tonometry, perimetry, and optic disc structural evaluation have each advanced, significant developments in one area have emphasized that aspect of glaucoma. The most recent technological improvements in objective optic disc and retinal nerve fiber layer (RNFL) assessment have moved our focus once again to the underlying neurological consequences of this group of diseases. We must remember: Technological capabilities drive our definitions and concepts of the glaucomas and their management.

Most glaucomas are chronic and relatively slowly progressive; technological advances occur faster than we can evaluate them critically. In every area, there is continued exponential growth. This could lead us to lose sight of our first call as clinicians: All these advances are ultimately for the benefits of individual patients, for whom management strategies need to balance potential benefits against possible risks of harm. Understanding of a patient's quality of life (QOL), independence, and personal dignity must also advance, so that progress has a meaningful human application. Physical, emotional, and financial considerations are part of this.

Currently, we define the glaucomas as an optic neuropathy (with multifactorial risk factors that include increased IOP, increasing age, and genetic predisposition) characterized by recognizable patterns of optic disc and retinal nerve fiber structural and visual field functional damage. Glaucomatous optic neuropathy is not the disease; it is the end-result of several as yet unidentified cellular disease processes. Unlike almost all other optic neuropathies, contour changes of the optic nerve head ("cupping") with progressive loss of the retinal nerve fiber layer and associated functional deficits are features of the disease; this results from accelerated retinal ganglion cell apoptosis, initiated by damaging processes that target the axons of these cells as they leave the globe. Thus, the definition varies with the perspective of the definer: retinal ganglion cell apoptosis to a scientist, optic neuropathy to a clinician, and fear of blindness for a patient.

## 1.2 What Are the Challenges We Face in the Twenty-First Century and Beyond?

We have to meet the challenge to find those with glaucoma who are undiagnosed.

Population studies have yielded a wealth of data about glaucoma prevalence, incidence, and risk factors in Caucasian, Latino, African-American, Afro-Caribbean, Indian sub-continental, and Oriental populations (see Fig. 1.1). Second only to cataract, globally the glaucomas are the

**Table 1.1** History of Glaucoma[2-8]

*Understanding of glaucoma*

Between the time of Hippocrates and the middle of the nineteenth century, glaucoma was very poorly understood. Any disease that was not diagnosable externally may have been labeled "glaucoma." Hippocrates is credited for the term "glaucosis," which translates to "sea green eye," but the differentiation of glaucoma from other diseases, especially cataract, took many centuries.

The word "glaucoma" is derived from the word "glaukos" and this means blue hue in Greek.

There were a few notable observations: during the middle ages, Arabian physicians gave some descriptions of glaucoma.

- Tenth century – At Tabari in the "Hippocratic writings" described inflammation and raised eye pressure.
- 1348 – Sams ad Din of Cairo described an eye condition with hardness of the eyeball, hemicrania, reduced vision, and dilated pupil.

Thereafter, understanding of glaucoma did not progress much until the 1800s.

- 1622 – Richard Banister, in the first ophthalmology textbook in English, *Banister's Breviary*, noted that the eye was hard in some morbid eye conditions. He also translated William Guillemeau's 1585 text, "A treatise of one hundred and thirteen diseases of the eyes, and eye-lids," which had incorporated information from Arabic and Greek sources.
- 1709 – Michel Brisseau differentiated glaucoma from lens disorders; he attributed glaucoma to the vitreous. This view prevailed until direct disc viewing was possible.
- 1818 – Antoine-Pierre Demours gave a good description of glaucoma and first described colored rings around lights.
- 1823 – George James Guthrie labeled the disease "glaucoma."
- 1830 – William Mackenzie, author of the first comprehensive English book on ophthalmology, *A Practical Treatise on the Diseases of the Eye*, noted "the eyeball always in glaucoma feels firmer than natural." The role of IOP in glaucoma was now firmly established.
- 1850s – Albrecht von Graefe differentiated acute, chronic, and secondary glaucoma.
- 1866 – Donders labeled cases with no congestive symptoms, with raised IOP "simple glaucoma;" this misleading label persisted for a century.
- 1938 – Jonas S. Freidenwald showed that aqueous was actively produced by the ciliary body and was not solely a dialysate of plasma.
- 1941 – Aqueous veins connecting the canal of Schlemm and the episcleral veins were described for the first time by K. W. Ascher.
- 1959 – A. E. Maumenee's advanced insights into congenital glaucoma.
- 1969 – Cup/disc ratio increase as a sign of the damaging effect of raised IOP, in eyes with normal visual fields, was reported in a paper by Mansour F. Armaly and Roger E. Sayegh. Armaly's cup/disc ratio gained widespread use in glaucoma management.
- 1970 – Stephen Drance associated disc hemorrhage with nerve fiber layer defects.
- 1973 – William Hoyt described nerve fiber layer defects as the earliest sign of glaucoma.
- 1982 – Harry Quigley reported that 40% of nerve fibers could be lost without visual field loss detected by quantitative kinetic perimetry.

*Investigations of glaucoma*
- Early 1800s – Ophthalmologists performed digital tonometry.
- 1860s – Several scleral tonometers were introduced, but use was not widespread.
- 1850 – Invention of ophthalmoscope by Hermann Ludwig Ferdinand (von) Helmholtz; disc cupping seen by Albrecht von Graefe, Mueller and the idea that glaucoma was a vitreous disorder was finally abandoned.
- 1856 – Albrecht von Graefe used a primitive campimeter, a row of dots on a sheet of paper, to plot peripheral visual field defects.
- 1889 – Quantitative perimetry. Jannik Petersen Bjerrum used his office door to plot field defects, thereby inventing the tangent screen. This became the dominant form of perimetry for 50 years. He described the arcuate scotoma, a hallmark of glaucoma.
- 1905 – Hjalmar Schiötz invented the first reliable indentation tonometer. Corneal tonometers were possible with the introduction of cocaine in 1884.
- Early 1900s – Iridocorneal angle was directly visualized by Trantas (1900), Salzmann (1915), Troncosco (1921).
- 1928 – Schmidt used the water-drinking test in glaucoma patients.
- 1916 – Biomicroscopes were invented in the 1890s. Allvar Gullstrand was the first to use slit illumination. In 1916, Zeiss combined these two principles, thus giving rise to the first slit lamp biomicroscope.
- 1935–1940 – Barkan popularized gonioscopy as an essential part of eye examination using the Koeppe direct gonioscopy lens.
- 1950 – W. Morton Grant described the tonographic method of measuring facility of outflow and rate of aqueous outflow.
- 1954 – Hans Goldmann invented his quantitative perimeter.
- 1955 – Hans Goldmann invented his tonometer, an unsurpassed instrument, based on the Imbert-Fick law. For once, patients could have IOP measurements sitting up. It remains the gold standard today and despite its limitations, it is a widely available and most commonly used tool.
- 1970s – Computerized perimeters are introduced and developed by Humphrey and Octopus.

*Drug treatment of glaucoma*
- 1862 – Calabar bean found to cause miosis by Sir Thomas Richard Fraser. The Calabar bean, native to West Africa, was growing in the Royal Botanic Gardens in Edinburgh from seeds brought back by missionaries. In 1864, physostigmine (eserine) was isolated from the Calabar bean.
- 1875 – Ludwig Laquer described the use of physostigmine for his own glaucoma.

(continued)

**Table 1.1** (continued)

- 1873-6 – Symphronio Coutinho, a Brazilian doctor, took samples of Jaborandi (*Pilocarpus pennatifolius*, a shrubby tree native to America) leaf to Europe. Systemic effects were noted and by 1876, Adolf Weber was using the isolated alkaloid, pilocarpine, in the treatment of glaucoma.
- 1925 – Epinephrine was reported by Gradle and Hamburger to reduce IOP, but after elevating IOP in some cases it was not used until the 1940s when gonioscopy identified narrow angles and thus patients who should not use it. R. Weekers reported on the use of epinephrine in 1954 and it was reintroduced.
- 1950s – Hyperosmotics – mannitol and urea.
- 1954 – Acetozolamide, initially used as a diuretic in congestive heart failure, was reported by Bernard Becker to reduce IOP very effectively when used orally.
- 1967 – Phillips reported IOP lowering with oral propranolol; in 1977, Zimmerman used timolol for glaucoma.

*Surgical treatment of glaucoma*
- 1857 – Surgical iridectomy used "to reduce aqueous production" by Albrecht von Graefe. An amazing advance in the treatment of glaucoma, this operation cured many cases of angle closure, but not by reducing aqueous production!
- 1859 – Iridectomy with iris inclusion-Coccius
- 1876 – Scleral trephination-Argyll-Robertson
- 1878 – Anterior sclerectomy-Louis De Wecker
- 1903 – Iridosclerectomy-Bader and Lagrange
- 1905 – Cyclodialysis-Heine
- 1906 – Iridenclesis-Soren Holth. This procedure was associated later with sympathetic ophthalmia.
- 1909 – Elliot published "Sclero-corneal Trephining in the Operative Treatment of Glaucoma," describing his first 900 cases. Corneoscleral trephination became the preferred operation, but was associated with thin blebs.
- 1920 – Curran and Banzinger (1922) described separately the use of iridectomy to relieve "congestive glaucoma," but the concept was ignored for 20 years until gonioscopy reliably allowed detection of pupil block angle closure.
- 1924 – Preziozi used electrocautery to create a full thickness fistula between the anterior chamber and the subconjunctival space.
- 1936 – Otto Barkan described goniotomy for chronic glaucoma in adults. It remains the operation of choice in congenital glaucoma, but is not used in adults.
- 1940s – Barkan rediscovered the mechanism of pupil block; keen gonioscopists (Kronfeldt, Chandler, and Shaffer) popularized iridectomy for pupil block.
- 1956 – Meyer-Schwickerath reported on laser iridotomy with a xenon arc photocoagulator.
- 1958 – Harold Scheie reported a full-thickness fistulizing procedure for glaucoma. He modified Preziozi's procedure by entering the eye with a knife and then using cautery to extend the scleral wound and to keep it open. Most common problems were hypotony and cataract.
- 1968 – Trabeculectomy. J. E. Cairns described a guarded procedure removing a rectangular section of trabecular meshwork and deep cornea. He aimed to remove a block of the canal of Schlemm to get aqueous to flow freely into its cut ends. A bleb formed in about a third of cases.
- 1968 – Anthony Molteno invented a glaucoma drainage device that shunted aqueous from the anterior chamber into a maintained episcleral reservoir.
- 1976 – Theodore Krupin invented the first valved glaucoma drainage tube, at first without a reservoir.
- 1979 – James B. Wise and Stanton L. Witter treated the trabecular meshwork with Argon laser to increase facility of outflow: "trabeculoplasty."
- 1982 – Robert Ritch described iridoplasty for acute angle closure crisis unresponsive to medication.
- 1983 – Chen Wu Chen used Mitomycin C as an adjunctive in trabeculectomy. Published in a minor journal, a decade passed before it became popular.
- 1984 – 5-Fluorouracil was first reported in an animal model and in a pilot study in glaucoma filtering surgery.

leading cause of visual disability. As the damage caused is irreversible, but mostly avoidable by treatment, the glaucomas are the leading cause of *preventable* blindness. As prevalence increases exponentially with increasing age, the glaucomas are set to become increasingly and relentlessly a worldwide public health issue as populations gray.

In all communities, glaucoma is under-diagnosed. In developed countries, such as Australia, half of all glaucoma cases are undiagnosed.[9,10] The percentage undiagnosed is far greater in underprivileged communities: up to 90% of glaucoma patients are not diagnosed.[11,12] Access to eye care is not the only issue: In an Australian study, up to 50% of the undiagnosed patients had seen either an ophthalmologist or an optometrist (or both) in the previous 12 months.[13] In the Melbourne Visual Impairment Project (VIP), 97% of undiagnosed glaucoma cases that had seen an eye professional within the last 12 months had a visual field defect on standard automated perimetry: these were not early, subtle cases. Professional education is an issue. The challenge to find undiagnosed cases is very real, and multiple strategies are needed to overcome this challenge.

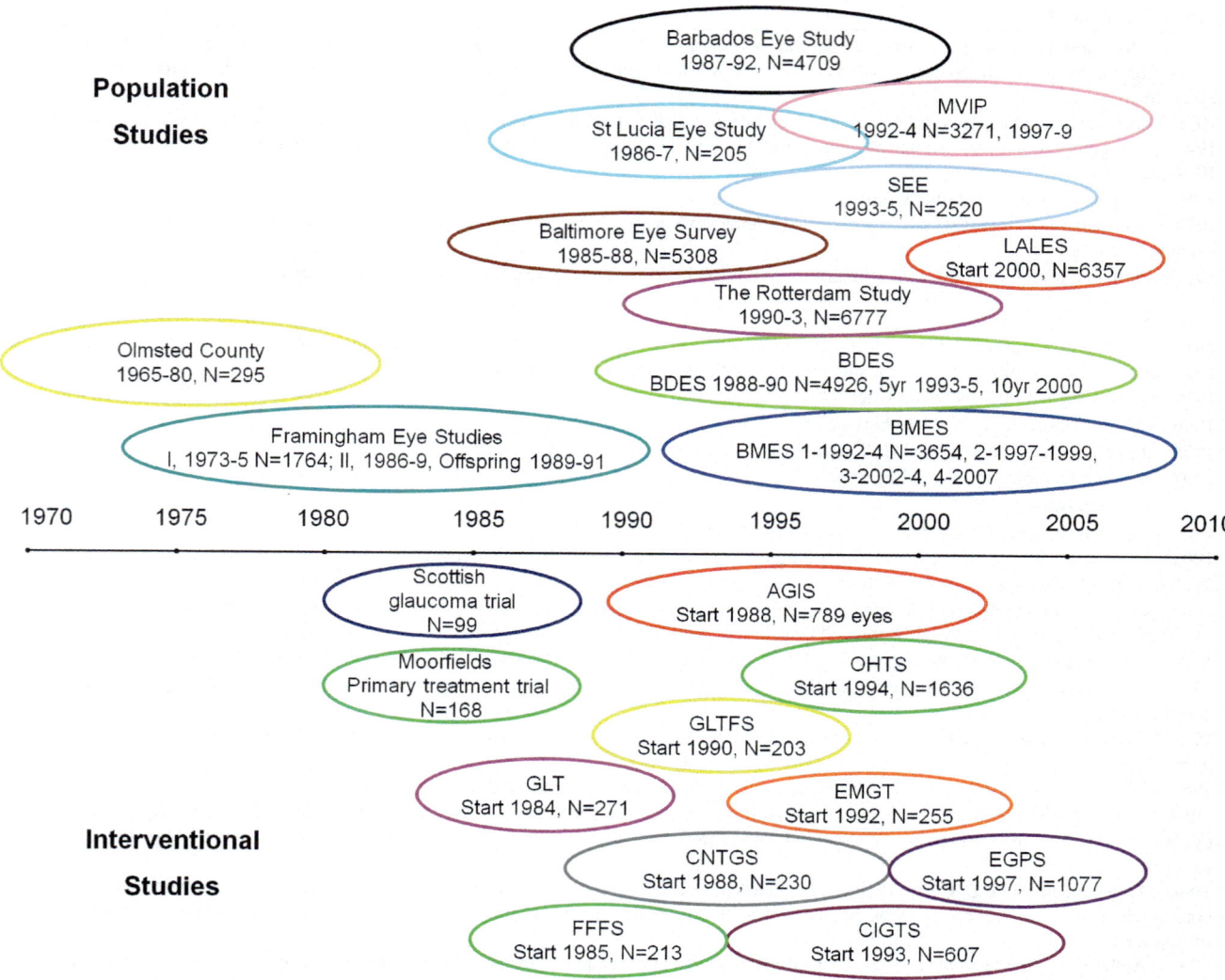

**Fig. 1.1** The studies timeline – important population and interventional studies in glaucoma. (Dates are recruitment or start dates and "*N*" is number of people unless stated as eyes). *AGIS* Advanced Glaucoma Intervention Study, multicenter USA.[20] *BDES* Beaver Dam Eye Study, Wisconsin, USA.[21] *BMES* Blue Mountains Eye Study, Blue Mountains, Australia.[9] *CIGTS* Collaborative Initial Glaucoma Study, multicenter USA.[22] *CNTGS* Collaborative Normal Tension Glaucoma Study, multicenter USA.[23] *EGPS* European Glaucoma Prevention Study, multicenter Europe.[24] *EMGT* Early Manifest Glaucoma Trial, Sweden.[25] *FFFS* Fluorouracil Filtering Surgery Study, multicenter USA.[26] *GLT* Glaucoma Laser Trial, multicenter USA.[27] *GLTFS* Glaucoma Laser Trial Follow Up Study, multicenter USA.[27] *LALES* Los Angeles Latino Eye Study, Los Angeles, USA.[11] *MVIP* Melbourne Visual Impairment Project, Melbourne, Australia.[10] *OHTS* Ocular Hypertension Treatment Study, multi-center USA.[28] *SEE* Salisbury Eye Evaluation Project, Maryland, USA[29]

### 1.2.1 Population-Based ("Universal") Screening

Screening is the use of a test or tests on a target population to find cases of disease. There are different types of screening: targeted and mass population screening. Tools used for screening should fulfill certain criteria. There is no one good mass-screening test for glaucoma. As stated by the World Health Organization in 1968, the principles of screening are [14]:

1. The condition should be an important health problem.
2. There should be an accepted treatment for the patients with recognized disease.
3. Facilities for diagnosis and treatment should be available.
4. There should be a recognizable latent or early symptomatic stage.
5. There should be a suitable test or examination.
6. The test should be acceptable to the population.

7. The natural history of the condition, including development from latent to declared disease should be adequately understood.
8. There should be an agreed policy on whom to treat as patients.
9. The cost of case finding (including diagnosis and treatment of patients diagnosed) should be economically balanced in relation to possible expenditure on medical care as a whole.
10. Case-finding should be a continuing process and not a "once and for all" project.

Population-based screening for glaucoma for long has been handicapped by an undue reliance on IOP levels. An IOP greater than 21 mmHg became so integral to the definition of glaucoma that this alone became synonymous with glaucoma. Another failing was the arbitrary cut-off of 21 mmHg to differentiate "high pressure from "low pressure" or "normal tension" glaucoma, as if they were two different diseases.[15]

The number 21 mmHg as the borderline between normal and abnormal began with Leydhecker's groundbreaking study in 1958 when the IOP of 20,000 eyes was measured with Schiotz tonometry, and a mean of 15.5 mmHg with a standard deviation of 2.57 mmHg was found.[16] By the time Hollows and Graham published their Welsh population data in 1966, the idea of 21 mmHg was so well established that a bias for *not* finding an IOP of 21 mmHg (the "decision effect") was seen.[17] In their population (40–75 years), the IOP was 15.9 (SD~3) mmHg in men and 16.6 (SD~3) mmHg in women. The distribution of IOP was non-Gaussian with a skew to the right (i.e., more individuals with higher IOP than predicted) in those older than 60 years. Elevated IOP is not glaucoma, and ocular hypertension does not lead invariably to glaucomatous optic neuropathy. This arbitrary differentiation is obsolete, although, because of its usefulness as a defined cut-off, it still remains part of ophthalmology outcome terminology. What is the current role of IOP in diagnosis and treatment of glaucoma? Although IOP is not part of the definition of glaucoma, its reduction remains the only proven and approved means of treatment, and is the single most important modifiable risk factor. To cause glaucomatous optic neuropathy, there is a complex interaction between IOP and other risk factors.

IOP is not a useful screening test for glaucoma. A single office measurement does not reflect an individual's pressure range; it cannot be the basis for diagnosis. Many cases of glaucoma have been missed or diagnosed late by reliance on IOP for screening. David Eddy recognized this.[18] David Eddy and John Billings also challenged the glaucoma world with their 1987 report that found "not a single book, chapter or paper that systematically reviewed the evidence on the effectiveness of treatment" of glaucoma.[19] While some clinicians became "glaucoma treatment skeptics," a larger group set out to obtain the best evidence for IOP reduction in glaucoma care. What resulted were a number of National Eye Institute-funded prospective, randomized, controlled, multicenter clinical trials of management of ocular hypertension and glaucoma (see Fig. 1.1): AGIS, CIGTS, CNTGS, EMGT, EPGS, and OHTS.

Is there a test or a group of tests that is good enough to detect the disease and is it a cost-effective exercise? In general, the cost considered is economic and not emotional or societal. A recent review of glaucoma screening in the United Kingdom[30] concluded that while population screening for glaucoma alone is not efficient or cost-effective generally, targeted screening of "at risk" groups is (such as family members of glaucoma patients), screening older populations for more than one eye disease simultaneously, or for systemic conditions as well, changes the economic parameters dramatically.

The 2005 report by the US Agency for Healthcare Research & Quality, US Preventative Services Task Force[31] stated that there is no good single test at present to conduct population screening. However, in 2008, the World Glaucoma Association (WGA) devoted their fifth Consensus meeting to glaucoma screening[32] for open-angle and angle-closure glaucomas. Their findings are summarized in Table 1.2.

### 1.2.2 Case Detection ("Opportunistic Screening")

Case detection or opportunistic screening is the process of finding asymptomatic cases as they present to the eye professional for other reasons. Currently, this consistently fails to find all cases of glaucoma, as demonstrated repeatedly in population studies. The most likely reason we fail to find all of the cases is an incomplete "comprehensive" examination, in which the optic disc and angle configuration have not been assessed properly. In agreement with the Melbourne VIP, a mass screening study in Malmö, Sweden,[33] found that of the cases of glaucoma newly diagnosed by the screening program, 62% had seen an ophthalmologist at some stage previously, with 17% having seen one in the preceding 2 years.

Many more cases of glaucoma would be diagnosed if ophthalmologists and optometrists competently and conscientiously examined the optic nerve, performed gonioscopy (and if necessary, performed a visual field test) in *all* adult patients, regardless of the presenting problem. This is particularly so in older patients where the disease is more prevalent. Eye care professionals need to be skilled to perform these tasks better.

Patients might wonder why the examiner is looking at their optic nerve when they came in with another problem.

**Table 1.2** WGA consensus on glaucoma screening (2008)

*Open-angle glaucoma*

1. Is Open Angle Glaucoma an important health issue?   YES
   - Glaucoma is the leading cause of preventable and irreversible blindness.
   - The goal of glaucoma screening is to prevent visual impairment, and to preserve both quality of life and visual functioning.
   - Each society should determine its own criteria, including the stage of disease, for the allocation of an affordable proportion of its resources for glaucoma care and screening.
   - The prevalence of open-angle glaucoma has been determined for some populations of European, African, and Asian ancestry.
   - Long-term data shows substantial frequency of glaucoma blindness in some populations.
2. Is there an accepted and effective treatment?   YES
   - High quality randomized trials (treatment versus no treatment) and meta-analyses have shown that topical ocular hypotensive medication is effective in delaying both onset and progression of open-angle glaucoma.
   - Treatments are effective, easy to use, and well tolerated.
   - It is not known whether postponing ocular hypotensive therapy affects the rate of subsequent conversion from ocular hypertension to open-angle glaucoma, or the rate of progression of visual field loss once open-angle glaucoma has developed.
   - It is not known whether the reduction in progression rate from IOP lowering therapy varies according to disease stage.
   - Current evidence suggests that glaucoma therapy itself is not associated with a measurable reduction of quality of life.
   - Patients' perceived vision-related quality of life (VRQOL) and visual function is correlated with visual field loss, especially binocular visual field loss, in open-angle glaucoma.
3. Are facilities for diagnosis and treatment available?   YES
   - The resources for diagnosis and treatment of glaucoma vary worldwide.
   - Fewer resources are required to diagnose glaucoma at moderate to advanced asymptomatic stages when compared with very early stages.
   - Treatment of glaucoma requires facilities for regular long-term monitoring.
   - There is a need to study barriers to access for glaucoma care so that available facilities can be used optimally.
4. Is there an appropriate screening test?   POTENTIALLY
   - The best single test or group of tests for open-angle glaucoma screening is yet to be determined.
   - Optimal screening test criteria are not yet known.
   - Diagnostic test accuracy may vary according to the severity of the disease.
   - The tests available and effective for case-finding are not necessarily the same as those for population-based glaucoma screening, which requires a very high specificity to be cost-effective.
5. Is the natural history adequately understood?   YES
   - Open-angle glaucoma incidence rates are known for untreated and treated patients with ocular hypertension.
   - Open-angle glaucoma progression rates vary greatly among patients.
   - Progression event rates for patients (in clinical trials, under clinical care or observation) in terms of percent of patients/eyes progressing per year are available both for open-angle glaucoma and ocular hypertension.
   - Progression data expressed as rate of disease progression, (i.e., expressed in dB/year or in % of full field/year) are very sparse.
6. Is the cost of case finding economically balanced?   POTENTIALLY
   - The best evidence to date, based on two modeling studies, suggests:
     1. Screening of high-risk subgroups could be more cost-effective than screening the entire population.
     2. Screening may be more cost-effective as glaucoma prevalence increases.
     3. The optimal screening interval is not yet known.
     4. Screening may be more cost-effective when initial assessment is a simple strategy that could be supervised by nonmedical technicians.
   - Population-based screening studies are required to determine optimal screening strategies and their cost-effectiveness.
   - Multi-eye disease screening needs to be evaluated as to whether it would be more cost-effective than glaucoma-only screening.

*Angle-closure glaucoma*

1. Are angle-closure and angle-closure glaucoma important health problems?   YES
   - Primary angle-closure glaucoma (PACG) accounts for approximately 25% of all glaucomatous optic neuropathy worldwide, but 50% of bilateral glaucoma blindness.
   - Visual impairment from Primary Angle Closure (PAC) and PACG can result from ocular damage other than glaucomatous optic nerve damage (e.g., corneal decompensation, cataract, and ischemic optic neuropathy).
   - Some Asian populations have a high prevalence of advanced angle closure glaucoma.
   - PACG is predominantly asymptomatic.
   - PACG is a problem of sufficient magnitude that public health intervention should be evaluated.
2. Is there an accepted and effective treatment?   YES
   - Angle closure is a progressive condition that can lead to glaucoma.
   - Iridectomy/iridotomy is the preferred initial treatment for cases of PAC and PACG.

(continued)

**Table 1.2** (continued)

- There is no evidence to support medical treatment alone for ACG in the absence of iridectomy/iridotomy.
- Medical treatment may be indicated for lowering IOP after iridectomy/iridotomy, following risk assessment.
- Iridectomy/iridotomy will not always alleviate irido-trabecular apposition since mechanisms other than pupillary block may be present, such as plateau iris or phacomorphic angle closure.
- There is good evidence that preventive iridectomy/iridotomy will eliminate the risk of acute angle closure when performed on the fellow eye of patients who have experienced unilateral acute angle closure.
- There is insufficient evidence for deciding which PACG patients should undergo lens extraction alone (without trabeculectomy).
- Although commonly performed, there is limited evidence about the effectiveness of combined cataract extraction and trabeculectomy in eyes with PACG.

3. Are facilities for diagnosis and treatment available?   YES
   - There is a need for a systematic assessment of the clinical capacity to identify and treat angle closure.
   - Gonioscopy is essential for diagnosis and treatment.
4. Is there an appropriate screening test?   POTENTIALLY
   - There is evidence that limbal anterior chamber depth (LCD) may be an appropriate screening test for angle closure.
   - Clinic-based case-detection should target established primary angle closure (PAC) and primary angle closure glaucoma (PACG) as blindness can still be prevented when interventions are implemented at these stages.
   - Gonioscopy is the current gold standard for angle examination and is the appropriate test for diagnosing angle closure.
   - For accuracy of clinic-based case detection of PAC and PACG to improve, there needs to be a significant increase in the level and use of gonioscopy and disc examination training for ophthalmologists.
5. Is the natural history adequately understood?   YES
   - An episode of symptomatic ("acute") angle closure places the unaffected fellow eye at high risk of a similar fate.
   - The current best estimate for progression from PACS to PAC, or from PAC to PACG is approximately 20–30% over 5 years.
   - Asymptomatic angle closure is associated with later presentation and more advanced loss of vision than symptomatic angle closure, where facilities for treatment are readily available.
6. Is the cost of case finding economically balanced?   POTENTIALLY
   - In assessing the cost-effectiveness of a screening program for PAC and PACG, we must consider fully the costs and benefits of the program.
   - Evaluation must consider the perspective of the decision maker, the incremental cost of the proposed program versus current programs and how we measure effectiveness.
   - A thorough cost-effectiveness analysis is not possible at present.

We explain this by saying, "Now that I have assessed you for your problem, I want to do a full eye examination for you, so you can be confident there is nothing else wrong with your eyes." This is an important public health message to reinforce to all our colleagues. As the Asia Pacific Glaucoma Guidelines stress: Use IOP levels, dilated optic disc examination, angle estimation by gonioscopy (and visual field testing as needed) on all adults over 35 years old presenting to eye specialists *for any reason,* to detect glaucoma (see Table 1.3.).[34]

### 1.2.3 Community Education and Awareness: Patient Support Groups

General community awareness of glaucoma, and increased understanding of their disease and the goals of treatment amongst our glaucoma patients, desperately needs improvement around the world. This is a challenge for all eye health practitioners. Although glaucoma patients have more knowledge of glaucoma than the general public, they also have significant misconceptions about glaucoma.[35] One in three new glaucoma patients, one in four established glaucoma patients, and almost one in two of the general public have been reported to believe that most patients with glaucoma go blind from it. Not surprisingly, diagnosis of glaucoma drops quality of life immediately, even in asymptomatic patients.[36] We must allay our patients' fears, balancing this with knowledge to encourage adherence to therapy. As glaucoma patients obtain their knowledge primarily from their treating physician, we must inform and educate them appropriately. As this information and support may need to be given repeatedly over a prolonged period, lack of professional time can be a major challenge. Patient support organizations are vital.

Community groups at national levels are foundation stones for the world glaucoma patient community. Lay glaucoma organizations, such as Glaucoma Australia, are our interface with the wider community. They celebrated their 20th birthday in 2008 (see Fig. 1.2a, b). Glaucoma Australia's mission is to minimize visual disability from glaucoma. It accomplishes this by increasing community awareness

**Table 1.3** Case detection guidelines

| Test | Ideal | Acceptable | Less than ideal | Comments |
|---|---|---|---|---|
| Tonometry | Applanation tonometry | Tonopen, ocular response analyser, rebound tonometers | Pneumotonometer, Shiotz tonometer, Phosphene tonometers | |
| Dilated evaluation of the optic disc | Dilated stereoscopic slit lamp biomicroscopy or fundus photography | Direct ophthalmoscope | Optic disc or RNFL computerized analysis alone | New technologies complement and do not replace clinical assessment |
| Slit lamp biomicroscope and van herick | NA | NA | NA | If flashlight (FL) or van Herick (VH) test is positive, confirmation with gonioscopy is necessary. FL and VH do not diagnose or exclude angle closure. If FL is negative (<1/3 on the nasal side of pupil shadowed) AND VH is negative (ACD>1/4 of peripheral cornea), occludable angle is unlikely. If VH is positive AND IOP is elevated, >99% likelihood of PAC |
| Gonioscopy | Indentation gonioscopy using a Sussman, Zeiss or Posner lens | Goldmann or Magna View lens using "manipulation" | | Mandatory in all glaucoma suspects. Should have both types of lenses available. To increase accuracy, gonioscopy is a "dark" art – dim room illumination, thin, short slit lamp beam, avoid light in pupil |
| Visual field examination if IOP>21 or disc is suspicious | A full threshold test using a standard automated achromatic perimetry | Frequency Doubling (FDP), Henson's perimetry or Bjerrum's screen | | A trained technician must perform Goldmann, Henson's and Bjerrum's screen |

Modified from Asia Pacific Glaucoma Guidelines by SEAGIG (South East Asian Glaucoma Interest Group), 2003[34]

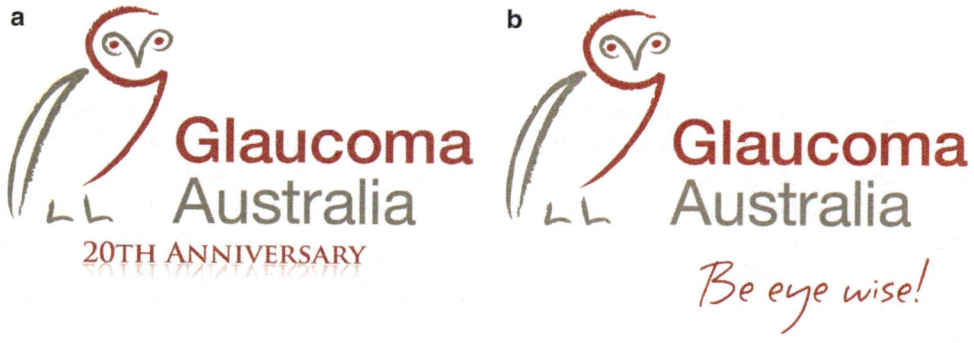

**Fig. 1.2** Glaucoma Australia – Australia's patient support organization. (**a**) Glaucoma Australia's 20th anniversary and (**b**) "be eye wise" logo. *Courtesy of Glaucoma Australia Inc*

and understanding of glaucoma and the need for regular eye checks (strategies include an annual National Glaucoma Week, regular articles in the popular press and magazines, and radio interviews with TV stories); by supporting glaucoma patients and their families, especially with information and dialogue; and by funding glaucoma research. It conducts information meetings for the public, supports a Web site, and produces glaucoma education pamphlets.

Globally, the World Glaucoma Association (WGA) links glaucoma professional associations. The WGA has helped to bring into being the World Glaucoma Patient Association (WGPA) to improve the lives of glaucoma patients by encouraging the establishment of and cooperation among glaucoma patient organizations worldwide. It was launched in October 2004.

The first World Glaucoma Day, a worldwide joint initiative of the World Glaucoma Association and the World Glaucoma Patient Association, took place on March 6, 2008. The day aimed to increase worldwide awareness of glaucoma so that more individuals would have their eyes checked, permitting earlier diagnosis and thus a chance for more effective therapy. Other initiatives such as the JULeye initiative in Australia strive to bring corporate and private sponsors, the public, eye professionals, and eye researchers together for a designated month to raise money for research, and to increase public awareness of eye diseases so that more are diagnosed (http://www.juleye.com.au/). Advocacy should also be encouraged at the government level. The first American Glaucoma Society Advocacy Day in March 2008 demonstrated how the profession could increase government awareness and, therefore, involvement in glaucoma care and blindness prevention. Ophthalmologists should be involved in these activities.

When and if patients do lose significant vision from glaucoma, we as physicians should guide them to low vision and rehabilitation support groups such as Vision Australia. As a profession, our record in offering this guidance is poor.

### 1.2.4 Patient Involvement to Spread Information to Their Families and Friends

Family history is an important risk factor for glaucoma. One effective way of finding new cases of glaucoma is to discuss family history with our patients. While many patients are ignorant of a positive family history, by encouraging extended family dialogue, new information may emerge, as well as urging other family members to be tested regularly. Also, when relatives accompany your glaucoma patient, ask them if they have had a comprehensive eye examination and encourage them to do so. "Don't lose sight of your family!" is an important message to all our glaucoma patients.

Self-reported recall of family history is known to be inaccurate. Even with this inaccuracy, family history of glaucoma is associated with a threefold excess age-adjusted risk of OAG (RR 3.14, 95% CI 2.32–4.25).[30] The Glaucoma Inheritance Study in Tasmania (GIST), Australia, has looked carefully at self-reporting of family history and compared this with true family history. About a third of people were unaware of their positive family history of glaucoma.[37] Patients were more aware of their parents' ophthalmic history than their siblings'. Cross-sectional studies report a positive family history of 10–50%. This emphasizes the need for us to engage in discussion of family history with our patients and the need to do this *repeatedly*. This starts the conversation with parents, children, siblings, and extended family to help detect other cases of glaucoma. To ask, ask, and ask again is the message for acquiring family history. In the GIST study, about 60% of glaucoma was familial.[38]

### 1.2.5 Genetic Testing

Genetic testing may be appropriate. Some familial glaucoma is more aggressive and requires early surgery. Knowing what mutation affects a patient may help this decision. There are other implications to genetic testing; genetic counseling must be available. Tests may not yet be specific enough to be much more than a research tool. While a good screening test needs to be highly specific (to avoid many false-positives that would overwhelm available resources), a good diagnostic test needs to be extremely sensitive (to avoid missing established cases).

Some of the genes available for testing are:

- Myocilin (MYOC)
- Optineurin (OPTN)
- Cytochrome P450 1B1 (CYP1B1)
- LOXL1 for pseudoexfoliation syndrome[39]

While the discovery of genes associated with different glaucomas opens a new and exciting era, one must remain cautious. It is the predictive value that indicates the true worth of a test, and predictive value depends on the prevalence of the disease. Used indiscriminately, a test might yield many more false than true positives: with no way to disprove the imminence of disease apart from passage of time, this could reduce the quality of life and do more harm than good. Progress in genetic research, such as the recent association of LOXL1 mutations with pseudoexfoliation syndrome, will unravel the underlying cellular mechanisms of glaucoma.[39]

In known family pedigrees of aggressive glaucoma such as familial juvenile-onset open angle glaucoma, characterized by high IOP and a rapidly progressive clinical course, testing for a known mutation in the myocilin gene is beneficial; it facilitates the decision to early surgery. Using gene testing in known pedigrees increases the likelihood that a positive test is a true positive and therefore is more meaningful.

Jamie Craig's Australian and New Zealand Registry of Advanced Glaucoma has started to collect information on patients with advanced glaucoma (at least one blind eye from glaucoma). Current known genes will be sought and perhaps new genes for blinding glaucoma will be found.[1]

## 1.3 We Have to Find Ways of Better and More Accurate Methods of 24-h IOP Measurement

IOP is the only truly modifiable risk factor in glaucoma. A precise measure of an individual's range of IOP would guide management. This is particularly so in patients whose

---

[1] Personal communication

glaucoma continues to worsen when "control" has been achieved on the basis of "office hours" IOP measurements. Fluctuations in IOP remain an unknown risk factor for glaucoma onset and progression. What fluctuations are important? Inter-visit fluctuations over months? Short-term fluctuations over hours and days? Very short-term fluctuations in seconds or fractions of a second? Diurnal fluctuations in IOP may be a glaucoma progression risk, independent of average IOP.[40] What parameters of IOP are important? Peak IOP? The area under the IOP curve? Mean IOP? Is ocular perfusion pressure (blood pressure – IOP) more important? If so, what aspects of perfusion pressure?

### 1.3.1 Phasing of IOP

To try to obtain more information about a patient's IOP levels, sometimes it is measured several times during the day; this is inconvenient for all. Although this diurnal curve is useful, it is only part of the information. "In office" tests may not detect peak IOP, and early morning and supine IOP levels are missing.

Another way to estimate this range is to see a patient at different times of the day on successive office visits. This is easier and more practical. Admitting a patient to hospital to measure IOP through day and night yields a fuller picture, but is impractical and costly.

Home tonometry is difficult to teach. Even though the Proview phosphene tonometer (Bausch & Lomb, Rochester, New York) allows for self-testing without local anesthesia, using an entopic phenomenon of the pressure-induced phosphene to measure IOP, it has poor correlation with Goldmann applanation tonometry (GAT), which does not improve with experience.[41,42] The Rebound tonometer (ICare, Tiolat Oy, Helsinki, Finland) might have the potential: It is easy to use, requires no anesthetic, can be performed by relatively inexperienced tonometrists[43], and correlates reasonably with GAT.[43]

### 1.3.2 The Water-Drinking Test

Recently, interest has returned to the water-drinking test (WDT).[44-46] Originally used as a tool to detect glaucoma,[47,48] the WDT might estimate the diurnal IOP curve.[44] Relatively easy to do and requiring no additional equipment, either a set volume of water (e.g., 1 L) or a bodyweight-related volume of water (e.g., 10 mL water per kg weight)[46] is imbibed in a few minutes. IOP is measured every 15 min for 1 h or until IOP has returned to baseline. Peak WDT IOP and peak diurnal IOP correlate, as do the fluctuations in IOP diurnally and following the WDT.

IOP fluctuations were significantly less in glaucoma patients controlled following surgery when compared with those on medical treatment.[45] If ongoing research shows WDT validity, reliability, and reproducibility to estimate the diurnal curve, this test could become an important clinical tool.

### 1.3.3 IOP Telemetry

Several forms of IOP telemetry are in various stages of development. A contact lens telemetry system has been used successfully in a small group of people.[49] Implantable IOP telemetry systems are in the stage of animal testing in rabbits and nonhuman primates. Sensors have been implanted on tube-shunts and intraocular lenses.[50,51] Ultimately, biocompatibility and sustained reliability will determine their long-term use.

## 1.4 We Have to Find Ways to Measure Progression So We Can Determine Who is at Risk in Their Lifetime to Lose Vision-Related QOL

For each patient, we need to determine as best we can who may lose quality of life from glaucoma. This entails three variables: the individual life expectancy, the extent of visual damage already, and the measured rate of visual decline.

The glaucoma continuum (see Fig. 1.3) facilitates our concepts of the glaucomas as they progress from undetectable through asymptomatic to manifest glaucoma.

There are a few provisos:

- Sometimes patients can have asymptomatic disease at a later stage of damage, while others can be symptomatic very early on due to bilateral disease with overlapping damaged areas
- Many people do not progress through the whole continuum
- The speed of decline is very individual
- Individual life expectancy is important
- Most patients are in the left part of the continuum rather than in the right
- Some people develop functional changes before structural. In the EMGT, changes were almost entirely functional[25] whilst in OHTS, 50% of the incident glaucoma was on the basis of structural changes only.[53] Their significant variability partly depends on the methods of assessment of structure and function.

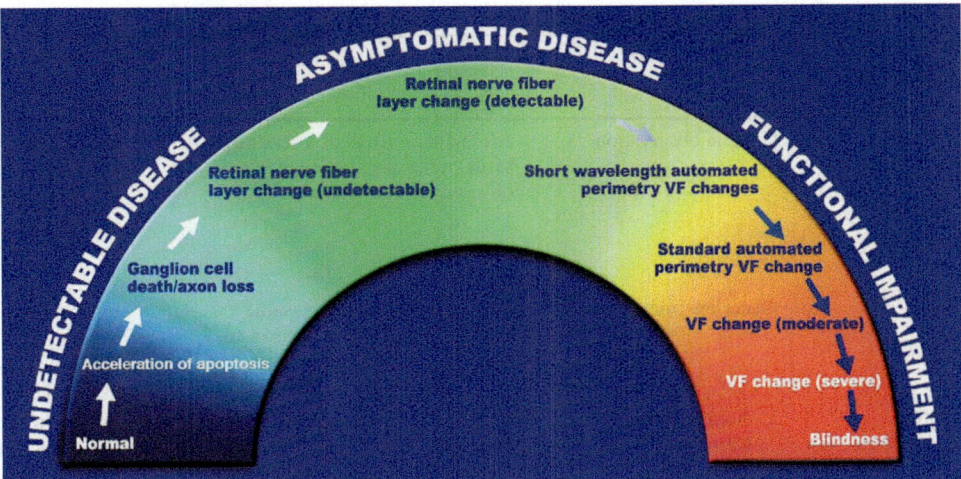

**Fig. 1.3** The glaucoma continuum. Reprinted from ref. 52, with permission from Elsevier

### 1.4.1 Structural Tests

Clinical examination detects structural progression. Objective testing with computerized nerve fiber layer and optic disc analyzers are supplementary to our clinical examination and *does not* replace it. Up-skilling eye care colleagues to recognize an abnormal optic disc and retinal nerve fiber layer and to detect changes clinically are vital. Repeated optic disc and RNFL stereophotography facilitates structural assessment and detection of progressive damage.

Major technological advances have occurred in the computerized objective assessment and follow-up of disc and RNFL structure. The Heidelberg Retina Tomograph (HRT, Heidelberg Engineering GmbH, Heidelberg, Germany), GDX (Laser Diagnostic Technologies, San Diego, California, USA) and Optical Coherence Tomograph (OCT, Stratus and Cirrus OCT; Carl Zeiss Meditec, Dublin, California, USA) have all improved.

Each technology has its strengths and weaknesses; ultimately, none is as good at detecting glaucoma as are a group of experts. However, each has a valuable place in glaucoma management. As they measure different aspects of structure, they are likely to be complementary to one another, rather than "one technology fits all." Any objective information that is reliable, reproducible, and is quantitative is useful and adds to management.

Every technology comes at a cost; even digital stereophotography is not affordable to all. It remains more important to document an optic disc clinically with a detailed, careful drawing than it is to own multiple expensive technologies.

### 1.4.2 Functional Tests

Visual field analysis is not precise to detect progressive glaucoma damage. Because of individual variability, several tests are needed to be sure of real change. For example, to detect a true difference of 4 dB in mean deviation over 2 years, three visual field tests are needed per year.[54] Most clinicians assess perimetric progression by simply "eye-balling" rather than applying scientific rigor. As more information is available than can be easily processed by "clinical judgment," any formalization is a bonus.

Clinicians managing glaucoma need to be familiar with methods to detect visual field progression. There are four main ways to do so: clinical judgment, defect classifications systems, and event or trend analyses (see Table 1.4.).

The perimetric progression analyses have to be accessible and user-friendly to *all* ophthalmologists. The Guided Progression Analysis and the Visual Field Index are being bundled with Humphrey software and may facilitate this. The other visual field analyzer in regular use is the Octopus system. Some, but not all of the above, can be used with the Octopus analyzer.

### 1.4.3 Effects of Visual Loss on Societal Functionality (e.g., Driving) and Independence

As most patients highly value their ability to drive, fear of losing independence by losing their driver's license markedly reduces quality of life. The link between visual field

**Table 1.4** Visual field progression analysis[55]

| Type of field progression analysis | Types | Description | Advantages | Disadvantages |
|---|---|---|---|---|
| Clinical judgment | Clinical observation | • All the parameters of a series of visual fields are studied by the observer and compared | • Easy to do<br>• No extra cost<br>• Can be used with all perimeters | • Non-scientific<br>• Poor reliability<br>• Poor reproducibility<br>• Large inter-observer variation<br>• Observer-dependant |
| | Overview printout | • Several fields are on the same printout page for comparison | • Easy to do<br>• No extra cost<br>• Faster than looking at individual fields | • Non-scientific |
| Defect classification systems | 1. Auhorn and Karmeyer[56]<br>2. Hodapp-Parrish-Anderson (Bascom Palmer Grading System[57]<br>3. Glaucoma Staging System & GSS 2[58]<br>4. Brusini's GSS & GSS 2[59]<br>5. AGIS Score[60]<br>6. CIGTS Score[60] | 1. Five descriptive stages for the kinetic perimeter<br>2. Three glaucoma stages: early, moderate, severe, based on MD, number of points affected and proximity to fixation<br>3. Six stage system based on MD, proximity to fixation and number of points affected<br>4. Six to seven stage system based on MD and PSD, can be used on Humphrey and Octopus visual fields; is provided on the printout of the Oculus visual field<br>5. Score 1–20, uses the total deviation plot of 24-2, threshold values<br>6. Score 1–20, uses the total deviation plot of 24-2, probability values | • Better defined<br>• Validated techniques<br>• Good reproducibility<br>• Correlates well to disease | • Stages are not necessarily linear to disease<br>• 2–6 do not provide spatial information about the defect<br>• 5,6 score calculations are time consuming and not suitable for normal clinical practice<br>• Not sensitive to small increments of progression |
| Trend analysis | • Mean deviation (defect) index (MDI)-change analysis (Humphrey), Peritrend (Interzaag) | • First index to be used for progression<br>• Linear regression on mean deviation | • Humphrey and octopus<br>• Age-matched normative data | • Affected by cataract |
| | • Glaucoma progression index (GPI)[61]/Visual field index | • Part of GPA printout<br>• Pattern deviation probability maps are used<br>• Central weighting | • Reported as a % of age-corrected normal<br>• More resistant to cataract formation<br>• Automated and included in Statpac | • May underestimate generalized reduction in sensitivities from glaucoma |
| | • Peridata[62] | • Progression analysis with box plot curve<br>• Trend Analysis with significance for every point | • Can be used with any perimeter<br>• Also simulates binocular fields<br>• Based on a statistical approach | • Additional software<br>• Data needs transferring to another computer<br>• Additional cost & time |
| | • Progressor | • Linear regression analysis of pointwise threshold data | • Uses all of the threshold information<br>• Represents the data at the point<br>• Also simulates binocular fields<br>• Based on a statistical approach | • Additional software<br>• Data needs transferring to another computer<br>• Additional cost & time<br>• Watch statistical significance versus clinical significance |

(continued)

**Table 1.4** (continued)

| Type of field progression analysis | Types | Description | Advantages | Disadvantages |
|---|---|---|---|---|
| Event analysis | • Delta program<br>• CNTGS | • Uses paired *t* test<br>• Defined as reduction in threshold by 10 dB or three time short-term fluctuation | • Relatively simple<br>• Relatively simple | • Octopus only<br>• Relatively simple |
| | • Glaucoma change probability (GCP, Statpac 2) | • Uses two baseline tests and compares the current total deviation at a point to baseline<br>• Flagged if outside the test-retest variation of a stable glaucoma patient (5–95%) | • Gives spatial and progression information<br>• Only three tests are needed to get a GCP result but this is not specific enough | • Needs reliable baseline<br>• It does not use all of the data available from previous tests<br>• Two confirming fields are required |
| | • Guided progression analysis (GPA) | • Similar to GCP but uses pattern deviation probability plots<br>• Tested in EMGT | • More resistant to cataract<br>• Flags "Possible Progression" and "Likely Progression" | • Needs reliable baseline, baseline can be reset<br>• It does not use all of the data available from previous tests<br>• May miss some fields progressive general loss i.e., underestimate progression[63] |

loss and driving capability is weak. Most countries have visual standards to be able to drive. In Australia, an unrestricted, noncommercial license holder must have a horizontal visual field of 120°, 10° above and below the horizontal axis. The Esterman visual field test (EVFT) has been the main way to estimate the visual field and suitability to drive. It has disadvantages: it involves further testing, and the central 7° of the visual field is not tested. Owen et al have looked at binocular integrated visual field (IVF) to predict which patients will lose visual function to a level below the legal standard for driving.[64] With IVF produced by simulating monocular Humphrey visual fields with the Progressor program,[65] they have described a method that simulates better than does the EVFT what patients see binocularly, using available threshold information. This can identify, even from initial diagnosis, which of our patients are at most risk to lose their driver's license. With this information, we may be able to determine which patients need more aggressive treatment to prevent such an outcome. The Peridata program also merges uniocular visual fields to yield binocular field information.[62]

The benefit of a program such as the Progressor is that all the threshold information that is recorded in normal follow-up testing can be merged to get the binocular data. No additional testing is required, as binocular information can be accessed with uniocular tests. This saves time and encourages routine access of binocular fields information; patients at risk may be found earlier, allowing more aggressive treatment. Figure 1.4 shows an example of a case of a visual field that is "passed fit for driving" on the EVFT that failed on the Progressor IVF analysis.

Another method of assessing the vision used for driving is the UFOV® (Useful field of view).[65] This is the amount of binocular visual field that is seen with both eyes open without moving the eyes or head. The UFOV has been shown to correlate with a history of car accidents in the previous 5 years, and a poor reading of four or five was shown in a prospective study to double the relative risk of involvement in a car accident in the following 3 years. The UFOV is influenced by other factors such as cognitive function and training can improve it.

### 1.4.4 Axon "Screamometer": Future Studies of Retinal Ganglion Cell and Optic Nerve Function

Paul Palmberg coined the term "axon screamometer" to describe a theoretical clinical device that would allow the detection of a single axon dying, or under glaucomatous attack. Working with ocular hypertensive and early glaucoma patients, Ventura and Porciatti have used the pattern electroretinogram (PERG) response to stress retinal ganglion cells, thereby identifying those under reversible attack.[66,67]

Francesca Codeiro has developed a noninvasive real-time imaging technique using confocal laser-scanning ophthalmoscopy to visualize single nerve cell apoptosis in vivo.[68] If an "axon screamometer" were shown to be accurate, decisions to initiate or to accelerate treatment would become far more scientific.

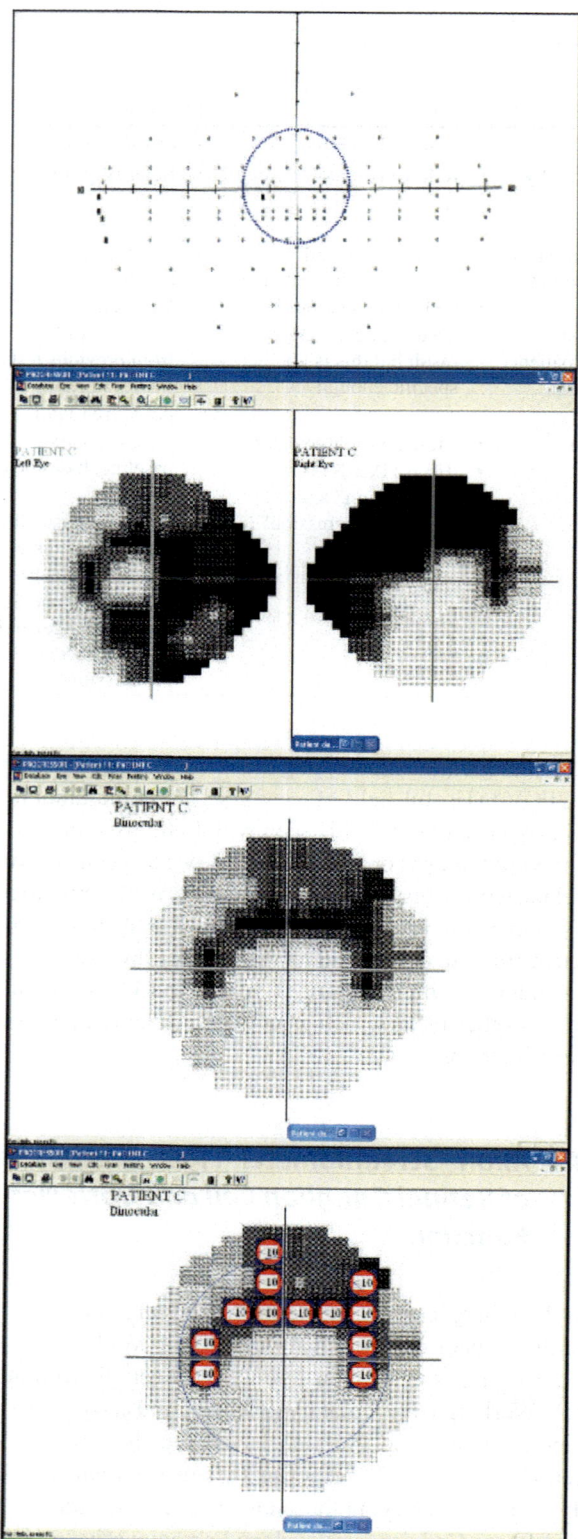

**Fig. 1.4** A comparison of the Esterman binocular visual field, individual Humphrey visual fields and the Progressor binocular visual field in a patient. While the patient satisfies the Esterman criteria for driving, the Progressor field indicates a significant defect and failure. Reprinted from ref.65 with permission of BMJ Publishing Group

## 1.5 We Need to Find Effective Ways of Treating Glaucoma that Are More Tolerable to Our Patients

What is on the horizon for treatment for our patients?

### 1.5.1 Medications with Minimal Side Effects with Which Adherence, Dyscompliance, and Perseverance Are Not Issues

Over the past decade, new classes of IOP-lowering medications have reduced the frequency of instillation and increased potency. With more types of eye drops and fixed combinations, adherence to and perseverance with a medication regimen have become greater issues. With eye drops, physical barriers to instillation success remain a challenge. While newer drug classes with high potency and low side effect potential will be welcomed, improved drug delivery systems might enhance the therapeutic index. For example, punctual plug delivery system technology[69] and anterior juxtascleral depot (AJD) injections[70] could well enhance the treatment.

Medications to arrest the disease by strategies other than IOP reduction would open new paradigms for treatment.

### 1.5.2 Effective Lasers with Minimal Side Effects

Newer lasers that appear to cause little or no structural damage to trabecular connective tissue (e.g., selective laser trabeculoplasty [SLT]) seem to be effective and repeatable. SLT is being used increasingly in earlier treatment. Even though the Glaucoma Laser Trial showed the effectiveness of Argon laser trabeculoplasty, its uptake as primary treatment was not high.[27] Now that we have an equally effective laser with very few side effects, the treatment paradigm is shifting (see Fig. 1.5).

### 1.5.3 Surgical Techniques Without Long-Term Consequences

Glaucoma surgery faces the challenges of overcoming surgical failure (short- and long-term) and complications related to the formation of a bleb, including blebitis and dysesthesia.

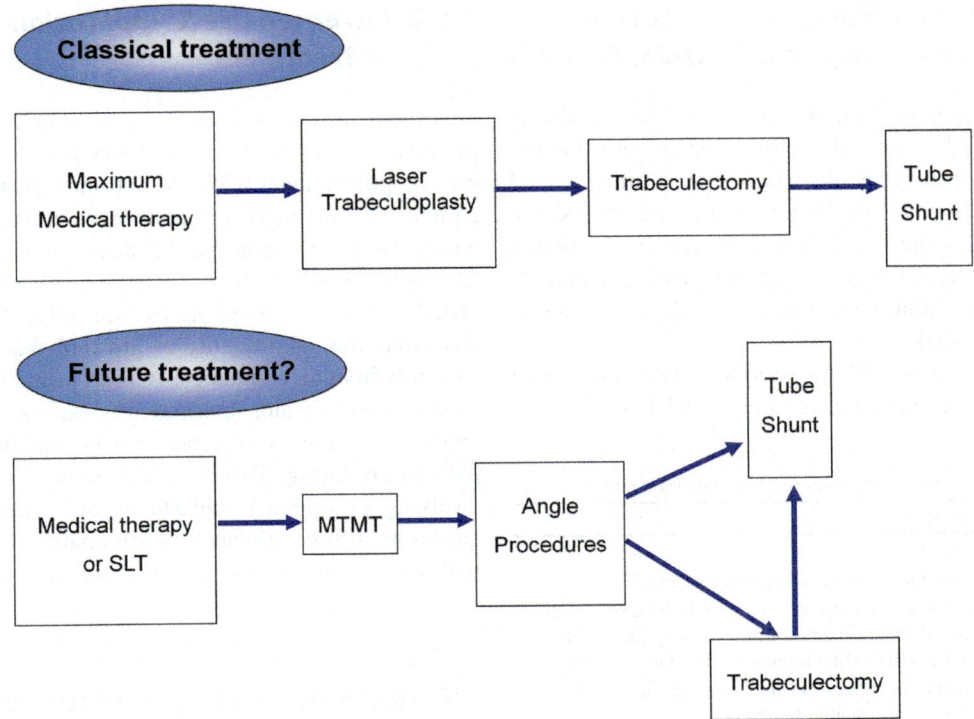

**Fig. 1.5** The classical treatment paradigm versus possible future treatment paradigm. *MTMT* maximum tolerated medical therapy, *SLT* selective laser trabeculoplasty

Trabeculectomy techniques are improving to try to produce diffuse, slightly elevated, normal vascularity, normal thickness, and comfortable blebs that last a lifetime and do not create a lifetime risk of blebitis and endophthalmitis. Peng Khaw's "Moorfields Safer Surgery System" with a fornix-based conjunctival flap, large area mitomycin C application, and adjustable releasable suture has improved safety.

Many newer surgical strategies represent variations to make a bleb. This includes the Express shunt procedure and the nonpenetrating glaucoma surgeries (deep sclerectomy, viscocanalostomy, Aqua Flow collagen glaucoma drainage device). The character of the blebs might be lower in profile and more diffuse; further studies are warranted.

Novel procedures that do not form a bleb are the Trabectome, I-stent micro bypass, Eye Pass procedure, and the SOL-X shunt. The Eye Pass, SOL-X shunt, and I-stent procedures involve the insertion of a device. The Eye Pass and the I-stent are shunts from the anterior chamber to Schlemm's canal, while the SOL-X is from the anterior chamber to the suprachoroidal space. The Trabectome and I-stent procedures have no conjunctival or scleral incisions; if they fail, trabeculectomy could be performed on "virginal" conjunctiva.

Glaucoma Drainage Devices (GDD) might be useful for earlier stages of glaucoma. Traditionally, they have been reserved for very damaged eyes when several other procedures have failed; it might be easier to teach and to perform than trabeculectomy, and reduce bleb-related complications. An ongoing study of trabeculectomy versus tubes (TVT study) should yield valuable information.[71]

In the next few decades, we may see changes in our treatment paradigm (see Fig. 1.5) with lasers being offered earlier, angle procedures being included in the treatment armamentarium, and possibly tube shunt procedures being performed earlier.

## 1.6 We Have to Measure QOL More Reliably and Use it to Help Patients More Appropriately

We have clinical endpoints to manage our patients. IOP, optic disc and retinal nerve fiber layer assessment, and visual field parameters have been our main outcomes. In the twenty-first century, we should focus on the patient as a whole, not only in research but also in clinical practice. To do this, we need to use quality of life measures in our day-to-day patient assessment and management.

### 1.6.1 Increase Familiarity of Profession with QOL Measure (e.g., NEI-VFQ-25, GQL-15)

There are four types of tools for quality of life measuring tools (see Table 1.5.): general health measurements, vision-specific instruments, glaucoma-specific instruments, and utility assessments. Some of these measures are not specific to glaucoma and some are designed for use in a research study setting. The types of quality-of-life measurement tools that are the most useful, clinically short, self-administered, reliable, and validated.

The NEI-VFQ-51 is a 51-question tool, which has been validated, as has a 25-question version: NEI-VFQ-25.

**Table 1.5** Quality of life instruments used in glaucoma patients

| Instrument | Description |
|---|---|
| General health instruments | |
| SIP | Modified to be more specific for glaucoma |
| SF-36 | 36 items, eight subscales (general health, physical/social functions, role limitations by physical/mental disability, mental health, vitality, pain) |
| MOS-20 | 20 items, six subscales (physical/role/social functioning, mental health, health perceptions, pain) |
| Vision-specific instruments | |
| ADVS | Developed to assess impact of cataract; 20 activities, subscales include day/night/far/near vision, glare impact, overall vision |
| VF-14 | Developed to assess impact of cataract; 14 vision-related activities from reading various print sizes to driving |
| VAQ | Assesses ten areas of vision, including peripheral vision, contrast sensitivity, acuity, impact of glare and low illumination, light/dark adaptation |
| NEI-VFQ | 51 items; developed to assess the impact of a broad range of eye problems; similar 25-item instrument (NEI-VFQ-25) developed later |
| IVI | 32 items, five domains: leisure/work, consumer/social interaction, household/personal care, mobility, emotional reaction to vision loss |
| Glaucoma-specific instruments | |
| GSS | Symptom checklist, ten items, two subscales |
| Viswanathan et al | Ten queries related to decreased visual ability |
| SIG | 43 items, 4 subscales: visual ability (visual function), local eye, systemic, and psychological |
| GHPI | Six items, glaucoma impact on physical, emotional, social, and cognitive components of health, stress associated with glaucoma and blindness worries |
| GQL-15 | 15-most glaucoma-specific queries selected from a starting list of 50 by factor analysis |
| Utility assessments | |
| Time trade-off | How much lifespan to trade for perfect vision? |
| Thermometer | Vision assessment of 0–100, transformed to death/health scale of 0–100 |
| Choice-based conjoint analysis | Choices between visual disability outcomes |

Based on ref. 72 with permission of Elsevier

### 1.6.2 Increased Use & Application to Treatment

Quality-of-life measures in glaucoma suffer the same predicament as do other clinical outcome measures: There is no true gold standard. We do not know how our glaucoma patients *really* feel. Therefore, we validate our instruments to a surrogate outcome such as the degree of visual field defect. The GQL-15, for example, correlates well with the degree of visual field loss. The GQL-15 (see Table 1.6.) has all the characteristics of a quality-of-life tool that could be used routinely in clinical practice. A 15-question tool, it could be used at baseline and intermittently during the course of a patient's disease to gain better understanding of how our patients are faring. There are five "seeing" questions, seven "walking or mobility" questions, and three "adjustment" questions in this validated questionnaire. It correlates well with visual field severity in glaucoma patients.

## 1.7 Find Safe and Appropriate Way to Share Care with Other Eye Care Professionals: Proper Use of Available Human Resources

Screening, case detection, professional and community education, promulgation of information, liaison with our communities, and tackling global blindness and visual disability are some ways we could train and work with other eye care professionals. With more work needed than human power or skills available, a safe sharing of this burden is necessary for success. This interface must be dynamic and under the leadership of ophthalmologists.

As populations age, so will the burden of glaucoma increase. Different sharing models include a system in some United Kingdom hospital centers, where medical practitioners not formally ophthalmically trained (associate specialists) and optometrists work side by side under the supervision of an ophthalmologist. This significantly reduces the manpower burden.[74] While using nonmedical optometric staff could reduce the burden, it could also increase it if unnecessary return visits results. That this depends on training and on supervision was shown by a formal comparison of the clinical decision skills of assistant optometrists in a glaucoma clinic at Moorfields Eye Hospital, London, with associate specialists.[74] There was no difference demonstrated.

In a rigorous randomized study assessing patient outcomes, the Bristol shared care glaucoma project compared hospital eye care with that of community optometrists.[75] At 2 years, while there was no difference to patient outcomes,

**Table 1.6** The glaucoma quality of life – 15 questionnaire

*The glaucoma quality of life – 15 questionnaire:*
*List of daily activities with the strongest relationship with visual field loss in glaucoma*[a]

Patient instruction: Please circle the correct answer on the scale ranging from 1 to 5 where [1] stands for no difficulty, [2] for a little bit of difficulty, [3] for some difficulty, [4] for quite a lot of difficulty, and [5] for severe difficulty. If you do not perform any of the activities for other than visual reasons, please circle [0].

Does your vision give you any difficulty, even with glasses, with the following activities?

| | None | A little bit | Some | Quite a lot | Severe | Do not perform for nonvisual reasons |
|---|---|---|---|---|---|---|
| Reading newspapers | 1 | 2 | 3 | 4 | 5 | 0 |
| Walking after dark | 1 | 2 | 3 | 4 | 5 | 0 |
| Seeing at night | 1 | 2 | 3 | 4 | 5 | 0 |
| Walking on uneven ground | 1 | 2 | 3 | 4 | 5 | 0 |
| Adjusting to bright lights | 1 | 2 | 3 | 4 | 5 | 0 |
| Adjusting to dim lights | 1 | 2 | 3 | 4 | 5 | 0 |
| Going from light to dark room or vice versa | 1 | 2 | 3 | 4 | 5 | 0 |
| Tripping over objects | 1 | 2 | 3 | 4 | 5 | 0 |
| Seeing objects coming from the side | 1 | 2 | 3 | 4 | 5 | 0 |
| Crossing the road | 1 | 2 | 3 | 4 | 5 | 0 |
| Walking on steps/stairs | 1 | 2 | 3 | 4 | 5 | 0 |
| Bumping into objects | 1 | 2 | 3 | 4 | 5 | 0 |
| Judging distance of foot to step/curb | 1 | 2 | 3 | 4 | 5 | 0 |
| Finding dropped objects | 1 | 2 | 3 | 4 | 5 | 0 |
| Recognizing faces | 1 | 2 | 3 | 4 | 5 | 0 |

Reprinted from ref. 73 with permission of Lippincott
[a]Based on the results of this study

community was more costly than hospital care. The optometrists involved were keen volunteers with specialized training; this group might not represent results in the general optometric community. The opportunities for collaboration are there. With appropriate training, supervision, and lines of responsibility, our patients and communities could be better served.

## 1.8 Conclusion

Glaucoma concepts and management are changing rapidly. In this new millennium, we need to find those with glaucoma as yet unidentified so that they can receive treatment; we need to focus on the therapeutic, emotional, and societal needs of the individual patient; we need to understand IOP levels and fluctuations better; we need to find effective strategies to protect individuals from visual disability beyond lowering IOP; we need to find more specific and more sensitive ways to diagnose glaucoma and to detect its progression; and we need to find safe, responsible ways of working collaboratively with other eye care workers, for the benefits of our patients and our communities.

## References

1. Shaffer RN. The centennial history of glaucoma (1896–1996), American Academy of Ophthalmology. *Ophthalmology*. 1996;103(8 Suppl):S40–S50.
2. Shaffer RN. Fifty years in ophthalmology. *Surv Ophthalmol*. 1990;35(3):236–239.
3. Nathan J. Hippocrates to Duke-Elder: an overview of the history of glaucoma. *Clin Exp Optom*. 2000;83(3):116–118.
4. Frezzotti R. The glaucoma mystery from ancient times to the 21st century, The glaucoma mystery: ancient concepts. *Acta Ophthalmol Scand Suppl* 2000;(232):14–18
5. Keeler R. Antique ophthalmic instruments and books: the Royal College Museum. *Br J Ophthalmol*. 2002;86(7):712–714.
6. Andersen SR. The history of the Ophthalmological Society of Copenhagen 1900–1950. *Acta Ophthalmol Scand Suppl*. 2002;234:6–17.
7. Dellaporta A. Historical notes on gonioscopy. *Surv Ophthalmol*. 1975;20(2):137–149.
8. Ritch R, Caronia RM, eds, Classic Papers in Glaucoma, Kugler Publications, The Netherlands, 2000.
9. Mitchell P, Smith W, Attebo K, Healey PR. Prevalence of open-angle glaucoma in Australia. The Blue Mountains Eye Study. *Ophthalmology*. 1996;103(10):1661–1669.
10. Wensor MD, McCarty CA, Stanislavsky YL, et al. The prevalence of glaucoma in the Melbourne Visual Impairment Project. *Ophthalmology*. 1998;105(4):733–739.
11. Varma R, Ying-Lai M, Francis BA, et al. Prevalence of open-angle glaucoma and ocular hypertension in Latinos: the Los Angeles Latino Eye Study. *Ophthalmology*. 2004;111(8):1439–1448.
12. Sakata K, Sakata LM, Sakata VM, et al. Prevalence of glaucoma in a South brazilian population: Projeto Glaucoma. *Invest Ophthalmol Vis Sci*. 2007;48(11):4974–4979.
13. Wong EY, Keeffe JE, Rait JL, et al. Detection of undiagnosed glaucoma by eye health professionals. *Ophthalmology*. 2004;111(8):1508–1514.
14. Wilson JMG, Jungner G. Principles and practice of screening for disease. *WHO Chron*. 1968;22:473.
15. Wilson MR. The myth of "21". *J Glaucoma*. 1997;6(2):75–77.
16. Leydhecker W, Akiyama K, Neumann HG. Intraocular pressure in normal human eyes. *Klin Monatsblatter Augenheilkd Augenarztl Fortbild*. 1958;133(5):662–670.
17. Hollows FC, Graham PA. Intra-ocular pressure, glaucoma, and glaucoma suspects in a defined population. *Br J Ophthalmol*. 1966;50(10):570–586.

18. Eddy DM, Sanders LE, Eddy JF. The value of screening for glaucoma with tonometry. *Surv Ophthalmol.* 1983;28(3):194–205.
19. Eddy DM, Billings J. The quality of medical evidence: implications for quality of care. *Health Aff (Millwood).* 1988;7(1):19–32.
20. The Advanced Glaucoma Intervention Study (AGIS): 7. The relationship between control of intraocular pressure and visual field deterioration. The AGIS Investigators. *Am J Ophthalmol.* 2000;130(4):429–440
21. Klein BE, Klein R, Sponsel WE, et al. Prevalence of glaucoma. The Beaver Dam Eye Study. *Ophthalmology.* 1992;99(10):1499–1504.
22. Feiner L, Piltz-Seymour JR. Collaborative Initial Glaucoma Treatment Study: a summary of results to date. *Curr Opin Ophthalmol.* 2003;14(2):106–111.
23. Comparison of glaucomatous progression between untreated patients with normal-tension glaucoma and patients with therapeutically reduced intraocular pressures. Collaborative Normal-Tension Glaucoma Study Group. *Am J Ophthalmol* 1998;126(4):487–497
24. Miglior S, Zeyen T, Pfeiffer N, et al. Results of the European Glaucoma Prevention Study. *Ophthalmology.* 2005;112(3):366–375.
25. Heijl A, Leske MC, Bengtsson B, et al. Reduction of intraocular pressure and glaucoma progression: results from the Early Manifest Glaucoma Trial. *Arch Ophthalmol.* 2002;120(10):1268–1279.
26. Five-year follow-up of the Fluorouracil Filtering Surgery Study. The Fluorouracil Filtering Surgery Study Group. *Am J Ophthalmol* 1996;121(4):349–366
27. The Glaucoma Laser Trial (GLT) and glaucoma laser trial follow-up study: 7. Results. Glaucoma Laser Trial Research Group. *Am J Ophthalmol* 1995;120(6):718–731
28. Gordon MO, Beiser JA, Brandt JD, et al. The Ocular Hypertension Treatment Study: baseline factors that predict the onset of primary open-angle glaucoma. *Arch Ophthalmol* 2002;120(6):714–720; discussion 829–830
29. Friedman DS, Jampel HD, Munoz B, West SK. The prevalence of open-angle glaucoma among blacks and whites 73 years and older: the Salisbury Eye Evaluation Glaucoma Study. *Arch Ophthalmol.* 2006;124(11):1625–1630.
30. Burr JM, Mowatt G, Hernandez R, et al. The clinical effectiveness and cost-effectiveness of screening for open angle glaucoma: a systematic review and economic evaluation. *Health Technol Assess* 2007;11(41):iii–iv, ix–x, 1–190
31. Fleming C, Whitlock E, Biel T, Smit B. Primary care screening for ocular hypertension and primary open-angle glaucoma: Evidence Synthesis. No. 34. Agency for Healthcare Research & Quality, US Preventative Services Task Force; 2005. Available at: http://www.ahrq.gov/clinic/uspstf05/glaucoma/ glaucsyn.pdf. Accessed June 2008
32. Weinreb RN, Healey PR and Topouzis Glaucoma Screening, WGA consensus series 5, Kugler Publications, 2008 The Netherlands
33. Grodum K, Heijl A, Bengtsson B. A comparison of glaucoma patients identified through mass screening and in routine clinical practice. *Acta Ophthalmol Scand.* 2002;80(6):627–631.
34. South East Asia Glaucoma Interest Group Guidlines, published online at www.seagig.org
35. Danesh-Meyer HV, Deva NC, Slight C, et al. What do people with glaucoma know about their condition? A comparative cross-sectional incidence and prevalence survey. *Clin Experiment Ophthalmol.* 2008;36(1):13–18.
36. Odberg T, Jakobsen JE, Hultgren SJ, Halseide R. The impact of glaucoma on the quality of life of patients in Norway. I. Results from a self-administered questionnaire. *Acta Ophthalmol Scand.* 2001;79(2):116–120.
37. McNaught AI, Allen JG, Healey DL, et al. Accuracy and implications of a reported family history of glaucoma: experience from the Glaucoma Inheritance Study in Tasmania. *Arch Ophthalmol.* 2000;118(7):900–904.
38. Green CM, Kearns LS, Wu J, et al. How significant is a family history of glaucoma? Experience from the Glaucoma Inheritance Study in Tasmania. *Clin Experiment Ophthalmol.* 2007;35(9):793–799.
39. Marx J. Genetics. High-risk glaucoma gene found in Nordic studies. *Science.* 2007;317(5839):735.
40. Asrani S, Zeimer R, Wilensky J, et al. Large diurnal fluctuations in intraocular pressure are an independent risk factor in patients with glaucoma. *J Glaucoma.* 2000;9(2):134–142.
41. Danesh-Meyer HV, Niederer R, Gaskin BJ, Gamble G. Comparison of the Proview pressure phosphene tonometer performed by the patient and examiner with the Goldmann applanation tonometer. *Clin Experiment Ophthalmol.* 2004;32(1):29–32.
42. Gunvant P, Lievens CW, Newman JM 3rd, et al. Evaluation of some factors affecting the agreement between the Proview Eye Pressure Monitor and the Goldmann applanation tonometer measurements. *Clin Exp Optom.* 2007;90(4):290–295.
43. Abraham LM, Epasinghe NC, Selva D, Casson R. Comparison of the ICare rebound tonometer with the Goldmann applanation tonometer by experienced and inexperienced tonometrists. *Eye.* 2008;22(4):503–506.
44. Susanna R Jr, Vessani RM, Sakata L, et al. The relation between intraocular pressure peak in the water drinking test and visual field progression in glaucoma. *Br J Ophthalmol.* 2005;89(10):1298–1301.
45. Danesh-Meyer HV, Papchenko T, Tan YW, Gamble GD. Medically controlled glaucoma patients show greater increase in intraocular pressure than surgically controlled patients with the water drinking test. *Ophthalmology.* 2008;115(9):1566–1570.
46. Kumar RS, de Guzman MH, Ong PY, Goldberg I. Does peak intraocular pressure measured by water drinking test reflect peak circadian levels? A pilot study. *Clin Experiment Ophthalmol.* 2008;36(4):312–315.
47. Schmidt K. Untersuchungen über Kapilarendothelstörungen bei Glaukoma simplex. *Arch Augenheilkd* 1928(98):569–581
48. Leydhecker W. The water-drinking test. *Br J Ophthalmol.* 1950;34(8):457–479.
49. Pitchon E, Leonardi M, Renaud P, et al. First in vivo human measure of the intraocular pressure fluctuation and ocular pulsation by a wireless soft contact lens sensor. Abstracts of the Association for Research in Vision and Ophthalmology 2008 Annual Meeting; April 27–May 1, 2008; Fort Lauderdale, Florida. Abstract 687, 2008.
50. Downs J, Burgoyne CF, Liang Y, Sallee VL. A new implantable system for telemetric IOP monitoring in nonhuman primates (NHP). Program and abstracts of the Association for Research in Vision and Ophthalmology 2008 Annual Meeting. Fort Lauderdale, Florida. Abstract 2043, 2008
51. Aebersold J, Jackson D, Crain M, et al. Development of an implantable, RFID-based intraocular pressure sensing system for glaucoma patients. Program and abstracts of the Association for Research in Vision and Ophthalmology 2008 Annual Meeting. Fort Lauderdale, Florida. Abstract 688, 2008
52. Weinreb RN, Friedman DS, Fechtner RD, et al. Risk assessment in the management of patients with ocular hypertension. *Am J Ophthalmol.* 2004;138(3):458–467.
53. Kass MA, Heuer DK, Higginbotham EJ, et al. The Ocular Hypertension Treatment Study: a randomized trial determines that topical ocular hypotensive medication delays or prevents the onset of primary open-angle glaucoma. *Arch Ophthalmol* 2002;120(6):701–713; discussion 829–830
54. Chauhan BC, Garway-Heath DF, Goni FJ, et al. Practical recommendations for measuring rates of visual field change in glaucoma. *Br J Ophthalmol.* 2008;92(4):569–573.
55. Spry PG, Johnson CA. Identification of progressive glaucomatous visual field loss. *Surv Ophthalmol.* 2002;47(2):158–173.

56. Aulhorn E, Karmeyer H. Frequency distribution in early glaucomatous visual field defects. *Doc Ophthalmol Proc Ser.* 1977;14:75–83.
57. Hodapp E, Parrish RI, Anderson D. *Clinical decisions in glaucoma, 52–61 ed.* St. Louis, MO: CV Mosby; 1993.
58. Mills RP, Budenz DL, Lee PP, et al. Categorizing the stage of glaucoma from pre-diagnosis to end-stage disease. *Am J Ophthalmol.* 2006;141(1):24–30.
59. Brusini P, Filacorda S. Enhanced glaucoma staging system (GSS 2) for classifying functional damage in glaucoma. *J Glaucoma.* 2006;15(1):40–46.
60. Katz J. Scoring systems for measuring progression of visual field loss in clinical trials of glaucoma treatment. *Ophthalmology.* 1999;106(2):391–395.
61. Bengtsson B, Heijl A. A visual field index for calculation of glaucoma rate of progression. *Am J Ophthalmol.* 2008;145(2):343–353.
62. Peridata. Available at: http://www.peridata.org. Accessed September 4, 2008
63. Artes PH, Nicolela MT, LeBlanc RP, Chauhan BC. Visual field progression in glaucoma: total versus pattern deviation analyses. *Invest Ophthalmol Vis Sci.* 2005;46(12):4600–4606.
64. Owen VM, Crabb DP, White ET, et al. Glaucoma and fitness to drive: using binocular visual fields to predict a milestone to blindness. *Invest Ophthalmol Vis Sci.* 2008;49(6):2449–2455.
65. Crabb DP, Fitzke FW, Hitchings RA, Viswanathan AC. A practical approach to measuring the visual field component of fitness to drive. *Br J Ophthalmol.* 2004;88(9):1191–1196.
66. Ventura LM, Sorokac N, De Los Santos R, et al. The relationship between retinal ganglion cell function and retinal nerve fiber thickness in early glaucoma. *Invest Ophthalmol Vis Sci.* 2006;47(9):3904–3911.
67. Ventura LM, Porciatti V. Restoration of retinal ganglion cell function in early glaucoma after intraocular pressure reduction: a pilot study. *Ophthalmology.* 2005;112(1):20–27.
68. Cordeiro MF, Guo L, Luong V, et al. Real-time imaging of single nerve cell apoptosis in retinal neurodegeneration. *Proc Natl Acad Sci USA.* 2004;101(36):13352–13356.
69. http://clinicaltrials.gov/ct2/show?term=xalatan&rank=35 2008.
70. http://clinicaltrials.gov/ct2/show/NCT00451152?term=anecortave&rank=18;2008
71. Gedde SJ, Schiffman JC, Feuer WJ, et al. Treatment outcomes in the tube versus trabeculectomy study after one year of follow-up. *Am J Ophthalmol.* 2007;143(1):9–22.
72. Spaeth G, Walt J, Keener J. Evaluation of quality of life for patients with glaucoma. *Am J Ophthalmol.* 2006;141(1 Suppl):S3–S14.
73. Nelson P, Aspinall P, Papasouliotis O, et al. Quality of life in glaucoma and its relationship with visual function. *J Glaucoma.* 2003;12(2):139–150.
74. Banes MJ, Culham LE, Bunce C, et al. Agreement between optometrists and ophthalmologists on clinical management decisions for patients with glaucoma. *Br J Ophthalmol.* 2006;90(5):579–585.
75. Gray SF, Spry PG, Brookes ST, et al. The Bristol shared care glaucoma study: outcome at follow up at 2 years. *Br J Ophthalmol.* 2000;84(5):456–463.

# Chapter 2
# An Evidence-Based Approach to Glaucoma Care

Louis R. Pasquale

Put several glaucoma specialists in a room and solicit opinions on just about any clinical issue and you are bound to receive multiple opinions on how to manage the problem. For example, a patient presents with shallow angles on van Herrick screening. What gonioscopic features would prompt you to perform a laser iridotomy? Would you perform a dark room provocative test to confirm your impression that the angle was potentially occludable? Do you perform a pharmacological challenge test before proceeding to prophylactic laser iridotomy? Would you order an ultrasound biomicroscopic test to confirm your impression? If you do decide that prophylactic laser iridotomy is indicated, what is the best surgical technique for achieving patency? Is there evidence to support a "best approach" to the patient with the narrow angle? In this chapter, we discuss how evidence-based medicine (EBM) can be used to provide the very best answers to questions such as these. This approach can be applied not only to glaucoma problems, but also to any clinical problem in medicine.

## 2.1 An Introduction to Evidence-Based Medicine

The era of evidence-based medicine is upon us. The Cochrane Collaboration (a large collection of volunteers who use a systematic approach to evaluate the efficacy and safety of medical interventions)[1] has outmuscled the senior, distinguished, and experienced collection of dinner speakers (the so-called members of "eminence-based medicine")[2] whisked in from afar by pharmaceutical companies to tell us what is best for our patients. Today, even when "thought leaders" (a buzzword that finds its origin in the business world used to denote someone held in high regard because of his or her trendsetting ideas or the appearance of his or her names on mail-in surveys) are recruited to speak about a medical product by industry, continuing medical education guidelines dictate that they must provide a balanced and evidence-based presentation.

Yet there is considerable confusion regarding EBM. An article in *Time* magazine stated that EBM was "a hard, cold empirical look at what works, what doesn't and how to distinguish between the two."[3] This statement about EBM suggests that all patient problems have straightforward solutions and EBM helps find those solutions fairly readily. Clearly, we commonly encounter glaucoma problems that are not straightforward at all. For instance, should we commit a European-derived Caucasian male patient with thin corneas, intraocular pressure (IOP) in the high-teens, glaucoma-like discs, and unreliable visual field findings to medical therapy for glaucoma? The Ocular Hypertension Treatment Study (OHTS), a randomized control trial (RCT) comparing IOP-lowering therapy versus observation in the prevention of primary open-angle glaucoma (POAG) in patients with ocular hypertension (OHTN), found thinner central corneal thickness (CCT) to be a risk factor for conversion to POAG among patients with OHTN[4]; but while our patient has thin CCT, his IOP is normal. The Barbados Eye Study[5] found that thinner CCT was an independent risk factor for POAG in a population of African descent, where subjects had a spectrum of IOP ranging from normal to high; however, this patient is Caucasian, which raises the question of whether the data are specifically applicable to his situation. Furthermore, there are absolutely no data to suggest that such treatment would be cost-effective at this time. Finally, there are patient-specific issues that may make the answer to this question even more difficult to arrive at. For example, if the patient is 80 years old and has a pill-rolling tremor secondary to Parkinson's disease and is already taking eight other oral agents for other systemic illnesses, then the physician may opt to observe the patient. On the other hand, if the patient is 53 years old, expresses anxiety about glaucoma blindness, and has a strong family history for the disease, then the physician may be inclined to initiate treatment.

Dr. David Sackett, often regarded as the father of EBM, defines EBM as "the conscientious, explicit and judicious use of current best evidence in making decisions about the care of individual patients."[6] EBM is a *process* and there is nothing cold and calculating about it. The process starts with a patient in your exam lane. Typically that patient has a clinical problem that cannot be answered by consulting an ophthalmology textbook or a single paper in the literature, unless that paper happens to be an EBM review on the topic. For example, a 45-year-old African-American female with a positive family history of glaucoma blindness presents with intraocular pressure (IOP) of 24 mmHg OU, central corneal thicknesses of 545 μm OU, and CDR = 0.4, OU. A standard automated perimetry test is performed and is reliable and normal in both eyes. Do we treat this patient? If we do treat her, what would be the best initial approach? First, we assemble what is called the "evidence cart." Admittedly, the cart may not be loaded with items (as it might be if we were dealing with breast cancer or myocardial infarction), but the items that are there may be quite appropriate for that patient sitting in your exam lane. Then, we need to examine the quality of the evidence in that cart. Finally, we apply that evidence to our patient as best as we can, given the medical and nonmedical circumstances related to her case. Later in this chapter, we will demonstrate the EBM process in detail.

## 2.2 Evidence-Based Medicine: An Interesting Story

In the year 2000, a glaucoma specialist was asked to give a talk on basic eye emergencies directed to primary care physicians. For a glaucoma specialist with a tertiary level glaucoma referral practice, delivering a talk on this subject seemed like a relatively easy task. During the talk, the glaucoma specialist pointed out that the best way to manage a traumatic corneal abrasion was to instill an antibiotic ointment and Cyclogyl 1% drops topically, pressure patch the eye, and follow-up with the patient the next day. A very clear rationale for this approach was provided: The antibiotic provided coverage against microbial invasion of the corneal stroma during the time when there was a breach in the overlying epithelial barrier; the cycloplegic agent reduced uveal spasm induced by the highly innervated cornea; and the pressure patch immobilized the lid to allow corneal limbal stem cells to resurface the epithelial break and settle onto the underlying Bowman's membrane. How could that possibly be the wrong way to manage garden-variety corneal abrasions? At the end of the lecture, one of the course attendees politely approached the glaucoma specialist and stated that he might not be practicing EBM and that most abrasions could be treated without patching. This sounded like heresy to the glaucoma specialist. After all, the patch made the patient comfortable, and theoretically it should enhance resurfacing of the cornea epithelial defect – it had to be the correct approach! That night, the glaucoma specialist did a literature search on the management of cornea abrasions, and to his amazement he found a meta-analysis published in 1998 synthesizing the results of five randomized clinical trials comparing the patch versus no patch approach to managing traumatic corneal abrasions. The meta-analysis concluded that there was no advantage to patching as long as the patient was treated with a topical antibiotic, topical cycloplegia, and topical nonsteroidal anti-inflammatory agent.[7] In fact, two randomized clinical trials (RCTs) published after this systematic literature review reached similar conclusions.[8,9] Of course, it did not mean patching corneal abrasions was akin to malpractice; but it did indicate that this glaucoma specialist who completed his ophthalmology residency in 1990 and was not treating corneal abrasions on a regular basis anymore did not stay up-to-date in the management of traumatic corneal abrasion. He was not aware that one could manage corneal abrasions without resorting to patching the eye prior to delivering a lecture of the subject in year 2000. Oh by the way, I was that glaucoma specialist and that was the "ah-hah" moment that sparked my interest in EBM.

### 2.2.1 The Evolution of Evidence-Based Medicine

While the origin of EBM can be traced back to medieval times,[10] the trends in medical care that resulted in the current embrace of EBM can be traced back to the American Revolution, starting with a physician-signer of the Declaration of Independence, Dr. Benjamin Rush. Dr. Rush's approach to disease was to zealously attack and conquer it. After all, it was this philosophy that allowed the colonists to ultimately prevail over a seemingly formidable British adversary. Unfortunately, there were no real tools to address most of the medical problems encountered; and the attacks fervently employed by Dr. Rush (limited exsanguinations, the induction of emesis, blistering, etc.) typically took a "one-size-fits-all" approach, without evidence that they actually helped patients.[11] Ultimately Dr. Rush's ardent medical philosophy was supplanted by the realization that most medical therapies of the time were largely ineffective. The highly influential Sir William Osler popularized this latter philosophy. His approach to disease can be summed up in one of his more famous aphorisms: *One of the first duties of the physician is to educate the masses not to take medicines.*[12] Sir Osler, regarded as the father of modern medicine, stated that the role of the physician was to provide accurate diagnoses, prognoses, and palliative care for most conditions. Beginning

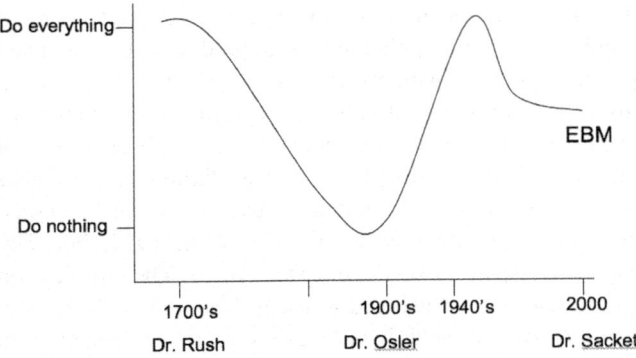

**Fig. 2.1** The medical profession's approach to treatment interventions over time

in the early 1940s, the field of medicine witnessed the antibiotic revolution, the introduction of chemotherapy agents, and the discovery of prednisone. These agents looked like miraculous substances compared to what treatments were available to address medical conditions in the early 1900s (see Morrris[13] for a historical account of the impact of antibiotic therapy in the 1940s). Nonetheless, initial enthusiasm for these new tools led to their indiscriminate and often ill-advised use that did not necessarily translate into clinical benefit for our patients. In the mid 1990s, Dr. David Sackett introduced the idea that we should evaluate the literature with an eye toward finding the best evidence to guide clinical decision-making. The relation between the degrees of intervention for medical illness as a function of time dating from the late 1700s to present is illustrated in Fig. 2.1.

### 2.2.2 Evidence-Based Medicine: Why Bother?

There are compelling reasons to use the EBM process in the delivery of health care. First, there is an increasing volume of evidence available to address clinical problems, and the EBM approach helps keep the clinician abreast of this evidence in a way that allows them to deliver the best care for patients. For example, a major innovation in managing patients with OHTN involves using risk calculators to assess the chance of developing POAG. An estimate of the risk can be an important factor in deciding whether an OHTN patient should be committed to medical therapy for glaucoma. Mansberger introduced a glaucoma risk calculator to estimate the probability of converting from OHTN to POAG in 2003 using data from OHTS.[14] In 2005, Medeiros and colleagues confirmed the function of a similar calculator in an independent sample of patients with OHTN.[15] In 2007, researchers from the United States and Europe introduced a revised calculator based on the combined results of OHTS and the European Glaucoma Prevention Study (EGPS).[16] The EGPS, was a placebo-controlled RCT that compared dorzolamide (a topical carbonic anhydrase inhibitor) versus placebo in the prevention of POAG among patients with OHTN. The EGPS has similar characteristics to OHTS, allowing investigators to pool the data from both trials in estimating the risk of developing POAG. The latest calculator represents a significant revision from the earlier tools in that it does not use diabetes status in estimating the risk of converting from OHTN to POAG. The initial versions of the calculator assigned a reduced risk of conversion from OHTN to POAG among diabetic patients because the OHTS found that a self-report of diabetes mellitus was associated with a reduced risk of converting from OHTN to POAG. However, when data from OHTS were combined with the EGPS, diabetes was no longer related with conversion from OHTN to POAG. Hence, the latest calculator provides the most updated assessment of risk. Certainly, more refinements of the glaucoma risk calculator are forthcoming, such as adjustment for life expectancy, and if you practice EBM, you will be familiar with these refinements because EBM engages you in following new developments in managing disease.

Another reason to practice EBM is that learning the principles of EBM will make you a perpetual student of medicine; and, after all, was not lifelong learning about disease one of the reasons we entered this noble profession in the first place? You can begin practicing EBM now. You can review the medical decision-making that you make during the course of a day in your office and follow the EBM process to see what the consensus of evidence suggests is the best way to arrive at a particular management decision. You will be surprised that more often than not, the literature does not address your particular patient problem. While one may view this as a shortcoming of the EBM approach, it may also represent an opportunity to perform research to advance clinical knowledge in a particular area.

There are other benefits to practicing EBM. It gives you a sense of control because you decide what questions are important and relevant (because they involve your patients) and you can find out the answer to these questions (if there are any answers). It provides a way for you to question the status quo. Does lowering IOP really slow the progression of visual field loss when we critically review the evidence? What is the ideal second-line treatment for POAG? What is the best surgical approach for a patient with pseudophakia and uncontrolled IOP? Many of these questions will be addressed in the subsequent chapters of this textbook. Finally, practicing EBM allows you to challenge seemingly authoritative expert opinion. If a learned glaucoma expert comes to your town espousing a statement like, "Visual field progression from POAG can be completely halted with the addition of new agent X," then you can use the EBM process to see if such a statement is justified.

### 2.2.3 The Evolution of Glaucoma Care

Since EBM centers on using published evidence to guide clinical decision-making, it is useful to review how ophthalmic advances influenced our managerial approach to the glaucoma patient. It is difficult to treat a disease if you do not even know what type of condition it is. It is somewhat ironic that the word glaucoma has its origins in the Greek language and it roughly means "grayish gleam" – hardly a term associated with an optic nerve disease. It originally was a term referring to elderly people with seemingly white and quiet eyes and a dull appearance on external inspection that was associated with visual disability from multiple causes including mature cataract. Thus, prior to the invention of the ophthalmoscope by Hemholtz[17] (before 1851), visual disability from glaucoma was frequently confused with other conditions. The *postophthalmoscope era* afforded the clinician an ability to inspect the optic nerve and identify a group of visually disabled people who had white and quiet eyes, relatively clear media, and excavated optic nerve heads. Palpation of the globes of many (but not all) of these patients suggested that the IOP was elevated (the Schiotz tonometer had not been invented yet). These observations established that glaucoma was an optic nerve disease, but the frequent association with a firm globe to palpation suggested that glaucoma was a condition of elevated IOP that produced pathologic optic nerve changes; it is now known that glaucoma can occur across a spectrum of IOP values that include those in the statistically normal range. Nonetheless, the invention of the ophthalmoscope allowed clinicians to direct IOP-lowering treatment to patients with pathologically cupped optic nerves and elevated IOP. Intuitively it made sense to lower IOP in these patients with the limited therapies available to achieve such an effect. No one dared to question that an RCT might be needed to confirm that patients would benefit from such treatment.

A clear understanding that glaucoma existed in an angle-closure form and an open-angle form was not apparent until after the gonioscope was embraced as an important diagnostic tool. The *postgonioscopic era* began around 1920 when Koeppe and others perfected the technique of evaluating the filtration apparatus with the patient in the seated position.[18] Ultimately, this technique allowed physicians to more accurately identify patients with angle closure glaucoma who would benefit from iridectomy. Interestingly, despite the clear-cut importance of gonioscopy in a glaucoma work-up, available evidence suggests that gonioscopy is relatively underutilized in the management of glaucoma patients today.[19,20]

Prior to the launch of timolol, ophthalmologists had fairly limited tools to lower IOP in glaucoma patients. The treatments available had either undesirable side-effect profiles or poor efficacy. Pilocarpine, which has reasonable efficacy and has been available for more than 130 years to treat glaucoma,[21] requires frequent application and produces a constricted pupil. In younger patients, these drugs produced significant myopic shift because of induced accommodation of the lens, and in myopic patients, they would occasionally cause retinal breaks.[22] Topical epinephrine had a slightly better ocular side-effect profile but limited efficacy. Systemic carbonic anhydrase inhibitors were available from 1954, but they exposed the patient to systemic side effects. The introduction of timolol in 1978 ushered in the *golden age of the topical beta-blocker*. Topical beta-blockers were welcomed with open arms because while they did have some systemic side effects, they were tolerable and these drugs provided acceptable efficacy with once-daily or twice-daily dosing. With relatively few published placebo-controlled masked trials using IOP lowering and safety parameters as the outcomes,[23] timolol's superiority over epinephrine and pilocarpine became apparent and it instantly became the first-line treatment for glaucoma. In this era, no one questioned whether topical beta-blockers should be used as a first-line agent for glaucoma unless there was a contraindication to using a beta-blocker.

The 1990s witnessed *the polypharmacy era*, characterized by a significant expansion of the pharmacological armamentarium in treating glaucoma. The drugs that were introduced (topical carbonic anhydrase inhibitors[24], alpha agonists[25], and prostaglandin analogs[26]) created more treatment options for glaucoma patients. In fact, prostaglandin analogs offered the possibility of once-daily dosing, the virtual absence of systemic side effects, and IOP-lowering superior to timolol. In the 1990s, the balance had shifted from having limited options for lowering IOP to having a confusing number of ways of dealing with glaucoma, especially when one considers that parallel advances in laser trabeculoplasty and guarded sclerostomy surgery threatened to rival medical therapy in the treatment of glaucoma. This time period shares some parallels to the 1940s in general medicine when multiple tools were available to address disease (see Fig. 2.1).

A dark cloud was building over the entire field of glaucoma sometime after the golden age of beta-blockers and just before the polypharmacy era when a public policy official (Dr. David Eddy) questioned whether many medical treatments for many diseases (his article did not specifically single out glaucoma treatment) were really benefiting patients.[27] The glaucoma field was particularly vulnerable to this criticism because it narrowly focused on IOP as an outcome with precious few studies focused on whether our treatments preserved optic nerve structure and function. This shift in emphasis from considering IOP outcomes to vision-preserving outcomes ushered in the *randomized clinical trial era* of the 1990s. These trials help establish that lowering IOP helped to prevent development of POAG among patients with the OHTS[28] and slow disease progression in those with early manifest open-angle glaucoma (the Early Manifest Glaucoma Trial).[29] In order to refine which IOP-lowering modalities were best for our patients, other RCTs compared a medicine-first approach to laser-first (the Glaucoma Laser Trial)[30] and medicine-first to surgery-first (the Collaborative Initial Glaucoma Treatment Study) in managing open-angle glaucoma.[31] These trials will be the subject of later chapters, but they can be summarized by stating that overall there is currently no clear-cut advantage to using one modality to lower IOP when compared with another for glaucoma. Nonetheless, I will demonstrate that the EBM process can be used to inform clinicians about the management of individual glaucoma patients.

What will the future hold for glaucoma care and how will EBM help shape it? To answer this question, it is important to hark back to the time before the "postophthalmoscope" era. Initially, we did not even know that glaucoma was a disease of the optic nerve. Today, POAG – the most common form of glaucoma in the Western world – is a condition that is described in terms of risk factors rather than pathoetiologic elements. Similarly, primary angle closure glaucoma (PACG) – a common form of glaucoma in the Eastern world – is also poorly understood at a fundamental level. Thus, the next wave in glaucoma management will stem from a more complete understanding of the combination of genetic and environmental factors that dictate the etiology of all forms of glaucoma. As the various combinations of genetic determinants and environmental influences that dictate disease are published and confirmed, they will become the basis for genotype-specific tailored therapies, which may presage the *"individualized medicine era of glaucoma."* EBM will be useful to determine if novel genotype-specific strategies to treat glaucoma are superior to conventional approaches of managing the condition. Initially, genotype-specific strategies may not be embraced (initially, there was resistance to accept Schiotz tonometry as a replacement for finger palpation of the globe in the assessment of IOP), but RCTs will pressure physicians to adopt these approaches if they are truly superior to the way we practice currently.

In the interim, we will see modifications of the current ocular hypertension risk calculator and the emergence of new risk calculators that estimate the risk of developing glaucoma and the risk of progressing to more severe forms of the disease. Such knowledge will be based on a more complete understanding of the natural history of disease and how it is modified by current treatment. Such knowledge will, of course, be evidence-based. We will also see an increase in the use of *meta-analysis* to synthesize the rapidly accumulating evidence regarding our current glaucoma treatments. Meta-analysis is really a formal statistical approach to review the literature on a subject. First, the quality of the evidence is assessed so that only worthwhile reports are included. Then, statistical methods are applied to determine which studies from disparate centers can be combined. Models are then formulated to convert a series of small trials into a single large trial. The advantage of this approach is particularly apparent if some of the smaller trials actually contradict one another, or if the individual trials conclude that one treatment is similar to another, but each individual study is actually underpowered to detect any real difference between the treatments. For example, a meta-analysis of nine RCTs concluded that bimatoprost and travoprost are slightly more effective in lowering IOP than latanoprost.[32] This finding is consistent with another meta-analysis of 13 RCTs that concluded that bimatoprost was superior to latanoprost in lowering IOP.[33]

Nevertheless, more work is needed as still another literature synthesis has pointed out that no individual medical agent has been shown to preserve optic nerve function as measured by automated perimetry, and only beta-blockers have been shown to slow disease progression.[34] The absence of such evidence does not mean that our current therapies are not effective at preserving vision, but more clinical research is needed to optimize our treatments for glaucoma.

## 2.3 The Evidence-Based Medicine Process

### 2.3.1 Formulation of a Clinical Problem

Assume a 70-year-old white female presented to your office today with difficulty driving at night. Your examination leads you to conclude that the patient's symptoms are related to mild cataract formation, but an incidental finding was the presence of exfoliation precipitates in the anterior segment of both eyes, IOPs of 26 mmHg OD and 21 mmHg OS, and open angles on gonioscopy. Furthermore, the cup-disc ratio is 0.8 OD and 0.55 OS. On Humphrey visual field testing, there is a superior arcuate defect and inferior nasal step in the right eye and a shallow superior nasal step in the left eye. The Snellen acuity is 20/30 OU in both eyes. After you explain that cataracts were making it difficult to drive at night, the patient opts to defer cataract extraction because she was not critically disabled by her visual complaint. She was actually relieved to know the major source of her vision problem was potentially fixable. Nonetheless, she was not prepared to discover she had glaucoma. You inform the patient about the diagnosis of exfoliation glaucoma and, without much reflection on the matter, initiate treatment with travoprost 0.004% ophthalmic solution dosed one drop at bedtime in both eyes. The patient readily accepts this treatment; but in a quieter moment, you wonder whether such treatment was the optimized approach to her case. This moment of reflection represents the genesis of the EBM process: formulation of a clinical question. In this case, the question is what is the best first-line treatment for this elderly lady with new-onset exfoliation glaucoma?

### 2.3.2 Assembling the Evidence Cart: From Textbooks to Systematic Reviews

After crystallizing a clinical problem based on a patient encounter, the next task is assembling the available evidence that addresses this particular issue. Your question really is: "If I am committing this patient to medical therapy, is travoprost really the best choice for her?" Stated another way: Is there a prostaglandin analog that is particularly effective for exfoliation glaucoma? The meta-analyses referenced in the last section indicating that travoprost and bimatoprost were superior to latanoprost did not stratify their results by open-angle glaucoma subtype (i.e., exfoliation glaucoma versus other types of glaucoma).[32,33] This reformulation of the question assumes that medical therapy, as opposed to laser trabeculoplasty or incisional surgery, represents the best initial approach to managing her condition – an issue we will return to later. Furthermore, in thinking about the answer to this question, we must also consider the ocular side-effect profile of each agent.

In general, there are many potential resources available to potentially address your patients' problems, and oftentimes, these sources contain conflicting information. They include textbooks, "blue ribbon panels" convened by cost-conscious third-party payers, consensus panels handpicked by pharmaceutical companies, journal articles, online search engines such as PubMed, or online databases that search multiple articles and synthesize the literature on a particular subject. Where would you go first to find the answer to your question?

Thomas Kuhn in his highly influential treatise entitled, *The Structure of Scientific Revolutions*,[35] points out that, "Textbooks aim to communicate the vocabulary and syntax of a contemporary scientific language." For example, a typical glaucoma textbook is useful to learn the basics about exfoliation glaucoma and will address disease management in general terms, but it is unlikely to guide you on the specifics of optimum management of your 70-year-old lady with newly diagnosed exfoliation glaucoma. You may seek the assistance of the personal library of journal articles that you subscribe to and read faithfully every month, but it will become obvious very quickly that scouring them will not be a terribly efficient way to find the answer to your question. The logical way to address this problem is to use a general online search engine like PubMed to find studies that address your particular question. In order to use PubMed, your patient encounter, which has been transformed to a relevant clinical question, must be transformed again into "keywords" that can be searched. If we had used the keywords *therapy* and *exfoliation glaucoma* (other synonyms such pseudoexfoliation glaucoma should also be tried) on June 21, 2008, there would be 319 references and most of these would not be relevant to this patient's individual clinical situation. In reviewing this list of publications, we find five articles[36–40] that are relevant to our clinical problem.

While we were able to find relevant information about our patient problem on PubMed, this is a somewhat time-consuming process. Is there a better way? The short answer is: not at the current time. Theoretically, the Cochrane Collaboration,[1] an organization that provides up-to-date reviews on healthcare interventions in all areas of medicine, would be the ideal shortcut to get the answer to our patient-related question. Essentially, the Cochrane Collaboration searches for articles that perform the kind of literature search outlined above and summarizes the results in one article. At this time, a search using keywords *therapy* and *exfoliation glaucoma* or *exfoliation glaucoma* alone did not yield any relevant results since no one has written an evidence-based review on the subject of optimum medical therapy for exfoliation glaucoma. In fact, the keyword *glaucoma* will yield a list of 86 meta-analytical articles on glaucoma in all.

### 2.3.3 Evaluating the Quality of the Evidence

Once the evidence cart for our clinical question has been assembled, we must examine the quality of that evidence. Certainly, if the five articles we found related to our patient were of poorly designed studies, then they would not be useful in guiding our decision-making process with respect to our patient. Cochrane reviews would ordinarily do the quality analysis for us, but again there are no such reviews related to our patient. It is recommended that when the evidence cart is assembled that one looks for the RCTs first, as they represent a gold standard level of evidence for any particular intervention. Then one needs to ask the following questions about these RCTs:

- Is the allocation to treatment arms random and, if possible, are the investigators masked to the interventions employed in the study?
- Are the baseline attributes of each treatment arm clearly stated? A particularly useful study design incorporates a crossover paradigm. In crossover studies, each patient serves as his or her own control and is exposed to each treatment after an adequate washout period. This addresses any difference in baseline attributes between groups and also serves to increase the power of the study.
- Is the study adequately powered to find a difference between treatment groups? Look for a mention of an

*a priori* power calculation in the methods section of the paper.
- Do the authors present an intention-to-treat (ITT) analysis? There is an important dictum in clinical trials: once randomized, always analyzed. Patients who switch treatment arms or who drop out are always analyzed in the groups they were allocated to at the time of randomization.
- Are withdrawals adequately reported and is the dropout rate reasonable (below 10%)?
- Is there industry sponsorship for the study? Industry sponsorship does not mean the study is tainted but it is important to take note of such sponsorship. It is almost certain that industry sponsorship creates a certain publication bias, whereby results that do not show a product in a favorable light are suppressed. New rules about registering clinical trials with the Food and Drug Administration (FDA) are trying to minimize such publication bias.

Let us look at the evidence we have accrued for our particular clinical question. All five studies are randomized clinical trials. The majority of studies involve Greek nationals, raising some concerns about the generalizability of the data to other populations. A summary of the quality of each article is provided in Table 2.1. Each article gets a point each if the masking is judged to be adequate, power calculations are provided, an intent-to-treat analysis is performed, the withdrawal rate is less than 10% (somewhat arbitrary), and industry support is declared. If the study is free from industry sponsorship, then a score of two points is given. More formal grading systems of papers can be performed, but since the purpose is not to perform a meta-analysis but to get a rough idea that the data in the paper are believable, a simplified grading system looking for these particular attributes is recommended. For the evidence, we have accumulated for our question, we have five studies with quality scores ranging from 1 to 6 on a scale of 0 to 6, with most studies having scores of 4 or more. Therefore, the quality of the evidence that we have accumulated is generally quite good.

### 2.3.4 Applying the Evidence to Our Case

After assessing the overall quality of the evidence assembled, it is important to ascertain the outcome of these studies. All of these studies looked at either diurnal IOP or IOP at one time point as the main efficacy outcome. There are no data regarding whether any of the treatment options available to treat our particular patient are more effective in preserving vision. In looking at the IOP outcomes, it is also important to distinguish between statistical significance and clinical significance. Regulatory agencies state that differences in IOP of 1.5 mmHg or more constitute clinical significance, although there is no evidence to refute the notion that smaller differences in IOP that are statistically significant may also be clinically significant. The side-effect profile of the various treatment options should also be considered in making a decision about our patient.

In summary, the evidence (summarized in Table 2.2) indicates that for exfoliation glaucoma, both travoprost and bimatoprost produce statistically significant lowering of diurnal IOP versus latanoprost, but the differences in IOP lowering are less than 1.5 mmHg. Latanoprost produced significant reduction in diurnal IOP versus timolol that was greater than 1.5 mmHg. Two studies indicated that fixed combination timolol 0.5%–dorzolamide 2% was superior to travoprost and latanoprost in terms of IOP lowering, but the difference was <1.5 mmHg. Furthermore, one of these studies did not receive a high quality score and the other only used 10 AM IOP as the outcome of interest. From a clinical perspective, it might not be a good idea to start newly diagnosed patients on fixed combination therapy because it exposes a newly diagnosed patient to the side effects of two classes of medicines. Overall, no major safety issues were raised in any of these studies. So the decision to start the patient on travoprost was reasonable, but one could not be faulted for starting any of the prostaglandin analogs for our newly diagnosed exfoliation glaucoma patient.

Is it reasonable to consider laser trabeculoplasty or trabeculectomy for our patient? There are no RCTs designed to compare medical therapy to laser trabeculoplasty

**Table 2.1** Quality scores for randomized clinical trials assessing the effectiveness of medical therapy for exfoliation glaucoma

| Study | Masking adequate? | Study design | Power adequate? | ITT analysis performed? | Withdrawal rate | Industry sponsorship delineated? | Quality score |
|---|---|---|---|---|---|---|---|
| Konstas et al[36] | Yes | Cross-over; N=40 | Yes | Yes | 5% | None provided | 6 |
| Konstas et al[37] | Yes | Cross-over; N=129 | Yes | Yes | 5% | Provided | 5 |
| Parmaksiz et al[38] | No | Parallel; N=50 | Not assessed | Yes | 16% | Unclear | 1 |
| Konstas et al[39] | Yes | Parallel; N=103 | Yes | Yes | 5.5% | Partial | 5 |
| Konstas et al[40] | Yes | Cross-over; N=65 | Not assessed | No | 16% | None provided | 4 |

*ITT* intent to treat

**Table 2.2** Randomized clinical trials assessing the effectiveness of medical therapy for exfoliation glaucoma

| Study | Quality score | Outcome measured | Efficacy | Magnitude of effect |
|---|---|---|---|---|
| Konstas et al[36] | 6 | Diurnal IOP | Travatan>Latanoprost | <1.5 mmHg difference |
| Konstas et al[37] | 5 | Diurnal IOP | Bimatoprost>Latanoprost[a] | <1.5 mmHg difference |
| Parmaksiz et al[38] | 1 | Diurnal IOP | Dorzolamide-Timolol fixed combination> Travoprost>Latanoprost | <1.5 mmHg difference |
| Konstas et al[39] | 5 | Diurnal IOP | Latanoprost>Timolol | >1.5 mmHg difference |
| Konstas et al[40] | 4 | 10 AM IOP | Dorzolamide-Timolol fixed combination>Latanoprost | No |

[a]Favors industry-sponsored product

(performed with either the argon or selective laser unit) in exfoliation glaucoma. Nonetheless, one can refer to the Glaucoma Laser Trial, which showed that argon laser trabeculoplasty was as effective as medical therapy (during the golden age of beta-blockers) in the treatment of open-angle glaucoma.[30] Thus, if there are unusual circumstances that prevent adherence or if the patient and the physician simply prefer a laser-first approach after an appropriate informed consent process, it is reasonable to proceed with laser trabeculoplasty to manage the case. With respect to surgery, the Collaborative Initial Glaucoma Study evaluated whether glaucoma filtration surgery or medicine is the optimal initial approach to manage newly diagnosed OAG.[31] The interim study results showed that visual acuity and visual field outcomes were similar in both groups after 4 years of follow-up, prompting the study investigators to conclude that physicians should not change their practice patterns of routinely not offering patients surgery as the first option to manage OAG.

### 2.3.5 The Basic Calculus of Evidence-Based Medicine

A typical RCT will report the main outcomes of a study and discuss the side effects associated with one intervention versus another. For example, in the OHTS, which assessed whether prophylactic treatment of OHTN prevented people from developing POAG, it was reported that the rate of conversion from OHTN to POAG was reduced from 9.5 to 4.5% with ocular hypotensive therapy after 5 years.[28] These data suggest that lowering IOP in OHTN helps people generally, but can we get a deeper understanding of the trial results? Furthermore, how do we use these data to guide treatment decisions for individual glaucoma patients? The terms *absolute risk reduction*, *relative risk reduction*, and *the number needed to treat*[41] help us assess exactly how effective ocular hypotensive therapy is in reducing conversion from OHTN to POAG.

The *absolute risk reduction* (ARR) is the difference in outcome rate between treatment option 1 and treatment option 2 in a clinical trial. In the OHTS, 9.5% of patients with OHTN who were observed converted to a diagnosis of POAG, while only 4.5% of those under treatment converted to the same diagnosis. The ARR is 9.5–4.5 or 5%. The *relative risk reduction* (RRR) is the proportional reduction in event rates (failure to respond to treatment) between treatment option 1 and treatment option 2 in a clinical trial. In the OHTS, treatment did not completely prevent patients with OHTN from developing glaucoma. In fact, treatment resulted in a 4.5/9.5 or 50% RRR. Most diseases have low rates of occurrence; therefore, RRR tends to inflate the apparent benefit of any given treatment and ARR tends to underestimate it. Thus, another term has been introduced into the calculus of EBM to put the relative effectiveness of treatment into perspective, and that term is the *number needed to treat* (NNT). The NNT is the number of patients who need to be treated in order for one patient to receive benefit (such as the prevention of one case of POAG from developing among a group of patients with OHTN). The NNT is calculated as 1/ARR, rounded to the next highest whole number.

For the OHTS, the NNT is 20 – that means one would have to treat 20 patients with OHTN to prevent one case of POAG from developing. A lower value for the NNT is desirable for any treatment intervention and an NNT in the range of 2–5 is generally regarded as indicative of an effective treatment (the NNT for the Early Manifest Glaucoma Trial where newly diagnosed OAG patients were randomized to treatment versus observation was 6),[29] but a higher NNT may be acceptable for prophylactic treatments. The OHTS can be considered a prophylactic or preventive trial.

Interestingly, if the RRR stays constant, but the number of people reaching an endpoint increases, then the NNT goes down. A case in point regards the subset of African-Americans enrolled in the OHTS. The 5-year risk of converting from OHTN to POAG for African-Americans in the OHTS was 8.4% in the medical therapy arm and 16.1% in the observation arm.[42] Thus, the ARR is 16.1–8.4 or 7.7% and the RRR is 8.4/16.1 or 48%. Overall, the NNT is 1/0.077 or 13. So among African-Americans, one would have to treat 13 patients with OHTN to prevent one case of POAG.

The ARR, RRR, and NNT provide quantitative insights into the results of RCTs yielding a global estimate of treatment effectiveness, but they do not tell us which individual patient requires treatment. The reader should be cautioned from concluding that all African-Americans with OHTN should be treated because the NNT is 13 when compared with an NNT of 20 overall. The decision to treat individual OHTN patients is better guided by the glaucoma risk calculator. The calculator, which has been validated in patients outside the OHTS[15], accounts for important risk factors that predict conversion from OHTN to POAG and provides a 5-year risk estimate of converting from OHTN to POAG. The parameters that go into the calculation are age, mean IOP, central corneal thickness, vertical cup-disc ratio, and mean defect on the Humphrey visual field. Race is not entered into the calculator because multivariable analysis indicated that race was not an independent risk factor for conversion from OHTN to POAG. So a 48-year-old patient with mean IOP of 24 mmHg, OU; CCT of 520 μm OU; CDR = 0.4 OU; and PSD of 1.5 dB OD and 1.7 dB OS has a 5-year risk of converting to POAG of 15%. If one uses the calculator to stratify patients into low (≤5% in 5 years), medium (5–15% risk in 5 years) or high (>15% risk in 5 years) risk of converting to POAG, then this person, regardless of race, would have a moderate-to-high increased risk of converting to POAG. As it turns out, African-Americans will tend to fall into the high-risk category by virtue of the fact that they tend to have thinner corneas than their Caucasian counterparts. Nonetheless, an African-American subject with thick corneas does not necessarily have to go on treatment because the NNT for African-Americans overall is 13. Ultimately, the risk calculator should not be viewed as the instrument that rigidly guides treatment decisions, as that is an individual decision between the patient and doctor.

All treatment interventions have side effects relative to observation without therapy or an alternative treatment. Thus, it is useful to place an adverse effect profile in quantitative perspective as well when considering treatment for the individual patient. The term *number needed to harm* (NNH) is the number of patients that need to be treated to harm one patient. In the Collaborative Initial Glaucoma Treatment Study (CIGTS), patients with newly diagnosed OAG were randomized to treatment with medical therapy or surgery to lower IOP. Both treatments were equally effective in stabilizing vision and the visual field over a 5-year period. In fact, both treatments seem to have equivalent impact on quality-of-life measures. Nevertheless, 9% of patients in the medical therapy arm developed cataracts requiring surgical intervention, while 20% of patients in the surgical arm required cataract extraction.[31] Thus, the NNH is calculated as 1/0.2–0.09 or 9. Thus in treating nine newly diagnosed patients with surgery first, the clinician would induce one extra cataract requiring surgical removal. A low NNH is not desirable, especially when the treatment inducing harm is not better than the alternative therapy (in this case medicine first). With that said, the "harm" in this case was a cataract that produces vision loss that is reversible with cataract extraction. In fact, CIGTS researchers show that cataract surgery in patients with prior filtration surgery is quite successful.[43]

While the NNT and NNH provide quantitative interpretation of RCT results in terms of how they benefit patients, they do not tell us if treatment is cost-effective. Cost-effectiveness is a somewhat controversial term because it indicates there is a cost above which society cannot bear the burden of treating a specific condition. We like to think that ideally we should spare no cost in preventing glaucoma, but in reality, resources are limited and must be distributed judiciously such that the most treatable conditions are addressed on a societal level. Certainly, we would not want to spend so much money on treating OHTN that there are no resources available to care for patients with cataract or progressive POAG. The costs of healthcare have risen by about 20% per year from 1998 to 2004, and society needs to allocate finite resources for the most cost-effective treatments.[44] The National Institute for Clinical Excellence has set a ceiling for annual costs associated with treating any disease, which reflects the resources available in an affluent country. Basically, if the incremental cost-effectiveness ratio (ICER) is greater than a societal cutoff for willingness to pay, the treatment is regarded as not cost-effective. The upper limit for ICER may be much lower in countries of more limited means. The ICER is calculated using RCT data, the actual costs of treating or observing the condition in question, and accounting for the number of years of life people would be willing to swap in order to remain free of the condition in question. The ICER for treating all OHTN patients is approximately $89,000.[45] That means the incremental cost of treating all OHTN patients to prevent one case of POAG is $89,000, a value that is of borderline cost-effectiveness even for a highly developed country like the United States. If we limit treatment, for example, to those patients with CCT 40 μm below the norm (550 μm), then the ICER is close to $37,000. Similarly, it is cost-effective to treat OHTN patients over the age of 76 (two decades above the age of 56), IOP >29 mmHg (4 mmHg above the IOP of 25 mmHg), and with vertical CDR of 0.6 or more (0.2 units above 0.4) because in each case the ICER is less than $50,000.

### 2.3.6 What Do We Do When There Is Little or no Evidence?

You are a busy glaucoma specialist and you are emotionally shaken because in the past 2 months you have performed two combined cataract extractions with trabeculectomy procedures that resulted in suprachoroidal hemorrhage – one occurred intraoperatively and one occurred postoperatively.

In both instances, the patients developed excruciating pain, and in one instance, the vision went to light perception (LP) and did not improve. You are trying to decide whether there are preoperative measures to consider to prevent this from ever happening to you again. The experience has been devastating for the patients and for you. Your question is quite simple: What can be done to prevent suprachoroidal hemorrhage from developing? Very quickly you discover that there are no trials designed to answer this question. In fact, it is likely that there will never be a trial to answer this question because suprachoroidal hemorrhage is a relatively rare event and a trial would have to include a large number of patients in order to be adequately powered to determine if a particular intervention reduced the rate of suprachoroidal hemorrhage. While suprachoroidal hemorrhage is rare, it seems like a common event when it happens to one of your patients. So you hope to find some evidence that can help you. In this instance, the best source of evidence that can provide the answer to your question is observational studies. Observational studies may point to risk factors for the development of suprachoroidal hemorrhages. Those risk factors may lead you to adopt some strategies to minimize the development of suprachoroidal hemorrhage.

The source of bleeding in suprachoroidal hemorrhages is the posterior ciliary arteries that bridge the sclera and enter the choroidal tissue. The literature review indicates that the risk factors for suprachoroidal hemorrhage can be divided into systemic and ocular risk factors. Systemic risk factors include older age, hypertension, atherosclerosis, and intraoperative tachycardia.[46–48] The insight that you gain from this list is that patients need to have their cardiovascular status maximized at the time of surgery. If a patient is running a very high blood pressure on the day of surgery, it might be better to defer the operation to another day. Ocular risk factors include longer axial length, aphakia, intraoperative vitrectomy, and multiple prior surgeries. In reviewing this list of ocular risk factors, you realize that low IOP, lack of lens support, and absence of ocular turgor provided by the vitreous gel may tug on the bridging posterior ciliary vessels causing them to rupture. Thus, you decide that in future you will be careful to maintain control over the anterior chamber depth intraoperatively during all anterior segment procedures. You will avoid outflow procedures in aphakic patients unless they are absolutely necessary and even then perform them in a guarded fashion. Finally, for your trabeculectomies, whether they are combined with cataract surgery or not, you will use laser suture lysis and releasable sutures in a judicious fashion avoiding extreme hypotony, which could trigger a postoperative suprachoroidal hemorrhage. These maneuvers intuitively make sense and while they may not completely prevent a suprachoroidal hemorrhage, they may reduce the chance of encountering one.

## 2.4 Conclusion

One of the wonderful things about the study of medicine is that the learning process continues for a lifetime. Adhering to EBM is like maintaining your continuing medical education. Physicians will benefit from engaging in the EBM process throughout their career. It allows one to track emerging practice trends (such as the intraocular injection of anti-angiogenic agents in the management of neovascular glaucoma[49]) and make rational decisions about adopting new management schema. One shortcoming is bringing EBM to the exam lane. The EBM process is not an exercise that can be performed when the patient is in our exam chair; however, once we have gone through the EBM process, it will certainly be absorbed into our practice patterns and help the next patients who present with similar problems. Furthermore, most of the searches for evidence are manual ones because ophthalmic meta-analytic topic reviews are just beginning to appear in the Cochrane database. At the current time, many glaucoma management issues cannot be resolved with the EBM process. The emergence of the electronic medical record, which requires a computer hooked up to the Internet in every exam lane, certainly helps us perform real-time calculations of risk for developing POAG in OHTN patients. In the end, the EBM process is about delivering the very best care for our patients.

---

Clinical Pearls

- EBM is a *process* whereby the best medical evidence in the literature is applied to patients with specific clinical problems.
- The EBM process involves four steps: (1) formulation of a clinical question, (2) assembly of the evidence that addresses that question, (3) an assessment of the quality of available evidence, and (4) application of the evidence to a particular patient.
- The absolute risk reduction, relative risk reduction, and number needed to treat represent quantitative measures to assess efficacy of an intervention in a RCT. The number needed to harm represents a quantitative measure to assess the adverse effects of an intervention in a randomized clinical trial.
- Most clinical challenges in glaucoma do not have a directly applicable randomized trial that addresses the problem.

# References

1. The reliable source of evidence in health care. In: Julian PT, Higgins, Sally, eds. *The Cochrane Handbook for Systematic Reviews of Interventions*. Wiley, Interscience, Sussex England; 2008.
2. Bhandari M, Zlowodzki M, Cole PA. From eminence-based practice to evidence-based practice: a paradigm shift. *Minn Med*. 2004;87:51–54.
3. Gorman C. Are doctors just playing hunches? *Time*. 2007;169(9):52–54.
4. Gordon MO, Beiser JA, Brandt JD, et al. The ocular hypertension treatment study: baseline factors that predict the onset of primary open-angle glaucoma. *Arch Ophthalmol*. 2002;120:714–720. discussion 829–830.
5. Leske MC, Wu SY, Hennis A, Honkanen R, Nemesure B. Risk factors for incident open-angle glaucoma: the Barbados Eye Studies. *Ophthalmology*. 2008;115:85–93.
6. Sackett DL, Rosenberg WM, Gray JA, Haynes RB, Richardson WS. Evidence based medicine: what it is and what it isn't. *BMJ*. 1996;312:71–72.
7. Flynn CA, D'Amico F, Smith G. Should we patch corneal abrasions? A meta-analysis. *J Fam Pract*. 1998;47:264–270.
8. Michael JG, Hug D, Dowd MD. Management of corneal abrasion in children: a randomized clinical trial. *Ann Emerg Med*. 2002;40:67–72.
9. Le Sage N, Verreault R, Rochette L. Efficacy of eye patching for traumatic corneal abrasions: a controlled clinical trial. *Ann Emerg Med*. 2001;38:129–134.
10. Daly WJ, Brater DC. Medieval contributions to the search for truth in clinical medicine. *Perspect Biol Med*. 2000;43:530–540.
11. North R. Benjamin Rush, MD: assassin or beloved healer? *Proc (Bayl Univ Med Cent)*. 2000;13:45–49.
12. Bean RB. *Sir William Osler. Aphorisms*. Springfield: Blackwell; 1961:164
13. Morris JN. Recalling the miracle that was penicillin: two memorable patients. *J R Soc Med*. 2004;97:189–190.
14. Mansberger SL. A risk calculator to determine the probability of glaucoma. *J Glaucoma*. 2004;13:345–347.
15. Medeiros FA, Weinreb RN, Sample PA, et al. Validation of a predictive model to estimate the risk of conversion from ocular hypertension to glaucoma. *Arch Ophthalmol*. 2005;123:1351–1360.
16. Gordon MO, Torri V, Miglior S, et al. Validated prediction model for the development of primary open-angle glaucoma in individuals with ocular hypertension. *Ophthalmology*. 2007;114:10–19.
17. von Helmholtz HLF. *Beschreibung eines Augen-Spiegels*. Berlin, Germany: A Förstner'sche Verlagsbuchhandlung; 1851.
18. Dellaporta A. Historical notes on gonioscopy. *Surv Ophthalmol*. 1975;20:137–149.
19. Hertzog LH, Albrecht KG, LaBree L, Lee PP. Glaucoma care and conformance with preferred practice patterns. Examination of the private, community-based ophthalmologist. *Ophthalmology*. 1996;103:1009–1013.
20. Coleman AL, Yu F, Evans SJ. Use of gonioscopy in medicare beneficiaries before glaucoma surgery. *J Glaucoma*. 2006;15:486–493.
21. Kronfeld P. Eserine and pilocarpine: our 100-year-old allies. *Surv Ophthalmol*. 1970;14:479.
22. Beasley H, Fraunfelder FT. Retinal detachments and topical ocular miotics. *Ophthalmology*. 1979;86:95–98.
23. Zimmerman TJ, Kass MA, Yablonski ME, Becker B. Timolol maleate: efficacy and safety. *Arch Ophthalmol*. 1979;97:656–658.
24. Lippa EA, Carlson LE, Ehinger B, et al. Dose response and duration of action of dorzolamide, a topical carbonic anhydrase inhibitor. *Arch Ophthalmol*. 1992;110:495–499.
25. Derick RJ, Robin AL, Walters TR, et al. Brimonidine tartrate: a one-month dose response study. *Ophthalmology*. 1997;104:131–136.
26. Camras CB, Schumer RA, Marsk A, et al. Intraocular pressure reduction with PhXA34, a new prostaglandin analogue, in patients with ocular hypertension. *Arch Ophthalmol*. 1992;110:1733–1738.
27. Eddy DM, Billings J. The quality of medical evidence: implications for quality of care. *Health Aff (Millwood)*. 1988;7:19–32.
28. Kass MA, Heuer DK, Higginbotham EJ, et al. The ocular hypertension treatment study: a randomized trial determines that topical ocular hypotensive medication delays or prevents the onset of primary open-angle glaucoma. *Arch Ophthalmol*. 2002;120:701–713. discussion 829–830.
29. Heijl A, Leske MC, Bengtsson B, Hyman L, Bengtsson B, Hussein M. Reduction of intraocular pressure and glaucoma progression: results from the Early Manifest Glaucoma Trial. *Arch Ophthalmol*. 2002;120:1268–1279.
30. The Glaucoma Laser Trial (GLT). 2. Results of argon laser trabeculoplasty versus topical medicines. The Glaucoma Laser Trial Research Group. *Ophthalmology* 1990;97:1403–1413
31. Lichter PR, Musch DC, Gillespie BW, et al. Interim clinical outcomes in the Collaborative Initial Glaucoma Treatment Study comparing initial treatment randomized to medications or surgery. *Ophthalmology*. 2001;108:1943–1953.
32. Denis P, Lafuma A, Khoshnood B, Mimaud V, Berdeaux G. A meta-analysis of topical prostaglandin analogues intra-ocular pressure lowering in glaucoma therapy. *Curr Med Res Opin*. 2007;23:601–608.
33. Cheng JW, Wei RL. Meta-analysis of 13 randomized controlled trials comparing bimatoprost with latanoprost in patients with elevated intraocular pressure. *Clin Ther*. 2008;30:622–632.
34. Vass C, Hirn C, Sycha T, Findl O, Bauer P, and Schmetterer L. Medical interventions for primary open angle glaucoma and ocular hypertension. *Cochrane Database Syst Rev* 2007: CD003167
35. Kuhn TS. *The structure of scientific revoluations, 3rd ed*. Chicago: The University of Chicago Press; 1996:212
36. Konstas AG, Kozobolis VP, Katsimpris IE, et al. Efficacy and safety of latanoprost versus travoprost in exfoliative glaucoma patients. *Ophthalmology*. 2007;114:653–657.
37. Konstas AG, Hollo G, Irkec M, et al. Diurnal IOP control with bimatoprost versus latanoprost in exfoliative glaucoma: a crossover, observer-masked, three-centre study. *Br J Ophthalmol*. 2007;91:757–760.
38. Parmaksiz S, Yuksel N, Karabas VL, Ozkan B, Demirci G, Caglar Y. A comparison of travoprost, latanoprost, and the fixed combination of dorzolamide and timolol in patients with pseudoexfoliation glaucoma. *Eur J Ophthalmol*. 2006;16:73–80.
39. Konstas AG, Mylopoulos N, Karabatsas CH, et al. Diurnal intraocular pressure reduction with latanoprost 0.005% compared to timolol maleate 0.5% as monotherapy in subjects with exfoliation glaucoma. *Eye* 2004;18:893–899
40. Konstas AG, Kozobolis VP, Tersis I, Leech J, Stewart WC. The efficacy and safety of the timolol/dorzolamide fixed combination vs latanoprost in exfoliation glaucoma. *Eye*. 2003;17:41–46.
41. Barratt A, Wyer PC, Hatala R, et al. Tips for learners of evidence-based medicine: 1. Relative risk reduction, absolute risk reduction and number needed to treat. *CMAJ*. 2004;171:353–358.
42. Higginbotham EJ, Gordon MO, Beiser JA, et al. The Ocular Hypertension Treatment Study: topical medication delays or prevents primary open-angle glaucoma in African American individuals. *Arch Ophthalmol*. 2004;122:813–820.
43. Musch DC, Gillespie BW, Niziol LM, et al. Cataract extraction in the collaborative initial glaucoma treatment study: incidence, risk factors, and the effect of cataract progression and extraction on clinical and quality-of-life outcomes. *Arch Ophthalmol*. 2006;124:1694–1700.

44. Pasquale LR, Dolgitser M, Wentzloff JN, et al. Health care charges for patients with ocular hypertension or primary open-angle glaucoma. *Ophthalmology*. 2008;115(4):633–638.
45. Kymes SM, Kass MA, Anderson DR, Miller JP, Gordon MO. Management of ocular hypertension: a cost-effectiveness approach from the Ocular Hypertension Treatment Study. *Am J Ophthalmol*. 2006;141:997–1008.
46. Speaker MG, Guerriero PN, Met JA, Coad CT, Berger A, Marmor M. A case-control study of risk factors for intraoperative suprachoroidal expulsive hemorrhage. *Ophthalmology*. 1991;98:202–209. discussion 210.
47. Obuchowska I, Mariak Z. Risk factors of massive suprachoroidal hemorrhage during extracapsular cataract extraction surgery. *Eur J Ophthalmol*. 2005;15:712–717.
48. Moshfeghi DM, Kim BY, Kaiser PK, Sears JE, Smith SD. Appositional suprachoroidal hemorrhage: a case-control study. *Am J Ophthalmol*. 2004;138:959–963.
49. Ehlers JP, Spirn MJ, Lam A, Sivalingam A, Samuel MA, Tasman W. Combination intravitreal bevacizumab/panretinal photocoagulation versus panretinal photocoagulation alone in the treatment of neovascular glaucoma. *Retina*. 2008;28:696–702.

# Chapter 3
# Glaucoma Risk Factors: Intraocular Pressure

Nils A. Loewen and Angelo P. Tanna

## 3.1 Intraocular Pressure is Causatively Linked to Glaucoma: A Brief History

For the first time, glaucoma was described as a blinding disease associated with high intraocular pressure (IOP) by the Persian physician Ali ibn Rabban at-Tabari (810–861 C.E.) in the writings *Firdaws al hikma* (Paradise of Wisdom).[1] This association was later pointed out by Richard Banister of England in his 1622 *A treatise of one hundred and thirteen diseases of eye:* "If one feele the Eye by rubbing upon the Eie-lids, that the Eye be growne more solid and hard than naturally it should be...the humour settled in the hollow nerves be growne to any solid or hard substance, it is not possible to be cured."[2] In the 1800s, the Dutch ophthalmologist Franciscus C. Donders coined the expression "simple glaucoma" for increased IOP occurring without any inflammatory symptoms.

In population-based surveys, intraocular pressure (IOP) has been consistently shown to be a continuous, positive risk factor for the prevalence of glaucoma, even through the normal range of IOP. The association of IOP and open angle glaucoma was first confirmed in studies in the 1990s, although still not in the form of a cause-effect relationship. In the Baltimore Eye Survey[3] and the Barbados Eye Study[4], IOP was found to be an important factor in glaucoma that correlated with increased prevalence and incidence.[5]

Statistically, elevated IOP does not equate with the diagnosis of glaucoma, and conversely, normal IOP does not exclude the diagnosis of glaucoma. From the standpoint of the management of individual patients, the significance of this is that the diagnosis of glaucoma must be based primarily on the examination of the optic discs and retinal nerve fiber layer and the evaluation of visual function. This often differs from the diagnosis of an individual at risk of converting to glaucoma, which includes other factors as reflected in glaucoma risk calculators (see *Clinical Pearl: Predicting Glaucoma Risk*).

Although IOP has been causatively linked to glaucoma development and progression, the value of IOP reduction in the treatment of glaucoma was passionately disputed until recently when the results of large randomized clinical trials of the late 1990s became available[6,7] (Fig. 3.1). These studies demonstrated beyond correlation that a true causal relationship existed, by showing that lowering IOP can slow or prevent POAG progression. The two most noteworthy trials in this regard are the Ocular Hypertension Treatment Study (OHTS),[8] which demonstrated that IOP reduction reduces the risk of conversion to glaucoma among ocular hypertensives, and the Early Manifest Glaucoma Trial (EMGT),[9] which demonstrated that IOP reduction lowers the risk of glaucoma progression. Today, these studies have direct practical implications for daily patient care and are summarized in the following. While there are other risk factors for glaucoma, IOP remains the only modifiable variable used to prevent or delay progression. Other strategies, such as vascular,[10,11] neuroprotective,[11-14] or metabolic management[15] appeared promising in animal experimentation or were recognized as risk factors (reviewed in[10,16]), but their influence on the course of glaucoma has not been established in randomized clinical trials.

## 3.2 IOP as a Function of Aqueous Humor Production and Outflow

Intraocular pressure can be expressed using the modified Goldmann equation,[17] which consists of four elements:

$$IOP = F/C + Pv - U$$

whereas $F$ is the aqueous humor formation rate in microliters per minute, $C$ is the facility of outflow in microliters per minute per millimeter of mercury, Pv is the episcleral venous pressure in millimeters of mercury, and $U$ is the rate of outflow of

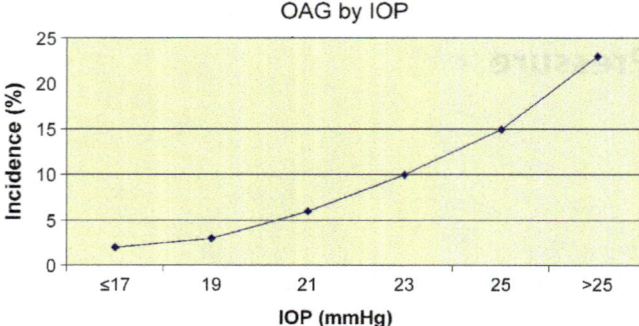

**Fig. 3.1** Graph showing the incidence of open-angle glaucoma by intraocular pressure (IOP)[7]

aqueous humor via all channels that are intraocular pressure independent.

Aqueous humor is produced by the ciliary body.[18] The ciliary processes contain a fibrovascular core and are covered by a bi-layered epithelium. This double layer is the result of the optic cup invagination during embryogenesis. As it is joined apically, the basement membrane of the inner, non-pigmented epithelium is facing the posterior chamber. The vasculature is connected to the major circle of the iris.[19] Blood flows toward the network of choroidal veins and exits through the vortex veins. A sphincter-like system regulates blood flow that allows adjustment of filtration pressure and, consequentially, aqueous humor production to some extent.[20–22] The capillaries from the anterior arteriole in the stromal core of the ciliary processes are lined by fenestrated endothelial cells, allowing the passage of macromolecules, ions, and water. The ciliary nonpigmented epithelium in contrast has zonulae occludentes, adherentes, and desmosomes[23,24] constituting the blood-aqueous barrier of the ciliary body.[25] It is primarily the epithelium at the tip of the ciliary processes that contains carbonic anhydrase and Na-K-ATPase to actively produce aqueous humor.

Aqueous humor leaves the eye via two routes: (1) the conventional outflow tract by passing through trabecular meshwork (TM) into Schlemm's canal and subsequently following circuitous channels toward the surface of the sclera into the episcleral vasculature, and (2) the uveoscleral outflow tract by absorption into uveal tissues.[26,27]

Most regard the juxtacanalicular meshwork or the inner wall of Schlemm's canal as the primary source of outflow resistance.[28] Past suggestions that increase in outflow resistance in primary open angle glaucoma (POAG) derive from the accumulation of extracellular matrix material in the open spaces of the uveal and corneoscleral trabecular meshwork have recently been shown to be problematic as these decrease with age and in POAG.[29,30] Aqueous humor passes through the juxtacanalicular trabecular meshwork and the inner wall of Schlemm's canal through micropores and unique giant vacuoles that form in a pressure-dependent and energy-independent fashion.[31,32] Around 30 external collector channels drain from the outer wall of Schlemm's canal toward the scleral surface into a deep scleral plexus that leads to the deep scleral veins and eventually to the episcleral veins. Despite this small caliber vascular network and its ability to regulate flow,[33] this effect is relatively insignificant. Several unique vessels, termed the aqueous veins of Ascher, bypass the deep scleral plexus directly into the episcleral veins.[34]

Under physiological conditions, 70–95% of outflow occurs through the trabecular meshwork and is pressure dependent.[35–38] The pressure independent uveoscleral outflow can increase significantly during inflammation to 60%.[26,27] Pharmacologic enhancement of uveoscleral outflow into the supraciliary space was first demonstrated in humans with prostaglandin acid prodrugs[39] and prostamides.[40] Despite increased leakiness of the ciliary body vasculature, intraocular pressure is usually decreased during intraocular inflammation because of increased uveoscleral outflow and disappearance of gap junctions that serve intercellular metabolic and electronic coupling of ciliary epithelial, resulting in decreased aqueous humor production.[41,42]

IOP can be decreased through carbonic anhydrase inhibitor mediated reduction of aqueous humor production,[43] beta-adrenergic antagonists,[44] and alpha-adrenergic agonists.[45] The only medication class that addresses the primary pathology of reduced conventional outflow, the parasympathomimetics,[46] has been all but abandoned because of its side effects and potential to reduce uveoscleral outflow.[26] Trabeculoplasty has been employed to lower intraocular pressure by inducing remodeling of the TM and extracellular matrix.[47] However, the extent of pressure reduction is much smaller than can be achieved with filtering procedures. Complete disruption of the TM and wall of Schlemm's canal has recently been achieved with the trabectome,[48] but this disruption is irreversible, creating a permanently open connection to the downstream drainage system. Therapies for advanced glaucoma traditionally attempt to lower intraocular pressure surgically by circumventing the outflow resistance of the TM by shunting aqueous humor to the sub-Tenon space (e.g., trabeculectomy, aqueous drainage device).[49] These filtering procedures have a high rate of complication and failure[50] despite the introduction of antifibrotics and improvement of drainage device design, respectively.

## 3.3 Important Randomized Clinical Trials

### 3.3.1 Collaborative Normal Tension Glaucoma Study

Before the Collaborative Normal Tension Glaucoma Study (CNTGS),[51] it was not known whether IOP that was in the normal statistical range was at all involved in glaucomatous optic nerve damage and visual field loss. During the study it became apparent that – similar to simple POAG – participating patients had a slower glaucoma progression (no progression in 5 years) when IOP was lowered by 30%. The most treatment benefits were observed in patients of female gender, with family history of glaucoma, without family history of stroke, without personal history of cardiovascular disease, and with mild disk excavation.[52] Risk factors were female gender, migraine headaches, and optic disc hemorrhages.[51,52] The natural course as well as the response to treatment can be highly variable, and treatment has to be individualized according to the stage of disease and rate of progression if the mentioned risk factors are not present.[52,53]

### 3.3.2 Advanced Glaucoma Intervention Study

The Advanced Glaucoma Intervention Study (AGIS)[54] has to be seen in its historical context. The goal of AGIS was to compare trabeculectomy with argon laser trabeculoplasty (ALT) in eyes that had failed medical management at a time when it was not established that ALT was less effective than trabeculectomy. Before 1980, trabeculectomy was the usual intervention for medically failing advanced glaucoma. AGIS established a benefit from lowering IOP in glaucoma by trabeculectomy[55]: Eyes with early average intraocular pressure greater than 17.5 mmHg had more progression than eyes with average intraocular pressure less than 14 mmHg. When IOP was less than 18 mmHg during all visits over 6 years in a separate analysis, mean changes from baseline in visual field defect scores were close to zero. A shortcoming is that AGIS was not originally designed to detect prevention of glaucoma progression but that preventative effects noted were detected in an after analysis.

### 3.3.3 Collaborative Initial Glaucoma Treatment Study

The Collaborative Initial Glaucoma Treatment Study (CIGTS)[56] compared treatment of newly diagnosed POAG with standard medical treatment (typically initial beta-blocker) versus filtration surgery. In the medication treatment arm, additional topical medications could be added, followed by ALT and filtration surgery if needed. In the surgical treatment arm, failed trabeculectomy could be followed by ALT. The surgical group had IOPs that were 2–3 points lower than the medical group. Surprisingly, despite the lower IOP, the surgical group had more visual field and more visual acuity loss than the medical group in the first 3 years, but this difference disappeared in the follow-up.[57] There were 3.8-fold more cataract extractions in the surgical group[58] in the initial 5 years after trabeculectomy but not thereafter. While the surgical group complained about foreign body sensation at the bleb site, the medical group experienced more systemic symptoms. Results from CIGTS did not support altering treatment practices of initial medical management of patients with primary open-angle glaucoma.[59]

### 3.3.4 Ocular Hypertension Treatment Study and the European Glaucoma Prevention Study

The purpose of the Ocular Hypertension Treatment Study (OHTS)[8] was to determine whether the pharmacological reduction of elevated IOP can prevent glaucoma and to define risk factors for glaucoma development. Topical ocular hypotensive medication was effective in delaying or preventing onset of POAG in individuals with elevated IOP by about 50%. Results to date have shown an approximate 50% reduction in conversion from OHT to POAG, with a 20% reduction in intraocular pressure.[60] OHTS demonstrated that medical treatment of people with intraocular pressure of ≥24 mmHg reduces the risk of the development of primary open-angle glaucoma (POAG) by 60%.[61]

Factors that predicted the development of POAG included older age, race (African-American), sex (male), larger vertical cup–disc ratio, larger horizontal cup–disc ratio, higher intraocular pressure, greater Humphrey visual field (VF) pattern standard deviation, heart disease, and thin central corneal thickness.[62] Reduction in IOP in the medication group was 22.5 ± 9.9% versus 4.0 ± 11.6% in the observation group. At 60 months, the overall probability of developing POAG was 4.4% in the medication group and 9.5% in the observation group.[60] Of African-American participants, 8.4% developed POAG in the medication group when compared with 16.1% in the observation group.[63] The occurrence of an optic disc hemorrhage was associated with an increased risk of developing a POAG end point in participants in the OHTS. However, most eyes (86.7%) in which a disc hemorrhage developed have not developed POAG to date. The 96-month cumulative incidence of POAG in the eyes without optic disc hemorrhage was 5.2%, when compared with 13.6% in the eyes with optic disc hemorrhage.[64]

The same predictors for the development of POAG were identified independently in both the OHTS observation group and the European Glaucoma Prevention Study (EGPS)[65]: placebo group-baseline age, intraocular pressure, central corneal thickness, vertical cup-to-disc ratio, and Humphrey VF pattern standard deviation.[66] There was no evidence for a general effect of topical ocular hypotensive medication on lens opacification or visual function.[67] Results of EGPS have to be interpreted with caution as several design problems might have caused the odd finding that IOP was lowered in the placebo-control group as well: (1) a high patient drop-out rate, especially in the dorzolamide arm; (2) commitment to dorzolamide treatment regardless of therapeutic effect; and (3) determination of baseline pressure with just two readings that could have been merely 2 h apart.[68]

### 3.3.5 Early Manifest Glaucoma Trial

The Early Manifest Glaucoma Trial (EMGT)[9] compared how glaucoma progression was affected by immediate combined medical (betaxolol) and laser therapy for newly diagnosed OAG with normal or moderately elevated IOP versus late or no treatment. Treatment caused an average reduction of IOP of about 5 mmHg (25%), which reduced glaucoma progression to 45% when compared with 62% in the control group and occurred later. These benefits were preserved after stratifying for age, ethnicity, and POAG stage and type. The percent of patient follow-up visits with disc hemorrhages was also related to progression (hazard ratio = 1.02 per percent higher).[69] Progression risk decreased by about 10% with each millimeter of mercury of IOP reduction from baseline to the first follow-up visit (HR = 0.90 per millimeter of mercury decrease).[69,70] Elevated IOP was a strong factor for glaucoma progression, but intraocular pressure fluctuation was not.[70] Higher IOP, exfoliation, bilateral disease, and older age were progression factors previously known.[71] New baseline predictors were lower ocular systolic perfusion pressure (≤160 mmHg; HR 1.42), cardiovascular disease history (HR 2.75) in patients with higher baseline IOP, and lower systolic blood pressure (BP) (≤125 mmHg; HR 0.46; 95% CI 0.21–1.02) in patients with lower baseline IOP. Thinner central corneal thickness (CCT) (HR 1.25 per 40 micrometer lower) was a new significant factor, a result observed in patients with higher baseline IOP.

### 3.3.6 Conclusion from Randomized Trials

Lower intraocular pressure does delay or prevent progression of POAG as evidenced by delay or prevention of development of optic nerve damage from ocular hypertension, visual field defects from existing optic nerve changes, and reduced progression of existing visual field defects. However, another conclusion is that despite good IOP control in many actively treated patients, POAG can still progress and can result in blindness in an unacceptably large number of patients.[72,73]

## 3.4 IOP as Risk Factor for Glaucoma Development

The role of IOP in the diagnosis of glaucoma is different from its role in treatment. Because of the wide range of IOP that can be found inter-individually as well as intra-individually (as will be discussed), a single IOP measurement above the expected average has little merit. Glaucoma risk calculators reflect the complexity of multiple other glaucoma risk factors that bear equal or greater significance. At least one variable – central corneal thickness (CCT) – influences IOP measurements directly and must be taken into account when judging IOP that was measured clinically with the most common technique: Goldmann applanation tonometry. In addition, CCT may be an independent risk factor reflecting overall ocular rigidity, including that of the lamina cribrosa. One recent histological study questioned this theory when no correlation was found in nonglaucomatous human globes between CCT and lamina cribrosa and peripapillary scleral thickness.[74] Histologic artifact and sectioning methods could partially account for the lack of a predicted association. CCT instead inversely correlates to optic disc size in Caucasians[75] suggesting that – following Laplace's law – a disc with a larger radius would be more deformable and vulnerable than a small one.

### 3.4.1 Clinical Pearl 3.1: Predicting Glaucoma Risk

Ophthalmologists can show a high range of estimates for the probability of developing glaucoma in the same ocular hypertensive patients. In comparison to OHTS glaucoma risk calculations, treating physicians underestimated the risk of developing glaucoma by almost twofold on average.[76] This can lead to either under- or over-treatment of patients. Clinicians need a more exact method to determine the probability of glaucoma from ocular hypertension. Gordon et al have recently developed a point system (Table 3.1) that can be more easily used than risk calculators for estimating the 5-year risk of developing POAG.[66]

**Table 3.1** Glaucoma risk calculator

| Baseline predictor | Points for baseline predictor | | | | |
|---|---|---|---|---|---|
| | 0 | 1 | 2 | 3 | 4 |
| Age (years) | <45 | 45 to <55 | 55 to <65 | 65 to <75 | ≥75 |
| Mean IOP (mmHg) | <22 | 22 to <24 | 24 to <26 | 26 to <28 | ≥28 |
| Mean CCT (μm) | ≥600 | 576–600 | 551–575 | 526–550 | ≤525 |
| Mean vertical cup-to-disc ratio by contour | <0.3 | 0.3 to <0.4 | 0.4 to <0.5 | 0.5 to <0.6 | ≥0.6 |
| Mean PSD (dB) | <1.8 | 1.8 to <2.0 | 2.0 to <2.4 | 2.4 to <2.8 | ≥2.8 |
| Sum of points | 0–6 | 7–8 | 9–10 | 11–12 | >12 |
| Estimated 5-year risk of POAG | ≤4.0% | 10% | 15% | 20% | ≥33% |

Eye-specific variables are the mean of right and left eyes

*CCT* central corneal thickness, *dB* decibels, *IOP* intraocular pressure, *PSD* pattern standard deviation

## 3.5 How to Measure Intraocular Pressure

### 3.5.1 Clinical Pearl 3.2: Instruments to Measure IOP

- Goldmann applanation tonometry (GAT) is the gold standard.
- Central corneal thickness (CCT) should be determined at one of the first visits.
- No direct correction of GAT by central corneal thickness is possible. GAT IOP and CCT can be integrated using a pressure-to-cornea index (IOP/(CCT^3); normal PCI = 120–140). CCT can also be classified as thin, normal, or thick.
- The latest generation Tono-Pen is as precise as GAT and can easily be integrated in the workup by support staff prior to patient-physician contact.
- Acquire an invaluable skill by practicing transpalpebral scleral IOP palpation after measuring IOP with an instrument.
- Dynamic contour tonometry takes the CCT out of the equation and might become the future standard. Its use remains limited mainly because of costs. Recording of the pulse amplitude can be useful in select cases, but its significance in daily practice is marginal.
- The latest noncontact air puff tonometry devices are almost as accurate as GAT and can be used with little training. Measurements create potentially infectious aerosol. The anticipation of the puff is uncomfortable to most patients and can produce lid artifacts from squeezing.
- Pneumatonometry and Schiotz tonometry are best employed as reserve techniques when other instruments are not available.

### 3.5.2 Goldmann Applanation Tonometry

Goldmann applanation tonometry (GAT, Haag Streit AG, Bern, Switzerland) is the standard method of measuring IOP[77,78] to which all other ones are compared. GAT was introduced by Goldmann in 1954[79,80] and applies the Imbert-Fick law that describes the applanation force of an ideal sphere to applanation of the cornea – a method that is more accurate than older indentation systems. GAT produces precise and repeatable IOP readings with an inter-observer variation of 11% and an intra-observer variation of 9% when compared with a single measurement.[81] It has remained the standard because it is simple and widely available with a popular slit-lamp system that allows comparison of historical measurements including ones obtained by others. GAT can be integrated well into the exam algorithm, as the fluorescein that is used is also helpful in evaluating the ocular surface. GAT displaces only about 0.5 μL of fluid, while Schiotz and other indentation techniques displace about 15–20 μL, depending on ocular rigidity. GAT is influenced by central corneal thickness, curvature, structure, and ocular axial length.[82]

No reliable nomogram exists that converts GAT and CCT into true IOP, although attempts have been made to develop a conversion factor.[83–85] Doughty et al found in a meta-analysis that a 10% difference in CCT would result in a $3.4 \pm 0.9$ mmHg difference in IOP in 133 data sets of all eyes but only $1.1 \pm 0.6$ mmHg in healthy eyes.[84] Others could not confirm a systematic error that would allow direct conversion of applanation tonometry readings with increasing CCT when compared to intracameral measurements.[86] GAT IOP and CCT (thin, normal, and thick) are best treated as two independent risk factors or integrated without calculation of "true" IOP. This can be done, for instance, by using a recently described pressure-to-cornea index (PCI).[87] PCI can be calculated as IOP/CCT^3. A PCI range of 120–140 is proposed as the upper normal limit.

The influence of CCT on GAT can be especially challenging after refractive surgery. Other disadvantages of GAT are that it requires more user skill than other methods, can be falsely high in anxious or obese patients second to Valsalva maneuver, and the device must be sent in for calibration when a preset weight indicates inaccurate readings. GAT readout is also user-dependent: Most examiners will use the IOP during the ocular pulse diastole, while others choose to estimate IOP between systole and diastole.

### 3.5.3 Tono-Pen Tonometry

A small handheld device, the Tono-Pen AVIA (Mentor, Santa Barbara, California, USA) uses the same principle as GAT and its development has a comparably long history, dating back to the Mackay-Marg tonometer in 1960.[88,89] While prior studies comparing Tono-Pen tonometry with other methods produced mixed results,[90] measurements with the later generation of Tono-Pen strongly correlate with GAT.[91] In addition to IOP, the Tono-Pen determines the confidence interval of several measurements. Because of a smaller area of applanation (2.36 mm$^2$) than GAT (7.35 mm$^2$), the Tono-Pen is less dependent on CCT in theory,[92] allows valid intraocular pressure measurements in the presence of corneal edema and irregularities,[93] and has even been used to measure through soft contact lenses.[94,95] Measurements can be performed while the patient rests back in the chair, avoiding false high readings from increased intra-abdominal pressure; e.g., in obese patients when leaning forward. In contrast to GAT, which cannot be adjusted by the user, the Tono-Pen self-calibrates. Support staff can obtain accurate readings with ease prior to physician encounter.

### 3.5.4 Dynamic Contour Tonometry

In dynamic contour tonometry (DCT) (Pascal dynamic contour tonometer; Swiss Microtechnology AG, Port, Switzerland), both IOP and ocular pulse amplitude can be read on a display. It uses a solid-state pressure sensor built into the center of a contoured, concave tip surface. The contour surface is designed to minimize distortion and to direct all forces acting within the cornea to the pressure sensor surface. The tonometer head allows the cornea to assume the shape it naturally adopts when pressure on both sides of the cornea are equal, which constitutes the measurement endpoint. A microprocessor determines the intraocular pressure and the ocular pulse amplitude. DCT is very similar to GAT, but does not vary with decreased CCT and has a lower intra- and inter-observer variability.[96] This is of particular interest after LASIK when GAT, but not DCT, produces lower IOP readings due to a thinner and more oblate cornea.[97] DCT does not have any benefit over GAT in thick corneas, however.[98]

### 3.5.5 Transpalpebral Scleral Palpation

Transpalpebral intraocular pressure estimation by palpation of the sclera in down gaze is an invaluable tool that has many advantages: It requires little patient cooperation, circumvents corneal pathology, is fast, and can be used without any equipment. In the operating room, direct corneal palpation might be the only available form of tonometry. Experienced observers are able to estimate IOP surprisingly accurately within only 2 mmHg[99] to 5 mmHg[100] median deviation from GAT, although IOPs below 14 mmHg may be overestimated.[99] In other hands, palpation may only be helpful in identifying IOPs above 30 mmHg.[101] It is best to practice and correlate palpation and GAT in daily practice.

### 3.5.6 Noncontact Air Puff Tonometry

A cited advantage of air puff tonometry is the absence of contact with the measured eye, which in theory makes the exam more comfortable as no anesthetic drops are needed, and there is no risk of a corneal abrasion by untrained personnel. In reality, many patients find the anticipation of multiple puffs uncomfortable, which can lead to false high-pressure measurements because of lid pressure. The air puff generates aerosol that potentially distributes infectious agents.[102] While earlier noncontact tonometry was inaccurate when compared with Goldman tonometry, earning the method a bad reputation, recent devices have a high accuracy that approaches GAT.[103–105] Noncontact tonometry is more influenced by CCT than other methods.[106] It has been reported to be performed with sufficient accuracy over soft contact lenses of less than 0.30 mm thickness and less than +3D power.[107]

### 3.5.7 Pneumatonometry

The pneumatonometer (Model 30 Classic Pneumatonometer, Reichert Ophthalmic Instruments, Depew, New York, USA) is a high displacement tonometer[108] that can also be used to measure outflow facility.[109] It must not be confused with the noncontact air puff tonometer. Its accuracy is exceeded by that of the Goldmann tonometer.[110] IOP measurements have only half the standard deviation of the Perkins handheld applanation tonometer[111] and are better than the Schiotz tonometer.[112] Another advantage is that – similar to an electrocardiogram strip – a live printout of IOP over time can be obtained that allows measuring and visualizing IOP fluctuations. The pneumatonometer tends to underestimate IOP above 40 mmHg.[113] IOP measurements are independent of the central corneal thickness after LASIK[114] and not significantly affected by bandage contact lenses.[115]

## 3.5.8 Schiotz Tonometry

The Schiotz tonometer[116] is another displacement tonometer that is less accurate, and influenced by the curvature and thickness of the cornea as well as by overall ocular rigidity. Because it is a small handheld, sterilizable full metal instrument that requires no batteries, it may be useful in the operating room or as a backup instrument.

## 3.6 Distribution of IOP and Factors Influencing IOP

### 3.6.1 Distribution of IOP Within the Population

IOP has a non-Gaussian distribution and is skewed to higher pressures (especially among subjects over 45 years of age,[117] and more markedly so in women.[118])

In a primarily Caucasian population in the United States, mean IOP was 16 mmHg (SD ±3 mmHg)[117] The Baltimore Eye Survey found no difference in IOP among normal African-Americans when compared with normal Caucasian subjects.[6] In the Barbados Eye Study, IOP was found to be higher among African-Caribbeans [18 mmHg (SD 4 mmHg)][119] when compared with Caucasians, 14.5 mmHg (SD 2.6 mmHg) in Iran,[120] 16.11 mmHg (SD 3.39 mmHg) in Northern China,[121] 11.7 mmHg (SD 2.5 mmHg) in Japan[122], and 15.5 mmHg[123] in West Africa. Myopic and more darkly pigmented subjects also have a higher average IOP.[120]

There is no upper IOP that can be defined as safe for the entire population below which no glaucomatous optic neuropathy occurs. This is exemplified by an average IOP of 15.4 mmHg (SD 2.8 mmHg) of Japanese POAG subjects in the Tajimi study[124] that is below or similar to the previously mentioned groups. There was a surprisingly high prevalence of POAG (3.9%) among participants, 92% of whom had an IOP of 21 mmHg or less.

### 3.6.2 Factors Influencing Intraocular Pressure

IOP is influenced by various external and internal factors that include time of the day and year, heartbeat, respiration, exercises, and fluid intake. Systemic medications and topically applied drugs can also have an impact. Measurement of IOP by the widespread Goldmann applanation tonometry is dependent on the central corneal thickness as detailed previously.

### 3.6.3 Clinical Pearl 3.3: Factors Influencing Intraocular Pressure

- IOP measurements are significantly dependent on central corneal thickness in Goldmann applanation tonometry: A thick cornea will lead to over- and a thin cornea to under-estimation.
- Variations of IOP by season, cardiac pulse wave, or respiration are of no practical clinical significance to the practitioner. A diurnal pressure curve can be utilized to get a better idea of the range of IOP an eye is subjected to. Always note the time of the day with each IOP measurement.
- Be aware that you are measuring office IOP, which may be lower than IOP at home as a result of increased compliance before the visit.
- Optimization of exercise, cessation of recreational drugs, and improvement of nutrition should always be encouraged, but must never be falsely prioritized.
- The possibility of progressive visual field defects secondary to Valsalva maneuvers when playing high-resistance wind instruments or during extreme postural changes such as in yoga should be pointed out clearly to glaucoma patients. IOP measured in the supine position allows estimation of nocturnal IOP in untreated glaucoma patients.
- The water drinking test can be used to estimate the highest naturally occurring IOP, but must be used with caution in cardiac or renal patients as fluid overload and electrolyte shifts can occur rapidly.
- Nightly systemic hypotension may result in cerebral and optic nerve hypoperfusion. Consider using topical beta-blockers only in the morning in such individuals and discuss the option of using systemic beta-blockers only in the morning in individuals who take them not primarily for blood pressure control (congestive heart failure, migraine prophylaxis).
- In the absence of any available medication, a good Scotch or other high percentage alcoholic beverage can be consumed to emergently treat acutely vision-threatening high IOP.

### 3.6.4 Circadian and Seasonal Variation

The diurnal (daytime) IOP varies by 2–6 mmHg in normal individuals. Pressure peaks most commonly occur in the morning hours but may be seen in the afternoon, evening, or sleep, especially if one measures IOP in the habitual position (sitting during the day, supine at night). Some individuals have no reproducible pattern. Generally, higher amplitude fluctuations are seen in higher mean IOP and in individuals with POAG,[125] and greater in progressive visual field loss than in the presence of stable fields.[126] The reason for higher IOP during the day is that the rate of aqueous humor formation has a circadian variation as well and is twice as high during the day as at night[127] as a result of endogenous cathecolamines.[128,129] Measurements of fluctuations to create a diurnal curve can be used to detect normal tension glaucoma, in which pressure peaks may contribute to progressive glaucomatous optic neuropathy, despite well-controlled average pressures at prior office visits. However, fluctuation itself is not significantly associated with a higher risk of progression to glaucoma in untreated ocular hypertensives.[130] In contrast to this study, Lee et al found in a cohort study that each unit increase in IOP standard deviation resulted in an approximately five times higher risk of glaucoma progression.[131] Although variations of IOP in the left and right eye are similar, the strength of association is only moderate, which makes one-eye therapeutic trials difficult to assess by single pairs of right and left IOP measurements.[132] IOP is higher in winter months by about 3 mmHg and within the range of the diurnal variations.[133]

### 3.6.5 Cardiac Pulse Wave

As the cardiac pulse wave is transmitted by the carotids to the ocular circulation it manifests in the choriocapillaris as pulse-synchronous IOP oscillations. The relationship between ocular perfusion pressure and intraocular pressure is more complicated because of auto-regulation within a physiological range of optic nerve head circulation, central retinal artery, and choroidal perfusion. This dynamic auto-regulation is impaired in glaucoma.[134] Counterintuitively, IOP might decrease, rather than increase with increased perfusion pressure.[135] This is different from other tissues (e.g., the kidney) because active secretion vastly exceeds passive filtration in aqueous humor production. It is difficult to study this relationship because ocular perfusion pressure cannot be changed selectively without affecting ocular blood return, ciliary body tension, etc. in vivo by pharmacological or physical means.

### 3.6.6 Respiration and Valsalva Maneuver

Short-term IOP changes occur with breathing as the result of acute changes of perfusion pressure.[136] With higher pressure than normal breathing – e.g., from high-resistance wind instruments (trumpet, oboe) – uveal engorgement becomes the major factor.[137] This increase is not trivial: Professional high-resistance musicians who are exposed to frequent and longer lasting, high amplitude IOP spikes, have a significantly greater incidence of visual field loss with characteristic glaucomatous damage.[137] During only 12 s, IOP can rise from 24 to 46 mmHg.[137] In contrast, decreased venous drainage from increased episcleral venous pressure as a result of high intra-abdominal pressure would be driven by aqueous humor production and would take 10–16 min in theory.[137]

### 3.6.7 Postural Changes

IOP also varies with postural changes as a result of increased episcleral venous pressure[138] as well as increased choroidal volume by vascular engorgement.[139] The relationship between the head-down body position and increased IOP is well known.[140-144] Nocturnal IOP in untreated glaucoma patients can be estimated during routine office visits by measuring the supine position.[145] Upside-down body changes such as in certain yoga poses can cause extreme IOPs and can result in visual field progression.[138,146]

### 3.6.8 Physical Exercise

The IOP decreases significantly after dynamic exercise, although heart rate and systolic artery pressure increase.[147] Different from the sustained high intrathoracic pressure when playing wind instruments, IOP increases only by about 4 mmHg with breath holding in resistance training (e.g., bench press) compared to about 2 mmHg with normal breathing.[148] While there is an immediate IOP spike after exercise, decrease is seen 30 min later and lasts for 2 h after exercise.[149] During aerobic exercise, duration of the systolic and diastolic phases of the intraocular pulse shortens, and the pulse amplitude and volume decrease, and total ocular blood flow increases by 18%.[135]

### 3.6.9 Fluid Intake

IOP and hydration status are related. While low IOP in hypovolemia can be used to estimated extent of dehydration,[150] a fluid bolus intake can increase IOP. The water drinking test has been used for a long time to detect peak IOPs that can be elusive during the day in the diagnosis of glaucoma.[151] Because recent studies have demonstrated that the amplitude of fluctuation correlates to the severity of glaucoma[152] and to visual field progression[153] this test has regained interest. Water drinking test peak pressures, and peak pressures seen in a normal diurnal pressure curve correlate.[5,154,155] Change of IOP after the water drinking test is one identified significant risk factor as are outflow facility, age, IOP, and cup-to-disc ratio.[5] Yoshikawa et al[154] found that the water drinking test could predict the progression of visual field loss also in normal tension glaucoma.

### 3.6.10 Nutrition and Recreational Substances

Patients frequently ask about the influence of nutrition, recreational substances (caffeine, alcohol, nicotine, marijuana) or blood pressure on IOP. Although there is evidence for a minimal but statistically significant increase of IOP after high amounts of caffeine[156] and smoking,[157] this has not been proven to be a significant factor in the context of glaucoma. There is a large school of thinking focused on improving optic nerve head perfusion with smoking cessation, aspirin, calcium antagonist, ginkgo extracts, or magnesium supplements, but this is not supported by convincing data. Alcoholic beverages can lower IOP and have been used to break acute pressure spikes; e.g., in angle closure.[158,159] Cannabinoids also have a moderate effect and lower IOP by about 5 mmHg for 4–6 h.[160–162]

## 3.7 Medications Influencing Intraocular Pressure

### 3.7.1 Clinical Pearl 3.4: Drug-Induced Intraocular Hypertension and Glaucoma

- Corticosteroids increase IOP in up to 36% of healthy and up to 92% of POAG patients. This may not be reversible after cessation.
- This can occur via all routes of exposure, not just ocular or oral.
- More potent steroids cause a faster and higher IOP increase. From low to high[163]: medrysone 1.0% = 1.0 mmHg, tetrahydrotriamcinolone 0.25% = 1.8 mmHg, hydrocortisone 0.5% = 3.2 mmHg, fluorometholone 0.1% = 6.1 mmHg, dexamethasone 0.005% = 8.2 mmHg, prednisolone 1.0% = 10.0 mmHg, and dexamethasone 0.1% = 22 mmHg.

### 3.7.2 Corticosteroids

The list of topical and systemic drugs that can increase IOP and cause glaucoma is long. The most notorious ones are corticosteroids (glucocorticosteroids more than mineralocorticosteroids) no matter their route of application: steroid-induced ocular hypertension has been reported following topical application to the eyelids,[164] chronic nasal or inhaled steroid,[165] subconjunctival,[166] and sub-Tenon's injection of steroid.[167–169] Endogenous corticosteroids can have the same effect.[170] Corticosteroid-induced glaucoma was first described in 1950 after administration of adrenocorticotropic hormone and cortisone.[171] Eighteen to 36% of healthy individuals and 46–92% of patients with POAG will respond with an elevation of IOP within 2–4 weeks.[172] Relatives of patients with POAG, angle recession, patients with diabetes mellitus, high myopia, and connective tissue disease (rheumatoid arthritis in particular) have a higher risk of steroid-induced intraocular hypertension. Thirty-one percent of children who receive prednisone for inflammatory bowel disease have a significant increase of IOP but respond well to dose reduction.[172]

Chances of steroid-induced ocular hypertension increase with steroid potency. It is very low with rimexolone, loteprednol etabonate, fluorometholone, and medrysone, but this risk and extent of IOP rise increase with steroid potency[163]: (medrysone 1.0% = 1.0 ± 1.3 mmHg, tetrahydro-triamcinolone 0.25% = 1.8 ± 1.3 mmHg, hydrocortisone 0.5% = 3.2 ± 1.0 mmHg, fluorometholone 0.1% = 6.1 ± 1.4 mmHg, dexamethasone 0.005% = 8.2 ± 1.7 mmHg, prednisolone 1.0% = 10.0 ± 1.7 mmHg, and dexamethasone 0.1% = 22.0 ± 2.9 mmHg). Physicians must be aware that steroid-induced ocular hypertension might not be reversible after discontinuation of steroid therapy.

The pathophysiology of steroid-induced ocular hypertension is localized in the trabecular meshwork, but the mechanism is incompletely understood. More than 1,000-fold upregulation of myocilin (Myoc – originally termed trabecular meshwork inducible glucocorticoid response [TIGR]) can be observed in trabecular meshwork with accompanying accumulation of polymerized glycosaminoglycans in the extracellular matrix.[173] It has been hypothesized but not proven that the primary means of action is a decreased funneling of aqueous humor toward the juxtacanalicular trabecular meshwork.[174] This mechanism is debated because myocilin mutants of some glaucomas act intracellularly and not primarily extracellularly.[175,176] Other proposed mechanisms include direct swelling of TM cells from inhibition of Na-K-Cl cotransporter that is regulated in TM cells,[177] decreased production of tissue plasminogen activator, collagenase IV, and stromelysin.[178–182]

### 3.7.3 Pupillary Block from Anticholinergics

Antipsychotics, antidepressants, antihistamines, anti-Parkinson medications, antispasmolytic agents, mydriatics, sympathomimetica, antiasthma medications (ipratropium),[183] and botulinum toxin (botulinum toxin can produce mydriasis if the ciliary ganglion is affected[184)] are drug classes that have the potential to increase IOP by angle closure secondary to their anticholinergic properties (except botulinum toxin). The prevalence of occludable angles in Caucasians 55 years of age or older in the Framingham study is 3.8%,[185] but the risk of this in a Vietnamese population was estimated to be as high as 47.8%.[186]

### 3.7.4 Pupillary Block from Phacomorphic Changes or Ciliary Body Rotation

Promethazine HCl, an H1 antihistamine, has been documented to also produce swelling of the lens[187] in addition to mydriasis. Salbutamol, an inhalation agent used in asthma, can raise IOP by increased production of aqueous humor by about 38%.[188] Pupillary dilation may trigger the release of pigment and trabecular obstruction.[189] Other drugs that can induce phacomorphic changes or anterior rotation of the ciliary body are: sulfa drugs such as acetazolamide,[190–192] sulfamethoxazole/trimethoprim,[191] indapamide, promethazine, spironolactone, isosorbide dinitrate, and bromocriptine[192]; tetracycline[191,192]; corticosteroids; hydrochlorothiazide; penicillamine; quinine; metronidazole; isotretinoin; and aspirin.[192] Recently, bilateral angle closure glaucoma with uveal effusions, forward rotation of the iris–lens diaphragm, transient myopia, and secondary angle closure has been associated with topiramate.[193,194] Topiramate is an antiepileptic that is also used as a secondary agent in the treatment of migraine, depression, and neuropathic pain. Similar to other sulfa drugs, it can produce swelling and forward displacement of the ciliary body, resulting in shallowing of the anterior chamber and angle closure,[194–196] which usually occurs within 2 weeks of therapy. It is possible that increased prostaglandin levels and ciliary body edema cause this. Because angle closure is not caused by pupillary block in this case, attacks must be broken by discontinuing topiramate and medically lowering IOP to allow IOP to return to normal levels within hours to days.[196]

### 3.7.5 General Anesthetics

Succinylcholine, ketamine, and chloral hydrate – agents that are used for general anesthesia – increase intraocular muscle tone and can temporarily elevate IOP.[197] IOP should be checked immediately after anesthesia induction to avoid falsely high readout.

## 3.8 Target IOP in Clinical Practice

### 3.8.1 Clinical Pearl 3.5: Target IOP

- Define a target IOP range at which no glaucoma progression is expected to occur. A good starting point is 20–30% IOP reduction followed by 15–20% reduction if progression persists.
- Alternatively, calculate target pressure range as [Initial IOP $\times$ (1 – Initial IOP/100) – $Z$ – $Y$] $\pm$ 1 mmHg.

Target pressure is an IOP range at which no glaucoma progression is expected to occur. Defining such a target pressure in clinical practice is a crucial element that helps guide glaucoma therapy in clinical practice. As IOP is the only variable that can alter the course of glaucoma to a measurable extent, target pressure establishes a treatment goal that can be evaluated and adjusted during future visits. For this, target IOP must be correlated to the structure and function of the optic nerve.

The concept of target pressure is old,[198] but could not be implemented well as the effect of IOP lowering therapy had not been studied in a stringent way using randomized clinical trials. The now outdated concept of a threshold IOP of 21 mmHg was originally derived from a study in 1987[199] in which patients with an IOP above 21 mmHg progressed more often than with IOP less than 14. Grant suggested in 1982 that different states of glaucoma require different target pressures,[200] but in a more contemporary view this might only be reflective of our present inability to detect glaucoma progression early enough. A nerve with advanced glaucomatous optic nerve cupping in a later stage of the disease would have likely required the same low IOP at an earlier state to prevent progression. On the other hand, there is experimental support that advanced axonal loss can lead to increased shear forces and disadvantageous biomechanical properties at the lamina cribrosa.[201–203] In addition, instead of a percentage attrition resulting in an asymptotic decay curve, the rate of retinal ganglion cell loss in glaucoma accelerates with progressive disease at least in animal models.[204] It is obvious that advanced optic nerve damage does not allow much time to evaluate pressure-lowering therapy that is only moderately effective.

Many different factors should be taken into account when defining a target pressure: pretreatment IOP, disease status, central corneal thickness, rate of progression, course of the other eye, ethnicity, family history, and past medical history. OHTS applied an initial reduction of 20–30% and additional 15–20% if progression persisted. Jampel recommends calculating target pressure using the formula:

$$\text{target pressure range} = [\text{Initial IOP} (1 - \text{Initial IOP}/100) - Z - Y] \pm 1 \text{ mmHg}$$

whereas $Z$ is optic nerve damage and $Y$ is a burden of therapy factor, each of which are determined on a scale of 0–3.[205]

The use of a target range rather than a single number allows taking into account the various factors of IOP fluctuations without having to proceed to more aggressive therapy. Burden of therapy must be taken very seriously as it can be challenging to adhere to frequent applications of topical medication and may present the reason for a failing therapy.

## 3.9 Conclusion

Intraocular pressure is a major risk factor for the development of glaucoma. It remains an important parameter in the diagnosis – and the only proven means to reduce the risk of progression – and the treatment of glaucoma. Randomized clinical trials, most notably the Ocular Hypertensive Treatment Study (OHTS) and Early Manifest Glaucoma Trial (EGMT) have established the protective role of lowering IOP in preventing conversion from ocular hypertension to glaucoma as well as progression of glaucoma. An IOP target range of at least 30% lower than initial presentation is helpful in setting treatment goals but requires individual adjustment.

In contrast to other tests, IOP can be determined objectively. It is best determined with Goldmann applanation tonometry, the gold standard of measuring intraocular pressure, which is widespread and allows comparison with historical data. Tono-Pen, dynamic contour, and even latest generation non-contact tonometry also produce accurate and repeatable results that rival or exceed Goldmann applanation. Where accurate IOP is not crucial or a tonometer not available, the experienced examiner can use scleral palpation to estimate IOP.

Within the population, IOP has a non-Gaussian distribution with an average of about 16 mmHg (worldwide range 11–18 mmHg). Examiners should be aware that IOP has 2–6 mmHg diurnal variation, with the maximum in the morning. The water drinking test has regained interest because it can be used to estimate peak pressures and risk of glaucoma.

IOP can be influenced by numerous medications that increase outflow resistance (steroids) or cause angle closure from anticholinergic action or forward rotation of the ciliary body. IOP increase from steroids may not be reversible. Patients with at least moderate glaucoma should be made aware that high-resistance wind instruments as well as extreme body postures can contribute to progression and should be avoided.

## References

1. Meyerhof M. *Ali at-Tabari's "Paradise of Wisdom," One of the Oldest Arabic Compendiums of Medicine.* Cambridge: Cambridge University Press; 1921:37–40.
2. Sorsby A. *Modern Ophthalmology.* Washington, DC: Butterworth; 1963.
3. Sommer A, Tielsch JM, Katz J, et al. Relationship between intraocular pressure and primary open angle glaucoma among white and black Americans. The Baltimore Eye Survey. *Arch Ophthalmol.* 1991;109:1090–1095.
4. Leske MC, Connell AM, Wu SY, Hyman LG, Schachat AP. Risk factors for open-angle glaucoma. The Barbados Eye Study. *Arch Ophthalmol.* 1995;113:918–924.
5. Armaly MF, Krueger DE, Maunder L, et al. Biostatistical analysis of the collaborative glaucoma study. I. Summary report of the risk factors for glaucomatous visual-field defects. *Arch Ophthalmol.* 1980;98:2163–2171.
6. Eddy DM, Sanders LE, Eddy JF. The value of screening for glaucoma with tonometry. *Surv Ophthalmol.* 1983;28:194–205.
7. Nemesure B, Honkanen R, Hennis A, Wu SY, Leske MC. Incident open-angle glaucoma and intraocular pressure. *Ophthalmology.* 2007;114:1810–1815.
8. Gordon MO, Kass MA. The Ocular Hypertension Treatment Study: design and baseline description of the participants. *Arch Ophthalmol.* 1999;117:573–583.
9. Leske MC, Heijl A, Hyman L, Bengtsson B. Early Manifest Glaucoma Trial: design and baseline data. *Ophthalmology.* 1999;106:2144–2153.
10. Ritch R. Complementary therapy for the treatment of glaucoma: a perspective. *Ophthalmol Clin North Am.* 2005;18:597–609.
11. Liu S, Araujo SV, Spaeth GL, Katz LJ, Smith M. Lack of effect of calcium channel blockers on open-angle glaucoma. *J Glaucoma.* 1996;5:187–190.
12. Yucel YH, Gupta N, Zhang Q, Mizisin AP, Kalichman MW, Weinreb RN. Memantine protects neurons from shrinkage in the lateral geniculate nucleus in experimental glaucoma. *Arch Ophthalmol.* 2006;124:217–225.
13. Hare WA, WoldeMussie E, Lai RK, et al. Efficacy and safety of memantine treatment for reduction of changes associated with experimental glaucoma in monkey, I: Functional measures. *Invest Ophthalmol Vis Sci.* 2004;45:2625–2639.
14. Hare WA, WoldeMussie E, Weinreb RN, et al. Efficacy and safety of memantine treatment for reduction of changes associated with experimental glaucoma in monkey. II. Structural measures. *Invest Ophthalmol Vis Sci.* 2004;45:2640–2651.
15. Sheldon WG, Warbritton AR, Bucci TJ, Turturro A. Glaucoma in food-restricted and ad libitum-fed DBA/2NNia mice. *Lab Anim Sci.* 1995;45:508–518.
16. Rhee DJ, Katz LJ, Spaeth GL, Myers JS. Complementary and alternative medicine for glaucoma. *Surv Ophthalmol.* 2001;46:43–55.
17. Goldmann H. Out-flow pressure, minute volume and resistance of the anterior chamber flow in man. *Docu Ophthalmol.* 1951; 5–6:278–356.
18. Haddad A, De Almeida JC, Laicine EM, Fife RS, Pelletier G. The origin of the intrinsic glycoproteins of the rabbit vitreous body: an immunohistochemical and autoradiographic study. *Exp Eye Res.* 1990;50:555–561.
19. Morrison JC, Van Buskirk EM. Anterior collateral circulation in the primate eye. *Ophthalmology.* 1983;90:707–715.
20. Morrison JC, Van Buskirk EM. Ciliary process microvasculature of the primate eye. *Am J Ophthalmol.* 1984;97:372–383.
21. Funk R, Rohen JW. SEM studies of the functional morphology of the ciliary process vasculature in the cynomolgus monkey: reactions after application of epinephrine. *Exp Eye Res.* 1988;47:653–663.
22. Funk R, Rohen JW. Scanning electron microscopic study on the vasculature of the human anterior eye segment, especially with respect to the ciliary processes. *Exp Eye Res.* 1990;51:651–661.
23. Raviola G, Raviola E. Intercellular junctions in the ciliary epithelium. *Invest Ophthalmol Vis Sci.* 1978;17:958–981.
24. Hirsch M, Montcourrier P, Arguillere P, Keller N. The structure of tight junctions in the ciliary epithelium. *Curr Eye Res.* 1985;4:493–501.

25. Freddo TF. Shifting the paradigm of the blood-aqueous barrier. *Exp Eye Res*. 2001;73:581–592.
26. Bill A, Phillips CI. Uveoscleral drainage of aqueous humour in human eyes. *Exp Eye Res*. 1971;12:275–281.
27. Weinreb RN. Uveoscleral outflow: the other outflow pathway. *J Glaucoma*. 2000;9:343–345.
28. Maepea O, Bill A. Pressures in the juxtacanalicular tissue and Schlemm's canal in monkeys. *Exp Eye Res*. 1992;54:879–883.
29. Knepper PA, Farbman AI, Telser AG. Aqueous outflow pathway glycosaminoglycans. *Exp Eye Res*. 1981;32:265–277.
30. Knepper PA, Goossens W, Hvizd M, Palmberg PF. Glycosaminoglycans of the human trabecular meshwork in primary open-angle glaucoma. *Invest Ophthalmol Vis Sci*. 1996;37:1360–1367.
31. Grierson I, Lee WR. Pressure-induced changes in the ultrastructure of the endothelium lining Schlemm's canal. *Am J Ophthalmol*. 1975;80:863–884.
32. Ethier CR, Coloma FM, Sit AJ, Johnson M. Two pore types in the inner-wall endothelium of Schlemm's canal. *Invest Ophthalmol Vis Sci*. 1998;39:2041–2048.
33. de Kater AW, Spurr-Michaud SJ, Gipson IK. Localization of smooth muscle myosin-containing cells in the aqueous outflow pathway. *Invest Ophthalmol Vis Sci*. 1990;31:347–353.
34. Ascher KW. Aqueous veins and their significance for pathogenesis of glaucoma. *Arch Ophthal*. 1949;42:66–76.
35. Bill A. Uveoscleral drainage of aqueous humor: physiology and pharmacology. *Prog Clin Biol Res*. 1989;312:417–427.
36. Bill A. Some aspects of aqueous humour drainage. *Eye*. 1993;7 (Pt 1):14–19.
37. Jocson VL, Sears ML. Experimental aqueous perfusion in enucleated human eyes. Results after obstruction of Schlemm's canal. *Arch Ophthalmol*. 1971;86:65–71.
38. Toris CB, Koepsell SA, Yablonski ME, Camras CB. Aqueous humor dynamics in ocular hypertensive patients. *J Glaucoma*. 2002;11:253–258.
39. Toris CB, Camras CB, Yablonski ME. Effects of PhXA41, a new prostaglandin F2 alpha analog, on aqueous humor dynamics in human eyes. *Ophthalmology*. 1993;100:1297–1304.
40. Brubaker RF, Schoff EO, Nau CB, Carpenter SP, Chen K, Vandenburgh AM. Effects of AGN 192024, a new ocular hypotensive agent, on aqueous dynamics. *Am J Ophthalmol*. 2001;131:19–24.
41. Green K, Bountra C, Georgiou P, House CR. An electrophysiologic study of rabbit ciliary epithelium. *Invest Ophthalmol Vis Sci*. 1985;26:371–381.
42. Edelman JL, Sachs G, Adorante JS. Ion transport asymmetry and functional coupling in bovine pigmented and nonpigmented ciliary epithelial cells. *Am J Physiol*. 1994;266:C1210–C1221.
43. Grant WM, Trotter RR. Diamox (acetazoleamide) in treatment of glaucoma. *AMA Arch Ophthalmol*. 1954;51:735–739.
44. Yablonski ME, Zimmerman TJ, Waltman SR, Becker B. A fluorophotometric study of the effect of topical timolol on aqueous humor dynamics. *Exp Eye Res*. 1978;27:135–142.
45. Lee DA, Brubaker RF. Effect of phenylephrine on aqueous humor flow. *Curr Eye Res*. 1982;2:89–92.
46. Grierson I, Lee WR, Abraham S. The effects of topical pilocarpine on the morphology of the outflow apparatus of the baboon (Papio cynocephalus). *Invest Ophthalmol Vis Sci*. 1979;18:346–355.
47. Rolim de Moura C, Paranhos A Jr, Wormald R. Laser trabeculoplasty for open angle glaucoma. *Cochrane Database Syst Rev* 2007;CD003919
48. Francis BA, See RF, Rao NA, Minckler DS, Baerveldt G. Ab interno trabeculectomy: development of a novel device (Trabectome) and surgery for open-angle glaucoma. *J Glaucoma*. 2006;15:68–73.
49. Gedde SJ, Schiffman JC, Feuer WJ, Herndon LW, Brandt JD, Budenz DL. Treatment outcomes in the tube versus trabeculectomy study after one year of follow-up. *Am J Ophthalmol*. 2007;143:9–22.
50. Edmunds B, Thompson JR, Salmon JF, Wormald RP. The National Survey of Trabeculectomy. III. Early and late complications. *Eye*. 2002;16:297–303.
51. Anderson DR. Collaborative normal tension glaucoma study. *Curr Opin Ophthalmol*. 2003;14:86–90.
52. Anderson DR, Drance SM, Schulzer M. Factors that predict the benefit of lowering intraocular pressure in normal tension glaucoma. *Am J Ophthalmol*. 2003;136:820–829.
53. Anderson DR, Drance SM, Schulzer M. Natural history of normal-tension glaucoma. *Ophthalmology*. 2001;108:247–253.
54. The Advanced Glaucoma Intervention Study (AGIS): 1. Study design and methods and baseline characteristics of study patients. Control Clin Trials 1994;15:299–325
55. The Advanced Glaucoma Intervention Study (AGIS): 7. The relationship between control of intraocular pressure and visual field deterioration. The AGIS Investigators. Am J Ophthalmol 2000; 130:429–440.
56. Musch DC, Lichter PR, Guire KE, Standardi CL. The Collaborative Initial Glaucoma Treatment Study: study design, methods, and baseline characteristics of enrolled patients. *Ophthalmology*. 1999;106:653–662.
57. Lichter PR, Musch DC, Gillespie BW, et al. Interim clinical outcomes in the Collaborative Initial Glaucoma Treatment Study comparing initial treatment randomized to medications or surgery. *Ophthalmology*. 2001;108:1943–1953.
58. Musch DC, Gillespie BW, Niziol LM, et al. Cataract extraction in the collaborative initial glaucoma treatment study: incidence, risk factors, and the effect of cataract progression and extraction on clinical and quality-of-life outcomes. *Arch Ophthalmol*. 2006;124:1694–1700.
59. Feiner L, Piltz-Seymour JR. Collaborative Initial Glaucoma Treatment Study: a summary of results to date. *Curr Opin Ophthalmol*. 2003;14:106–111.
60. Kass MA, Heuer DK, Higginbotham EJ, et al. The Ocular Hypertension Treatment Study: a randomized trial determines that topical ocular hypotensive medication delays or prevents the onset of primary open-angle glaucoma. *Arch Ophthalmol*. 2002;120:701–713. discussion 829–730.
61. Kymes SM, Kass MA, Anderson DR, Miller JP, Gordon MO. Management of ocular hypertension: a cost-effectiveness approach from the Ocular Hypertension Treatment Study. *Am J Ophthalmol*. 2006;141:997–1008.
62. Gordon MO, Beiser JA, Brandt JD, et al. The Ocular Hypertension Treatment Study: baseline factors that predict the onset of primary open-angle glaucoma. *Arch Ophthalmol*. 2002;120:714–720. discussion 829–730.
63. Higginbotham EJ, Gordon MO, Beiser JA, et al. The Ocular Hypertension Treatment Study: topical medication delays or prevents primary open-angle glaucoma in African American individuals. *Arch Ophthalmol*. 2004;122:813–820.
64. Budenz DL, Anderson DR, Feuer WJ, et al. Detection and prognostic significance of optic disc hemorrhages during the Ocular Hypertension Treatment Study. *Ophthalmology*. 2006;113:2137–2143.
65. Miglior S, Zeyen T, Pfeiffer N, Cunha-Vaz J, Torri V, Adamsons I. The European glaucoma prevention study design and baseline description of the participants. *Ophthalmology*. 2002;109:1612–1621.
66. Gordon MO, Torri V, Miglior S, et al. Validated prediction model for the development of primary open-angle glaucoma in individuals with ocular hypertension. *Ophthalmology*. 2007;114:10–19.
67. Herman DC, Gordon MO, Beiser JA, et al. Topical ocular hypotensive medication and lens opacification: evidence from the ocular hypertension treatment study. *Am J Ophthalmol*. 2006;142:800–810.

68. Quigley HA. European glaucoma prevention study. *Ophthalmology*. 2005;112:1642–1643.
69. Leske MC, Heijl A, Hussein M, Bengtsson B, Hyman L, Komaroff E. Factors for glaucoma progression and the effect of treatment: the early manifest glaucoma trial. *Arch Ophthalmol*. 2003;121:48–56.
70. Bengtsson B, Leske MC, Hyman L, Heijl A. Fluctuation of intraocular pressure and glaucoma progression in the early manifest glaucoma trial. *Ophthalmology*. 2007;114:205–209.
71. Leske MC, Heijl A, Hyman L, Bengtsson B, Dong L, Yang Z. Predictors of long-term progression in the early manifest glaucoma trial. *Ophthalmology*. 2007;114:1965–1972.
72. Oliver JE, Hattenhauer MG, Herman D, et al. Blindness and glaucoma: a comparison of patients progressing to blindness from glaucoma with patients maintaining vision. *Am J Ophthalmol*. 2002;133:764–772.
73. Hattenhauer MG, Johnson DH, Ing HH, et al. The probability of blindness from open-angle glaucoma. *Ophthalmology*. 1998;105: 2099–2104.
74. Jonas JB, Holbach L. Central corneal thickness and thickness of the lamina cribrosa in human eyes. *Invest Ophthalmol Vis Sci*. 2005;46:1275–1279.
75. Pakravan M, Parsa A, Sanagou M, Parsa CF. Central corneal thickness and correlation to optic disc size: a potential link for susceptibility to glaucoma. *Br J Ophthalmol*. 2007;91:26–28.
76. Mansberger SL, Cioffi GA. The probability of glaucoma from ocular hypertension determined by ophthalmologists in comparison to a risk calculator. *J Glaucoma*. 2006;15:426–431.
77. Wessels IF, Oh Y. Tonometer utilization, accuracy, and calibration under field conditions. *Arch Ophthalmol*. 1990;108:1709–1712.
78. van der Jagt LH, Jansonius NM. Three portable tonometers, the TGDc-01, the ICARE and the Tonopen XL, compared with each other and with Goldmann applanation tonometry*. *Ophthalmic Physiol Opt*. 2005;25:429–435.
79. Moses RA. The Goldmann applanation tonometer. *Am J Ophthalmol*. 1958;46:865–869.
80. Goldmann H. Schmidt T [Applanation tonometry]. *Ophthalmologica*. 1957;134:221–242.
81. Dielemans I, Vingerling JR, Hofman A, Grobbee DE, de Jong PT. Reliability of intraocular pressure measurement with the Goldmann applanation tonometer in epidemiological studies. *Graefes Arch Clin Exp Ophthalmol*. 1994;232:141–144.
82. Whitacre MM, Stein R. Sources of error with use of Goldmann-type tonometers. *Surv Ophthalmol*. 1993;38:1–30.
83. Ehlers N, Bramsen T, Sperling S. Applanation tonometry and central corneal thickness. *Acta Ophthalmol*. 1975;53:34–43.
84. Doughty MJ, Zaman ML. Human corneal thickness and its impact on intraocular pressure measures: a review and meta-analysis approach. *Surv Ophthalmol*. 2000;44:367–408.
85. Shimmyo M, Ross AJ, Moy A, Mostafavi R. Intraocular pressure, Goldmann applanation tension, corneal thickness, and corneal curvature in Caucasians, Asians, Hispanics, and African Americans. *Am J Ophthalmol*. 2003;136:603–613.
86. Feltgen N, Leifert D, Funk J. Correlation between central corneal thickness, applanation tonometry, and direct intracameral IOP readings. *Br J Ophthalmol*. 2001;85:85–87.
87. Iliev ME, Meyenberg A, Buerki E, Shafranov G, Shields MB. Novel pressure-to-cornea index in glaucoma. *Br J Ophthalmol*. 2007;91:1364–1368.
88. Mackay RS, Marg E. Fast, automatic, electronic tonometers based on an exact theory. *Acta Ophthalmol*. 1959;37:495–507.
89. Mackay RS, Marg E, Oechsli R. Automatic tonometer with exact theory: various biological applications. *Science*. 1960;131:1668–1669.
90. Eisenberg DL, Sherman BG, McKeown CA, Schuman JS. Tonometry in adults and children. A manometric evaluation of pneumatonometry, applanation, and TonoPen in vitro and in vivo. *Ophthalmology*. 1998;105:1173–1181.
91. Li J, Herndon LW, Asrani SG, Stinnett S, Allingham RR. Clinical comparison of the Proview eye pressure monitor with the Goldmann applanation tonometer and the Tonopen. *Arch Ophthalmol*. 2004;122:1117–1121.
92. Orssengo GJ, Pye DC. Determination of the true intraocular pressure and modulus of elasticity of the human cornea in vivo. *Bull Math Biol*. 1999;61:551–572.
93. Rootman DS, Insler MS, Thompson HW, Parelman J, Poland D, Unterman SR. Accuracy and precision of the Tono-Pen in measuring intraocular pressure after keratoplasty and epikeratophakia and in scarred corneas. *Arch Ophthalmol*. 1988;106:1697–1700.
94. Panek WC, Boothe WA, Lee DA, Zemplenyi E, Pettit TH. Intraocular pressure measurement with the Tono-Pen through soft contact lenses. *Am J Ophthalmol*. 1990;109:62–65.
95. Scibilia GD, Ehlers WH, Donshik PC. The effects of therapeutic contact lenses on intraocular pressure measurement. *CLAO J*. 1996;22:262–265.
96. Kaufmann C, Bachmann LM, Thiel MA. Comparison of dynamic contour tonometry with goldmann applanation tonometry. *Invest Ophthalmol Vis Sci*. 2004;45:3118–3121.
97. Kaufmann C, Bachmann LM, Thiel MA. Intraocular pressure measurements using dynamic contour tonometry after laser in situ keratomileusis. *Invest Ophthalmol Vis Sci*. 2003;44: 3790–3794.
98. Doyle A, Lachkar Y. Comparison of dynamic contour tonometry with goldman applanation tonometry over a wide range of central corneal thickness. *J Glaucoma*. 2005;14:288–292.
99. Troost A, Yun SH, Specht K, Krummenauer F, Schwenn O. Transpalpebral tonometry: reliability and comparison with Goldmann applanation tonometry and palpation in healthy volunteers. *Br J Ophthalmol*. 2005;89:280–283.
100. Rubinfeld RS, Cohen EJ, Laibson PR, Arentsen JJ, Lugo M, Genvert GI. The accuracy of finger tension for estimating intraocular pressure after penetrating keratoplasty. *Ophthalmic Surg Lasers*. 1998;29:213–215.
101. Baum J, Chaturvedi N, Netland PA, Dreyer EB. Assessment of intraocular pressure by palpation. *Am J Ophthalmol*. 1995;119:650–651.
102. Britt JM, Clifton BC, Barnebey HS, Mills RP. Microaerosol formation in noncontact 'air-puff' tonometry. *Arch Ophthalmol*. 1991;109:225–228.
103. Regine F, Scuderi GL, Cesareo M, Ricci F, Cedrone C, Nucci C. Validity and limitations of the Nidek NT-4000 non-contact tonometer: a clinical study. *Ophthalmic Physiol Opt*. 2006;26:33–39.
104. Ogbuehi KC. Assessment of the accuracy and reliability of the Topcon CT80 non-contact tonometer. *Clin Exp Optom*. 2006; 89:310–314.
105. Gupta V, Sony P, Agarwal HC, Sihota R, Sharma A. Inter-instrument agreement and influence of central corneal thickness on measurements with Goldmann, pneumotonometer and noncontact tonometer in glaucomatous eyes. *Indian J Ophthalmol*. 2006;54:261–265.
106. Tonnu PA, Ho T, Newson T, et al. The influence of central corneal thickness and age on intraocular pressure measured by pneumotonometry, non-contact tonometry, the Tono-Pen XL, and Goldmann applanation tonometry. *Br J Ophthalmol*. 2005;89:851–854.
107. Patel S, Illahi W. Non-contact tonometry over soft contact lenses: effect of contact lens power on the measurement of intra-ocular pressure. *Cont Lens Anterior Eye*. 2004;27:33–37.
108. Brubaker RF. Tonometry. In: Tasman W, Jaeger EA, eds. *Duane's Clinical Ophthalmology*. Philadelphia, PA: Lippincott Williams & Wilkins; 1993.
109. Feghali JG, Azar DT, Kaufman PL. Comparative aqueous outflow facility measurements by pneumatonography and Schiotz tonography. *Invest Ophthalmol Vis Sci*. 1986;27:1776–1780.
110. Quigley HA, Langham ME. Comparative intraocular pressure measurements with the pneumatonograph and Goldmann tonometer. *Am J Ophthalmol*. 1975;80:266–273.

111. Gudmundson LE. The pneumatonograph and Perkins' tonometer. A clinical study of the reproducibility in glaucomatous eyes. *Acta Ophthalmol.* 1984;62:731–738.
112. Wheeler NC, Lee DA, Cheng Q, Ross WF, Hadjiaghai L. Reproducibility of intraocular pressure and outflow facility measured by pneumatic tonography and Schiotz tonography. *J Ocul Pharmacol Ther.* 1998;14:5–13.
113. Gelatt KN, Peiffer RL Jr, Gum GG, Gwin RM, Erickson JL. Evaluation of applanation tonometers for the dog eye. *Invest Ophthalmol Vis Sci.* 1977;16:963–968.
114. Bayraktar S, Bayraktar Z. Central corneal thickness and intraocular pressure relationship in eyes with and without previous LASIK: comparison of Goldmann applanation tonometer with pneumatonometer. *Eur J Ophthalmol.* 2005;15:81–88.
115. Rubenstein JB, Deutsch TA. Pneumatonometry through bandage contact lenses. *Arch Ophthalmol.* 1985;103:1660–1661.
116. Schiotz H. Ein neues Tonometer. *Arch Augenheilkd.* 1905;52:401–424.
117. Colton T, Ederer F. The distribution of intraocular pressures in the general population. *Surv Ophthalmol.* 1980;25:123–129.
118. Qureshi IA. Intraocular pressure: a comparative analysis in two sexes. *Clinical Physiol.* 1997;17:247–255.
119. Leske MC, Connell AM, Wu SY, Hyman L, Schachat AP. Distribution of intraocular pressure. The Barbados Eye Study. *Arch Ophthalmol.* 1997;115:1051–1057.
120. Hashemi H, Kashi AH, Fotouhi A, Mohammad K. Distribution of intraocular pressure in healthy Iranian individuals: the Tehran Eye Study. *Br J Ophthalmol.* 2005;89:652–657.
121. Xu L, Li J, Zheng Y, et al. Intraocular pressure in Northern China in an urban and rural population: the Beijing eye study. *Am J Ophthalmol.* 2005;140:913–915.
122. Nomura H, Shimokata H, Ando F, Miyake Y, Kuzuya F. Age-related changes in intraocular pressure in a large Japanese population: a cross-sectional and longitudinal study. *Ophthalmology.* 1999;106:2016–2022.
123. Ntim-Amponsah CT. Mean intraocular pressure in Ghanaians. *East Afr Med J.* 1996;73:516–518.
124. Iwase A, Suzuki Y, Araie M, et al. The prevalence of primary open-angle glaucoma in Japanese: the Tajimi Study. *Ophthalmology.* 2004;111:1641–1648.
125. Drance SM. The significance of the diurnal tension variations in normal and glaucomatous eyes. *Arch Ophthalmol.* 1960;64:494–501.
126. Zeimer RC, Wilensky JT, Gieser DK, Viana MA. Association between intraocular pressure peaks and progression of visual field loss. *Ophthalmology.* 1991;98:64–69.
127. Reiss GR, Lee DA, Topper JE, Brubaker RF. Aqueous humor flow during sleep. *Invest Ophthalmol Vis Sci.* 1984;25:776–778.
128. Maus TL, McLaren JW, Shepard JW Jr, Brubaker RF. The effects of sleep on circulating catecholamines and aqueous flow in human subjects. *Exp Eye Res.* 1996;62:351–358.
129. Topper JE, Brubaker RF. Effects of timolol, epinephrine, and acetazolamide on aqueous flow during sleep. *Invest Ophthalmol Vis Sci.* 1985;26:1315–1319.
130. Medeiros FA, Weinreb RN, Zangwill LM, et al. Long-term intraocular pressure fluctuations and risk of conversion from ocular hypertension to glaucoma. *Ophthalmology.* 2008;115(6):934–940.
131. Lee PP, Walt JW, Rosenblatt LC, Siegartel LR, Stern LS. Association between intraocular pressure variation and glaucoma progression: data from a united states chart review. *Am J Ophthalmol.* 2007;144(6):901–907.
132. Liu JH, Sit AJ, Weinreb RN. Variation of 24-hour intraocular pressure in healthy individuals: right eye versus left eye. *Ophthalmology.* 2005;112:1670–1675.
133. Qureshi IA, Xiao RX, Yang BH, Zhang J, Xiang DW, Hui JL. Seasonal and diurnal variations of ocular pressure in ocular hypertensive subjects in Pakistan. *Singapore Med J.* 1999;40:345–348.
134. Tutaj M, Brown CM, Brys M, et al. Dynamic cerebral autoregulation is impaired in glaucoma. *J Neurol Sci.* 2004;220:49–54.
135. Lovasik JV, Kergoat H. Consequences of an increase in the ocular perfusion pressure on the pulsatile ocular blood flow. *Optom Vis Sci.* 2004;81:692–698.
136. Cooper RL, Beale DG, Constable IJ, Grose GC. Continual monitoring of intraocular pressure: effect of central venous pressure, respiration, and eye movements on continual recordings of intraocular pressure in the rabbit, dog, and man. *Br J Ophthalmol.* 1979;63:799–804.
137. Schuman JS, Massicotte EC, Connolly S, Hertzmark E, Mukherji B, Kunen MZ. Increased intraocular pressure and visual field defects in high resistance wind instrument players. *Ophthalmology.* 2000;107:127–133.
138. Bertschinger DR, Mendrinos E, Dosso A. Yoga can be dangerous–glaucomatous visual field defect worsening due to postural yoga. *Br J Ophthalmol.* 2007;91:1413–1414.
139. Rosen DA, Johnston VC. Ocular pressure patterns in the Valsalva maneuver. *Arch Ophthalmol.* 1959;62:810–816.
140. Krieglstein GK, Waller WK, Leydhecker W. The vascular basis of the positional influence of the intraocular pressure. *Albrecht Von Graefes Arch Klin Exp Ophthalmol.* 1978;206:99–106.
141. Kaskel D, Muller-Breitenkamp R, Wilmans I, Rudolf H, Jessen K. The influence of changes in body position on intraocular pressure, episcleral venous pressure, and blood pressure (author's transl). *Albrecht Von Graefes Arch Klin Exp Ophthalmol.* 1978;208:217–228.
142. Chiquet C, Custaud MA, Le Traon AP, Millet C, Gharib C, Denis P. Changes in intraocular pressure during prolonged (7-day) head-down tilt bedrest. *J Glaucoma.* 2003;12:204–208.
143. Linder BJ, Trick GL. Simulation of spaceflight with whole-body head-down tilt: influence on intraocular pressure and retinocortical processing. *Aviat Space Environ Med.* 1987;58:A139–A142.
144. Linder BJ, Trick GL, Wolf ML. Altering body position affects intraocular pressure and visual function. *Invest Ophthalmol Vis Sci.* 1988;29:1492–1497.
145. Mosaed S, Liu JH, Weinreb RN. Correlation between office and peak nocturnal intraocular pressures in healthy subjects and glaucoma patients. *Am J Ophthalmol.* 2005;139:320–324.
146. Baskaran M, Raman K, Ramani KK, Roy J, Vijaya L, Badrinath SS. Intraocular pressure changes and ocular biometry during Sirsasana (headstand posture) in yoga practitioners. *Ophthalmology.* 2006;113:1327–1332.
147. Iester M, Torre PG, Bricola G, Bagnis A, Calabria G. Retinal blood flow autoregulation after dynamic exercise in healthy young subjects. *Ophthalmologica.* 2007;221:180–185.
148. Vieira GM, Oliveira HB, de Andrade DT, Bottaro M, Ritch R. Intraocular pressure variation during weight lifting. *Arch Ophthalmol.* 2006;124:1251–1254.
149. Dane S, Kocer I, Demirel H, Ucok K, Tan U. Long-term effects of mild exercise on intraocular pressure in athletes and sedentary subjects. *Int J Neurosci.* 2006;116:1207–1214.
150. Hao-Hui C. Dehydration therapy and hypotension in post-resuscitation cerebral oedema, and application of intra-ocular pressure measurement – a review of resuscitation work, part I. *Resuscitation.* 1980;8:195–209.
151. Schmidt K. Untersuchungen über Kapillarendothelstörungen bei Glaukoma simplex. *Arch Augenheilkd.* 1928;98:569–581.
152. Susanna R Jr, Hatanaka M, Vessani RM, Pinheiro A, Morita C. Correlation of asymmetric glaucomatous visual field damage and water-drinking test response. *Invest Ophthalmol Vis Sci.* 2006;47:641–644.
153. Susanna R Jr, Vessani RM, Sakata L, Zacarias LC, Hatanaka M. The relation between intraocular pressure peak in the water

drinking test and visual field progression in glaucoma. *Br J Ophthalmol*. 2005;89:1298–1301.
154. Yoshikawa K, Inoue T, Inoue Y. Normal tension glaucoma: the value of predictive tests. *Acta Ophthalmol*. 1993;71:463–470.
155. Cartwright MJ, Anderson DR. Correlation of asymmetric damage with asymmetric intraocular pressure in normal-tension glaucoma (low-tension glaucoma). *Arch Ophthalmol*. 1988;106:898–900.
156. Chandrasekaran S, Rochtchina E, Mitchell P. Effects of caffeine on intraocular pressure: the Blue Mountains Eye Study. *J Glaucoma*. 2005;14:504–507.
157. Lee AJ, Rochtchina E, Wang JJ, Healey PR, Mitchell P. Does smoking affect intraocular pressure? Findings from the Blue Mountains Eye Study. *J Glaucoma*. 2003;12:209–212.
158. Houle RE, Grant WM. Alcohol, vasopressin, and intraocular pressure. *Invest Ophthalmol*. 1967;6:145–154.
159. Kolker AE. Hyperosmotic agents in glaucoma. *Invest Ophthalmol*. 1970;9:418–423.
160. Tomida I, Azuara-Blanco A, House H, Flint M, Pertwee RG, Robson PJ. Effect of sublingual application of cannabinoids on intraocular pressure: a pilot study. *J Glaucoma*. 2006;15:349–353.
161. Beilin M, Neumann R, Belkin M, Green K, Bar-Ilan A. Pharmacology of the intraocular pressure (IOP) lowering effect of systemic dexanabinol (HU-211), a non-psychotropic cannabinoid. *J Ocul Pharmacol Ther*. 2000;16:217–230.
162. Naveh N, Weissman C, Muchtar S, Benita S, Mechoulam R. A submicron emulsion of HU-211, a synthetic cannabinoid, reduces intraocular pressure in rabbits. *Graefes Arch Clin Exp Ophthalmol*. 2000;238:334–338.
163. Kersey JP, Broadway DC. Corticosteroid-induced glaucoma: a review of the literature. *Eye*. 2006;20:407–416.
164. Cubey RB. Glaucoma following the application of corticosteroid to the skin of the eyelids. *Br J Dermatol*. 1976;95:207–208.
165. Garbe E, LeLorier J, Boivin JF, Suissa S. Inhaled and nasal glucocorticoids and the risks of ocular hypertension or open-angle glaucoma. *JAMA*. 1997;277:722–727.
166. Kalina RE. Increased intraocular pressure following subconjunctival corticosteroid administration. *Arch Ophthalmol*. 1969;81:788–790.
167. Huang SY, Tsai YY, Lin JM, Hung PT. Intractable glaucoma following posterior sub-tenon's triamcinolone acetonide for central retinal vein occlusion in a young adult. *Eye*. 2006;20:1458–1459.
168. Hanson RJ, Downes S. Conservative management of refractory steroid-induced glaucoma following anterior subtenon steroid injection. *Clin Experiment Ophthalmol*. 2007;35:197–198. author reply 198.
169. Jea SY, Byon IS, Oum BS. Triamcinolone-induced intraocular pressure elevation: intravitreal injection for macular edema and posterior subtenon injection for uveitis. *Korean J Ophthalmol*. 2006;20:99–103.
170. Bayer JM, Neuner HP. Cushing's syndrome and increased intraocular pressure. *Dtsch Med Wochenschr*. 1967;92:1791–1799.
171. Goldmann H. Cortisone glaucoma. *Arch Ophthalmol*. 1962;68:621–626.
172. Tripathi RC, Parapuram SK, Tripathi BJ, Zhong Y, Chalam KV. Corticosteroids and glaucoma risk. *Drugs Aging*. 1999;15:439–450.
173. Francois J, Victoria-Troncoso V. Corticosteroid glaucoma. *Ophthalmologica*. 1977;174:195–209.
174. Hayasaka S. Lysosomal enzymes in ocular tissues and diseases. *Surv Ophthalmol*. 1983;27:245–258.
175. Joe MK, Sohn S, Hur W, Moon Y, Choi YR, Kee C. Accumulation of mutant myocilins in ER leads to ER stress and potential cytotoxicity in human trabecular meshwork cells. *Biochem Biophys Res Commun*. 2003;312:592–600.
176. Yam GH, Gaplovska-Kysela K, Zuber C, Roth J. Aggregated myocilin induces russell bodies and causes apoptosis: implications for the pathogenesis of myocilin-caused primary open-angle glaucoma. *Am J Pathol*. 2007;170:100–109.
177. Putney LK, Brandt JD, O'Donnell ME. Effects of dexamethasone on sodium-potassium-chloride cotransport in trabecular meshwork cells. *Invest Ophthalmol Vis Sci*. 1997;38:1229–1240.
178. Yun AJ, Murphy CG, Polansky JR, Newsome DA, Alvarado JA. Proteins secreted by human trabecular cells. Glucocorticoid and other effects. *Invest Ophthalmol Vis Sci*. 1989;30:2012–2022.
179. Steely HT, Browder SL, Julian MB, Miggans ST, Wilson KL, Clark AF. The effects of dexamethasone on fibronectin expression in cultured human trabecular meshwork cells. *Invest Ophthalmol Vis Sci*. 1992;33:2242–2250.
180. Dickerson JE Jr, Steely HT Jr, English-Wright SL, Clark AF. The effect of dexamethasone on integrin and laminin expression in cultured human trabecular meshwork cells. *Exp Eye Res*. 1998;66:731–738.
181. Snyder RW, Stamer WD, Kramer TR, Seftor RE. Corticosteroid treatment and trabecular meshwork proteases in cell and organ culture supernatants. *Exp Eye Res*. 1993;57:461–468.
182. Samples JR, Alexander JP, Acott TS. Regulation of the levels of human trabecular matrix metalloproteinases and inhibitor by interleukin-1 and dexamethasone. *Invest Ophthalmol Vis Sci*. 1993;34:3386–3395.
183. Malani JT, Robinson GM, Seneviratne EL. Ipratropium bromide induced angle closure glaucoma. *N Z Med J*. 1982;95:749.
184. Kupfer C. Selective block of synaptic transmission in ciliary ganglion by type A botulinus toxin in rabbits. *Proc Soc Exp Biol Med*. 1958;99:474–476.
185. Leibowitz HM, Krueger DE, Maunder LR, et al. The Framingham Eye Study monograph: an ophthalmological and epidemiological study of cataract, glaucoma, diabetic retinopathy, macular degeneration, and visual acuity in a general population of 2631 adults, 1973–1975. *Surv Ophthalmol*. 1980;24:335–610.
186. Nguyen N, Mora JS, Gaffney MM, et al. A high prevalence of occludable angles in a Vietnamese population. *Ophthalmology*. 1996;103:1426–1431.
187. Bard LA. Transient myopia associated with promethazine (phenegan) therapy: report of a case. *Am J Ophthalmol*. 1964;58:682–686.
188. Miichi H, Nagataki S. Effects of pilocarpine, salbutamol, and timolol on aqueous humor formation in cynomolgus monkeys. *Invest Ophthalmol Vis Sci*. 1983;24:1269–1275.
189. Kristensen P. Mydriasis-induced pigment liberation in the anterior chamber associated with acute rise in intraocular pressure in open-angle glaucoma. *Acta Ophthalmol*. 1965;43:714–724.
190. Hook SR, Holladay JT, Prager TC, Goosey JD. Transient myopia induced by sulfonamides. *Am J Ophthalmol*. 1986;101:495–496.
191. Bovino JA, Marcus DF. The mechanism of transient myopia induced by sulfonamide therapy. *Am J Ophthalmol*. 1982;94:99–102.
192. Krieg PH, Schipper I. Drug-induced ciliary body oedema: a new theory. *Eye*. 1996;10(Pt 1):121–126.
193. Sankar PS, Pasquale LR, Grosskreutz CL. Uveal effusion and secondary angle-closure glaucoma associated with topiramate use. *Arch Ophthalmol*. 2001;119:1210–1211.
194. Rhee DJ, Goldberg MJ, Parrish RK. Bilateral angle-closure glaucoma and ciliary body swelling from topiramate. *Arch Ophthalmol*. 2001;119:1721–1723.
195. Banta JT, Hoffman K, Budenz DL, Ceballos E, Greenfield DS. Presumed topiramate-induced bilateral acute angle-closure glaucoma. *Am J Ophthalmol*. 2001;132:112–114.
196. Fraunfelder FW, Fraunfelder FT, Keates EU. Topiramate-associated acute, bilateral, secondary angle-closure glaucoma. *Ophthalmology*. 2004;111:109–111.
197. Katz RL, Eakins KE. Mode of action of succinylcholine on intraocular pressure. *J Pharmacol Exp Ther*. 1968;162:1–9.
198. Chandler PA. Long-term results in glaucoma therapy. *Am J Ophthalmol*. 1960;49:221–246.
199. Odberg T, Riise D. Early diagnosis of glaucoma. II. The value of the initial examination in ocular hypertension. *Acta Ophthalmol*. 1987;65:58–62.

200. Grant WM, Burke JF Jr. Why do some people go blind from glaucoma? *Ophthalmology*. 1982;89:991–998.
201. Miller KM, Quigley HA. The clinical appearance of the lamina cribrosa as a function of the extent of glaucomatous optic nerve damage. *Ophthalmology*. 1988;95:135–138.
202. Quigley HA, Hohman RM, Addicks EM, Massof RW, Green WR. Morphologic changes in the lamina cribrosa correlated with neural loss in open-angle glaucoma. *Am J Ophthalmol*. 1983;95:673–691.
203. Quigley HA, Addicks EM. Regional differences in the structure of the lamina cribrosa and their relation to glaucomatous optic nerve damage. *Arch Ophthalmol*. 1981;99:137–143.
204. Danias J, Lee KC, Zamora MF, et al. Quantitative analysis of retinal ganglion cell (RGC) loss in aging DBA/2NNia glaucomatous mice: comparison with RGC loss in aging C57/BL6 mice. *Invest Ophthalmol Vis Sci*. 2003;44:5151–5162.
205. Jampel HD. Target pressure in glaucoma therapy. *J Glaucoma*. 1997;6:133–138.

# Chapter 4
# Glaucoma Risk Factors: Fluctuations in Intraocular Pressure

Felipe A. Medeiros

Intraocular pressure (IOP) has been consistently demonstrated to be associated with incidence, prevalence, and progression of glaucoma. However, although there is strong evidence to support mean IOP as a risk factor for both development and progression of the disease, there is uncertainty with regard to the role of IOP fluctuations in glaucoma. One of the difficulties in investigating this relationship comes from the concept of IOP fluctuation. Some authors define fluctuation as variation in IOP during the diurnal period. Others include the nocturnal period as well and point out that one should look at 24-h fluctuation as an important parameter for glaucoma progression. Finally, others have defined IOP fluctuation as the variability in IOP measurement between visits, which is often called long-term fluctuation.[1] The role of very short-term fluctuations in IOP is explored in Sidebar 4.1.

Two studies have recently addressed the relationship between long-term IOP fluctuations and progression of glaucoma with conflicting results. As part of the Advanced Glaucoma Intervention Study (AGIS), Nouri-Mahdavi et al[2] found that long-term IOP fluctuations were a statistically significant risk factor associated with visual field progression. The AGIS[3] was a long-term study designed to evaluate the clinical course of medically uncontrolled open-angle glaucoma by two surgical treatment sequences. Of 591 patients, 789 eyes were randomized to a treatment sequence of (1) argon laser trabeculoplasty, trabeculectomy, and trabeculectomy (ATT) or (2) trabeculectomy, argon laser trabeculoplasty, and trabeculectomy (TAA). To be eligible for the AGIS, eyes had to meet specific criteria consisting of combinations of uncontrolled IOP with medications, glaucomatous visual field defect, and/or optic disc damage. During follow-up, surgical interventions were supplemented by medical therapy with the goal of reducing IOP to less than 18 mmHg. Long-term IOP fluctuation was calculated as the standard deviation of all available IOP measurements during follow-up, after the initial surgical procedure. In a multivariate logistic regression model, each 1 mmHg higher IOP fluctuation was associated with 31% higher odds of developing progression. According to the study, eyes with an IOP fluctuation <3 mmHg remained stable over time, whereas eyes with an IOP fluctuation ≥3 mmHg demonstrated significant progression.

As part of the Early Manifest Glaucoma Trial (EMGT), Bengtsson et al[4] did not find long-term IOP fluctuations to be associated with visual field progression. The EMGT enrolled 255 newly diagnosed, previously untreated, open-angle glaucoma patients who had reproducible visual field defects at baseline (median MD = −4 dB). Patients with advanced visual field loss or IOP greater than 30 mmHg at baseline were excluded. Patients were randomized to 360° trabeculoplasty plus betaxolol vs. no treatment. Eyes stayed in their allocation arms unless significant progression occurred. If the IOP in treated eyes exceeded 25 mmHg at two consecutive follow-ups or 35 mmHg in control eyes, latanoprost was added. Patients were followed for a median of 6 years with excellent retention. The definition of long-term IOP fluctuation in the EMGT was also based on the standard deviation of IOP measurements over time. However, IOP measurements were only included up to the date of progression (for progressors) or last follow-up visit (for nonprogressors). The analysis involved 255 patients with a median follow-up time of 8 years. Mean long-term IOP fluctuations were 2.02 mmHg and 1.78 mmHg in patients who progressed and in patients who did not progressed, respectively. In a multivariate Cox regression model, IOP fluctuation was not a significant risk factor for progression (adjusted HR = 1.0; 95% CI: 0.81–1.24; $P = 0.999$). The model was adjusted for mean IOP, age, baseline IOP, presence of exfoliation, severity of visual field loss at baseline, and whether one or both eyes were eligible for the study. Mean IOP was significantly associated with the risk of progressive visual field loss. Each 1 mmHg higher mean IOP was associated with 11% increase in risk. Similar results were identified when treated and control patients were analyzed separately.

### SIDEBAR 4.1. Rapid oscillations in intraocular pressure

W. Daniel Stamer and Renata F. Ramos

Because pathology associated with ocular hypertension resides in the conventional drainage pathway, research studies have focused on understanding how resistance to outflow is regulated in order to develop better pharmacological treatments for glaucoma. Much of the work to date has examined functional, morphological, and biochemical changes in conventional drainage tissues, including the trabecular meshwork and Schlemm's canal, in response to elevated IOP. Unfortunately, little is known about the contribution of dynamic changes in pressure to outflow resistance regulation.

As the name implies, aqueous humor dynamics are not static, but an orchestra of physiological processes in the human eye responsible for aqueous humor circulation and the generation of IOP. These dynamic processes result in pressure changes that occur over second- to day time scales to regulate IOP. Unfortunately, most studies to date have only examined physiological consequences of static IOP elevations and neglected IOP alterations during the day (circadian rhythm), with each heartbeat (ocular pulse), with changes in posture (sitting vs. standing), with changes in ciliary muscle tone (accommodation), and with other daily activities (blinking, sneezing, squeezing, eye movement, etc.). Interestingly, depending upon the activities/processes, IOP can be transiently or repetitively altered between 3 and 100 mmHg in seconds (Fig. 4.1).

The conventional drainage tissues are thought to be responsible for regulating outflow facility, both accommodating to rapid changes in pressure (short-term regulation) as well as maintaining IOP within a narrow range on the order of days to decades (long-term regulation). While the contribution of physiological IOP oscillations to long-term regulation of conventional outflow is unknown, recent data shows that IOP oscillations similar in magnitude to ocular pulsations in vivo (3 mmHg at 1 Hz) significantly alter outflow facility (IOP) in both porcine and human eyes (Fig. 4.2). Studies using organ-cultured anterior eye segments showed a 30% decrease in conventional outflow facility in response to fluctuations in IOP over the span of a few hours. The decrease in outflow facility was shown not to be due to damage to conventional tissues. In fact, the cellularity of conventional drainage tissues exposed to IOP oscillations was significantly greater than that of tissues exposed to a static IOP gradient, suggesting that cells are both healthy and functionally respond to mechanical stress. In terms of mechanism of action, it appears that ocular pulse modifies the level of contractility (tone) of trabecular meshwork cells (Ramos and Stamer, unpublished data) to decrease the outflow facility (increase resistance). In retrospect, such a result was not surprising, considering the importance of trabecular meshwork cell contractility in outflow facility regulation and its potential usefulness as a target of novel glaucoma therapeutics currently in clinical trials.

Similar to known importance of repetitive cyclic mechanical stress in controlling homeostasis in other tissues (i.e., cardiovascular and bone physiology), it appears that the conventional outflow pathway is no different. Ocular pulse (and likely other stimuli like circadian changes in IOP) appears important in "grooming" conventional outflow cells to help set contractile tone and subsequently impact the IOP setting. An interesting area of research for the future is to understand whether people who develop ocular hypertension and ultimately glaucoma have aberrant responses of conventional outflow tissues (and possibly optic nerve head tissues) over time to such repetitive mechanical queues.

This affords us another way of looking at glaucoma. Is repetitive mechanical stimulation important in the maintenance of IOP? The data here provides some of the first evidence that moment to moment changes in eye pressure may actually be important. Physiologically, this makes a great deal of sense. Further, clinicians often forget that accommodation, blinking, squeezing, and even saccades all have an effect on IOP. All of these may be important in maintaining eye pressure, and some have even speculated that such fluctuations are important in maintaining the health of other ocular structures such as the optic nerve.

## Bibliography

Cai S, Liu X, Glasser A, et al. Effect of latrunculin-A on morphology and actin-associated adhesions of cultured human trabecular meshwork cells. *Mol Vis.* 2000;6:132–143.

Coleman DJ, Trokel S. Direct-recorded intraocular pressure variations in a human subject. *Arch Ophthalmol.* 1969;82:637–640.

Epstein DL, Rowlette LL, Roberts BC. Acto-myosin drug effects and aqueous outflow function. *Invest Ophthalmol Vis Sci.* 1999;40:74–81.

Ethier CR, Read AT, Chan DW. Effects of latrunculin-B on outflow facility and trabecular meshwork structure in human eyes. *Invest Ophthalmol Vis Sci.* 2006;47:1991–1998.

Gabelt BT, Hu Y, Vittitow JL, et al. Caldesmon transgene expression disrupts focal adhesions in HTM cells and increases outflow facility in organ-cultured human and monkey anterior segments. *Exp Eye Res.* 2006;82: 935–944.

Peterson JA, Tian B, Bershadsky AD, et al. Latrunculin-A increases outflow facility in the monkey. *Invest Ophthalmol Vis Sci.* 1999;40:931–941.

Peterson JA, Tian B, Geiger B, Kaufman PL. Effect of latrunculin-B on outflow facility in monkeys. *Exp Eye Res.* 2000;70:307–313.

Ramos RF, Stamer WD. Effects of cyclic intraocular pressure on conventional outflow facility. *Invest Ophthalmol Vis Sci.* 2008;49:275–281.

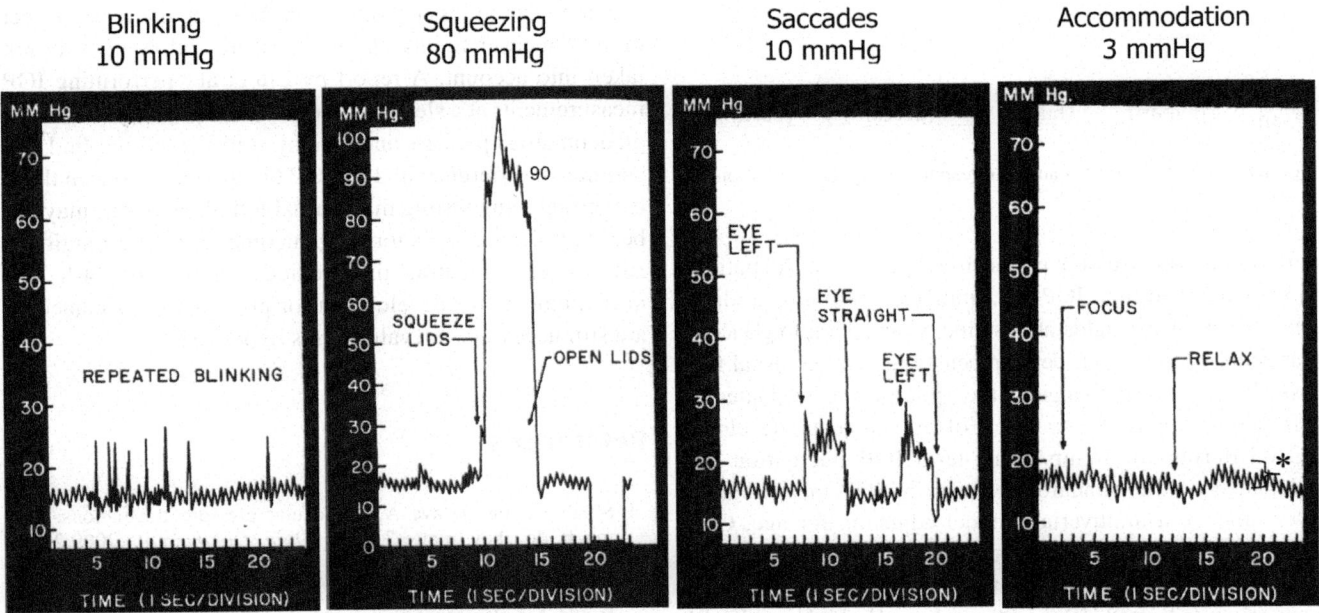

**Fig. 4.1** Intraocular pressure oscillations recorded from a living human eye during different ocular activities. *Bracket* marked by *asterisk* in *right panel* highlights ocular pulse that is prevalent throughout measurements. Modified from Singh and Shrivastava[1]

Several factors have been proposed to explain the different results with regard to the role of IOP fluctuation in the EMGT and the AGIS,[5] including different study designs, different populations, and outcomes. Although both studies calculated long-term IOP as the standard deviation of measurements over time, the AGIS calculations of IOP fluctuation included measurements obtained after progression had occurred, whereas in the EMGT, measurements were obtained only up to the study endpoint. After progression occurred, it is possible that treatment would have been intensified and resulted in further IOP lowering and a consequent increase in IOP fluctuation. This could have resulted in spurious positive relationship between IOP fluctuation and risk of progression in the AGIS investigation. In fact, when the EMGT data was reanalyzed including postprogression IOP measurements in the calculation of fluctuation, the authors also found IOP fluctuation to be related to progressive visual field damage.[4] A subsequent study by the AGIS investigators was performed to reanalyze the data and investigate this issue.[6] The authors suggested that IOP fluctuation was a relatively more important predictor of progression in patients with low IOP and that mean IOP was perhaps more relevant in those with higher IOP. The authors postulated that large IOP fluctuations could potentially cause a loading and unloading of stresses, which might be responsible for the damage seen in glaucoma patients. However, no conclusive evidence to support this hypothesis has been presented and Singh et al[1] suggested that the opposing argument could easily be made that periodic decrease in IOP below the mean with large fluctuations could actually relieve stress on the optic nerve leading to less damage.

Both the AGIS and the EMGT included only patients with definite glaucoma diagnosis at baseline. It is possible that the role of long-term IOP fluctuation as a risk factor for glaucoma development could be different than for glaucoma progression. Results from the OHTS and EGPS evaluating the role of IOP fluctuation have not been published yet. A recent study by Medeiros et al[7] involving 126 ocular hypertensive patients followed for an average time of 7 years did not find long-term IOP fluctuation to be significantly associated with the risk of

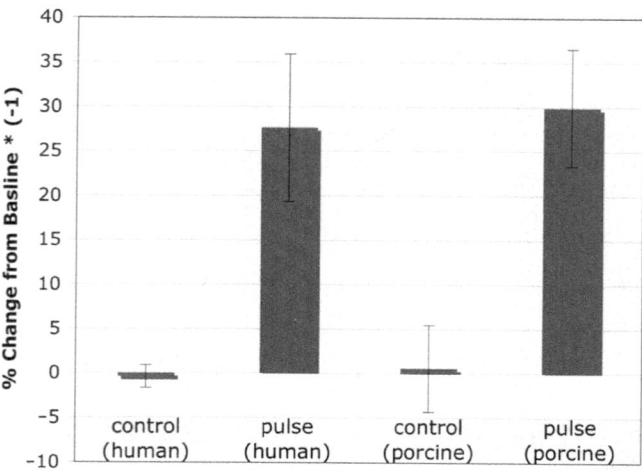

**Fig. 4.2** Outflow facility changes in response to cyclic oscillations

conversion from ocular hypertension to glaucoma. All patients in the study had high IOP (>22 mmHg), normal optic discs, and normal visual fields at baseline. Conversion to glaucoma was defined based on the development of repeatable visual field loss or progressive change to the optic disc as evaluated by stereophotographs. Forty eyes of 31 subjects developed POAG during follow-up. Long-term IOP fluctuation was calculated as the standard deviation of IOP measurements over time. In a multivariate model adjusting for age, CCT, PSD, vertical cup/disc ratio, and mean IOP, long-term IOP fluctuation was not significantly associated with glaucoma conversion (adjusted HR = 1.08 per 1 mmHg higher; 95% CI: 0.79–1.48; $P = 0.620$). Mean IOP was significantly associated with glaucoma conversion (adjusted HR = 1.20 per 1 mmHg higher; 95% CI: 1.06–1.36; $P = 0.005$).

In another study, Bengtsson and Heijl[8] followed high risk ocular hypertensive patients for 10 years as part of a prospective investigation (Malmö Ocular Hypertension Study) to compare the rates of development of glaucomatous visual field loss in patients treated with timolol compared to placebo. Patients were followed every 3 months with Goldmann tonometry measurements obtained at 8:00 A.M., 11:30 A.M., and 3:30 P.M. No association was found between parameters measuring long-term IOP fluctuation and risk of glaucoma development.

In the study of the relationship between IOP fluctuation and risk of glaucoma development and progression, it is important to observe that fluctuation is usually correlated with the level of mean IOP. Eyes with higher mean IOP tend to have higher fluctuations. Therefore, when investigating the risk attributable to IOP fluctuation, it becomes important to adjust for mean IOP level.

A few retrospective studies have investigated the role of diurnal (24 h) IOP fluctuations and risk of glaucoma progression. Asrani et al[9] found that diurnal IOP fluctuation, as measured by home self-tonometry, was a significant risk factor for progression. In their study, home tonometry measurements were obtained at baseline and their association with the risk of progression over time was investigated. The authors found a significant hazard ratio for diurnal IOP fluctuation in a model adjusting for office IOP (mean of two measurements at baseline), age, race, gender, and severity of visual field loss at baseline. The study, however, was based on retrospective chart review with lack of well-defined criteria for visual field progression, and large number of patients excluded due to loss of follow-up. Also, the predictive effect of IOP measurements obtained during follow-up was not taken into account. A report by Liu et al[10] performing IOP measurements at a sleep lab over the 24-h period in untreated glaucomatous patients and healthy subjects did not find any significant difference in 24-h IOP fluctuations between these two groups, suggesting that diurnal IOP fluctuations may not be a significant risk factor for glaucoma. However, longitudinal studies evaluating the predictive ability of 24-h IOP measurements for development or progression of glaucoma are still necessary to evaluate this hypothesis.

## References

1. Singh K, Shrivastava A. Intraocular pressure fluctuations: how much do they matter? *Curr Opin Ophthalmol*. 2009;20(2): 84–87.
2. Nouri-Mahdavi K, Hoffman D, Coleman AL, et al. Predictive factors for glaucomatous visual field progression in the Advanced Glaucoma Intervention Study. *Ophthalmology*. 2004;111(9): 1627–1635.
3. The AGIS Investigators. The Advanced Glaucoma Intervention Study (AGIS): 7. The relationship between control of intraocular pressure and visual field deterioration. *Am J Ophthalmol*. 2000; 130(4):429–440.
4. Bengtsson B, Leske MC, Hyman L, Heijl A. Fluctuation of intraocular pressure and glaucoma progression in the early manifest glaucoma trial. *Ophthalmology*. 2007;114(2):205-209.
5. Palmberg P. What is it about pressure that really matters in glaucoma? *Ophthalmology*. 2007;114(2):203–204.
6. Caprioli J, Coleman AL. Intraocular pressure fluctuation a risk factor for visual field progression at low intraocular pressures in the advanced glaucoma intervention study. *Ophthalmology*. 2008; 115(7):1123–1129.
7. Medeiros FA, Weinreb RN, Zangwill LM, et al. Long-term intraocular pressure fluctuations and risk of conversion from ocular hypertension to glaucoma. *Ophthalmology*. 2008;115(6): 934–940.
8. Bengtsson B, Heijl A. Diurnal IOP fluctuation: not an independent risk factor for glaucomatous visual field loss in high-risk ocular hypertension. *Graefes Arch Clin Exp Ophthalmol*. 2005;243(6):513–518.
9. Asrani S, Zeimer R, Wilensky J, et al. Large diurnal fluctuations in intraocular pressure are an independent risk factor in patients with glaucoma. *J Glaucoma*. 2000;9(2):134–142.
10. Liu JH, Zhang X, Kripke DF, Weinreb RN. Twenty-four-hour intraocular pressure pattern associated with early glaucomatous changes. *Invest Ophthalmol Vis Sci*. 2003;44(4):1586–1590.

# Chapter 5
# Glaucoma is a 24/7 Disease

Amish B. Doshi, John H.K. Liu, and Robert N. Weinreb

IOP is typically measured while sitting during office hours by Goldmann applanation tonometry (GAT). A patient with glaucoma may have two to six IOP measurements by GAT over the course of a year as part of follow-up or to determine response to treatment. As the magnitude of IOP measurements may not differ much, a patient may have the impression that IOP is a static value not prone to significant fluctuations. Instead, IOP is a dynamic physiologic value which at least follows a circadian (24-h) pattern.[1] Short-term fluctuations in IOP are typical within a 24-h (24H) period.[2] These changes in IOP may be important in the diagnosis and management of a patient with glaucoma.

Several different strategies have been employed in clinical practice to quantify these changes in IOP, each with practical limitations. The first involves diurnal measurement of IOP. The definition of diurnal IOP, however, varies between clinicians and is typically used to indicate either IOP during daylight hours or IOP during 3–5 office hours. Nevertheless, these diurnal curves can be obtained by taking several IOP measurements over time.[3] The entire nocturnal period, indicating either the 8 h of sleep or 12 h after a 12 h diurnal period, is not included during these measurements. Yet these nocturnal measurements may offer substantial insight into the disease process in a number of glaucoma patients. Larger short-term fluctuations in IOP are more common in glaucoma (OAG), normal tension glaucoma (NTG), and ocular hypertension (OHTN) patients.[4] Yet fully one-third to one-half of the circadian period is not included in the usual diurnal measurements obtained during office hours. Moreover, each person typically spends one-third of the day in a recumbent position. GAT can measure a diurnal IOP curve in the seated position, but the relationship of these measures to physiologic IOP during a 24H period has only recently been elucidated.

under strictly controlled conditions. The methodology approximates a 24H IOP curve with every 2 h measurements and can provide a comparison of supine and seated IOP in both young and elderly individuals. IOP often is higher during the nocturnal period in both groups of individuals.[1,5,6] This finding is in large part explained by the change in body position from upright to supine. While supine body positioning changes hydrostatic and perfusion pressures in the eye, the exact cause for this IOP change is not fully known. It has been hypothesized that it is caused partially by a rise in episcleral venous pressure.[7] When left in a supine position over 24 h, however, nocturnal IOP is still higher than diurnal IOP.[1,5] Therefore, increased episcleral venous pressure alone is unlikely to be the sole factor causing increased nocturnal IOP. Change in ambient lighting has no effect on this finding.[8] While nocturnal changes in IOP have been well documented, the significance of a high nocturnal IOP is not known as there are other physiologic changes that occur simultaneously that could influence optic nerve health including changes in ocular blood flow.

There are several differences between 24H IOP curves in healthy and glaucomatous eyes (Fig. 5.1.).[4] In glaucoma, both diurnal and nocturnal IOP are higher when compared to age-matched healthy eyes, while the absolute change from the diurnal to nocturnal period is less. The difference in IOP between the two groups is reduced at night. The supine IOP curves between the two groups diverge between 5:30 AM and 7:30 AM. In healthy eyes, IOP peaks at 5:30 AM and subsequently falls. In glaucoma, IOP continues to rise between 5:30 and 7:30 AM before falling during the diurnal period. This phase shift in the 24H IOP curve between healthy eyes and glaucoma may be related to pathogenesis.

## 5.1 Nocturnal and Diurnal IOP

The 24H sleep laboratory at the Hamilton Glaucoma Center at the University of California, San Diego has incorporated a method of 24H IOP measurement using pneumatonometry

## 5.2 Medication Efficacy

Clinicians make several assumptions regarding the efficacy and dosing schedule of a medication. First, they assume that diurnal measurements of IOP are an adequate method of

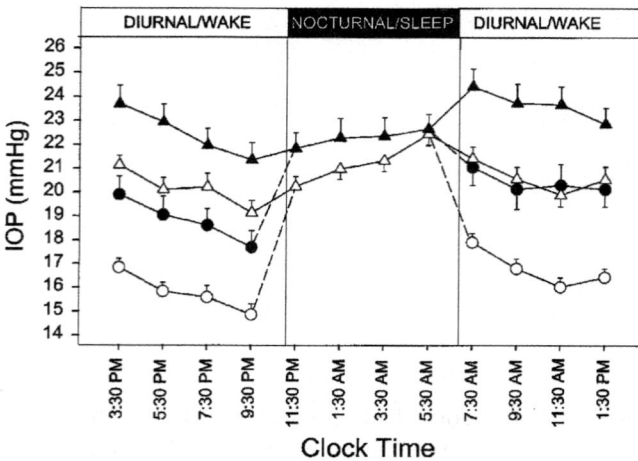

**Fig. 5.1** Twenty-four-hour intraocular pressure (IOP) patterns in normal and glaucoma patients. Untreated patients with glaucoma (*filled symbols*) have a higher IOP in the seated (*circle*) and supine (*triangle*) position than age-matched controls (*open symbols*). The 24-h pattern diverges between 5:30 AM and 7:30 AM with normal patients experiencing a decrease in IOP while glaucoma patients have an increase. Peak IOP is at 5:30 AM in normal patients and at 7:30 AM in glaucoma patients. Supine measurements are consistently higher than seated values. This may be due to an increase in episcleral venous pressure when supine

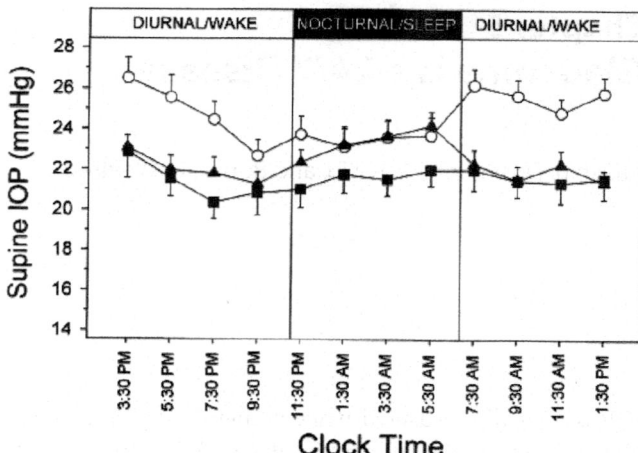

**Fig. 5.2** Twenty-four-hour supine intraocular pressure (IOP) patterns on glaucoma monotherapy. Topical latanoprost (*filled square*) causes uniform decrease in IOP during the diurnal and nocturnal period relative to untreated controls (*open circles*). Timolol (*filled triangle*) causes a significant decrease in diurnal IOP with no significant nocturnal effect

determining response to therapy. Yet, IOP is significantly higher during the nocturnal period. Habitual positioning during the nocturnal period also has a significant effect on IOP. Second, monocular trials are felt to be a practical means for determining both the IOP lowering effect of a medication and the subsequent binocular effect when added to the untreated eye. Asymmetry in IOP is common; however, in OAG and fellow eye response has not extensively been studied. Third, they assume standard dosing regimens based on the pharmokinetics of a medication effectively lower IOP at all time points during the 24H period. Nocturnal measurements of IOP in a variety of clinical scenarios can offer important insight into dosing regimens. While nocturnal measurement of IOP remains impractical in a clinical setting, a 24H sleep laboratory may test several working hypotheses.

IOP is determined by aqueous production, outflow facility, and episcleral venous pressure. Aqueous production diminishes during the nocturnal period despite a rise in IOP.[9,10] Thus, aqueous suppressants such as a beta-adrenergic antagonist would theoretically have a lower effect during the nocturnal period. The nocturnal rise in IOP has been hypothesized to result from changes in outflow facility which are not well understood. Indeed, the beta-blocker, timolol has been found to be almost exclusively effective in the diurnal period[11] while prostaglandin analogs, latanoprost and travoprost, have both a diurnal and nocturnal effect in habitual positions (Fig. 5.2.).[12] The limited nocturnal effect of timolol may be related to a decreased bioavailability of the medication and increased outflow resistance during the nocturnal period. Prostaglandin analogs, which improve uveoscleral outflow, achieve a near uniform flattening of the normal peaks and valleys observed during the 24H period.[11,13] The nocturnal effect of the prostaglandin travoprost is sustained over 48 h.[13] Dorzolamide, a carbonic anhydrase inhibitor, has been shown to be effective during the nocturnal period.[14] Dosing of these medications may need to be adjusted based on these results. As an example, a second dose of timolol in the evening may be unnecessary.

Young, healthy subjects show similar 24H IOP patterns between eyes with the right eye having a slightly higher IOP than the left.[15,16] Association between eyes in OAG patients is not as strong, possibly due to fluctuations in IOP secondary to variability in outflow facility. Correlation of IOP between eyes is fairly weak at a single time point in the day, but becomes more strongly associated when measured at multiple time points during the same day.[17] These results cast doubt on the current method of performing the monocular drug trial in glaucoma patients which assumes symmetry between eyes.

## 5.3 Clinical Import

How should office measurements of IOP be interpreted? 24H IOP studies suggest a paradigm shift in managing OAG. Target IOP may be exceeded throughout the day if clinical measurements of IOP are performed in the afternoon: low afternoon readings in IOP may mislead the patient and clinician as morning and night-time IOP should be significantly higher. Indeed, 20% of Japanese patients with NTG may exceed an IOP of 21 mmHg during the nocturnal period.[18] Seated GAT readings also offer little insight into supine, nocturnal IOP values. Monocular drug trials in glaucoma may have little physiologic basis. Current standard dosing schedules for topical hypotensive agents may unnecessarily increase costs without improving efficacy. If short-term fluctuations in peak IOP lead to glaucomatous damage, nocturnal values may be most critical in determining response to therapy. NTG patients may also have substantially higher IOP readings or lower ocular perfusion during the nocturnal period.

Continuous IOP measuring devices could definitively address these issues. Until these devices are clinically available, several modifications in management of OAG patients can be made: to maximize the likelihood of measuring peak IOP, IOP can be measured at the beginning of the day; supine measurements can be taken to approximate peak nocturnal IOP[6]; several diurnal IOP readings may be taken to determine second eye response to a medication[17]; dosing of medications can be altered based on 24H effect.[13] Choice of therapy in the future may be determined by 24H efficacy rather than an isolated diurnal lowering effect. For example, recent evidence suggests that laser trabeculoplasty may lower IOP more consistently during the nocturnal period than diurnal period.[19]

## 5.4 Conclusion

IOP is a significant risk factor in the development and progression of glaucoma.[20] IOP peaks in the early morning period before awakening and supine IOP is higher than seated IOP. While OAG is associated with a phase-shift in the 24H IOP curve with a continued rise in IOP in the morning relative to healthy eyes, the relevance of this difference on pathogenesis is not known. Certain medications, including beta-blockers, have limited efficacy during the nocturnal period, while prostaglandins may have a sustained effect even after missing a dose. Dosing of medications may need to be adjusted to reflect these observations. Monocular drug trials may also not be a reliable method of predicting fellow eye response as measurements between glaucomatous eyes often do not correlate. IOP measured in the office should be interpreted based on the positioning of the patient, time of day, and current medication regimen. These factors may offer insight into peak IOP and the effect of therapy on peak values. Still, the importance of short-term fluctuations in IOP is not well known especially in the subset of patients with NTG. Continuous methods of IOP measurement could offer insight into the importance of fluctuation and peak IOP in clinical decision-making.

## References

1. Liu JH, Kripke DF, Twa MD, et al. Twenty-four-hour pattern of intraocular pressure in the aging population. *Invest Ophthalmol Vis Sci.* 1999;40(12):2912–2917.
2. Liu JH. Diurnal measurement of intraocular pressure. *J Glaucoma.* 2001;10(5 Suppl 1):S39–S41.
3. David R, Zangwill L, Briscoe D, et al. Diurnal intraocular pressure variations: an analysis of 690 diurnal curves. *Br J Ophthalmol.* 1992;76(5):280–283.
4. Liu JH, Zhang X, Kripke DF, Weinreb RN. Twenty-four-hour intraocular pressure pattern associated with early glaucomatous changes. *Invest Ophthalmol Vis Sci.* 2003;44(4):1586–1590.
5. Liu JH, Kripke DF, Hoffman RE, et al. Nocturnal elevation of intraocular pressure in young adults. *Invest Ophthalmol Vis Sci.* 1998;39(13):2707–2712.
6. Mosaed S, Liu JH, Weinreb RN. Correlation between office and peak nocturnal intraocular pressures in healthy subjects and glaucoma patients. *Am J Ophthalmol.* 2005;139(2):320–324.
7. Friberg TR, Sanborn G, Weinreb RN. Intraocular and episcleral venous pressure increase during inverted posture. *Am J Ophthalmol.* 1987;103(4):523–526.
8. Liu JH, Kripke DF, Hoffman RE, et al. Elevation of human intraocular pressure at night under moderate illumination. *Invest Ophthalmol Vis Sci.* 1999;40(10):2439–2442.
9. Brubaker RF. Flow of aqueous humor in humans [The Friedenwald Lecture]. *Invest Ophthalmol Vis Sci.* 1991;32(13):3145–3166.
10. Koskela T, Brubaker RF. The nocturnal suppression of aqueous humor flow in humans is not blocked by bright light. *Invest Ophthalmol Vis Sci.* 1991;32(9):2504–2506.
11. Liu JH, Kripke DF, Weinreb RN. Comparison of the nocturnal effects of once-daily timolol and latanoprost on intraocular pressure. *Am J Ophthalmol.* 2004;138(3):389–395.
12. Mishima HK, Kiuchi Y, Takamatsu M, et al. Circadian intraocular pressure management with latanoprost: diurnal and nocturnal intraocular pressure reduction and increased uveoscleral outflow. *Surv Ophthalmol.* 1997;41(Suppl 2):S139–S144.
13. Sit AJ, Weinreb RN, Crowston JG, et al. Sustained effect of travoprost on diurnal and nocturnal intraocular pressure. *Am J Ophthalmol.* 2006;141(6):1131–1133.
14. Orzalesi N, Rossetti L, Invernizzi T, et al. Effect of timolol, latanoprost, and dorzolamide on circadian IOP in glaucoma or ocular hypertension. *Invest Ophthalmol Vis Sci.* 2000;41(9):2566–2573.
15. Liu JH, Sit AJ, Weinreb RN. Variation of 24-hour intraocular pressure in healthy individuals: right eye versus left eye. *Ophthalmology.* 2005;112(10):1670–1675.
16. Realini T, Barber L, Burton D. Frequency of asymmetric intraocular pressure fluctuations among patients with and without glaucoma. *Ophthalmology.* 2002;109(7):1367–1371.
17. Sit AJ, Liu JH, Weinreb RN. Asymmetry of right versus left intraocular pressures over 24 hours in glaucoma patients. *Ophthalmology.* 2006;113(3):425–430.
18. Hara T, Hara T, Tsuru T. Increase of peak intraocular pressure during sleep in reproduced diurnal changes by posture. *Arch Ophthalmol.* 2006;124(2):165–168.
19. Lee AC, Mosaed S, Weinreb RN, et al. Effect of laser trabeculoplasty on nocturnal intraocular pressure in medically treated glaucoma patients. *Ophthalmology.* 2007;114(4):666–670.
20. Medeiros F, Brandt JD, Liu JHK, Sehi M, Weinreb RN, Susanna R. *IOP as a Risk Factor for Glaucoma Development and Progression.* Amsterdam: Kugler Publications; 2007:16.

# Chapter 6
# Continuous Monitoring of Intraocular Pressure

Ron E.P. Frenkel, Max P.C. Frenkel, and Shamim A. Haji

To date, the only way to directly measure intraocular pressure (IOP) is by manometry. The true pressure inside the eye cannot be determined by pressing on the outside of the eye (tonometry). At present, there are two problems with our current clinical methods of measuring IOP: namely, the lack of true accuracy and the inability to detect variations.

Since lowering IOP is presently the only widely accepted known treatment for glaucoma[1,2], it is essential not only to accurately measure IOP but also to have a device that will continuously monitor IOP. The limitation of not measuring IOP accurately and the inability to detect variations are particularly troublesome in glaucoma patients with "normal" IOP and those who respond poorly to IOP-lowering therapy. Most studies suggest a progression rate of about 10% annually despite IOP-lowering therapy; and 12% of patients in the Normal Tension Glaucoma Study progressed in spite of "controlled" IOP, based on measurements made in a physician's office.[3]

## 6.1 Challenges in Diagnosing and Managing Glaucoma

Since often we cannot accurately measure IOP clinically or know in great detail how it changes over time, we are handicapped in our ability to correlate IOP to optic nerve damage in diagnosing patients with glaucoma. The importance of diurnal variation has been pointed out elsewhere in this text. Once the diagnosis of glaucoma is made, the first step in treating patients usually involves the use of medications to reduce IOP. Each medication has varying mechanisms of action as well as different peak and trough times of efficacy. When these variable effects of medications are superimposed on an individual patient's circadian rhythm, which may itself be variable, the resulting effect on IOP is even more complex and difficult to predict.

The efficacy of glaucoma medications in the short term is primarily determined by the measurement of IOP in doctor's office during normal work hours, which typically consists of three or four measurements over the course of a year. These measurements provide only a snapshot of a parameter that is known to change significantly over hours, minutes, and even seconds. These isolated measurements of IOP do not provide a complete picture of the state of the patient. This is analogous to looking at a few individual frames from a movie and trying to understand the meaning of the entire picture – it is a rather difficult deduction.

Often when the visual field progressively worsens, the physician is unsure whether this is due to noncompliance, non-IOP factors (such as poor blood flow), or undetected IOP spikes. Since IOP is the only known treatable factor in glaucoma, the clinician assumes that the IOP has been too high and lowers it further. Essentially, the clinician is determining the adequacy of therapy in a retrospective fashion after irreversible damage has occurred. Unfortunately, this is a common occurrence in the treatment of glaucoma patients. Often, further progressive optic nerve or visual field damage occurs before the clinician is willing to use laser and, particularly, surgical treatment on a patient. Before progressive visual field damage is documented, there must already be significant damage to the optic nerve. Until we have a method of more accurately measuring circadian IOP, this problem is likely to endure.

### 6.1.1 Current Methods of Measuring IOP and Their Limitations

Current measurements of IOP are based on relating the deformation of the optical globe to the force responsible for the deformation. The current gold standard, Goldmann applanation tonometry, is both inaccurate and unable to detect most variations since it requires the patient to be in the doctor's office. This method is limited in that it factors into its calculations of IOP a fixed resistance of the cornea, which varies in individual eyes. Additionally, accurate external IOP measurements are difficult to make due to differences between eyes in their corneal steepness, rigidity, hydration, scleral thickness, axial length, aqueous volume, and vitreous consistency. Furthermore, we know that IOP varies with posture, sleep, diurnal variations, and bodily activity, but none of these are detected during usual readings in the office.

Goldmann and Schmidt reported that Goldmann applanation tonometric IOP can be affected by corneal thickness, modulus of elasticity, and tear film.[4] Algorithms have been developed that attempt to modify the true IOP reading based on the influence of corneal thickness. Although there have been numerous "correction algorithms" to compensate for corneal thickness, there is wide disagreement among investigators as to whether any of them are valid and many feel they cannot be used clinically. We continue to try and find the best tonometer, but none of them are completely accurate. Tonometers either rely on mechanical indentation,[5] mechanical flattening,[6] or air[7] to deform the globe. While the accuracy of all three types of devices is reasonable for clinical use, they all have a fundamental limitation – they only provide an isolated measurement of IOP. The isolated nature of these pressure measurements deprives the clinician of the knowledge of the dynamics of IOP changes. They neither provide a way to assess changes that occur between individual measurements, nor a way to assess changes that result from various activities in a patient's daily routine, such as reading, watching television, exercising, or REM sleep.

Newer methods of measuring IOP have been developed to compensate for such differences between eyes. For example, the Pascal Dynamic Contour Tonometer (DCT) utilizes contour matching, which is believed to be independent of corneal curvature, biomechanical properties, diameter, and appositional force. However, the DCT does not appear to be clinically advantageous over the Goldmann tonometer in patients with thick corneas.[8] Another device, the Reichert Ocular Response Analyzer takes into account corneal hysteresis. Although IOP measurements with this method are pachymetry-independent, they are not significantly different from measurements obtained with a Goldman or a standard noncontact tonometer.[9] ICare is yet another tonometer that takes into account corneal properties such as corneal hysteresis and corneal resistance factor, but not corneal thickness.[10]

## 6.2 The Necessity of Continuous IOP Monitoring

Lazlo Z. Bito, the developer of Xalatan, has stated "I have also regarded and still regard continuous IOP-monitoring devices as the most important single step with respect to understanding the true role of IOP in glaucomatous damage."

IOP fluctuation during follow-up is associated with a higher probability of VF progression.[11,12] Large diurnal fluctuations in intraocular pressure are an independent risk factor in patients with glaucoma.[13] Hence, the care of patients with advancing glaucoma should include measurement of long-term IOP fluctuation. Even short-term IOP fluctuation is not accurately measured by three IOP measurements during typical office hours (8 AM to 5 PM).[14] A continuous monitoring technique is necessary to accurately document a patient's baseline IOP and the extent of intervisit fluctuations. The continuous monitoring technique must be able to sample IOP quickly enough to capture its dynamic behavior. This technique is vital for many reasons, such as (1) determining factors associated with elevated IOP; (2) understanding circadian variations of IOP, especially during sleep; (3) understanding the complex peak and trough effects of combined glaucoma medications; (4) understanding IOP effects of patient compliance; and (5) guiding the treatment of elevated IOP.

Our understanding of the factors associated with changes in IOP is rather limited. The links between IOP and race,[15,16] genetics,[17,18] age,[19,20] sex,[19] pulse rate,[21] obesity,[22] and blood pressure[23,24] have been examined, but are not well understood. A continuous IOP monitoring system would, for example, allow the relationship between pulse rate, blood pressure and intraocular pressure to be evaluated during and immediately following exercise.

Circadian variations in IOP were first recorded by Sidler-Huguenin in 1898.[25] These variations typically range from 3 to 6 mmHg in normal eyes[26,27] and can exceed 30 mmHg in glaucomatous eyes.[28] Understanding these variations in IOP are important for two reasons. First, they raise the possibility that a single reading taken in the physician's office is not an accurate representation of the patient's normal pressure level.[29] Second, the magnitude of the variation itself is believed to be important for the diagnosis, treatment, and prognosis of glaucoma.[30] IOP measurements can be made at regular intervals ranging from seconds to hours. Many glaucoma patients' IOP increases more than 5–10 mmHg during sleep. One study of diurnal variations in IOP concluded that if elevated IOPs are present for any considerable period of time, it could require a complete reassessment of how IOP is monitored in glaucoma patients[31]. Other diurnal studies show that peak IOP may be nocturnal, IOP may vary in different stages of sleep,[32] and IOP may decrease substantially upon waking.[33] Current methods of measuring IOP at night cause the patient to be awakened, which precludes the true determination of IOP during sleep. This measurement is important because the hours of sleep make up a significant portion of a patient's 24-h cycle. A system that measures IOP during sleep without disturbing the patient is necessary in determining the significance of this information void. Correlation between nocturnal IOP and nocturnal blood pressure would be possible. Continuous monitoring of IOP is the best way to assess whether medical therapy is producing the desired effect, particularly in patients with "normal" or borderline IOP. In these patients, the presence of pressure peaks and the degree of fluctuation is considered to be an important indicator of continued risk for glaucomatous damage.[34–40]

For patients who are on multiple medications, compliance is known to be poor. Because they tend to take their medications more regularly prior to their visit to the eye doctor, in-office IOP measurements may not be reflective of what is happening in the real world. Furthermore, when patients are taking multiple medications either at the proper or improper time, or not at all, the peak and trough effects are difficult to predict. A continuous IOP sensor would allow the physician to know the exact result of the drug effects combined with the compliance effects. Such information would be extremely difficult and cumbersome to gather, if it were at all possible, by traditional means.

The problems of current IOP monitoring technology are exacerbated by the growing realization that the magnitude of temporal fluctuations in IOP has clinical significance. Asrani's study showed that in glaucoma patients whose office-IOP was in the normal range, large fluctuations in diurnal IOP were a significant risk factor, independent of parameters obtained in the office.[13] The study also concluded that fluctuations in IOP may be important in managing patients with glaucoma and that development of methods to control fluctuation in IOP rather than just IOP itself may be warranted. Technical innovations that enable continuous IOP monitoring promise to increase our understanding of the mechanisms responsible for such fluctuations in IOP and will in turn lead to better treatment strategies for patients with glaucoma and ocular hypertension. Such a device will also be of value in evaluating new pharmacological agents for the treatment of elevated IOP.

## 6.3 Home Tonometers

Home tonometers have been designed in order to make a preliminary assessment of a patient's IOP in their natural environment as well as circadian variations in IOP. These instruments fall into two classes: those that require patient assistance in performing the measurement and those that are intended for self-use. One such home tonometer developed by Ziemer and colleagues[37,38] has yielded acceptable measurements in a number of patients, but is not appropriate for those with poor vision (worse than 20/200), heavy blinking, insufficient eyelid clearance, and head instability.

Another home tonometer, the Proview, made by Bausch and Lomb, was introduced based on phosphene perception after eyelid indentation. Unfortunately, this device was found to be neither accurate nor repeatable enough to be used effectively in the management of glaucoma.[39] Although these home tonometers are helpful, they suffer from three primary drawbacks. First, patients and relatives are typically elderly and often not willing or skilled enough to make accurate measurements.[30] Second, there exists a possibility for complications such as corneal abrasions.[40] And third, most patients are unwilling to repeat the measurements with sufficient frequency to fully characterize circadian IOP changes, as some of these changes may be so brief as to render them virtually undetectable by intermittent IOP measurements.

## 6.4 Continuous IOP Monitoring Devices Under Development

Several attempts are being made to develop an implantable continuous IOP sensor. One example is by Chen and colleagues who have developed a wireless, passive IOP sensor implanted at the pars plana or iris, using Parylene as the biocompatible structural material for intraocular implantation.[41] In animal studies, their sensor was stable intraocularly for more than 150 days and demonstrated high sensitivity.

We currently are working on an implantable continuous IOP monitoring device, which consists of an entirely passive transducer that is flexible and changes volume in response to changes in IOP. The transducer is an integrated module that consists of a parallel plate capacitor and a discrete inductor connected in series to form an L-C circuit (Fig. 6.1). As the pressure surrounding the capacitor changes, the separation of the capacitor plates is varied and the resonant frequency of the L-C circuit changes. Noncontact pressure readings are made by measuring the resonant frequency of the coil using radio frequency (RF) energy from an external probe. The measured natural frequency of our micro-fabricated pressure sensor and inductor correlates well with pressure (Fig. 6.2).

The external probe consists of an antenna that can be mounted onto an eyeglass frame, and a probe, small enough to be worn on the patient's waist, which will store all data including pressure waveforms, maximum and minimum IOP values, and their time of occurrence for up to 30 days. This information can then be electronically transferred to a physician's office using a standard telephone modem or via the Internet. This system will have an initial target accuracy of 2 mmHg over a pressure range of 0–60 mmHg. Evaluation of the biocompatibility of this device with a Parylene coating is underway.

Bäcklund and co-workers[42–44] have designed a similar implantable device that contains a passive transensor, but differs from our approach in several important ways. Their design utilizes an external inductive coil, rather than an internal coil. The external coil requires the use of a biocompatible material before implantation and increases the overall size of the device. Our design, which uses an internal coil, results in a smaller

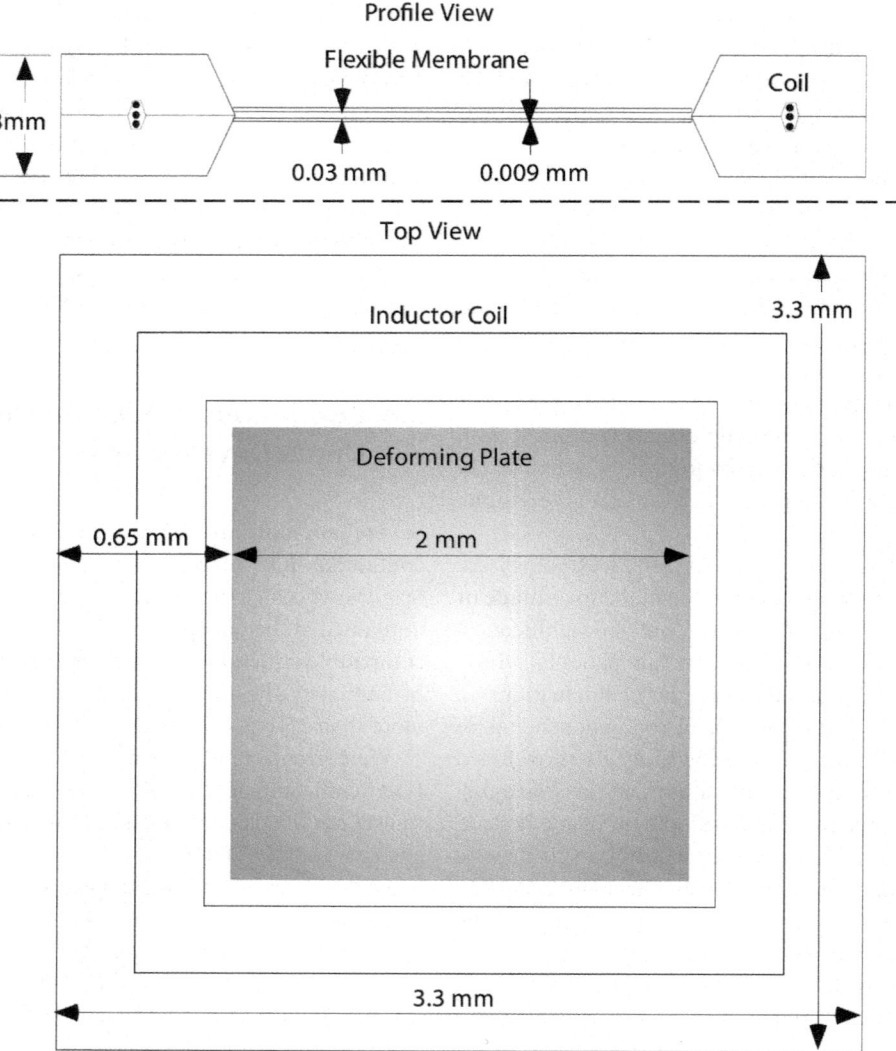

**Fig. 6.1** Implantable pressure transducer. A capacitor is formed by the air gap between the coated flexible membranes. A hand-wound inductor coil is mounted within the structure and connected electrically in series with the capacitor

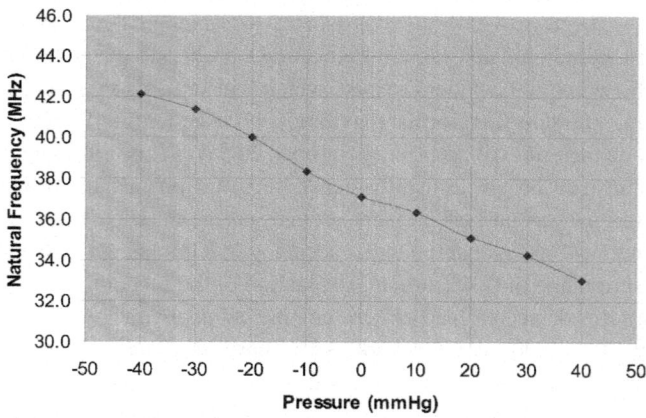

**Fig. 6.2** Measured natural frequency of pressure sensor and wire-wound inductor as a function of pressure. These data show that the natural frequency of the LC circuit formed by our pressure sensitive capacitor and our wire-wound inductor can be measured. The total pressure change is approximately 10 MHz for 80 mmHg

size and is more appropriate for intraocular implantation. Also, their design is based on a single deflectable membrane, rather than two deflectable membranes, which results in half of the sensitivity of our design. However, in spite of the design limitations, Bäcklund's approach did demonstrate that it was possible to build a transensor with a high Q (over 100) and to make noncontact measurements of the resonant frequency of the implanted transensor.

Others are working to develop contact lenses to continuously monitor IOP, such as Sensimed's Contact Lens Sensor and the "Smart" Contact Lens.[45] These contact lenses reportedly measure IOP by detecting changes in the corneoscleral curvature induced by changes in IOP. The "Smart" Contact Lens is made of a polydimethylsiloxane (PDMS). Powdered silver is placed on the lens in a precise pattern that creates conductive wires. An external reader would be used to record IOP data. These have yet to be studied in human glaucoma patients.

Attempts at creating a device for continuous IOP measurement are still in progress. Before they become available for clinical use, they must prove to be both safe for long-term use and to be functional for a useful period of time, if not indefinitely. At present it is too early to accurately speculate how soon such a device will become available. However, there is no doubt that when we have such a device it will fundamentally change our understanding of IOP, and the diagnosis and treatment of glaucoma.

## References

1. Leske MC. The epidemiology of open-angle glaucoma: a review. *Am J Epidemiol.* 1983;118:166–191.
2. Sommer A. Intraocular pressure and glaucoma. *Am J Ophthalmol.* 1989;107:186–188.
3. Collaborative Normal-Tension Glaucoma Study Group. Comparison of glaucomatous progression between untreated patients with normal-tension glaucoma and patients with therapeutically reduced intraocular pressures. *Am J Ophthalmol.* 1998;126(6):487–497.
4. Goldmann H, Schmidt TH. Über applanations tonometrie. *Ophthalmologica.* 1957;134:221–242.
5. Moses RA, Tarkkanen A. Tonometry: the pressure–volume relationship in the intact human eye at low pressures. *Am J Ophthalmol.* 1937;20:985.
6. Moses RA. The Goldmann applanation tonometer. *Am J Ophthalmol.* 1958;46:865.
7. Grolman B. A new tonometer system. *Am J Optom Arch Am Acad Optom.* 1972;49:646.
8. Detry-Morel M, Jamart J, Detry MB, et al. Clinical evaluation of the Pascal dynamic contour tonometer. *J Fr Ophthalmol.* 2007;20:260–270.
9. Montard R, Kopito R, Touzeau O, et al. Ocular response analyzer: feasibility study and correlation with normal eyes. *J Fr Ophthalmol.* 2007;30:978–984.
10. Brusini P, Salvetat M, Zeppieri M, et al. Comparison of ICare tonometer with Goldmann applanation tonometer in glaucoma patients. *J Glaucoma.* 2006;15:213–217.
11. Nouri-Mahdavi K, Hoffman D, Coleman AL, et al. Predictive factors for glaucomatous visual field progression in the Advanced Glaucoma Intervention Study. *Ophthalmology.* 2004;111:1627–1635.
12. Caprioli J. Intraocular pressure fluctuation: an independent risk factor for glaucoma? *Arch Ophthalmol.* 2007;125:1124–1125.
13. Asrani S, Zeimer R, Wilensky J, Gieser D, Vitale S, Lindenmuth K. Large diurnal fluctuations in intraocular pressure are an independent risk factor in patients with glaucoma. *J Glaucoma.* 2000;9(2):134–142.
14. Mosaed S, Liu J, Weinreb RN. Correlation between office and peak nocturnal intraocular pressures in healthy subjects and glaucoma patients. *Am J Ophthalmol.* 2005;139(2):320–324.
15. Wilensky JT, Gandhi N, Pan T. Racial influences in open-angle glaucoma. *Ann Ophthalmol.* 1978;10:1398.
16. David R, Livingston D, Luntz MH. Ocular hypertension: a comparative follow-up of Black and White patients. *Br J Ophthalmol.* 1978;62:676.
17. Armaly MF. The genetic determination of ocular pressure in the normal eye. *Arch Ophthalmol.* 1967;78:187.
18. Armaly MF, Monstavicius BF, Sayegh RE. Ocular pressure and aqueous outflow facility in siblings. *Arch Ophthalmol.* 1968;80:354.
19. Armaly MF. On the distribution of applanation pressure. I. Statistical features and the effect of age, sex, and family history of glaucoma. *Arch Ophthalmol.* 1965;73:11.
20. Ruprecht KW, Wulle KG, Christl HL. Applanation tonometry within medical diagnostic "check-up" programs. *Klin Monatsbl Augenheilkd.* 1976;169:754.
21. Carel RS, Korczyn AD, Rock M, Goya I. Association between ocular pressure and certain health parameters. *Ophthalmology.* 1984;91:311.
22. Shoise Y, Kawase Y. A new approach to stratified normal intraocular pressure in a general population. *Am J Ophthalmol.* 1986;101:714.
23. Schulzer M, Drance SM. Intraocular pressure, systemic blood pressure, and age: a correlation study. *Br J Ophthalmol.* 1987;71:245.
24. Shoise Y. The aging effect on intraocular pressure in an apparently normal population. *Arch Ophthalmol.* 1984;102:883.
25. Sidler-Huguenin A. Die Spaterfolge der Glaukombehandlung bei 76 Privatpatienten von Prof Haab. *Beitr Z Augenheilkd.* 1898;32:1.
26. Katavisto M. The diurnal variations of ocular tension in glaucoma. *Acta Ophthalmol Suppl.* 1964;78:1–130.
27. Kitazawa Y, Horie T. Diurnal variation of intraocular pressure in primary open-angle glaucoma. *Am J Ophthalmol.* 1975;79:557.
28. Newell FW, Krill AE. Diurnal tonography in normal and glaucomateous eyes. *Trans Am Ophthalmol Soc.* 1964;62:349.
29. Wilensky JT, Gieser DK, Mori MT, et al. Self-tonometry to manage patients with glaucoma and apparently controlled intraocular pressure. *Arch Ophthalmol.* 1987;105:1072.
30. Zeimer R. Circadian variations in intraocular pressure. In: Ritch R, Shields MB, Krupin T, eds. *The Glaucomas.* St Louis: C.V. Mosby; 1989.
31. Wilensky JT. Diurnal variations in intraocular pressure. *Trans Am Ophthalmol Soc.* 1991;89:757–790.
32. Noel C, Kabo AM, Romanet JP, Montmayeur A, Buguet A. Twenty-four-hour time course of intraocular pressure in healthy and glaucomatous Africans: relation to sleep patterns. *Ophthalmology.* 2001;108(1):139–144.
33. Zeimer RC, Wilensky JT, Gieser DK. Presence and rapid decline of early morning intraocular pressure peaks in glaucoma patients. *Ophthalmology.* 1990;97(5):547–550.
34. Drance SM. The significance of the diurnal tension variations in normal and glaucomateous eyes. *Arch Ophthalmol.* 1960;64:494.
35. Drance SM. Diurnal variation of intraocular pressure in treated glaucoma: significance in patients with chronic simple glaucoma. *Arch Ophthalmol.* 1963;70:302.
36. Starrels ME. The measurement of intraocular pressure. *Int Ophthalmol Clin.* 1979;19:9.
37. Zeimer RC, Wilensky JT. An instrument for self-measurement of intraocular pressure. *IEEE Trans Biomed Eng.* 1982;29:178.
38. Zeimer RC, Wilensky JT, Gieser DK, Mori MM, Baker JP. Evaluation of a self-tonometer for home use. *Arch Ophthalmol.* 1983;101:1791.
39. Herse P, Hans A, Hall J, et al. The proview eye pressure monitor: influence of clinical factors on accuracy and agreement with the Goldmann tonometer. *Ophthalmic Physiol Opt.* 2005;25:416–420.
40. Jensen AD, Maumenee AE. Home tonometry. *Am J Ophthalmol.* 1973;76:929.
41. Chen P, Rodger D, Saati S, Humayun M, Tai Y. Implantable parylene-based wireless intraocular pressure sensor. In: *MEMS*; 2008:58–61.
42. Backlund Y, Rosengren L, Hok B, Svedbergh B. Passive silicone transensor intended for biomedical, remote pressure monitoring. *Sens Actuators.* 1990;A21–A23:58–61.

43. Eklund A, Linden C, Backlund T, et al. Evaluation of applanation resonator sensors for intra-ocular pressure measurement: results from clinical and in vitro studies. *Med Biol Eng Comput.* 2003;41:190–197.
44. Hallberg P, Linden C, Backlund T, Eklund A. Symmetric sensor for applanation resonance tonometry of the eye. *Med Biol Eng Comput.* 2006;44:54–60.
45. Pressure-Sensing Contact Lenses. A tiny electrical circuit built into contact lenses may provide 24-hour monitoring for glaucoma. Available at: http://www.technologyreview.com/biomedicine/21170/.

# Chapter 7
# Aqueous Veins and Open Angle Glaucoma

Murray Johnstone, Annisa Jamil, and Elizabeth Martin

## 7.1 What Are the Aqueous Veins?

The aqueous veins are visible on the surface of the eye and contain aqueous being returned to the general circulation. Aqueous veins are of great importance because aqueous outflow system models can be judged by their ability to predict and explain properties of directly visible aqueous flow. Aqueous humor circulation through the anterior segment of the eye involves one of the vascular circulatory loops that is driven down a continuous pressure gradient initially set up by the heart. Aqueous exits the eye by passing through the trabecular meshwork to Schlemm's canal. After entering Schlemm's canal, aqueous enters collector channels that have a lumen in communication with the aqueous veins. The aqueous vein lumen in turn communicates with episcleral veins that return blood to the general circulation.

## 7.2 Why Are Aqueous Veins Clinically Important Now?

We owe so much to the discovery of the aqueous veins. All current ideas about glaucoma have been placed on a solid foundation by the recognition of these unique vessels; it is a remarkable story for a simple reason; their recognition was what established a powerful concept. Aqueous flows! The concept underlies all current approaches to treatment of both open and closed angle glaucoma. Aqueous flows; that remarkably simple premise was the subject of great dispute until Ascher's[1] and Goldmann's[2] independent discovery of the aqueous veins in the early 1940s. The concept of a stagnant aqueous held such sway that it was not until the 1970s that the concept was eliminated from discussion.[3]

The idea that aqueous flows was little more than speculation until such flow was identified in the aqueous veins. Although some laboratory studies suggested aqueous flows,[4] the evidence involved indirect measurements that were not sufficiently definitive to permit development of a consensus opinion. In the absence of a consensus about aqueous flow, the concept of using peripheral iridectomy for treatment of angle closure was on shaky ground. Furthermore, efforts to improve aqueous outflow in open angle glaucoma did not have a satisfactory rationale.

Direct observation of flow through the aqueous veins eliminated uncertainty, it changed everything. Gonioscopy to characterize the status of the aqueous outflow apparatus suddenly became relevant. Advocates of peripheral iridectomy could point to a very clear rationale for their recommendations; the approach was rapidly accepted worldwide. The mechanism of action of glaucoma drugs could be placed within a rational context. Specific microsurgical procedures could be envisioned because they could be tied to a clear goal of the restoration of normal flow. Procedures that owe their genesis to the concept of aqueous flow include goniotomy, trabeculotomy, sinusotomy, and newer procedures including trabectome, the Glaukos shunt, non-penetrating surgery, and trabecular tightening.

## 7.3 Why Will the Aqueous Veins be Clinically Important in the Future?

Where else can we directly observe and measure return of an extravascular fluid to the vascular system? How remarkable that we can see the behavior involved in normal outflow! How remarkable that we can also directly observe outflow system abnormalities in glaucoma! How remarkable that we can directly observe the effect of drugs that restore aqueous outflow to normal! What a wonderful gift, what a wonderful opportunity to gain new insights. Direct observation is the investigative tool which is the most reliable and the most powerful in the hierarchy of methodologies that establish the validity of evidentiary claims. Because of the aqueous veins, we no longer need to rely entirely on indirect measurements. No longer need our scope of thought be limited by the need to base claims entirely on assumptions made following the examination of fixed tissues.

Theories of aqueous outflow mechanisms can be subjected to the intense scrutiny made available by the observations of numerous clinical observers. Theories no longer need to be limited by laboratory techniques, assumptions, and calculations that are the province of only a small group of investigators. Theories of aqueous flow can be validated and reconciled with observations readily available to clinicians. Is a proposed theory of flow consistent with such clinical observations? Does a medication improve flow through the aqueous veins? Does a proposed surgical procedure make sense in light of the requirements of aqueous outflow system physiology as revealed by flow patterns in the aqueous veins? Does a surgical procedure designed to restore normal flow actually improve flow through the aqueous veins? Direct observation of aqueous vein flow provides a powerful probe to answer these questions. Simple observation and measurement of flow through aqueous veins provides a remarkable window, a window that if fully exploited may well provide the tools to solve the riddle of glaucoma.

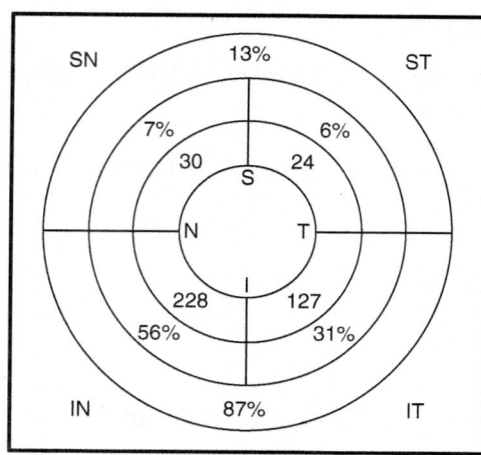

**Fig. 7.1** Aqueous vein distribution. Figure derived from data of DeVries[6]

## 7.4 Where Are the Aqueous Veins and How Many Are There?

Aqueous veins originate from the depths of the limbus in about one-half of cases. The rest originate from more anterior limbal loops and from more posterior scleral emissaries. The aqueous veins range in length from fractions of a millimeter to as much as a centimeter before joining episcleral veins.[1,5]

Two to three aqueous veins are typically visible in an eye.[6] However, four to five aqueous veins are visible in a few eyes while there may be a maximum of six.[6] Aqueous vein distribution around the limbus is not symmetrical. Aqueous veins are most commonly present in the inferior nasal quadrants (285 of 409 in one study) with most of the rest in the inferior temporal quadrants (Fig. 7.1).[6]

Intrascleral mixing of aqueous and blood occurs in some eyes.[7] The intrascleral mixing prevents easy identification of clear aqueous veins on the surface of such eyes.[8] The reported occurrence of visible aqueous veins in patients was reported to be ~75% by Goldmann[2] although Ascher[7] observes, "With high power magnification they can be seen in almost every eye." Aqueous veins have a diameter ranging from 20 to 100 µm with an average of about 50 µm.[6,9,10] Aqueous vein appearance is indistinguishable from that of regular conjunctival and episcleral veins histologically.[11–13] Aqueous flow when present is subject to direct observation providing a powerful tool for analysis of aqueous outflow mechanisms.[7]

## 7.5 Aqueous Veins, Mixing Veins, and Episcleral Veins: A Continuum

Aqueous veins generally contain clear aqueous at their origins. Aqueous veins eventually join recipient episcleral vessels that contain blood. Vessels in these transitional regions of mixing may be more appropriately called mixing veins since they contain a spectrum of aqueous and blood in varying proportions.[6,14]

The transitional area of mixing varies in the same vein complex in an eye and is dependent on the vigor of aqueous discharge.[6,14] For example, the vascular region involved in mixing of aqueous and blood may be near the aqueous vein origin when flow is not vigorous. With increasing vigor of pulsatile flow, for example after administration of an outflow improving medication, a much longer region of the recipient vein may fill with aqueous[15] in a manner like that seen in Fig. 7.2.

When the aqueous-filled portion of the vessel moves distally, the region of mixing also moves distally in the same vessel complex. Diurnal changes[16–18] and water drinking[14] that raises intraocular pressure (IOP) cause similar more distal changes in location within the vascular complex in which aqueous mixing occurs. Although the pulsatile aqueous column may advance or retreat along a vascular complex of aqueous and recipient episcleral veins, the anatomic features of an aqueous, mixing, and episcleral vein complex remain stable for many years and probably a lifetime.[7]

Aqueous veins near their origins often have small episcleral tributaries that intermittently discharge small amounts of blood into the stream of clear aqueous. When an aqueous vein joins an episcleral vein of comparable size to create a single vessel, stratification or lamination occurs in the joined vessel[1,6,8] (Fig. 7.2). Within the single joined vessel a clear layer of

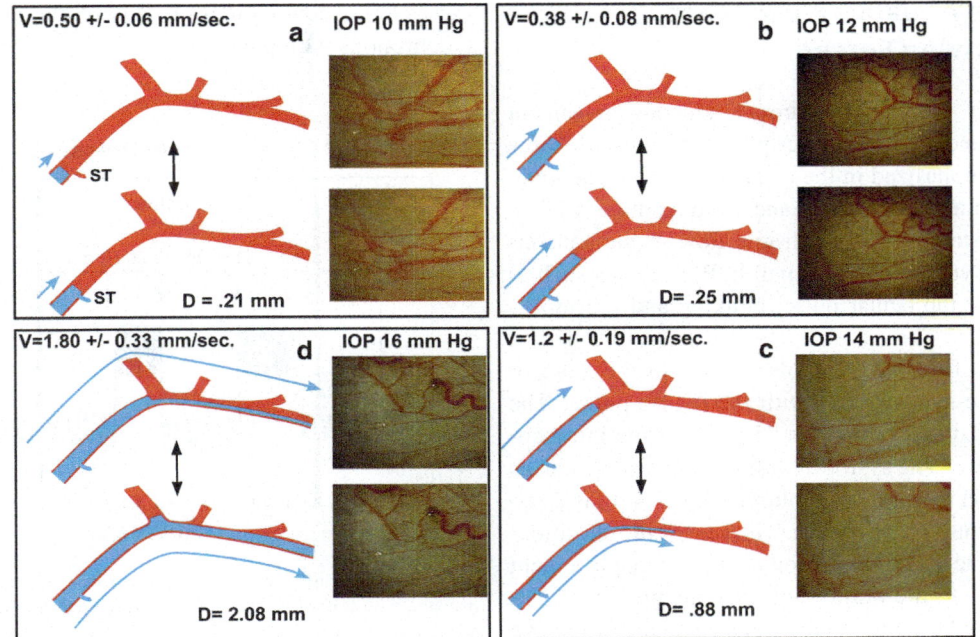

**Fig. 7.2** Illustrations and related still frames from video images of 59-year-old male. Increase in intraocular pressure (IOP) follows a water drinking test but typifies findings seen with a stroke volume increase from other causes such as medications. (**a**) Baseline IOP, velocity (*V*) is low, aqueous pulse wave travel (*D*) with each stroke is small. A standing transverse wave oscillates resulting in systolic discharge of aqueous into a small venous tributary (ST). (**b**) An increased distance of travel of the oscillatory aqueous pulse wave. (**c**) Increased velocity and travel of the aqueous pulse wave. At each systole a lamina of clear aqueous discharges into an episcleral vein. (**d**) Further velocity increase and increase in travel of the pulse wave. Continuous oscillating laminar flow is present in a more distal episcleral vein. Two hours after drinking water, IOP was again 10 mmHg and stroke volume returned to appearance seen in (**a**)

aqueous from the aqueous vein streams alongside a layer of blood from the episcleral vein. Stratification can persist for a long distance because of the differences of specific gravity, surface tension, and viscosity between blood and aqueous.[8] Often an aqueous vein will empty into the mid portion of the junction of two episcleral veins. Aqueous entry then creates multiple laminations called trilaminar flow with a central aqueous column and two peripheral columns of blood.

## 7.6 How Do We Recognize Aqueous Veins?

Stratification of lamina of aqueous and blood as discussed above and pulsatile aqueous flow into the veins to be discussed later, provide two of the most effective tools for identifying aqueous veins. Veins that intermittently contain aqueous may be primarily carrying blood at the time of examination leaving the identity uncertain. A useful identification tool in such vessels involves gentle digital pressure through the lids to raise IOP slightly. The resulting transient elevation of pressure will cause a transient bolus of aqueous to enter and at time completely fill the recipient vessel. A change from a blood-filled lumen like that seen in Fig. 7.2a to that of aqueous-filled lumen like that seen in Fig. 7.2d occurs in a matter of seconds.

Veins containing clear aqueous can be similarly difficult to identify. By applying gentle digital pressure through the lid, pressure becomes elevated transiently forcing extra aqueous out through the aqueous vein. Following release of pressure, there is a transient interval when IOP is reduced below the homeostatic setpoint. Aqueous transiently fails to flow into the aqueous veins because pressure is correspondingly lower.

The reduced aqueous pressure transiently favors flow of episcleral blood into the vein previously containing clear aqueous; this blood influx suddenly makes the presence of the aqueous vein apparent. In a matter of seconds, IOP rises to the homeostatic setpoint and aqueous again enters the vein forcing blood out of the vessel. Once such veins are identified, careful examination generally demonstrates the origin of the aqueous vein emissary. Small episcleral venous tributaries just distal to the aqueous vein scleral emissary then are often identified that are discharging blood into the clear aqueous vein. Continued examination of the region will often permit identification of a well defined network of aqueous veins.

## 7.7 Pulsatile Aqueous Flow: What is the Driving Force?

Pulsatile flow is a salient feature of aqueous movement through the aqueous veins; descriptions of pulsatile flow were strongly emphasized in the original independent aqueous vein descriptions of Ascher[1] and Goldmann[2] as well as many later investigators.[6,10,19] Pulsatile flow in the aqueous veins occurs in synchrony with small IOP transients such as those induced by the ocular pulse, blinking and eye movements (Fig. 7.3).[7,14]

What driving force causes pulse waves in the anterior chamber that are synchronous with the ocular pulse? The choroidal vasculature contributes 85–95% of the intraocular blood volume.[20] The systolic cardiac pulse wave induces a rapid expansion of choroidal volume (Fig. 7.4) thus causing choroidal pulsations.[21] The increase in choroidal blood volume "acts like the piston of a fluid displacement pump in relation to the outflow of aqueous humor."[21] The expanding choroidal volume in the closed space of the eye causes a transient increase in IOP of about 3 mmHg that is synchronous with the cardiac pulse (Fig. 7.5).[22]

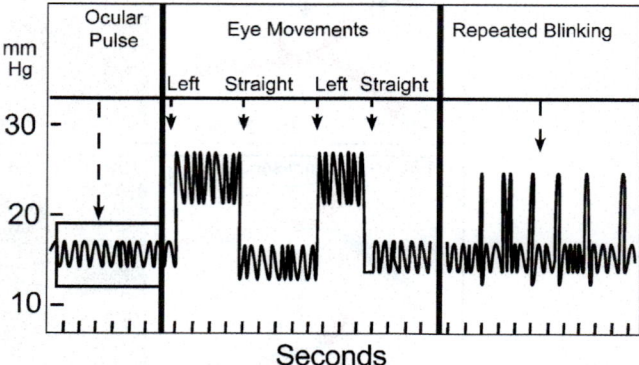

**Fig. 7.3** Illustration of effect of the force of physiologic pressure transients on IOP oscillations. Derived from data reported by Coleman and Trokel[22]

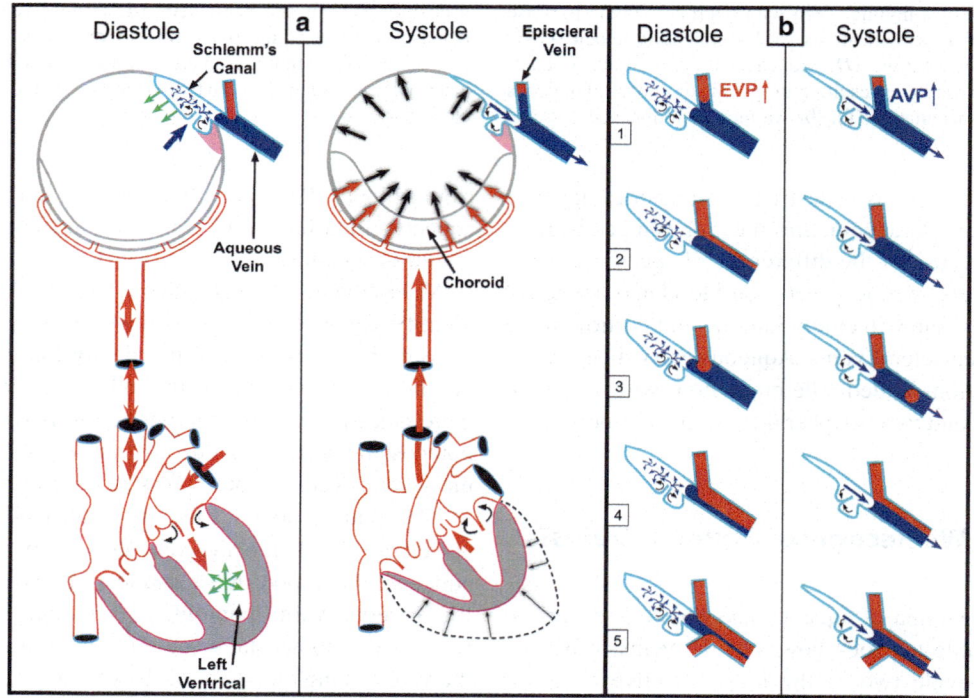

**Fig. 7.4** (**a**) (*right side*) Cardiac source of pulsatile flow. Systole-induced choroidal vasculature expansion (*red arrows*). Transient IOP increase (*large black arrows*). Aqueous pulse wave distends the trabecular meshwork (TM) forcing it outward into Schlemm's canal (SC). Distention of the TM into SC reduces SC volume. SC pressure increases. Aqueous pulse wave then enters the aqueous vein. Backflow (*small curved black arrows*) is prevented by inlet valves (SC pores or tubes). (**a**) (*left side*) Blood enters the left ventricle (*green circle of arrows*). Absence of a pressure wave in diastole is indicated by *double arrows*. Aqueous enters SC during diastole (*green arrows*). Large and small *blue arrows* denote aqueous entry into and out of SC. (**b**) During diastole episcleral venous pressure (EVP) is slightly higher than aqueous vein pressure (AVP), resulting in a relative EVP ↑. The EVP ↑ causes ESV blood to move toward (**b1**) or into (**b2–5**) the aqueous mixing vein. The next systole causes a transient AVP ↑. The following oscillatory pulsatile flow manifestations result. The AVP ↑ causes transient movement of a standing aqueous wave into a tributary ESV (**b1**), transient elimination of a lamina of blood (**b2**), a bolus of blood swept into the increased aqueous stream (**b3**), an oscillating increase in diameter of the aqueous component of a persistent laminar (**b4**) or trilaminar (**b5**) aqueous flow wave

**Fig. 7.5** Aqueous vein systolic stroke volume determinates. (Structural requirements imposed by pulsatile flow. These relationships must be characterized to understand pulsatile flow abnormalities in glaucoma.)

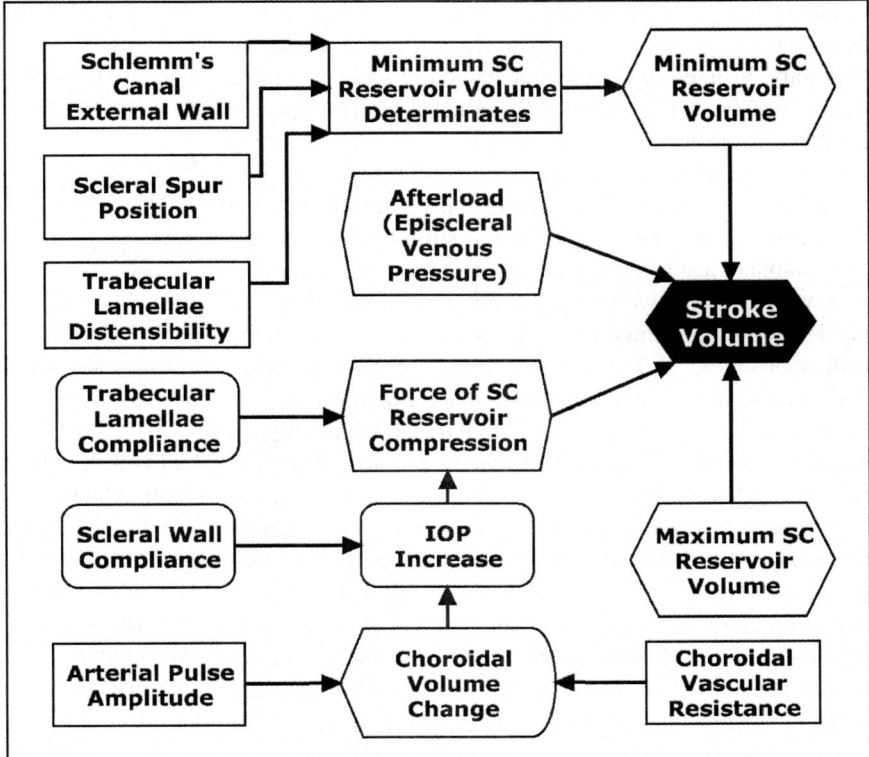

## 7.8 Where Does Pulsatile Flow in the Aqueous Veins Originate?

Schlemm's canal is the origin of pulsatile aqueous flow.[8,14] Direct observation by Stegmann of pulsatile flow in the collector channels just distal to SC provides the most convincing evidence of the origin of pulsatile flow in aqueous veins.[14,23] Episcleral venous pulse waves are not implicated for the following reasons. The aqueous wave propagates distally from its aqueous vein origin on the surface of the eye. The waveform has a steep ascending and slow descending limb characteristic of an arterial rather than a venous pulse wave. The propagating aqueous wave moves distally at a faster speed than episcleral blood in the same vessel. Furthermore, aqueous also displaces episcleral blood both within the primary vessel and within tributary vessels as it moves forward. No pulsatile behavior is observed in adjacent episcleral veins. In addition, the rate of propagation of the aqueous pulse wave is more rapid than the continuous flow observed in adjacent episcleral vessels.

When potential venous pressure waves are prevented, pulsatile aqueous flow increases.[1,5,6,24–26] Temporary occlusion of a distal recipient episcleral vein with a glass rod precludes any episcleral vein pulse wave from entering the aqueous vein. The temporary episcleral vein occlusion causes the amplitude and velocity of the aqueous pulse wave in the aqueous vein to increase. Blood previously present in areas of laminar flow is displaced by aqueous. Pulsating columns of aqueous also fill small proximal episcleral vein tributaries. The aqueous veins become distended and even tense taking on a "glass rod" appearance.[8]

## 7.9 How Do We Validate Theories of Aqueous Outflow System Structure and Function?

Medical and surgical approaches to treatment of glaucoma are predicated on the basis of an underlying theoretical framework. Because sight and enormous costs to society are involved glaucoma theories need to be subjected to open debate and rigorous examination. Such theories can be validated by their ability to predict and explain what can be directly observed in vivo[27] in the aqueous veins.

For example, there are very different and incompatible theories or paradigms, one passive[28] the other dynamic[14] that purport to explain control of aqueous flow from the eye. Which paradigm is correct? Because very different medical and especially surgical approaches depend on the answer, the question is highly relevant to those treating glaucoma.

The theoretical framework or paradigm of a passive outflow system acting as a geometrically stable sieve was developed long ago based on studies of enucleated eyes. In the absence of knowledge of the importance of IOP on TM appearance, enucleated eyes were typically fixed under conditions of hypotony. In hypotony the juxtacanalicular space appeared narrow and the extracellular material in the region appeared compact. Microscopists from the era are cited[29,30] as noting "the presence of many cells and a complete absence of trabecular spaces."[31] A reasonable conclusion at the time was that the region acts as a passive filter that is sufficiently geometrically stable to act as a resistance controlling mechanism.

A very different dynamic paradigm posits a model involving TM movement and outflow resistance resulting from SC wall apposition.[32-37] The dynamic paradigm also proposes that aqueous flow is driven by trabecular tissue movement in response to ocular transients.[14,23,38] The dynamic paradigm is based on evidence accumulated using the tools of biomechanics.[27,39] Biomechanics is the study of tissue responses to an applied load, in this case IOP. Tissues resisting a loading force undergo deformation thus revealing their resistance properties. The newer evidence involves systematic fixation over a range of physiologic pressures especially fixation of still living eyes with normal ciliary body tone and episcleral venous pressure.[34,40-43] These biomechanics studies have led to the knowledge that the trabecular meshwork is not a geometrically stable structure but is rather highly mobile.

This new evidence demonstrates that the juxtacanalicular space is not geometrically stable and thus is unable to explain resistance characteristics of the outflow system; rather the juxtacanalicular space undergoes orders of magnitude (300%) change in dimensions in response to physiologic pressure changes.[34,40,42] Modern histologic studies further emphasize the absence of sufficient extracellular matrix material in the juxtacanalicular space to account for resistance.[44-46] Furthermore, several studies indicate that it is trabecular meshwork outward movement leading to apposition of SC walls that is a major factor in resistance and may be the proximate causal factor in glaucoma.[32,33,37]

Among rival and clearly distinct paradigms how may we determine whether the passive or dynamic model is correct? In the language of biomechanics, "in vivo tissue loading" is the validation criteria to which theoretical models must be held accountable.[27] The aqueous veins are constantly subjected to such in vivo tissue loading; clinical investigators can see it and can study it. The validity of different paradigms can be evaluated and their relevance to the treatment of glaucoma assessed.

## 7.10 What Outflow System Properties Must be Present to Permit Pulsatile Aqueous Flow?

Direct observation of pulsatile flow in the aqueous veins tells us a great deal about structural and functional behavior that must be present in SC and the trabecular meshwork.

**Table 7.1** Physiologic design requirements imposed by pulsatile flow

| General requirements | Specific requirements | Outflow system counterparts |
|---|---|---|
| Reservoir or chamber | Inlet | Channels from JCT to SC |
| | Outlet | Collector channels |
| Oscillatory compressive force | Physiologic driving force | Cardiac pulse |
| | | Blinking |
| | | Eye movement |
| Changing reservoir dimensions | Pressure and volume change | Schlemm's canal |
| Deforming tissue | Ability to distend and recoil | Trabecular meshwork |

General design principles in physiology provide a series of requirements that must be met to permit pulsatile flow[47-49] (Table 7.1). A reservoir must be present; SC provides such a reservoir. The reservoir must have an inlet and outlet; such an inlet requirement is fulfilled by channels across SC inner wall endothelium and the collector channels. The reservoir must change shape. Therefore deformable tissues must surround the reservoir. Since the outer wall of SC is rigid collagen, the trabecular meshwork must deform.

An oscillating force must also be present to induce shape changes in the reservoir. The cardiac pulse, blinking and eye movements provide the transient oscillatory forces.[22] Some type of valves must also be present at the SC inner wall endothelium to prevent backflow.[47-49] Collapsible tubes acting by the widely utilized principle of a Starling resistor system have been proposed to act as valves in SC to maintain a large pressure drop between the anterior chamber and the venous system.[14] Collapsible tubes in the venous system of the eye maintain a comparable large pressure drop between the interior and exterior of the eye.[50] Schlemm's canal inner wall endothelium may contain pores that could conceivably fulfill the pressure regulatory role. However, authorities point out that "the inner-wall pores could be responsible for, at most, a modest fraction of total outflow resistance."[51,52] Thus pores are unlikely to fulfill a role as components of a resistance that could control flow. Authorities also point out that we have reason to question the existence of pores based on recent evidence suggesting that pores are artifacts caused by fixative perfusion techniques.[53]

## 7.11 What Does Pulsatile Flow in the Aqueous Veins Tell Us About SC and the TM?

Pulsatile flow observed in aqueous veins originates in SC. Since pulsatile flow originates in SC, pressure and volume changes must occur in the canal. Since pressure and volume changes occur in SC, a local mechanism must be present that causes the pressure and volume changes.

The external wall of SC is composed of dense collagen.[31] Since the trabecular tissues are the only structural elements capable of inducing pressure and volume changes in SC, they must undergo changes in configuration. Trabecular tissues must also undergo sufficiently large excursions to alter both pressure and volume. Furthermore, since pulsatile flow is synchronous with pulse transients such as the cardiac pulse,[22] the trabecular tissues must be capable of undergoing sufficiently rapid changes in configuration to induce the pressure and volume changes. Evidence from in vivo studies of the aqueous veins demonstrates the need for requirements that cannot be easily fulfilled by the traditional passive outflow model because the passive model can neither predict nor explain pulsatile flow in the aqueous veins.

## 7.12 How Does Pulsatile Flow in Aqueous Veins Change During Systole and Diastole?

Pulsatile flow manifestations result from a dynamically poised equilibrium between pressure in the aqueous veins, mixing veins, and episcleral veins. The oscillating equilibrium shifts to a higher aqueous pressure in the mixing vein during the transient IOP increase associated with cardiac systole. The equilibrium then shifts to a higher episcleral venous pressure during diastole (Figs. 7.2 and 7.4b).

During the diastolic phase where episcleral venous pressure is higher than aqueous vein pressure, blood moves toward or into the aqueous mixing vein. The next systole results in an oscillatory transient increase in aqueous venous pressure. The resulting transient increase in aqueous flow also causes transient alterations in the relationship between the distribution and movement of both the blood and aqueous components. Although they represent a spectrum of findings, authors have divided the oscillating relationships between blood and aqueous in the aqueous veins into distinct categories.[6,8]

## 7.13 Pulsatile Aqueous Flow: What Does It Look Like?

The first category (Fig. 7.4b1) of pulsatile flow is oscillatory distal movement of a standing aqueous wave into an episcleral vein tributary during systole. The second category (Fig. 7.4b2) involves a proximal tributary of the aqueous vein having sufficiently high pressure to cause entry of a laminar column of blood into an aqueous vein during diastole. During the next systole, there is sufficient pressure driving the aqueous wave to completely eliminate blood entry into the aqueous vein. However, the lamina of blood is swept forward in the pulse wave of aqueous moving forward in the vein. The third category (Fig. 7.4b3) involves a proximal tributary of an aqueous vein having sufficient pressure during diastole to force a discreet bolus of blood into the aqueous stream. During the next systole, pressure in the aqueous vein is high enough to again stop blood flow into the aqueous vein. However, the bolus of blood deposited in the aqueous vein is swept along in the aqueous vein during the next systolic pulse wave.

A fourth and fifth category involve alterations resulting from oscillations of persisting laminar components in the same vessel. The forth category (Fig. 7.4b4) results from an oscillating increase in diameter of the aqueous component of a persistent lamina of aqueous and blood. The fifth category (Fig. 7.4b5) is trilaminar flow; such a pattern of flow results from the rather common entry of an aqueous vein at the apex of the junction of two episcleral vein. Aqueous then forms a central clear column with a laminar column of blood on each side. Oscillatory increases in pressure of the aqueous column result in oscillatory trilaminar flow.

Many and often all of the above manifestations of pulsatile flow are commonly seen in one aqueous vein region as the aqueous wave propagates through it (Fig. 7.2). For example, in small proximal episcleral vein tributaries oscillatory movement of aqueous within the vessel, a transient lamina of blood or a bolus of blood are typically seen. More distally, where the aqueous vein joins a comparable sized recipient episcleral vein, oscillating laminar and trilaminar flow are encountered along the course of the same vessel.

## 7.14 What Causes Pulsatile Flow in the Aqueous Veins to Increase?

Prior to spontaneous diurnal reductions in IOP, pulsatile flow increases.[16–18,54] Similarly, before a diurnal rise in IOP pulsatile flow into the aqueous veins slows or stops.[16–18,54] Pressure on the side of the eye[9] and ophthalmodynamometry[6] temporarily raise IOP that is accompanied by an increase in pulsatile aqueous flow. The temporary artificially induced rise in pressure results in an IOP lower than the prior baseline IOP once external pressure is eliminated. Pulsatile flow into the aqueous veins stops for a period of time until pressure rises to the baseline setpoint present prior to application of external pressure.[6,55]

Water drinking that raises IOP also causes an increase in pulsatile aqueous outflow[14] (Fig. 7.2). The increase in pulsatile flow caused by water drinking persists until IOP returns to its baseline level. Three classes of medications cause an increase in pulsatile aqueous outflow that precedes the reduction in IOP. Occlusion of distal episcleral vessels causes the appearance of more vigorous pulsatile aqueous inflow into proximal tributary episcleral vessels and filling of the vessel with aqueous resulting in exclusion of the lamina of blood in the vessel.[1,5,19,24]

## 7.15 What Does an Increase in Aqueous Flow Look Like? (Stroke Volume Increases)

The concept of stroke volume is used to characterize pulsatile flow in the arterial system and serves as a surrogate for functional efficiency of the cardiac pump.[27,56] Structural and functional parameters that determine stroke volume place study of cardiac output on a rational basis. Less well known is that "stroke volume" is employed to describe and characterize pulsatile flow in returning loops of the circulatory system such as the veins and lymphatics.[56] The transient IOP increase associated with systole causes an aqueous volume to discharge from SC at each oscillatory cycle. The aqueous volume discharged can thus also be described as a stroke volume. Structural and functional parameters that define stroke volume in the normal aqueous outflow system are the same parameters that must become abnormal in glaucoma; the concept of stroke volume is thus of great importance.

Stroke volume varies greatly (Fig. 7.2) within the same group of aqueous veins, tributary veins, mixing veins, and distal episcleral veins depending on physiologic status[8] and pharmacologic exposure.[8,15,57] At a resting homeostatic setpoint, visible aqueous vein pulsations are often of low amplitude with a small stroke volume. The small stroke volume leads to the appearance of an interface of blood and aqueous that generates an oscillating transverse wave within the recipient episcleral vein (Fig. 7.2). A progressive increase in aqueous stroke volume manifests itself as a spectrum of findings (Fig. 7.2).

Forces that raise IOP such as pressure on the side of the eye[1,2,6,58] ophthalmodynamometry[6] and water drinking[14] increase stroke volume. Pharmacologic exposure that precedes an IOP fall to a new homeostatic set point is accompanied by the same characteristic spectrum of changes associated with an increase stroke volume.[1,2,7,15,25,59,60] A diurnal reduction in IOP is regularly preceded by an increasing clear aqueous content associated with an increasing stroke volume, while an increasing blood content precedes a diurnal IOP rise.[16,18]

Appearance of an increased stoke volume initially involves distal movement of oscillating transverse waves (Fig. 7.5) A wider aqueous lamina develops in stratified aqueous veins. A greater velocity and a steeper amplitude of the rising phase of the aqueous wave are seen. The increased stroke volume is accompanied by an oscillating aqueous wave that enters proximal tributary episcleral veins previously filled with blood. Standing transverse oscillating waves of blood and aqueous also become apparent in those more distal vessels.

In association with the greater stroke volume, progressive complete filling by aqueous occurs in vessels previously containing lamina of aqueous and blood. The stroke volume increase is sufficient to cause a progressive advance of the pulsatile aqueous lamina along the episcleral vein previously containing only blood. Distal tributary episcleral vessels previously containing only blood now have an oscilatory discharge of aqueous into them during each systolic wave (Fig. 7.5).

A study found that a higher ocular pulse amplitude strongly correlated with a higher IOP in a group of normals and ocular hypertensives.[21] An increase in pulse amplitude in response to an increase in IOP may provide a simple mechanical coupling able to act as short-term feedback mechanism to regulate stroke volume and thus regulate IOP.

## 7.16 Can Aqueous Veins Account for all of Aqueous Outflow?

The aqueous veins are typically ~50 μm in diameter. By measuring vein diameter and velocity of flow, Stepanik found the minute volume of a single aqueous vein to average 1.08 μl/min[10]; Ascher points out that flow through two aqueous veins can easily account for all of aqueous outflow.[8]

## 7.17 What Pulsatile Flow Abnormalities Are Present in Glaucoma?

Ascher's treatise provides a clear description of several pulsatile flow abnormalities in glaucoma that are supported by a number of studies[8] (Table 7.2). When IOP is raised in normal eyes by ophthalmodynamometry, pulsatile aqueous flow increases markedly but in glaucoma eyes, pulsatile flow is attenuated or stopped[19,61]; the technique has been named the "compensation maximum test."

Aqueous influx occurs in subjects when a distal episcleral vein is intentionally occluded by external compression and has been named the aqueous influx phenomenon. The aqueous influx phenomenon occurs in about one-half of all normals while a blood influx phenomenon occurs in the rest.[8] Normally an equilibrium is present in which a pulse wave of aqueous enters episcleral veins in systole and blood from the episcleral veins enters aqueous veins in diastole. Distal occlusion of a recipient aqueous vein results in more vigorous pulsatile flow in the proximal portion of the aqueous vein with increased velocity, increased amplitude of the aqueous lamina, and a steeper wave form. Aqueous enters and then fills proximal episcleral vein tributaries that formerly contained blood. This constellation of findings has been the subject of extensive study.[1,5,6,24,26]

In contrast, a "blood influx phenomenon" is seen in almost all glaucoma eyes."[6,62-64] Occlusion of a distal recipient vessel results in influx of blood into the aqueous veins from tributary episcleral vessels proximal to the occlusion. Blood influx leads to complete filling of the aqueous even causing blood to enter the scleral emissaries. In one study of six patients with unilateral glaucoma, all showed aqueous reflux in the normal eye and blood reflux in the glaucoma eye.[62] The lack of vigorous pulsatile aqueous flow and blood reflux into aqueous veins are thought to be manifestations of an outflow system abnormality in open angle glaucoma.[8] In glaucoma eyes administration of pilocarpine to enlarge SC can cause the blood influx phenomenon to change into an aqueous influx phenomenon.[6]

## 7.18 Why Does Pulsatile Aqueous Vein Flow Become Abnormal in Glaucoma?

Consideration of fundamental design principles in physiology can again help answer the question of abnormalities that may explain progressive reduction and eventual absence of pulsatile aqueous flow in glaucoma (Table 7.2). The progressively more abnormal changes in pulsatile flow indicate that oscillatory forces necessary to permit changes in SC volume and pressure are progressively compromised. Something must happen to prevent the trabecular meshwork from transferring the oscillatory pressure transients present in the anterior chamber into a change in SC volume and pressure.

To transfer oscillatory forces to SC in a way that permits rapid changes in volume and pressure, the trabecular tissues must retain their capability to distend and recoil. The progressive reduction in pulsatile flow indicates that some abnormality develops that leads to a slowing and an eventual absence of TM excursions; is there any such direct evidence?

## 7.19 TM Tissue Abnormalities: An Explanation for Failure of Pulsatile Flow in Glaucoma?

Again, the highest quality evidence, that evidence which comes from direct clinical observation comes to our aid. This evidence was gathered in an era when many of the best minds in glaucoma research relied heavily on conclusions that could be confirmed by directly observable phenomena (Table 7.2). Blood normally refluxes rapidly into SC during gonioscopy in response to techniques that cause episcleral venous pressure to be higher than IOP. Similarly, blood normally empties rapidly from SC when pressure gradients are normalized.

If the TM was sufficiently rigid to function as a geometrically stable structure, there would be no enlargement of SC and no reason for reduction in SC pressure that would permit flow. The presence of blood reflux requires the presence of trabecular tissue movement to enlarge the volume of SC with a corresponding reduction in SC pressure. Reflux of

**Table 7.2** Clinically visible and inter-related outflow system abnormalities in glaucoma

| Location | Finding | Details | Proposed explanation |
| --- | --- | --- | --- |
| Aqueous veins | Pulsatile flow decreased or absent (manifest as reduced stroke volume) | Few aqueous veins visible | Loss of TM tissue motion results in inability to generate volume and pressure changes in SC |
| | Aqueous influx changes to blood influx | Follows occlusion of distal recipient AV | |
| | "Compensation maximum" | Ophthalmodynamometry | |
| | Normal increase of pulsatile AV flow caused by pressure on eye is reduced | | |
| | Medications cause marked increase in pulsatile aqueous flow until new IOP homeostatic setpoint is reached | When effect of medication is lost pulsatile flow slows and IOP rises | |
| Schlemm's canal | *Mild glaucoma* Slowed blood entry and exit from SC *Moderate glaucoma* Progressive slowing of blood Entry into and exit from SC *Advanced glaucoma* Blood entry very slow with patchy filling of SC *Severe glaucoma* Blood entry to SC absent | Gonioscopic findings after blood reflux into SC by compression gonioscopy, suction gonioscopy or aqueous withdrawal from anterior chamber | TM tissue sclerosis results in progressive loss of ability to undergo rapid movement. Loss of TM ability to distend, and especially to recoil, results in eventual apposition and final adhesion of SC walls |

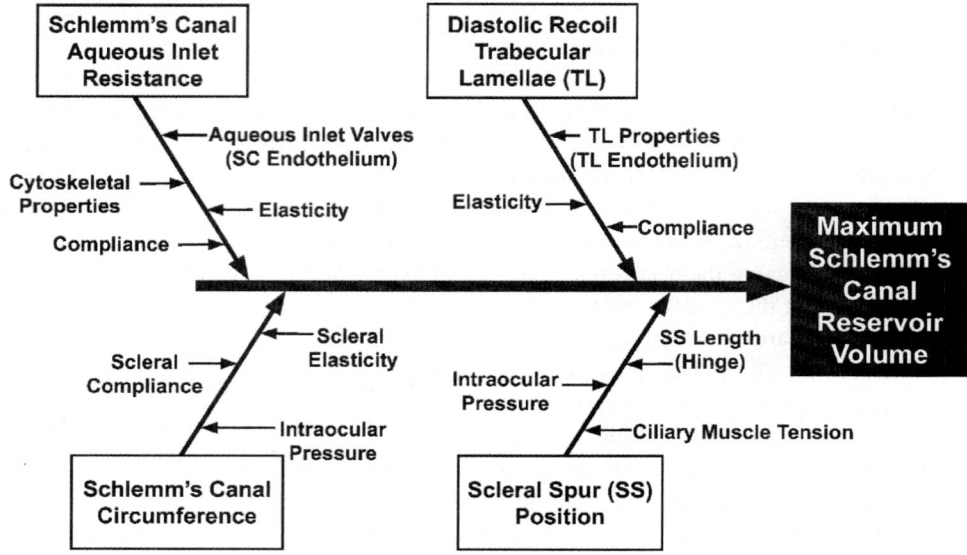

**Fig. 7.6** Maximum effective SC diastolic volume determinates. Important structural considerations imposed by pulsatile flow that further frame and identify structural issues that must be characterized to define pulsatile flow abnormalities in glaucoma

blood into SC thus functions as a surrogate for trabecular meshwork movement. Trabecular meshwork movement with very large changes in the volume of SC have been well-documented in living normal primate eyes in which IOP is reduced below episcleral venous pressure before in vivo fixation.[14,34,41] Such pressure gradient changes and associated filling of SC with blood are a normal physiologic response to a head down position.[65]

Progressive glaucoma severity leads to a progressive decrease in the speed of blood reflux into and emptying of blood from SC.[66–70] Several authors conclude that the inability to reflux blood is a result of loss of trabecular compliance related to trabecular sclerosis that initially causes a slow filling and emptying of the canal.[66,69,71] Ascher has made the association between the alterations in SC filling and emptying abnormalities in glaucoma eyes and pulsatile flow abnormalities in these same eyes suggesting that they are related phenomena.[8]

In advanced glaucoma, blood only enters patchy areas of SC, and in far advanced glaucoma, it becomes impossible to reflux blood into the canal. The complete inability to fill the canal in advanced glaucoma is thought to result from eventual adhesion of SC walls.[66,70,71] The conclusion is supported by histologic studies in glaucomatous eyes demonstrating trabecular sclerosis and obliteration of SC lumen.[72]

Well-defined principles characterize cardiovascular system systolic pumps and provide a means of assessing functional status,[27,56,73] considerations that may be of importance in aqueous outflow system function. Pulsatile flow optimization in the return loops of the circulation are subject to the same principles and functional analysis. These principles include the concept of stroke volume (Fig. 7.5) determined by diastolic distending pressure, the highly important effective diastolic reservoir maxima (Fig. 7.6) as well as the ejection fraction. The principles also include a pressure–volume cycle as well as afterload associated with downstream pressure gradients.[56] These parameters, especially stroke volume determinates provide a framework in which to place structural and functional abnormalities in the eye in glaucoma.

## 7.20 What Medications Increase Pulsatile Flow in the Aqueous Veins

Pulsatile aqueous outflow has been reported to increase in response to three classes of medications (Table 7.3); the first is miotics[1,5,6,15,17,55,59,74], the second is adrenergics,[1,2,5,6,15,38,60,75] and the third is prostaglandins.[38,76] The typical onset of a directly observable increase in pulsatile flow is about 5 min with epinephrine and brimonidine, 5–20 min with miotics, and 20–30 min with prostaglandins. Videography that identifies movement of a bolus of blood permits measuring velocity of aqueous flow within aqueous veins (Fig. 7.4b3) and also aqueous stratum diameter (Fig. 7.4b4). These measurements provide the ability to measure volume of aqueous flow. An increase in stroke volume and velocity as seen in Fig. 7.4 results from instillation of each of the above agents.

If alterations in stroke volume act as a common pathway to increase aqueous outflow, then agents which increase outflow may be expected to do so through the same pathway. In fact, it is evident from the above studies that more than

**Table 7.3** Medications that increase pulsatile aqueous outflow (increased pulse amplitude and velocity or "stroke volume")

| Medication class | Onset (min) | Proposed mechanism of action |
|---|---|---|
| Miotics | 5–20 | Ciliary muscle contraction rotates scleral spur, SC enlarges, TM spaces enlarge, TM under greater tension distends and recoils more forcefully to ocular transients |
| Adrenergics | 5 | Precapillary arterioles constrict, reduced blood flow through capillary beds, reduced flow and pressure in aqueous veins, aqueous pulse waves face reduced pressure head or "afterload" |
| Prostaglandins | 20–30 | Increased amplitude of ocular pulse, increase of volume blood entering choroid during systole resulting from vasorelaxation of choroidal vasculature |

one class of medication can act through a pulsatile flow mechanism. Although the final common pathway that causes an increase in pulsatile aqueous flow may be the same, mechanisms by which drug classes increase stroke volume may prove to be quite different.

For example, adrenergic agents such as brimonidine have been recently shown in the laboratory to rapidly reduce episcleral venous pressure with a time course of episcleral venous pressure reduction that corresponds to the onset of increased stroke volume of aqueous seen with adrenergic agents.[77] Veins are primarily compliance vessels lacking a significant adrenergic innervation. Adrenergic agents primarily act on precapillary arterioles to reduce the volume of flow to the capillary beds.[78] A reduction of blood flow from the capillary bed to the venous system can be anticipated. These considerations suggest that the adrenergic mechanism of action may be to reduce episcleral venous pressure that normally limits the volume of pulsatile aqueous discharge into the recipient episcleral vein.

Pilocarpine causes ciliary muscle contraction that increases tension on the scleral spur. Increased scleral spur tension causes a rotation that pulls the trabecular tissues further from the external wall of Schlemm's canal and enlarges the canal lumen.[37] The scleral spur movement causes lengthening of the distance between the TM attachments to Schwalbe's line and scleral spur thus altering length–tension relationships. Ciliary muscle contraction also enlarges spaces between trabecular lamellae.[37] These altered structural relationships move the trabecular meshwork up the length–tension curve so that a pressure rise during systole induces greater tension and stores more energy to permit greater recoil during diastole.

Prostaglandins have been shown in four studies[79–82] to cause an increase in the ocular pulse, which has been suggested to result from latanoprost-induced vasorelaxation of the choroidal vasculature.[79,80] Although a complete explanation is likely to involve complex interactions of a number of factors, the suggested mechanisms illustrate that various classes of outflow drugs acting by different mechanisms may each result in an increase in stroke volume of the aqueous pulse wave.

## 7.21 Does Episcleral Vein Pressure Change with Posture? What About the Starling Resistor?

The collapsible veins of the neck illustrate a widely used mechanism in physiology that prevents flow down what would otherwise be a simple hydrostatic pressure gradient. The neck veins act as collapsible tubes while turgor in the tissues surrounding the veins act like an external pressure reservoir. The behavior is modeled as a Starling resistor (Fig. 7.7) and is also referred to as the "vascular waterfall

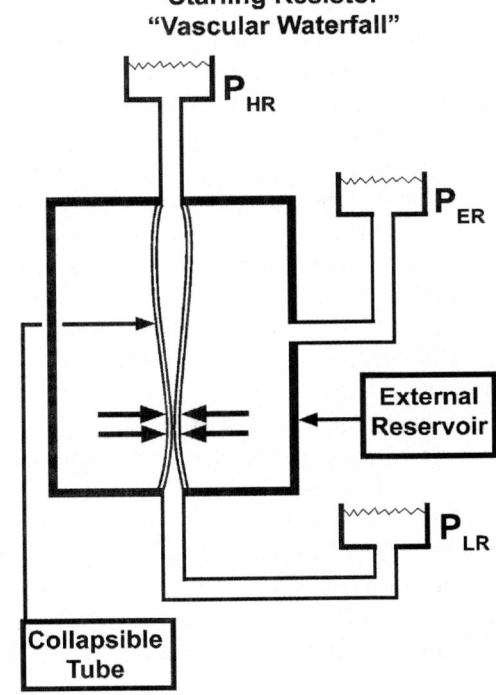

**Fig. 7.7** Starling resistor or "vascular waterfall." General design principle widely utilized throughout physiology. The mechanism controls episcleral venous pressure, intraocular venous pressure, and possibly IOP. Collapsible tube passes through an external surrounding chamber. Pressure in the surrounding chamber is controlled by pressure in an external reservoir ($P_{ER}$). A higher reservoir ($P_{HR}$) is connected to the upper end and a lower reservoir ($P_{LR}$) is connected to the lower end of the collapsible tube. Flow occurs when $P_{LR}$ exceeds $P_{ER}$ because the tube is inflated at its end. Flow stops when $P_{ER}$ exceeds $P_{LR}$ because the tube collapses at its end (*double arrows*). Flow becomes virtually independent of the lower reservoir $P_{LR}$ height. No matter how low the lower reservoir is placed, no flow occurs. See text for physiologic examples in eye and elsewhere

phenomenon."[39,50,83–85] For these reasons, little change in episcleral venous pressure may be expected in changing from the supine to upright position.

The generalizability of the Starling resistor principle is emphasized by employment in control of coronary artery and pulmonary vein flow as well as the pulmonary airways, the urethra, and the eustachian tube.[84] Vascular waterfall mechanisms involving collapsible tubes are important for autoregulation of fluid flow to many tissues including liver, intestines, brain, kidney, skeleton, and heart muscle,[86] emphasizing widespread utilization of the design principle in physiology.

Collapsible tubes are of great importance to the eye because they not only maintain venous pressure above the neck, but also maintain venous pressure in the choroidal and retinal circulation inside the eye at a level substantially above the venous pressure outside the eye.[50] Collapsible vortex vein collectors also act as collapsible tubes as they cross the choroid and pass through the sclera. Similarly collapsible central retinal veins act as collapsible tubes as they exit the optic nerve.

The intraocular venous system is poised at an equilibrium with intraocular pressure.[85] Non-uniform pressure induced by oscillatory transients leads to intermittent one-way fluid discharge in collapsible tubes acting as Starling resistors.[85] Examination of the central retinal veins regularly reveals oscillatory collapse of the lumen demonstrating that they are collapsible tubes acting as a Starling resistor system.[87]

The Starling resistor autoregulatory mechanism that maintains intraocular venous pressure above IOP functions over a wide range of IOPs and thus maintains a comparably wide range of differences between intraocular and episcleral venous pressure.[50,84] "Partial collapse of veins… is an important factor in maintaining arterial pressure gradients in the brain, drainage of cerebrospinal fluid and maintenance of correct intraocular pressure."[84]

It would be attractive to place control of aqueous outflow system pressure within the realm of widely utilized design principle of collapsible tubes used for fluid pressure control in other fluid compartments above the heart. Pressure in the anterior chamber is typically maintained at a considerably higher pressure (~16 mmHg) than that in the episcleral veins (~8 mm). Pulsatile aqueous outflow provides convincing evidence that transient pressure changes occur in SC. If collapsible tubes discharged fluid into SC, then such tubes would provide a mechanism to both control flow and to induce wave propagation. A number of different types of studies provide evidence that aqueous-filled collapsible tubes span across SC.[14,23,34,38,88–90] These collapsible tubes have in fact been proposed as a mechanism to act as one-way valves, to enable pulsatile flow and to provide a means of autoregulation of the pressure gradient between the anterior chamber and the episcleral veins.[14,38]

## 7.22 The Future: Can Aqueous Vein Studies Provide New Outflow Mechanism Insights?

Studies of the aqueous veins hold great future promise. In the hierarchy of evidence, direct in vivo observation provides the standard by which theories and models of aqueous outflow can best be judged. Such evidence does not require reliance on assumptions associated with indirect measurements nor does it require making assumptions about in vivo behavior that are derived from non-living tissues fixed under non-physiologic conditions.

Conclusions drawn in the laboratory about control of pressure and flow at the level of the trabecular meshwork and Schlemm's canal can be reconciled with directly observable outflow behavior in living eyes. Direct examination provides a means to ensure that such theories predict, explain, and adequately reflect observable physiologic behavior. Studies of abnormalities of aqueous vein flow in glaucoma can add new insights into the nature of outflow abnormalities at the level of the trabecular meshwork and Schlemm's canal.

Medication effects and mechanisms of action can be assessed by means of directly observable changes in aqueous vein flow. Surgical procedures that purport to restore normal aqueous flow can be assessed by direct examination of their ability to restore normal flow patterns in the aqueous veins. Aqueous veins studies have provided enormously important insights in the past and provide a unique promise of providing new insights in the future.

## References

1. Ascher KW. Aqueous veins. *Am J Ophthalmol*. 1942;25:31.
2. Goldmann H. Abfluss des Kammerwassers beim Menschen. *Ophthalmologica*. 1946;111:146–152.
3. Bill A. Basic physiology of the drainage of aqueous humor. *Exp Eye Res*. 1977;25(suppl):291–304.
4. Kinsey VE, Reddy DV. Chemistry and dynamics of aqueous humor. In: Prince JH, ed. *The Rabbit in Eye Research*. Springfield: Thomas; 1964:218–219.
5. Ascher KW. Physiologic importance of the visible elimination of intraocular fluid. *Am J Ophthalmol*. 1942;25:1174–1209.
6. De Vries S. *De Zichtbare Afvoer Van Het Kamerwater*. 1st ed. Amsterdam: Drukkerij Kinsbergen; 1947.
7. Ascher KW. *The Aqueous Veins: Biomicroscopic Study of Aqueous Humor Elimination*. Springfield, IL: Charles C. Thomas; 1961.
8. Ascher KW. *The Aqueous Veins*. Vol 1. Springfield, IL: Charles C. Thomas; 1961.
9. Goldmann H. Weitere Mitteilung über den Abfluss des Kammerwassers beim Menschen. *Ophthalmologica*. 1946;112: 344–346.
10. Stepanik J. Measuring velocity of flow in aqueous veins. *Am J Ophthalmol*. 1954;37:918.
11. Thomassen TL, Bakken K. Anatomical investigations into the exit canals of aqueous humor. *Acta Ophthalmol*. 1951;29:257.

12. Ashton N. Anatomical study of Schlemm's canal and aqueous veins by means of neoprene casts, Part I. *Br J Ophthalmol.* 1951;35:291.
13. Ashton N. Anatomical study of Schlemm's canal and aqueous veins by means of neoprene casts, Part II, Aqueous veins. *Br J Ophthalmol.* 1952;36:265.
14. Johnstone MA. The aqueous outflow system as a mechanical pump: evidence from examination of tissue and aqueous movement in human and non-human primates. *J Glaucoma.* 2004;13:421–438.
15. Ascher KW. Local pharmacologic effects on aqueous veins. *Am J Ophthalmol.* 1942;25:1301.
16. Ascher KW. Backflow phenomena in aqueous veins. *Am J Ophthalmol.* 1944;27:1074.
17. Thomassen TL. On aqueous veins. *Acta Ophthalmol.* 1947;25:369–378.
18. Thomassen TL, Perkins ES, Dobree JH. Aqueous veins in glaucomatous eyes. *Br J Ophthalmol.* 1950;34:221.
19. Kleinert H. The compensation maximum: a new glaucoma sign in aqueous veins. *Arch Ophthalmol.* 1951;46:618.
20. Bill A. Blood circulation and fluid dynamics in the eye. *Physiol Rev.* 1975;55:383–417.
21. Phillips CI, Tsukahara S, Hosaka O, Adams W. Ocular pulsation correlates with ocular tension: the choroid as piston for an aqueous pump? *Ophthalmic Res.* 1992;24(6):338–343.
22. Coleman DJ, Trokel S. Direct-recorded intraocular pressure variations in a human subject. *Arch Ophthalmol.* 1969;82:637–640.
23. Johnstone MA. A new model describes an aqueous outflow pump and explores causes of pump failure in glaucoma. In: Grehn H, Stamper R, eds. *Essentials in Ophthalmology: Glaucoma II.* Vol 2. Heidelberg: Springer; 2006.
24. Ascher KW, Spurgeon WM. Compression tests on aqueous veins of glaucomatous eyes; application of hydrodynamic principles to the problem of intraocular-fluid elimination. *Am J Ophthalmol.* 1949;32(Part II):239.
25. Vries S. *De zichtbare Afvoer von het Kamerwater.* Amsterdam: Drukkerij Kinsbergen; 1947.
26. Weinstein P. New concepts regarding anterior drainage of the eye. *Br J Ophthalmol.* 1950;34:161.
27. Humphrey JD. *Cardiovascular Solid Mechanics: Cells, Tissues, and Organs.* 1st ed. New York: Springer; 2002.
28. Kaufman PL. Pressure-dependent outflow. In: Ritch R, Shields MB, Krupin T, eds. *The Glaucomas,* vol. 1. St. Louis: Mosby; 1996:307–333.
29. Flocks M. The anatomy of the trabecular meshwork as seen in tangential section. *Arch Ophthalmol.* 1957;56:708–718.
30. Fine BS. Structure of the trabecular meshwork and the canal of Schlemm. *Trans Am Acad Ophthalmol Otolaryngol.* 1966;70(5):777–790.
31. Hogan MJ, Alvarado J, Weddell JE. *Histology of the Human Eye, and Atlas and Textbook.* Philadelphia: Saunders; 1971.
32. Ellingsen BA, Grant WM. The relationship of pressure and aqueous outflow in enucleated human eyes. *Invest Ophthalmol.* 1971;10(6):430–437.
33. Ellingsen BA, Grant WM. Trabeculotomy and sinusotomy in enucleated human eyes. *Invest Ophthalmol.* 1972;11(1):21–28.
34. Johnstone MA, Grant WM. Pressure-dependent changes in structure of the aqueous outflow system in human and monkey eyes. *Am J Ophthalmol.* 1973;75:365–383.
35. Van Buskirk EM, Grant WM. Lens depression and aqueous outflow in enucleated primate eyes. *Am J Ophthalmol.* 1973;76(5):632–640.
36. Van Buskirk EM. Changes in facility of aqueous outflow induced by lens depression and intraocular pressure in excised human eyes. *Am J Ophthalmol.* 1976;82(5):736–740.
37. Van Buskirk EM. Anatomic correlates of changing aqueous outflow facility in excised human eyes. *Invest Ophthalmol Vis Sci.* 1982;22(5):625–632.
38. Johnstone MA. Aqueous outflow: the case for a new model. *Rev Ophthalmol.* 2007;14:79–84.
39. Fung YC. *Biomechanics: Circulation.* New York: Springer; 1996.
40. Grierson I, Lee WR. The fine structure of the trabecular meshwork at graded levels of intraocular pressure. (1) Pressure effects within the near-physiological range (8–30 mmHg). *Exp Eye Res.* 1975;20(6):505–521.
41. Grierson I, Lee WR. The fine structure of the trabecular meshwork at graded levels of intraocular pressure. (2) Pressures outside the physiological range (0 and 50 mmHg). *Exp Eye Res.* 1975;20(6):523–530.
42. Grierson I, Lee WR. Changes in the monkey outflow apparatus at graded levels of intraocular pressure: a qualitative analysis by light microscopy and scanning electron microscopy. *Exp Eye Res.* 1974;19(1):21–33.
43. Lee WR, Grierson I. Relationships between intraocular pressure and the morphology of the outflow apparatus. *Trans Ophthalmol Soc U K.* 1974;94(2):430–449.
44. Gong H, Ruberti J, Overby D, Johnson M, Freddo TF. A new view of the human trabecular meshwork using quick-freeze, deep-etch electron microscopy. *Exp Eye Res.* 2002;75(3):347–358.
45. Freddo TF, Gong H. Anatomy of the ciliary body and outflow pathways. In: Duane's Clinical Ophthalmology, William Tasman, ed., *Lipincott Williams and Wilkins.* 2007;3:1–18.
46. Gong H, Underhill CB, Freddo TF. Hyaluronan in the bovine ocular anterior segment, with emphasis on the outflow pathways. *Invest Ophthalmol Vis Sci.* 1994;35(13):4328–4332.
47. LaBarbera M, Vogel S. The design of fluid transport systems in organisms. *Am Sci.* 1982;70:54–60.
48. LaBarbera M. Principles of design of fluid transport systems in zoology. *Science.* 1990;249(4972):992–1000.
49. Zamir M, Ritman E. *The Physics of Pulsatile Flow.* New York: Springer; 2000.
50. Ethier CR, Johnson M, Ruberti J. Ocular biomechanics and biotransport. *Annu Rev Biomed Eng.* 2004;6:249–273.
51. Ethier CR, Coloma FM, Sit AJ, Johnson M. Two pore types in the inner-wall endothelium of Schlemm's canal. *Invest Ophthalmol Vis Sci.* 1998;39(11):2041–2048.
52. Bill A, Svedbergh B. Scanning electron microscopic studies of the trabecular meshwork and the canal of Schlemm – an attempt to localize the main resistance to outflow of aqueous humor in man. *Acta Ophthalmol.* 1972;50(3):295–320.
53. Johnson M, Chan D, Read AT, Christensen C, Sit A, Ethier CR. The pore density in the inner wall endothelium of Schlemm's canal of glaucomatous eyes. *Invest Ophthalmol Vis Sci.* 2002;43(9):2950–2955.
54. Stepanik J. Diurnal tonographic variations and their relation to visible aqueous outflow. *Am J Ophthalmol.* 1954;38:629.
55. Thomassen TL. The venous tension of eyes suffering from simple glaucoma. *Acta Ophthalmol.* 1947;25:221.
56. Levick JR. *Cardiovascular Physiology.* 3rd ed. London: Arnold; 2003.
57. Gartner, S. Blood vessels of the conjunctiva. *Arch. Ophthamol.* 1944;32:464–476.
58. Goldmann H. Weitere Mitteilung uber den Abfluss des Kammerwassers beim Menschen. *Ophthalmologica.* 1946;112:344.
59. Cambiaggi A. Effeto della jaluronidasi sulla pressone intraocular e sull'asetto della vene dell'accqueo. *Boll Soc Biol Sper.* 1958;34:1–7.
60. Kleinert H. Uber das Zustandekommen der augendrucksenkenden Wirkung des Adrenalins und anderer gefassverengender Pharmaka. *Von Graefes Arch Ophthalmol.* 1955;157:24–30.
61. Kleinert H. Das durch Druck auf das Auge erzielte Ruckflussphanomen in den Kammerwasservenen. *Klin Monatsbl Augenheilkd.* 1951;122:726.
62. Ascher KW. Glaucoma and the aqueous veins. *Am J Ophthalmol.* 1942;25(11):1309–1315.

63. Goldmann H. Uber Abflussdruck und Glasstab-phanomen. Pathogenese des einfachen Glaukoms. *Ophthalmologica*. 1948;116:193.
64. Miyata N. Study of aqueous vein. II. Study of aqueous vein in glaucoma. *Acta Soc Ophthalmol Jpn*. 1957;61:253.
65. Friberg TR, Sanborn G, Weinreb RN. Intraocular and episcleral venous pressure increase during inverted posture. *Am J Ophthalmol*. 1987;103(4):523–526.
66. Kronfeld PC, McGarry HT, Smith HE. Gonioscopic study on the canal of Schlemm. *Am J Ophthalmol*. 1942;25:1163.
67. Schirmer KE. Reflux of blood in the canal of Schlemm quantitated. *Can J Ophthalmol*. 1969;4:40–44.
68. Schirmer KE. Gonioscopic assessment of blood in Schlemm's canal. Correlation with glaucoma tests. *Arch Ophthalmol*. 1971;85(3):263–267.
69. Smith R. Blood in the canal of Schlemm. *Br J Ophthalmol*. 1956;40:358.
70. Suson EB, Schultz RO. Blood in Schlemm's canal in glaucoma suspects. A study of the relationship between blood-filling pattern and outflow facility in ocular hypertension. *Arch Ophthalmol*. 1969;81(6):808–812.
71. Kronfeld PC. Further gonioscopic studies on the canal of Schlemm. *AMA Arch Ophthalmol*. 1949;41:393.
72. Dvorak-Theobald G, Quentin K. Aqueous pathways in some cases of glaucoma. *Trans Am Ophthalmol Soc*. 1955;53:301–315.
73. Nichols WM, O'Rourke MF. *McDonald's Blood Flow in Arteries*. 5th ed. London: Hodder Arnold; 2005.
74. Hodgson TH, MacDonald RK. Slitlamp studies on the flow of aqueous humor. *Br J Ophthalmol*. 1954;38:266.
75. Johnstone MA, Martin E, Mills R. Brimonidine-dependent pulsatile aqueous discharge to the episcleral veins. *Invest Ophthalmol Vis Sci*. 2006;47S:253.
76. Johnstone MA, Martin E, Jamil A. Latanoprost instillation results in a rapid directly measurable increase in conventional aqueous outflow. *Invest Ophthalmol*. 2007;48:76.
77. Reitsamer HA, Posey M, Kiel JW. Effects of a topical alpha2 adrenergic agonist on ciliary blood flow and aqueous production in rabbits. *Exp Eye Res*. 2006;82(3):405–415.
78. Katzung BG. *Basic and Clinical Pharmacology*. 10th ed. New York: McGraw-Hill; 2007.
79. Georgopoulos GT, Diestelhorst M, Fisher R, Ruokonen P, Krieglstein GK. The short-term effect of latanoprost on intraocular pressure and pulsatile ocular blood flow. *Acta Ophthalmol Scand*. 2002;80(1):54–58.
80. Geyer O, Man O, Weintraub M, Silver DM. Acute effect of latanoprost on pulsatile ocular blood flow in normal eyes. *Am J Ophthalmol*. 2001;131(2):198–202.
81. Liu CJ, Ko YC, Cheng CY, Chou JC, Hsu WM, Liu JH. Effect of latanoprost 0.005% and brimonidine tartrate 0.2% on pulsatile ocular blood flow in normal tension glaucoma. *Br J Ophthalmol*. 2002;86(11):1236–1239.
82. McKibbin M, Menage MJ. The effect of once-daily latanoprost on intraocular pressure and pulsatile ocular blood flow in normal tension glaucoma. *Eye*. 1999;13(Pt 1):31–34.
83. Shapiro AH. Steady flow in collapsible tubes. *J Biomech Eng*. 1977;99:126–147.
84. Shapiro AH. Physiological and medical aspects of flow in collapsible tubes. In: *Proceedings of Sixth Canadian Congress of Applied Mechanics*. Vancouver, BC; 1977.
85. Kamm RD. Flow in collapsible tubes. In: Skalak R, Chien S, eds. *Hanbook of Bioengineering*. New York: McGraw-Hill; 1987.
86. Holt JP. Flow through collapsible tubes and through in situ veins. *IEEE Trans Biomed Eng*. 1969;16:274–283.
87. Hedges TR, Baron EM, Hedges TR, Sinclair SH. The retinal venous pulse: its relation to optic disc characteristics and choroidal pulse. *Ophthalmology*. 1994;101:542–547.
88. Johnstone MA. Pressure-dependent changes in configuration of the endothelial tubules of Schlemm's canal. *Am J Ophthalmol*. 1974;78(4):630–638.
89. Johnstone MA, Tanner D, Chau B. Endothelial tubular channels in Schlemm's canal. *Invest Ophthalmol Vis Sci*. 1980;19:123.
90. Smit BA, Johnstone MA. Effects of viscoelastic injection into Schlemm's canal in primate and human eyes: potential relevance to viscocanalostomy. *Ophthalmology*. 2002;109(4):786–792.

# Chapter 8
# Glaucoma Risk Factors: The Cornea

Lionel Marzette and Leon Herndon

## 8.1 Central Corneal Thickness

It has long been accepted that elevated intraocular pressure (IOP) is a key parameter in the diagnosis of glaucoma. IOP is used in the assessment of disease progression and response to treatment. In fact, it is the only modifiable risk factor for glaucoma. Therefore, its accurate measurement is critical. For over half a century, Goldmann applanation tonometry (GAT) has been the most widely used method of measuring IOP. In their seminal article, Goldmann and Schmidt[1] determined that, in accordance with the Imbert-Fick Law, IOP is equal to the force necessary to flatten a spherical surface, divided by the surface area of that flattened surface (the cornea). GAT utilizes a cone that applanates a circular area of the corneal surface with a diameter of 3.06 mm. With this circular applanation area, the force necessary to overcome the resistance of the cornea to flattening is equal to the surface tension of the tear film. This allows the force applied to equal the IOP.

Goldmann and Schmidt believed that central corneal thickness (CCT) was very similar among individuals in the normal population. However, they acknowledged that when large variations in CCT did occur, the accuracy of the GAT readings could be affected. Corneas that were thicker than normal would require greater force to flatten and thinner corneas would require less. This meant that thicker corneas yielded an overestimation of IOP, whereas thinner corneas gave an underestimation. It has since been demonstrated definitely that significant variations do occur in a normal population.

### 8.1.1 Case Presentation

A 59-year-old white female has been followed as a glaucoma suspect for 30 years. At the time of her initial glaucoma specialist evaluation, intraocular pressure (IOP) was measured using three different methods: Goldmann tonometry 22 mmHg OD, 24 mmHg OS; Direct Contour Tonometry (DCT) 19.1 mmHg OD (OPA 3.8; Q1), 21.6 mmHg OS (OPA3.9; Q1); and Ocular Response Analyzer (ORA) 24.9 OD, 29.55 OS. Corneal hysteresis was 13 mmHg OD and 11.25 mmHg OS. Central Corneal Thickness (CCT) was 627 µm OD and 621 µm OS. Dilated funduscopic examination showed a vertical cup-to-disc ratio of 0.35 with mild temporal sloping OD (Fig. 8.1a) and 0.3 with an intact neural rim OS (Fig. 8.1b). Humphrey visual fields showed scattered inferior depression OU (Fig. 8.2a, b). Optical Coherence Tomography (OCT) was within normal limits OU. She was taking three different glaucoma medications.

The landmark Ocular Hypertension Treatment Study[2] (OHTS) was the first to prospectively demonstrate that a decreased CCT predicts the development of primary open angle glaucoma (POAG). Ocular hypertensive participants with a CCT of 555 µm or less were three times more likely to progress to glaucoma than those with a CCT of greater than 588 µm. The OHTS also supported other clinical investigations that showed significant racial differences in CCT.[3–6] There are no significant gender differences in the CCT of men and women.

In the 1970s, Ehlers et al[7–9] performed a number of studies assessing the effect of CCT on IOP. They cannulated 29 otherwise normal eyes undergoing cataract surgery and correlated corneal thickness with errors in GAT. They found that GAT most accurately reflected "true" intracameral IOP when CCT was 520 µm, and that deviations from this value resulted in an over- or underestimation of IOP by as much as 7 mmHg per 100 µm.

Across populations, patients with normal eyes have a CCT of approximately 540 µm. Patients with ocular hypertension have been found to have CCT values that are increased about 50 µm compared to glaucoma patients or controls.[10,11] This means that many individuals have been falsely labeled as having ocular hypertension, when in fact they have normal IOP once CCT is taken into account.

Several studies have shown that some patients with normal tension glaucoma have thinner corneas than patients with normal eyes.[12,13] Therefore, if CCT is taken into account, these patients may have elevated IOP with "high pressure" glaucoma. This underscores the importance of taking CCT measurements in all patients who have ocular hypertension or glaucoma.

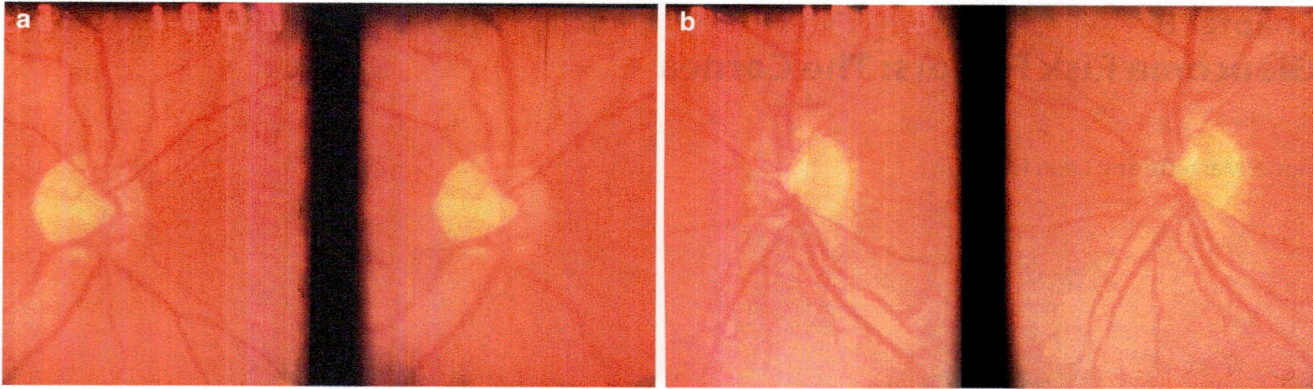

**Fig. 8.1** (a) Funduscopic view of right optic nerve. (b) Funduscopic view of left optic nerve

## 8.2 Differences in CCT

### 8.2.1 Racial Differences

Blacks with glaucoma have CCT values that are on the order of 20 μm less than that of whites. Blacks have a six times higher incidence of POAG than whites. It is also known that the disease has an earlier onset in life and is more aggressive in its course among blacks. These differences in CCT may explain the more advanced progression of glaucomatous disease at a relatively lower measured IOP among blacks. Other evidence supports that this racial difference is not just among glaucoma patients, but also among normal subjects. LaRosa et al[3] reported thinner CCT values among normal black male veterans (mean thickness 530 μm) compared to their white counterparts (545 μm). In another study of patients at a large refractive surgery center, black patients also had thinner CCT values than white patients seeking surgery.[5] Further support of the racial differences can be found in one study that showed subjects who were of mixed black and white descent had CCT values that were intermediate between blacks and whites.[14] Hispanics[15] and Mongolians[16] have also been shown to have lower CCT values than their white counterparts.

### 8.2.2 Age-Related Differences

CCT increases beginning at infancy up to ages 2–4, at which time it reaches its adult thickness.[17] At some point in adulthood, CCT begins to decrease in at least some individuals.[18] The decrease appears to occur more markedly in glaucoma patients than in the normal population. One longitudinal study showed up to a 23 μm decrease over an 8-year period in glaucoma patients.[19] Therefore, not only should CCT be measured at the onset of suspicion or diagnosis of glaucoma, consideration should be given to measuring it approximately every 5 years thereafter to ensure proper management.

### 8.2.3 Corneal Refractive Surgery

At least one million LASIK surgeries are preformed each year on predominately young to middle-aged myopic patients. Myopia is recognized to be a strong risk factor for glaucoma.[20] Many of these LASIK patients are therefore genetically destined to develop glaucoma within a few decades of their procedure. In a patient who has had his cornea artificially thinned by LASIK, an IOP measurement taken by GAT can grossly underestimate the true value. Hence the importance of doing CCT measurements on glaucoma patients and repeating them if a patient has any procedure that may compromise the CCT, such as LASIK. Tonometers that measure IOP independently of corneal thickness are generally more accurate than GAT in taking IOP in patients with corneas thinned by LASIK. One such tonometer is the Dynamic Contour Tonometer (DCT; Ophthalmic Development Company (ODC) AG Zurich, Switzerland). DCT (Fig. 8.3) is a continuously recording type of tonometry that gives IOP and ocular pulse amplitude (OPA).[21] The OPA is a measurement of blood flow entering the eye. The OPA is pulsatile and has maximum and minimum measurements, in association with the heart's pumping action.

This DCT has a central gauge surrounded by a contoured plastic tip. This tip contacts the cornea and creates a tight-fitting shell, but does not applanate the cornea. The DCT compensates for all forces exerted upon the cornea. An electronic sensor measures IOP independently of corneal properties.

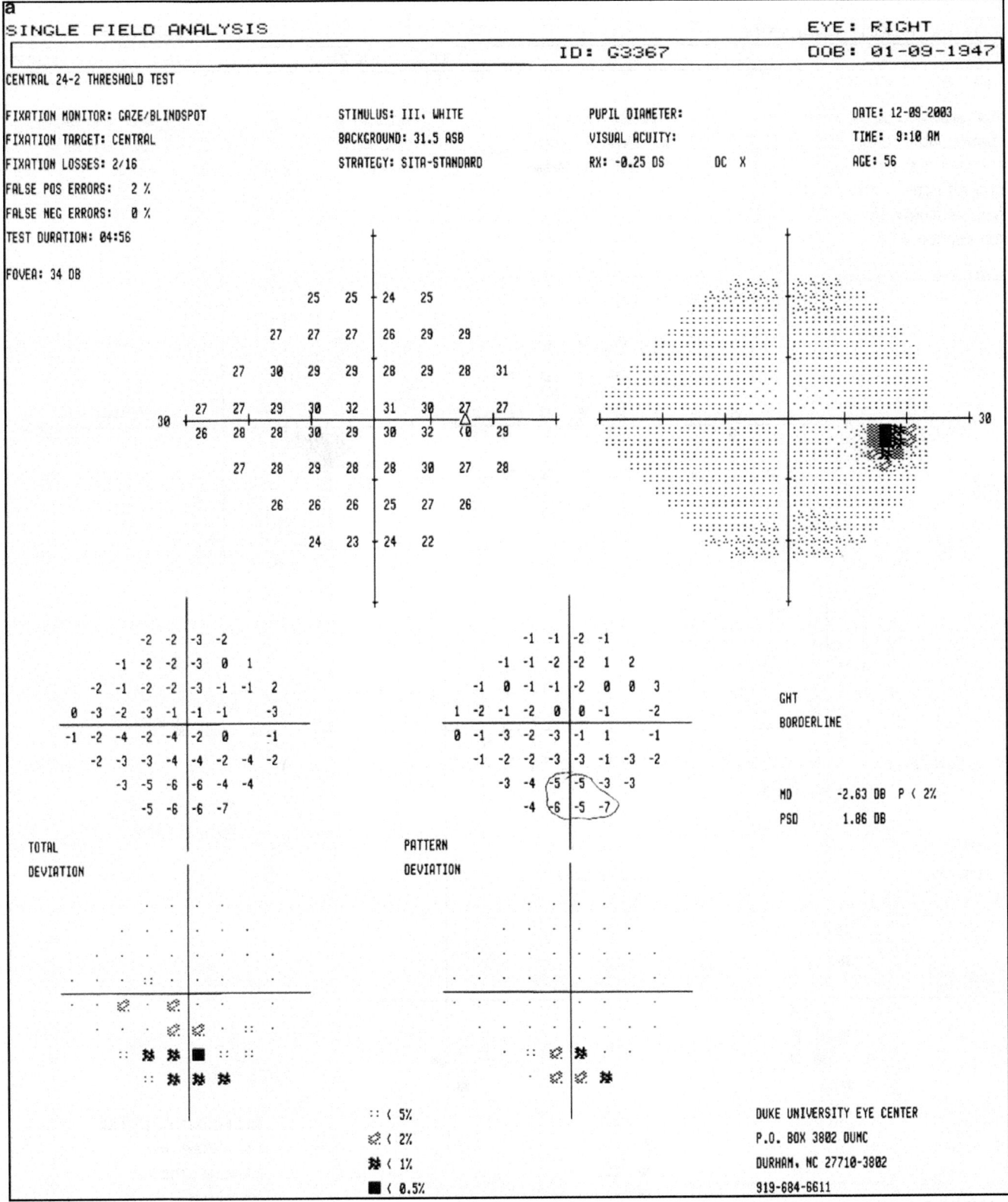

**Fig. 8.2** (a) Humphrey visual field of right eye.

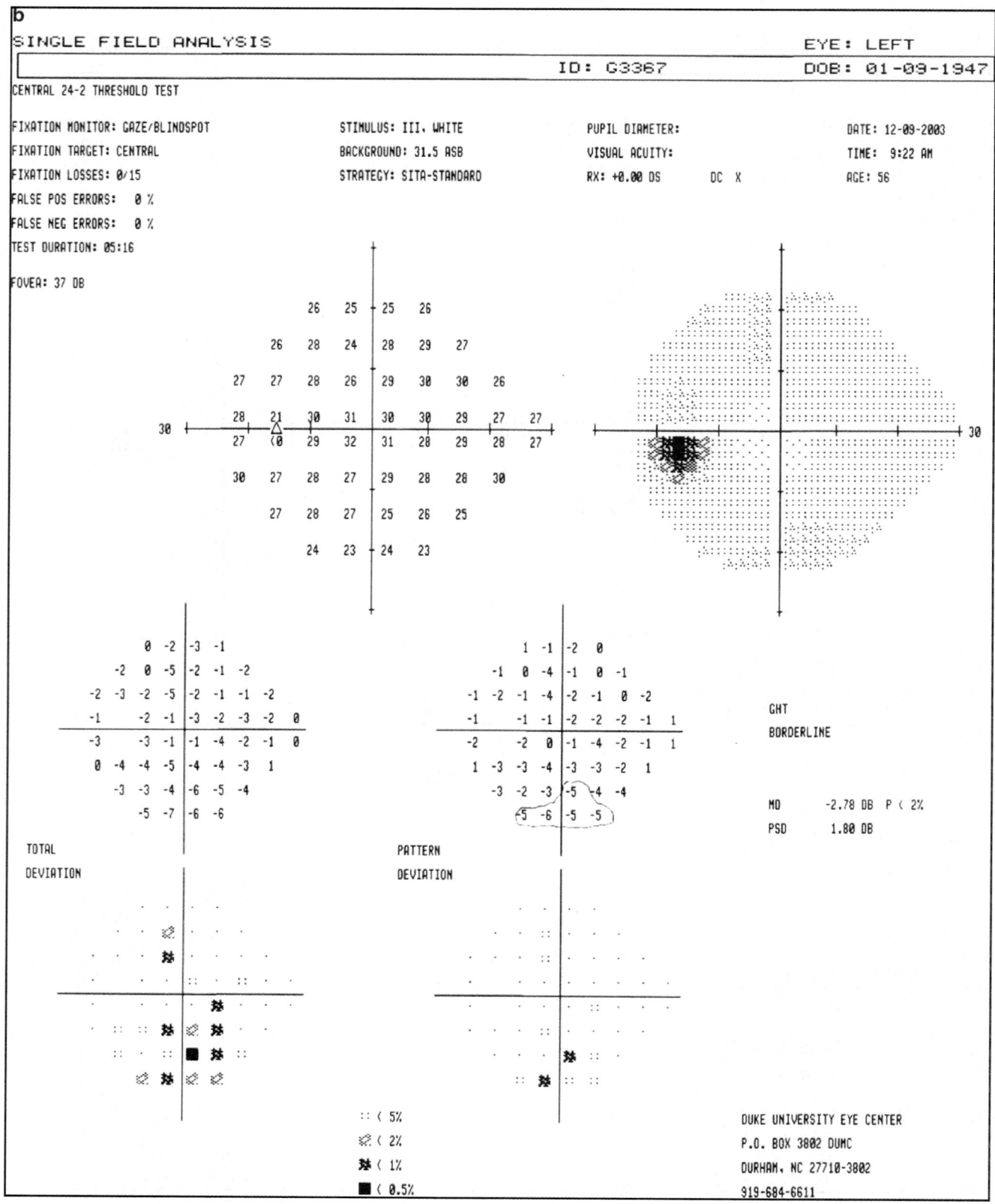

**Fig. 8.2** (continued) (**b**) Humphrey visual field of left eye

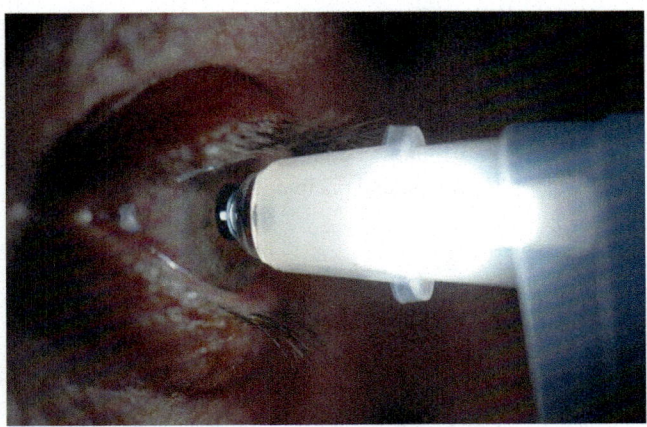

**Fig. 8.3** The dynamic contour tonometer (DCT) (Ophthalmic Development Company (ODC) AG Zurich, Switzerland)

A pilot study[22] was conducted that compared IOP measurements using GAT with DCT in patients who had undergone first-time LASIK with a median ablation of 90 µm. Preoperative and postoperative IOPs were measured. GAT was found to postoperatively underestimate IOP by as much as 5 mmHg, whereas DCT measurements did not change from the pre- to postoperative periods.

### 8.2.4 Other Factors

CCT may show diurnal variations with values highest in the mornings and progressively decreasing throughout the day. A single measurement taken between 11 AM and 2 PM captures the best estimate of a patient's mean CCT.[23]

Despite earlier concerns, CCT does not appear to be significantly affected in the long term by either phacoemulsification[24] or trabeculectomy.[25]

CCT may be influenced by estrogen. Estrogen receptors are found in the human cornea. One study showed that CCT was thickest in women at the time of ovulation and at the end of the menstrual cycle than it was at the beginning.[26,27] There is also evidence that CCT increases during pregnancy, another time when estrogen levels are elevated.

Disease processes can sometimes affect CCT. In the OHTS, subjects with diabetes were found to have slightly increased CCT values compared to their nondiabetic counterparts.[19] Diabetic patients who have had the disease for greater than 10 years may have abnormalities of the corneal endothelium, including a lower cell density and a greater variation of cell size than normal.[28] Diabetes may also cause corneal edema that can also contribute to an increased CCT.

### 8.2.5 Lamina Cribrosa

The lamina cribrosa is a sieve-like cartilaginous tissue in the posterior portion of the sclera through which the optic nerve and retinal vessels traverse. It is thought to be the site where damage from glaucoma primarily occurs.[29] Patients with larger optic discs also have a larger lamina cribrosa. Axonal damage and excavation of the inferior and superior disc areas are associated with higher lamina cribrosa pore-to-disc area ratio and thinner connective tissue support.[30] When the disc size is smaller, the pore-to-disc area ratio is also smaller, which allows for greater tissue support.

In addition, with all other factors being equal, the deformability of the optic disc with a smaller radius is less than that of one with a larger radius, in accordance with LaPlace's Law. A study by Pakaravan et al found that eyes with increased CCT were associated with smaller discs, and thus a more robust optic nerve head.[31] It can therefore be implied that patients with lamina cribrosa with high pore-to-disc ratios (and greater lamina tissue) have thinner CCT values. This may make such patients more susceptible to glaucoma. However, this is an area where more research should be conducted before any firm conclusions can be drawn. A study of 111 enucleated eyes in patients without glaucoma showed no association between corneal thickness and lamina cribrosa thickness.[32] However, the lack of association may be secondary to postmortem- and preparation-induced changes. The cornea and the lamina cribrosa arise from similar tissues embryologically (the ectoderm). It therefore stands to reason that pathogenetic influences might affect them both.[33]

## 8.3 Present Methods of Measuring CCT

Ultrasonic pachymetry is currently the most commonly used method for measuring the CCT. It entails the use of a probe that makes contact with the cornea and sends out an ultrasound signal that ultimately returns to the probe for analysis of corneal thickness. This technique has been shown to be both accurate and reliable.[34] Since the probe must come into contact with the cornea, local anesthesia is required. Also, there is a risk of infection and corneal indentation. Ultrasound measurements can be affected by the fluctuations in corneal hydration.

Modern methods of optical pachymetry use a camera that takes a series of three-dimensional images of the cornea to calculate the CCT. One example of this is the Oculus Pentacam (Oculus Inc. Lynnwood, Washington), which uses a rotating Scheimpflug camera that yields the CCT and other information from the anterior corneal surface to the posterior crystalline capsule.[35]

The Orbscan system (Bausch and Lomb Inc., Rochester, New York) is another type of non-contact pachymetry that scans the anterior segment to provide maps that give CCT as well as anterior and posterior corneal topography measurements and elevation maps. The Orbscan has been shown to underestimate CCT in corneas with haze, particularly after LASIK.[36]

Anterior segment optical coherence tomography (AS-OCT) obtains high resolution cross-sectional images of the cornea and anterior segment. It allows for both central and regional pachymetry and for assessment of other anterior segment structures. It has been found to consistently give decreased CCT values relative to ultrasound pachymetry[37] (see Sidebar 8.1).

---

### Sidebar 8.1. Pachymeters for measuring central corneal thickness

Odette Callender

Pachymetry is an important piece of the puzzle in evaluating glaucoma suspects and is recommended by the American Academy of Ophthalmology (Primary Open-angle Glaucoma Suspect Preferred Practice Pattern). A thin central corneal thickness (CCT) was found to be an independent risk factor for the development of glaucoma in the Ocular Hypertension Treatment Study (OHTS), European Glaucoma Prevention Study (EGPS), and the Barbados Eye Study. Ocular hypertensive patients with visual field loss, detected by either frequency doubling technology perimetry (FDT) or short-wavelength automated perimetry (SWAP), have significantly thinner corneas than those without such defects and in a study by Meideros et al, a thin CCT was a significant predictor for the development of visual field loss in patients with preperimetric glaucomatous optic neuropathy.

Pachymetry may also be important in patients already diagnosed with glaucoma as some studies suggest that a thin CCT is a risk factor for the severity of glaucomatous disease. Glaucoma patients with thinner corneas have been reported to be more likely to present with more advanced glaucomatous optic nerve damage, increased vertical cup to disc ratios, greater visual field changes including more negative mean deviation and higher Advanced Glaucoma Intervention Study (AGIS) score and use more glaucoma medications. This may be secondary to the higher risk of progression from ocular hypertension to glaucoma in patients with thinner corneas or it may represent a selection artifact in that patients with thinner corneas tend to have lower intraocular pressures and are therefore at greater risk for delayed detection of glaucomatous disease. Of five population based studies, including the Barbados Eye Study, only the Rotterdam Study demonstrated an association between CCT and glaucoma suggesting that pachymetry is likely *not* a good screening tool for the presence of disease. Once present, progression of glaucomatous disease appears to be *independent* of central corneal thickness.

In summary, a thin CCT is associated with an increased risk of developing glaucoma (from ocular hypertension) and perhaps the severity of glaucoma at the time of presentation but NOT with the PROGRESSION of glaucoma.

There are numerous pachymetry techniques available – ultrasound, Orbscan, partial coherence interferometry (PCI), the Pentacam Scheimpflug imaging system (Oculus) optical low-coherence reflectometer (OLCR), and anterior segment optical coherence tomography (AS-OCT). Of these, ultrasound is the current gold standard and is the technique utilized in OHTS, EGPS, and Barbados Eye study. The results of these devices are not interchangeable as there may be significant differences in the pachymetry measurements obtained with each.

Measurements with optical pachymetry are generally thinner than with ultrasound. While multiple studies have shown that readings obtained with Orbscan are significantly thicker than ultrasound, one study found the opposite to be true.

Dedicated noncontact anterior segment Optical Coherence Tomography (AS-OCT) devices produce high resolution cross-sectional imaging of the cornea and can be used for pachymetry (in either automatic or manual modes). The SL-OCT (Heidelberg Engineering, Heidelberg, Germany) and Visante (Carl Zeiss Meditec, Dublin, California) are the two AS-OCT devices currently available and although similar in design and working principles differ in their CCT results and from ultrasound pachymeter readings. Studies by Kima et al and Zhaoa et al found that CCT with either the SL-OCT or the Visante OCT were significantly thinner that CCT obtained with ultrasound. Li et al further demonstrated that results with these instruments can vary depending on whether measurements are obtained in automatic vs. manual mode. In their study, there was no significant difference in CCT between ultrasound and SL-OCT automatic or manual measurements. However, automatic Visante results were significantly less than ultrasound measurements while the manual Visante numbers were significantly higher than ultrasound.

Partial coherence interferometry and Pentacam Scheimpflug imaging system produce smaller measurements than ultrasound. Rainer et al found that even with ultrasound technology, different units can produce different results. They evaluated three different ultrasound pachymeters (DGH 500, DGH Technology Inc.; SP 2000, Tomey Inc.; Paxis, Biovision Inc.) and although the differences among the three devices were within 6.0 μm, they were statistically significant. The mean CCT values with the DGH 500, SP 2000, and Paxis were 541.0, 539.2, and 545.1 μm, respectively.

In the OHTS study, patients with a CCT < 555 μm (<558 μm in EGPS) were at greater risk for progressing to glaucoma irregardless of intraocular pressure or vertical cup to disc ratio. However, a value of 555 with Orbscan, anterior segment OCT, or optical pachymetry is NOT the same as a value of 555 with ultrasound. There is no known conversion factor to extrapolate measurements with one technique to a predicted value with ultrasound. Given the differences in results from the various pachymetry techniques, to interpret central corneal thickness measurements based on OHTS or EGPS data you must use an ultrasound pachymeter realizing that even different ultrasound units can produce dissimilar results. If you have multiple offices, you should use the same type and brand of pachymeter throughout for consistency.

Despite the use of ultrasound pachymetry, the 555 μm OHTS or 558 μm EGPS threshold should only be applied to patients who meet the same criteria as participants of either study. The mean central corneal thickness of OHTS patients was 573 μm, with 24% of them having a CCT > 600 μm. Doughty et al showed that the average CCT in the normal population is 535–545 μm with only approximately 5% patients having a CCT > 600 μm. The patient in your chair with a CCT of 540 μm may just be normal and not necessarily at increased risk of progressing to glaucoma.

In addition to method of measurement induced differences, pachymetry results are affected by refractive surgery, after contact lens wear for up to 2 weeks, and corneal drying decreasing by 3.0% after 60 s of non-blinking. There are conflicting reports as to whether or not there is significant diurnal or long term variation in CCT. Falsely increased measurements can result with ultrasound pachymetry if the probe tip is not placed straight and in the center of the cornea.

It is generally accepted that when using Goldmann applanation tonometry (GAT), IOP will tend to be higher than measured in thicker corneas and lower in thinner ones. In light of this, many have tried to correct IOP based on CCT readings. However, the Barbados Eye study did not reveal clear trends in the relationship between corneal thickness with increasing IOP. In that study, there was a significant positive correlation between CCT and IOP in the white participants but not in the black and mixed race participants (even after omitting patients with OAG) who tended to have a thinner CCT but a higher IOP. A review of the literature reveals that the relationship of CCT on IOP is not linear with proposed correction factors varying from 1.1 to 7.14 mmHg IOP for every 100 μm in CCT. There is currently no standard nomogram for correcting applanation IOP measurements for central corneal thickness that has been fully validated. Even if there were a validated algorithm to correct IOP for CCT, recent work suggests that the effect of corneal thickness is less important than corneal elasticity on IOP measurements. Work by Liu and Roberts shows that while CCT accounts for 2.87 mmHg difference in predicted IOP readings, corneal elasticity accounts 17.26 mmHg. According to Dr. James Brandt, "two individuals can have the same pachymetry but one with a stiff cornea and the other with a soft cornea. Each has a large error, but in opposite directions; it is therefore possible to adjust IOP in the wrong direction in individuals with the same pachymetry measurement." The amount of corneal elasticity/stiffness (corneal hysteresis) can be measured by the Reichert Ocular Response Analyzer, a bi-directional applanation process that utilizes a rapid air impulse to apply force to the cornea. The resultant amount of corneal deformation is then measured by an electro-optical system. Glaucoma patients have significantly lower corneal hysteresis and a much wider range than normals. Corneal hysteresis is only weakly correlated with CCT, is independent of IOP and a lower corneal hysteresis was associated with VF progression in a recent study at Wilmer.

Glaucoma can occur with both low and high eye pressures, and patients with similar values do not progress in the same way. Our treatment goal is a percentage reduction (30–50%) in IOP (irregardless of the starting pressure) NOT an absolute IOP number. Therefore, correcting the pressure, by whatever influence the corneal thickness may have on measured GAT IOP generally will not significantly alter our treatment strategies. "Additionally, in the vast majority of patients, the 'rule of thumb' correction factor for CCT is only 1 or 2 mmHg, within the range of the repeatability of tonometry."

Pachymetry is a piece of the puzzle in glaucoma management. It is helpful in identifying patients that are at greater risk for progressing from ocular hypertension to glaucoma but does NOT identify which patients with glaucoma are at risk for progression of their disease. A thin central cornea (e.g., 490 μm) may explain visual field loss or optic nerve damage in an eye despite normal applanation IOP. Conversely, a thick central cornea (e.g., 610 μm) may explain longstanding normal visual field and optic nerve despite a high IOP. However, given the variability in CCT measurements between instruments and the multiple factors that can affect results, it is best to categorize values as thin, thick, or average instead of using exact numbers in an attempt to classify risk or adjust treatment. Although there are no specifically defined numbers for these various categories, a general guideline would be thin (less than 510 μm), average (510–570 μm), and thick (greater than 570 μm).

## Bibliography

American Academy of Ophthalmology Glaucoma Panel. Preferred practice pattern (primary open-angle glaucoma suspect). In: San Francisco: American Academy of Ophthalmology; 2005:7–8. Available at: http://www.aao.org/ppp. Accessed July 7, 2008.

American Academy of Ophthalmology Glaucoma Panel. Preferred practice pattern (Primary open-angle glaucoma). In: San Francisco: American Academy of Ophthalmology; 2005:9–10. Available at: http://www.aao.org/ppp. Accessed July 2, 2008.

Brandt JD, Beiser JA, Kass MA, Gordon MO, the Ocular Hypertension Treatment Study (OHTS) Group. Central corneal thickness in the ocular hypertension treatment study (OHTS). *Ophthalmology*. 2001;108:1779–1788.

Congdon NG, Broman A, Bandeen-Roche K, et al. Central corneal thickness and corneal hysteresis associated with glaucoma damage. *Am J Ophthalmol*. 2006;141:868–875. Available at: http://www.ajo.com/article/S0002-9394(05)01292-4/abstract. Accessed July 11, 2008.

Dayani V, Sakarya R, Ozcura F, et al. Effect of corneal drying on central corneal thickness. *J Glaucoma*. 2004;1:6–8.

Doughty MJ, Zaman ML. Human corneal thickness and its impact on intraocular pressure measures: a review and meta-analysis approach. *Surv Ophthalmol*. 2000;44:367–408.

Dueker DK, Singh K, Lin SC, et al. Corneal thickness measurement in the management of primary open-angle glaucoma. *Ophthalmology*. 2007;114:1779–1787.

EGPS Study Group. The Ocular Hypertension Treatment Study: baseline factors that predict the onset of primary open-angle glaucoma. *Ophthalmology*. 2007;114:3–9.

Fogagnolo P, Rossetti L, Mazzolani F, et al. Circadian variations in central corneal thickness and intraocular pressure in patients with glaucoma. *Br J Ophthalmol*. 2006;90:24–28.

Giraldez Fernandez MJ, Diaz Rey A, Cervino A, Yebra-Pimentel E. A comparison of two pachymetric systems: slit-scanning and ultrasonic. *CLAO J*. 2002;28(4):221–223.

Gordon MO, Beiser JA, Brandt JD, Heuer DK, et al, for the Ocular Hypertension Treatment Study Group. The Ocular Hypertension Treatment Study: baseline factors that predict the onset of primary open-angle glaucoma. *Arch Ophthalmol*. 2002;120:714–720.

Harper CL, Boulton ME, Bennett D. Diurnal variations in human corneal thickness. *J Ophthalmol*. 1997;81:175. Available at: http://bjo.bmjjournals.com/cgi/content/abstract/80/12/1068. Accessed July 12, 2008.

Herndon LW, Weizer JS, Stinnett SS. Central corneal thickness as a risk factor for advanced glaucoma damage. *Arch Ophthalmol*. 2004;122:17–21.

Brandt J. Available at: http://www.modernmedicine.com/modernmedicine/article/articleDetail.jsp?id=379903&pageID=1&sk=& date. Accessed July 13, 2008.

Jonas JB, Stroux A, Velten I, et al. Central corneal thickness correlated with glaucoma damage and rate of progression. *Invest Ophthalmol Vis Sci*. 2005;46:1269–1274. Available at: http://www.iovs.org/cgi/content/abstract/46/4/1269. Accessed June 2, 2008.

Kima HY, Budenz DL, Lee PS, et al. Comparison of central corneal thickness using anterior segment optical coherence tomography vs ultrasound pachymetry. *Am J Ophthalmol*. 2008;145;228–232.

Lackner B, Schmidinger G, Pieh S, et al. Repeatability and reproducibility of central corneal thickness measurement with Pentacam, Orbscan, and ultrasound. *Optom Vis Sci*. 2005;82:892–899.

Leske MC, Wu S-Y, Hennis A, Honkanen R, Nemesure B, BESs Study Group. Risk factors for incident open-angle glaucoma: the Barbados Eye Studies. *Ophthalmology*. 2008;115:85–93.

Li H, Shun Leung CK, Wong L, et al. Comparative study of central corneal thickness measurement with slit-lamp optical coherence tomography and visante optical coherence tomography. *Ophthalmology*. 2008;115(5):796–801

Liu J, Roberts CJ. Influence of corneal biomechanical properties on intraocular pressure measurement: quantitative analysis. *J Cataract Refract Surg*. 2005;31:146–155.

Medeiros FA, Sample PA, Weinreb RN. Corneal thickness measurements and frequency doubling technology perimetry abnormalities in ocular hypertensive eyes. *Ophthalmology*. 2003;110:1903–1908.

Marsich MM, Bullimore MA. The repeatability of corneal thickness measures. *Cornea*. 2000;19:792–795.

Medeiros FA, Sample PA, Weinreb RN. Corneal thickness measurements and visual function abnormalities in ocular hypertensive patients. *Am J Ophthalmol*. 2003;135:131–137.

Medeiros FA, Sample PA, Zangwill LM, et al. Corneal thickness as a risk factor for visual field loss in patients with preperimetric glaucomatous optic neuropathy. *Am J Ophthalmol*. 2003;136: 805–813.

Mills, R. If intraocular pressure measurement is only an estimate – then what? *Ophthalmology*. 2000;107:1807–1808

Módis L Jr, Langenbucher A, Seitz B. Corneal thickness measurements with contact and noncontact specular microscopic and ultrasonic pachymetry. *Am J Ophthalmol*. 2001;132:517–521.

Nemesure B, Wu SY, Hennis A, Leske MC, for the Barbados Eye Study Group. Corneal thickness and intraocular pressure in the Barbados Eye Studies. *Arch Ophthalmol*. 2003;121: 240–244.

Nourouzi H, Rajavi J, Okhovatpour MA. Time to resolution of corneal edema after long-term contact lens wear. *AJO*. 2006;142: 671–673.

Rainer G, Findl O, Petternel V, et al. Central corneal thickness measurements with partial coherence interferometry, ultrasound, and the Orbscan system. *Ophthalmology*. 2004;111:875–879.

Rainer G, Petternel V, Findl O, et al. Comparison of ultrasound pachymetry and partial coherence interferometry in the measurement of central corneal thickness. *J Cataract Refract Surg*. 2002;28:2142–2145.

Shah S. Accurate intraocular pressure measurement – the myth of modern ophthalmology? [editorial]. *Ophthalmology*. 2000;107: 1805–1806.

Shah S, Spedding C, Bhojwani R, et al. Assessment of the diurnal variation in central corneal thickness and intraocular pressure for patients with suspected glaucoma. *Ophthalmology*. 2000;107:1191–1193.

Weizer JS, Stinnett SS, Herndon LW. Longitudinal changes in central corneal thickness and their relation to glaucoma status: an 8 year follow up study. *Br J Ophthalmol*. 2006;90: 732–736.

White Paper – Reichert ocular response analyzer measures corneal biomechanical properties and IOP. David Luce, Ph.D. and David Taylor; March 2006. Available at: http://www.ocularresponseanalyzer.com/Ocular%20Response%20Analyzer%20White%20Paper.pdf. Accessed July 11, 2008.

Wickham L, Edmunds B, Murdoch IE. Central corneal thickness: will one measurement suffice? *Opthalmology*. 2004;112:225–228.

Zhaoa PS, Wongabc TY, Won W-L, et al. Comparison of central corneal thickness measurements by visante anterior segment optical coherence tomography with ultrasound pachymetry. *Am J Ophthalmol*. 2007;143:1047–1049.

## 8.4 Correction Factors

Since a study by Ehlers et al[9] in the 1970s in which 29 human eyes were cannulated to find true IOP compared to that obtained by GAT, correction factors have been used. They found that a correction factor of 5 mmHg to every 70 μm difference in CCT from an average 520 μm could be used. Doughty and Zaman[38] calculated a correction of 2.5 mmHg for each 50 μm difference in CCT (from a mean of 535 μm). Another study[39] found a correction of 2 mmHg for each 100 μm difference in CCT (from a mean CCT of 537 μm). The clinician should be cautious in rigidly extrapolating any linear algorithm into practice. For example, when using Ehlers' correction on patients with both very thin corneas and low IOPs, a negative IOP value could be obtained! A general recommendation supported by the data so far is that one can take far better care of patients simply by categorizing corneas as "thin (<500 μm), average (500–600 μm), or thick (>600 μm)," just as it is important to recognize that optic discs come in "small, medium, and large" sizes, allowing the clinician to interpret disc configurations accordingly.

## 8.5 Drug Effect on CCT

Prostaglandin analogs, which are generally very effective medications used in the treatment of glaucoma, have been associated with a significant reduction in CCT. In a prospective study[40] of travoprost, 6 weeks of treatment was found to cause a 6.9 μm CCT decrease. Another study[41] found latanoprost also lowered CCT. However, this lowering was found to have little to no effect on the measured IOP reduction. While it is not completely understood why this drug-induced reduction in CCT occurs, it could be due to activation of matrix metalloproteinases in the cornea by prostaglandin analogs.

Topical dorzolamide has been shown to cause up to 14.4% increase in CCT in patients with cornea guttata.[42] It has been suggested that patients with severe corneal guttata or a highly compromised endothelial cell layer may have a higher risk of corneal decompensation after prolonged use of dorzolamide.

However in normal human eyes, several studies have shown that dorzolamide causes a small decrease in CCT that is clinically insignificant.[43,44] Topical beta-blockers appear to cause a similar decrease in CCT that dorzolamide does in normal subjects.

## 8.6 Corneal Hysteresis

IOP is derived from the force measurement indirectly, based on a number of assumptions about corneal deformability. Corneal deformability in turn represents a summation of the cornea's curvature, elastic properties, surface tension, and the intraocular pressure.[45] A model of corneal biomechanics indicates that CCT and corneal properties should be considered as the clinician obtains a picture of the true IOP.[44] While CCT is probably the major component of corneal elasticity, it is likely not the only component. The cornea mix of collagen types, corneal hydration, packing density of collagen fibrils, extra-cellular matrix, and other factors undoubtedly vary among individuals. In some patients these other factors may dwarf the effect of CCT on the accuracy of IOP estimation.

Corneal hysteresis (CH) is a measurement that reflects the viscoelastic properties of the cornea and gives an indication of its biomechanical integrity. Patients with primary open angle glaucoma (POAG) and normal tension glaucoma (NTG) have decreased values of corneal hysteresis. The Ocular Response Analyzer (ORA) (Reichert Corp., Buffalo, New York) uses a rapid air pulse to record two applanation pressures (Fig. 8.4).[46] One is recorded while the cornea is moving inward and another when moving outward. These two pressures are different because of resistance properties of the cornea that cause delays in the inward and outward applanation. The difference between the two pressures is CH. This key measurement is a result of viscous damping of corneal tissue and yields important information about the biomechanical properties of the cornea.

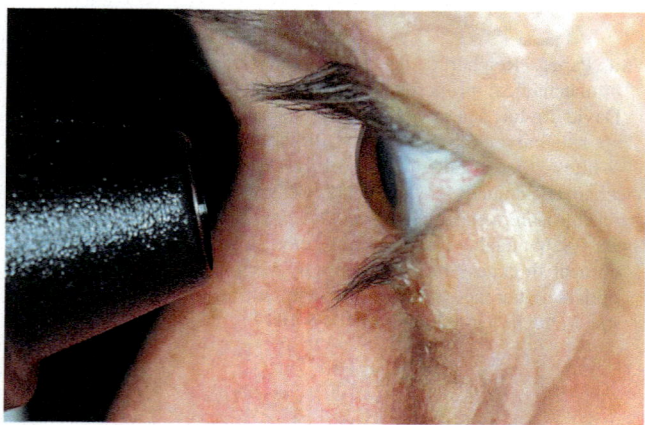

**Fig. 8.4** The ocular response analyzer (ORA) (Reichert Corp. Buffalo, New York)

A study by Bochmann et al[47] showed that POAG patients with acquired pit of the optic nerve (APON) had significantly lower CH values compared to glaucoma patients without APON (mean CH 8.89 and 10.2 mmHg, respectively). In another study by Congdon and coworkers,[48] a lower CH was associated with progressive visual field worsening.

Unlike IOP, CH shows little variation throughout the day.[49]

## 8.7 Practical Aspects

It is now clear that CCT is the most predictive factor for progression of ocular hypertension to glaucoma.[2] There are also data to support the fact that patients with POAG and decreased CCT tend to have more severe glaucomatous damage.[6] As such, all patients with glaucoma or ocular hypertension should have CCT measured. This measurement should be undertaken at the initial diagnosis. Because the cornea thins with time in many patients, consideration should be given to repeat it every 5 years. Also, all patients who have eye surgeries that compromise the CCT, particularly LASIK, should have repeat CCT values taken afterward.

At this time, CCT correction factors or nomograms are not recommended as no algorithm can sufficiently adjust for IOP on the basis of CCT alone, nor do they account for differences in corneal biomechanics between eyes. Categorizing CCT as thin, average, or thick is best at the present. This undoubtedly means that clinicians should more aggressively treat some patients with normal tension glaucoma who have thinner CCT values. Likewise, treatment might be simplified in many patients who have ocular hypertension and thicker CCT values.

### 8.7.1 Case Revisited

On Goldmann applanation, this patient's IOP values are elevated above the normal range. However, it can also be noted that she has increased CCT in both eyes with values greater than 600 μm. Her IOP as measured by DCT of 19.1 mmHg OD is within normal limits, and her IOP OS of 21.6 mmHg is only mildly elevated. The Ocular Pulse Amplitude was normal at 3.8 mmHg OD and 3.9 mmHg OS, indicating relatively good ocular perfusion. A quality value of Q1 indicates good test reliability. Her corneal hysteresis values were within the normal range (8–16 mmHg) at 13 OD mmHg and 11.25 mmHg OS.

This patient's most reliable IOP values can likely be obtained from her DCT measurement, as DCT takes IOP without being affected by CCT. A manometric study showed that DCT IOP values are closer to "true intraocular pressure."[50]

Her fundus exam is relatively normal with good cup-to-disc ratios and normal macular and periphery exams. The Humphrey visual fields showed no significant field defects.

Our patient was actually taken off her glaucoma medications, with instructions to have follow-up clinic visits every 4–6 months.

### 8.7.2 Clinical Pearls

1. CCT measurement is a necessary part of the evaluation and management of glaucoma suspects and glaucoma patients. It should be measured in all such patients at the time of diagnosis.
2. Blacks with glaucoma have CCT values that are on the order of 20 μm less than that of their white counterparts.
3. CCT can decrease in some patients significantly as they age. Therefore, consideration should be given to measuring CCT every 5 years after it is initially measured at diagnosis.
4. Diurnal variations may occur in CCT. CCT is best measured between 11 AM and 2 PM.
5. DCT (Dynamic Contour Tonometer) is the truest noninvasive method of measuring IOP. It should be used when an accurate IOP measurement is needed independent of corneal properties. It is particularly useful when measuring IOP in patients after LASIK.
6. Ultrasonic pachymetry is currently the method with the highest test reliability for measuring CCT.
7. Prostaglandin analogs can modestly decrease CCT.
8. CCT should be categorized as "thin (<500 μm), average (500–600 μm), or thick" (>600 μm). No correction factor currently adequately corrects IOP on a population level.
9. A thin CCT is the most predictive factor for progression of ocular hypertension to glaucoma.

## References

1. Goldmann H, Schmidt T. Applanation tonometry [German]. *Ophthalmologica.* 1957;134:221–242.
2. Gordon MO, Beiser JA, Brandt JD, et al. The Ocular Hypertension Treatment Study: baseline factors that predict the onset of primary open-angle glaucoma. *Arch Ophthalmol.* 2002;120:714–720.
3. LaRosa FA, Gross RL, Orengo-Nania S. Central corneal thickness of Caucasians and African Americans in glaucomatous and nonglaucomatous populations. *Arch Ophthalmol.* 2001;119:23–27.
4. Nemesure B, Wu SY, Hennis A, et al. Corneal thickness and intraocular pressure in the Barbados eye studies. *Arch Ophthalmol.* 2003;121:240–244.
5. Shimmyo M, Ross AJ, Moy A, et al. Intraocular pressure, Goldmann applanation tension, corneal thickness, and corneal curvature in Caucasians, Asians, Hispanics, and African Americans. *Am J Ophthalmol.* 2003;136:603–613.
6. Herndon LW, Weizer JS, Stinnett SS. Central corneal thickness as a risk factor for advanced glaucoma damage. *Arch Ophthalmol.* 2004;122:17–21.
7. Ehlers N, Hansen FK, Aasved H. Biometric correlations of corneal thickness. *Acta Ophthalmol (Copenh).* 1975;53:652–659.
8. Ehlers N, Hansen FK. Corneal thickness in low-tension glaucoma. *Acta Ophthalmol (Copenh).* 1974;52:740–746.
9. Ehelers N, Bramsen T, Sperling S. Applanation tonometry and central corneal thickness. *Acta Ophthalmol (Copenh).* 1975;53(1):34–43.
10. Argus WA. Ocular hypertension and central corneal thickness. *Ophthalmology.* 1995;102:1810–1812.
11. Herndon LW, Choudhri SA, Cox T, et al. Central corneal thickness in normal, glaucomatous, and ocular hypertensive eyes. *Arch Ophthalmol.* 1997;115:1137–1141.
12. Copt RP, Thomas R, Mermoud A. Central thickness in ocular hypertension, primary open-angle glaucoma, and normal tension glaucoma. *Arch Ophthalmol.* 1999;117:14–16.
13. Emara BY, Tingey DP, Probst LE, et al. Central corneal thickness in low-tension glaucoma. *Can J Opthalmol.* 1999;34:319–324.
14. Nemesure B, Wu S, Hennis A, et al. Corneal thickness and intraocular pressure in the Barbados eye studies. *Arch Opthalmol.* 2003;121:240–244.
15. Hahn S, Azen S, Ying-Lai M, et al. Central corneal thickness in Latinos. *Invest Ophthalmol Vis Sci.* 2003;44:1508–1512.
16. Foster PJ, Baasanhu J, Alsbirk PH, et al. Central corneal thickness and intraocular in a Mongolian population. *Ophthalmology.* 1998;105:969–973.
17. Hamilton KE, Pye DC, Aggarwala S, et al. Diurnal variation of central corneal thickness and Goldmann applanation tonometry estimates of intraocular pressure. *J Glaucoma.* 2007;16:29–35.
18. Brandt JD, Beiser JA, Kass MA, et al. Central corneal thickness in the ocular hypertension treatment study. *Ophthalmology.* 2001;108:1779–1788.
19. Weizer JS, Stinnett SS, Herndon LW. Longitudinal changes in central corneal thickness and their relation to glaucoma status: an 8 year follow up study. *Br J Ophthalmol.* 2006;990:732–736.
20. Mitchell P, Hourihan F, Sandbach J. The relationship between glaucoma and myopia: the Blue Mountains Eye Study. *Ophthalmology.* 2000;107:1026–1027.
21. Kaufmann C, Bachmann LM, Robert YC, et al. Ocular pulse amplitude in healthy subjects as measured by dynamic contour tonometry. *Arch Ophthalmol.* 2006;124:1104–1108.
22. Kaufmann C, Bachmann LM, Thiel MA. Intraocular pressure measurements using dynamic contour tonometry after laser in situ keratomileusis. *Invest Ophthalmol Vis Sci.* 2003;44:3790–3794.
23. Hara T, Hara T. Postoperative change in the corneal thickness of the pseudophakic eye: amplified diurnal variation and consensual increase. *J Cataract Refract Surg.* 1987;13:325–329.
24. Ventura AC, Wälti R, Böhnke M. Corneal thickness and endothelial density before and after cataract surgery. *Br J Ophthalmol.* 2001;85:18–20.
25. Cunliffe IA, Dapling RB, West J, et al. A prospective study examining the changes in factors that affect visual acuity following trabeculectomy. *Eye.* 1992;6:618–622.
26. Giuffrè G, Di Rosa L, Fiorino F, et al. Variations in central corneal thickness during the menstrual cycle in women. *Cornea.* 2007;26:144–6.
27. Suzuki T, Kinoshita Y, Masayoshi T, et al. Expression of sex steroid hormone receptors in human cornea. *Curr Eye Res.* 2001;22:28–33.
28. Lee JS, Oum BS, Choi HY, et al. Differences in corneal thickness and corneal endothelium related to duration in diabetes. *Eye.* 2006;20:315–318.
29. Anderson DR, Hendrickson A. Effect of intraocular pressure on axoplasmic transport in monkey optic nerve. *Invest Ophthalmol.* 1974;13:771–783.
30. Jonas JB, Mardin CY, Schlotzer-Schrehardt U, et al. Morphometry of the lamina cribrosa surface. *Invest Ophthalmol Vis Sci.* 1991;32:401–405.
31. Pakravan M, Parsa A, Sanagou M, et al. Central corneal thickness and correlation to optic disc size: a potential link for susceptibility to glaucoma. *Br J Ophthalmol.* 2007;91:26–28.
32. Jonas JB, Hobach L. Central corneal thickness and thickness of the lamina cribrosa in human eyes, *Invest Ophthalmol Vis Sci.* 2005;46:1275–1279.
33. Azar NF, Davis EA. Embryology of the eye. In: Yanoff M, Duker JS, Augsburger JJ, et al., eds. *Ophthalmology.* Amsterdam: Elsevier; 2004.
34. Gunvant P, Broadway DC, Watkins RJ. Reliability and reproducibility of the BVI ultrasonic pachymeter. *Eye.* 2003;17:825–828.
35. Oculus Pentacam. Oculus ophthalmic diagnostic devices. Available at: http://www.oculus.de/us/sites/detail_ger.php?page=322. Accessed March 24, 2008.
36. Kim SW, Byun YJ, Kim EK, et al. Central corneal thickness measurements in unoperated eyes and eyes after PRK for myopia using Pentacam, Orbscan II, and ultrasonic pachymetry. *J Refract Surg.* 2007;23:888–894.
37. Zhao PS, Wong TY, Wong WL, et al. Comparison of central corneal thickness measurements by Visante Anterior Segment Optical Coherence Tomography with ultrasound pachymetry. *Am J Ophthalmol.* 143:1047–1049.
38. Doughty MJ, Zaman ML. Human corneal thickness and its impact on intraocular pressure measures. *Surv Ophthalmol.* 2000;44:367–408.
39. Wolfs RC, Klaver CC, Vingerling JR, et al. Distribution of central corneal thickness and its association with intraocular pressure: The Rotterdam Study. *Am J Ophthalmol.* 1997;123:767–772.
40. Harasymowycz PJ, Pappamatheakis DG, Ennis M, et al. Relationship between travoprost and central corneal thickness in ocular hypertension and open-angle glaucoma. *Cornea.* 2007;26:34–41.
41. Lass JH, Eriksson GL, Osterling L, et al. Comparison of the corneal effects of latanoprost, fixed combination latanoprost-timolol, and timolol, and timolol: a double-masked randomized, one year study. *Ophthalmology.* 2001;108:264–271.
42. Wirtitsch MG, Findl O, Heinz H, et al. Effect of dorzolamide hydrochloride on central corneal thickness in humans with cornea guttata. *Arch Ophthalmol.* 2007;125:1345–1350.
43. Lass JH, Khosrof SA, Laurence JK, et al. A double-masked, randomized, 1-year study comparing the corneal effects of dorzolamide, timolol, and betaxolol. *Arch Ophthalmol.* 1998;116:1003–1010.
44. Egan CA, Hodge DO, McLaren JW, et al. Effect of dorzolamide on corneal endothelial function in human eyes. *Invest Ophthalmol Vis Sci.* 1998;39:23–29.

45. Liu J, Roberts CJ. Influence of corneal biomechanical properties on intraocular pressure measurement quantitative analysis. *J Cataract Refract Surg.* 2005;31:146–155.
46. Available at: http://www.ocularresponseanalyzer.com/how.html. Accessed March 24, 2009.
47. Bochmann F, Ang GS, Azuara-Blanco A. Lower corneal hysteresis in glaucoma patients with acquired pit of the optic nerve (APON). *Graefes Arch Clin Exp Ophthalmol.* 2008; Epub ahead of print.
48. Congdon NG, Broman AT, Bandeen-Roche K, et al. Central corneal thickness and corneal hysteresis associated with glaucoma damage. *Am J Ophthalmol.* 2006;141:495–505.
49. Laiquzzaman M, Bhojwani R, Cunliffe I, et al. Diurnal variation of ocular hysteresis in normal subjects: relevance in clinical context. *Clin Exp Ophthalmol.* 2006;34:114–118.
50. Kniestedt C, Nee M, Stamper RL. Dynamic contour tonometry: a comparative study on human cadaver eyes. *Arch Ophthalmol.* 2004;122:1287–1293.

# Chapter 9
# Glaucoma Risk Factors: Family History – The Genetics of Glaucoma

John R. Samples

## 9.1 Introduction

Who goes blind with glaucoma? People with a family history of blindness go blind with glaucoma. The association of open angle glaucoma and family history has been known for years[1]; the lifetime risk for first-degree relatives of affected individuals to develop open angle glaucoma is 22% when compared with a 2% risk in controls,[2] but clinicians routinely overlook this fact when interviewing and evaluating patients. Patients are rarely accurate in reporting family history. Three genetic loci for glaucoma were first found in a single glaucoma practice in Portland, Oregon – GLC1C, GLC1F, and GLC1G – because of repeated and persistent inquiries about affected relatives. Asking a patient only once about his or her family history is rarely effective; patients tend to confuse macular degeneration, cataracts, and glaucoma.

The purpose of this chapter is to call attention to family history as a critical risk factor and provide a basis for those interested in gaining a basic understanding of the currently known genetics of glaucoma and its implications on patient care. A complete course in human genetics is beyond the scope of this chapter; selected genes, loci, phenotypes, associations, and salient references are presented here to enable the reader to take an inquiry to the next step if they wish to do so and to answer the most common questions posed by patients.

Perhaps the most important concept in discussing glaucoma genetics is to point out that it is likely both monogenic and polygenic. Instances where a single gene causes glaucoma (monogenic) have emerged (e.g., the *myocilin* and *optineurin* genes), but in other instances glaucoma is much more likely the result of multiple genes (polygenic). Being polygenic makes a disease substantially more difficult to study. Unique susceptibility genes and genetic variants also likely play a significant role in glaucoma. The value in testing for these genes will ultimately be based on their clinical utility; while the test also needs to be cost-effective.

Terminology is important in a discussion of this topic. The genetic loci for open angle glaucomas are termed GLC1, the narrow angle glaucomas are termed GLC2, and the congenital glaucomas are termed GLC3. Many of the secondary glaucomas have their own designations. Table 9.1 details selected genes, loci, phenotypes, and associations. Ultimately, glaucoma may be defined in genetic terms rather than anatomically or biochemically, but because of the complications of the influence of risk factors, the concept of susceptibility, and the polygenic nature of the disease, it is unlikely that this will occur in the immediate future.

## 9.2 Definitions and Nomenclature

Humans have 23 pairs of chromosomes with two copies of most genes; one donated from the maternal side and one donated from the paternal side. Each location that generates a protein is termed a gene, and each gene consists of numerous sequences of DNA that may have mutations or single nucleotide substitutions (SNPs). The term *exon* refers to specific regions of DNA that encodes for messenger RNA. Genes have their own taxonomy. They may be grouped into families or into functional classes. Gene families may be regulatory or structural. Genes have alternate forms called alleles. Alternate alleles at a single genetic locus are known as polymorphisms.

The first polymorphism to be described in humans was for the ABO blood groups in 1901.[28] Many polymorphisms have been subsequently identified in human populations. Polymorphisms may be considered "usually normal" variations; they are not necessarily indicative of pathology. Linkage data (information gathered from medical and research reporting) following transmission of a disease gene with specific chromosome markers through a family of affected individuals can be used to narrow the initial field of more than 20,000–25,000 human genes to a chromosomal subregion containing several hundred genes.

The three basic modes of inheritance are autosomal dominant in which a gene is passed and a single gene prevails on generating a protein whenever it is present; autosomal recessive in which two copies of the same gene

**Table 9.1** Selected genes and loci associated with glaucoma

| Loci | Gene | Chromosome | Phenotype | Comment | References |
|---|---|---|---|---|---|
| GLC1A | MYOC | 1q23-24 | JOAG, POAG | GLC1A maps to chromosome 1 | Stone[3]; Sheffield[4] |
| GLC1B | – | 2cen-q13 | POAG | GLC1B maps to chromosome 2 and has been associated with relatively low pressures | Stoilova[5] |
| GLC1C | – | 3q21-24 | POAG | GLC1C on chromosome 3 appears to produce a high pressure glaucoma which has a late onset and a moderate response to medications, very typical of the usual type of open angle glaucoma | Wirtz[6] |
| GLC1D | – | 8p23 | POAG | GLC1D is associated with a high pressure glaucoma and maps to the long arm of chromosome 8 | Trifan[7] |
| GLC1E | OPTN | 10p13-15 | LTG, POAG | GLC1E may be associated with glaucoma with lower pressures and like GLC1B may render the optic nerve to be more sensitive at lower pressures | Rezaie[8]; Sarfarazi[9] |
| GLC1F | – | 7q35-36 | POAG | There is an association of pigmentary dispersion syndrome with a chromosome distal to GLC1F | Wirtz[10] |
| GLC1G | WDR36 | 5q22.1 | POAG | GLC1G has been mapped | Monemi[11]; Kramer[12] |
| GLC1H | – | 2p16.3-p15 | POAG | GLC1H, GLC1I, GLC1J, GLC1K, GLC1M, and GLC1N have all been described, and it is likely that there will be additional genetic loci for open angle glaucoma in the future | Lin[13,14]; Suriyapperuma[15] |
| GLC1I | – | 15q11-q13 | POAG | | Allingham[16] |
| GLC1J | – | 9q22 | JOAG | | Wiggs[17] |
| GLC1K | – | 20p12 | JOAG | | Wiggs[17] |
| GLC1L | – | 3p22-p21 | POAG | | Baird[18] |
| GLC1M | – | 5q22.1-q32 | JOAG | | Pang[19] |
| GLC1N | – | 15q22-q24 | JOAG | | Wang[20] |
| GLC3A | CYP1B1 | 2p21 | PCG | | Sarfarazi[21] |
| GLC3B | – | 1p36 | PCG | | Akarsu[22] |
| GLC3C | – | 14q24.3 | PCG | | Stoilov[23] |
| RIEG1 (IRID2) | PITX2 | 4q25-27 | Axenfeld-Reiger, iridogoniodysgenesis | | Kulak[24] |
| RIEG2 | – | 13q14 | Axenfeld-Reiger | | Lin[13] |
| IRID1 | FOXC1 (FKHL7) | 6p25 | Axenfeld-Reiger, PCG | | Raymond[25] |
| PAX6 | PAX6 | 11p13 | Anirida, Peters, Axenfeld-Reiger | | Hanson[26] |
| LOXL1 | LOXL1 | 15q24 | Pseudoexfoliation glaucoma | | Thorleifsson[27] |

*JOAG* juvenile open angle glaucoma; *LTG* low tension glaucoma; *PCG* primary congenital glaucoma; *POAG* primary open angle glaucoma.

have to be present before it is expressed; and sexlinked, in which case it may appear if an individual is male, XY, but not XY if the individual is female, in which case they are XX.

Mutations occurring in DNA result in phenotypes that include both aberrant RNA and protein products. A phenotype is any characteristic or train of an organism (e.g., its morphology), development, or biochemical properties. Conceptually, phenotypes result from gene expression as well as environmental factors, and possible interactions of the two. In glaucoma, environmental factors affecting glaucoma might include oscillations and pulsations that may be of physiologic importance (see Sidebar 4.1), nutrition (see Chaps. 56 and 60) and blood flow (see Chap. 11).

There are several major categories of mutation including the following:

- Genome mutations that affect the total number of chromosomes in the cells (monosomy, trisomy, etc.).
- Chromosome mutations that are microscopically visible and are often studied in human genetics laboratories, such as the deletion, duplication, inversion, and translocations.
- Gene mutations where alterations occur in the discrete sequences of coding and noncoding DNA – for example, single nucleotide polymorphisms. (This last type of mutation gives rise to the highest number of known genetic diseases.)

Mutations may arise de novo in germ cells and appear without warning in an affected child (e.g., as is sometimes seen in pediatric glaucoma), or may not be manifested until adulthood. Most new mutations are found in x-linked recessive conditions and in severe conditions with autosomal dominant inheritance. If the affected individual reproduces, the new mutation will be inherited according to the usual rules of Mendelian transmission. Mutations may also arise in differentiated tissues.

Targeted mutagenesis (artificial genetic mutation) is a laboratory technique in which mutations are made to elucidate the function of a particular gene, and has been successfully used in mice. The phenotype exhibited by mutant mice can be used to research the literature for individuals with a similar disorder. This procedure, called *gene knockout technology*, is useful and many gene knockouts have been created. Most common human diseases, including glaucoma, are thought to result from mutations in multiple genes, and the knockout technique may be particularly useful in studying how particular combinations of mutations interact with one another. Because of the genetic differences between mice and humans, some mutations known to cause disease in humans do not result in a similar phenotype in mice. Thus, knockouts are not always informative.

There are a number of strategies for finding genes causing human disease:

- The *candidate gene* approach assumes that it is known which gene is likely to be abnormal.
- *Linkage analysis*, which is basically a fishing expedition with success dependent upon the number of individuals that are found. Linkage analysis can be difficult for diseases with late onset such as primary open angle glaucoma and macular degeneration.
- Using clues from chromosomal abnormalities.
- Whole genome-wide association studies.

Although the initial discoveries of glaucoma loci appeared to be monogenic, very few human diseases are monogenic, and currently the prevailing wisdom is that glaucoma is highly complex and that a variety of pathological processes are involved. It is likely that each of the open angle glaucomas have different yet subtle phenotypic characteristics. The direct implication of this is that some may respond better to medicines, while others ought to have surgery because of the aggressive nature of the disease since the diseases may vary in terms of their time course and their tendency to progress. Other major phenotypic differences may exist with regard to corneal thickness, diurnal fluctuation, appearance of the optic nerve head (perhaps detected by an optic nerve analyzer before clinical glaucoma is actually detected) (Table 9.2).

*Transcription factors* are one example of a functional class of genes that have potential importance for glaucoma. These are genes that alter the production of messenger RNA by other genes. Transcription factors bind directly to promoters that are specific DNA sites in the genes that the factors regulate. These factors are proteins that bind DNA sequence, and thereby control the transfer of genetic

**Table 9.2** Potential phenotypic differences for OAG

Potential phenotypic differences at each genetic loci for open angle glaucoma
Anterior
  Corneal thickness
  Corneal compliance
  Fine angle structures
  Insertion of the iris
  Transillumination defects at the route of the iris
  Prominence of Schwalbe's line
  Schlemm's canal and collector channels (requires UBM)
Posterior
  Optic nerve
  Geometric aspects of cupping
  Peripapillary atrophy
  Optic nerve head size
  Optic nerve head blood vessel positioning
  Nerve fiber hemorrhages
Vascular
  Blood flow in the optic nerve
  Peripapillary blood flow
  Nerve fiber layer
  Patterns of thickness variation
Drug responses
  Alpha agonist drugs
  Beta blockers
  Carbonic anhydrase inhibitors
  Prostaglandins
  New agents
Other
  Pattern of diurnal pressure fluctuation
  Potential markers for glaucoma in aqueous
  CD44
  Matrix metalloproteinases (in aqueous)
  Proteoglycans
  Other potential biochemical markers

information from DNA to RNA. They may either do this alone or in combination with other proteins in the form of a complex. There are many genes that encode for DNA binding transcription factors. Technology at the time of this writing is about to make array testing of many transcription factors available, and in so doing, may substantially transform our understanding of glaucoma (Genefac, Portland Oregon). A second important type of gene is the *homeobox genes*. The homeobox is a 180 base pair DNA sequence that is highly conserved among the genes of all vertebrates. A third important type of gene is the *zinc-finger* gene. Here the DNA binding motif consists of a small loop of amino acids held together by a single zinc atom.

Single nucleotide polymorphisms SNPs are variations in single nucleotides resulting in a DNA sequence variation that may generate complicated protein changes and may themselves be associated with diseases. Numerous SNP associations have been found with diseases, and it is now possible to do a cheek swab test and submit ones' own genes for testing to any of several services available on the Web (e.g., http://www.navigenic.com and http://www.23andMe.com). Indeed, some of these services actually provide an annual subscription to provide updates as clinically important SNPs are found. At the time of this writing, none offer glaucoma-related testing but that is likely to change in the near future. SNPs can be assigned a minor allele frequency, the lowest frequency at a locus that is observed with a particular population. An SNP allele that is found in one geographic or ethnically defined group may be much rarer than in another. SNPs found in a coding sequence will not always change the amino acid sequence of the protein that is produced since there is some degeneracy in the genetic code. An SNP in which both forms lead to the same peptide sequence is termed *synonymous*. If a different polypeptide is produced, as in the case of exfoliation, then it is termed *nonsynonymous*. SNPs that are not in specific protein coding regions may still have substantial consequence for transcription factor binding and for gene splicing. While it is obvious that DNA sequences can affect how humans respond to chemical drugs and vaccines, they are useful in comparing groups of individuals with specific diseases.[29]

## 9.3 Early Findings

Kass and Becker[1] were among the first to observe a relationship between family history and glaucoma, and focused their research on the cup-to-disc ratio, elevated pressure, and the glucocorticoid response. Their early investigations into hereditary aspects of glaucoma noted that there was a relationship between family history and the presence of glaucoma, but that it seemed to defy simple genetic analysis.

Becker, and later Armaly,[30] found that glucocorticoid treatment re-elevated IOP more often in glaucoma patients than in other individuals. Testing of family members showed that this response was usually inherited as an autosomal recessive trait. Subsequently, Polansky[31] theorized that the mutations of these genes in the trabecular meshwork were associated with a corticoid steroid response. He called the specific induced proteins "*Trabecular meshwork Inducible Glucocortoid Response protein*" (TIGR), the same protein later being termed "*Myocilin*". Initially, this protein was thought to be associated uniquely with juvenile glaucoma, but later, it was found to be associated with up to 3% of the glaucomas in the general population. The myocilin gene was subsequently mapped to chromosome 1. Since then, a number of additional genetic loci have been identified that are associated with open angle glaucoma. They all appear to be autosomal dominant.

## 9.4 Types of Glaucoma and Genetics

Open angle glaucoma is the most common form of glaucoma affecting more than 33 million people world-wide.[32] Although many types of subdivisions are possible, for our purposes, open angle glaucomas may be divided into adult or primary open angle glaucomas (POAG), juvenile open angle glaucomas (JOAG), and low-tension glaucomas (LTG) – also referred to as normal tension glaucoma The reasons for the distinction between LTG and POAG is addressed elsewhere in the text (see Chaps. 34 and 35), but the distinction may be somewhat artificial, especially from a genetic perspective. However, the lack of distinction between JOAG and POAG is very important. JOAG is defined as having an earlier age of onset, in the range of age 3 to age 25, as discrete from pediatric glaucoma, which is discussed in Chap. 50. JOAG seems to be an autosomal dominant disorder, whereas POAG seems to be an inherited as autosomal dominant with incomplete penetrance.

The first gene found for open angle glaucoma, GLC1A or myocilin, has both juvenile and adult phenotypes, depending on which mutation is present. At the time of this writing in 2009, there are 14 well documented chromosomal loci for POAG that are listed by the Human Genome Organization (HUGO), which can be accessed at http://www.genenames.org/index.html. Most loci were elucidated using genetic linkage analysis in families. Table 9.3 lists selected loci and genes for open angle glaucoma; although it is not comprehensive as the list continues to expand, and in some instances, loci designations have been claimed without full publication or disclosure at the time of this writing, but it is quite likely that this list will lengthen and that additional detail will be available in the near future.

**Table 9.3** Selected gene variants which have been associated with glaucoma

Select genetic variants associated with glaucoma[a]

| Gene | Chromosome | Phenotype | Association | Reference |
| --- | --- | --- | --- | --- |
| ANP | 1p36.2 | POAG | Atrial natriuretic polypeptide | Tunny[33] |
| CDH-1 | 16q22.1 | POAG | Cadherin 1 | Lin[34] |
| CYP1B1 | 2p22-p21 | POAG | Cytochrome P450, 1B1 | Bhattacharjee[35]; Melki[36] |
| HSPA1A | 6p21.3 | POAG, NTG | Heat shock 70 kDa protein 1A | Tosaka[37] |
| IGF2 | 11p15.5 | POAG | Insulin-type growth factor 2 | Lin[34] |
| IL1α | 2q14 | POAG | Interleukin-1α | Wang[38] |
| IL1β | 2q14 | POAG | Interleukin-1β | Lin[39] |
| MTHFR | 1p36.3 | NTG, POAG | Methylenetetrahydrofolate | Junemann[40] |
| NOS3 | 7q36 | POAG with migraine | Nitric oxide synthase 3 | Tunny[41] |
| OLFM2 | 19p13.2 | POAG | Olfactomedin 2 | Funayama[42] |
| OPA1 | 3q28-q29 | NTG | Optic atrophy 1 | Liu[14] |
| P21 | 6p21.2 | POAG | p53 signaling pathway | Lin[34] |
| PON1 | 7q21.3 | NTG | Paraoxonase 1 | Inagaki[43] |
| TAP1 | 6p21.3 | POAG | ABC transporter, MHC 1 | Lin[39] |
| TNFα | 6p21.3 | POAG | Tumor necrosis | Lin[44] |

[a]Selected for relevance to cytokines, growth factors and potential interesting proteins.

### 9.4.1 Genetic Loci of Glaucoma

While it is known that major gene defects cause glaucoma in specific individuals, the proportion of glaucoma patients affected by one or several major genes remains unknown; unpublished estimates of the frequency vary from as little as a few percent to 50%. This is likely due to the complex nature of glaucoma and (potentially) the interaction with environmental factors; the relative contribution of environmental and genetic factors remains unknown at this point. It is exciting to contemplate that there are different phenotypic characteristics associated with specific loci and mutations. Understanding which differences are associated with which proteins could lead to major breakthroughs in diagnostics and treatment. The prevalence of glaucoma, enlarged cup-disc ratios, and elevated intraocular pressure (IOP) are all much higher in siblings and offspring of patients with glaucoma than in the general population. A positive family history remains a major risk factor for the development of POAG although some have misinterpreted the Ocular Hypertension Treatment Study (OHTS) study as suggesting that this is not the case. That study evaluated patients with intraocular pressure elevation without glaucoma and provided a simple query about family history of glaucoma. A detailed approach is required to elicit family history in patients.

### 9.4.2 Gene Variants

Numerous gene variants, as discrete from mutations, have been associated with glaucoma and are presented in Table 9.3.

The list presented here is a only a partial one. From a pathophysiologic viewpoint, some of these are quite interesting. Tumor necrosis factors alpha and interleukin 1, both cytokines which play an important role in laser trabeculoplasty, have been associated with open angle glaucoma. The gene optic atrophy 1, OPA, has also been associated with glaucoma in some populations but not others.[14]

### 9.4.2.1 GLC1A (Myocilin, TIGR)

The first reported locus for POAG, at chromosome 1, was initially described by Stone[45] at the locus GLC1A. This is the location for the production of myocilin. Myocilin was concurrently described by Polansky as being glucocorticoid inducible and termed Trabecular meshwork Inducible Glucocortoid Response protein, or more commonly TIGR.[31] To date, GLC1A is the most studied of the glaucoma genes.

Myocilin/TIGR consists of a protein with myoscin-like sequences at one end and olfactomedin at the C-terminus end. Myocilin is not unique to the eye and is found in many tissues and organs.[46] The sequence homology is not 100% for myosin and olfactomedin, though it is sometimes erroneously said to be so. The N-terminal of myocilin is encoded by exon 1 and has approximately 25–30% amino acid homology with myosin heavy chain.[46]

Prevalence of all myocilin mutations has been between 3 and 5%; it has one promoter region and three exons with approximately 40 mutations having been described to date. The protein is expressed throughout the body.[47]

All of the known genetic POAGs are autosomal dominant and myocilin is no exception. Approximately 90% of myocilin carriers are said to develop glaucoma.[48] Individuals who are homozygous for some of the mutations do not get glaucoma, but this is not the case with all of the mutations.[49]

Introduction of mycollin protein appears to increase outflow resistance in organ explant systems where eyebank eyes are subjected to flow.[50,51] Paradoxically perhaps, Caballero et al[52] has shown that overexpression of the N terminal domain of myocilin results in an increase of outflow facility perfused anterior segment system that is not the effect one would, at first glance, expect from a "glaucoma causing" protein. The mechanism by which myocilin is implicated in glaucoma remains unclear and the subject of substantial speculation. Intracellular accumulation of misfolded proteins appears to be the result of a disease-associated form of myocilin being present. Myocilin is associated with the shedding of small vesicles, exosomes, in the aqueous. Exosomes have ligands that are involved in paracrine and autocrine signaling and play a role in cellular homeostasis.[53]

Pigmentary, pseudoexofoliation, angle closure, and mixed-mechanism glaucoma have been associated with myocilin mutations.[54,55] The report of a family with mixed-mechanism glaucoma having a myocilin mutation is intriguing since it suggests that two gene interactions, one for open angle glaucoma and one for narrow angle glaucoma, can both lead to glaucoma. One mutation (Gly399Val MYOC) led to adult POAG with a mean age of onset of 51. When this mutation occurred in combination with a CYP1B1 mutation (Arg368His), there was a mean age of onset of 27 years. Digenic and polygenic interactions such as this may explain much of the present complexity of open angle glaucoma.

An excellent and interesting source of further information will be found at www.myocilin.com. This chapter would not be complete without noting that there has been a long-standing controversy about the role of a promoter mutation for GLC1A, which may have particular clinical utility.[56]

The second gene to be discovered was on the fifth identified locus 17.[8] Optineurin is located on GLC1E at chromosome 10. Some of these patients, but not all, appear to have a low tension-like phenotype.[8] Estimates on the frequency of optineurin have varied substantially, with the original report identifying 16 open angle glaucoma patients as having the disease.[8] GLC1E has numerous mutations. Low tension patients who have E50K have a more severe form of glaucoma when compared with those who do not have the mutation.[57,58] It has been suggested that those with the mutation appear to have more advanced cupping and require more frequent surgical intervention.[59] A synonymous variant Thr34Thr was associated with glaucoma in Japan.[60] This paper is particularly interesting because certain TNF alpha variants in combination with optineurin OPTN variants occurred more frequently in POAG patients. This also suggests that several genes may be associated with POAG.

Optineurin localizes to several ocular tissues including the trabecular meshwork (TM), retina, and nonpigmented ciliary epithelium.[8] Optineurin may have a role in TNF alpha signaling pathways and has also been implicated in modulation of cellular cytokeleoin of TM cells.

### 9.4.2.2 WDR36

WDR36 was initially linked to the GLC1G locus at chromosome 5 and subsequently linked to the gene, WDR 36.[11,12] The original family that established linkage to the GLC1G locus did not demonstrate any WDR36 mutations, and thus suggested that another gene might be at the GLC1G locus.

## 9.5 Exfoliation Glaucoma

It is well known that exfoliation syndrome varies among ethnic groups as detailed elsewhere (see Chap. 39). From a genetics perspective, genomic-wide associations identified a locus on 15q24 that is strongly associated with exfoliation. The gene has been identified as lysyl oxidase-like 1 (LOXL1) and it is strongly associated with exfoliation. Two single nucleotide polymorphisms in the first exon of the gene and one single-nucleotide polymorphism in the first intron were identified. The two variants, GLY153Asp and AR141Leu, cause mis-sense changes in the LOXL1 protein and account for nearly all the observed cases of exfoliation in Icelandic and Swedish cohorts.[27] Common sequence variants in the LOXL1 gene confer susceptibility to exfoliation glaucoma.[27] All exfoliation patients have LOXL1 polymorphisms, whether they have glaucoma or not, suggesting that other factors are involved in the development of glaucoma.

## 9.6 Congenital Glaucoma

Primary congenital glaucoma is described elsewhere in this text (see Chap. 50). Three genetic loci have been found, they are GLC3A at locus 2p21,[21] GLC3 B at chromosome locus 1p36,[22] and GLC3C at locus 14q24.3.[23] CYP1B1 is regarded as the most important enzyme of the human cytochrome p450 pathway and is the gene at GLC3A.[9] Mutations of this gene have been reported in 20–30% of ethnically mixed populations and nearly 100% of highly consanguineous groups.[61,62] This enzyme is involved in the metabolism of drug and dietary compounds. Mutations are likely to profoundly disturb some aspects of development.

## 9.7 Mesodermal Dysgenesis Syndromes

Mesodermal dysgensis syndromes occur in a range from posterior embryotoxin with its anteriorly placed Schwalbe's line to Axenfeld-Rieger anomaly found with iris hypoplasia, polycoria, and correctopia. Axenfeld-Rieger's syndrome consists of the anomaly with systemic findings that are primarily skeletal. Two transcription factors have been identified as causative PITX2, which is at the REIG1 locus.[63,64]

Peters anomaly is characterized by corneal leukoma and defects in Descemet's membrane with iridocorneal adhesions. Numerous mutations have been reported in the PAX6 gene for Aniridia.[26]

## 9.8 Angle Closure Glaucoma and Genetic Defects

Angle closure glaucoma has long been known to run in families, clinicians find that it defies simple genetic analysis. A group in Taiwan which included the author of this chapter reported a single nucleotide polymorphism for angle closure involving MMP9.[65] Others have not yet been able to replicate this work.[66] The reason for failure to replicate may be that different populations were studied. Further work in the genetics of angle closure is needed, since it could be an extremely useful predictor for who is going to develop angle closure. It seems likely possible that there are phenotypic variations among angle closure patients that have not yet been fully appreciated, which may be discovered through working with families. A non-ophthalmic gene (NNO1) in which the angle is closed due to the distortion of the anterior segment has been described.[67]

## 9.9 Future for Gene Therapy

In instances where glaucoma appears to be monogenic or where it is polygenic and all of the genes are known, there is a prospect for gene therapy. To date, no gene therapy trials have been performed in humans for glaucoma, but trabecular meshwork has been transfected.[68] It should be noted that finding a gene in glaucoma does not necessarily implicate exclusively either the trabecular meshwork or the optic nerve; one or both may be involved. Conceivably, a gene could involve the ciliary body, the collector channels or even the aqueous veins. Where there is high intraocular pressure, it is likely that the deep trabecular meshwork is involved.

## 9.10 Future for Genetic Testing

It is likely that the genes causing glaucoma vary in their phenotypic expression. For instance, corneal thickness may be a manifestation of phenotype. There is a distinct possibility that optic nerves having varying phenotypic characteristics among the glaucoma genes, for instance in the presence of peripapillary nerve change or other specific parameters.

A commercial genetic test for three of the lesser mutations for GLC1A has been available in the United States for some time. This test evaluated three lesser exons and one promoter gene. Genetic testing in the United *States was dramatically altered by the Genetic Privacy Act of 2008* (110th Congress 2008), which prevents insurance from discriminating against applicants on the basis of genetic findings alone.[69]

Table 9.4 ABC transporters and glaucoma loci. Adapted from Knepper[74]

| ABC transporters and glaucoma loci | | | |
|---|---|---|---|
| Symbol | Location | Name | Function |
| ABCA1 | 9q21-22 | GLC1J (JOAG) – Wiggs[17] | Cholesterol efflux onto HDL |
| ABCA2 | 9q34 | JOAG – Knepper[70] | Multidrug resistance |
| ABCA5,6,8,9,10 | 17q24 | Wiggs[71] | Unknown |
| ABCB1 | 7p21 | Alzheimer/POAG Knepper[70] | Multidrug resistance (MDR) |
| ABCB2 | 6p21 | POAG polymorphism/Lin[44,72] | Peptide transport |
| ABCB8 | 7q35-36 | GLC1F Wirtz/Samples/Acott[10] | Unknown |
| ABCF2 | | Pigment dispersion syndrome | |
| ABCC8 | 11p15 | Charcot–Marie with early onset glaucoma[73] | Multidrug resistance |
| ABCG5 | 2p21 | JOAG | Sterol transport |
| ABCG8 | | CYP1B1 (causative gene)[35] | Multidrug resistance |
| | 15q11-13 | GLC1I Allingham/Wiggs[16] | ATPase class V modifier of ABC |

## 9.11 Pharmacogenetics

With the finding of individual loci for open angle glaucoma, it has been apparent that patients with some genetic glaucomas respond differently to medications from others. Many of the genes may point to a single class of proteins, called ABC transporter proteins some of which are involved in drug metabolism (Table 9.4). This is an area of significant future research since it may be that the genes found in glaucoma patients will predict how they behave clinically. Genetic differences in the response to systemic beta blockers are well established. Ultimately, the usefulness of this approach will depend upon how widespread the different genetic loci are actually found to be. Unpublished estimates vary from a low of 3% to a high of 50%, and it is likely that the truth lies somewhere in the middle.

This act is likely to eliminate the possibility of patients who are found to have glaucoma genes from undergoing significant discrimination.

## References

1. Kass MA, Becker B. Genetics of primary open-angle glaucoma. *Sight Sav Rev.* 1978;48:21–28.
2. Wolfs RC, Klaver CC, Ramrattan RS, Van Duijn CM, Hofman A, De Jong PT. Genetic risk of primary open-angle glaucoma. Population-based familial aggregation study. *Arch Ophthalmol.* 1998;116:1640–1645.
3. Stone MA, Fingert JH, Alward WL, et al. Identification of a gene that causes primary open angle glaucoma. *Science.* 1997;275: 668–670.
4. Sheffield VC, Stone EM, Alward WL, et al. Genetic linkage of familial open angle glaucoma to chromosome 1q21-q31. *Nat Genet.* 1993;4:668–670.
5. Stoilova D, Child A, Trifan OC, Crick RP, Coakes RL, Sarfarazi M. Localization of a second locus (GLC1B) for adult-onset primary open angle glaucoma to the 2cen-q13 region. *Genomics.* 1996;36:142–150.
6. Wirtz MK, Samples JR, Kramer PL, et al. Mapping a gene for adult-onset primary open-angle glaucoma to chromosome 3q. *Am J Hum Genet.* 1997;60:296–304.
7. Trifan OC, Traboulsi EI, Stoilova D, et al. A third locus (GLC1D) for adult-onset primary open-angle glaucoma maps to the 8q23 region. *Am J Ophthalmol.* 1998;126(1998):17–28.
8. Rezaie T, Child A, Hitchings R, et al. Adult-onset primary open-angle glaucoma caused by mutations in optineurin. *Science.* 2002;295:1077–1079.
9. Sarfarazi M, Stoilov I, Schenkman JB. Genetics and biochemistry of primary congenital glaucoma. *Ophthalmol Clin North America.* 2003;16:543–544.
10. Wirtz MK, Samples JR, Rust K, et al. GLC1F, a new primary open-angle glaucoma locus, maps to 7q35-q36. *Arch Ophthalmol.* 1999;117:237–241.
11. Monemi S, Spaeth G, DaSilva A, et al. Identification of a novel adult-onset primary open-angle glaucoma (POAG) gene on 5q22.1 the 1p36 region. *Hum Mol Genet.* 2005;14:725–733.
12. Kramer PL, Samples JR, Monemi S, Sykes R, Sarfarazi M, Wirtz MK. The role of the WDR36 gene on chromosome 5q22.1 in a large family with primary open-angle glaucoma mapped to this region. *Arch Ophthalmol.* 2006;124:1328–1331.
13. Lin Y, Liu T, Li J, et al. A genome-wide scan maps a novel autosomal dominant juvenile-onset open-angle glaucoma locus to 2p15-16. *Mol Vis.* 2008;14:739–744.
14. Liu Y, Schmidt S, Qin X, et al. No association between OPA1 polymorphisms and primary open-angle glaucoma in three different populations. *Mol Vis.* 2007;13:2137–2141.
15. Suriyapperuma SP, Child A, Desai T, et al. A new locus (GLC1H) for adult-onset primary open-angle glaucoma maps to the 2p15-p16 region. *Arch Ophthalmol.* 2007;125:86–925.
16. Allingham RR, Wiggs JL, Hauser ER, et al. Early adult-onset POAG linked to 15q11-13 using ordered subset analysis. *Invest Ophthalmol Vis Sci.* 2005;46:2002–2005.
17. Wiggs JL, Lynch S, Ynagi G, et al. A genomewide scan identifies novel early-onset primary open-angle glaucoma loci on 9q22 and 20p12. *Am J Hum Genet.* 2004;74(6):1314–1320.
18. Baird PN, Richardson AJ, Craig JE, Mackey DA, Rochtchina E, Mitchell P. Analysis of optineurin (OPTN) gene mutations in subjects with and without glaucoma: the Blue Mountains Eye Study. *Graefes Arch Clin Exp Ophthalmol.* 2004;32:518–522.
19. Pang CP, Fan BJ, Canlas O, et al. A genome-wide scan maps a novel juvenile-onset primary open angle glaucoma locus to chromosome 5q. *Mol Vis.* 2006;12:85–92.
20. Wang DY, Fan BJ, Chua JKH, et al. A genome-wide scan maps a novel juvenile-onset primary open-angle glaucoma locus to 15q. *Invest Ophthalmol Vis Sci.* 2006;47:5315–5321.
21. Sarfarazi M, Akarsu AN, Hossain A, et al. Assignment of a locus (GLC3AGLC3B) for primary congenital glaucoma (Buphthalmos) to 2p21 and evidence for genetic heterogeneity. *Genomics.* 1995;30:171–177.
22. Akarsu AN, Turacli ME, Aktan SG, et al. A second locus (GLC3B) for primary congenital glaucoma (Buphthalmos) maps to the 1p36 region. *Hum Mol Genet.* 1996;5:1199–1203.
23. Stoilov IR, Safarazi M. The Third Genetic Locus (GLC3C) for primary congenital glaucoma (PCG) maps to chromosome 14q24.3. *Invest Ophthalmol Vis Sci.* 2002. Available at: http://abstracts.iovs.org/cgi/content/abstract/43/12/3015. Accessed May 15, 2009.
24. Kulak SC, Kozlowski K, Semina EV, Pearce WG, Walter MA. Mutation in the RIEG1 gene in patients with iridogoniodysgenesis syndrome. *Hum Mol Genet.* 1998;7:1113–1117.
25. Raymond V, Dubois S, Rodrigue MA, et al. Chromosomal duplication at the IRID1 locus on 6p25 associated with wide variability of the glaucoma phenotypes. *Invest Ophthalmol Vis Sci.* 2002. Available at: http://abstracts.iovs.org/cgi/content/abstract/43/12/3016. Accessed May 15, 2009.
26. Hanson IM, Fletcher JM, Jordan T, et al. Mutations at the PAX 6 locus are found in heterogenous anterior segment malformations including Peters' anomaly. *Nat Genet.* 1994;6:163–173.
27. Thorleifsson G, Magnusson KP, Sulem P, et al. Common sequence variants in the LOXL1 gene confer susceptibility to exfoliation glaucoma. *Science.* 2007;317:1397–1400.
28. Beckman L. ABO bloodtypes reported racial & ethnic distribution sorted by population groups. ABO Blook. July 13, 2008. Available at: http://www.aboblood.com/. Accessed May 20, 2009.
29. Carlson B. SNPs – a shortcut to personalized medicine; medical applications are where the market's growth is expected. Genetic Engineering & Biotechnology News. June 15, 2008. Available at: http://www.genengnews.com/articles/chitem.aspx?aid=2507. Accessed May 10, 2009.

30. Armaly MF. Inheritance of dexamethasone hypertension and glaucoma. *Arch Ophthalmol.* 1967;77:747–751.
31. Nguyen TD, Chen P, Huang WD, Chen H, Johnson D, Polansky JR. Gene structure and proteins of TIGR, an olfactomedin-related glycoprotein cloned from glycocortiocid-induced trabecular meshwork cells. *J Biol Chem.* 1998;273:6341–6350.
32. Quigley HA. Number of people with glaucoma worldwide. *Br J Ophthalmol.* 1996;80:389–393.
33. Tunny TJ, Xu L, Richardson KA, Stowasser M, Gartside M, Gordon RD. Insertion/deletion polymorphism of the angiotensin-converting enzyme gene and loss of the insertion allele in aldosterone-producing adenoma. *J Hum Hypertens.* 1996;10(12):827–830.
34. Lin HJ, Tsai FJ, Hung P, et al. Association of E-cadherin gene 3'-UTR C/T polymorphism with primary open angle glaucoma. *Ophthalmic Res.* 2006;38(1):44–48.
35. Bhattacharjee A, Banerjee D, Mookherjee S, et al. Variation Consortium. Leu432Val polymorphism in CYP1B1 as a susceptible factor towards predisposition to primary open-angle glaucoma. *Mol Vis.* 2008;14:841–850.
36. Melki R, Colomb E, Lefort N, Brézin AP, Garchon HJ. CYP1B1 mutations in French patients with early-onset primary open-angle glaucoma. *J Med Genet.* 2004;41(9):647–651.
37. Tosaka K, Mashima Y, Funayama T, Ohtake Y, Kimura I, Glaucoma Gene Research Group. Association between open-angle glaucoma and gene polymorphism for heat-shock protein 70–1. *Jpn J Ophthalmol.* 2007;51(6):417–423.
38. Wang CY, Shen YC, Lo FY, et al. Polymorphism in the IL-1alpha (-889) locus associated with elevated risk of primary open angle glaucoma. *Mol Vis.* 2006;12:1380–1385.
39. Lin HJ, Tsai CH, Tsai FJ, Chen WC, Chen HY, Fan SS. Transporter associated with antigen processing gene 1 codon 333 and codon 637 polymorphisms are associated with primary open-angle glaucoma. *Mol Diagn.* 2004;8(4):245–252.
40. Jünemann AG, von Ahsen N, Reulbach U, et al. C677T variant in the methylentetrahydrofolate reductase gene is a genetic risk factor for primary open-angle glaucoma. *Am J Ophthalmol.* 2005;139(4):721–723.
41. Tunny TJ, Richardson KA, Clark CV. Association study of the 5' flanking regions of endothelial-nitric oxide synthase and endothelin-1 genes in familial primary open-angle glaucoma. *Clin Exp Pharmacol Physiol.* 1998;25(1):26–29.
42. Funayama T, Mashima Y, Ohtake Y, et al, Glaucoma Gene Research Group. SNPs and interaction analyses of noelin 2, myocilin, and optineurin genes in Japanese patients with open-angle glaucoma. *Invest Ophthalmol Vis Sci.* 2006;47(12):5368–5375.
43. Inagaki Y, Mashima Y, Funayama Y, et al. Paraoxonase 1 gene polymorphisms influence clinical features of open-angle glaucoma. *Graefes Arch Clin Exp Ophthalmol.* 2006;244(8):984–990.
44. Lin HJ, Tsai FJ, Chen WC, Shi YR, Hsu Y, Tsai SW. Association of tumour necrosis factor alpha-308 gene polymorphism with primary open-angle glaucoma in Chinese. *Eye.* 2003;17(1):31–34.
45. Stone EM, Fingert JH, Alward WL, et al. Identification of a gene that causes primary open angle glaucoma. *Science.* 1997;275(5300):668–670.
46. Ortego J, Escribano J, Coca-Pardos M. Cloning and characterization of subtracted cDNAs from a human ciliary body library encoding TIGR, a protein involved in juvenile open angle glaucoma with homology to myosin and olfactomedin. *FEBS Lett.* 1997;413(2):349–35.
47. Fingert JH, Stone EM, Sheffield VC, Alward WL. Myocilin glaucoma. *Surv Ophthalmol.* 2002;147:547–561.
48. Alward WL, Fingert JH, Coote MA, et al. Clinical features associated with mutations in the chromosome 1 open-angle glaucoma gene (GLC1A). *N Engl J Med.* 1998;338(15):1022–1027.
49. Hewitt AW, Bennett SL, Dimasi DP, Craig JE, Mackey DA. A myocilin Gln368STOP homozygote does not exhibit a more severe glaucoma phenotype than heterozygous cases. *Am J Ophthalmol.* 2006;141:402–403.
50. Fautsch MP, Bahler CK, Jewison DJ, Johnson DH. Recombinant TIGR/MYOC increases outflow resistance in the human anterior segment. *Invest Ophthalmol Vis Sci.* 2000;41:4163–4168.
51. Fautsch MP, Bahler CK, Vrabel AM, et al. Perfusion of his-tagged eukaryotic myocilin increases outflow resistance in human anterior segments in the presence of aqueous humor. *Invest Ophthalmol Vis Sci.* 2006;47:213–221.
52. Caballero LL, Rowlette T, Borras T. Altered secretion of a TIGR/MYOC mutant lacking the olfactomedin domain. *Biochim Biophys Acta.* 2000;1502:447–460.
53. Hardy KM, Hoffman EA, Gonzalez P, McKay BS, Stamer WD. Extracellular trafficking of myocilin in human trabecular meshwork cells. *J Biol Chem.* 2005;280:28917–28926.
54. Faucher M, Anctil JL, Rodrigue MA, et al. Founder TIGR/myocilin mutations for glaucoma in the Quebec population. *Hum Mol Genet.* 2002;11: 2077–2090.
55. Vincent AL, Billingsley G, Buys Y, et al. Digenic inheritance of early-onset glaucoma: CYP1B1, a potential modifier gene. *Am J Hum Genet.* 2002;70(2):448–460.
56. Polansky JR, Juster RP, Spaeth GL. Association of the myocilin mt.1 promoter variant with the worsening of glaucomatous disease over time. *Clin Genet.* 2003;64(1):18–27.
57. Hauser MA, Sena DF, Flor J, et al. Distribution of optineurin sequence variations in an ethnically diverse population of low-tension glaucoma patients from the United States. *J Glaucoma.* 2006;15:358–363.
58. Ayala-Lugo RM, Pawar H, Reed DM, et al. Variation in optineurin (OPTN) allele frequencies between and within populations. *Mol Vis.* 2007;13:151–163.
59. Aung T, Rezaie T, Okada K, et al. Clinical features and course of patients with glaucoma with the E50K mutation in the optineurin gene. *Invest Ophthalmol Vis Sci.* 2005;46:2816–2822.
60. Funayama K, Ishikawa K, Ohtake Y, et al. Variants in optineurin gene and their association with tumor necrosis factor-alpha polymorphisms in Japanese patients with glaucoma. *Invest Ophthalmol Vis Sci.* 2004;45:4359–4367.
61. Chakrabarti S, Kaur K, Komatireddy S, et al. Gln48H is the prevalent myocilin mutation in primary open angle and primary congenital glaucoma phenotypes in India. *Mol Vis.* 2005;11:111–113.
62. Chakrabarti S, Kaur K, Kaur I, et al. Globally, CYP1B1 mutations in primary congenital glaucoma are strongly structured by geographic and haplotype backgrounds. *Invest Ophthalmol Vis Sci.* 2006;47:43–47.
63. Semina EV, Reiter R, Leysens NJ, et al. Cloning and characterization of a novol biocoid related homeobox transcription factor gene, RIEG, involved in Rieger syndrome. *Nat Genet.* 1996;14:392–399.
64. Mears AJ, Jordan T, Mirzzayans F, et al. Mutations of the forkhead/winged-helix gene FKHL7 in patients with Axenfeld Rieger anomaly. *Am J Hum Genet.* 1998;63:1316–1328.
65. Wang IJ, Chiang TH, Shih YF, et al. The association of single nucleotide polymorphisms in the MMP-9 gene with susceptibility to acute primary angle closure glaucoma in Taiwanese patients. *Mol Vis.* 2006;12:1223–1232.
66. Aung T, Yong VH, Lim MC, et al. Lack of association between the rs2664538 polymorphism in the MMP-9 gene and primary angle closure glaucoma in Singaporean subjects. *J Glaucoma.* 2008;17:257–258.
67. Othman MI, Sullivan SA, Skuta GL, et al. Autosomal dominant nanophthalmos (NNO1) with high hyperopia and angle-closure glaucoma maps to chromosome 11. *Am J Hum Genet.* 1998;63(5):1411–1418.
68. Filla MS, Liu X, Nguyen TD, et al. In vitro localization of TIGR/MYOC in trabecular meshwork extracellular matrix and binding to fibronectin. *IOVS.* 2002;43:151–161.

69. 110th Congress. H.R. 493 Genetic Information Nondiscrimination Act of 2008. Available at: http://www.govtrack.us/congress/bill.xpd?bill=h110-493&tab=summary. Accessed May 15, 2009.
70. Knepper PA, Nolan MJ, Wirtz MK, et al. Regulation of ABC transporters and glaucoma: new ideas. ARVO 2006; poster.
71. Wiggs JL, Allingham RR, Hossain A, et al. Genome-wide scan for adult onset primary open angle glaucoma. *Hum Mol Genet.* 2000;9(7):1109–1117.
72. Lin HJ, Tsai SC, Tsai FJ, Chen WC, Tsai JJ, Hsu CD. Association of interleukin 1beta and receptor antagonist gene polymorphisms with primary open-angle glaucoma. *Ophthalmologica.* 2003;217(5):358–64.
73. Azzedine H, Bolino A, Taïeb T, et al. Mutations in MTMR13, a new pseudophosphatase homologue of MTMR2 and Sbf1, in two families with an autosomal recessive demyelinating form of Charcot–Marie–Tooth disease associated with early-onset glaucoma. *Am J Hum Genet.* 2003;72(5):1141–1153.
74. Knepper PA, Nolan MJ, Wirtz MK, Samples JR, Allingham RR, Wiggs JL, and Yue BYJT. Regulation of ABC Transporters and Glaucoma: New Ideas invest. *Ophthalmol Vis. Sci.* 2006;47: E-Abstract 174.

# Chapter 10
# Glaucoma Risk Factors: Ethnicity and Glaucoma

M. Roy Wilson and Mark Gallardo

The diagnosis of glaucoma of primary open-angle glaucoma requires the evaluation of multiple ophthalmic characteristics. Additionally, it is usefully to identify accompanying demographic factors that suggest populations at risk for the disease. The risk of the development and/or the progression of glaucoma can be influenced by the patient's race, age, family history of glaucoma, intraocular pressure, central corneal thickness, and presence of certain systemic diseases. Epidemiologic studies have enabled us to better understand those features that place a patient at increased risk for the development of glaucomatous optic neuropathy.[1–18] Studies have also highlighted that racial differences not only exist in the prevalence and incidence of glaucoma but also in those ophthalmic features that are critical in glaucoma detection. Succeeding chapters will focus explicitly on the diagnosis and management of various forms of glaucoma. In this chapter, we describe how the results of various epidemiologic studies, particularly as they relate to race and ethnicity, maybe used in the evaluation of the individual patient.

## 10.1 Race/Ethnicity and Prevalence of Glaucoma

That the prevalence of primary open-angle glaucoma (POAG) differs by race and ethnicity is universally accepted. Yet there is considerable confusion as to definitions of race and ethnicity. These terms are not synonymous, but nonetheless they are often substituted for each other.

Race is admittedly an inaccurate label for genetic variations that a given individual might or might not possess. Though not universally agreed upon, the concept of race is founded in genetics. Generally, three major groups are recognized: White, Black, and Asian/American Indian. The concept of ethnicity, on the other hand, is concerned with learned behavior, and ethnic groups are culturally distinct. As with race, what constitutes an ethnic group is often difficult to define.

It is important to keep these distinctions in mind in interpreting results of studies of prevalence of POAG in different populations. For example, on the basis of the results of the landmark Baltimore Eye Survey, it is generally accepted that black-Americans have a prevalence of POAG that is three to four times that of white-Americans.[1] However, this assertion is undoubtedly incorrect for all black populations or all white populations. Both the black and white populations in this study were from East Baltimore, and they likely, but not necessarily, are representative of black-Americans and white-Americans in the United States. Two population-based studies performed in the West Indies island countries of Barbados and St. Lucia found glaucoma developed at an earlier age, and the overall prevalence of POAG in those black populations was closer to six to seven times than that of the white-American population of East Baltimore.[2,3] The black-American and black-Caribbean populations are ethnically distinct, and the reported prevalence of POAG among the Caribbean black population is almost twice than that of the U.S. black population. Whether this difference in prevalence is due to genetic factors (greater genetic admixture with whites among black-Americans than among black-Caribbeans) or to cultural factors is still undetermined.

Similarly, there are many ethnic populations among whites. For example, results from a large population-based study in Greece indicate that the prevalence of open-angle glaucoma (primary open-angle glaucoma and pseudoexfoliation glaucoma) in that population is considerably higher than in the white-American population.[4]

Recent reports have indicated that Hispanics or Latinos have a prevalence of POAG that is intermediate between that of black-Americans and white-Americans.[5,6] However, these studies were performed in Mexican-Americans. "Hispanics" do not constitute a racial grouping, but rather comprise heterogeneous subgroups differing in geographical origin and cultural factors. Hispanics can be racially white or black. Although not confirmed through research, there exists a strong clinical impression that the prevalence of POAG among black Hispanics is likely to be higher than among white Hispanics. Thus, a more accurate statement would be that "Mexican-Americans have a prevalence of POAG that is intermediate between that of black-Americans and non-Hispanic white-Americans" (see Sidebar 10.1).

**SIDEBAR 10.1. Glaucoma in Latinos**

Elizabeth Salinas-Van Orman

Many population-based studies have documented the higher prevalence of open angle glaucoma (OAG) in African Americans relative to non-Hispanic white populations in the US and worldwide. However, few studies have focused on Latinos, the largest and fastest growing minority in the US Census 2000 data reveal that 12.5% of the residents in the US are Latino or Hispanic (35 million people) and projections estimate that, by 2050, 25% of the US population will be of Hispanic origin. Therefore, it is important to identify the risk factors associated with glaucoma and other ocular problems to prevent and treat Latinos.

The Los Angeles Latino Eye Study (LALES), which evaluated the largest Latino group in the U.S., primarily of Mexican ancestry (94.7%), reported a prevalence of OAG of 4.74%. The prevalence of OAG in Latinos 80 years or older was 16 times higher (21.76%) that that in Latinos 40–49 years old (1.32%). Ocular hypertension (OHT), a risk factor for glaucoma, was present in 3.56% of the participants examined. The prevalence of OHT was also higher (threefold) in older Latinos (≥80 years old) relative to the younger ones (40–49 years).

Proyecto VER, a population-based study of Hispanics living in Nogales and Tucson, found a lower prevalence of OAG (1.97%) than the LALES (4.74%). The age-specific prevalence of OAG increased nonlinearly from 0.50% in those aged 41–49 years to 12.63% in those 80 years and older.

Although both studies were of Latino individuals, approximately 40% of the Proyecto VER participants had some Native American ancestry compared with only 5.3% of the LALES participants. These genetic and hereditary differences between the two populations of Proyecto VER and the LALES, along with differences in study design and recruitment methodology as well as variations in definitions of OAG could explain the variability in the results reported.

An analysis of risk factors done by Doshi et al in 2008 suggests that older age, male gender, nonmarried status, and positive family history among first-degree relatives are significant independent factors that lead to a greater risk of having glaucoma.

It is important to note that over 75% of the participants with OAG in the LALES, and 62% in Proyecto VER were unaware of their glaucoma at the time they were included in the study. Such high prevalence of under diagnosis highlights the need to develop and assess early detection and treatment programs directed at Latinos. The fact that Latinos with OAG have a low prevalence of high intraocular pressure (IOP > 21 mmHg) indicates the limited usefulness of IOP for the screening and diagnosis of glaucoma. According to the data obtained in Proyecto VER, screening results with an intraocular pressure higher than 22 mmHg (in the eye with a higher pressure) would miss 80% of the OAG cases. Among the participants with OAG in the LALES, the mean IOP was 17.3 mmHg, with 82% having an IOP of ≤21 mmHg. Higher systolic blood pressure, higher central corneal thickness, and diabetes mellitus were the major factors associated with elevated IOP in this study.

The prevalence of OAG was 40% higher in participants with type 2 diabetes mellitus (T2DM) than in those without T2DM in the LALES. Trend analysis revealed that a longer duration of T2DM was associated with a higher prevalence of OAG. Proyecto VER found no association between primary OAG and a history of T2DM. The relatively high prevalence of DM and OAG in this group presents significant public health implications.

While OAG is generally a disease that occurs bilaterally, over half (53%) of all persons with OAG in the LALES had only unilateral glaucomatous optic nerve damage at the time of examination, and 58% had OHT in one eye and no OAG or OHT in the other eye. The central corneal thickness (CCT) among persons with OAG was less than that of those with ocular hypertension (OAG, 545 μm; ocular hypertension, 568 μm).

Prevalences of visual impairment in persons with and without OAG were 6.6 and 1.07%, respectively. Prevalences of legal blindness in persons with and without OAG were 1.04 and 0.37%, respectively.

Overall, findings from the LALES regarding the causes of low vision are similar to those from Proyecto VER despite known demographic differences such as the LALES population being slightly younger, having fewer female participants (58% vs. 65%), and lesser Native American ancestry (5.3% vs. 40%). In addition to demographic differences, other factors may contribute to differences, including environmental exposure, accessibility and use of eye care services, and patterns of surgical practice in the two communities.

The LALES results, as compared with those from the Proyecto VER study, show a striking similar percentage of vision loss from cataract (49.% vs. 46.7%), diabetic retinopathy (17.3% vs. 13%), and age-related macular degeneration (14.8% vs. 14.1%) together accounting for 82% of the low vision cases identified in the LALES. Contrary to the Proyecto VER study, LALES did not find glaucoma to be a major cause of blindness in Latinos, instead found age-related macular degeneration, diabetic retinopathy, and myopic degeneration to be more of a concern in this population, accounting for 62.5% of the cases of blindness. This may suggest that the severity of glaucomatous damage is less advanced or that the diagnosis was made at an earlier stage of the disease. In addition, this population of Latinos on average is younger than those in other population-based studies, and the course of their glaucoma over time remains to be determined.

Even though the LALES data are applicable to the largest ethnic subgroup of Latinos who live in the United States, Latino persons of Mexican origin, they do not necessarily apply to other Latino subgroups such as Cubans, Puerto Ricans, or Dominicans.

The data reported by the LALES suggest that Latinos with a predominantly Mexican ancestry have rates of OAG comparable to those of US blacks and significantly higher than those seen in non-Hispanic whites, and a high prevalence of ocular hypertension. Due to the fact that Latinos are the fastest-growing segment of the US population and vision loss from glaucoma can be prevented with early diagnosis and timely treatment, there is a need for directing additional resources toward preventing and treating glaucoma in the Latino population.

## Bibliography

Chopra V, Varma R, Francis BA, et al. Type 2 diabetes mellitus and the risk of open-angle glaucoma. The Los Angeles Latino Eye Study. *Ophthalmology*. 2008;115:227–232.

Cotter SA, Varma R, Ying-Lai M, et al. Causes of low vision and blindness in adult latinos. The Los Angeles Latino Eye Study. *Ophthalmology*. 2006;113:1574–1582. www.nei.nih.gov/latinoeyestudy/.

Doshi V, Ying-Lai M, Azen SP, et al. Sociodemographic, family history, and lifestyle risk factors for open-angle glaucoma and ocular hypertension. The Los Angeles Latino Eye Study. *Ophthalmology*. 2008;115:639–647.

Leske MC. The epidemiology of open-angle glaucoma: a review. *Am J Epidemiol*. 1983;118:166–191.

Memarzadeh F, Ying-Lai M, Azen SP, et al. Associations with intraocular pressure in Latinos: The Los Angeles Latino Eye Study. *Am J Ophthalmol*. 2008;146:69–76.

Quigley HA, West S, Rodriquez J, et al. The prevalence of glaucoma in a population-based study of Hispanic subjects (Proyecto VER). *Arch Ophthalmol*. 2001;119:1819–1826.

Rodriguez J, Sanchez R, Munoz B, et al. Causes of blindness and visual impairment in a population-based sample of U.S. Hispanics. *Ophthalmology*. 2002;109:737–743.

Tielsch JM, Sommer A, Katz J, et al. Racial variations in the prevalence of primary open-angle glaucoma. The Baltimore Eye Survey. *JAMA*. 1991;266:369–374.

U.S. Census Bureau. (NP-T4-F) Projections of the total resident population by 5-year age groups, race and Hispanic origin with special age categories: middle series, 2025 to 2045. Available at: http://www.census.gov/population/projections/nation/summary/np-t4-f.pdf. Accessed February 4, 2004.

U.S. Census Bureau. Current population reports. Population projections of the United States by age, sex, race and Hispanic origin: 1995 to 2050. P25-1130. 1996. Available at: http://www.census.gov/prod/1/pop/p25-1130/p251130.pdf. Accessed February 4, 2004.

Varma R, Ying-Lai M, Francis BA, et al. Prevalence of open-angle glaucoma and ocular hypertension in Latinos: The Los Angeles Latino Eye Study. *Ophthalmology*. 2004;111:1439–1448.

West SK, Munoz B, Klein R, et al. Risk factors for type II diabetes and diabetic retinopathy in a Mexican-American population; Proyecto VER. *Am J Ophthalmol*. 2002;134:390–398.

---

Likewise, Asians comprise many ethnicities, and findings in one group of Asians do not necessarily generalize to another group of Asians. For example, a nationwide Japanese glaucoma survey reported a prevalence of POAG that is intermediate between that of black-Americans and white-Americans, and a POAG to primary angle-closure glaucoma (PACG) proportion that is similar to that in western populations.[7] In contrast, PACG is the predominant type of glaucoma in some Asian populations such as the Chinese.[8]

The Japanese have also been found to have a higher prevalence of POAG with lower intraocular pressures compared to other populations.[7] The average intraocular pressure for patients with untreated POAG in this population was calculated to be approximately 15 mmHg. A population-based study of descendents of Japanese living in the United States has not been conducted to confirm that this finding also applies to the Japanese-American population. However, clinical impression supports a similarity with the native Japanese population, at least among first-generation Japanese-Americans.

Aside from giving us clues as to which populations are at greater risk for developing glaucoma, prevalence studies have provided insight into the differences between and within various ethnicities/races.[1-15] Table 10.1 illustrates the variability in POAG prevalence among various races/ethnicities.

Whenever possible, we use the more restricted nomenclature of "black-American" when the data have been derived from studies performed only in this specific population. When the data are fairly consistent over several different black populations, the more general designation of "black" is used. Likewise, "Mexican-American" is used rather than the more general term "Hispanic." Either "white-Americans" or "non-Hispanic whites" are used rather than the more general designation of "white." Studies in Asia may look at very specific regional or ethnic groups with very well-defined populations.[15]

## 10.2 Race/Ethnicity and Incidence of Glaucoma

As has been noted, a number of population-based studies of prevalence in relation to glaucoma have been conducted. Incidence studies, however, have been few in number and of variable quality. Furthermore, direct comparison of the various population groups studied in the available incidence studies is difficult as study design, patient selection, duration of study, and definitions of disease differed. What we can gather from these published studies is that like prevalence the incidence of glaucoma is higher in blacks.[16–19]

## 10.3 Race/Ethnicity, Age, and Glaucoma

Race/ethnicity is only one of many factors to take into account when evaluating a patient for a possible diagnosis of glaucoma. As people age, the prevalence and incidence of glaucoma increases in all races and ethnicities (refer to Tables 10.1 and 10.2). This finding is consistent among all major population-based epidemiologic studies evaluating age as a risk factor for glaucoma. It is important to note that the finding of higher POAG prevalence with advancing age is more pronounced in blacks and Mexican-Americans compared to non-Hispanic whites.

In the Baltimore Eye Study, as an example, the prevalence of POAG in black-Americans between the ages of 40–49 was 1.2% and increased to 11.3% in those above 80 years of age.[1] The same study estimated a prevalence of 0.9% and only 2.2% in the same age groups for white-Americans. This accelerated prevalence with age was also seen, yet more pronounced, in Caribbean blacks in Barbados and St. Lucia.[2,3] The prevalence studies conducted on Mexican-Americans living in both Southern California[5] and Arizona[6] revealed a similar pattern of increased prevalence compared

**Table 10.1** Age-specific prevalence of definite primary open-angle glaucoma

| | Black | | | White | | | Hispanic | | Asian | |
|---|---|---|---|---|---|---|---|---|---|---|
| | Baltimore[1] | Barbados[2] | St. Lucia[3] | Baltimore[1] | Melbourne[9] | Thessa-loniki[4] | Proyecto[6] | LALES[5] | Tajimi[7] | Liwan District[15] |
| | American | Caribbean | Caribbean | American | Australian | Greek | Mexican-American | Mexican-American | Japanese | Chinese |
| Age (years) | | | | | | | | | | |
| 30–39 | | | 4 | | | | | | | |
| 40–49 | 1.23 | 1.4 | 7.3 | 0.92 | 0.1 | | 0.5 | 1.32 | 2 | |
| 50–59 | 4.05 | 4.1 | 8.7 | 0.41 | 0.6 | | 0.59 | 2.92 | 2.7 | 1.1 |
| 60–69 | 5.51 | 6.7 | 15.2 | 0.88 | 1.9 | 2.6 | 1.73 | 7.36 | 4.7 | 2.9 |
| 70–79 | 9.15 | 14.8 | | 2.89 | 5.2 | 4.9 | 5.66 | 14.72 | 8.2 | 5.5 |
| 70+ | | | 9.5 | | | | | | | |
| 80–89 | | | | | 5.5 | | 12.02 | | | |
| 80+ | 11.26 | 23.2 | | 2.16 | | 4.3 | 20 | 21.76 | 6 | 12 |
| 90+ | | | | | 11.8 | | | | | |
| All | 4.74 | 6.8 | 8.76 | 1.29 | 1.7 | 3.8 | 2 | 4.74 | 3.9 | 3.9 |

**Table 10.2** Age-specific incidence of definite primary open-angle glaucoma

| Black | | | White | | | | | | |
|---|---|---|---|---|---|---|---|---|---|
| Barbados Eye Study | | | Melbourne VIP Project | | Rotterdam Eye Study | | Blue Mountain Eye Study | | |
| Age (years) | (4-year incidence) | (9-year incidence) | Age (years) | (5-year incidence) | Age (years) | (5-year incidence) | Age (years) | (10-year incidence) |
| 40–49 | 1.2 | 2.2 | 40–49 | 0 | 55–59 | 1.4 | | |
| 50–59 | 1.5 | 3.6 | 50–59 | 0.1 | 60–64 | 0.6 | <60 | 2 |
| 60–69 | 3.2 | 6.6 | 60–69 | 0.6 | 65–69 | 1.8 | 60–69 | 3.7 |
| 70+ | 4.2 | 7.9 | 70–79 | 1.4 | 70–74 | 2.4 | >70 | 10.3 |
| | | | 80+ | 4.1 | 75–79 | 2.6 | | |
| | | | | | 80+ | 2.6 | | |
| Total | 2.2 | 4.4 | Total | 0.5 | Total | 1.8 | Total | 4.5 |
| Annual incidence | 0.55 | 0.489 | | 0.1 | | 0.36 | | 0.45 |

to white-Americans. The Los Angeles Latino Eye Study estimated a prevalence of 1.32% in Latinos of Mexican descent in the 40- to 49-year-old age group and 21.76% in those who were 80 years old or older – the most pronounced increase of prevalence in any population group studied thus far. We have clear evidence that the probability and risk of developing POAG increases with age through both prevalence and incidence studies. This information is useful in evaluating patients with suspected glaucoma as it can influence treatment patterns for patients. As glaucoma in all races/ethnicities is rare prior to the age of 40, a patient's age should be considered a risk factor for open-angle glaucoma. Simply stated, the older the patient is, the higher the risk. Further, the risk profile as a function of age is accentuated in blacks and Mexican-Americans.

## 10.4 Race/Ethnicity and Ocular Risk Factors

### 10.4.1 Intraocular Pressure

We know from various studies that intraocular pressure (IOP) is a major risk factor for the development of and the progression of glaucoma.[1,20–22] However, there is no magical value of intraocular pressure at which patients are either absolutely protected from or absolutely certain to developing glaucoma. Historically, there was a range of intraocular pressures of 10–21 mmHg that was considered "normal." Being within this "normal" range, however, does not protect one from developing or having glaucoma, or from having an individual patient's disease progress. Also, being above this IOP range does not necessarily mean that one will develop glaucoma or have glaucoma. So how does intraocular pressure matter in relation to glaucoma? Lowering the intraocular pressure in those patients suffering from POAG definitively reduces the incidence of disease progression.[23–26] And lowering the intraocular pressure in certain patients with ocular hypertension also reduces the risk of progression to POAG.[23]

When comparing blacks and whites, there are conflicting reports in the medical literature, discussing differences in baseline IOPs in nonglaucomatous,[1,20,27,28] ocular hypertensive,[29,30] or POAG[31–33] eyes. But there may be a racial difference in patient susceptibility to developing optic nerve head damage for a given intraocular pressure. In one study, optic nerve head and visual field progression were more prevalent in untreated black-Americans than in untreated white-Americans with POAG despite having identical IOP levels.[32] Additionally, a study in South Africa reported that while only 5.4% of whites with ocular hypertension progress to POAG, 18.1% of blacks with ocular hypertension progress to POAG.[29]

Given this information, we may be more prone to initiate treatment earlier in black patients with ocular hypertension and may even be more aggressive in our degree of IOP reduction compared to our non-Hispanic white patients. The role of central corneal thickness and race in the measurement of IOP will be discussed more fully, but it may be that most clinical studies done before the turn-of-the-century failed to account for IOP measurement errors that might vary systematically (on average) in different racial/ethnic populations.

As previously mentioned, the Japanese have been found to have a much higher prevalence of POAG, with intraocular pressures 21 mmHg or lower compared to other populations.[7] In addition, the population sample in this study had a higher prevalence of POAG with pressures 21 mmHg or lower (3.6%) compared to that of POAG with an intraocular pressure greater than 21 mmHg (0.3%). This higher prevalence of POAG with lower intraocular pressures might be accounted for by the known thinner central corneal thickness in the Japanese population.

This information, however, does not automatically translate into an increased prevalence of "low-tension" glaucoma among other Asian populations. Further prevalence studies are required in different Asian populations to determine if other Asian populations are at greater risk for developing glaucoma in the face of lower intraocular pressures.

### 10.4.2 Central Corneal Thickness

For decades, Goldmann applanation has been considered the gold standard for measuring intraocular pressure. We do know, however, that the measurement of intraocular pressure can be influenced by the thickness of the central cornea. It is thought that thinner corneas may underestimate and thicker corneas may overestimate the actual intraocular pressure.[34–36] The importance of this phenomena is not clearly understood and there are differing opinions on the necessity to correct the intraocular pressure based on the thickness of the central cornea. Central corneal thickness (CCT) does become important when dealing with patients suffering from ocular hypertension because those with thinner CCT measurements (<555 µm) have a higher risk of progression to POAG.[37] Indeed, it was the publication of the Ocular Hypertension Treatment Study[37] in 2001 that first made many clinical ophthalmologists aware of the importance of measuring central corneal thickness in their glaucoma and ocular hypertension patients. In patients suffering from POAG, there is conflicting evidence as to whether patients with thinner CCT measurements are at higher risk for disease progression.[38]

Differences have been seen in CCT measurements in patients with normal eyes, OHT, POAG, and normal tension glaucoma (NTG). Patients with normal tension glaucoma tend to have thinner corneas than the general population and in those with POAG.[39] Conversely, those with ocular hypertension tend to have thicker corneas.[37,39] There is also a racial difference in CCT measurements. In the Ocular Hypertension Treatment Study (OHTS), black-Americans with ocular hypertension had an average central corneal thickness of 557.7 μm while non-Hispanic white-Americans with ocular hypertension had an average central corneal thickness of 579.0 μm. Black-Americans were also found to have thinner corneas in normal eyes and in those suffering from POAG compared to white-Americans. Because most ophthalmologists did not determine central corneal thickness until after the publication of the OHTS article in 2001, it is possible that black patients may have been consistently undertreated for many years as we did not have better estimates of their IOPs because of the thinner corneas they have on average compared to white patients.

Several studies have reported that Asian patients have intermediate CCT values when compared to white and black-Americans.[7,40,41] Given this intermediate value of CCT, one can conclude that corneal thickness would not account for the higher prevalence of NTG in Japanese patients. It is also not known with certainty if a thinner CCT value in Asians with ocular hypertension is considered a risk factor as the Ocular Hypertension Study had a very small Asian patient population.

The importance of obtaining a CCT measurement is clear in ocular hypertensive patients. There are conflicting reports on the clinical usefulness for obtaining a CCT measurement in all patients, particularly since the association of CCT and glaucoma progression has not been unequivocally established. For established open angle glaucoma patients who have been followed for many years without progression, it may not be necessary to obtain a CCT measurement as it is unlikely the physician will act on this information in a truly stable patient.

### 10.4.3 Optic Nerve Head and Retinal Nerve Fiber Layer Anatomy

As pointed out elsewhere in this text, glaucoma is defined as a progressive optic neuropathy with characteristic structural changes of the optic nerve head and associated characteristic visual field loss. Despite what risk factors a patient may or may not have, evaluation of the optic nerve head is the single most important component of the glaucoma evaluation. Abnormally appearing optic nerve heads provide cause for suspicion of the presence of glaucoma and the need for subsequent evaluation of optic nerve head structure and function.

Clinically, the changes of the optic nerve head are characterized by enlargement of the optic nerve head cup and thinning of the neural retinal rim. Ocular hypertensive patients have been shown to have a 1.4-fold increase in progression to POAG for every 0.1-unit increase from the baseline cup-to-disc ratio.[42] Furthermore, there is an increased incidence of glaucomatous visual field defects in patients with larger cup-to-disc ratios.[43–45]

There are racial differences in the various optic nerve head parameters assessed in glaucoma. Several studies have observed black-Americans to have larger optic disc areas compared to white-Americans in both normal[46–49] and glaucomatous[28] eyes. This finding may account for the inherent larger cup volumes,[46,48,49] cup-to-disc ratio,[46,49,50] and smaller neural retinal rim area-to-disc area ratios seen in blacks.[49] It is unclear if patients with large optic discs have an increased or decreased susceptibility to developing glaucoma as there are conflicting reports and theories for basis of disease.[46,50–52]

Because loss of retinal ganglion cells and thinning of the peripapillary retinal nerve fiber layer (RNFL) precedes changes in the optic nerve head, it has become customary to assess the RNFL in patients suspected of or suffering from glaucoma. Although early reports indicated that blacks had a thinner mean RNFL compared to non-Hispanic whites,[53,54] a more recent study found a trend for black-Americans to have a thicker mean RNFL than white-Americans.[55]

### 10.4.4 Refractive Error

Population-based surveys in white,[56,57] black,[58] and Japanese[59] populations have provided some evidence to the commonly held belief that myopia is associated with an increased risk for POAG, although other studies did not lend support to this notion. The Early Manifest Glaucoma Trial (EMGT) did not find myopic patients with ocular hypertension to have a higher incidence of glaucoma nor did myopic patients have a greater risk of progression when suffering from glaucoma.[60]

Because of the anatomic changes seen in the optic nerve heads of patients with moderate to high myopia, it is often difficult to evaluate these patients for glaucoma on the basis of the structural appearance of their optic nerves. For these patients, distinguishing between a glaucoma suspect and a patient suffering from glaucoma is a challenge to the physician. When compared to emmetropic or hyperopic patients, high myopes tend to have a larger optic nerve head with larger areas of peripapillary atrophy.[61] Peripapillary atrophy or degeneration of the neurosensory retina and underlying retinal pigmented epithelium has been shown to be associated with glaucoma.[62–64] Though indistinguishable by direct clinical exam, retinal nerve fiber layer imaging studies may aid in the differentiation between myopic and glaucomatous peripapillary changes. A recent study of nonglaucomatous, myopic Chinese found no difference of mean retinal nerve fiber layer thickness when compared to controls.[65] Retinal nerve fiber layer imaging may provide a useful tool for following myopic patients with glaucoma. Further investigation is needed to determine similar characteristics in various ages and races/ethnicities.

## 10.5 Race/Ethnicity and Non-ocular Risk Factors

The prevalence of several systemic factors, most notably diabetes mellitus and blood pressure, is known to differ among various racial/ethnic populations. Both of these factors have also been suggested to increase the risk of developing glaucoma. However, the results of the various studies have not been consistent in this regard.[66-68]

None of the major population-based studies in black populations have found an association between diabetes mellitus and POAG,[66,67] and reports of an association of diabetes mellitus and POAG in Mexican-Americans and non-Hispanic whites have been conflicting.[6,68] Associations of systemic hypertension and POAG have been reported as positive, negative, or none.[69-72] A stronger relationship has been seen with low diastolic perfusion pressure. Population-based studies have noted an increased prevalence of POAG in patients with low perfusion pressure, but an effect of race/ethnicity on this association has not yet been described.

## 10.6 Conclusion

The diagnosis of glaucoma is determined not by a single factor, but rather on the integration of various aspects of a patient's history and examination. Epidemiologic studies have guided us in identifying patient characteristics that may lead to increased risk of disease. Race/ethnicity is one of these factors. Such knowledge may assist in the monitoring of patients who have not yet developed glaucoma, as well as assist in the clinical management of those who have the disease. For example, since POAG develops at younger ages in blacks than in non-Hispanic whites, it is important to begin detection efforts earlier in this population. Further, because a larger proportion of black patients with ocular hypertension convert to glaucoma than do non-Hispanic whites, more frequent monitoring may also be warranted.

The pathogenic mechanisms that render race as a risk factor for glaucoma are not understood. However, some of the parameters that influence glaucoma diagnosis – optic nerve head appearance, central corneal thickness, and intraocular pressure – differ by race. When assessing a patient, it is important to take all these factors into account when making a diagnosis of a lifelong, chronic disease.

## References

1. Tielsch JM, Sommer A, Katz J, et al. Racial variations in the prevalence of primary open-angle glaucoma: the Baltimore Eye Survey. *JAMA*. 1991;226:369–374.
2. Leske MC, Connell AM, Schachat AP, et al. The Barbados Eye Study: prevalence of open-angle glaucoma. *Arch Ophthalmol*. 1994;112:821–829.
3. Mason RP, Kosoko O, Wilson MR, et al. National survey of the prevalence and risk factors of glaucoma in St Lucia, West Indies. Part 1: prevalence findings. *Ophthalmology*. 1989;96:1363–1368.
4. Topouzis F, Wilson MR, Harris A, et al. Prevalence of open-angle glaucoma in Greece: the Thessaloniki Eye Study. *Am J Ophthalmol*. 2007;144(4):511–519.
5. Varma R, Ying-Lai M, Francis BA, et al. The Los Angeles Latino Eye Study: prevalence of open-angle glaucoma and ocular hypertension in Latinos. *Ophthalmology*. 2004;111:1439–1448.
6. Quigley HA, West SK, Rodriguez J, et al. The prevalence of glaucoma in a population-based study of Hispanic subjects: Proyecto VER. *Arch Ophthalmol*. 2001;119:1819–1826.
7. Iwase A, Suzuki Y, Araie M, et al. The prevalence of primary open-angle glaucoma in Japanese: The Tajimi Study. *Ophthalmology*. 2004;111:1641–1648.
8. Hu Z, Zhao ZL, Dong FT, et al. An epidemiologic investigation of glaucoma in Beijing and Shun-yi County. *Chin J Ophthalmol*. 1989;25:115–118.
9. Wensor MD, McCarty CA, Stanislavsky YL, et al. The prevalence of glaucoma in the Melbourne Visual Impairment Project. *Ophthalmology*. 1998;105:733–739.
10. Vijaya L, George R, Baskaran M, et al. Prevalence of primary open-angle glaucoma in an urban south Indian population and comparison with a rural population: The Chennai Glaucoma Study. *Ophthalmology*. 2008;115(4):648–654.
11. Mitchell P, Smith W, Attebo K, et al. Prevalence of open-angle glaucoma in Australia: The Blue Mountains Eye Study. *Ophthalmology*. 1996;103:1661–1669.
12. Eye Diseases Prevalence Research Group. Prevalence of open-angle glaucoma among adults in the United States. *Arch Ophthalmol*. 2004;122:532–538.
13. Friedman DS, Jampel HD, Munoz B, et al. The prevalence of open-angle glaucoma among blacks and white 73 years and older: The Salisbury Eye Evaluation Glaucoma Study. *Arch Ophthalmol*. 2006;124:1625–1630.
14. Klein BE, Klein R, Sponsel WE, et al. Prevalence of glaucoma: The Beaver Dam Eye Study. *Ophthalmology*. 1992;22:1499–1504.
15. He M, Foster P, Ge J, et al. Prevalence and clinical characteristics of glaucoma in adult Chinese: a population-based study in Liwan District, Guangzhou. *Invest Ophthalmol Vis Sci*. 2006;47:2782–2788.
16. Leske MC, Wu SY, Honkanen R, et al. Nine-year incidence of open-angle glaucoma in the Barbados Eye Studies. *Ophthalmology*. 2007;114:1058–1064.
17. Mukesh BN, McCarty A, Rait J, et al. Five-year incidence of open-angle glaucoma: The Visual Impairment Project. *Ophthalmology*. 2002;109:1047–1051.

18. deVoogd S, Ikram MK, Wolfs RC, et al. Incidence of open-angle glaucoma in a general elderly population: The Rotterdam Study. *Ophthalmology*. 2005;112:1487–1493.
19. Mitchell P, Lee AJ, Rochtchina E, et al. 10-Year incidence and progression of open-angle glaucoma in an older population: the Blue Mountains Eye Study. Invest Ophthalmol Vis Sci 2006;47: E-Abstract 2342.
20. Sommer A, Tielsch JM, Katz J, et al. Relationship between intraocular pressure and primary open angle glaucoma among white and black Americans. The Baltimore Eye Survey. *Arch Ophthalmol*. 1991;109:1090–1095.
21. Sommer A. Glaucoma: facts and fancies. *Eye*. 1996;10:295–301.
22. Wormald RPL, Basauri E, Wright LA, et al. The African Caribbean eye survey: risk factors for glaucoma in a sample African Caribbean people living in London. *Eye*. 1994;8:315–320.
23. Kass MA, Heuer DK, Higginbotham EJ, et al. The Ocular Hypertension Treatment Study: a randomized trail determines that topical ocular hypotensive medication delays or prevents the onset of primary open-angle glaucoma. *Arch Ophthalmol*. 2002;120:701–713.
24. Heijl A, Leske C, Bengtsson B, et al. Reduction of intraocular pressure and glaucoma progression: results from the Early Manifest Glaucoma Trial. *Arch Ophthalmol*. 2002;120:1268–1279.
25. Collaborative Normal Tension Glaucoma Study Group. The effectiveness of intraocular pressure reduction in the treatment of normal-tension glaucoma. *Am J Ophthalmol*. 1998;126:498–505.
26. The Advanced Glaucoma Intervention Study (AGIS): 7. The relationship between control of intraocular pressure and visual field deterioration. The AGIS Investigators. Am J Ophthalmol 2000;130: 429–440.
27. Coulehan JL, Helzlsouer KJ, Rogers KD, et al. Racial differences in intraocular tension and glaucoma surgery. *Am J Epidemiol*. 1980;111:759–768.
28. Martin MJ, Sommer A, Gold EB, et al. Race and primary open-angle glaucoma. *Am J Ophthalmol*. 1985;99:383–387.
29. David R, Livingston D, Luntz MH. Ocular hypertension: a comparative follow-up of black and white patients. *Br J Ophthalmol*. 1978;62:676–678.
30. Gordon MO, Kass MA. The Ocular Hypertension Treatment Study: design and baseline description of the participants. *Arch Ophthalmol*. 1999;117:573–583.
31. Leske MC, Connell AM, Wu SY, et al. Risk factors for open-angle glaucoma. The Barbados Eye Study. *Arch Ophthalmol*. 1995;113:918–924.
32. Wilson R, Richardson TM, Hertzmark E, et al. Race as a risk factor for progressive glaucomatous damage. *Ann Ophthalmol*. 1985;17: 653–659.
33. AGIS: The Advanced Glaucoma Intervention Study (AGIS): 3. Baseline characteristics of black and white patients. Ophthalmol 1998;105:1137–1145.
34. Johnson M, Kass MA, Moses RA, et al. Increased corneal thickness stimulating elevated intraocular pressure. *Arch Ophthalmol*. 1978;96: 664–665.
35. Doughty MJ, Zaman ML. Human corneal thickness and its impact on intraocular pressure measures: a review and metaanalysis approach. *Surv Ophthalmol*. 2000;44:367–408.
36. Kniestedt C, Lin S, Choe J, et al. Clinical comparison of contour and applanation tonometry and their relationship to pachymetry. *Arch Ophthalmol*. 2005;123:1532–1537.
37. Brandt JD, Beiser JA, Kass MA, et al. Central Corneal thickness in the Ocular Hypertension Treatment Study (OHTS). *Ophthalmology*. 2001;108:1779–1788.
38. Ducker DK, Singh K, Lin SC, et al. Corneal thickness measurement in the management of primary open-angle glaucoma; a report by the American Academy of Ophthalmology. *Ophthalmology*. 2007;114: 1779–1787.
39. LaRosa FA, Gross RL, Orengo-Nania S. Central corneal thickness of caucasians and African Americans in glaucomatous and non-glaucomatous populations. *Arch Ophthalmol*. 2001;119:23–27.
40. Suzuki S, Suzuki Y, Iwase A, et al. Corneal thickness in an ophthalmologically normal Japanese population. *Ophthalmology*. 2005; 112:1327–1336.
41. Lee ES, Kim CY, Ha SJ, et al. Central corneal thickness of Korean patients with glaucoma. *Ophthalmology*. 2007;114:927–930.
42. Gordon MO, Breiser JA, Brandt JD, et al. The Ocular Hypertension Treatment Study: baseline factors that predict the onset of primary open-angle glaucoma. *Arch Ophthalmol*. 2002;120:714–720.
43. Armaly MF, Krueger DE, Maunder L, et al. Biostatistical analysis of the collaborative glaucoma study. I. Summary report of the risk factors for glaucomatous visual-field defects. *Arch Ophthalmol*. 1980;98:2163–2171.
44. Hart WM, Yablonski M, Kass MA, Becker B. Multivariate analysis of the risk of glaucomatous visual field loss. *Arch Ophthalmol*. 1979;97:1455–1458.
45. Yablonski ME, Zimmerman TJ, Kass MA, Becker B. Prognostic significance of optic disc cupping in ocular hypertensive patients. *Am J Ophthalmol*. 1980;89:585–592.
46. Chi T, Ritch R, Stickler D, et al. Racial differences in optic nerve head parameters. *Arch Ophthalmol*. 1989;107:836–839.
47. Mansour AM. Racial variation of optic disc size. *Ophthalmic Res*. 1991;23:67–72.
48. Tsai CS, Zangwill L, Gonzalez C, et al. Ethnic differences in optic nerve head topography. *J Glaucoma*. 1995;4:248–257.
49. Varma R, Tielsch JM, Qjuigley HA, et al. Race-, age-, gender-, and refractive error-related differences in normal optic disc. *Arch Ophthalmol*. 1994;112:1068–1076.
50. Beck RW, Messner DK, Musch DC, et al. Is there a racial difference in physiologic cup size? *Ophthalmology*. 1985;92:873–876.
51. Jonas JB, Gusek GC, Naumann GO. Optic disc, cup and neuroretinal rim size, configuration and correlations in normal eyes. *Invest Ophthalmol Vis Sci*. 1988;29:1151–1158.
52. Caprioli J, Miller JM. Optic disc rim area is related to disc size in normal subjects. *Arch Ophthalmol*. 1987;105:1683–1685.
53. Poinooswmy D, Fontana L, Wu JX, et al. Variations of nerve fiber layer thickness measurements with age and ethnicity by scanning laser polarimetry. *Br J Ophthalmol*. 1997;81:350–354.
54. Tjon-Fo Sang MJ, Lemij HG. Retinal nerve fiber layer measurements in normal blacks subjects as determined with scanning laser polarimetry. *Ophthalmology*. 1998;105:78–81.
55. Racette L, Boden C, Kleinhandler SL. Differences in visual function and optic nerve structure between healthy eyes of blacks and whites. *Arch Ophthalmol*. 2005;123:1547–1553.
56. Mitchell P, Hourihan F, Sandbach J, et al. The relationship between glaucoma and myopia: the Blue Mountains Eye Study. *Ophthalmology*. 1999;106:2010–2015.
57. Wong TY, Klein BE, Klein R, et al. Refractive errors, intraocular pressure, and glaucoma in a white population. *Ophthalmology*. 2003;110:211–217.
58. Wu SY, Nemesure B, Leske MC. Barbados Eye Study Group. Refractive errors in black a black adult population: the Barbados Eye Study. *Invest Ophthalmol Vis Sci*. 1999;40:2179–2184.
59. Suzuki Y, Iwase A, Araie M, et al. Risk factors for open-angle glaucoma in a Japanese population. The Tajimi Study. *Ophthalmology*. 2006;113:1613–1617.
60. Leske MC, Heijl A, Hussein M, et al. Factors for glaucoma progression and the effect of treatment: the Early Manifest Glaucoma Trial. *Arch Ophthalmol*. 2003;121(1):48–56.
61. Jonas JB, Gusek GC, Naumann GO. Optic disk morphometry in high myopia. *Graefes Arch Clin Exp Ophthalmol*. 1998;226:587–590.
62. Jonas JB, Nguyen XN, Gusek GC, Naumann GOH. Parapapillary chorioretinal atrophy in normal and glaucoma eyes. I. Morphometric date. *Invest Ophthalmol Vis Sci*. 1989;30:908.
63. Primrose J. Early signs of glaucomatous disc. *Br J Ophthalmol*. 1971;55:820.
64. Wilensky JT, Kolker AE. Peripapillary changes in glaucoma. *Am J Ophthalmol*. 1976;81:341.

65. Hoh S, Lim MC, Seah SK. Peripapillary retinal nerve fiber layer thickness variation in myopia. *Ophthalmology*. 2006;113:773–777.
66. Tielsch JM, Katz J, Quigley HA, et al. Diabetes, intraocular pressure, and primary open-angle glaucoma in the Baltimore Eye Survey. *Ophthalmology*. 1995;102:48–53.
67. Leske MC, Wu S, Hennis A. Risk factors for incident open-angle glaucoma: the Barbados Eye Studies. *Ophthalmology*. 2008;115(1):85–93.
68. Chopra V, Varma R, Francia BA. Type 2 diabetes mellitus and the risk of open-angle glaucoma: the Los Angles Latino Eye Study. *Ophthalmology*. 2008;115(2):227–232.
69. European Glaucoma Prevention (EGPS) Group. Predictive factors for open-angle glaucoma among patients with ocular hypertension in the European Glaucoma Prevention Study. *Ophthalmology*. 2007;114:3–9.
70. Leske MC, Wu SY, Nemesure B, et al. Incident open-angle glaucoma and blood pressure. *Arch Ophthalmol*. 2002;120:954–959.
71. Tielsch JM, Katz J, Sommer A, et al. Hypertension, perfusion pressure, and primary open-angle glaucoma; a population based assessment. *Arch Ophthalmol*. 1995;113:216–221.
72. Mitchell P, Lee AJ, Rochtchna E, et al. Open-angle glaucoma and systemic hypertension; the Blue Mountains Eye Study. *J Glaucoma*. 2004;13:319–326.

# Chapter 11
# Glaucoma Risk Factors: Ocular Blood Flow

Brent Siesky, Alon Harris, Rita Ehrlich, Nisha Kheradiya, and Carlos Rospigliosi Lopez

The prevalence of glaucoma is 0.7% among 40–49-year-olds and rises over subsequent decades to 7.7% amongst those over 80 years of age.[1] As the population of the United States ages, the number of patients with open angle glaucoma (OAG) is expected to increase by 50% to 3.36 million in the year 2020.[2] OAG represents an emerging disease with increasing costs and negative impacts.

Elevated intraocular pressure (IOP) is the only major risk factor approved by the United States Food and Drug Administration (FDA) at the time of this writing for treatment in glaucoma management. Despite the medical or surgical interventions to lower IOP, some glaucoma patients continue to experience disease progression. In the Early Manifest Glaucoma Trial (EMGT), the disease progression rate in the treatment group was 45% as compared to 62% in the control arm.[3] In the Collaborative Initial Glaucoma Treatment Study (CIGTS), substantial visual field loss occurred in 10–13.5% of participants during 5 years of follow-up.[4] Specifically, increased incidence of visual field deterioration occurs with older age (increased risk of visual field loss by 40% every 10 years), race (nonwhites had a 50% increased risk relative to whites), and diabetes (59% increased risk relative to non-diabetic patients).[4] In a similar capacity, 20% of normal tension glaucoma (NTG) patients show continued visual field loss even after 5 years of IOP reduction.[5]

Among other often-discussed OAG risk factors, reductions in ocular blood flow and faulty vascular autoregulation continue to emerge as possibly contributing to OAG disease pathophysiology. For many years, vascular abnormalities have been reported as contributing factors to glaucomatous optic neuropathy.[6] Prospective clinical trials have demonstrated blood flow deficiencies of OAG patients in the retinal,[7] choroidal,[8] and retrobulbar[9–12] circulations, and (regional) ischemia has been shown to correspond with areas of glaucomatous visual field loss.[13] Furthermore, OAG has been found to be associated with ocular perfusion pressure,[14,15] blood pressure,[16] nocturnal hypotension,[17] aging of the vasculature,[18] optic disc hemorrhage,[19] migraine, and diabetes.[19] Reduced ocular perfusion may be secondary to IOP elevation or represent a primary insult to the optic nerve in glaucoma. In this capacity, chronic ocular ischemia may be due to faulty vascular autoregulation and/or the inability of the vasculature to overcome elevated IOP to maintain consistent adequate perfusion.

## 11.1 Ischemia and Glaucomatous Optic Neuropathy

The human eye offers a unique opportunity to directly view and thus study hemodynamics without invasive measurement techniques. It is the only location in the body where capillary blood flow may be observed and recorded in humans without invasive intervention. The study of ocular blood flow in relation to glaucomatous optic neuropathy dates back over 100 years when Wagemann and Salzmann first observed vascular sclerosis in glaucoma patients.[20] Since then, numerous researchers have documented reductions in the capillary beds, sclerosis of nutritional vessels, vascular lesions and degeneration, and other circulatory pathologies in many eye diseases including glaucoma.[21–25] A century of observation and circumstantial evidence suggesting a vascular component in the pathogenesis of glaucoma is now supported by direct evidence.

In glaucoma, low ocular blood flow is one possible mechanism by which retinal ganglion cells can be damaged. In recent years, chronic optic nerve ischemia has been shown to induce retinal ganglion cell loss independent of IOP.[26] In animal models with glaucoma, retinal ganglion cells die via apoptosis (programmed cell death), a process in which ischemia may play a central role.[27–33] Models[27,34,35] of retinal ischemic/reperfusion injury emphasize the critical impact of loss of nutrient delivery, especially to the highly sensitive retinal ganglion cells. In this context, it is possible that "neuroprotection" of these cells may be accomplished by improving blood flow. Figure 11.1 shows how it is logical to consider relief of ischemia (and increased oxygen levels) as a prime and under-explored route to neuroprotection of ganglion cells in glaucoma management.

## Retinal Ganglion Cell Death

**Fig. 11.1** Shows how ocular ischemia can result in loss of retinal ganglion cells independent of intraocular pressure (IOP)

Advances in imaging technologies have allowed for an increased focus on ocular hemodynamics in glaucoma. As evidence-based medicine has taken on significant importance over the past several years, large population-based studies have begun to contribute evidence of vascular-related pathophysiology in glaucoma. Specifically, glaucoma has been associated with low ocular perfusion pressure, defined as 2/3 (mean arterial pressure) IOP in many studies. Low perfusion pressure has been identified in large population-based investigations of glaucoma including the Baltimore Eye Survey, Egna–Neumarkt Glaucoma Study, Long Island Case Control Study, Barbados Eye Studies, and Proyecto VER investigations. These studies have linked decreased diastolic ocular perfusion pressure with the prevalence[36,37] and incidence[38] of glaucoma. Recently, Leske et al[39] presented data on predictors of long-term progression in the Early Manifest Glaucoma Trial (EMGT). Lower systolic perfusion pressure, lower systolic blood pressure, and cardiovascular disease history emerged as new predictors, suggesting a vascular role in glaucoma progression.[39] The Thessaloniki Eye Study[40] similarly associated decreased diastolic blood pressure with increased cupping and decreased rim area of the optic disc in nonglaucomatous individuals.

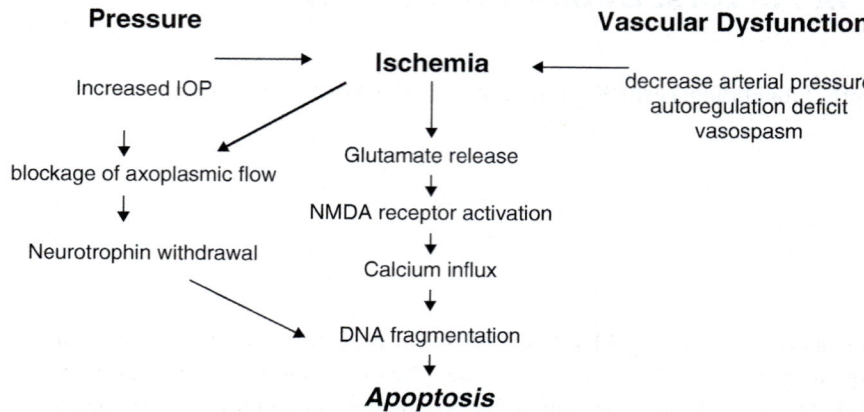

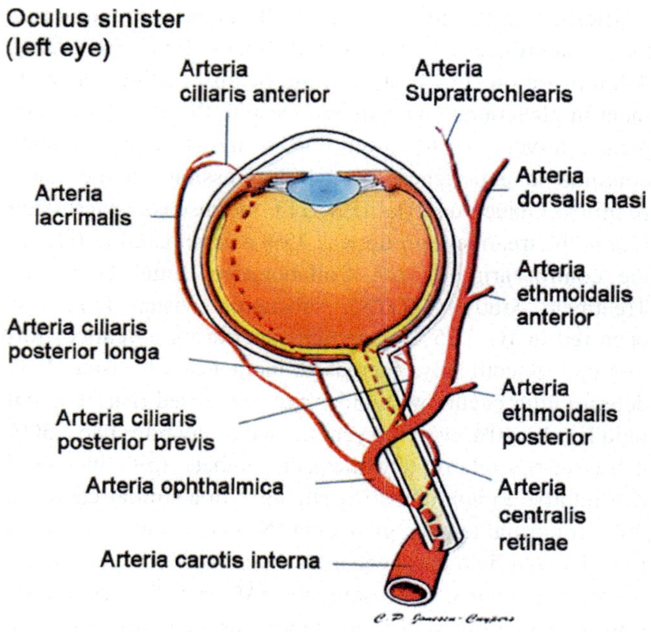

**Fig. 11.2** Ocular blood supply arises primarily from the ophthalmic artery, the first branch of the internal carotid artery. Reprinted with permission from Harris et al[111]

## 11.2 Anatomy of Ocular Blood Flow

The blood supply to the eye is comprised of two distinct systems: the retinal and the uveal. Ocular blood supply arises primarily from the ophthalmic artery, the first branch of the internal carotid artery (Fig. 11.2). The ophthalmic artery enters the orbit via the optic canal and runs inferolaterally to the optic nerve. As the ophthalmic artery courses nasally and anteriorly, it then runs superior to the optic nerve and gives off most of its major branches.[41] Its major branches include those to extraocular muscles, the central retinal artery, and the posterior ciliary arteries.[42]

The retinal system is supplied by the central retinal artery and sustains the inner two-thirds of the retina, the superficial nerve fiber layer of the optic nerve head (ONH), and contributes to the supply of the retrolaminar optic nerve. The central retinal artery branches off the ophthalmic artery to pierce the ventral surface of the optic nerve sheath approximately 10–15 mm posterior to the lamina cribrosa.[43] The central retinal artery courses adjacent to the central retinal vein through the center of the optic nerve, then emerges from the optic nerve within the globe, where it branches into four major vessels. These four vessels include the arteriola nasalis retinae superior, arteriola nasalis retinae inferior, arteriola temporalis retinae superior, and arteriola temporalis retinae inferior.

The uveal system, which supplies blood to the iris, ciliary body, and choroid, is supplied by one to five posterior ciliary arteries. In most individuals, a medial and lateral posterior ciliary artery branch from the ophthalmic artery in the posterior orbit. Each posterior ciliary artery then divides into one long posterior ciliary artery and seven to ten short posterior ciliary arteries before penetrating the sclera surrounding insertion of the optic nerve. The two long posterior ciliary arteries pierce the sclera about 3–4 mm nasally and temporally from the optic nerve and travel anteriorly within the suprachoroidal space, along the horizontal meridians of the globe. They then typically divide in the vicinity of the ora serrata, sending recurrent branches posteriorly to supply the anterior choriocapillaris in concert with the anterior ciliary arteries. The short posterior ciliary arteries supply the posterior choriocapillaris, peripapillary choroid, and the majority of the anterior optic nerve. The choriocapillaris underneath the fovea is supplied by the lateral posterior ciliary artery. Often, a noncontinuous arterial circle exists within the perineural sclera, the circle of Zinn–Haller. This structure is formed by the convergence branches from the short posterior ciliary arteries. The circle of Zinn–Haller provides blood for various regions of the anterior optic nerve, the peripapillary choroid, and the pial arterial system.[44–51]

## 11.3 Optic Nerve Vascular Anatomy

The anterior optic nerve may be divided into four anatomic regions: the superficial nerve fiber layer, the prelaminar region, the lamina cribrosa, and the retrolaminar region[52,53] (Fig. 11.3). The anterior-most region of the superficial nerve fiber layer is continuous with the nerve fiber layer of the ret-

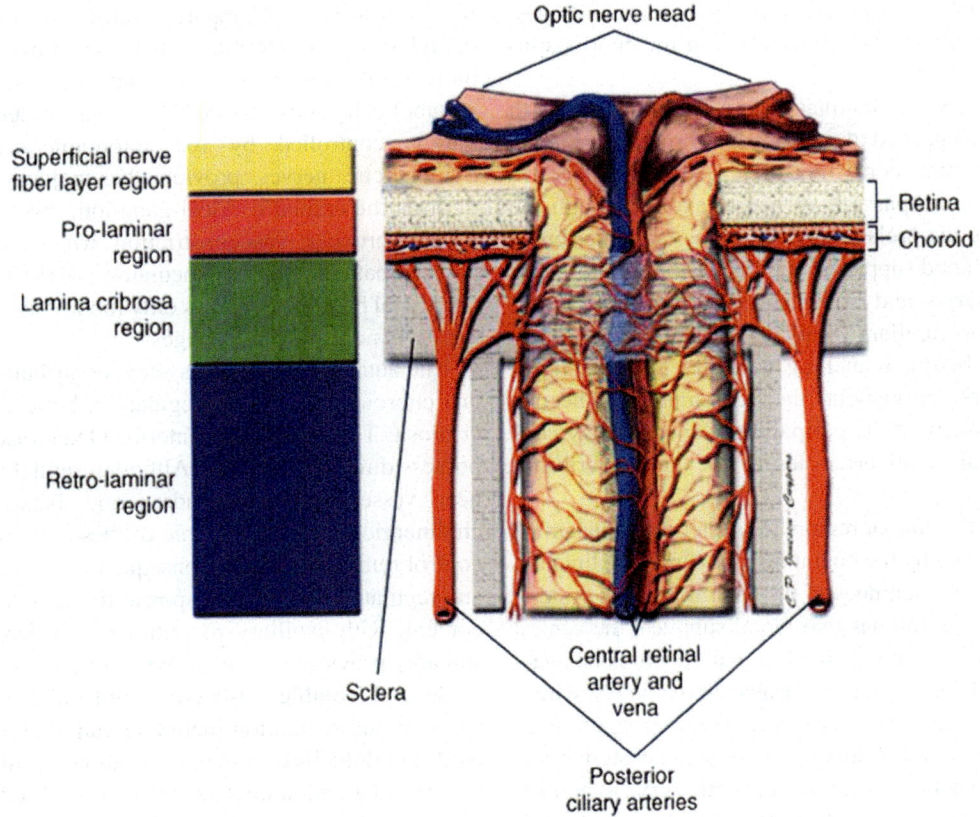

**Fig. 11.3** The anterior optic nerve may be divided into four anatomic regions: the superficial nerve fiber layer, the prelaminar region, the lamina cribrosa, and the retro-laminar region. Reprinted with permission from Harris et al[111]

ina and is the only nerve head structure visible by the routine fundus exam. It is supplied by retinal arterioles arising from the branches of retinal arteries. These small vessels originate in the surrounding nerve fiber layer and run toward the center of the optic nerve head. They have been referred to as "epipapillary vessels." The temporal nerve fiber layer may receive additional blood from a cilioretinal artery when it is present. No direct choroidal or choriocapillaris contribution is observed in the superficial nerve fiber layer.[44–54]

Immediately posterior to the nerve fiber layer is the prelaminar region, which lies adjacent to the peripapillary choroid. In this region, ganglionic axons group into bundles for passage through the lamina cribrosa. The prelaminar region is supplied primarily by branches of the short posterior ciliary arteries and by branches of the circle of Zinn–Haller, though some investigators have observed a vascular contribution to the prelaminar region from peripapillary choroidal arterioles. The amount of choroidal contribution may be difficult to ascertain, as there are branches from both the circle of Zinn–Haller and from the short posterior ciliary arteries that course through the choroid and ultimately supply the optic nerve in this region. These vessels do not originate in the choroid, but merely pass through it. The direct arterial supply to the prelaminar region arising from the choroidal vasculature is minimal. This minimal contribution from the choroidal vasculature is limited to small arterioles. There is no known vascular contribution of the choriocapillaris to the region.[52–56]

More posteriorly, the laminar region is continuous with the sclera and is composed of the lamina cribrosa. The lamina cribrosa is a structure consisting of fenestrated connective tissue that allows the passage of neural axons through the scleral coat. Like the prelaminar region, the lamina cribrosa also receives its blood supply from branches of the short posterior ciliary arteries and branches of the circle of Zinn–Haller. These precapillary branches perforate the outer lamina cribrosa before branching centrally and forming a capillary network throughout the fenestrated connective tissue. Larger vessels of the peripapillary choroid may contribute occasional small arterioles to the lamina cribrosa region.[44–59]

Finally, the retro-laminar region lies posterior to the lamina cribrosa and, marked by the beginning of axonal myelination, is surrounded by the meninges of the central nervous system. The retro-laminar region has two blood supplies: the central retinal artery and the pial system. The pial system is an anastomosing network of capillaries located immediately within the pia mater. The pial system originates at the circle of Zinn–Haller and may also be fed directly by the short posterior ciliary arteries. Its branches extend into the optic nerve to nourish the axons. The central retinal artery may provide several small intraneural branches in the retro-laminar region. Some of these blood vessel branches anastomose with the pial system.

This typifies the complex nature of the vascular system supplying the various regions of the optic nerve.[44–59]

The venous drainage of the anterior optic nerve is almost exclusively via a single vein: the central retinal vein (CRV).[60] In the nerve fiber layer, blood is drained directly into the retinal veins, which then join to form the CRV. In the prelaminar, laminar, and retro-laminar regions, venous drainage also occurs via the central retinal vein or axial tributaries to the central retinal vein.[58,60]

## 11.4 Regulation of Ocular Blood Flow

Blood flow is controlled by blood vessels via two separate system pathways: extrinsic and intrinsic controls.[61] Extrinsic controls include hormones and stimulation from the autonomic nervous system while intrinsic controls involve chemicals produced by cells in the immediate vicinity of the blood vessels. Intrinsic controls are often known as autoregulatory controls, which will be discussed. Extrinsic controls maintain the body's systemic blood pressure and are very important in the control of the choroid.[61]

Typically, retinal blood flow remains relatively constant over a substantial range of intraocular pressure and systemic blood pressure.[62,63] Compared with the choroidal circulation (a high flow, variable-rate system), the retinal circulation is a more stable, lower flow, constant-rate system supplying a metabolically active tissue.[62] Vascular resistance in the choroid is controlled by the autonomic nervous system. Sympathetic nerves provide the majority of regulation through the cranial cervical ganglion, involve neuropeptide Y, and provoke vasoconstriction when stimulated.[64] The parasympathetic system mediates poorly defined control. Choroidal blood flow shows only modest autoregulation during perfusion pressure changes.

The autonomic nervous system contributes to retrobulbar and choroidal circulatory regulation, but ends at the lamina cribrosa. The retinal and anterior ONH vasculature do not possess direct innervation. Although retinal and optic nerve head vessels have alpha-adrenergic, beta-adrenergic, and cholinergic receptors, the role of these receptors in vascular control remains unclear. Consequently, retinal blood flow is autoregulated locally in response to variable blood oxygen content, with capillary recruitment and derecruitment presumably providing constant oxygen delivery.[65]

Several soluble vasoactive molecules mediate retinal vascular autoregulation including endothelial-derived nitric oxide, endothelins, superoxide anions, renin–angiotensin, and vascular endothelial growth factor (VEGF). Nitric oxide is produced by two endothelial enzymes, constitutive nitric oxide synthase (membrane bound) and inducible nitric oxide synthase (cytosolic), both of which oxidize L-arginine to produce nitric oxide.[66] Endothelial cell nitric oxide diffuses to the pericyte or smooth muscle cell surface, where it binds to guanylate cyclase, causing intracellular cyclic guanosine monophosphate (cGMP) accumulation and subsequent vasodilation. Nitric oxide production is directly stimulated by increased local shear force, bradykinins, insulin-like growth factor 1, acetylcholine, thrombin, and various platelet products.[67] In addition to its vasodilatory actions, nitric oxide protects vessels by inhibiting platelet aggregation, platelet granule secretion, leukocyte adhesion, and possibly smooth muscle cell proliferation.[67]

Endothelins, another group of vasoactive molecules, are released by endothelial cells and bind to receptors on adjacent pericytes and smooth muscle cells.[56,68,69] Endothelins (ET1, ET2, and ET3, each 21 amino acids) are the most potent vasoconstrictor agents known. Endothelin-dependent contraction is mediated by three receptor subtypes (ETR A, B, and C).[56,68,69] Human studies show that vasoconstriction following intravenous injection of ET1 is mediated through ETR-A. Several in vitro studies, using tissues from a variety of species, demonstrate that endothelins are involved in retinal microvascular control; and animal experiments substantiate in vitro findings that ocular blood flow can be profoundly influenced by endothelin activity.[56,68,69] For instance, intravitreal injection of synthetic ET1 causes retinal vasoconstriction and decreased ocular blood flow, with no change in iris, ciliary, or choroidal blood flow.[56,68–70]

In addition to nitric oxide and endothelins, superoxide anions play a role in retinal microvascular autoregulation. Superoxide anions inactivate nitric oxide, thereby inhibiting vasodilatory capacity. The vascular endothelium generates basal levels of superoxide anions and can be stimulated to produce deleterious amounts of these molecules during many pathologic conditions. This pathologic inhibition may mediate vascular changes found in hypertension, hypercholesterolemia, retinopathy of prematurity, diabetes, and ischemia/reperfusion injury.[61-70]

Another component of the retinal microvascular autoregulatory system is the renin–angiotensin pathway. Angiotensin-converting enzyme (ACE) on the luminal endothelial cell surface rapidly converts angiotensin I to angiotensin II, and ACE inactivates bradykinin. Angiotensin II stimulates retinal vasoconstriction via smooth muscle cells and pericytes. Isolated porcine ophthalmic arteries vasoconstrict in response to angiotensin II, and relax in response to bradykinin via a nitric oxide-dependent mechanism. ACE-inhibitors used in this model prevent angiotensin-mediated constriction and potentiate bradykinin relaxation. After intravenous infusion of angiotensin II, cerebral and ocular blood flow was examined in healthy subjects by Doppler sonography and fundus pulsation amplitudes and demonstrated little decrease in choroidal or optic nerve head blood flow. Angiotensin II decreased the resistive index and fundus pulsation amplitude and increased the mean flow velocities in both the ophthalmic and the middle cerebral arteries; however, when compared to systemically measured parameters of mean arterial pressure, the intraocular vessels are relatively insensitive to angiotensin II.[61-70]

These complex and dynamic mechanisms by which ocular blood flow is regulated are also influenced by disease processes and may be vulnerable to the effects of aging and medications. It is therefore important to understand the effects of topical and systemic medications on ocular blood flow.

## 11.5 Vascular Risk Factors for Open-Angle Glaucoma

### 11.5.1 Systemic Hypertension and Hypotension

Along with specific ocular vascular tissue dysfunction, systemic hypertension and hypotension have both been reported as potential risk factors in glaucoma.[15,17,71–77] Chronic hypertension may cause microvascular damage, interference with autoregulatory mechanisms, and atherosclerotic changes, while hypotension may reduce local perfusion and lead to ischemic injury. Both of these mechanisms lead glaucomatous progression in the face of IOP elevation or poor vascular autoregulation of blood flow.[15,71–77] A decrease in blood pressure can lead to perfusion pressure below critical limits in the optic nerve head resulting in repeated ischemic insults.[17] It has been further speculated that ocular perfusion instability, rather than a steady reduction of ocular blood flow, might contribute to glaucomatous optic neuropathy. The combination of low blood pressure and high IOP can result in significant drops in ocular perfusion pressure and contribute to ocular ischemia. Recently, Leske et al[39] found lower systolic blood pressure, lower systolic perfusion pressure, and cardiovascular disease history as new predictors of glaucoma progression in the Early Manifest Glaucoma Trial (EMGT).

Although many studies show an association between blood pressure and IOP,[16,75–77] the information available on high blood pressure and OAG continues to be complex and inconclusive. In the Egna–Neumarkt study,[14] a positive correlation was found between systemic blood pressure and diagnosis of OAG as well as to IOP, unrelated to age. The Baltimore Eye Study demonstrated that patients with systolic blood pressure higher than 130 mmHg have greater risk for OAG.[15] Further analysis found that in patients under 60 years of age, systemic hypertension has a protective effect, while patients over 70 years old were adversely affected by systemic hypertension.

Contrasting this, however, the Barbados Incidence Study of Eye Diseases (BISED)[38] researched a large, predominantly African-origin population finding that persons with hypertension had a statistically significant decreased risk of OAG. One explanation is that higher blood pressure in the early stages can protect the optic nerve by maintaining the ocular perfusion pressure, while at later stages, chronic systemic hypertension may lead to dysfunctional regulation.

Medically lowered blood pressure may not be compensated for by local factors that maintain constant ocular perfusion. For instance, a subset of 3,842 participants of the Rotterdam Study participants using calcium channel antagonists had a 1.8-fold (95% confidence interval [CI], 1.04–3.2; $P=0.037$) higher risk of developing incident open-angle glaucoma while beta-blockers were associated with a nonsignificant risk reduction (odds ratio, 0.6; 95% CI, 0.3–1.02; $P=0.060$).[78] The European Glaucoma Prevention Study (EGPS) found that use of systemic diuretics (HR 2.41, 95% CI 1.12–5.19) were associated with the development of OAG.[79] In addition, the Thessaloniki eye study found that treatment with antihypertensive medication in nonglaucoma subjects was associated with increased cup-to-disc ratio of the optic nerve head.[40] The Rotterdam study[80] also reported an association between high tension glaucoma and high pulse pressure accompanied by arterial stiffness as well as with low diastolic perfusion pressure in patients receiving treatment for systemic hypertension. Increased vascular stiffness may contribute to the impaired autoregulation in certain glaucoma patients. These studies suggest that there is need for heightened awareness of medication regimens in glaucoma patient populations, especially medications that may interact with systemic blood pressure.

As abnormal vascular autoregulation has been reported in some glaucoma patients, blood pressure-related decreases in ocular perfusion pressure may have a direct effect on ocular blood flow. Gherghel et al reported lower mean blood pressure and lower end diastolic blood flow velocities in the central retinal artery in patients with progressing OAG compared to controls.[81] The mean perfusion pressure correlated positively with end diastolic blood flow velocities in the ophthalmic artery and central retinal artery and negatively with Pourcelot's resistive index in the ophthalmic and central retinal arteries.[81] Ocular blood flow in POAG patients may be compromised during fluctuating blood pressure, IOP, and perfusion pressure as a result of faulty autoregulation.

### 11.5.2 Nocturnal Hypotension

Circadian rhythms play an important role in maintaining homeostasis in the human body. Numerous recent studies have attempted to associate glaucoma risk with nocturnal hypotensive events. Studies indicate that blood pressure (BP) normally decreases at night, during sleep, to levels 10–20% below the diurnal average.[82,83] When a patient's mean daytime BP falls by more than 10% at night, they are often considered "dippers," while "nondippers" demonstrate a nocturnal decline that is absent or blunted.[82] Roughly two-thirds of individuals in the general healthy population have been characterized as dippers, indicating the physiologic nature of the nocturnal decline in blood pressure.[84] Tokunaga et al classified the dipper group as "physiologic dippers" and both the nondippers and extreme dippers as "nonphysiologic dippers." They found that nonphysiologic dippers had a higher incidence of visual field progression over a 4-year period.[85] Few studies, however, have attempted to investigate ocular blood flow at night in glaucoma patients. Harris et al[86] investigated whether reductions in nocturnal BP are linked to retrobulbar blood flow perturbations in glaucoma patients. They found that maximal posture-corrected nocturnal BP reductions were similar (~10%) in patients and controls, suggesting that in patients with nonprogressing glaucoma, there was no evidence of cerebral or retrobulbar hemodynamic abnormalities during nocturnal BP dips.[86] Although few conflicting data remain, the majority of studies point to a correlation between nocturnal hypotension and glaucoma.

The use of certain medications to reduce blood pressure may exacerbate OAG. This may be a concern especially during nocturnal dips in blood pressure. Hayreh et al noted that both glaucoma patients using topical beta-blockers[87] and hypertensive patients on oral beta-blocker therapy[88] had greater nocturnal dips than other patients. Although some studies purposefully excluded patients with known cardiovascular disease or ocular beta-blocker therapy, none have further expounded on the relationship between nocturnal hypotension and medical management, indicating an important avenue of research in glaucoma risk assessment.

In summary, cumulative data support the idea that systemic hypertension and nocturnal declines in blood pressure are potential risk factors for glaucoma. Recent studies also demonstrate the importance of assessing hypotensive episodes before initiating systemic antihypertensive therapy, in order to maintain consistent adequate perfusion to the optic nerve head and retinal ganglion cells.

### 11.5.3 Ocular Perfusion Pressure

Perfusion pressure is defined as the difference between arterial and venous pressure. In the eye, venous pressure is equal to or slightly higher than IOP. Ocular perfusion pressure (OPP) can therefore be defined as the difference between arterial blood pressure and IOP, and is calculated by taking two-thirds of mean arterial pressure minus IOP. This can be further broken down into diastolic perfusion pressure (diastolic blood pressure − IOP) and systolic perfusion pressure (systolic blood pressure − IOP). Hence, ocular perfusion pressure can be decreased by elevating IOP or reducing blood pressure. Ocular perfusion pressure is directly proportional to ocular blood flow (OBF), since ocular blood flow is equal to ocular perfusion pressure divided by vascular resistance.

Ocular blood flow, and subsequently ischemic injury to the optic nerve head, is dependent on ocular perfusion pressures and vascular resistance. Therefore, changes in ocular perfusion pressures (via blood pressure or IOP fluctuations) or vascular resistance (via autoregulatory dysfunction) affect ocular blood flow. Vascular autoregulation in healthy individuals provides consistent OBF over a wide range of perfusion pressures.[89] Glaucomatous patients, however, may experience vascular regulatory dysfunction, which causes fluctuations in OPP (via changes in either systemic blood pressure or IOP) to change retinal and optic nerve head perfusion.[90] Evidence supporting a relationship between OPP and glaucoma can be found in several large, population-based studies. The Baltimore Eye Study determined that patients with diastolic perfusion pressures lower than 30 mmHg were at greater risk for OAG; therefore, diastolic perfusion pressure below 50 mmHg is an important emerging risk factor for OAG.[15] Recently, the Early Manifest Glaucoma Trial found that low systolic perfusion pressures increase the risk of glaucoma by 50%, suggesting that glaucoma may be influenced by altered circulation at the optic disc.[39] A population-based study of Hispanic subjects found that the lower the diastolic perfusion pressure, the more likely the subjects were to have OAG.[91] Furthermore, those with perfusion pressures lower than 50 mmHg had a four times greater risk of OAG than those with perfusion pressures of 80 mmHg.[91] In the Barbados Incidence Study of Eye Diseases (BISED),[38] patients of African origin had the highest incidence of OAG with low ocular perfusion pressures: lower systolic perfusion pressure more than doubled the relative risk and lower diastolic perfusion pressure (<55 mmHg) more than tripled the relative risk of OAG. Reduced diastolic perfusion pressure below 55 mmHg is emerging as an important risk factor for OAG.

Although patients with high diastolic blood pressures of 85 mmHg or higher have an increased risk of NTG, surprisingly, patients with low diastolic perfusion pressure have a significantly lower risk of NTG.[92] Bonomi et al[14] investigating vascular risk factors for primary open-angle glaucoma in the Egna–Neumarkt Study found an association between decreased perfusion pressure and increased prevalence of glaucoma. Additionally, ocular perfusion pressure fluctuations have been shown to be related to visual field progression.[92]

It is always important to remember that as IOP increases, OPP decreases proportionally without concurrent changes in blood pressure. Within this context, several studies have shown that it is not the greatest elevations in IOP or greatest declines in OPP that increase the risk of glaucoma, but instead it is associated with greater fluctuations in IOP or OPP.[93,94] In one clinical setting where 24-h IOP monitoring replaced standard one-time evaluations, identification of IOP fluctuations, and spikes led to patient management changes in 79.3% of cases.[95] Choi et al noted that wider circadian OPP fluctuations in glaucoma patients were associated with excessive nocturnal blood pressure dipping and with worse visual field indices.[92] A more recent study further identified diurnal OPP fluctuation as the most consistent clinical risk factor for glaucoma severity.[96] The authors found that both anatomic (retinal nerve fiber layer thickness) and functional (visual field) outcome variables were significantly worse in glaucoma patients with wider circadian OPP fluctuation.[96] They attributed glaucoma progression to daily repetitive ischemic insults followed by reperfusion injury in eyes with defective autoregulatory mechanisms that could not maintain consistent OPP.

In summary, diurnal variations in IOP and blood pressure can cause decreased nocturnal OPP and wider diurnal OPP fluctuations in glaucoma patients (see Sidebar 11.1). Evidence has linked these OPP fluctuations with increased clinical severity and disease progression. The mechanism thought to be responsible for these poor functional outcomes in certain glaucoma patients may involve defective autoregulation of OBF, resulting in ischemic injury when challenged with fluctuating IOP and blood pressure.

### Sidebar 11.1. Ocular perfusion pressure and glaucoma: another view

Edney R. Moura Filho and Arthur J. Sit

Intraocular pressure (IOP) is currently the most important risk factor associated with glaucoma and its reduction remains the only proven therapy for glaucoma. However, the existence of patients with low IOP developing glaucomatous disc and visual field changes and patients with primary open-angle glaucoma (POAG) continuing to progress despite apparently adequate IOP have indicated the need to glaucoma identify risk factors other than increased IOP. One possible factor is inadequate blood flow to the optic nerve head. Numerous studies have identified circulatory abnormalities in the eyes of glaucoma patients, but the clinical significance of these specific changes remains to be demonstrated. Ocular perfusion pressure (OPP) is a clinical measure that has been suggested as a measure of the blood flow to the eye and possible risk for glaucoma.

OPP is a calculated value based on the systolic and diastolic blood pressure, and IOP. Different definitions of OPP are used depending on the particular study leading to some difficulty in the interpretation of results. Further complicating the calculation of OPP is the fact that changes in IOP as well as hemodynamics occur with changes in posture. The appropriate way to account for these changes in OPP calculations is controversial. Nevertheless, most calculations of OPP involve determining the average blood pressure and subtracting the IOP. OPP can be further subdivided into systolic perfusion pressure (SPP) and diastolic perfusion pressure (DPP).

Low DPP has been found to be a consistent risk factor for glaucoma in several epidemiological studies. In the Baltimore Eye Survey, the prevalence of open angle glaucoma (OAG) was constant at DPP above 50 mmHg, but increased dramatically with a decrease in DPP to below 50 mmHg. The age-and sex-adjusted Odds Ratio for OAG was six times higher in subjects with DPP<30 mmHg. In the Egna–Neumarkt Study, glaucoma prevalence was found to be higher in the population with DPP less than 70 mmHg. In the Rotterdam Study, the odds ratio for open angle glaucoma was 4.68 in subjects with DPP<50 mmHg, compared with subjects with DPP>65 mmHg. In the Barbados Eye Study, Leske et al reported a mean DPP of 63.2 mmHg in healthy subjects, and of 53.8 mmHg in subjects with open angle glaucoma. For the population with DPP<55 mmHg, there was a 2.2 times increased risk of OAG after a 9-year follow-up.[16]

The association between primary OAG and SPP is less clear. Mitchell et al reported only a marginal association between increasing SPP and OAG prevalence while Orzalesi et al reported that SPP was only minimally higher in subjects with OAG compared with normal subjects. However, the Barbados Eye Study found a relative risk for glaucoma in the population with low SPP of 2.6 and 2.1 at the 4- and 9-year follow-ups, respectively. In addition, the Early Manifest Glaucoma Trial found lower SPP to be a significant risk factor for glaucomatous progression, with baseline SPP≤125 mmHg associated with an almost 50% increase in risk for glaucomatous progression.

The role of OPP in normal tension glaucoma is of particular interest due to the absence of a clearly abnormal IOP as a causative factor. Choi et al examined the circadian variations in IOP and BP in a group of normal tension glaucoma patients. They found that the circadian mean OPP fluctuation was a consistent risk factor for glaucomatous damage. As well, the magnitude of OPP fluctuations appeared to be independent of IOP fluctuations, indicating a role of blood pressure fluctuations.

An increased risk of glaucoma progression with low OPP suggests the possibility that dysregulation of blood flow may contribute to disease progression. Autoregulation of blood flow in the optic nerve head would presumably compensate at least partially for changes in OPP. Insufficient autoregulation may contribute or exacerbate the decreased OPP, resulting in optic nerve head ischemia in susceptible individuals. However, vascular dysregulation as a clinical entity is difficult to define. Its diagnosis is mainly based on clinical clues obtained from the history, and there is no consensus regarding the value of specific diagnostic tests. Furthermore, effective treatment and the benefit from therapy for vascular dysregulation have not been shown.

Whether or not OPP will be useful in the clinical management of glaucoma remains to be demonstrated. One of the criticisms of research into OPP is that it is calculated based on measurements of blood pressure and IOP, and does not reflect the true vascular pressure in the optic nerve head. While this is true, it does not necessarily decrease its potential value in glaucoma research and possibly clinical management. It is conceivable that OPP may be the primary risk factor, and IOP is a secondary factor for glaucoma. However, the most direct treatment for low OPP at this time is reduction of IOP. Systemic treatment of low OPP is clearly an area in need of further investigation. Until more definitive results are available, treatment of glaucoma patients with ocular vasoprotective therapy remains controversial.

## Bibliography

Bonomi L, Marchini G, Marraffa M, et al. Vascular risk factors for primary open angle glaucoma: the Egna-Neumarkt Study. *Ophthalmology*. 2000;107(7):1287–1293.

Choi J, Kim KH, Jeong J, et al. Circadian fluctuation of mean ocular perfusion pressure is a consistent risk factor for normal-tension glaucoma. *Invest Ophthalmol Vis Sci*. 2007;48(1):104–111.

Delaney Y, Walshe TE, O'Brien C. Vasospasm in glaucoma: clinical and laboratory aspects. *Optom Vis Sci*. 2006;83(7):406–414.

Deokule S, Weinreb RN. Relationships among systemic blood pressure, intraocular pressure, and open-angle glaucoma. *Can J Ophthalmol*. 2008;43(3):302–307.

Dielemans I, Vingerling JR, Algra D, et al. Primary open-angle glaucoma, intraocular pressure, and systemic blood pressure in the general elderly population. The Rotterdam Study. *Ophthalmology*. 1995;102(1):54–60.

Flammer J, Orgul S. Optic nerve blood-flow abnormalities in glaucoma. *Prog Retin Eye Res.* 1998;17(2):267–89.

Flammer J, Orgul S, Costa VP, et al. The impact of ocular blood flow in glaucoma. *Prog Retin Eye Res.* 2002;21(4):359–393.

Grieshaber MC, Flammer J. Blood flow in glaucoma. *Curr Opin Ophthalmol.* 2005;16(2):79–83.

Grunwald JE, Piltz J, Hariprasad SM, DuPont J. Optic nerve and choroidal circulation in glaucoma. *Invest Ophthalmol Vis Sci.* 1998;39(12):2329–2336.

Grunwald JE, Piltz J, Hariprasad SM, et al. Optic nerve blood flow in glaucoma: effect of systemic hypertension. *Am J Ophthalmol.* 1999;127(5):516–522.

Hennis A, Wu SY, Nemesure B, Leske MC. Hypertension, diabetes, and longitudinal changes in intraocular pressure. *Ophthalmology.* 2003;110(5):908–914.

Leske MC, Connell AM, Wu SY, et al. Risk factors for open-angle glaucoma. The Barbados Eye Study. *Arch Ophthalmol.* 1995;113(7):918–924.

Leske MC, Heijl A, Hyman L, et al. Predictors of long-term progression in the early manifest glaucoma trial. *Ophthalmology.* 2007;114(11):1965–1972.

Leske MC, Wu SY, Hennis A, et al. Risk factors for incident open-angle glaucoma: the Barbados Eye Studies. *Ophthalmology.* 2008;115(1):85–93.

Liu JH, Gokhale PA, Loving RT, et al. Laboratory assessment of diurnal and nocturnal ocular perfusion pressures in humans. *J Ocul Pharmacol Ther.* 2003;19(4):291–297.

Michelson G, Groh MJ, Langhans M. Perfusion of the juxtapapillary retina and optic nerve head in acute ocular hypertension. *Ger J Ophthalmol.* 1996;5(6):315–321.

Mitchell P, Lee AJ, Rochtchina E, Wang JJ. Open-angle glaucoma and systemic hypertension: the blue mountains eye study. *J Glaucoma.* 2004;13(4):319–326.

Nicolela MT, Hnik P, Drance SM. Scanning laser Doppler flowmeter study of retinal and optic disk blood flow in glaucomatous patients. *Am J Ophthalmol.* 1996;122(6):775–783.

Orzalesi N, Rossetti L, Omboni S. Vascular risk factors in glaucoma: the results of a national survey. *Graefes Arch Clin Exp Ophthalmol.* 2007;245(6):795–802.

Piltz-Seymour JR. Laser Doppler flowmetry of the optic nerve head in glaucoma. *Surv Ophthalmol.* 1999;43 Suppl 1:S191–S198.

Piltz-Seymour JR, Grunwald JE, Hariprasad SM, Dupont J. Optic nerve blood flow is diminished in eyes of primary open-angle glaucoma suspects. *Am J Ophthalmol.* 2001;132(1):63–69.

Rojanapongpun P, Drance SM, Morrison BJ. Ophthalmic artery flow velocity in glaucomatous and normal subjects. *Br J Ophthalmol.* 1993;77(1):25–9.

Tielsch JM, Katz J, Sommer A, et al. Hypertension, perfusion pressure, and primary open-angle glaucoma. A population-based assessment. *Arch Ophthalmol.* 1995;113(2):216–221.

Ulrich WD, Ulrich C, Bohne BD. Deficient autoregulation and lengthening of the diffusion distance in the anterior optic nerve circulation in glaucoma: an electro-encephalo-dynamographic investigation. *Ophthalmic Res.* 1986;18(5):253–259.

## 11.6 Signs and Conditions Associated with Decreased Perfusion

### 11.6.1 Disc Hemorrhages

A flame- or splinter-shaped hemorrhage that is radially oriented across the optic disc margin to the adjacent peripapillary retina is considered to be related to the glaucomatous process if it occurs in the absence of any retinovascular abnormalities. These hemorrhages commonly occur at the upper and lower poles of the optic nerve head.[97] Within the glaucoma population, disc hemorrhages have been positively related to NTG.[19] Specifically, patients with the presence of a disc hemorrhage at baseline had a 2.7 times greater risk of experiencing glaucomatous progression than patients without hemorrhage at baseline.[19] Further, Rasker et al[98] reported that 80–89% of glaucoma patients with optic disc hemorrhages experienced glaucomatous progression as opposed to 32% of patients who did not have disc hemorrhage (mean follow-up of 9 years). Of note, OAG patients with diabetes and those using aspirin were reported to have a higher risk of having optic disc hemorrhage.[99] The Early Manifest Glaucoma Trial (EMGT) also reported that patients with frequent disc hemorrhages had increased progression of glaucoma.[100] It was also reported that NTG patients without baseline disc hemorrhage responded better to treatment than patients with baseline disc hemorrhage.[101] Lowering eye pressure may not make disc hemorrhages resolve.[102]

While it is not clear how disc hemorrhages are involved in the disease pathophysiology of glaucoma, they represent a vascular anomaly that continues to be strongly correlated to glaucoma disease and progression.

### 11.6.2 Migraines

Migraine as a disease may reflect a more generalized vasospastic tendency that can further affect ocular blood flow, possibly contributing to glaucoma pathology. Migraine has been reported to increase the risk of progression in patients with NTG. The reported risk ratio of patients with migraine to experience disease progression was 2.58 times greater than patients without migraine.[19] Migraine is significantly more common in patients with NTG compared with control subjects and patients with high-pressure glaucoma.[103] In the NTG study group, untreated female patients with migraine experienced faster visual function deterioration than those without migraine.[101]

Although inconclusive at this time, migraine may represent a more generalized vascular disease that can manifest itself in other diseases such as glaucoma. In this capacity, migraine may represent a vasospastic disease that can contribute to glaucoma in susceptible individuals. Patients with ocular hypertension were found to have a normal vasodilatory response within the retrobulbar vasculature during hypercapnia resulting in increased volumetric blood flow to the retina while patients with glaucoma did not, suggesting there is vasospasm at or downstream from the central retinal artery, which may result in decreased volumetric blood flow to the retina.[104] This builds upon previous research by Harris et al that found that NTG patients had reversible vasospasm apparent in the retrobulbar blood vessels.[11]

### 11.6.3 Diabetes

Diabetes, a disease with many vascular complications, has been reported to be related to glaucoma.[105] The prevalence of OAG was 40% higher in participants of the Los Angeles Latino Eye Study with type 2 diabetes mellitus than in those without (age/gender/intraocular pressure-adjusted odds ratio, 1.4; 95% confidence interval, 1.03–1.8; $P = 0.03$).[106] However, consistent evidence for diabetes as a contributing factor in OAG pathology is currently lacking. Population-based studies, such as the Baltimore eye survey,[107] the Barbados eye study,[108] and the Rotterdam study[109] have failed to support an association between diabetes and glaucoma. While some studies have found increased glaucomatous risk with diabetes, the majority of large population-based studies have failed to correlate diabetes with glaucoma risk. Due to the multitude of vascular changes in diabetes, more prospective evidence is required before definitive conclusions can be made regarding diabetes and glaucoma.

## 11.7 Prospective Ocular Blood Flow Studies in Glaucoma Patients

As previously discussed, reduced ocular blood flow may be secondary to IOP elevation or represent a primary insult to the optic nerve in glaucoma regardless of IOP. Chronic ocular ischemia may be due to faulty vascular autoregulation, and the inability of the vasculature to overcome elevated IOP or changes in blood pressure to maintain adequate perfusion. Regardless, chronic optic nerve ischemia has been shown to induce retinal ganglion cell loss independent of IOP.[26] The cascade of events involving reduction of ocular blood flow leading to retinal ganglion cell apoptosis is shown in Fig. 11.1.[110]

There are a multitude of various small prospective studies that have demonstrated blood flow deficiencies of OAG patients in the retinal,[7] choroidal,[8] and retrobulbar[9-12] circulations. Importantly, reductions in ocular blood flow have also been shown to correspond with areas of glaucomatous visual field loss.[13] The studies and evidence mentioned previously are just a sample of the many different ocular blood flow imaging technologies utilized in an attempt to reveal blood flow deficits in glaucoma. Each imaging technology has various limitations and is tissue-specific[111] within the eye's vasculature and will be discussed in detail in the next section. What is important to note is that the overwhelming amount of evidence from the various imaging techniques in the retinal, choroidal, and retrobulbar vascular beds point to a vascular role in OAG pathophysiology.

It is important to consider, however, that the direct and indirect evidence for ocular ischemia in OAG represents a surrogate for retinal metabolism and oxygenation. In this capacity, it is not a lack of blood flow per se but a consequential reduction in tissue oxygen and/or build-up of waste products that jeopardizes retinal ganglion cells. The direct measurement of retinal tissue oxygenation would reveal the true nature of ischemia's impact on retinal ganglion cell health and function. Currently, ocular blood flow investigations suggest that retinal tissue may be experiencing a lack of oxygenation and this hypoxia is contributing to OAG disease. New and emerging metabolic assessment tools may help reveal how reductions in ocular blood flow and ocular tissue hypoxia are related[112] and will be discussed further in the next section.

## 11.8 Methods for Measuring Ocular Blood Flow

This section provides detailed information on the most commonly used imaging technologies employed to investigate ocular blood flow: color Doppler imaging, confocal scanning laser ophthalmoscopic angiography with fluorescein and indocyanine green dye, the Canon laser blood flowmeter, scanning laser Doppler flowmetry, pulsatile ocular blood flow meter, retinal vessel analyzers, and retinal photographic oximetry. Understanding the tissue-specific nature and various limitations of each ocular imaging technology is essential to interpreting ocular hemodynamic study results. Currently, no single imaging device is capable of evaluating ocular blood flow in all of the relevant ocular tissue beds. Producing a comprehensive ocular hemodynamic evaluation therefore requires the use of several separate imaging modalities, each with its specific limitations.[110] By describing how these various imaging technologies function, we hope to contribute to the clinician's ability to differentiate ocular blood flow outcome measures and understand how they influence ocular health and disease.

### 11.8.1 Color Doppler Ultrasound Imaging

B-scan ultrasound is capable of producing detailed grayscale images of ocular anatomy. Color Doppler imaging (CDI) is an ultrasound technique[113-116] that combines B-scan grayscale imaging with color representation of blood flow measured by the Doppler shift in frequency of returning sound waves and pulsed-Doppler measurements of blood flow velocities. The motion of blood through the vessels is represented by a color-coded overlay placed on the familiar B-scan grayscale image of ocular anatomy. Most units code red-to-white for motion toward the probe and blue-to-white for motion away from the probe Fig. 11.4.

Measurements of Doppler-shifted sound frequencies correspond to the tissue within the sampling window. The CDI unit plots flow velocity data against time, with the peak and trough of the wave identified by the operator. From these, the computer calculates peak systolic velocity (PSV) and end diastolic velocity (EDV). In addition, Pourcelot's resistive index (RI), a measure of downstream vascular resistance, can be calculated according to the formula[117]:

$$RI = \frac{PSV - EDV}{PSV}$$

Values of this index range from zero to one, with higher values indicating higher distal vascular resistance.

In vitro studies have established the validity of Doppler ultrasound measures of blood flow velocity.[118] Using CDI, retrobulbar blood vessels such as the ophthalmic, central retinal, and nasal and temporal short posterior ciliary arteries are easily imaged. Reproducibility of retrobulbar blood vessel imaging is available in detail elsewhere, with the best reproducibility found in the ophthalmic artery.[65]

CDI measurements in glaucoma require careful interpretation, as reports in normal healthy individuals have shown reductions in blood flow to the optic nerve with increasing age.[18] Nevertheless, studies of retrobulbar blood velocities in POAG and NTG patients have found increased resistance to

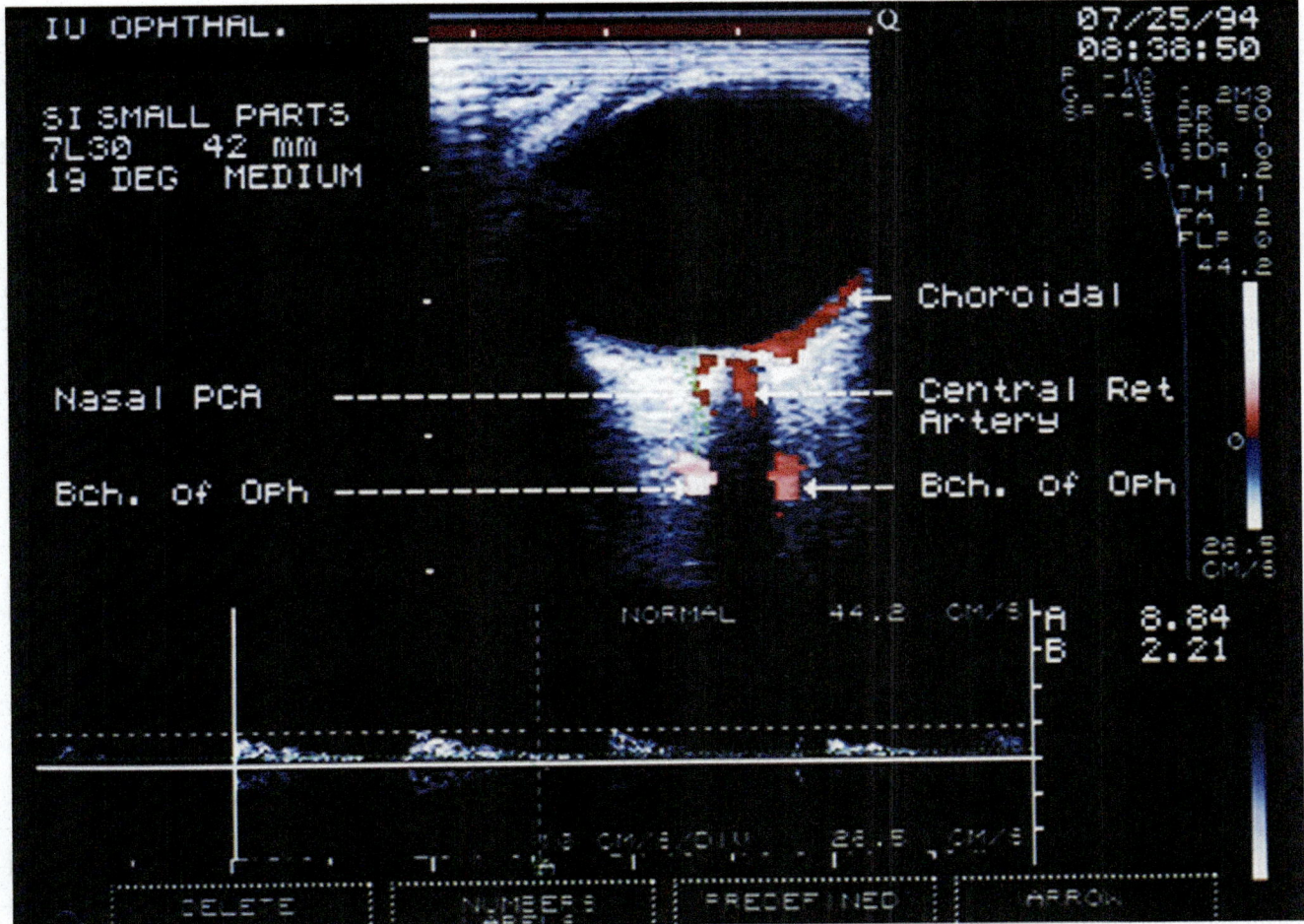

**Fig. 11.4** Color Doppler imaging plots flow velocity data against time, with the peak and trough of the wave identified by the operator. From these, the computer calculates peak systolic velocity (PSV) and end diastolic velocity (EDV) and Pourcelot's resistive index (RI)

blood flow and reduced blood flow velocities.[86,119–122] It has also been suggested that the existence of reduced retrobulbar hemodynamics in glaucoma patients may be associated with poor disease prognosis.[123] In a 7-year follow-up of POAG patients, increased resistive index in the ophthalmic artery was associated with an approximately sixfold increase in the likelihood of visual field deterioration compared with a cohort of POAG patients with a lower resistive index and stable fields.[124]

Reduced blood flow velocity and increased resistance to flow is not limited to the ocular vasculature, but has also been observed in the middle cerebral artery of patients with pseudoexfoliation glaucoma. This concept is further supported by reports of vascular regulatory dysfunction in both the retrobulbar vasculature and throughout the entire body in these patients.[11,125] In this capacity, the cerebral and ocular circulations may be related, and evidence suggests that systemic vascular regulatory dysfunction may also exist in NTG and POAG patients.[104,126] Furthermore, an ultrasound study of cerebral hemodynamics found diminished central visual function to be one manifestation of widespread cerebrovascular insufficiency in glaucoma.[127]

The vascular dysfunction in the retrobulbar blood vessels measured by CDI may also appear as an observable vasospasm in certain glaucoma patients.[104] Vasospasm within the blood vessels supplying the optic nerve head and retinal ganglion cells may lead to accelerated loss of visual function and increased rates of glaucomatous disease progression.[123,128] Specifically, Plange et al found that asymmetric glaucomatous visual field loss was associated with asymmetric flow velocities in the central retinal and ophthalmic arteries in POAG patients.[123] In addition, POAG patients with greater visual field damage displayed reduced flow velocities in the retrobulbar vessels.

In summary, CDI allows assessment of retrobulbar vasculature blood flow that supplies the eye and orbit. Reduced blood flow velocities and increased vascular resistance using this technology have been observed in these vessels in glaucoma patients. Retrobulbar vascular dysfunction is therefore apparent in glaucomatous disease in certain patients.

## 11.8.2 Scanning Laser Ophthalmoscopic Angiography

The scanning laser ophthalmoscope (SLO) increases the capabilities of quantitative angiography by enhancing image contrast and temporal resolution. The incandescent light source used in photographic and video techniques is replaced by a low-power scanning argon laser beam providing excellent penetration of lens and corneal opacities. Since the laser beam only illuminates a single spot on the retina at any moment, overall retinal illumination is reduced and contrast is improved. The exceptional optics and pure laser light sources of the SLO are currently most often used in spectral retinal analysis and microperimetry.[129–131]

The SLO is free from many of the deficiencies of the well established techniques of photographic and video angiography. Through the application of confocal optics, light reflected from the fundus exits the eye, passing through an aperture at the exterior principal focus of the lens before reaching a solid-state detector.[132–134] The detector generates a voltage proportional to the intensity of incoming light. The detector voltage level, measured in real time, creates a standard video signal. Scattered light and light reflected from sources outside the focal plane cannot enter the confocal aperture, which is fully open in angiography mode. The signal is generally passed through a video timer and then into an S-VHS video recorder. The resulting images not only have the high temporal resolution of those obtained with standard video angiography, but also possess superior spatial resolution and contrast.

The SLO can be used for fluorescein or indocyanine green angiography,[135–137] as discussed as follows. Excitation provided by a 488 nm argon blue laser and a 530 nm barrier filter are used for fluorescein angiography.[138,139] A 790-nm infrared diode laser with an 830-nm barrier filter is used for indocyanine green angiography.[140]

### 11.8.2.1 Scanning-Laser Ophthalmoscopic Fluorescein Angiography

Macro and micro retinal hemodynamics evaluated by the SLO fluorescein angiography system are usually quantified by arteriovenous passage (AVP) time and capillary transit velocities (CTV)[132–134] (Figs. 11.5 and 11.6). AVP time is analogous to mean circulation time and is equal to the difference in the time of dye arrival in a retinal artery and corresponding retinal vein (Fig. 11.5).[132–134]

Utilizing SLO video technology, reduced retinal hemodynamics have been observed in patients with glaucoma,[141] as evidenced by prolonged AVP times.[142] It has also been demonstrated that areas corresponding to more severe visual field damage have prolonged AVP time compared with areas of less damage.[143] Schulte found AVP deficits in glaucomatous eyes, and questioned whether blood flow reductions are primary or secondary to IOP increases.[143] This concern is ubiquitous, and it remains unclear whether there is a primary vascular component that leads to OAG, if the vascular component of OAG is secondary to increased IOP, or if OAG represents a combination of vascular dysregulation and increased IOP. Regardless of primary or secondary origin, the clinical impact of reduced retinal blood flow can manifest itself in accelerated loss of neuroretinal tissue.[144]

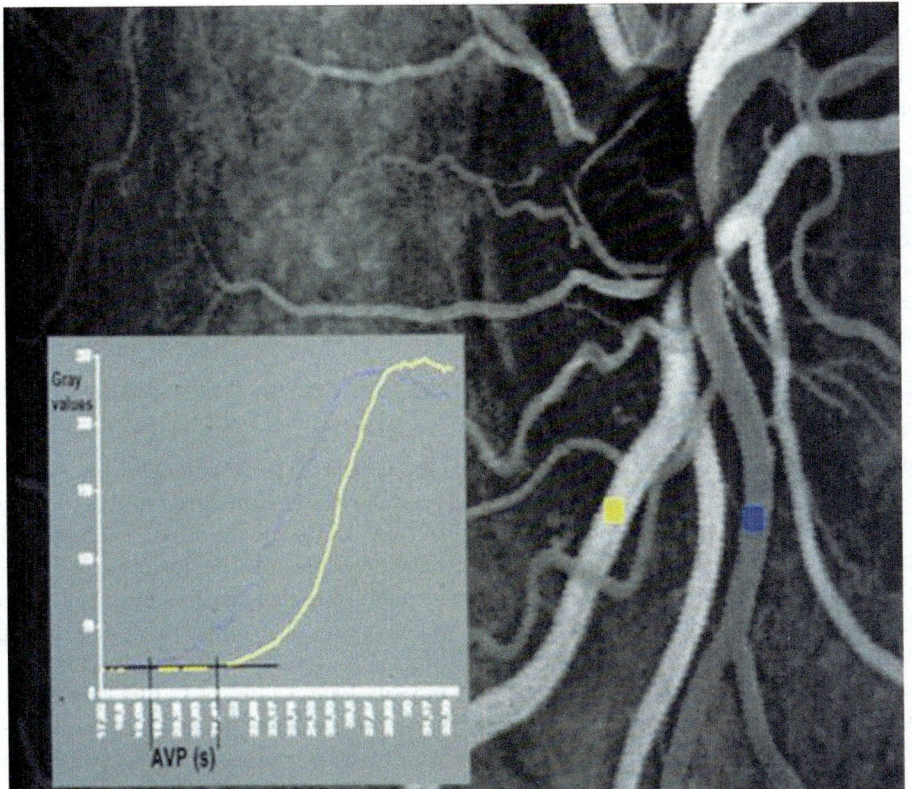

**Fig. 11.5** Macro and micro retinal hemodynamics evaluated by the SLO fluorescein angiography system are usually quantified by arteriovenous passage (AVP) time. AVP time is analogous to mean circulation time and is equal to the difference in the time of dye arrival in a retinal artery and corresponding retinal vein. Reprinted with permission from Harris et al[111]

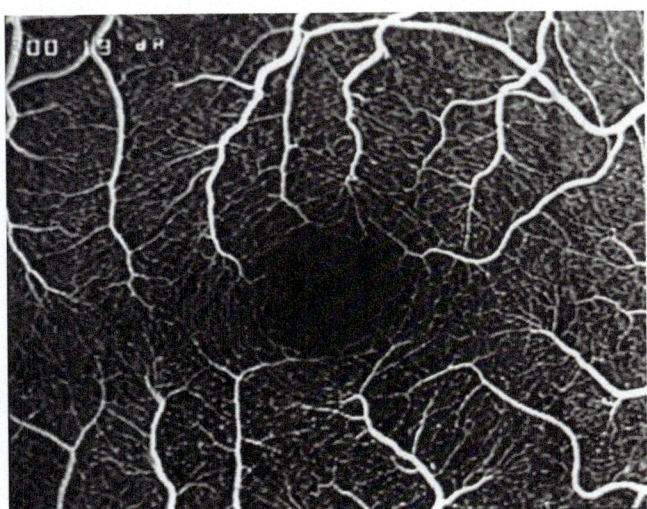

**Fig. 11.6** Capillary transit velocities (CTV) evaluated by the SLO fluorescein angiography system. Reprinted with permission from Harris et al[111]

In addition to measuring AVP times, the SLO's high temporal resolution permits visualization of hyper- and hypofluorescent segments in the perimacular and peripapillary capillary circulation. These light and dark segments are readily visible as they pass through the capillaries, thus allowing for CTV assessment. Using an image analysis system and customized software, it is possible to quantify CTV by measuring the distance traveled in a sequence of frames divided by the time taken to cover that distance.[139,145] This technique has also demonstrated optic disc capillary dropout in patients with glaucoma, which has been shown to correlate with visual field loss and morphometric damage in these patients.[146] As with other hemodynamic parameters, it is not known if capillary depletion was involved in the loss of tissue and function, or merely an epiphenomenon of disease progression.

### 11.8.2.2 Scanning-Laser Ophthalmoscopic Indocyanine Green Angiography

The bulk of ocular blood flow, especially flow to the outer retinal layers and optic nerve, is derived via the choroid. It is therefore important to have a method to evaluate the vasculature of this region. The application of SLO indocyanine green (ICG) angiography overcomes some of the limitations of fluorescein angiography in the study of choroidal blood flow (Fig. 11.7).[147] The near-infrared light used for scanning laser ICG angiography penetrates the pigmented layers of the fundus more efficiently than the shorter-wavelength light used in fluorescein angiography.[136,140] ICG has a high affinity for plasma proteins, with approximately 98% of the dye within the circulation binding to plasma albumin or lipoprotein.[148,149] As a result, ICG diffuses slowly out of the fenestrated choriocapillaris, in contrast to the swiftly diffusing fluorescein dye, and allows higher resolution of choroidal vasculature.[136,140]

Utilizing Indiana University Glaucoma Research and Diagnostic Center's software applications,[150,151] it is possible to produce the quantification of SLO choroidal ICG angiography. The entire 40° captured in an ICG angiogram is divided into a number of small regions, and dye-dilution curves are created for each region (Fig. 11.7). Six locations on the image, each at 6° square, are identified for analysis.[150,151] The average brightness of the area contained in each box is computed for each frame of the angiogram. Area dye-dilution analysis identifies three parameters from the dye-dilution curves: 10% filling time, the slope of the curve, and maximum brightness. The 10% filling time is the amount of time required to reach intensity 10% above baseline values. This parameter describes the rapidity of filling in the early choroidal filling phase. Slope of the filling curve is calculated by (1) noting the difference between the intensity at 10% filling and that at 90% filling, and (2) dividing the difference by the number of frames during that time, where each frame represents a known time interval. Hence, the slope represents the overall speed of blood flow as it enters the choroid.[150,151] Initial studies utilizing this technique suggest that some glaucomatous eyes present with select regions of slow choroidal filling and sluggish movement of blood into and out of the choroid.[150,151]

### 11.8.3 Canon Laser Blood Flowmetry

The Canon laser Doppler flowmeter (CLBF) is a modified fundus camera equipped with two lasers: one measuring blood velocity and the other simultaneously measuring vessel diameter while tracking its location[152,153] (Fig. 11.8). Utilizing a fixation target, the technician positions the desired measurement site into the center of a circular image. With the vessel of interest centered, a green line made by a 544-nm laser scanning the retina is rotated to lie across the vessel. After positioning the fundus, the technician initiates the measurement. A red laser dot appears on the center of the vessel of interest and automated vessel tracking software holds the laser in position to compensate for any eye movements during data acquisition.

As with other technologies, the CLBF has been used to demonstrate dysfunctional vascular regulation of the retinal vessels in glaucoma. For instance, a significant difference was observed in the variance of blood flow response to posture change between POAG patients and controls, suggesting underlying autoregulatory dysfunction in the glaucoma patients.[154] However, as with each previous technique, care must be taken in the interpretation of CLBF flow measurements. Although several studies report reproducible CLBF measurements of retinal blood flow in normal patients,[152,153,155] an in vitro model suggests that increasing densities of cataract create increasing levels of error in the vessel diameter measurement.[156] The CLBF, like the SLO with fluorescein angiography, has provided evidence that retinal blood flow is abnormal in glaucoma patients. Whether retinal blood flow is reduced due to faulty autoregulation or generalized ischemia is yet to be fully understood.

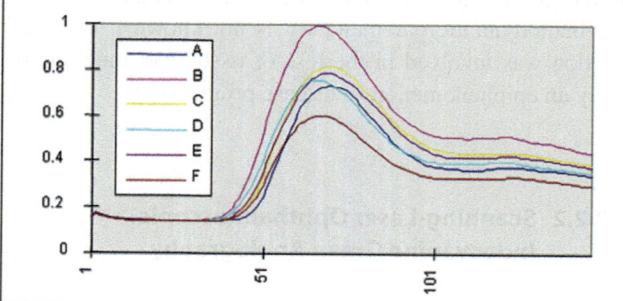

**Fig. 11.7** The entire 40° captured in an SLO ICG angiogram is divided into a number of small regions, and dye-dilution curves are created for each region and six locations on the image, each a 6° square, are identified for analysis. The average brightness of the area contained in each box is computed for each frame of the angiogram

### 11.8.4 Laser Doppler Flowmetry

The Laser Doppler Flowmeter (LDF) is a laser Doppler device consisting of a modified fundus camera and computer.[147] Unlike the CLBF, the LDF measures volumetric flow in the capillary beds of retinal and choroidal tissue. Though no longer

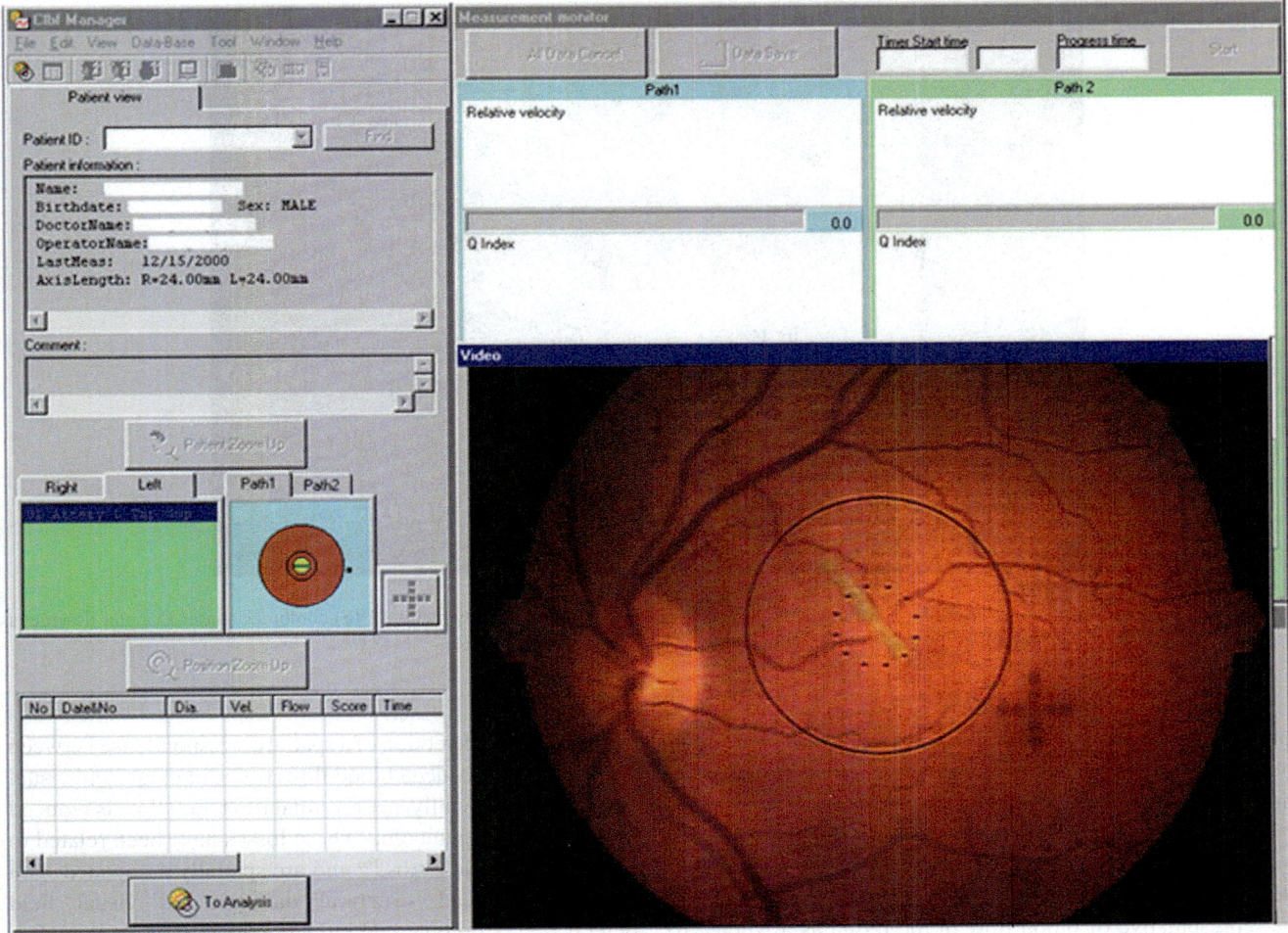

**Fig. 11.8** The Canon laser Doppler flowmeter (CLBF) is a modified fundus camera equipped with two lasers: one measuring blood velocity and the other simultaneously measuring vessel diameter while tracking its location. Reprinted with permission from Harris et al[111]

commercially available, data from the experimental Oculix LDF is well represented in the medical literature. Specifically, Boehm found decreased blood flow of the temporal neuroretinal rim compared with nasal blood flow in normal healthy subjects, suggesting a potential vulnerability of the temporal neuroretinal rim to ischemic insult.[157]

In addition to no longer being commercially available, it is difficult to interpret LDF data, as the source of measured Doppler shifts may be both the retinal and choroidal vasculature.[158] LDF is now, therefore, most often used to measure choroidal blood flow in the foveal avascular zone.[159]

### 11.8.5 Confocal Scanning Laser Doppler Flowmetry

The confocal scanning laser Doppler flowmeter (CSLDF) or Heidelberg retinal flowmeter (HRF) combines a laser Doppler flowmeter with a confocal scanning laser tomograph.[160–162] The instrument obtains images of a $2,560 \times 640 \times 400\,\mu m$ deep region of the retina or optic nerve head with a measurement accuracy of $10\,\mu m$ (Fig. 11.9). A 790-nm laser scans every line of the target at a line sampling rate of 4,000 Hz.[162] Upon completion of the scan, the HRF computer performs a fast Fourier transformation to extract the point by point Doppler frequency shift of reflected light. A frequency spectrum is calculated for each point of the scan. Each frequency location on the x-axis of the spectrum represents a blood velocity, and the height of the spectrum at each point is a function of the number of blood cells giving rise to the observed intensity of emission. Integrating the spectrum yields a value for total blood flow. On its default setting, the instrument analyzes a 10 pixel × 10 pixel ($100 \times 100\,\mu m$) region of tissue.[160,162,164]

The HRF has been shown to accurately measure blood flow in an artificial capillary tube and operators have obtained coefficients of reliability near 0.85 for acutely repeated volume, velocity, and flow measurements from 10 pixel × 10 pixel sampling areas[164,165] (Fig. 11.9). Reproducibility from these

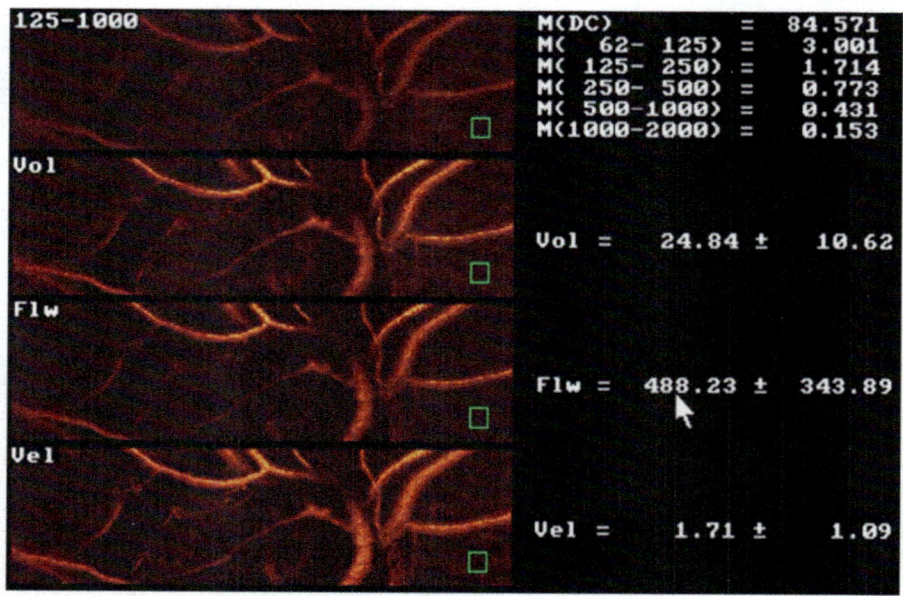

**Fig. 11.9** The confocal scanning laser Doppler flowmeter (CSLDF) or Heidelberg retinal flowmeter (HRF) combines a laser Doppler flowmeter with a confocal scanning laser tomography measuring retinal blood flow

small sampling boxes, however, has been demonstrated to be time dependent, with the coefficients of variation of measurements taken each week for 4 weeks averaging 30% of the mean.[163]

It has been suggested that perfusion of the conventional/default 10 pixel by 10 pixel area for data collection may not be representative of blood flow in the retina as a whole. To overcome these limitations, the Glaucoma Research and Diagnostic Center of Indiana University has developed a pixel-by-pixel analysis method in which individual qualifying pixels from the entire 256 pixel×64 pixel image are examined.[163] Large vessels, atrophic peripapillary regions, and image areas interrupted by movement saccades are avoided with this technique. In processing the HRF data, the total number of pixels in the image is determined, an average flow value is calculated, and a histogram of blood flow data is produced. Flow, volume, and velocity data at the 25th, 50th, 75th and 90th percentiles are the derived characteristics used for analysis of total retinal capillary blood flow (Fig. 11.10). The percentage occurrence of zero flow pixels within the image is also calculated. Broadening the analysis to include every qualifying pixel within the entire image improves test/retest reliability and reduces the coefficient of variation for repeated weekly measurements to 15% for selected portions of the flow histogram.

Similar to the aforementioned ocular vascular imaging technologies, prospective studies using HRF have found reductions in blood flow in both POAG and NTG patients. The ability of HRF to measure blood flow in precise locations (including the peripapillary areas) of the optic nerve head allows for detection of a spatial correspondence between the location of reduced blood flow, tissue damage, and visual field loss. Specifically, neuroretinal rim blood flow is reduced in persons with glaucoma. These losses have been related to larger cup-to-disc ratios,[166] and are spatially associated with optic nerve head structural damage and visual field defects.[167,168] Combined with the previous technologies' data on retinal blood flow, HRF measurements point to a reduction in retinal blood supply in ophthalmic disease such as glaucomatous optic neuropathy.

### 11.8.6 Pulsatile Ocular Blood Flow

Blood surges into the blood vessels of the eye during systole and continues to flow in more gradually during diastole. Similarly, blood pulses out of the ocular vessels throughout the cardiac cycle, though somewhat delayed relative to the inward flow from the arteries. Utilizing this principle, it has been proposed that real time measurements of IOP can be used to calculate the pulsatile component of blood flow.[169-172] The pulsatile ocular blood flow (POBF) devices (Paradigm systems and others) (Fig. 11.11) utilize a pneumatonometer that measures IOP in real time. It is based on the principle that blood volume in the eye increases with the systolic pulse and decreases during diastole. When the volume increases, eye pressure also increases. If the relationship between eye pressure and eye volume is similar throughout the patient population, then transient changes in IOP can be used to

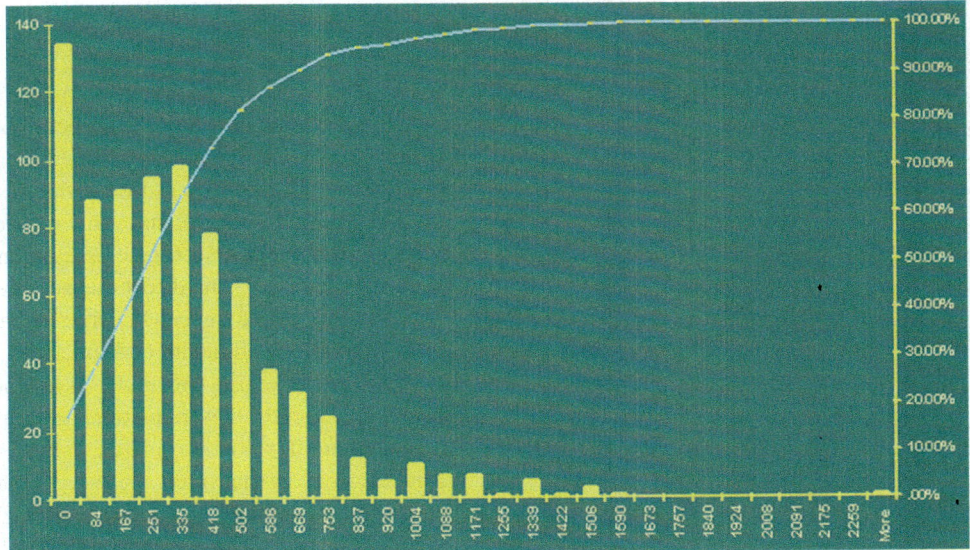

**Fig. 11.10** In processing the HRF data, the total number of pixels in the image is determined, an average flow value is calculated and a histogram of blood flow data is produced. Flow, volume and velocity data at the 25th, 50th, 75th and 90th percentiles are the derived characteristics used for analysis of total retinal capillary blood flow. Reprinted with permission from Harris et al[111]

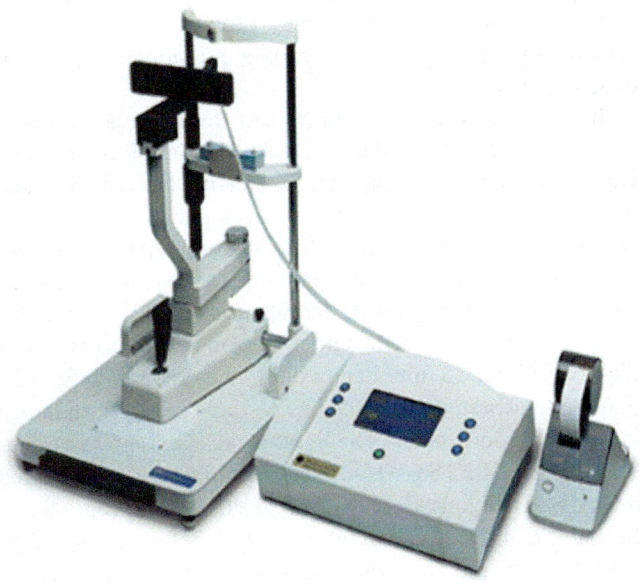

**Fig. 11.11** The pulsatile ocular blood flow (POBF) devices (Paradigm systems and others) utilize a pneumotonometer that measures IOP in real time. The IOP pulse wave is transformed into an ocular volume wave using the presumed universal relationship. The change in volume over time is reported as the POBF value

calculate absolute transient changes in ocular volume. The IOP pulse wave is transformed into an ocular volume wave using the presumed universal relationship. The change in volume over time is reported as the POBF value.

The POBF instrument is used in a similar capacity to a Goldmann applanation tonometer (Fig. 11.12). A pressurized tip is positioned in contact with the cornea and air pressure within the tip is increased until the cornea is indented. By measuring the level of air pressure required to indent the cornea, IOP is measured. Individual pressure readings are taken at a rate of 200 per second. When the measurement is complete, the waveforms observed on the display can be printed, along with a detailed report containing the average IOP, IOP range, ocular pulse amplitude (OPA), and calculated POBF.

There are advantages and disadvantages associated with the POBF technique. The greatest advantage is that the system is relatively inexpensive and affordable for the average clinical practice. The greatest disadvantage of POBF is that it is not a direct measurement of blood flow. IOP is measured, and several assumptions about scleral rigidity and a universal IOP/eye volume relationship are made. As with a leaking tire, however, the true volume of blood entering the eye is unknown. The rate of venous flow (the leak) is not measured, is unknown, and varies between individual eyes. Furthermore, large arteries and veins may provide large volumetric blood flow, which is indistinguishable from a lesser flow through smaller vessels.

Clinically, reduced POBF and OPA values have been found in glaucoma patients when compared to healthy normal subjects. For instance, POBF values were found to be significantly lower in juvenile glaucoma patients,[173] POAG patients,[174] and high risk ocular hypertensive patients[175] compared with normal subjects. Because of the obtuse nature of POBF and OPA readings, reductions in these variables may indicate generalized ischemia in ocular tissues that appears as retinal and choroidal defects when examined with more precise imaging technologies.

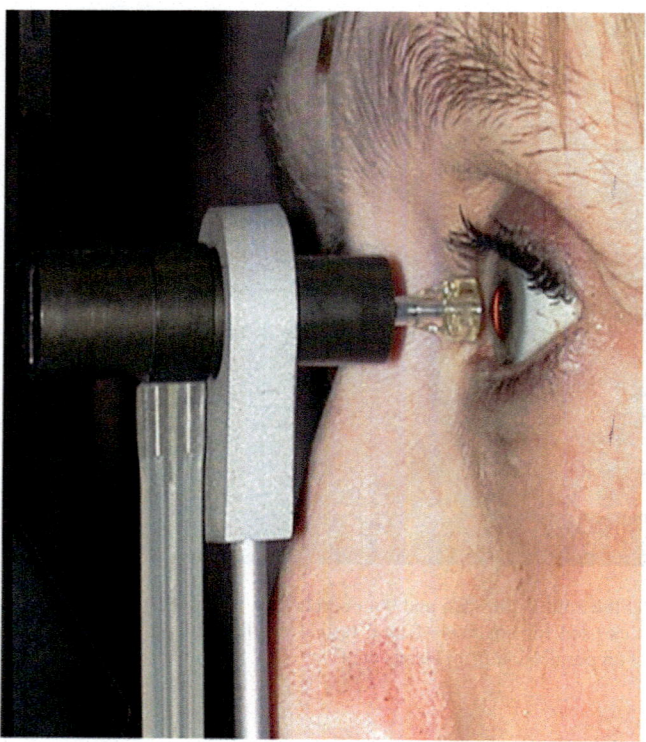

**Fig. 11.12** The POBF instrument is used in a similar capacity to a Goldmann applanation tonometer. Reprinted with permission Harris et al[111]

### 11.8.7 Retina Vessel Analyzer

In an attempt to limit the assumptions made in blood flow imaging techniques, the Retina Vessel Analyzer (RVA) from Imedos GmbH (Jena, Germany) was developed to produce real-time measurements of large retinal vessels with a spatial resolution less than 1 μm.[176] This is accomplished by averaging hundreds of individual measurements acquired at 250 per second. Despite a physical resolution of 17 μm per pixel, a floating average allows the RVA to accurately monitor the pulsation of retinal vessels throughout the cardiac cycle.[176]

Using the RVA, Nagel et al found that the retinal vein diameter autoregulatory response to acute IOP elevation is diminished in patients with primary open angle glaucoma.[177] Garhofer found that the autoregulatory response to flicker-induced vasodilation of retinal veins is significantly diminished in patients with glaucoma compared with healthy volunteers.[178] The authors suggest that the regulation of retinal vascular tone is impaired in patients with early glaucoma; however, as with Nagel's findings, differences were not significant in arteries.[178] As with other imaging technologies, RVA measurements suggest that ocular (retinal) circulation is abnormal in ophthalmic disease such as glaucoma. Further improvements in metabolic imaging technologies, such as retinal oximetry, may help tie together the various findings of these technologies as they relate to tissue hypoxia.

### 11.8.8 Retinal Oximetry

Each of the hemodynamic assessment technologies previously presented quantify some aspect of ocular blood flow. It is impossible, however, to interpret the impact of any single blood flow parameter measured within a single vascular bed on total retinal metabolism. The measurement of ocular blood flow is only a surrogate assessment of the metabolic status of the retina. The direct measurement of retinal tissue oxygenation would reveal the true impact of ischemia on retinal ganglion cell health and function.

New and emerging metabolic assessment tools may help reveal specifically how reductions in ocular blood flow and ocular tissue hypoxia are related.[112] For instance, a study by Michelson et al measured the oxygen saturation in retinal arterioles and venules in patients with glaucomatous optic neuropathy using imaging spectrometry.[179] In all examined eyes, the arteriolar oxygen saturation and the retinal arteriovenous differences in oxygen correlated significantly with the patient's rim area. Eyes with NTG, but not those with POAG, showed significantly decreased arteriolar oxygen saturation. These metabolic assessment tools, while still undergoing improvements,[180] may provide the next step in specifically assessing retinal hypoxia, possibly as a result of ocular ischemia.

In response to the continued need for noninvasive metabolic measurements in the eye, the Glaucoma Research and Diagnostic Center at Indiana University has collaborated with the University of Iceland to develop a dual wavelength retinal spectral oximeter.[180] This photographic oximeter (Fig. 11.13) consists of a modified Topcon 50VT fundus camera containing a top Polaroid mount fitted with a 1:4 image splitter (Optical Insights, Tucson, Arizona) and four dichroic filters (5 nm bandwidth) centered at 542, 558, 586 nm (isosbestic), and 605 nm. A single xenon flash image is split into four frames. The light in each band is then quantified using a SBIG ST-7 16-bit scientific digital charge coupled device (CCD) camera (Santa Barbara Imaging Group, Santa Barbara, California). This clinical tool is being utilized to expand upon the surrogate measurements of ocular blood flow to further understand hypoxia's role in ocular health and disease. While still undergoing improvements, this kind of photographic retinal oximetry may provide the next step in specifically assessing retinal hypoxia experienced as a result of ocular ischemia.[180]

Another recent application of oximetry involves Fourier domain optical coherence tomography (OCT) data to assess retinal blood oxygen saturation.[181] Three-dimensional disc-centered retinal tissue volumes were assessed in 17 normal healthy subjects. A difference between arterial and venous blood saturation was detected, suggesting that retinal oximetry may possibly be added as a metabolic measurement in structural imaging devices.[181] Once ocular tissue metabolism

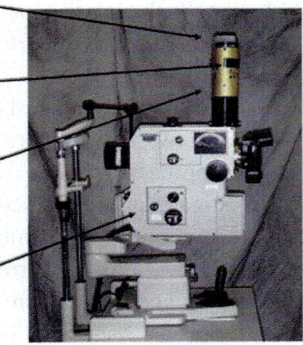

## Oximetry

- **Digital camera port**
  - Quantifies light scattered by the fundus
- **Four individual band-pass filters**
  - Isolate the frequencies of interest
- **1:4 Image Splitter**
  - Create four equal images from a single fundus flash photo
- **Standard Fundus Camera**

**Fig. 11.13** This photographic oximeter consists of a modified Topcon 50VT fundus camera containing a top Polaroid mount fitted with a 1:4 image splitter (Optical Insights, Tucson, AZ) and four dichroic filters (5 nm bandwidth) centered at 542, 558, 586 nm (isosbestic) and 605 nm. A single xenon flash image is split into four frames. The light in each band is then quantified using a SBIG ST-7 16 bit scientific digital charge coupled device (CCD) camera (Santa Barbara Imaging Group, Santa Barbara, CA). This clinical tool is being utilized to expand upon the surrogate measurements of ocular blood flow to further understand hypoxia's role in ocular health and disease

measurements are fully apparent, our understanding of disease pathophysiology will greatly improve as will our understanding of disease treatments and potentially result in earlier patient diagnosis.

## 11.9 Relationship Between Ocular Blood Flow, Visual Function, and Structure

The relationship between ocular blood flow, visual function, and structure has begun to emerge in the literature. Various measures of ocular perfusion pressure and directly assessed ocular blood flow have been found to be related to measures of glaucomatous visual field loss and structural changes. For instance, ocular perfusion pressure fluctuations have been shown to be related to visual field progression.[92] A more recent study further identified diurnal ocular perfusion pressure (OPP) fluctuation as the most consistent clinical risk factor for glaucoma severity.[96] The authors found that both anatomic (retinal nerve fiber layer thickness) and functional (visual field) outcome variables were significantly worse in glaucoma patients with greater fluctuation of perfusion pressure.

Directly assessed ocular blood flow has also been associated with glaucoma and glaucoma progression. In the retrobulbar vasculature, reductions in ocular blood flow using CDI have been shown to correspond with areas of glaucomatous visual field loss.[13,182] Yamazaki and Drance[183] reported an association between abnormal retrobulbar ocular blood flow and glaucoma. They found that NTG patients with progressive visual field defects had significantly impaired retrobulbar blood flow parameters compared to those with clinically stable visual fields. These findings are especially significant because blood flow velocity measurements more closely approximate true volumetric blood flow changes when peak systolic and end diastolic velocities change in tandem.[184] Another significant finding from the visual field studies was that the resistive index of the ophthalmic artery might be used as a predictor of glaucoma progression. In a 7-year follow-up of POAG patients, increased resistive index in the ophthalmic artery was associated with an approximately sixfold increase in the likelihood of visual field deterioration compared with a cohort of POAG patients with a lower resistive index and stable fields.[124] Martinez and Sanchez[185] also found that having an ophthalmic artery resistive index of greater than 0.82 gave a positive posttest probability of 90.5% for progression.

Plange et al found that asymmetric glaucomatous visual field loss was associated with asymmetric flow velocities in the central retinal and ophthalmic arteries in POAG patients.[123] In addition, POAG patients with more severe visual field damage displayed reduced flow velocities in the retrobulbar vessels. Additionally, Zeitz et al found glaucoma progression to be associated with decreased blood flow velocities in the short posterior ciliary arteries.[128] Finally, Zink et al found an association between lower optic nerve laser Doppler blood volume measurements and glaucomatous visual field progression.[186]

In addition to worsening visual fields, progressive structural changes in the optic nerve head have also been related to abnormal ocular blood flow in glaucoma patients. Neuroretinal rim blood flow has also been shown to be reduced in persons with glaucoma. These losses have been related to larger cup-to-disc ratios,[166] and are spatially associated with optic nerve head structural damage and visual field defects.[167,168] Specifically, Logan et al[167] found decreased capillary flow in areas of the retina associated with abnormal optic disc segments. In contrast, normal optic disc segments from these same glaucoma patients were not associated with compromised retinal flow. Scanning laser ophthalmoscopy has also demonstrated optic disc capillary dropout in patients with glaucoma, which has been shown to correlate with visual field loss and morphometric damage in these patients.[146] A recent study also found association between decreased retrobulbar blood flow and progressive structural damage to the retinal nerve fiber layer.[187]

It remains unclear whether there is a primary vascular component that leads to OAG, if the vascular component of OAG is secondary to increased IOP, or if OAG represents a combination of vascular dysregulation and increased IOP. Regardless of primary or secondary origin, the clinical impact of reduced retinal blood flow may manifest itself as accelerated loss of neuroretinal tissue, structural damage, and glaucomatous visual field loss. However, the exact relationship between abnormal ocular blood flow and structural/functional outcomes needs to be more completely defined.

## 11.10 Conclusion

Advances in ocular blood flow and metabolism imaging technologies continue to help reveal the multifactorial etiology of glaucomatous optic neuropathy. It is clear from population-based studies that controlling IOP alone is not enough to prevent progression in some glaucoma patients. In addition to IOP, vascular risk factors continue to be confirmed as possibly contributing to glaucoma disease prevalence, incidence, and progression. Low OPP remains a vital consideration in glaucoma management as demonstrated by multiethnic large population-based studies. In this capacity, it is strongly suggested that blood pressure measurements be taken during ophthalmic examinations and be evaluated in relation to IOP. Direct evidence of low ocular blood flow in glaucoma patients compared with controls compliment the large population-based studies on ocular perfusion pressure, although it remains unclear why some patients exhibit lower blood flow values than other patients.

There remains a lack of clear association between blood flow deficiencies and optic nerve head or visual field progression in glaucoma patients. Several large, prospective, controlled, long-term studies are needed to fill this gap. Such studies must use multiple technologies to assess the breadth of ocular blood flow parameters that may change in glaucoma. Hemodynamics should also be monitored throughout the 24-h period to allow association of circadian changes in perfusion pressure with blood flow changes and ultimately with glaucomatous progression. The preliminary studies presented in this chapter highlight the initial evidence upon which further research should be built. In this capacity, methods of assessing ocular blood flow need to be standardized, streamlined, and adapted to clinical ophthalmology.

New strategies to enhance ocular blood flow and potentially slow the progression of disease need to be designed and implemented into treatment protocols. Work in this realm has already begun by studying the effects of current IOP-lowering medications on ocular hemodynamics. To impact ocular circulation, topical glaucoma medications need to possess three basic principles of physiology: (1) ocular penetration, (2) accumulation of sufficient physiochemical concentration, and (3) the ability to interact with ocular vascular tissues to cause vasodilation. It is vital to evaluate current and new medications used in glaucoma management to understand the possible impacts they have on ocular circulation.

### 11.10.1 Clinical Pearls

1. Low perfusion pressure and large fluctuations in intraocular pressure may be important prognostic factors for glaucomatous progression.
2. No current gold standard exists for measuring total ocular blood flow; we therefore strongly suggest a comprehensive approach utilizing several imaging technologies to investigate multiple vascular beds.
3. It is important to remember that measurements of ocular blood flow remain a surrogate assessment for tissue oxygenation and metabolism. Future advances in tissue oxygenation assessment will improve our understanding of glaucomatous disease pathophysiology.
4. Systemic medications such as antihypertensives have been associated with the development of open angle glaucoma (OAG), indicating a need for heightened awareness of medication regimens in the glaucoma patient population.

## References

1. National Eye Institute. Statistics and Data. Prevalence of Blindness Data. Data Tables. http://www.nei.nih.gov/eyedata/pbd_tables.asp. Accessed on September 18, 2007.
2. Eye Diseases Prevalence Research Group. Prevalence of open-angle glaucoma among adults in the United States. *Arch Ophthalmol.* 2004;122(4):532–538.
3. Heijl A, Leske MC, Bengtsson B, Hyman L, Bengtsson B, Hussein M; Early Manifest Glaucoma Trial Group. Reduction of intraocular pressure and glaucoma progression: results from the Early Manifest Glaucoma Trial. *Arch Ophthalmol.* 2002;120(10):1268–1279.
4. Lichter PR, Musch DC, Gillespie BW, et al. Interim clinical outcome in the collaborative initial glaucoma treatment study comparing initial treatment randomized to medications or surgery. *Ophthalmology.* 2001;108:1943–1953.
5. Collaborative Normal-Tension Glaucoma Study Group. The effectiveness of intraocular pressure reduction in the treatment of normal-tension glaucoma. *Am J Ophthalmol.* 1998;126:498–505.
6. Flammer J, Orgül S, Costa VP, et al. The impact of ocular blood flow in glaucoma. *Prog Retin Eye Res.* 2002;21:359–393.
7. Chung HS, Harris A, Kagemann L, Martin B. Peripapillary retinal blood flow in normal tension glaucoma. *Br J Ophthalmol.* 1999;83:466–469.
8. Yin ZQ, Vaegan, Millar TJ, et al. Widespread choroidal insufficiency in primary open-angle glaucoma. *J Glaucoma.* 1997;6:23–32.
9. Butt Z, McKillop G, O'Brien C, et al. Measurement of ocular blood flow velocity using colour Doppler imaging in low tension glaucoma. *Eye.* 1995;9:29–33.
10. Galassi F, Sodi A, Ucci F, et al. Ocular haemodynamics in glaucoma associated with high myopia. *Int'l Ophthalmol.* 1998;22:299–305.
11. Harris A, Sergott RC, Spaeth GL, et al. Color Doppler analysis of ocular vessel blood velocity in normal-tension glaucoma. *Am J Ophthalmol.* 1994;118:642–649.

12. Rojanapongpun P, Drance SM, Morrison BJ. Ophthalmic artery flow velocity in glaucomatous and normal subjects. *Br J Ophthalmol.* 1993;77:25–29.
13. Breil P, Krummenauer F, Schmitz S, Pfeiffer N. [The relationship between retrobulbar blood flow velocity and glaucoma damage] [German]. *Ophthalmologe.* 2002;99:613–616.
14. Bonomi L, Marchini G, Marraffa M, et al. Vascular risk factors for primary open-angle glaucoma: the Egna-Neumarkt Study. *Ophthalmology.* 2000;107:1287–1293.
15. Tielsch JM, Katz J, Sommer A, et al. Hypertension, perfusion pressure, and primary open-angle glaucoma. A population based assessment. *Arch Ophthalmol.* 1995;113:216–221.
16. Leighton DA, Phillips CI. Systemic blood pressure in open-angle glaucoma, low tension glaucoma, and the normal eye. *Br J Ophthalmol.* 1972;56:447–453.
17. Hayreh SS, Zimmerman MB, Podhajsky P, Alward WL. Nocturnal arterial hypotension and its role in optic nerve head and ocular ischemic disorders. *Am J Ophthalmol.* 1994;117:603–624.
18. Harris A, Harris M, Biller J, et al. Aging affects the retrobulbar circulation differently in females and males. *Arch Ophthalmol.* 2000;118:1076–1080.
19. Drance S, Anderson DR, Schulzer M. Risk factors for progression of visual field abnormalities in normal-tension glaucoma. *Am J Ophthalmol.* 2001;131:699–708.
20. Wagemann A, Salzmann P. Anatomische Untersuchungen uber einseitige Retinitis Haemorrhagica mit Secundar-Glaucom nebst Mittheilungen uber dabei beobachtete Hypopyon-Keratitis. *Arch Ophthalmol.* 1892;38:213.
21. Elschnig. *Hendbuch der speziellen pathologiseher Anatomie und Histologie.* Vol 1. Berlin: Julius Springs; 1928.
22. Lauber H. Treatment of atrophy of the optic nerve. *Arch Ophthalmol.* 1936;16:555–568.
23. Reese AB, McGavic JS. Relation of field contraction to blood pressure in chronic primary glaucoma. *Arch Ophthalmol.* 1942;27:845–850.
24. Duke-Elder WS. *Textbook of Ophthalmology,* vol. 3. St. Louis: CV Mosby Company; 1940:3354.
25. Loewenstein A. Cavernouos degeneration, necrosis and other regressive processes in optic nerve with vascular disease of eye. *Arch Ophthalmol.* 1945;34:220–225.
26. Cioffi GA, Wang L, Fortune B, et al. Chronic ischemia induces regional axonal damage in experimental primate optic neuropathy. *Arch Ophthalmol.* 2004;122:1517–1525.
27. Pease ME, McKinnon SJ, Quigley HA, Kerrigan-Baumrind LA, Zack DJ. Obstructed axonal transport of BDNF and its receptor TrkB in experimental glaucoma. *Invest Ophthalmol Vis Sci.* 2000;41:764–774.
28. Quigley HA, Nickells RW, Kerrigan LA, Pease ME, Thibault DJ, Zack DJ. Retinal ganglion cell death in experimental glaucoma and after axotomy occurs by apoptosis. *Invest Ophthalmol Vis Sci.* 1995;36:774–786.
29. Nickells RW. Retinal ganglion cell death in glaucoma: the how, the why, and the maybe. *J Glaucoma.* 1996;5:345–356.
30. Chen J, Graham SH, Nakayama M, et al. Apoptosis repressor genes Bcl-2 and Bcl-x-long are expressed in the rat brain following global ischemia. *J Cereb Blood Flow Metab.* 1997;17:2–10.
31. Gillardon F, Lenz C, Waschke KF, et al. Altered expression of Bcl-2, Bcl-x, Bax, and c-Fos colocalizes with DNA fragmentation and ischemic cell damage following middle cerebral artery occlusion in rats. *Brain Res Mol Brain Res.* 1996;40:254–260.
32. Macaya A. Apoptosis in the nervous system. *Rev Neurol.* 1996;24:1356–1360.
33. Romano C, Price MT, Almli T, Olney JW. Excitotoxic neurodegeneration induced by deprivation of oxygen and glucose in isolated retina. *Invest Ophthalmol Vis Sci.* 1998;39:416–423.
34. Katai N, Yoshimura N. Apoptotic retinal neuronal death by ischemia-reperfusion is executed by two distinct caspase family proteases. *Invest Ophthalmol Vis Sci.* 1999;40:2697–2705.
35. Ju WK, Kim KY, Hofmann HD, et al. Selective neuronal survival and upregulation of PCNA in the rat inner retina following transient ischemia. *J Neuropathol Exp Neurol.* 2000;59:241–250.
36. Sommer A, Tielsch JM, Katz J, et al. Relationship between intraocular pressure and primary open angle glaucoma among white and black Americans. The Baltimore Eye Survey. *Arch Ophthalmol.* 1991;109:1090–1095.
37. Collaborative Normal-Tension Glaucoma Study Group. Comparison of glaucomatous progression between untreated patients with normal-tension glaucoma and patients with therapeutically reduced intraocular pressures. *Am J Ophthalmol.* 1998;126:487–497.
38. Leske MC, Connell AM, Wu SY, et al. Incidence of open-angle glaucoma: the Barbados Eye Studies. *Arch Ophthalmol.* 2001;119:89–95.
39. Leske MC, Heijl A, Hyman L, Bengtsson B, Dong L, Yang Z. Predictors of long-term progression in the early manifest glaucoma trial. *Ophthalmology.* 2007;114(11):1965–1972.
40. Topouzis F, Coleman AL, Harris A, et al. Association of blood pressure status with the optic disk structure in non-glaucoma subjects: the Thessaloniki eye study. *Am J Ophthalmol.* 2006;142:60–67.
41. Hayreh SS, Dass R. The ophthalmic artery. II: intra-orbital course. *Br J Ophthalmol.* 1962;46:165–185.
42. Hayreh SS. The ophthalmic artery. III: branches. *Br J Ophthalmol.* 1962;46:212–247.
43. Bignell J. Investigations into the blood supply of the optic nerve with special reference to the lamina cribrosa region. *Trans Ophthalmol Soc Aust.* 1952;12:105.
44. Hayreh SS. Structure and blood supply of the optic nerve. In: Heilmann K, Richardson KT, eds. *Glaucoma: Conceptions of a Disease: Pathogenesis, Diagnosis, Therapy.* Stuttgart: Georg Thieme; 1978:78–96.
45. Olver JM, Spalton DJ, McCartney ACE. Microvascular study of the retrolaminar optic nerve head in man: the possible significance in anterior ischaemic optic neuropathy. *Eye.* 1990;4:7.
46. Onda E, Cioffi GA, Bacon DR, Van Buskirk EM. Microvasculature of the anterior human optic nerve. *Am J Ophthalmol.* 1996;121(4):452–453.
47. Anderson DR, Braverman S. Reevaluation of the optic disc vasculature. *Am J Ophthalmol.* 1976;82:165.
48. Haller A. Arteriarum oculi historia et tabulae arteriarum oculi. Gottigen, 1754. Cited by Francois et al. in *Br J Ophthalmol.* 1954;38:472.
49. Ko MK, Kim DS, Ahn YK. Morphological variations of the peripapillary circle of Zinn-Haller by flat section. *Br J Ophthalmol.* 1999;83(7):862–866.
50. Lieberman MF, Maumenee AE, Green WR. Histologic studies of the vasculature of the anterior optic nerve. *Am J Ophthalmol.* 1976;82:405.
51. Zinn IG. *Descriptio Anatomica Oculi Humani.* 1st ed. Gottingen: Abrami Vandenhoeck; 1755:216.
52. Anderson DR. Ultrastructure of human and monkey lamina cribrosa and optic nerve head. *Arch Ophthalmol.* 1969;82:800.
53. Anderson DR, Hoyt WF. Ultrastructure of the intraorbital portion of human and monkey optic nerve. *Arch Ophthalmol.* 1969;82:506.
54. Anderson DR. Vascular supply to the optic nerve of primates. *Am J Ophthalmol.* 1970;70:341.
55. Olver JM, Spalton DJ, McCartney ACE. Quantitative morphology of human retrolaminar optic nerve vasculature. *Invest Ophthalmol Vis Sci.* 1994;35(11):3858–3866.
56. Steele EJ, Blunt MJ. The blood supply of the optic nerve and chiasma in man. *J Anat.* 1956;90(4):486–493.

57. Alm A. Ocular circulation. In: Hart WM, ed. *Alder's Physiology of the Eye*. 6th ed. St. Louis: C.V. Mosby; 1992:198.
58. Hayreh SS. The central artery of the retina – Its role in the blood supply of the optic nerve. *Br J Ophthalmol*. 1963;47:651–663.
59. Cioffi GA, Van Buskirk EM. Microvasculature of the anterior optic nerve. *Surv Opthalmol*. 1994; 38 suppl:S107–S116; discussion.
60. Ernest JT, Potts AM. Pathophysiology of the distal portion of the optic nerve. II. Vascular relationships. *Am J Ophthalmol*. 1968;66(3):380–387.
61. Rhodes R, Tanner G. *Medical Physiology*. New York, NY: Little Brown and Co; 1995.
62. Bill A, Sperber GO. Control of retinal and choroidal blood flow. *Eye*. 1990;4:319–325.
63. Hayreh S. Factors influencing blood flow in the optic nerve head. *J Glaucoma*. 1997;6:412–425.
64. Wetter JJ, Schachar RA, Ernest JT. Control of intraocular blood flow. II. Effects of sympathetic tone. *Invest Ophthalmol*. 1973;12:332–334.
65. Williamson T, Harris A. Ocular blood flow measurement. *Br J Ophthalmol*. 1994;78:939–945.
66. Lowenstein C, Dinerman J, Snyder S. Nitric oxide: a physiologic messenger. *Ann Intern Med*. 1994;120:227–237.
67. Buga GM, Gold ME, Fukuto JM, Ignarro LJ. Shear stress-induced release of nitric oxide from endothelial cells grown on beads. *Hypertension*. 1991;25:831–836.
68. Kadel KA, Heistad DD, Faraci FM. Effects of endothelium on blood vessels in the brain and choroids plexus. *Brain Res*. 1990;518:78–82.
69. Brian JE Jr, Faraci FM, Heistad DD. Recent insights into the regulation of cerebral circulation. *Clin Exp Pharmacol Physiol*. 1996;23:449–457.
70. Cioffi GA, Sullivan P. The effect of chronic ischemia on the primate optic nerve. *Eur J Ophthalmol*. 1999; 9 Suppl 1:S34–S36.
71. Wong T, Mitchell P. The eye in hypertension. *Lancet*. 2007;369:425–435.
72. Graham SL, Drance SM, Wijsman K, et al. Ambulatory blood pressure monitoring in glaucoma patients. The nocturnal dip. *Ophthalmology*. 1995;102:61–69.
73. Graham SL, Fraco MS, Drance SM. Nocturnal hypotension: role in glaucoma progression. *Surv Ophthalmol*. 1999;43(Suppl):S10–S16.
74. Grieshaber MC, Flammer J. Blood flow in glaucoma. *Curr Opin Ophthalmol*. 2005;16:79–83.
75. Mcleod SD, West SK, Quigley HA, Fozard JL. A longitudinal study of the relationship between intraocular and blood pressure. *Invest Ophthalmol Vis Sci*. 1990;31:2361–2366.
76. Dielemans I, Vingerling JR, Algra D, et al. Primary open-angle glaucoma, intraocular pressure, and systemic blood pressure in the general elderly population. The Rotterdam Study. *Ophthalmology*. 1995;102:54–60.
77. Flammer J. The vascular concept of glaucoma. *Surv Ophthalmol*. 1994; 38 Suppl:S3–S6.
78. Müskens RP, de Voogd S, Wolfs RC, et al. Systemic antihypertensive medication and incident open-angle glaucoma. *Ophthalmology*. 2007;114(12):2221–2226.
79. Miglior S, Torri V, Zeyen T, Pfeiffer N, Vaz JC, Adamsons I; EGPS Group. Intercurrent factors associated with the development of open-angle glaucoma in the European glaucoma prevention study. *Am J Ophthalmol*. 2007; 144(2):266–275.
80. Hulsman CAA, Vingerling JR, Hofman A, et al. Blood pressure, arterial stiffness and open angle glaucoma. The Rotterdam study. *Arch Ophthalmol*. 2007;125:805–812.
81. Gherghel D, Orgul S, Gugleta K, et al. Relationship between ocular perfusion pressure and retrobulbar blood flow in patients with glaucoma with progressive damage. *Am J Ophthalmol*. 2000;130:597–605.
82. O'Brien E, Murphy J, Tyndall A, et al. Twenty-four hour ambulatory blood pressure in men and women aged 17 to 80 years: The Allied Irish Bank Study. *J Hypertens*. 1991;9:355–360.
83. Staessen J, Pagard R, Lijnen P, Thija L, Van Hoof R, Amary A. Mean and range of the ambulatory pressure in normotensive subjects from a meta-analysis of 23 studies. *Am J Cardiol*. 1991;67:723–727.
84. Verdecchia P, Schillaci G, Porcellati C. Dippers versus nondippers. *J Hypertens*. 1991;9(Suppl):S42–S44.
85. Tokunaga T, Kashiwagi K, Tsumura T, et al. Association between nocturnal blood pressure reduction and progression of visual field defect in patients with primary open-angle glaucoma or normal-tension glaucoma. *Jpn J Ophthalmol*. 2004;48:380–385.
86. Harris A, Evans D, Martin B, et al. Nocturnal blood pressure reduction: effect on retrobulbar hemodynamics in glaucoma. *Graefes Arch Clin Exp Ophthalmol*. 2002;240(5):372–378.
87. Hayreh SS, Podhajsky P, Zimmerman MB. Beta-blocker eyedrops and nocturnal arterial hypotension. *Am J Ophthalmol*. 1999;128:301–309.
88. Hayreh SS, Podhajsky P, Zimmerman MB. Role of nocturnal arterial hypotension in optic nerve head ischemic disorders. *Ophthalmologica*. 1999;213:76–96.
89. Liu JH, Gokhale PA, Loving RT, et al. Laboratory assessment of diurnal and nocturnal ocular perfusion pressures in humans. *J Ocul Pharmacol Ther*. 2003;19:291–297.
90. Harris A, Jonescu-Cuypers C, Martin B, et al. Simultaneous management of blood flow and IOP in glaucoma. *Acta Ophthalmol Scand*. 2001;79:336–341.
91. Quigley HA, West SK, Rodriguez J, et al. The prevalence of glaucoma in a population based study of Hispanic Subjects. Proyecto VER. *Arch Ophthalmol*. 2001;119:1819–1826.
92. Choi J, Jeong J, Cho HS, Kook MS. Effect of nocturnal blood pressure reduction on circadian fluctuation of mean ocular perfusion pressure: a risk factor for normal tension glaucoma. *Invest Ophthalmol Vis Sci*. 2006;47:831–836.
93. Asrani S, Zeimer R, Wilensky J, et al. Large diurnal fluctuations in intraocular pressure are an independent risk factor in patients with glaucoma. *J Glaucoma*. 2000;9:134–142.
94. Nouri-Mahdavi K, Hoffman D, Coleman AL, et al. Predictive factors for glaucomatous visual field progression in the Advanced Glaucoma Intervention Study. *Ophthalmology*. 2004;111:1627–1635.
95. Hughes E, Spry P, Diamond J. 24-hour monitoring of intraocular pressure in glaucoma management: a retrospective review. *J Glaucoma*. 2003;12:232–236.
96. Choi J, Kim KH, Jeong J, et al. Circadian fluctuation of mean ocular perfusion pressure is a consistent risk factor for normal-tension glaucoma. *Invest Ophthalmol Vis Sci*. 2007;48:104–111.
97. Drance SM. Disc hemorrhages in the glaucomas. *Surv Ophthalmol*. 1989;33(5):331–337.
98. Rasker MT, van den Enden A, Bakker D, Hoyng PF. Deterioration of visual fields in patients with glaucoma with and without optic disc hemorrhages. *Arch Ophthalmol*. 1997;115:1257–1262.
99. Soares AS, Artes PH, Andreou P, et al. Factors associated with optic disc hemorrhages in glaucoma. *Ophthalmology*. 2004;111:1653–1657.
100. Leske MC, Heijl A, Hyman L, et al. Factors for progression and glaucoma treatment: the Early Manifest Glaucoma Trial. *Curr Opin Ophthalmol*. 2004;15:102–106.
101. Anderson DR, Drance SM, Schulzer M; Collaborative Normal-Tension Glaucoma Study Group. Factors that predict the benefit of lowering intraocular pressure in normal tension glaucoma. *Am J Ophthalmol*. 2003;136:820–829.
102. Bengtsson B, Leske MC, Yang A, et al. Disc hemorrhages and treatment in the Early Manifest Glaucoma Trial. *Ophthalmology*. 2008;115:2044–2048.
103. Cursiefen C, Wisse M, Cursiefen S, et al. Migraine and tension headache in high-pressure and normal pressure glaucoma. *Ophthalmology*. 1998;105:216–223.
104. Sines D, Harris A, Siesky B, et al. The response of retrobulbar vasculature to hypercapnia in primary open-angle glaucoma and ocular hypertension. *Ophthalmic Res*. 2007;39:76–80.

105. Nielsen NV. The prevalence of glaucoma and ocular hypertension in type 1 and type 2 diabetes mellitus. *Arch Ophthalmol.* 1983;61:662–672.
106. Chopra V, Varma R, Francis BA, Wu J, Torres M, Azen SP; Los Angeles Latino Eye Study Group. Type 2 Diabetes Mellitus and the Risk of Open-angle Glaucoma The Los Angeles Latino Eye Study. *Ophthalmology.* 2008;115(2):227–232.
107. Tielsch JM, Katz J, Quigley HA, et al. Diabetes, intraocular pressure and primary open angle glaucoma in the Baltimore eye survey. *Ophthalmology.* 1995;102:48–53.
108. Leske MC, Connell AMS, Wu SY. et al; the Barbados eye study group. Risk factors for open angle glaucoma. *Arch Ophthalmol.* 1995;113:918–924.
109. de Voogd S, Ikram MK, Wolfs RC, et al. Is diabetes mellitus a risk factor for open-angle glaucoma? The Rotterdam Study. *Ophthalmology.* 2006;113:1827–1831.
110. Harris A, Rechtman E, Siesky B, et al. The role of optic nerve blood flow in the pathogenesis of glaucoma. *Ophthalmol Clin North Am.* 2005;18:345–353.
111. Harris A, Jonescu-Cuypers CP, Kagemann L, Ciulla TA, Krieglstein G. *Atlas of Ocular Blood Flow – Vascular Anatomy, Pathophysiology, and Metabolism.* Philadelphia: Butterworth-Heinemann; 2003:19–70.
112. Harris A, Dinn RB, Kagemann L, Rechtman E. Review of methods for human retinal oximetry. *Ophthalmic Surg Lasers Imaging.* 2003;34:152–164.
113. Oksala A, Jaaslahti SL. Experimental observations on the acoustic shadow in B-scan examination of the eye. *Acta Ophthalmol (Copenh).* 1971;49:151–158.
114. Byrne SR, Glaser JS. Orbital tissue differentiation with standardized echography. *Ophthalmology.* 1983;90:1071–1090.
115. Guthoff R, Berger RW, Helmke K, Winckler B. Doppler sonographic findings in intraocular tumors. *Fortschr Ophthalmol.* 1989;86:239–241.
116. Guthoff RF, Berger RW, Winkler P, Helmke K, Chumbley LC. Doppler ultrasonography of the ophthalmic and central retinal vessels. *Arch Ophthalmol.* 1991;109:532–536.
117. Pourcelot L. Indications of Doppler's ultrasonography in the study of peripheral vessels. *Rev Prat.* 1975;25:4671–4680.
118. von Bibra H, Stempfle HU, Poll A, et al. [Accuracy of various Doppler technics in recording blood flow velocity. Studies in vitro]. *Z Kardiol.* 1990;79:73–82.
119. Galassi F, Nuzzaci G, Sodi A, Casi P, Vielmo A. Color Doppler imaging in evaluation of optic nerve blood supply in normal and glaucomatous subjects. *Int Ophthalmol.* 1992;16:273–276.
120. Sergott RC, Aburn NS, Trible JR, Costa VP, Lieb WE Jr, Flaharty PM. Color Doppler imaging: methodology and preliminary results in glaucoma. *Surv Ophthalmol.* 1994;38 Suppl:S65-S70; discussion S70-S71, S65-S70.
121. Nicolela MT, Walman BE, Buckley AR, Drance SM. Various glaucomatous optic nerve appearances. A color Doppler imaging study of retrobulbar circulation. *Ophthalmology.* 1996;103:1670–1679.
122. Roff EJ, Harris A, Chung HS, et al. Comprehensive assessment of retinal, choroidal and retrobulbar haemodynamics during blood gas perturbation. *Graefes Arch Clin Exp Ophthalmol.* 1999;237:984–990.
123. Plange N, Kaup M, Arend O, Remky A. Asymmetric visual field loss and retrobulbar haemodynamics in primary open-angle glaucoma. *Graefes Arch Clin Exp Ophthalmol.* 2006;244:978–983.
124. Galassi F, Sodi A, Ucci F, Renieri G, Pieri B, Baccini M. Ocular hemodynamics and glaucoma prognosis: a color Doppler imaging study. *Arch Ophthalmol.* 2003;121:1711–1715.
125. Akarsu C, Unal B. Cerebral haemodynamics in patients with pseudoexfoliation glaucoma. *Eye.* 2005;19:1297–1300.
126. Atalar PT, Atalar E, Kilic H, et al. Impaired systemic endothelial function in patients with pseudoexfoliation syndrome. *Int Heart J.* 2006;47:77–84.
127. Harris A, Siesky B, Zarfati D, et al. Relationship of cerebral blood flow and central visual function in primary open-angle glaucoma. *J Glaucoma.* 2007;16:159–163.
128. Zeitz O, Galambos P, Wagenfeld L, et al. Glaucoma progression is associated with decreased blood flow velocities in the short posterior ciliary artery. *Br J Ophthalmol.* 2006;90:1245–1248.
129. Springer C, Volcker HE. Rohrschneider K [Static fundus perimetry in normals. Microperimeter 1 versus SLO]. *Ophthalmologe.* 2006;103:214–220.
130. Rohrschneider K, Springer C, Bultmann S, Volcker HE. Microperimetry – comparison between the micro perimeter 1 and scanning laser ophthalmoscope – fundus perimetry. *Am J Ophthalmol.* 2005;139:125–134.
131. Seth R, Gouras P. Assessing macular pigment from SLO images. *Doc Ophthalmol.* 2004;108:197–202.
132. Wolf S, Toonen H, Arend O, et al. Quantifying retinal capillary circulation using the scanning laser ophthalmoscope. *Biomed Tech (Berl).* 1990;35:131–134.
133. Arend O, Wolf S, Schulte K, Jung F, Bertram B, Reim M. Conjunctival microcirculation and hemorheology in patients with venous occlusions of the retina. *Fortschr Ophthalmol.* 1991;88:243–247.
134. Wolf S, Arend O, Toonen H, Bertram B, Jung F, Reim M. Retinal capillary blood flow measurement with a scanning laser ophthalmoscope. Preliminary results. *Ophthalmology.* 1991;98:996–1000.
135. Arend O, Remky A, Elsner AE, Wolf S, Rein M. Indocyanine green angiography in traumatic choroidal rupture: clinicoangiographic case reports. *Ger J Ophthalmol.* 1995;4:257–263.
136. Wolf S, Remky A, Elsner AE, Arend O, Reim M. Indocyanine green video angiography in patients with age-related maculopathy-related retinal pigment epithelial detachments. *Ger J Ophthalmol.* 1994;3:224–227.
137. Wolf S, Arend O, Reim M. Measurement of retinal hemodynamics with scanning laser ophthalmoscopy: reference values and variation. *Surv Ophthalmol.* 1994;38 Suppl:S95–S100.
138. Mainster MA, Timberlake GT, Webb RH, Hughes GW. Scanning laser ophthalmoscopy. Clinical applications. *Ophthalmology.* 1982;89:852–857.
139. Tanaka T, Muraoka K, Shimizu K. Fluorescein fundus angiography with scanning laser ophthalmoscope. Visibility of leukocytes and platelets in perifoveal capillaries. *Ophthalmology.* 1991;98:1824–1829.
140. Scheider A. [Indocyanine green angiography with an infrared scanning laser ophthalmoscope. Initial clinical experiences]. *Ophthalmologe.* 1992;89:27–33.
141. Sonty S, Schwartz B. Two-point fluorophotometry in the evaluation of glaucomatous optic disc. *Arch Ophthalmol.* 1980;98:1422–1426.
142. Wolf S, Arend O, Haase A, Schulte K, Remky A, Reim M. Retinal hemodynamics in patients with chronic open-angle glaucoma. *Ger J Ophthalmol.* 1995;4:279–282.
143. Schulte K, Wolf S, Arend O, Harris A, Henle C, Reim M. Retinal hemodynamics during increased intraocular pressure. *Ger J Ophthalmol.* 1996;5:1–5.
144. Bjarnhall G, Tomic L, Mishima HK, Tsukamoto H, Alm A. Retinal mean transit time in patients with primary open-angle glaucoma and normal-tension glaucoma. *Acta Ophthalmol Scand.* 2007;85:67–72.
145. Harris A, Arend O, Kopecky K, et al. Physiological perturbation of ocular and cerebral blood flow as measured by scanning laser ophthalmoscopy and color Doppler imaging. *Surv Ophthalmol.* 1994;38 Suppl:S81–S86.
146. Plange N, Kaup M, Huber K, Remky A, Arend O. Fluorescein filling defects of the optic nerve head in normal tension glaucoma, primary open-angle glaucoma, ocular hypertension and healthy controls. *Ophthalmic Physiol Opt.* 2006;26:26–32.
147. Pournaras CJ, Riva CE. Studies of the hemodynamics of the optic head nerve using laser Doppler flowmetry. *J Fr Ophthalmol.* 2001;24:199–205.

148. Takase S, Takada A, Matsuda Y. Studies on the pathogenesis of the constitutional excretory defect of indocyanine green. *Gastroenterol Jpn*. 1982;17:301–309.
149. Keiding S, Ott P, Bass L. Enhancement of unbound clearance of ICG by plasma proteins, demonstrated in human subjects and interpreted without assumption of facilitating structures. *J Hepatol*. 1993;19:327–344.
150. Harris A, Chung HS, Ciulla TA, Kagemann L. Progress in measurement of ocular blood flow and relevance to our understanding of glaucoma and age-related macular degeneration. *Prog Retin Eye Res*. 1999;18:669–687.
151. Harris A, Kagemann L, Chung HS, et al. The use of dye dilution curve analysis in the quantification of indocyanine green angiograms of the human choroid. *Ophthamic Imaging Diagn*. 1998;11:331–337.
152. Feke GT. Laser Doppler instrumentation for the measurement of retinal blood flow: theory and practice. *Bull Soc Belge Ophthalmol*. 2006;171–184.
153. Yoshida A, Feke GT, Mori F, et al. Reproducibility and clinical application of a newly developed stabilized retinal laser Doppler instrument. *Am J Ophthalmol*. 2003;135:356–361.
154. Feke GT, Pasquale LR. Retinal blood flow response to posture change in glaucoma patients compared with healthy subjects. *Ophthalmology*. 2008;115(2):246–252.
155. Guan K, Hudson C, Flanagan JG. Variability and repeatability of retinal blood flow measurements using the Canon Laser Blood Flowmeter. *Microvasc Res*. 2003;65(3):145–151.
156. Azizi B, Buehler H, Venkataraman ST, Hudson C. Impact of simulated light scatter on the quantitative, noninvasive assessment of retinal arteriolar hemodynamics. *J Biomed Opt*. 2007;12:034021.
157. Boehm AG, Pillunat LE, Koeller U, et al. Regional distribution of optic nerve head blood flow. *Graefes Arch Clin Exp Ophthalmol*. 1999;237:484–488.
158. Petrig BL, Riva CE, Hayreh SS. Laser Doppler flowmetry and optic nerve head blood flow. *Am J Ophthalmol*. 1999;127:413–425.
159. Riva CE, Cranstoun SD, Grunwald JE, Petrig BL. Choroidal blood flow in the foveal region of the human ocular fundus. *Invest Ophthalmol Vis Sci*. 1994;35:4273–4281.
160. Hollo G, Greve EL, van den Berg TJ, Vargha P. Evaluation of the peripapillary circulation in healthy and glaucoma eyes with scanning laser Doppler flowmetry. *Int Ophthalmol*. 1996;20:71–77.
161. Michelson G, Groh MJ, Langhans M. Perfusion of the juxtapapillary retina and optic nerve head in acute ocular hypertension. *Ger J Ophthalmol*. 1996;5:315–321.
162. Michelson G, Schmauss B, Langhans MJ, Harazny J, Groh MJ. Principle, validity, and reliability of scanning laser Doppler flowmetry. *J Glaucoma*. 1996;5:99–105.
163. Kagemann L, Harris A, Chung HS, Evans D, Buck S, Martin B. Heidelberg retinal flowmetry: factors affecting blood flow measurement. *Br J Ophthalmol*. 1998;82:131–136.
164. Chauhan BC, Smith FM. Confocal scanning laser Doppler flowmetry: experiments in a model flow system. *J Glaucoma*. 1997;6:237–245.
165. Tsang AC, Harris A, Kagemann L, Chung HS, Snook BM, Garzozi HJ. Brightness alters Heidelberg retinal flowmeter measurements in an in vitro model. *Invest Ophthalmol Vis Sci*. 1999;40:795–799.
166. Hafez AS, Bizzarro RL, Rivard M, Lesk MR. Changes in optic nerve head blood flow after therapeutic intraocular pressure reduction in glaucoma patients and ocular hypertensives. *Ophthalmology*. 2003;110:201–210.
167. Logan JF, Rankin SJ, Jackson AJ. Retinal blood flow measurements and neuroretinal rim damage in glaucoma. *Br J Ophthalmol*. 2004;88:1049–1054.
168. Sato EA, Ohtake Y, Shinoda K, Mashima Y, Kimura I. Decreased blood flow at neuroretinal rim of optic nerve head corresponds with visual field deficit in eyes with normal tension glaucoma. *Graefes Arch Clin Exp Ophthalmol*. 2006;244:795–801.
169. Friedenwald JS. Contribution to the theory and practice of tonometry. *Am J Ophthalmol*. 1937;20:985–1024.
170. Silver DM, Farrell RA, Langham ME, et al. Estimation of pulsatile ocular blood flow from intraocular pressure. *Acta Ophthalmol*. 1989;191(Suppl):25–29.
171. Walker RE, Litovitz TL, Langham ME. Pneumatic applanation tonometer studies. II. Rabbit corneal data. *Exp Eye Res*. 1972;13:187–193.
172. Harris A, Kagemann L, Cioffi GA. Assessment of human ocular hemodynamics. *Surv Ophthalmol*. 1998;42(6):509–533.
173. Mrugacz M, Sredzi ska-Kita D, Bakunowicz-Lazarczyk A, Pawłowski P. Pulsatile ocular blood flow in patients with juvenile glaucoma. *Klin Oczna*. 2004;106(1-2 Suppl):209–210.
174. Zhang MZ, Fu ZF, Liu XR, Zheng C. [A comparison study of pulsitile ocular blood flow in normal eyes and primary open angle glaucoma]. *Zhonghua Yan Ke Za Zhi*. 2004;40(4):250–253.
175. Kerr J, Nelson P, O'Brien C. Pulsatile ocular blood flow in primary open-angle glaucoma and ocular hypertension. *Am J Ophthalmol*. 2003;136(6):1106–1113.
176. Blum M, Bachmann K, Wintzer D, Riemer T, Vilser W, Strobel J. Noninvasive measurement of the Bayliss effect in retinal autoregulation. *Graefes Arch Clin Exp Ophthalmol*. 1999;237:296–300.
177. Nagel E, Vilser W, Lanzl IM. Retinal vessel reaction to short-term IOP elevation in ocular hypertensive and glaucoma patients. *Eur J Ophthalmol*. 2001;11:338–344.
178. Garhofer G, Zawinka C, Resch H, Huemer KH, Schmetterer L, Dorner GT. Response of retinal vessel diameters to flicker stimulation in patients with early open angle glaucoma. *J Glaucoma*. 2004;13:340–344.
179. Michelson G, Scibor M. Intravascular oxygen saturation in retinal vessels in normal subjects and open-angle glaucoma subjects. *Acta Ophthalmol Scand*. 2006;84:289–295.
180. Hardarson SH, Harris A, Karlsson RA, et al. Automatic retinal oximetry. *Invest Ophthalmol Vis Sci*. 2006;47:5011–5016.
181. Kagemann L, Wollstein G, Wojtkowski M, et al. Spectral oximetry assessed with high-speed ultra-high-resolution optical coherence tomography. *J Biomed Opt*. 2007;12(4):041212.
182. Satilmis M, Orgul S, Doubler B, Flammer J. Rate of progression of glaucoma correlates with retrobulbar circulation and intraocular pressure. *Am J Ophthalmol*. 2003;135:664–669.
183. Yamazaki Y, Drance SM. The relationship between progression of visual field defects and retrobulbar circulation in patients with glaucoma. *Am J Ophthalmol*. 1997;124:287–295.
184. Spencer JA, Giussani DA, Moore PJ, Hanson MA. In vitro validation of Doppler indices using blood and water. *J Ultrasound Med*. 1991;10:305–308.
185. Martinez A, Sanchez M. Predictive value of colour Doppler imaging in a prospective study of visual field progression in primary open-angle glaucoma. *Acta Ophthalmol Scand*. 2005;83:716–722.
186. Zink JM, Grunwald JE, Piltz-Seymour J, Staii A, Dupont J. Association between lower optic nerve laser Doppler blood volume measurements and glaucomatous visual field progression. *Br J Ophthalmol*. 2003;87:1487–1490.
187. Janulevičienė I, Sliesoraitytė I, Siesky B, Harris A. Diagnostic compatibility of structural and haemodynamic parameters in open-angle glaucoma patients. *Acta Ophthalmol*. 2008;86(5):552–557.

# Chapter 12
# Glaucoma Risk Factors: Sleep Apnea and Glaucoma

Rick E. Bendel and Janet A. Betchkal

An association between obstructive sleep apnea syndrome (OSA) and glaucoma was described in 1982 when physicians identified a family whose members had OSA and glaucoma, with the severity of the glaucoma correlating with the severity of the OSA.[1] Since this first recognized possible association, several case reports and case series, studies, and other reports have described a variable association of OSA with glaucoma. Most reports found an association, but some reports did not. This chapter discusses all of these findings, and the reader will see that a possible/probable – but not definite – association with OSA and glaucoma exists.

Sleep apnea is diagnosed by the apnea/hypopnea index (AHI), where apnea is the obstruction of airflow at the level of the oropharynx for at least 10 s, and hypopnea is the reduction of airflow by at least 30% associated with arousal or oxyhemoglobin desaturation by at least 3%. AHI is the number of these events per hour. An early prevalence study in 1993 defined OSA by an AHI>5 with daytime hypersomnolence or an AHI>15 with/without symptoms. A prevalence of 2% of women and 4% of men aged 30–60 was found.[2] The prevalence of OSA has been increasing due to the increasing obesity and awareness of the disorder. A recent synopsis of four major prevalence studies found a range of 7–26% in men and 2–28% in women above 20 years of age.[3] OSA has been identified as a risk factor for hypertension, cardiovascular and cerebrovascular disease, pulmonary hypertension, and overall mortality.[3-10] With the far-reaching systemic consequences of OSA, it would not be surprising if some ophthalmic effects were also present. The association of Floppy Eyelid Syndrome and OSA is fairly well established.[11-17] The association of papilledema and nonarteritic anterior ischemic optic neuropathy and OSA has also been made.[18-24] A look at reports investigating the association of OSA and glaucoma follows.

In 1982, Walsh and Montplaisir described the first report of possible association with OSA and glaucoma.[1] They described five patients from two generations of a family who had sleep apnea and glaucoma, and the more severe the sleep apnea, the more severe the glaucoma. In 1999, Mojon et al found a glaucoma prevalence of 7.2% (5/69) in patients who were diagnosed with OSA, and none of the patients (0/45) who were not diagnosed with OSA had glaucoma.[25] The study involved 114 consecutive patients referred for evaluation in a sleep study lab for OSA. They found a positive correlation of AHI with intraocular pressure, visual field loss, and optic nerve changes. In 2000, Mojon et al diagnosed OSA in 20% of patients known to have primary open glaucoma (6/30) using overnight oximetry.[26] The investigators concluded that sleep apnea syndrome was associated with glaucoma. In 2002, Mojon et al performed polysomnography in 16 consecutive patients with normal-tension glaucoma (NTG) and found that in patients older than 45, more than 50% (8/14) were found to have sleep apnea syndrome and concluded that NTG patients should be screened for OSA.[27]

In 2000, Onen et al administered a questionnaire that indicated the presence of sleep disordered breathing (SDB) in 212 glaucoma patients and 218 normal controls. Patients with glaucoma had a significantly higher percentage of SDB, and in those most likely to have OSA the rate was 14.6% of glaucoma patients vs. 7.8% of controls.[28] OSA was not confirmed with any sleep studies in this report. Another historical interview-based diagnosis of OAS in NTG patients, with limited subsequent confirmation of OSA by polysomnography, was completed by Marcus et al in 2001.[29] They found a positive history in 57% (13/23) of NTG patients, and 43% (6/14) in NTG suspects vs. 1% (1/30) of controls. Some of the patients consented to polysomnography and confirmation were found in 79% (7/9) of the NTG group, 100% (4/4) NTG suspects, and 100% (1/1) of controls. They recommended obtaining sleep histories from NTG patients as it may be a risk factor.

Of the studies exploring an association of sleep apnea and glaucoma, only two have found no relationship. In 2003, Geyer et al evaluated 228 of 390 newly diagnosed sleep apnea syndrome (SAS) patients and found that 2% (5/228) had glaucoma – the same percentage one would expect in the general population.[30] The AHI for diagnosis of SAS was >10 and glaucoma patients had visual field and optic nerve changes. Girkin et al looked at a diagnostic database at a US Veterans Affairs healthcare center for limited sleep apnea diagnostic codes in 667 newly diagnosed glaucoma patients and matched them with 6,667 controls. Although glaucoma patients were more likely to have a previous diagnosis of OSA, when controlling for other possible risk factors there was no significant association.[31]

In 2007, Sergi et al examined 51 OSA patients for glaucoma compared to 40 controls and found a positive diagnosis of NTG in 5.9% (3/51) of OSA patients and in none of the controls.[32] The severity of OSA correlated with intraocular pressure, the mean deviation of the visual field, the cup/disk ratio, and the mean of the retinal nerve fiber layer thickness. They concluded that OSA may be an important risk factor for NTG. In 2008, Bendel et al reported a case series of 100 newly diagnosed OSA patients within 48 h of their new OSA diagnosis and found glaucoma in 27%. In this study, as opposed to all previous studies, glaucoma diagnosis was made in 9% with optic nerve changes alone with normal visual fields. Fourteen percent had optic nerve and visual field changes and 4% had a previous glaucoma diagnosis.[33]

Abnormal findings in visual field and nerve fiber layer thickness in OSA patients have been reported. In 2005, Kargi et al found that 34 newly diagnosed OSA patients had a thinner retinal nerve fiber layer (RNFL) than 20 controls and that the severity of OSA correlated with the decrease of the RNFL.[34] Also in 2005, Tsang et al compared 41 newly diagnosed OSA patients to 35 controls and found abnormalities of the optic nerve four times as often in OSA patients (26.4% vs. 6.7%) and that OSA patients had significantly more visual field defects.[35] In 2008, Karakucuk et al explored the difference in ocular perfusion between 31 OSA patients and 25 controls and found a positive correlation between resistance in ophthalmic and central retinal arteries and visual field mean defect.[36] The eye examinations and visual fields done as part of the study revealed glaucoma in 12.9% (4/31) of OSA patients all of whom had more severe OSA. Variable reports on IOP in OSA patients have been reported in all the studies previously discussed, and Goldblum et al measured IOPs during sleep apneic episodes and found no difference compared to normal respirations.[37]

Finally, regarding the treatment of OSA and glaucoma progression, very little is known. The literature has two reports of three patients with improvement or lack of further progression once the treatment of OSA was begun. In 2003, Kremmer et al reported 2 patients whose glaucoma progressed despite low IOP, with successful medical treatment and/or trabeculectomy.[38] Sleep apnea treatment with continuous positive airway pressure (CPAP) halted visual field (VF) progression for up to 4 years at the time they published their cases. In 2006, Sebastian et al[39] found that a patient with suspicious glaucomatous VF changes was diagnosed with severe OSA and had continued improvement in VF over 2 years once CPAP was begun.

The association of glaucoma and sleep apnea turns out to be a positive one in nearly all studies looking for the association except for two. We think that all of the studies have methodological problems limiting the power of the findings as well as variable definitions of glaucoma and sleep apnea throughout the discussed literature. Until a definitive, controlled, large-scale study is done, it is reasonable to look for sleep apnea in our glaucoma patients and to look for glaucoma in patients with sleep apnea, but it is too early in our investigations to make this the standard of care. A further discussion of this topic appears at the end of Chap. 60.

## References

1. Walsh JT, Montplaisir J. Familial glaucoma with sleep apnea: a new syndrome? *Thorax*. 1982;37:845–849.
2. Young T, Palta M, Dempsey J, Skarrud J, Weber S, Badr S. The occurrence of sleep-disordered breathing among middle aged adults. *N Engl J Med*. 1993;328:1230–1235.
3. Parish J, Somers V. Obstructive sleep apnea syndrome and cardiovascular disease. *Mayo Clin Proc*. 2004;79(8):1036–1046.
4. Olson EJ, Moore WR, Morgenthaler TI, et al. Obstructive sleep apnea–hypopnea syndrome. *Mayo Clin Proc*. 2003;78:1545–1552.
5. Yumino D, Tsurumi Y, Takagi A, et al. Impact of obstructive sleep apnea syndrome on clinical and angiographic outcomes following percutaneous coronary intervention in patients with acute coronary syndrome. *Am J Cardiol*. 2007;99:26–30.
6. Wang H, Parker JD, Newton GE, et al. Influence of obstructive sleep apnea syndrome on mortality in patients with heart failure. *J Am Coll Cardiol*. 2007;49:1625–1631.
7. Lattimore JL, Celermajer DS, Wilcox I. Obstructive sleep apnea syndrome and cardiovascular disease. *J Am Coll Cardiol*. 2003;41:1429–1437.
8. Yaggi HK, Concato J, Kernan WN, et al. Obstructive sleep apnea syndrome as a risk factor for stroke and death. *N Eng J Med*. 2005;353:2034–2041.
9. Peppard PE, Young T, Palta M, Skatrud J. Prospective study of the association between sleep-disordered breathing and hypertension. *N Eng J Med*. 2000;342:1378–1384.
10. Chobanian AV, Bakris GL, Black HR, et al. The seventh report of the joint national committee on prevention, detection, evaluation, and treatment of high blood pressure: the JNC 7 report. *JAMA*. 2003;289:2560–2572.
11. McNab AA. Floppy eyelid syndrome and obstructive sleep apnea. *Ophthal Plast Reconstr Surg*. 1997;13(2):98–114.
12. Woog JJ. Obstructive sleep apnea syndrome and the floppy eyelid syndrome. *Am J Ophthalmol*. 1990;110(3):314–315.
13. Leibovitch I, Selva D. Floppy eyelid syndrome: clinical features and the association with obstructive sleep apnea. *Sleep Med*. 2006;7:117–122.
14. Karger RA, White WA, Park W, et al. Prevalence of the floppy eyelid syndrome in obstructive sleep apnea–hypopnea syndrome. *Ophthalmology*. 2006;113:1669–1674.
15. Mojon DS, Goldblum D, Fleischauer J, et al. Eyelid, conjunctival and corneal findings in sleep apnea syndrome. *Ophthalmology*. 1999;106:1182–1185.
16. Robert PY, Adenis JP, Tapie P, Melloni B. Eyelid hyperlaxity and obstructive sleep apnea syndrome (O.S.A.) syndrome. *Eur J Ophthalmol*. 1997;7(3):211–215.
17. McNab AA. Reversal of floppy eyelid syndrome with treatment of obstructive sleep apnea. *Clin Exp Ophthalmol*. 2000;28:125–126.
18. Mojon DS, Mathis J, Zulauf M, et al. Optic neuropathy associated with sleep apnea syndrome. *Ophthalmology*. 1998;105:874–877.
19. Li J, McGwin G, Vaphiades MS, et al. Nonarteritic anterior ischemic optic neuropathy and presumed sleep apnea syndrome

screened by the sleep apnea scale of the sleep disorders questionnaire (SA-SDQ). *Br J Ophthalmol.* 2007;91(11):1524–1527.
20. Mojon DS, Hedges TR, Ehrenberg B, et al. Association between sleep apnea syndrome and nonarteritic anterior ischemic optic neuropathy. *Arch Ophthalmol.* 2002;120:601–605.
21. Behbehani R, Mathews MK, Sergott RC, Savino PJ. Nonarteritic anterior ischemic optic neuropathy in patients with sleep apnea while being treated with continuous positive airway pressure. *Am J Ophthalmol.* 2005;139:518–521.
22. Palombi K, Renard E, Levy P, et al. Non-arteritic ischaemic optic neuropathy is nearly systematically associated with obstructive sleep apnoea. *Br J Ophthalmol.* 2006;90:879–882.
23. Bucci FA, Krohel GB. Optic nerve swelling secondary to the obstructive sleep apnea syndromes. *Am J Ophthalmol.* 1988;105(4):428–430.
24. Purvin VA, Kawasaki A, Yee RD. Papilledema and obstructive sleep apnea syndromes. *Arch Ophthalmol.* 2000;118:1626–1630.
25. Mojon DS, Hess CW, Goldblum D, et al. High prevalence of glaucoma in patients with sleep apnea syndrome. *Ophthalmology.* 1999;106:1009–1012.
26. Mojon DS, Hess CW, Goldblum D, et al. Primary open-angle glaucoma is associated with sleep apnea syndrome. *Ophthalmologica.* 2000;214:115–118.
27. Mojon DS, Hess CW, Goldblum D, et al. Normal-tension glaucoma is associated with sleep apnea syndrome. *Ophthalmologica.* 2002;216:180–184.
28. Onen SH, Mouriaux F, Berramdane L, et al. High prevalence of sleep-disordered breathing in patient with primary open-angle glaucoma. *Acta Ophthalmol Scand.* 2000;78:638–641.
29. Marcus DM, Costarides AP, Gokhale P, et al. Sleep disorders: a risk factor for normal-tension glaucoma? *J Glaucoma.* 2001;10:177–183.
30. Geyer O, Cohen N, Segev E, et al. The prevalence of glaucoma in patients with sleep apnea syndrome: same as in general population. *Am J Ophthalmol.* 2003;136:1093–1096.
31. Girkin CA, McGwin G, McNeal SF, Owsley C. Is there an association between pre-existing sleep apnoea and the development of glaucoma? *Br J Ophthalmol.* 2006;90:679–681.
32. Sergi M, Salerno DE, Rizzi M, et al. Prevalence of normal tension glaucoma in obstructive sleep apnea syndromes patient. *J Glaucoma.* 2007;16:42–46.
33. Bendel RE, Kaplan J, Heckman M, et al. Prevalence of glaucoma in patients with obstructive sleep apnoea-a cross-sectional case-series. *Eye.* 2008;22(9):1105–1109.
34. Kargi SH, Altin R, Koksal M, et al. Retinal nerve fibre layer measurements are reduced in patients with obstructive sleep apnoea syndrome. *Eye.* 2005;19:575–579.
35. Tsang CSL, Chong SL, Ho CK, Li MF. Moderate to severe obstructive sleep apnoea patients is associated with a higher incidence of visual field defect. *Eye.* 2006;20:38–42.
36. Karakucuk S, Goktas S, Aksu M, et al. Ocular blood flow in patients with obstructive sleep apnea syndromes. *Graefes Arch Clin Exp Ophthalmol.* 2008;246(1):129–134.
37. Goldblum D, Mathis J, Bohnke M, et al. Nocturnal measurements of intraocular pressure in patients with normal-tension glaucoma and sleep apnea syndrome. *Klin Monatsbl Augenheilkd.* 2000;216(5):246–249.
38. Kremmer S, Niederdraing NM, Ayertey HD, et al. Obstructive sleep apnea syndromes, normal tension glaucoma, and nCPAP therapy – a short note. *Sleep.* 2003;2:161–162.
39. Sebastian RT, Johns S, Gibson RA. Treating obstructive sleep apnoea syndrome: does it improve visual field changes? *Eye.* 2006;20:116–118.

# Chapter 13
# Evaluating Ophthalmic Literature

Dan Eisenberg and Paul N. Schacknow

Over the past two decades, we have heard an increasing demand for practicing evidence-based medicine.[1] The medical literature is the core of our knowledge base in ophthalmology. The so-called "hierarchy of evidence" has caused much unresolved controversy about the nature of evidence that is truly most relevant for the practice of glaucoma.[2-5] While systematic reviews and meta-analyses synthesize the information in a broad range of studies, the highest level of basic research is still considered the "randomized clinical trial (RCT)."

There are many other types of scientific studies as shown in Table 13.1. Unfortunately, many physicians do not have the training for adequately evaluating studies that appear in our professional journals. Often, physicians assume that if a study is published in a peer-reviewed journal, its results must be valid. In a phrase, "published equals proof."

What are the criteria that journal editors use in deciding whether a study gets published or rejected? Did a study concern an important or trivial scientific problem? What hypothesis is to be tested, and is it clearly stated? Is it original or does it merely replicate the work of others? Was the method adequate to address the scientific question that was at issue? Were the conclusions justified by the data? Were the statistical techniques employed appropriate for data analysis? Was there a financial conflict of interest between the authors and the makers of drugs or devices used in the study? Many of our colleagues assume that each scientific journal employs in-house statisticians and highly qualified panels of experts who fully review every article considered for publication. Further, it is assumed that only articles that pass this gauntlet of statistical and subject matter experts get published. Nothing could be further from the truth. Scientific publishing reviewers are volunteers chosen from the scientific community.

It is the job of the journal editor to find reviewers who are experts in the subject matter being reviewed. It is difficult to always get the best people – whose professional lives are busy. A thoughtful review can take hours of work, all without reimbursement. Journals may have editorial review boards with subject matter experts who agree to serve for periods of months to several years, but often scientific articles are reviewed by physicians with only moderate familiarity with the subject matter. Editors are pressed to meet deadlines and are often forced to use any available and willing reviewer. It is often the case that a true expert in the area of investigation is available for review, but there is no guarantee that this is so for every article. Most importantly, even physicians and scientists who are experts in certain subject matters may not be highly trained with respect to statistics and experimental methodology.

It may be true that many good studies are published and some good studies are rejected. It is not true that most of everything published is worthy and most of everything rejected is not. There is much that is published that should have been rejected, or at least altered. In the end, it is the reader of a scientific article who must determine its value based both on the subject matter and the credibility of the methods used to collect and analyze the data. It is the reader who must be the final judge of the quality of the literature appearing in our scientific journals. The reader is the ultimate arbiter of "scientific truth."

This chapter will describe the structure of typical journal articles and introduce statistical concepts for understanding the analysis of data. Basic statistical principles needed to properly read and evaluate a scientific article are not difficult to acquire by the average physician. In this chapter, we have used a simplified outline of the format used in many ophthalmology journals. For an example of an "author's guide" that is a more elaborate version of the structure discussed in this chapter, see the style guide used for the peer-reviewed journal *Ophthalmology*.[6]

## 13.1 The Introduction

Why is this research being done? What question(s) is(are) being asked? That's it. The Introduction section must clearly describe the nature of the scientific questions being studied. A solid introduction includes a brief description of prior

**Table 13.1** The hierarchy of levels of evidence

| 1. | A | Systematic reviews/meta-analyses |
|---|---|---|
|  | B | RCTs |
|  | C | Experimental designs |
| 2. | A | Cohort control studies |
|  | B | Case-control studies |
| 3. | A | Consensus conference |
|  | B | Expert opinion |
|  | C | Observational study |
|  | D | Other types of study, e.g., interview-based, local survey |
|  | E | Quasi-experimental, qualitative design |
| 4. |  | Anecdotal |

work on similar questions. This should lead into a discussion of how the present study will add important information going beyond previous work in the field. All key variables to be studied should be declared. When you have finished reading the introduction, you should easily be able to determine whether the research is useful to the scientific community and you should know which variables are going to be investigated. If you are not yet convinced of the need for the research, or cannot determine the important items being studied, then the introduction may have failed. Often the introduction is trivialized. Authors may present a topic and then proceed immediately into the body of the paper. This is not inappropriate, but rather is a lost opportunity to fully explain the purpose of the research. The introduction is the perfect area to organize the study, like a table of contents in prose.

## 13.2 The Methods Section

Methods are the actual steps taken in the organization, collection, and analysis of the data identified in the introduction. What data are to be included? How are these data to be collected? What data will be excluded, and why? How much or how long are data to be collected? How will patients be selected or excluded? How many patients will be chosen and how many different groups and/or conditions will be used? What instruments will be used to obtain measurements? How will the data be recorded? The statistical methods to be used to evaluate the data should be described along with the appropriateness of each test for the kind of data obtained. All variables declared in the introduction must be fully defined here. New variables should not be introduced.

The Methods section must include enough information for future authors to replicate the study, and for reviewers and readers to confirm the analysis chosen. In the future, some journals or research-granting agencies may require that the raw data be published online for access by anyone who would like to replicate or extend the analysis. Because print publishing space is so expensive, it is also common to omit information that is considered generally known to the scientific community if it is not directly under investigation in the present study. For example, a study of cataract surgery could simply state that Goldmann applanation tonometry – a standard technique to measure intraocular pressure (IOP) – was used without explaining the mechanics of the tonometer. Yet a study of a new phacoemulsification system for removing cataracts should include technical details of its unique design and improved operation. Professional judgment is needed to determine how much or how little to include when describing topics likely well known by the typical reader of the specific journal. Usually this expertise is supplied by the editor who may shorten parts of the manuscript.

A common error is for authors to discuss results in the Methods section, and doing so may reflect the scientific maturity of the author. For example, the actual sample size for a variable in the study should appear in the "Results" section, while the desired or proposed sample size (perhaps based on the calculation of "statistical power" – as defined later in this manuscript) properly belongs in the "Methods" section. The Methods section might state: "44 patients are needed for Group A based on power estimates." It should not, however, read: "44 patients were enrolled in the study." The Methods section must introduce the planned statistical analysis and include the rationale for the choice of statistics used. The single greatest issue to require evaluation in the Methods section is the adequacy of the sampling method or randomization. Sample size determination is also vitally important and must be explained in Methods section.

### Methodology

The term *methodology* means the science and study of methods. It is not a fancy synonym for the word "methods" and must not be used unless the study is about methods. In order to advance any science, there must be an accepted methodology for performing research. Researchers do not have to agree on the meaning of any given set of data, but must agree on the methods used to collect, analyze, and present the data. Without this fundamental agreement there can be no improvement on prior work. In our methodology, we believe in publishing papers that are structured around four topics: introduction, methods, results, and discussion. Each section has very specific requirements. We will review these in detail, as many authors blur the lines between topics or fail to follow the accepted structure. It is possible to present good data with poor organization, but lack of such creates concern about lapses in other critical areas.

## 13.3 The Results Section

This is the most straightforward part of the paper to write. Results should show only the data, all of the data, and nothing but the data. The data should not be interpreted in the Results section. This is not the place for the authors to offer opinions or qualifications. Yet how data are presented can profoundly affect how they are perceived.

The data in the Results section should be presented in a way that is clear and obvious to the reader. Presenting just the data alone in this section would seem simple to do. Yet many papers do contain some subtle interpretation of the data in the Results section. Because of limitations on publication space, sometimes important data must be left out. The data that are chosen and the data that are omitted will always reflect the bias of the authors who hope to convince the reader that their hypotheses are confirmed. Papers with positive results are more likely to be published than those with negative findings.

It is not uncommon to see authors declaring that the results of statistical analysis show that the observed findings are "almost (statistically) significant" or that they "trend toward significance." From a mathematical perspective, both of these statements have no meaning. Both statements show a bias in favor of the outcome that did not happen. A probability that is not statistically significant (e.g., >5%) should be rejected. There is no meaning to phrases such as "sort of," "almost," and "maybe-a-little" significant. Without a hard delineation for statistical significance, the concept becomes useless and statistical analysis itself becomes meaningless.

When performing analysis of a paper, subtle omission of data by arbitrary "cutoffs" is another common problem that occurs when results are presented. Surgical studies commonly use arbitrary definitions of success and only present results for those patients that yield data meeting these arbitrary values. Glaucoma drug studies commonly present graphs with a limited range of values that exaggerate small differences in pressure – this makes small changes seem to be of great clinical importance. Scientific truth requires that all data associated with an investigation are presented without regard to the success or failure of the underlying hypotheses.

Finally, the Results section should not introduce new experimental variables. Only variables described in the introduction and defined critically in the Methods section should be presented in the Results section. Ex post facto introduction of interesting variables is forbidden in the Results section. If the data analysis discovers interesting new variables for study, they should be described in the "Discussion" section and considered for future experiments.

### Statistical Significance

There is a distinction between the way significance is used in the biological sciences and the use in engineering. In the biological sciences, experiments are typically done once and only once. Even when repeated, there are usually modifications. Therefore the 5% cutoff for significance is usually considered an absolute. This is the Neyman–Pearson model[7] and how we will use the term "significance" throughout this chapter. It should be noted that in engineering and other physical sciences, experiments can be very short and repeated many times. Under these circumstances, the concept of "almost significant" does take on meaning. If an experiment is performed ten times and the $p$ value is 0.08, and then after another ten replicates the $p$ value is 0.07, and so on, at some point in the series the direction toward significance will be clear. In this situation, the concept of almost significant can take on meaning. The replication now becomes an important variable and allows significance to be predicted. In fact, the ability to predict the outcome of an experiment, with less than 5% uncertainty, was Fisher's original concept of statistical significance.[8] The engineers' version of significance is much closer to Fisher's original description of significance than is the biologic sciences. For our purposes, we will restrict significance to the 5% cutoff as an absolute delineation.

## 13.4 The Discussion Section

The "Discussion" is where authors are allowed to show their creativity in interpreting the meaning of the data. If they favor certain outcomes, it is here in this section where it is permitted for them to say why the data did or did not support the experimental hypotheses. How do the results relate to other similar work? This is the place for intellectual interpretation of the data. What were the unique strengths and weaknesses of this study? What went right? What went wrong? Would the results have been different if the methods were changed in some ways? Were there any surprising findings? What do these results mean for scientific advancement (e.g., better patient outcomes)? Do these results suggest the design of future studies?

The Discussion section should not just repeat the data presented in the Results section. Also, new data not found in the Results section should not be introduced. Although some of the relevant past literature can be presented in the introduction, the discussion should contain a review of the obtained data and analysis as compared to other studies. Do these data extend or contradict the current knowledge base on this topic?

After reading the Discussion section, the reader should understand the study findings and be able to integrate them into the body of scientific literature on this topic. What did the study show? What caveats must be remembered? What advancement was achieved?

## 13.5 Figures, Tables, and Graphs

While raw data are critical for the statistical analysis done in the study (and for future generations to mine as well), tables and lists of numbers can be difficult to interpret. Well-designed graphics engage the readers and allow them to see comparisons between groups and summary statistics (measures of central tendency and variability) that are not immediately obvious from the raw data tables or text descriptions.

Graphics can highlight important findings in the data, but they can also be used to mislead the interpretation of the facts. Selection bias is common in graphics that appear in scientific papers. Including only those patients with an IOP of less than 21 mmHg may leave out a large number of patients for whom the experimental drug did not reduce IOP very much at all. The reader must have access to all the data – positive and negative. This last item is especially important as it is very easy to mislead with clever choices for the graph parameters or data exclusion. The concept also applies to choice of graph scale. It is easy to compress a difference not wanted, or expand the apparent difference if wanted, by choice of scale. Imagine a 1.5 mmHg difference in IOP between two groups, 17.5 mmHg vs. 16 mmHg. If graphed on a scale from 0 through 30 mmHg, this difference would appear trivial, but change the scale to 15–18 mmHg and the difference appears very large. By constraining the $Y$ axis far from zero the reader is misled by the graphic into thinking that the small numerical difference in mean IOP between the two groups of patients is "large" and important.

## 13.6 Citations

Scientific publications that are evidenced-based need to contain references for all the statements found throughout each of the formal sections of the paper. It is very common for authors to assume that information that is generally well known by scientists in the specific field does not need to be referenced. Nonetheless, although not strictly required, it is helpful to have references to all the things we have learned by interacting with our colleagues and our teachers, which we just assume are "given" in our special field.

It is best to find primary sources rather than secondary sources such as textbooks and discussions from literature when listing references and bibliography. Secondary sources (a reference that discusses another reference that contains the issue under discussion) may propagate errors contained in the secondary source. The ideal citation is to find the very first presentation of a concept.

## 13.7 Statistic Essentials

Our scientific methodology assumes that there is a truth, a reality, that there really is an "answer." Our job, as scientists, is to find this truth. To do so we must remove our own biases as much as possible and we must attempt to observe nature in its purest, most undistorted form possible. Random sampling of data is the method that best achieves these goals.

### 13.7.1 The Box of Truth

Think of the reality we seek to discover by research as a something inside a box. We may reach into the box of truth and grab something, pull it out and examine it, but we cannot directly see into the box. We do not know if what we have grabbed is representative or unusual of the items contained in the box. We do not even know if we have altered or damaged the item by our grabbing it for examination. We do not know the size of the box or how many pieces it may contain. All we have is what we grab, a *sample* from the total *population* (or universe) of items within the box. We may grab again, but it yields nothing more than another piece of the something inside. Should we grab again? If so, how many more times? What do we do with what we grab? The art and science of statistics is our guide to understanding samples and populations and also gives us guidance for understanding the truth of our research data.

The building blocks of statistics are samples. Sampling is the act of taking a measurement. It is well known, from fields as disparate as quantum mechanics (Heisenberg's uncertainty principle[9]) to factory production (Hawthorne effect[10]), that the act of measurement may itself change what is being measured. Using sampling methods we can determine the number of grabs that are likely needed to characterize the population accurately and evaluate the resulting pieces that have been grabbed (samples). Two critical concepts result from this idea. The first is that the act of sampling must be regulated. This process of sampling in a regulated fashion is called randomization. Randomization is done to reduce our selection bias when choosing samples (see section titled "Bias"). Second is that we may plot the results of sampling to see what sort of grouping or a shape may be formed to summarize the data. Such a graph is called a sampling distribution.

The distribution obtained from a regulated (randomized) sampling process is the foundation of all statistical tests. Mathematicians have developed different statistical tests for each of many different kinds (shapes) of sampling distributions. It is imperative to have some idea of the type of distribution exhibited by our research data so that we can select the appropriate statistical tests for analysis.

Also note that unregulated sampling, not randomized, yields what is formally called *anecdotal data* and has little value for scientific enquiry designed to determine "truth." The exception is when the anecdote negates the generalization. If we declare all bacteria susceptible to antibiotic X, and someone presents a bacterium that is not, then this anecdote provides great value. The reverse, presenting a positive finding and declaring it as generalized, is completely inappropriate and will lead to dangerously wrong solutions. The example would be presenting a single bacterium sensitive to antibiotic X and then declaring all bacteria susceptible to X.

> **Bias**
>
> Bias, in the statistical sense, is not a pejorative term. It is the acknowledgment that we cannot possibly perform an experiment without outside influence. Selection bias is a necessity. We do not randomly enter peoples' homes to begin a research study. Rather, patients who we wish to enroll in a study present to us in a medical setting. We do not hijack people off the street and randomize them into having one of two different kinds of glaucoma surgery. We enroll those who present to us, meet explicit criteria, and agree to enter the study. There is very little randomness about this selection process. Yet once a patent qualifies for surgery and is willing to enter the study, we may then randomize them to either of the two treatments and we can thereby reduce some of the unnaturalness, or bias, of the selected group.
>
> Opinion bias of the researcher is also mandatory. If a researcher were to have zero bias regarding a research interest, then there would be no stimulus for the physician to perform the research. The researcher would not care enough about the result to justify the effort of doing the study. The entire reason a study is done is because someone believes in something strongly enough, is biased enough, to perform all the work required of a study. Researcher bias is the driving force of research. It is just that while the scientist may hope for a certain outcome, he/she must do everything to ensure that such bias has the least influence humanly possible on the design of the experiment, the choice of statistical analyses used, and the interpretation of the data obtained.

## 13.8 Randomization

Why is randomization so important? The long answer lies deep within probability theory and has its ancient roots in gambling.[11] If we return to our "box of truth," we would not want to grab all the samples from only one corner of the box. We want to know the truth, a representation of the entire contents of the box. Therefore, we would want to grab samples from all over the entire volume of the box. The "all over" part describes randomization. The more randomly we can place our grabs, the better our samples will represent what is really in the box. This is the reason randomization is so important, and why it is critical to inspect the Methods section of an article very carefully. Salsburg discussed R.A. Fisher's analysis of 90 years of nonrandomized fertilizer crop data. It was found completely useless because it was collected in a nonrandomized way.[7]

This demonstrates the concept that randomization is more important than sample size when searching for the truth. A small (number of subjects), well-randomized study is much more likely to yield quality results than a large, poorly randomized study. It is often assumed that large is good, small is not, but this is incorrect. The randomization is the primary determinant of study quality. One should evaluate the methods carefully to understand the care used in the randomization process. Many studies fail at this step. If randomization is not done appropriately, the rest of the paper will describe worthless observations. Poor randomization might lead to good results by chance alone, but more often will produce poor results with limited value.

Key elements found in strong randomization methods include: (1) study designs purposely biased against the hypothesis, (2) masking, (3) independent analysis, and (4) post hoc evaluation of randomness. As noted, all studies have a research hypothesis or bias. If the hypothesis is that drug A works better than drug B, then the study design should purposely aid drug B. Imagine two glaucoma drugs, each given to a different group of patients. If the mean starting IOP of group 1 is 26.7 mmHg, and the mean starting IOP of group 2 is 26.3 mmHg then drug B should be assigned to group 2, assuming final mean IOP was the endpoint. The very small, 0.4 mmHg, IOP advantage should go to drug B, because this is *appropriately* biased against the researcher's hypothesis. Doing this helps balance the presumed natural advantage of the favored drug A.

Because both subjects and scientists are biased, both consciously and unconsciously by what they observe, it is key to design research with *double-masked* experimental treatments and outcomes wherever possible. For example, using drugs in identical masked containers (labeled drug A and drug B) or having one investigator manipulate the dial on a Goldmann Tonometer but another observer reading and recording the measurement without announcing values helps protect against such bias.

Although a luxury, having the statistical analysis performed by an independent entity (e.g., a centralized reading center in a multicenter study for optic nerve head photos or visual fields) also helps reduce bias if the data sets (i.e., treatment groups for photos and fields) are masked to the analysts. This is not always possible for both economic and other pragmatic reasons. Alternatively, it would be best if separate members of the research team analyze the data, distinct from those who conduct the project and examine patients and administer treatments. At the very least, the statistical database should be encoded to mask the data identity.

Finally, because even the best randomization plans may end up with nonrandom results, post hoc analysis of the randomization plan is useful and easy to do. If two experimental groups of patients are created from one large group, it is a simple task to determine if the variance of the sample is the same as the variances of the randomized groups. If not, then the study analysis must be changed to accept this situation. This will be explained later. It is important to realize that even the best randomization methods do not guarantee randomized results. Probability theory dictates that a nonrandom-appearing result will occur in a small percentage of trials. This result alone does not imply poor randomization.

## 13.9 Scales of Measurement: Data Types

Data resulting from observations made in research studies fall along four kinds of *measurement scales* called nominal, ordinal, interval, and ratio. Each succeeding scale represents a higher degree of measurement (as described in this section), with more powerful statistical tests being available as we progress from nominal to ratio data.

*Nominal data* is named data – data that may be classified into categories. Examples of nominal classification include color (values: red, yellow, green, etc.), gender (values: male, female), and musical genre (values: classical, rock-and-roll, hip-hop, etc.). Nominal data are commonly found in the ophthalmology literature. We classify subjects in glaucoma experiments by race, gender, and presence or absence of a disease. Even pre-op and post-op classifications are nominal categories. Beware of tortured nominal data, artificial categories such as "less than 21 mmHg" vs. "greater than 21 mmHg," that are arbitrary and easily manipulated. Intraocular pressure is measured along an interval scale (discussed below) and such data should not be arbitrarily divided into coerced nominal categories and then treated statistically as if it were nominal data. There is a difference between what we measure and what we describe. A description is a nominal or categorical result. A measurement is a continuous result.

*Ordinal data* produce a ranking such as: $A>B>C$, but the magnitude between entries is not regular or not even known: $A-B \neq B-C$. Example: $20/20>20/40>20/100$ is a ranked result of visual acuity with unequal differences between the items. We often need ranked data when trying to evaluate subjective findings such as hyperemia, irritation, pain, or the degree of cataract. Anything that cannot be precisely measured, but can be graded or ranked, yields ordinal data. These forms of data are very common in ophthalmic research. Most of the symptoms patients describe as symptoms or the signs we see during examining them are graded as ordinal data. The patient is asked to describe pain on a scale of 1–10, but nuclear sclerotic cataracts are graded 1–4+.

*Interval data* are numbered (and thus able to be ranked) with the numbers evenly spaced, but there is no natural zero. Here $A>B>C$, and $A-B=B-C$. The majority of our studies use interval data. Eye pressure and blood pressure in mmHg and the Fahrenheit and Celsius temperature scales measured in degree units are examples of interval scale data. Wait, you say, all four of these scales have a zero. They do, but it is not a natural, physical zero, representing "none" of the quantity being measured. All of these examples have possible measurements that are less than the scale zero, that is, negative values are possible. For the pressure scales, both eye pressure and blood pressure measurements are relative to earth's atmospheric pressure, not the vacuum of outer space (true zero pressure). The two temperature scales have arbitrary zero values, different for each scale.

*Ratio data* are interval scale data but with a natural, physical, zero. Temperature in Kelvin degrees is a ratio scale measurement. It represents true zero because it is the temperature at which molecular motion stops. Time measured from *start* is on a ratio scale of measurement, but *timeline* data are interval scale because the numbers relate to each other but not a true zero. Very few biological metrics are ratio scale. The good news is that the distinction between interval and ratio measurement is mostly unimportant for us as data analysts performing research. That's because all major statistical tests are designed for interval scale measurements and remain statistically valid for ratio scale measurements as well.

A special note about data that are "counted items." It is tempting to consider counted data as interval data, but this is not correct and leads to bizarre and unclear outcomes. For example, we commonly see studies that report that the patients used 2.6 drops per day, or the typical family has 2.5 children. Clearly neither the drops nor the children are likely to be partial, non-integer, entities. Counted data are special and require special handling or else impossible findings occur. Think of counted data as groups of nominal data. We first name what we find and then count how many of each type is found. This is clearly not the same as taking a continuous measurement.

Assuming data on the wrong scale of measurement may lead to the use of inappropriate statistical tests and yield invalid conclusions. Unfortunately this is more commonplace than might be expected. Some tests, however, are mathematically robust enough to handle data that they were not designed to evaluate. Note that the term "robust" in statistics means essentially "flexibility." A robust test is able to tolerate deviations from the ideal and still produce valid results. It is valid, but not always desirable, to use statistical tests designed for lower scales on higher scale data, *but not the reverse*. Higher scale tests cannot be used with lower scale data. For example, it is possible and valid to use an ordinal scale test, such as the Mann–Whitney *U*-test, on interval scale data, like intraocular pressure. Discrimination ability (statistical power) will be lost, and this might make it an unwise choice, but still technically correct. The problem here is not that it is wrong to use the lower form of statistical test. It is just that the chances of finding meaningful (statistically significant) differences are lessened when the less-powerful test is applied to higher-scale data.

But let us emphasize that a test developed for a higher scale of measurement uses underlying assumptions that render it useless for analysis of lower scale data. For example, the very commonly used "Student's *t*-test" should not be used to compare the mean Snellen visual acuity between two groups of subjects, because it assumes interval or ratio scale of measurements, while Snellen data are ordinal scale metrics. Using the *t*-test on these data is wrong and any results will be incorrect. (Interestingly, this popular test was developed in 1908 by William Gossett to aid in evaluating the Guinness brewing process. His employer forbid publishing and so he used the pseudonym "Student" to protect his identity.)

It is mathematically possible to analyze counted data with a *t*-test, but the results are undefined and likely to be misleading. You can do various statistical tests on any set of numbers, but if the assumptions underlying the test are violated, the results are not valid.

## 13.10 Distributions: Part I

Distributions are the way we visualize and organize the results of our grabs (samples). Say we grab ten samples and all ten items come out red. Our nominal distribution, sorted by color, would have a single column labeled red, ten units high. We could be very comfortable declaring that the stuff in the box was very likely red and our next grab would most likely be red. If we then examine a blue item we could declare that it was unlikely to have come from our box. However, if we grabbed ten items from another box and we obtained two red, two blue, two yellow, two green, and two pink items, then our distribution, sorted by color, would be flat. We would have no good way to predict the color obtained by the next grab. Another blue item could likely come from this box. Statistical testing is the method of comparing one distribution to another, and estimating the *likelihood or probability* that they are one and the same set of data. All statistical tests that sample data produce results that are expressed as probabilities. This is not to be vague or indecisive, but to illustrate that we never really know the contents of the box. Some boxes have a very large, unknowable or even infinite content. We can only sample a small portion of the contents, hopefully in a representative fashion. Everything we do in statistics, and life, is but a sampling of the total possibilities of the universe (population) of data. The term "likely" is a reminder that we are only making estimates of the truth based on our sampled data.

Statistical testing is usually stated in terms of the "null hypothesis ($H_0$)," although it may seem like a counterintuitive way to go about comparing alternatives. This concept was first developed by the legendary geneticist and mathematician Sir Ronald Fisher in 1925.[8] The null hypothesis assumes that any kind of difference you see in the data between (among) two or more groups is due to chance and chance alone. This "chance and chance alone" is the presumed source of the findings until a statistical test rejects it, thus the double negative "reject the null hypothesis." The confusing triple negative "fail to reject the null hypothesis" indicates the inability to reject and therefore a passive "acceptance" of chance as the main actor. We never accept the null hypothesis, or any other hypothesis, because we can never know the truth. This philosophical view is our scientific methodology. Mathematicians Jerzy Neyman and Egon Pearson, developed an alternate hypothesis (H1) model that is used in comparative study designs where one treatment is placed against another treatment, instead of against placebo.[7] This alternate hypothesis model allows statistical power calculations.

The term *statistical power* is an important term also related to distributions. The formal meaning of power is the degree of ability to correctly reject the null hypothesis, that is, to find a *true positive* result. For example, if a study has 80% power to find a true difference of 2 mmHg IOP between two samples, then a found difference of 2 mmHg will be correctly declared significant 80% of the time, and incorrectly declared not significant 20% of the time. We will not discuss the calculation of statistical power here, but it is important to note that it is heavily dependent on sample size and sample variability. Therefore, an otherwise excellently designed, masked, randomized controlled clinical trial may fail to show the desired outcome if the sample size (number of patients enrolled in the study) is too small and thus the power of the statistical testing is low relative to the degree of treatment effect. Put another way, if two drugs that truly have great differences in their ability to lower IOP were tested in two small groups of patients, you would likely find this large difference a "true" effect. But in order to find a statistical difference between two glaucoma medications with only slight differences in their ability to lower IOP, you would need much larger numbers of patients in each treatment group than in the first example. Large treatment effects are easier to demonstrate with smaller samples, while small treatment effects usually require larger samples. See Table 13.2 for an example of the interrelationship of power, statistical significance, and sample size.

Power is especially important for negative studies because a low power test will have a large false-negative percentage finding "not significant" when in truth significance was correct. The obtained results in the low-powered test are then either truly negative, or, the study was underpowered and not able to discriminate the true difference that really exists between the groups. Power estimates, even post hoc, are therefore mandatory on all negative findings; otherwise the reader is unable to interpret the result. Overpowered studies, too large a sample size, are likely to declare trivial differences as "significant." Correct study power balances false positive (Type I error) and false negative (Type II error) with respect to treatment effect and variability of the sample measurements as shown in Table 13.3.

**Table 13.2** Interrelationship of power, statistical significance, and sample size

Original Neyman–Pearson model

| N | p | Power | Significant | Sample size |
|---|---|---|---|---|
| 90 | 0.001 | 0.92 | Yes | Over (Error I) |
| 80 | 0.002 | 0.88 | Yes | Over (Error I) |
| 70 | 0.004 | 0.84 | Yes | Correct |
| 60 | 0.007 | 0.78 | Yes | Correct |
| 50 | 0.01 | 0.70 | Yes | Borderline |
| 40 | 0.03 | 0.60 | Yes | Borderline |
| 30 | 0.06 | 0.48 | No | Under (Error II) |
| 20 | 0.12 | 0.34 | No | Under (Error II) |

Difference of 1.5 mmHg, SD=3.0, 2-tailed $z$ test, power from $t$ distribution.

**Table 13.3** Correct study power balances false positive (Error I) and false negative (Error II) with respect to treatment effect and variability of the sample measurements

Significance and power

| Choice | If null hypoth TRUE | If null hypoth FALSE |
|---|---|---|
| Not significant (same) | Correct | Error II false negative |
| | 1-Alpha% | 1-Power% |
| Significant (different) | Error I false positive | Correct |
| | Alpha (5%) | Power (80%) |

Error I = declare significant when not: false positive (alpha%).
Error II = declare not significant when it is: false negative (1-power%).
Without power nothing can be said about case where null is false.
We never really know the actual value of the null hypothesis.
Adapted from Mandel J. *Statistical Analysis of Experimental Data*. Mineola, NY: Dover; 1984.

## 13.11 Distributions: Part II

The shapes of the population and sampling distributions are the keys to understanding the data. To describe the shape of a distribution there are a number of key metrics. Most distributions have a *density function* that describes all aspects of the curve exactly. These density functions are very complex. For our purpose it is enough to know that they exist and that they are used to generate probabilities. Density functions themselves are never used in biologic reporting. Instead we more commonly see certain *descriptive statistics* to describe the data.

Distributions of data are first described by *measures of central tendency*, various kinds of "averages." You are most familiar with the *arithmetic mean*, hereafter called the *mean* unless otherwise indicated. (There are also a *geometric* and a *harmonic mean*, but these will not be described here.) It is calculated by adding up all the interval or ratio measurements and dividing the sum by the number of measurements. But the mean may not be the centermost point in the distribution, as it will be distorted if the distribution is not 100% symmetrical. Data points that are skewed to the right or left of the center will influence the calculation and shift the calculation of the mean toward the side of the distribution with the most and/or largest value measurements. For example, if 85 out of the 100 patients in a sample have IOPs between 18 and 22 mmHg, but 15 of the patients have IOPs of 50 mmHg, the mean will be 24.5 and not a good descriptor of the majority of the population. Outlying data influence the value of the mean. The mean tells us where the center of gravity lies for all of the values in the distribution, but it does not tell anything about the shape of the curve (symmetrical or nonsymmetrical).

The *median* is defined as the measure of central tendency that is the point on an interval or ratio scale above and below exactly half of the data – truly the middle point. It is not influenced by large-value outlying measurements, only the rank order. More powerful statistical tests are possible on the mean as compared to the median.

The *mode* is a meager descriptor of central tendency, defined as the most common value in the distribution. It is not used directly in statistical analysis but is a descriptive statistic used with nominal data, e.g., the most common name in a group of 150 middle school girls might be Brittany – the modal value.

*Measures of variability* describe the shape of the distribution. The *range* is a simple statistic taken as the difference between the largest and smallest measurements. It is rarely used to describe the data in ophthalmic research except for very small size pilot studies and the presentation of patient ages. Similarly the *mean deviation*, which is the sum of the absolute (without regard to sign) differences of each measurement from the arithmetic mean of the distribution, divided by the number of measurements, is rarely used in statistical testing on higher-order data. The two most commonly used measures of variability used in statistical tests are the *variance* (*V*) and the *standard deviation* (*SD*), which is calculated as the square root of the variance. The variance is calculated by taking the sum of squares of deviations about the mean divided by the number of observations. (This eliminates the sign of each deviation from the mean.) The variance is a statistical value in squared units. The standard deviation is not in squared units and is more useful as a descriptive statistic while the variance is more useful in statistical calculations. The SD helps to describe the spread of the distribution relative to its mean. Is it tight and tall or wide and low? If we see one group has IOP of 24 mmHg with an SD of 4, compared to another group mean of 24 mmHg and SD of 7, we can know that the first group was a tighter set of measurements.

The variance of data sets can and should directly be compared to determine if the two (or more) data sets are similar or have different variances. It is important to realize that many statistical tests are invalid if the variances of the groups to be compared are significantly different! It is unreasonable to simply assume that all sets of measurements result in equivalent variances. Of course there are methods designed to handle unequal variances (heteroscedastic in statistical speak). Also note that the SD, by itself, must be interpreted only with reference to the shape (type) of the underlying distribution. The SD only has meaning with respect to a specific kind of distribution. Fortunately, most biologic data are "*t*-shaped" or "normally (Gaussian)" distributed. Realize that by declaring the statistical tests you will use in the Methods section, you have by definition indicated that you know the distribution shape of the underlying experimental data. Some data sets that occur under less common experimental designs may not be normally or *t*-shaped in distribution. Examples include the Poisson and the related binomial distributions. These are discrete probability distributions that are useful for analysis of rare events. Using the Poisson distribution for statistical testing will be described later in this chapter.

## 13.12 Statistical Testing

In scientific research, we formulate a hypothesis and conduct a randomized, double-masked clinical trial in an attempt to see if it is "true." The data are interpreted by subjecting them to one or more appropriate statistical tests. These tests all state their conclusions in probabilistic terms. The results are described by the investigator not as certainties, but associated with some degree of doubt, even if the degree of doubt is small. We propose a null hypothesis that treatment one is no better than treatment two, or placebo. We then estimate the likelihood of finding a difference equal to or larger than the one that was found. If this probability is small, say less than 5%, we "reject" the null hypothesis of no difference in treatment outcomes and assert that the alternative hypothesis of differences in outcome for the two treatment conditions is true (significant). If the probability of the null hypothesis is not very small (>5%), we say that the treatment groups *probably* do not differ in response to the two medications (not significant, or formally, we "fail to reject" the null hypothesis). Results and interpretation of experimental findings are described in probabilistic terms. The degree of probability for rejecting the null hypothesis is described as the *level of statistical significance* (5% in the example above).

Statistical testing, as used in clinical studies, is usually of the inferential type. This was the type of testing described earlier, where the goal was to predict the outcome of the next grab (sample). An *inference* is a statistical prediction of the population (the contents of the box) made on the basis of the characteristics of the sample. The way all statistical tests work is to compare the actual outcome to an estimated, theoretical outcome. The actual outcome is exactly what we have grabbed or sampled. The estimated outcome is our expected contents of the box (population) under investigation. In clinical terms, we hope that the limited observations made on the patients in the experimental groups reflect the true situation in the much larger population of all glaucoma patients, or at least those glaucoma patients with demographic characteristics similar to those patients in the study.

These calculations for different kinds of distributions have been extensively worked out by mathematicians specializing in probability theory. You do not have to understand the details of the calculations to work with and interpret statistical tests. The concept of "statistically significantly different" means that the grabs (samples) obtained in one group is unlikely to have come from the same box as the other group, and that there are at least two different boxes. Formally we say there is less than a 5% chance that these distributions are really the same. Note that the exact nature of the measurement is not important. We do not care if the samples are intraocular pressure, phacoemulsification time, or any other defined parameter of interest. All measurements are converted into distributions, and then the distributions are compared to each other. (Of course this is the foundation of parametric statistics. Nonparametric or distribution free tests use alternate methods.) The final probability only declares the relationship of the distributions to each other. The exact method (i.e., the appropriate and most powerful statistical test) used to compare distributions does depend on the type of measurement in use.

The statistician decides among the different tests available based on the characteristics of the (sampled) data set. As was mentioned when discussing measurement scales, each scale has an appropriate set of distributions and these distributions have appropriate sets of tests. There is some flexibility in which tests are chosen to analyze a specific set of data, but one must not "shop" for the test that gives the desired experimental outcome as statistically significant. The appropriate tests are determined a priori, before the data are analyzed, not a posteriori or "selected" after trying out several of them and seeing which gives the "best" results consistent with the researchers' hypothesis. In short, looking for the test that gives the best statistical results is cheating!

Let us explore the concept of "degrees of statistical significance" in some more detail. Some physicians and textbooks promote the idea that lower probabilities for the level of significance are associated with more important or stronger (more true) outcomes. For example, a probability ($p$) interpretation for the level of significance, like $p<0.05$ is *significant*, $p<0.01$ is *very significant*, and $p<0.001$ is *highly significant*. This entire idea is completely incorrect, and demonstrates a poor understanding of the concept of statistical significance in the biological sciences. It also has nothing to do with the magnitude of the experimental effect. The actual p value of any statistical test is determined by the differences between the sample means, the variances of the samples and the sample sizes. Because the sample sizes are arbitrarily determined and easily manipulated by the researcher, any p value obtained could likely be made smaller by simply increasing the sample sizes for any experiment. For an example, see Fig. 13.1.

The p value, in itself, carries no meaning of clinical significance at all, and must be interpreted within the context of the study power and design. In summary, the 5% level of statistical significance means that the obtained difference among the means of the experimental groups *could* have occurred by chance alone – randomly – without the treatment having any effect, one time in 20, if the same experiment had been repeated 20 times. By rejecting the null hypothesis we declare the results likely correct (true) but acknowledge that there is still a 5% chance that we are wrong. This 5% cutoff is arbitrary but commonly used in biological sciences as it balances the risk of rejecting true results with the risks of accepting false results. Other cutoffs may be chosen and this choice should be well documented in the Methods section.

"Study power" incorporates the meaningful difference between sample measurements (means) and determines the appropriate sample size. For example, the US Food and Drug Administration (FDA) has somewhat arbitrarily declared a 2 mmHg difference in IOP pressure readings as a meaningful *clinical* difference. This value now has experimental meaning and if used in a power equation would lead to a sample size with meaning, and therefore a p value with meaning per the 2 mmHg difference. Yet even in this circumstance, a very small probability is still just "significant" and no more. Significance is essentially an all or none phenomenon. The null hypothesis of no difference among the groups is accepted or rejected, not almost accepted or almost rejected. The probability cannot be used as a measurement implying better or worse outcomes.

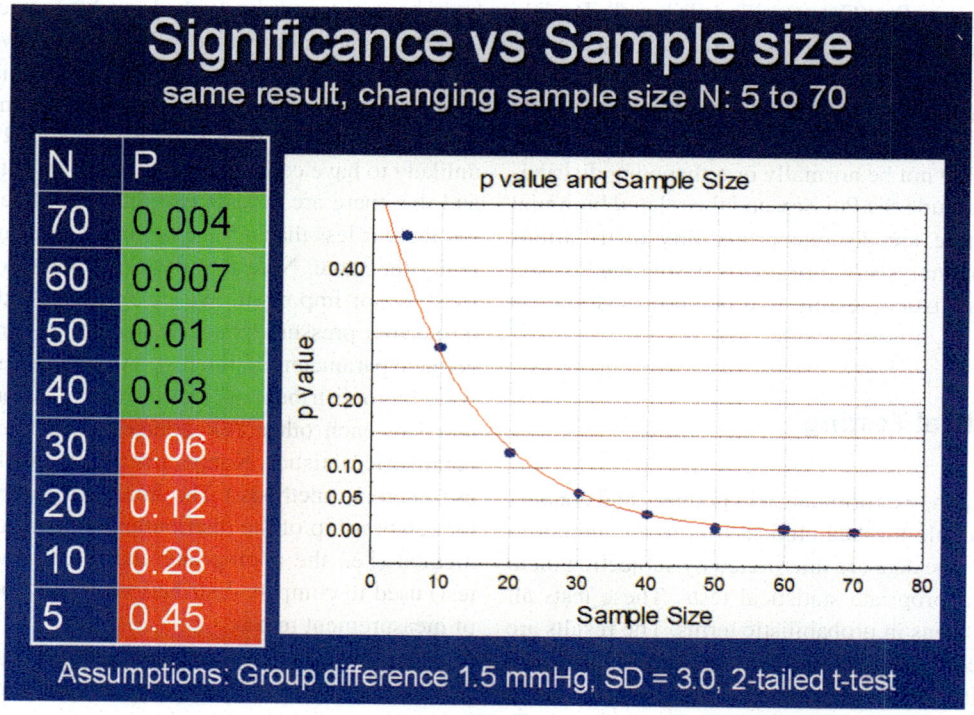

**Fig. 13.1** Changing sample size changes significance level of result

Likewise, if one study can reject the null hypothesis (finds "statistical significance") at a $p<0.05$ level and another study finds $p<0.01$ level, both studies carry equal clinical weight as the concept of "more significant" rejection of the null hypothesis does not exist, it is a meaningless idea in biological sciences. Comparative significance within a single study may yield valid comparisons if the same hypothesis is being tested in limited circumstances (see section titled "Expectation").

Finally, remember it is the physician who determines if the magnitude of the experimental effect on the observed differences in the means of the groups is *clinically significant*. The statistical significance of the experimental tells us nothing at all about the clinical importance of the outcome, only that is more likely than not (19:1 chance) to be real, but may or may not be important to the patient's welfare.

**Expectation**

Many wonder how to interpret mathematical "statistical significance," in some real world way. Because statistical significance is a yes/no construct, it is or is not, the concept of "greater or more significant" is undefined. The application of statistical findings to real problems can be found in the gambling world where it is known more formally as *expectation*.[12]

Expectation takes the probability of an occurrence and multiplies it by the numerical magnitude or worth of the occurrence to obtain a value. Gambling provides us with an easily understood example of this concept. A lottery ticket is truly worth, monetarily, the amount of money in the prize award times the likelihood of winning (which is related to the number of outstanding tickets.). Usually this value is a very small fraction of one cent. (The psychological, not monetary, value of the ticket – at least before the prize winner is announced – may be very great indeed.) Another application of *expectation theory* is glaucoma therapy. If we take the typical pressure reduction of a drug, and multiply by the probability of compliance based on the number of applications needed per day, we now have the expected effectiveness of the drug. For example, topical beta blockers are used once daily and typically reduce IOP by 25%. A once-daily drug has about 90% compliance; therefore the expected pressure reduction is about 22%. Contrast this to pilocarpine, used four times daily with about 35% pressure reduction. Four times daily drugs have about 25% compliance yielding an expected reduction of only 9%. This expectation estimate demonstrates that a more potent drug can have worse real-world outcomes, and this nicely agrees with the clinical popularity of timolol compared to pilocarpine.

## 13.13 Common Tests and Common Errors

### 13.13.1 Parametric vs. Non-parametric Statistical Tests

Knowing the shape and characteristics (the density function) of the data distributions relevant to our experiment enables us to use *parametric statistical tests* that rely on the characteristics of the known distributions. These tests are applied to data that fall along interval or ratio scales of measurement. Sometimes our clinical trial compares data that at best fall along an ordinal scale of measurement, where data are simply ranked but where the true quantitative measurement interval between numbered observations cannot be determined. This condition prevents the distribution of the data from being determined. These data may be analyzed with less powerful non-parametric (distribution free) statistical tests. What this means is that for the same sample sizes, the parametric tests are less likely to show statistical significance than would the non-parametric tests. If you do not know or cannot make a very good educated case about the nature of measurement scale for your data, you are obliged to use the less powerful non-parametric testing procedures.

### 13.13.2 Parametric Tests

Most ophthalmologists have some familiarity with the normal or Gaussian or "z" curve of probability distribution. It is also called the "bell-shaped" curve because of its shape. Further it is known mathematically that "the sampling distribution of the sample mean is approximately normal, even if the distribution of the population from which the sample is taken is not normal." Imagine a collection of sample groups from the same population. The mean of the each of the means (mean of the means) is the same as the population mean and the SD of the means is normally distributed.[13] This is known as the central limit theorem and is very helpful in those experiments where the population distribution is not normally distributed, because obtaining the means of multiple different samples allows parametric statistics to be used.

Physicians may be less familiar with the *t*-probability distribution. The *t*-distribution is a modification of the bell-shaped curve that better describes the probability distribution when using small sample sizes. Student's *t*-test allows us to compare the means of two groups. Interestingly, most probability distributions used in statistical testing are modifications of the normal distribution. Key features of the *t*-distribution are that it is useful for small but not very small samples sizes, and that it merges with the z distribution for large sample sizes. Small is typically five or more measurements.

Large is considered greater than 30 measurements. This may seem surprising, but generally about 30 sample measurements produce similar results whether a test uses underlying $t$ or $z$ distributions.

While many understand the need to use a $t$-test for small sample sizes, few understand the need to have equal variances, independent samples, and $t$-distributed data. Few authors check the variance of their groups ($F$-test) prior to working with the $t$-test. Let us discuss these requirements in more detail. Equal variance for each of the two groups is the easiest to verify. The $F$-ratio of variances developed by R. A. Fisher (mentioned earlier) yields a known probability distribution. This can be used to determine if there is too much discrepancy between the two groups with respect to variance. A significant $F$-test indicates that the variances deviate by too large an amount to be considered equivalent. (Of course there are special $t$-tests designed to handle this condition of unequal variance or heteroscedastic groups, but they are beyond the discussion level of this chapter.) Also note that tests that employ unequal variance models are less powerful than those that assume equal variance for the groups. The samples must be grabbed independently, without the data being interrelated (*confounded*). The $t$-test assumes the data in the two groups are not confounded, if they are, the test should not be used (see section "Confounding"). Unfortunately, there is no fix for confounded data.

In most cases, researchers do not test to see if the sampled data for the small groups in their experiment are in fact arranged in a $t$-distribution. In some cases, we know the data are not normally or $t$-distributed, like IOP by Goldmann tonometer.[14] Other times we do not know the distribution. It is relatively simple to check the distribution by one of the statistical measures. All is not lost if the data are found not normally distributed as this may be an interesting finding in itself.

Another common $t$-test issue is to use the test on the means of counted data. For example, preoperative glaucoma medications average 2.8 per patient compared to a postoperative average of 1.7. These means would be used in a $t$-test and usually found to be statistically significant. In many cases, the result really is statistically significant, but the $t$-test is too likely to yield a falsely positive result when used on this type (counted) of data.

The other major $t$-test error is to apply multiple $t$-tests to the same data set. If each test has a 5% chance of wrongly rejecting the null hypothesis, then multiple tests increase the chance that one test will turn significant simply by chance alone. If you do ten such tests at the 5% level of significance, you have a 40% probability of having observed a random occurrence (rejection of the null hypothesis) not due to any treatment effect but chance alone. Researchers like the $t$-test because of its simplicity in application, comparing group A with group B. Yet we often see test protocols such as A vs. B, A vs. C, A vs. D, and so on. Because each test has a false positive and negative probability, doing multiple tests increase the chances of both kinds of false results. Multiple comparisons among different groups within the same data set are usually best handled by multifactor statistical tests that are designed for just such comparisons.

### 13.13.3 Analysis of Variance for Multiple Group Comparisons

In terms of its mathematical derivation, Student's $t$-test between the means of two groups of subjects is actually the limiting condition of the more general statistical test that is used to compare means among multiple (three or more) groups *called analysis of variance* (ANOVA). ANOVA uses the F distribution of population probabilities and becomes equivalent to the $t$-distribution when only two groups are compared simultaneously. Analysis of variance allows for "repeated measures" research designs.

It is important to understand that a correct use of the $F$-test requires that all cells in the comparison have an equal and independent chance at the same outcome. The $F$-test is often used incorrectly in the glaucoma literature. For example, some researchers have taken serial measurements of IOP over time, but have used both IOP and time as "independent variables." This is not appropriate because each measurement of IOP is not truly independent but more likely related to the value of the most recently obtained previous IOP value. The "next" IOP is likely related to the "previous" IOP reading. The data cells in this experiment are related and their values are somewhat determined by the amount of time that has passed between the measurements. This "interaction" between cells or conditions violates the assumption of statistical independence underlying the ANOVA sampling distribution. There are mathematical techniques for modifying standard ANOVA to allow for these interactions but their details are outside the discussion of basic statistical techniques described in this chapter.

It is important to note that the variance of the sampling distributions for each cell (experimental condition or each different test group) must be equal (homoscedastic) for the assumptions behind ANOVA to be valid. If the variance among the groups is unequal (heteroscedastic) the ANOVA test must be modified. Similarly, accurate "power" calculations designed to determine how many subjects might be needed for the clinical trial to likely reject the null hypothesis will be wrong if between-group variances are unequal.

### 13.13.4 Confounding of Variables in Clinical Trial Design

*Confounding* is a specific statistical term that means that the variance of one data set is somehow linked to and influenced by the other data set in an immeasurable way. If this is true, then the statistical test cannot differentiate among the different sources of variance. Thus the confounded data sets are impossible to separate mathematically and the ANOVA test cannot be applied.

A good ophthalmic example of confounding may be found in the Ocular Hypertension Treatment Study (OHTS).[15,16] In this study, central corneal thickness (CCT) was analyzed along with many other subject-related variables. CCT was found to correlate with conversion from glaucoma suspect status to definite glaucoma by several objective criteria (visual field and optic nerve head changes by photography). Yet the Goldmann applanation tonometer used to measure IOP in the study is known to change its measured value in relation to the CCT of the subject being examined. Therefore the CCT and the Goldmann IOP are *confounded variables* that cannot be separated statistically (mathematically). Unfortunately, some respected colleagues who do not fully appreciate this fact have in print referred to CCT as an independent risk factor, independent from IOP level, for glaucoma suspects converting to glaucoma patients. This statement is simply untrue for all current technologies used in the clinic to measure IOP. All tonometers in community-based clinics are influenced by CCT. Until we have a truly cornea-independent method of doing tonometry in the community setting, or an additional new technology that can reliability separate corneal influence from tonometer readings, the actual independent influence of CCT on glaucoma progression remains unknown. No amount of additional studies can change this fact; they will all have confounding of CCT and IOP measurements, even when thousands of patients are employed to ensure large "power" to find small effects.

Also note that *confounding* and *covariance* are different concepts. Variables that are confounded cannot be separated from each other with respect to their influence on another variable. Covariance, on the other hand, refers to variables that are together influenced (vary) base on a common third factor. Covariance can be isolated and accounted for by appropriate statistical methods, as long as it is searched for and noted in the experimental design. Experimental factors that co-vary may also be said to be *correlated*. Covariance may be positive (both variables tend to increase in magnitude together) or negative (when one variable gets larger the other gets smaller). For example, there is a positive covariance or correlation between the amount of water consumed at the beach on a sunny day and the amount of sunscreen block applied while visiting that beach. Yet neither drinking water causes the use of sunscreen nor does the use of sunscreen cause the imbibing of water; both of these actions co-vary with a third variable, namely the amount of sunshine at the beach. The more sunshine, the more water is consumed (it's hot outside), and the more sunscreen lotion that is applied (you don't want to get a sunburn).

### 13.13.5 Nonparametric Testing

The most powerful statistical tests are able to reject the null hypothesis and find small clinical differences between groups even with small numbers of subjects, because they rely on the known density functions of the underlying probability sampling and population distributions. Put another way, they know the shape and defining parameters of these curves. Statistical tests based on these known distributions are called *parametric tests*.

When we work with experimental data that are at best rank ordered (ordinal scale) we often do not know the exact nature of the distributions involved. Statistical tests have been developed to reject null hypotheses on just such data, although they are not as powerful (likely to reject the null hypothesis) as the tests based on interval or ratio scaled data with known distribution properties. These mathematical techniques are called "nonparametric" statistical tests. Nonparametric simply means that we do not know the distribution or we do know that it is not normally distributed. The Mann–Whitney $U$-test is the nonparametric $t$-test used the most frequently. Conceptually, the nonparametric tests typically have less discriminating ability (power) than the parametric tests. Thus it is possible that the experimental or treatment condition might truly have an effect on the subjects, but the non-parametric test might not conclude so. Simply put, non parametric tests may require larger sample sizes (bigger groups) to find the same magnitude of statistically significant difference than would a parametric test like Student's $t$-test. If the non-parametric test concludes significance, then the sample size was adequate, but if it does not then may be the sample was inadequate in size or underpowered.

A common error is to apply the Mann–Whitney $U$-test to higher scale data. This is not technically incorrect but may produce results different from the standard $t$-test. That is, because the non parametric test is inherently less able to discriminate among true mean differences between groups than a parametric test, which uses more information, you may falsely conclude that there is no difference between the experimental and control groups in your clinical trial. Be especially alert for a negative finding (not significant) with the $U$-test applied to interval scale data. For example, the $U$-test should not be used for intraocular pressure measurement comparisons, because these are interval data and more powerful tests can be applied to the data.

One other technical note about ordinal data before we leave the subject of parametric vs. nonparametric testing. Sometimes data along an ordinal scale may be mathematically converted to a distribution with a known density function, especially the normal distribution. For examples, Snellen visual acuities as commonly taken (e.g., 20/20, 20/40, etc.) do not represent equal intervals between measurement and as such cannot be mathematically averaged in a *mean*ingful (pun intended!) way. However, by doing a logarithmic conversion on these scores (the "logMar" visual acuity – defined as the logarithm of the minimum angle of resolution) the resulting logMar values do fall on an interval scale of measurement and are normally distributed. Parametric (e.g., $t$-tests or ANOVA) may then be applied to these data. After the statistical tests are done, the data are converted back to their original form for presentation in the Results section of the article. While these conversions may seem like some sleight of hand, they are entirely legitimate mathematical procedures used to increase the power of the statistical test applied to the data.

### 13.13.6 Nominal and Binomial Scale Distributions

With nominal (categorical) data we often have a simple situation where we measure the presence or absence of a single property, a so-called *binomial distribution*. Many biological (ophthalmological) variables may be described in this form. For example, male or female, dieting or not dieting, alive or dead. Fisher's exact test is a suitable statistical test for examining such data, very useful for small samples sizes, generally less than 10 in each group. The data are presented in a 2 by 2 cell contingency table. As with ordinal data, the log of a binomial distribution is also normally distributed. Therefore it is common to take a binomial, log transform, and then insert into a linear regression. This is called log-linear regression, or logistic regression. For example, if we were to evaluate gender and IOP we would log transform gender (male, female) and then use the transformed data in a linear regression against IOP. The result is a log-linear relationship that needs to be reversed for presentation (anti-log). The most common error is to create arbitrary nominal categories such as "success" and then apply Fisher's Exact Test. Because the cutoff for defining the category is arbitrary, virtually any result may be achieved by changing the dividing line (value that defines "success").

When there are categorical data with more than two categories and at least ten exemplars in each cell, requirements are likely to be met for the chi square distribution and associated statistical test. First developed by Karl Pearson in the early 1900s,[17] *Pearson's Chi Square* test has been modified by Yates[18] (correction for continuity) when one cell has fewer than five observations.

It is not acceptable to use a measured result as a percentage (such as a percentage of postoperative IOP decrease) and use it in a chi-square test. It is also not appropriate to create arbitrary subdivisions (arbitrary categories) of a measured result and then place the counts into a chi-square analysis. The underlying chi square distribution is only valid for discrete counted events >5 per cell. The most common error is the overextension of chi square into rare events (<5 counts). The test is invalid in this range.

### 13.13.7 Rare Events

Rare events are often studied in ophthalmology, such as endophthalmitis, cystoid macular edema, retinal detachment, and (hopefully) other surgical complications. Any discrete event too rare to use the chi-square distribution falls into the Poisson distribution and should be analyzed with the Poisson test. The Poisson test only needs the counts of the events per some unit – usually time. The actual denominator is not needed and is a unique feature of the test. For example, we can study endophthalmitis rate per year without knowing how many surgeries were performed.

## 13.14 Example Evaluation of a Journal Article

The exercise presented here is meant to illustrate the process of reviewing a published clinical trial. The sample research provided comes from a real study that was never published, with the authors' identities hidden. This non-published paper is being used for instructional purposes only and cannot be found in print or online. Any resemblance to an actual published work is purely a coincidence.

The stated purpose of the article was to investigate two different methods of tonometry to determine if they produced different results on the same eyes. A prospective, masked trial was declared. Influence of central corneal thickness (CCT) was a primary variable of interest in explaining the difference in measurement results.

### 13.14.1 Comment

The premise is very reasonable and appropriate. It is a little odd that prior literature or a pilot study was not discovered first.

If the two instruments do not differ then the entire hypothesis is lost. Overall the introduction was minimal and only moderately convincing.

## 13.15 Methods

A reasonable randomization of eyes was presented along with inclusion and exclusion criteria. The study presented the sample size obtained, a result, in the Methods section without any explanation of how the size was determined. This is likely the most common error. The sample size needed should be based on a priori statistical power calculation based on expected variance and expected mean differences between the groups. This is a basic requirement that should be done before the research protocol is finalized (and funded). The sample size actually studied is a result, not part of the method used.

A detailed explanation of the tonometry techniques was presented. A paired $t$-test was the stated statistic for the tonometry measurement, a reasonable choice of test. Sometimes the results of a $t$-test are shown incorrectly. Paired data need to show the mean of the differences with the variance of the differences. Many authors present the means and standard deviation of the individual groups. Then the authors use linear regression to assess (correlate) other variables, including CCT, as they relate to the tonometry results. The problem with this approach is that the authors do not know if the resulting data are linear in relationship. Linear regression only determines degree of linear (first-order degree) relationship, not the influence of one variable on another. This is another common error. Linear regression is easy to use incorrectly as a large sample size will often have a statistically significant linear component. This does not describe the influence of the factors, only that the slope of the resulting line deviates from zero. There may be no clinical meaning at all in the finding even though it has a statistically significant linear component. (A full discussion of this and other common graphical errors is described by Krummenauer et al.[19]) So far as we look at this research, we have a relatively vague study goal, a statistic that is often presented incorrectly (paired results) and a relational analysis that is very sensitive to sample size if not constrained by clinical meaning.

## 13.16 Results

In the Results section, the authors present a statistically significant finding on the paired $t$-test between the two tonometry methods. The paired data were presented correctly as mean and standard deviation of the differences. They present the regression slope of 0.60 with $r^2$ (proportion of explained variance) of 0.30 for the tonometries. This means one tonometer is reading about 60% of the other, but with only 30% of the variance explained by the linear relationship. There are several problems here, even though 30% was "statistically significant," we are not comforted that 70% of the data remain unexplained. The authors should have performed alternate tests to evaluate more of the relationship. To their credit they do a Bland–Altman analysis and show that the spread is very large and not related to measured IOP. The Bland–Altman is a critical method of determining relationships that vary in some systematic way. For example, a graph of the differences in tonometry ($Y$ axis) vs. the CCT ($X$ axis) would show any influence of CCT on tonometry differences. This very powerful method is underutilized. In this study, the authors used the mean of the tonometries as the $X$ to show the differences in tonometry did not change in a predictable way. Unfortunately, they did not do the example cited: difference vs. CCT. Because this was one of the key goals of the study this omission is difficult to understand. Instead, a linear regression was used with CCT, as noted previously this will not appropriately address the influences on the tonometry. Negative linear regression findings were presented, which do not mean there was no influence, but only that there was no linear association. At this point, we can stop reading as the main objective of the study was not addressed. We can conclude that this study design did not achieve the stated goals.

## 13.17 Conclusion

Reading and evaluating clinical research papers is within the skill set of all ophthalmologists who are willing to use logic, common sense, and a bit of statistical knowledge. Here we have described the formal structure of peer-reviewed randomized clinical trials, dabbled a bit into the concepts behind statistical analysis, and briefly applied these concepts to evaluate a sample research study. The analysis of the data should be carefully planned long before the study is undertaken. Off-the-cuff post hoc analytical methods rarely contribute valid or useful clinical findings for the management of our patients. The scales of measurement and the design of the experiment constrain the conclusions that can be drawn from data obtained. Important discoveries in science favor not only the prepared mind, but careful planning and design of clinical research.

## References

1. Eddy DM, Billings J. The quality of medical evidence: implications for quality of care. *Health Aff (Millwood)*. 1988;7(1):19-32.
2. Sackett DL. Rules of evidence and clinical recommendations on the use of antithrombotic agents. *Chest*. 1986;89:2s-3s.

3. Sackett DL, Haynes RB, Guyatt GH, Tugwell P. *Clinical Epidemiology: A Basic Science for Clinical Medicine*. London: Little, Brown; 1991.
4. Sackett DL, Richardson WS, Rosenberg WMC, Haynes RB. *Evidence-Based Medicine: How to Practice and Teach EBM*. London: Churchill-Livingstone; 1996.
5. Guyatt GH, Sackett DL, Sinclair JC, Hayward R, Cook DJ, Cook RJ. Users' guides to the medical literature. IX. A method for grading health care recommendations. *JAMA*. 1995;274:1800-1804.
6. Available at: http://ophsource.org/periodicals/ophtha/authorinfo. Accessed April 8, 2009.
7. Salsburg D. *The Lady Tasting Tea: How Statistics Revolutionized Science in the Twentieth Century*. New York: W. H. Freeman & Co; 2001.
8. Fisher RA. *Statistical Methods for Research Workers*. Edinburgh: Oliver and Boyd; 1925.
9. Heisenberg W. *Physikalische Prinzipien der Quantentheorie*. Leipzig: Hirzel. English translation: *The Physical Principles of Quantum Theory*. Chicago: University of Chicago Press; 1930.
10. Adair G. The Hawthorne effect: a reconsideration of the methodological artifact. *J Appl Psychol*. 1984;69(2):334-345.
11. David FN. *Games, Gods & Gambling: A History of Probability and Statistical Ideas*. unabridged ed. Mineola, NY: Dover; 1998.
12. Malmuth M. *Gambling Theory and Other Topics*. 6th ed. Las Vegas, NV: Two Plus Two Publishing; 2004.
13. Rice J. *Mathematical Statistics and Data Analysis*. 2nd ed. Belmont, CA: Wadsworth Publishing Co.; 1995.
14. Colton T, Ederer F. The distribution of intraocular pressure in the general population. *Surv Ophthalmol*. 1980;25(3):123-129.
15. Kass MA, Heuer DK, Higginbotham EJ, et al, for the Ocular Hypertension Treatment Study Group. The Ocular Hypertension Treatment Study: a randomized trial determines that topical ocular hypotensive medication delays or prevents the onset of primary open-angle glaucoma. *Arch Ophthalmol*. 2002;120:701-713.
16. Gordon MO, Beiser JA, Brandt JD, et al, for the Ocular Hypertension Treatment Study Group. The Ocular Hypertension Treatment Study: baseline factors that predict the onset of primary open-angle glaucoma. *Arch Ophthalmol*. 2002;120:714-720.
17. Pearson K. On the criterion that a given system of deviations from the probable in the case of a correlated system of variables is such that it can be reasonably supposed to have arisen from random sampling. *Philos Mag.*. 1900;50(5):157-175. Reprinted in K. Pearson 1956; 339-357.
18. Yates F. Contingency table involving small numbers and the $\chi^2$ test. *J R Stat Soc*. 1934;1(suppl):217-235.
19. Krummenauer F, Storkebaum K, Dick HB. Graphic representation of data resulting from measurement comparison trials in cataract and refractive surgery. *Ophthalmic Surg Lasers Imaging*. 2003;34:240-244.

# Chapter 14
# Indications for Therapy

George L. Spaeth

## 14.1 Indications for Treatment

This chapter will broadly examine considerations about how to approach the treatment of those who wish to remain healthy or have their existing disease eliminated, or, at the least, prevented from getting worse. Those seeking care will be called "patients," even though that word itself implies that the patient is less knowledgeable and less powerful than the physician, which results in a self-fulfilling prophecy: specifically, that doctors act as if they know more and patients act as if they know less. There are aspects related to health and disease about which physicians are expected to be more knowledgeable than patients. However, only the patient knows what he or she wants, and only the patient has the power to care for himself or herself. As such, then, patients have many powers that physicians do not have; recognizing this is essential for both the patient and the physician if the appropriate goal – health – is to be achieved. Nevertheless, not being able to use the word "patient" introduces such awkwardness in language that there is no other practical option.

### 14.1.1 The Purposes of Treatment

There is only one overarching purpose of medical treatment, specifically the health of the patient. This could involve prevention of illness, maintenance of health, or restoration of health. Because health is difficult to define and its definition differs from patient to patient and doctor to doctor, getting a proper understanding of what health means is not easy. Additionally, different patients and different doctors are likely to emphasize different aspects of health and deemphasize others. Furthermore, the development of the specific areas of expertise has made consideration of the whole patient by physicians, and even by patients themselves, problematical. Patients often consult physicians for specific reasons, such as poor vision or pain, and often do not think of themselves in a broad, holistic, unspecialized way. Because of these problems, physicians and patients alike tend to concentrate on specific measurables, such as blood pressure, fasting blood sugar, intraocular pressure, or decibels of mean visual field defect. Such markers, however, are rarely valid indicators of the patient's health. However, because they do relate to health, they often become transformed into the desired outcome measures themselves. It is hard to remember that measurements such as blood pressure, fasting blood sugar, intraocular pressure, or mean defect are but lighthouses, illuminating landmarks of health. It is easy to forget that these surrogate markers are not the desired destination. That destination is the broad consideration of the health of the patient; and without keeping that destination clearly in mind, the physician is not likely to be able to help the patient achieve such an important goal.

The purpose of treatment, then, is health, and the physician helps the patient achieve that by creating an environment that encourages health.

Physicians want to recognize factors that predispose to disease and eliminate or minimize their consequences. Patients want the same thing. There is understandably great interest in those things that predispose to illness, and they have come to be called "risk factors." Unfortunately, most of the so-called risk factors related to glaucoma have never been studied in terms of their relationship to the development of decreased quality of life or decreased ability to perform the activities of daily living. There are some studies that have started looking at this issue and find that patients with severe glaucoma have a decreased quality of life, are more prone to fall, have difficulty reading, and have other similar problems.[1-7] While there is an obvious relationship between loss of visual field and the ability to function – those with far-advanced visual field loss being more disabled by their loss of vision than those with no visual field loss – the relationship in the intermediate amounts is more complex.[7] Many patients with poor visual fields, for example, can perform very well, sometimes far better than those with minimal visual field loss. For example, it is not true that a person with 5 dB of visual field loss will be more able to perform the activities of daily living than a person with a decrease of 10 dB. A great deal of work needs to be done in this regard.

### 14.1.2 The Primacy of History Taking

The point, however, is that physicians and patients alike must recognize the primacy of the history-taking aspect of the examination of the patient. It is in the history-taking that both patient and physician come to the most accurate assessment of the patient's quality of life and actual ability to perform those activities the patient wishes to perform. There is simply no substitute for an accurate, quantitative, compassionate, knowledgeable discussion with the patient. It is this discussion that informs and guides all the subsequent parts of the evaluation and of the treatment. Instruments are presently available to evaluate the quality of life. However, it is important to recognize that none of these has been externally validated. Because they are by definition subjective, it is my opinion that such instruments provide little benefit beyond a carefully taken history. In contrast, performance-based measures are objective, and are starting to come into their own. One comprehensive, performance-based measure has been developed, tested, and found to be a valid indicator of what patients can do[1] and others can do in specialized areas.[3] It is certain that in the future these will become more widely utilized.

### 14.1.3 Individualizing Indications for Treatment

In the game of Bridge, one of the four players wins the contract to play the cards, usually in one of the four suits: spades, hearts, diamonds, or clubs. That chosen suit then becomes the "trump" suit, that is, a card in that suit is more powerful than any card in any other suit. For example, if the trump suit is clubs, then whenever a club is played, it "takes the trick." Consider the situation in which the first of the four players plays the queen of spades, the second follows with the king of spades (which, being more powerful than the queen, would be expected to take the trick), the third plays the ace of spades (which is even more powerful than the king), but the fourth plays the lowly two of clubs. The trick is won by the player with the two of clubs. That would ordinarily be the least powerful card in the deck, were it not that clubs were, in this situation, trumps. And so it is in considering the appropriate indications for treatment. The critical issue is considering what indication trumps all the others. The answer is straightforward, but tends to be forgotten.

Table 14.1 lists the reasons frequently given for justifying treatment. All of these can be defended, but all are subsidiary to the reason that trumps all others. This most appropriate reason to treat requires consideration of at least six different factors (Table 14.2), and all six require the acquisition of data and of knowledge that tends to be inadequately considered by most physicians, or considered too difficult to obtain. The result is that other reasons are advanced without recognizing that those apparent justifications are "trumped up" (to use "trump" in a different sense). Let us consider in more detail the reasons listed in Table 14.1.

1. "I treated the patient because she has glaucoma." Many patients with glaucoma will never develop any disability whatsoever from their glaucoma, but will immediately develop a decrease in quality of life and some disability from the treatment.
2. "I treated the patient because he may have glaucoma and I would have felt terrible if he got worse." This is an even less justifiable reason than #1.
3. "The patient had risk factors indicating that she would develop visual field loss." How long would it take that field loss to develop? Would the field loss be sufficient to cause symptoms? If not, how can one justify treatment?
4. "The patient was one of those people who is likely to sue, and therefore I started treatment." Physicians have been found guilty of malpractice for treating unnecessarily as well as for not treating. The best defenses against suit are to hold out realistic expectations to oneself and to the

**Table 14.1** Reasons to justify treatment

1. The patient has glaucoma
2. The patient may have glaucoma
3. The patient will develop visual field loss
4. The physician is fearful of being sued
5. The patient is more likely to return for a check-up if treated
6. The patient wants to be treated
7. The physician wants to receive a fee
8. The patient will develop additional field loss
9. Treatment will prevent the patient from getting worse

**Table 14.2** Speculations predicting the rate of change in glaucoma[a]

| Amount of existing nerve damage | | | |
|---|---|---|---|
| Level of IOP (mmHg) | None | Mild/marked | Advanced |
| 100 | 1 min | 1 min | 1 min |
| 50 | 4 weeks | 2 weeks | 1 week |
| 35 | 12 months | 6 months | 1 month |
| 15 | 20 years | 10 years | 5 years |

[a]These estimates are based on personal clinical examination combined with the small amount of published material dealing with rate of change and susceptibility of change related to stage of disease and level of intraocular pressure. These rates do *not* apply to patients with increased propensity to damage, such as those with hemoglobin S, or those already known to have developed damage at the IOP in question.

patient, and to provide good care that is appropriate for the patient.

5. "It has been shown that patients who are treated are more likely to return for their visit." Indeed, Bigger[8] did show that patients who are treated are more likely to return. However, that in itself is not a justification for treatment. It takes time to explain to patients why they need to return, but a thoughtful discussion is probably more likely to result in developing a good doctor–patient relationship than simply starting the patient on treatment. Thoughtful patients will wonder whether treatment was really justified, and may elect another physician who seems more thorough.

6. "But the patient wanted to be treated." Few patients, of course, want to get worse. Therefore, many patients, as is true for many doctors, take a default position of believing that treatment is preferable to no treatment. They forget that treatments often cause problems that are greater than those the treatment is designed to prevent or alleviate. It is understandable that patients may prefer to be treated. However, when it is explained to patients that a treatment has a greater likelihood of causing problems than deferring a treatment, most patients choose not to be treated. There may be, however, some patients who are so strongly fearful of getting worse that it is appropriate to use a treatment, indicating to the patient that the need for the treatment will be carefully reconsidered in the future and perhaps stopped.

7. Though rarely consciously articulated, all caregivers know that treatments generate fees. It is reasonable for all caregivers, including physicians, to expect some reimbursement for their services. However, the reimbursement should be related to the value of the service. Moreover, it is not proper to treat because one gets reimbursed, but rather because the treatment is appropriate, and in doing the appropriate thing, one deserves to get reimbursed.

8. "But the patient already has visual field loss and may develop more field loss." This is starting to sound reasonable. When patients already have definite glaucomatous visual field loss, they are at risk for developing more visual field loss, and in such a situation treatment is likely to be justified, but not always.

9. "Treatment will prevent the patient from getting worse." Aha! Here is the only justifiable reason for treating.

The reason that trumps all other reasons regarding treatment, specifically, the only justifiable reason for treatment *is the certainty that treatment will prevent the patient from getting worse*. Preventing visual field loss is not in itself a justifiable reason for treatment. Improving visual acuity is in itself not a justifiable reason for treatment. Lowering intraocular pressure by itself is certainly not a justifiable reason to treat (unless it is at a level certain to make the person worse), nor is prevention of a development of glaucomatous cupping, that is, worsening of the optic neuropathy that has, unfortunately, become the *sine qua non* of the diagnosis of glaucoma. It is well established that patients can have marked narrowing of the neuroretinal rim of the optic nerve head without developing any detectable visual loss. Lowering intraocular pressure is only of value if it relieves pain, prevents a vascular occlusion, or has some other direct beneficial effect on the person's quality of life. Even if the risk attendant to improving visual acuity is minimal, it is still unjustifiably great if the person is already entirely satisfied with his or her vision. As far as visual field loss is concerned, mild field loss rarely is associated with any symptomatology and even moderate bilateral visual field loss may not cause any disability. All of these characteristics of glaucoma are important and need to be monitored, because they are helpful in establishing a rate of change, but they all too frequently become inadvertent surrogates for the person himself or herself.

### 14.1.4 Predictors of the Future

Accurate predictors come primarily in two forms: (1) a single marker that is almost always a sign of things to come,[9,10] or (2) a trend that will almost always continue.[11] "Almost" is present in this sentence, because accurate prediction of a future assumes that there is a future. For example, an intraocular pressure (IOP) of 100 mmHg will almost always cause optic nerve damage; the "almost" is added because an IOP of 100 mmHg probably does not cause damage when it is momentary, as it is when using digital massage following a filtering procedure, or as it is in some types of refractive surgery, or when the person will die 30 s after the pressure becomes 100 mmHg. The "almost" is there because it is usually necessary to consider the duration of the causative force. More on that later. Single markers that are highly predictive of making the person worse as a result of glaucoma then must be combined with information about rate of change and duration of change. For some situations, such as an IOP greater than 100 mmHg, the rate of change is usually a minute or even seconds, so a duration of, say, 5 min is of concern. Table 14.2 gives rough guidelines for IOP-producing damage that takes into account the amount of damage already present, as well as the duration of time involved to cause the damage. The estimates shown in Table 14.2 have not been established, but they are conceptual guidelines of some importance. Because accurate prediction of the future is important in decision-making, there has long been an interest in so-called risk factors, that is, findings that increase the risk of change occurring.

Standard risk factors for developing visual field loss in glaucoma are listed in Table 14.3. It should be noted that

**Table 14.3** Risk factors for developing or worsening of glaucomatous visual field loss

| Finding | Significance |
|---|---|
| Acquired pit of the optic nerve | Always |
| Narrowing of the neuroretinal rim in excess of that occurring related to aging | Almost always |
| Aging | May not be a predictive factor, but is related to loss of nerve cells |
| Intraocular pressure | The higher the IOP, the greater the predictive value |
| Family history | The more positive, the greater the predictive value |
| Myopia | The more myopic, the greater the predictive value |
| Disc hemorrhage | Not definitely an independent factor for worsening |
| Age | May be merely associated |
| Pigment dispersion syndrome | Probably not an independent risk factor other than its relationship to intraocular pressure and myopia |
| Exfoliation syndrome | Probably not an independent risk factor except for its relationship to intraocular pressure, but this is not certain |

these are not factors for developing disability, but rather for developing field loss. Except for acquired pit of optic nerve or rim narrowing, all of these factors are relative. That is, their significance is relative to their severity. Though age is frequently listed as a risk factor, age in itself may not be a valid risk factor for the development of glaucomatous visual field loss. As persons age, they lose visual field due to lost neurons; that is, the process of aging is itself associated with progressive visual field loss. This loss tends to be global; it does not appear to follow the pattern of glaucomatous visual field loss (limited initially to one hemifield, a nasal step, an inferior paracentral scotoma, an arcuate pattern, etc.), though this needs better investigation. Because glaucoma involves loss of neurons and aging involves loss of neurons, aging probably contributes to the process of glaucomatous nerve loss. But it is far less clear that age itself plays a role. Mean values can be misleading in this regard. For example, Caprioli's group showed that age was highly significantly related to further visual field loss, but, when considering the range of the ages, the oldest patients did not have any field loss.[11]

The most reliable predictor of the future often is a trend that is likely to continue. It is for this reason that patients with glaucoma and without known glaucoma, need to be followed, in order to permit the accumulation of enough data points to allow establishing a reliable trend. The number of such data points that are required relates to the accuracy of the data and the rapidity of change. Because changes in the optic disc and retinal nerve fiber layer usually precede changes in the visual field,[12,13] and because changes in the disc and nerve fiber layer can be obtained relatively objectively, it would be ideal to record this information for every person around the age of 15 to serve as a baseline measurement for future comparisons. Once visual field loss is present, the more frequently visual field examinations are repeated, and the less noisy those examinations are, the more quickly a valid trend can be established. A minimum of two visual fields per year is probably a rough guideline for most patients with glaucoma, but more frequent fields will establish a trend more rapidly.[14] Any reproducible change in the width of the neuroretinal rim within a period of 5 years is probably clinically significant, and a change of 2 dB per year of mean defect is also probably indicative of change that exceeds that occurring normally.

### 14.1.5 Colored Glaucoma Graph

Figure 14.1 shows a graphic way of considering the issues just discussed from a clinical point of view.[15,16] This "colored glaucoma graph" is used by me every day in my clinical practice. The vertical axis concerns units of glaucoma damage and the horizontal axis units of time (duration). The surest way to predict the future, then, is to extrapolate from valid observations of what has already happened.

Because what the physician and the patient want to know relates to what is going to happen to the patient's ability to perform the activities of daily living (ADL), plotting a reliable course of change in ADL would in some ways be ideal. However, by the time such changes have occurred, the amount of glaucoma damage is already either moderate or marked and neither the doctor nor the patient wants to await further change in ability to perform ADL before deciding whether treatment is necessary. Early visual field changes precede loss of functional ability. Also, early visual field changes are often variable and may be seriously misleading. Once definite loss of field is present, and especially in patients in whom the testing results are highly reproducible, then serial visual fields can be of great value. Were it possible to count retinal ganglion cells, that might be the ideal unit to place on the "Y" axis of the patient's clinical course, that is, a measurement of the deterioration in the patient's stage. Though this is still not possible today, it probably will be in time. That will be a great step ahead! Estimates of nerve fiber layer thickness are a surrogate for retinal ganglion cells, but may not yet be sufficiently reliable or reproducible measures of number of ganglion cells. Furthermore, it seems likely that in many cases a structural change in the topography of the optic nerve is the initiating event, causing the damage to the neurons and thus preceding change in nerve fiber layer thickness or, for that matter, ganglion cell loss.

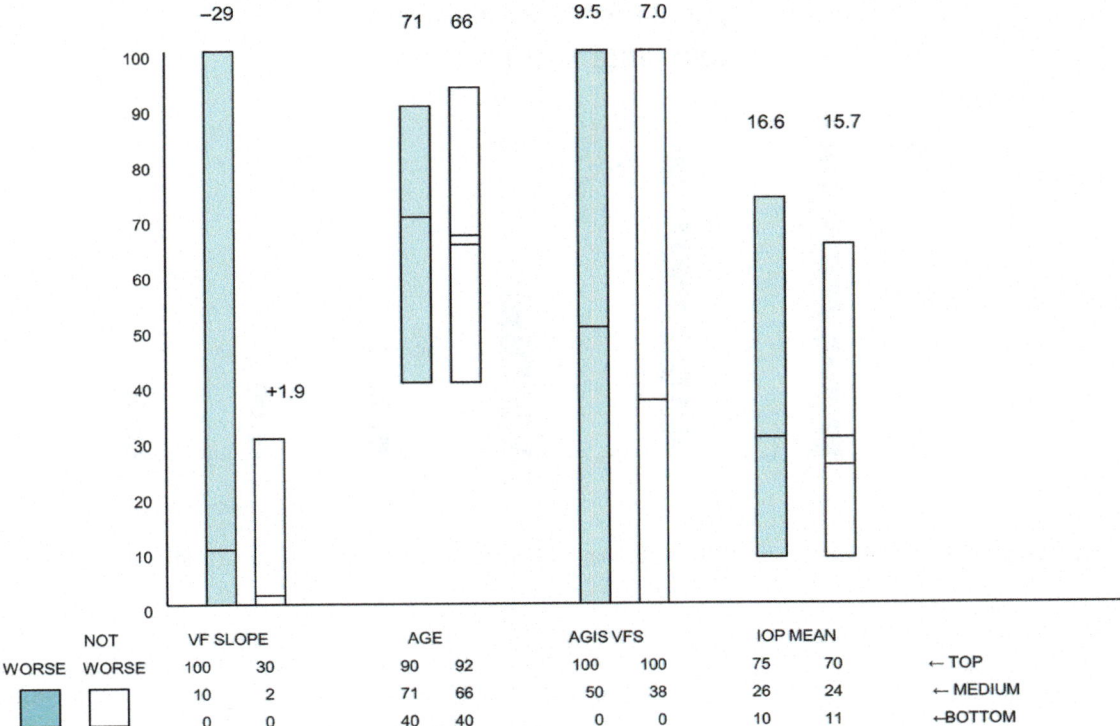

**Fig. 14.1** The *darker blue bars* represent patients who showed progressive visual field loss in the Advanced Glaucoma Intervention Study (modified from Ref. [10]). The Y axis has arbitrary units designed to include the majority of the range of values. The figures on top of the bars indicate the actual numbers. For the left-hand column, this represents the slope of the visual field, the *left-hand bar* indicating a rapidly deteriorating slope and the *right-hand bar* – one which was slightly positive. The mean values are indicated by the *lines* crossing the eight bars. The highest value of the range is indicated by the figures entitled, "Top." Thus, when considering age, the mean age of patients getting worse is 71, and the mean age of patients not getting worse is 66. The oldest patient getting worse is 90, and the oldest patient not getting worse is 92. *VF* visual field; *AGIS* Advanced Glaucoma Intervention Study; *VFS* visual field score; *IOP* intraocular pressure

It is possible that in some patients ganglion cell damage precedes optic nerve topography change, but this has not been established and seems unlikely. Some measure, however, of perimetric damage is appropriate, and the more valid and quantitative that is the better.

Except for the extraordinarily rare situation in which a child is born with glaucomatous nerve damage, nobody starts with glaucoma damage. That is, glaucoma damage is acquired. This gives the physician and the patient the opportunity to detect the damage in its early stages and plot changes prior to the time that sufficient functional damage has occurred that the glaucomatous process can be established with certainty as being present. Obtaining two, or preferably three, reliable evaluations in which the separation between the points exceeds the noise and biological variability of the points allows establishing points that can be used to estimate the future results of accuracy. Hitchings and others believe the course of glaucoma occurs in a linear pattern.[17] However, it is probably wise to recognize the limits of an extrapolated projection and use each new point to refine the previously defined curve, recognizing the variability of the point caused by noise and short-term fluctuations. In actual practice, one is looking for a trend that will indicate whether the condition is roughly stable or significantly deteriorating. As shown by Caprioli, the rate of change is an excellent prognostic indicator, far better than amount of field loss, level of intraocular pressure, or fluctuation of intraocular pressure[11] (Fig. 14.2).

The course of glaucoma can be roughly divided into three: (1) early or questionable tissue damage; (2) definite but still asymptomatic damage; and (3) sufficient visual loss to cause disability. The initial stages of glaucoma, then, are in the period of time when changes cannot at a single examination be determined to be signs of pathology or variations of normal. While cup/disc ratios can be helpful in detecting change, they are of almost no help in establishing the presence or absence of glaucoma, unless the cup/disc ratio is greater than 0.8. This is because the cup/disc ratio system does not take into account the position of the cup[18] or the size of the disc.[19] A cup/disc ratio of 0.5 with a concentrically placed cup is not likely to be a sign of glaucoma; but a cup/disc ratio of 0.5 that is eccentrically placed, so that the rim is absent in one area, is a highly reliable sign of glaucomatous damage (Fig. 14.3). A cup/disc ratio of 0.5 in a large disc with a vertical diameter of 3 mm is not likely to be a sign of pathology, whereas a

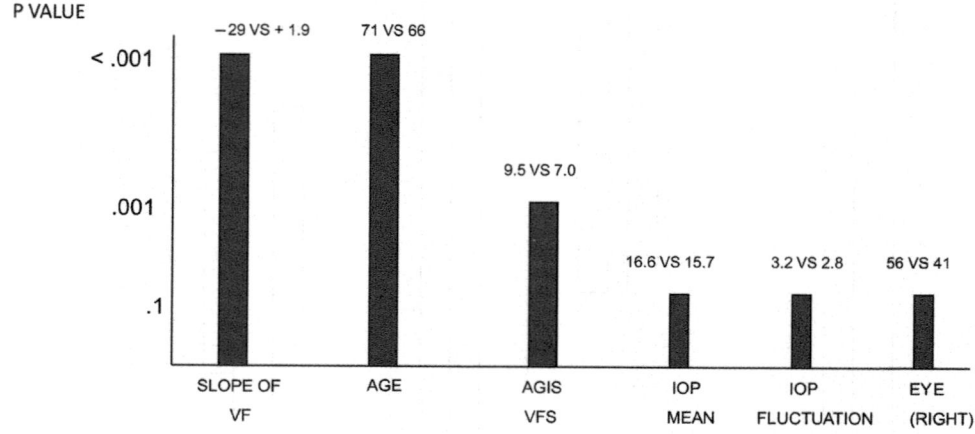

**Fig. 14.2** Likelihood that characteristics of patients in the AGIS study were related to worsening of the visual field[10]

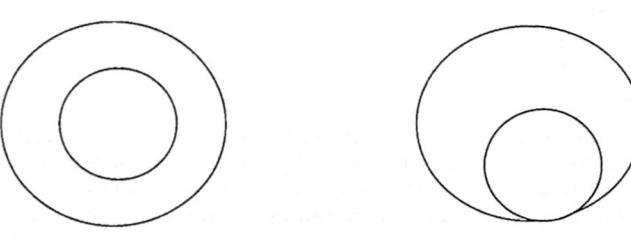

**Fig. 14.3** The position of the cup and the width of the rim are usually more valid indicators of the presence of glaucoma than the size of the cup of the optic disc

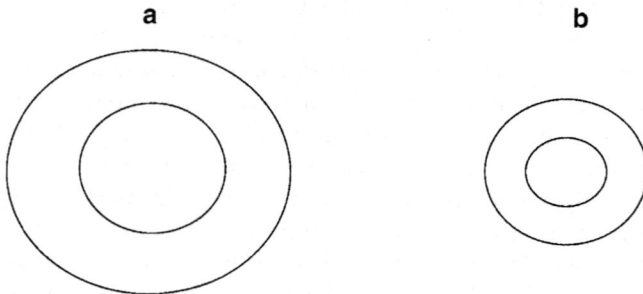

**Fig. 14.4** The size of the cup of the optic disc and the width of the rim are related to the size of the optic disc itself. Though both discs have a cup-to-disc ratio of 0.5, Disc **a** is probably healthy, while **b** may well be pathologic

cup/disc ratio of 0.5 in a small disc of 1 mm vertical diameter is a disturbing finding (Fig. 14.4). The Heidelberg Retinal Tomography Moorfields Regression Analysis can provide help, but it takes neither pattern nor disc size into sufficient account to be a highly reliable diagnostic tool. In contrast, the Disc Damage Likelihood Sale (Fig. 14.5) takes into account the width of the neuroretinal rim and the size of the disc and correlates better the visual field loss than the Heidelberg Retinal Tomography parameters.[15,20-24] It can, then, serve as a useful guide to the "*Y*" axis of any graph depicting the course of glaucoma.

In the Disc Damage Likelihood Scale (DDLS) scores of 1–4 cannot by themselves be considered pathologic, though if the DDLS has worsened by two units, say from 1 to 3, that is a definite sign of pathology. Often it is possible to be quite sure of a 1 unit change. Only very rarely would a DDLS of 5 not represent pathology and not be associated with a visual field loss. Stages 6–10 are unquestionably pathologic; it is not until a stage of 7 or usually 8 is reached that the patient has sufficient field loss that he or she is symptomatic. Thus, it is possible to consider stages 1–4 as usually within normal limits. Stages 7 or greater are almost always associated with awareness of disability. Because symptomatology is highly subjective, some individuals may notice changes earlier and others later in the course of their deterioration.

When patients are in the latter third of their clinical course, they know that they are damaged, and any deterioration, even though slight, is associated with an increase in troublesome symptomatology. A major goal of the treating physician is to try to keep patients from achieving this stage, which we can call the red zone of glaucoma. When patients are already in the red zone, the goal must be to prevent *any* further deterioration. In this red zone, it is neither necessary nor appropriate to try to determine the rate of change, because any deterioration is associated with worsening of the patient.

In contrast to the situation in which patients are in the red zone, in the early stages of glaucoma it may be impossible to answer in any meaningful way the patient's question, "Do I have glaucoma?" There is so much variability in the findings, and the classic risk factors are associated with such low

## THE DISC DAMAGE LIKELIHOOD SCALE

| DDLS Stage | Narrowest width of rim (rim/disc ratio) | | | DDLS Stage | Examples | | |
|---|---|---|---|---|---|---|---|
| | For Small Disc <1.50 mm | For Average Size Disc 1.50–2.00 mm | For Large Disc >2.00 mm | | 1.25 mm optic nerve | 1.75 mm optic nerve | 2.25 mm optic nerve |
| 1 | .5 or more | .4 or more | .3 or more | 0a | | | |
| 2 | .4 to .49 | .3 to .39 | .2 to .29 | 0b | | | |
| 3 | .3 to .39 | .2 to .29 | .1 to .19 | 1 | | | |
| 4 | .2 to .29 | .1 to .19 | less than .1 | 2 | | | |
| 5 | .1 to .19 | less than .1 | 0 for less than 45° | 3 | | | |
| 6 | less than .1 | 0 for less than 45° | 0 for 46° to 90° | 4 | | | |
| 7 | 0 for less than 45° | 0 for 46° to 90° | 0 for 91° to 180° | 5 | | | |
| 8 | 0 for 46° to 90° | 0 for 91° to 180° | 0 for 181° to 270° | 6 | | | |
| 9 | 0 for 91° to 180° | 0 for 181° to 270° | 0 for more than 270° | 7a | | | |
| 10 | 0 for more than 180° | 0 for more than 270° | | 7b | | | |

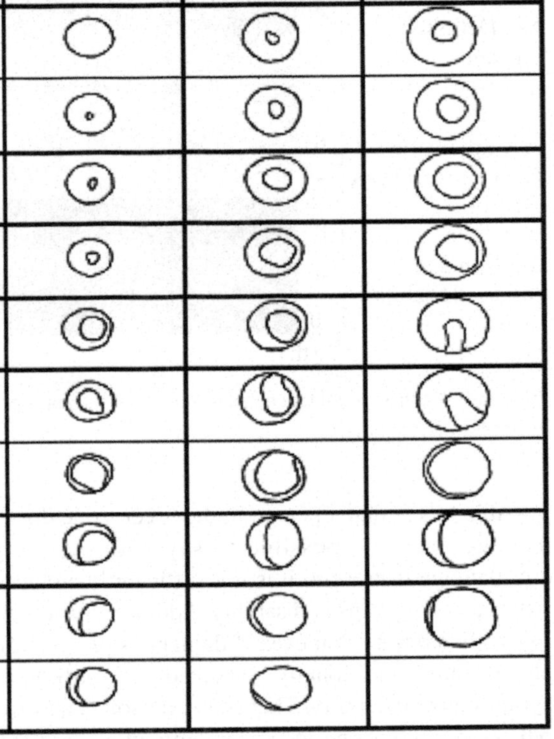

**Fig. 14.5** The Disc Damage Likelihood Scale (DDLS) nomogram.[15,18–23] The *left-hand column* shows the current DDLS score system. The *fifth column* indicates the scores that were part of the first version of the DDLS

probability and certainty, that in many cases the only way to determine whether a patient actually has the glaucomatous process is to document progressive deterioration.

There are many reasons why patients are treated. This is true for patients with glaucoma, as well as for all other conditions. However, there is only one appropriate reason why a person with any condition *should* be treated. That justifiable reason is: "The person will develop a disability or troublesome symptoms or have a worsening of existing disability or symptoms unless effective, adequately safe treatment is provided." This treatment must, of course, be directed toward the condition causing the symptoms or disability. The determination of these justifiable indications for treatment is made by establishing whether the person already has symptoms or disability by taking a careful history or conducting a performance-based test such as Assessment of Function Related to Vision (AFREV)[1,7]; or, if the person is presently asymptomatic and without any disability related to the condition, by establishing a trend based on the rate and duration of change of the condition (Table 14.4, Fig. 14.2). The discussion thus far has dealt primarily with rate of change (item number 1 on Table 14.3). We will now consider the other issues.

**Table 14.4** Factors that must be considered in deciding on the justification to treat

1. The rate of change of the disease in the absence of treatment
2. The stage of the disease
3. The duration that the worsening of the disease will continue
4. The effectiveness of treatment (that is, the rate of change when treated appropriately)
5. The problems caused by the treatment
6. A wide variety of socioeconomic factors

## 14.2 Stage of the Disease

Figure 14.6 shows a graph with three zones that symbolize the early, moderate, and advanced stages of any disease, in this particular instance, glaucoma. The green zone signifies uncertain damage; that is, there are no-definite signs. It is not

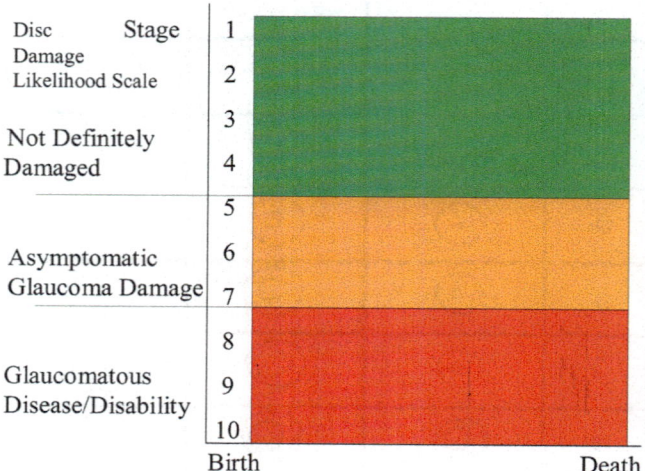

**Fig. 14.6** An instrument that helps to determine the appropriateness of treatment[15,16]

possible to say that a person in the green zone does not have damage, but it is possible to say with certainty that if any damage is present, it is not sufficiently advanced that it will cause symptoms or disability. Additionally, it is possible to say with certainty that even if damage is present, the person can become additionally damaged and still not develop symptoms or disability. That is, the person can move into the buffer or yellow zone. A person without visual field loss but with a higher intraocular pressure in the eye with the more suspicious appearing disc would be in the green zone.

The yellow zone signifies that area in which a person has definite damage, but not enough damage that it has yet caused symptomatology. In the yellow zone, an individual might have a definite nasal step in the visual fields in both eyes, or an unquestionable notch of the optic nerve associated with unilateral paracentral field loss, but either of those persons would have to be completely unaware that there was any limitation whatsoever on their activity. They would not have any disability as determined by history or studied by a performance-based measure such as the Assessment of Function Related to Vision.[1,7]

The red zone signifies that an individual already has symptoms or disability related to the condition under consideration. The best way to determine whether or not a person is in the red zone is to ask. Taking a valid history is a great art, but one that can be learned, and for which there is no substitute. Performance-based measures can quantitate the amount of disability.[1,7]

Within each of these three zones – the green, the yellow, and the red zones – there are subdivisions best quantitated objectively. In the field of glaucoma, probably the ideal units for the $Y$ axis, that is the amount of damage, would be the number of retinal ganglion cells that have died or have become damaged. A suitable surrogate for this is some other quantitative measure of optic nerve damage, such as the Disc Damage Likelihood Scale,[15] or the results of an imaging technique such as Heidelberg retinal tomography (HRT) or optical coherence tomography (OCT). Regarding HRT and OCT, however, at present there is no accepted staging system, and it is unclear as to which units to use. Furthermore, how loss correlates with disability has not been well established.

Visual field assessment is not appropriate to use on the $Y$ axis, because visual field changes occur relatively late in most types of glaucoma, and thus one would not be able to chart the early stages of the disease, which is essential as discussed in the next section. Intraocular pressure is also not appropriate as it is not related in any meaningful way to the stage of a patient's glaucoma.

Assigning a stage of disease to a patient with glaucoma has at least two purposes. In the first place, staging the disease gives the physician a good idea of how much that disease is actually affecting the patient's quality of life and ability to perform the activities of daily living. This certainly applies to patients with glaucoma. Staging also provides an excellent estimate of how likely a person is to get worse. When patients are in the "green zone," that is they have no visual field loss and the reason to suspect the possible presence of glaucoma may be a slightly suspicious disc or an elevated intraocular pressure, the likelihood that they will develop a disability from the glaucoma is probably in the single digits, perhaps as low as around 2%. This estimate is based on a conversion rate from ocular hypertension to glaucoma of around 1% a year, coupled with the belief that a great majority of those developing early visual field loss can be prevented from developing symptomatic damage by the initiation in that early stage of appropriate anti-glaucoma treatment.[25,26] In contrast, patients in the yellow zone have developed sufficient damage that they all have visual field loss, so that they have demonstrated that they have a disease that effectively damages their retinal ganglion cells. Because the nature of most primary glaucomas is to progress, it is appropriate to assume that such damage will be progressive. Although the rate of change and the duration that the change will continue are still important considerations, for patients in the yellow zone it seems prudent to assume that all such cases will get worse unless there is a strong reason to believe that the cause for their glaucoma is no longer active, as would be the case in previous steroid-induced glaucoma or some other types of secondary glaucoma. As such, most patients in the yellow zone need to be treated, unless there is compelling reason not to do so. Once in the red zone, patients are already symptomatic from their glaucoma. Any further deterioration makes all such patients even more symptomatic – that is it makes the patients worse. They have a decrease in their quality of life and/or their ability to perform the activities of daily living. Thus, when patients are in an advanced stage of glaucoma, specifically the red zone, it is appropriate to use treatments that are designed to prevent any further deterioration at all, and, if possible, cause some improvement.[27] As such, treatments of relatively high risk are frequently acceptable in such patients.

## 14.3 Duration

Regarding the duration of disease, the usual appropriate consideration is the number of years the patient is expected to live. Most primary glaucomas last for the duration of a patient's life. There are some self-limited types of glaucoma where this is not the case, such as steroid-induced glaucoma and a few of the secondary glaucomas. "Life expectancy" is a rather confusing term, and for many people connotes the age at which the person is likely to die. However, "number of years remaining" is a more easily understood and direct phrase. The number of years remaining can be quite reliably estimated[28] (Table 14.5). While age is a consideration, it is by no means the most important. Estimates of average life expectancy cannot be meaningfully generalized to individuals. For example, if the average life expectancy of an American female was 77 years, it would not be correct to assume that she would die the following year. In fact, the average number of years remaining for such a 77-year-old woman would be closer to 11 than 0. The range of remaining years for such a 77-year-old woman, of course, would be much greater, from 0 to 30 or more years. In contrast, the expected number of years remaining for a 35-year-old woman with metastatic ovarian cancer is much closer to 2 than the "expected" 42. Consider another example: The likelihood that a 92-year-old healthy woman will live to age 97 is far greater than the likelihood that a 40-year-old, overweight hypertensive man who has already had a heart attack will live to age 45.

When estimating the anticipated number of years a patient still has to live, it is appropriate to take into account the patient's age, but only as one of the factors that needs to be combined with others such as gender, body weight index, history of smoking, significant cardiac or pulmonary disease, family history, age to which parents and siblings lived, patterns of behavior, and lifestyle factors such as use of certain drugs. Because an individual's state of health may change from time to time, so also the anticipated number of years remaining will change from time to time. Thus, fresh estimates of the anticipated years remaining must be made at each encounter when the need to treat is being considered.

## 14.4 Effectiveness and Safety of Treatment

The effectiveness and safety of treatment also play major roles in deciding whether treatment is indicated. For example, with regard to treatment of primary angle-closure in those of European extraction, treatment is close to 100% effective and safe when applied appropriately; in contrast, surgery for neovascular glaucoma is frequently ineffective and often associated with serious complications. The threshold for treatment of anterior chamber angles considered occludable, then, is in a totally different and lower range than the threshold for treatment of neovascular glaucoma, in which the threshold is high. One must also know the relative effectiveness of treatment. For example, primary open-angle glaucoma (POAG) as treated in the Early Manifest Glaucoma Trial Group (EMGTS) was likely to progress (Fig. 14.7),[26] whereas

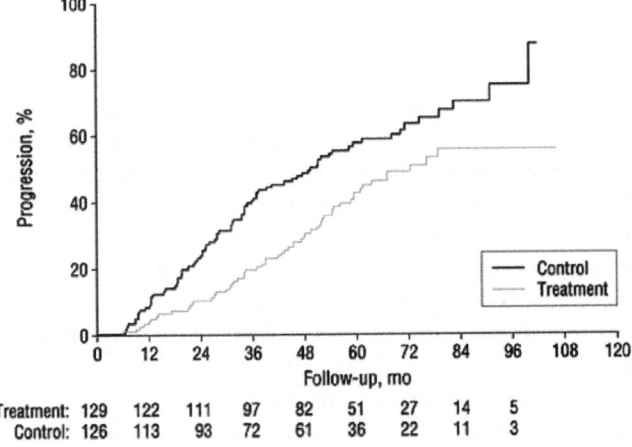

**Fig. 14.7** The rate of development of visual field loss in patients with early manifest glaucoma. The *darker line* represents those who are untreated, and the *lighter line* those who were treated with betaxolol and argon laser trabeculoplasty. Reproduced with permission from Heijl A, Leske C, Bengtsson B, Hyman L, Bengtsson B, Hussein M, Early Manifest Glaucoma Trial Group. Reduction of intraocular pressure and glaucoma progression. *Arch Ophthalmol.* 2002;120:1268-1279.[26] Copyright © 2002 American Medical Association. All rights reserved

**Table 14.5** Expected years of remaining life[28]

| Life expectancy factors | Points for each factor |
|---|---|
| Age | 1 point for every 4 years over 60 |
| Gender | 2 points if male |
| DM | 1 point, BMI: 1 point <25 |
| Cancer | 2 points |
| Heart disease | 2 points |
| Lung disease | 2 points; current smoker 2 points |
| Difficulty bathing | 2 points |
| Managing finances | 2 points |
| Pulling/pushing heavy objects | 1 point |
| Expected 4-year mortality rate | Total points |
| 3% | 0–5 |
| 15% | 6–9 |
| 40% | 10–13 |
| 67% | 14+ |

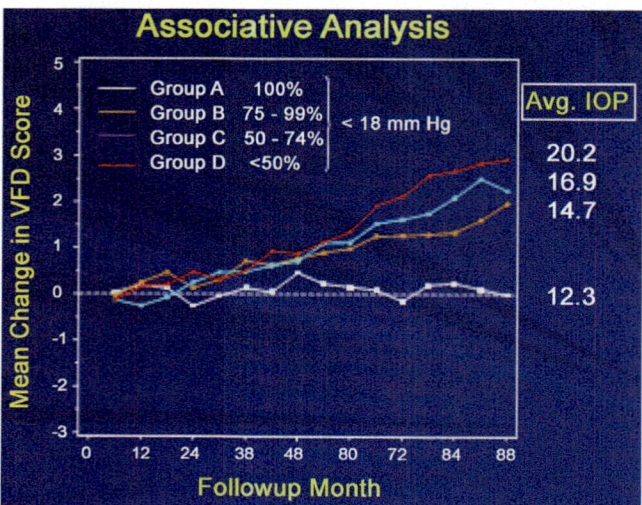

**Fig. 14.8** Graph depicting the rate of deterioration of visual fields in patients in the Advanced Glaucoma Intervention Study. The patients were subdivided according to the control of intraocular pressure, the *top bar* being the subdivision of the least satisfactory control, and the *bottom bar* the group of the most satisfactory control. The average intraocular pressure in the four groups is indicated on the *right*. The units on the *left* are measures of the amount of visual field loss according to the AGIS visual field scoring system, which ranged from 0 to 20. Modified from Ref.[29]

in the Advanced Glaucoma Intervention Study (AGIS) – and the Collaborative Initial Glaucoma Treatment Study (CIGTS) – the course was far more likely to be stable (Fig. 14.8).[28–30]

## 14.5 Socioeconomic Factors

Finally, it is essential that the patient's socioeconomic, cultural, geographical, and sociologic status be meticulously and thoroughly considered and responded to appropriately. For example, a person in good health and with moderate glaucoma who is a poor, self-observant intelligent farmer living in a remote area, who also has a great deal of resourcefulness and has demonstrated an ability to care for himself, may be a suitable candidate for medicinal therapy, whereas his next-door neighbor – another farmer with the same amount of glaucoma, but who has neither the intelligence nor the drive to care for himself well – is far more likely to be a candidate for surgery. These socioeconomic and cultural factors are frequently the most important considerations regarding the need and type of treatment.

This discussion of the proper indications for treatment has stressed, among other things, the importance of determining the rate of change. Obviously to determine this requires more than one point on the graph. Furthermore, the measurements are often not precise. Given such considerations, how can one care for a patient properly? The answer is appropriate knowledgeable individualization, including recognition of the clinical significance associated with waiting and with the possibility that one could be wrong.

There is to date no evidence that the development of early changes of the optic disc or retina in glaucoma predispose the affected person to more rapid development of changes in the future. The occurrence of damage is enormously important, because it signals the fact that damage is likely to continue unless there is some effective change. There are compelling suggestions that eyes with advanced optic nerve damage are more likely to develop further damage than eyes with moderate or early damage.[31] But, there is, to date, no evidence that early damage actually facilitates continuing damage or that it makes treatment less effective.

This discussion leads, however, to an extremely important issue; specifically, "What if I am wrong?" When considering a patient who already is in the red zone, if the physician is wrong about the adequacy of treatment, the patient will become systematically worse. That is, inadequate therapy will be associated with increasing disability. In contrast, if the physician is wrong about what constitutes adequate treatment of a person in the green zone (and certainly patients in the green zone sometimes need treatment) and the person becomes more damaged because the treatment is inadequate, the patient still does not become symptomatic. Thus, the significance of that wrong decision is far greater for a person in the red zone than it is for a person in the green zone.

This discussion, then, is not intended to suggest that any existing algorithm is adequate to apply to individual, specific patients. "Risk calculators"[28–32] can be very rough guidelines, but only that. Such algorithms are not good rules to indicate which patients need to be less vigorously treated or which more vigorously treated. The point I hope to make is quite the opposite. This discussion suggests that treatment be individualized, based on the likelihood that a person will develop some type of symptomatology or disability. It also stresses the need to take into account the patient's socioeconomic, cultural, and personality characteristics. It should be added here that "art of care" factors must also be considered. A person in the green zone who has virtually no likelihood of developing disability if not treated, but who is presently using three different types of medications because her physician told her she needed them all, should not be told that the first physician was wrong or that the treatment is unnecessary. Such a patient could, however, be told that possibly it was not necessary to use all three medications and that it might be possible gradually to wean the patient off medications. At the other end of the spectrum of treatment – serious under-treatment – it is deeply saddening to see patients develop increasing disability because of inadequate treatment, often associated with the physician not listening to the patient, misreading the visual fields, or lacking confidence in his or her surgical ability.

## 14.6 Conclusion

This chapter has dealt broadly with indications for treatment, and also specifically with indications of treatment for patients with glaucoma or suspected glaucoma. The essential point is that the proper outcome must always be kept in mind; specifically, what is most likely to benefit the patient from the point of view of the patient's general health. In order to accomplish this one must take into account the current stage of the disease, the rate of change of the disease in the absence of treatment, the duration that the change in the disease will continue, how effective treatment is, the problems caused by treatment, and a wide variety of socioeconomic issues. Considering all of these, the decision as to whom to treat can be made quite rationally.

## References

1. Altangerel U, Spaeth GL, Steinmann WC. Assessment of function related to vision (AFREV). *Ophthalmic Epidemiol.* 2006;13:67–80.
2. Gutierrez P, Wilson MR, Johnson C, et al. Influence of glaucomatous visual field loss on health-related quality of life. *Arch Ophthalmol.* 1997;115:777–784.
3. West SK, Munoz B, et al. Function and visual impairment in a population-based study of older adults. The SEE project. Salisbury Eye Evaluation. *Invest Ophthalmol Vis Sci.* 1997;38(1):72–82.
4. Freeman EE, Muñoz B, West SK, Jampel HD, Friedman DS. Glaucoma and quality of life: the Salisbury Eye Evaluation. *Ophthalmology.* 2008;115:233–238.
5. Klein BE, Klein R, Lee KE, Cruickshanks KJ. Performance-based and self-assessed measures of visual function as related to history of falls, hip fractures, and measured gait time. The Beaver Dam Eye Study. *Ophthalmology.* 1998;105(1):160–164.
6. Lamoreux EL, Chong E, Wang JJ, et al. Visual impairment, causes of vision loss, and falls: the Singapore Malay Eye Study. *Invest Ophthalmol Vis Sci.* 2008;49:528–533.
7. Lorenzana L, Lankaranian D, Dugar J, et al. A new method of assessing ability to perform activities of daily living: design, methods and baseline data. *Ophthalmic Epidemiol.* 2009;16(2):107–114.
8. Bigger JF. A comparison of patient compliance in treated versus untreated ocular hypertension. *Trans Sect Ophthalmol Am Acad Ophthalmol Otolaryngol.* 1976;81(2):277–285.
9. Nouri-Mahdavi K, Hoffman D, Coleman AL, et al. Predictive factors for glaucomatous visual field progression in the Advanced Glaucoma Intervention Study. *Ophthalmology.* 2004;111:1627–1635.
10. Jonas JB, Martus P, Horn FK, Jünemann A, Korth M, Budde WM. Predictive factors of the optic nerve head for development or progression of glaucomatous visual field loss. *Invest Ophthalmol Vis Sci.* 2004;45(8):2613–2618.
11. Nouri-Mahdavi K, Hoffman D, Gaasterland D, Caprioli J. Prediction of visual field progression in glaucoma. *Invest Ophthalmol Vis Sci.* 2008;49:528–533.
12. Read RM, Spaeth GL. The practical clinical appraisal of the optic disc in glaucoma: the natural history of cup progression and some specific disc-field correlations. *Trans Am Acad Ophthalmol Otolaryngol.* 1974;78:OP255–OP274.
13. Quigley HA, Dunkelberger GR, Green WR. Retinal ganglion cell atrophy correlated with automated perimetry in human eyes with glaucoma. *Am J Ophthalmol.* 1989;107(5):453–464.
14. Chauhan BC, Garway-Heath DF, Goñi FJ, et al. Practical recommendations for measuring rates of visual field change in glaucoma. *Br J Ophthalmol.* 2008;92:569–573.
15. Spaeth GL, Henderer J, Steinmann W. The Disc Damage Likelihood Scale (DDLS): its use in the diagnosis and management of glaucoma. *Highlights Ophthalmol.* 2003;31:4–19.
16. Caprioli J, Garway-Heath DF, International Glaucoma Think Tank. A critical reevaluation of current glaucoma management: International Glaucoma Think Tank. July 27–29, 2006, Taormina, Sicily. *Ophthalmology.* 2007;114(suppl):S1–S41.
17. Fitzke FW, Hitchings RA, Poinoosawmy D, McNaught AI, Crabb DP. Analysis of visual field progression in glaucoma. *Br J Ophthalmol.* 1996;80(1):40–48.
18. Armaly MF. The optic cup in the normal eye. I. Cup width, depth, vessel displacement, ocular tension and outflow facility. *Am J Ophthalmol.* 1969;68(3):401–407.
19. Jonas JB, Stürmer J, Papastathopoulos KI, Meier-Gibbons F, Dichtl A. Optic disc size and optic nerve damage in normal pressure glaucoma. *Br J Ophthalmol.* 1995;79(12):1102–1105.
20. Henderer JD, Liu C, Kesen M, et al. Reliability of the Disk Damage Likelihood Scale. *Am J Ophthalmol.* 2003;135(1):44–48.
21. Bayer A, Harasymowycz P, Henderer JD, Steinmann WG, Spaeth GL. Validity of a new disk grading scale for estimating glaucomatous damage: correlation with visual field damage. *Am J Ophthalmol.* 2002;133(6):758–763.
22. Spaeth GL, Henderer J, Liu C, et al. The Disc Damage Likelihood Scale: reproducibility of a new method of estimating the amount of optic nerve damage caused by glaucoma. *Trans Am Ophthalmol Soc.* 2002;100:181-185. discussion 5–6.
23. Danesh-Meyer H, Ku J, Papchenko T, Jayasundera T, Hsiang J, Gamble G. Regional correlation of structure and function in glaucoma, using the Disc Damage Likelihood Scale, Heidelberg retina tomograph, and visual fields. *Ophthalmology.* 2006;113:603–611.
24. Hornova J, Kuntz Navarro JBV, Prasad A, Freitas DGJ, Nunes CM. Correlation of Disc Damage Likelihood Scale, visual field and Heidelberg retina tomograph II in patients with glaucoma. *Eur J Ophthalmol.* 2008;18:739–747.
25. Kass MA, Heuer DK, Higginbotham EJ, et al. The Ocular Hypertension Treatment Study: a randomized trial determines that topical ocular hypotensive medication delays or prevents the onset of primary open-angle glaucoma. *Arch Ophthalmol.* 2002;120:701–713.
26. Heijl A, Leske C, Bengtsson B, Hyman L, Bengtsson B, Hussein M, Early Manifest Glaucoma Trial Group. Reduction of intraocular pressure and glaucoma progression. *Arch Ophthalmol.* 2002;120:1268–1279.
27. Glaucoma Laser Trial Research Group. The glaucoma laser trial (GLT) and glaucoma laser trial follow-up study: 7. Results. *Am J Ophthalmol.* 1995;120(6):718.31.
28. Lee SJ, Lindquist K, Segal MR, Coninsky KE. Development and validation of a prognostic index for 4-year mortality in older adults. *JAMA.* 2006;295:801–808.
29. AGIS Investigators: Advanced Glaucoma Intervention Study (AGIS): 4. Comparison of treatment outcomes within race: 7 yr results. *Ophthalmology.* 1998;105:1146–1164.
30. Lichter PR, Musch DC, Gillespie BW, et al. CIGTS Study Group: Interim Clinical Outcomes in the Collaborative Initial Glaucoma Treatment Study (CIGTS) comparing initial treatment randomized to medications or surgery. *Ophthalmology.* 2001;108:1943–1953.
31. Grant WM, Burke JF. Why do some people go blind from glaucoma? *Ophthalmology.* 1982;89:991-998.
32. Weinreb RN, Friedman DS, Fechtner RD, et al. Risk assessment in the management of patients with ocular hypertension. *Am J Ophthalmol.* 2004;138(3):458–467.

# Part II
# The Examination

# Part II
## The Examination

# Chapter 15
# Clinical Examination of the Optic Nerve

Scott J. Fudemberg, Yuanjun Zhao, Jonathan S. Myers, and L. Jay Katz

## 15.1 Anatomy

The optic nerve is a confluence of retinal ganglion cell axons that traverse the scleral canal to exit the eye. It ends as these axons merge with axons of the contralateral optic nerve at the optic chiasm. The optic nerve can be divided into (1) the intraocular part, comprising the retinal ganglion cell layer, the retinal nerve fiber layer, and the optic disc, and (2) the retrobulbar part, consisting of the intraorbital portion (about 25 mm long), the intracanalicular part within the osseous optic canal (4–20 mm), and the intracranial portion (about 10 mm), at which point the nerve fibers merge into the optic chiasm and the post-chiasmal optic tracts.[1]

### 15.1.1 Retinal Nerve Fiber Layer

The retinal nerve fiber layer (RNFL) is composed primarily of ganglion cell axons, astrocytes, retinal vessels, and Müller cell processes. Astrocytes and Müller cells surround the nerve fibers and add a structural framework that supports the neural elements. The Müller cells occupy a significant portion of the retinal space and form the inner limiting membrane, which covers the nerve fiber layer on its vitreal surface. Astrocyte processes envelop all nerve fibers and add nutritional as well as structural support. In combination with pericytes, the astrocytes cover retinal capillaries, isolating the retinal ganglion cells and their axons from the retinal blood flow. The ganglion cell axons extend from their cell body toward the optic disc. Axons of ganglion cells in the temporal fundus stream in an arcuate course around the fovea. At the fovea, different axons separate into a superior temporal and an inferior temporal bundle, touching each other at the temporal raphe that extends from the foveola to the temporal periphery of the retina. In general, the thickness of the nerve fiber layer increases from the fundus periphery to the optic disc. However, regional differences do exist. For example, the nerve fiber layer surrounding the optic disc is thicker at the vertical poles and thinner at the temporal and nasal poles of the disc.

### 15.1.2 Optic Disc

Retinal ganglion cell axons leave the eye through the posterior scleral foramen, which forms a truncated cone with a narrow neck internally and a broad base externally.[1] The narrow internal neck of this cone is clinically visualized as the optic disc. The scleral ring surrounding the optic nerve is termed the *peripapillary ring of Elschnig*.

### 15.1.3 Intralaminar Part of the Optic Nerve

In this portion, the lamina cribrosa divides the optic nerve head into prelaminar, laminar, and postlaminar portions. The neuroretinal rim consists of bundles of axons that pass from the nerve fiber layer, making a right-angled turn into the scleral canal. Extensions from the inner one-third of adjacent sclera over the posterior scleral foramen create a sieve-like network of tunnels or pores through which the ganglion cell axon bundles pass. The human lamina cribrosa contains about 500–600 of these pores.[2] Rather than cross the posterior scleral foramen, fibers of the outer two-thirds of the sclera turn at right angles to blend with the fibers of the dura, which covers the optic nerve.

Just behind the globe, the posterior ciliary arteries (branches of the ophthalmic artery) penetrate the sclera in a circumferential fashion around the optic nerve. At the level of the choroid, these vessels form an incomplete anastomotic ring called the circle of Zinn–Haller, supplying blood to the choroidal circulation and optic nerve head. Additionally, the central retinal artery passes through the innermost area of the optic nerve head and contributes to the optic nerve's blood supply.

## 15.1.4 Retrobulbar Optic Nerve

Myelin, supplied by oligodendrocytes, forms a sheath around the retinal ganglion cell axons as they emerge from the lamina cribrosa. At this junction, the posterior lamina blends into the connective tissue, or septae, of the retrolaminar optic nerve, and runs parallel to the nerve fiber bundles. The retrobulbar optic nerve is covered by the pia, arachnoid, and dura mater. The dura fuses with the sclera anteriorly and with the periosteum at the sphenoid bone posteriorly. Arachnoid and pia fuse with the dura at the sclera and are continuous with the meninges of the brain at the optic canal.

The intracanalicular portion of the optic nerve measures roughly 10 mm from the entrance of the optic foramen, in the lesser wing of the sphenoid, to the intracranial cavity. The optic canal itself extends medially and superiorly before entering the intracranial cavity and is separated from the sphenoid sinus by a thin wall of bone. The vascular supply of the intraorbital optic nerve is more robust than that of the optic nerve head. Branches of the ophthalmic artery serve numerous longitudinal pial vessels on the surface of the optic nerve, which in turn yield penetrating vessels that extend toward the center of the nerve. The central retinal artery enters the nerve about 10 mm behind the globe, also contributing to the vascular supply of the proximal intraorbital optic nerve. Medial and lateral paraoptic short posterior ciliary arteries anastomose to form an elliptical arterial circle around the optic nerve, and to supply the retrolaminar optic nerve.

## 15.1.5 The Normal Optic Disc

The normal optic disc is round or oval and pink in color. Its diameter varies in size from 0.95 to 2.9 mm, with the average dimensions being 1.9 mm vertically and 1.7 mm horizontally.[3,4] Typically, it is flat or mildly elevated on the periphery, which is called the neuroretinal rim, with a central depression called the cup.

Five basic rules have been proposed ("the 5 Rs")[5] for the assessment of a normal optic disc:

1. Observe the scleral *R*ing to identify the limits of the optic disc and its size.
2. Identify the size of the *R*im.
3. Examine the *R*etinal nerve fiber layer.
4. Examine the *R*egion outside the disc for parapapillary atrophy.
5. Watch for *R*etinal and optic disc hemorrhage.

In the normal eye, the width of neuroretinal rim tissue varies by quadrant and normally follows the ISNT rule, which was originally described by Jonas et al[6] They calculated rim thickness measurements of normal eyes using optic disc photographs. The rim thickness of a healthy optic disc generally varies by sector with the Inferior (I) typically being thickest, followed by the Superior (S), Nasal (N), and Temporal (T) regions. Likewise, the parapapillary retinal nerve fiber layer is thickest superiorly and inferiorly. The optic cup of a healthy optic disc that follows the ISNT rule typically appears as a horizontal oval. Loss of neuroretinal rim in glaucoma most often starts at the inferior and superior poles, so violation of the ISNT rule is a clue to glaucomatous optic neuropathy. However, it should be noted that 20% or more of normal eyes may not follow the ISNT rule, and that 25% of glaucomatous eyes may follow the ISNT rule.[7]

## 15.2 Examining the Optic Disc and Surrounding Area

Evaluation of the optic disc is central to the diagnosis and management of glaucoma. Data about the optic disc is collected by visualization as well as measurement of disc characteristics by instrumentation. A variety of techniques are used to gather detailed information during clinical examination of the optic nerve, including direct and indirect ophthalmoscopy, stereoscopic fundus photography, and imaging of the optic disc and RNFL.

### 15.2.1 Direct Ophthalmoscopy

The direct ophthalmoscope yields a real, upright image of the optic disc. Assuming an emmetropic model eye with a refracting power of +60 D, the magnification of a direct ophthalmoscope is 15×. The highly magnified view through a direct ophthalmoscope may be essential for delineating subtle changes in the neuroretinal rim and/or areas of rim loss in advanced disc damage. The direct ophthalmoscope is also useful for easy estimation of disc size. The commonly used Welch–Allyn direct ophthalmoscope (on the middle aperture size setting) illuminates a cone angle of 5°, and projects a circle of light with a diameter of 1.5 mm and an area of 1.8 mm on the retina when it is held in the usual range.[8] The spot may be aligned over or adjacent to the optic disc, and then the size of the optic disc is compared to the size of the spot of light. If the optic nerve head is smaller than the spot of light, the disc can be estimated as small. If the optic nerve head is more than 1.5 times the size of the light spot, the optic disc is large.

The direct ophthalmoscope is a monocular tool and, therefore, limited by its inability to provide any stereopsis. Also, it has a small field of view, so patient cooperation and dilation are important to performing a successful exam. It is uniquely useful for following individual vessels as they radiate from the optic nerve, to look for emboli and vascular changes associated with hypertension.

## 15.2.2 Indirect Ophthalmoscopy

Indirect ophthalmoscopy may be performed with a binocular headset or a slit-lamp biomicroscope. This technique provides a magnified, stereoscopic view of the optic nerve. Contact and non-contact lenses are used to focus a virtual image of the optic disc. The Goldmann three-mirror lens is a contact lens that yields an erect, virtual image of the optic disc. Although the Goldmann lens itself provides little magnification, 16× magnification and greater may be achieved using the slit-lamp optical systems.[9] Coupling solution, with the Goldmann lens, and corneal contact are necessary to resolve an image. Thus, this lens may be somewhat uncomfortable for the patient and inconvenient for the examiner. After using the lens, further examination may be limited by disruption of the corneal epithelium from contact lenses and viscous coupling agents. The Hruby lens is a non-contact plano-concave lens (−55 D) that is available as an attachment to most slit lamps. It produces an erect, virtual image of the optic disc. In addition to having the advantage of being non-contact, it leaves the examiner's hands free and facilitates disc drawing during biomicroscopy. However, using this lens is a challenge because it provides only a small field of view. Biconvex high power aspheric lenses (+60–90 D) are non-contact lenses that produce an inverted, virtual image of the optic disc. They are relatively easy to use and provide a larger field of view than the Hruby lens. They have become the lenses of choice, used by most ophthalmologists when examining the optic nerve head, with the 78 D version and 90 D versions being the most common. Magnification of the biconvex aspheric lenses is calculated by multiplying the magnification of the lens by that of the slit lamp. For example, transverse magnification of the aerial image is the ratio of the power of the patient's eye to that of the condensing lens. For an emmetropic model eye of power +60 D, the transverse magnification of a +90 D lens is about 0.667×. The low magnification setting on a typical Haag-Streit slit lamp is 10×, so the total magnification of disc imaged with a +90 D lens using low magnification on the slit lamp is about 6.67×. The Biconvex aspheric lenses may be used to measure the optic disc diameter. The slit lamp beam is adjusted to a trapezoid of light in which the vertical and horizontal borders are dialed to the largest vertical and horizontal diameter of the optic disc respectively. The size of the vertical disc diameter is read in millimeters from the aperture height scale on the slit lamp . Correction factors for lenses to account for the influence of magnification on the measured disc diameter are available. The correction factor should be multiplied by the measured aperture height value to determine the disc diameter.

For example, a +90 D lens carries a correction factor of about 1.3. Using a +90 D lens, a measured disc diameter of 1.5 mm would yield a corrected disc size of 1.95 mm. A +66 D lens carries a correction factor of 1, so measurements on the slit lamp scale should correspond directly with the size of the disc diameter for this lens. One disadvantage of biconvex aspheric lenses is the inverted nature of their image, which is less convenient for the examiner. This is similar to the view provided by binocular indirect ophthalmoscopy.

Importantly, all comments about magnification using the different types of lenses are based on assumptions that do not completely hold true in clinical use. Likewise, correction factors provided by lens manufacturers are based on assumptions that do not completely apply in clinical practice. Although these numbers are good estimates, they should not be taken as absolutely correct.

## 15.2.3 Optic Disc Photography

Capturing an image of the optic disc with a fundus camera yields an objective record of the optic disc appearance. However, interpretation of photographs is subjective. Also, photographs are subject to variations in technique and quality. Traditionally, fundus cameras required dilation, and images were recorded on film. Now, non-mydriatic and digital fundus cameras are available. A stereoscopic camera produces two slightly dissimilar images by photographing the optic disc from two different angles. When the two photographs are viewed simultaneously through a stereoscopic viewer, the image appears 3-dimensional.

## 15.2.4 Retinal Nerve Fiber Layer Examination

Retinal ganglion cell axons make up the RNFL and the optic nerve. RNFL loss has been shown to precede glaucomatous visual field loss in patients with elevated intraocular pressure.[10] Therefore, examination of the RNFL may play an important role in the diagnosis and management of glaucoma and should be part of an optic disc examination. In a healthy eye, the RNFL appears slightly opaque with radially oriented striations, which have been likened to "horsehair."[11] Fibers of RNFL follow an arcuate pattern above and below the macula and are typically brighter along the superior and inferior arcuate bundles than the nasal and temporal bundles.[11] Although defects in the RNFL may be visualized ophthalmoscopically with white light, applying the red-free filter (green appearing light) may enhance contrast and facilitate their identification. Photography of the RNFL follows the same principle. The use of high contrast film and a red-free filter improves the diagnostic yield.

## 15.2.5 Retinal Nerve Fiber Layer and Optic Disc Analyzers

Three main techniques are currently used for computerized optic nerve and retinal nerve fiber layer analysis. First, confocal scanning laser ophthalmoscopy (Heidelberg Retina Tomograph (HRT); Heidelberg Engineering, Heidelberg, Germany) generates up to 64 transaxial laser scans through the optic nerve head and peripapillary retina to reconstruct a high resolution 3-dimensional image.[12] Second, scanning laser polarimetry (GDxVCC; Carl Zeiss Meditec, Dublin, CA, USA) measures peripapillary RNFL thickness by sending a laser beam to the posterior retina and assessing changes in the polarization of the reflected beam.[12] Third, optical coherence tomography (OCT; Carl Zeiss Meditec, Dublin, CA, USA) is an axial cross-section of tissues based on the optical backscattering of low-coherence laser light (850 nm) as it passes through layers of different optical density.[12] Recent improvements in OCT technology called Fourier-domain OCT yield up to five times higher resolution with 60 times faster imaging speed than conventional time-domain OCT.[13]

In 2007, the American Academy of Ophthalmology published an Ophthalmic Technology Assessment that evaluated the literature on optic disc and RNFL analyzers. Based on evidence published from 2003 to 2006, the group concluded that these devices provide quantitative information as a complement to optic nerve and RNFL examination as well as other tests for glaucoma. Comparison of the studies was limited by differences in patient populations, definitions of glaucoma, and algorithms for detection. No single device was superior in distinguishing glaucoma patients from controls. Few studies addressed detection of glaucoma progression. All three machines were determined to be useful adjuncts in glaucoma care, with emphasis on familiarization with the device and placing the results in an appropriate perspective within the clinical context.[12] These technologies are constantly being updated, with respect to both hardware and software. It is expected that as digital imaging analyzers continue to improve, they may become the standard of care for optic nerve and RNFL examinations over the next decade.

## 15.3 Evaluating and Monitoring the Optic Disc

Practical application of information about the optic disc requires an accurate, precise, and reproducible way to document and follow its appearance. Characteristics of optic disc appearance from a clinical examination are recorded using drawings and disc photographs. Optic disc and RNFL digital image analyzers create printouts that may be compared over time.

Disc drawing is a quick, inexpensive, and valid method of following the optic nerve in patients with glaucoma. However, intraobserver and interobserver variability may limit the accuracy and precision of this method. Also, drawings of the optic disc based on examination through an undilated pupil often sacrifice detail and may be misleading. Regular drawings of the optic nerve based on findings of a dilated examination are important therefore in following patients by disc drawings. Several features of the optic nerve are systematically examined to formulate a composite picture of the optic nerve: (1) the shape of the outer margin of the optic disc, (2) the width of the neuroretinal rim as well as its color and shape, (3) the depth and dimension of the cup, (4) the peripapillary area, and (5) comparison of the discs between the two eyes. The optic nerve is typically drawn by sketching the cup as an inner circle within a larger circle representing the outer edge of the disc. The margins of both the outer edges of the disc may be difficult to discern, especially in cases with peripapillary atrophy. Also, the width of the neuroretinal rim may be unclear in cases of advanced rim loss and sloping (gradual incline) of the optic disc cup. Sloping may be represented by hash marks perpendicular to the drawn border of the neuroretinal rim or by multiple concentric lines of decreasing circumference. The relatively high magnification afforded by a direct ophthalmoscope may be helpful in identifying details of the optic nerve. Disc blood vessels may be good indicators of the border of the cup because they often travel along the superficial tissue of the optic disc. Therefore, blood vessels change direction at points of significant change in the contour of the optic disc cup. For example, at the juncture of the base of the optic disc cup and the face of its peripheral wall, blood vessels often bend abruptly. In addition, blood vessels bend sharply as they crest the wall of the optic disc cup, which is often a reliable marker of the neuroretinal rim margin. The cup is determined entirely by contour, and not by color. However, the color of the neuroretinal rim may be used to determine important information about the health of the optic nerve. The neuroretinal rim is supplied by a rich network of small blood vessels that give it an orange and/or pink color (Fig. 15.1). Loss of healthy neuroretinal rim, with its orange/pink color, and enlargement of optic disc cup make the optic disc look paler overall. However, an intact but pale neuroretinal rim indicates greater likelihood of non-glaucomatous optic neuropathy.[14]

There are different systems to classify the optic nerve appearance in a standardized manner. Armaly first mentioned the cup-to-disc ratio as a method of optic nerve head classification in 1969.[15] After recognizing the margin of the disc and cup, the optic nerve is divided into tenths, and the cup is compared to the entire optic disc to obtain the cup-to-disc ratio, vertically and horizontally. Loss of the neuroretinal rim

# 15 Clinical Examination of the Optic Nerve

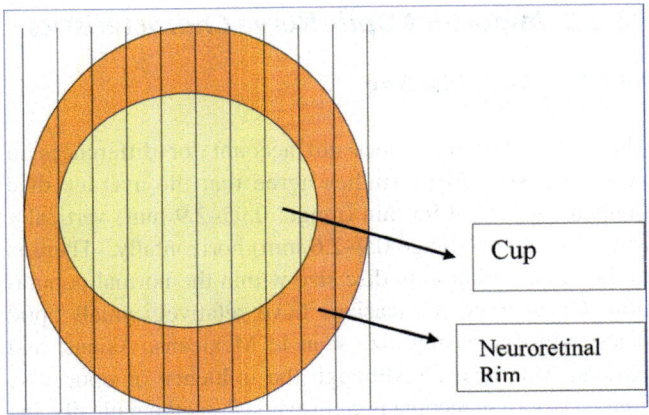

**Fig. 15.1** Neuroretinal ring

one contains loss of the neuroretinal rim, such as a notch, and one does not (see Fig. 15.2).

Since the cup-to-disc ratio may not reflect the true rim loss if there is a localized notch, the Disc Damage Likelihood Scale (DDLS) was designed in an attempt to provide a more accurate and reproducible method of defining glaucomatous optic nerve damage.[10,18] Briefly, the scale is based on the appearance of the neuroretinal rim of the optic disc, corrected for the disc diameter; gradations in the scale depend on the degree of rim loss rather than enlargement of the optic disc cup. Essentially, the examiner determines the smallest rim-to-disc ratio in any area of the nerve; the extent, if any, of circumference with no rim; and the size of the optic nerve. The DDLS has ten stages, ranging from no damage to far-advanced damage.

with a corresponding increase in cupping, results in an increase in the cup/disc ratio. Because the optic disc is vertically oval and the optic cup is horizontally oval, the cup-to-disc ratios in normal eyes are larger horizontally than vertically. Less than 10% of normal eyes have a smaller horizontal cup-disc ratio than their vertical cup-disc ratio.[14,16] In early and moderate stages of glaucoma, rim loss typically occurs at the superior and inferior poles of the disc first. Thus, enlargement of the vertical cup-to-disc ratio rapidly overtakes enlargement of the horizontal cup-to-disc ratio.[14]

Cup-to-disc ratios greater than 0.6 or cup-to-disc asymmetry greater than 0.2 between fellow eyes are suggestive of glaucoma.[17] However, interpretation of optic disc appearance depends on factors not specified in the cup-to-disc system. Notching of the neuroretinal rim, optic disc pits, intraretinal hemorrhage crossing the rim of the optic disc, rim loss, and localized pallor may all be signs of glaucomatous optic neuropathy. None of these signs are included in the cup-to-disc classification system. For example, two different optic discs may accurately be rated a 0.5 cup-to-disc ratio, though

### 15.3.1 Determining the DDLS: Step by Step

*Step 1.* Perform dilation, if necessary. The pupils must be sufficiently enlarged to allow a clear view of the fundus.

*Step 2.* Obtain a measurement of the vertical size of the patient's optic nerve via a slit lamp biomicroscope that indicates the size in millimeters. Multiply this figure by 0.9 for a +60 D lens, by 1 for a +66 D, or by 1.3 for a +90 D lens.

*Step 3.* Examine the optic disc for an area where its outer edge is clearly distinguished from other ocular tissue such as sclera, and determine the full circumference of the outer edge.

*Step 4.* Define the inside edge of the neuroretinal rim (outer edge of the cup). To obtain an estimate of the rim-to-disc ratio, compare the width of the neuroretinal rim with that of the disc diameter on the same axis. Repeat this comparison using several clock positions. If the rim-to-disc ratio is different at various parts of the rim, find the narrowest section of the rim and calculate the rim-to-disc ratio at that point.

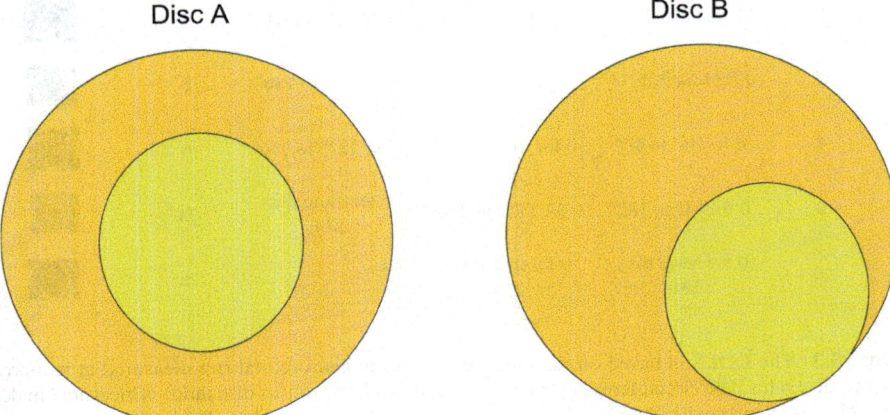

**Fig. 15.2** Two optic nerves with cup-to-disc ratio of 0.5 – Disc B has a notch with neuroretinal rim loss inferior temporally while Disc A does not

*Step 5.* Draw the shape of the optic disc. When sketching the neuroretinal rim's inner edge, indicate areas of clear demarcation by drawing a thick line and those of less clear demarcation with thin or hatched lines. Make a note of the course of the blood vessels that help determine the rim's width and any pertinent features of the disc, such as notches, pallor, hemorrhage, etc.

*Step 6.* To determine the DDLS, use your disc drawing, the narrowest rim-to-disc ratio, the disc size, and compare to the DDLS nomogram (Fig. 15.3). If the nerve is smaller or larger than average, adjust the DDLS score appropriately. An easy adjustment method is to stage the nerve as if it were of average size, and then increase the stage by one if the nerve is small or decrease the stage by one if it is large.

DDLS scores of 1–3 are rarely associated with glaucomatous visual field loss. However, any disc graded stage 5 or higher will almost always be pathologic, although it may not be glaucomatous.

For Caucasians without high myopia, mean optic disc area can range from 2.1 mm$^2$ to about 2.8 mm$^2$ in different studies. In healthy subjects, the size range for a normal optic nerve head is between 1.3 and 2.7 mm in diameter, with 1.9 mm considered to be average.

### 15.3.2 Important Optic Nerve Characteristics

#### 15.3.2.1 Optic Disc Size

The cup-to-disc ratio does not account for differences in optic disc size. Most studies agree that the average disc diameter is 1.85–1.95 mm (range: 0.95–2.9 mm) vertically and 1.7–1.8 mm (range 0.9–2.6 mm) horizontally.[2] There is tremendous variation in disc size within the normal population. On average, Caucasians have relatively small optic discs, with increasing size seen in Mexicans, Asians, and African-Americans.[19] Although the influence of optic disc area on risk of glaucoma is controversial, mathematically, the larger the optic disc area, the larger the neuroretinal rim area, despite a consistent cup-to-disc ratio. Conversely, smaller optic disc area confers smaller neuroretinal rim area despite consistent cup-to-disc ratio. This seems to indicate that vision loss from glaucoma in large optic nerves would require more rim loss than in small optic nerves. Also, large optic nerves have a larger cup volume than small optic nerves despite proportional cup-to-disc ratios. This characteristic draws attention and sometimes predisposes physiologically cupped large optic nerves to an erroneous diagnosis of glaucoma.

| DDLS Stage | Narrowest width of rim (rim/disc ratio) | | | DDLS Stage | Examples | | |
|---|---|---|---|---|---|---|---|
| | For Small Disc <1.50 mm | For Average Size Disc 1.50–2.00 mm | For Large Disc >2.00 mm | | 1.25 mm optic nerve | 1.75 mm optic nerve | 2.25 mm optic nerve |
| 1 | .5 or more | .4 or more | .3 or more | 0a | | | |
| 2 | .4 to .49 | .3 to .39 | .2 to .29 | 0b | | | |
| 3 | .3 to .39 | .2 to .29 | .1 to .19 | 1 | | | |
| 4 | .2 to .29 | .1 to .19 | less than .1 | 2 | | | |
| 5 | .1 to .19 | less than .1 | 0 for less than 45° | 3 | | | |
| 6 | less than .1 | 0 for less than 45° | 0 for 46° to 90° | 4 | | | |
| 7 | 0 for less than 45° | 0 for 46° to 90° | 0 for 91° to 180° | 5 | | | |
| 8 | 0 for 46° to 90° | 0 for 91° to 180° | 0 for 181° to 270° | 6 | | | |
| 9 | 0 for 91° to 180° | 0 for 181° to 270° | 0 for more than 270° | 7a | | | |
| 10 | 0 for more than 180° | 0 for more than 270° | | 7b | | | |

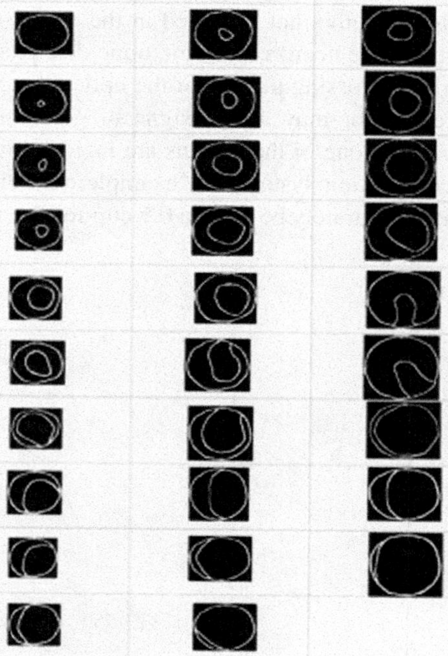

**Fig. 15.3** The DDLS is based on the radial width of the neuroretinal rim measured at its narrowest point. The unit of measurement is the rim-to-disc ratio. The circumferential extent of absent rim (zero rim-to-disc ratio) is measured in degrees. Reprinted with permission from Spaeth GL. The disc damage likelihood scale. *Glaucoma Today.* 2005; Bryn Mawr Publishing

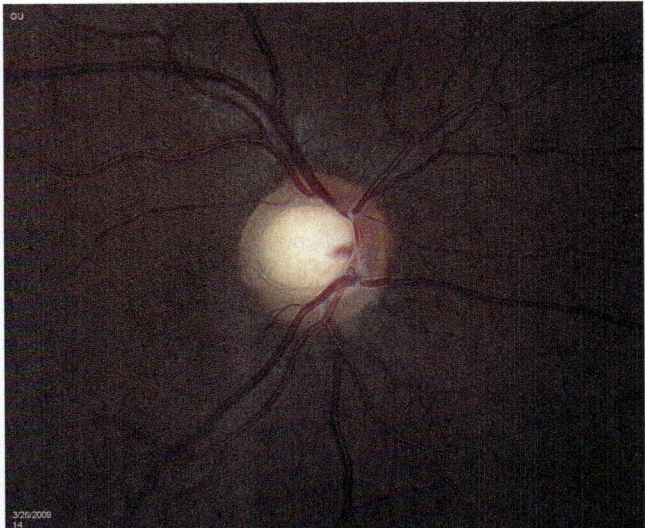

**Fig. 15.4** Glaucomatous optic neuropathy with intact but thin neuroretinal rim

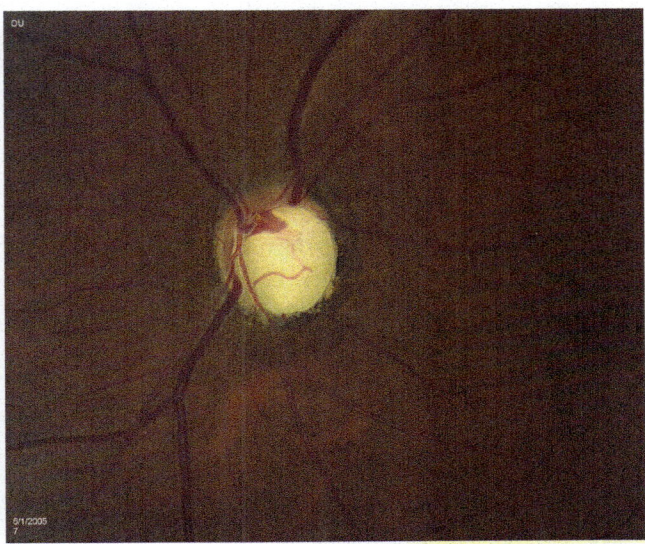

**Fig. 15.5** Glaucomatous optic neuropathy with significant neuroretinal rim loss

The converse may also be true. Small optic nerves with proportionately small cups may be underappreciated. Finally, optic disc size is correlated with refractive error. Eyes with greater than 8 D of myopia have increasing optic disc area and those with more than 4 D of hyperopia have decreasing disc area. Between −8 and +4 D of refractive error, optic disc size varies independent of refractive error.[20]

### 15.3.2.2 Neuroretinal Rim Size and Shape

The neuroretinal rim width is the distance between the borders of the optic disc delimited by the scleral ring and the inner edge of the rim as it turns posteriorly to create the cup. Neuroretinal rim loss is critically important because it correlates well with loss of visual function.[21] Also, loss of the neuroretinal rim is helpful in separating glaucoma patients from normals as well as ocular hypertensives.[21,22] The wide range in size of the optic disc cup in normal populations may make cupping less valuable for diagnosis of glaucoma than neuroretinal rim loss.[19] Particularly in patients with focal neuroretinal rim loss, the location of the visual field defect should easily correspond to the location of rim loss. For example, given the arcuate nature of RNFL axon bundles as they stream to the vertical poles of the optic disc, loss of superior and inferior neuroretinal rim will match an inferior or superior arcuate visual field defect respectively. When focal neuroretinal rim loss adopts a crescent-shaped configuration, it may be termed a notch. Typically, notches are circular or oval in appearance, but with a steeper curvature than the larger internal edge of the neuroretinal rim[1] (Figs. 15.4 and 15.5).

### 15.3.2.3 Neuroretinal Rim Pallor

Pallor of the neuroretinal rim increases the likelihood that a non-glaucomatous optic neuropathy is present, especially when the pallor is more prominent than the cupping.[18] In 1980, Trobe et al published a study in which three experienced ophthalmologists evaluated stereoscopic optic disc photographs of "unknowns" with glaucomatous and non-glaucomatous optic neuropathy. They found that neuroretinal rim pallor was 94% specific for non-glaucomatous atrophy, while focal or diffuse obliteration of the neuroretinal rim was 87% specific for glaucoma. Thinning of the rim was more common in glaucoma than in non-glaucomatous damage, but was only 47% specific for glaucoma.[23] Therefore, both neuroretinal rim pallor and neuroretinal rim thinning should be placed into perspective with other findings when separating non-glaucomatous from glaucomatous optic neuropathy.

### 15.3.2.4 Disc Asymmetry

Asymmetry of optic disc cupping between fellow eyes may be an indicator of unilateral glaucoma, asymmetric but bilateral glaucoma, or non-glaucomatous optic neuropathy.

In general, the cup-to-disc ratio in a normal subject will not differ between fellow eyes by more than 0.2.[24] However, data regarding disc size, cup-to-disc ratio, and degree of asymmetry is varied among published glaucoma surveys in different populations.

#### 15.3.2.5 Optic Disc Hemorrhages

Retinal nerve fiber layer hemorrhages at the disc margin have been associated with increased risk of glaucoma progression, especially in average pressure glaucoma.[25] Disc hemorrhages are detected in about 4–7% of eyes with glaucoma.[26] Usually, they extend from the disc tissue across the disc margin. They may overlie an adjacent peripapillary zone of choroidal or retinal pigment epithelium atrophy, but have at least one end touching the disc margin. Disc hemorrhages may be small and located near blood vessels, making detection difficult. They typically occur in areas of localized RNFL defects and notches of the neuroretinal rim.[14] Reports indicate that disc hemorrhages rarely occur in conditions other than glaucoma. Therefore, although they are poorly sensitive, disc hemorrhages are highly specific for glaucoma.[14] Generally, hemorrhages are transient and visible only for days to months, but they may recur. Concurrent retinal changes may help make non-glaucomatous etiology of disc hemorrhage obvious. Diabetic retinopathy, retinal vein occlusion, and papillitis may occur with disc hemorrhage. Acute posterior vitreous detachment may cause disc hemorrhage as well (Fig. 15.6).

#### 15.3.2.6 Peripapillary Chorioretinal Atrophy

Peripapillary atrophy (PPA) refers to the thinning, misalignment, irregularity, and degeneration of the retinal pigment epithelium, choriocapillaris, choroid, and sclera just outside of the optic disc. PPA has an association with the development and progression of glaucoma.[18] Among ocular hypertensives, studies have shown that 50–75% of patients who converted to glaucoma also experienced progression of peripapillary atrophy. Among those patients who did not develop glaucoma, 10–14% experienced progressive PPA.[27,28] PPA may also be a congenital anomaly in which the neurosensory retina terminates short of the optic disc.[1] Ophthalmoscopically, the regions of peripapillary chorioretinal atrophy may be divided into a peripheral zone (alpha zone) and a central zone (beta zone).[14] Bordered by retina peripherally and sclera centrally, zone alpha is characterized by irregular hyper- and hypopigmentation indicative of chorioretinal thinning. Choroidal vessels and sclera may be clearly visible in zone alpha. Zone beta is marked by significant atrophy of the retinal pigment epithelium and choriocapillaris, with more clear visibility of the choroidal vessels and sclera than in the alpha zone. If both alpha and beta zones are present, the beta zone is always closer to the optic disc than the alpha zone.[14] Some authors suggest that disc damage is more likely in areas adjacent to PPA. However, PPA occurs to a variable degree in normal eyes and may not be directly related to glaucoma[29] (Fig. 15.7, Sidebar 15.1).

### 15.4 Other Structural Changes

#### 15.4.1 Blood Vessel Changes

Retinal vessels that emerge from the optic nerve may undergo changes in their appearance with progressive glaucomatous damage. In areas of neuroretinal rim loss, blood vessels that once rested on the rim may bridge a part of the cup. This phenomenon is called "overpass." "Baring" of a vessel is when space or pallor exists between the inner cup

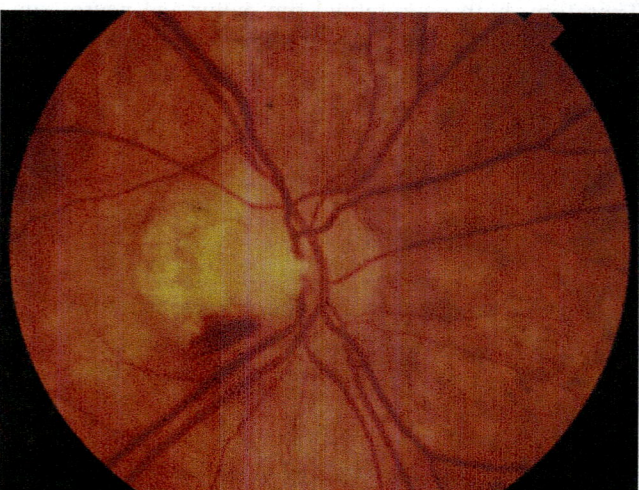

**Fig. 15.6** Nerve fiber layer hemorrhage along inferior temporal optic disc margin

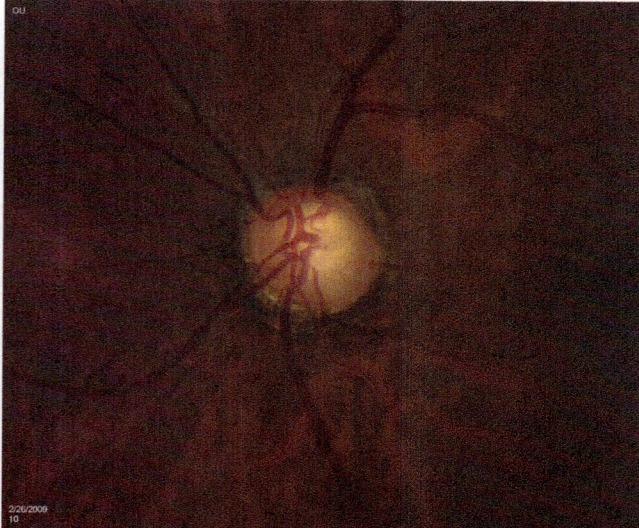

**Fig. 15.7** Glaucomatous optic neuropathy and peripapillary chrioretinal atrophy

### Sidebar 15.1 Alpha–beta peripapillary atrophy

S. Fabian Lerner

Observation and documentation of the peripapillary atrophy (PPA) is part of the fundus examination in patients with glaucoma. PPA can be divided into an alpha and a beta zone. Alpha zone is used to describe an area with both hypo- and hyper-pigmentation; beta zone is characterized by atrophy of the retinal pigment epithelium and the choriocapillaris, with visible sclera and large choroidal vessels. If both zones are present, beta zone is central to alpha zone: beta is between the optic nerve and the alpha zone (Fig. 15.1-1).

The presence of these zones is not pathognomonic of glaucoma. The alpha zone may be common in normal eyes, while the beta zone may be present in up to 20% of normal eyes. However, both zones are larger and more common in patients with glaucoma than in normal subjects. PPA is larger next to the area of the nerve that is more damaged. It is also largest in the more distant area close to the exit of the central vessel trunk through the lamina cribrosa. In visual field exams, the alpha zone corresponds to a relative scotomas, while the beta zone correlates with an absolute scotoma.

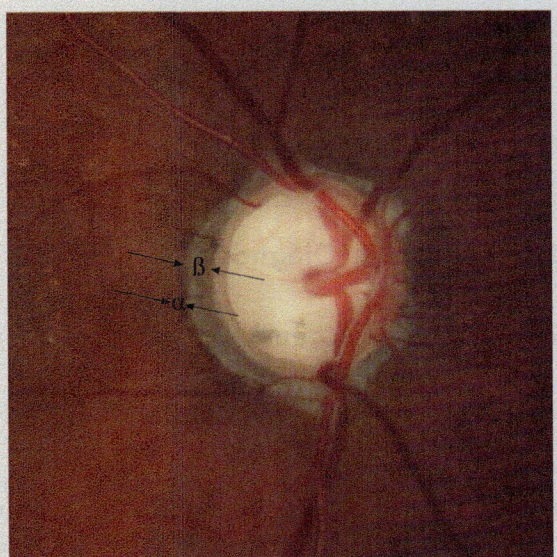

**Fig. 15.1-1** Alpha and beta zone peripapillary atrophy of the optic disc. Courtesy of Dr. Matthew kay, Golden Beach, FL

This concept should be kept in mind when examining a patient, because a correlation between function and structure should include not only the nerve and the RNFL but the PPA as well when comparing with visual field abnormalities.

The size of the beta zone was reported to vary among different glaucoma diagnoses. Using optic disc photographs and a morphometrical analysis, Jonas et al reported that the beta zone was larger in sclerotic primary open-angle glaucoma (POAG), followed by exfoliation glaucoma, "ordinary" POAG, focal normal pressure glaucoma, and juvenile glaucoma.

The presence of PPA may be a risk factor for a disc hemorrhage in patients with glaucoma. Law et al investigated the optic nerve features that had more probabilities to antedate the appearance of an optic disc hemorrhage. PPA was the most frequent attribute (79%) to antedate a hemorrhage. Ahn et al reported PPA as an independent risk factor for a hemorrhage in a multivariate analysis. So, in patients with PPA, one must be alert to the appearance of an optic disc hemorrhage.

Jonas et al described the sizes of alpha and beta zones of PPA as less useful parameters to differentiate between normal subjects and individuals with pre-perimetric glaucoma. PPA was therefore considered a second order parameter for early detection of glaucoma. Interestingly, in a retrospective study of ocular hypertension patients who have been carefully followed-up, the progression of PPA during the ocular hypertension period corresponded with the location and extension of visual field defects that developed late.

PPA is considered to be stable in non-glaucomatous optic neuropathies, such as in anterior ischemic optic neuropathy or in optic neuritis. In glaucomatous eyes, PPA zone beta was discovered to increase, but the frequency of this finding was low. In patients with open-angle glaucoma, PPA zone beta enlarged in 1.6% of the eyes after $3.9 \pm 2.6$ (0.6–9.1) years. After the eyes with myopia greater than $-3$ D were excluded, the increase in PPA zone beta was found more frequently in progressive glaucoma (6.2%) compared with non-progressive glaucoma (0.8%).

Clinically, an alpha zone broader than 0.2 mm in the temporal horizontal area, the presence of alpha zone in the nasal region or the finding of beta zone anywhere, were all found more frequently in glaucomatous eyes damaged early than in normal eyes.

**Sidebar 15.1** (continued)

***Clinical Pearls***

- Two zones: alpha (hyperpigmented and peripheral) and beta (hypopigmented and central).
- Look for it next to the most damaged area of the nerve.
- Alpha zone: relative scotoma in the visual field.
- Beta zone: absolute scotoma in the visual field.
- Look for hemorrhages next to the PPA.
- PPA progression may precede visual field defects in ocular hypertensive eyes.
- Progression may occur in PPA in glaucoma, but its frequency is low.
- PPA in non-glaucomatous optic neuropathies is stable.
- PPA is a second-order parameter in the diagnosis of glaucoma.

**Bibliography**

Ahn JK, Kang JH, Park KH. Correlation between a disc hemorrhage and peripapillary atrophy in glaucoma patients with a unilateral disc hemorrhage. *J Glaucoma.* 2004;13:9–14.

Budde WM, Jonas JB. Enlargement of parapillary atrophy in follow-up of chronic open-angle glaucoma. *Am J Ophthalmol.* 2004;137:646–654.

Jonas JB. Clinical implications of peripapillary atrophy in glaucoma. *Curr Opin Ophthalmol.* 2005;16:84–88.

Jonas JB, Nguyen XN, Gusek GC, Naumann GOH. Parapapillary chorioretinal atrophy in normal and glaucoma eyes. *Invest Ophthalmol Vis Sci.* 1989;30:908–918.

Jonas JB, Gusek GC, Fernández MC. Correlation of the blind spot size to the area of the optic disc and parapapillary atrophy. *Am J Ophthalmol.* 1991;111:559–565.

Jonas JB, Fernández MC, Naumann GOH. Glaucomatous parapapillary atrophy: occurrence and correlations. *Arch Ophthalmol.* 1992;110:214–222.

Jonas JB, Budde W, Panda-Jonas S. Ophthalmoscopic evaluation of the optic nerve head. *Surv Ophthalmol.* 1999;43:293–320.

Jonas JB, Budde WM, Lang PJ. Parapapillary atrophy in the chronic open-angle glaucomas. *Graefe's Arch Clin Exp Ophthalmol.* 1999;237:793–797.

Jonas JB, Bergua A, Schmitz-Valckenberg P, et al. Ranking of optic disc variables for detection of glaucomatous optic nerve damage. *Invest Ophthalmol Vis Sci.* 2000;41:1764–1773.

Law SK, Choe R, Caprioli J. Optic disk characteristics before the occurrence of disk hemorrhage in glaucoma patients. *Am J Ophthalmol.* 2001;132:411–413.

Rath EZ, Rehany U, Linn S, Rummelt S. Correlation between optic disc atrophy and aetiology: anterior ischaemic optic neuropathy vs optic neuritis. *Eye.* 2003;17:1019–1024.

Tezel G, Dorr D, Kolker AE, et al. Concordance of parapapillary chorioretinal atrophy in ocular hypertension with visual field defects that accompany glaucoma development. *Ophthalmology.* 2000;107:1194–1199.

---

edge and a retinal blood vessel. Sudden angulation of a blood vessel as it changes direction is called "bayoneting." Blood vessels often bend dramatically as they reach the top of the steep wall of a cupped disc and change direction to traverse over the neuroretinal rim. Thus, bayoneting may be an important indicator of the margin of the optic disc cup.

### 15.4.2 Optic Disc Pits

Acquired pits of the optic nerve (APON) may be associated with glaucoma. Severe and highly localized tissue loss in the optic disc may result in disc pitting. Theoretically, a focal structural weakness or abnormality in the lamina cribrosa could exacerbate glaucomatous disc cupping in one area yielding an APON. Most commonly located at the inferior temporal pole of the disc, pits often produce visual field defects close to fixation. An APON may also be referred to as a pseudopit, and should be differentiated from congenital optic disc pits (see section 15.5.5).

## 15.5 Differential Diagnosis

### 15.5.1 Anterior Ischemic Optic Neuropathy

Anterior ischemic optic neuropathy (AION) typically occurs in the middle-aged and the elderly. Like glaucoma, AION commonly presents with painless loss of vision, afferent papillary defect, and visual field defects. However, the onset of AION is sudden, whereas glaucoma is most often a chronic condition with gradually progressive vision loss. Visual field defects may be similar in glaucoma and AION, with nasal and arcuate scotomas common in both diseases. Altitudinal defects, especially inferior, are often seen in AION, but are far less common in glaucoma.[30] AION is subdivided into non-arteritic AION (NAION) and arteritic AION (AAION). The distinction is

### Sidebar 15.2 Relative afferent pupillary defects in glaucoma patients

Edney R. Moura Filho and Rajesh K. Shetty

Levantin in 1959, first described the relative afferent pupillary defect (RAPD) as an indicator of an asymmetric loss of neuronal function in many optic nerve and retinal disorders. Although primary open-angle glaucoma usually affects both eyes, it is also often an asymmetric disease. George Spaeth et al reported that the detection of a RAPD may precede apparent optic disc and visual field damage. In some cases, the presence of an RAPD may be the only objective indicator of the presence of glaucomatous optic neuropathy.

The normal pupillary light reflex during the swinging flashlight test consists of an initial contraction followed by redilation as the light source is moved across the nose. Then, a new contraction is seen when the other eye is illuminated (the consensual response). The swinging flashlight test starts with the patient fixating at a distant target. Distance fixation is stressed to the patient to avoid pupillary changes from near accommodation should the patient attempt to look at the flashlight itself. The examiner turns the slit lamp or a flashlight on and off to observe baseline *efferent* pupillary motor function (dilation and constriction). This is done for both eyes. Pupil size, response, and symmetry are noted. The examiner looks at one eye with the illumination light off, as he swings the light from one eye to the other. First, the light is shined directly into the eye viewed, allowing observation of pupil constriction. While continuing to monitor the same pupil, the light is then directed to the other eye to elicit the consensual response. The light is swung rapidly from one eye to the other and should remain on each eye for approximately 3 s to allow for pupillary stabilization. In the presence of a RAPD, both pupils will constrict as the light is shifted to the normal or better eye and dilate once the light is shined back into the abnormal or worse eye. If a RAPD is present in the worse eye and it has an non-reactive pupil, then the observed contralateral pupil will constrict to light and dilate when the light is shined in the worse eye.

The basis for all pupillary reactions to light is the underlying neuroanatomy of the eyes, the optic nerves and the brain structures to which they connect. The afferent pathway starts with the photoreceptors in the retina inner layers, which in turn connect with the bipolar and retinal ganglion cells (RGCs). The axons of the RGCs traverse the optic nerve; the impulses then travel to the pretectal nuclei in the dorsal midbrain, ending the afferent arc of this pupillary reflex. From there, they go via the intermediate neurons to the Edinger–Westphal subnucleus of the ocular motor nucleus, and finally reach the iris constrictor muscles along the efferent arc via the oculomotor nerve and the short ciliary nerves. The Edinger–Westphal subnucleus simply sums the afferent input from either or both optic nerves (both eyes) and does not distinguish if the light stimulus is present in one or both eyes. The efferent motor output, which causes pupil constriction, goes equally to each eye, regardless of the symmetry or asymmetry of the afferent stimulation from the two eyes (Fig. 15.2-1).

The presence of an RAPD in the illuminated eye is indicated by any of the three findings: a small initial momentary constriction followed by greater dilation, initially no apparent change followed by dilation, or initial immediate dilation.

The alternating (swinging) flashlight test should be a routine part of any ophthalmic examination. This test can be done quickly in the office or at the bedside; however, it is not without problems: end-point determination, unequal retinal illumination, and examiner bias adversely affect reliability. Small relative afferent pupillary defects are often difficult to detect in patients with relatively mild differences in optic nerve dysfunction. Dark irides and sluggish or miotic pupils also add to the difficulty in diagnosis. Sometimes, physiological *hippus*, a rhythmic low frequency irregular dilation and contraction of the pupil by the sphincter and dilator muscles, can confuse the examiner testing for RAPDs. It is possible to discern hippus by its relatively rapid periodicity.

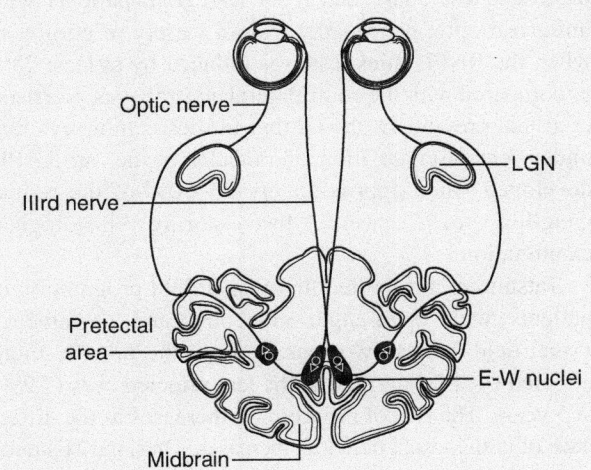

**Fig. 15.2-1** Pupillary pathways. E-W: Edinger–Westphal subnucleus

**SIDEBAR 15.2** (continued)

One may be able to correlate the presence of a relative afferent pupillary defect with visual field changes. The eye showing the RAPD should also be the eye with relatively worse nerve fiber bundle defects on the visual field printouts. In fact, if this is not the case, then the examiner should question the findings of the swinging flashlight test and repeat it, perhaps in the presence of a second observer.

Glazer-Hockstein et al suggested using the magnification provided by a slit-lamp biomicroscope for the purpose of a better detection of small changes. A modified swinging flashlight test with magnification, using a +20-D lens, proposed by Spaeth et al, increases the sensitivity of the test in detecting an RAPD. Using infrared pupillography, they found an RAPD in 39 (56%) of 70 glaucoma subjects. Using magnification, they found an RAPD in 42 (60%) of 70 glaucoma subjects and in 20 (29%) of 70 glaucoma subjects using the standard swinging flashlight method.

Various other techniques have also been described to quantify or measure RAPDs. These include the use of neutral density filters, cross-polarized filters, and infrared computerized pupillometry. The latter method can be used to detect optic neuropathy in glaucoma with high sensitivity and specificity, although it is not something that would lend itself to routine use in a community-based practice.

RAPD is directly associated with the difference in average RNFL thickness in patients with asymmetric GON and is clinically detectable when the average peripapillary RNFL is reduced by 27% in the more affected eyes compared with the less affected. The swinging flashlight test could detect an RAPD in patients with unilateral optic neuropathy from a variety of etiologies when the RNFL thickness was reduced by at least 25% as compared with the contralateral control eyes. Kerrison et al had previously shown that in rhesus monkeys that underwent laser ablation of macular tissue, an RAPD developed when approximately 25–50% of the retinal ganglion cells were lost during histological examination.

Tatsumi et al reported that visual field progression in patients with open-angle glaucoma and asymmetric visual field damage worsens faster in the initially more affected eyes (25%) than in the less affected eyes (7.2%) at 5 years. The risk of progression increases as the difference of initial visual field loss increases. Thus, the existence of an RAPD may be indicative not only of a substantial difference in the RNFL thickness between eyes but also of the risk of future visual field progression in the eyes with the RAPD.

In summary, an asymmetric pupillary light reflex or RAPD is an objective, inexpensive, and efficient method to detect significant retinal or optic nerve disease, including glaucomatous optic neuropathy. It provides an accurate method to determine the eye with the worse disease and with the higher risk of becoming blind.

## Bibliography

Bell RA, Waggoner PM, Boyd WM, et al. Clinical grading of relative afferent pupillary defects. *Arch Ophthalmol.* 1993;111:938–942.

Bergamin O, Zimmerman MB, Kardon RH. Pupil light reflex in normal and diseased eyes: diagnosis of visual dysfunction using waveform partitioning. *Ophthalmology.* 2003;110:106–114.

Chen PP, Park RJ. Visual field progression in patients with initially unilateral visual field loss from chronic open-angle glaucoma. *Ophthalmology.* 2000;107:1688–1692.

Digre KB. Principles and techniques of examination of the pupils, accommodation, and lacrimation. In: Miller NR, Newman NJ, eds. *Walsh and Hoyt's Clinical Neuro-Ophthalmology.* 6th ed. Baltimore: Lippincott Williams & Wilkins; 2005:715–737.

Glazer-Hockstein C, Brucker AJ. The detection of a relative afferent pupillary defect. *Am J Ophthalmol.* 2002;134:142–143.

Kalaboukhova L, Fridhammar V, Lindblom B. Relative afferent pupillary defect in glaucoma: a pupillometric study. *Acta Ophthalmol Scand.* 2007;85:519–525.

Kawasaki A, Moore P, Kardon RH. Variability of the relative afferent pupillary defect. *Am J Ophthalmol.* 1995;120:622–633.

Kerrison JB, Buchanan K, Rosenberg ML, et al. Quantification of optic nerve axon loss associated with a relative afferent pupillary defect in the monkey. *Arch Ophthalmol.* 2001;119:1333–1341.

Lagreze WD, Kardon RH. Correlation of relative afferent pupillary defect and estimated retinal ganglion cell loss. *Graefes Arch Clin Exp Ophthalmol.* 1998;236:401–404.

Lankaranian D, Altangerel U, Spaeth GL, Leavitt JA, Steinmann WC. The usefulness of a new method of testing for a relative afferent pupillary defect in patients with ocular hypertension and glaucoma. *Trans Am Ophthalmol Soc.* 2005;103:200–208.

Levatin P. Pupillary escape in disease of the retina or optic nerve. *Arch Ophthalmol.* 1959;62:768–779.

Nakanishi Y, Nakamura M, Tatsusmi Y, et al. Quantification of retinal nerve fiber layer thickness reduction associated with a relative afferent pupillary defect. *Graefe's Arch Clin Exp Ophthalmol.* 2006;244:1480–1484.

Rosenberg ML, Oliva A. The use of crossed polarized filters in the measurement of the relative afferent pupillary defect. *Am J Ophthalmol*. 1990;110:62–65.

Tatsumi Y, Nakamura M, Fujioka M, Nakanishi Y, Kushuara A, Maeda H, Negi A. Quantification of retinal nerve fiber layer thickness reduction associated with a relative afferent pupillary defect in asymmetric glaucoma. *Br J Ophthalmol*. 2007;91:633–637.

Thompson HS, Corbett JJ, Cox TA. How to measure the relative afferent pupillary defect. *Surv Ophthalmol*. 1981;26:39–42.

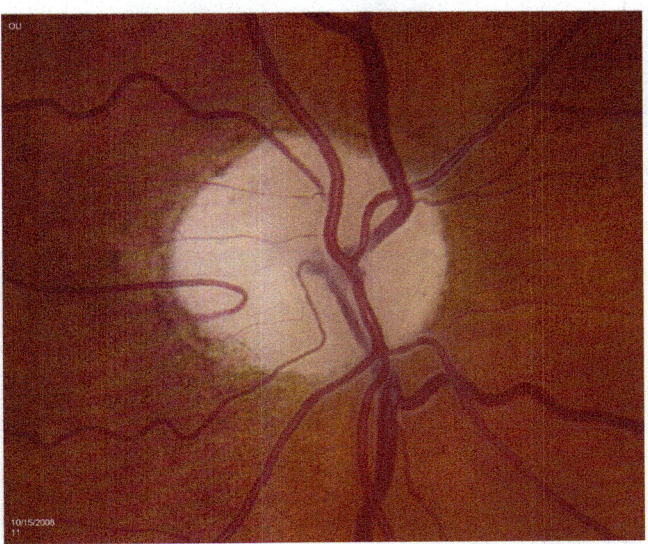

**Fig. 15.8** Optic disc pallor and atrophy following ischemic optic neuropathy

important because AAION is caused by vasculitis, such as giant cell arteritis, and must be diagnosed emergently to prevent the spread of ischemic damage to the other structures, including the fellow eye. Non-arteritic AION occurs more often in the "disc at risk," which is a small optic disc with small optic cup and crowded or full appearance (Fig. 15.8).[31]

### 15.5.2 Optic Disc Drusen

Optic disc drusen (ODD) are thought to be the remnants of the axonal transport system of degenerated retinal ganglion cells. Disc drusen have been found clinically in 0.3% of the white population, with up to 91% presenting bilaterally.[32] The evolution of disc drusen is a dynamic process.[33] In infancy, visible disc drusen are rare, but by childhood, the disc adopts a "full" appearance and may become tan or straw colored. Later, subtle excrescences emerge on the disc surface, predominantly nasally, and the disc margin may become irregular and scalloped. As the drusen enlarge, they may deflect blood vessels, causing an irregular branching pattern.

Ultimately, the disc flattens and becomes pale.[33] Buried drusen may be detected by various imaging modalities: fluorescein angiography, red-free photography, B-scan ultrasonography, or CT scan (Fig. 15.9a and b).

Visual field defects have been reported in as many as 75% of patients with optic disc drusen and may be indistinguishable from those of glaucoma.[34] Field loss may correspond with RNFL loss just like in glaucoma. There is no correlation between the location of visible disc drusen and the pattern of visual field loss in these patients. Diagnosis and treatment of glaucoma in patients with disc drusen may be exceedingly difficult, secondary to distortion of the disc and cup. However, despite the evolutionary nature of the disc appearance in patients with drusen, the symptoms related to drusen are not usually progressive.

### 15.5.3 Optic Neuritis

Optic neuritis is inflammation of the optic nerve and its myelin sheath. The initial attack is unilateral in 70% of adult patients and bilateral in 30%, and the resulting vision loss is rapid and progressive, but usually temporary. Optic neuritis is predominantly a disease in young women. There is a strong association between optic neuritis and multiple sclerosis. Retrobulbar optic neuritis occurs in roughly two-thirds of cases, so the optic nerve head often appears normal on examination. If the intraocular portion of the optic nerve is affected, disc swelling occurs. When disc swelling resolves, pallor and atrophy may remain as indicators of a past episode of optic neuritis (Fig. 15.10).

### 15.5.4 Morning Glory Syndrome

Morning glory syndrome is a congenital optic disc anomaly in which much of the excavated colobomatous optic disc is filled with glial tissue. An elevated chorioretinal pigment abnormality occurs in the circumpapillary area.[2] On examination, the optic disc appears funnel-shaped, with retinal vessels arising from the periphery of the disk and running an abnormally straight course over the peripapillary retina (Fig. 15.11).

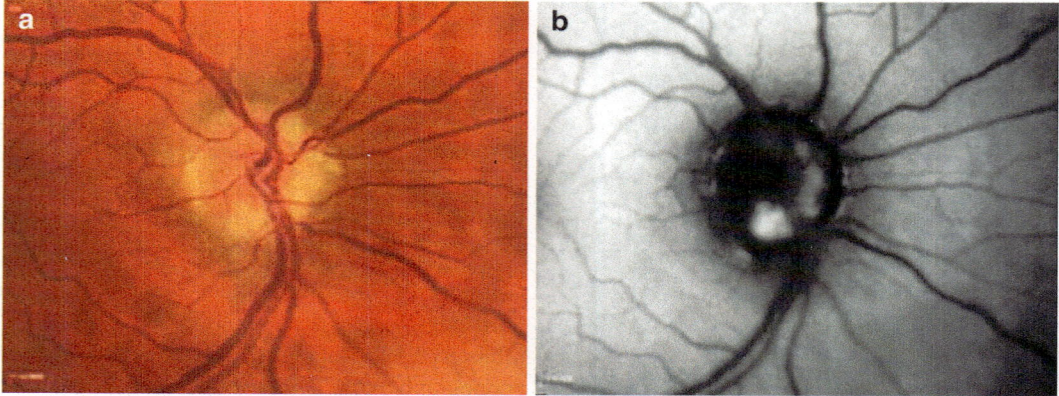

**Fig. 15.9** (a) Color photo of optic disc drusen. (b) Autofluorescence of optic disc drusen

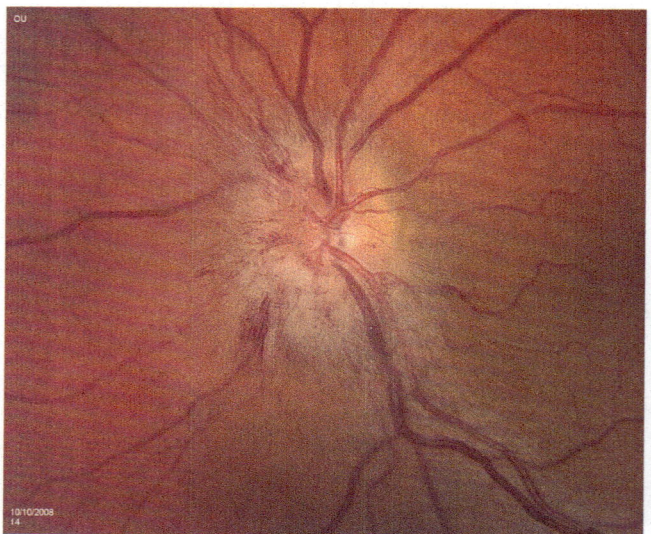

**Fig. 15.10** Optic disc edema in a patient with optic neuritis

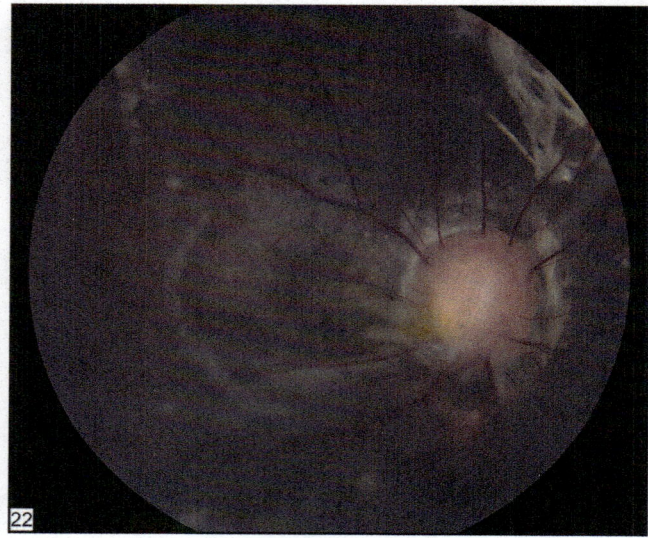

**Fig. 15.11** Morning glory disc anomaly

### 15.5.5 Congenital Optic Disc Pits

Optic disc pit is a congenital excavation of the optic nerve head resulting from a malformation during development of the eye (Fig. 15.12). It may be associated with other abnormalities of the optic nerve and peripapillary retina. Optic pits along the rim of the optic disc are most likely to lead to serous detachments of the retina and associated full-thickness or laminar retinal holes, retinal pigment epithelium mottling, and general cystic changes. Optic pits may remain asymptomatic unless complicated by macular lesions, such as edema, schisis, or serous detachment. Congenital pits range greatly in size and, in severe cases, may occupy most of the optic disc. They appear as small, hypopigmented, grayish, oval or round excavated depressions in the optic nerve head and do not change appearance with time. Enlarged blind spot and arcuate scotomas may occur in patients with congenital disc pits. Fluorescein angiography and an electroretinogram test are usually unremarkable in cases of optic pits. Additional technology, like OCT, can demonstrate a marked reduction in the thickness of the RNFL in the quadrant corresponding to the optic pit, and may be helpful in supporting a diagnosis.

### 15.5.6 Compressive Optic Neuropathy

This condition is rare, but crucial to recognize. Compression of the optic nerve may occur in cases of thyroid orbitopathy, trauma, and tumors of the pituitary, orbit, optic nerve, and

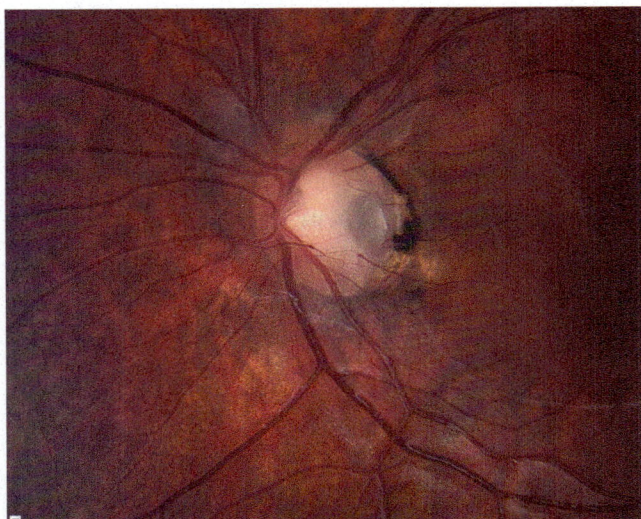

**Fig. 15.12** Congenital optic disc pit

skull base. Patients with thyroid orbitopathy may have increased resistance to retropulsion and tight orbits, as well as extraocular motility deficits and proptosis. Orbital tumors may cause resistance to retropulsion and displacement of the globe. Pituitary tumors are not associated with orbital signs, but may lead to uni- or bilateral nerve pallor, depending on whether their location is more anterior or posterior. Field defects may range from enlargement of the blind spot to junctional scotomas and bitemporal defects. These patterns of field loss warrant neuro-imaging. Unilateral optic disc swelling or pallor may be an initial sign of compressive optic neuropathy. Optic atrophy and optociliary shunt vessels may also occur in patients with a compressive etiology.

Evaluation of the optic nerve is critical in glaucoma. While non-ophthalmologists continue to use direct ophthalmoscopy, glaucoma specialists continue to prefer the convenience of evaluating the optic nerve with the 78 and 90 D inverted lenses. In small pupil situations and to estimate the size of the optic nerve, an ophthalmologist may find the direct ophthalmoscope useful. In many ways the two techniques are complimentary, and it may be wisest to use both in the evaluation of the routine patient.

# References

1. Varma RV, Spaeth GL. *The Optic Nerve in Glaucoma*. Philadelphia, PA: J.B. Lippincott Co.; 1993.
2. Ritch R, Shields MB, Krupin T. *The Glaucomas: Basic Sciences*. 2nd ed. Mosby: St. Louis; 1996:152.
3. Quigley HA, Brown AE, Morrison JD, Drance SM. The size and shape of the optic disc in normal human eyes. *Arch Ophthalmol*. 1990;108(1):51–57.
4. Caprioli J, Miller JM. Optic disc rim area is related to disc size in normal subjects. *Arch Ophthalmol*. 1987;105(12):1683–1685.
5. Fingeret M, Medeiros FA, Susanna R Jr, Weinreb RN. Five rules to evaluate the optic disc and retinal nerve fiber layer for glaucoma. *Optometry*. 2005;76(11):661–668.
6. Jonas JB, Gusek GC, Naumann GO. Optic disc, cup and neuroretinal rim size, configuration and correlations in normal eyes. *Invest Ophthalmol Vis Sci*. 1988;29(7):1151–1158.
7. Harizman N, Oliveira C, Chiang A, et al. The ISNT rule and differentiation of normal from glaucomatous eyes. *Arch Ophthalmol*. 2006;124(11):1579–1583.
8. Gross PG, Drance SM. Comparison of a simple ophthalmoscopic and planimetric measurement of glaucomatous neuroretinal rim areas. *J Glaucoma*. 1995;4:314–316.
9. Choplin NT, Lundy DC, eds. *Atlas of Glaucoma*. London: Martin Dunitz, Ltd; 1998:68.
10. Sommer A, Katz J, Quigley HA, et al. Clinically detectable nerve fiber atrophy precedes the onset of glaucomatous field loss. *Arch Ophthalmol*. 1991;109:77–83.
11. Ritch R, Shields MB, Krupin T, eds. *The Glaucomas: Basic Sciences*. 2nd ed. Mosby: St. Louis; 1996:626–627.
12. Lin SC, Singh K, Jampel HD, et al. Optic nerve head and retinal nerve fiber layer analysis: a report by the American Academy of Ophthalmology. *Ophthalmology*. 2007;114(10):1937–1949.
13. Menke MN, Knecht P, Sturm V, Dabov S, Funk J. Reproducibility of nerve fiber layer thickness measurements using 3D Fourier-domain OCT. *Invest Ophthalmol Vis Sci*. 2008;49(12):5386–5391.
14. Jonas JB, Budde WM. Diagnosis and pathogenesis of glaucomatous optic neuropathy: morphological aspects. *Prog Retin Eye Res*. 2000;19(1):1–40.
15. Armaly MF, Sayegh RE. The cup-disc ratio. The findings of tonometry and tonography in the normal eye. *Arch Ophthalmol*. 1969;82(2):191–196.
16. Carpel EF, Engstrom PF. The normal cup-disk ratio. *Am J Ophthalmol*. 1981;91(5):588–597.
17. Armaly MF. The correlation between appearance of the optic cup and visual function. *Trans Am Acad Ophthalmol Otolaryngol*. 1969;78:898.
18. Spaeth GL, Henderer J, Liu C, et al. The disc damage likelihood scale: reproducibility of a new method of estimating the amount of optic nerve damage caused by glaucoma. *Trans Am Ophthalmol Soc*. 2002;100:181–185. discussion 5–6.
19. Susanna R Jr, Vessani RM. New findings in the evaluation of the optic disc in glaucoma diagnosis. *Curr Opin Ophthalmol*. 2007;18(2):122–128.
20. Jonas JB. Optic disk size correlated with refractive error. *Am J Ophthalmol*. 2005;139(2):346–348.
21. Balazsi AG, Drance SM, Schulzer M, Douglas GR. Neuroretinal rim area in suspected glaucoma and early chronic open-angle glaucoma. Correlation with parameters of visual function. *Arch Ophthalmol*. 1984;102(7):1011–1014.
22. Caprioli J, Miller JM, Sears M. Quantitative evaluation of the optic nerve head in patients with unilateral visual field loss from primary open angle glaucoma. *Ophthalmology*. 1987;94:1484–1487.
23. Trobe JD, Glaser JS, Cassady J, et al. Nonglaucomatous excavation of the optic disc. *Arch Ophthalmol*. 1980;98:1046–1050.
24. Armaly MF. Genetic determination of cup/disc ratio of the optic nerve. *Arch Ophthalmol*. 1967;78(1):35–43.
25. Drance S, Anderson DR, Schulzer M, for the Collaborative Normal-Tension Glaucoma Study Group. Risk factors for progression of visual field abnormalities in normal-tension glaucoma. *Am J Ophthalmol*. 2001;131(6):699–708.
26. Healey PR, Mitchell P, Smith W, Wang JJ. Optic disc hemorrhages in a population with and without signs of glaucoma. *Ophthalmology*. 1998;105(2):216–223.

27. Tezel G, Kolker AE, Wax MB, et al. Parapapillary chorioretinal atrophy in patients with ocular hypertension. II. An evaluation of progressive changes. *Arch Ophthalmol*. 1997;115:1509–1514.
28. Uchida H, Ugurlu S, Caprioli J. Increasing peripapillary atrophy is associated with progressive glaucoma. *Ophthalmology*. 1998;96:16.
29. Morrison JC, Pollack IP. *Glaucoma: A Clinical Guide*. China: Thieme; 2003:99.
30. Levin LA, Arnold AC. *Neuro-Ophthalmology: The Practical Guide*. China: Thieme; 2005:110.
31. Doro S, Lessell S. Cup-disc ratio and ischemic optic neuropathy. *Arch Ophthalmol*. 1985;103(8):1143–1144.
32. Aumiller MS. Optic disc drusen: complications and management. *Optometry*. 2007;78(1):10–16.
33. Miller NR, Walsh FB, Hoyt WF, Newman NJ, Biousse V, Kerrison JB. *Walsh and Hoyt's Clinical Neuro-Ophthalmology: The Essentials*. Baltimore: Lippincott Williams & Wilkins; 2007:91.
34. Susanna R, Drance S, Medeiros FA. *The Optic Nerve in Glaucoma*. Amsterdam: Kugler Publications; 1995:130.

# Chapter 16
# Clinical Cupping: Laminar and Prelaminar Components

Claude F. Burgoyne, Hongli Yang, and J. Crawford Downs

## 16.1 The Optic Nerve Head

While glaucomatous damage to the visual system likely includes important pathophysiologies within the retinal ganglion cell (RGC) body,[1-6] photoreceptors,[7-11] lateral geniculate body,[12-14] and visual cortex,[14] strong evidence suggests that damage to the retinal ganglion cell axons within the lamina cribrosa of the optic nerve head (ONH)[15-20] is the central pathophysiology underlying glaucomatous vision loss. Recent studies in the monkey[19-26] and rat[27-29] support the importance of the ONH, by describing profound alterations within the prelaminar, laminar, and peripapillary scleral tissues of the ONH at the earliest detectable stage of experimental glaucoma.

The ONH tissues make up a dynamic environment, wherein 1.2–2.0 million retinal ganglion cell axons converge, turn, and exit the eye through the inner (Bruch's Membrane opening) and outer (scleral) portions of the neural canal (Fig. 16.1). Within the scleral portion of the canal, the bundled axons pass through a 3-dimensional (3D) meshwork of astrocyte-covered, capillary-containing, connective tissue beams known as the lamina cribrosa. Within the lamina, axonal nutrition is dependent upon the movement of oxygen and nutrients from the laminar capillaries, through the laminar beam extracellular matrix, across the astrocyte basement membrane into the astrocyte, finally reaching the peripheral and central axons of each bundle via cell processes.[30]

The connective tissue beams of the lamina cribrosa are anchored via the neural canal wall to a circumferential ring of collagen and elastin fibers within the peripapillary sclera[31-33] and are presumed to bear the forces generated by intraocular pressure (IOP). However, while IOP[34-37] has been shown to play a causative role in glaucomatous ONH damage at all levels of IOP, no agreement exists on the effects of IOP within the tissues of the ONH, no data exist that would allow one to predict a safe level of IOP for a given ONH, and there are no accepted explanations for the varied clinical manifestations of glaucomatous damage,[38] glaucomatous cupping, and glaucomatous visual field loss.

## 16.2 ONH Cupping

"Cupping" is a clinical term used to describe enlargement of the ONH cup in all forms of optic neuropathy[39-46] (Fig. 16.2). However, "cupping" is also used as a synonym for the pathophysiology of glaucomatous damage to the ONH.[18,47-49] Because the clinical and pathophysiologic contexts for "cupping" are seldom clarified, there is confusing literature regarding the presence, importance, and meaning of "cupping" in a variety of optic neuropathies.[50-64]

## 16.3 ONH Biomechanics

We propose that ONH Biomechanics provides a framework for explaining how IOP-related stress (force/cross-sectional area of the tissue experiencing that force) and strain (a measure of local deformation of a tissue induced by applied stress) within the load-bearing tissues of the ONH (Fig. 16.3) influence the physiology and pathophysiology of all three ONH tissue types (Fig. 16.4). These include: (1) the connective tissues (load-bearing connective tissues of the peripapillary sclera, scleral canal wall, and lamina cribrosa), (2) the neural tissues (retinal ganglion cell axons), and (3) the cells that exist alone or in contact with both 1 and 2 (astrocytes, glial cells, endothelial cells, and pericytes and their basement membranes).[65-67] ONH Biomechanics, so defined, is simply the engineering of these tissues and, in our view, is the likely link by which non-IOP-related risk factors such as ischemia, inflammation, auto-immunity, astrocyte, and glial molecular biology are influenced by or interact with the effects of IOP. ONH biomechanics attempts to combine these factors with laminar and peripapillary scleral connective tissue geometry and material properties (strength, stiffness, structural rigidity, compliance, and nutrient diffusion properties) to explain the physiology of normal ONH aging, ONH susceptibility to IOP, and the clinical manifestation of all forms of optic neuropathy. ONH biomechanics holds as a central principle

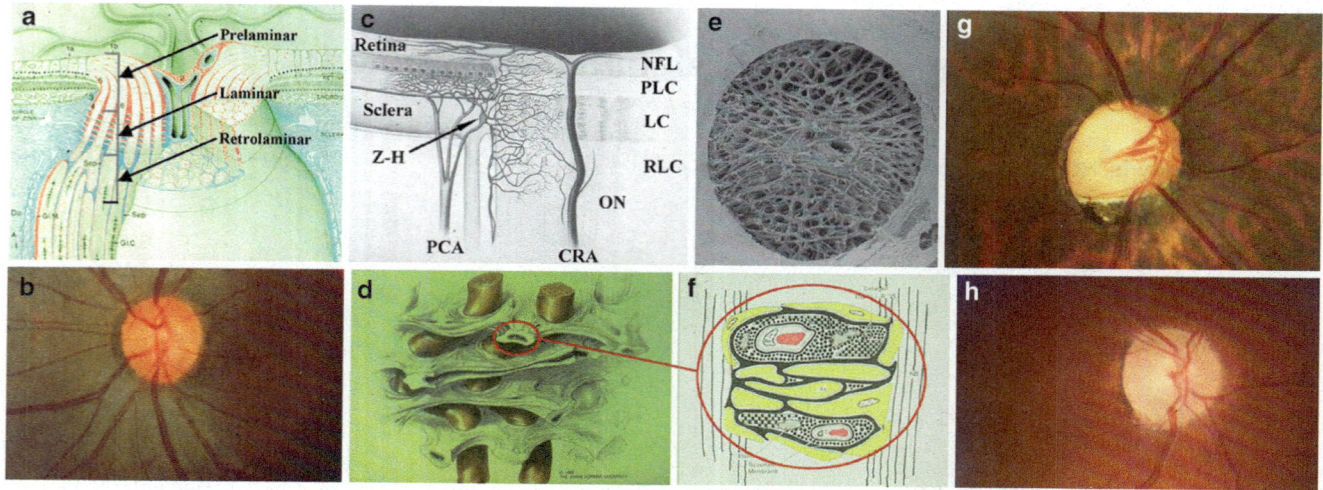

**Fig. 16.1** The optic nerve head (ONH) is centrally influenced by IOP-related stress and strain. The ONH is made up of prelaminar, laminar, and retrolaminar regions (**a**). Within the clinically visible surface of the normal ONH (referred to as the optic disc) (**b**), central retinal vessels enter the eye and RGC axons appear *pink* due to their capillaries, which are principally supplied by branches from the posterior ciliary arteries (PCA) in (**c**). The primary site of RGC axon insult in glaucoma is within the lamina cribrosa schematically depicted with axon bundles in (**d**), isolated by trypsin digest in a scanning electron micrograph in (**e**) and drawn with stippled extracellular matrix (ECM), central capillary (*red*), and surrounding astrocytes (*yellow* with basement membranes in *black*) (**f**). Blood flow within the ONH, while controlled by autoregulation, can be affected by non-IOP-related effects such as systemic blood pressure fluctuation and vasospasm within the retrobulbar portion of the PCAs. Additional IOP-induced effects may include compression of PCA branches within the peripapillary sclera (due to scleral stress and strain) and compression of laminar beam capillaries reducing laminar capillary volume flow (**c** and **f**).[125] There is no direct blood supply to the axons within the laminar region. Axonal nutrition within the lamina (**f**) requires diffusion of nutrients from the laminar capillaries, across the endothelial and pericyte basement membranes, through the ECM of the laminar beam, across the basement membranes of the astrocytes, into the astrocytes, and across their processes to the adjacent axons (*vertical lines*). Chronic age-related changes in the endothelial cell and astrocyte basement membranes, as well as IOP-induced changes in the laminar ECM and astrocyte basement membranes may diminish nutrient diffusion to the axons in the presence of a stable level of laminar capillary volume flow. The clinical manifestation of IOP-induced damage to the ONH is most commonly "deep cupping" (**g**) but in some eyes cupping can be shallower accompanied by pallor (**h**). *Z-H* circle of Zinn–Haller; *PCA* posterior ciliary arteries; *NFL* nerve fiber layer; *PLC* prelaminar region; *LC* lamina cribrosa; *RLC* retrolaminar region; *ON* optic nerve; *CRA* central retinal artery. (**a**) Reprinted with permission from Anderson DR. Ultrastructure of human and monkey lamina cribrosa and optic nerve head. *Arch Ophthalmol.* 1969;82:800-814, Copyright © 1969, American Medical Association. All rights reserved. (**b, g,** and **h**) Reprinted with permission from Burgoyne C. Premise and prediction – how optic nerve head biomechanics underlies the susceptibility and clinical behavior of the aged optic nerve head. *J Glaucoma.* 2008;17:318-328, Wolters Kluwer Health. (**c**) Reprinted with permission from Cioffi GA, Van Buskirk EM. Vasculature of the anterior optic nerve and peripapillary choroid. In: Ritch R, Shields MB, Krupin T, eds. *The Glaucomas.* St. Louis, Mosby: Basic Sciences; 1996:177-197, Elsevier. (**d**) Reprinted with permission from Quigley H. Overview and introduction to session on collective tissue. In: Drance S, ed. *Optic Nerve in Glaucoma.* Amsterdam: Kugler; 1995:15-36. (**e**) Reprinted with permission from Quigley HA, Brown AE, Morrison JD, Drance SM. The size and shape of the optic disc in normal human eyes. *Arch Ophthalmol.* 1990;108:51-57, Copyright © 1990, American Medical Association. All rights reserved. (**f**) Reprinted with permission from Morrison JC, L'Hernault NL, Jerdan JA, Quigley HA. Ultrastructural location of extracellular matrix components in the optic nerve head. *Arch Ophthalmol.* 1989;107:123-129, Copyright © 1989, American Medical Association. All rights reserved

**Fig. 16.2** All clinical cupping, regardless of etiology, is a manifestation of underlying "prelaminar" and "laminar" pathophysiologic components. (**a**) Normal ONH. To understand the two pathophysiologic components of clinical cupping, start with (**b**) a representative digital central horizontal section image from a postmortem 3D reconstruction of this same eye (white section line in (**a**)) – vitreous top, orbital optic nerve bottom, lamina cribrosa between the sclera and internal limiting membrane (ILM) delineated with *green dots*. (**c**) The same section is delineated into principle surfaces and volumes (*black* – ILM; *purple* – prelaminar neural and vascular tissue; *cyan blue line* – Bruch's membrane opening (BMO)-zero reference plane cut in section; *green outline* – Post-BMO total prelaminar area or a measure of the space below BMO and the anterior laminar surface). (**d**) Regardless of the etiology, clinical cupping can be "shallow" (**e**) or "deep" (**f**) (these clinical photos are representative and are not of the eye in (**a**)). A prelaminar or "shallow" form of cupping (**g**, *black arrows*) is primarily due to loss (thinning) of prelaminar neural tissues without important laminar or ONH connective tissue involvement. Laminar or "deep" cupping (**h**, *small white arrows* depict expansion of the *green shaded space*) follows ONH connective tissue damage and deformation that manifests as expansion of the total area beneath BMO, but above the lamina. Notice in (**h**) that while a laminar component of cupping predominates (*white arrows*), there is a prelaminar component as well (*black arrows*). While prelaminar thinning is a manifestation of neural tissue damage alone, we propose that laminar deformation can only occur in the setting of ONH connective tissue damage followed by permanent (fixed) IOP-induced deformation. (Reprinted with permission from Yang H, Downs JC, Bellezza A, Thompson H, Burgoyne CF. 3-D histomorphometry of the normal and early glaucomatous monkey optic nerve head: prelaminar neural tissues and cupping. *Invest Ophthalmol Vis Sci.* 2007;48:5068-5084.)

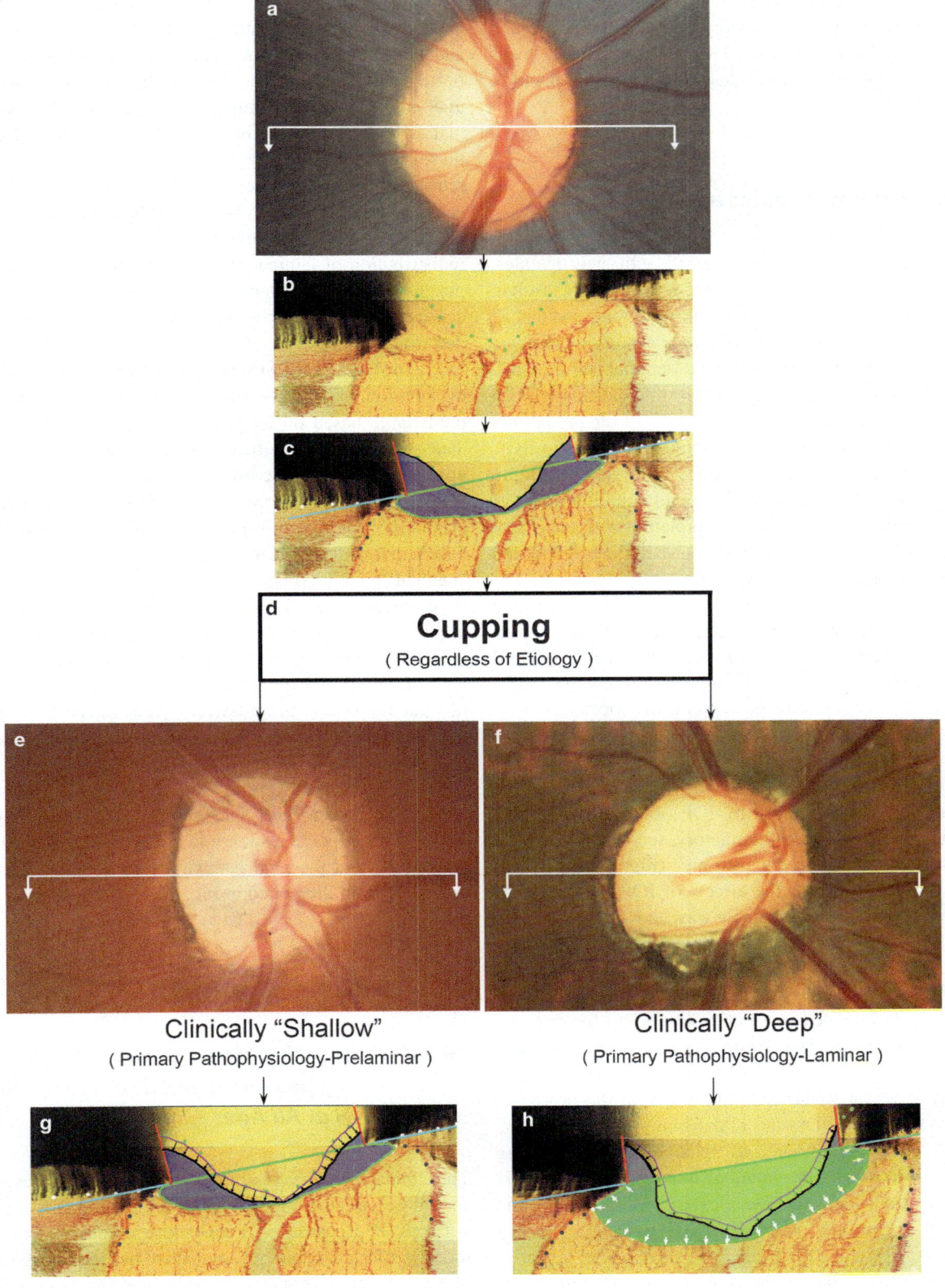

that while IOP may not always be the primary risk factor contributing to an optic neuropathy, it is always present and its effects are likely to be substantial even at normal levels of IOP. These ideas have been described in greater detail in previous reports.[67-71]

## 16.4 ONH Biomechanics and Cupping

We have previously proposed[24] that all optic neuropathies, regardless of the location and etiology of the primary insult to the visual system can demonstrate clinical cupping, and that all forms of *clinical* cupping have two principal *pathophysiologic* components: "prelaminar thinning" and "laminar deformation" (Fig. 16.2). "Prelaminar thinning" is that portion of cup enlargement that results from net thinning of the prelaminar tissues because of physical compression and/or loss of RGC axons even in the presence of gliosis.[72-75] In this paradigm, prelaminar thinning results in a clinically shallow form of cupping[76,77] (being limited to the prelaminar tissues) that occurs in all forms of RGC axon loss (including aging) and is therefore nonspecific to glaucoma.

"Laminar deformation" is that portion of cup enlargement that results from lamina cribrosa and peripapillary scleral connective tissue damage followed by permanent, IOP-induced deformation (Fig. 16.3).[19,20,22,23,67] Laminar deformation results in a clinically deeper form of cupping that occurs only in those optic neuropathies in which the ONH connective tissues have been damaged and have become susceptible to permanent IOP-induced deformation. Whether the ONH connective tissues are primarily damaged by IOP or some other insult (ischemic, auto-immune, inflammatory, secondary astrocyte activation, or genetic predisposition[67] (Fig. 16.4), if they deform, they do so under the effects of IOP (whether it is normal or elevated) in a predictable way, and this deformation underlies "laminar" or "deep" or "glaucomatous" cupping (Fig. 16.3). The previous sentence contains two important ideas. First, it is possible for the ONH to be primarily damaged by non-IOP-related processes and end up looking and behaving in a manner we comfortably call "glaucomatous." Second, even in this setting, IOP-related connective tissue stress and strain (at whatever level) still drive the processes that cause the damaged tissues to deform.

Thus, "deep," "laminar," or "glaucomatous" cupping are terms referring to the clinical manifestation of ONH connective tissue damage, i.e., posterior deformation and excavation. It can only occur when IOP-related connective tissue stress and strain are actively involved (as either a 1° or 2° process). Hayreh[78,79] has argued that primary ischemia to the retrolaminar optic nerve could cause a fibrotic response that pulls the lamina posteriorly into a form that is indistinguishable from glaucomatous cupping. However, we see no evidence for this in early experimental glaucoma monkeys (16–30% axon loss) which demonstrate profound posterior deformation and thickening of the lamina and expansion of the scleral portion of the neural canal.[19,20,22-24] These deformations occur after only 4–8 weeks of minimal to moderate IOP elevations.

Early glaucomatous thickening of the lamina cribrosa in these same eyes may be due in part to recruitment of the retrolaminar septal connective tissues through the process of active remodeling.[26] However, we believe this phenomenon, if present, occurs in response to RGC axonal loss and/or the redistribution of laminar load to the retrolaminar septa and pia. Understood as such, it is a response to, rather than a cause of, laminar, peripapillary scleral, and scleral canal wall deformation.

Central tenets of structural engineering hold that the distribution of stress within any load-bearing structure is predictable based on its geometry and material properties. The structure will deform (generating strain within its constituent parts) according to its constituent material properties, and the structure will yield (stretch beyond its elastic limit) and/or fail (pull apart) in a predictable manner based on this distribution of strain. We have proposed that in "laminar" cupping (Figs. 16.2 and 16.3), individual connective tissue trabeculae of the anterior lamina cribrosa yield, transferring the force they were resisting to the immediately adjacent trabeculae, which increases their load for the same level of IOP. Thus, even under a constant level of IOP, adjacent laminar trabeculae progressively yield as the IOP-induced load is spread over a continually decreasing cross-sectional area of connective tissue.

While new findings in early experimental glaucoma suggest that the lamina deforms (yields), thickens,[23,25] and may recruit retrolaminar septa in response to initial damage (Fig. 16.5),[26] we believe that the final pathway to profound deformation and excavation illustrated in Fig. 16.4[80,81] still holds.

## 16.5 Clinical Implications

### 16.5.1 Connective Tissue Stiffness Underlies the Appearance and Behavior of the ONH at All Ages

The clinical manifestation of glaucomatous damage at all ages should be variable depending upon ONH connective tissue stiffness.[53,82] Because aged connective tissues are most commonly stiffer than younger connective tissues,[83-95] age should be a reasonable surrogate for ONH connective tissue stiffness. Stiffer ONH connective tissues should lead to a shallower form of cupping in both the young and old patient.[53] While a stiff lamina will always be more resistant to deformation, in

# 16 Clinical Cupping: Laminar and Prelaminar Components

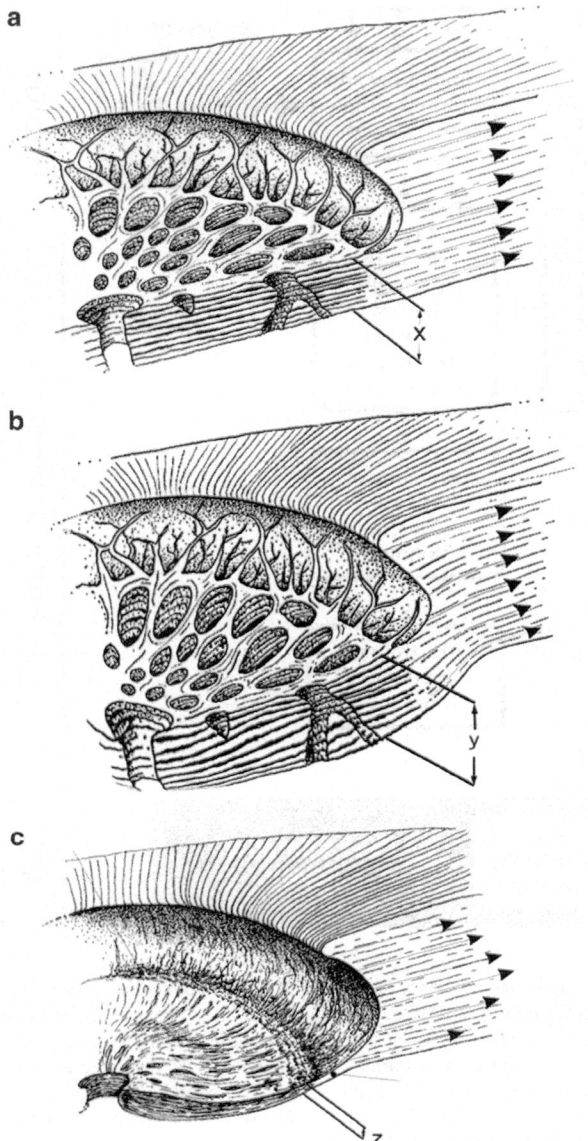

**Fig. 16.3** Our central hypothesis regarding ONH connective tissue damage in "laminar" cupping: "Deep," "laminar," or "glaucomatous" cupping is a manifestation of ONH connective tissue damage that can be caused by either IOP-related or non-IOP related insults (see Fig. 16.5). However, regardless of the primary insult to the ONH connective tissues, their deformation (if present) is driven by IOP-related connective tissue stress and strain. Thus, the presence of ONH connective tissue deformation in any optic neuropathy is evidence that the level of IOP at which it occurred (whether normal or elevated) is too high for the connective tissues in their present condition. (**a**) Schematic of normal laminar thickness ($x$) within the scleral canal with scleral tensile forces acting on the scleral canal wall. (**b**) Early IOP-related damage in the monkey eye[19–24] includes posterior bowing of the lamina and peripapillary sclera accompanied by neural canal expansion (mostly within the posterior (outer) scleral portion) and thickening (not thinning) of the lamina ($y$). In our studies to date, this appears to represent mechanical yield (permanent stretching) rather than mechanical failure (physical disruption) of the laminar beams and may include recruitment of retrolaminar optic nerve septa.[26] (**c**) Progression to end-stage damage includes profound scleral canal wall expansion (clinical excavation) and posterior deformation and thinning of the lamina ($z$) by mechanisms that are as yet

the aged patient, the laminar trabeculae may also become brittle (i.e., deform less as stress increases, but fail at lower levels of strain). Thus, the aged lamina may be less likely to deform posteriorly because of its increased structural stiffness, but more susceptible to catastrophic failure (rather than yield).

## 16.5.2 The Susceptibility and Clinical Behavior of the Aged Optic Nerve Head

A variety of data suggest that the ONH becomes more susceptible to progressive glaucomatous damage as it ages, though this concept remains unproven through direct experimentation and may not be true for every aged eye. These data can be summarized as follows. First, in most,[96–100] but not all,[101,102] population-based studies, IOP either does not increase with age, or if it does, the magnitude of increase is not likely to be clinically important. Thus, the fact that the prevalence of the neuropathy increases with age[103] is likely explained by a greater susceptibility to IOP and other non-IOP-related risk factors, rather than a higher prevalence of IOP elevation with increasing age.

Second, in an extensive review of the literature, we can find only a few reports of the onset and progression of normal tension glaucoma (NTG) in infants, children, and young adults.[104] While we acknowledge that accurate NTG prevalence estimates require long-term telemetric characterization of untreated IOP and rigorous population-based ONH and visual field examinations, all existing studies suggest that NTG is most commonly a disease of the elderly[105–110] and by most measures exists only rarely in the young.[104] Third, age is an independent risk factor for both the prevalence[111] and progression of the neuropathy at all stages of damage.[112–114]

## 16.5.3 The Clinical Behavior of the Aged ONH

Apart from the issue of ONH susceptibility, we predict that if all aspects of insult are equal (alterations in IOP, the volume flow of blood, and nutrient transfer from the laminar capillary to the ONH astrocytes are all of the same magnitude, duration, and fluctuation), the aged eye will demonstrate clinical cupping that is on average shallow and pale (at all stages of field loss)

---

uncharacterized.[80,81] If all other aspects of the neuropathy are identical, the stiffer the lamina, the more resistant it will be to deformation. Whether this is better or worse for the adjacent axons is a separate question that remains to be determined. (Modified from Ref.[67]).

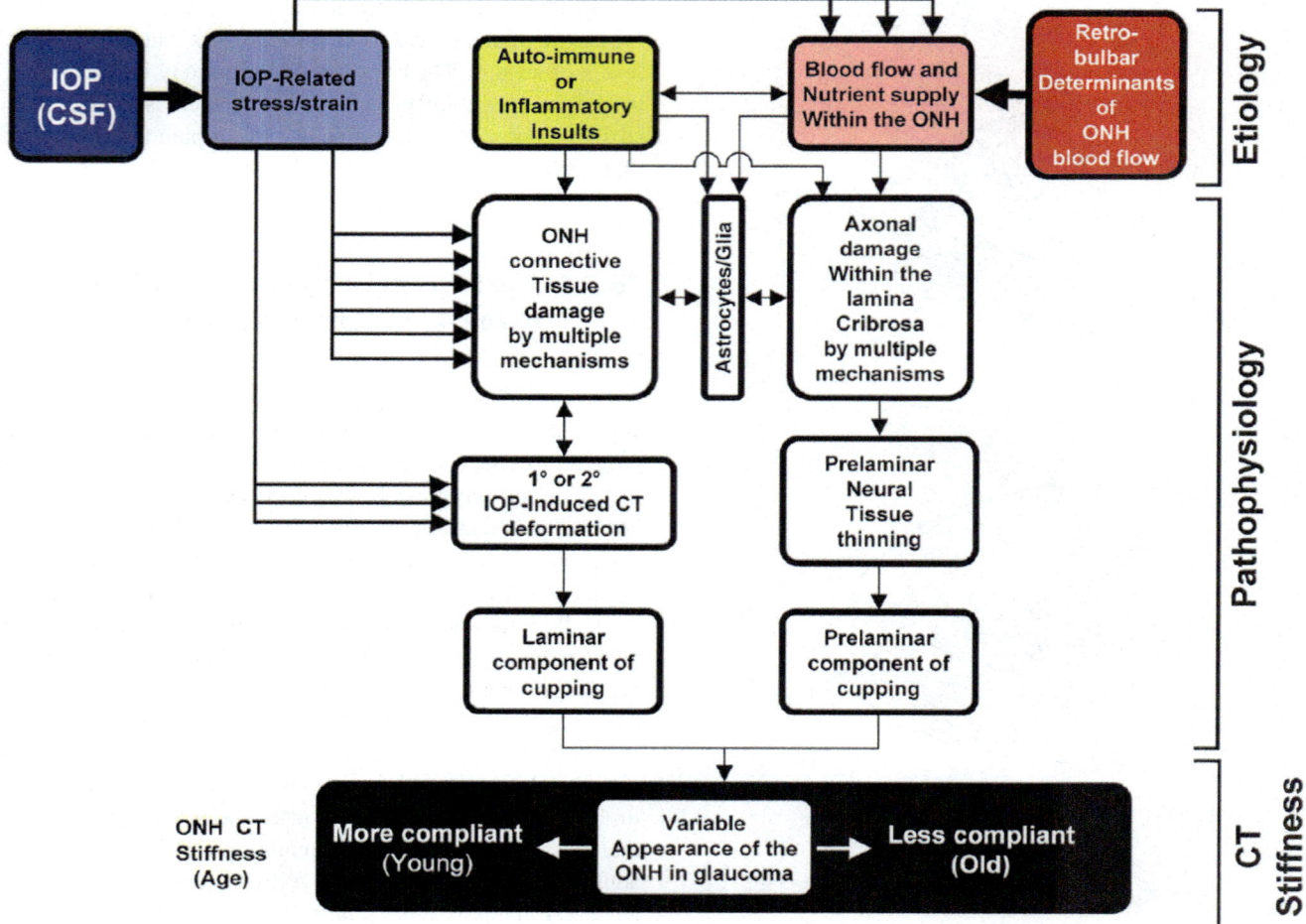

**Fig. 16.4** While damage to the neural and connective tissues of the ONH is multifactorial, ONH appearance in the neuropathy is importantly influenced by connective tissue stiffness. In our biomechanical paradigm, IOP-related strain influences the ONH connective tissues and the volume flow of blood (primarily) and the delivery of nutrients (secondarily), through chronic alterations in connective tissue stiffness and diffusion properties (explained in Fig. 16.1). Non-IOP related effects such as auto-immune or inflammatory insults (*yellow*) and retrobulbar determinants of ocular blood flow (*red*) can primarily damage the ONH connective tissues and/or axons, leaving them vulnerable to secondary damage by IOP-related mechanisms at normal or elevated levels of IOP. Once damaged, the ONH connective tissues can become more or less rigid depending upon lamina cribrosa astrocyte and glial response. If weakened, ONH connective tissues deform in a predictable manner (Fig. 16.3), which underlies a laminar component of clinical cupping (Fig. 16.2). (Adapted and reprinted with permission from Burgoyne C. Premise and prediction – how optic nerve head biomechanics underlies the susceptibility and clinical behavior of the aged optic nerve head. *J Glaucoma*. 2008;17:318-328, Wolters Kluwer Health.)

compared with the eye of a child or young adult. This clinical behavior in its most recognizable form is described as senile sclerotic cupping.[38,53,115–119]

### 16.5.4 Implications for Clinical ONH Imaging in Glaucoma

At present, all forms of clinical imaging in glaucoma assess either the thickness of the peripapillary retinal nerve fiber layer or the surface architecture of the prelaminar neural tissues for glaucomatous damage or progression. Our concept of ONH Biomechanics and its proposed links to ONH aging and ONH appearance suggest that new, "subsurface" targets for clinical ONH imaging are necessary to predict ONH susceptibility and detect early glaucomatous damage.[69,120] Our concepts of ONH aging additionally suggest that these deeper imaging strategies will also be necessary to characterize the differences in the neuropathy with age.

### 16.5.5 Early Detection of Subsurface Structural Change in Ocular Hypertension

Our recent reports on early experimental glaucoma[22–25] utilized high-resolution, digital, 3D histomorphometry to describe not only laminar deformation and thickening, but also prelaminar

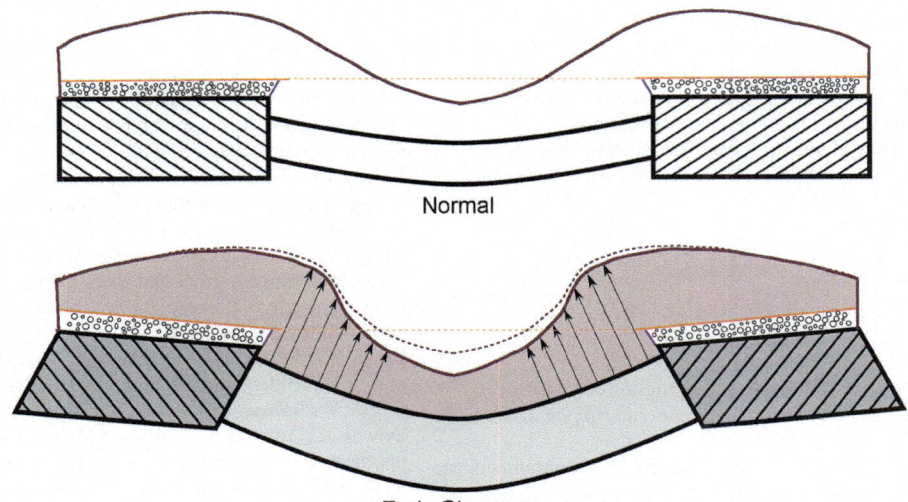

**Fig. 16.5** Profound subsurface structural change accompanies the onset of CSLT-detected clinical cupping in the young adult monkey eye, but this may be different in the old monkey eye. *Upper*: normal lamina cribrosa (unhatched), scleral flange (hatched), prelaminar tissue (beneath the internal limiting membrane – *brown line*), Bruch's membrane (*solid orange line*), Bruch's membrane opening (BMO) zero reference plane (*dotted orange line*), Border tissue of Elschnig (*purple line*), choroid (*black circles*) are schematically represented in the upper illustration. *Lower*: overall changes in the ONH surface and subsurface architecture at the onset of CSLT-detected ONH surface change in experimental ocular hypertension in young adult monkey eyes are depicted below. Posterior bowing of the lamina and peripapillary scleral flange, thickening of the lamina and thickening (*arrows*) not thinning of the prelaminar neural tissues (*brown shading*) underlie posterior deformation of the ONH and peripapillary retinal surface (*dotted brown* to *solid brown* ILM). Thus, while expansion of the clinical cup and deformation of the surface are clinically detectable at this early stage of the neuropathy, because they occur in the setting of prelaminar tissue thickening (not thinning), clinical cupping in experimental ocular hypertension in these young adult eyes is "laminar" in origin, without a significant "prelaminar" component (Fig. 16.3). Because aged eyes will have (on average) stiffer connective tissues, we predict that they will demonstrate less laminar and more prelaminar cupping at the onset of clinically detectable ONH surface change. (Adapted from Yang H, Downs JC, Bellezza A, Thompson H, Burgoyne CF. 3-D histomorphometry of the normal and early glaucomatous monkey optic nerve head: prelaminar neural tissues and cupping. *Invest Ophthalmol Vis Sci.* 2007;48:5068-5084.)

neural tissue thickening, posterior deformation of the scleral flange, and the peripapillary sclera; and expansion of the scleral portion of the neural canal beneath Bruch's Membrane opening at the onset of Confocal Scanning Laser Tomographic (CSLT)-detected optic nerve head surface change. All of these "subsurface" structural changes may eventually be detectable with high-resolution OCT, or other next-generation technologies for clinical imaging.[121–124]

If true in humans, these data suggest that all ocular hypertensive patients might one day be followed to detect an increase in prelaminar neural tissue volume or thickening of the lamina cribrosa, which precedes significant visual field and peripapillary nerve fiber layer (NFL) loss. Our concepts of ONH aging additionally suggest that the ratio of "prelaminar" to "laminar" alterations at the onset of glaucomatous ONH damage may be different in young vs. old (compliant vs. stiff) human eyes (Fig. 16.5). The clinical importance of this difference is that ONH surface change may reflect more axon loss in the aged than in the young ONH. If true, visual field loss may precede clinically detectable ONH surface change more commonly in the aged (stiff) ONH.

Finally, beyond changes that are early in the neuropathy, clinical characterization of all stages of clinical cupping into laminar and prelaminar components[24] should provide quantitative definitions for common clinical descriptions such as "shallow," "deep," senile sclerotic," "thinned," "tilted," and "excavated."

## 16.6 Conclusion

We propose that the characterization of all forms of clinical cupping into prelaminar and laminar components will add a precision to the discussion of clinical cupping that does not currently exist, and eventually aid in the assessment of etiology in all forms of optic neuropathy including those that may be age-related.[24] Using the next generation of ONH imaging devices in this way should create a significant refinement in categorizing glaucomas and dividing them into better understood phenotypes. They may also lead to the early detection of ONH axonal and connective changes in ocular hypertension.

**Acknowledgement** Portions of this chapter have appeared previously in two publications.[24,69]

Supported in part by USPHS grant R01EY011610 (CFB) from the National Eye Institute, National Institutes of Health, Bethesda, Maryland; unrestricted research support from Heidelberg Engineering; a grant from the American Health Assistance Foundation, Rockville, Maryland (CFB); a grant from The Whitaker Foundation, Arlington, Virginia (CFB); a Career Development Award (CFB) from Research to Prevent Blindness, Inc., New York, New York and unrestricted support from The Sears Trust, Mexico MO.

# References

1. Asai T, Katsumori N, Mizokami K. Retinal ganglion cell damage in human glaucoma. 2. Studies on damage pattern. *Nippon Ganka Gakkai Zasshi.* 1987;91:1204–1213.
2. Garcia-Valenzuela E, Shareef S, Walsh J, Sharma SC. Programmed cell death of retinal ganglion cells during experimental glaucoma. *Exp Eye Res.* 1995;61:33–44.
3. Quigley HA, Nickells RW, Kerrigan LA, et al. Retinal ganglion cell death in experimental glaucoma and after axotomy occurs by apoptosis. *Invest Ophthalmol Vis Sci.* 1995;36:774–786.
4. Weber AJ, Kaufman PL, Hubbard WC. Morphology of single ganglion cells in the glaucomatous primate retina. *Invest Ophthalmol Vis Sci.* 1998;39:2304–2320.
5. Quigley HA, McKinnon SJ, Zack DJ, et al. Retrograde axonal transport of BDNF in retinal ganglion cells is blocked by acute IOP elevation in rats. *Invest Ophthalmol Vis Sci.* 2000;41:3460–3466.
6. Quigley HA. Ganglion cell death in glaucoma: pathology recapitulates ontogeny. *Aust NZ J Ophthalmol.* 1995;23:85–91.
7. Wygnanski T, Desatnik H, Quigley HA, Glovinsky Y. Comparison of ganglion cell loss and cone loss in experimental glaucoma. *Am J Ophthalmol.* 1995;120:184–189.
8. Panda S, Jonas JB. Decreased photoreceptor count in human eyes with secondary angle-closure glaucoma. *Invest Ophthalmol Vis Sci.* 1992;33:2532–2536.
9. Kendell KR, Quigley HA, Kerrigan LA, Pease ME, Quigley EN. Primary open-angle glaucoma is not associated with photoreceptor loss. *Invest Ophthalmol Vis Sci.* 1995;36:200–205.
10. Nork TM, Ver Hoeve JN, Poulsen GL, et al. Swelling and loss of photoreceptors in chronic human and experimental glaucomas. *Arch Ophthalmol.* 2000;118:235–245.
11. Janssen P, Naskar R, Moore S, Thanos S, Thiel HJ. Evidence for glaucoma-induced horizontal cell alterations in the human retina. *Ger J Ophthalmol.* 1996;5:378–385.
12. Yucel YH, Zhang Q, Gupta N, Kaufman PL, Weinreb RN. Loss of neurons in magnocellular and parvocellular layers of the lateral geniculate nucleus in glaucoma. *Arch Ophthalmol.* 2000;118:378–384.
13. Yucel YH, Zhang Q, Weinreb RN, Kaufman PL, Gupta N. Atrophy of relay neurons in magno- and parvocellular layers in the lateral geniculate nucleus in experimental glaucoma. *Invest Ophthalmol Vis Sci.* 2001;42:3216–3222.
14. Yucel YH, Zhang Q, Weinreb RN, Kaufman PL, Gupta N. Effects of retinal ganglion cell loss on magno-, parvo-, koniocellular pathways in the lateral geniculate nucleus and visual cortex in glaucoma. *Prog Retin Eye Res.* 2003;22:465–481.
15. Gaasterland D, Tanishima T, Kuwabara T. Axoplasmic flow during chronic experimental glaucoma. 1. Light and electron microscopic studies of the monkey optic nervehead during development of glaucomatous cupping. *Invest Ophthalmol Vis Sci.* 1978;17:838–846.
16. Minckler DS, Bunt AH, Johanson GW. Orthograde and retrograde axoplasmic transport during acute ocular hypertension in the monkey. *Invest Ophthalmol Vis Sci.* 1977;16:426–441.
17. Quigley HA, Addicks EM, Green WR, Maumenee AE. Optic nerve damage in human glaucoma. II. The site of injury and susceptibility to damage. *Arch Ophthalmol.* 1981;99:635–649.
18. Quigley HA, Green WR. The histology of human glaucoma cupping and optic nerve damage: clinicopathologic correlation in 21 eyes. *Ophthalmology.* 1979;86:1803–1830.
19. Bellezza AJ, Rintalan CJ, Thompson HW, et al. Deformation of the lamina cribrosa and anterior scleral canal wall in early experimental glaucoma. *Invest Ophthalmol Vis Sci.* 2003;44:623–637.
20. Burgoyne CF, Downs JC, Bellezza AJ, Hart RT. Three-dimensional reconstruction of normal and early glaucoma monkey optic nerve head connective tissues. *Invest Ophthalmol Vis Sci.* 2004;45: 4388–4399.
21. Downs JC, Suh JK, Thomas KA, et al. Viscoelastic material properties of the peripapillary sclera in normal and early-glaucoma monkey eyes. *Invest Ophthalmol Vis Sci.* 2005;46:540–546.
22. Downs JC, Yang H, Girkin C, et al. Three dimensional histomorphometry of the normal and early glaucomatous monkey optic nerve head: neural canal and subarachnoid space architecture. *Invest Ophthalmol Vis Sci.* 2007;48:3195–3208.
23. Yang H, Downs JC, Girkin C, et al. 3-D histomorphometry of the normal and early glaucomatous monkey optic nerve head: lamina cribrosa and peripapillary scleral position and thickness. *Invest Ophthalmol Vis Sci.* 2007;48(10):4597–4607.
24. Yang H, Downs JC, Bellezza AJ, Thompson H, Burgoyne CF. 3-D histomorphometry of the normal and early glaucomatous monkey optic nerve head: prelaminar neural tissues and cupping. *Invest Ophthalmol Vis Sci.* 2007;48:5068–5084.
25. Yang H, Downs JC, Burgoyne CF. Physiologic inter-eye differences in monkey optic nerve head architecture and their relation to changes in early experimental glaucoma. *Invest Ophthalmol Vis Sci.* 2009;50: 224–234.
26. Roberts MD, Grau V, Grimm J, et al. Remodeling of the connective tissue microarchitecture of the lamina cribrosa occurs early in experimental glaucoma in the monkey eye. *Invest Ophthalmol Vis Sci.* 2009;50:681–690.
27. Johnson EC, Morrison JC, Farrell S, et al. The effect of chronically elevated intraocular pressure on the rat optic nerve head extracellular matrix. *Exp Eye Res.* 1996;62:663–674.
28. Johnson EC, Deppmeier LM, Wentzien SK, Hsu I, Morrison JC. Chronology of optic nerve head and retinal responses to elevated intraocular pressure. *Invest Ophthalmol Vis Sci.* 2000;41:431–442.
29. Cepurna WO, Kayton RJ, Johnson EC, Morrison JC. Age related optic nerve axonal loss in adult Brown Norway rats. *Exp Eye Res.* 2005;80:877–884.
30. Anderson DR. Ultrastructure of human and monkey lamina cribrosa and optic nerve head. *Arch Ophthalmol.* 1969;82:800–814.
31. Morrison JC, Jerdan JA, L'Hernault NL, Quigley HA. The extracellular matrix composition of the monkey optic nerve head. *Invest Ophthalmol Vis Sci.* 1988;29:1141–1150.
32. Quigley HA, Dorman-Pease ME, Brown AE. Quantitative study of collagen and elastin of the optic nerve head and sclera in human and experimental monkey glaucoma. *Curr Eye Res.* 1991;10:877–888.
33. Hernandez MR. Ultrastructural immunocytochemical analysis of elastin in the human lamina cribrosa. Changes in elastic fibers in primary open-angle glaucoma. *Invest Ophthalmol Vis Sci.* 1992;33:2891–2903.
34. Investigators A: The Advanced Glaucoma Intervention Study (AGIS): 7. The relationship between control of intraocular pressure and visual field deterioration. *Am J Ophthalmol.* 2000;130:429–440.
35. Kass MA, Heuer DK, Higginbotham EJM, et al. The Ocular Hypertension Treatment Study: a randomized trial determines that topical ocular hypotensive medication delays or prevents the onset of primary open-angle glaucoma. *Arch Ophthalmol.* 2002;120: 701–713.

36. Leske MC, Heijl A, Hussein M, et al. Factors for glaucoma progression and the effect of treatment: the early manifest glaucoma trial. *Arch Ophthalmol.* 2003;121:48–56.
37. Anderson DR, Drance SM, Schulzer M. Factors that predict the benefit of lowering intraocular pressure in normal tension glaucoma. *Am J Ophthalmol.* 2003;136:820–829.
38. Nicolela MT, Drance SM. Various glaucomatous optic nerve appearances: clinical correlations. *Ophthalmology.* 1996;103:640–649.
39. Pederson JE, Anderson DR. The mode of progressive disc cupping in ocular hypertension and glaucoma. *Arch Ophthalmol.* 1980;98:490–495.
40. Pederson JE, Gaasterland DE. Laser-induced primate glaucoma. I. Progression of cupping. *Arch Ophthalmol.* 1984;102:1689–1692.
41. Johns KJ, Leonard-Martin T, Feman SS. The effect of panretinal photocoagulation on optic nerve cupping. *Ophthalmology.* 1989;96:211–216.
42. Klein BE, Klein R, Lee KE, Hoyer CJ. Does the intraocular pressure effect on optic disc cupping differ by age? *Trans Am Ophthalmol Soc.* 2006;104:143–148.
43. Sponsel WE, Shoemaker J, Trigo Y, et al. Frequency of sustained glaucomatous-type visual field loss and associated optic nerve cupping in Beaver Dam, Wisconsin. *Clin Exp Ophthalmol.* 2001;29:352–358.
44. Greenfield DS, Siatkowski RM, Glaser JS, Schatz NJ, Parrish RK II. The cupped disc. Who needs neuroimaging? *Ophthalmology.* 1998;105:1866–1874.
45. Bianchi-Marzoli S, Rizzo JF III, Brancato R, Lessell S. Quantitative analysis of optic disc cupping in compressive optic neuropathy. *Ophthalmology.* 1995;102:436–440.
46. Schwartz JT, Reuling FH, Garrison RJ. Acquired cupping of the optic nerve head in normotensive eyes. *Br J Ophthalmol.* 1975;59:216–222.
47. Kalvin NH, Hamasaki DI, Gass JD. Experimental glaucoma in monkeys. I. Relationship between intraocular pressure and cupping of the optic disc and cavernous atrophy of the optic nerve. *Arch Ophthalmol.* 1966;76:82–93.
48. Vrabec F. Glaucomatous cupping of the human optic disk: a neurohistologic study. *Albrecht Von Graefes Arch Klin Exp Ophthalmol.* 1976;198:223–234.
49. Anderson DR, Cynader MS. Glaucomatous optic nerve cupping as an optic neuropathy. *Clin Neurosci.* 1997;4:274–278.
50. Quigley H, Anderson DR. Cupping of the optic disc in ischemic optic neuropathy. *Trans Am Acad Ophthalmol Otolaryngol.* 1977;83:755–762.
51. Trobe JD, Glaser JS, Cassady J, Herschler J, Anderson DR. Nonglaucomatous excavation of the optic disc. *Arch Ophthalmol.* 1980;98:1046–1050.
52. Hayreh SS, Jonas JB. Optic disc morphology after arteritic anterior ischemic optic neuropathy. *Ophthalmology.* 2001;108:1586–1594.
53. Jonas JB, Grundler A. Optic disc morphology in "age-related atrophic glaucoma". *Graefes Arch Clin Exp Ophthalmol.* 1996;234:744–749.
54. Hall ER, Klein BE, Knudtson MD, Meuer SM, Klein R. Age-related macular degeneration and optic disk cupping: the Beaver Dam Eye Study. *Am J Ophthalmol.* 2006;141:494–497.
55. Piette SD, Sergott RC. Pathological optic-disc cupping. *Curr Opin Ophthalmol.* 2006;17:1–6.
56. Alward WL. Macular degeneration and glaucoma-like optic nerve head cupping. *Am J Ophthalmol.* 2004;138:135–136.
57. Danesh-Meyer HV, Savino PJ, Sergott RC. The prevalence of cupping in end-stage arteritic and nonarteritic anterior ischemic optic neuropathy. *Ophthalmology.* 2001;108:593–598.
58. Ambati BK, Rizzo JF III. Nonglaucomatous cupping of the optic disc. *Int Ophthalmol Clin.* 2001;41:139–149.
59. Greenfield DS. Glaucomatous versus nonglaucomatous optic disc cupping: clinical differentiation. *Semin Ophthalmol.* 1999;14:95–108.
60. Sharma M, Volpe NJ, Dreyer EB. Methanol-induced optic nerve cupping. *Arch Ophthalmol.* 1999;117:286.
61. Manor RS. Documented optic disc cupping in compressive optic neuropathy. *Ophthalmology.* 1995;102:1577–1578.
62. Orgul S, Gass A, Flammer J. Optic disc cupping in arteritic anterior ischemic optic neuropathy. *Ophthalmologica.* 1994;208:336–338.
63. Sonty S, Schwartz B. Development of cupping and pallor in posterior ischemic optic neuropathy. *Int Ophthalmol.* 1983;6:213–220.
64. Votruba M, Thiselton D, Bhattacharya SS. Optic disc morphology of patients with OPA1 autosomal dominant optic atrophy. *Br J Ophthalmol.* 2003;87:48–53.
65. Fechtner RD, Weinreb RN. Mechanisms of optic nerve damage in primary open angle glaucoma. *Surv Ophthalmol.* 1994;39:23–42.
66. Burgoyne CF, Morrison JC. The anatomy and pathophysiology of the optic nerve head in glaucoma. *J Glaucoma.* 2001;10:S16–S18.
67. Burgoyne CF, Downs JC, Bellezza AJ, Suh JK, Hart RT. The optic nerve head as a biomechanical structure: a new paradigm for understanding the role of IOP-related stress and strain in the pathophysiology of glaucomatous optic nerve head damage. *Prog Retin Eye Res.* 2005;24:39–73.
68. Downs JC, Burgoyne CF. Mechanical strain and restructuring of the optic nerve head. In: Shaarawy T, Sherwood MB, Hitchings RA, et al., eds. *Glaucoma.* 1st ed. London: W. B. Saunders; 2009.
69. Burgoyne CF, Downs JC. Premise and prediction – how optic nerve head biomechanics underlies the susceptibility and clinical behavior of the aged optic nerve head. *J Glaucoma.* 2008;17:318–328.
70. Sigal IA, Roberts MD, Girard M, Burgoyne CF, Downs JC. Biomechanical changes of the optic disc. In: Levin LA, Albert DM, ed. *Ocular Disease: Mechanisms and Management.* New York: Elsevier; 2009.
71. Downs JC, Roberts MD, Burgoyne CF. Mechanical environment of the optic nerve head in glaucoma. *Optom Vis Sci.* 2008;85:425–435.
72. Quigley HA, Addicks EM. Chronic experimental glaucoma in primates. II. Effect of extended intraocular pressure elevation on optic nerve head and axonal transport. *Invest Ophthalmol Vis Sci.* 1980;19:137–152.
73. Hernandez MR. The optic nerve head in glaucoma: role of astrocytes in tissue remodeling. *Prog Retin Eye Res.* 2000;19:297–321.
74. Agapova OA, Kaufman PL, Lucarelli MJ, Gabelt BT, Hernandez MR. Differential expression of matrix metalloproteinases in monkey eyes with experimental glaucoma or optic nerve transection. *Brain Res.* 2003;967:132–143.
75. Johnson EC, Jia L, Cepurna WO, Doser TA, Morrison JC. Global changes in optic nerve head gene expression after exposure to elevated intraocular pressure in a rat glaucoma model. *Invest Ophthalmol Vis Sci.* 2007;48:3161–3177.
76. Jonas JB, Dichtl A. Optic disc morphology in myopic primary open-angle glaucoma. *Graefes Arch Clin Exp Ophthalmol.* 1997;235:627–633.
77. Fernandez MC, Jonas JB, Naumann GO. Para-papillary chorioretinal atrophy in eyes with shallow glaucomatous optic disk cupping. *Fortschr Ophthalmol.* 1990;87:457–460.
78. Hayreh SS. Pathogenesis of cupping of the optic disc. *Br J Ophthalmol.* 1974;58:863–876.
79. Hayreh SS, Pe'er J, Zimmerman MB. Morphologic changes in chronic high-pressure experimental glaucoma in rhesus monkeys. *J Glaucoma.* 1999;8:56–71.
80. Emery JM, Landis D, Paton D, Boniuk M, Craig JM. The lamina cribrosa in normal and glaucomatous human eyes. *Trans Am Acad Ophthalmol Otolaryngol.* 1974;78:OP290–OP297.
81. Quigley HA, Hohman RM, Addicks EM, Massof RW, Green WR. Morphologic changes in the lamina cribrosa correlated with neural loss in open-angle glaucoma. *Am J Ophthalmol.* 1983;95:673–691.

82. Jonas JB, Grundler A. Optic disc morphology in juvenile primary open-angle glaucoma. *Graefes Arch Clin Exp Ophthalmol.* 1996;234:750–754.
83. Albon J, Purslow PP, Karwatowski WS, Easty DL. Age related compliance of the lamina cribrosa in human eyes. *Br J Ophthalmol.* 2000;84:318–323.
84. Morrison JC, Jerdan JA, Dorman ME, Quigley HA. Structural proteins of the neonatal and adult lamina cribrosa. *Arch Ophthalmol.* 1989;107:1220–1224.
85. Pena JD, Roy S, Hernandez MR. Tropoelastin gene expression in optic nerve heads of normal and glaucomatous subjects. *Matrix Biol.* 1996;15:323–330.
86. Quigley HA. Childhood glaucoma: results with trabeculotomy and study of reversible cupping. *Ophthalmology.* 1982;89:219–226.
87. Hernandez MR, Luo XX, Andrzejewska W, Neufeld AH. Age-related changes in the extracellular matrix of the human optic nerve head. *Am J Ophthalmol.* 1989;107:476–484.
88. Jeffery G, Evans A, Albon J, et al. The human optic nerve: fascicular organisation and connective tissue types along the extra-fascicular matrix. *Anat Embryol (Berl).* 1995;191:491–502.
89. Albon J, Karwatowski WS, Easty DL, Sims TJ, Duance VC. Age related changes in the non-collagenous components of the extracellular matrix of the human lamina cribrosa. *Br J Ophthalmol.* 2000;84:311–317.
90. Bailey AJ, Paul RG, Knott L. Mechanisms of maturation and ageing of collagen. *Mech Ageing Dev.* 1998;106:1–56.
91. Brown CT, Vural M, Johnson M, Trinkaus-Randall V. Age-related changes of scleral hydration and sulfated glycosaminoglycans. *Mech Ageing Dev.* 1994;77:97–107.
92. Albon J, Karwatowski WS, Avery N, Easty DL, Duance VC. Changes in the collagenous matrix of the aging human lamina cribrosa. *Br J Ophthalmol.* 1995;79:368–375.
93. Friedenwald J. Contribution to the theory and practice of tonometry. *Am J Ophthalmol.* 1937;20:985–1024.
94. Kotecha A, Izadi S, Jeffrey G. Age related changes in the thickness of the human lamina cribrosa. *Br J Ophthalmol.* 2006;90:1531–1534.
95. Albon J, Farrant S, Akhtar S, et al. Connective tissue structure of the tree shrew optic nerve and associated ageing changes. *Invest Ophthalmol Vis Sci.* 2007;48:2134–2144.
96. Rochtchina E, Mitchell P, Wang JJ. Relationship between age and intraocular pressure: the Blue Mountains Eye Study. *Clin Exp Ophthalmol.* 2002;30:173–175.
97. Nomura H, Ando F, Niino N, Shimokata H, Miyake Y. The relationship between age and intraocular pressure in a Japanese population: the influence of central corneal thickness. *Curr Eye Res.* 2002;24:81–85.
98. Nomura H, Shimokata H, Ando F, Miyake Y, Kuzuya F. Age-related changes in intraocular pressure in a large Japanese population: a cross-sectional and longitudinal study. *Ophthalmology.* 1999;106:2016–2022.
99. Klein BE, Klein R, Linton KL. Intraocular pressure in an American community. The Beaver Dam Eye Study. *Invest Ophthalmol Vis Sci.* 1992;33:2224–2228.
100. Weih LM, Mukesh BN, McCarty CA, Taylor HR. Association of demographic, familial, medical, and ocular factors with intraocular pressure. *Arch Ophthalmol.* 2001;119:875–880.
101. Leske MC, Connell AM, Wu SY, Hyman L, Schachat AP. Distribution of intraocular pressure. The Barbados Eye Study. *Arch Ophthalmol.* 1997;115:1051–1057.
102. Wu SY, Leske MC. Associations with intraocular pressure in the Barbados Eye Study. *Arch Ophthalmol.* 1997;115:1572–1576.
103. Suzuki Y, Iwase A, Araie M, et al. Risk factors for open-angle glaucoma in a Japanese population: the Tajimi Study. *Ophthalmology.* 2006;113:1613–1617.
104. Geijssen HC. *Studies on Normal Pressure Glaucoma.* Kugler: Amstelveen; 1991.
105. Drance SM, Sweeney VP, Morgan RW, Feldman F. Studies of factors involved in the production of low tension glaucoma. *Arch Ophthalmol.* 1973;89:457–465.
106. Levene RZ. Low tension glaucoma: a critical review and new material. *Surv Ophthalmol.* 1980;24:621–664.
107. Chumbley LC, Brubaker RF. Low-tension glaucoma. *Am J Ophthalmol.* 1976;81:761–767.
108. Goldberg I, Hollows FC, Kass MA, Becker B. Systemic factors in patients with low-tension glaucoma. *Br J Ophthalmol.* 1981;65:56–62.
109. Klein BE, Klein R, Sponsel WE, et al. Prevalence of glaucoma. The Beaver Dam Eye Study. *Ophthalmology.* 1992;99:1499–1504.
110. Shiose Y. Prevalence and clinical aspects of low-tension glaucoma. In: Henkind P, ed. *Acta 24th International Congress of Opthalmology.* Philadelphia: Lippincott; 1983.
111. Tielsch JM, Sommer A, Katz J, et al. Racial variations in the prevalence of primary open-angle glaucoma. The Baltimore Eye Survey [see comments]. *JAMA.* 1991;266:369–374.
112. Gordon MO, Beiser JA, Brandt JD, et al. The Ocular Hypertension Treatment Study: baseline factors that predict the onset of primary open-angle glaucoma. *Arch Ophthalmol.* 2002;120:714–720. discussion 829–830.
113. Nouri-Mahdavi K, Hoffman D, Coleman AL, et al. Predictive factors for glaucomatous visual field progression in the Advanced Glaucoma Intervention Study. *Ophthalmology.* 2004;111:1627–1635.
114. Heijl A, Leske MC, Bengtsson B, Hussein M. Measuring visual field progression in the Early Manifest Glaucoma Trial. *Acta Ophthalmol Scand.* 2003;81:286–293.
115. Broadway DC, Nicolela MT, Drance SM. Optic disk appearances in primary open-angle glaucoma. *Surv Ophthalmol.* 1999;43(Suppl 1):S223–S243.
116. Nicolela MT, Drance SM, Broadway DC, et al. Agreement among clinicians in the recognition of patterns of optic disk damage in glaucoma. *Am J Ophthalmol.* 2001;132:836–844.
117. Nicolela MT, McCormick TA, Drance SM, et al. Visual field and optic disc progression in patients with different types of optic disc damage: a longitudinal prospective study. *Ophthalmology.* 2003;110:2178–2184.
118. May CA. The optic nerve head region of the aged rat: an immunohistochemical investigation. *Curr Eye Res.* 2003;26:347–354.
119. Nicolela MT, Walman BE, Buckley AR, Drance SM. Various glaucomatous optic nerve appearances. A color Doppler imaging study of retrobulbar circulation. *Ophthalmology.* 1996;103:1670–1679.
120. Burgoyne CF, Yang H, Reynaud J, et al. New optical coherence tomography (OCT) targets for optic nerve head imaging in glaucoma. In: Green A, ed. *US Ophthalmic Review.* vol 3. London: Touch Briefings; 2008.
121. Guo L, Tsatourian V, Luong V, et al. En face optical coherence tomography: a new method to analyse structural changes of the optic nerve head in rat glaucoma. *Br J Ophthalmol.* 2005;89:1210–1216.
122. Van Velthoven ME, Faber DJ, Verbraak FD, van Leeuwen TG, de Smet MD. Recent developments in optical coherence tomography for imaging the retina. *Prog Retin Eye Res.* 2007;26:57–77.
123. Srinivasan VJ, Adler DC, Chen Y, et al. Ultrahigh-speed optical coherence tomography for three-dimensional and en face imaging of the retina and optic nerve head. *Invest Ophthalmol Vis Sci.* 2008;49(11):5103–5110.
124. Strouthidis NG, Yang H, Fortune B, Downs JC, Burgoyne CF. Detection of the optic nerve head neural canal opening within three-dimensional histomorphometric and spectral domain optical coherence tomography data sets. *Invest Ophthalmol Vis Sci.* 2009;50(1):214–223.
125. Langham M. The temporal relation between intraocular pressure and loss of vision in chronic simple glaucoma. *Glaucoma.* 1980;2:427–435.

# Chapter 17
# Disc Hemorrhages and Glaucoma

David J. Palmer

## 17.1 Definition of a Disc Hemorrhage

A disc hemorrhage (DH) represents an isolated flame or splinter-shaped bleeding site with radial orientation perpendicular to the disc margin on the optic disc tissue (Fig. 17.1). Alternatively, the DH may be present in the peripapillary retina reaching the disc rim, usually within one disc diameter of the disc margin. Though often associated with glaucoma, the DH may be caused by other conditions such as vascular occlusive disease, diabetic retinopathy, or ischemic optic neuropathy.

The optic disc exam is often performed with a high magnification convex lens and stereoscopic slit lamp biomicroscopy. Documentation of the findings is accomplished by drawing the hemorrhage location, and taking stereoscopic disc photographs. According to the Ocular Hypertensive Treatment Study (OHTS),[1] disc hemorrhages were identified more on disc photographs (84%) compared with the clinical exam and photographic review (16%). Optic disc imaging currently cannot document disc hemorrhages and highlights the need for the clinical exam to complement testing results.[2]

## 17.2 Ocular Blood Flow

In young, healthy, normal individuals, ocular hemodynamics are autoregulated to maintain constant tissue perfusion despite the variability in blood pressure (BP) and intraocular pressure (IOP). In glaucoma patients, it is theorized that autoregulation of ocular blood flow results in ischemic damage and reperfusion injury, which is possibly exacerbated by dips in diastolic perfusion pressure, mean perfusion pressure, and systolic perfusion pressure[3–6] (Table 17.1). In normal tension glaucoma (NTG), Yamakazi and Drance[7] found that those patients with progressive visual field defects had significantly impaired retrobulbar blood flow parameters compared with those with mostly stable visual fields. Another study demonstrated that an increased ophthalmic artery resistive index was associated with a sixfold greater rate of visual field deterioration and may be a predictor of glaucoma progression.[8] Additionally, Harris postulated that vasospasm is more frequent in NTG,[9] and that there are subgroups of patients with reversible vasospasm by $CO_2$ inhalation, which can potentially improve visual function.

Peripapillary atrophy (PPA) is thought to be related to local blood flow insufficiency and is clinically subdivided into the alpha zone and the beta zone (Fig. 17.2), which represents the obliteration of the choroidal blood vessels and dissolution of the retinal pigment epithelium. The presumed absence or dysfunction of the short posterior ciliary artery branches in the peripapillary region may also impair the integrity of the vascular walls in or around the disc causing a DH.[10]

## 17.3 Prevalence of Optic Disc Hemorrhages

In a cross-sectional, population-based study,[11] Healey et al found a 1.4% overall DH prevalence in the primary open angle glaucoma (POAG), NTG, and ocular hypertension (OHT) population in one or both eyes. Subdivided, 8% POAG, 25% NTG, and 1.5% OHT had disc hemorrhages, suggesting a threefold greater prevalence in the NTG group. Diehl et al[12] investigated an unselected glaucoma population in a longitudinal study and reported a baseline DH prevalence of 0% in normal subjects, 0.44% in OHT subjects, and 2.44% in glaucomatous eyes. The authors concluded that the low DH prevalence limits its usefulness as a screening tool for glaucoma. In another longitudinal study over 7 years, Hendrickx et al[13] also detected a threefold higher cumulative incidence of disc hemorrhages in NTG patients (35% NTG, 10.3% POAG, and 10.4% OHT patients). Collectively in these studies, DH associations included increased vertical disc cupping, increased or decreased IOP, systolic hypertension, pseudoexfoliation, more nerve fiber layer atrophy, worse visual fields (VFs), and a female preponderance. Other relationships have included cardiac and cerebral insufficiency and migraines.[14]

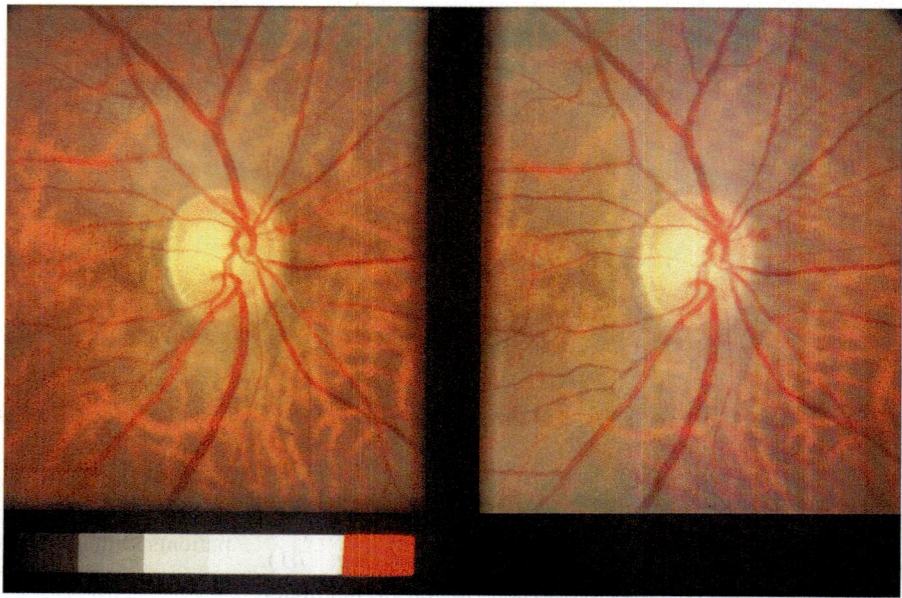

**Fig. 17.1** Disc hemorrhage located at 2:00 on the margin (Photo courtesy of Robert Weinreb, M.D.)

**Table 17.1** Ocular perfusion pressure definitions

| Parameter | Calculation |
| --- | --- |
| Mean arterial pressure (MAP) | ⅔ Diastolic BP + Systolic BP |
| Mean perfusion pressure | MAP − IOP |
| Systolic perfusion pressure | Systolic BP − IOP |
| Diastolic perfusion pressure | Diastolic BP − IOP |

In several retrospective studies,[15,16] VF loss was detected in 63–89% with disc hemorrhages occurring a mean 16.8–36 months later compared with 24–32% without DHs. Optic disc changes were evident in 79% with DH (versus 22% without) a mean 23.8 months later while the timing of DH recurrences was observed a mean 21.5 months later. The majority of disc hemorrhages were in the inferotemporal quadrant, and VF changes primarily corresponded with the site of the DH, especially if recurrent.[15–17] Conversely, another study cited no difference in VF loss between single and recurrent hemorrhages.[18]

## 17.4 Morphologic Relationships

The relationship between disc hemorrhages, the disc, and the retinal nerve fiber layer (RNFL) have been assessed by photographic and imaging studies. Imaging studies of the optic disc and adjacent RNFL have been performed in eyes with and without disc hemorrhages. Localized wedge-shaped defects are increased in NTG and POAG patients versus controls in patients with DH as compared to those without using scanning laser tomography.[19]

Similar tomographic studies in patients with disc hemorrhages documented a smaller neuroretinal rim area and rim volume, especially in the inferotemporal area,[20,21] and polarimetry suggests RNFL thinning is not restricted to the DH sector.[22] Disc hemorrhages appeared to be independent of disc size.[23] In a mostly NTG cohort, PPA, specifically zone beta, appeared larger and more prevalent in DH eyes versus contralateral controls, irrespective of a small neuroretinal rim area and volume.[21] In contrast, PPA did not correlate with the development of unilateral disc hemorrhages among POAG subjects.[24]

## 17.5 Consequences of Disc Hemorrhages

Among subjects in the OHT study with disc hemorrhages,[1] 14% developed disc cupping and/or visual field endpoints over 8 years, representing a 3.7-fold increased POAG risk in a multivariate analysis. Siegner and Netland retrospectively studied 91 patients over a mean of 41.9 months during which VF loss was detected in 63% with disc hemorrhages (versus 24% without DHs) occurring a mean 16.8 months later. Optic disc changes were observed in 79% with disc hemorrhages (versus 22% without) a mean 23.8 months later. Disc hemorrhages mostly involved the inferotemporal quadrants, and were recurrent in 22% of the subjects a mean 21.5 months later.[15] Another retrospective analysis involving 70 subjects over a mean 5.6 years related disc hemorrhages, especially

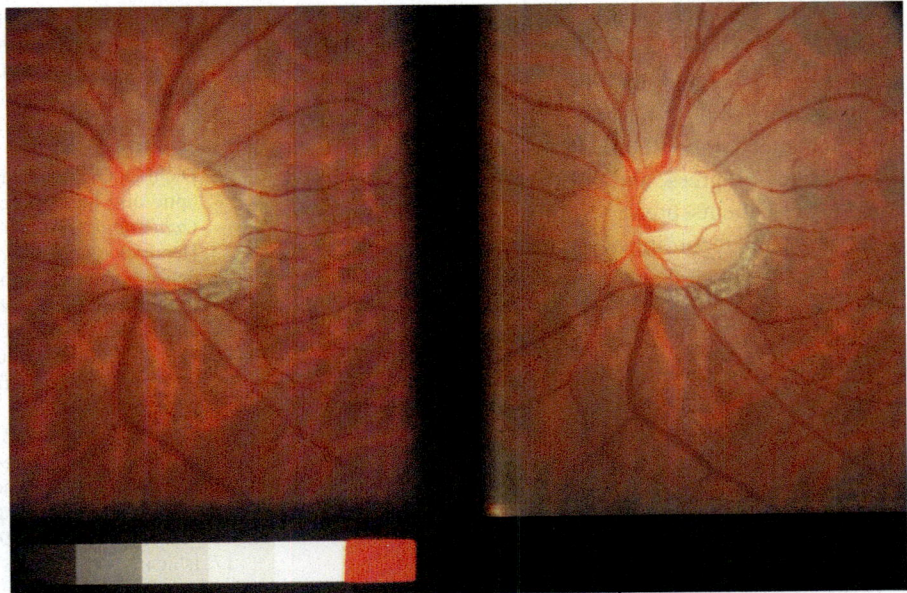

**Fig. 17.2** Peripapillary atrophy of the disc. The lighter area closest to the disc margin is the beta zone (Photo courtesy of Robert Weinreb, M.D.)

recurrent, to progressive mean deviation deterioration or change in probability analysis on Humphrey VF testing. The DH location corresponded with VF changes in the majority of instances.[16] Kim and Park, however, cited no difference in VF loss between single and recurrent hemorrhages.[18]

## 17.6 Disc Hemorrhages and Pressure Reduction

The Collaborative NTG Study[25] was designed to determine whether lowering eye pressure more than 30% versus no treatment altered VF progression times between the groups. A secondary analysis of the study was also performed to determine if pressure-lowering benefits varied according to certain traits. By univariate analysis, treatment benefits occurred in patients without baseline disc hemorrhages, of female gender, especially with a migraine history, with a family history of glaucoma, without a family history of stroke, without a personal history of cardiovascular disease, and with mild disc excavation. Investigating the effects of trabeculectomy with adjunctive mitomycin-C on DH frequency in POAG patients, Miyake et al[26] found the cumulative probability of detecting a DH postsurgery in POAG declined from 33% to 5.5%, and in NTG from 42.1% to 23.1%. The authors concluded that IOP reduction significantly decreased DH frequency in both groups. Conversely, in the Early Manifest Glaucoma Trial (EMGT), Bengtsson et al[6] observed that IOP-reducing treatment was unrelated to the presence or frequency of DHs with a median 8-year follow-up. The authors suggested that disc hemorrhages may not be a sign that a patient is receiving suboptimal IOP-lowering treatment and that glaucoma progression cannot be totally halted by IOP reduction in eyes with disc hemorrhages.

## 17.7 Conclusions

Disc hemorrhages are reportedly related to localized vascular disturbances in the optic disc with possible systemic condition influences. The exact etiology of disc hemorrhages,

**Table 17.2** Local and systemic DH associations

| |
|---|
| *Local factors* |
| Vasospasm |
| Impaired retrobulbar blood flow |
| Reduced ocular perfusion pressure |
| Increased vertical cup/disc ratio |
| Increased or decreased IOP |
| Pseudoexfoliation |
| RNFL atrophy |
| Peripapillary atrophy (zone Beta) |
| Reduced neuroretinal rim and volume |
| *Systemic factors* |
| Nocturnal diastolic hypotension |
| Systolic hypertension |
| Cardiac and cerebral insufficiency |
| Female gender |
| Migraine |
| Diabetes |
| Aspirin use |

however, is not fully understood. Prognostically, single or recurrent disc hemorrhages are related to VF deterioration, a loss in the neuroretinal rim area and rim volume, larger PPA, or alterations in the RNFL as seen by photographic and digital imaging techniques. Fortunately, not all patients with disc hemorrhages progress, and only a minority of OHT, NTG, and POAG patients present with disc hemorrhages. Close observation and recording of disc, PPA, and VF changes, and early, significant IOP reduction may prevent continued vision, disc, or VF loss with or without a DH history. Further understanding of the relationships between blood pressure, blood flow, vasospasm, and hematologic properties (such as elevated anticardiolipin antibody levels[27]) to disc hemorrhages may also benefit treatment strategies and lead to diagnostic instrumentation refinements. Table 17.2 summarizes some of the local and systemic factors associated with disc hemorrhages.

## References

1. Budenz D, Anderson D, Feuer W. Detection and prognostic significance of optic disc hemorrhages during the ocular hypertension treatment study. *Ophthalmology*. 2006;113:2137–2143.
2. Greenfield D, Weinreb R. Role of optic disc imaging in glaucoma clinical practice and clinical trials. *Am J Ophthalmol*. 2008;145:598–603.
3. Harris A, Werner A, Cantor L. Vascular abnormalities in glaucoma: from population-based studies to the clinic? *Am J Ophthalmol*. 2008;145:595–597.
4. Bonomi L, Marchini G, Bernardi P, et al. Vascular risk factors for POAG: the Egna-Neumarkt Study. *Ophthalmology*. 2000;107:1287–1293.
5. Heijl A, Leske MC, Bengtsson B, Early Manifest Glaucoma Trial Group, et al. Reduction of intraocular pressure and glaucoma progression: results from the Early Manifest Glaucoma Trial. *Arch Ophthalmol*. 2002;120:1268–1279.
6. Bengtsson B, Leske MC, Yang A, et al. Disc hemorrhages and treatment in the Early Manifest Glaucoma Trial. *Ophthalmology*. 2008;115:2044–2048.
7. Yamakazi Y, Drance S. The relationship between progression of visual field defects and retrobulbar circulation in patients with glaucoma. *Am J Ophthalmol*. 1997;124:287–295.
8. Galassi F, Sodi A, Ucci F, et al. Ocular hemodynamics and glaucoma prognosis: a color Doppler imaging study. *Arch Ophthalmol*. 2003;121:1711–1715.
9. Harris A, Sergott R, Spaeth G, et al. Color Doppler analysis of ocular vessel blood velocity in normal tension glaucoma. *Am J Ophthalmol*. 1994;118:642–649.
10. Kitazawa Y, Hayakawa T, Sugiyama K, et al. Epidemiology of normal tension glaucoma and the incidence of optic disc hemorrhage. In: Pullinat L, Harris A, Anderson D, Greve E, eds. *Current Concepts of Ocular Blood Flow*. Kugler Publications: The Hague, Netherlands; 1999:63–69.
11. Healey P, Mitchell P, Smith W, et al. Optic disc hemorrhages in a population with and without signs of glaucoma. *Ophthalmology*. 1998;105:216–223.
12. Diehl D, Quigley H, Miller N, et al. Prevalence and significance of optic disc hemorrhage in a longitudinal study of glaucoma. *Arch Ophthalmol*. 1990;108:545–550.
13. Hendrickx K, van den Enden A, Rasker M, et al. Cumulative incidence of patients with disc hemorrhages in glaucoma and the effect of therapy. *Ophthalmology*. 1994;101:1165–1172.
14. Drance S, Anderson D, Schulzer M, Collaborative Normal-Tension Glaucoma Study Group. Risk factors for progression of visual field abnormalities in normal tension glaucoma. *Am J Ophthalmol*. 2001;131:699–708.
15. Siegner S, Netland P. Optic disc hemorrhages and progression of glaucoma. *Ophthalmology*. 1996;103:1014–1024.
16. Rasker M, van den Enden A, Bakker D, et al. Deterioration of visual fields in patients with glaucoma with and without disc hemorrhages. *Arch Ophthalmol*. 1997;115:1257–1262.
17. Ishida K, Yamamoto T, Sugiyama K, et al. Disc hemorrhage is a significantly negative prognostic factor in normal-tension glaucoma. *Am J Ophthalmol*. 2000;129:796–797.
18. Kim S, Park K. The relationship between recurrent optic disc hemorrhage and glaucoma progression. *Ophthalmology*. 2006;113:598–602.
19. Sugiyama K, Uchida H, Tomita G, et al. Localized wedge-shaped defects of retinal nerve fiber layer and disc hemorrhage in glaucoma. *Ophthalmology*. 1999;106:1762–1767.
20. Liou S, Sugiyama K, Uchida H, et al. Morphometric characteristics of optic disk with disk hemorrhage in normal-tension glaucoma. *Am J Ophthalmol*. 2001;132:618–625.
21. Ahn J, Kang J, Park K. Correlation between a disc hemorrhage and peripapillary atrophy in glaucoma patients with a unilateral disc hemorrhage. *J Glaucoma*. 2004;13:9–14.
22. Gunvant P, Zheng Y, Essock E, et al. Predicting subsequent visual field loss in glaucomatous subjects with disc hemorrhage using retinal nerve fiber layer polarimetry. *J Glaucoma*. 2005;14:20–25.
23. Jonas J, Martus P, Budde W, et al. Morphologic predictive factors for development of optic disc hemorrhages in glaucoma. *Invest Ophthalmol Vis Sci*. 2002;43:2956–2961.
24. Jonas JH, Martus P, Budde W. Inter-eye differences in chronic open-angle glaucoma patients with unilateral disc hemorrhages. *Ophthalmology*. 2002;109:2078–2083.
25. Anderson D, Drance S, Schulzer M, Collaborative Normal-Tension Glaucoma Study Group. Factors that predict the benefit of lowering intraocular pressure in normal tension glaucoma. *Am J Ophthalmol*. 2003;136:820–829.
26. Miyake T, Sawada A, Yamamoto T, et al. Incidence of disc hemorrhages in open-angle glaucoma before and after trabeculectomy. *J Glaucoma*. 2006;15:164–171.
27. Balwantray C, Mikelberg F, Balaszi A, Canadian Glaucoma Study Group, et al. Canadian Glaucoma Study. 2. Risk factors for the progression of open-angle glaucoma. *Arch Ophthalmol*. 2008;126:1030–1036.

# Chapter 18
# Some Lessons from the Disc Appearance in the Open Angle Glaucomas

Stephen M. Drance

In a 1973[1] study of risk factors, it was shown that the condition very rarely progressed for normal pressure glaucoma patients with a history of a major shock-like state preceding the diagnosis of their glaucoma; whereas patients without such a history of shock usually did have their glaucoma worsen over time.

In 1977, Spaeth,[2] reporting on fluorescein angiography studies of glaucomatous eyes, suggested the existence of four groups of glaucoma patients. The first group, categorized with primary hyperbaric glaucoma, was characterized by progressive nerve changes with high intraocular pressures (IOPs) in the absence of fluorescein appearances of ischemia. These discs showed symmetric, round enlargement of the optic cups, and the laminae cribrosa were bowed backward. The second group was identified as having primary ischemic loss with glaucoma-like involvement of the optic nerve in the absence of a high IOP. These patients had a well-defined area of absolute hypofluorescence on their discs, usually inferotemporally located with eccentrically placed cupping. Linear hemorrhages were often seen in the damaged part of the disc, and they had dense, often absolute, paracentral scotomas, which were often noticed by the patients, in the upper portion of the visual field. The third group was classified with secondary ischemic glaucoma; it showed inferotemporal or superotemporal cupping with arcuate scotomas and optic nerve hypoperfusion, on fluorescein angiography that changed in size and density with IOP levels. The fourth group consisted of cases that did not fall into the previous three groups.

In 1982, Greve and Geijssen[3] described an optic nerve appearance that they called the "senile sclerotic low-tension glaucoma disc." Geijssen[4] then studied the differences between four groups of normal pressure glaucoma patients with myopic normal pressure glaucomatous discs, focal ischemic normal pressure glaucoma discs, senile sclerotic normal pressure glaucoma discs, and finally a group of discs showing a generalized enlargement of the optic cup.

They found no clear differences between the glaucoma patients with elevated IOP and those with normal pressure, but there were clear-cut differences in their four subgroups.

Details of our study of glaucoma patients with the same four "pure" phenotypic disc appearances have been fully described in the literature[5,6] and included patients whose IOP had never been recorded above 21-mm Hg. The different disc appearances are shown in Fig. 18.1.

Stereo optic disc photographs of 1,870 subjects with chronic open angle glaucoma (COAG), or a suspicion of glaucoma, were first reviewed in a masked fashion by the investigators to find optic nerve heads featuring the pure forms of the four types of glaucomatous appearance named by Geijssen and Greve (Fig. 18.1).

1. Focal ischemic: A disc with localized tissue loss (polar notching) within the superior and/or inferior pole and an otherwise relatively intact neuroretinal rim. In many cases, the notch was associated with a small, localized area of peripapillary atrophy.
2. Myopic disc with glaucoma: A tilted, obliquely implanted disc with a myopic temporal crescent of peripapillary atrophy and additional evidence of glaucomatous damage such as thinning of the superior and/or inferior neuroretinal rim in the absence of degenerative myopia.
3. Senile sclerotic disc: A saucerized, shallow cup and gently sloping sides; a "moth-eaten" appearance and peripapillary atrophy surrounding the nerve and often with some choroidal sclerosis.
4. Verifiable generalized enlargements of the optic cup were characterized by a uniformly enlarged, round cup, and no localized thinning of the neuroretinal rim. The enlargement of the cup had to be confirmed over time, usually from previous photographs, or the glaucomatous nature of the enlarged cup had to be confirmed by a glaucoma-like visual field defect.

Only 123 optic disc photographs of the 1,870 could be classified as pure focal ischemic glaucoma ($n=38$), myopic glaucoma ($n=37$), senile sclerotic glaucoma ($n=24$), and glaucoma with verifiable generalized enlargement of the optic cup ($n=24$) and were available for study. Most discs could not be classified because either the very advanced glaucomatous

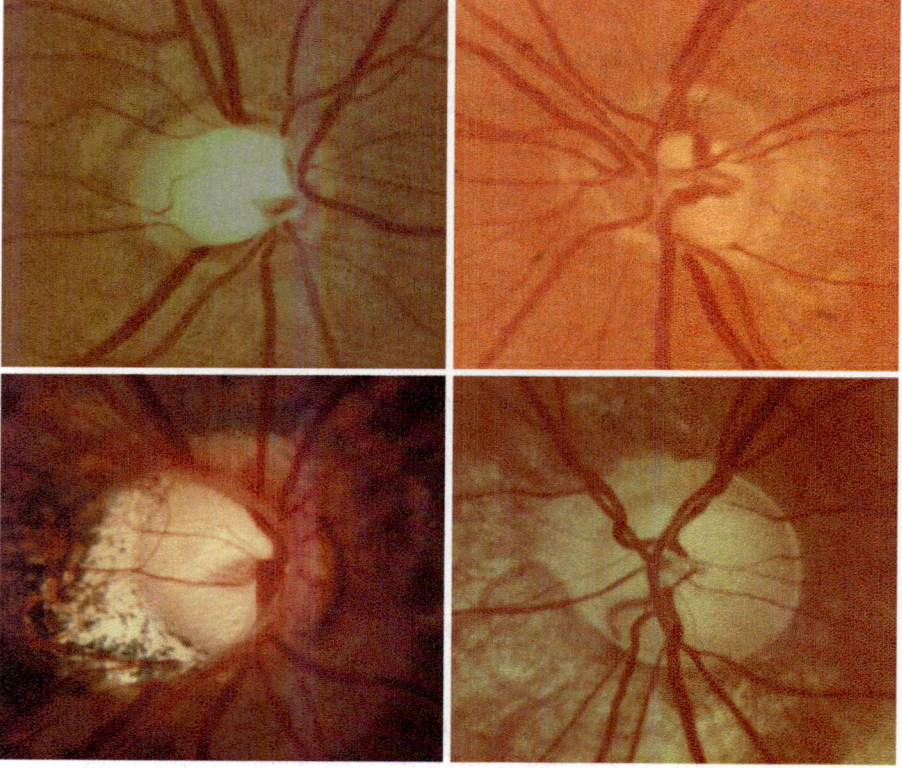

**Fig. 18.1** The appearances of the four types of glaucomatous discs. The generalized enlargement of the cup is seen (*top left*) while the focal ischemic disc shows the localized inferior rim defect (*top right*). The myopic glaucomatous disc appearance is seen (*bottom left*) and the senile sclerotic (atrophic) disc can be seen (*bottom right*)

damage could not be classified or because they had mixtures of more than one grouping. When there was any disagreement in disc classification between the investigators, the patients were not included in the study.

The following information was then collated from the clinical charts of the 123 patients: age; sex; race; ocular data including family history of glaucoma; visual acuity; visual field data; the highest untreated, recorded IOPs measured by applanation tonometry; and the mean of the three highest treated or untreated, recorded IOPs. The presence of migraine, cold hands/feet, vascular hypertension, ischemic heart disease, cerebral ischemic disease, hemodynamic crises, diabetes, and thyroid disease were noted, and drug and smoking histories were ascertained. The patients included those with COAG as well as those with normal-tension glaucoma (NTG).

The analysis showed the group of patients with myopic glaucoma was significantly younger than the groups with the other optic disc appearances. Patients with senile sclerotic glaucoma were significantly older than those with other optic disc appearances. There was a significant excess of men in the myopic glaucoma group, and more women in the focal ischemic group. The level of IOP, both as the highest untreated recorded pressure and the mean of the three highest recorded pressures, was significantly greater in the group of eyes with generalized enlargement of the optic cup. The visual field defects were densest in the focal ischemic group in comparison with either senile sclerotic glaucoma or the group with evidence of generalized cup enlargement. A known family history of glaucoma was not significantly different between the groups.

Both a peripheral vasospastic response to temperature change and the subjective complaint of cold extremities were significantly more common in the focal ischemic group and significantly less common in the group with generalized cup enlargement. Migraine was also more prevalent in the focal ischemic group in comparison with the other groups. The overall mean vasospastic score for the focal ischemic group was significantly higher than in the other groups. There was a tendency for the vasospastic parameters to be more prevalent in the myopic glaucoma group.

Hypertension and ischemic heart disease were far more prevalent in the senile sclerotic group in comparison with the other groups. Diabetes and cerebral ischemic disease were also more common in the senile sclerotic group, but the differences were not statistically significant. The overall mean cardiovascular disease score was significantly higher in the senile sclerotic group when compared with the others. Thyroid disease (mainly hypothyroidism) was also found to be more prevalent in the senile sclerotic group.

It should be noted that patients who had verifiable evidence of a generalized neuroretinal rim diminution with increase of the overall cupping always had markedly elevated IOPs and statistically less evidence of vasospastic disease than the other groups. There may, of course, be other disc appearances yet to be recognized, which might manifest other risk factors that fail to be detected when an overall multifactorial disease such as glaucoma is studied without breaking it down by phenotypes.

While the "pure" forms of the four disc appearances are relatively uncommon, patients who show manifestations of more than one recognizable phenotypic disc appearance are common (Fig. 18.2). It is quite possible that some patients with such mixed disc appearances may have pressure sensitive disease and later develop pressure independent changes when they develop ischemic vascular disease.

It should be noted that the focal ischemic, senile sclerotic, and the myopic groups could have somewhat elevated or normal IOPs, whereas the generalized cup enlargements were always associated with high IOPs.

In 1990,[7] we reported two glaucoma populations by principal component analysis. One was related to vasospasticity to cold, the presence of cold hands and feet, migrainous attacks, and somewhat low blood pressure. In this group, there was a linear relationship between the highest IOP and the amount of visual field loss, while the other group had virtually no vasospasm but showed the presence of biochemical abnormalities usually associated with small vessel disease. This latter group showed no relationship between the highest recorded IOP and the amount of field defect. All patients whose electrocardiograms showed evidence of ischemic heart disease, that were not part of the grouping, were in fact in the ischemic cluster. It was therefore clear that the open angle glaucoma patients belonged to either a vasospastic pressure-dependent cluster or to a nonpressure-dependent ischemic vascular cluster. Both clusters contained the so-called normal tension patients and those in whom the IOP was elevated.

## 18.1 Conclusion

Between 1998 and 2003, the multicenter Normal Tension Glaucoma Study[8–12] published five papers reporting its findings. The clinically and statistically significant findings were:

1. Thirty percent or greater IOP reduction altered the progression of the disease and was beneficial to the treated patients when cataracts were taken into account.
2. Twenty percent of the patients who had major IOP reductions continued to progress.
3. Fifty percent of the untreated patients did not show progression, as defined by the study, even though their IOPs remained untreated and at their previous IOP levels. In 45% of these untreated patients, progression occurred rather slowly, but in 5%, the progression was rapid.
4. The risk factors for a more rapid progression in the untreated patients were female gender, history of migraine, and the presence of disc hemorrhages at the baseline examinations. An oriental background determined a more benign course than in Caucasians.
5. In a univariate analysis, the factors, which reduced the effectiveness of IOP reduction, appeared to be male gender, a history of ischemic cardiovascular disease, a family history of cerebrovascular disease, and the presence of disc hemorrhages.
6. The author estimates that even in NTG patients, 65% have an IOP sensitive disease.

The three studies show that there are at least two glaucoma populations: one vasospastic and related to IOP levels, and the other predominantly with occlusive vascular disease, which was IOP independent. There is a large group (65%), even among the normal tension glaucoma patients, who have pressure-sensitive disease that responds well to IOP lowering. There were, however, some 20% who continued to progress in spite of the greater than 30% IOP reduction. The fact that some 50% of NTG patients in whom the IOP was not therapeutically reduced showed no obvious progression of their field defects over prolonged time also suggests that their disease might not be pressure sensitive. In 50% of untreated NTG patients, there

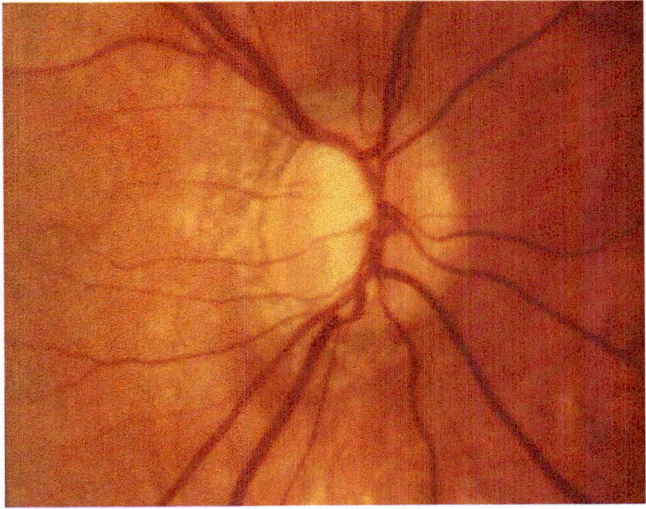

**Fig. 18.2** A mixed focal ischemic and senile sclerotic disc that suggests IOP sensitive disease, which should respond to IOP reduction. The senile sclerotic components probably indicate a cardiovascular origin that might be IOP insensitive. IOP reduction might stabilize the disease but may later be followed by progression in spite of IOP reduction

was no measurable progression. Progression takes place most steeply in women and in migraineurs, who also have the most favorable benefit from IOP reduction. Males, patients with a history of occlusive vascular disease, those with a family history of stroke, and those with disc hemorrhages derived least benefit from IOP reduction. The disc appearances are related to the same risk factors and should be clinically helpful in a more rational management of the disease.

A lot of study should now be focused on these and other yet-to-be-discovered, nonpressure-related risk factors and their interrelationships with one another and with IOP to best understand and manage this complex and enigmatic disease.

The author has no proprietary interest in any of the findings reported in this article.

## References

1. Drance SM, Sweeney VP, Morgan RW, Feldman F. Studies of factors involved in the production low-tension glaucoma. *Arch Ophthalmol*. 1973;89:457–465.
2. Spaeth GL. Fluorescein angiography: Its contributions towards understanding the mechanisms of visual loss in glaucoma. *Trans Am Ophthalmol Soc*. 1975;73:491–553.
3. Greve EL, Geijssen HC. The relation between excavation and visual field in glaucoma patients with high and with low intraocular pressure. *Doc Ophthalmol Proc Series*. 1982;35:35–424.
4. Geijssen HC. *Studies on normal pressure glaucoma*. Amsterdam: Kugler Publications; 1991.
5. Nicolela MT, Drance SM. Various glaucomatous optic nerve appearances: clinical correlations. *Ophthalmology*. 1996;103:640–649.
6. Broadway DC, Nicolela MT, Drance SM. Disc appearance in primary open angle glaucoma. *Surv Ophthalmol*. 1999;43:S223–S243.
7. Schulzer M, Drance SM, Carter CJ, Brooks DE, Douglas GR, Lau W. Biostatistical evidence for two distinct chronic open angle glaucoma populations. *Br J Ophthalmol*. 1990;74:196–200.
8. Collaborative Normal Tension Glaucoma Study Group. Comparison of glaucomatous progression between untreated patients with normal-tension glaucoma and patients with therapeutically reduced intraocular pressures. *Am J Ophthalmol*. 1998;126:487–497.
9. Collaborative Normal-tension Glaucoma Study Group. The effectiveness of intraocular pressure reduction in the treatment of normal-tension glaucoma. *Am J Ophthalmol*. 1998;126:498–505.
10. Collaborative Normal-tension Glaucoma Study Group. Natural history of normal-tension glaucoma. *Ophthalmology*. 2001;108:247–257.
11. Anderson DR, Drance SM, Schulzer M. As writing committee for the Collaborative Normal Tension Glaucoma Study Group. Risk factors for progression of visual field abnormalities in normal tension glaucoma. *Ophthalmology*. 2001;131:699–708.
12. Anderson DR, Drance SM, Schulzer M. As writing committee for the Collaborative Normal Tension Glaucoma Study Group. Factors that predict the benefit of lowering IOP in normal tension glaucoma. *Am J Ophthalmol*. 2003;136:820–829.

# Chapter 19
# Evaluating the Optic Nerve for Glaucomatous Progression

Felipe A. Medeiros

Identification of progressive glaucomatous damage to the optic disc is one of the most important aspects of glaucoma management, yet it remains largely subjective and imprecise. Progressive change in the appearance of the optic disc or retinal nerve fiber layer (RNFL) often precedes the development of visual field defects in glaucoma.[1-10] Because visual field defects on standard automated perimetry may only be detected after a substantial number of nerve fibers has been lost, assessment of the optic disc and RNFL is essential for monitoring the initial stages of the disease. Before the development of visual field defects, structural changes in the optic disc or RNFL may be the only evidence for the ophthalmologist that the glaucoma is progressing and treatment needs to be intensified. Even in the presence of visual field defects, progression of optic disc damage may occur without any detectable evidence of functional deterioration.[11-17]

Because of the wide variability of the optic disc appearance in the normal population, it is frequently not possible to establish the diagnosis of glaucoma based on a single examination of the optic disc. This is especially true in the early stages of the disease. For some patients, a confirmed diagnosis can only be established by demonstrating change during follow-up. Change here means alteration of the appearance of the optic disc in comparison with its previous appearance. Therefore, demonstration of change requires continued monitoring and documentation of the optic disc and RNFL appearance.

## 19.1 Clinical Assessment of Progressive Damage to the Optic Disc and RNFL

In clinical practice, the optic disc and RNFL are routinely assessed through either direct ophthalmoscopy or fundus biomicroscopy using high magnification lens (e.g., Volk 78D). The ophthalmologist then records his or her observations in a drawing or description based on the clinical examination. The description of the optic disc examination using only a simple measure such as the cup/disc ratio is insufficient for this purpose. Even a good optic disc drawing is of limited value when comparing examinations over time. Glaucomatous changes in the optic disc occur slowly over several years, and even very well-drawn representations or detailed descriptions of the optic disc can be insufficient to detect small progressions of the glaucomatous lesion. Besides, assessment of the structural characteristics of the optic disc, such as the cup/disc ratio, is subjective and can vary widely among different examiners. Objective recording of the appearance of the optic disc is therefore essential to monitor a patient with glaucoma or suspect of having the disease.

Optic disc photographs remain the gold standard for documentation and monitoring of optic disc appearance. Monocular photographs often fail to provide enough information on the contour of the optic disc cup to permit an adequate assessment of progressive changes. Whenever possible, stereophotographs should be used to document the optic disc appearance.[18] Stereophotographs can be either simultaneous or nonsimultaneous (pseudo-stereophoto). Although simultaneous stereoscopic photographs are preferable, sequential pseudo-stereophotos are generally sufficient for adequate monitoring of the patient. If stereoscopic photographs are impossible to obtain, monocular photographs are still preferable to a simple schematic drawing or description of the appearance of the optic nerve.

Among the limitations of the use of stereophotography for optic disc monitoring is the lack of consistency in the quality of photographs over time and the subjectivity involved in their interpretation. The comparison of photographs for detection of progression can be largely influenced by the examiner skills. To reduce the subjectivity of optic disc evaluation, several objective imaging methods have been developed such as confocal scanning laser ophthalmoscopy, scanning laser polarimetry, and optical coherence tomography. These methods, and their use for evaluation of glaucoma progression, are discussed in detail elsewhere in this book.

Evaluation of serial optic disc photographs for detection of optic disc change should follow a predefined scheme covering all the important points. Signs of glaucoma progression on the optic disc can be very subtle and easily overlooked unless a meticulous examination is performed. Initially, the ophthalmologist should evaluate the quality of the photographs available for comparison. Is the quality good enough to permit an adequate assessment of optic disc progression? Is the stereopsis consistent among photographs? Differences in magnification, focus, illumination, color or stereopsis can influence the comparison between photographs, resulting in either false-positives or false-negatives assessments of glaucoma progression. Changes in the color of photographs can produce changes in the rim color giving a false impression of progression.

After quality evaluation, the examiner should carefully compare the characteristics of the neuroretinal rim and optic disc cup between photographs. This comparison should be performed in each sector of the optic disc. Progressive changes in the position of blood vessels are useful "clues" to detect progressive rim loss. The position and location of deflection of blood vessels should be compared across all available photographs to uncover changes that may indicate neuroretinal rim loss in a specific sector. Baring of the circumlinear vessel or progressive nasalization of vessels can also occur with progression.

Progressive neuroretinal rim loss in glaucoma can occur in either a diffuse or a localized pattern. With diffuse neuroretinal rim loss, all sectors show progressive thinning (Fig. 19.1a and b), and there is concentric enlargement of the cup. Although neuroretinal rim loss can be observed in all sectors, the progression can be more marked in one sector than the other. The term temporal unfolding is used to describe a subtype of concentric enlargement of the cup in which the major neuroretinal rim loss occurs away from the central vascular trunk, extending superiorly and inferiorly, as well as temporally (Fig. 19.2a and b).

With localized neuroretinal rim loss, the progression occurs in a specific sector, usually affecting the inferior temporal or superior temporal rim (Fig. 19.3a and b). The development of a notching is a type of localized rim loss. It should be noted that, although localized progression is more commonly seen in the superior and inferior poles of the optic disc, in some cases the damage is most prominent at the nasal sector. Therefore, the examiner should pay attention to all disc sectors when comparing photographs for progression.

After evaluation of changes in the neuroretinal rim and optic disc cup, the exam should be directed toward the RNFL. Changes in the RNFL can frequently precede changes in the optic disc in patients with glaucoma progression.[1] *Red-free RNFL photographs* provide a permanent record of the RNFL aspect, permitting comparisons over time and evaluation of diffuse or localized RNFL loss. However, these photographs are generally difficult to obtain and are rarely used in clinical practice. Although not ideal, color stereoscopic optic disc photographs can be used instead of red-free photographs for RNFL assessment. When evaluating serial photographs, the examiner should compare the brightness and striations of the RNFL to detect the presence of diffuse or localized loss. Diffuse RNFL loss appears as a diffuse reduction in the brightness and loss of normal striations. This pattern of RNFL loss is difficult to detect using color photographs.

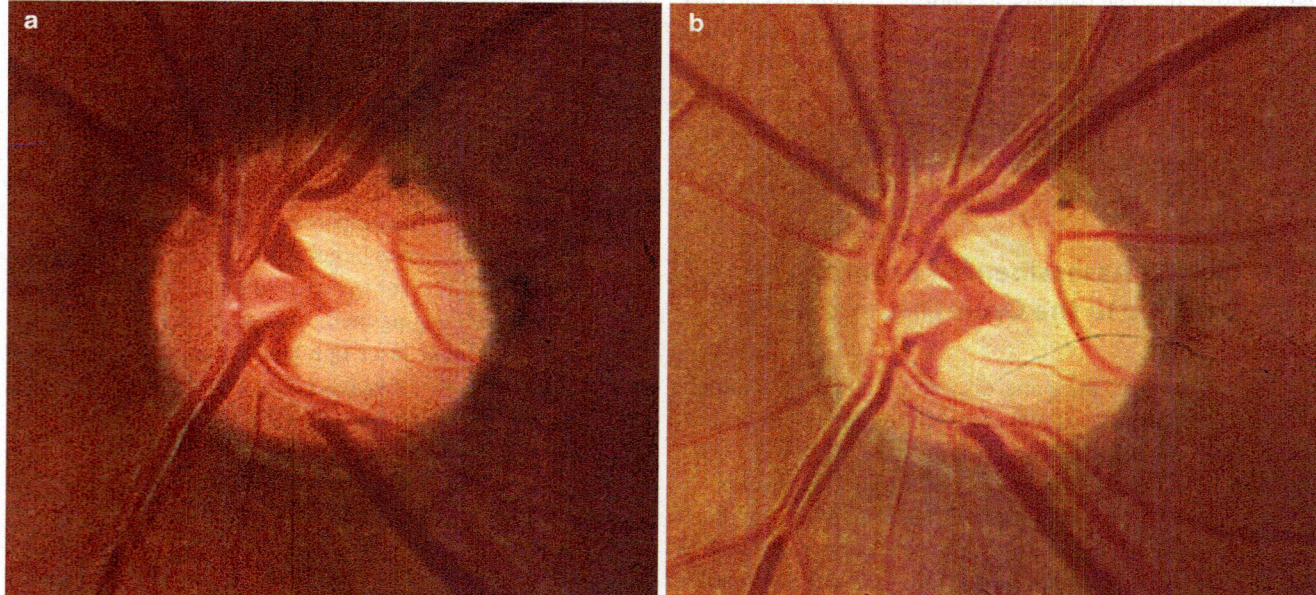

**Fig. 19.1** (**a**) Diffuse neuroretinal rim loss. (**b**) All sectors show progressive thinning and there is concentric enlargement of the cup

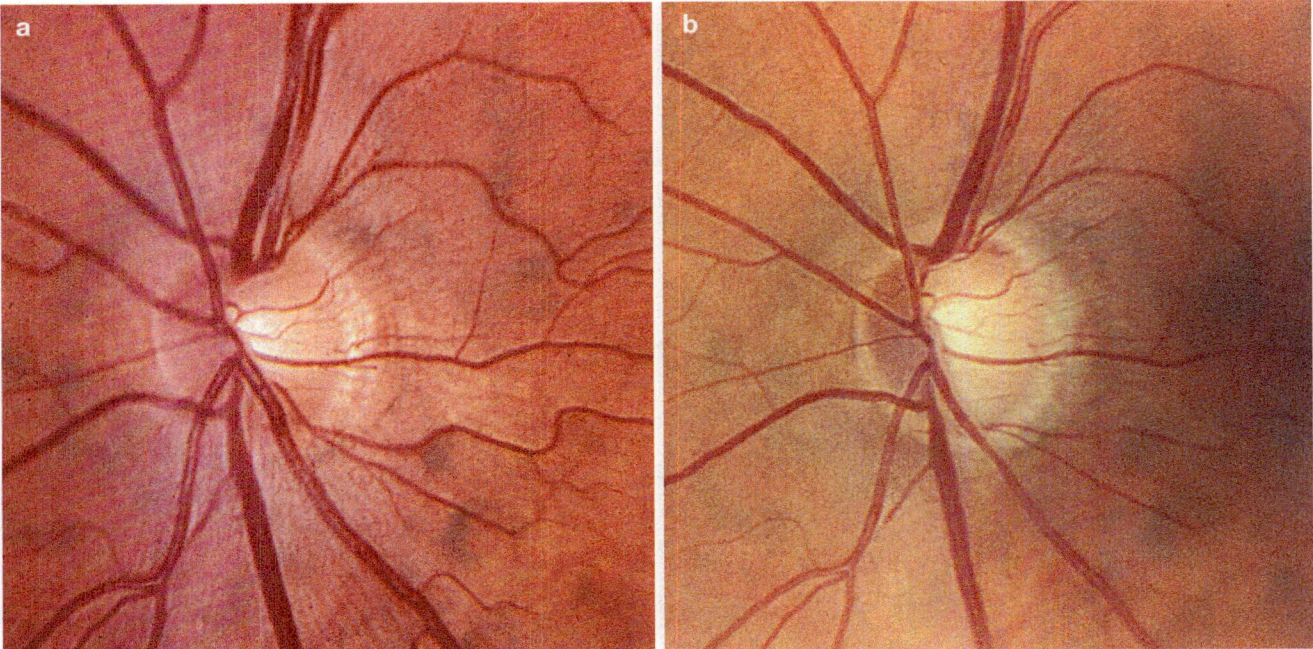

**Fig. 19.2** (a) Temporal unfolding is a subtype of concentric enlargement of the cup in which the major neuroretinal rim loss occurs away from the central vascular trunk, (b) extending superiorly and inferiorly, as well as temporally

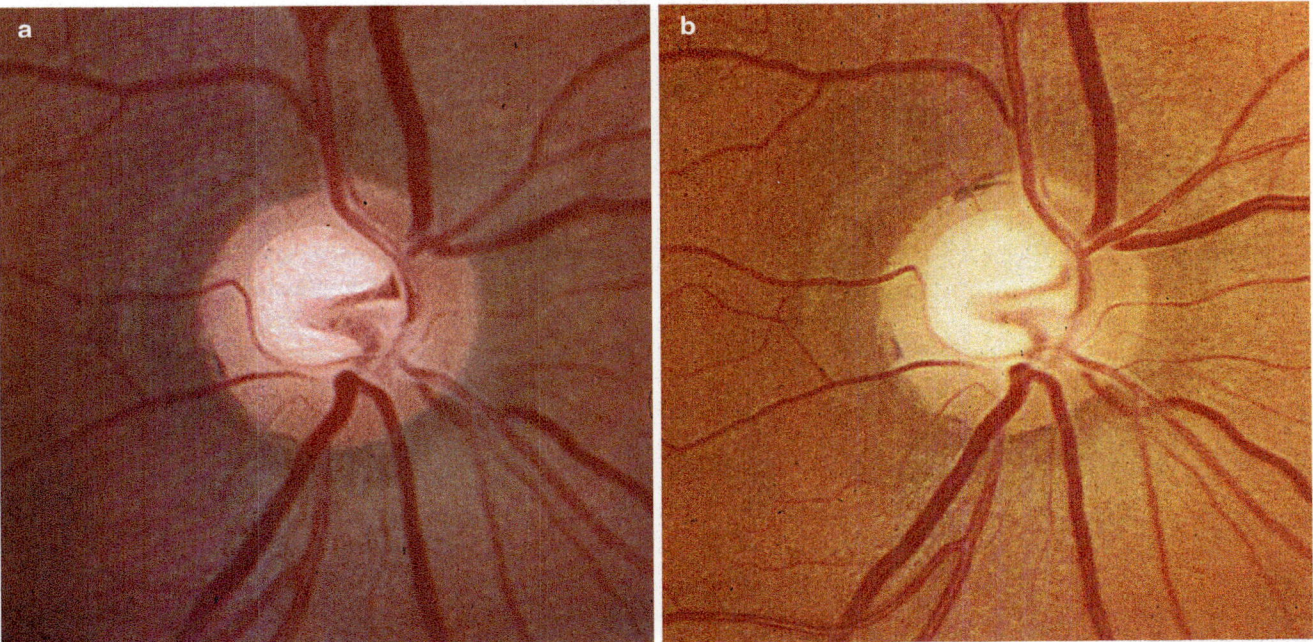

**Fig. 19.3** (a) With localized neuroretinal rim loss, the progression occurs in a specific sector, (b) usually affecting the inferior temporal or superior temporal rim

Localized RNFL loss is easier to detect and appears as wedge-shaped defects extending from the optic disc. The photographs should be compared for development of new wedge-shaped defects or enlargement of previously existing ones. Whenever a wedge-shaped defect is present, it is very important that the examiner compare its extension between the available photographs (Fig. 19.4a and b). The retinal blood vessels can be used as landmarks to evaluate

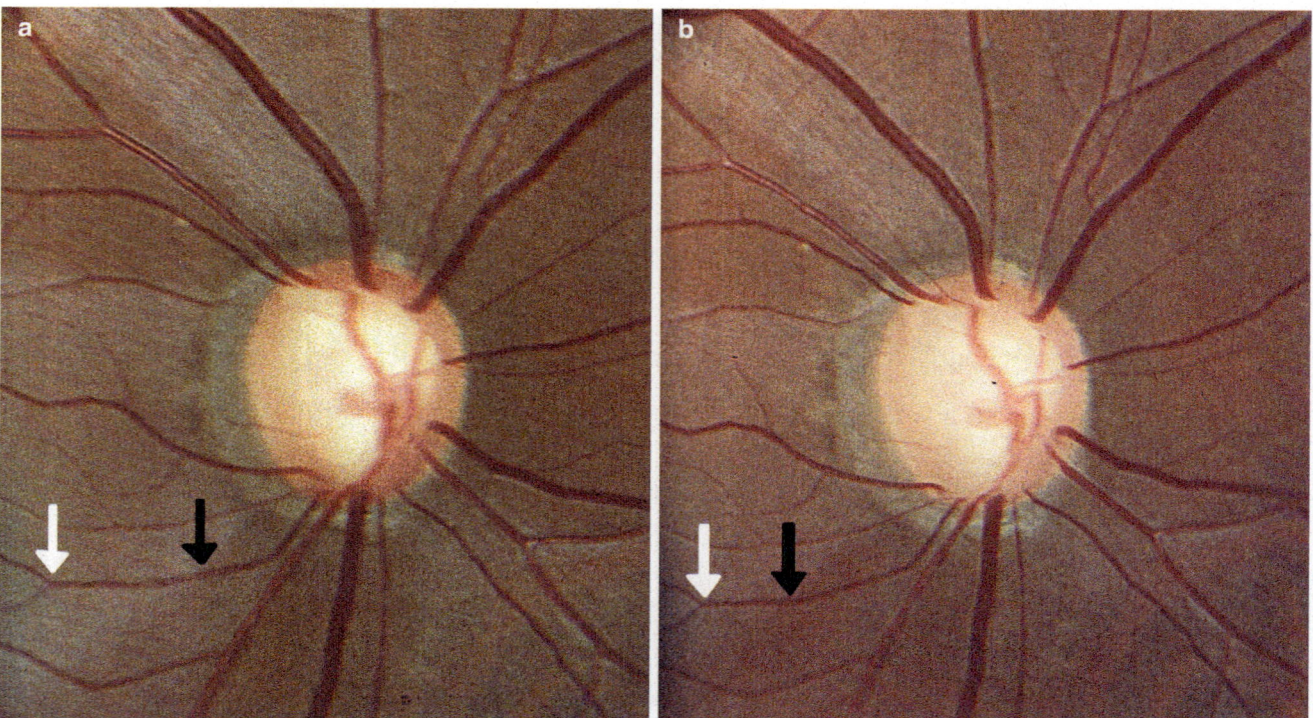

**Fig. 19.4** (a) Localized RNFL loss appears as wedge-shaped defects extending from the optic disc. (b) Whenever a wedge-shaped defect is present, the examiner should compare its extension between the available photographs

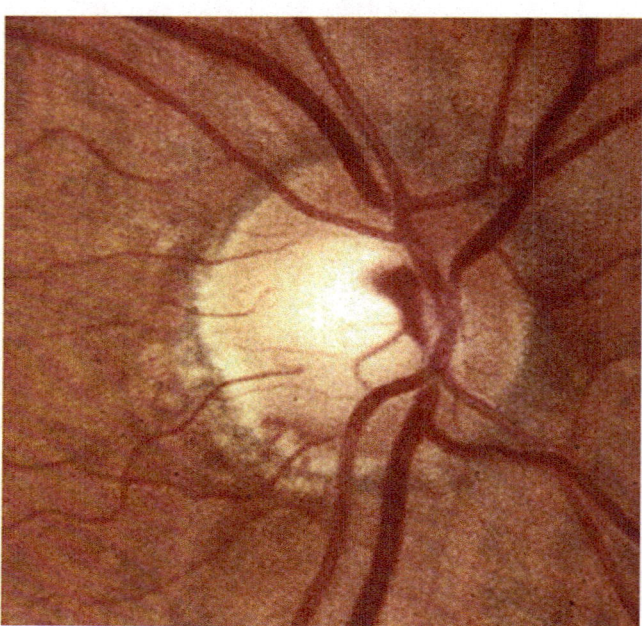

**Fig. 19.5** Optic disc hemorrhage

the position of the wedge-shaped defect margins. Broadening of a previously existing RNFL defect is a commonly overlooked sign of glaucomatous progression.

Special attention must be given for the presence of optic disc hemorrhages (Fig. 19.5). Disc hemorrhages constitute one of the main risk factors for progression of glaucoma.[28–32] Whenever a disc hemorrhage is seen, the examiner should look carefully at the corresponding area of neuroretinal rim and RNFL. Disc hemorrhages are commonly followed by neuroretinal rim loss and progression of RNFL defects.[33]

When evaluating disc photographs for progression, it is also important to observe the changes in the area of parapapillary atrophy, especially in the β zone. Progression of parapapillary atrophy can indicate progressive glaucomatous damage to the optic nerve.[19–25] An increase in the β zone of parapapillary atrophy is associated with progressive neuroretinal rim loss in the corresponding optic disc sector and with progression of visual field defects in glaucoma.[19–27]

## 19.2 Conclusion

Careful examination and objective documentation of the optic disc and RNFL appearance over time are necessary for identification of glaucomatous progression. The examination should follow a series of systematic steps including evaluation of the neuroretinal rim area and RNFL, search for optic disc hemorrhages and evaluation of regions of parapapillary atrophy.

# References

1. Quigley HA, Katz J, Derick RJ, Gilbert D, Sommer A. An evaluation of optic disc and nerve fiber layer examinations in monitoring progression of early glaucoma damage. *Ophthalmology*. 1992;99:19–28.
2. Quigley HA, Reacher M, Katz J, Strahlman E, Gilbert D, Scott R. Quantitative grading of nerve fiber layer photographs. *Ophthalmology*. 1993;100:1800–1807.
3. Sommer A, Miller NR, Pollack I, Maumenee AE, George T. The nerve fiber layer in the diagnosis of glaucoma. *Arch Ophthalmol*. 1977;95:2149–2156.
4. Sommer A, Pollack I, Maumenee AE. Optic disc parameters and onset of glaucomatous field loss. I. Methods and progressive changes in disc morphology. *Arch Ophthalmol*. 1979;97:1444–1448.
5. Sommer A, Katz J, Quigley HA, et al. Clinically detectable nerve fiber atrophy precedes the onset of glaucomatous field loss. *Arch Ophthalmol*. 1991;109:77–83.
6. Tuulonen A, Airaksinen PJ. Initial glaucomatous optic disk and retinal nerve fiber layer abnormalities and their progression. *Am J Ophthalmol*. 1991;111:485–490.
7. Tuulonen A, Lehtola J, Airaksinen PJ. Nerve fiber layer defects with normal visual fields. Do normal optic disc and normal visual field indicate absence of glaucomatous abnormality? *Ophthalmology*. 1993;100:587-597; discussion 597–598.
8. Pederson JE, Anderson DR. The mode of progressive disc cupping in ocular hypertension and glaucoma. *Arch Ophthalmol*. 1980;98:490–495.
9. Airaksinen PJ, Heijl A. Visual field and retinal nerve fibre layer in early glaucoma after optic disc haemorrhage. *Acta Ophthalmol (Copenh)*. 1983;61:186–194.
10. Zeyen TG, Caprioli J. Progression of disc and field damage in early glaucoma. *Arch Ophthalmol*. 1993;111:62–65.
11. Chauhan BC, McCormick TA, Nicolela MT, LeBlanc RP. Optic disc and visual field changes in a prospective longitudinal study of patients with glaucoma: comparison of scanning laser tomography with conventional perimetry and optic disc photography. *Arch Ophthalmol*. 2001;119:1492–1499.
12. Tan JC, Franks WA, Hitchings RA. Interpreting glaucoma progression by white-on-white perimetry. *Graefes Arch Clin Exp Ophthalmol*. 2002;240:585–592.
13. Katz J, Gilbert D, Quigley HA, Sommer A. Estimating progression of visual field loss in glaucoma. *Ophthalmology*. 1997;104:1017–1025.
14. Katz J, Congdon N, Friedman DS. Methodological variations in estimating apparent progressive visual field loss in clinical trials of glaucoma treatment. *Arch Ophthalmol*. 1999;117:1137–1142.
15. Katz J. Scoring systems for measuring progression of visual field loss in clinical trials of glaucoma treatment. *Ophthalmology*. 1999;106:391–395.
16. Lee AC, Sample PA, Blumenthal EZ, Berry C, Zangwill L, Weinreb RN. Infrequent confirmation of visual field progression. *Ophthalmology*. 2002;109:1059–1065.
17. Hitchings R, Varma R, Poinoosawmy D. Optic disc photographs. In: Varma R, Spaeth GL, eds. *The optic nerve in glaucoma*. Philadelphia: Lippincott; 1993.
18. Odberg I, Ruse D. Early diagnosis of glaucoma. The value of successive stereophotography of the optic disc. *Acta Ophthalmol (Copenh)*. 1985;63:257–263.
19. Tezel G, Siegmund KD, Trinkaus K, Wax MB, Kass MA, Kolker AE. Clinical factors associated with progression of glaucomatous optic disc damage in treated patients. *Arch Ophthalmol*. 2001;119:813–818.
20. Tezel G, Dorr D, Kolker AE, Wax MB, Kass MA. Concordance of parapapillary chorioretinal atrophy in ocular hypertension with visual field defects that accompany glaucoma development. *Ophthalmology*. 2000;107:1194–1199.
21. Tezel G, Kolker AE, Wax MB, Kass MA, Gordon M, Siegmund KD. Parapapillary chorioretinal atrophy in patients with ocular hypertension. II. An evaluation of progressive changes. *Arch Ophthalmol*. 1997;115:1509–1514.
22. Tezel G, Kolker AE, Kass MA, Wax MB, Gordon M, Siegmund KD. Parapapillary chorioretinal atrophy in patients with ocular hypertension. I. An evaluation as a predictive factor for the development of glaucomatous damage. *Arch Ophthalmol*. 1997;115:1503–1508.
23. Uchida H, Ugurlu S, Caprioli J. Increasing peripapillary atrophy is associated with progressive glaucoma. *Ophthalmology*. 1998;105:1541–1545.
24. Daugeliene L, Yamamoto T, Kitazawa Y. Risk factors for visual field damage progression in normal-tension glaucoma eyes. *Graefes Arch Clin Exp Ophthalmol*. 1999;237:105–108.
25. Quigley HA, Enger C, Katz J, Sommer A, Scott R, Gilbert D. Risk factors for the development of glaucomatous visual field loss in ocular hypertension. *Arch Ophthalmol*. 1994;112:644–649.
26. Jonas JB, Martus P, Budde WM, Junemann A, Hayler J. Small neuroretinal rim and large parapapillary atrophy as predictive factors for progression of glaucomatous optic neuropathy. *Ophthalmology*. 2002;109:1561–1567.
27. Martinez-Bello C, Chauhan BC, Nicolela MT, McCormick TA, LeBlanc RP. Intraocular pressure and progression of glaucomatous visual field loss. *Am J Ophthalmol*. 2000;129:302–308.
28. Anderson DR, Drance SM, Schulzer M. Natural history of normal-tension glaucoma. *Ophthalmology*. 2001;108:247–253.
29. Sonnsjo B, Dokmo Y, Krakau T. Disc haemorrhages, precursors of open angle glaucoma. *Prog Retin Eye Res*. 2002;21:35–56.
30. Piltz-Seymour J. Disc hemorrhages and glaucoma management. *J Glaucoma*. 2000;9:273–277.
31. Ishida K, Yamamoto T, Kitazawa Y. Clinical factors associated with progression of normal-tension glaucoma. *I Glaucoma*. 1998;7:372–377.
32. Jonas JB, Budde WM, Panda-Jonas S. Ophthalmoscopic evaluation of the optic nerve head. *Surv Ophthalmol*. 1999;43:293–320.
33. Greenfield DS. Optic nerve and retinal nerve fiber layer analyzers in glaucoma. *Curr Opin Ophthalmol*. 2002;13:68–76.

# Chapter 20
# Digital Imaging of the Optic Nerve

Shan Lin and George Tanaka

Why do we need measures of the optic nerve head (ONH) and/or the retinal nerve fiber layer (RNFL) in clinical glaucoma management?

The reason is that glaucoma is a disease of the optic nerve characterized by retinal ganglion cell death and corresponding nerve fiber layer loss. Glaucomatous damage may eventually result in characteristic visual field (VF) loss and ultimately cause blindness. However, studies have shown that a substantial percentage of retinal ganglion cells in the retina and axons in the optic nerve can be lost before functional defects are exhibited on VF testing.[1,2] Moreover, in the Ocular Hypertension Treatment Study more than half of those who reached an end point (glaucoma) were diagnosed based on optic nerve progression.[3] Thus, the ability to detect glaucomatous change prior to visual field damage may lead to early treatment and prevention of future field loss.

In the past, the reference standard for structural documentation of optic nerve head damage has been stereophotography of the ONH. The advantages of this technique include a permanent, reproducible record; potential quantitative assessment of ONH and RNFL parameters; demonstrated correlation with visual field loss; and ability to detect subtle optic disc hemorrhages. However, limitations include limited diagnostic accuracy by itself for screening, expert grading typically required, and difficulty in attaining true stereophotographs in about half of subjects.

Over the past decade, high-resolution ONH and RNFL analyzers have gained widespread use for the diagnosis and follow-up of patients with, and at risk for, glaucoma. However, it is important to investigate whether these devices have been validated as effective for the detection of glaucoma, particularly in cases of preperimetric glaucoma in which visual field loss has not yet occurred and diagnosis is often unclear. Also, are these devices effective in detecting progression of established glaucoma?

## 20.1 Digital Imaging Devices

The devices that will be reviewed here are the confocal scanning laser ophthalmoscope (CSLO), the optical coherence tomography (OCT) machine, and the scanning laser polarimeter (SLP). Brief descriptions of the three technologies will be provided. Normative data have been accumulated for each device. These data are then automatically compared to the clinical patient to aid in determining whether the obtained images represent normal structure or likely glaucomatous optic neuropathy.

### 20.1.1 Confocal Scanning Laser Ophthalmoscopy

The CSLO device generates up to 64 transaxial scans through the ONH/peripapillary retina, and creates a 3-dimensional reconstruction of those tissues. The emitting source is a 670-nm diode laser that creates a beam focused in the $x$-axis and $y$-axis (horizontal and vertical dimensions) of the ONH, perpendicular to the $z$-axis (axis along the optic nerve). The reflected image from this plane is captured as a 2-dimensional scan. Depending on the cup depth, up to 64 successive equidistant images are obtained in order to form a 3-dimensional construct of the ONH region. Surfaces of the optic cup, optic rim, and peripapillary retina are determined by a change in reflectance intensity along the $z$-axis at each point. This allows for the creation of a topographic map from which parameters such as cup-to-disc (C/D) ratio, rim area, and other optic disc can be calculated.

In this chapter, we will focus on the CSLO devices from Heidelberg Engineering (Heidelberg, Germany): the Heidelberg Retina Tomographs I and II (HRT I and HRT II).

The HRT III has the same hardware as the HRT II but also includes a software algorithm for assessing the optic nerve.

The HRT I is able to image 10°, 15°, or 20° of width. The HRT II images at only 15°, and provides better resolution than the HRT I at that width (384×384 pixels, 11-μm lateral resolution). Moreover, the HRT II has more automated features such as serial scans, averaging of the scans, and fine focus and scan depth. User input is required for both devices in the form of drawing the disc margin. The recently released HRT III has an operator-independent assessment of the disc, but evidence-based data on this function remains limited. Optic disc parameters are then quantified relative to the reference plane (defined as that plane 50 μm below the neuroretinal rim as measured along the contour line at the inferior papillomacular bundle). Change analysis does not require user input. Software algorithms in the HRT II and HRT III automatically align and normalize the entire topographic maps. Statistically significant changes in the local surface height relative to the baseline examination are then highlighted and quantified.

### 20.1.2 Optical Coherence Tomography

The OCT obtains axial cross sections of tissues based on optical backscattering, akin to ultrasound technology. The optical backscattering of low-coherence laser light (850 nm) as it passes through layers of differing optical density is recorded by an interferometer and amplified to construct a 2-dimensional image of the scanned area. In the evaluation of glaucoma, scans of the macula, optic disc, and RNFL may be utilized. The RNFL scan images a circle of 3.4 mm diameter centered on the optic disc. The "double hump" of the RNFL is compared to the normative database, to look for diffuse and/or focal defects. A macular thickness map can be created by performing a series of radial scans through the foveola. Recently, the optic disc algorithm was developed that provides a 3-dimensional reconstruction of the ONH. It is based on three axial scans through the center of the disc.

The current model in most clinical use is the third-generation Stratus OCT (aka, OCT III) (Zeiss Meditec, Inc., Dublin, California). It delivers resolution at the 7–8 μm level. Recently Fourier-domain (also known as spectral domain) OCTs from various companies have been approved for clinical use. The resolution of these new devices is in the 4–5 μm range.

### 20.1.3 Scanning Laser Polarimetry

The SLP (GDx, Zeiss Meditec, Inc., Dublin, California) measures the RNFL thickness by assessing the change in polarization (retardation) of the reflected laser beam (780 nm). The microtubules with the RNFL axons cause proportional change in the polarization of the laser. A high-resolution image of 256×256 pixels is created of the optic nerve and peripapillary retina. Three serial scans are generated with each test. The "calculation circle" for the RNFL is 3.2 mm in diameter, centered on the optic disc. It is 8-pixel-wide and is graphically represented as the "double hump" for comparison to the normal range of age-matched controls. The inferior and superior poles represent the thickest portions of the RNFL in normal controls. Some of the parameters presented are based on the RNFL thickness measurements of the calculation circle; however, the nerve fiber indicator (NFI, a summary value that is intended to represent the likelihood of glaucomatous RNFL loss) is based on the entire RNFL thickness map. Also, an available progression algorithm utilizes data based on the entire image, not just the calculation circle.

Currently, the SLP incorporates a compensation mechanism for the cornea (GDx-Variable Corneal Compensator (VCC)), as the cornea was discovered to provide a significant contribution to the polarization detected by the device. This corneal component is often variable and could change with age or surgery.

## 20.2 Are These Devices Able to Detect Glaucoma?

A recent evidence-based assessment of ONH and RNFL analyzers was conducted and published by the Ophthalmic Technology Assessment Committee (OTAC) of the American Academy of Ophthalmology (AAO).[4] In the vast majority of publications, the glaucomatous ("diseased") group was comprised of patients who had visual field loss. As described previously, glaucoma that has advanced to a stage in which visual field loss has occurred is at a more severe stage. The ability of the devices to distinguish normal from such advanced glaucoma is biased toward greater detectability. In practice, the devices have more potential usefulness when they can detect glaucoma before visual field loss has occurred.

Published evidence will be provided as follows for each device. The ability of a test to distinguish between pathologic and normal states is often described in the literature by the area under the receiver operator curve (AUC). It is a graphic representation of the sensitivity plotted against (1-specificity). Values for the area under the ROC range from 0.5 to 1, with the latter value representing the ideal test to discriminate disease from normal.

## 20.3 CSLO

Numerous studies have demonstrated the ability of the HRT I to discriminate glaucoma associated with VF loss from normal[5–9] (Fig. 20.1a–f). In a paper by Miglior et al.,[7] the

**a**

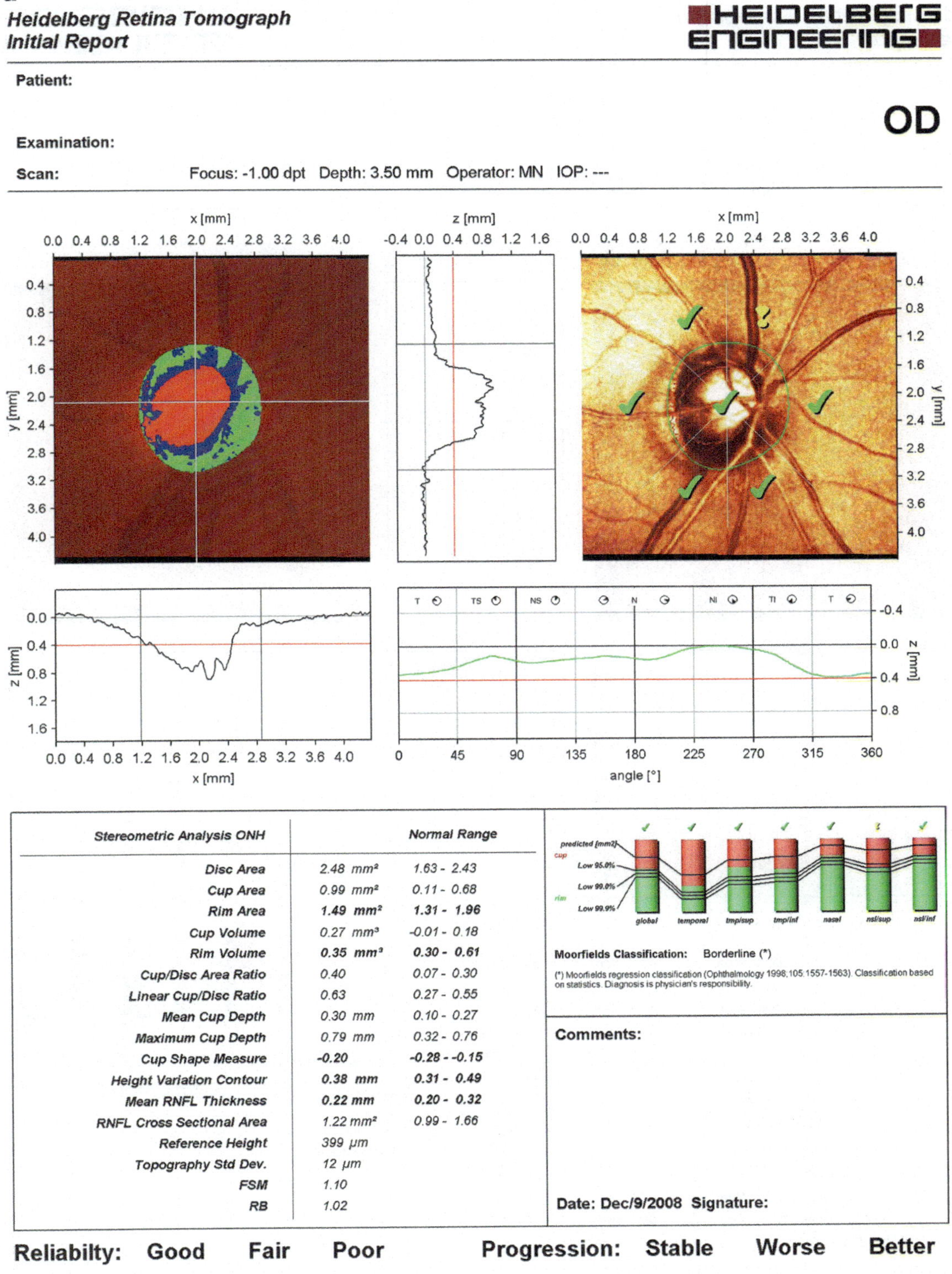

*Heidelberg Retina Tomograph*
*Initial Report*

**HEIDELBERG ENGINEERING**

Patient:

OD

Examination:

Scan:   Focus: -1.00 dpt   Depth: 3.50 mm   Operator: MN   IOP: ---

| Stereometric Analysis ONH | | Normal Range |
|---|---|---|
| Disc Area | 2.48 mm² | 1.63 - 2.43 |
| Cup Area | 0.99 mm² | 0.11 - 0.68 |
| Rim Area | 1.49 mm² | 1.31 - 1.96 |
| Cup Volume | 0.27 mm³ | -0.01 - 0.18 |
| Rim Volume | 0.35 mm³ | 0.30 - 0.61 |
| Cup/Disc Area Ratio | 0.40 | 0.07 - 0.30 |
| Linear Cup/Disc Ratio | 0.63 | 0.27 - 0.55 |
| Mean Cup Depth | 0.30 mm | 0.10 - 0.27 |
| Maximum Cup Depth | 0.79 mm | 0.32 - 0.76 |
| Cup Shape Measure | -0.20 | -0.28 - -0.15 |
| Height Variation Contour | 0.38 mm | 0.31 - 0.49 |
| Mean RNFL Thickness | 0.22 mm | 0.20 - 0.32 |
| RNFL Cross Sectional Area | 1.22 mm² | 0.99 - 1.66 |
| Reference Height | 399 μm | |
| Topography Std Dev. | 12 μm | |
| FSM | 1.10 | |
| RB | 1.02 | |

Moorfields Classification:   Borderline (*)

(*) Moorfields regression classification (Ophthalmology 1998;105:1557-1563). Classification based on statistics. Diagnosis is physician's responsibility.

Comments:

Date: Dec/9/2008   Signature:

**Reliabilty:** Good   Fair   Poor       **Progression:** Stable   Worse   Better

**Fig. 20.1** This is a 53-year-old patient with normal-tension glaucoma. These are the confocal scanning laser ophthalmoscopy (CSLO) images of the optic nerves showing (**a**) significant loss in the supero-nasal region of the right eye and

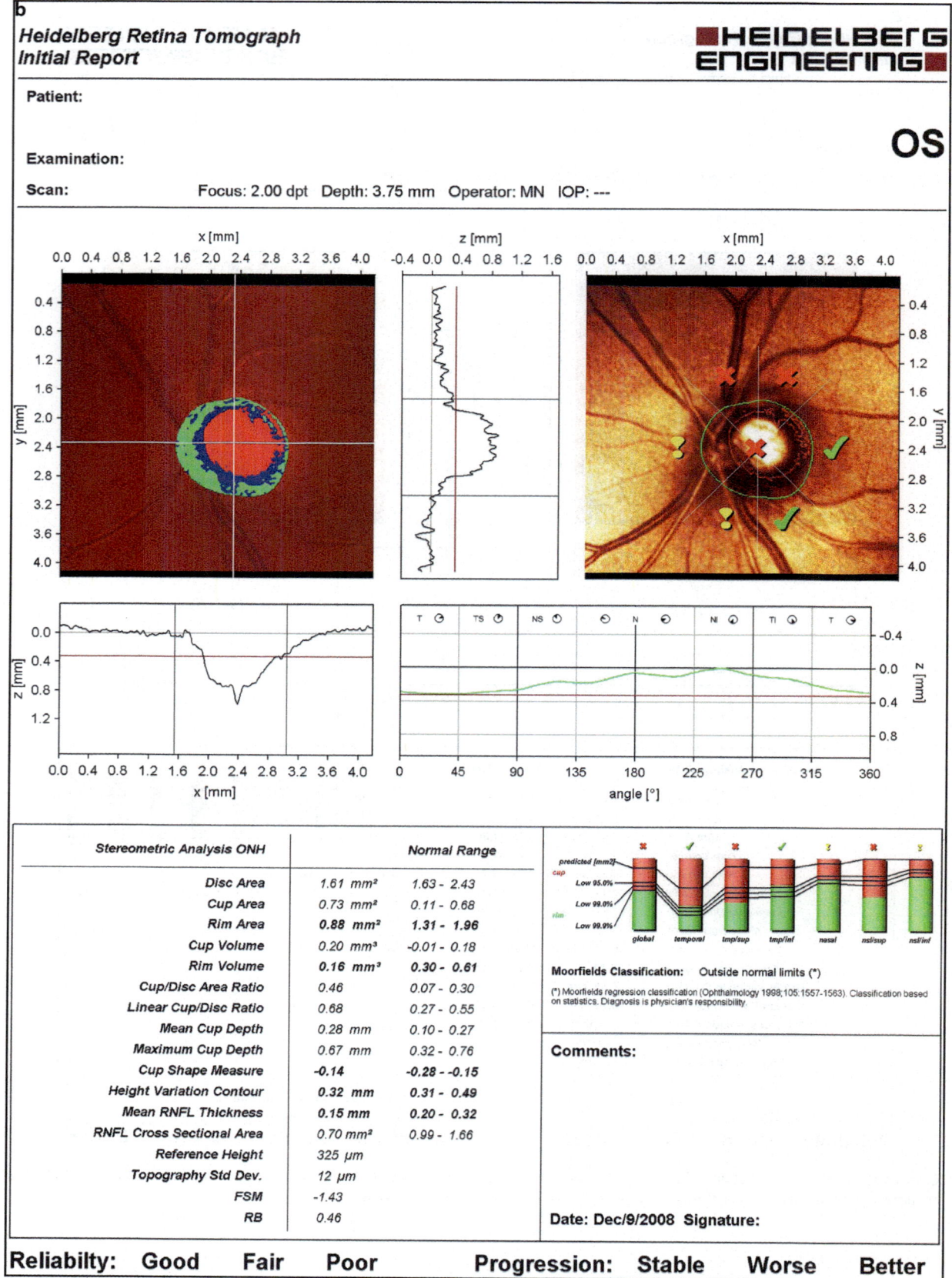

**Fig. 20.1** (continued) (**b**) substantial loss in the superior regions of the left eye. The visual fields demonstrate corresponding loss in

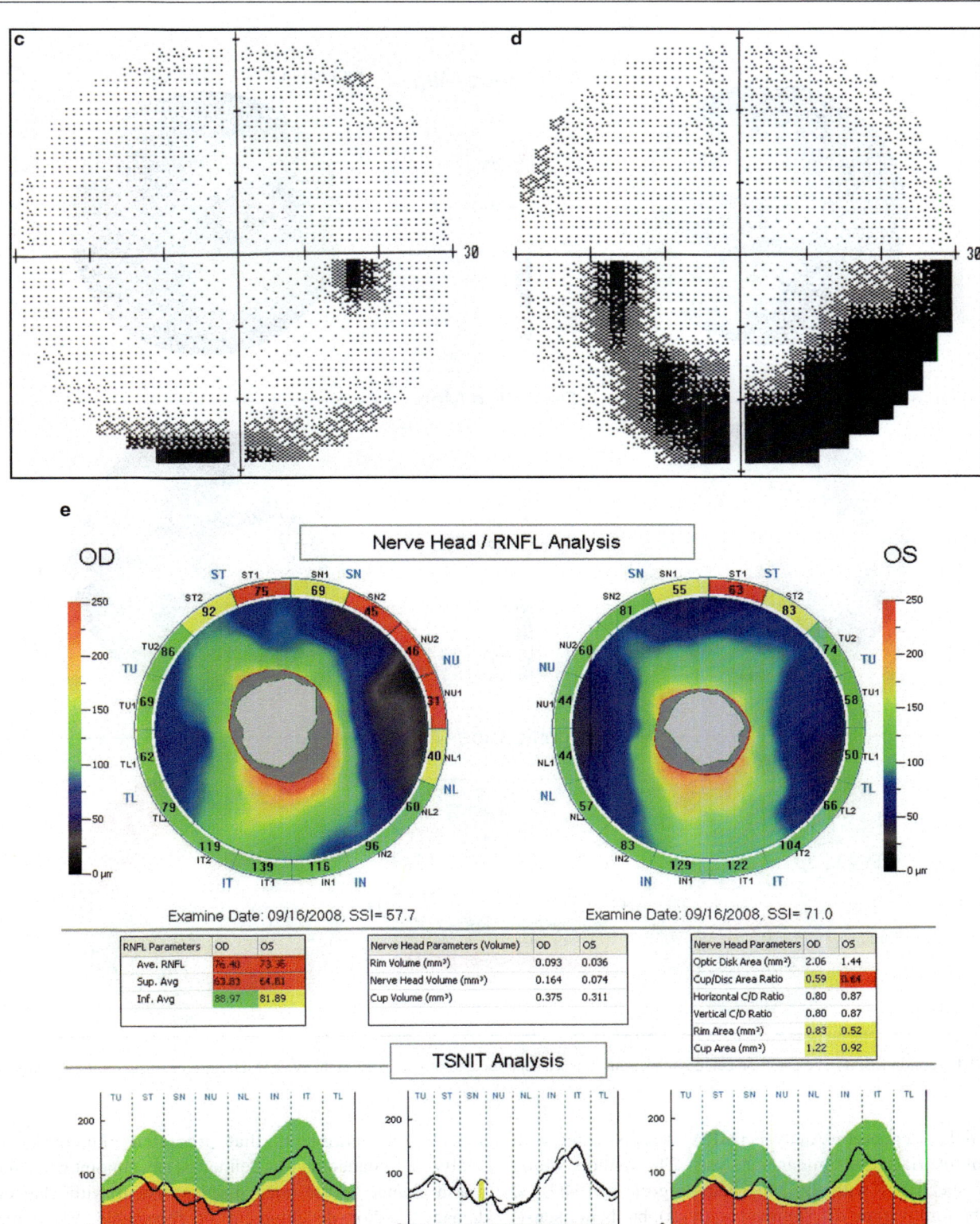

**Fig. 20.1** (continued) (**c**) the inferior field of the right eye and (**d**) dense inferior arcuate loss in the left eye. (**e**) The spectral domain optical coherence domain (SD-OCT) (RTVue, Optovue, Inc., Fremont, CA) imaging of the retinal nerve fiber layer shows loss of the supero-nasal loss in the right eye and superior loss in the left eye

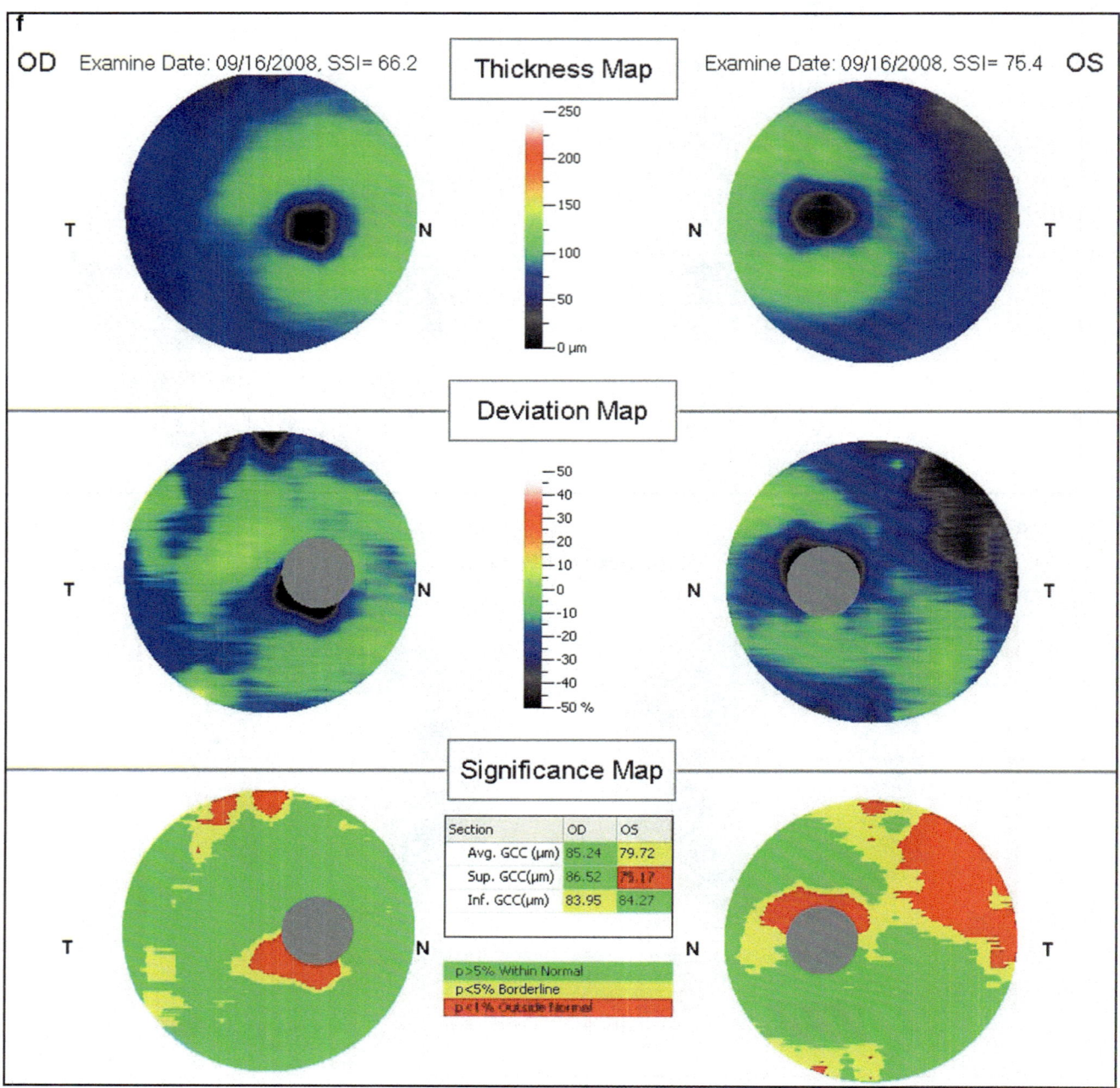

**Fig. 20.1** (continued) (**f**) The ganglion cell complex scan shows a superior area of loss in the right eye and a large area of superior loss in the left

Moorfields Regression Analysis (MRA) was compared with the multivariate discriminant analysis. The authors found better specificity with the Moorfields algorithm (94% vs. 75% by multivariate discriminant analysis), but better sensitivity using the multivariate analysis (83% vs. 74% by MRA). Others have also used different software algorithms to separate glaucomatous from control cases with varying success.[5,6,9]

In the Ocular Hypertension Treatment Study, the HRT I was used in a subset of the participating sites and a retrospective analysis of parameters that predicted glaucoma were analyzed.[10] Glaucoma was defined as an endpoint when there was a change in the optic disc consistent with glaucoma damage, and/or development of repeatable VF defects. Parameters that were associated with glaucoma development included larger C/D area ratio, mean cup depth, mean height contour, cup volume, and reference plane height and smaller rim area, rim area-to-disc area ratio, and rim volume. The most predictive values were mean height contour, rim area, and mean cup depth.

Studies on HRT II and III have also shown very good distinction of perimetric glaucoma (associated with visual field loss).[11–13] The HRT III analysis does not require user input. Harizman et al. compared the MRA of the HRT II and the Glaucoma Probability Score (GPS) for the detection of perimetric glaucoma.[13] Sensitivity and specificity were 77% and 90% for GPS, and 71% and 92% for MRA, respectively.

## 20.4 OCT

Studies have evaluated RNFL measurement by OCT and its relationship to glaucoma diagnosis or VF loss[14–21] (Fig. 20.2). Quadrants that correlated with the highest AUCs were the superior and inferior quadrants (0.79–0.952, superior; 0.863–0.971, inferior) for distinguishing eyes with glaucomatous VF loss from controls.[14,15,17–19] When individual clock hours were assessed, the 6, 7, 11, and 12 clock hours (in right eyes), representing the inferior/inferior–temporal and superior/superior–temporal areas of the optic nerve, had higher AUCs than other clock hours.[15,17,19] Overall, OCT III had higher AUCs than OCT II. Studies comparing controls versus glaucoma suspects found lower AUCs than for perimetric glaucoma.[17–19]

Recently Lalezary et al. found that thinner RNFLs on baseline OCT2 are predictive of glaucomatous change in glaucoma suspects.[22]

ONH and macular scans with the OCT have also been studied for their effectiveness in detecting glaucoma.[23–28] Overall, RNFL and ONH scans were superior to macular scans in distinguishing glaucoma.[25,27,28] ONH parameters such as C/D ratio and rim area performed very well, with AUCs similar to the best parameters of the RNFL.

No published data on commercially available Fourier-domain OCTs and glaucoma was available at the time of this writing.

## 20.5 GDx

Studies comparing the uncompensated GDx and the GDx VCC revealed better discriminate function with the VCC.[29–32]

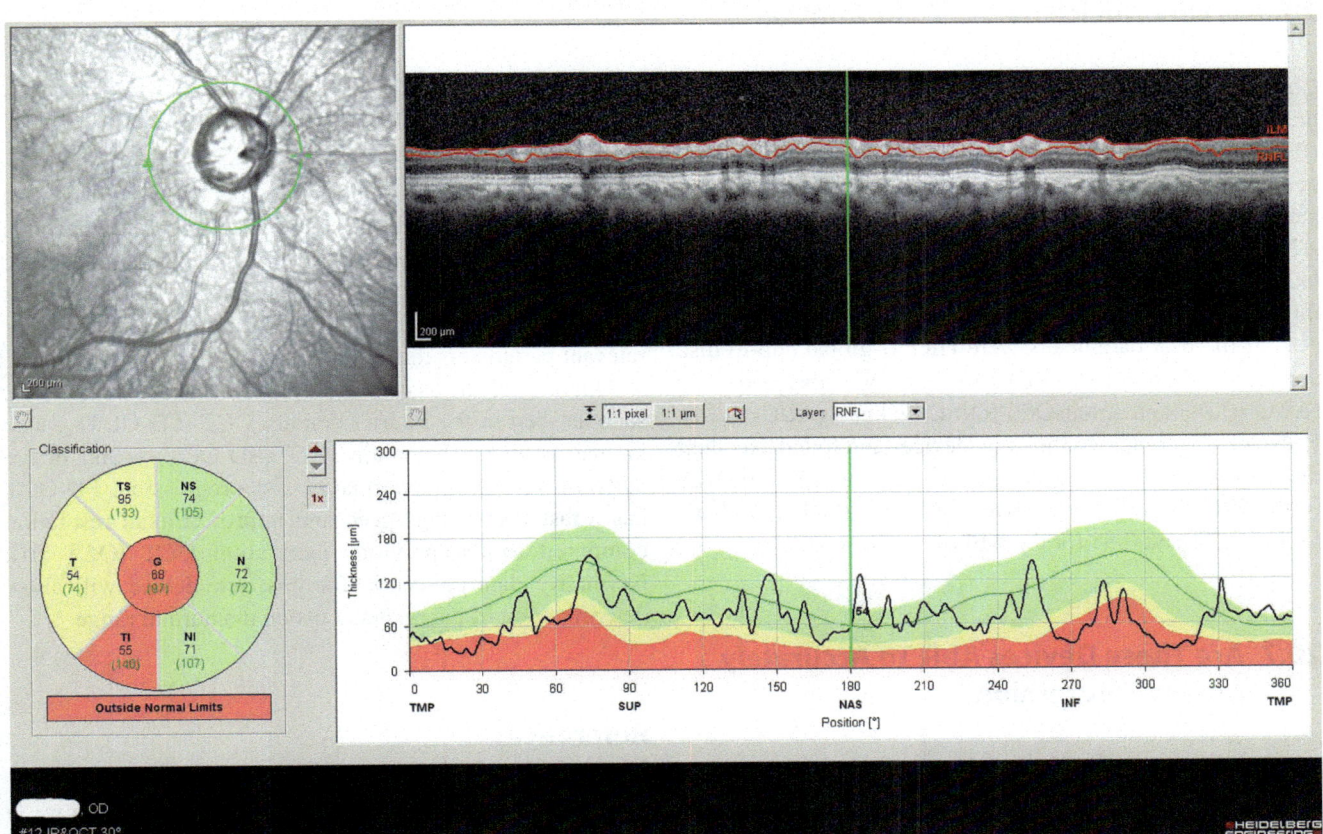

**Fig. 20.2** Spectral domain optical coherence tomography (SD-OCT) (Spectralis OCT, Heidelberg Engineering, Heidelberg, Germany) imaging of the retinal nerve fiber layer (RNFL) in a patient with advanced glaucoma. The irregularity of the circular scan contour likely represents the very high resolution details of the RNFL

One explanation is that inadequate corneal compensation can lead to widening of the normal range, thus masking true glaucomatous defects in the RNFL.[32]

Using various parameters or algorithms, the GDx VCC has shown an excellent ability to detect glaucoma.[33–37] Bowd et al.[33] used two machine learning classifiers that both had similar AUCs (0.90 and 0.91). Essock et al.[34] and Medeiros et al.[35] evaluated Fourier-based algorithms that yielded high AUCs (0.938–0.978) for glaucoma detection. In a separate paper, Medeiros et al.[36] compared GDx VCC parameters with RNFL photography scores. Both methods demonstrated good correlations for damage in corresponding hemiretinas, although the best GDx VCC parameter had an AUC (0.91 for NFI) higher than the best RNFL photography score (0.84 for global score). A subsequent publication by Medeiros et al.[37] used ONH progression by stereoscopic disc photographs as the criterion for glaucoma diagnosis. Again the NFI was the best parameter, with an AUC of 0.94 for eyes with perimetric loss at the baseline and 0.89 for preperimetric eyes. Among standard GDx VCC parameters the NFI provided the highest AUCs (0.87–0.94) in the majority of studies.[29,36,37]

## 20.6 Is One Device Better Than Another?

Comparative studies of OCT III, GDx VCC, and/or HRT II have revealed minimal or no significant differences (REFs-Leung IV, Meideros, DeLeon-Ortega). Medeiros et al.[38] compared the three main devices in use today and found similar AUCs for the best parameters from each instrument – NFI for the GDx VCC (AUC=0.91), inferior quadrant for OCT III (AUC=0.92), and linear discriminant function of the HRT II (AUC=0.86). In the study by DeLeon-Ortega et al.,[12] the best parameters were HRT II global cup-to-disc area ratio (AUC=0.86), GDx VCC Nerve Fiber Indicator (AUC=0.84), and Stratus OCT RNFL thickness (AUC=0.84). Pueyo et al.[39] compared the same devices and found excellent discriminate ability for each device: AUC of 0.90 for MRA of the HRT II, 0.91 for the average RNFL thickness of the StratusOCT, and 0.88 for the NFI of the GDx VCC.

## 20.7 Are These Devices Able to Accurately Assess Progression?

There is limited available data on the ability of these devices to detect glaucoma progression. Overall there is significant overlap in the detection of progression by structural and functional tests (REFS), but there are also substantial percentages of glaucoma patients who progress by only one of the techniques.

For the HRT I, comparison with perimetric tests found that although there was considerable overlap of eyes that were identified as having progressed by the visual field and the HRT tests, significant numbers of eyes were found to have progressed by only functional or structural (HRT) criteria.[40] It may be that these tests represent independent indicators of progression. In a study[41] that evaluated glaucoma progression among four groups with different glaucomatous disc types (focal, myopic, senile sclerotic, and generalized), progression rates by HRT (44–82%) were greater than those by standard automated perimetry (33–57%), echoing the groups' earlier reported results.[42] Moreover, there were similarly high rates of progression by either test alone (20–61%) across the groups. A more recent study found that the HRT II also detected a higher rate of glaucomatous progression when compared to visual field.[43]

With regard to the OCT, Wollstein II[44] also reported higher rates of progression when the structural test was used (25%) as compared with standard automated perimetry (12%), although their study population included glaucoma suspects and preperimetric glaucoma patients in addition to patients with baseline VF defects. It is unclear if this represents greater sensitivity for progression or hypersensitivity (false positives) of the structural test.

## 20.8 Conclusion and Future Directions

ONH/RNFL imaging devices provide useful quantitative information for the diagnosis and management of glaucoma. There are no studies that have clearly shown that one single device outperforms the others in diagnostic ability. Results from these devices should be analyzed in conjunction with other relevant parameters that define glaucoma and progression.

Ongoing advances include improvements in the hardware, such as seen in the Fourier-domain OCT (FD-OCT) – also known as spectral domain OCT (SD-OCT) – and in the software to assess abnormality and progression. FD-OCT has a faster scanning speed and improved axial resolution compared to the previous generation OCT (OCT III). Normative data collection for this new device will allow determination of parameters outside the normal range.

## References

1. Quigley HA, Addicks EM, Green WR. Optic nerve damage in human glaucoma III. Quantitative correlation of nerve fiber loss and visual field defect in glaucoma, ischemic neuropathy, papilledema, and toxic neuropathy. *Arch Ophthalmol.* 1982;100:135–146.
2. Kerrigan-Baumrind LA, Quigley HA, Pease ME, Kerrigan DF, Mitchell RS. Number of ganglion cells in glaucoma eyes compared

with threshold visual field tests in the same persons. *Invest Ophthalmol Vis Sci.* 2000;41(3):741-748.
3. Kass MA, Heuer DK, Higginbotham EJ, et al. The Ocular Hypertension Treatment Study: a randomized trial determines that topical ocular hypotensive medication delays or prevents the onset of primary open-angle glaucoma. *Arch Ophthalmol.* 2002;120:701-713, discussion 829-830.
4. Lin SC, Singh K, Jampel HD, et al, American Academy of Ophthalmology, Ophthalmic Technology Assessment Committee Glaucoma Panel. Optic nerve head and retinal nerve fiber layer analysis: a report by the American Academy of Ophthalmology. *Ophthalmology.* 2007;114(10):1937-1949.
5. Ford BA, Artes PH, McCormick TA, et al. Comparison of data analysis tools for detection of glaucoma with the Heidelberg Retina Tomograph. *Ophthalmology.* 2003;110:1145-1150.
6. Mardin CY, Hothorn T, Peters A, et al. New glaucoma classification method based on standard Heidelberg Retina Tomograph parameters by bagging classification trees. *J Glaucoma.* 2003;12:340-346.
7. Miglior S, Guareschi M, Albe' E, et al. Detection of glaucomatous visual field changes using the Moorfields regression analysis of the Heidelberg retina tomograph. *Am J Ophthalmol.* 2003;136:26-33.
8. Miglior S, Guareschi M, Romanazzi F, et al. The impact of definition of primary open-angle glaucoma on the cross-sectional assessment of diagnostic validity of Heidelberg retinal tomography. *Am J Ophthalmol.* 2005;139:878-887.
9. Zangwill LM, Chan K, Bowd C, et al. Heidelberg retina tomograph measurements of the optic disc and parapapillary retina for detecting glaucoma analyzed by machine learning classifiers. *Invest Ophthalmol Vis Sci.* 2004;45:3144-3151.
10. Zangwill LM, Weinreb RN, Beiser JA, et al. Baseline topographic optic disc measurements are associated with the development of primary open-angle glaucoma: the Confocal Scanning Laser Ophthalmoscopy Ancillary Study to the Ocular Hypertension Treatment Study. *Arch Ophthalmol.* 2005;123:1188-1197.
11. De León-Ortega JE, Sakata LM, Monheit BE, McGwin G Jr, Arthur SN, Girkin CA. Comparison of diagnostic accuracy of Heidelberg Retina Tomograph II and Heidelberg Retina Tomograph 3 to discriminate glaucomatous and nonglaucomatous eyes. *Am J Ophthalmol.* 2007;144(4):525-532.
12. Deleón-Ortega JE, Arthur SN, McGwin G Jr, Xie A, Monheit BE, Girkin CA. Discrimination between glaucomatous and nonglaucomatous eyes using quantitative imaging devices and subjective optic nerve head assessment. *Invest Ophthalmol Vis Sci.* 2006;47(8):3374-3380.
13. Harizman N, Zelefsky JR, Ilitchev E, Tello C, Ritch R, Liebmann JM. Detection of glaucoma using operator-dependent versus operator-independent classification in the Heidelberg retinal tomograph-III. *Br J Ophthalmol.* 2006;90(11):1390-1392. Epub 2006 Jul 26.
14. Bourne RR, Medeiros FA, Bowd C, et al. Comparability of retinal nerve fiber layer thickness measurements of optical coherence tomography instruments. *Invest Ophthalmol Vis Sci.* 2005;46:1280-1285.
15. Budenz DL, Michael A, Chang RT, et al. Sensitivity and specificity of the StratusOCT for perimetric glaucoma. *Ophthalmology.* 2005;112:3-9.
16. Hougaard JL, Heijl A, Krogh E. The nerve fibre layer symmetry test: computerized evaluation of human retinal nerve fibre layer thickness as measured by optical coherence tomography. *Acta Ophthalmol Scand.* 2004;82:410-418.
17. Kanamori A, Nakamura M, Escano MF, et al. Evaluation of the glaucomatous damage on retinal nerve fiber layer thickness measured by optical coherence tomography. *Am J Ophthalmol.* 2003;135:513-520.
18. Leung CK, Yung WH, Ng AC, et al. Evaluation of scanning resolution on retinal nerve fiber layer measurement using optical coherence tomography in normal and glaucomatous eyes. *J Glaucoma.* 2004;13:479-485.
19. Nouri-Mahdavi K, Hoffman D, Tannenbaum DP, et al. Identifying early glaucoma with optical coherence tomography. *Am J Ophthalmol.* 2004;137:228-235.
20. Mok KH, Lee VW, So KF. Retinal nerve fiber loss pattern in high-tension glaucoma by optical coherence tomography. *J Glaucoma.* 2003;12:255-259.
21. Mok KH, Lee VW, So KF. Retinal nerve fiber loss in high- and normal-tension glaucoma by optical coherence tomography. *Optom Vis Sci.* 2004;81:369-372.
22. Lalezary M, Medeiros FA, Weinreb RN, et al. Baseline optical coherence tomography predicts the development of glaucomatous change in glaucoma suspects. *Am J Ophthalmol.* 2006;142(4):576-582.
23. Ishikawa H, Stein DM, Wollstein G, et al. Macular segmentation with optical coherence tomography. *Invest Ophthalmol Vis Sci.* 2005;46:2012-2017.
24. Lederer DE, Schuman JS, Hertzmark E, et al. Analysis of macular volume in normal and glaucomatous eyes using optical coherence tomography. *Am J Ophthalmol.* 2003;135:838-843.
25. Burgansky-Eliash Z, Wollstein G, Chu T, et al. Optical coherence tomography machine learning classifiers for glaucoma detection: a preliminary study. *Invest Ophthalmol Vis Sci.* 2005;46:4147-4152.
26. Choi MG, Han M, Kim YI, Lee JH. Comparison of glaucomatous parameters in normal, ocular hypertensive and glaucomatous eyes using optical coherence tomography 3000. *Korean J Ophthalmol.* 2005;19:40-46.
27. Medeiros FA, Zangwill LM, Bowd C, et al. Evaluation of retinal nerve fiber layer, optic nerve head, and macular thickness measurements for glaucoma detection using optical coherence tomography. *Am J Ophthalmol.* 2005;139:44-55.
28. Wollstein G, Schuman JS, Price LL, et al. Optical coherence tomography (OCT) macular and peripapillary retinal nerve fiber layer measurements and automated visual fields. *Am J Ophthalmol.* 2004;138:218-225.
29. Bowd C, Zangwill LM, Weinreb RN. Association between scanning laser polarimetry measurements using variable corneal polarization compensation and visual field sensitivity in glaucomatous eyes. *Arch Ophthalmol.* 2003;121:961-966.
30. Brusini P, Salvetat ML, Parisi L, et al. Discrimination between normal and early glaucomatous eyes with scanning laser polarimeter with fixed and variable corneal compensator settings. *Eur J Ophthalmol.* 2005;15:468-476.
31. Schlottmann PG, De Cilla S, Greenfield DS, et al. Relationship between visual field sensitivity and retinal nerve fiber layer thickness as measured by scanning laser polarimetry. *Invest Ophthalmol Vis Sci.* 2004;45:1823-1829.
32. Weinreb RN, Bowd C, Zangwill LM. Glaucoma detection using scanning laser polarimetry with variable corneal polarization compensation. *Arch Ophthalmol.* 2003;121:218-224.
33. Bowd C, Medeiros FA, Zhang Z, et al. Relevance vector machine and support vector machine classifier analysis of scanning laser polarimetry retinal nerve fiber layer measurements. *Invest Ophthalmol Vis Sci.* 2005;46:1322-1329.
34. Essock EA, Zheng Y, Gunvant P. Analysis of GDx-VCC polarimetry data by Wavelet-Fourier analysis across glaucoma stages. *Invest Ophthalmol Vis Sci.* 2005;46:2838-2847.
35. Medeiros FA, Zangwill LM, Bowd C, et al. Fourier analysis of scanning laser polarimetry measurements with variable corneal compensation in glaucoma. *Invest Ophthalmol Vis Sci.* 2003;44:2606-2612.
36. Medeiros FA, Zangwill LM, Bowd C, et al. Comparison of scanning laser polarimetry using variable corneal compensation and retinal nerve fiber layer photography for detection of glaucoma. *Arch Ophthalmol.* 2004;122:698-704.
37. Medeiros FA, Zangwill LM, Bowd C, et al. Use of progressive glaucomatous optic disk change as the reference standard for

38. Medeiros FA, Zangwill LM, Bowd C, Weinreb RN. Comparison of the GDx VCC scanning laser polarimeter, HRT II confocal scanning laser ophthalmoscope, and Stratus OCT optical coherence tomograph for the detection of glaucoma. *Arch Ophthalmol.* 2004;122:827-837.
39. Pueyo V, Polo V, Larrosa JM, Ferreras A, Pablo LE, Honrubia FM. Diagnostic ability of the Heidelberg retina tomograph, optical coherence tomograph, and scanning laser polarimeter in open-angle glaucoma. *J Glaucoma.* 2007;16(2):173-177.
40. Artes PH, Chauhan BC. Longitudinal changes in the visual field and optic disc in glaucoma. *Prog Retin Eye Res.* 2005;24:333-354.
41. Nicolela MT, McCormick TA, Drance SM, et al. Visual field and optic disc progression in patients with different types of optic disc damage A longitudinal prospective study. *Ophthalmology.* 2003;110:2178-2184.
42. Chauhan BC, McCormick TA, Nicolela MT, LeBlanc RP. Optic disc and visual field changes in a prospective longitudinal study of patients with glaucoma: comparison of scanning laser tomography with conventional perimetry and optic disc photography. *Arch Ophthalmol.* 2001;119:1492-1499.
43. Hudson CJ, Kim LS, Hancock SA, Cunliffe IA, Wild JM. Some dissociating factors in the analysis of structural and functional progressive damage in open-angle glaucoma. *Br J Ophthalmol.* 2007;91(5):624-628.
44. Wollstein G, Schuman JS, Price LL, et al. Optical coherence tomography longitudinal evaluation of retinal nerve fiber layer thickness in glaucoma. *Arch Ophthalmol.* 2005;123:464-470.

(References 1-37 continued from previous page; entry preceding 38: evaluation of diagnostic tests in glaucoma. *Am J Ophthalmol.* 2005;139:1010-1018.)

# Chapter 21
# Clinical Utility of Computerized Optic Nerve Analysis

Neil T. Choplin

This chapter emphasizes the point that glaucoma is a disease of retinal nerve fibers and their ganglion cells. The diagnosis and management of glaucoma requires the ability to detect the loss of retinal nerve fibers (i.e., determining if an individual has less nerve fibers than he/she is supposed to have based upon the population from which he/she comes) and to determine if the loss of retinal nerve fibers occurs at a rate greater than what is expected from normal aging. The "traditional" method for doing this has been through direct ophthalmoscopy and the determination of the cup-to-disc ratio, with the assumption that "cupping" represents the loss of nerve fibers from the neuroretinal rim. The problem with the traditional method is that it has no way of accounting for the large structural variability of human optic nerve heads. A cup-to-disc ratio of 0.6, for example, may be quite normal in an axial myope, but may be quite pathological if it was 0.3 ten years before the patient was ever seen by the eye care provider. Likewise, it may be quite normal if the disc is large, and abnormal if the disc is small. Plus, the determination of cup-to-disc ratio only provides an (subjective) indirect measure of the retinal nerve fiber layer, the tissue of interest in glaucoma. Small changes in cup-to-disc ratio may be very difficult to detect by ophthalmoscopy, and progression may go unnoticed for years. Hence, better methods are required and, as outlined in this chapter, have been developed.

Functional testing in glaucoma, particularly white-on-white computerized automated perimetry, is currently the gold standard for detecting glaucomatous damage. It has been estimated that a large percentage of retinal nerve fibers (30–50%) may be lost before a visual field defect is detectable.[1] Why should this matter? Could we not wait until visual field loss has begun and then start treatment? The problem with this approach is that by the time we begin to see functional damage, a considerable portion of retinal nerve fibers may have been lost. Treating glaucoma by adequate lowering of intraocular pressure may eliminate the accelerated (compared to normal aging) loss of nerve fibers that occurs in the disease, but will not eliminate natural loss due to aging, and our populations continue to age and live much longer than we ever expected. A well "controlled" glaucoma patient may thus continue to show progression and even functional blindness if the disease started at an early age, a large number of nerve fibers were lost, and they lived into the 1990s or beyond. The key to preventing blindness from glaucoma in an ever-aging population is to detect retinal nerve fiber layer damage early, and this requires technology that goes beyond ophthalmoscopic observation.

Computerized scanning imaging is the term we should be using while discussing machines that are used to analyze the structure of the optic nerve head and retinal nerve fiber layer in the living eye. All the machines described in this chapter have in common the incorporation of a computer system to control image acquisition, analyze the data obtained, and manage the patient database. They all incorporate the ability to scan an area of the retina (including or excluding the optic nerve head), obtaining data pixel by pixel and constructing two or three dimensional images. The three main devices discussed in the chapter, confocal scanning laser ophthalmoscopy (CSLO), scanning laser polarimetey (SLP), and optical coherence tomography (OCT), differ significantly from each other in how they work, what they are capable of imaging, and what information they provide to us as clinicians. They all have the ability to provide us with high resolution (compared to the direct ophthalmoscope) images, bypass moderate media opacities, provide objective quantitative information that is fairly reproducible, make comparisons to normative databases and provide statistical analysis, limit bias in the observations, and, because of good reproducibility, detect changes over time that, if they exceed a defined statistical inter-measurement variability, are most likely due to disease progression. Computerized scanning imaging thus provides us with a number of significant clinical advantages. First, in an eye suspected of having glaucoma, usually based upon "elevated" intraocular pressure readings, large cup-to-disc ratio, or asymmetrical cups, a "normal" scan can confirm the absence of abnormalities and prevent unnecessary treatment. Next, the ability to provide objective, quantitative information about optic disc or retinal nerve fiber layer structure allows the detection of small abnormalities that might otherwise go undetected, allowing appropriate intervention before functional damage occurs. Finally, the ability to determine significant change over time allows for earlier changes in treatment before significant functional damage occurs or progresses.

The interpretation of data provided by a computerized scanning imaging machine requires the user to thoroughly understand what the machine was designed to do, how it may have been adapted to do other things beyond its original intent, and, most importantly, the underlying operating principles of the device including its limitations.

The computerized scanning imaging technologies that have emerged for assessing the optic nerve, the retinal nerve fiber layer, and the peripapillary retina over the past 10–15 years discussed in this chapter are still evolving. Many of them have branched out into providing information for which they were never originally designed. CSLO, epitomized by the Heidelberg Retinal Tomograph, was designed to obtain a three-dimensional image of the optic nerve and peripapillary retina by taking multiplanar images (by means of a moving pinhole aperture). Information regarding the retinal nerve fiber layer is indirect, since only the retinal nerve fiber layer contour is determined by drawing a line above a predefined "reference plane," or, in the latest iteration, comparing the overall surface contour to a normative database and estimating the probability that the retinal nerve fiber layer is abnormal. Optical Coherence Tomography (OCT) was designed to provide an in vivo cross-sectional view of the retina by measuring the echo time delay of a back-scattered laser light compared to an "unaltered" reference light ray by a principle known as interferometry. Using "segmentation" algorithms, quantitative information about the thickness of the retina and retinal nerve fiber layer have been derived, but again, the retinal nerve fiber layer is not directly measured. The latest iteration of OCT, spectral-domain or Fourier domain OCT may offer an advantage over time domain, since analysis of the waveform contained in the individual A-scans should detect the different reflectivity from the retinal nerve fiber layer compared to the other retinal structures, and thus may be a more accurate measure. The very high scanning speed afforded by spectral domain OCT compared to time domain OCT (26,000 A-scans per second compared to 400) allows for the acquisition of retinal nerve fiber layer data outside of a single peripapillary circle, thus providing much more clinical information. Scanning laser polarimetry was designed to provide quantitative information about the retinal nerve fiber layer by measuring the phase shift (retardation) of a polarized laser light passing through the naturally birefringent tissues of the eye, using some sort of compensation to remove the portion of the signal attributed to the anterior segment. Limitations of these measurements are usually due to the reflection of light from the sclera or other structures or residual anterior segment birefringence. The phase shift is measured in angular degrees (theta), yet the output is expressed in microns based upon a primate study that showed one degree of phase shift was equivalent to 7.4 μm of tissue thickness.[2] In addition, removal of the portion of the signal attributed to the anterior segment is required to properly assess the retinal nerve fiber layer, and understanding how this compensator works is essential to interpreting SLP output. Without an understanding of what the machines were designed to do, how they do things for which they were not originally designed, sources of artifact, limitations of normative databases, etc., interpretation of data could lead to false conclusions regarding the clinical situation.

One other thing to consider: perhaps the structural measures provided by computerized scanning imaging devices are not merely structural measures per se, but an indirect measure of function as well. Scanning laser polarimetry, for example, derives its signal from birefringence, which in the retinal nerve fiber layer is attributed to microtubules as demonstrated in a beautiful non-human primate study presented at the Association for Research in Vision and Ophthalmology.[3] In this study, intravitreal colchicine, which destroys microtubules, caused decreases in polarimetry measurements but not those from OCT within 2 h of injection, and histology showed the microtubules were indeed decreased. Hence, the decrease in apparent retinal nerve fiber layer "thickness" may be attributed to the decrease in microtubule density, a sign of nerve fiber dysfunction, and not an actual decrease in tissue "thickness." Treatment to restore the nerve fibers to health may allow regeneration of microtubules and an increase in signal on repeat testing, something that has been reported with both scanning laser polarimetry and optical coherence tomography (although it was reported as an increase in retinal nerve fiber layer "thickness").[4,5] Again, knowing what is being measured allows the proper conclusion regarding the finding, and not the false conclusion that the retinal nerve fiber layer has become "thicker." It is probably better to think in terms of "signal" when evaluating the output of a computerized scanning imaging device and not the reported output measure.

Computerized scanning imaging devices have not yet become the standard of care, but their role in patient care is increasing. Users of these devices, researchers reporting the results of studies employing these devices, and readers of those studies should and must understand the underlying technologies to properly interpret the printouts of the results of the patients and that of the studies.

## References

1. Quigley HA, Addicks EM, Green WR. Optic nerve damage in human glaucoma III. Quantitative correlation of nerve fiber loss and visual field defect in glaucoma, ischemic neuropathy, papilledema, and toxic neuropathy. *Arch Ophthalmol*. 1982;100:135–146.
2. Weinreb RN, Dreher AW, Coleman A, et al. Histopathologic validation of Fourier-ellipsometry measurements of retinal nerve fiber layer thickness. *Arch Ophthalmol*. 1990;108:557–560.
3. Fortune, B, Wang, G, Cull, Cioffi GA. Intravitreal colchicine causes decreased retinal nerve fiber layer thickness measured by scanning laser polarimetry but not by optical coherence tomography in non-human primates. *Inv Vis Sci*. 2007;(48), Abstract no. 2877.
4. Yamada N, Tomita G, Yamamoto T, Kitazawa Y. Changes in the nerve fiber layer thickness following a reduction of intraocular pressure after trabeculectomy. *J Glaucoma*. 2000;9(5):371–375.
5. Aydin A, Wollstein G, Price LL, Fujimoto JG, Schuman JS. Optical coherence tomography assessment of retinal nerve fiber layer thickness changes after glaucoma surgery. *Ophthalmology*. 2003;110(8):1506–1511.

# Chapter 22
# Photography of the Optic Nerve

Roy Whitaker Jr. and Von Best Whitaker

Characteristic glaucomatous damage to the optic nerve and nerve fiber layer (NFL) are definitive structural features for the diagnosis of glaucoma. Clinical evaluation of the nerve may be difficult when the patient is blinking, moving, avoiding the examining light, and with ocular saccades.

The purposes of optic nerve photography are multi-fold. Initially, it provides a still, permanent image of the optic nerve and surrounding retina that allows the physician to carefully document the appearance of the optic nerve and to establish a benchmark. Secondly, photographs provide a serial comparison of the optic nerve over time with visual documentation of stability or progression of the optic nerve head. A magnified photographic view allows the detection of subtle signs of glaucomatous damage in a way that has not yet been accomplished by optic nerve analyzers. The position and appearance of retinal vessels and abnormalities such as peripapillary hemorrhages are documented with the photo. The magnified photographic image may reveal subtle changes such as a shift in the retinal vessels, which are not detected during the clinical exam with the patient. Asymmetry of the nerves between the two eyes of the same individual can also be detected and documented with photography better than with image analyzers.

## 22.1 Cameras for Optic Nerve Photography

The first fundus camera for commercial use was available in 1926 and was developed by Nordinson in Upsala.[1,2] This camera required a one-half second exposure time using color film. Subsequent fundus cameras were developed based on that original camera. Current analog cameras use aspheric objective lenses aligned with 35-mm single reflex camera bodies.[3] Most commercially available digital fundus cameras today use charge coupled detection systems.

There are a large number of fundus cameras currently marketed for both retinal and glaucoma subspecialists.

The cameras suitable for optic nerve head photography should be able to take simultaneous stereo photographs. As of early 2009, the current cameras most suitable for this task include the Canon CR-1 45° nonmydriatic retinal camera, Nidek AFC-230-210, Discam (Marcher Enterprises Ltd., Hereford, UK), and Topcon TRC-50DX.

## 22.2 Types of Optic Nerve Photographs

### 22.2.1 Black-and-White Photography

High quality black-and-white photography is useful to observe fine detail of the retinal nerve fiber layer. Black-and-white photography enables easy measurement of vessels with large and constant magnification. These photos lend themselves to excellent imagery on photographic paper as well as on Kodachrome slides. The photographic print is an excellent source of documentation that can easily be stored in the patient chart.[3,4]

Concomitant with the advent of digital fundus photography, the black-and-white print or the black-and-white computer image is excellent for viewing on the computer monitor.

### 22.2.2 Retinal Nerve Fiber Layer Photography

The retinal nerve fiber layer (RNFL) is composed of retinal ganglion cell axons. The axonal layer becomes thinner in the glaucomatous eye. Areas of retinal nerve fiber layer loss become less brightly reflective and show up as dark bands radiating out from the optic disc. The RNFL can be visualized with fundus photography. In addition to images of the optic nerve head, black-and-white photography is very useful for documenting the structure of the retinal nerve fiber layer.

Identification of retinal nerve fiber layer defects can be more challenging on standard color photographs.[5]

Special photographic techniques may be used to enhance the appearance of the NFL. Monochromatic red-free photography is used with black-and-white film such as FP4, FP5, TRI-X, and Panatomic-XH.[2] High quality red-free photos are more difficult to obtain because of wide angle requirement and the scarcity of photographers skilled in this technique. This technique is more widely used in research settings but not widely used in general practice in the community setting.[3]

### 22.2.3 Monocular Photography

Clinical assessment of the optic nerve can be performed utilizing two-dimensional viewing. This occurs when the clinician utilizes a direct ophthalmoscope to observe the optic nerve. Monocular fundus cameras are less expensive than stereo fundus cameras. Two-dimensional imaging of the optic nerve can be provided by monocular fundus cameras. The two images of the retina are obtained by changing the eye fixation relative to the camera. The monocular system has not been found suitable for three-dimensional evaluation of the optic nerve. Stereo photography is much preferred for optic nerve evaluation.[6]

### 22.2.4 Stereo Color Photography

Color stereo photography remains the most widely used and accepted photographic technique for documentation of the optic nerve head.[2,7–10] Stereo fundus cameras are available in two types: The images are captured either by sequential stereoscopic photography or by simultaneous photography.

Sequential stereoscopic optic disc photography is usually performed by using a manual shift of the camera joystick to obtain stereo images through opposite sides of the pupil. Alternatively, most current fundus cameras have an Allen stereo separator to create stereo optical disk images. The Allen stereo separator was developed by Lee Allen in 1964.[11] The stereo separator in modern units consists of a motorized device that fits over the photographic tube of a fundus camera such as the Zeiss fundus camera. Stereo separation of images is created by optically directing light toward the alternate areas of the dilated pupil, by swiveling a glass plate that is suspended over the front camera lens. This method allows for good reproducibility of the photographs because the shifting technique is standardized. A drawback to this technique is the requirement of a widely dilated pupil of approximately 6 mm. This is not always achievable in all eyes, especially patients with a previous history of iritis or patients who are on chronic miotic therapy.[7]

The manual shift technique may be performed with any fundus camera and is probably the most widely utilized technique of stereoscopic fundus imaging. In this technique, after obtaining wide dilation of the pupil, the camera is focused on the optic disc in the center of the pupil, and a photographic image is obtained. Then the camera is shifted to the right and to the left to capture the second image of a stereo pair. The photographer may obtain a central image and a right and left image to determine each stereo pair – choosing the right central or the left central for the best stereo viewing. However, the shift technique may be among the least reproducible of all stereographic photographic techniques because it does not employ features to augment reproducibility of the stereo base in contrast to the Allen stereo separator.

In simultaneous stereoscopic optic disc photography, the fundus camera captures stereo images with a single exposure. The Donaldson stereo fundus camera introduced in 1964 was the first simultaneous stereoscopic camera to produce truly reliable images.[12] The Donaldson stereo camera has been considered the standard for simultaneous fundus photography. Unfortunately, the Donaldson camera is not commercially available, which prevents its widespread use.

Both the simultaneous and sequential stereo photography of the optic nerve can reveal excellent photographs. In general, the sequential method is considered inferior to the simultaneous method because it requires maintaining equal focus and illumination between images and maintaining a uniformed stereo base between photographic sessions, which is very difficult to do in practice. The sequential method requires a manual shift, which makes it difficult to compare the photographs over time. Changes in the magnitude of the shift between baseline and follow-up photographs can introduce artifacts in the perceived depth of the optic nerve when comparing the photographs.[3,7] Several studies report better reproducibility with the simultaneous method compared with sequential stereophotography.[13–15]

Two current simultaneous fundus cameras are the Nidek 3Dx and the Topcon TRC-SS2.

The Nidek 3Dx camera was introduced by Nidek in 1999 (Fig. 22.1). The Nidek camera catches simultaneous stereoscopic images with a 32° view of the fundus. The camera has an adjustable binocular eyepiece. The split frame images obtained with the unit are typically prepared on a 35-mm slide with two adjacent stereoscopic images of the optic nerve on the same slide (Fig. 22.2a, b). The images are viewed stereoscopically utilizing a specialized viewing system such as the stereo viewer II (Asahi-Pentax Co, Englewood Colorado) (Fig. 22.3). Investigators have demonstrated that simultaneous stereoscopic slides obtained with the Nidek 3Dx provides significantly more interobserver consistency for judgments of cup depth and overall stereo effect than

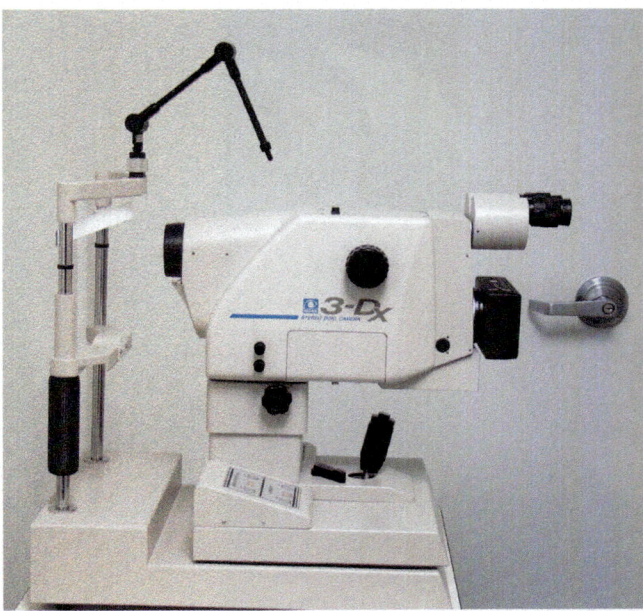

**Fig. 22.1** The Nidek 3Dx camera catches simultaneous stereoscopic images with a 32° view of the fundus

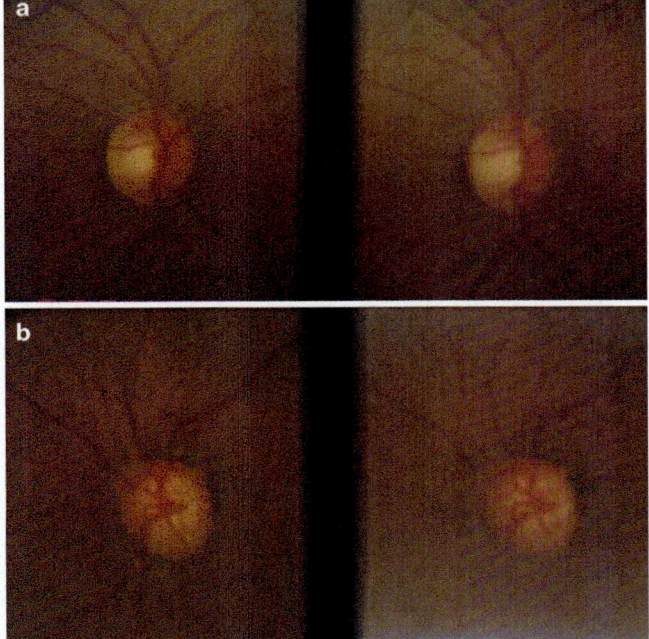

**Fig. 22.2** (**a, b**) Stereoscopic images obtained with the Nidek 3Dx camera

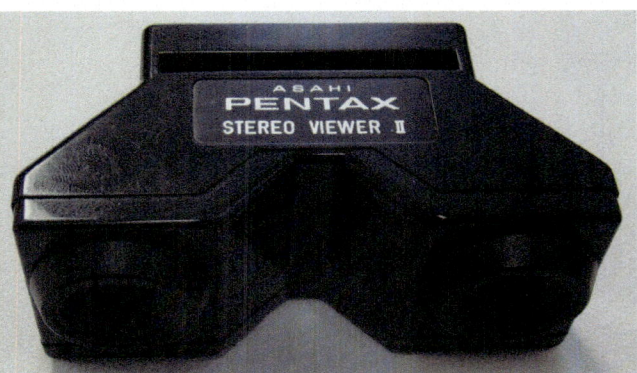

**Fig. 22.3** Asahi-Pentax Stereo Viewer II used to view stereoscopic images

sequential stereo slides.[14] Green and colleagues demonstrated that the Nidek 3Dx fundus camera produced significantly better stereoscopic images than the Donaldson fundus camera.[16]

The Topcon TRC-SS2 is similar to the Nidek camera. The Topcon camera produces simultaneous stereo images in the form of a split frame image. Both cameras produce high quality images with a photographic magnification of 2.6× and both cameras are equipped to perform retinal nerve fiber layer photography. The Topcon camera utilizes a monocular eyepiece. The viewing magnification of the Topcon is reduced 16.5× compared with 24.1× with the Nidek camera. The Topcon fundus camera is capable of producing high-resolution reproducible simultaneous stereoscopic images of the optic nerve.

An additional digital optic nerve head analysis system (the "image net stereometric analysis system") is available for the Topcon camera at an additional cost.[7] This system allows computerized measurements of optic nerve parameters and stereo viewing.

Unfortunately, the Nidek 3Dx fundus camera and the Topcon TRC-SS2 are no longer commercially available.

The fundus camera back may record the images on either 35 mm analog or digital media. Photographic film used is typically 35-mm color slide film such as Ektachrome 100 or a comparable brand. Thirty-five millimeter film has a theoretical resolution of 6,000 dots per inch (dpi).[17] Scanning such a 35-mm slide would yield a resolution image of 144 megapixels. The current scanning software rarely requires resolution this high (fine). The resolution of a 6.1 megapixel digital camera would be equivalent to scanning a 35-mm slide at 1,200 dpi.[18] Investigators have found no significant differences in the evaluation of cup-to-disk ratio when simultaneous optic disc stereo photographs obtained with 35-mm film is compared to digital images obtained with a 6.1 megapixel camera.[19]

### 22.2.5 Digital Fundus Photography

Several digital fundus cameras are currently available for taking stereo photographs of the optic nerve. These cameras will be more widely used as more eye doctors employ electronic health records. Digital imaging technologies and

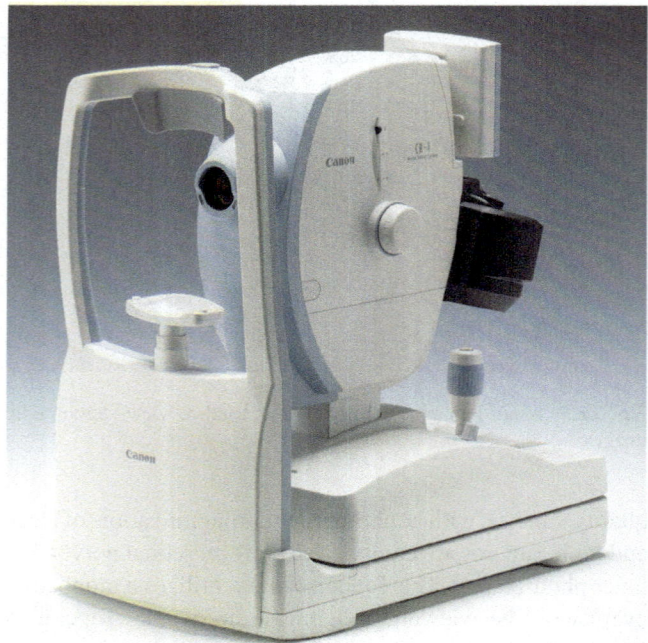

**Fig. 22.4** The Canon CR-1, a 45° non-mydriatic retinal camera

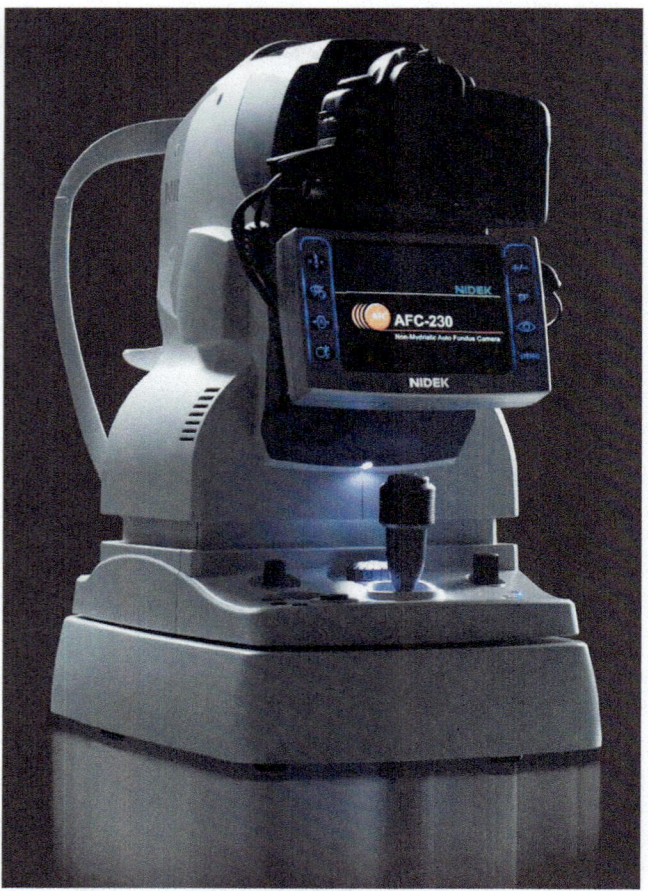

**Fig. 22.5** The Nidek AFC-230-210 camera

recording media will continue to evolve with time. The images from these cameras will be incorporated into legally mandated electronic health records of the present and future. Such storage will save paper records. They are readily available for viewing by physicians at multiple office locations. Digitized images may be analyzed by software programs that are constantly being updated and improved. With an appropriately equipped office, digital fundus images may be viewed in each office examination room and reviewed with the patient.

As of early 2009, there were several digital fundus cameras on the market. These include the Canon CR-1, a 45° nonmydriatic retinal camera (Fig. 22.4), the Nidek AFC-230-210 (Fig. 22.5), the Discam (Marcher Enterprises Ltd., Hereford, UK), and the Topcon TRC-50DX (Fig. 22.6). It is also possible to retrofit a digital camera back to some of the existing stereo fundus cameras such as the Nidek 3Dx. These retrofit projects do require additional software and computer technology expertise. None of the currently available digital fundus cameras perform simultaneous photography. The Topcon TRC-50DX obtains stereo images of the optic nerve by manually taking one image to the right and left of the nerve. This camera contains a stereo lock that limits X/Y plate movement, thus the stereo images can be reproduced more easily.

The Nidek nonmydriatic camera may be particularly useful when dilation of the eye is not convenient, ill advised, or not possible. It is particularly useful for nondilated glaucoma screening situations. The current model has several automatic functions including autofocus, automatic stereo mode, and automatic acquisition of the image once the image of the optic nerve is optimal. Disc area measurements with the Nidek 900 camera are similar to measurements obtained with the Heidelberg Retina Tomograph. Excellent repeatability and substantial agreement with the HRT and stereoscopic digital images obtained with the Nidek 900 camera have been demonstrated.[20,21]

The Discam system (Marcher Enterprises Ltd., Hereford, UK) is a digital semi automatic, charge-coupled device camera. Charge coupled image recording devices work better at low levels of light than older digital image processing technologies. This camera captures 20° by 20° optic nerve head photographs. It can automatically measure vertical cup-to-disc ratios and horizontal cup-to-disc ratios. The computer-assisted evaluation of the optic nerve using the Discam digital camera has been shown to compare favorably to the HRT and stereo photography using the Nidek 3DX with glaucoma specialist assessment for detection of glaucoma. There was no significant difference in the sensitivity

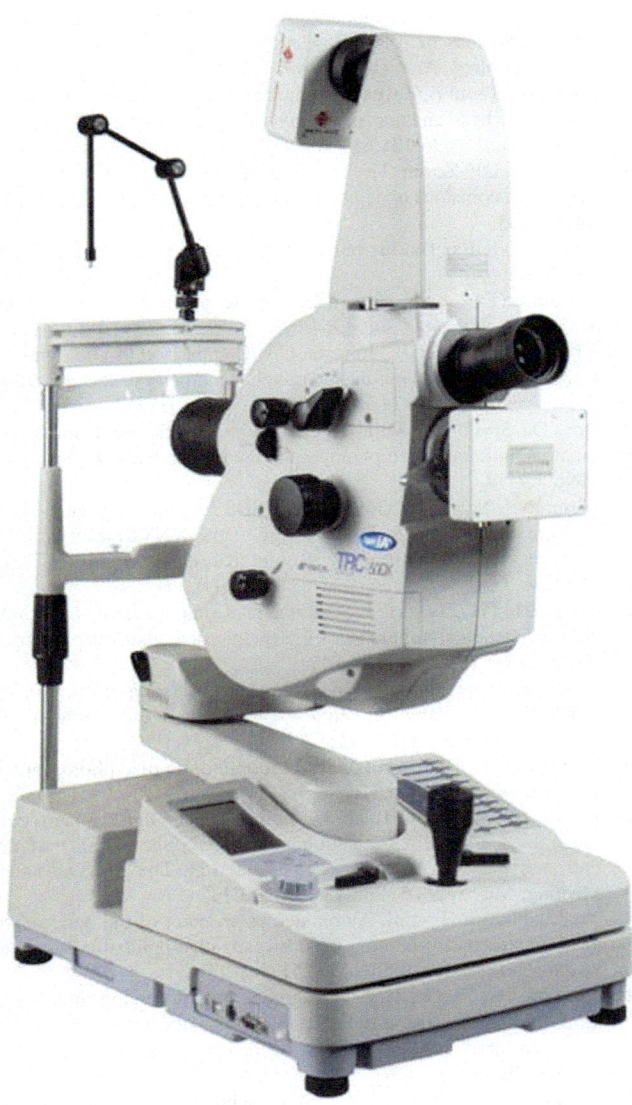

**Fig. 22.6** The Topcon TRC-50DX camera

and specificity of glaucoma detection utilizing the three techniques.[22]

Digital images may be compared for changes in the optic nerve head by using the technique of flicker chronoscopy. The observer sees a series of digital images that "flicker" back and forth to compare two images. This technique is highly sensitive for detecting small changes in optic disc topography.[23,24]

Digital stereo photography has many advantages: (1) instant preview of the image capture by the camera, (2) the ability to review the photograph on the computer screen with the patient (3) electronic storage without the requirement for scanning and (4) its potential use for telemedicine. At the present time, however, digital cameras have less resolution compared with 35-mm slide film.

### 22.2.6 Polaroid Photography

These cameras provide an "instant" image that is stored in the patient's paper chart. Unfortunately, the image quality is low resolution.[3] The Polaroid Corporation has recently (late 2008) announced that it will soon discontinue manufacturing this specialized film. Polaroid photography will soon only be of historic interest.

## 22.3 Frequency of Optic Nerve Head Photography and Glaucoma

The glaucoma patient and the glaucoma suspect should have a color photograph, in stereo when possible, of the optic nerve at the baseline visit. A similar photo for comparison should be repeated every 1–2 years[25] or whenever a change is noted such as the occurrence of an optic nerve hemorrhage. Although many different fundus cameras may be available in a large or multi office practice, it is important to attempt to follow the patient with the same fundus camera in order to accurately document progression. Serial photographs should be taken with the same camera if possible because changing the magnification may affect the appearance of sloping of the optic nerve.

### 22.3.1 Viewing Stereo Images

The photographs should be viewed in stereo with commercial viewers or with high magnification (+10 diopter lenses) to note changes in the neural retinal rim, peripapillary retina and choroid, retinal vessels and contour of the optic nerve cup. Digital photographs on a computer screen will require a special stereo viewer. If the viewing device is not available, the images will not easily be seen in stereo.

It is preferable to review the photograph in the office with the patient to compare the photograph to the current appearance of the optic nerve head whenever the patient's eye is dilated. The stereo photograph may also be reviewed prior to the patient visit to compare with old photographs. A handwritten or keyboard typed note should interpret the photography and be added to the patient's medical record. Copies of printed photographs should be provided, whenever possible, when medical records are given to the patient or other physicians.

A drawing of the optic nerve is particularly useful for immediate feedback to the patient, especially if the photograph made on 35-mm film will not be immediately processed for viewing. (Most practices send their film out for developing and printing.) This drawing may be scanned into the electronic health record and can supplement a stereo photograph.

In an office utilizing electronic medical records, the drawing may be done on an electronic drawing pad that allows the drawing to be directly saved as part of the patient's electronic health record. In these circumstances, the drawing might be displayed "live" on an LCD computer screen in the examination room to provide education and feedback to the patient. The digitized display may be compared with standardized photos of optic nerve appearance at various stages of glaucoma that can be displayed in the examination room. This is very useful to help demonstrate glaucoma progression to the patient. This is also an advantage of the digital stereo camera which allows the patient to see an immediate image of their optic nerve.

Stereo color photography is still the current gold standard for initial and serial documentation of the optic nerve head in patients with ocular hypertension or frank glaucoma. While digital image analyzers with sophisticated software programs may someday supplant the role of the fundus camera in this regard, most offices at current may not be able to have the latest and most advanced of such continually evolving technologies. Photography should continue to play an important role in the care of glaucoma patients for the foreseeable future.

## References

1. Nordenson JW. Augencamera zum stanionaren Ophthalmoskop Von Gulstrand. *Der Dtsch Ophthalmol Ges*. 1925;45:278.
2. Hitchings RA, Varma R, Poinoosawmy D. Optic photographs. In: Varma R, Spaeth GL, Parker JW, eds. *The Optic Nerve in Glaucoma*, Philadelphia: Lippincott-Raven; 1993.
3. Bowd C, Weinreb RN, Zangwill LM. Evaluating the optic disc and retinal nerve fiber layer in glaucoma. I: Clinical examination and photographic methods. *Semin Ophthalmol*. 2000;15(4):194–205.
4. Riedel H. Photography. In: Heilmann K, Richardson KT, eds. *Glaucoma: Conceptions of a Disease*. Philadelphia: WB Saunders; 1978:241–263.
5. Towsend KA, Wollstein G, Schuman JS. Imaging of the retinal nerve fibre layer for glaucoma. *Br J Ophthalmol*. 2009;93(2):139–143.
6. Martinello M, Favaro P, et al. 3D Retinal surface inference: stereo or monocular fundus camera? Proceedings of the 29th Annual International Conference of the IEEE EMBS Cite Internationale, Lyon, france August 23–26, 2007.
7. Greenfield DS. Stereoscopic optic disc. In: Schulman JS, ed. *Imaging in Glaucoma*. Thorofare, NJ: SLACK; 1997:3–14.
8. Sommer A, Pollack I, Maumenee AE. Optic disc parameters in onset of glaucomatous field loss. I. Methods and progressive changes in disc morphology. *Arch Ophthalmol*. 1979;97:1444–1448.
9. Caprioli J, Prum B, Zeyen T. comparison of methods to evaluate the optic nerve head and nerve fiber layer for glaucomatous change. *Am J ophthalmol*. 1996;121:659–667.
10. O'connor DJ, Zeyen T, Caprioli J. Comparisons of methods to detect glaucomatous optic nerve damage. *Ophthalmology*. 1993;100: 1498–1503.
11. Allen L. Ocular fundus photography. *Am J Ophthalmol*. 1964; 57:13–28.
12. Donaldson DD. A new camera for stereoscopic funduus photography. *Trans Am Ophthalmol Soc*. 1964;6:6.
13. Krohn MA, Keltner JL, Johnson CA. Comparison of photographic techniques and films use in stereophotogrammetry of the optic disc. *Am J Ophthalmol*. 1979;88:859–863.
14. Boes Da, Spaeth GL, Mills RP, et al. Relative optic cup depth assessment using three stereo photograph viewing methods. *J Glaucoma*. 1996;5:9–14.
15. Weinreb R, Nelson M, Goldbaum M, et al. Digital image analysis of optic disc topography. Proceedings of the XXVth international Congress of ophthalmology. Rome: Kugler & Ghedini; 1986: 16–221.
16. Greenfield DS, Zacharia P, Schuman JS. Comparison of Nidek 3Dx and Donaldson simultaneous stereoscopic disc photography. *Am J Ophthlamol*. 1993;116:741–747.
17. Accurate image manipulation for desktop publishing. Silver Halide Resolution. Available at: http://www.aim-dtp.net/aim/technology/silver_halide/index.htm.
18. McKinnon SJ. The value of stereoscopic optic disc photography. *J Glaucoma*. 2005;3(6):31.
19. Khouri AS, Szirth BC, Realini T, Fechtner RD. Digital images correlate well with film for simultaneous stereophotography of the optic nerve in glaucoma. Paper presented at: The ARVO Annual Meeting; May 5, 2005; Fort Lauderdale, FL.
20. Xu J, Ishikawa H, et al. Automated assessment of the optic nerve head on stereo disc photographs. Investigative ophthalmology and visual science June 2008;2512–2517.
21. Lamourex EL, Lo K, et al. The agreement between the Heidelberg retina tomograph and a digital non-midget attic retinal camera in assessing area cup to disc ratio. *Invest Ophthalmol Vis Sci*. 2006;47:93–98.
22. Correnti AJ, Wollstein G, Price LL, Schuman JS. Comparison of optic nerve head assessment with a digital stereoscopic camera (discam), scanning laser ophthalmoscopy, and stereophotography. *Ophthalmology*. 2003;110(8):1499–1505.
23. Heijl A, Bengtsson B. Diagnosis of early glaucoma with flicker comparisons of serial disc photographs. Invest Ophthalmol Vis Sci. 1989;30:2376–2384.
24. Parkin B, Shuttleworth G, Costen M, et al. A comparison of stereoscopic and monoscopic evaluation of optic disc topography using a digital optic disc stereo camera. *Br J Ophthalmol*. 2001; 85:1347–1351.
25. Stamper RL, Lieberman MF, Drake M. *Becker-Shaffer's Diagnosis and Therapy of the Glaucomas*. St. Louis: Mosby; 1999.

# Chapter 23
# Detecting Functional Changes in the Patient's Vision: Visual Field Analysis

Chris A. Johnson

The ability to evaluate visual function is one of several important clinical components for the detection, management, and treatment of glaucoma. The structural integrity of the optic nerve head and retinal nerve fiber layer, risk factors for development and progression of glaucoma, intraocular pressure (IOP), and other factors are key elements in the clinical assessment of glaucoma. The status of visual function is vital for examining the efficacy of therapy and disease progression as well as for determining the impact of visual damage on a patient's quality of life and activities of daily living.[1-8] Although contrast sensitivity, vernier acuity, and many other visual functions have been studied in glaucoma patients, perimetry and visual field testing are the primary visual function tests that are useful for glaucoma.[9-14] This chapter provides an overview of perimetry and visual field testing with regard to its use in the clinical assessment of glaucoma.

## 23.1 Structural Versus Functional Methods: Techniques to Assess Glaucomatous Damage to the Optic Nerve

Recent clinical, technologic, and methodological advances have dramatically enhanced the ability to monitor glaucomatous damage and its consequences for patients with this disease. Although there are many factors that are critical for evaluating a patient's status (e.g., IOP, risk factors, general medical health, visual function, optic nerve, and retinal nerve fiber layer integrity), two significant components are the structural and functional properties of the visual system and the pathophysiological alterations produced by glaucoma. Many laboratories are presently evaluating the relationship between structural and functional damage produced by glaucoma, although this relationship remains an enigma.[15-22] It is generally accepted that both optic nerve structure and function provide important and useful clinical information, and that both are necessary to provide a complete assessment of a glaucoma patient's ocular status.

Ophthalmoscopy, optic disc photography, and new imaging techniques (e.g., scanning laser ophthalmoscopy, optical coherence tomography, and retinal nerve fiber layer birefringence) are common methods of determining the clinical assessment of structural properties of the glaucomatous optic nerve head and retinal nerve fiber layer. These topics are covered in other chapters of this book, and will therefore not be discussed in this section.

For functional evaluation, there are now many different methods for performing perimetry and visual field testing (e.g., short wavelength automated perimetry (SWAP), frequency doubling technology (FDT) perimetry, rarebit perimetry, motion perimetry, flicker perimetry, ring perimetry), and other psychophysical test procedures (e.g., contrast sensitivity, flicker-defined form, vernier acuity). Although many of these procedures are described, this chapter emphasizes standard automated (white-on-white) perimetry because it is the most common method of currently determining functional impairment produced by glaucoma.

### 23.1.1 The Hill of Vision and Its Clinical Relevance

Perimetry and visual field testing are methods that are designed to evaluate a patient's peripheral field of view to determine and measure the status of the visual field. Although there have been a number of studies that have examined different test conditions for perimetry (adaptation level, stimulus configuration, testing strategy, stimulus duration, kinetic versus static presentation, etc.),[23-25] the most common procedure has been to use a 31.5 asb (10 cd/m$^2$) background luminance and stimulus sizes originally determined by Goldmann (sizes 0 through V) for performing projection (increment threshold) perimetry.[23-25] The 31.5 asb background is a low photopic luminance level that the eye can rapidly adapt to, can produce the most reliable and stable response properties within and between subjects, and is most resistant to the confounding influence of stimulus, physiological, and attention factors on visual sensitivity. The target sizes (0 through V) provide logarithmic increases in stimulus area that create approximately constant changes in the subject's responses. Other properties such as stimulus duration, inter-stimulus interval, and related factors have also been designed to optimize the clinical utility, reliability, sensitivity, specificity, efficiency, and accuracy of these techniques when used as a diagnostic instrument.[23–25]

Under standard conditions (31.5 asb background, size III stimulus size), the sensitivity profile of the visual field for a normal eye is illustrated in Fig. 23.1, which presents the stimulus luminance increment (increment threshold) or visual field sensitivity that can just be detected on the uniform background luminance. When normal visual sensitivity is plotted as a function of visual field eccentricity, the three-dimensional representation has a shape that is similar to a hill or an island, with the highest sensitivity (the peak) occurring at the fovea. Sensitivity becomes reduced with increasing eccentricity until it reaches a plateau (iso-sensitivity region) in the mid-periphery, followed by a steeper decline in sensitivity at greater peripheral eccentricities. The sensitivity gradient is more gradual for the inferior visual field than the superior visual field, and for the temporal visual field as compared to the nasal visual field. It should be noted that these coordinates (nasal, temporal, superior, inferior) refer to the patient's view of the world, which is opposite to the location of stimuli on the retina (the examiner's view into the eye), and hence, the inferior visual field projects to the superior retina and vice versa, and the nasal visual field projects to the temporal retina and vice versa.

Sensitivity losses produced by ocular or neurologic pathology, stimulus characteristics, or other conditions can be diffuse or widespread, localized, or a combination of diffuse and localized loss (Fig. 23.2). The pattern, location, and shape of visual field sensitivity loss, in combination with monocular or binocular visual field deficits, are useful diagnostic clues used for detection, diagnosis, localization, and monitoring of pathologic conditions affecting the visual pathways. In this view, visual field information can be a powerful clinical tool for determining the specific location of damage to the visual system because the patterns of visual field loss mimic the anatomical arrangement of nerve fiber pathways throughout the visual system. Although this chapter emphasizes visual field losses produced by glaucoma, there are a variety of other references that provide a thorough assessment of patterns of visual field loss associated with different ocular and neurologic disorders affecting the visual system.[26]

A representative sample of visual field deficits associated with glaucoma is shown in Fig. 23.3. The retinal ganglion cell nerve fibers enter the optic nerve head to form the optic nerve in three distinct patterns: (1) the papillomacular bundle, which is a candle flame-shaped group of nerve fibers subserving the region between the optic nerve head (visual field blind spot) and the macula; (2) superior and inferior arcuate nerve fiber bundles, which enter the upper and lower portion of the optic nerve head; and (3) nerve fibers that enter the nasal portion of the optic nerve head (temporal visual field) in a radial pattern. In most instances, the papillomacular bundle is not affected until late in the glaucomatous disease process, so visual field deficits for this region are uncommon. Because the superior and inferior arcuate nerve fiber bundles are most often damaged during the early phases of glaucoma, the visual field deficits (Fig. 23.3) produced by this damage correspond to all or part of these nerve fiber bundles in the form of nasal steps, paracentral defects, partial arcuate, complete arcuate, or double arcuate defects. Damage to the radial nerve fiber bundles is infrequent, but can lead to temporal wedge visual field defects.

Most of the current automated perimeters are able to provide an immediate quantitative comparison of an individual's test results to those of a population with normal visual function, taking into account normal aging effects, variations in sensitivity for different visual field locations, reproducibility within the normal population, response reliability, and related factors. Additionally, changes in the visual fields of the same individual over repeated tests can also be accomplished and compared to results obtained from normal individuals and individuals with visual field loss but stable findings over a short period of time. Analysis of single and multiple visual field results will be presented in a later section of this chapter, although Fig. 23.4 presents a representative example of glaucomatous visual field progression.

### 23.1.2 Methods of Testing the Hill of Vision: Brief Descriptions

There are many different methods of testing the peripheral visual field. Although confrontation visual field testing (using fingers, hands, pencils, medicine bottle caps, or related objects to qualitatively map the visual field) is often performed, the

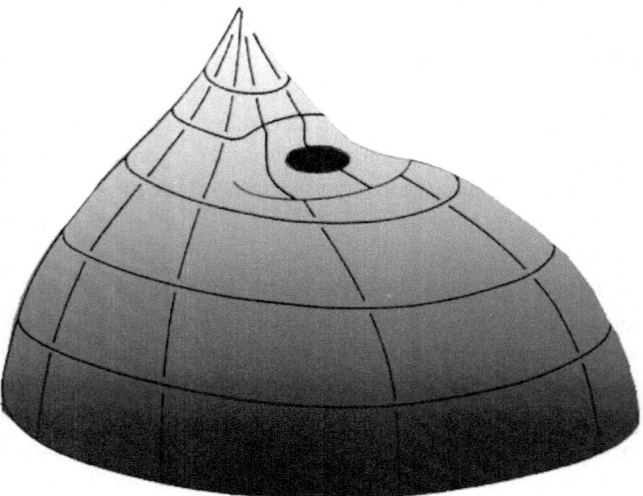

**Fig. 23.1** A schematic representation of the hill of vision for a normal right eye. Sensitivity is plotted as a function of visual field location. The dark oval represents the location of the blind spot and the peak of the hill of vision represents the fovea

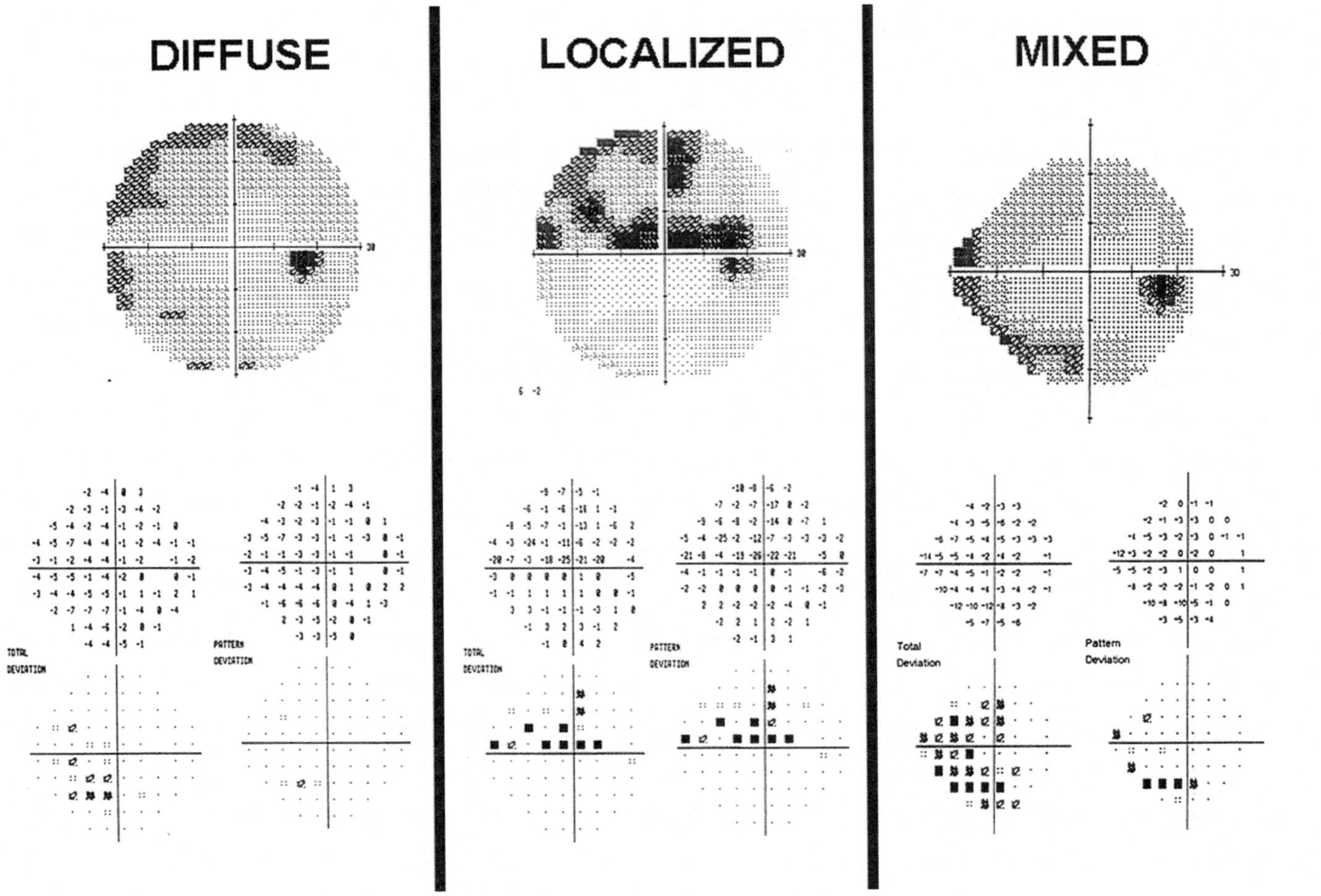

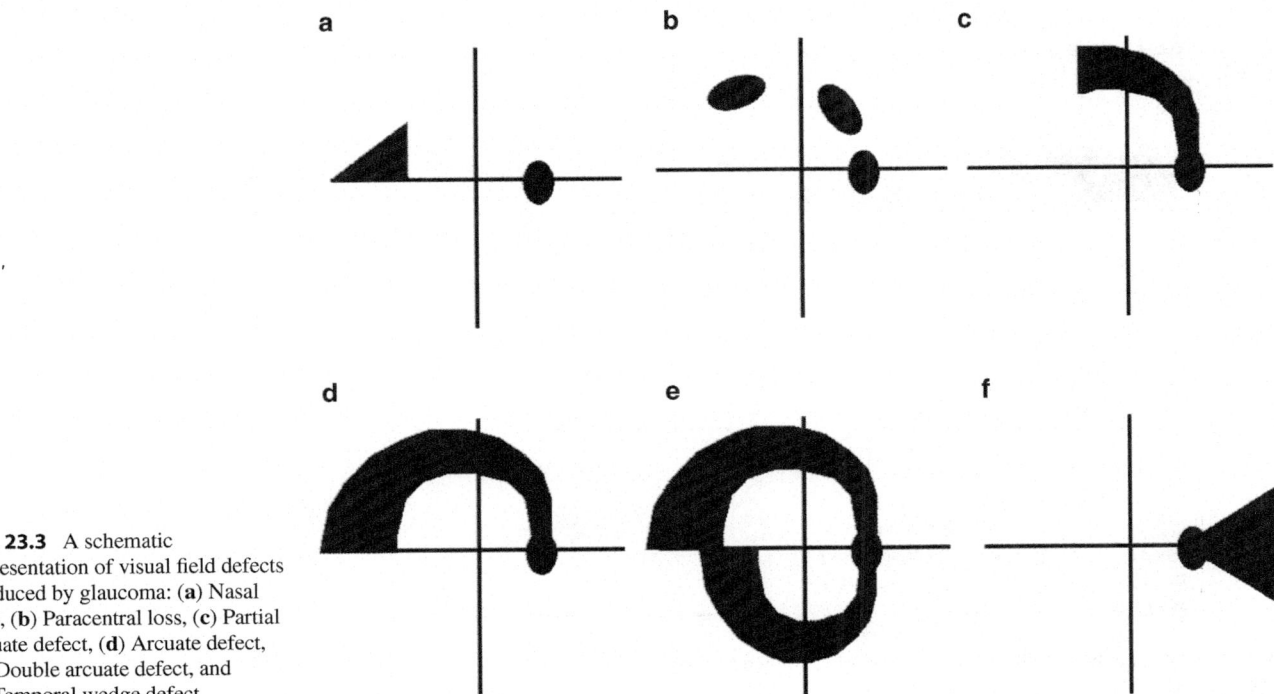

**Fig. 23.2** Humphrey Field Analyzer visual field results for the right eye that demonstrates predominantly diffuse or widespread visual field loss (*left panel*), predominantly localized visual field loss (*center panel*) and a mixed combination of diffuse and localized visual field loss (*right panel*)

**Fig. 23.3** A schematic representation of visual field defects produced by glaucoma: (**a**) Nasal step, (**b**) Paracentral loss, (**c**) Partial arcuate defect, (**d**) Arcuate defect, (**e**) Double arcuate defect, and (**f**) Temporal wedge defect

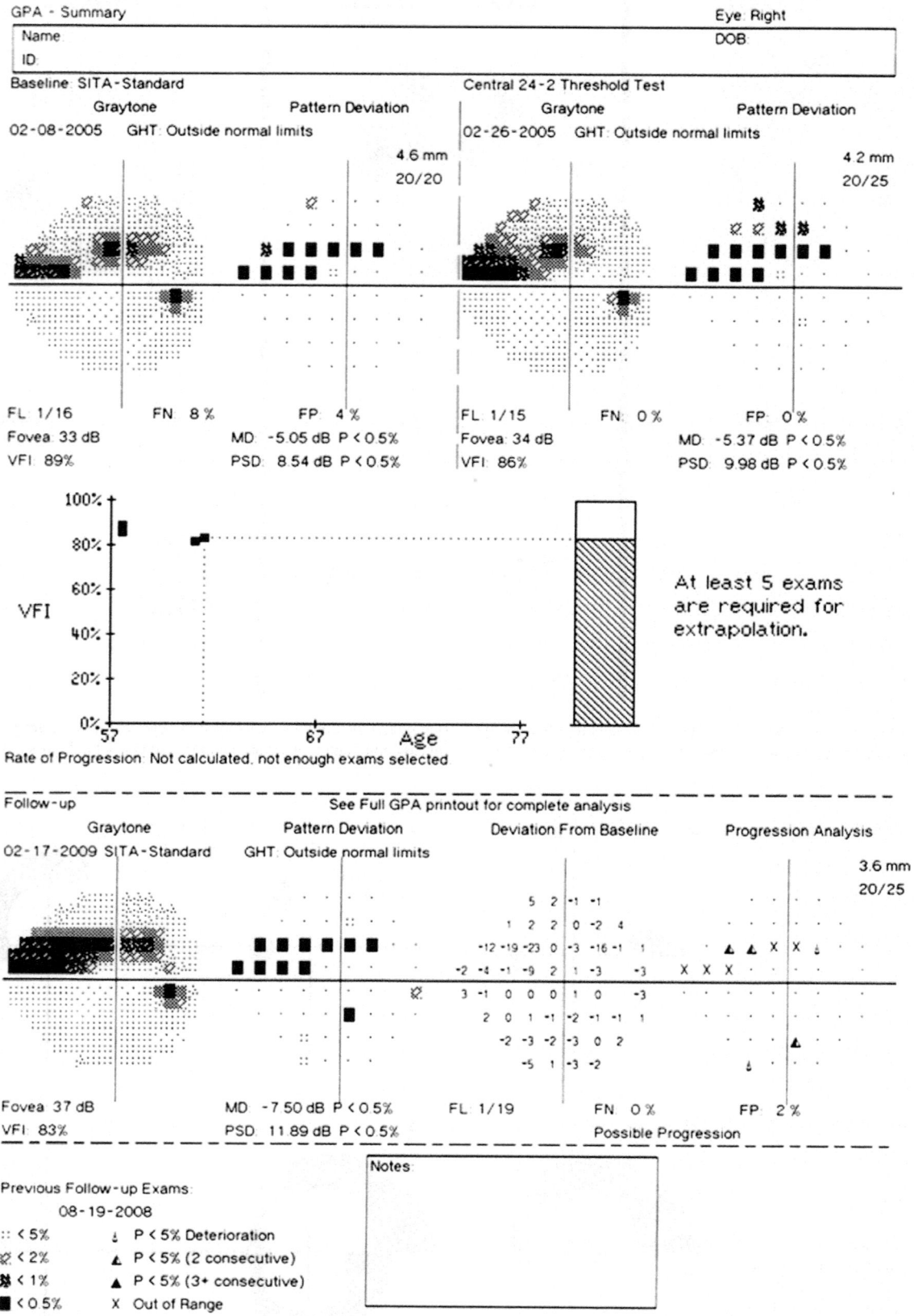

**Fig. 23.4** An example of visual field progression as shown by the Glaucoma Progression Analysis (GPA) printed output for the right eye of a glaucoma patient tested with the Humphrey Field Analyzer II

most common form of testing consists of detecting a small white stimulus that is superimposed on a uniform white background known as projection perimetry. Kinetic, static, and suprathreshold static perimetry can be performed in this manner. Kinetic perimetry is usually conducted manually, although an automated perimetry program is now available on the Octopus perimeter.[27] Static and suprathreshold static perimetry can be performed in a manual or automated fashion. For each of these forms of perimetry, testing is normally performed on one eye that has a proper refractive correction for the testing distance, with the other eye occluded.

It is also important to perform quality control assessment procedures to minimize the influence of nonpathologic factors affecting the test results. There are a number of artifactual test results (lens rim artifacts, droopy eyelids, misalignment, blind spot mislocalization, etc.) that can be avoided by carefully observing the patient during testing[28] (see Sidebar 23.1) It has also been reported that unreliable

---

**SIDEBAR 23.1  Lens induced artifacts during visual field testing**

Andrew C. S. Crichton

Correct lens selection and proper lens placement are paramount in promoting accurate and useful visual field studies. Lens artifacts can occur with either manual or automated perimetry.

The first and most obvious mistake is using the incorrect power of lens. Using too much plus power can artificially enlarge the field. Too much minus power can artificially minify the field. In both cases, the image seen by the patient may be blurry enough to cause an overall generalized depression of the field.

Another source of lens selection error during visual field testing, is not noticing that the patient's refraction may have changed since the last time the visual field exam was performed. The patient may have an unnoticed significant change in refractive error such as can occur after cataract surgery or in a patient under 60 years of age whose pupils are dilated. In these cases, the lens selected for visual field testing might be significantly different from what is needed. Patients should be asked at each exam if they have received new glasses or new contact lenses and of course if they have had any eye surgeries since the last visual field exam. It is always useful to measure their current spectacle correction with a lensometer.

Uncorrected astigmatism may also cause visual field artifacts. A significant amount of uncorrected astigmatism can result in blurry vision causing an overall depression in the field. Also, a lens set at an incorrect axis will blur the patient's vision and produce incorrect field results.

In addition to selecting the correct power and setting the correct axis, the lens must be positioned properly in its holder in front of the patient. The first concern is centering the lens. A lens that is off center can restrict the field on the side, where the edge of the lens is closest to the visual axis. A second error is the possibility of induced prism from a decentered lens. Prentice's Rule describes this effect as:

Induced Prism (PD) = lens power (D) × optical center displacement

This effect is more pronounced the larger the power of the lens being used. For example, a −8.00 lens displaced by 2 cm will induce 16 PD. This effect could shift the field and potentially mask small central or paracentral scotomata. These positioning defects may result not from the location of the lens itself in the lens holder, but rather from the seated position of the patient who is not centered directly behind the lens.

A lens that is sitting too far from the eye can cause the characteristic rim defect, as seen in (Fig. 23.1-1), because of an artifactual constriction of the field. A second effect from the distance a lens sits from the eye concerns vertex distance. The power of the lens for perimetry is generally determined from a patient's spectacle refraction set at a certain vertex distance. If the trial lens during perimetry is not set at the same distance, the effective power can be different than intended. For lenses less than 4 diopters, the effective change in power is negligible. For minus lenses over 4 diopters, the effective power is reduced if the lens is sitting too close to the eye and increased if it is sitting too far. For plus lenses, the effective power is increased if it is sitting too close to the eye and reduced if too far. As with induced prism, the effect is larger with higher powered lenses.

In summary, the proper power of the lens and the proper position of the lens are very important when performing perimetry in order to have artifact free results. Both technicians and physicians must know how to avoid lens related visual field artifacts and also how to spot them when they do occur. These tips and caveats apply when performing and interpreting both manual and automated perimetry.

## Bibliography

Cassin B. *Fundamentals for Ophthalmic Technical Personnel.* Philadelphia: Saunders; 1995:148.
Cassin B. *Fundamentals for Ophthalmic Technical Personnel.* Philadelphia: Saunders; 1995:342.

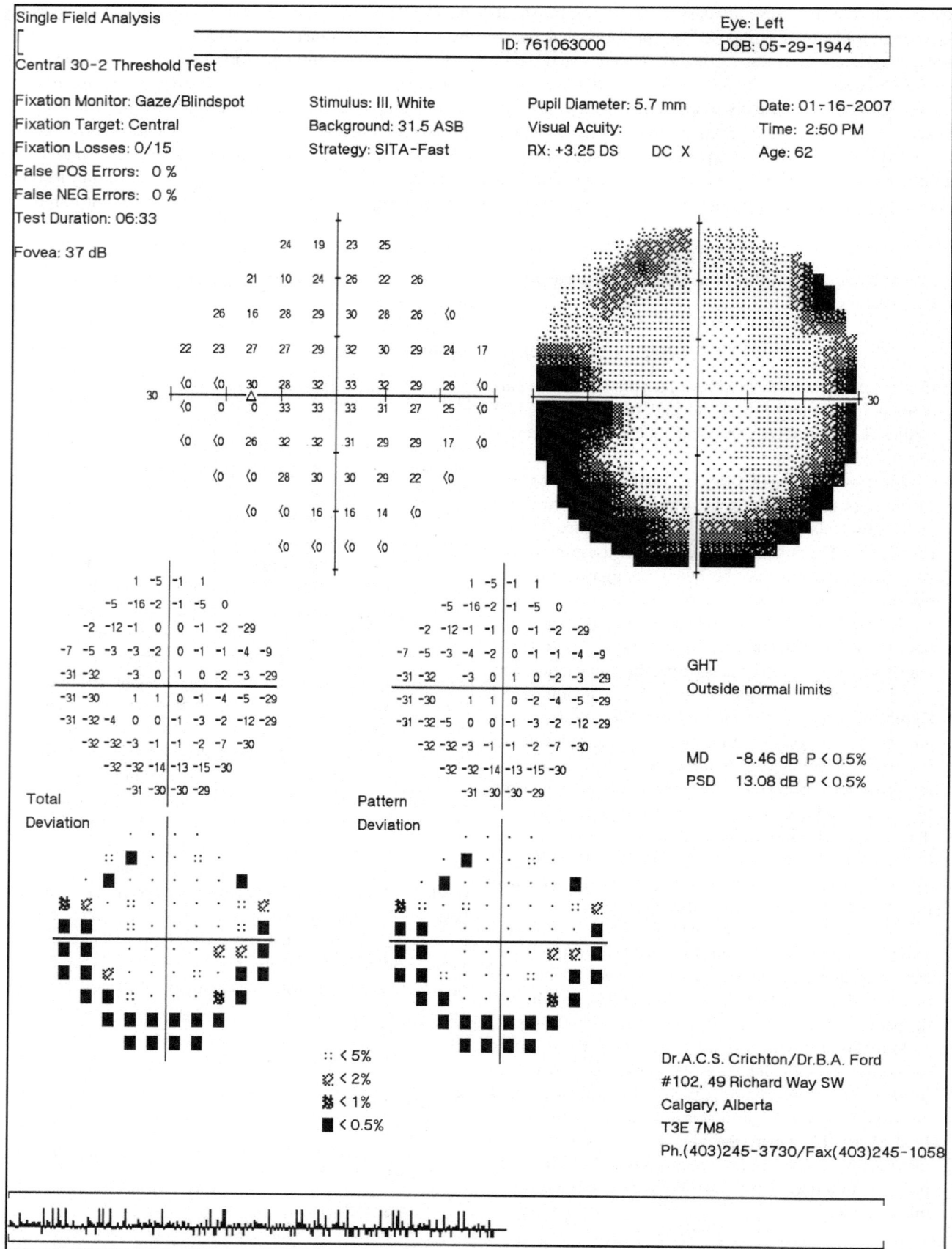

**Fig. 23.1-1** Characteristic rim defects due to an artifactual constriction of the field caused by a lens that is sitting too far from the eye

# 23 Detecting Functional Changes in the Patient's Vision

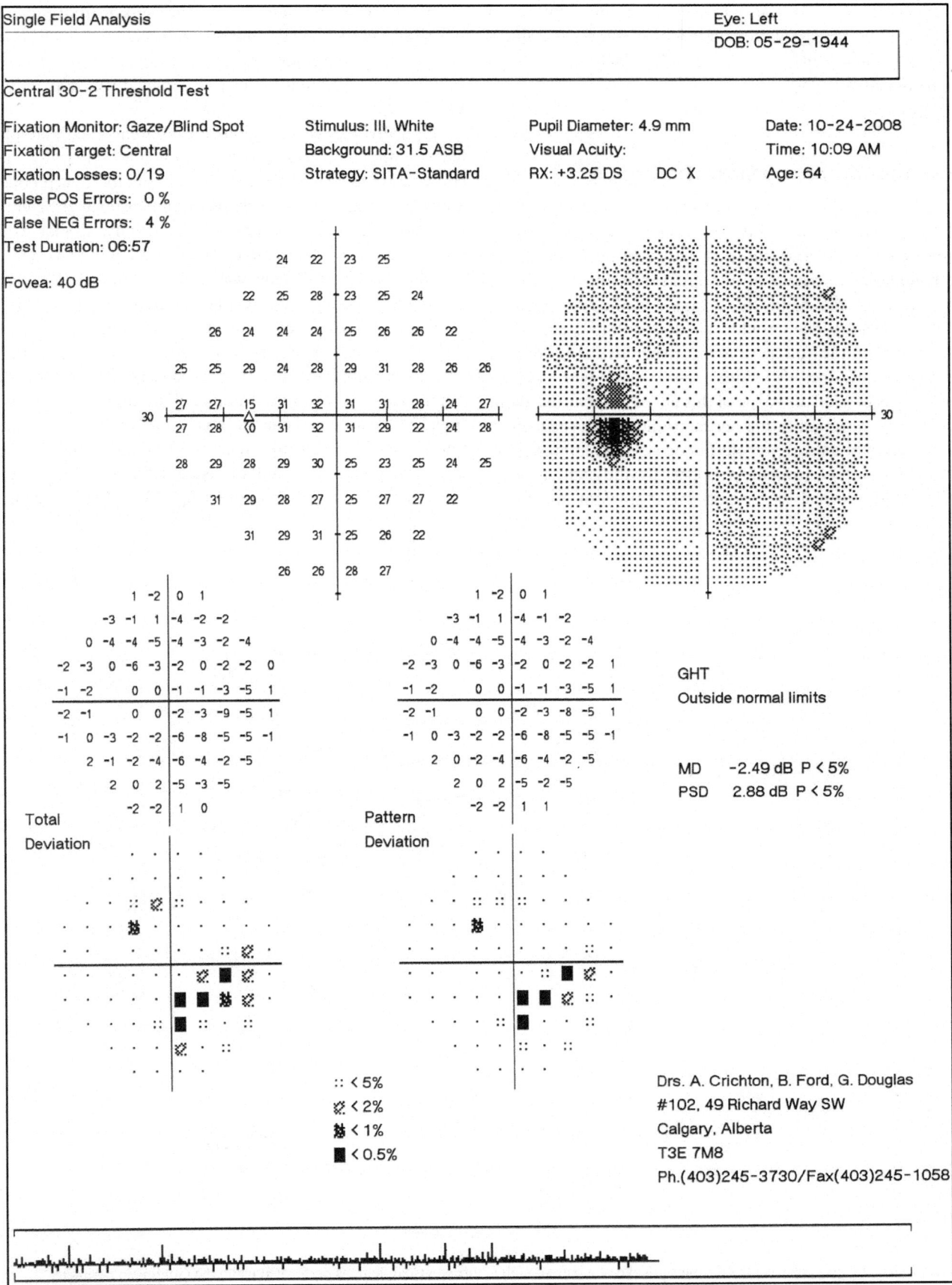

**Fig. 23.1-1** (continued)

visual field results can be obtained in patients with visual field loss,[29] but when quality control assessment procedures have been implemented, unreliable and artifactual test results can be mostly avoided.[30,31]

## 23.2 Kinetic versus Static Perimetry

Kinetic perimetry involves the movement of a stimulus from a nonseeing to a seeing region of the visual field to map out the boundaries of detection of stimuli differing in size and luminance. In the hands of a highly skilled perimetrist, kinetic perimetry can provide an outstanding quantitative assessment of the full peripheral visual field. A detailed description of the techniques associated with kinetic perimetry is beyond the scope of this chapter, but an excellent review may be found in the perimetry book by Anderson.[32] Basically, a stimulus of predetermined size and luminance is moved (2°/s to 5°/s) from the periphery toward fixation along different radii to map out seeing and regions of nonseeing inside of the seeing boundaries. The iso-sensitivity regions of seeing a particular stimulus are connected to form isopters, and similarly, the nonseeing regions are connected to form scotomas for different targets, as depicted schematically in Fig. 23.5.

Typically, the seeing regions for different stimuli are plotted in different colors, and the nonseeing regions for each stimulus are filled with the corresponding color. This produces a two-dimensional plot of the three-dimensional structure of the visual field's differential light sensitivity, similar to the topographic geological survey maps used for landscape. In this view, the three-dimensional structure of visual field sensitivity (see Fig. 23.1) has often been referred to as the "hill of vision" or the "island of vision in a sea of blindness."

Static perimetry involves a group of stationary targets whose threshold for detection is measured by varying its luminance. A collection of points along different meridians (Fig. 23.6) in polar coordinates, or grids in Cartesian coordinates, may be used to determine sensitivity to light. This provides an alternate view of the hill of vision in the form of grayscale plots or profile representations (Fig. 23.7). Static perimetry

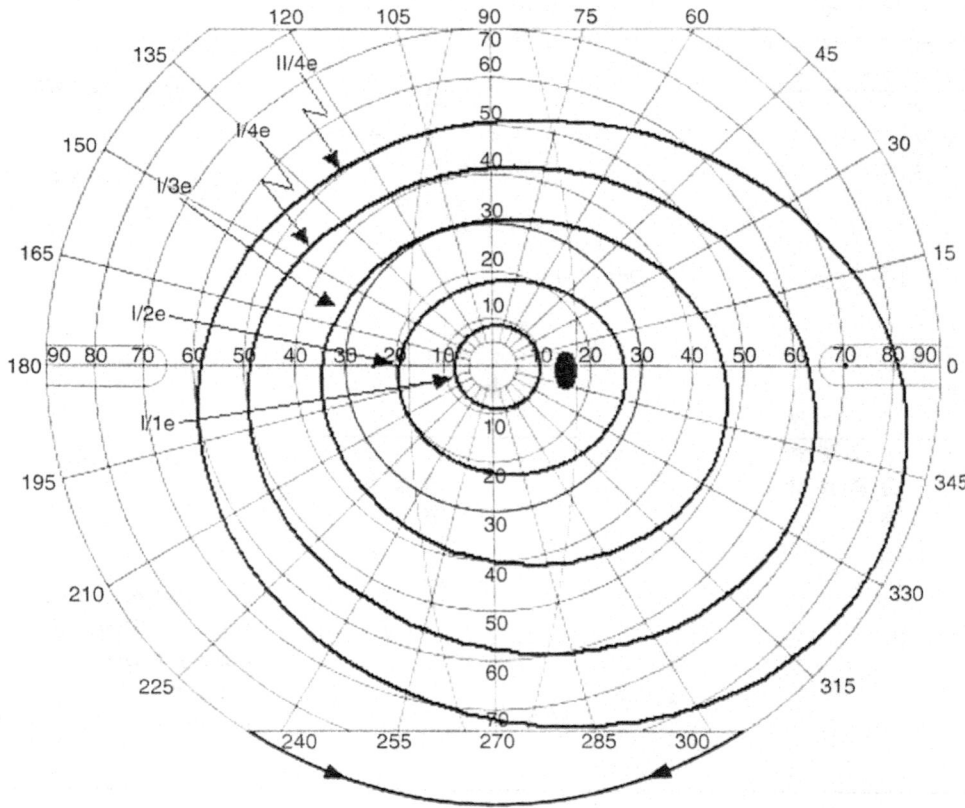

**Fig. 23.5** Kinetic perimetry results for the right eye of a patient with a normal visual field, as performed using the Goldmann perimeter

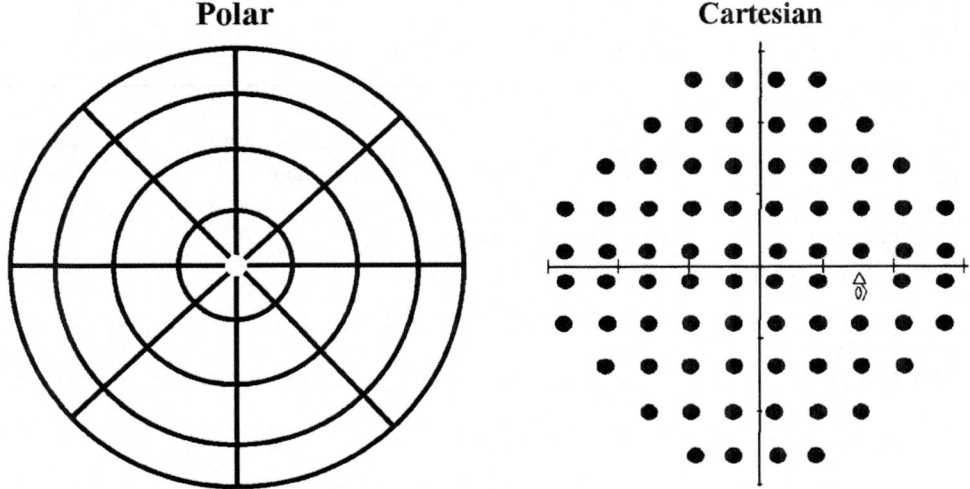

**Fig. 23.6** A schematic representation of polar and Cartesian coordinate systems used for performing perimetry and visual field testing. Representation for a right eye is shown in this figure

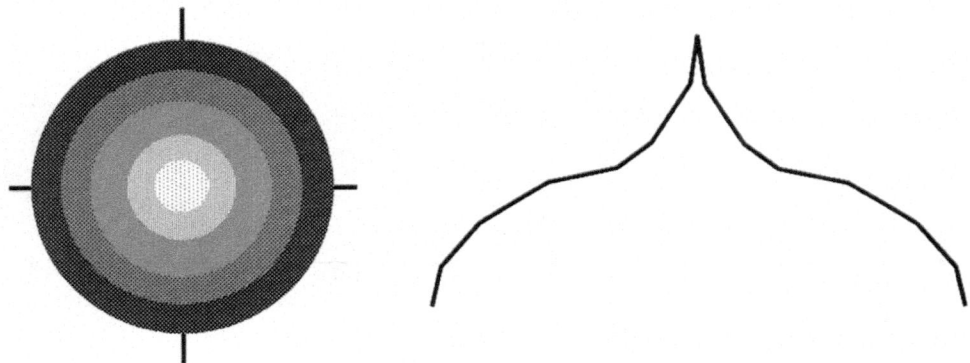

**Fig. 23.7** A schematic representation of grayscale (*left*) and profile (*right*) sensitivity plots for perimetry test results

is currently the most common form of quantitative visual field testing performed by eye care specialists.

Suprathreshold static perimetry is a procedure that is primarily used as a screening technique to determine whether different locations of the visual field are within normal limits or are below normal limits (Fig. 23.8). In some instances, a rough estimate of the amount of abnormality can also be derived. Usually, these procedures are able to provide visual field information more rapidly than quantitative (kinetic and static) techniques, although research on these procedures has been limited to only a few clinical laboratories.[33–39] At the present time, there are a very large number of visual field screening procedures that are available, there is sparse information concerning the performance capabilities of these procedures, comparisons among different screening methods are rare, and their clinical significance is somewhat indeterminate. Additionally, the cost-effectiveness and societal–medical value of glaucoma screening has been a topic of debate among many investigators.[40,41]

In some instances – such as determining an individual's fitness to drive, evaluating visual performance capabilities, assessing quality of life and activities of daily living issues, and related topics – it is important to measure an individual's binocular visual field. Most perimetric devices do not have the ability to easily perform binocular visual field testing. However, several investigators have proposed methods of combining monocular visual field information to estimate the binocular visual field.[42,43] For conjugate points in the visual field for the two eyes, the most sensitive threshold value and probability summation of sensitivity values between the two eyes can usually provide reasonably accurate estimates of binocular visual field threshold sensitivity.[42,43] These procedures have now been employed by several laboratories for these purposes.[8,42–46]

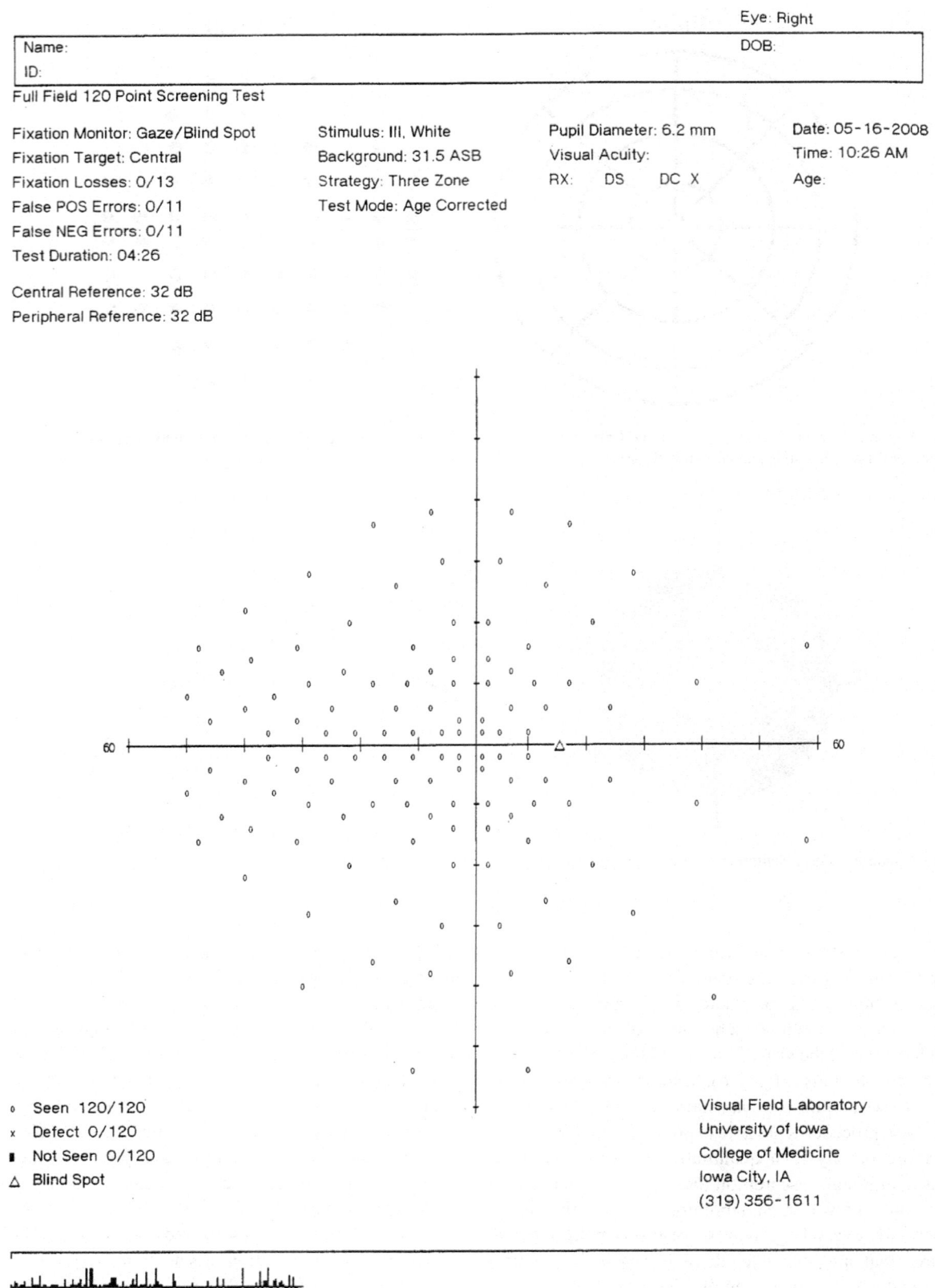

**Fig. 23.8** Printed output for the 120 point visual field screening test for a right eye, as performed on the Humphrey Field Analyzer. The three zone test strategy is shown

### Is It Useful to Perform Visual Field Screening for Glaucoma?

Screening for glaucoma has been a controversial topic, primarily because of the low prevalence and incidence of glaucoma, the high cost of performing screening, and the relatively low incidence of significant disabling visual impairment and binocular blindness.[179] In addition, recent investigations have demonstrated that compliance and adherence to medical glaucoma therapy is poor.[180,181] On the other hand, recent multicenter trials indicate that treatment is effective in delaying or preventing glaucomatous damage,[182–186] the impact of glaucoma on quality of life and activities of daily living occur at early stages of the disease,[1–8,187,188] half or more of the individuals who have glaucoma remain undiagnosed,[188] and certain populations are more susceptible to developing undiagnosed glaucoma.[189,190] The value of early glaucoma detection has been succinctly and elegantly stated by Javitt, Lee, and Lum.[41] Until further information is available, the best alternatives for glaucoma screening today should be directed toward the assessment of risk factors for developing glaucoma, performing screening in populations at higher risk for developing glaucoma or who have limited access to traditional health care, and selecting test procedures that provide the best performance (sensitivity, specificity, predictive value) for detecting glaucoma. Additionally, a screening procedure that is directed toward many major ocular and neurologic disorders rather than just glaucoma would also be helpful.

## 23.3 Modern Methods of Checking the Visual Field and Their Relevance

In the previous section, various methods for performing standard (white-on-white) perimetric testing have been described. However, there are many other techniques for performing visual field testing that evaluate a variety of visual functions. Some of these test procedures have not provided much clinically useful information, whereas others have demonstrated an ability to detect glaucomatous damage at an earlier stage, predict future glaucomatous loss, provide better information about glaucomatous progression, generate a more objective measure of glaucomatous loss, and determine visual status in subjects with limited ability to perform conventional perimetric testing. In this chapter, only those procedures that have demonstrated the capabilities of providing helpful clinical information will be discussed.

### 23.3.1 Short Wavelength Automated Perimetry

Stiles[47] developed a technique known as the two-color increment threshold technique, wherein it was possible to selectively isolate and measure the sensitivity of individual color vision mechanisms by using a chromatic background field (to adapt the other color vision mechanisms and reduce their sensitivity) and a different chromatic stimulus (to selectively measure the sensitivity of a single color vision mechanism). In this view, short-wavelength-sensitive (blue) mechanisms can be isolated by using a high-luminance, broadband, middle-wavelength (yellow) background to adapt and suppress the other (middle wavelength or "green" and long wavelength or "red") color vision mechanisms in combination with a large (Goldmann size V) narrow band short wavelength ("blue") stimulus. Kitahara[48] and Kranda and King-Smith[49] were among the initial investigators to evaluate the efficacy of this procedure for evaluating short wavelength sensitivity loss in glaucoma and other ocular and neurologic diseases. Unfortunately, complex calibration issues, long examination times, and difficult response characteristics precluded the implementation of this procedure for routine clinical use.

Sample and colleagues[50–59] and Johnson and collaborators[60–69] were able to modify the existing automated perimeters to perform SWAP. Cross-sectional and longitudinal investigations from these laboratories were able to establish that SWAP was capable of characterizing glaucomatous visual field defect patterns,[50–53,60–64] could detect glaucomatous visual field loss up to 10 years earlier than standard perimetric testing,[70] could predict future glaucomatous damage on conventional perimetric testing,[55–57,60–66] and was able to determine a greater amount of progressive glaucomatous loss as compared to standard perimetric testing.[52,55,61,68]

A collaborative study was able to determine the optimal clinical test procedures for SWAP, which consisted of a high-luminance (100 cd/m$^2$) broadband yellow background with a dominant wavelength of 530 nm (OG 530 Kodak Wratten filter), a narrow band (10 nm) large (Goldmann Size V) "blue" stimulus (dominant wavelength of 440 nm, Omega filter) presented for 200 ms.[54] These conditions were able to minimize the effect of lens attenuation of short wavelength light, maximize the dynamic range of SWAP, and provide the greatest amount of isolation of short wavelength sensitive mechanisms. Subsequent investigations were able to adapt Bayesian forecasting test procedures to SWAP to diminish testing time to 3–4 min per eye, expand the dynamic range by more than 4 dB, and slightly reduce variability while maintaining similar measurement procedures to the original SWAP procedure.[71–74] Several publications provide a review of SWAP findings in glaucoma.[58,59,66,67] Additionally, many other characteristics were identified for SWAP, and it was also determined that SWAP was useful for characterizing damage from other ocular and neurologic disorders.[75] Several references have provided excellent review of the use of SWAP for evaluating visual field properties of patients with glaucoma and other ocular and neurologic conditions.[58,59,67] Figure 23.9 presents an example of SWAP results in the right eye of a patient with early glaucomatous visual field loss.

### 23.3.2 Frequency Doubling Technology Perimetry

When a low spatial frequency (less than two cycles per degree) sinusoidal grating undergoes high temporal frequency (greater than 15 Hz) counterphase flicker, the stimulus appears to have twice as many alternating light and dark bars in the grating (i.e., its spatial frequency appears to be doubled). The frequency doubling effect was reported many years ago by Kelly[76,77] and other investigators,[78–82] but it was not until Maddess and Henry indicated that this psychophysical procedure could be used to characterize and evaluate glaucomatous visual field loss that it was considered for clinical ophthalmic diagnostic purposes.[83] Rather than evaluating the doubled appearance of this stimulus, they indicated that the contrast sensitivity for detecting the stimulus was the appropriate method of measuring FDT responses. Shortly thereafter, Johnson and Samuels reported a perimetric method of performing FDT testing that appeared to perform very well for detecting glaucomatous visual field loss, consisting of 19 large ($10° \times 10°$) targets distributed over the central $20°–30°$ radius.[84]

Several modifications were made to the original FDT perimeter (including the use of the Modified Binary Search (MOBS) procedure, an adaptive staircase method of measuring contrast sensitivity values).[84] FDT perimetry was evaluated in ocular and neurologic conditions other than glaucoma,[85–89] and the underlying basis and visual pathway location responsible for generating the FDT effect[90,91] have been reported. A review of findings for FDT perimetry may be found in the literature.[92]

Recently, a second-generation FDT perimeter has been developed that is referred to as the Humphrey Matrix. The Humphrey Matrix provided a number of enhancements to FDT perimetry, including: the use of Zippy Estimation of Sequential Threshold (ZEST), a Bayesian forecasting procedure for estimating detection sensitivity; smaller ($5° \times 5°$) targets with a number of different stimulus configurations (30-2, 24-2, and ($2° \times 2°$) targets) 10-2 and Macula tests); direct monitoring of eye position using a video camera display system; a more extensive analysis and test printout system; a greater amount of statistical analysis; enhanced storage and data transfer procedures; and many additional features.[93–98] The development of the Humphrey Matrix and the normative database and statistical analysis package has been published,[93] and performance characteristics of the Humphrey Matrix has been reported for glaucoma and other ocular and neurologic conditions.[94–98]

Primers that give a brief description of the FDT and Matrix tests, their underlying basis, and an assortment of results for different ocular and neurologic conditions have been made available for interested users for both instruments.[99,100] The FDT testing procedure is preferred by most individuals over conventional perimetric test procedures. Additionally, it has been reported that there is a much lower amount of increase in variability in damaged visual field areas when compared to conventional perimetry, with the Matrix showing essentially equivalent reproducibility throughout the entire dynamic range of the instrument.[101] The FDT perimetry test has also been used for rapid screening of pathologic ocular and neurologic conditions, with one method that emphasizes high sensitivity and another method that emphasizes high specificity.[102,103] Both procedures have been reported to offer very good performance and provide two alternatives for rapid testing of individuals, depending on the needs of the examiner. For both procedures, the testing can be performed in 30 s or less per eye for individuals with normal vision and in less than 2 min per eye for individuals with visual field loss.[102] Overall, the FDT perimetry test procedure has been shown to have clinical value. Figure 23.10 presents Humphrey Matrix results for the left eye of a patient with moderate glaucomatous visual field loss.

### 23.3.3 Motion Perimetry

The ability to detect target movement is a salient aspect of visual function in the periphery. Although movement perception has been a topic of interest to psychophysicists and physiologists for many years, it has only been in recent times that motion detection has been used as a clinical ophthalmic diagnostic tool.[104–117] There are two basic methods of conducting motion detection thresholds. One method evaluates the minimum spatial displacement of a target on a uniform background[104–106] and the other uses a variable size random cluster of small dots that either move in the same direction while other dots are stationary (size thresholds)[107–109] or a proportion of dots move coherently in the same direction while other dots are moving randomly (coherence thresholds).[110–116] Each of these procedures have been reported to be effective in detecting early glaucomatous visual field loss.

This visual field test procedure is quite robust, being minimally affected by the effects of moderate amounts of blur,

# 23 Detecting Functional Changes in the Patient's Vision

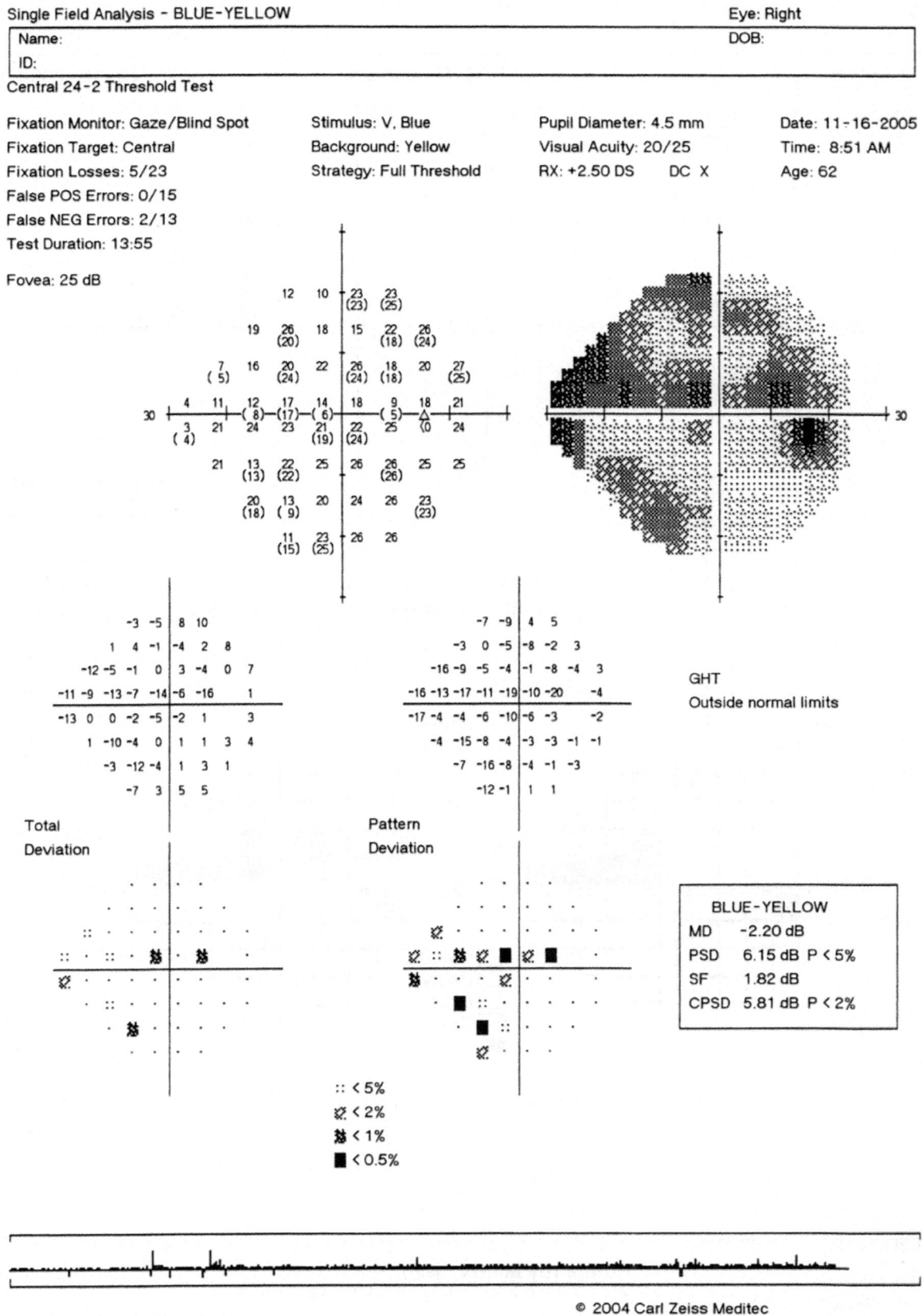

**Fig. 23.9** Short Wavelength Automated Perimetry (SWAP) for the right eye of a patient with superior and inferior glaucomatous visual field loss

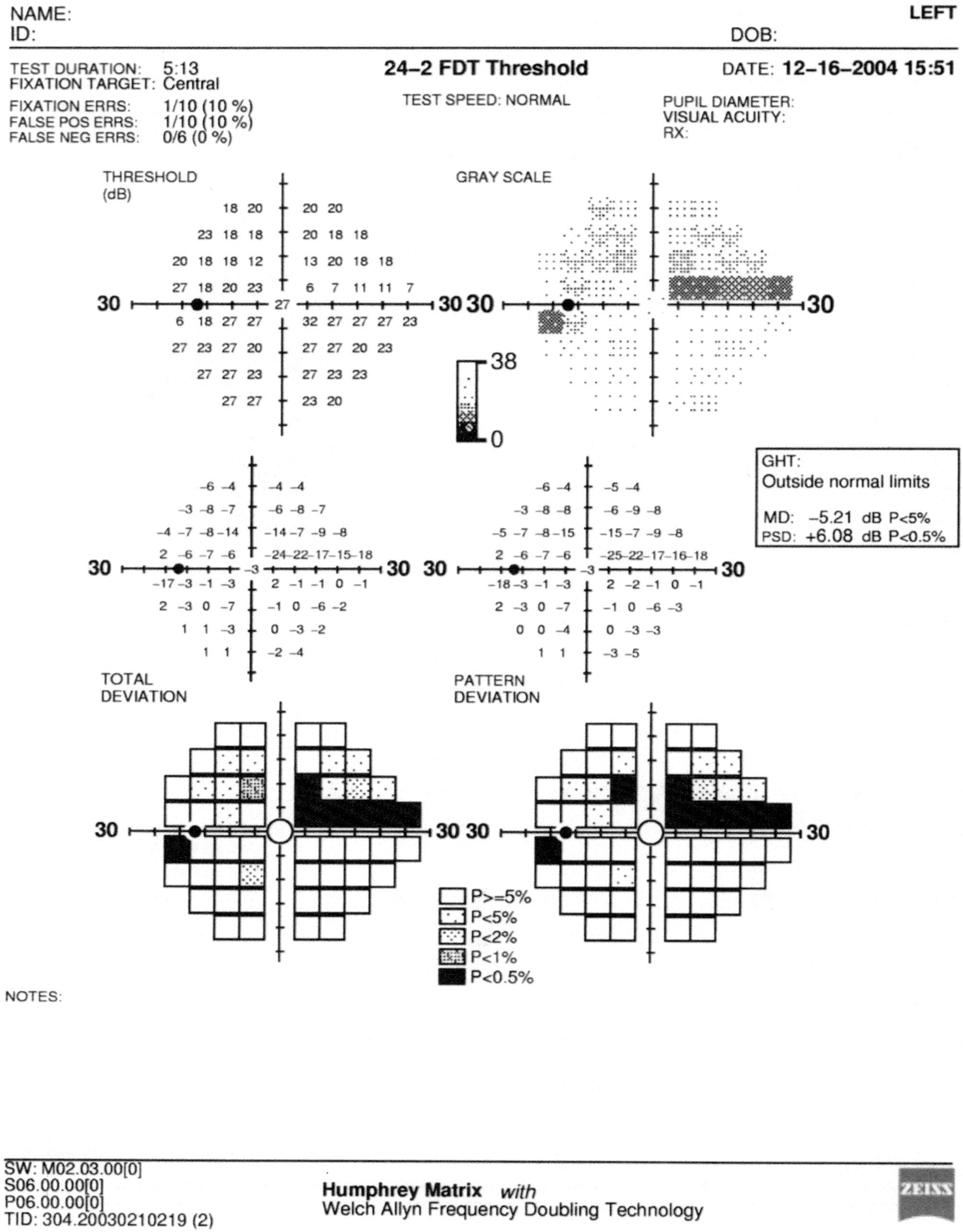

**Fig. 23.10** Results for the left eye of a patient with superior arcuate visual field loss as performed on the Humphrey Matrix Frequency Doubling perimeter using the 24-2 threshold test procedure

# 23 Detecting Functional Changes in the Patient's Vision

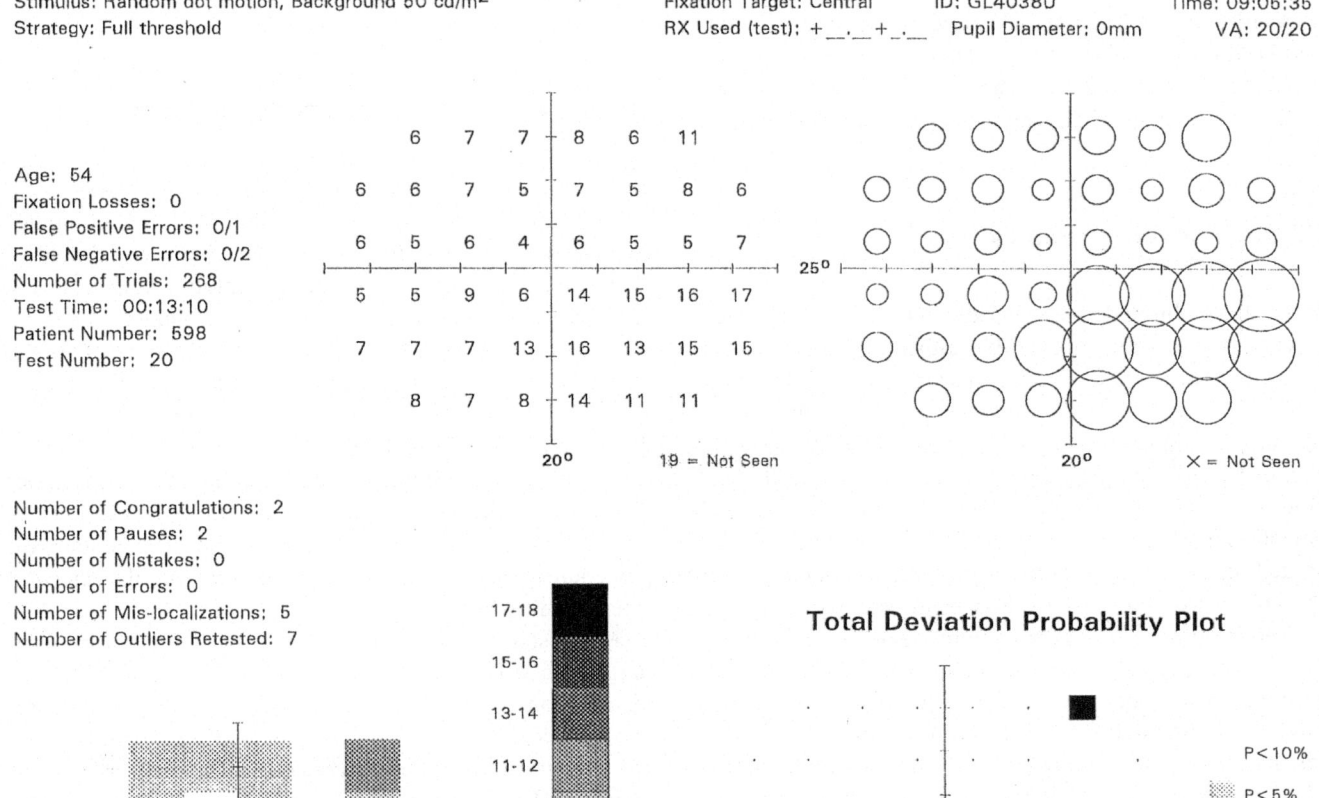

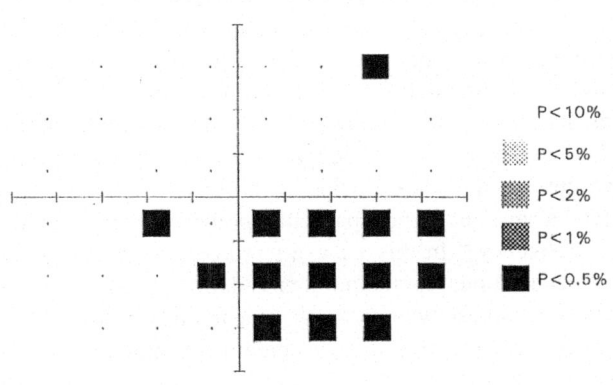

**Fig. 23.11** Motion perimetry results for the left eye of a patient with inferior arcuate glaucomatous visual field loss

contrast variations, and background luminance levels.[118] In addition, motion detection thresholds are a simple response property for peripheral visual function assessment, and most subjects prefer this procedure to standard automated perimetry methods. The reliability and reproducibility of motion perimetry is also quite good. Figure 23.11 presents an example of motion perimetry obtained in the left eye of a patient with glaucomatous visual field loss, using the techniques that present motion of a cluster of dots within a larger group of stationary dots.

### 23.3.4 Flicker Perimetry

When a stimulus undergoes periodic light and dark alternation (flicker), it is possible to determine either the highest temporal frequency that can be distinguished from a steady light stimulus (critical flicker fusion) or to evaluate the minimum amount of flicker amplitude needed to detect alternation of the stimulus (temporal modulation perimetry) at a fixed rate of flicker.[119] Both of these procedures have been used effectively in the detection of glaucomatous visual field loss and have demonstrated the ability to provide earlier detection of damage and the ability to predict future loss using standard automated perimetry tests.[68,119–125] A direct comparison of the two procedures that tested the same normal controls and glaucoma patients using both techniques suggested that temporal modulation perimetry provided slightly better separation of results from normal control subjects in comparison to glaucoma patients.[119] Although it has been reported that high temporal frequencies provide the best results,[121] more recent studies have not found a particular preference for any temporal frequency.[68] In this view, a temporal frequency of 8 Hz has been adopted for temporal modulation perimetry because it has the largest dynamic range (due to higher sensitivity), is less affected by other stimulus parameters that affect flicker, and appears to be the most reliable.[68] An example of temporal modulation perimetry in the left eye of a patient with glaucoma is presented in Fig. 23.12.

Similar to motion perimetry, flicker perimetry results are quite resistant to the influence of blur and other testing variables, but can be affected by changes in pupil size and many other physiologic and pathophysiologic factors.[126] Flicker perimetry testing must therefore be performed carefully and with consideration of confounding variables.

Two recent methods that employ flicker as a stimulus attribute include luminance pedestal flicker and flicker-defined form. The luminance pedestal flicker presents a flickering stimulus that is superimposed onto a steady pedestal of light, and the subject's task is to determine whether the stimulus appears to be flickering or steady.[127–129] Flicker-defined form presents a number of stimuli that are undergoing rapid temporal alternation, except that one of the targets is flickering in counterphase to the others (i.e., is dark when the others are light and vice versa).[130,131] This procedure has been incorporated into the Edge perimeter manufactured by Heidelberg Engineering. At the present time, there is insufficient data to determine the clinical value of these approaches for detection of glaucomatous visual field loss.

### 23.3.5 High Pass Resolution Perimetry

High pass resolution perimetry (HPRP) uses a series of ring stimuli varying in size that are displayed on a computer monitor at various locations within the central visual field.[132] The stimuli resemble visual acuity optotypes such as the Landolt C and consist of a dark ring surrounding a central circular white region. Contrast of the HPRP rings is approximately 85%, and the targets are constructed digitally by high-pass spatial frequency filtering of the ring stimulus.[132,136] The stimuli were designed to make detection and resolution threshold for the stimulus to be approximately equivalent. The subject's task is to press the response button each time a stimulus is detected, and the program performs a staircase procedure to increase and decrease target size until a detection threshold is achieved.

Many studies have demonstrated that HPRP is a useful diagnostic test procedure for characterizing visual field loss in glaucoma and other ocular and neurologic disorders, and glaucomatous deficits are detected approximately 18 months prior to those observed for standard automated perimetry.[132–141] HPRP has a number of desirable characteristics, including: (1) a rapid test procedure, (2) interactive communication with the patient, (3) feedback to the patient concerning performance, (4) good ability to detect visual field loss in glaucoma and other ocular and neurologic disorders, (5) ability to determine visual field progression earlier than standard automated perimetry, and (6) an easy to follow test procedure.[132–141] Unfortunately, the commercial availability of HPRP at the present time is very limited. An example of HPRP conducted for the right eye of a patient with glaucomatous visual field loss is presented in Fig. 23.13.

### 23.3.6 Rarebit Perimetry

Rarebit perimetry is a relatively new visual field test procedure that has a somewhat limited record of clinical performance to date.[142–146] A computer display is used to present one or two small white dots (pixels) on a uniform background that are located in a small area of the visual field. The subject's task is to indicate whether one or two dots were detected for each stimulus presentation. High density maps of stimulus dots are constructed for subsequent stimulus trials, and the Rarebit procedure uses correct and incorrect responses as a

| Patient ID | Test Date | Eye | OD |
|---|---|---|---|
| *Flicker* | DOB | | |

| | | |
|---|---|---|
| MD | -6.186 | |
| MD Prob | 0.020 | |
| PSD | 5.396 | |
| PSD Prob | 0.980 | |

**Raw Data**

|      |      |      |      |      |      |      |      |
|------|------|------|------|------|------|------|------|
|      |      | 10.0 | 19.0 | 16.0 | 16.0 |      |      |
|      | 12.0 | 16.0 | 16.5 | 12.0 | 16.5 | 14.0 |      |
| 12.0 | 7.5  | 14.0 | 16.5 | 19.0 | 14.0 | 16.5 | 24.5 |
| 12.0 | 14.0 | 14.0 | 14.0 | 24.5 | 18.5 | 21.5 | 21.5 |
| 12.0 | 12.0 | 10.0 | 3.0  | 21.0 | 21.5 | 23.5 | 19.0 |
| 12.0 | 7.5  | 8.5  | 5.0  | 12.0 | 1.0  | 12.0 | 18.5 |
|      | 12.0 | 10.0 | 7.5  | 12.0 | 14.0 | 16.5 |      |
|      |      | 14.0 | 10.0 | 13.5 | 19.0 |      |      |

**Age Adjusted Data**

|      |      |      |      |      |      |      |      |
|------|------|------|------|------|------|------|------|
|      |      | 11.5 | 20.3 | 17.4 | 17.4 |      |      |
|      | 12.6 | 18.1 | 17.5 | 13.0 | 17.7 | 15.7 |      |
| 12.4 | 8.0  | 15.5 | 17.2 | 20.1 | 15.3 | 17.0 | 26.0 |
| 12.2 | 15.0 | 15.1 | 14.5 | 25.1 | 18.8 | 22.7 | 22.3 |
| 13.1 | 13.1 | 10.6 | 3.8  | 21.4 | 22.7 | 24.5 | 20.6 |
| 12.8 | 8.9  | 9.6  | 6.0  | 12.8 | 2.8  | 13.1 | 20.0 |
|      | 13.6 | 11.5 | 8.6  | 12.7 | 15.2 | 17.7 |      |
|      |      | 15.4 | 11.3 | 15.5 | 20.2 |      |      |

**Total Threshhold Deviation**

|      |      |      |       |       |       |       |      |
|------|------|------|-------|-------|-------|-------|------|
|      |      | -7.5 | 0.8   | -1.2  | -0.8  |       |      |
|      | -6.2 | -3.7 | -4.8  | -6.1  | -3.5  | -4.4  |      |
| -6.6 | -12.7| -7.9 | -5.5  | -2.2  | -7.4  | -4.3  | 5.5  |
| -6.0 | -5.3 | -7.3 | -9.4  | 0.1   | -5.6  | -1.5  | 1.0  |
| -6.0 | -8.2 | -12.4| -19.5 | -2.9  | -2.4  | 1.3   | -1.2 |
| -7.5 | -13.0| -12.4| -17.4 | -10.4 | -19.6 | -9.2  | -0.7 |
|      | -6.4 | -8.9 | -13.4 | -8.2  | -6.5  | -2.9  |      |
|      |      | -5.0 | -8.6  | -5.5  | 0.2   |       |      |

**Pattern Threshhold Deviation**

|      |       |       |       |      |       |      |      |
|------|-------|-------|-------|------|-------|------|------|
|      |       | -6.8  | 1.5   | -0.5 | -0.1  |      |      |
|      | -5.5  | -3.0  | -4.1  | -5.4 | -2.8  | -3.7 |      |
|      | -5.9  | -12.0 | -7.2  | -4.8 | -1.5  | -6.7 | -3.6 | 6.2 |
| -5.3 | -4.6  | -6.6  | -8.7  | 0.8  | -4.9  | -0.8 | 1.7  |
| -5.3 | -7.5  | -11.7 | -18.8 | -2.2 | -1.7  | 2.0  | -0.5 |
| -6.8 | -12.3 | -11.7 | -16.7 | -9.7 | -18.9 | -8.5 | 0.0  |
|      | -5.7  | -8.2  | -12.7 | -7.5 | -5.8  | -2.2 |      |
|      |       | -4.3  | -7.9  | -4.8 | 0.9   |      |      |

**Total Threshhold Deviation Probability**

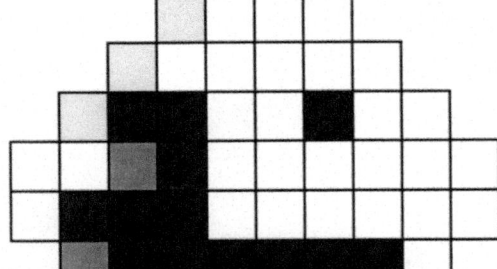

**Pattern Deviation Probability**

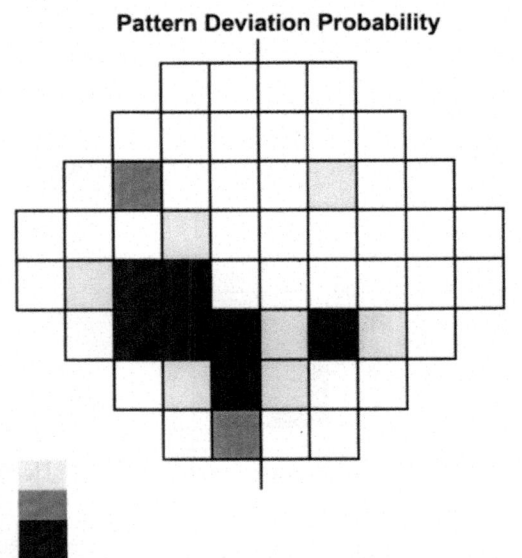

P < 5%
P < 2%
P < 1%
P < 0.5%

**Fig. 23.12** Flicker perimetry results for the left eye of a patient with inferior arcuate glaucomatous nerve fiber bundle visual field loss. For this procedure the amplitude of flicker is varied for a constant flicker frequency of 8 Hz

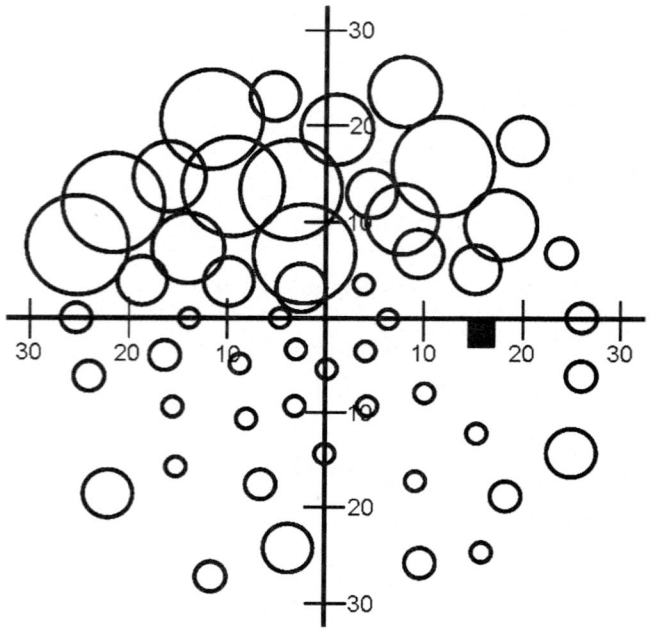

**Fig. 23.13** High pass resolution perimetry results for the right eye of a glaucoma patient with superior arcuate visual field loss. Note that *larger circles* indicate lower sensitivity and *smaller circles* reflect higher sensitivity

basis for determining normal and abnormal regions of the visual field in this manner by finding gaps and discontinuities in response performance. Theoretically, this type of mapping procedure is able to generate high density topographic profiles of the visual field and identify small regions of functional loss produced by random or clustered dropout of visual mechanisms.

To date, Rarebit perimetry has been found to be useful for characterizing visual field loss in glaucoma and other ocular and neurologic diseases, although most of the findings have come from a small number of laboratories. Figure 23.14 presents an example of Rarebit perimetry for the right eye of a patient with glaucoma.

### 23.3.7 Multifocal Electroretinograms

In the past, electrophysiological evaluation of glaucomatous damage has not been widely used, particularly for assessing the functional status of the peripheral visual field. Standard electroretinogram (ERG) measures are able to separate out rod and cone responses and identify damage to specific regions of the retina. However, the response has been a gross

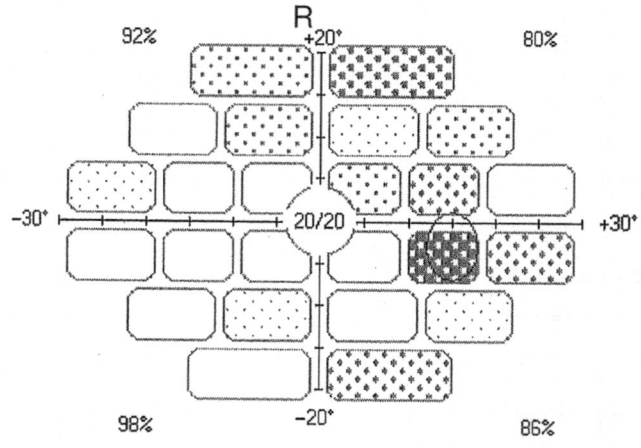

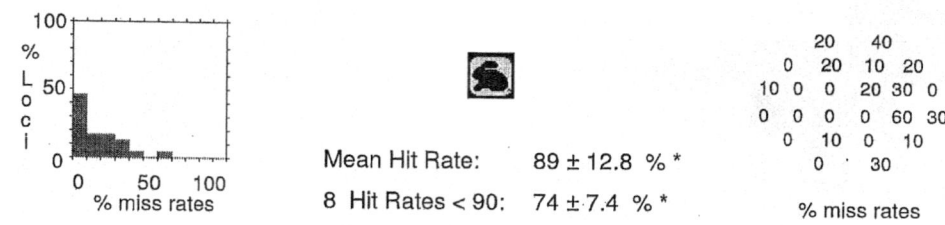

**Fig. 23.14** Rarebit perimetry results for the right eye of a patient with superior and inferior arcuate visual field loss. *Lighter rectangles* indicate higher sensitivity and *darker rectangles* reflect lower sensitivity

(mass) potential from the entire retina, so localized information could not be obtained. Sutter and colleagues[147] developed a new technique that was able to overcome this problem to provide localized information about ERG and visual evoked potential (VEP) measures. As with conventional ERG testing, a contact lens electrode (electrically coupled to the retina) is employed to measure changes in the retina's electrical potential in response to alternating stimuli. By performing a complex mathematical approach that incorporated a modified binary M-sequence for stimulus presentations and an autocorrelation function to extract localized signals, they were able to obtain ERG-like waveforms from a number of locations throughout the central visual field. Many investigators have found that this procedure is most helpful in evaluating retinal disorders and in distinguishing between retinal and optic nerve pathology.

The multifocal ERG (mfERG) approach has a number of advantages over conventional electrophysiological approaches for clinical use, including the ability to provide information about the functional status of localized retinal locations, fewer attention and cooperation demands for the subject, more objective assessment of visual function, and related issues.[147–151] Unfortunately it takes longer to perform mfERG than other visual field procedures, and its dynamic range is more limited.[147–151] Figure 23.15 presents an example of mfERG responses from the both eyes of a patient with glaucoma (see Chap. 24 for further discussion).

### 23.3.8 Multifocal Visual Evoked Potentials

Similar to the mfERG procedure, multifocal visual evoked potentials (mfVEPs) are obtained by using a modified binary M-sequence to alternate a series of checkerboard displays at various locations within the central visual field by means of a computer monitor. A series of four electrodes are placed on the scalp in and around the occipital lobe region at well-identified anatomical landmarks. The mfVEP analysis is able to display responses from a number of visual field locations. Figure 23.16 presents an example of multifocal VEP responses obtained from both eyes of a patient with glaucomatous visual field loss in the left eye. Note that the waveform becomes inverted when going from the inferior to the superior visual field hemisphere, due largely to the folding pattern of occipital cortex. Many investigators have found that mfVEP visual field measures correlate quite well with standard automated perimetry results, can be accomplished in some patients who are not able to perform standard automated perimetry, and has a relatively constant amount of variability for all levels of glaucomatous damage in the visual fields.[152–158] As with mfERG, the procedure is rather time consuming in comparison to standard automated perimetry, maintaining good attention is critical (daydreaming and inattention can invoke Alpha waves, which resemble mfVEP responses), and has a limited response range. Its clinical utility at this point is still therefore limited, but it is a most valuable research tool.

### 23.4 Testing Strategies for The Glaucoma Patient

Perimetric testing strategies consist of procedures that are designed for screening (suprathreshold static perimetry) and quantitative procedures to measure threshold sensitivity (kinetic and static perimetry). This chapter will provide a brief overview of these procedures, although thorough descriptions of screening and threshold visual field test procedures are available in other literature sources.[23-26,32–39,159–161] A number of visual field test procedures and analysis techniques have been designed to evaluate glaucomatous visual field loss, and these methods have been promoted by many investigators as an efficient means of evaluating glaucoma patients. However, it is also useful to remember a quote by Abraham Maslow, "If the only tool you have is a hammer, you tend to see every problem as a nail." Eye care specialists should be cautioned that patients referred to them for glaucoma or patients with glaucoma can also have other conditions that affect vision. Thus, there are both potential advantages and disadvantages of using a perimetric test procedure that is designed specifically for glaucoma.

### 23.4.1 Visual Field Screening (Suprathreshold Static Perimetry)

Screening procedures for perimetry are designed to address two purposes: (1) rapid population-based screening of large numbers of individuals to identify persons who may have glaucoma but not be aware of it, or be at risk for having glaucoma; and (2) methods for performing rapid clinic-based visual field evaluations to determine whether a patient requires more extensive clinical evaluation for glaucoma. A number of screening procedures are available for evaluating the visual field using a fixed stimulus luminance and size for all test locations, using a stimulus luminance or size that is a fixed amount above the expected normal threshold for all locations, or by identifying normal and abnormal regions and subsequently quantitatively for all

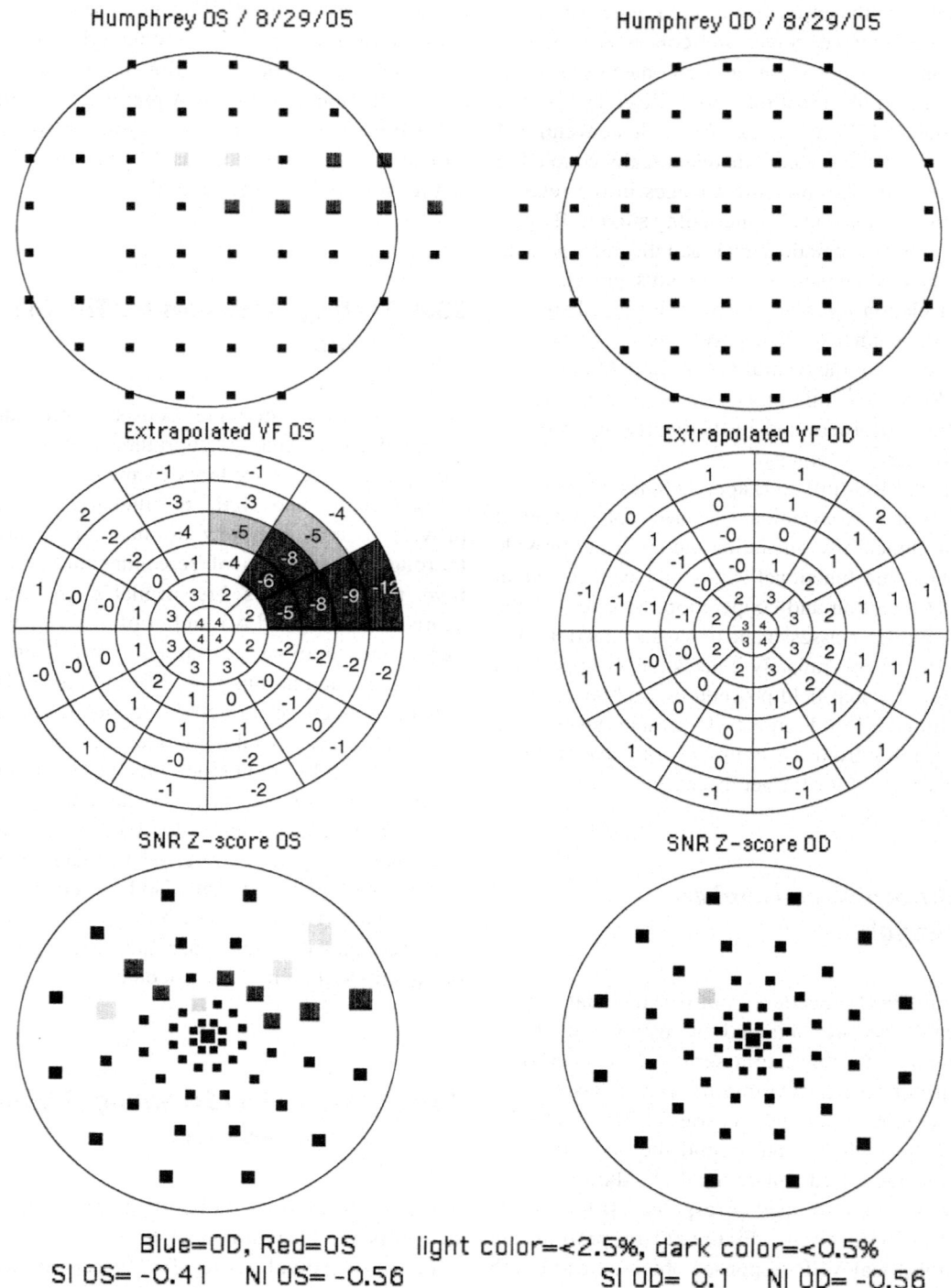

**Fig. 23.15** Multifocal visual evoked potential (VEP) results for the left and right eyes of a patient with a superior nasal step visual field defect in the left eye. In the *bottom panels*, *larger squares* indicate smaller VEP signals (lower sensitivity) and *smaller squares* indicate larger VEP signals (higher sensitivity)

locations, or by identifying normal and abnormal regions and subsequently quantitatively testing the abnormal locations to determine the amount of loss. Unfortunately, there has been considerably less research time and effort devoted to studying and evaluating visual field screening procedures in comparison to quantitative threshold techniques. An example of visual field screening results was presented in Fig. 23.8.

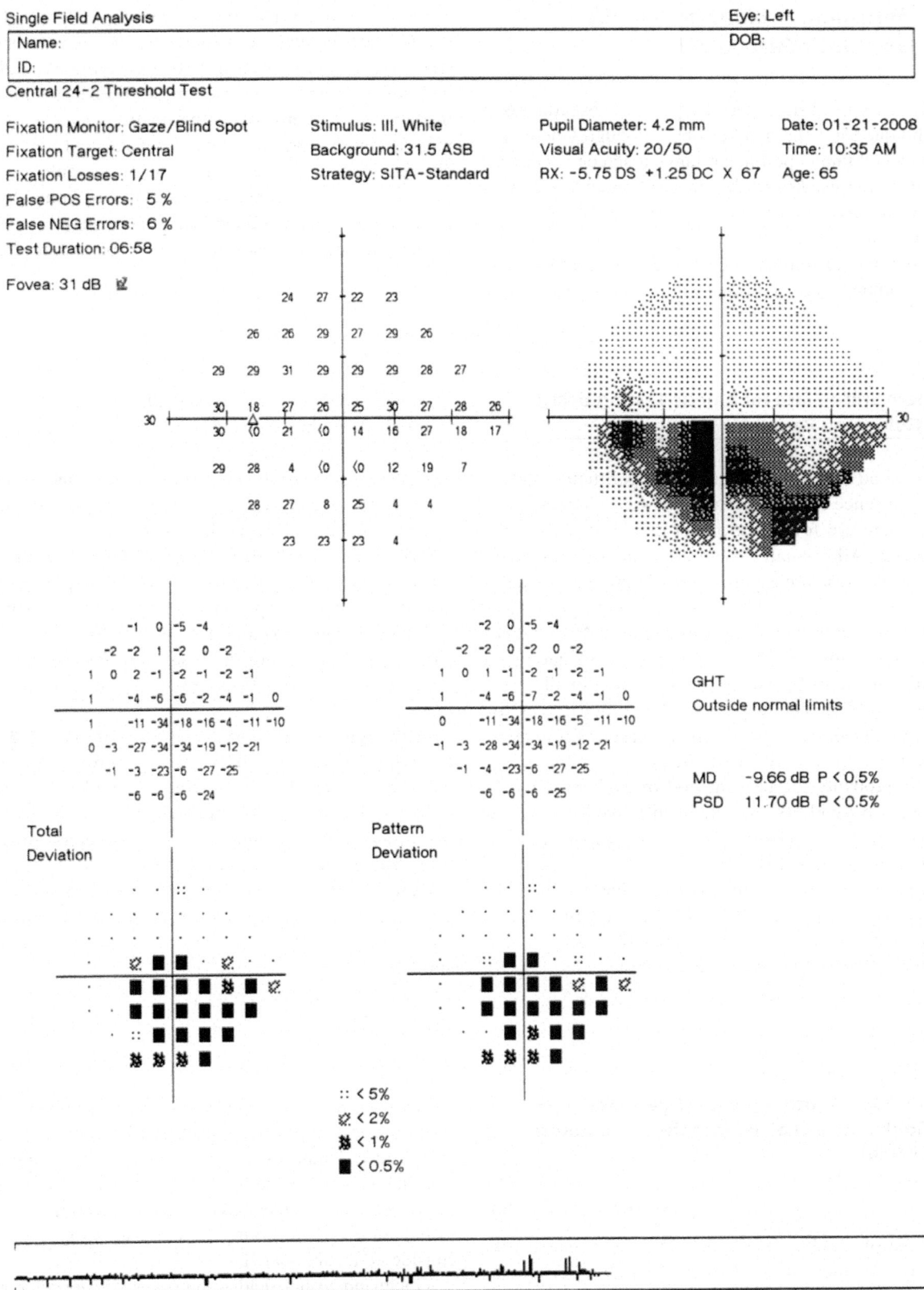

**Fig. 23.16** Visual field results for standard automated perimetry (white-on-white) for the left eye of a patient with inferior arcuate glaucomatous visual field loss

### 23.4.2 Threshold Evaluation (Kinetic and Static Perimetry)

Currently, automated static perimetry is the most commonly used technique for visual field testing; although kinetic testing using a Goldmann perimeter, tangent screen, or devices of similar design used to be the standard procedure and are still in use in many clinics today (see Sidebar 23.2). Kinetic perimetry is a flexible, interactive procedure between the patient and the examiner, which requires a tremendous amount of knowledge, skill, and ability on the part of the examiner. In one sense, it is essentially a means of testing and verifying hypotheses concerning the type of visual field characteristics, their shape, their underlying etiologies, and their relationship to other portions of the eye examination. In the hands of a highly skilled perimetrist, one can obtain the most accurate representations of visual field damage in an efficient manner. However, there is considerable variation in the perimetric performance abilities demonstrated by different examiners, so automated static perimetry can provide a greater degree of standardization in procedure from one clinic to another.

---

**Is There Still a Place for Kinetic Testing Using The Goldmann Perimeter?**

With the advent of automated static perimetry, and the recent absence of manufacturing new Goldmann perimeters, there are fewer and fewer clinics that have this capability. Additionally, there are a smaller number of perimetrists who are capable of performing high quality kinetic visual field testing. It is becoming a skill that is rarely encountered in today's eye clinics. Nonetheless, there is probably no better method of evaluating the visual field than by means of an exceptionally well-trained, skilled, and experienced perimetrist. In this view, I believe that there are many reasons for continuing to perform Goldmann kinetic perimetry, including:

It is probably the best method of evaluating the far periphery beyond 30°, and this can be very helpful for characterizing the pattern, extent, and locus of involvement for visual field loss.

Kinetic perimetry is highly interactive, which therefore makes it especially useful when testing children, adults with attentional and/or cognitive deficits, and patients with other medical complications.

Kinetic perimetry is essentially an active search (through hypothesis testing) of possible underlying causes of the visual field loss.

Kinetic perimetry is often able to detect and evaluate visual field losses that are not commonly assessed properly by automated static perimetric procedures.

With kinetic perimetry, it is possible to alter the test strategy during the procedure if patient responses suggest that a different approach would be more informative (e.g., characterizing retinal versus optic nerve pathology contributing to visual field loss, evaluating the possibility of functional (malingering) visual field loss).

Although kinetic perimetry is most often performed manually, there are a few manufacturers who have made automated kinetic testing available. The most sophisticated automated kinetic perimetry procedure is now available on some Octopus perimeters. In addition to achieving accurate control of many stimulus parameters and standardizing the test methodology, this procedure is able to measure and correct for individual differences in reaction time from one patient to another.

---

**SIDEBAR 23.2 Another perspective on the need for Goldmann visual fields in the era of automated visual fields**

Andrew C. S. Crichton

The role of Goldmann visual field testing seems to be increasingly questioned. Indeed, for some Goldmann visual fields are simply a memory. As patient volumes increase and financial considerations become more of a concern, diagnostic testing that is time consuming, labor intensive, and requires highly trained technicians, may be considered unnecessary. In our institution, technicians learning Goldmann perimetry spend 6 months with a senior Goldmann technician. What, therefore, is the justification for preserving testing with what could be considered an antiquated test?

Goldmann visual field testing was developed around 1946. It allowed evaluation of the field of vision by both static and kinetic testing. This was the gold standard until the computer-assisted field analyzers were developed in the early 1980s. The wealth of information provided and the objective reproducibility were very attractive features of this new technology. Additionally, the test time became shorter, and the performance of the examination became less technician-dependent. With time, the statistical packages assessing change improved markedly. Many publications have validated the results and Humphrey field-testing has become the gold standard for clinical trials.

After the introduction of automated perimetry, there were several initial publications comparing the new technology Humphrey Field Analyzer (HFA) with the gold standard of the time, Goldmann perimetry (Fig. 23.2-1). Trope and Britton compared Humphrey with Goldmann perimetry in glaucoma patients. Sensitivity and specificity were comparable, therefore validating the use of automated perimetry. The patients preferred the manual (Goldmann) perimetry, whereas the technicians preferred the automated field machinery. Testing was done with the 30-2 program, however, and would therefore be more taxing on the patient than the more efficient programs commonly used today. Nevertheless the major limitations of accurate fixation, maintenance of concentration, and fatigue, are still relevant for the shorter programs (Figs. 23.2-2 and 23.2-3). The authors also highlighted that defects may fall into the 6° spaces between the tested points. Also, additional tests are required to evaluate the field beyond 30°.

In another paper by Beck et al that included glaucoma, neurologic and normal patients, defects were found by the HFA that were not found by the Goldmann perimetry. Again, fixation problems led to more unreliability for automated perimetry.

Katz evaluated a group of patients followed for years and found to have progression by manual perimetry. Post hoc, the changes were suggested 1 year earlier by automated perimetry using the glaucoma hemifield test.

Since the introduction of automated perimetry and the recognition of some of the limitations, improvements have been made to try to address some of the problems. 24° fields and shorter programs (Fastpac,

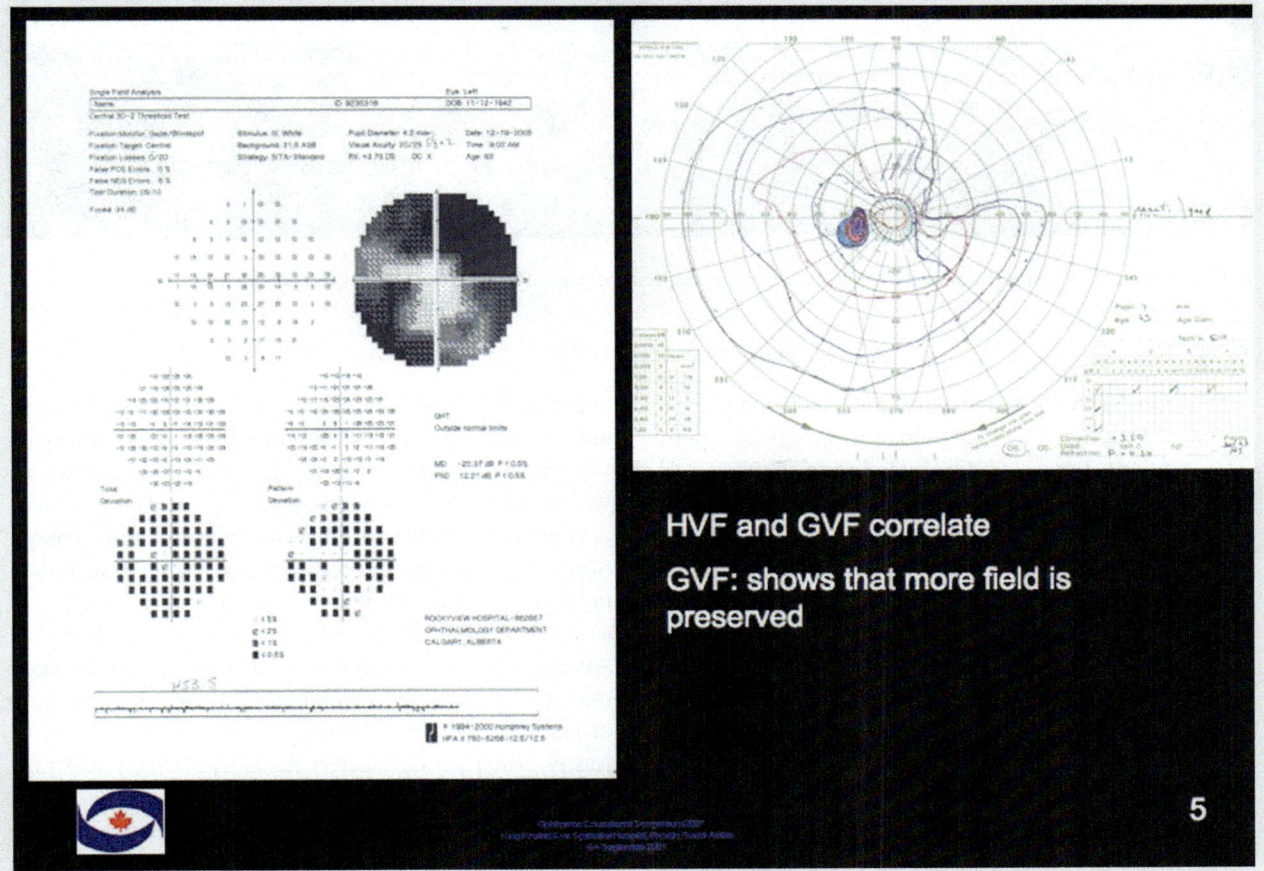

**Fig. 23.2-1** Humphrey visual field and Goldmann visual field (GVF) correlate. GVF shows that more field is preserved

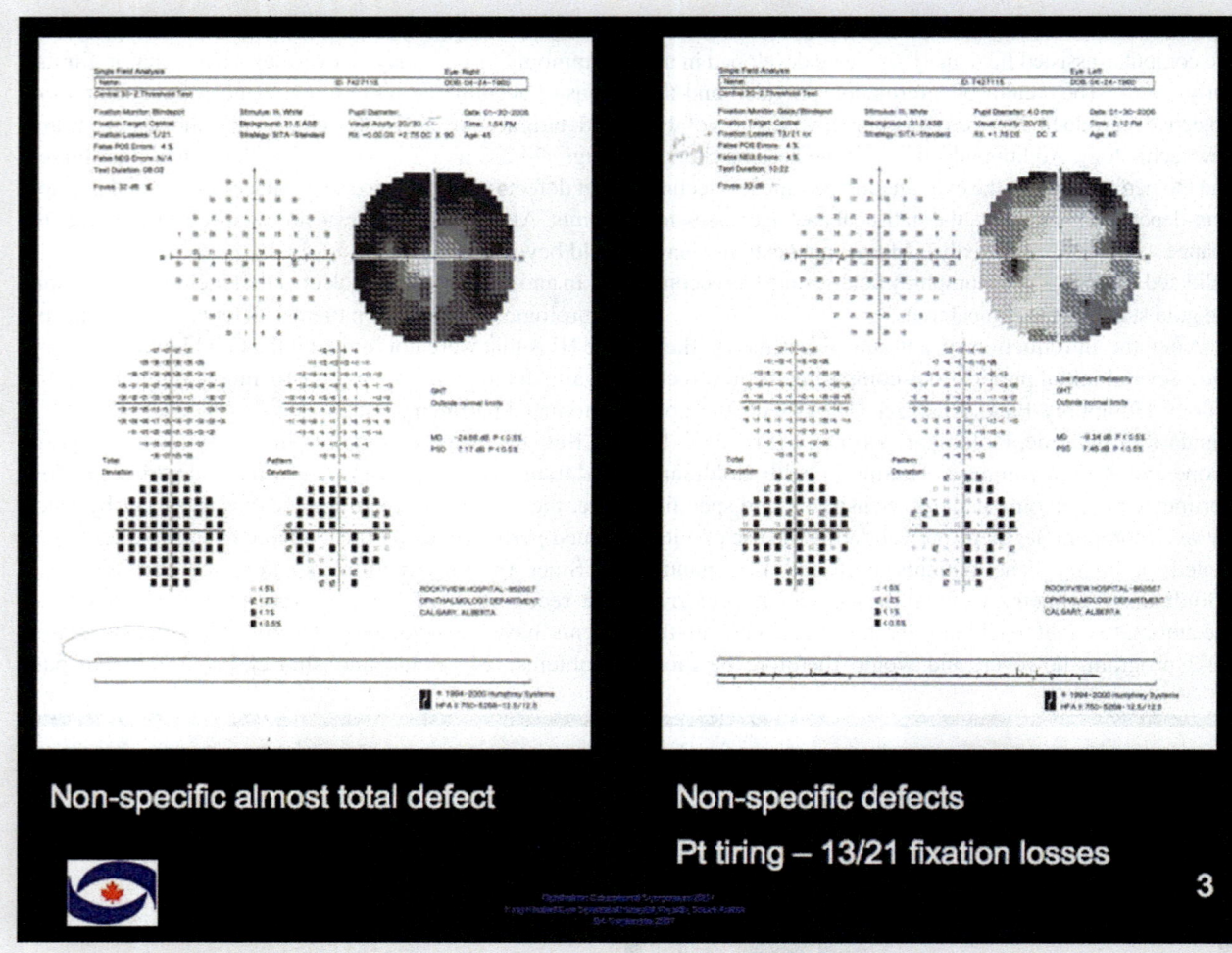

**Fig. 23.2-2** (*left*) Nonspecific almost total defect. (*right*) Nonspecific defects. Patient tiring – 13/21 fixation losses

SITA and SITA Fast) partially addressed the issue of fatigue. Programs with 2° separation between points (10-2) allowed more precise mapping of the defect and decreased the chance of a defect falling in a gap between testing points. The use of larger targets (Size V Stimulus) assisted in providing useful information in moderately to severely damaged fields. Improved statistical packages allowed a more objective assessment of progression.

Despite these improvements, however, there still remains a place for Goldmann visual field tests in the management of glaucoma patients. As highlighted previously, issues of unreliability were seen more commonly with automated perimetry. This was seen even in patients deemed reasonable to approach for participation in a clinical trial. There are many patients for whom issues of attention are even more of a problem. In these situations, automated perimetry can be virtually useless. Although with manual perimetry there may still be some patients with totally unreliable fields, a caring and patient technician is usually able to elicit some useful information. Some information can be gathered in patients with nystagmus. Patients with severe glaucoma may be left with a small central island and a large temporal island. Although the 10-2 field of the HFA provides very good information centrally, a Goldmann field at a single testing can provide a superior overview as to the visual function. Lastly, some patients detest fields so strongly that they may be unwilling to return for any follow-up at all if the field-testing is required. Again, a compassionate technician may allow a manual test with more patient interaction to be performed.

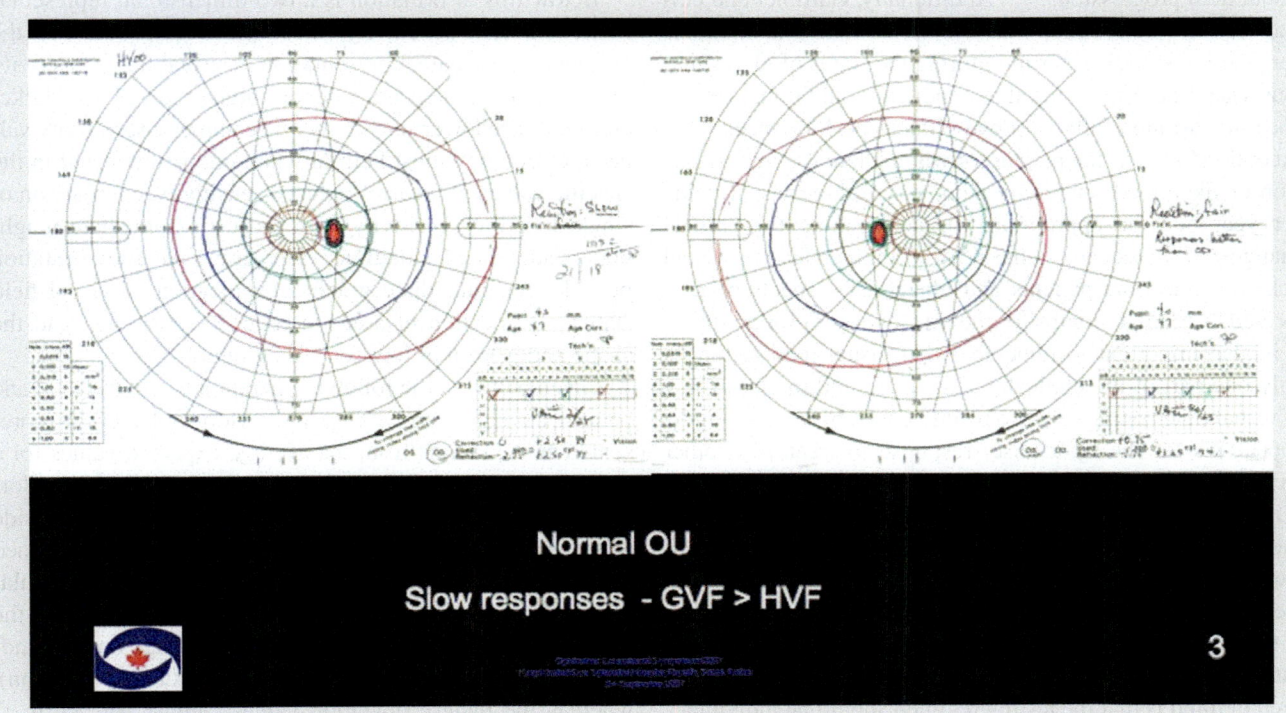

**Fig. 23.2-3** Normal OU. Slow responses – GVF>HFV

## Conclusion

Although it would be tempting from a financial, logistical, and staff satisfaction point of view to eliminate Goldmann visual field testing from clinics and offices, the information provided is too valuable for too many patients, especially in a tertiary care setting. For optimal patient care, both manual and automated perimetry should be available and the appropriate test ordered for the suitable patient.

## Bibliography

Beck RW, Bergstrom TJ, Lichter PR. A clinical comparison of visual field testing with the new automated perimeter, the Humphrey Field Analyzer, and the Goldmann perimeter. *Ophthalmology*. 1985;92:77–82.

Katz J, Tielsch JM, Quigley HA, Sommer A. Automated perimetry defects visual field loss before manual Goldmann perimetry. *Ophthalmology*. 1995;102:21–26.

Trope GE, Britton R. A comparison of Goldmann and Humphrey automated perimetry in patients with glaucoma. *Br J Ophthalmology*. 1987;71:489–493.

## 23.5 The Humphrey Visual Field

### 23.5.1 How Many, How Often?

The question of how many visual fields to perform for a patient suspected of developing glaucoma or who has already been diagnosed with glaucoma has been a question of interest to practitioners for many years. Primary open angle glaucoma (the most common form of glaucoma in most parts of the world) typically demonstrates a slow, progressive visual field loss in the presence of considerable variability. In moderately damaged visual field locations, variability can be up to 300–400% greater than in visual field areas with normal sensitivity, spanning a range of sensitivity values that encompasses nearly the entire dynamic range of the visual field device. These factors make it a significant challenge to determine whether a patient's glaucoma is stable or is undergoing progression, and there is no clear consensus as to which method of evaluating visual field progression is the best choice. There are differences among the many approaches for analyzing visual field progression, but most of them agree that a minimum of 5–7 visual fields are necessary to achieve good clinical performance in the assessment of glaucomatous visual field progression.[163,164] Additionally, Gardiner and colleagues have determined that two visual field examinations per year are sufficient for monitoring the status of glaucomatous visual field loss, and that conducting additional testing does not meaningfully improve clinical performance.[162] An exception to this is the patient for whom there is a high suspicion or likelihood for progression, where three visual fields per year may be appropriate for determining the earliest changes. More recently, it has been recommended that visual fields in glaucoma patients and glaucoma suspects be performed every 3–4 months for the first 2 years of follow-up.[165] It is also important to remember that visual field testing is only one part of the clinical examination, and the frequency of visual field testing can also be influenced by changes in the appearance of the optic disc, response to treatment, other medical conditions, age, and other factors. As a general rule, it is helpful to keep in mind that a visual field examination should be repeated if there is a suspicion that progression of the visual field has occurred, or the current visual field results are equivocal. There are large variations among practitioners in terms of the frequency of visual field testing for glaucoma patients and glaucoma suspects. Perhaps, the best thing to keep in mind is that the testing regimen should be individualized for each patient, taking into account their age, stamina, reliability, clinical condition, and related factors. There is no universal rule that can be applied to every patient.

### *23.5.2 Interpreting the HVF: A Beginner's Guide*

#### 23.5.2.1 Single Field Analysis

The test strategies, stimulus configuration, and stimulus presentation patterns are important for evaluating glaucomatous visual function damage by means of perimetry. However, it is also important that the information derived from these procedures be rapidly and easily analyzed by eye care practitioners, especially within a busy clinical setting. Of greatest importance are the shape, location, and extent of visual field loss. Figure 23.16 presents the printout of an example of visual field results obtained for the left eye of a patient with glaucomatous field loss, who was examined using the HFA. All of the information presented on this printout is important. At the top of the printout is information about the test conditions that were employed (stimulus size and color, background luminance, test strategy, fixation monitoring method, pupil size, date and time of testing, and fixation target used), patient characteristics (name, ID, visual acuity, refractive correction used, age and date of birth) and other information (fixation losses, false positive errors, false negative errors, test duration, foveal threshold value).

Below this information is a two-dimensional representation of numeric sensitivity values (in decibels (dB)) on the left, and a grayscale representation of visual field sensitivity on the right (lighter areas denote higher sensitivity, darker areas indicate lower sensitivity). The numeric sensitivity values are probably most helpful when one is interested in the specific values of areas of reduced sensitivity, comparison of single location sensitivity with those of immediate neighbors, and related situations. The grayscale representation provides an immediate graphical indication of visual field status, the location of areas of reduced sensitivity, and the shape and pattern of low-sensitivity regions.

Given below in the following paragraphs are the total and pattern deviation probability plots (left and center) represented as deviations from the average expected values for a normal individual of the same age (top) and probability plots indicating whether the results are within (dots) or outside (dithered squares) the normal limits by a predetermined amount (lower than 5, 2, 1, and 0.5% of the normal population of the same age). The total deviation results indicate the deviation of the current results from an average normal findings for individuals of the same age (location by location), whereas the pattern deviation values "adjust" or "correct" the total deviation values by the average amount of loss, the General Height value (determined by the location with the sensitivity corresponding to the upper 85th percentile). This provides a means of evaluating diffuse (widespread) and localized sensitivity losses and is a significant means of evaluating the visual field information.

For diffuse or widespread loss (as produced by media opacities and other factors), the total deviation plot will show many locations with reduced sensitivity and dithered probability patterns, while the pattern deviation plot will have few or no locations outside of normal limits. Localized losses will appear with identical or near identical patterns for both the total and pattern deviation plots. Combined diffuse and localized loss will be represented by a mixture of these patterns for the total and pattern deviation plots. Finally, when the total deviation plot has little or no locations outside the normal limits, but the pattern deviation plots have many dithering patterns throughout the visual field, it is usually because the patient has been "trigger happy" or a "happy clicker" (pressing the response button too often), and false positive errors and fixation losses are also typically beyond the normal expected limits. A brief glimpse of this portion of the visual field printout can provide useful clinical information in a most efficient manner.

To the right of the total and pattern deviation probability plots, visual field indices are presented. These consist of: (1) Mean Deviation (MD), which represents the average deviation of the visual field from average normal results for individuals of the same age; (2) Pattern Standard Deviation (PSD), which is the root mean square deviation of values from the normal slope of the sensitivity gradient for normals; and (3) Glaucoma Hemifield Test (GHT) results, which compare sensitivity of five clusters of points (nerve fiber bundle segments) in the superior and inferior visual field. Because glaucomatous visual field loss is typically asymmetric for the superior and inferior hemifields, this analysis is particularly useful for detecting these types of visual field abnormalities. Five determinations are given: (1) within normal limits (superior and inferior hemifield differences are small and within expected normal values), (2) borderline (superior and inferior hemifield asymmetries are larger than the 3% probability level), (3) outside normal limits (superior and inferior hemifield asymmetries are larger than the 1% probability level), (4) general reduction in sensitivity (when both the superior and inferior hemifield sensitivities are below the 0.5% level for normal), and (5) abnormally high sensitivity (when the General Height value is better than 99.5% of the normal population of that age). Together, these indices provide helpful information concerning diffuse, localized, and glaucomatous visual field losses.

The final portion of the single field printout is represented by gaze tracking, which essentially presents a timeline of activity throughout the testing sequence. The gaze tracker uses an infrared light source to obtain a diffuse reflection from the retina (the retinal reflex) that illuminates the pupil and a specular reflection from the anterior surface of the cornea (the corneal reflex). By monitoring the relative position and continuity of these reflexes, the gaze tracker indicates alignment deviations (upward deflections of the timeline) produced by head and eye movements, and blinks or ptosis (downward deflections of the timeline) throughout the test procedure. This is a most helpful index. Examples of different gaze-tracking results can be found in the book by Anderson and Patella.[24] By observing this gaze-tracking timeline, it is possible to determine when a patient becomes drowsy, fatigued, or fidgety, as well as other factors during perimetric testing.

It is important to note that all of the information that is presented on the printout is important and that none of it should be ignored or disregarded. A careful perusal of all of the information that is available can assist in preventing unnecessary retesting of patients, minimization of improper or misleading test conditions, and misinterpretation of visual field test results.

In a busy clinical setting, it is sometimes difficult to interpret visual field information properly, and if it is a subspecialty glaucoma clinic, there is a tendency to view all visual fields from the perspective of glaucomatous loss. However, it is important to recognize visual field loss due to other ocular and neurologic problems, and to properly identify artifactual test results. In this view, a multistep process is presented to assist in rapidly being able to interpret visual field information:

**Step 1.** Place the visual fields in front of you, with the left eye findings to your left and the right eye results to your right. Determine whether the visual fields of both eyes are within or outside of normal limits. If both eyes are within the normal limits, then your task is complete; otherwise, proceed to step 2.

**Step 2.** Determine whether the visual field results are outside the normal limits for one eye or both eyes. If only one eye is outside of normal limits, then the deficit is anterior to the chiasm (optics, retina, or optic nerve). If both eyes are involved, then the deficit is either chiasmal or retrochiasmal, or the patient has bilateral disease.

**Step 3.** If both eyes have visual field loss, determine the general location of the deficit (superior, inferior, binasal, bitemporal, nasal in one eye, temporal in the other). If there is extensive visual field loss, determine the general location of the predominant amount of visual field loss. Deficits that are bitemporal suggest that the deficit is located at the chiasm, where the crossing fibers from the nasal retina (temporal visual field) are damaged. Binasal deficits are commonly associated with diseases of the optic nerve (glaucoma, anterior ischemic optic neuropathy, or other optic neuropathies) and retinal disorders. A deficit that occurs in the nasal visual field of one eye and the temporal visual field of the other eye often represents a deficit produced by damage to the optic radiations (retrochiasmal lesions). By simply following this step, it is possible to refine the location of the deficit producing the visual field loss. This is an especially important step, because retinal, chiasmal and retrochiasmal deficits can be misinterpreted as glaucomatous losses.

**Step 4.** Evaluate the shape of the defect. There are certain features that appear in the visual field output that can be crucial to determining the potential sites of pathological involvement within the visual pathways. It is beyond the scope of this chapter to provide a detailed illustrative set of visual field patterns that are associated with pathology to various locations within the visual pathways, although there are literature sources that provide good examples of noteworthy patterns of visual field loss.[23–26,32–39,159–161] Briefly, it should be remembered that visual field losses usually correspond to the anatomic arrangement of nerve fibers at different locations within the visual pathways.

Diffuse, widespread, or generalized visual field sensitivity loss can most often be associated with cataract and other ocular media opacities, although this can also infrequently occur for glaucoma, retinal, and optic nerve disorders (Fig. 23.17). Localized defects are more common. Visual field losses that appear to be irregular and inconsistent with anatomical arrangements are usually characteristic of retinal dysfunction. If the far periphery (beyond 30° eccentricity) is evaluated, retinal disorders can frequently have a scalloped edge and gradually sloping contours to the defect. A full or

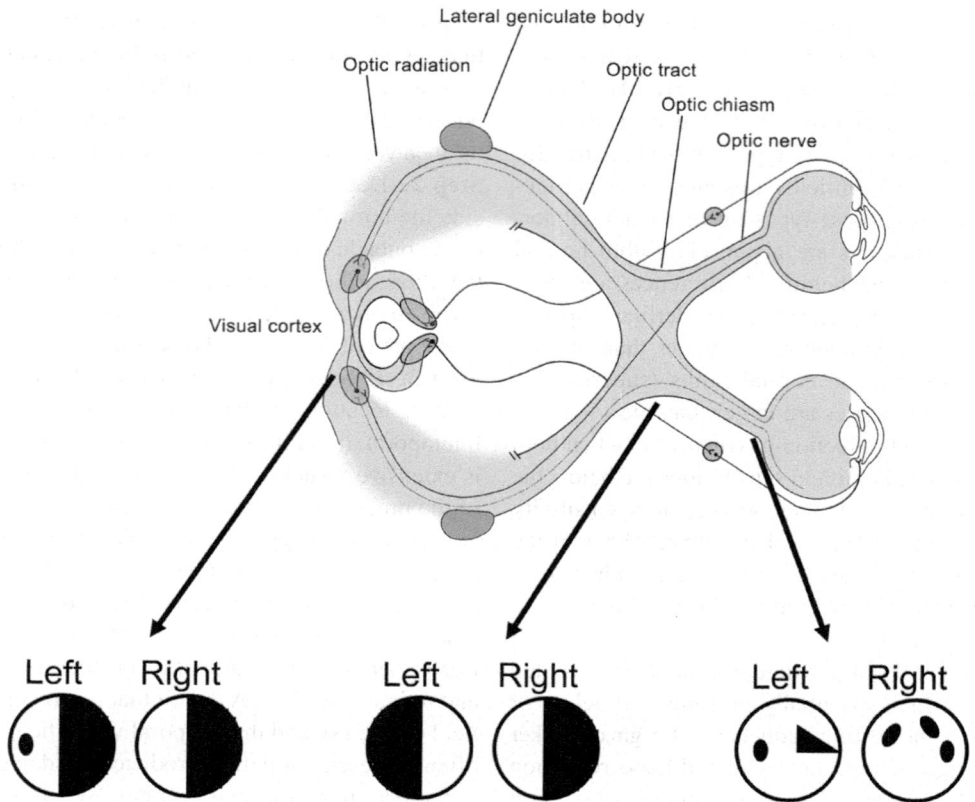

**Fig. 23.17** Representation of the visual field for lesions affecting different portions of the visual pathways

partial ring scotoma (area of nonseeing to a specific target) is frequently associated with retinitis pigmentosa. Some retinal vascular disorders (e.g., branch artery occlusion) will demonstrate visual field losses that are similar to those that occur in glaucoma (respecting the horizontal meridian, depicting a fan-shaped arcuate pattern of loss). Diseases that primarily affect central vision (e.g., age-related macular degeneration) will manifest a central scotoma. In most instances, the form of visual field loss will be considerably different for the two eyes if retinal disease is the cause of visual field sensitivity loss.

Glaucoma is an ocular disease, in which damage to the retinal ganglion cells produces characteristic visual field loss that usually corresponds to the underlying anatomic arrangement of retinal ganglion cells (Fig. 23.17). As the retinal ganglion cells exit the eye at the optic nerve head to travel back to the brain, there are three patterns of fiber arrangements: (1) the papillomacular bundle, (2) the superior and inferior arcuate retinal nerve fibers, and (3) the temporal visual field (nasal retina) radial fibers. The papillomacular bundle subserves the region between the blind spot and fixation, enters the temporal portion of the optic nerve head (nasal visual field) and consists of many small nerve fibers that are relatively unaffected by glaucoma until late stages of the disease process. The superior and inferior arcuate nerve fiber bundles enter the top and bottom of the optic nerve head, and are especially susceptible to glaucomatous damage. The nerve fiber bundles are laminated structures that accumulate the axons of nerve fibers from different discrete locations in the retina. These fiber bundles splay out in a fan-shaped pattern progressively away from the optic nerve head. The superior and inferior nerve fiber bundles terminate in a distinct manner along the nasal visual field meridian (raphe), so that there is a sharp transition of superior and inferior nerve fibers. Visual field defects associated with this bundle of fibers thus show a distinct transition in sensitivity along the horizontal meridian (the visual field defects "respect the horizontal"). The radial nerve fibers enter the nasal portion of the optic nerve head (temporal visual field). Visual field losses from glaucoma mimic these nerve fiber bundle patterns, revealing temporal wedges (radial fibers), nasal steps, paracentral defects, and partial and total arcuate deficits (superior and inferior arcuate nerve fiber bundles). Additionally, there is often asymmetry in the amount of loss observed for the superior and inferior visual fields, and between the two eyes.

Pathologic insults to the optic chiasm produce bitemporal visual field defects. This is due to the fact that the nerve fibers from the nasal retina (temporal visual field) cross over to the opposite cortical hemisphere (i.e., the left half of the visual field is relayed to the right hemisphere and vice versa). Additionally, because the transition in nerve fibers from nasal and temporal retina occurs along the vertical meridian, there is a distinct transition in sensitivity at this location (the visual field deficits "respect the vertical"). Beyond the chiasm, the nerve fibers from the nasal visual field of one eye combine with the temporal fibers of the other eye, so that the right side of the visual field from both eyes is transmitted to the left hemisphere and vice versa. Because the visual field defects are occurring on the same side of vision, the deficits are referred to as homonymous. The visual field losses also respect the vertical meridian. There are several other features that are useful for visual field deficits that are produced by damage to the optic radiations beyond the chiasm. First, the more congruous (similar) are the defects between the two eyes, the deficit is located farther back in the optic radiations (near or at the occipital lobe). Conversely, the greater the amount of congruity, the more anterior is the insult to the optic radiations. Secondly, "pie in the sky" (a wedge or piece of pie removed from the visual field) is more closely associated with temporal lobe lesions, whereas "pie on the floor" is more consistent with parietal lobe lesions. Third, a "cookie cutter punched out lesion" is typical of occipital lobe damage. Finally, it should be noted that a total homonymous hemianopsia indicates that the deficit can only be localized to the region beyond the chiasm because it indicates that all of the nerve fibers have been damaged (note that the most likely locations are the occipital lobe and just beyond the chiasm because these locations have the densest spatial packing of nerve fibers).

**Step 5.** Correlate the visual field results with other clinical findings and correlations with the appearance of the retina, optic disc, retinal nerve fiber layer, and neuro-imaging findings. In most cases, your visual field assessment will be refined by correlating structural features and clinical information with visual field results. If you are uncertain about a particular visual field result and have done the recommended clinical and structural correlations, it is best to repeat the visual field test to confirm the visual field findings. You should adopt a heuristic method of combining visual field and other clinical information to logically deduce the most likely locus of involvement (and those that are unlikely), what additional tests or observations could be helpful, and what the opinions of others are able to yield.

Clearly, there will always be exceptions to these general principles, so it will sometimes occur that visual field loss does not follow these guidelines. However, the steps that are mentioned will be able to properly direct you through the majority of cases dealing with proper visual field interpretation. Perhaps, the most common errors occur when a practitioner interpreting the visual field results skips one or more steps, or performs them in the wrong order.

### 23.5.3 Analysis of Multiple Visual Fields

Two factors that are critical to monitoring the status of glaucoma patients is ascertaining whether their visual field loss has progressed and, consequently, the rate of progression, because this can assist in determining the efficacy of treatment. Unfortunately, there is presently no consensus for the proper method of evaluating visual field progression. Several investigators have made comparisons of different methods to evaluate glaucomatous visual field progression and have found the following common issues: (1) there is only modest agreement (40–60%) among the various methods to evaluate progression, using a variety of approaches; (2) when there are less than six visual fields available for analysis, evaluation of visual field progression is difficult, irrespective of the analysis method used; (3) the amount of time and/or visual field examinations needed to determine progression with good performance varies greatly among the various analysis methods; and (4) comparisons among different analysis techniques typically indicate more discordance than concordance in results for the final outcome.[164–175] There are many techniques that are available for evaluating visual field progression, and there is presently no consensus among experts as to which method is the one that is preferred for evaluation of glaucomatous visual field progression. In many instances, the most appropriate technique to use depends on the specific question that is being asked. Hopefully, with the use of machine classifiers, multivariate analyses and related procedures, we will be able to achieve agreement on useful clinical techniques. Progressor (linear regression) and the Glaucoma Progression Analysis (GPA – comparison of current visual field results to the average of two baseline exams, or event analysis) are the most commonly used techniques for evaluation of glaucomatous visual field progression.

Rate of progression is perhaps the most important feature for practitioners monitoring glaucoma patients to determine whether current treatment is effective or needs to be altered.[176] Unfortunately, little work has been conducted on this topic at the present time. One feature that has been recently introduced is the Glaucoma Progression Index (GPI), which is a rate of progression indicator that is now available for the HFA.[177] It is basically a linear regression procedure that has been adjusted to minimize the influence of cataract formation and to account for other factors.

### 23.6 Conclusion

In recent years, there have been a number of new visual field test procedures that have been developed for the evaluation of glaucoma, some of which have been clinically useful and some of which have not. In this chapter, the emphasis has been placed on those test procedures that have demonstrated clinical benefit and have merited further exploration. Automated static perimetry using small white targets superimposed on a uniform white background and a Bayesian forecasting test strategy is currently the most common method of visual field testing for glaucomatous loss. However, it should be kept in mind that kinetic, chromatic, spatial, temporal, spatiotemporal, electrophysiologic, and other forms of perimetry can also be useful in many circumstances. Some test procedures are better suited for rapid screening, some are more sensitive to early changes, some are more suitable for young children and older patients with limited attention capabilities, some have more consistent reproducibility throughout the entire spectrum of glaucomatous damage, some are more interactive, some are more resistant to external and confounding influences, some have better statistical and mathematical analysis procedures, and some are more highly preferred by patients. In summary, there is no single visual field solution that is applicable to all patients and clinical circumstances. Perimetry is both an art and a science, and while the quantitative, technologic, and scientific basis of visual field testing has undergone tremendous changes in recent times, it is still the judgment, skills, expertise, and "art" of the clinical practitioner to decide which of these options (or combinations of options) are most appropriate for monitoring and following individual patients.

## 23.7 Clinical Pearls

1. Many studies have reported that when a visual field change is suspected, it is best to confirm this suspicion. A large majority of visual field changes are not reproduced by the next visual field test.[178] Confirmation of the change can be accomplished by repeating the visual field examination at another time, correlating it with concomitant structural alterations, evaluating it within the context of other aspects of the eye examination, reviewing the patient's history, determining the patient's response to IOP, lowering medications or surgery, comparing with risk factors for glaucoma, and other clinical issues.

   It is always helpful to remember that patients who are referred to a clinic for one purpose (e.g., evaluation of a suspicion of glaucoma) may have another ocular or neurologic condition that is producing the visual field loss, or may have more than one medical condition. There are many other conditions that can produce visual field deficits that are similar to those produced by glaucoma, such as artifactual test results (trial lens rim visual field obstruction, droopy eyelid, alignment difficulties and fixation losses, etc.) and pathology to other portions of the visual pathways. A common occurrence is inappropriately interpreting a chiasmal visual field defect (bitemporal visual field loss that respects the vertical meridian) as glaucomatous loss. Thus, it is always useful to keep an open, objective mind when interpreting visual fields, use the five-step approach outlined in this chapter (in the proper order) to conduct the visual field interpretation, and to independently evaluate the visual field information prior to conducting any comparisons with other clinical findings.

2. It is useful to keep in mind that "automated perimetry" means that the test procedure and stimulus conditions that are selected can be run with minimal intervention on the part of the examiner. However, it does not mean that the examiner can just press a button, start the test, and then walk away. In keeping with most clinical procedures, it is important for the examiner to maintain an active approach to perimetry. Many problems associated with unreliable, artifactual, or nonphysiologic test results can be avoided or minimized by maintaining an interactive and attentive approach to the patient during visual field testing. Fatigue, drowsiness, attentional difficulties, misalignment, head and eye movements, anxiety, boredom, and other factors can be identified by the examiner in this manner. In addition to minimizing problems associated with these circumstances, this approach will also reinforce the impression of caring, concern, quality assurance, and confidence on the part of the patient.

3. The five-step process for evaluation of visual fields:

   (a) Is the field normal or abnormal (both eyes)?
   (b) Is the deficit in one eye or both eyes?
   (c) Where is the most prominent visual field loss (superior, inferior, nasal, temporal)?
   (d) What is the pattern and shape of visual field loss? How does it compare to previous results?
   (e) How do the visual field results correlate with other clinical findings and management?

**Acknowledgments** I am indebted to Patricia Duffel and Tuyet Dorau for their invaluable assistance in the preparation of figures for this book chapter.

## References

1. Guitierrez P, Wilson MR, Johnson C, et al. Influence of glaucomatous visual field loss on health-related quality of life. *Arch Ophthalmol.* 1997;115:777–784.
2. Parrish RK, Gedde SJ, Scott IU, et al. Visual function and quality of life among patients with glaucoma. *Arch Ophthalmol.* 1997;115:1447–1455.
3. Mills RP, Janz NK, Wren PA, Guire KE. Correlation of visual field with quality-of-life measures at diagnosis in the Collaborative Initial Glaucoma Treatment Study (CIGTS). *J Glaucoma.* 2001;10:192–198.

4. Iester M, Zingirian M. Quality of life in patients with early, moderate and advanced glaucoma. *Eye*. 2002;16:44–49.
5. Nelson P, Aspinall P, Papasouliotis O, Worton B, O'Brien C. Quality of life in glaucoma and its relationship with visual function. *J Glaucoma*. 2003;12:139–150.
6. Ringsdorf L, McGwin G, Owlsey C. Visual field defects and vision-specific health-related quality of life in African Americans and whites with glaucoma. *J Glaucoma*. 2006;15:414–418.
7. Freeman EE, Munoz B, West SK, Jampel HD, Friedman DS. Glaucoma and quality of life: the Salisbury Eye evaluation. *Ophthalmology*. 2008;115:233–238.
8. McKean-Cowdin R, Wang Y, Wu J, Azen SP, Varma R, Los Angeles Latino Eye Study Group. Impact of visual field loss on health-related quality of life in glaucoma: the Los Angeles Latino Eye Study. *Ophthalmology*. 2008;115:941–948.
9. Piltz JR, Swindale NV, Drance SM. Vernier thresholds and alignment bias in control, suspect and glaucomatous eyes. *J GAlaucoma*. 1993;2:87–95.
10. McKendrick AM, Johnson CA, Anderson AJ, Fortune B. Elevated vernier acuity thresholds in glaucoma. *Invest Ophthalmol Vis Sci*. 2002;43:1393–1399.
11. Sponsel WE, DePaul KL, Martone JF, Shields MB, Ollie AR, Stewart WC. Association of Vistech contrast sensitivity and visual field findings in glaucoma. *Br J Ophthalmol*. 1991;75:558–560.
12. McKendrick AM, Sampson GP, Walland MJ, Badcock DR. Contrast sensitivity changes due to glaucoma and normal aging: low-spatial-frequency losses in both magnocellular and parvocellular pathways. *Invest Ophthalmol Vis Sci*. 2007;48:2115–2122.
13. Hot A, Dul MW, Swanson WH. Development and evaluation of a contrast sensitivity perimetry test for patients with glaucoma. *Invest Ophthalmol Vis Sci*. 2008;49:3049–3057.
14. Sun H, Swanson WH, Arvidson B, Dul M. Assessment of contrast gain signature in inferred magnocellular and parvocellular pathways in patients with glaucoma. *Vision Res*. 2008;48(26):2633–2641.
15. Caprioli J. Correlation of visual function with optic nerve and nerve fiber layer structure in glaucoma. *Surv Ophthalmol*. 1989;33(suppl):319–330.
16. Johnson CA, Cioffi GA, Liebmann JR, Sample PA, Zangwill L, Weinreb RN. The relationship between structural and functional alterations in glaucoma: a review. *Semin Ophthalmol*. 2000;15: 221–233.
17. Garway-Heath D, Poinoosawmy D, Fitzke F, Hitchings R. Mapping the visual field to the optic disc in normal tension glaucoma eyes. *Ophthalmology*. 2000;107:1809–1815.
18. Gardiner SK, Johnson CA, Cioffi GA. Evaluation of the structure-function relationship in glaucoma. *Invest Ophthalmol Vis Sci*. 2005;46:3712–3717.
19. Strouthidis NG, Vinciotti V, Tucker AJ, Gardiner SK, Crabb DP, Garway-Heath DF. Structure and function in glaucoma: the relationship between a functional visual field map and an anatomic retinal map. *Invest Ophthalmol Vis Sci*. 2006;47:5356–5362.
20. Racette L, Medieros FA, Bowd C, Zangwill LM, Weinreb RN, Sample PA. The impact of the perimetric measurement scale, sample composition, and statistical method on the structure-function relationship in glaucoma. *J Glaucoma*. 2007;16:676–684.
21. Harwerth RS. Charles F. Prentice Award Lecture 2006: a neuron doctrine for glaucoma. *Optom Vis Sci*. 2008;85:436–444.
22. Hood DC, Kardon RH. A framework for comparing functional and structural measures of glaucomatous damage. *Prog Retin Eye Res*. 2007;26:688–710.
23. Greve EL. Single and multiple stimulus static perimetry in glaucoma; the two phases of perimetry. *Doc Ophthalmol*. 1973;36:1–355.
24. Anderson DR, Patella VM. *Automated static perimetry*. St Louis: CV Mosby; 1990.
25. Harrington DO, Drake MV. *The visual fields – text and atlas of clinical perimetry*. St Louis: CV Mosby; 1990.
26. Wall M, Johnson CA. Principals and techniques of the examination of the visual sensory system. In: Miller NR, Newman NJ, eds. *Walsh and Hoyt's Textbook of Neuro-Ophthalmology*. Vol 1. Philadelphia: Lippincott, Williams and Wilkins; 2005:83–149.
27. Dolderer J, Vonthein R, Johnson CA, Schiefer U, Hart W. Scotoma mapping by semi-automated kinetic perimetry – The effects of stimulus properties and the speed of subjects'responses. *Acta Ophthalmol Scand*. 2006;84:338–344.
28. Keltner JL, Johnson CA, Cello KE, et al. Classification of visual field abnormalities in the ocular hypertension treatment study. *Arch Ophthalmol*. 2003;121:643–650.
29. Katz J, Sommer A. Reliability indexes of automated perimetric tests. *Arch Ophthalmol*. 1988;106:1252–1254.
30. Keltner JL, Johnson CA, Beck RW, Cleary PA, Spurr JO, Optic Neuritis Study Group. Quality control functions of the Visual Field Reading Center (VFRC) for the Optic Neuritis Treatment Trial (ONTT). *Control Clin Trials*. 1993;14:143–159.
31. Keltner JL, Johnson CA, Cello KE, et al. Visual field quality control in the Ocular Hypertension Treatment Study (OHTS). *J Glaucoma*. 2007;16:665–669.
32. Anderson DR. *Perimetry with and without automation*. St Louis: CV Mosby; 1987.
33. Artes PH, Henson DB, Marper R, McLeod D. Multisampling Suprathreshold perimetry: a comparison with conventional suprathreshold and full-threshold strategies by computer simulation. *Invest Ophthalmol Vis Sci*. 2003;44:2582–2587.
34. Henson DB, Artes PH. New developments in Suprathreshold perimetry. *Ophthalmic Physiol Opt*. 2002;22:462–468.
35. Henson DB. Visual field screening and the development of a new screening program. *J Am Optom Assoc*. 1989;60:893–898.
36. Langerhorst CT, Bakker D, Raakman MA. Usefulness of the Henson Central Field Screener for the detection of visual field defects, especially in glaucoma. *Doc Ophthalmol*. 1989;72:279–285.
37. Johnson CA, Keltner JL. Automated suprathreshold static perimetry. *Am J Ophthalmol*. 1980;89:731–741.
38. Johnson CA, Keltner JL, Balestrery FG. Suprathreshold static perimetry in glaucoma and other optic nerve disease. *Ophthalmology*. 1979;86:1278–1286.
39. Araujo ML, Feuer WJ, Anderson DR. Evaluation of baseline-related suprathreshold testing for quick determination of visual field nonprogression. *Arch Ophthalmol*. 1993;111:365–369.
40. Hernandez R, Rabindranath K, Fraser C, et al. Screening for open angle glaucoma: systematic review of cost-effectiveness studies. *J Glaucoma*. 2008;17:159–168.
41. Javitt J, Lee P, Lum F. The value of regular examinations to detect glaucoma and other chronic conditions among older Americans. *Ophthalmology*. 2007;114:833–834.
42. Nelson-Quigg JM, Cello KE, Johnson CA. Predicting binocular visual field sensitivity from monocular visual field results. *Invest Ophthalmol Vis Sci*. 2000;41:2212–2221.
43. Crabb DP, Viswanathan AC. Integrated visual fields: a new approach to measuring the binocular field of view and visual disability. *Graefes Arch Clin Exp Ophthalmol*. 2005;243:210–216.
44. Owen VM, Crabb DP, White ET, Viswanathan AC, Garway-Heath DF, Hitchings RA. Glaucoma and fitness to drive: using binocular visual fields to predict a milestone to blindness. *Invest Ophthalmol Vis Sci*. 2008;49:2449–2455.
45. Kotecha A, O'Leary N, Melmoth D, Grant S, Crabb D. The functional consequences of glaucoma for eye-hand coordination. *Invest Ophthalmol Vis Sci*. 2009;50(1):203–213.
46. Jampel HD, Friedman DS, Quigley H, Miller R. Correlation of the binocular visual field with patient assessment of vision. *Invest Ophthalmol Vis Sci*. 2002;43:1059–1067.
47. Stiles WS. Increment thresholds and the mechanisms of colour vision. *Doc Ophthalmol*. 1949;3:138–165.

48. Kitahara K, Tamaki R, Noji J, Kandatsu A, Matsuzaki H. Extrafoveal Stiles π mechanisms. *Doc Ophthalmol Proc Ser.* 1982;35:397–404.
49. Kranda K, King-Smith PE. What can color thresholds tell us about the nature of underlying detection mechanisms? *Ophthalmic Physiol Opt.* 1984;4:83–87.
50. Sample PA, Weinreb RN, Boynton RM. Isolating color vision loss of primary open angle glaucoma. *Am J Ophthalmol.* 1988;106:686–691.
51. Sample PA, Weinreb RN. Color perimetry for assessment of primary open angle glaucoma. *Invest Ophthalmol Vis Sci.* 1990;31:1869–1875.
52. Sample RA, Weinreb RN. Progressive color visual field loss in glaucoma. *Invest Ophthalmol Vis Sci.* 1992;33:2068–2071.
53. Sample PA, Martinezz GA, Weinreb RN. Short-wavelength automated perimetry without lens density testing. *Am J Ophthalmol.* 1994;118:632–641.
54. Sample PA, Johnson CA, Haegerstrom-Portnoy G, Adams AJ. Optimum parameters for short-wavelength automated perimetry. *J Glaucoma.* 1996;5:375–383.
55. Sample PA, Martinez GA, Weinreb RN. Color visual fields: a 5 year prospective study in eyes with rimary open angle glaucoma. In: Mills RP, ed. *Perimetry Update 1992/93.* New York: Kugler Publications; 1993:473–476.
56. Sample PA, Taylor JD, Martinez GA, Lusky M, Weinreb RN. Short wavelength color visual fields in glaucoma suspects at risk. *Am J Ophthalmol.* 1993;115:225–233.
57. Sample PA, Medieros FA, Racette L, et al. Identifying glaucomatous vision loss with visual-function-specific perimetry in the diagnostic innovations in glaucoma study. *Invest Ophthalmol Vis Sci.* 2006;47:3381–3389.
58. Racette L, Sample PA. Short-wavelength automated perimetry. *Ophthalmol Clin North Am.* 2003;16:227–236.
59. Sample PA. Short-wavelength automated perimetry: its role in the clinic and for understanding ganglion cell function. *Prog Retin Eye Res.* 2000;19:369–383.
60. Johnson CA, Adams AJ, Casson EJ, Brandt JD. Blue-on-Yellow perimetry can predict the development of glaucomatous visual field loss. *Arch Ophthalmol.* 1993;111:645–650.
61. Johnson CA, Adams AJ, Casson EJ, Brandt JD. Progression of early glaucomatous visual field loss for Blue-on-Yellow and standard White-on-White automated perimetry. *Arch Ophthalmol.* 1993;111:651–656.
62. Johnson CA, Brandt JD, Khong AM, Adams AJ. Short wavelength automated perimetry (SWAP) in low, medium and high risk ocular hypertensives: initial baseline findings. *Arch Ophthalmol.* 1995;113:70–76.
63. Johnson CA, Adams AJ, Casson EJ. Blue-on-yellow perimetry: a five year overview. In: Mills RP, ed. *Perimetry Update 1992/93.* New York: Kugler Publications; 1993:459–466.
64. Johnson CA. Selective vs nonselective losses in glaucoma. *J Glaucoma.* 1994;3:S32-S44. Feature Issue – Journal Supplement.
65. Demirel S, Johnson CA. Incidence and prevalence of Short Wavelength Automated Perimetry (SWAP) deficits in ocular hypertensive patients. *Am J Ophthalmol.* 2001;131:709–715.
66. Demirel S, Johnson CA. Isolation of short wavelength sensitive mechanisms in normal and glaucomatous visual field regions. *J Glaucoma.* 2000;9:63–73.
67. Demirel S, Johnson CA. Short Wavelength Automated Perimetry (SWAP) in ophthalmic practice. *J Am Optom Assoc.* 1996;67:451–456.
68. Casson EJ, Johnson CA, Shapiro LR. A longitudinal comparison of Temporal Modulation Perimetry to White-on-White and Blue-on-Yellow Perimetry in ocular hypertension and early glaucoma. *J Opt Soc Am.* 1993;10:1792–1806.
69. Lewis RA, Johnson CA, Adams AJ. Automated static visual field testing and perimetry of short-wavelength-sensitive (SWS) mechanisms in patients with asymmetric intraocular pressures. *Graefes Arch Clin Exp Ophthalmol.* 1993;231:274–278.
70. Sit AJ, Medieros FA, Weinreb RN. Short-wavelength automated perimetry can predict glaucomatous visual field loss by ten years. *Semin Ophthalmol.* 2004;19:122–124.
71. Turpin A, Johnson CA, Spry PGD. Development of a maximum likelihood procedure for Short Wavelength Automated Perimetry (SWAP). In: Wall M, Mills RP, eds. *Perimetry Update 2000/2001.* The Hague: Kugler Publications; 2001:139–147.
72. Bengtsson B. A new rapid threshold algorithm for short-wavelength automated perimetry. *Invest Ophthalmol Vis Sci.* 2003;44:1388–1394.
73. Bengtsson B, Heijl A. Normal intersubject threshold variability and normal limits of the SITA SWAP and full threshold SWAP perimetric programs. *Invest Ophthalmol Vis Sci.* 2003;44:5029–5034.
74. Bengtsson B, Heijl A. Diagnostic sensitivity of fast blue-yellow and standard automated perimetry in early glaucoma: a comparison between different test programs. *Ophthalmology.* 2006;113:1092–1097.
75. Keltner JL, Johnson CA. Short Wavelength Automated Perimetry (SWAP) in neuro-ophthalmologic disorders. *Arch Ophthalmol.* 1995;113:475–481.
76. Kelly DH. Frequency doubling in visual responses. *J Opt Soc Am A.* 1966;56:1628–1633.
77. Kelly DH. Nonlinear visual responses to flickering sinusoidal gratings. *J Opt Soc Am.* 1981;71:1051–1055.
78. Richards W, Felton DB. Spatial frequency doubling: retinal or central? *Vision Res.* 1973;13:2129–2137.
79. Tyler CW. Observations on spatial frequency doubling. *Perception.* 1974;3:81–86.
80. Virsu V, Nyman G, Lehtio PK. Diphasic and polyphasic temporal modulations multiply apparent spatial frequency. *Perception.* 1974;3:323–336.
81. Tolhurst DJ. Illusory shifts in spatial frequency caused by temporal modulation. *Perception.* 1975;4:331–335.
82. Virsu V, Laurinen P. Long-lasting afterimages caused by neural adaptation. *Vision Res.* 1977;17:853–860.
83. Maddess T, Henry H. Performance of nonlinear visual units in ocular hypertension and glaucoma. *Clin Vis Sci.* 1992;7:371–383.
84. Johnson CA, Samuels SJ. Screening for glaucomatous visual field loss using the frequency-doubling contrast test. *Invest Ophthalmol Vis Sci.* 1997;38:413–425.
85. Fujimoto N, Adachi-Usami E. Frequency doubling perimetry in resolved optic neuritis. *Invest Ophthalmol Vis Sci.* 2000;41:2558–2560.
86. Wall M, Neahring RK, Woodward KR. Sensitivity and specificity of frequency doubling perimetry in neuro-ophthalmic disorders: a comparison with conventional automated perimetry. *Invest Ophthalmol Vis Sci.* 2002;43:1277–1283.
87. Girkin CA, McGwin G, DeLeon-Ortega J. Frequency doubling technology perimetry in non-arteritic ischaemic optic neuropathy with altitudinal defects. *Br J Ophthalmol.* 2004;88:1274–1279.
88. Sheu SJ, Chen YY, Lin HC, Chen HL, Lee IY, Wu TT. Frequency doubling technology perimetry in retinal disease – preliminary report. *Kaohsiung J Med Sci.* 2001;17:25–34.
89. Parikh R, Naik M, Mathai A, Kuriakose T, Muliyil J, Thomas R. Role of frequency doubling technology perimetry in screening of diabetic retinopathy. *Indian J Ophthalmol.* 2006;54:17–22.
90. White AJ, Sun H, Swanson WH, Lee BB. An examination of physiological mechanisms underlying the frequency-doubling illusion. *Invest Ophthalmol Vis Sci.* 2002;43:3590–3599.
91. Zeppieri M, Demirel S, Kent K, Johnson CA. Perceived spatial frequency of sinusoidal gratings. *Optom Vis Sci.* 2008;85:318–329.

92. Anderson AJ, Johnson CA. Frequency doubling technology perimetry. *Ophthalmol Clin North Am.* 2003;16:213–225.
93. Anderson AJ, Johnson CA, Fingeret M, et al. Characteristics of the normative database for the Humphrey Matrix perimeter. *Invest Ophthalmol Vis Sci.* 2005;46:1540–1548.
94. Clement CI, Goldberg I, Graham S, Healey PR. Humphrey matrix frequency doubling perimetry for detection of visual field defects in open-angle glaucoma. *Br J Ophthalmol.* 2009;93(5):582–588.
95. Brusini P, Salvatet ML, Zeppieri M, Parisi L. Frequency doubling technology perimetry with the Humphrey Matrix 30-2 test. *J Glaucoma.* 2006;15:77–83.
96. Spry PG, Hussin HM, Sparrow JM. Clinical evaluation of frequency doubling perimetry using the Humphrey Matrix 24-2 threshold strategy. *Br J Ophthalmol.* 2005;89:1031–1035.
97. Taravati P, Woodward KR, Keltner JL, et al. Sensitivity and specificity of the Humphrey Matrix to detect homonymous hemianopias. *Invest Ophthalmol Vis Sci.* 2008;49:924–928.
98. Huang CQ, Carolan J, Redline D, et al. Humphrey Matrix perimetry in optic nerve and chiasmal disorders: comparison with Humphrey SITA standard 24-2. *Invest Ophthalmol Vis Sci.* 2008;49:917–923.
99. Johnson CA, Wall M, Fingeret M, Lalle P. *A Primer for Frequency Doubling Technology Perimetry.* Skaneateles, NY: Welch Allyn; 1998.
100. Spry PGD, Johnson CA, Anderson AJ, et al. *A Primer for Frequency Doubling Technology (FDT) Perimetry Using the Humphrey Matrix.* Skaneateles, NY: Welch Allyn; 2008.
101. Artes PH, Hutchison DM, Nicolela MT, LeBlanc RP, Chauhan BC. Threshold and variability properties of matrix frequency-doubling technology and standard automated perimetry in glaucoma. *Invest Ophthalmol Vis Sci.* 2005;46:2451–2457.
102. Johnson CA, Cioffi GA, Van Buskirk EM. Evaluation of two screening tests for frequency doubling technology perimetry. In: Wall M, Wild JM, eds. *Perimetry Update 1998/1999.* Amsterdam: Kugler Publications; 1999:103–109.
103. Spry PG, Hussin HM, Sparrow JM. Performance of the 24–2–5 frequency doubling technology screening test: a prospective case study. *Br J Ophthalmol.* 2007;91:1345–1349.
104. Ruben S, Fitzke F. Correlation of peripheral displacement thresholds and optic disc parameters in ocular hypertension. *Br J Ophthalmol.* 1994;78:291–294.
105. Johnson CA, Marshall D, Eng K. Displacement threshold perimetry in glaucoma using a Macintosh computer system and a 21 inch monitor. In: Wall M, Mills RP, eds. *Perimetry Update 1994/95.* Amsterdam: Kugler Publications; 2001:103–110.
106. Westcott MC, Fitzke FW, Hitchings RA. Abnormal motion displacement thresholds are associated with fine scale luminance sensitivity loss in glaucoma. *Vision Res.* 1998;38:3171–3180.
107. Wall M, Ketoff KM. Random dot motion perimetry in patients with glaucoma and in normal subjects. *Am J Ophthalmol.* 1995;120:587–596.
108. Wall M, Jennisch CS, Munden PM. Motion perimetry identifies nerve fiber bundlelike defects in ocular hypertension. *Arch Ophthalmol.* 1997;115:26–33.
109. Wall M, Jennisch CS. Random dot motion stimuli are more sensitive than light stimuli for detection of visual field loss in ocular hypertension patients. *Optom Vis Scci.* 1999;76:550–557.
110. Joffe KM, Raymond JE, Chrichton A. Motion coherence perimetry in glaucoma and suspected glaucoma. *Vision Res.* 1997;37:955–964.
111. Bosworth CF, Sample PA, Weinreb RN. Perimetric motion thresholds are elevated in glaucoma suspects and glaucoma patients. *Vision Res.* 1997;37:1989–1997.
112. Bosworth CF, Sample PA, Gupta N, Bathija R, Weinreb RN. Motion automated perimetry identifies early glaucomatous field defects. *Arch Ophthalmol.* 1998;116:1153–1158.
113. Silverman SE, Trick GL, Hart WM. Motion perception is abnormal in ptimary open angle glaucoma and ocular hypertension. *Invest Ophthalmol Vis Sci.* 1990;31:722–729.
114. Bullimore MA, Wood JA, Swenson K. Motion perception in glaucoma. *Invest Ophthalmol Vis Sci.* 1993;34:3526–3533.
115. Bosworth CF, Sample PA, Williams JM, Zangwill L, Kee B, Weinreb RN. Spatial relationships of motion automated perimetry and optic disc topography in patients with glaucomatous optic neuropathy. *J Glaucoma.* 1999;8:281–289.
116. Sample PA, Bosworth CF, Blumenthal EZ, Girkin C, Weinreb RN. Visual function-specific perimetry for indirect comparison of different ganglion cell populations in glaucoma. *Invest Ophthalmmol Vis Sci.* 2000;41:1783–1790.
117. Shabana N, Cornilleau PV, Carkeet A, Chew PT. Motion pereption in glaucoma patients: a review. *Surv Ophthalmol.* 2003;48:92–106.
118. Johnson CA, Scobey RP. Foveal and peripheral displacement thresholds as a function of stimulus luminance, line length and duration of movement. *Vision Res.* 1980;20:709–715.
119. Yoshiyama KK, Johnson CA. Which method of flicker perimetry is most effective for detection of glaucomatous visual field loss? *Invest Ophthalmol Vis Sci.* 1997;38:2270–2277.
120. McKendrick AM, Johnson CA. Temporal properties of vision. In: Alm A, Kaufmann P, eds. *Adler's Physiology of the Eye.* 10th ed. St. Louis: C.V. Mosby; 2002:511–530 [Section 9: Visual perception].
121. Tyler CW. Specific deficits of flicker sensitivity in glaucoma and ocular hypertension. *Invest Ophthalmol Vis Sci.* 1981;100:135–146.
122. Lachenmayr BJ, Drance SM, Douglas GR, Mikelberg FS. Light-sense, flicker and resolution perimetry in glaucoma: a comparative study. *Graefes Arch Clin Exp Ophthalmol.* 1991;229:246–251.
123. Lachenmayr BJ, Drance SM, Chauhan BC, House PH, Lalani S. Diffuse and localized glaucomatous field loss in light-sense, flicker and resolution perimetry. *Graefes Arch Clin Exp Ophthalmol.* 1991;229:267–273.
124. Casson EJ, Johnson CA. Temporal modulation perimetry in glaucoma and ocular hypertension. In: Mills RP, ed. *Perimetry Update 1992/93.* New York: Kugler Publications; 1993:443–450.
125. Matsumoto C, Takada S, Okuyama S, Arimura E, Hashimoto S, Shimomura Y. Automated flicker perimetry in glaucoma using Octopus 311: a comparative study with the Humphrey Matrix. *Acta Ophthalmol Scand.* 2006;84:866–872.
126. Swanson WH, Ueno T, Smith VC, Pokorny J. Temporal modulation sensitivity and pulse-detection thresholds for chromatic and luminance perturbations. *J Opt Soc Am A.* 1987;4:1992–2005.
127. Anderson AJ, Vingrys AJ. Interactions between flicker thresholds and luminance pedestals. *Vision Res.* 2000;40:2579–2588.
128. Anderson AJ, Vingrys AJ. Effect of eccentricity on luminance-pedestal flicker thresholds. *Vision Res.* 2002;42:1149–1156.
129. Anderson AJ, Vingrys AJ. Multiple processes mediate flicker sensitivity. *Vision Res.* 2001;41:2449–2455.
130. Quaid PT, Flanagan JG. Defining the limits of flicker defined form: effect of stimulus size, eccentricity and number of random dots. *Vision Res.* 2005;45:1075–1084.
131. Goren D, Flanagan JG. Is flicker-defined form (FDF) dependent on the contour? *J Vis.* 2008;8:15.1–15.11.
132. Frisen L. Acuity perimetry: estimation of neural channels. *Int Ophthalmol.* 1988;12:169–174.
133. Wall M, Lefante J, Conway M. Variability of high-pass resolution perimetry in normals and patients with idiopathic intracranial hypertension. *Invest Ophthalmol Vis Sci.* 1991;32:3091–3095.
134. Wall M, Conway MD, House PH, Alley R. Evaluation of sensitivity and specificity of spatial resolution and Humphrey automated perimetry in pseudotumor cerebri patients and normal subjects. *Invest Ophthalmol Vis Sci.* 1991;32:3306–3312.

135. Sample PA, Ahn DS, Lee PC, Weinreb RN. High-pass resolution perimetry in eyes with ocular hypertension and primary open-angle glaucoma. *Am J Ophthalmol.* 1992;113:309–316.
136. Frisen L. High-pass resolution perimetry: a clinical review. *Doc Ophthalmol.* 1993;83:1–25.
137. Chauhan BC, LeBlanc RP, McCormick TA, Mohandas RN, Wijsman K. Correlation between the optic disc and results obtained with conventional, high-pass resolution and pattern discrimination perimetry in glaucoma. *Can J Ophthalmol.* 1993;28:312–316.
138. Chauhan BC, House PH, McCormick TA, LeBlanc RP. Comparison of conventional and high-pass resolution perimetry in a prospective study of patients with glaucoma and healthy controls. *Arch Ophthalmol.* 1999;117:24–33.
139. Chauhan BC. The value of high-pass resolution perimetry in glaucoma. *Curr Opin Ophthalmol.* 2000;11:85–89.
140. Ennis FA, Johnson CA. Are high-pass resolution perimetry thresholds sampling limited or optically limited? *Optom Vis Sci.* 2002;79:506–511.
141. Wall M, Chauhan B, Frisen L, House PH, Brito C. Visual field of high-pass resolution perimetry in normal subjects. *J Glaucoma.* 2004;13:15–21.
142. Frisen L. New, sensitive window on abnormal spatial vision: rarebit probing. *Vision Res.* 2002;42:1931–1939.
143. Martin L, Wanger P. New perimetric techniques: a comparison between rarebit and frequency doubling technology perimetry in normal subjects and glaucoma patients. *J Glaucoma.* 2004;13:268–272.
144. Brusini P, Salvatet ML, Parisi L, Zeppieri M. Probing glaucoma visual damage by rarebit perimetry. *Br J Ophthalmol.* 2005;89:180–184.
145. Salvatet ML, Zeppieri M, Parisi L, Brusini P. Rarebit perimetry in normal subjects: test-retest variability, learning effect, normative range, influence of optical defocus, and cataract extraction. *Invest Ophthalmol Vis Sci.* 2007;48:5320–5331.
146. Yavas GF, Kusbeci T, Eser O, Ermis SS, Cosar M, Ozturk F. A new visual field test in empty sella syndrome: rarebit perimetry. *Eur J Ophthalmol.* 2008;18:628–632.
147. Bearse MA Jr, Sutter EE. Imaging localized retinal dysfunction with the multifocal electroretinogram. *J Opt Soc Am A.* 1996;13:634–640.
148. Chan HL, Brown B. Multifocal ERG changes in glaucoma. *Ophthalmic Physiol Opt.* 1999;19:306–316.
149. Hood DC, Zhang X. Multifocal ERG and VEP responses and visual fields: comparing disease-related changes. *Doc Ophthalmol.* 2000;100:115–137.
150. Fortune B, Bearse MA, Cioffi GA, Johnson CA. Selective loss of an oscillatory component from temporal retinal multifocal ERG responses in glaucoma. *Invest Ophthalmol Vis Sci.* 2002;43:2638–2647.
151. Chan HH. Detection of glaucomatous damage using multifocal ERG. *Clin Exp Optom.* 2005;88:410–414.
152. Graham SL, Klistorner AL, Grigg JR, Billson FA. Objective VEP perimetry in glaucoma: asymmetry analysis to identify early deficits. *J Glaucoma.* 2000;9:10–19.
153. Klistorner A, Graham SL. Objective perimetry in glaucoma. *Ophthalmology.* 2000;107:2283–2299.
154. Hood DC, Greenstein VC. Multifocal VEP and ganglion cell damage: applications and limitations for the study of glaucoma. *Prog Retin Eye Res.* 2003;22:201–251.
155. Graham SL, Klistorner AL. Goldberg. Clinical application of objective perimetry using multifocal visual evoked potentials in glaucoma practice. *Arch Ophthalmol.* 2005;123:729–739.
156. Grippo TM, Hood DC, Kandani FN, Greenstein VC, Liebmann JM, Ritch R. A comparison between multifocal and conventional VEP latency changes secondary to glaucomatous damage. *Invest Ophthalmol Vis Sci.* 2006;47:5331–5336.
157. Fortune B, Demirel S, Zhang X, et al. Comparing multifocal VEP and standard automated perimetry in high-risk ocular hypertensives and early glaucoma. *Invest Ophthalmol Vis Sci.* 2007;48:1173–1180.
158. Klistorner A, Graham SL, Martins A, et al. Multifocal blue-on-yellow visual evoked potentials in arly glaucoma. *Ophthalmology.* 2007;114:1613–1621.
159. Johnson CA, Keltner JL. Principals and techniques of the examination of the visual sensory system. In: Miller NR, Newman NJ, eds. *Walsh and Hoyt's Textbook of Neuro-Ophthalmology.* Baltimore: Williams and Wilkens; 1998:153–235.
160. Frisen L. *Clinical tests of vision.* New York: Raven Press; 1990.
161. Lachenmayr BJ, Vivell PMO. *Perimetry and its clinical correlations.* New York: Thieme; 1993.
162. Gardiner SK, Crabb DP. Frequency of testing for detecting visual field progression. *Br J Ophthalmol.* 2002;86:560–564.
163. Spry PGD, Johnson CA. Identification of progressive glaucomatous visual field loss. *Surv Ophthalmol.* 2002;47:158–173.
164. Vesti E, Johnson CA, Chauhan BC. Comparison of different methods for detecting glaucomatous visual field progression. *Invest Ophthalmol Vis Sci.* 2003;44:3873–3879.
165. Smith SD, Katz J, Quigley HA. Analysis of progressive change in automated visual fields in glaucoma. *Invest Ophthalmol Vis Sci.* 1996;37:1419–1428.
166. Åsman P, Heijl A. Glaucoma Hemifield Test: automated visual field evaluation. *Arch Ophthalmol.* 1992;110:812–819.
167. Heijl A, Lindgren G, Lindgren A, et al. Extended empirical statistical package for evaluation of single and multiple fields in glaucoma. Statpak 2. In: Mills RP, Heijl A, eds. *Perimetry Update 1990/91.* Amsterdam: Kugler and Ghedini; 1991:303–315.
168. Mayama C, Araie M, Suzuki Y, et al. Statistical evaluation of the diagnostic accuracy of methods used to determine the progression of visual field defects in glaucoma. *Ophthalmology.* 2004;111:2117–2125.
169. Katz J, Congdon N, Friedman DS. Methodological variations in estimating apparent progressive visual field loss in clinical trials of glaucoma treatment. *Arch Ophthalmol.* 1999;117:1137–1142.
170. Nouri-Mahdavi K, Hoffman D, Ralli M, Caprioli J. Comparison of methods to predict visual field progression in glaucoma. *Arch Ophthalmol.* 2007;125:1176–1181.
171. Boden C, Blumenthal EZ, Pascual J, et al. Patterns of glaucomatous visual field progression identified by three progression criteria. *Am J Ophthalmol.* 2004;138:1029–1036.
172. AGIS Investigators. The Advanced Glaucoma Intervention Study (AGIS): 14. Distinguishing progression of glaucoma from visual field fluctuations. *Ophthalmology.* 2004;111:2109–2116.
173. Schulzer M. Errors in the diagnosis of visual field progression in normal-tension glaucoma. *Ophthalmology.* 1994;101:1589–1594.
174. Heijl A, Bengtsson B, Chauhan BC, et al. A comparison of visual field progression criteria of 3 major glaucoma trials in Early Manifest Glaucoma Trial patients. *Ophthalmology.* 2008;115:1557–1565.
175. Broman AT, Quigley HA, West SK, et al. Estimating the rate of progressive visual field damage in those with open-angle glaucoma, from cross-sectional data. *Invest Ophthalmol Vis Sci.* 2008;49:66–76.
176. Bengtsson B, Heijl A. A visual field index for calculation of glaucoma rate of progression. *Am J Ophthalmol.* 2008;145:343–353.
177. Keltner JL, Johnson CA, Spurr JO, Kass MA, Ocular Hypertension Study Group. Confirmation of visual field abnormalities in the Ocular Hypertension Treatment Study (OHTS). *Arch Ophthalmol.* 2000;118:1187–1194.
178. Hattenhauer MG, Johnson DH, Ing HH, et al. The probability of blindness from open-angle glaucoma. *Ophthalmology.* 1998;105:2099–2104.
179. Friedman DS, Hahn SR, Gelb L, et al. Doctor-patient communication, health-related beliefs, and adherence in glaucoma results from the Glaucoma Adherence and Persistency Study. *Ophthalmology.* 2008;115:1320–1327.
180. Friedman DS, Quigley HA, Gelb L, et al. Using pharmacy claims data to study adherence to glaucoma medications: methodology and findings of the Glaucoma Adherence and Persistency Study (GAPS). *Invest Ophthalmol Vis Sci.* 2007;48:5052–5257.

181. The Advanced Glaucoma Intervention Study Group. The Advanced Glaucoma Intervention Study (AGIS): 4. Comparison of treatment outcomes within race. Seven-year results. *Ophthalmology*. 1998;105:1146–1164.
182. Feiner L, Piltz-Seymour JR, Collaborative Initial Glaucoma Treatment Study. Collaborative Initial Glaucoma Treatment Study: a summary of results to date. *Curr Opin Ophthalmol*. 2003;14:106–111.
183. Leske MC, Heijl A, Hussein M, et al. Factors for glaucoma progression and the effect of treatment: the early manifest glaucoma trial. *Arch Ophthalmol*. 2003;121:48–56.
184. Kass MA, Heuer DK, Higginbotham EJ, et al. The Ocular Hypertension Treatment Study: safety and efficacy of topical ocular hypotensive medication in preventing or delaying the onset of primary open angle glaucoma. *Arch Ophthalmol*. 2002;120:701–713.
185. Anderson DR, Drance SM, Schulzer M, Collaborative Normal-Tension Glaucoma Study Group. Factors that predict the benefit of lowering intraocular pressure in normal tension glaucoma. *Am J Ophthalmol*. 2003;136:820–829.
186. Hyman LG, Komaroff E, Heijl A, Bengtsson B, Leske MC, Early Manifest Glaucoma Trial Group. Treatment and vision-related quality of life in the early manifest glaucoma trial. *Ophthalmology*. 2005;112:1505–1513.
187. Jampel HD, Schwartz A, Pollack I, Abrams D, Weiss H, Miller R. Glaucoma patients' assessment of their visual function and quality of life. *J Glaucoma*. 2002;11:154–163.
188. Coleman AL. Glaucoma. *Lancet*. 1999;354:1803–1810.
189. Girkin CA. Primary open-angle glaucoma in African Americans. *Int Ophthalmol Clin*. 2004;44:43-60. Review.
190. Varma R, Ying-Lai M, Francis BA, et al. Prevalence of open-angle glaucoma and ocular hypertension in Latinos: the Los Angeles Latino Eye Study. *Ophthalmology*. 2004;111:1439-1448.

# Chapter 24
# Using Electroretinography for Glaucoma Diagnosis

Kevin C. Leonard and Cindy M. L. Hutnik

It has been suggested that up to 35% of retinal ganglion cells (RGCs) are lost before visual field defects become apparent.[1] Automated perimetric testing is the current gold standard for diagnosis.[1] This concept led to the theory of an "RGC reserve" with structural damage preceding functional loss in early glaucoma. However, as more advanced techniques for assessing both RGC structure and function have been developed, evidence has arisen indicating that RGC dysfunction may precede the structural loss of these cells. This suggests the potential for more effective early detection techniques. Digital imaging techniques (e.g., retinal tomography, scanning polarimetry, and optical coherence tomography) that attempt to detect structural changes in the optic nerve and RGC nerve fiber layer have become very popular as complimentary to functional perimetric testing for early glaucoma. In this chapter, however, we will discuss developments regarding electrophysiological measures of RGC loss or dysfunction to detect and monitor glaucoma. Glaucoma is a disease in which such early detection and early therapeutic intervention are critical for preventing progression and loss of vision.

Ocular hypertension is an important risk factor for primary open angle glaucoma (POAG). Many clinicians offer treatment to lower intraocular pressure (IOP) to prevent the conversion to disease. However, as it has been estimated that 20 patients need to be treated to prevent one conversion to glaucoma,[2] a test to identify the nonconverters would spare them from the cost and any side effects of IOP lowering treatment. This concept provides additional support for the development of a method for earlier detection of glaucomatous change before visual field defects arise.

Electroretinography is a rapid, noninvasive method of assessing retinal function that is useful in the diagnosis of various retinal disease processes. The flash electroretinogram (ERG) represents the summed electrical activity of different groups of retinal cells, and it is recorded from the corneal surface in response to a flash of light. The primary waveforms in the flash ERG are the a-wave and b-wave, which arise predominantly from the outer and middle retinal layers, respectively. The flash ERG is somewhat limited in terms of utility in the diagnosis or monitoring of glaucoma, where the pathology involves selective loss of RGCs. Some studies have revealed no difference in a-wave, b-wave, and implicit time between POAG and normal subjects.[3] Other studies have demonstrated that these parameters may be affected later in the disease, suggesting involvement of outer or middle retinal layers as the disease progresses.[4,5]

One feature of the flash ERG that has shown some utility in POAG is the photopic negative response (PhNR). This is a slow negative potential that follows the b-wave in response to a photopic stimulus and originates from the inner retina. It has been suggested that this waveform arises as a consequence of spiking activity of RGCs and, thus, may be a sensitive measure of retinal dysfunction in diseases that affect the inner retina.[3,6] The first study to demonstrate this in human glaucoma showed that PhNR amplitudes are consistently smaller in POAG patients and correlate with the mean deviation determined by static perimetry, even with mild visual field sensitivity losses.[3] A more recent study has shown that PhNR amplitudes correlate with decrease in function and morphology of retinal neurons in eyes with OAG, indicating that inner retinal function apparently declines proportionately with neural loss in glaucomatous eyes. The amplitude of the PhNR has been shown to decrease with an increase in visual field defects and is significantly correlated with the retinal nerve fiber layer thickness (RNFLT) and the rim area of the optic disc as well as the cup:disc ratio.[7] These results provide evidence against the RGC reserve theory mentioned previously and suggest that RGC dysfunction is detectable at least as early as the structural loss of these cells.

Pattern ERG (PERG) is another test that has been investigated as an early predictor of conversion to glaucoma. PERG provides a stimulus in the form of alternating gratings (i.e., checkerboard stimuli) at a constant mean luminance and is felt to represent a more focal response from a specific area of the retina being stimulated. Importantly, PERG has been shown to be a direct and objective measure of RGC function. Multiple studies have shown that PERG is significantly altered in glaucoma. A long-term prospective study designed to assess the predictive value of the PERG for the occurrence of visual field defects in patients with ocular hypertension revealed its ability to predict conversion more than 1 year before conversion was detected based on visual field testing.[8] Another recent study has shown that PERG amplitude correlates with RNFL thickness in early glaucoma but not ocular hypertension. PERG amplitude losses in early glaucoma and glaucoma suspects were substantially greater than the corresponding losses in RNFL thickness.[9] These results suggest some clinical utility for PERG in identifying patients who will progress to glaucoma prior to changes in structure of RNFL or visual field tests.

The multifocal ERG (mfERG) permits topographic display of retinal function and allows for much more detailed assessment of retinal function at specific areas affected by disease. The mfERG has been shown to be very useful in the assessment of outer retinal function, with the responses being very similar to photopic flash ERGs. However, with standard stimulation parameters, only a small reduction in amplitude and increase in latencies was identified for POAG patients.[10] More recently, its utility in assessing inner retinal function has been established with the identification of the optic nerve head component (ONHC), which is of inner retinal origin and is thought to arise in the vicinity of the optic nerve head. This component shows most relevance to the detection of early glaucoma because it has been shown that its propagation time correlates with the length of the ganglion nerve fibers and thus seems to be dependent on the nerve fiber layer.[11] This component differs from other typical components of the mfERG in both luminance and contrast sensitivity; thus, various modifications to the mfERG have been proposed and investigated to enhance this particular component. Several stimulus variations have been shown to increase the ONHC and facilitate the detection of change in early glaucoma, including interposing global flashes into the stimulation sequence,[12] slowing the stimulation sequence,[13] luminance modulation,[14] and assessing for selective effects on oscillatory potentials.[14,15] The development of multifocal pattern ERG (mfPERG) combines the PERG stimulation with the multifocal technique to achieve a topographic mapping of the PERG. Studies have demonstrated significant changes in the mfPERG of glaucoma patients, with components of the mfPERG significantly decreased, most distinctly in the central ring, and decreasing further with a progression of glaucoma stage.[16] While this seems promising, an early study showed little correlation between topographic PERG changes and visual field defects in glaucoma patients.[17]

Another electrophysiological technique that is distinct from ERG but showing some promise in the detection and monitoring of glaucomatous change is the visual evoked potential (VEP). In particular, the multifocal VEP (mfVEP) is a technique that measures the response to a stimulus arising from the visual cortex and parts of the optic nerve. Studies have shown that the mfVEP can detect early visual field changes not seen with standard automated perimetry.[18] Another benefit of mfVEP is its objective and reproducible visual field recordings, which eliminate the high test–retest variability seen in current perimetric tests, the latter becoming particularly problematic as visual fields worsen.[19] Further, a recent study has demonstrated mfVEP as a viable method for detecting the progression of glaucoma, based on a statistically significant change in several mfVEP parameters when reassessed after at least 6 months.[20] The mfVEP offers similar advantages to the various ERG modalities described, with the most obvious difference being the provision of objective and reproducible data regarding patients' visual fields as opposed to strictly retinal function.

## 24.1 Conclusion

The development of a noninvasive, rapid, and sensitive electrophysiological test for the early detection of glaucoma remains a work-in-progress at the current time. While the value of such a test would be immense, there is currently insufficient evidence to incorporate routine ERG or VEP testing into the care of glaucoma patients or suspects. The research in this technology is constantly evolving, and based on the success to date with the various modalities described, it seems likely that there will be such a test for the early detection of glaucoma in the future. The rationale behind this concept is sound, and the success in these early studies has provided evidence that RGC dysfunction is likely detectable prior to structural changes or changes in psychometric testing (i.e., visual fields). Further study and refinement of these technologies will likely allow for more reliable testing and identification of early glaucomatous change.

## References

1. Kerrigan-Baumrind LA, Quigley HA, Pease ME, Kerrigan DF, Mitchell RS. Number of ganglion cells in glaucoma eyes compared with threshold visual field tests in the same persons. *Invest Ophthalmol Vis Sci*. 2000;41(3):741–748.
2. Kass MA, Heuer DK, Higginbotham EJ, et al. The ocular hypertension treatment study: a randomized trial determines that topical ocular hypotensive medication delays or prevents the onset of primary open-angle glaucoma. *Arch Ophthalmol*. 2002;120(6): 701–713; discussion 829–730.
3. Viswanathan S, Frishman LJ, Robson JG, Walters JW. The photopic negative response of the flash electroretinogram in primary open angle glaucoma. *Invest Ophthalmol Vis Sci*. 2001;42(2): 514–522.
4. Velten IM, Korth M, Horn FK. The a-wave of the dark adapted electroretinogram in glaucomas: are photoreceptors affected? *Br J Ophthalmol*. 2001;85(4):397–402.

5. Velten IM, Horn FK, Korth M, Velten K. The b-wave of the dark adapted flash electroretinogram in patients with advanced asymmetrical glaucoma and normal subjects. *Br J Ophthalmol.* 2001;85(4):403–409.
6. Viswanathan S, Frishman LJ, Robson JG, Harwerth RS, Smith EL 3rd. The photopic negative response of the macaque electroretinogram: reduction by experimental glaucoma. *Invest Ophthalmol Vis Sci.* 1999;40(6):1124–1136.
7. Machida S, Gotoh Y, Toba Y, Ohtaki A, Kaneko M, Kurosaka D. Correlation between photopic negative response and retinal nerve fiber layer thickness and optic disc topography in glaucomatous eyes. *Invest Ophthalmol Vis Sci.* 2008;49(5):2201–2207.
8. Bach M, Unsoeld AS, Philippin H, et al. Pattern ERG as an early glaucoma indicator in ocular hypertension: a long-term, prospective study. *Invest Ophthalmol Vis Sci.* 2006;47(11):4881–4887.
9. Falsini B, Marangoni D, Salgarello T, et al. Structure-function relationship in ocular hypertension and glaucoma: interindividual and interocular analysis by OCT and pattern ERG. *Graefes Arch Clin Exp Ophthalmol.* 2008;246(8):1153–1162.
10. Palmowski AM, Ruprecht KW. Follow up in open angle glaucoma. A comparison of static perimetry and the fast stimulation mfERG. Multifocal ERG follow up in open angle glaucoma. *Doc Ophthalmol.* 2004;108(1):55–60.
11. Sutter EE, Bearse MA Jr. The optic nerve head component of the human ERG. *Vision Res.* 1999;39(3):419–436.
12. Palmowski-Wolfe AM, Todorova MG, Orguel S, Flammer J, Brigell M. The "two global flash" mfERG in high and normal tension primary open-angle glaucoma. *Doc Ophthalmol.* 2007;114(1):9–19.
13. Palmowski-Wolfe AM, Allgayer RJ, Vernaleken B, Schotzau A, Ruprecht KW. Slow-stimulated multifocal ERG in high- and normal-tension glaucoma. *Doc Ophthalmol.* 2006;112(3):157–168.
14. Chu PH, Chan HH, Brown B. Glaucoma detection is facilitated by luminance modulation of the global flash multifocal electroretinogram. *Invest Ophthalmol Vis Sci.* 2006;47(3):929–937.
15. Fortune B, Bearse MA Jr, Cioffi GA, Johnson CA. Selective loss of an oscillatory component from temporal retinal multifocal ERG responses in glaucoma. *Invest Ophthalmol Vis Sci.* 2002;43(8):2638–2647.
16. Stiefelmeyer S, Neubauer AS, Berninger T, Arden GB, Rudolph G. The multifocal pattern electroretinogram in glaucoma. *Vision Res.* 2004;44(1):103–112.
17. Klistorner AI, Graham SL, Martins A. Multifocal pattern electroretinogram does not demonstrate localised field defects in glaucoma. *Doc Ophthalmol.* 2000;100(2–3):155–165.
18. Hood DC, Thienprasiddhi P, Greenstein VC, et al. Detecting early to mild glaucomatous damage: a comparison of the multifocal VEP and automated perimetry. *Invest Ophthalmol Vis Sci.* 2004;45(2):492–498.
19. Chauhan BC, Johnson CA. Test-retest variability of frequency-doubling perimetry and conventional perimetry in glaucoma patients and normal subjects. *Invest Ophthalmol Vis Sci.* 1999;40(3):648–656.
20. Wangsupadilok B, Greenstein VC, Kanadani FN, et al. A method to detect progression of glaucoma using the multifocal visual evoked potential technique. *Doc Ophthalmol.* 2009;118(2):139–150.

# Chapter 25
# Glaucomatous Versus Nonglaucomatous Visual Loss: The Neuro-Ophthalmic Perspective

Matthew D. Kay, Mark L. Moster, and Paul N. Schacknow

The diagnosis of glaucoma is generally straightforward in the setting of elevated intraocular pressure (IOP), glaucomatous excavation of the disc, and characteristic nerve fiber bundle defects on visual field testing. However, one should always carry an index of suspicion for an alternative nonglaucomatous process and critically evaluate the optic nerves and visual fields. Is the degree of visual loss consistent with the optic nerve changes? Is the character of the visual field loss compatible with glaucomatous change? Are additional investigations warranted, and if so, what studies should be performed?

Any neuro-ophthalmologist can cite cases they have encountered of patients with bona fide glaucoma who have developed a superimposed nonglaucomatous optic neuropathy. These include compressive lesions such as a sphenoid wing meningioma or a pituitary adenoma, patients with ocular hypertension whose visual field loss from a compressive lesion or a prior ischemic event is attributed to glaucoma, or patients with physiologic cupping who have progressive visual loss from a compressive lesion. Some of these patients have undergone filtering/shunt procedures with excellent IOP control prior to the question being asked: *Is the progression of visual field loss out of proportion to the optic nerve changes regardless of the IOP?* This is the reason for obtaining baseline detailed drawings of the optic nerve, disc photographs, and the like, and for reevaluating them when there is progression of visual field loss. Serial ocular coherence tomography (OCT) of the nerve fiber layer is insufficient as an isolated imaging modality because any progressive optic neuropathy will lead to progressive thinning of the peripapillary nerve fiber layer. Following the optic nerve appearance in terms of cupping, excavation, and color of the neural rim is an essential aspect of monitoring glaucoma patients, particularly in the setting of progressive visual field loss.

## 25.1 Differentiating Glaucoma from Nonglaucomatous Optic Neuropathy

Patients are not infrequently referred to neuro-ophthalmologists by comprehensive ophthalmologists and glaucoma specialists in order to evaluate for the possibility of a nonglaucomatous optic neuropathy as the basis for a patient's optic nerve head changes and visual field defects. We need to identify those patients who may have an erroneous diagnosis of glaucoma who harbor neuro-ophthalmologic disorders requiring other investigations and treatment. Glaucoma is, in fact, just one of many anterior optic neuropathies, such as anterior ischemic optic neuropathy (AION), disc drusen, papillitis, and papilledema. Accordingly, glaucoma shares characteristic features inherent to these other optic neuropathies, including nerve fiber bundle defects on visual field testing, loss of retinal ganglion cells, retinal nerve fiber layer loss, and optic atrophy.[1] However, there are specific clinical features that help to distinguish glaucoma from other optic neuropathies.

The distinction between nonglaucomatous optic neuropathies and glaucoma generally takes into account the color of the optic nerve's residual neural rim, visual acuity, character of the visual field defects, and color vision. Of the multitude of optic neuropathies, glaucoma is unique because preservation of central acuity, intact color vision, and retained pink color of the residual neural rim is the rule. Nonglaucomatous optic neuropathies often involve central acuity early, produce dyschromatopsia, and result in pallor of the residual neural rim, the latter being evident in any chronic nonglaucomatous optic neuropathy. The visual field loss in glaucoma tends to be denser nasally and tends to spare central fixation until late in the disease, while compressive lesions of the optic chiasm will produce bilateral visual field loss, which is denser temporally. See Table 25.1.

Table 25.1 Features suggesting a nonglaucomatous diagnosis

| | Features suggesting a nonglaucomatous diagnosis |
|---|---|
| History | Young age |
| | Rapid onset |
| | Rapid progression |
| | Headache (other than typical migraine) |
| | Other neurologic symptoms |
| Exam | Loss of visual acuity or visual field out of proportion to cupping |
| | Severe dyschromatopsia |
| | Afferent pupillary defect without significant asymmetry of cupping |
| | Ocular motility or other neurologic defects |
| Visual field | Atypical visual field: temporal > nasal, respect of vertical meridian, inferior altitudinal defect, central scotoma |
| Optic disc | Pallor of preserved rim |

Although these clinical characteristics that separate glaucomatous from nonglaucomatous entities are generally readily assessed, there can be situations in which these distinctions become blurred. For example, normal tension glaucoma (NTG) can sometimes affect central vision early in the disease course. A study by Takeda et al. found that the superior central 5–10° of the visual field was significantly more depressed in patients with NTG as opposed to primary open angle glaucoma (POAG).[2] Another study found that for a given amount of visual field damage, the area just above the horizontal meridian was significantly more depressed in NTG patients, whereas those individuals with POAG exhibited more diffuse visual field loss.[3]

Glaucoma and ocular hypertension are relatively common eye diseases, with the prevalence increasing with advancing age. In the United States, glaucoma is estimated to be present in 5.2% of black individuals and 1.8% of the white population over the age of 40.[4] The prevalence of open angle glaucoma increases with advancing age and was found to be 4.7% in a white population 75 years of age or older.[5] The prevalence in Hispanic individuals is intermediate between black and white individuals, occurring in 1.97% of individuals over the age of 40 and increasing to 12.63% for people over the age of 80.[6] The prevalence of ocular hypertension in one study was 2.1% in a northern Italian population over the age of 40, while the prevalence was 3.56% in a similar-aged Hispanic population in the United States.[7,8]

Because of the relatively common occurrence of glaucoma and ocular hypertension, they may occur simultaneously or sequentially with other optic neuropathies. For example, one would expect roughly 4.7% of white individuals over the age of 75 harboring a pituitary adenoma or sphenoid wing meningioma to have coexisting glaucoma, as this is the prevalence of glaucoma in that patient population.

Thus, when rendering a diagnosis of glaucoma or diagnosing progression of known glaucomatous disease, it is most important to be certain that the patient's visual fields are consistent with the degree of optic nerve cupping and not related to an alternative process such as a compressive lesion.

In order to attribute visual field loss to glaucoma, corresponding optic nerve cupping must be present. Individuals with elevated IOP and visual field loss in the absence of cupping require evaluation for an alternative superimposed nonglaucomatous process to account for the visual field defects (e.g., disc drusen, retrobulbar compressive lesions, prior ischemic optic neuropathy, etc.). The visual field defects of glaucoma produce nerve fiber bundle defects as in any optic neuropathy, thus it is essential that the field defects are consistent with the optic nerve head changes. However, it should be noted that in the setting of advanced cupping from end-stage glaucoma, individuals may develop some pallor of the minimal residual rim. This tends to happen only when the cup-to-disc ratio is in the range of 0.9 or when there is extreme thinning of the neural rim in a region of focal notching or excavation. Any optic nerve pallor with a lesser degree of optic nerve excavation should be viewed with great suspicion as possibly representing an alternative nonglaucomatous process.

### 25.1.1 Cupping in Nonglaucomatous Optic Neuropathy

A particularly common referral to a neuro-ophthalmology practice is for the evaluation of a possible prior ischemic optic neuropathy as the basis for visual field loss and optic nerve changes prior to rendering a diagnosis of NTG. It is important to consider the possibility of neuro-ophthalmic disease in NTG because IOP is normal in both settings, while the visual field defects may also be identical. Additionally, cupping may occur in optic neuropathies other than glaucoma. However, the distinction between prior nonarteritic anterior ischemic optic neuropathy (NAION) and glaucoma is almost always straightforward as it would be most unusual to encounter a case of NAION in which there is a cup-to-disc ratio in excess of 0.2 either in the involved or fellow eye.[9]

The neural rim in NAION will become pale in either sectoral or diffuse fashion, often corresponding to the residual visual field defect, while there will be a conspicuous absence of cupping once the edema from the acute event resolves. It should be noted that any unexplained optic nerve pallor demands that imaging studies be performed in the absence of a prior documented history of optic nerve swelling, acute optic neuritis, etc. in order to exclude a retrobulbar compressive or infiltrative lesion.

However, in the setting of *arteritic* AION (A-AION) from giant cell arteritis, it has long been recognized that glaucomatous-like excavation of the optic nerve may develop once the edema has resolved[10] (Fig. 25.1). A more recent study by Danesh-Myer et al.[11] found optic nerve cupping to be present in 92% of patients with A-AION, whereas only 2% of patients with NAION developed cupping. This is generally associated with prominent pallor of the residual neural rim and often associated with severe visual field loss. The clinical history of acute unilateral or bilateral visual loss generally associated with systemic symptoms of giant cell arteritis should help sort out the diagnosis in this setting. Although Hayreh and Jonas[12] similarly noted common morphologic features of the optic disc cupping and neuroretinal rim loss in A-AION and glaucomatous optic neuropathy, they found that A-AION is distinguished from glaucomatous optic neuropathy by the absence of associated enlargement of the peripapillary retinal pigment epithelium (RPE) atrophy in the arteritis patients. Their findings notwithstanding, the patient's right optic nerve depicted in Fig. 25.1 clearly demonstrates relatively greater peripapillary retinal RPE atrophy temporally as compared to the unaffected eye.

Trobe et. al.[13] found that there is cupping in 20% of eyes with nonglaucomatous optic atrophy, with 6% of patients demonstrating typical glaucomatous excavation. Eight percent of individuals with longstanding compressive lesions of the optic nerve and/or chiasm developed glaucomatous-like cupping of the disc in that study. Other relatively common conditions that can lead to optic nerve cupping include central retinal artery occlusion (CRAO) and optic neuritis. A recent study assessed the cup-to-disc ratio in 50 individuals who had experienced unilateral optic neuritis and compared the affected eyes to the fellow nonaffected eyes and to 50 control eyes.[14] Cup-to-disc area ratio, vertical ratio, and horizontal ratio as assessed via OCT, were significantly larger in affected eyes when compared to both fellow and control eyes (Fig. 25.2). A relatively rare condition in which temporal excavation of

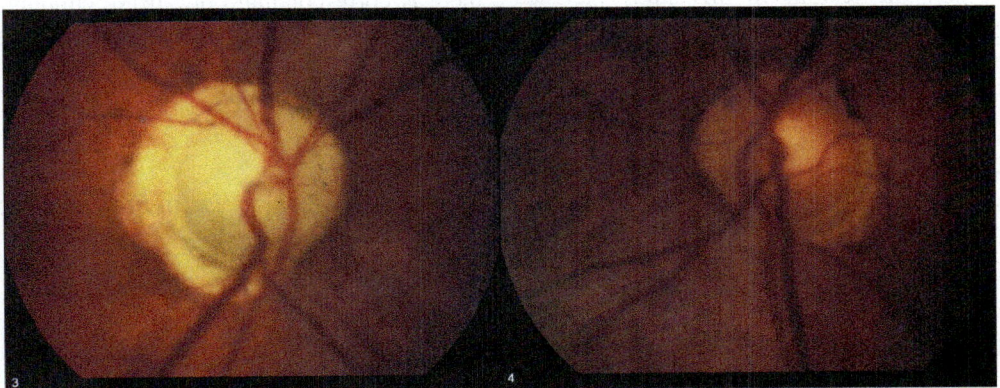

**Fig. 25.1** Glaucomatous-like excavation in giant cell arteritis (GCA). Right eye shows extensive cupping following episode of arteritic anterior ischemic optic neuropathy secondary to GCA, with normal disc in unaffected left eye. Note also pallor of residual neural rim, right eye, which would be atypical for glaucoma

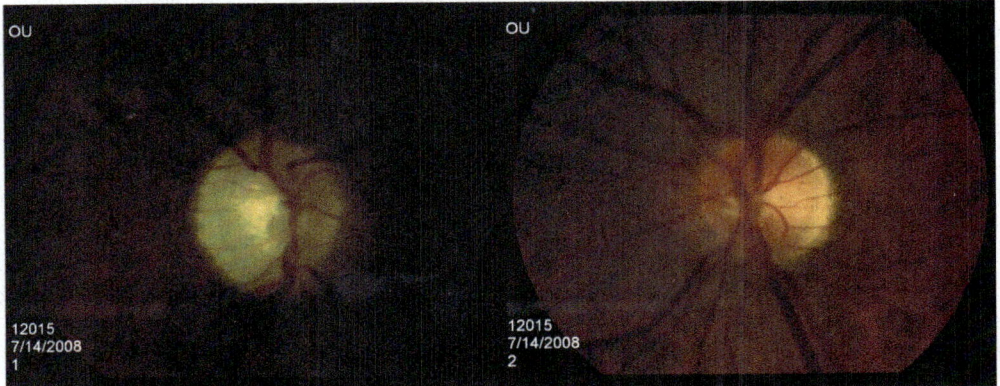

**Fig. 25.2** Glaucomatous-like excavation after episode of optic neuritis. Affected right eye demonstrates greater vertical and horizontal cupping as compared to non-affected left eye. Diffuse pallor seen in right eye is not consistent with glaucoma

the optic nerve is a characteristic feature is Dominant Optic Atrophy (DOA), although this is accompanied by pallor of the neural rim.[15]

Trobe et al. reviewed optic nerve photographs, using two glaucoma specialists and one neuro-ophthalmologist, with 44% of the nonglaucomatous cases being missed by at least one examiner. Pallor of the neural rim was found to be 94% specific for nonglaucomatous processes, while focal or diffuse rim obliteration was 87% specific for glaucoma. Thinning of the neural rim was only 47% specific for glaucoma.[16] Another study assessed disc cupping in the setting of a compressive optic neuropathy.[17] The eyes with a compressive lesion had a larger cup-to-disc ratio (C/D) than the controls, measuring 0.37 versus 0.10 respectively. In those patients with a unilateral compressive lesion of the optic nerve, the C/D in the involved eye was larger than in the fellow eye with a difference of 0.13, whereas the difference in the C/D in control eyes was only 0.04. This finding of intereye asymmetry in those individuals with unilateral compressive lesions of the optic nerve led the authors to conclude that the enlarged cup was an acquired feature. The responsible lesions in this study included pituitary adenomas, meningiomas, craniopharyngiomas, and aneurysms.

### 25.1.2 Afferent Pupillary Defects in Glaucoma

As the visual loss and cupping in glaucoma tends to be relatively symmetric, a relative afferent pupillary defect (APD) is infrequently encountered in glaucoma via standard clinical assessment with the swinging flashlight test. However, if there is asymmetric cupping in excess of 0.2–0.3, one may certainly encounter an APD. A study evaluating the incidence of an APD in the setting of asymmetric glaucoma found the mean difference in C/D for the APD group was 0.43 (range 0.2–0.6) while the mean difference in C/D in those patients with asymmetric glaucoma without an APD was 0.24 (range 0.2–0.3)[18] Therefore, the finding of an APD in a patient with presumed glaucoma that has asymmetric cupping of less than 0.3 should certainly raise concern for an underlying nonglaucomatous optic neuropathy. Although there was an overlap between the APD and nonAPD groups in those individuals with C/D asymmetry of ≤0.3, there was no overlap in the mean difference in visual field asymmetry between the fellow eyes. The mean difference in visual field asymmetry between the fellow eyes in the APD group ranged from 13 to 93%, while the mean difference in the nonAPD group ranged from 0 to 5.5%.

Although more sophisticated techniques for assessing pupillary reaction beyond the standard swinging flashlight test are not generally available in the clinical setting, an increased prevalence of an APD in glaucoma can be documented via such modalities. One study identified an APD in 56% of glaucoma patients via automated pupillography, whereas the sensitivity of detecting an APD in these same patients by the standard swinging flashlight test was only 41%.[19]

### 25.1.3 Nasal Step as Early Sign of Visual Field Loss in Nonglaucomatous Optic Neuropathy

A nasal step may be the earliest sign of visual loss in the setting of glaucoma, however, it is certainly not specific for this condition. In fact, any optic neuropathy may develop inferonasal depression as an early sign of visual loss including papilledema[20] and disc drusen.[21] Optic nerve hypoplasia with truncation of the disc may produce nerve fiber bundle defects as well.[22] Therefore, it is imperative to be certain that there is corresponding optic nerve cupping or notching to account for the visual field defect regardless of the IOP prior to attributing the visual loss to glaucoma.

### 25.1.4 Temporal Visual Field Defects and Glaucoma

Although temporal wedge defects are described as one of the types of visual field loss that may occasionally occur in glaucoma, the presence of a visual field defect that is denser temporally should always raise strong concern for a compressive or infiltrative process affecting the optic chiasm.[23]

The arcuate nerve fiber bundle defects of glaucoma are virtually always denser nasally, whereas pathology affecting the optic chiasm and occasionally the immediately prechiasmatic optic nerve will be denser temporally. Figure 25.3a–e depict the case history of a patient with both asymmetric glaucoma and a pituitary tumor. The patient has more cupping on the left, with both a bitemporal hemianopia and a left eye glaucomatous nerve fiber bundle defect. Pallor is more prominent in the left optic nerve. Postoperatively, the temporal hemianopic defect in each eye decreased, while the arcuate scotoma in the left is now seen to be predominately nasal, consistent with the patient's underlying glaucomatous optic neuropathy.

A peculiar exception to the location of the field defects can occur in the unusual setting of glaucoma in an individual with situs inversus of the retinal vessels One of

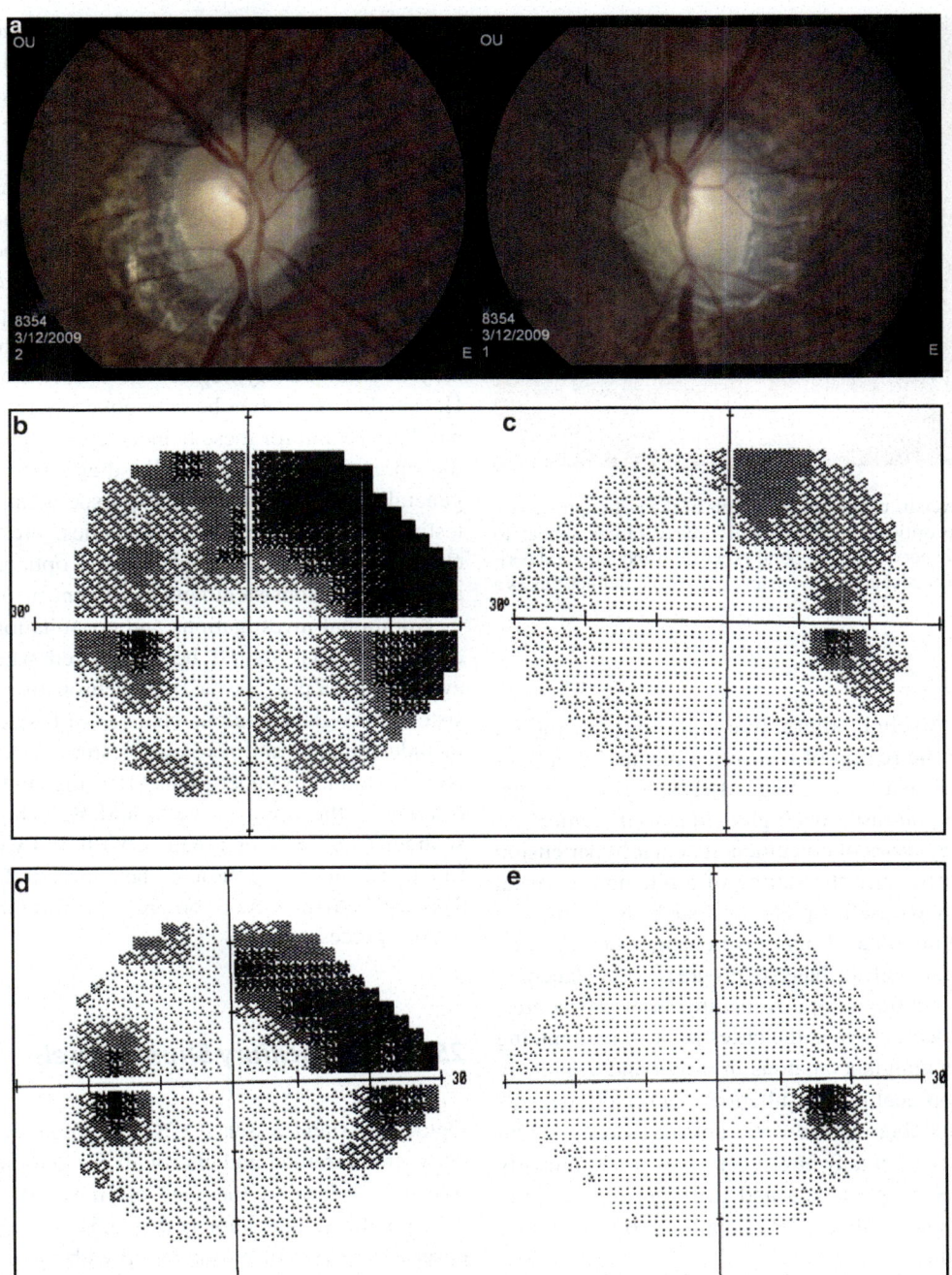

**Fig. 25.3** (a) Patient with pituitary adenoma and unilateral glaucoma, left eye. Left optic nerve shows increased vertical cupping consistent with glaucoma and pallor secondary to compression. The right eye remains pink. (b) Humphrey visual field, left eye, preoperatively. This field demonstrates what appears to be a dense superior arcuate scotoma and an infero-nasal defect. (c) Humphrey visual field, right eye, preoperatively. This field demonstrates a supero-temporal defect uncharacteristic for glaucomatous optic neuropathy. (d) Humphrey visual field, left eye, postoperatively. The field demonstrates significant improvement of the supero-temporal scotoma. What initially appeared to represent a dense superior arcuate scotoma has now resolved into a predominantly supero-nasal defect consistent with the patient's underlying glaucoma. (e) Humphrey visual field, right eye, postoperatively. This field demonstrates complete resolution of the scotoma seen in preoperative Fig. 25.3c

the authors (MDK) has encountered several of these cases over the years in which the retinal vessels emanate from the temporal aspect of the disc (for example, see Fig. 25.4), and the optic nerves become excavated nasally resulting in bitemporal visual field defects. Prior to attributing visual loss with predominant *temporal* field loss to glaucoma,

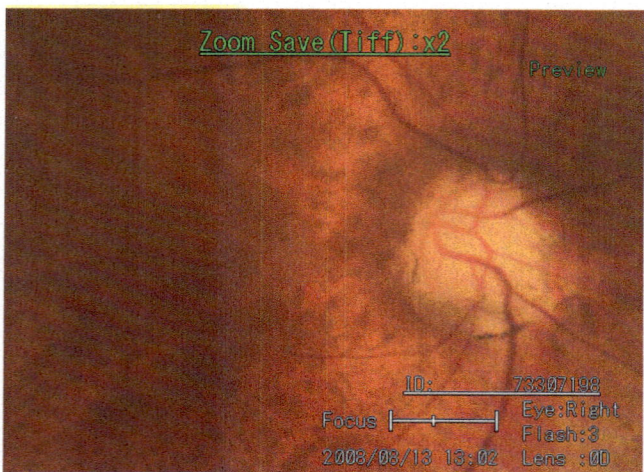

**Fig. 25.4** Situs inversus of the retinal vessels of the right optic nerve. Upon viewing the optic nerve alone, this image might appear to represent a left optic nerve with temporal excavation and temporal peripapillary atrophy. The location of the macula, however, defines this as a right optic nerve

it is essential to exclude alternative pathology, including a mass lesion in the region of the optic chiasm, by obtaining a magnetic resonance imaging (MRI) study of the sella, with and without contrast, on a high field closed scanner.

There are many cases of coincidental ocular hypertension or bona fide glaucoma in the setting of a bitemporal visual field defect from parasellar pathology such as a pituitary adenoma or meningioma. Progressive changes documented in serial visual fields and attributed to progression of glaucoma have resulted in additional topical therapy, laser procedures, and even trabeculectomy in some cases prior to recognizing the visual loss as nonglaucomatous in origin and ultimately obtaining neuro-ophthalmic consultation. Conversely, patients with mass lesions abutting the optic apparatus but without significant compression may have visual loss predominantly or entirely related to glaucoma and therefore may require additional treatment for their IOP as opposed to resection of their parasellar mass.

## 25.1.5 Peripapillary Nerve Fiber Hemorrhages

One finding that will occasionally be present either on the surface of or immediately adjacent to the optic disc is a nerve fiber layer hemorrhage. These tend to occur much more frequently in NTG as opposed to POAG, with a prevalence of 25% and 8% respectively.[24] Splinter hemorrhages on the surface or adjacent to the disc were found to be 100% specific for glaucoma in one study.[25] However, another report found that 70% of disc hemorrhages were not associated with glaucoma, although these authors did observe that the patients without glaucoma tended to demonstrate increased vertical cupping.[24] Of note, this study was conducted prior to the advent of nerve fiber analysis with modalities such as optical coherence tomography (OCT). Therefore, it is possible that these patients may have had preperimetric glaucoma. Often these hemorrhages are quite fine in caliber and may be immediately adjacent to one of the retinal vessels. Hence, they may often be overlooked. Scrutinizing the peripapillary region for these hemorrhages is most important as their presence often secures the diagnosis of glaucoma and generally obviates the need to pursue additional diagnostic testing such as neuroimaging studies, presuming that the character of the visual field loss and optic disc appearance are otherwise consistent with the diagnosis of glaucoma.

Additional investigations and consultation with a neuro-ophthalmologist should be considered whenever there is evidence for a progressive optic neuropathy felt to be inconsistent with glaucomatous change, with studies possibly to include imaging and serologic testing. Presuming that the patient is able to undergo an MRI, the study of choice for evaluating the optic nerve would be a high field closed scanner (1.0 Tesla or greater), with and without contrast, to include images up through the region of the optic chiasm. This will help to exclude compressive, infiltrative, and inflammatory processes.

## 25.1.6 Optociliary Shunt Vessels

Optociliary shunt vessels (OCSV) are venous communications between the retinal and choroidal circulations that occur on the disc surface in the face of impaired venous outflow through the retinal vein (Fig. 25.5). Although classically described as part of a triad along with optic disc pallor and progressive visual loss in the setting of an optic nerve sheath meningioma (ONSM),[26] OCSV are most commonly associated with central retinal vein occlusions (CRVO). OCSV may occur in both ischemic and nonischemic CRVOs. Notably, OCSV are reported to occur in the setting of chronic glaucoma as well.[27] As CRVOs occur with increased incidence in individuals with glaucoma, it is possible that some of the OCSVs observed in patients with glaucoma actually arose following a nonischemic CRVO that was not observed clinically secondary to preserved central acuity.

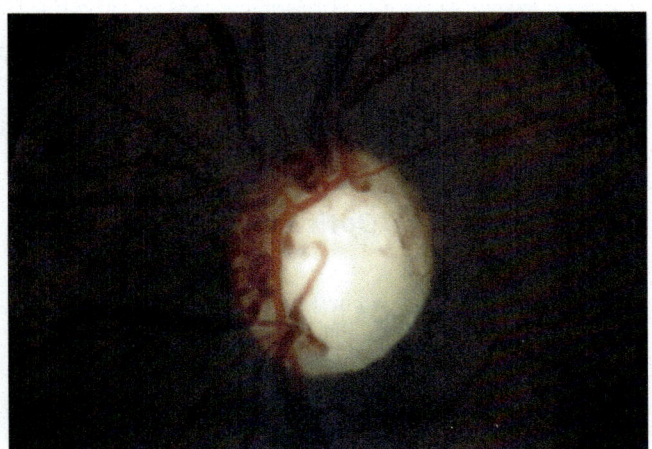

**Fig. 25.5** Optociliary shunt vessels, left optic nerve. Patient with previous central retinal vein occlusion and glaucoma

OCSVs are generally identified clinically and can be easily documented with color photography. Patients in whom OCSVs are identified should have a history taken regarding prior CRVO. If no prior history of such an event can be obtained, a contrast-enhanced MRI of the orbits on a high field closed scanner with fat saturation technique should be obtained in order to evaluate for a compressive lesion of the optic nerve such as an ONSM, before the physician may attribute the vessels to chronic glaucoma.

### 25.1.7 Failure to Diagnose Compressive Lesions of the Optic Apparatus

A study by Kupersmith[28] examined the frequency with which there was a delay in the diagnosis of compressive lesions of the optic nerves and/or chiasm. Sixteen out of 250 patients in whom there was visual compromise from a mass lesion had a delay in their diagnosis after presenting with visual symptoms. Five of them (30%) were misdiagnosed with NTG. Of note, all of these patients exhibited pallor of their neural rims. Cavernous degeneration by contour changes was noted in 25 out of 31 eyes. Most patients exhibited bitemporal field defects, while there was loss of visual acuity out of proportion to the degree of disc cupping in 12 (75%) patients. These lesions included eight pituitary tumors (50%), five meningiomas, two chiasmal gliomas, and one aneurysm.

A study by Greenfield et al.[25] evaluated the clinical features that would help to distinguish between glaucomatous and compressive optic neuropathies. All the patients with glaucoma had NTG and underwent neuro-imaging studies. None of the NTG patients exhibited a mass lesion to account for their visual field defects, whereas the control group had known compressive lesions of the optic apparatus. The patients with NTG demonstrated significantly greater vertical loss of the neural rim, better central acuity, more frequent disc hemorrhages, less neural rim pallor, and more nerve fiber bundle defects that obeyed the horizontal meridian. Features that were highly specific for nonglaucomatous cupping secondary to compressive lesions were visual acuity less than 20/40, visual field defects that were aligned along the vertical meridian, optic nerve pallor in excess of the degree of optic nerve cupping, and age younger than 50 years. Although it is certainly not necessary nor cost-effective to perform neuro-imaging on all patients with the presumed diagnosis of NTG, individuals with atypical features for glaucoma such as decreased central acuity, optic nerve pallor, predominantly central or temporal field loss, or progressive visual loss felt to be inconsistent with optic nerve head changes should undergo imaging of the optic nerve up through the chiasm.

Missing the diagnosis of neurologically related disease by ophthalmologists may not only be costly in terms of resultant permanent visual loss and potential loss of life, the failure to identify such pathology by ophthalmologists accounted for nearly 25% of large loss indemnity payments by the Ophthalmic Mutual Insurance Company.[29] In keeping with the findings in Kupersmith's article,[28] failure to identify pituitary gland and other endocrine tumors represented 53% of lesions that were alleged to have been missed on ophthalmologic exams. The average indemnity payment in such cases exceeded the average settlement of all ophthalmology cases by greater than 80%.

### 25.1.8 Shock-Induced Ischemic Optic Neuropathy

When taking a history on a patient suspected of having NTG, it is important to ask about any prior episodes of severe blood loss or hypotension. The so called "shock-induced" ischemic optic neuropathy may sometimes masquerade as glaucoma, with the visual loss not being recognized at the time of the acute event, particularly if central acuity has been preserved. Such patients may exhibit nerve fiber bundle defects typical for glaucoma or any other optic neuropathy. However, they will also exhibit optic nerve pallor in addition to any cupping present. It generally takes approximately 6 weeks to manifest disc pallor following the acute ischemic event because of the time required to develop retrograde axonal degeneration.[30] Shock-induced ischemic optic neuropathy has occurred as a complication of numerous surgical procedures, most commonly cardiac bypass and prolonged orthopedic procedures.[31]

### 25.1.9 Optic Nerve Excavation in Hereditary Optic Neuropathy

With the notable exception of Leber's hereditary optic neuropathy (LHON), most hereditary optic neuropathies are slowly progressive and develop pallor of the optic disc without cupping.[32] However, there are certainly patients with hereditary optic neuropathy who do develop cupping. The clues in this situation are that the rim is pale, the onset is early, the visual loss may be central, and there is a family history of similarly affected individuals.[15] For example, temporal excavation of the optic nerve head in DOA has long been a recognized clinical feature of this disorder many decades prior to the availability of genetic analysis to confirm the diagnosis serologically.[32] Although LHON can also result in optic nerve cupping, the clinical history of rapidly progressive severe central visual field and acuity loss affecting both eyes, either simultaneously or in relatively rapidly sequential fashion, should allow one to easily distinguish this latter entity from glaucoma.

While the optic disc morphology in DOA may lead to the erroneous diagnosis of NTG, there are several features that should be helpful in distinguishing between these two entities. The mean age at the time of diagnosis of DOA in two relatively recent studies was 28 (range, 11–62) and 37 years respectively,[15,33] whereas NTG tends to occur in older individuals.[34] Although temporal optic nerve excavation was present in 77–79% of eyes, this was associated with prominent optic nerve pallor in all cases either temporally or in diffuse fashion. A cup-to-disc ratio in excess of 0.5 was observed in at least one eye in 88% of the patients. Mean visual acuity was reduced to the 20/80 level in one of the studies. Other features that would be uncharacteristic for glaucoma would be the presence of primarily central visual field loss with conspicuous sparing of the peripheral field.

In LHON, 73% of eyes were characterized as being glaucomatous as assessed by HRT when evaluated in the atrophic phase[35] while another study found a C/D of 0.7–0.9 in 7 patients following the development of visual loss.[36]

Again, the clinical history should readily permit one to distinguish these patients from individuals with glaucoma.

### 25.1.10 Traumatic Optic Neuropathy

Optic neuropathy may occur after severe head injury and rarely following blunt trauma to the brow. Patients will demonstrate the typical features of an optic neuropathy, often with severe visual loss. Occasionally, shallow diffuse cupping of the optic nerve is seen.[13]

### 25.1.11 Optic Nerve Cupping in Alzheimer's Disease

There has been literature suggesting that glaucoma may be more common in Alzheimer's disease (AD) than in the general population.[37] However, our sense is that the degeneration seen in the optic nerve is more likely a function of neuronal degeneration in Alzheimer's disease than a secondary disease such as NTG. A study by Bayer et al.[37] found visual field defects or optic nerve cupping compatible with the diagnosis of glaucoma in 26% of 112 patients with Alzheimer's disease. Another study by Tsai[38] compared optic nerve variables in AD patient with controls. There was a significant increase in the mean cup-to-disc ratio (0.501 vs. 0.397) and cup volume (0.545 mm$^3$ vs. 0.300 mm$^3$) in the AD patients, while the rim area (1.226 mm$^2$ vs. 1.006 mm$^2$) was significantly greater in the controls. In a Danish study of 11,721 patients with POAG or NTG, no increased risk of AD was found.[39]

Several studies have found a decrease in peripapillary and/or macular nerve fiber layer thickness and macular volume as assessed via OCT in AD patients.[40-43] The reduction in macular volume was found to be related to the severity of cognitive impairment in one of the studies.[43] Morphologic description of the optic nerve cup was not provided in these reports.

### 25.1.12 Intermittent IOP Elevation

Some patients with visual loss and optic nerve changes attributed to NTG actually have intermittent elevation of IOP not noted on examination. Examples include musicians who play wind instruments; weight lifters; and people who stand on their head, use gravity inversion boots, rub their eyes aggressively, or have "popping eyes (voluntary anterior luxation of the globes)."[44-48]

## 25.2 Role of Prophylactic IOP Lowering in Nonglaucomatous Optic Neuropathy: An Unanswered Question

Ocular hypertension is certainly relatively common with prevalence in the range of 2–3% of the population over the age of 40.[7,8] A similar percentage of patients with optic atrophy secondary to an underlying compressive lesion, postinflammatory optic neuropathy, prior AION, etc., will have coincidental elevation of IOP. The role of lowering IOP in individuals with ocular hypertension who have an underlying nonglaucomatous optic neuropathy has never been studied in a randomized controlled trial. There has been a report of the potential benefit of IOP lowering in preventing visual loss in the setting of disc drusen in patients with normal IOP. The investigators found significantly less mean visual field progression in patients with disc drusen who were treated with topical IOP-lowering agents as compared to untreated patients during a mean follow-up of 21.4 months.[49] Another recent study found that visual field loss occurs more frequently in eyes with disc drusen and ocular hypertension as opposed to eyes with disc drusen and normal IOP. These authors recommended that close monitoring with appropriate treatment be initiated in order to prevent progressive visual field loss.[50] As it may be difficult to assess for the development or progression of glaucomatous field defects in the setting of an underlying nonglaucomatous optic neuropathy, prophylactic topical therapy to lower IOP in an ocular hypertensive with a coexisting nonglaucomatous optic neuropathy may be reasonable in some cases.

## 25.3 Neuroprotection in Nonglaucomatous Optic Neuropathies

As of yet, no studies have shown any neuroprotective benefit of pharmacologic therapy in human trials for glaucoma. There are several studies assessing neuro-protection in glaucoma using agents such as brimonidine and memantine and comparing these agents to other modalities such as ALT and other topical agents.[51] Similarly, there have been several studies that have investigated the neuroprotective role of these medications in other optic neuropathies.

Because of the theoretical neuroprotective benefit of the alpha-2 agonist, brimonidine, a trial of this agent in the setting of the acute onset of AION was initiated in order to determine whether there would be any benefit in terms of visual outcome over the natural history of this disorder. Thirty-six patients with NAION were randomized to treatment with either brimonidine or placebo within the first week of visual loss. However, there was no statistically significant benefit of treatment for the patients receiving brimonidine as compared to placebo.[52]

Memantine, an NMDA-type glutamatergic receptor antagonist used in the treatment of Alzheimer's disease, has been investigated as a potential neuro-protective agent in glaucoma and other optic neuropathies.[53-56] A primate study[56] found decreased lateral geniculate shrinkage in monkeys with experimental unilateral glaucoma when treated with memantine as compared with vehicle-only treated animals. Another study found that memantine was neuroprotective in a rat model of optic nerve injury.[54] Memantine has also been shown to be neuroprotective in an experimental rabbit model of optic nerve ischemia, with the authors raising the possibility that memantine may be of potential benefit in the management of other ischemic optic neuropathies including glaucoma.[53] However, the results of a recently concluded phase III clinical trial of memantine in patients with open angle glaucoma found that there was no treatment benefit when comparing memantine to placebo.[57]

## 25.4 Assessing for Glaucomatous Progression in the Presence of Coexisting Neurologic Field Defects

A particular dilemma occurs in the setting of glaucoma or ocular hypertension in an individual who has a superimposed homonymous hemianopia such as may occur from an occipital lobe stroke (Figs. 25.6a–d and 25.7a–c). As the nasal visual field in the eye ipsilateral to the involved occipital lobe will be compromised by the underlying neurologic process, assessing for glaucomatous change in this region will be impossible via standard perimetric techniques. This precludes one's ability to evaluate a patient for the development or progression of glaucomatous related visual field loss, which generally is more prominent in the nasal hemifield. Accordingly, careful monitoring of the optic nerve appearance and/or following serial nerve fiber layer analysis with modalities such as OCT or Heidelberg retinal tomography is essential.

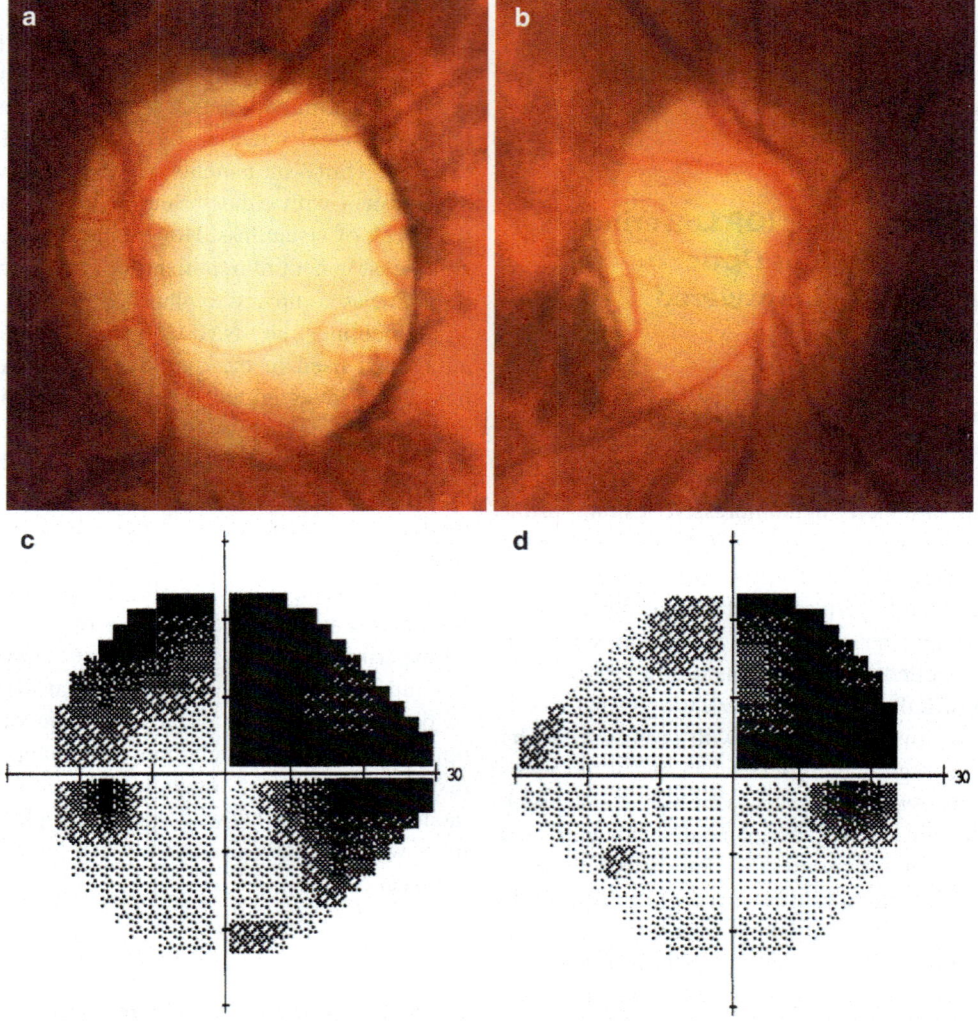

**Fig. 25.6** (**a**) Left and (**b**) right optic nerves in a patient with glaucoma and a right superior quadrantanopsia corresponding to a left occipital stroke affecting the lingual gyrus. Left optic nerve with vertical cupping of 0.75 and inferotemporal notching. Right eye has vertical cupping of 0.5 and subtle inferior notch. Humphrey visual fields corresponding to optic nerves in Fig. 25.6a and b. (**c**) Shows a field with superior arcuate scotoma and nasal depression. (**d**) However, note the absolute superior nasal defect corresponding to the homonymous superior quadrantic defect. (**d**) Shows a field with a right superior quadrantic defect with only mild supero-nasal (early arcuate) depression consistent with the subtle inferior notching of the neural rim in the right eye

## 25.5 Vascular Events Mimicking Glaucomatous Field Loss

The case study illustrated in Fig. 25.8a–c presents a patient with dense superior altitudinal visual field defects in both eyes and asymmetric optic nerve cupping. However, the visual field loss was felt to be out of proportion to the degree of optic nerve cupping. Furthermore, the visual field defect in the right eye is more depressed temporally, which would be most unusual for glaucoma alone. Accordingly, an MRI scan was obtained revealing bilateral infarcts of the inferior occipital lobes (lingual gyri) accounting for the observed visual field changes.

Figure 25.9a–e come from an 87-year-old woman with long-standing bilateral glaucoma. Serial visual fields demonstrated a superior arcuate defect that was present for many years in the left eye, an example of which is seen as Fig. 25.9a. On a routine glaucoma follow-up examination, repeat visual field testing showed significant worsening, with a new dense inferior scotoma as shown in

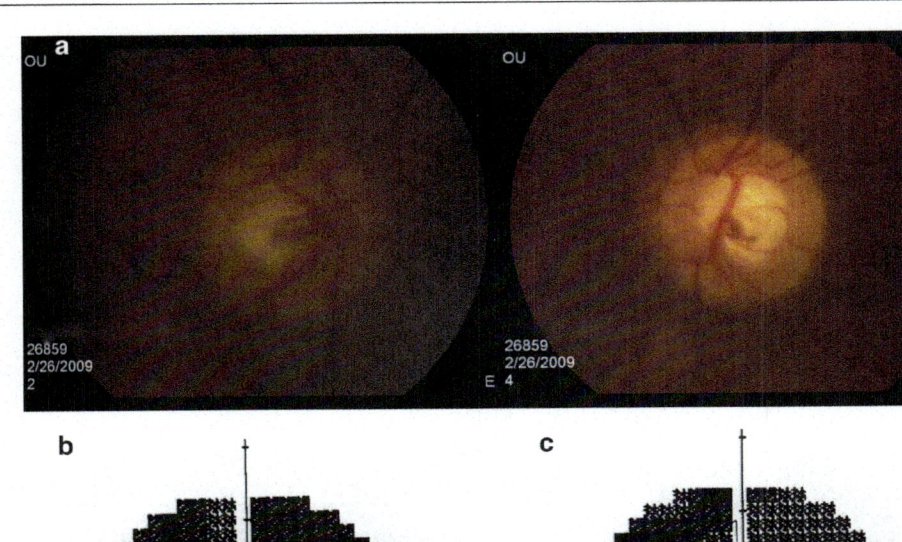

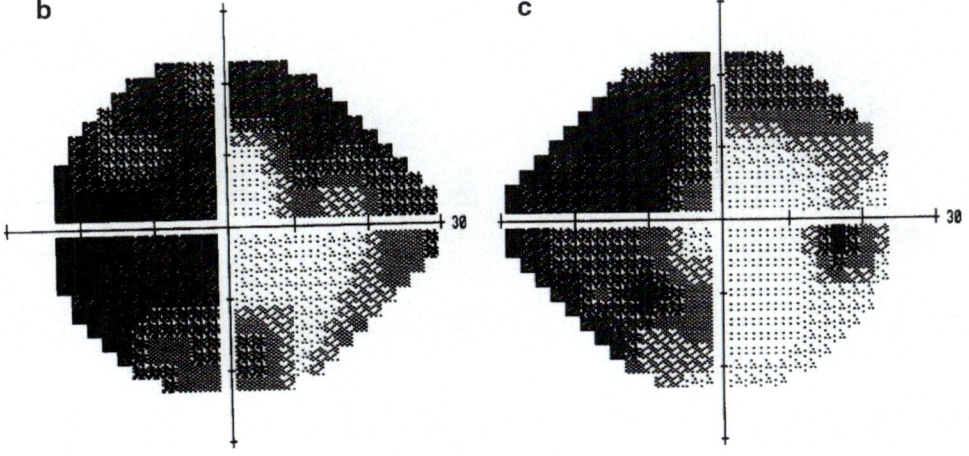

**Fig. 25.7** Glaucoma patient with right occipital stroke and left homonymous hemianopia. (**a**) Shows the patient's discs with asymmetric cupping, left eye greater than right. (**b**) Dense left homonymous hemianopia, (**c**) superimposed upon arcuate defects from glaucoma

Fig. 25.9b and c. Neuro-ophthalmologic exam identified the calcium emboli depicted in the superior vascular temporal arcade seen in Fig. 25.9d and e. These emboli produced retinal arteriole occlusions accounting for the progression of the field defect inferiorly that appeared to be glaucomatous.

## 25.6 Neuro-Imaging in the Evaluation of Optic Nerve Disorders

As the request to obtain an imaging study is essentially seeking a radiologic consultation, communication between the ophthalmologist and the radiologist is most important in order to be certain that the appropriate study is performed in order to best identify pathology accounting for a patient's visual loss. Although this does not necessarily mean that verbal communication is required, the imaging request should detail the clinical history and the suspected processes that you are entertaining (e.g., patient with progressive unilateral visual loss affecting the right eye in which a compressive lesion of the optic nerve is suspected). If available, it is preferable to have the films interpreted by a fellowship-trained neuro-radiologist, as they should not only be able to identify any pathology that is present, but will be well versed in providing an accurate differential diagnosis if any abnormalities are noted. The preferred imaging modality for evaluating an optic nerve lesion is an MRI scan of the orbits with and without contrast employing fat suppression technique. Images should extend posteriorly through the optic chiasm. The study must be performed on a closed high field scanner with a magnet strength of 1.0 Tesla or greater, as open scanners do not have fat suppression capability. If there are contraindications to an MRI such as the presence of a pacemaker, cardiac defibrillator, or a cochlear implant, a contrast-enhanced CT scan of the orbits can be obtained.

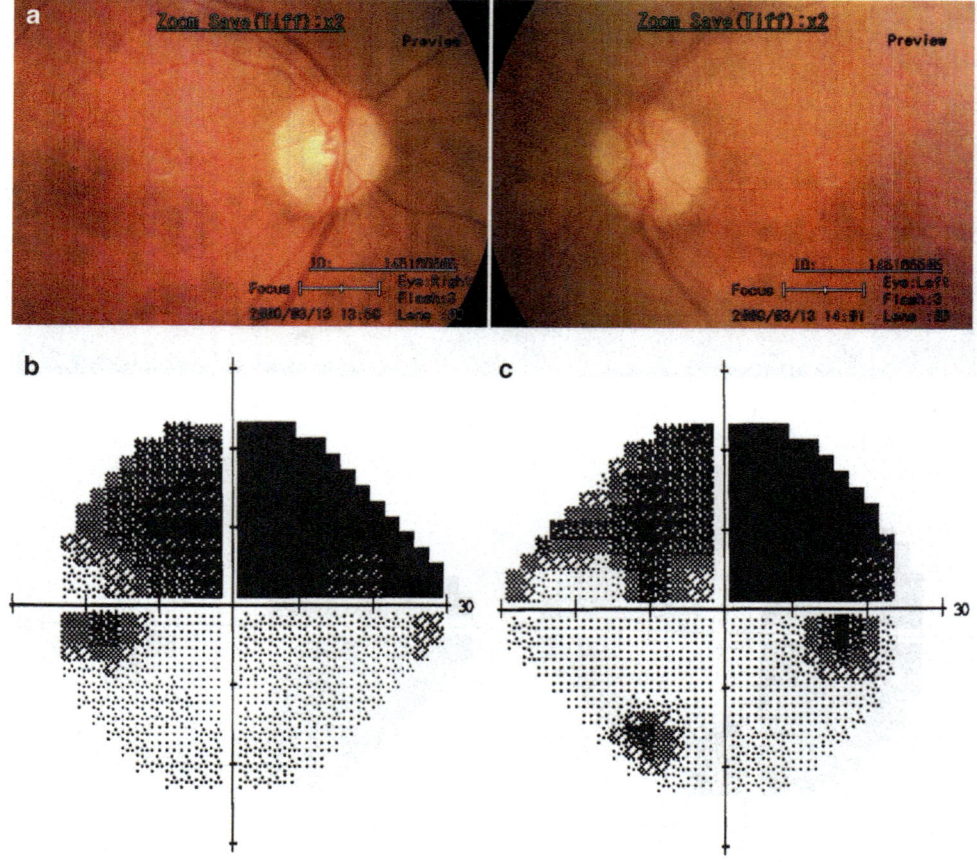

**Fig. 25.8** Bilateral, superior altitudinal visual field defects in a patient with bilateral inferior occipital lobe infarctions. (**a**) Depicts asymmetric cupping, right greater than left, with cup-to-disc ratio of approximately 0.30 in the right eye and a less than 0.1 cup-to-disc ratio in the left eye. This mild degree of cupping is inconsistent with the dense field loss seen. (**b**) Shows a complete right superior homonymous quadrantanopia. (**c**) Additionally, there is a congruent left superior homonymous quadrantanopia, with some relative sparing along the superior horizontal meridian peripherally

## 25.7 Serologic Evaluation of Nonglaucomatous Optic Atrophy

Serologic evaluation in and of itself would rarely be required to differentiate between glaucomatous and nonglaucomatous optic neuropathies. An extensive discussion of the differential diagnosis and evaluation of nonglaucomatous optic neuropathies is beyond the scope of this chapter. However, basic serologic testing for unexplained optic atrophy may include an antinuclear antibody (ANA) test in order to assess for underlying vasculitic disorders, rapid plasma regain (RPR) and Fluorescent Treponemal Antibody–Absorption (FTA-ABS) tests in order to evaluate for luetic optic neuropathy or to identify a false positive RPR related to collagen vascular disease, angiotensin converting enzyme for sarcoid optic neuropathy, and B12, folate, and complete blood count (CBC) for nutritional optic neuropathy. More specialized testing such as DNA analysis for LHON and DOA can be obtained based upon the patient's clinical presentation.

## 25.8 Conclusion

In conclusion, a high index of suspicion for the possibility of a nonglaucomatous process as the basis for a component of a patient's visual loss is essential in the setting of bona fide glaucoma or ocular hypertension whenever there is visual loss (field or acuity) out of proportion to changes in optic nerve cupping. As glaucoma and ocular hypertension are relatively common disorders, the presence of these entities coexisting in the setting of nonglaucomatous optic neuropathy is not rare.

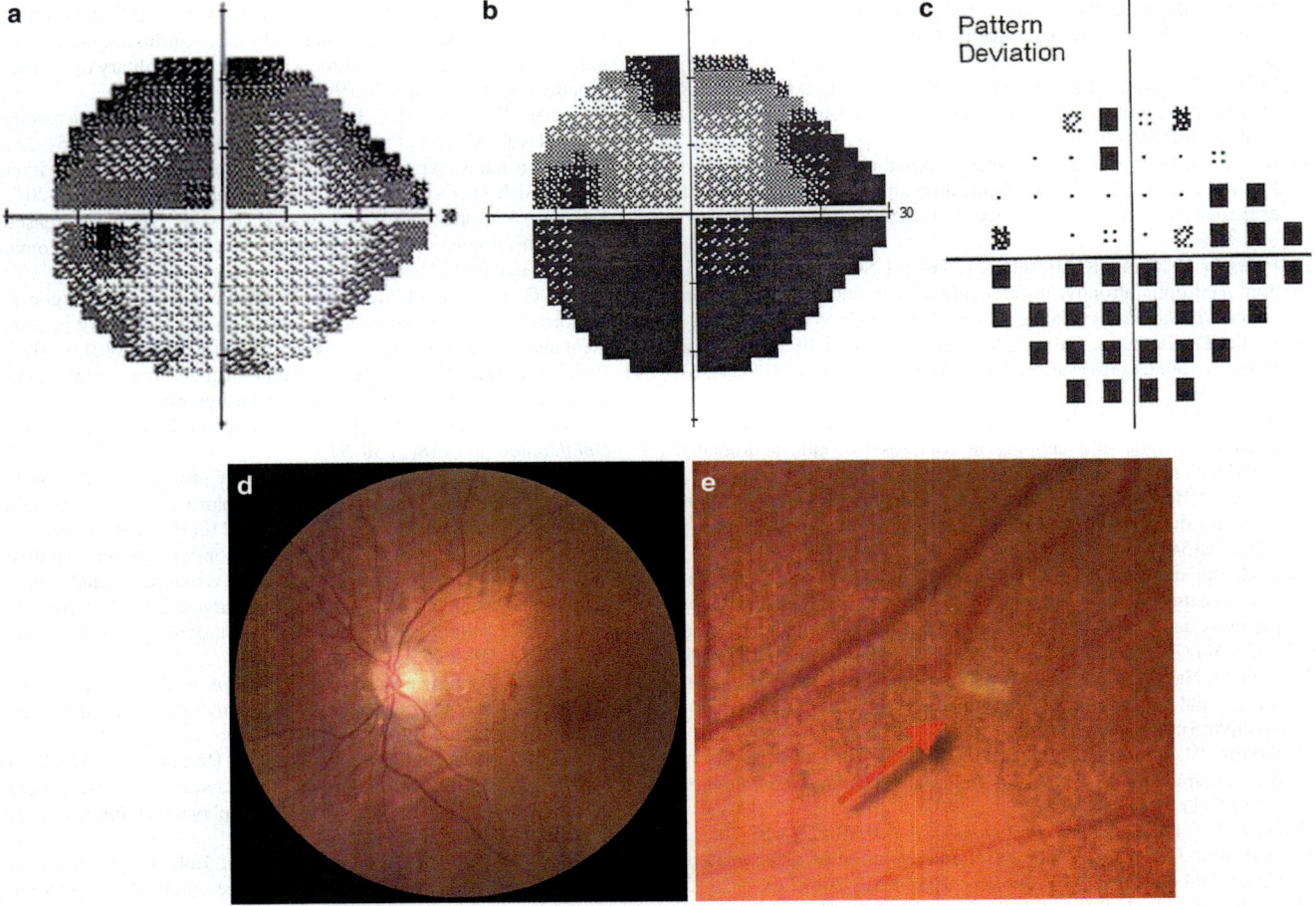

**Fig. 25.9** (a) Shows a visual field, left eye, with glaucoma, prior to occurrence of the vascular events. (b) Shows the same eye after the occlusion of two arterioles in the superior temporal arcade. (c) A new dense inferior defect is seen. Fundus photographs of left eye demonstrate multiple calcium emboli in the superior temporal vascular arcade. (d) A larger embolus is seen in a supero-temporal branch arteriole immediately beyond the first birfucation. (e) A smaller plaque is seen just supero-nasal to the fovea

## References

1. Levin L. Neurobiologic rationale for neuroprotection. In: Weinreb RN, ed. *Glaucoma Neuroprotection*. Philadelphia: Wolters Kluwer Health; 2006:1–7.
2. Takada M, Araie M, Suzuki Y, Koseki N, Yamagami J. The central visual field defects in low-tension glaucoma. A comparison of the central visual field defects in low-tension glaucoma with those in primary open angle glaucoma. *Nippon Ganka Gakkai Zasshi*. 1993;97(11):1320–1324.
3. Araie M, Yamagami J, Suziki Y. Visual field defects in normal-tension and high-tension glaucoma. *Ophthalmology*. 1993;100(12):1808–1814.
4. Quigley HA, Vitale S. Models of open-angle glaucoma prevalence and incidence in the United States. *Invest Ophthalmol Vis Sci*. 1997;38(1):83–91.
5. Klein BE, Klein R, Sponsel WE, et al. Prevalence of glaucoma. The Beaver Dam Eye Study. *Ophthalmology*. 1992;99(10):1499–1504.
6. Quigley HA, West SK, Rodriguez J, Munoz B, Klein R, Snyder R. The prevalence of glaucoma in a population-based study of Hispanic subjects: Proyecto VER. *Arch Ophthalmol*. 2001;119(12):1819–1826.
7. Bonomi L, Marchini G, Marraffa M, et al. Prevalence of glaucoma and intraocular pressure distribution in a defined population. The Egna-Neumarkt Study. *Ophthalmology*. 1998;105(2):209–215.
8. Varma R, Ying-Lai M, Francis BA, et al. Prevalence of open-angle glaucoma and ocular hypertension in Latinos: the Los Angeles Latino Eye Study. *Ophthalmology*. 2004;111(8):1439–1448.
9. Beck RW, Savino PJ, Repka MX, Schatz NJ, Sergott RC. Optic disc structure in anterior ischemic optic neuropathy. *Ophthalmology*. 1984;91(11):1334–7.
10. Sebag J, Thomas JV, Epstein DL, Grant WM. Optic disc cupping in arteritic anterior ischemic optic neuropathy resembles glaucomatous cupping. *Ophthalmology*. 1986;93(3):357–361.
11. Danesh-Meyer HV, Savino PJ, Sergott RC. The prevalence of cupping in end-stage arteritic and nonarteritic anterior ischemic optic neuropathy. *Ophthalmology*. 2001;108(3):593–598.

12. Hayreh SS, Jonas JB. Optic disc morphology after arteritic anterior ischemic optic neuropathy. *Ophthalmology*. 2001;108(9):1586–1594.
13. Trobe JD, Glaser JS, Cassady J, Herschler J, Anderson DR. Nonglaucomatous excavation of the optic disc. *Arch Ophthalmol*. 1980;98(6):1046–1050.
14. Rebolleda G, Noval S, Contreras I, Arnalich-Montiel F, Garcia-Perez JL, Munoz-Negrete FJ. Optic disc cupping after optic neuritis evaluated with optic coherence tomography. *Eye*. 2009;23(4):890–894
15. Fournier AV, Damji KF, Epstein DL, Pollock SC. Disc excavation in dominant optic atrophy: differentiation from normal tension glaucoma. *Ophthalmology*. 2001;108(9):1595–1602.
16. Trobe JD, Glaser JS, Cassady JC. Optic atrophy. Differential diagnosis by fundus observation alone. *Arch Ophthalmol*. 1980;98(6):1040–1045.
17. Bianchi-Marzoli S, Rizzo JF 3rd, Brancato R, Lessell S. Quantitative analysis of optic disc cupping in compressive optic neuropathy. *Ophthalmology*. 1995;102(3):436–440.
18. Brown RH, Zilis JD, Lynch MG, Sanborn GE. The afferent pupillary defect in asymmetric glaucoma. *Arch Ophthalmol*. 1987;105(11):1540–1543.
19. Lankaranian D, Altangerel U, Spaeth GL, Leavitt JA, Steinmann WC. The usefulness of a new method of testing for a relative afferent pupillary defect in patients with ocular hypertension and glaucoma. *Trans Am Ophthalmol Soc*. 2005;103:200–207; discussion 207–208.
20. Wall M, Hart WM Jr, Burde RM. Visual field defects in idiopathic intracranial hypertension (pseudotumor cerebri). *Am J Ophthalmol*. 1983;96(5):654–669.
21. Savino PJ, Glaser JS, Rosenberg MA. A clinical analysis of pseudopapilledema. II. Visual field defects. *Arch Ophthalmol*. 1979;97(1):71–75.
22. Dorrell D. The tilted disc. *Br J Ophthalmol*. 1978;62(1):16–20.
23. Hart WM Jr, Becker B. The onset and evolution of glaucomatous visual field defects. *Ophthalmology*. 1982;89(3):268–279.
24. Healey PR, Mitchell P, Smith W, Wang JJ. Optic disc hemorrhages in a population with and without signs of glaucoma. *Ophthalmology*. 1998;105(2):216–223.
25. Greenfield DS, Siatkowski RM, Glaser JS, Schatz NJ, Parrish RK, 2nd. The cupped disc. Who needs neuroimaging? *Ophthalmology*. 1998;105(10):1866–1874.
26. Moster ML. Detection and treatment of optic nerve sheath meningioma. *Curr Neurol Neurosci Rep*. 2005;5(5):367–75.
27. Varma R, Spaeth GL, Katz LJ, Feldman RM. Collateral vessel formation in the optic disc in glaucoma. *Arch Ophthalmol*. 1987;105(9):1287.
28. Kupersmith MJ, Krohn D. Cupping of the optic disc with compressive lesions of the anterior visual pathway. *Ann Ophthalmol*. 1984;16(10):948–953.
29. Ellis J. Risk Management Issues in Failure to Diagnose Neurologic Illness. *Omic Digest*; 1994.
30. Lundstrom M, Frisen L. Evolution of descending optic atrophy. A case report. *Acta Ophthalmol (Copenh)*. 1975;53(5):738–746.
31. Newman NJ. Perioperative visual loss after nonocular surgeries. *Am J Ophthalmol*. 2008;145(4):604–610.
32. Kline LB, Glaser JS. Dominant optic atrophy. The clinical profile. *Arch Ophthalmol*. 1979;97(9):1680–1686.
33. Votruba M, Thiselton D, Bhattacharya SS. Optic disc morphology of patients with OPA1 autosomal dominant optic atrophy. *Br J Ophthalmol*. 2003;87(1):48–53.
34. Werner E. Low tension glaucoma. In: Ritch R, Shields M, Krupin T, eds. *The Glaucomas*. Mosby: St. Louis;1989:804.
35. Mashima Y, Kimura I, Yamamoto Y, et al. Optic disc excavation in the atrophic stage of Leber's hereditary optic neuropathy: comparison with normal tension glaucoma. *Graefes Arch Clin Exp Ophthalmol*. 2003;241(2):75–80.
36. Ortiz RG, Newman NJ, Manoukian SV, Diesenhouse MC, Lott MT, Wallace DC. Optic disk cupping and electrocardiographic abnormalities in an American pedigree with Leber's hereditary optic neuropathy. *Am J Ophthalmol*. 1992;113(5):561–566.
37. Bayer AU, Ferrari F, Erb C. High occurrence rate of glaucoma among patients with Alzheimer's disease. *Eur Neurol*. 2002;47(3):165–168.
38. Tsai CS, Ritch R, Schwartz B, et al. Optic nerve head and nerve fiber layer in Alzheimer's disease. *Arch Ophthalmol*. 1991;109(2):199–204.
39. Kessing LV, Lopez AG, Andersen PK, Kessing SV. No increased risk of developing Alzheimer disease in patients with glaucoma. *J Glaucoma*. 2007;16(1):47–51.
40. Paquet C, Boissonnot M, Roger F, Dighiero P, Gil R, Hugon J. Abnormal retinal thickness in patients with mild cognitive impairment and Alzheimer's disease. *Neurosci Lett*. 2007;420(2):97–99.
41. Parisi V. Correlation between morphological and functional retinal impairment in patients affected by ocular hypertension, glaucoma, demyelinating optic neuritis and Alzheimer's disease. *Semin Ophthalmol*. 2003;18(2):50–57.
42. Parisi V, Restuccia R, Fattapposta F, Mina C, Bucci MG, Pierelli F. Morphological and functional retinal impairment in Alzheimer's disease patients. *Clin Neurophysiol*. 2001;112(10):1860–1867.
43. Iseri PK, Altinas O, Tokay T, Yuksel N. Relationship between cognitive impairment and retinal morphological and visual functional abnormalities in Alzheimer disease. *J Neuroophthalmol*. 2006;26(1):18–24.
44. Friberg TR, Weinreb RN. Ocular manifestations of gravity inversion. *JAMA*. 1985;253(12):1755–1757.
45. Slamovits T. Popping eyes. *Surv Ophthalmol*. 1989;33(4):273–280.
46. Pecora L, Sibony P, Fourman S. Eye-rubbing optic neuropathy. *Am J Ophthalmol*. 2002;134(3):460–461.
47. Schuman JS, Massicotte EC, Connolly S, Hertzmark E, Mukherji B, Kunen MZ. Increased intraocular pressure and visual field defects in high resistance wind instrument players. *Ophthalmology*. 2000;107(1):127–133.
48. Chromiak JA, Abadie BR, Braswell RA, Koh YS, Chilek DR. Resistance training exercises acutely reduce intraocular pressure in physically active men and women. *J Strength Cond Res*. 2003;17(4):715–720.
49. Schargus M, Gramer E. IOP-lowering therapy prevents visual field progression in patients with optic disc drusen, poster 560, page 248. *American Academy of Opthalmology*. Las Vegas, NV; 2006.
50. Grippo TM, Shihadeh WA, Schargus M, et al. Optic nerve head drusen and visual field loss in normotensive and hypertensive eyes. *J Glaucoma*. 2008;17(2):100–104.
51. Greenfield DS. Measuring neuroprotection in glaucoma clinical trials. In: Weinreb RN, ed. *Glaucoma Neuroprotection*. Philadelphia: Wolters Kluwer Health; 2006:73–81.
52. Wilhelm B, Ludtke H, Wilhelm H. Efficacy and tolerability of 0.2% brimonidine tartrate for the treatment of acute non-arteritic anterior ischemic optic neuropathy (NAION): a 3-month, double-masked, randomised, placebo-controlled trial. *Graefes Arch Clin Exp Ophthalmol*. 2006;244(5):551–558.
53. Kim TW, Kim DM, Park KH, Kim H. Neuroprotective effect of memantine in a rabbit model of optic nerve ischemia. *Korean J Ophthalmol*. 2002;16(1):1–7.
54. WoldeMussie E, Yoles E, Schwartz M, Ruiz G, Wheeler LA. Neuroprotective effect of memantine in different retinal injury models in rats. *J Glaucoma*. 2002;11(6):474–480.
55. Levin LA, Peeples P. History of neuroprotection and rationale as a therapy for glaucoma. *Am J Manag Care*. 2008;14(1 Suppl):S11–14.
56. Yucel YH, Gupta N, Zhang Q, Mizisin AP, Kalichman MW, Weinreb RN. Memantine protects neurons from shrinkage in the lateral geniculate nucleus in experimental glaucoma. *Arch Ophthalmol*. 2006;124(2):217–225.
57. Stuart A. Glaucoma neuroprotection research, part 2. *EyeNet*. 2008:29–31.

# Chapter 26
# Gonioscopy

Reid Longmuir

Gonioscopy is critical in the evaluation of all forms of glaucoma. It is unfortunately common that secondary forms of glaucoma are unrecognized because of the failure to perform gonioscopy. Not only is gonioscopy able to provide information about the potential causes of raised intraocular pressure, but it can also provide clues critical to the determination of therapy.

When light coming from the iridocorneal angle reaches the tear–air interface, it is reflected back into the eye. This is known as the principal of total internal reflection. The critical angle at which light from the angle structures can be seen is 46°.[1] In patients with keratoconus, the angle is sometimes open beyond this critical angle, and the iridocorneal angle can be seen with slit lamp biomicroscopy alone. In eyes with a normally vaulted cornea, a contact lens must be used to examine the iridocorneal angle. Two types of lenses are used: the direct lens and the indirect lens.

## 26.1 Direct Gonioscopy

Direct gonioscopy is performed with a convex lens, which modifies the tear–air interface and creates a view directly into the angle. The Koeppe lens (Fig. 26.1), which is a 50-diopter lens, is placed on the eye while the patient is supine. The examiner views the angle through a separate hand-held microscope. The Koeppe lens magnifies ×1.5. These lenses come in several sizes for infants and adults, but all are rarely used today.

Direct lenses are used to perform surgical procedures involving the iridocorneal angle, such as goniotomy. The Hoskins–Barkan (Fig. 26.2) and Swan–Jacobs (Fig. 26.3) lenses are commonly used. These lenses can also be used to examine sedated or anesthetized patients, either at the operating microscope or with a portable slit lamp, replacing the need for the Koeppe lens (Fig. 26.4).

## 26.2 Indirect Gonioscopy

The lenses used in indirect gonioscopy use mirrors to overcome total internal reflection. The mirror redirects light from the angle so that it exits the eye perpendicularly to the lens–air interface.

The Posner lens (Fig. 26.5) has four identical mirrors. This allows examination of all four quadrants of the angle while moving the slit lamp and with only minimal rotation of the lens to look in the areas skipped by each mirror. Because the lens has a small (9 mm) area of contact with the cornea, the angle can be deepened by pushing on the lens (indentation gonioscopy). A coupling agent is not required. The Sussman lens (Fig. 26.6) is very similar to the Posner lens, except that it has no handle. There are no particular advantages or disadvantages between these lenses and individual preference typically determines which is used.

The Goldmann three-mirror lens (Fig. 26.7a, b) has one mirror dedicated to viewing the angle. There are two additional mirrors for examination of the peripheral retina. The Goldmann lens is coupled to the cornea by means of a viscous methylcellulose fluid. The lens has a broad (12 mm) area of contact with the globe and can, under the application of pressure, artificially close the angle. It cannot be used to perform indentation gonioscopy, but provides an outstanding view of the angle. A single-mirror Goldmann lens has only the gonioscopic mirror.

## 26.3 Comparison of Direct and Indirect Gonioscopy

Both direct and indirect gonioscopy have advantages and disadvantages.

Although direct gonioscopy is no longer widely practiced outside the operating room, it does have certain advantages

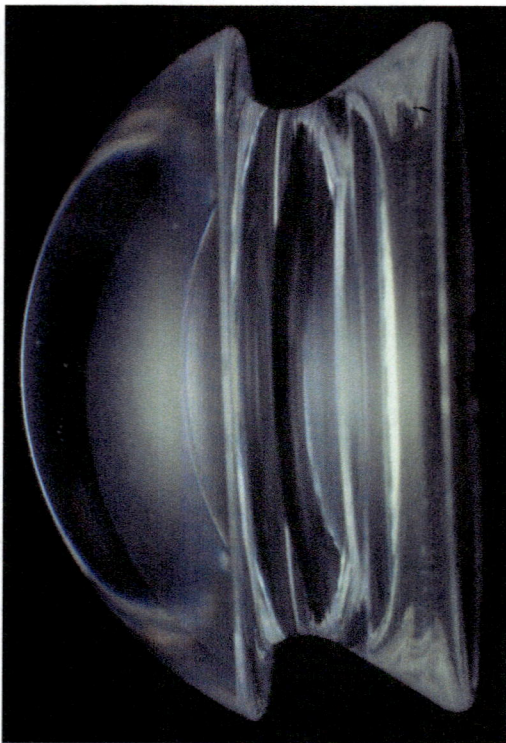

**Fig. 26.1** The Koeppe lens. Courtesy of Ocular Instruments Inc. Bellevue, Washington

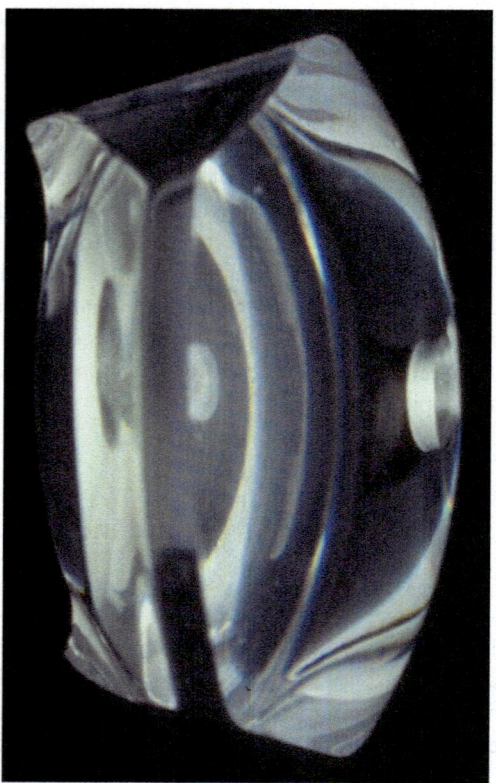

**Fig. 26.2** The Hoskins-Barkan lens. Courtesy of Ocular Instruments Inc. Bellevue, Washington

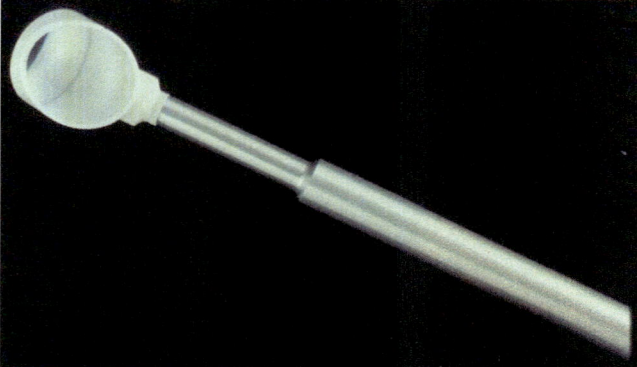

**Fig. 26.3** The Swan Jacobs lens. Courtesy of Ocular Instruments Inc. Bellevue, Washington

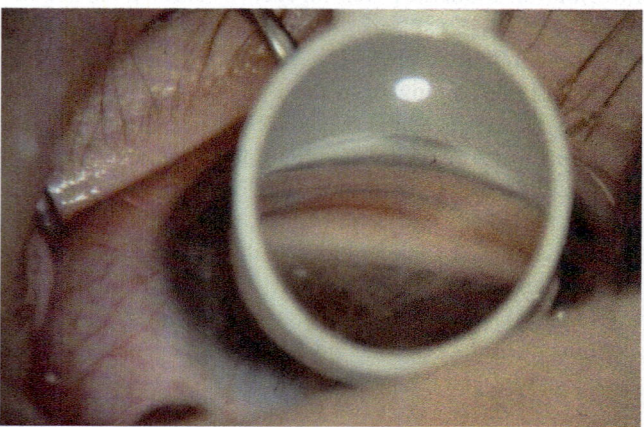

**Fig. 26.4** View of the pediatric angle through the Swan Jacobs lens. Reprinted with permission from Alward WLM and Longmuir RA. *Color Atlas of Gonioscopy*, second edition. San Francisco: American Academy of Ophthalmology

over indirect gonioscopy. Direct gonioscopy provides a straight-on view of the angle rather than the mirror image given by the indirect lenses. As a result, it is much easier to avoid becoming disoriented when documenting localization of findings. Direct gonioscopy permits the examiner to vary the angle of visualization more easily. Therefore, the examiner can look into a narrow angle to see if it is a steep approach to an open angle or a completely closed angle.

The major disadvantage of direct gonioscopy is its inconvenience. The patient has to lie supine, which is not compatible with the standard layout and patient scheduling in most outpatient eye clinics.

Indirect lenses have several advantages that have made them the preferred lenses for most ophthalmologists. The first advantage, specific to the four-mirror lenses, is that they do not require viscous coupling agents, which can

**Fig. 26.5** The Posner lens. Courtesy of Ocular Instruments Inc. Bellevue, Washington

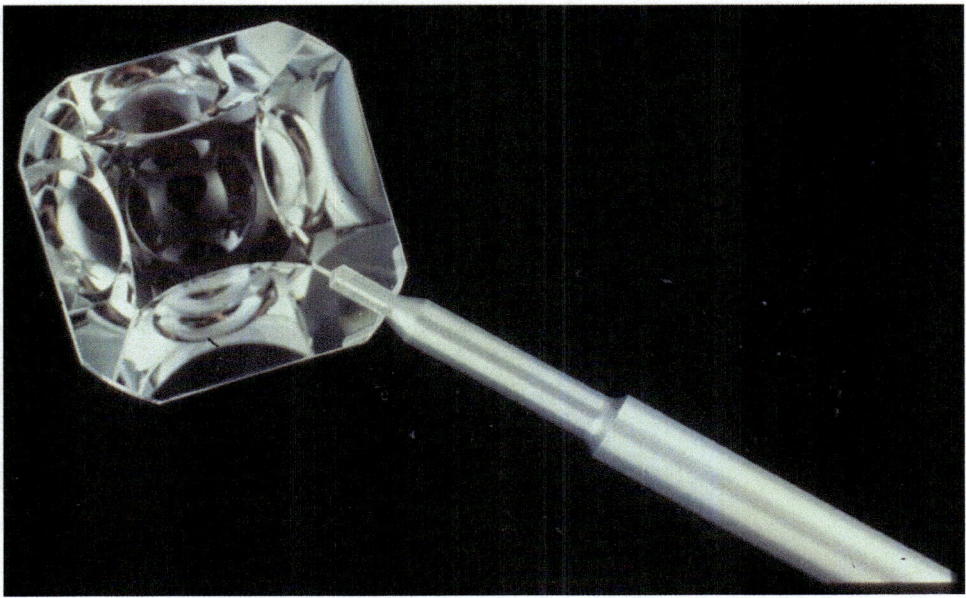

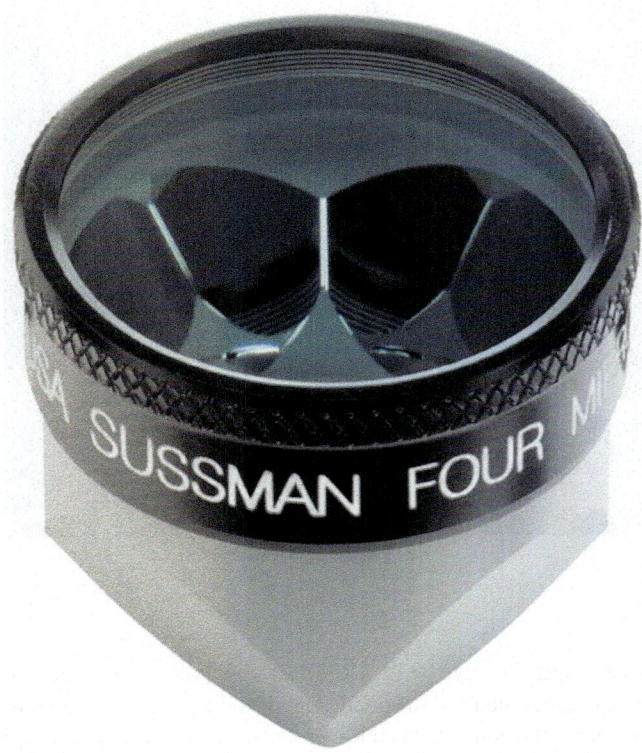

**Fig. 26.6** The Sussman lens. Courtesy of Ocular Instruments Inc. Bellevue, Washington

alter the view of the fundus and diminish photographic quality. Because only a topical anesthetic is required, one can perform applanation tonometry and then move directly to gonioscopic exam. The slit lamp serves as a source of variable magnification and illumination. The slit beam can create a corneal wedge to help to define the structures of the angle. Indentation gonioscopy can be performed with the Posner or Sussmann lens to distinguish appositional from synechial angle closure, allowing for a much more dynamic exam.

Indirect lenses have the disadvantage of giving a mirror-image view of the angle, which can be somewhat confusing until the technique has been practiced. This becomes relevant when trying to localize an angle mass, or an area of synechiae or angle recession. It is also easy to open or close the angle inadvertently by applying excessive pressure to the indirect lenses. These lenses may exaggerate the degree of angle narrowing and are less able to provide a view into the depths of a narrow angle.[2] This is also more common for beginners and becomes less problematic with experience.

## 26.4 Gonioscopy General Guidelines

The eye should be examined carefully with the slit lamp before beginning gonioscopy. Many clues exist on slit lamp exam to predict possible findings on the gonioscopic exam, such as corneal endothelial pigment, iris transillumination defects, or posterior embryotoxon. An estimation of chamber depth can be obtained at the slitlamp although an apparently

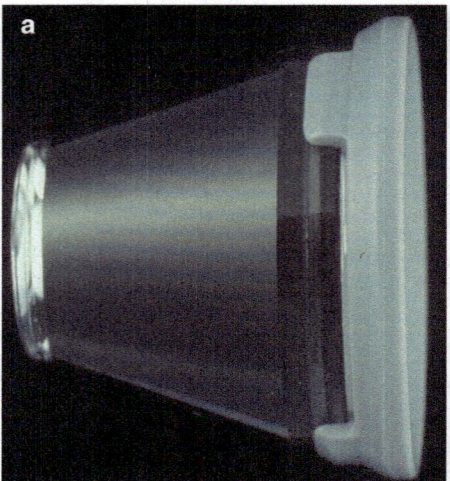
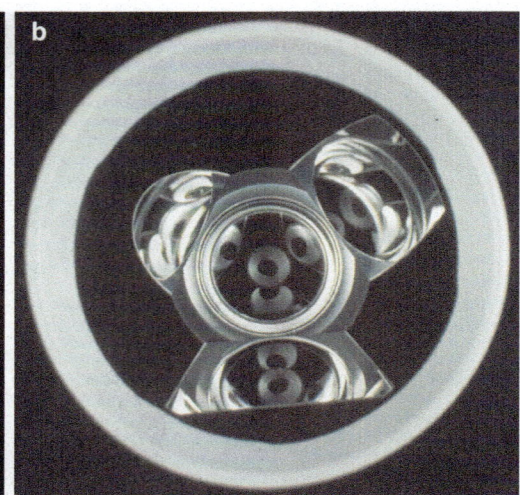

**Fig. 26.7** The Goldmann three-mirror lens. (**a**) Outside view. (**b**) Inside view. Courtesy of Haag-Streit, Koeniz, Switzerland

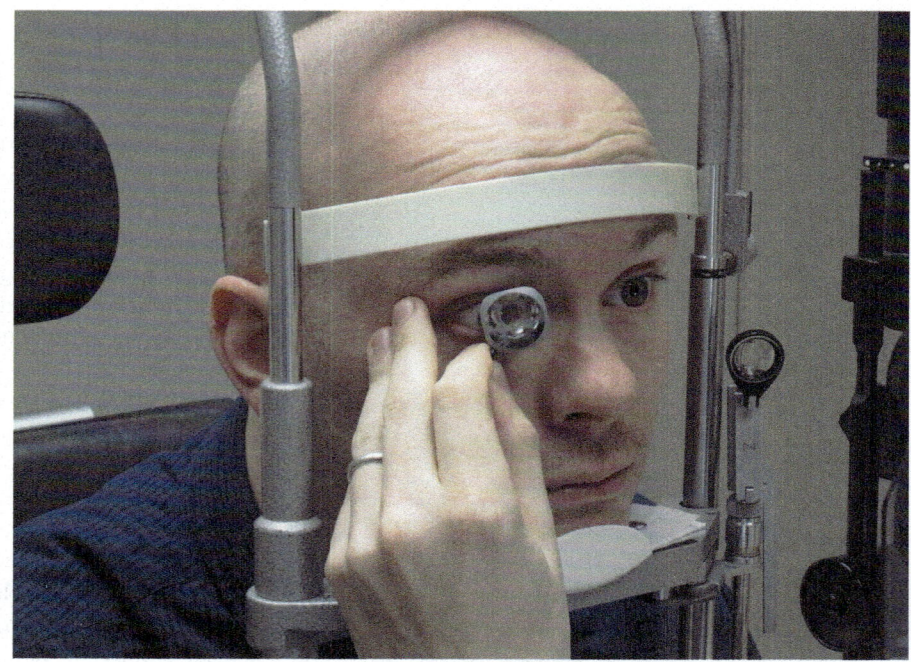

**Fig. 26.8** The Posner lens being placed on the eye, with the flat surfaces of the lens parallel with the eyelids to avoid discomfort

deep chamber should not exclude the need for gonioscopy. Tonometry should be performed prior to gonioscopy as pressure on the eye from the examining lens can temporarily lower the intraocular pressure.

The eye should be anesthetized with a topical agent. The patient must be comfortably positioned at the slit lamp. Align the lateral canthus of the patient's eye with the canthal marker of the slit lamp. It is inconvenient to have the patient's head too high or too low and have to pause the examination in order to reposition. The lens can then be gently placed on the surface of the eye (Fig. 26.8). If the patient is properly aligned, one can see all quadrants of the angle, only pausing to move the lens from one eye to the other. The examiner should try to brace his or her elbow on either the slitlamp table or an additional support. Often times a lens case will suffice (Fig. 26.9). Slit lamp magnification should start at low power as is typical for a standard slit lamp or fundus exam. Bright illumination can be employed to identify the key landmarks, and then the beam length should be decreased and narrowed in order to grade the angle. When the angle

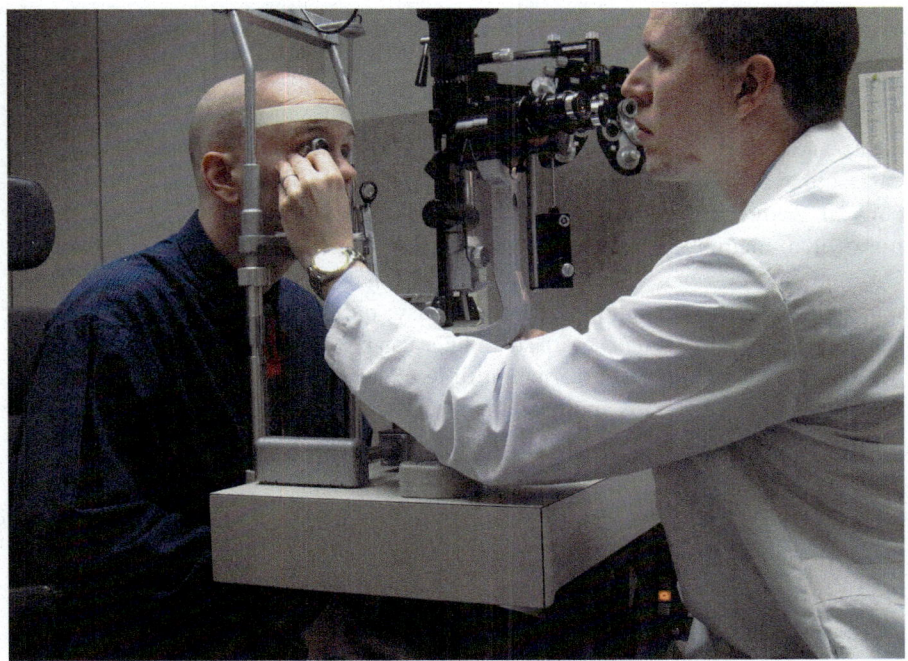

**Fig. 26.9** The elbow is braced against a lens case to provide stability

depth is being graded, light should not be allowed to enter the pupil as pupillary constriction will place the iris on stretch and may the angle appear more open than it is in dark conditions.

## 26.5 The View

When performing slit lamp gonioscopy, the examiner must remember that the image is a mirror image. As an example, the angle viewed in the temporal part of the superior mirror is really the temporal part of the inferior angle. This is often more difficult to remember for ophthalmologists in the context of having to recall the fundus exam as an inverted image.

By using a thin slit of light, offset from the oculars, two separate corneal reflections are perceived – one on the inner aspect of the cornea and the other on the outer. This is no different than that is seen with direct examination of the cornea, except that the mirror is involved. The unique benefit of generating these separate corneal reflections is that one can follow these reflections all the way down to the interface between the cornea and the face of the opaque sclera. These reflections form a wedge-shaped line termed the corneal wedge. The lines of the corneal wedge intersect at Schwalbe's line. Because Schwalbe's line indicates the most anterior portion of the trabecular meshwork, the corneal wedge can be used to locate the trabecular meshwork (Fig. 26.10) when no other clear landmarks are present. A key hint for beginners is to use brighter illumination with the thinnest beam possible in order to create the corneal wedge. By sliding the gonioscopy lens in the direction of the mirror being used, a better view is gained of the cornea and the corneal wedge will become more apparent.

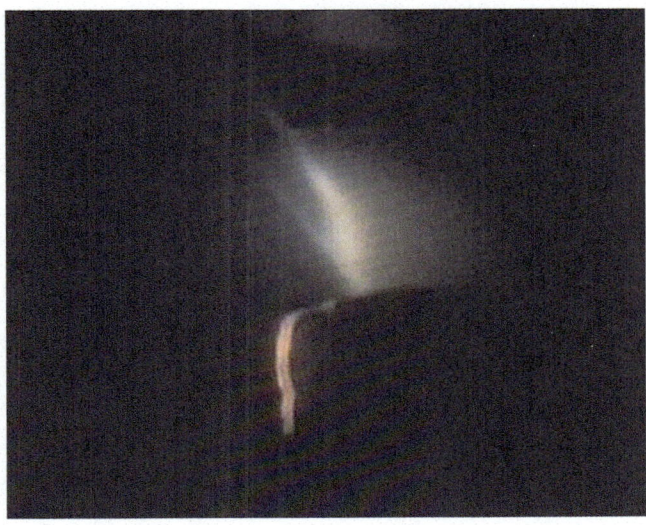

**Fig. 26.10** The corneal wedge. Courtesy of WLM Alward, MD

The corneal wedge is best identified in the superior or inferior mirror. An inclined horizontal slit beam can be obtained in the nasal and temporal mirrors but this requires additional manipulation of the slit lamp and is not usually necessary to define basic angle structures. It is usually easiest to examine the inferior angle first not only to obtain a corneal wedge, but also because it is the usually most pigmented, thereby revealing the trabecular meshwork. Once one has become oriented to the patient's anatomy the remainder of the examination is relatively easy; one should always proceed in the same pattern so findings can be remembered without having to perform multiple examinations. In patients with a steep iris approach to the angle, the patient should be instructed to look slightly toward the examining mirror. When in doubt about angle anatomy, indentation gonioscopy is very helpful, and is discussed below.

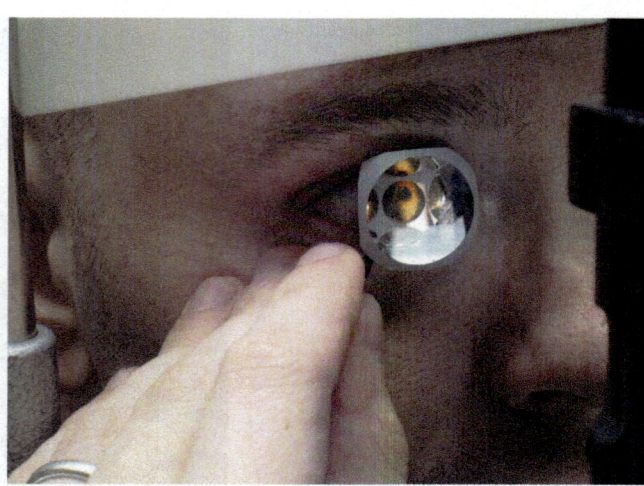

**Fig. 26.11** Demonstration of the proper technique for bracing the hand against the patient during gonioscopy when using the Posner lens

## 26.6 Goldmann Lens Technique

The Goldmann lenses and other similar lenses are all handled in a similar fashion to four mirror lenses, except for the use of a coupling agent. The concave face of the Goldmann lens should be filled with a methylcellulose coupling fluid before it is applied to the eye. Care should be taken to keep air bubbles out of the solution, typically accomplished by storing the bottle upside down, and by expressing a small amount of the solution onto a tissue before transferring the stream over to the lens surface.

While the patient is looking up, the lower edge of the Goldmann lens is brought into contact with the inferior sclera. As the patient looks straight ahead, the lens is brought forward over the cornea. A relative seal forms when the lens is pressed forward onto the globe. The angle is viewed through the shortest mirror on the three-mirror lens.

Holding the lens with three fingers of one hand, the examiner can rotate the lens easily, leaving the other hand free to operate the slit lamp. The thumb, index, and middle finger are used to hold the lens and the other two fingers are braced against the patient's cheek to enable the examiner to keep up with small movements of the head. The lens should be held lightly. Excessive pressure can cause reflux of blood into Schlemm's canal. The suction created by pulling on the lens may make the angle appear artificially deep. These lenses can be difficult to remove if a seal has formed between the lens and the globe. Very slight pressure with the index finger on the globe immediately adjacent to the lens will break the seal and the lens will pull away from the eye easily. Remaining viscous solution can be irrigated away at this point to improve the view for any further examination of the eye.

## 26.7 Four-Mirror Lenses

The Posner and Sussman lenses are normally used with only the tear film coupling them optically to the cornea. The Posner lens is used on a handle that is held between the thumb and forefinger with the remaining three fingers braced against the patient's face (Fig. 26.11). The lens should be applied with a very light touch. Folds seen in Descemet's membrane during the exam indicate that too much pressure is being applied. It is better to lose lens contact with the eye and reposition the lens, rather than to artificially open the angle with unintentional indentation.

## 26.8 Indentation Gonioscopy

In 1966 Forbes described using the Zeiss four-mirror lens to distinguish between angle closure due to synechiae and appositional closure.[3] Forbes recognized that indentation of the cornea caused aqueous to be pushed into the angle. This deepens an appositionally closed angle, allowing the examiner to see the trabecular meshwork (Fig. 26.12a, b). Conversely, angles closed by synechiae would not open with indentation (Fig. 26.13). When one performs indentation, folds in Descemet's membrane will occur, but they should not greatly limit the view of the angle. Indentation can often provide clarification of the more confusing angle anatomy. For example, finding the ciliary body face with indentation can help identify an angle as being open in someone who has no trabecular meshwork pigment and might otherwise appear closed. Similar

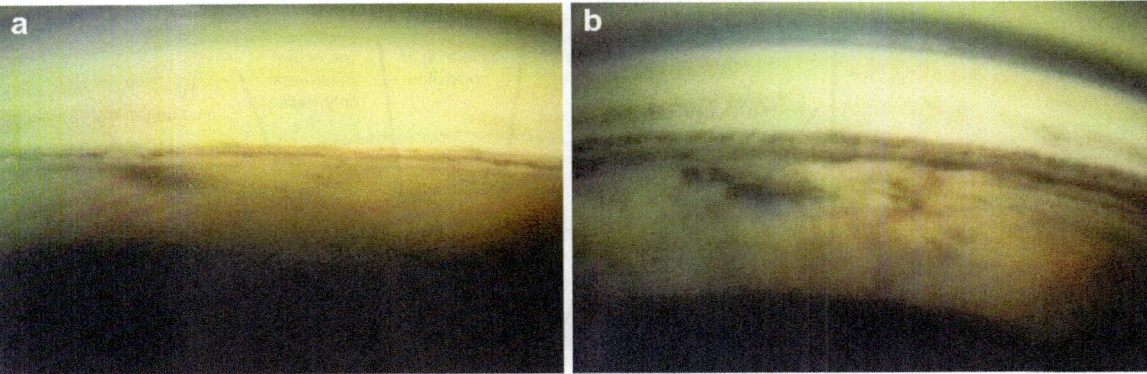

**Fig. 26.12** (a) Opening of a narrow angle via indentation gonioscopy. (b) Note that the scleral spur and trabecular meshwork are easily visible. Courtesy of WLM Alward, MD

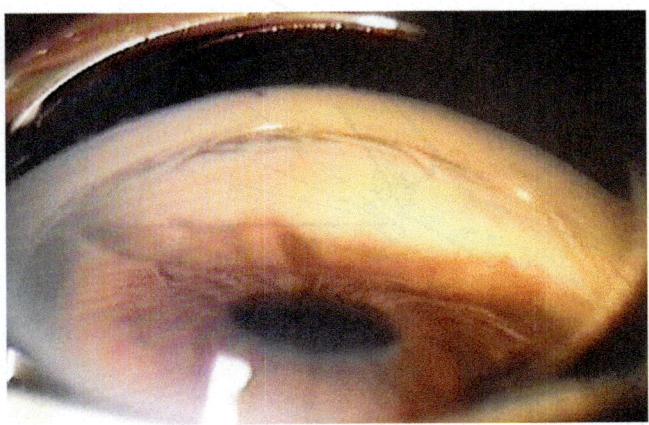

**Fig. 26.13** Peripheral anterior synechiae as seen during indentation gonioscopy. Note that the angle structures are still not visible. Courtesy of WLM Alward, MD

benefit comes from indenting to determine if a pigmented line is a Sampaolesi's line or the trabecular meshwork.

Indentation gonioscopy is effective with four-mirror lenses such as the Zeiss, Posner, and Sussman. The key similarity of these lenses is that they all have areas of contact which are smaller than the cornea. Lenses with large areas of contact, such as the Goldmann and Koeppe lenses, may make the angle shallower with indentation.

## 26.9 Gonioscopic Grading Systems

Grading systems are key to accurate recording of gonioscopic findings for future reference. Many systems for grading the angle exist. The three systems most commonly used for grading are the Scheie, Shaffer, and Spaeth systems.

## 26.10 Scheie System

In 1957, Scheie developed a grading system using Roman numerals to describe the angle.[4] One determines the angle structures that are visible on gonioscopy (Fig. 26.14) and higher numbers signify a narrower angle, with "IV" representing a closed angle. The term "wide" was used to describe an angle in which all structures were visible. Scheie also described angle pigmentation on a scale from 0 (no pigmentation) to IV (heavy pigmentation).

## 26.11 Shaffer System

Shaffer described a system that indicates the degree to which the angle is open rather than the degree to which it is closed.[2,5] The Shaffer system requires estimation of the angle at which the iris inserts relative to the plane of the trabecular meshwork (Fig. 26.15). An angle between the iris and the meshwork of 20° or greater is not considered to be at risk for closure. Angles at 20° or below are considered capable of closure if not already closed.

## 26.12 Spaeth System

In 1971, Spaeth proposed a system that separately grades the three major features of the angle's anatomy: the level of iris insertion, the width of the angle, and the configuration of the iris.[6] The goal of this system is to provide a more descriptive interpretation of the angle.

The level of iris insertion is represented by letters "A" through "E". If the iris inserts anterior to Schwalbe's line, it

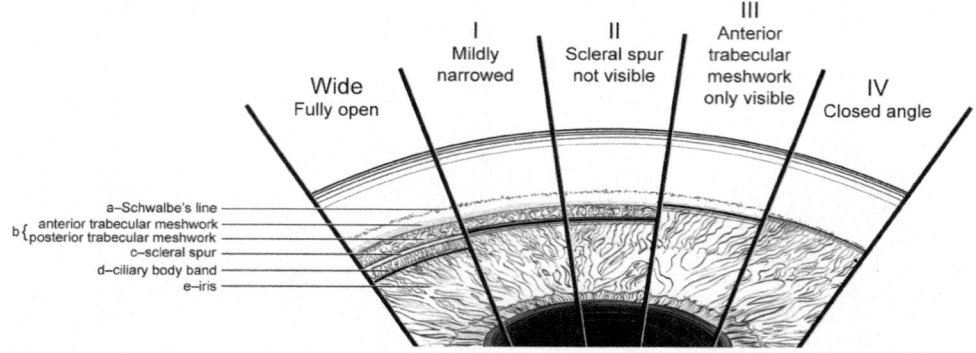

**Fig. 26.14** The Scheie angle grading system. *a* Schwalbe's line; *b* full trabecular meshwork; *c* scleral spur; *d* ciliary body face; *e* iris root

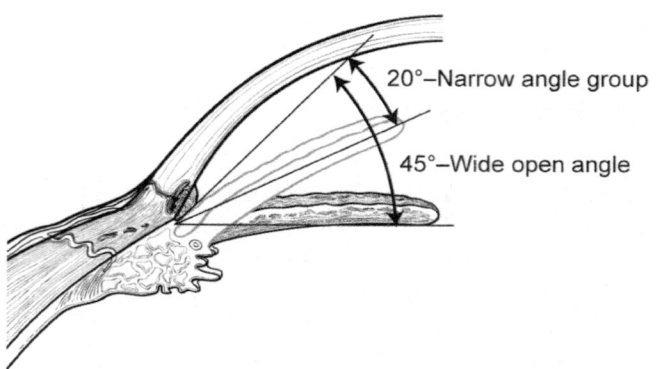

**Fig. 26.15** Shaffer's grading system

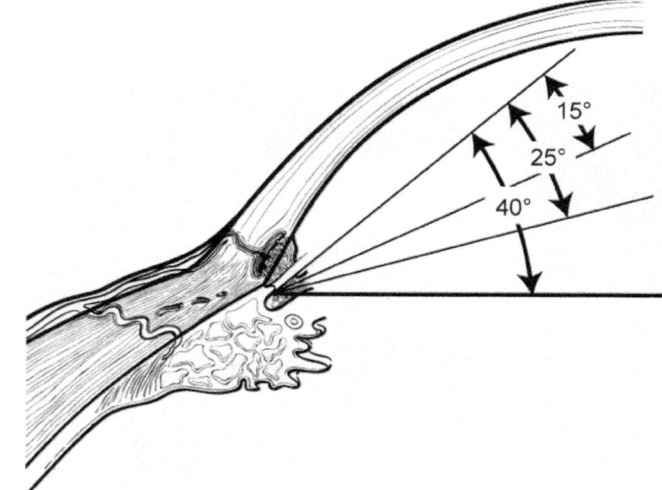

**Fig. 26.17** Spaeth's classification of the angle width

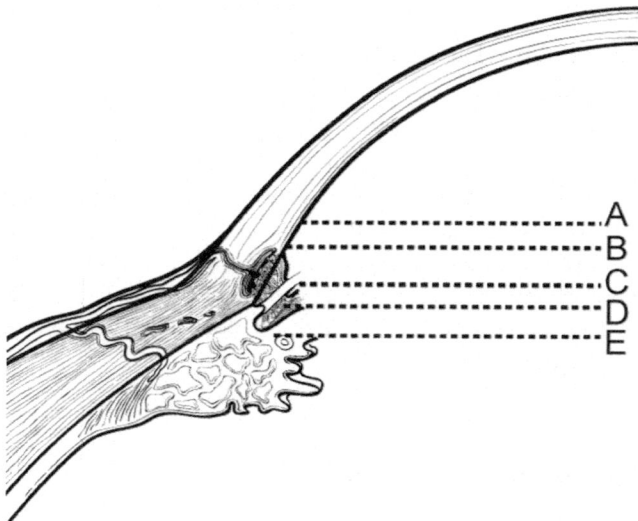

**Fig. 26.16** Spaeth's classification of the level of iris insertion. *A* Anterior to trabecular meshwork; *B* behind Schwalbe's line; *C* posterior to scleral spur; *D* deep, into ciliary body face; *E* extremely deep

is described as grade "A" (for "anterior"). If it inserts anterior to the posterior limit of the trabecular meshwork, it is grade "B" (for "behind" Schwalbe's line). If the insertion is posterior to the scleral spur, the iris is grade "C" (for the "c" in sclera). Insertion into the ciliary body face is recorded as grade "D" (for "deep") or grade "E" (for "extremely" deep) (Fig. 26.16).

Angular width is the estimated angle between a line tangential to the trabecular meshwork and a line tangential to the surface of the iris about one-third of the way from the periphery. The angle is expressed in degrees and no additional grade is assigned (Fig. 26.17).

The third characteristic that is described is the curvature of the peripheral iris: "r" for a regular or flat configuration, "s" for a steep curvature or iris bombé, and "q" for a "queer" or concave curvature (Fig. 26.18). This system was subsequently modified, using "f" to denote a flat configuration, "c" to describe the "concave" iris, "b" to describe the forwardly "bowed" iris, and "p" for a plateau iris configuration. The letter used to describe iris configuration in this way should be kept lowercase to avoid confusion with grading of the level of iris insertion.

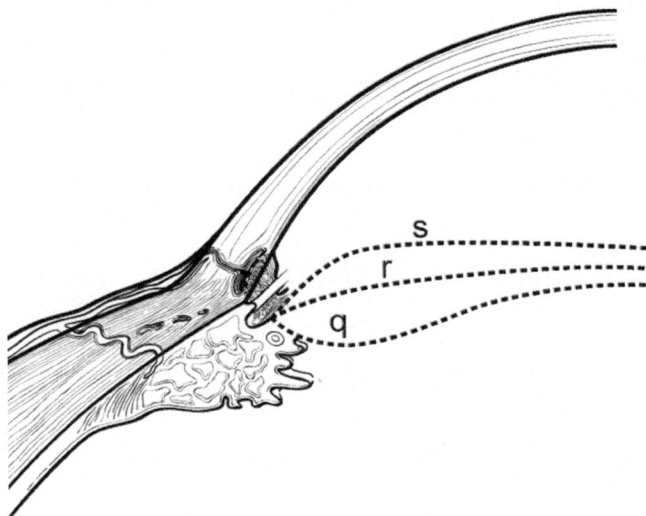

**Fig. 26.18** Iris configuration in the original Spaeth classification. *s* steep or convex; *r* regular or flat; *q* queer or concave

Spaeth also graded posterior pigmented meshwork in the 12 o'clock angle on a scale of 0 to 4+ and this grade is often assigned separately at the end of the gonioscopic description. An appropriate depiction of an open angle with 35° iris insertion at the ciliary body face and moderate meshwork pigmentation would read "D40f 2+". If indentation demonstrates that the insertion is a "D" when it originally appeared to be a "C," this would be indicated as "(C)D." Therefore, an angle is always defined by an alphanumeric description such as (C)D35b.[7]

# References

1. Shields MB. *Textbook of Glaucoma*. Baltimore: Williams & Wilkins; 1992.
2. Shaffer RN. *Stereoscopic Manual of Gonioscopy*. St Louis: C. V. Mosby; 1962.
3. Forbes M. Gonioscopy with indentation: a method for distinguishing between appositional closure and synechial closure. *Arch Ophthalmol*. 1966;76:488.
4. Scheie HG. Width and pigmentation of the angle of the anterior chamber. *Arch Ophthalmol*. 1957;58:510–512.
5. Shaffer RN. Gonioscopy, ophthalmoscopy, and perimetry. *Trans Am Acad Ophthalmol Otolaryngol*. 1960;64:112–125.
6. Spaeth GL. The normal development of the human anterior chamber angle: a new system of grading. *Trans Ophthalmol Soc UK*. 1971;91:709–739.
7. Spaeth GL. Distinguishing between the normally narrow, the suspiciously shallow, and the particularly pathological, anterior chamber chamber angle. *Perspect Ophthalmol*. 1977;1:205–214.

# Chapter 27
# Beyond Gonioscopy: Digital Imaging of the Anterior Segment

Robert J. Noecker

Evaluation of the angle is an essential part of the exam of the glaucoma patient. Gonioscopy is a somewhat subjective evaluation of the anterior chamber angle of the eye using a lens. Gonioscopy is essential to determine what subtype of glaucoma an individual may have. However, at times, it may be difficult to obtain consistent gonioscopic results because of factors related to the patient's eye and/or cooperation. Gonioscopy is never as objective as we would like for it to be.

The disease state that is most commonly encountered with an abnormal angle is the narrow angle. Primary angle-closure glaucoma is the predominant subtype of glaucoma in some regions of the world.[1-5] Treating narrow or occludable angle with laser peripheral iridotomy may prevent the development of angle closure glaucoma.[6]

Imaging of the anterior segment of the eye has become increasingly useful in gaining objective information about the anatomy of the angle and the structures around it. While gonioscopy is still the mainstay of clinical evaluation of the angle, it is a subjective test, and the findings can vary depending on patient cooperation, environmental lighting, and type of gonioscopy being performed.[7] Imaging of the anterior segment of the eye is a useful tool that complements the clinical exam and provides documentation of the anatomical status of the angle and anterior segment of the eye.[8]

It is important that clinicians understand the strengths and weaknesses of the various technologies available.[9,10] Ultrasound technologies in the form of the ultrasound biomicroscope (UBM) can provide information about structures deeper in the eye.[11-13] The trade off is that they need to be in contact with the eye to provide images. In contrast, optical coherence tomography is noncontact but does not provide information about more posterior or deeper structures in the eye.

## 27.1 UBM

The ultrasound biomicroscope uses relatively low frequency ultrasound to image the structures of the eye. A typical UBM unit (Paradigm Medical Industries, Salt Lake City, Utah) uses a 50-MHz transducer. This provides axial resolutions of 25 μm and lateral resolutions of 50 μm. At this frequency, the penetration depth is about 5 mm. The UBM produces a 5×5-mm field with 256-A-scans at a rate of 8 frames/s. Other UBM units such as one by OTI (Toronto, Canada) use a 35–50-MHz transducer, which records 40 s of video image at 25 frames/s. The screen resolution is optimized for 35-MHz transducer and provides lower screen resolution than the other units.

When the test is performed, the patient is placed in a supine position. A fixation target is on the ceiling for the patient. The operator must choose the right size of eyecup from among three sizes. Topical anesthetic is placed and the eyecup is inserted. Saline solution is used as a coupling medium. The OTI device has smaller eye cups and probe body with screw in transducer.

The resolution of the current UBM devices is fairly good, and be used to image the anterior chamber and also image the anterior lens, ciliary body, posterior iris, and materials that are placed behind the iris. Current UBM can also be used to image filtering blebs and filtering tubes on the surface of the eye.

A higher frequency UBM has become available in the past several years. This frequency permits imaging of Schlemm's canal as well as the angle. Due to the higher frequency, the images posterior to the iris are not as well visualized as with the higher frequency UBM. It is usable in the operating room or office (Iscience, Mountain View, California). This technology uses an 80-MHz probe that allows visualization of Schlemm's canal and trabecular meshwork. The system is optimized to evaluate the upper

2 mm of the anterior segment of the eye. Axial resolution is 25 μm. The video captures 7 frames/s also has a sterile imaging cap, which is of single use and disposable. Other manufacturers have begun to offer an imaging cap for the probes for use with the lower frequency devices.

## 27.2 OCT

Anterior segment OCT systems have become available in the past several years. These systems use the reflectance of light instead of ultrasound to provide high-resolution images of the anterior segment of the eye.[14–17] This technology is performed with the patient seated upright at a slit-lamp type of headrest. Because it can be performed in a noncontact fashion, patient comfort is greater than with UBM. This technique can also be performed faster than UBM, and less skill is required by the technician than with UBM. The superior eyelid position can sometimes limit the imaging of the angle, so most often, the cross sectional images are often obtained at oblique angles. Because of the lack of a coupling medium, image quality can be affected by the abnormalities in the anterior surface of the eye.[18,19]

The OCT gives excellent images of the cornea that can be exceptionally helpful in determining evaluating these patients after surgical procedures such as DSEK or LASIK. It can also give a measure of corneal curvature and corneal thickness.

The time domain OCT devices (Visante, Zeiss, Dublin, California) enable measurement of anterior chamber depth, angles, and diameter, as well as corneal thickness. It can measure corneal flap and stromal thickness. A 1,310 superluminescent LED is used as the light source. These devices use 256/line sampling with 0.125 second per line acquisition. The axial resolution is 18 μm and the transverse resolution is 60 μm. This wavelength allows imaging through an opaque cornea, but the wavelength is blocked by pigment.

The drawback in the area of glaucoma is that OCT does not provide information posterior to the iris (due to the pigment).[20] This is important in that the placement of the ciliary body can be important in confirming the diagnosis of plateau iris, ciliary body cysts, tumors, or ciliary effusions that may be the cause of a narrowed or closed angle.

HD-OCT devices have become available and have been recently introduced for imaging the retina and optic nerve. The devices use scanning rates 50–60 times faster than current time-domain OCT devices. These newer machines provide axial resolutions of 3–5 μm. Prototypes have been studied and have shown to have much higher resolution of both anterior structures and posterior segment structures. These devices provide scan rates of 27,000 a scans per second (versus 2,000/s). An image is acquired in as little as 0.04 s with less motion artifact as a result. The tissue depth of the scans is 2 mm or so depth in tissue. Axial resolution is about 5 mm. Rtvue (Optovue, Freemont, California) offers a commercially available device for anterior segment analysis.

Clinically, these devices offer the promise of even higher resolution than previously available. Studies have shown that in the angle, the agreement with other technologies is good and that the key structures of the trabecular meshwork and the scleral spur are even more easily visualized. Given the faster image acquisition time, it is easier for the patient to be examined with this newer technology. Also, faster scanning time permits more difficult populations to be imaged better than with the other technologies.[21–25]

## 27.3 The Normal Angle

In the normal eye, the cornea, iris, ciliary body, and anterior lens surface can be seen easily. In evaluating the angle, the easiest structure to identify is the scleral spur. It is the anatomical landmark from which all other evaluations are based. The scleral spur is best visualized by tracking the posterior curvature of the cornea to the junction where it meets the curvature of the sclera (Figs. 27.1 and 27.2).

The relationship of the iris to the scleral spur is the most important indicator of whether the angle is open or not. When the iris position is posterior to the scleral spur, the angle is open, if the iris is in front of the iris, then that portion of the angle is not open. The trabecular meshwork is located anterior to the scleral spur, as is Schwalbe's line. Posterior to the scleral spur is the ciliary body and iris root.

In the normal angle, the iris is fairly flat with minimal anterior bowing. The anterior chamber is wide with a lot of space between the iris and cornea. The shapes and locations

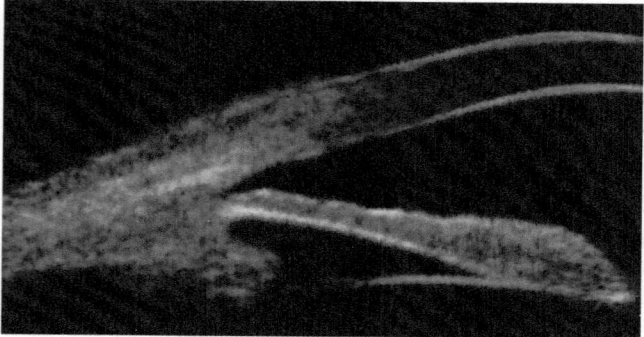

**Fig. 27.1** UBM of normal angle. The angle is wide open, the trabecular meshwork is not obstructed, and the iris is in a planar position. There is a normal ciliary sulcus present as well

**Fig. 27.2** OCT of normal angle of same patient. The widefield view over 180° provides information about two sides of the angle

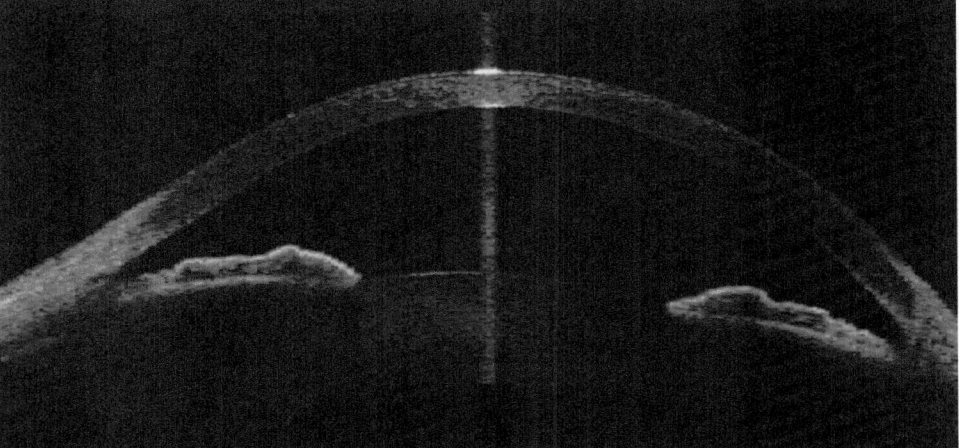

of structures such as the iris and lens can change in concert with environmental changes such as lighting or accommodation. As a result, controlling the testing conditions is important for accurate and reproducible measurement.

## 27.4 Angle Closure

This condition is defined as iris apposition to the trabecular meshwork due to a number of different disorders. Anterior segment imaging can be very helpful in evaluating the source of the underlying problem. Angle closure (see Chap. 36) can result with problems with the iris, the ciliary body, and the lens or posterior forces such as those seen in malignant glaucoma.

In determining whether an eye with a narrow angle is occludable or not, provocative testing can be useful. This is best performed with the UBM, as it is more difficult to standardize ambient lighting with a slit lamp or other imaging devices. Information can be provided about the angle under normal light conditions as well as the tendency to become occluded under dark conditions (Fig. 27.3).

## 27.5 Pupillary Block

This is the most common type of angle closure and is due to lens-iris contact, which in turn leads to a build up of, aqueous in the posterior chamber. This build up causes the iris to bow forward toward the cornea with narrowing of the angle. The other structures remain normal. Laser iridotomy equalizes the pressure in front of and behind the iris, flattening the iris, and widening the angle.

Primary angle closure can be confirmed with either UBM or anterior segment OCT. The important structure that needs to be identified is the scleral spur. Another helpful finding in primary angle closure is that there tends to be anterior bowing of iris because of the pupillary block component (Figs. 27.4 and 27.5).

## 27.6 Plateau Iris

Plateau iris is best diagnosed with UBM (Fig. 27.6). Because of the blockage of the light wavelength by pigment, the OCT cannot provide adequate information about the ciliary body or ciliary sulcus (Fig. 27.7). In plateau iris, the iris root is shortened and inserted anteriorly on the ciliary body resulting in loss of a ciliary sulcus. The central anterior chamber is usually moderately deep. On gonioscopy, a "double hump sign" may be seen, which corresponds to peripheral hump being the ciliary body holding up the iris and the central hump being the lens pushing on the iris. Laser gonioplasty can be helpful in thinning the peripheral iris and shrinking the ciliary body in order to widen the angle.

## 27.7 Other Causes of Angle Closure

In phacomorphic glaucoma, the angle may be narrowed due to anterior subluxation of the lens that pushes the iris forward toward the trabecular meshwork. In malignant glaucoma or aqueous misdirection, forces from the vitreous pushes the entire lens – iris diaphragm forward, so that all anterior segment structures are pressed up against the cornea with or without fluid in the supraciliary space. Iridociliary cysts

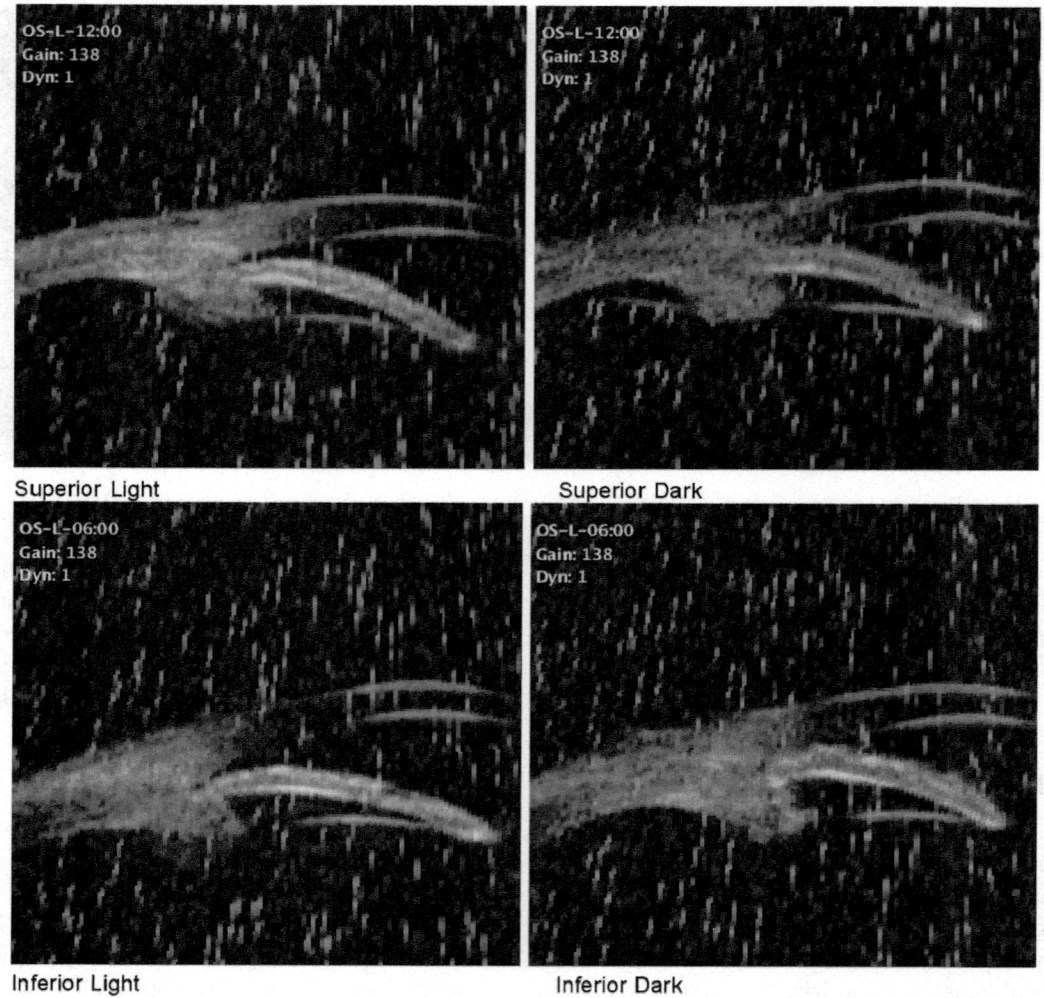

**Fig. 27.3** UBM of occludable angle under both light and dark conditions. The angle is narrow under light condition but closes under dark conditions

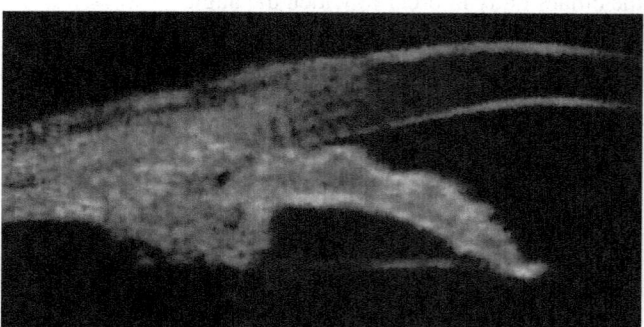

**Fig. 27.4** UBM of angle closure with pupillary block. The iris is significantly bowed forward due to the pressure gradient caused by iridolenticular touch

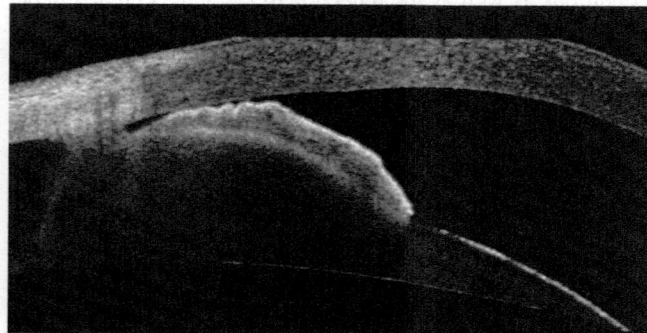

**Fig. 27.5** OCT of angle closure with pupillary block. The iris is significantly bowed forward due to the pressure gradient caused by iridolenticular touch. Note the higher resolution of the image but lack of posterior information

**Fig. 27.6** UBM of narrow angle with plateau component. The ciliary body is very prominent and anteriorly displaced. There is no ciliary sulcus evident

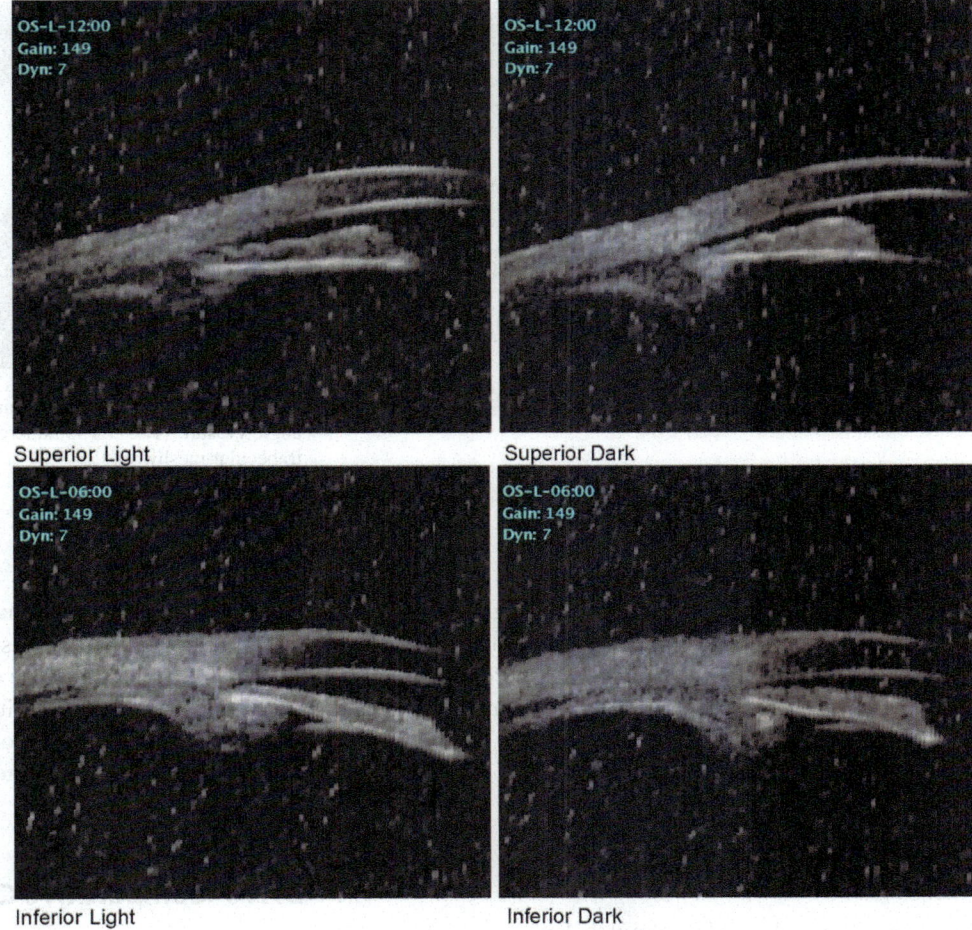

**Fig. 27.7** OCT of narrow angle with plateau component. The angle narrowing is easily seen but there is no information about the ciliary sulcus or ciliary body

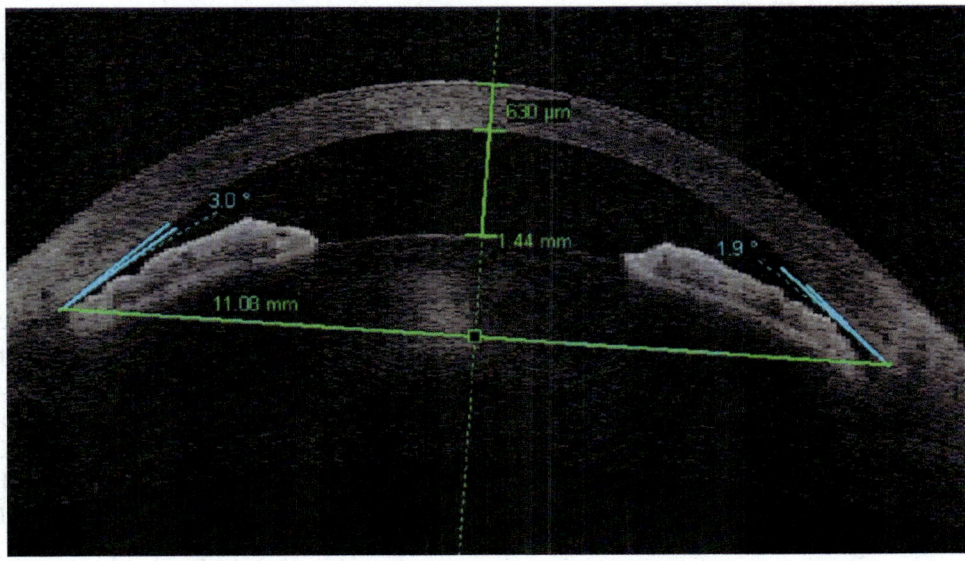

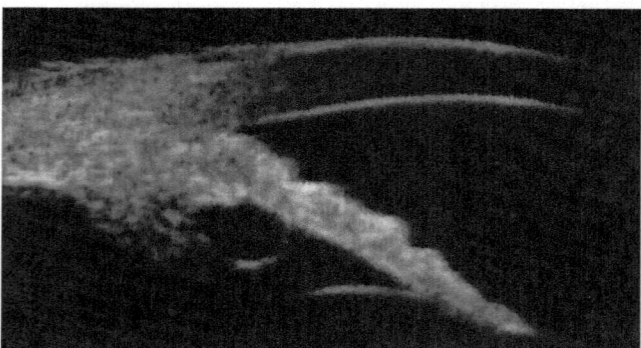

**Fig. 27.8** UBM of closed angle due to an iris cyst. The cyst is fluid filled which appears black on the UBM

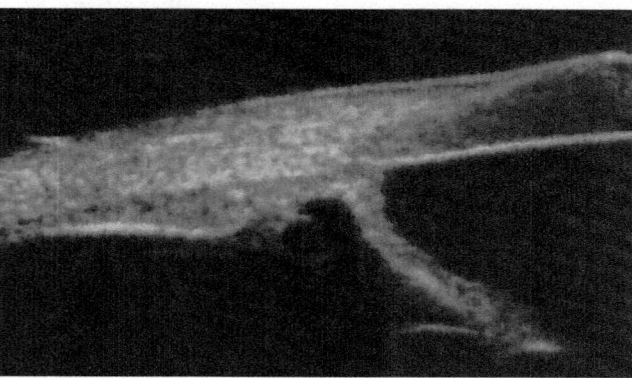

**Fig. 27.9** UBM of peripheral anterior synechiae in eye with chronic angle closure. The iris is adherent to the cornea and obstructing the trabecular meshwork

can cause narrowing or occlusion of the angle (Figs. 27.8). Tumors, ciliary body enlargement, or gas bubbles can also be responsible for secondary angle closure. Persistent iridocorneal touch can result in peripheral anterior synechiae and chronic angle closure (Fig. 27.9).

## 27.8 Open Angle Findings

Imaging of the angle can be helpful to demonstrate changes in the iris contour in pigmentary glaucoma. The iris in this condition tends to be floppy and bows posteriorly, so that it comes in contact with the ciliary body or zonules. The pigment from the posterior is released is distributed throughout the anterior chamber. Findings on imaging include a widely open angle with posterior iris bowing and increased lens-iris contact centrally (Figs. 27.10 and 27.11).

Eyes that have experienced ocular trauma have open but abnormal angles. Angle recession can be seen as a tear between the ciliary body and the iris insertion. The angle is wide open and the sclera and ciliary body are in contact. A cyclodialysis cleft, commonly seen in patients with hypotony, is a condition in which the ciliary body becomes detached from the scleral spur with a resulting direct pathway from the anterior chamber to the ciliary space (Fig. 27.12).

## 27.9 Findings Posterior to the Iris

Choroidal effusions or choroidal hemorrhages appear as space underneath the ciliary body. UBM is most effective for diagnosing these conditions when they are anterior or small.

OCT is also capable of imaging these if done through the sclera directly over the effusion or hemorrhage.

Foreign bodies, drainage devices, or intraocular lens position can also be best seen with UBM, The position and extent of these findings can be monitored quantitatively over time as can ciliary body and posterior iris masses (Fig. 27.13).

## 27.10 Comparative Clinical Performance

Studies have demonstrated that each of the technologies have fairly good agreement with each other as well as gonioscopy and pathology. While there are differences in terms of actual degrees measured between UBM and OCT, these differences are more due to differences in technique, position of the patient, and part of the angle measured than due to differences in technology capability. The only meaningful clinical difference between the technologies is the ability of UBM to provide information about structures posterior to the iris such as the ciliary body.

## 27.11 Conclusions

Imaging of the anterior segment of the eye continues to evolve. New technology continues to improve the resolution and ease of use. In combination with thorough clinical exams, these technologies provide quantitative information about anterior segment structures, especially the angle. As newer, noncontact technologies become more available, future uses can be foreseen in telemedicine and large population screenings.

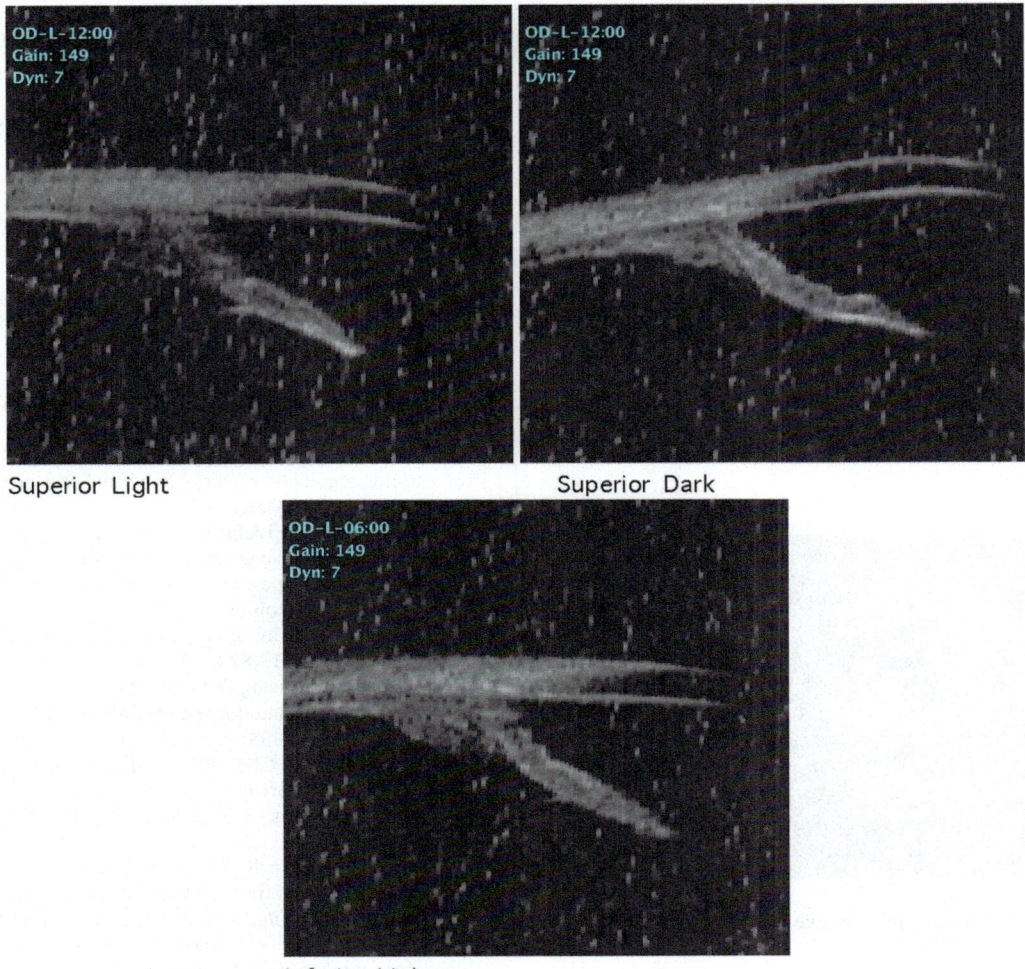

**Fig. 27.10** UBM of iris with pigment dispersion. Notable posterior iris bowing is evident, which changes slightly with changes in illumination. Contact of peripheral iris with ciliary body can be seen

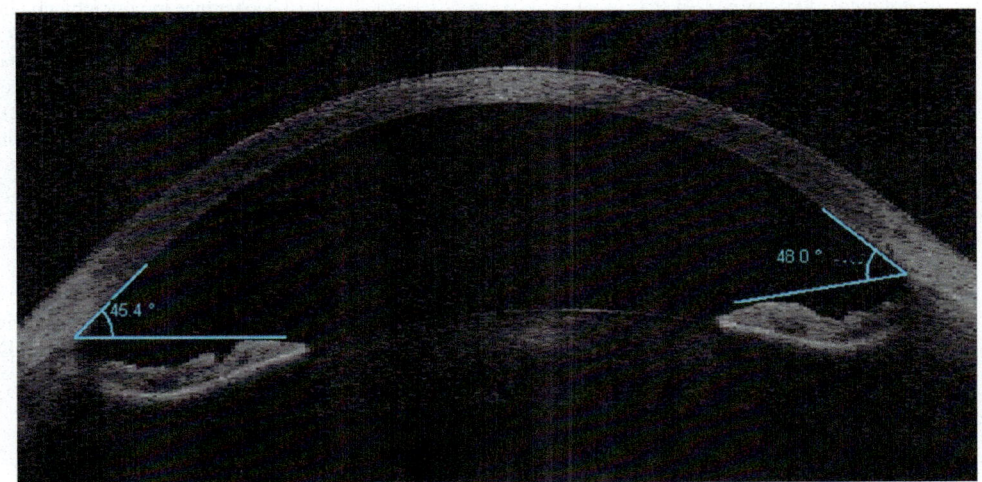

**Fig. 27.11** OCT of same patient with pigment dispersion. The iris bowing is easily seen, but, once again, the image does not provide information about posterior structures

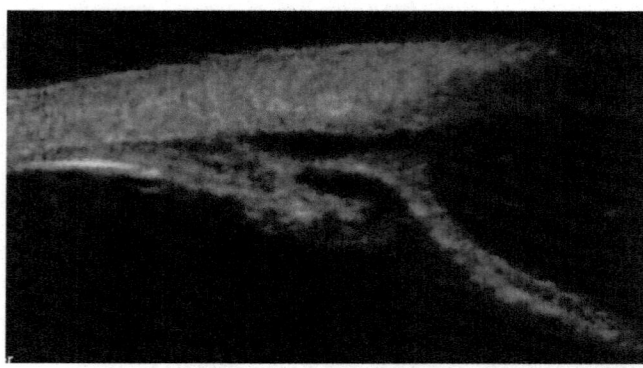

**Fig. 27.12** UBM of ciliary body cleft due to trauma. The IOP is low due to direct exit of aqueous into the supraciliary space

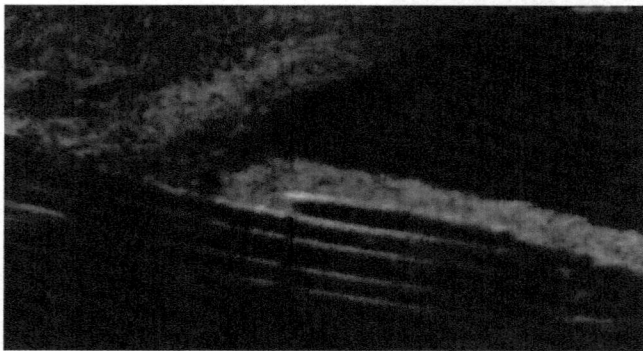

**Fig. 27.13** UBM of glaucoma drainage device in the ciliary sulcus posterior to the iris

## References

1. Erie JC, Hodge DO, Gray DT. The incidence of primary angle-closure glaucoma in Olmstead County, Minnesota. *Arch Ophthalmol.* 1997;115:177–181.
2. Foster PJ. Glaucoma in China: how big is the problem? *Br J Ophthalmol.* 2001;85:1277–1282.
3. Dandona L, Dandona R, Mandal P, et al. Angle-closure glaucoma in an urban population in southern India. The Andhra Pradesh eye disease study. *Ophthalmology.* 2000;107:1710–1716.
4. Foster PJ, Baasanhu J, Alsbirk PH, et al. Glaucoma in Mongolia: A population-based survey in Ho "vsgo" l Province, Northern Mongolia. *Arch Ophthalmol.* 1996;114:1235–1241.
5. Foster PJ, Oen FT, Machin D, et al. The prevalence of glaucoma in Chinese residents of Singapore: a cross-sectional population survey of the Tanjong Pagar district. *Arch Ophthalmol.* 2000;118:1105–1111.
6. Gazzard G, Friedman D, Devereux J, et al. A prospective ultrasound biomicroscopy evaluation of changes in anterior segment morphology after laser iridotomy in Asian eyes. *Ophthalmology.* 2003;110: 630–638.
7. Sakata LM, Lavanya R, Friedman DS, et al. Comparison of gonioscopy and anteriorsegment ocular coherence tomography in detecting angle closure in different quadrants of the anterior chamber angle. *Ophthalmology.* 2008;115:769–774.
8. Ishikawa H, Liebmann JM, Ritch R. Quantitative assessment of the anterior segment using ultrasound biomicroscopy. *Curr Opin Ophthalmol.* 2000;11(2):133–139.
9. Radhakrishnan S, Goldsmith J, Huang D, et al. Comparison of optical coherence tomography and ultrasound biomicroscopy for detection of narrow anterior chamber angles. *Arch Ophthalmol.* 2005;123(8):1053–1059.
10. Dada T, Sihota R, Gadia R et al. Comparison of anterior segment optical coherence tomography and ultrasound biomicroscopy for assessment of the anterior segment. *J Cataract Refract Surg.* 2007;33:837–840.
11. Pavlin CJ, Foster FS. Ultrasound biomicroscopy in glaucoma. *Acta Ophthalmologica.* 1992;(Suppl 204):7–9.
12. Pavlin CJ, Harasiewicz K, Foster FS. Ultrasound biomicroscopy of anterior segment structures in normal and glaucomatous eyes. *Am J Ophthalmol.* 1992;113:381–389.
13. Ishikawa H, Esaki K, Liebmann JM, et al. Ultrasound biomicroscopy dark room provocative testing: a quantitative method for estimating anterior chamber angle width. *Jpn J Ophthalmol.* 1999;43:526–534.
14. Radhakrishnan S, Rollins AM, Roth JE, et al. Real-time optical coherence tomography of the anterior segment at 1,310 nm. *Arch Ophthalmol.* 2001;119(8):1179–1185.
15. Radhakrishnan S, Huang D, Smith SD. Optical coherence tomography imaging of the anterior chamber angle. *Ophthalmol Clin North Am.* 2005;18(3):375–381.
16. Nolan WP, See JL, Chew PT, et al. Detection of primary angle closure using anterior segment optical coherence tomography in Asian eyes. *Ophthalmology.* 2007;114(1):33–39.2008; 115(5):769–774.
17. Sakata LM, Lavanya R, Friedman DS, et al. Assessment of the scleral spur in anterior-segment ocular coherence tomography images. *Arch Ophthalmol.* 2008;126(2):181–185.
18. Hoerauf H, Wirbelauer C, Scholz C, et al. Slit-lamp-adapted optical coherence tomography of the anterior segment. *Graefes Arch Clin Exp Ophthalmol.* 2000;238:8–18.
19. See JLS, Chew P, Smith S, et al. Changes in anterior segment morphology in Asian eyes: an anterior segment OCT study response to illumination and after laser iridotomy. *Br J Ophthalmol.* 2007;91: 1485–1489.
20. van den Berg TJTP, Spekreijse H. Near infrared light absorption in the human eye media. Vision Res 1997; 37:249–253 2007;91: 1485–1489.
21. Wong HT, Lim M, Friedman D, Aung T. High-definition optical coherence tomography imaging of the iridocorneal angle of the eye. *Arch Ophthalmol.* 2009;127(3):256–260.
22. Goldsmith JA, Li Y, Chalita MR, et al. Anterior chamber width measurement by highspeed optical coherence tomography. *Ophthalmology.* 2005;112(2):238–244.
23. Drexler W, Morgner U, Ghanta RK, Kärtner FX, Schuman JS, Fujimoto JG. Ultrahigh resolution ophthalmic optical coherence tomography. *Nat Med.* 2001;7(4):502–507.
24. Wojtkowski M, Bajraszewski T, Gorczynska I, et al. Ophthalmic imaging by spectral optical coherence tomography. *Am J Ophthalmol.* 2004;138(3):412–419.
25. Christopoulos V, Kagemann L, Wollstein G, et al. In vivo corneal high-speed, ultra high-resolution optical coherence tomography. *Arch Ophthalmol.* 2007;125(8):1027–1035.

# Chapter 28
# Office Examination of the Glaucoma Patient

Paul N. Schacknow

The initial examination of the patient with presumed glaucoma or glaucoma suspect status should be a problem-focused, enhanced version of the "new" patient set of clinical observations, diagnostic tests, and history taking routinely done by all ophthalmologists. My perspective in this chapter shall be that of a community-based glaucoma subspecialist, working in a group ophthalmology practice. I see patients referred for glaucoma-related diagnostic workup, consultation, and possible treatment. Everything I describe or recommend here should be well within the current or attainable skill sets of most eye care physicians and the facilities of average office environments. This chapter should serve as an informal guide for residents, fellows, and comprehensive ophthalmologists who wish to incorporate evidence-based diagnosis and patient management techniques into their glaucoma practices. I will also consider the occasional need for and use of advanced diagnostic technology that might be available for patients referred to academic medical centers, such as ultrasound biomicroscopy (UBM) and anterior segment ocular coherence tomography (AS-OCT).

## 28.1 The Appointment Booking Process

Like most branches of medicine, much of the information needed to guide diagnostic observations and testing may be gleaned from the patient's orally provided medical history and the medical records from physicians they have previously visited. As part of the telephone appointment booking process, have your office staff ask the new patient to obtain eye medical records from their previous physicians before the date of the appointment. They should request that visual fields, optic nerve head photos, and imaging reports (e.g., Scanning laser polarimetry based retinal nerve fiber analyzer (GDx), optical coherence tomography (OCT), and Heidelberg Retinal Tomograph (HRT)) be included when available. Usually 2 or 3 years' worth of medical records is sufficient. If another physician is referring the patient to you, the patient *also* should ask for a letter summarizing the reasons behind the request for consultation. For patients who are moving to your area from another locale, the previous physician might provide a brief written summary of the patient's ophthalmologic status in addition to medical records. A description of any eye surgeries should be included.

It is best to tell the patient to have their medical records sent directly to them and not to your office. We use facsimile or postal mail to send them a records-release form that they may sign and forward to their previous physician. (Sometimes their previous eye doctor requires the use of their own practice-specific records-release form.) Request that the patient bring the records with them to their first office visit with you. This helps to ensure that the records *have* been obtained in advance of the patient's arrival and that they haven't been received but misplaced by your office staff. I have had many patients very surprised that their previous doctors have not mailed or faxed the records to us even though the patient has requested that this be done. By asking the *patient* to obtain the records (rather than your office staff), and to bring them to the visit, they will themselves determine if a second records request is needed in advance of their scheduled appointment with you.

During the initial telephone conversation, the appointment-setting staff member should ask the patient to bring all of their glaucoma medications with them, bottles of drops as well as any pills in containers. Additionally, they should prepare a written list of all medications (with dosages) taken for their general health issues. By doing this at home with access to the medications, rather than when they come to the office, a patient's faulty memory is less likely to become an issue in this regard.

Patients are sometimes unaware of their medical problems. Noting from a written list that someone is taking Lanoxin (digoxin), for example, directs the ophthalmologist to consider diagnoses such as congestive heart failure versus atrial fibrillation. Topical beta-blocker therapy for glaucoma might be relatively contraindicated with the first diagnosis and more acceptable with the second condition. Patients taking diuretics may be at risk of potassium wasting if additionally prescribed an oral carbonic anhydrase inhibitor for their glaucoma. A phone call to the primary care physician, during the office visit, may help to clarify these issues in case the patient is unaware of why they are taking certain medications.

We ask that the patient bring in their most current distance spectacles, even if they routinely wear contact lenses. We use a lensometer with these spectacles to help determine the appropriate correction for initial visual field testing.

It is very useful to have a recent (less than 6-months-old) visual field print-out available during the initial patient visit. This might be contained in the patient's old medical records. For patients arriving without medical records, a phone call by your office staff may yield a recent visual field by facsimile (and perhaps a few pages of ophthalmology notes). Be prepared to fax a written records request to the previous physician because of privacy laws. It should be signed by the patient. This should all be done routinely, by trained office staff, before the patient sees the physician.

Generally, unless a recent visual field is available, we schedule a Zeiss-Humphrey visual field examination (HVF) to be performed by a technician the same day as the first office visit, before the patient is seen by the doctor. Nonetheless, in a high-volume glaucoma practice, it is often necessary to ask patients referred for glaucoma consultation to have their HVF examination done several days to a week earlier than their appointment with me, at times that I am not seeing patients. The appointments booking clerk explains to the patient that this is similar to having X-ray procedures or blood tests done before the patient sees their general medical practitioners. (Patients tend not to be happy about scheduling visual fields separately from their office examination visit!) Having the visual field done in advance of the patient's visit with the physician allows many more new and established patients to be seen by the doctor in a given day, because for us the HVF appointment slots are the rate-limiting resource in this process.

The appointments clerk verifies insurance information, reminds the patient to bring insurance documentation with them to the office visit, and requests that any "managed-care" or other insurance-related referral authorizations should be faxed to our office or brought with them. We determine if the patient needs or soon will need refill prescriptions for current glaucoma medications. If a "new" patient, whom we have not yet examined, requests refills, we direct them back to their previous eye physician, because we do not yet have a doctor–patient relationship. We have not yet reviewed their medical records nor examined them to determine the appropriateness of their current therapy. Also, we try to accommodate the situation by making an appointment to see them as quickly as possible.

We have an automated system that telephones the patient several days before their appointment to remind them of it and also to remind them to bring in insurance documentation and insurance referral authorizations. Instead of using automated telephone systems, some practices do appointment-reminding using clerical staff, while some use mailed postal cards.

## 28.2 Office Intake Process

Upon entering our office suite, new and established patients present themselves to a clerk who handles both the "check-in" and later "check-out" duties. The clerk verifies insurance documentation (making sure that it is current and updating our records as necessary) and insurance-related visit authorizations. Any medical records brought with the patient are added to the office chart.

Our long-established group practice still uses paper-based medical records. (See Chap. 30 for a discussion of electronic medical records.) Patients are given a set of intake documents to complete (perhaps with the help of accompanying family members) before being seen by an ophthalmic assistant. Samples of these intake documents are presented in the Appendices accompanying this chapter. Recently, we have uploaded these intake documents (in Adobe Acrobat PDF format) to a practice-based website. The appointments clerk encourages the patient to download this packet using a computer at home, and complete the forms before they come to the office. This helps ensure they will be seen in a timely manner when coming to the office, rather than first spending 15–20 min doing paperwork before seeing an ophthalmic assistant.

The clinically most important document in this packet is the Medical History Questionnaire (MHQ). This form (Appendix 1) meets Medicare legal coding requirements while providing the physician with information regarding both ophthalmology and general medical patient problems. Medications, both eye and general medical, should be listed on this form. Handwritten or typed lists of medications brought in by the patient may simply be stapled to the form.

Appendix 2 is an example of a "welcome to the practice" letter we use that describes the nature of the glaucoma examination the patient is about to undergo. Note that on the second page of this letter the patient is asked to acknowledge, by their signature, that they are aware of their responsibilities as a glaucoma patient or glaucoma suspect. Reading and signing this form makes them aware that glaucoma is a lifelong illness requiring follow-up with an appropriate physician. This involves them in the glaucoma care process and may provide some relief to the physician from potential medical liability for patients who do not return to your office as requested. I personally ask them to sign this portion of the form at the end of their examination, after I have discussed their diagnoses and my treatment recommendations.

There also is a space on this letter for signatures by a family member who might have accompanied the patient and for an office staff member as a witness to the signatures. A photocopy of this signed document is given to the patient and the original is placed within the medical chart. We encourage one or more family members to join the patient and the doctor in the examination room if the patient so desires.

Appendices 3 and 4 request the patient to give us permission to dilate their eyes on the first and subsequent examinations, and allow us to take fundus photos from time to time. We do provide patients with disposable sunglasses for use after dilated examinations. Other documents provided in the intake packet concern payment and insurance issues, medical record privacy issues, and describe general policies of our group practice. Each patient is also given a "physician's practice pamphlet" Appendix 5 that describes the doctor's academic training and clinical experience.

### 28.2.1 The Role of the Ophthalmic Assistant in Chart Review and Interviewing the Patient

The intake clerk places these completed forms into the medical chart that is then made available to an ophthalmic assistant. The assistant retrieves the chart and escorts the patient and accompanying family members into an examination lane. Lanes for both assistants and the physician are equipped in a similar manner. Each of our several examination lanes contains an eye chart projector, slit-lamp (various brands have been acquired over the years) and accompanying control console (with a direct ophthalmoscope and "muscle" light), a reclining examination chair, and one or two other small chairs for accompanying visitors. Examination lenses (high diopter, goniolenses) are kept in the physician's lab coat pockets. An indirect ophthalmoscope is in each lane used by the examining physician. Drops needed for diagnostic purposes, preprinted prescription forms, and various pamphlets and brochures are available in each exam room. Some rooms contain phoropters, although generally we defer refractions to nonglaucoma-related visits. In this regard, we often schedule the patient to visit separately with our practice-based optometrists.

The assistant interviews the patient regarding past medical history and current eye problems. Both the assistant and physician portions of the formal glaucoma examination are based upon a highly structured protocol that I have refined over the past 20 years of practice. We use a Glaucoma Consultation Report – New Patient form (Appendix 6) that guides the interviews and examinations and gives us a place to record the obtained information. This form helps to ensure that even newly trained assistants and busy, overwhelmed ophthalmologists systematically inquire about important signs and symptoms and conduct a thorough ophthalmic examination relevant to glaucoma diagnoses and other eye diseases. The version of Appendix 6 has been annotated with colored "boxes" to facilitate my description of how the form is used in our practice. The version of Appendix 6 used in our office does not contain any boxes. A similar form (Appendix 7, without annotations) is used for returning (established) patients.

After greeting the patient and their family members, the ophthalmic assistant determines if language translation will be necessary to conduct the interview and examination effectively. Various members of our office staff speak Spanish and French (which helps with our Haitian patients who speak Creole), but generally we find that patients will often bring family members who are bilingual in both their native language and in English. Deaf patients are often accompanied by a professional aid who is fluent in American Sign Language. Studies have shown that patients who require an interpreter may be at a disadvantage in interacting with medical personnel compared to patients who speak the same language as the interviewers; these patients offer fewer comments and are more likely to have their comments ignored.[1,2]

An experienced ophthalmic assistant verifies that all forms have been completed by the patient and aids them in making sure that the medical history questionnaire is complete. Both "leading" and "open-ended" questions are used to help obtain as accurate a description of the eye and general medical history as possible.[3]

The assistant asks why the patient has come to see the doctor (the so-called "chief complaint"). Sometimes we get answers like "I don't know," "my insurance changed," "my family doctor told me to," "I just moved here and I have glaucoma," and "the other eye doctor downstairs said I should see you but didn't tell me why." Most patients, however, do know why they have come for a glaucoma evaluation and many are well-versed about the details of their eye medical history. We teach our ophthalmic assistants to thoroughly review any previous chart notes from other ophthalmologists within our group practice, as well as any medical chart notes obtained from previous eye physicians. Many of our long-term assistants are very experienced in extracting important eye medical and surgical historical information and writing it into the appropriate sections of the glaucoma consultation form (Appendix 6) that I use for each new patient.

The assistant asks questions about any family history of glaucomatous disease. They try to determine whether there are any particular eye-related symptoms that led to the patient seeking ophthalmic care. They ask the patient about any eye drops or pills they are using for glaucoma or other eye diseases, and cross-reference this with the medical history questionnaire just completed. Spouses or other accompanying family members may help to provide this information.

The assistants are trained to ask at first only open-ended questions about ophthalmic medication usage for those patients who have not brought the medications themselves or a list of them to the office.[4] That is, we have learned that if you suggest to a patient that they are using a certain brand of medicine, a certain number of times per day (perhaps because the ophthalmic assistant has read that they are supposed to be doing so by looking at the medical chart notes), most patients tend to agree with whatever you have said to them. If you ask if they are using "pilocarpine four times a day" the answer will often be "yes." It is much better to ask what are the names of the drops and how many times are they being used, rather than suggesting this information to the patient. And please realize that "four times a day" may be breakfast time, lunch time, dinner time, and bed time, or it may be 9 A.M., 10 A.M., 11 A.M., and noon "to finish each day before I play my regular tennis game." In the real world, open-ended questions often yield no responses or blank stares. Directed questions may need to be used, but one should do so with escalating specificity only as needed. For example, the assistant might ask what the colors are of the bottle tops in an attempt to see if the patient was using the beta-blocker (yellow) previously prescribed or perhaps a prostaglandin analog medication (teal). Only as a last resort do I recommend that specific prompts such as "Are using Timoptic?" or "Is the bottle you are using once a day at night called Lumigan or Travatan or Xalatan?" be employed. Less experienced ophthalmic assistants are much more likely to use directed questions, because it takes some time to acquire the skill of effectively asking open-ended questions. A clinical pearl that we teach new assistants is to specifically inquire about the use of aspirin and related products, and the use of multivitamins and supplementary minerals and nutraceuticals (e.g., fish-oil, ginkgo biloba, bilberry). Many patients do not consider these substances to be medications. Some women do not mention they are taking birth control pills unless specifically asked about them. Finally, we note that there is a strong tendency for many ophthalmic assistants to simply copy into the current note the medications listed in the last note, without attempting to verify how and whether or not the patient has used them at home as prescribed.

Even though we attempt to obtain the previous medical records in advance of the office visit, the patient may not have received them and/or brought them to the office. Our ophthalmic assistants are trained to call the previous or referring physician's office before I see the patient, and request that the records be faxed to us. Alternatively, sometimes the assistant is able to get the previous or referring physician to come to the phone and speak with me briefly, so that I may make some handwritten notes in lieu of formal medical records.

## 28.2.2 The Ophthalmic Assistant's Role in Recording Information and in Examining the Patient

After helping to ensure the completeness of the MHQ and checking to see that all forms in the intake packet have been filled out and signed as necessary, the ophthalmic assistant begins the examination portion of his/her interaction with the patient. As mentioned previously, the interview and examination of the patient by the assistant is very structured. They follow a protocol based upon the Glaucoma Consultation Report – New Patient form (Appendix 6) and record their findings on the report form.

1. *Demographic Information:* Information from the initial interview process – including the patient's age, gender, race, and primary language – are recorded in Box 1 of the consult form. Epidemiological studies indicate that some of these demographic characteristics are associated with prevalence and severity of glaucoma.[5–11]
2. *Chief Complaint, Medical and Surgical History (glaucoma)*, and *Ocular Medical and Surgical History (nonglaucoma), Current Ocular Medications, Current Systemic Medications,* and *Medication Allergies*, are recorded in Boxes 2 through 7, respectively.

   When I review this information, I look for potential medication interactions with glaucoma drugs. I question the patient about medication allergies to see if they are really allergies such as skin rash or difficulty breathing, as compared to simply some gastrointestinal upset, and also to see if any glaucoma-related eye drops were discontinued because of mild irritation versus toxicity versus true allergies.

   The assistants are trained to go through the medical record and summarize relevant glaucoma surgical procedures, both incisional and laser-based. Details of procedures, such as which 180° of the anterior chamber angle was treated during argon laser trabeculoplasty, are helpful when subsequent laser treatment becomes necessary.

   Noting a family ocular history of relatives with glaucoma increases the risk of suspicion for those patients we are examining as "glaucoma suspects."
3. *Visual Acuity:* All patients, both new and established, have their visual acuity determined both with and without current spectacle correction. Pinhole vision, with correction, is also evaluated to see how much visual acuity is influenced by media opacity versus posterior segment pathology (Boxes 8 and 9). The assistant should make sure the patient is not using their reading glasses when assessing distance acuity using the Snellen chart in the examination lane! For established patients whose visual acuities have decreased by two or more lines since the previous visit, the assistants have been trained to dilate

the patients prior to my examining them. (These are for patients who have had previous recent gonioscopy to ensure their anterior chamber angles are not appositional.)

4. *Current Eyeglasses:* A lensometer is used to measure the refraction of the patient's current eyeglasses that were used when determining visual acuity (Box 10). This information is also useful for determining appropriate lenses for use with the automated visual field analyzer.

5. *Central Corneal Thickness (CCT):* If the patient has never had central corneal thickness determined, or if this measurement is not available to us, the assistant measures it twice for each eye using a portable pachymetry device (in my office we use the Pachmate Model DGH55, from DGH Technology, Inc., Exton, Pennsylvania). While government Medicare regulations in the United States will generally only pay for CCT pachymetry related to glaucoma management once in a patient's lifetime, we do these measurements even if they have been done previously in another physician's office because of their importance. This is a simple, noninvasive procedure, and we just repeat it and absorb the cost as part of the price of being ethical physicians. The assistant records the CCT values in Box 11 on the form, where the physician will review the measurements and also write some brief comments.

See Chap. 8 for discussion of CCT, corneal hysteresis, and other structural factors related to the cornea and glaucoma as well as the selection and use of various pachymeters for measuring the CCT. When the Ocular Hypertension Treatment Study[12-14] first highlighted the clinical significance of CCT in the diagnosis and management of glaucoma, many ophthalmologists began using various nomograms[15] to introduce correction factors for measuring Goldmann applanation tonometry readings. More recently, most glaucoma specialists, rather than introducing formal numerical correction factors, generally indicate in their chart notes that the measured CCTs are thin, average, or thick, and write a sentence or two indicating significance of this finding for the individual patient being examined. We find that this simple classification of CCT into *thin*, *average*, and *thick* categories gives us a pragmatic handle on interpreting Goldmann tonometry and making initial intraocular pressure (IOP) reduction target treatment goals.[16]

Some patients have been followed for many years in our group practice with stable, definitely nonprogressing glaucoma. These patients joined our practice before determining CCT became in vogue after the Ocular Hypertension Treatment Study was published in 2002. I do not feel it is necessary to routinely determine CCT for these patients. True, the Goldmann IOPs recorded for them in the chart may be a bit higher or lower than perhaps more accurate values based on their undetermined CCT. But there is no need to change their therapies, because their glaucomas are stable. For these patients, determining CCT would add information to the chart that will not result in a change of therapeutic management. I find determining CCT is useful for setting initial target treatment goals for new patients or in interpreting possible reasons why patients with presumed reasonable target pressures may be progressing. It is also possible that some patients classified with normal tension glaucoma might be more accurately categorized as primary open angle patients if they have very thin central corneas.

6. *Visual Fields:* If formal visual field testing has been performed, the assistant simply records the date, the examiner's initials, and the type of visual field (e.g., Humphrey 24-2, Goldmann) in Box 12. Brief comments regarding the visual field interpretation also will be entered by the physician after reviewing the visual field (Box 12).

For the great majority of my glaucoma suspects and known glaucoma patients, I employ the Zeiss-Humphrey, static, 24-2 visual field protocol, with the SITA-FAST testing algorithm. Most stable suspects and OAG patients get repeat visual field examinations at 6-month intervals, and occasionally at 12-month intervals for suspects. I rarely find it helpful to repeat visual field for patients at intervals shorter than 6 months, even for those patients with advanced visual field defects. I do sometimes repeat visual fields at shorter intervals, at no charge to the patient, when there is a finding inconsistent with previous visual fields. Sometimes the patient just has "a bad day" and is unable to pay careful attention to the demands of the testing procedure.

While the SITA-STANDARD protocol is somewhat more likely to show subtle field changes, the increased efficiency with the SITA-FAST test has led to its routine use in our high-volume glaucoma practice. We routinely employ "white-on-white" stimulus parameters, preserving the "blue–yellow" for select glaucoma suspects. Patients with advanced visual field loss are examined with 10-2 visual field protocols. The Humphrey FDT machine (in various forms) is only used by us for occasional community-based, glaucoma screening events.

Kinetic visual field testing with the classic Goldmann perimeter is rarely performed in our practice. Some state motor vehicle driver license bureaus require kinetic field testing and will not accept static Zeiss-Humphrey protocols. Unfortunately, in the twenty-first century, few ophthalmic assistants and technicians are proficient in performing manually based Goldmann field testing, because of the common use of the automated perimeters.

It is important for the ophthalmic physician to keep an open mind when examining visual field reports. While the retinal anatomy of nerve fiber bundles results in glaucomatous visual field defects that respect the horizontal meridian (arcuate scotomas), one must not ignore and should in fact search for other visual field findings suggestive of other pathologies. I have had several patients who had been followed by other ophthalmologists for glaucoma, who also had bitemporal hemianopsias that reflected chiasmal lesions (pituitary adenomas). They indeed had glaucomatous arcuate defects in their visual fields, but they had neurological field defects respecting the vertical meridians as well.

See Chap. 23 for a discussion of visual fields and other functional tests for glaucoma and Chap. 25 for interpretation of visual fields that are suggestive of nonglaucomatous optic neuropathy.

7. *Confrontation Visual Fields:* The assistant performs confrontation visual fields every time the patient is examined in our office, unless a recent formal Humphrey or Goldmann test report is available for physician review (Box 13).

8. *Pupillary Responses to Light:* A penlight is used to measure both direct and consensual pupillary responses to light in a darkened room. Although recorded on the second page of the exam form, this is among the first tasks the assistant does as part of the examination. The patient is asked to look toward a spot on a distant wall to avoid the near accommodation reflex that would constrict the pupils. The light beam is directed from slightly below the patient's visual axis, again to avoid near accommodation. The assistant reminds the patient to look in the distance should they attempt to look toward the penlight. The "swinging-flashlight test"[17] (described in Chap. 15) is used to determine the presence or absence of a relative afferent pupillary defect[17] (Relative Afferent Pupillary Defect (RAPD) or Marcus-Gunn pupil). Finding such a RAPD suggests asymmetric damage to the optic nerves, with the eye exhibiting the RAPD likely having more glaucomatous neuropathy. If the patient is new to my practice or if this is the first time an APD has been noticed in an established patient, the assistant asks me to personally observe this phenomenon before dilating drops are placed in the patient's eyes. The shape, size, and responsiveness to light are noted in the consult form on the chart in Boxes 18 and 19 on page 2.

If a RAPD is observed, the physician should briefly glance at the visual field printouts if available (before a more formal interpretation). There is generally good agreement between the comparative severity of visual field defects between the two eyes and the finding of a relative afferent pupillary defect in the eye with greater visual field loss.[18]

9. *Tonometry:* Assistants are trained not to perform tonometry on patients with symptoms suggesting ocular infection (e.g., conjunctivitis, contact lens-related corneal ulcer) or ocular trauma (e.g., corneal abrasion). These patients are first seen by the physician who will determine if tonometry is indicated or should be postponed. We routinely employ Goldmann applanation tonometry in our office and the assistant records these values in Box 17, page 2. The portable TonoPen device (Reichert Instruments, various distributors) is used for those patients who cannot be reliably applanated at the slit-lamp (e.g., very obese patients, patients with irregular corneas).

Assistants are encouraged to recheck any IOPs they are unsure of as to accuracy, by having a different assistant repeat the measurement or by asking the physician to do so. We train them not to put pressure on the globe when trying to hold eyelids open, and to make sure that the patient is not squeezing closed the eye that is not being applanated. Some patients have a psychological need for the physician rather than the assistant to perform tonometry and we accommodate them when they make such a request.

For established patients in the practice, we ask that the assistant request another assistant to recheck any IOPs that are higher or lower by two mmHg from the IOPs found on the patient's previous visit to our office, if no intervention (e.g., new medications, surgery) has occurred.

Newer forms of tonometry,[19] with technologies that incorporate "corrections" for central corneal thickness and corneal hysteresis (e.g., Dynamic Contour Tonometer, Ocular Response Analyzer) may eventually supplant the traditional Goldmann applanation technique that has been the gold standard for more than 100 years. More information about these devices is presented in Chap. 8.

Some physicians specifically write into the chart a single target value for IOP reduction[20,21] based on their examination. As discussed in Chap. 51 on medical therapy, we prefer and highly endorse the concept of a target IOP "range," which is reevaluated and modified each visit as the clinical situation warrants. I do not include a specific place on the consultation form for this information, rather it may be written into the physician's recommendations section in Box 21 on page 2.

Studies[22-24] by Robert Weinreb and his colleagues at the University of California San Diego suggest that patients may have their highest IOPs during the night when they are sleeping and supine. Dr. Weinreb (personal communication) feels that measuring the patient's IOP in the office environment, both sitting up and after 5 min of being recumbent in the examination chair, may simulate the situation that occurs when the patient is at home at night, sleeping and supine. It is necessary to use the same instrument for both measurements, for example, a TonoPen (community environment) or pneumotonometer (academic environment). In some patients, the supine IOP may be five or more mmHg higher than the IOP measured when the patient is sitting up. We find that this clinical pearl is useful for patients who have achieved what we felt were adequate target pressures, but who nonetheless were having their glaucoma progress. They may simply be having much higher pressures outside the office visit time than during their office examination.[25,26]

After performing tonometry the assistant escorts the patient to a waiting area. The medical chart is placed in the bin outside the examination lane being used by the physician.

### 28.2.3 The Role of the Physician in Interviewing and Examining the Patient

I personally escort the patient from the waiting area to one of my examining lanes. I introduce myself to new patients (e.g., "Good morning, Mrs. Johnson. I'm Dr. Schacknow and I'll be examining you after we go over your medical history and reasons for coming to see me."), shake their hand, and ask them to sit in the examining chair and have any accompanying person sit in a second chair we have in each lane. For established patients, my greeting remarks always include some questions about their general health, significant social events that may have transpired since their last visit to my office, and any specific questions they have about medication use or side effects and any change in their vision. For the new ("consult") patients, I thoroughly review the intake documents, the Glaucoma Consultation Report form sections completed by the ophthalmic assistant, and any visual fields. I may ask some questions about medication use and compliance, further elaborate on reputed medication allergies, clarify details about previous laser or incisional surgeries, and verbally review with the patient significant highlights of their medical history. I use Box 12 of the form to record my interpretation of the visual field report. Box 15 is used for notes, and additionally I write in any of the sections of the first page where something must be clarified or elaborated upon.

## 28.3 Slit-Lamp Examination: Part One

I begin my examination of the patient by asking them to remove their spectacles (if any) and place their chin into the chin-rest of the slit-lamp, with their forehead pressed against the plastic band. I make adjustments to the height of the slit-lamp and/or the examining chair as needed to ensure patient comfort and proper positioning for the examination. My observations about the anterior segment of each eye are recorded in the appropriate sections of page 2 of the Glaucoma Consultation Report form.

### 28.3.1 Extraocular Muscles

I note any strabismus or restrictive eye disease (thyroid orbitopathy[27]) that may relate to increased IOP in certain positions of gaze.

### 28.3.2 Lids

I manually lift each upper eyelid, looking for signs of previous eye surgery and any pathology. Lid margins are evaluated for blepharitis and trichiasis, findings that could potentially compromise glaucoma surgery and also indicate the presence of ocular surface disease. Hypertrichosis[28] is common in patients on hypotensive lipid (HL) therapy. Similarly, hyperpigmentation[29] of the periorbital skin is common with the HLs. Figure 28.1 shows a patient with hypertrichosis and periorbital skin changes and unilaterally using bimatoprost in the right eye.

### 28.3.3 Pupils

I review the notes made by the ophthalmic assistant regarding the pupils. I correlate any noted RAPD with visual field findings.[30] It is worth reviewing old photos, including those on a driver's license, for a history of anisocoria (unilateral

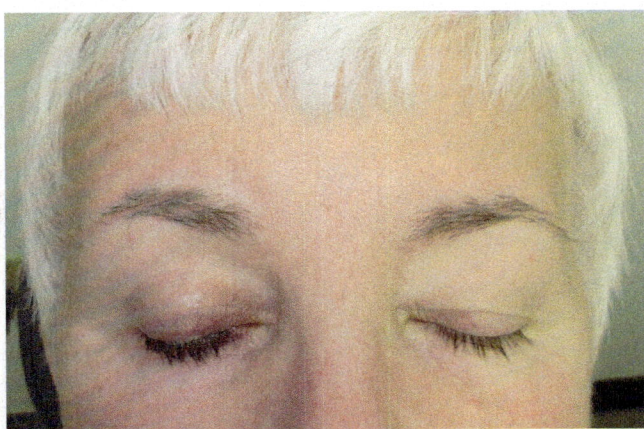

**Fig. 28.1** Patient using bimatoprost only in right eye. Periorbital skin changes and hypertrichosis are noted unilaterally. (Courtesy of Drs. T.A. Shazly and M.A. Latina)

use of miotics or dilating agents, old trauma, Horner's syndrome[31] (Fig. 28.2), Adie's tonic pupil[32]) or other unusual pupil findings. Pupils that do not readily dilate with drops may have had long-term exposure to miotics, posterior synechiae, or previous surgery or trauma. An attack of acute angle-closure glaucoma with very high IOP may result in a nonmotile iris even after the attack is broken.[33]

### 28.3.4 Iris

I note the presence (or absence) and location of iridotomies (previously narrow angles or acute angle closure); heterochromia (Fig. 28.3) (Fuch's heterochromic iridocylcitis[34,35] (Fig. 28.4), siderosis,[36] congenital Horner's syndrome,[37] unilateral use of HLs); rubeosis[38] (Fig. 28.5a, b) (neovascularization of the iris: CRVO, proliferative diabetic retinopathy, ischemic syndrome); transillumination defects[39] (pigmentary dispersion syndrome or glaucoma) (Fig. 28.6); pseudoexfoliation (Fig. 28.7a, b) material at the pupil margin[40]; moth-eaten appearance of the iris (iridocorneal-endothelial (ICE) syndrome[41] (Fig. 28.8) or related diseases); and nodules[42] (Koeppe nodules: inflammatory cell precipitates at the pupillary margin found in nongranulomatous as well and granulomatous uveitis; Bussaca nodules on the iris surface: which are pathognomonic for granulomatous uveitides such as sarcoidosis). Iris bombe (Fig. 28.9), a forward bowing of the iris, occurs when the pupil margin is completely bound down to the lens with posterior synechia. The forward pressure of the fluid in the posterior chamber causes the bowed appearance. Portions of the iris may be touching the corneal endothelium. Peripheral laser iridotomies, often needed in several places around the iris, will relieve this forward pressure and allow the iris to flatten to its normal position. Iris bombe may occur in both phakic and pseudophakic eyes with untreated uveitis.[43–45]

### 28.3.5 Conjunctiva

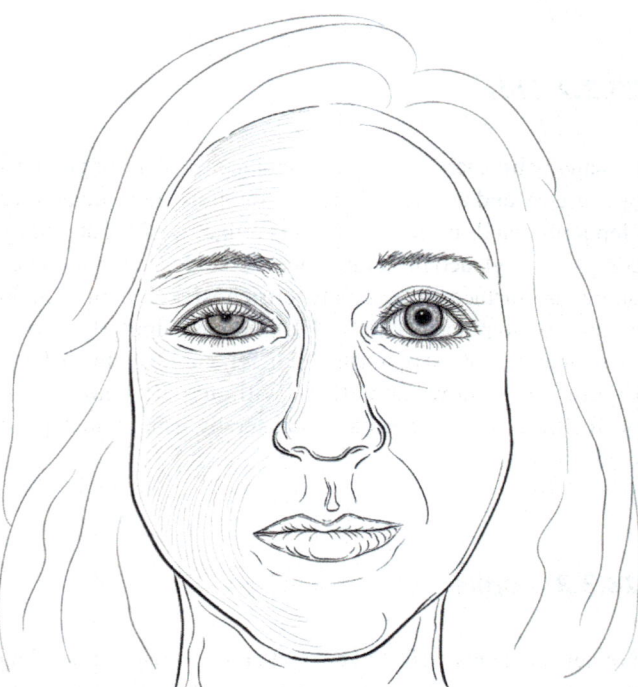

**Fig. 28.2** Horner's syndrome, *right side*. Note ptosis, miosis, and anhidrosis

The patient is requested to look downward while I simultaneously lift their upper lid. I inspect the superior conjunctiva

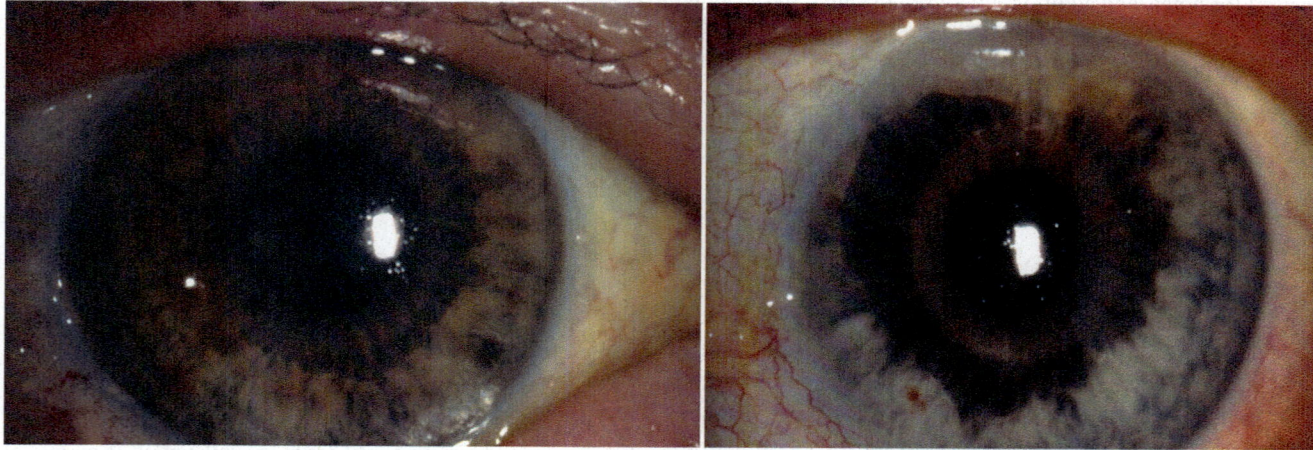

**Fig. 28.3** Heterochromia of irides. The right eye is darker than the left eye. (Image courtesy of http://www.medicalmediakits.com)

for the presence of a filtering bleb (Fig. 28.10), and if it is found, I note its location, size, shape, and quality (cystic, flat, overhanging the cornea, scarred, etc.) If glaucoma tube shunt surgery has occurred, I described the conjunctiva's appearance and the presence of any scleral patch graft. I notice if there are any leaks from either kind of glaucoma surgery (Seidel's test, using sterile fluorescein strips to "paint" the area of the bleb that appears to leak). I release their upper lid and ask them to look forward. I note any hyperemia, possible secondary to chronic use of glaucoma medications (and also ask about itching, burning, etc.). I look for the presence and location of any subconjunctival hemorrhages (Fig. 28.11) and review the patient's use of aspirin, Plavix, Coumadin, etc. I ask them to look upward and inspect the lower portion of the bulbar conjunctiva. Upper and lower palpebral conjunctival areas are examined if there is significant lid margin disease or symptomatic complaints by the patient. If glaucoma surgery is being contemplated I search for areas of "virgin" conjunctiva to place new incisions.

### 28.3.6 Cornea

The epithelial surface, stroma, and endothelial layers of the cornea are examined using both broad and thin slit beams. I have found it increasingly helpful to take the 15 s of extra "chair time" required to do a tear breakup time (TBUT)[46,47] test for each eye. Chronic exposure to glaucoma medications, which contain toxic benzalkonium chloride (BAK)[48] as well as the natural aging process, may lead to symptoms of ocular surface disease[49] and patient distress. Place a drop of

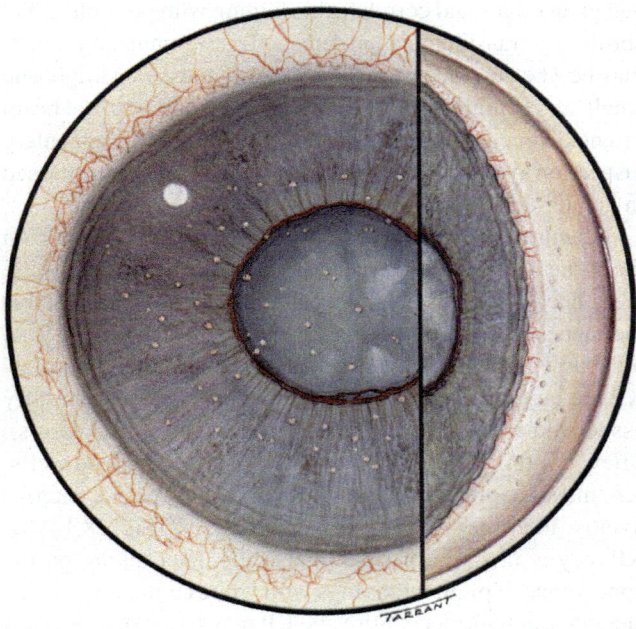

**Fig. 28.4** Fuch's heterochromic iridocyclitis. Stellate keratic precipitates are noted. (Courtesy of Terry Tarrant and Alcon Labs, Fort Worth, Texas)

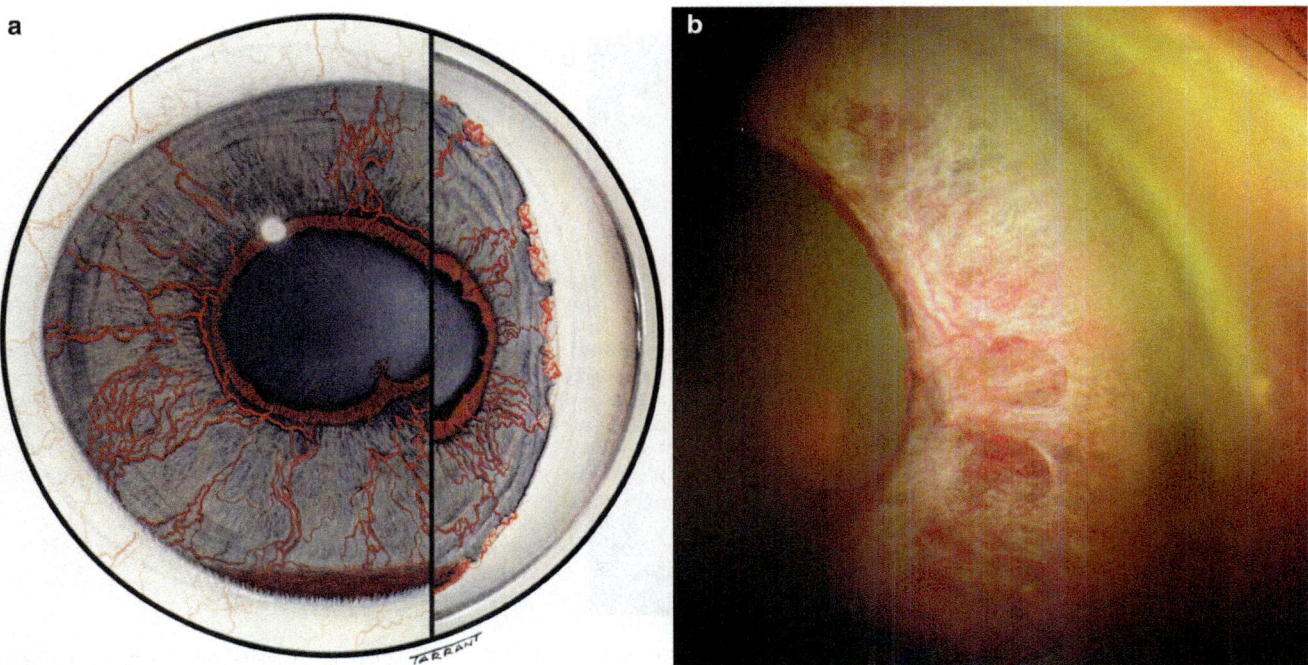

**Fig. 28.5** (**a**) Rubeosis iridis. Fragile blood vessels occur in the iris and anterior chamber angle. (**b**) Rubeosis iridis, clinical photo. Neovascularization of the iris is a response to ischemia. (Courtesy of Terry Tarrant and Alcon Labs, Fort Worth, Texas)

fluorescein with anesthesia on the eye, have the patient blink, and observe the corneal surface through the slit-lamp with the blue light engaged. Normal TBUTs are 10 s or longer in duration. Additionally, damaged epithelium may be detected using sterile lissamine green strips.[50] It stains devitalized corneal and conjunctival epithelium and is much gentler to the eye and patient friendly than rose bengal[51] solution.

We examine the endothelial surface for Krukenberg spindles[52] – an isosceles triangle-shaped deposition of melanin pigment found in the central posterior cornea (Fig. 28.12) associated with pigmentary dispersion syndrome (see Fig. 28.6) and glaucoma – and correlate this finding with possible radial slit-like iris transillumination defects. Transillumination defects may best be observed by making the slit-lamp beam bright and small, and shining it directly through the pupil with the beam oriented directly in front of the eye, not obliquely. Pigmentary dispersion syndrome and pigmentary glaucoma are discussed in greater detail in Chap. 38.

Inflammatory keratic precipitates (KP) (Fig. 28.13) seen on the corneal endothelial surface are indicative of uveitis. These are collections of inflammatory cells. When the uveitis is active they appear white. They may appear as pigmented residua from old, burned-out inflammatory disease. So-called "mutton-fat" KP are larger, have a greasy appearance, and are generally associated with granulomatous diseases (e.g., sarcoidosis). They contain both macrophages and epithelioid cells. KP may be present in all forms of nonspecific anterior uveitis. In Posner–Schlossman syndrome,[53,54] (Fig. 28.14) the KP may at first appear small and white, later taking on the appearance of pigmented rings with white centers. In Fuch's Heterochromic Iridocyclitis[55] the KP may be small and have a stellate appearance (Fig. 28.15). All forms of anterior segment inflammation may at first lead to increased intraocular pressure because of cellular debris and an inflamed trabecular

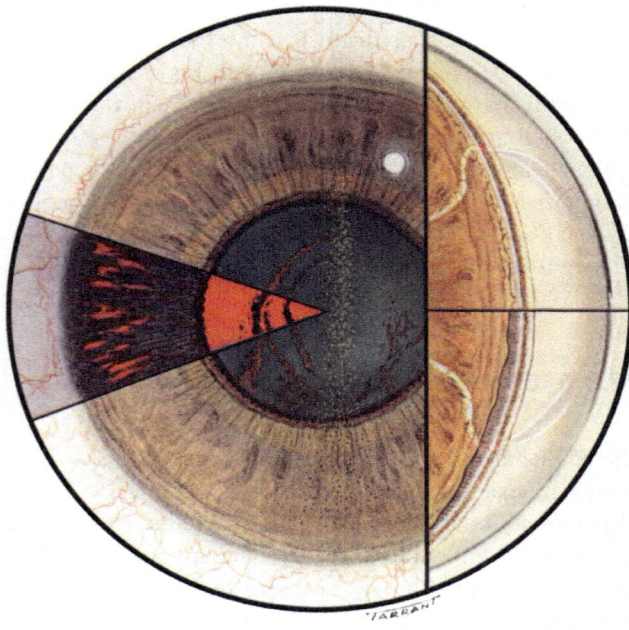

**Fig. 28.6** Pigmentary dispersion syndrome and glaucoma. Transillumination defects of the iris and a krukenberg pigment spindle are noted. (Courtesy of Terry Tarrant and Alcon Labs, Fort Worth, Texas)

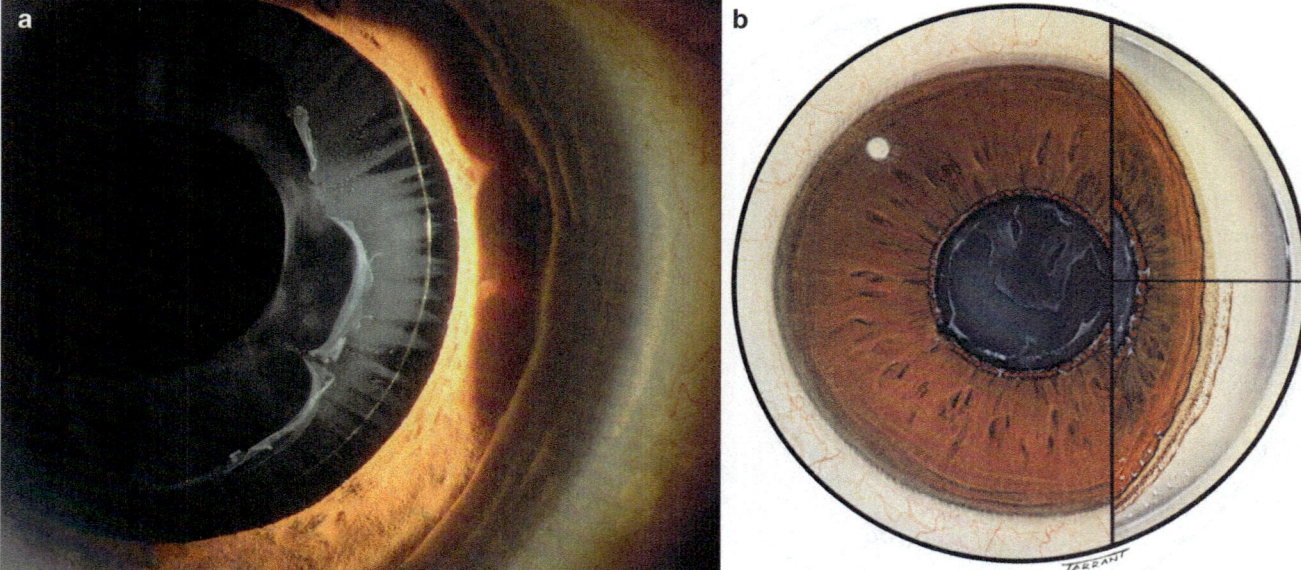

**Fig. 28.7** (a) Exfoliation syndrome, clinical photo. "Dandruff-like" pseudoexfoliation material is seen on the anterior lens capsule and pupillary margin. (Image courtesy of Michael P. Kelly, CPT, Duke Eye Imaging, Duke University Eye Center, Durham, North Carolina with permission of EyeNet, American Association of Ophthalmology.) (b) Exfoliation syndrome. Sampaolesi's line seen in the angle results from deposition of the exfoliative material anterior to Schwalbe's line. (Courtesy Terry Tarrant and Alcon Labs, Fort Worth, Texas)

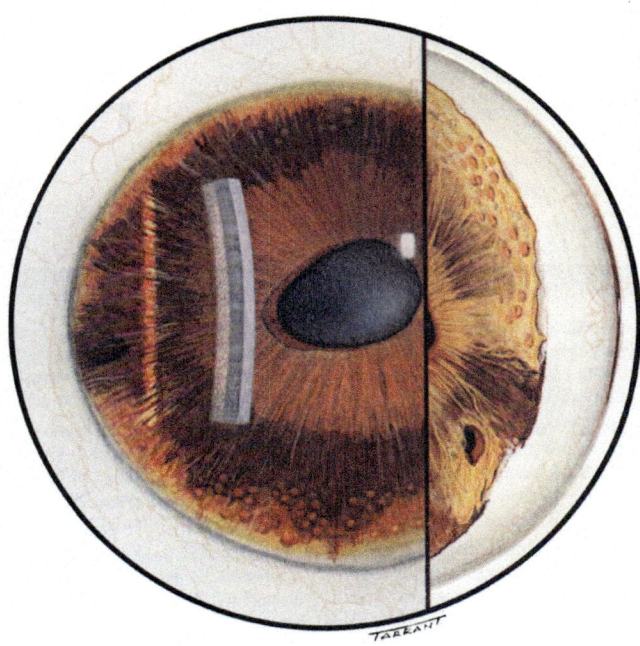

**Fig. 28.8** ICE (iridocorneal-endothelial) syndrome. Corneal edema, moth-eaten appearance of the iris, and difficult to control glaucoma are common features. (Courtesy Terry Tarrant and Alcon Labs, Fort Worth, Texas)

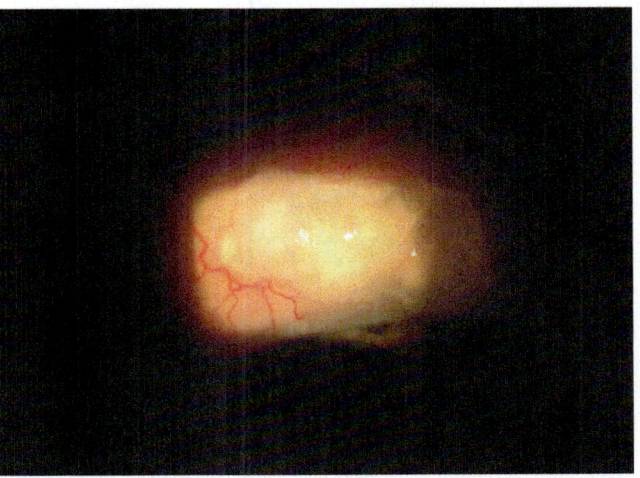

**Fig. 28.10** Filtering bleb. This bleb is fairly thin and cystic as may occur with the use of antimetabolites such as mitomycin-C. (Courtesy of Drs. T.A. Shazly and M.A. Latina)

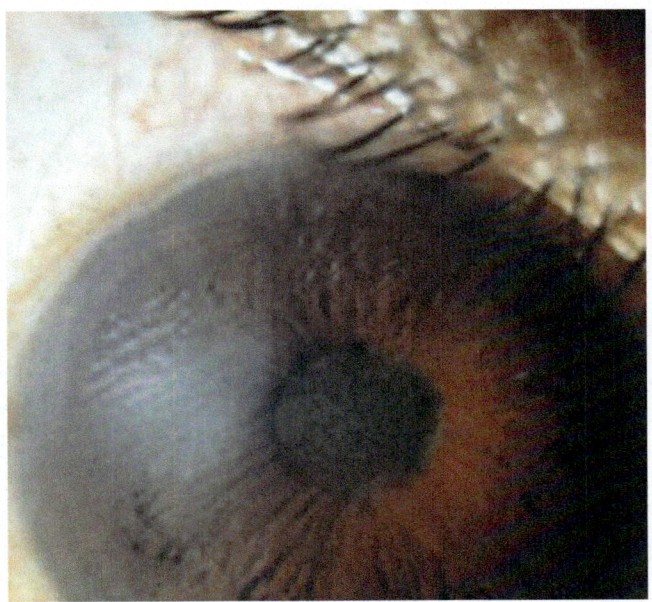

**Fig. 28.9** Iris bombe. Posterior synechia completed seclude the iris causing a forward bowing with resultant angle-closure glaucoma. Laser iridotomies are curative.

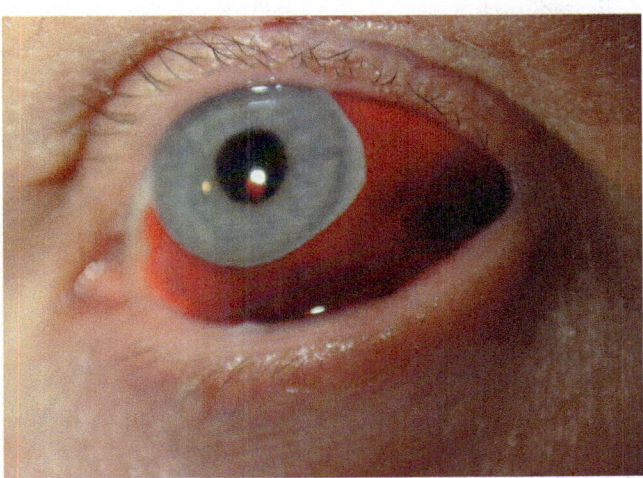

**Fig. 28.11** Subconjunctival hemorrhage. Painless accumulation of blood under the conjunctiva that usually results from rubbing, coughing, or Valsalva maneuver. Rarely related to blood dyscrasia. Frightening to patients who should be reassured that it is not sight threatening. (Image courtesy of http://www.medicalmediakits.com)

meshwork, while later inflammation of the ciliary body may lead to a decreased production of aqueous humor, and a fall in intraocular pressure.[56] Posner–Schlossman Syndrome is further discussed in Chap. 42, while Fuch's Heterochromic Iridocyclitis is elaborated upon in Chap. 43.

Aging changes of the corneal endothelium may appear as guttatae, focal thickenings of Descemet's membrane (Fig. 28.16). These may be indicative of early Fuchs' endothelial dystrophy[57–59] (Fig. 28.17), a dominantly inherited, usually bilateral disease more common in women than men, usually presenting in patients older than 60 years of age. Patients with early or late Fuchs' endothelial dystrophy may be more likely to suffer bullous keratopathy (corneal edema) after intraocular surgery (cataract or glaucoma filter). Younger, asymptomatic individuals may exhibit Hassall–Henle bodies,[60] wart-like guttatae at the peripheral regions of the corneal endothelium. Fuchs' endothelial dystrophy is more fully explored in Chap. 48.

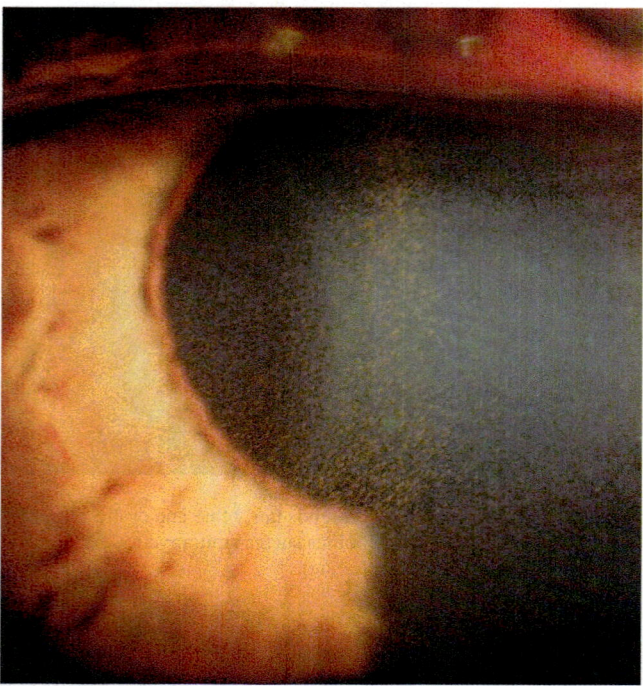

**Fig. 28.12** Krukenberg pigment spindle – "pine tree" shaped deposition of pigment on corneal endothelium. Comes from pigment liberated from rear of iris as it scrapes lens zonules in predisposed individuals. (Image courtesy of http://www.medicalmediakits.com)

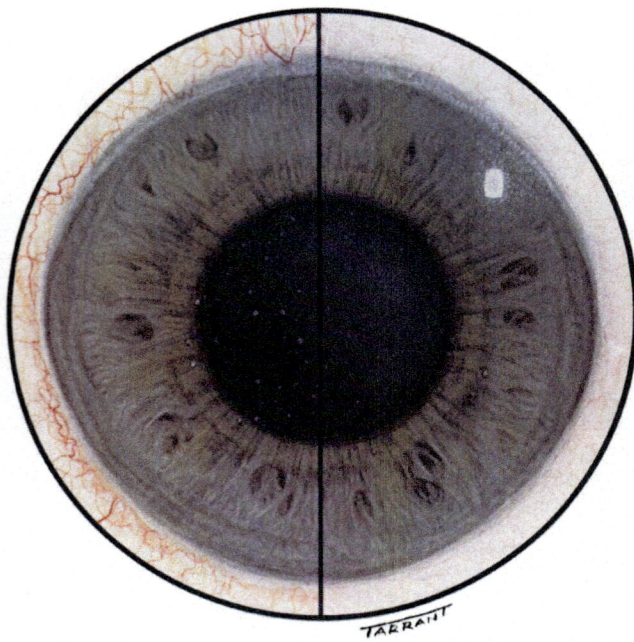

**Fig. 28.14** Posner–Schlossman syndrome (glaucomatocyclitic crisis). The morphology of the KP may vary with the stage of the disease. (Courtesy Terry Tarrant and Alcon Labs, Fort Worth, Texas)

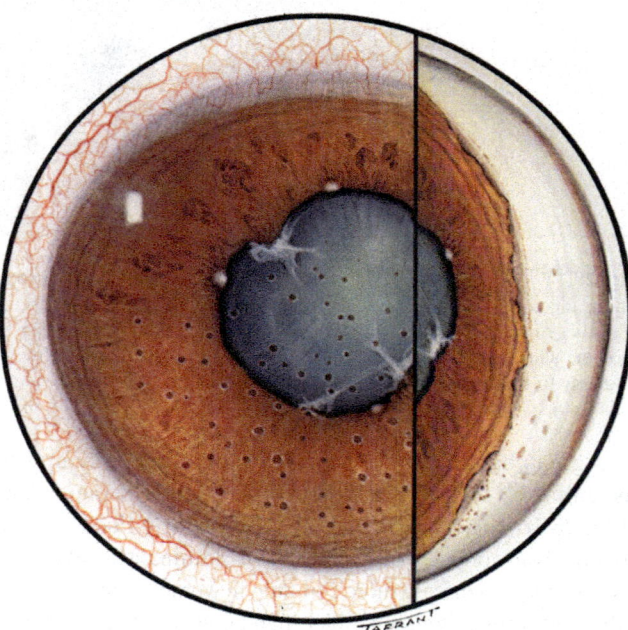

**Fig. 28.13** Inflammation of the anterior segment of the eye. Keratic precipitates form on the endothelium. (Courtesy Terry Tarrant and Alcon Labs, Fort Worth, Texas)

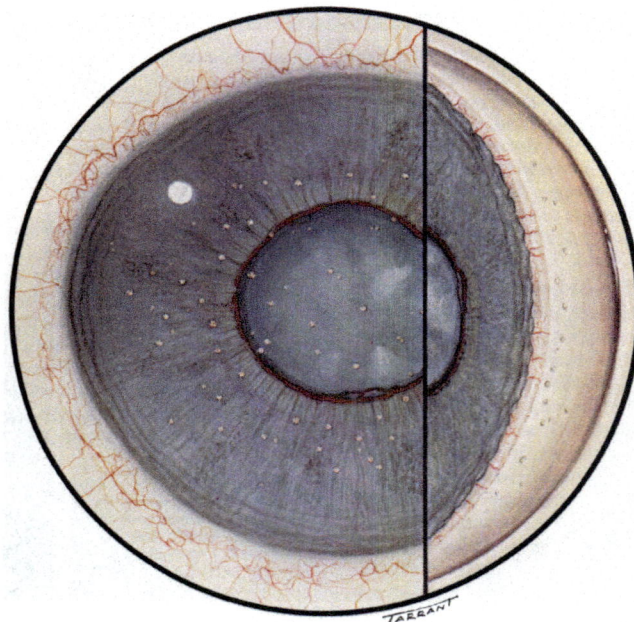

**Fig. 28.15** Fuch's heterochromic iridocylcitis – fine white stellate KP may be present. The affected eye appears hypopigmented compared to the patient's other eye. (Courtesy Terry Tarrant and Alcon Labs, Fort Worth, Texas)

If present, I comment on the appearance of an arcus senilis (Fig. 28.18), which represents lipid deposition in the peripheral corneal stroma. When opaque, an arcus may make it difficult to aim laser light through the cornea blocking the attempt to create a truly *peripheral* iridotomy for patients with narrow anterior chamber angles. Arcus may appear in

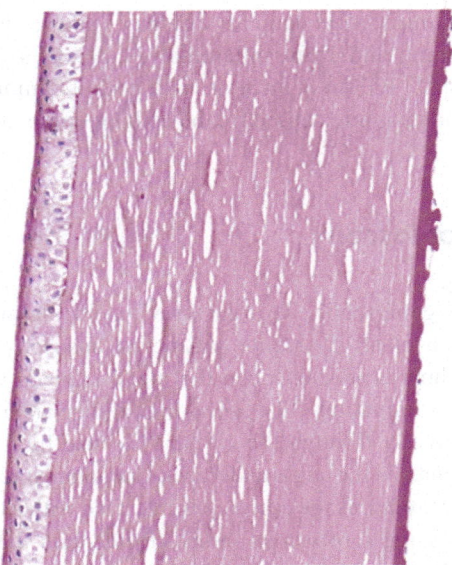

**Fig. 28.16** Guttata are excrescences on the surface of the corneal endothelium, often a sign of aging. Found commonly in Fuch's endothelial dystrophy. (Image courtesy of http://www.medicalmediakits.com)

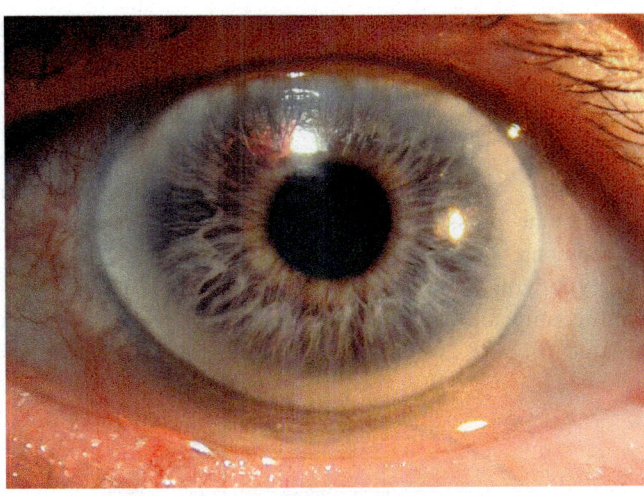

**Fig. 28.18** Arcus senilis is a *grayish-whitish* arc or ring found in the periphery of the cornea. It causes no visual symptoms. It is more common in older individuals. If found in young patients it may be associated with hypercholesterolemia, hyperlipidemia, or hyperlipoproteinemia. (Image courtesy of http://www.medicalmediakits.com)

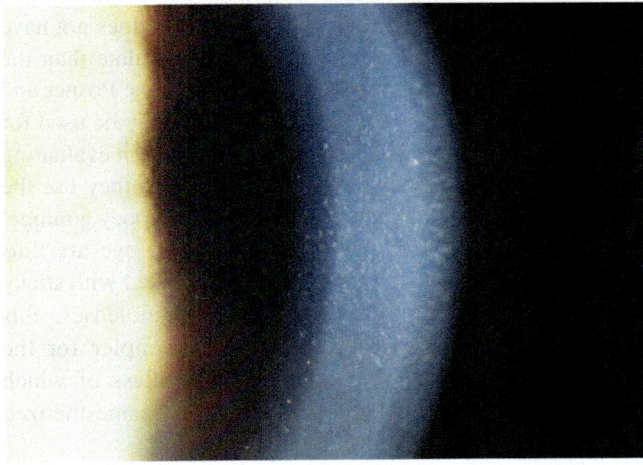

**Fig. 28.17** Fuch's endothelial dystrophy, clinical photo. Guttata are seen on the back of the corneal endothelium. (Image courtesy of http://www.medicalmediakits.com)

some persons at a young age (often associated with familiar hyperlipidemia), but is more commonly found in the elderly (hence the name).

Finally, I describe the condition (e.g., clear and compact, edematous, folds in Descemet's membrane, neovascularized, opaque) of any penetrating keratoplasty (PKP, corneal transplant) that may be present. The presence or absence of sutures, and whether or not the knots are buried, is described in the chart notes.

### 28.3.7 Anterior Chamber

The anterior chamber (AC) is evaluated for its depth (normal, shallow centrally, or peripherally) and whether or not inflammation is present. The presence and degree of cells, flare (protein), hyphema (blood), or hypopyon (layered white cells) are noted. Cells and flare are evaluated by using a thin and narrow slit-beam in a darkened room, to observe the Tyndall effect of light scattering off particles (cells) in a suspension. This is similar to the phenomenon of observing dust particles in the light beam of the projector in a darkened movie theater. Patients with uveitis are often light sensitive and are discomforted by light intensities that need be no stronger than that found in indoors with normal incandescent lighting levels. This patient symptom and complaint suggests uveitis and directs your examination to search for cell and flare. Uveitic glaucomas are more fully explored in Chap. 41.

Blood in the AC (hyphema) may be diffused or layered. Trauma is the most likely cause. Fragile abnormal blood vessels on the iris (rubeosis) or in the angle may bleed. This neovascularization may be due to proliferative diabetic retinopathy, following central retinal vessel occlusion, branch retinal vein occlusion, or ocular ischemic syndrome. Inquires must be made about blood dyscrasias (including sickle cell anemia) and the use of anticoagulants. Blood cells can clog the trabecular meshwork and raise intraocular pressure.[61] If the IOP is raised high enough and long enough, blood staining of the cornea may occur.[62]

Mechanical chaffing of the iris by an intraocular lens, usually an anterior chamber lens, can liberate blood and cause the so-called UGH syndrome (uveitis, glaucoma, and hyphema).[63,64]

Ghost cells – pale tan remnants of blood in the vitreous – may be seen in slit-beam or may layer inferiorly in the anterior chamber (Fig. 28.19). They may also clog the trabecular meshwork, usually transiently, and can cause a rise in intraocular pressure.[65] Chapter 47 elaborates on these phenomena.

Hypopyon – a layering of inflammatory cells inferiorly in the anterior chamber – may be sterile or infection related (Fig. 28.20). Hypopyon can result from infectious endophthalmitis, from neoplastic diseases such as leukemia or lymphoma and from inflammatory diseases of many etiologies.[66–72] IOP may increase with both inflammation of the TM and clogging caused by the cellular components.

## 28.4 Gonioscopy

I perform gonioscopy, in a darkened room, at the initial examination of all glaucoma patients or suspects, without regard to how obviously open the angle appears to be on slit-lamp examination. The anterior chamber angle cannot be seen directly through the cornea, because light coming from structures in the angle undergoes total internal reflection. A goniolens replaces the cornea–air interface with a different interface having a refractive index greater than that of the cornea. Direct gonioscopy provides a direct view of the angle and indirect gonioscopy shows a reflected image from a mirror of a portion of the angle across the anterior chamber. Direct gonioscopy using Keoppe lenses is rarely performed outside of the academic environment.

I prefer to use the indirect Posner goniolens (Fig. 28.21a, b) or the similar Zeiss goniolens. These have four mirrors and thin metal handles. The indirect Sussman lens does not have a handle. While a bit more difficult to manipulate than the more traditional three-mirror Goldmann lens, the Posner and Zeiss devices have two advantages: (1) they may be used for indentation gonioscopy,[73] especially helpful when evaluating narrow or slightly appositional angles; and (2) they use the patient's tear film as an interface, requiring no gooey goniogel coupling agent.[74] Further observations of the eye are thus unimpeded by a corneal surface that is *not* coated with sticky methylcellulose. With the Posner/Zeiss goniolenses, this portion of the glaucoma examination is simpler for the physician and easier for the patient. Regardless of which goniolens is used, the patient's eye must first be anesthetized with a topical agent such as proparacaine.

Please note that the silvered outer surface of these prisms may be scratched easily. When I first take possession of a new Posner or Zeis goiniolens, I coat the outer surface with two layers of clear nail polish that seals the surface and prevents scratches.

I take note of the following anterior chamber angle structures (Fig. 28.22):

*Ciliary Body Band (CBB):* This is the most posterior structure in the angle. Normal color variations include pink, gray, and brownish tints. The CBB tends to be wider in myopic eyes and narrower in hyperopic eyes. Angle recession may be observed after blunt trauma. There may be a history of hyphema. Angle recession results from tears to the ciliary body along the longitudinal and meridional muscles. (Increased IOP secondary to angle recession may occur many years

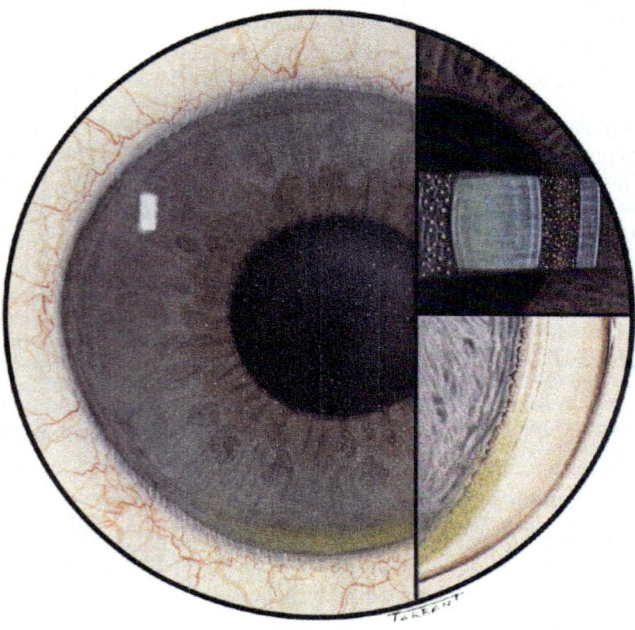

**Fig. 28.19** Ghost cell glaucoma. Pale cell membranes of old blood may be seen in the vitreous or anterior chamber. They may clog the trabecular meshwork and raise intraocular pressure. (Courtesy Terry Tarrant and Alcon Labs, Fort Worth, Texas)

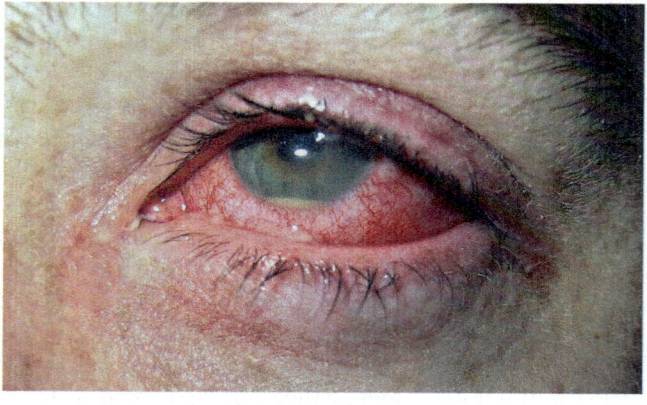

**Fig. 28.20** Hypopyon. Layered collections of white blood cells may be seen in the inferior portion of the anterior chamber in response to infection or severe inflammation. (Image courtesy of http://www.medicalmediakits.com)

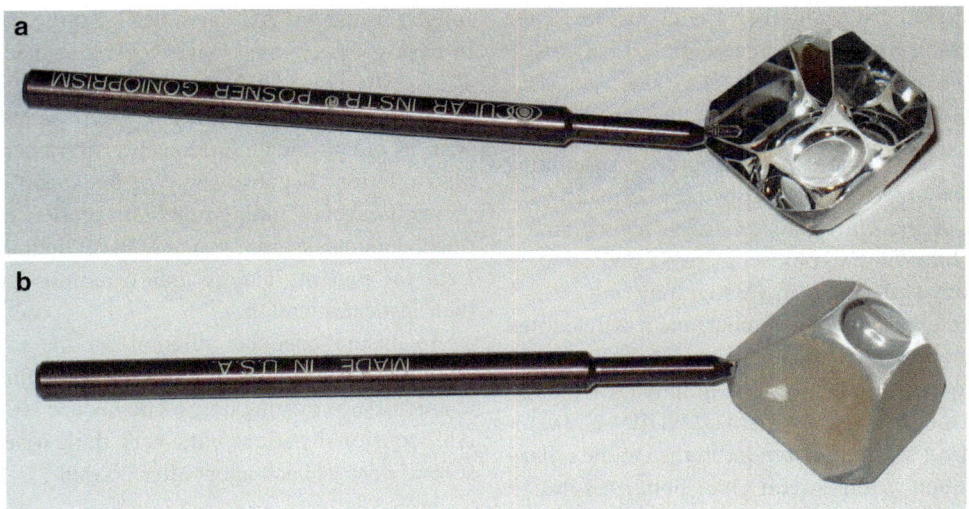

**Fig. 28.21** (a) Posner style goniolens – in this view the side facing the examiner is seen. This lens requires only the patient's tears as a coupling agent. (b) The outside surface of the lens has been coated with opaque "nail polish" to help prevent scratching of the material used to provide the mirrored surface.

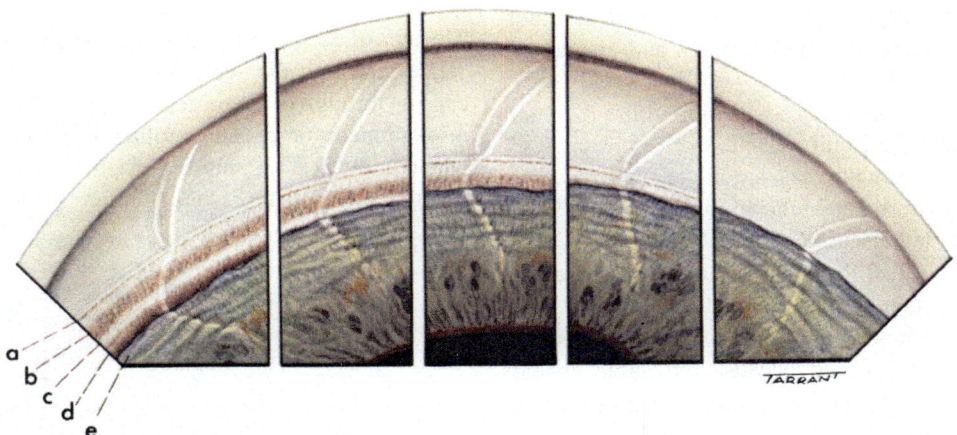

**Fig. 28.22** The normal anterior chamber angle as seen gonioscopically. (Courtesy Terry Tarrant and Alcon Labs, Fort Worth, Texas)

after the trauma – patients with angle recession should be made aware of this potential future problem and be examined every year.[75])

*Scleral Spur (SS):* This is the most anterior projection of the sclera. The longitudinal muscle of the ciliary body is attached to the scleral spur. On gonioscopy, SS is found just posterior to the trabecular meshwork. It appears as a narrow, whitish band.

*Trabecular Meshwork (TM):* The TM extends from the scleral spur to Schwalbe's line. The posterior section starting at the SS is pigmented, with a grayish-blue translucent hue. The anterior section begins at Schwalbe's line. It has a whitish color. Only the pigmented portion functions to pass aqueous from the eye. Increased pigmentation of the TM is observed often in patients with pigment dispersion syndrome[76] or pseudoexfoliation syndrome.[77]

*Schwalbe's Line:* This opaque line is the most forward structure of the anterior chamber angle. It arises from the anterior termination of the TM and the edge of the corneal Descemet's membrane. I note the presence of peripheral anterior synechiae, iris processes, the quantity and quality of trabecular meshwork pigmentation, presence or absence of Sampaolesi's Line[78] (pigment deposited anterior to Schwalbe's Line, often seen in pseudoexfoliation syndrome or pigment dispersion syndrome), abnormal appearance of angle vessels or neovascularization,[79] and occasionally the presence of a foreign body or neoplasm in the anterior chamber angle. I estimate the degree of angle width using a modified simple Shaffer system[80] I–IV notation, from slit to narrow (I) to wide open (IV). I report the findings in Box 16 on page 2 of the consult form.

There is an art as well as a science to appropriately examining the anterior chamber angle by gonioscopy (see Chap. 26). Dr. Wallace Alward, of the University of Iowa, has created a superb Website (http://www.gonioscopy.org/) dedicated to teaching gonioscopy skills through videography.

Gonioscopy is inexpensive, convenient, and a skill learned fairly easily. Academic medical centers may have access to anterior segment optical coherence tomography (AS-OCT)[81] and/or ultrasound biomicroscopy (UBM).[82,83] UBM can visualize anterior segment structures from the cornea to the ciliary body. Higher frequency ultrasound gives better resolution but poorer penetration. UBM employs immersion techniques similar to B-scan ultrasonography. AS-OCT has higher resolution than UBM but poorer penetration. Newer AS-OCT machines have good sensitivity and specificity for diagnosing appositional angles.[84]

These newer imaging modalities have been useful in examining anterior segment tumors[85,86] as well as elucidating mechanisms behind pupillary block and plateau iris syndrome.[87,88]

Each machine has proponents advocating its use for determining the potential occludability of anterior chamber angles.[89] Devices under development may automate the process of determining the depth of the anterior chamber angle.[90] See Chap. 27 for a detailed discussion of UBM and AS-OCT.

Our group has not had the luxury of using these various instruments in the community setting. Fortunately, laser peripheral iridotomy has a high benefit-to-risk ratio, so the occasional eye that is lasered because the angle appears occludable on gonioscopy but is not truly occludable, seems a reasonable price to pay for those many eyes that will avoid acute angle closure.

## 28.5 Dilation

Dilating drops are placed in the new patient's eyes after they have undergone the anterior segment slit-lamp exam (excluding the lens), gonioscopy, and visual field testing. The patient then sits in a waiting area for about 20 min to allow for maximum effect of the drops. Their chart is placed into a bin adjacent to one of the examining lanes being used by the physician.

I routinely have patients dilated every 6 months, and as signs and symptoms indicate. Established patients returning for periodic examinations, known to have normal depth to their anterior chambers, may be dilated by my assistants before I examine either their anterior or posterior segments. (This assistant is required to use the slit-lamp beam to get a rough estimate of AC depth before using the dilating drops, in case gross changes have occurred since the last exam.) This saves considerable time with the office routine in a high-volume practice, because each patient must only be seen by the physician once each visit, rather than before and after dilation. Because some patients skip or miss appointments, I have a standing rule that experienced assistants may dilate patients or order visual fields at their discretion, before I see the patient, if more than 6 months have passed since their last examination.

To ensure adequate dilation for the posterior segment examination, I routinely use phenylephrine 2.5% and tropicamide 1% as dilating drops. I do not use 10% phenylephrine. An occasional patient with very dark irises will require a second dose of each agent after 20 min.

## 28.6 Slit-Lamp Examination: Part Two

### 28.6.1 Lens

The lens of each eye is examined using a narrow slit-beam to "slice" through the sections of the lens from the anterior capsule through to the posterior capsule. The anterior capsule is examined for pseudoexfoliation material and pigment. Glaucomflecken[91] – small, grayish, anterior subcapsular or capsular opacities representing infarcts (Fig. 28.23) – may be

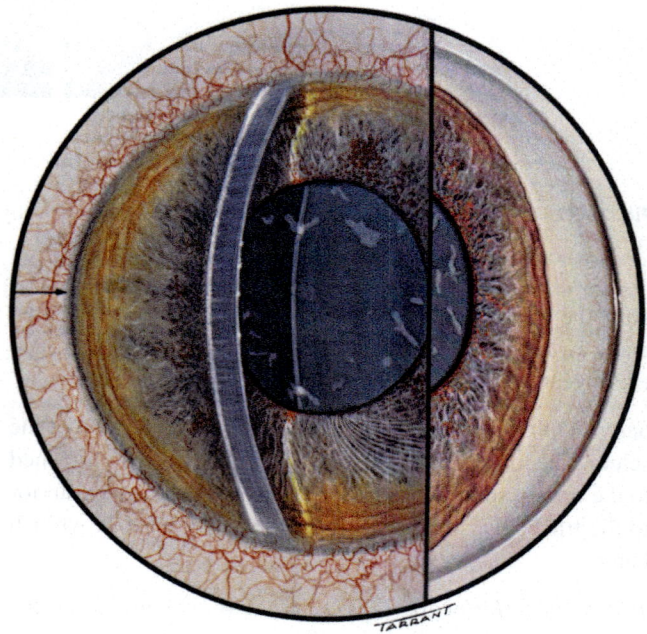

**Fig. 28.23** Acute angle-closure glaucoma sequellae – glaucomflecken represent infarcts of the lens capsule resulting from the acute high intraocular pressures. (Courtesy Terry Tarrant and Alcon Labs, Fort Worth, Texas)

present within the pupillary area (after high intraocular pressure secondary to acute angle-closure glaucoma). Posterior synechiae are noted and described. Cataract (anterior polar, nuclear sclerotic, posterior subcapsular) is indicated in the chart notes. The nature of any pseudophakic lens (anterior chamber, iris fixated, or posterior chamber) is described. Opacification of the posterior lens capsule is noted if present. The shape and extent of any posterior capsulotomy is described.

### 28.6.2 Posterior Segment: Macula to Midperipheral Retina

#### 28.6.2.1 Vitreous

The anterior portion of the vitreous is examined at the slit-lamp using a thin and intense beam of light. I look for floaters, asteroid hyalosis, hemorrhage, and pigment. The posterior vitreous (I look for posterior vitreous detachment (PVD)), macula, vessels, and optic nerve are usually examined with a 78+ diopter lens. Some glaucoma specialists prefer 60+ or 90+ diopter lenses, but I have found the 78+ diopter lens adequate for the fundus examination. The images are viewed with up–down and left–right reversal. I rarely use the direct ophthalmoscope unless a patient cannot be dilated.

#### 28.6.2.2 Macula

I note the presence of macula pathology, such as age-related macular degeneration, cystoid macular edema, retinal holes and epiretinal membranes.

#### 28.6.2.3 Midretina

Here I look for background or proliferative diabetic retinopathy, laser scars from photocoagulation, or other lesions. I carefully search for any pigmented or raised lesions.

### 28.6.3 Optic Nerve and Retinal Nerve Fiber Layer

Examination and documentation of the structure of the optic nerve is, of course, perhaps the most important part of the glaucoma examination performed by the physician. See Chap. 15 for an excellent discussion of the optic nerve and retinal nerve fiber layer and Chap. 18 for a further elaboration of the optic nerve head appearance; Chap. 16 discusses the laminar substrates of optic disk cupping; Chap. 19 teaches how to evaluate glaucomatous optic nerve progression and describes the significance of optic disk hemorrhages; and Chap. 25 considers evaluation of the optic nerve when changes may not be glaucomatous but neurological. Here I will just highlight some of the basic features of examining the optic nerve for glaucoma.

I note and record both the vertical and horizontal cup-to-disk ratios. I comment if the disk is much larger or smaller than average. I note signs of focal notching. The "ISNT rule"[92] is a useful rubric for looking at the thickness of the rim of the optic nerve: Generally, most healthy optic nerves have the thickest rim *inferiorly*, followed next by the *superior*, *nasal*, and *temporal* regions (thinnest). This rule is only a heuristic used to guide your examination, being accurate only about 60% of the time.[93] Arcuate visual field defects correspond to thinning of these rims, but with a left–right, up–down, reversed presentation. For example, thinning of the inferior rim of the optic disk results in a superior visual field defect.

The degree and location of pallor is observed.[94] Disk hemorrhages, peripapillary atrophy (alpha and beta zones), collateralized vessels (from ischemia), optociliary shunt vessels, optic disk pits, and optic disk drusen are noted. If the patient brings optic disk photos, or if I have them available from a previous visit to our office, I compare these images to the live examination findings with the high plus diopter lens.

I do not take red-free photos for examination of the retinal nerve fiber layer (RNFL). I have come to rely on the new digital imaging devices (GDx, OCT) for this kind of information, even though some of the finer details are lost. In this case the convenience of using the RNFL imaging devices has outweighed any information lost about localized wedge defects that might have been seen on the red-free photos.

### 28.6.4 Posterior Segment: Peripheral Retina

The peripheral retina is examined using a binocular indirect ophthalmoscope with a 20+ diopter lens. Patients whose history or examination requires them to have sclera depression for adequate peripheral retinal view are referred to retinal colleagues within my group practice.

After completing the exam and recording my findings on the consultation form, I summarize my observations for the patient and accompanying guests, along with my suggestions for further testing, if any, and a treatment plan. I also use page 2 of the consultation form to record brief observations about the mental status of the patient with respect to our interactions, and initial the space provided that indicates

I have talked with the patient and family members about their disease and course of treatment. I provide the patient with written information about glaucoma, medications use and side effects, and laser and incisional surgeries if these have been recommended.

Prescriptions for glaucoma medications are written on preprinted forms I have created (Fig. 28.24). These are kept in pads of 50 sheets each in a drawer at each examination lane. Use of these preprinted forms saves time and helps avoid medication errors due to poor handwriting by me or my assistants. On subsequent visits, the assistant inquires about the need for patient refills and prepares the appropriate prescriptions for my signature during the assistant's part of the exam. This also saves time for the physician. I occasionally have to discard one of these filled out prescriptions, because of medication intolerance or lack of efficacy and complete additional prescription forms reflecting new medications. But for the vast majority of established patient visits I simply review and sign the preprinted forms, for refills, completed by my assistants.

I use Box 22 on page 2 of the consultation form to schedule future visits and testing procedures. When seeing a returning patient, the assistant reviews this portion of the previous note to understand what testing is required before I examine the patient on that visit. The patient is then presented to the office clerk who schedules their next appointment and any testing (visual fields, image analysis). Finally, patients who are dilated and who need fundus photos are escorted to our technical department for optic nerve head photos. Charts containing photos are placed on my desk for review to be done by me at the end of the clinical day.

We thus conclude the protocol we generally use for all patients new to the practice that are being examined for glaucoma or for glaucoma suspect status. Returning or "established" stable patients are generally treated in much the same manner, usually seen every 3 or 4 months, with the scheduling of repeat visual fields at 6-month to 12-month intervals, dilation about every 6 months, and optic nerve head photos and/or digital imaging analysis of the optic nerve and retina at about 12-month intervals. We use the Established Patient Report form (Appendix 8), to direct the exam and record the findings. It is a modified version of the form used for the new patient (consult) examination. Patients with active glaucoma-related problems or uncontrolled intraocular pressure are seen as frequently as necessary to

**Your Practice Name and Logo Goes Here**

Patient ______________________ Phone ____________

Address ______________________ Date ____________

ALPHAGAN P 0.10 % 0.15%
AZOPT 1%
BETAGAN 0.25% 0.5%
BETIMOL 0.25% 0.5%
BETOPTIC 0.25%-S
BRIMONIDINE 0.2%
COMBIGAN
COSOPT
ISTALOL 0.5%
LUMIGAN 0.03%
OCUPRESS 1%
PILOCARPINE 1% 2% 4%
TIMOLOL 0.25% 0.5% GFS
TIMOPTIC 0.25% 0.5% XE
TRAVATAN Z 0.004%
TRUSOPT 2%
XALATAN 0.005%

DIAMOX 250 MG REGULAR / 500 MG SEQ NEPTAZANE 25 MG 50 MG
ALREX 0.2% LOTEMAX 0.5% VEXOL 1%
PREDNISOLONE ACETATE 0.125% / 1%
ATROPINE 1% CYCLOGYL 1%
TOBRADEX MAXITROL POLY-PRED DROPS / UNG
POLYSPORIN UNG VIGAMOX PATADAY 0.2% PATANOL 0.1%

**DISPENSE:** 2.5 ML 5 ML 10 ML 15 ML 30 60 #___ TABLETS
ONE TUBE 90 DAY SUPPLY **REFILLS:** 0 1 2 3 4 6 12
**SIG:** ONE GTT APPLY 1/4 INCH UNG RIGHT / LEFT / BOTH EYE(S)
QAM QHS BID TID QID EVERY 1 2 4 6 12 HOUR(S)
ONE TABLET BY MOUTH ***PLEASE LABEL CONTAINER***

***GOOD MAN, M.D., Chief of Glaucoma Services***
NY 00566008 *Brand Medically Necessary*

**Glaucoma, The Sneak Thief of Vision**
***"Working together we can safeguard the precious gift of sight."***
***Your Practice Name***
***5000 10th Avenue, North Somewhere, NY (564) xxx -0707***
***102 Jones Way Elsewhere, NY (564) xxx-1111***

**Fig. 28.24** An example of a preprinted prescription form

bring the disease under control, with medications, laser treatments, and incisional surgeries added to their treatment protocol as necessary.

## 28.7 Additional Considerations

### 28.7.1 Digital Image Analysis of the Optic Nerve and Retinal Nerve Fiber Layer

Astute observers will no doubt have noticed that we did not include provisions for using the newer digital image analysis machines in the protocol for examining new glaucoma patients or suspects. Generally, we prefer to get a visual field before or on the first office visit, and a film-based optic nerve head photo as well, rather than a digital image analysis. We do this for two reasons: first a pragmatic one of not wanting to exhaust the patient, and second the fiscal one, that most insurance entities (such as Medicare) will not pay for digital image analysis and optic nerve head photo (and, in some cases, visual field test) performed on the same day. Thus, for those patients in whom we feel one of these tests is appropriate, we schedule it to be done before or on a subsequent visit. I do not order digital image analysis routinely or periodically on all patients in my glaucoma practice. I have found the GDx machine helpful in making the decision about whether or not to begin treatment in glaucoma suspect patients with borderline intraocular pressures, borderline optic nerve head, and visual field changes.

Unlike some university centers, our ophthalmology group practice does not own each of the three image analysis machines (GDx, HRT, and Stratus-OCT). I mostly utilize the current incarnation (2008 version) of the GDx machine with variable corneal compensation. It employs scanning laser polarimetry of the retinal nerve fiber layer to produce images. Analysis is done by a neural network derived set of parameters with a normative database. Our retina service has a Stratus-OCT device that is available to me. Our practice does not have an HRT device available nor one of the new spectral domain optical coherence tomography machines.

Each apparatus has its champions and its usefulness. I have found the GDx machine helpful in making the decision as to whether or not to begin treatment in glaucoma suspect patients with borderline intraocular pressures, and borderline optic nerve head and visual field changes. In my conversations with glaucoma specialists around the globe, I have learned that most physicians are not yet ready to use these machines to judge glaucomatous progression. The hardware frequently changes, and, most importantly, the software is constantly upgraded. Normative and pathological databases are being added to the newer software packages all the time.

Clearly it is hoped that these objective, structural, digital analyzers would achieve sufficient standardization, reliability, and functionality to become in the future as valuable as digital visual field testing is currently. Further discussion of digital image analysis is provided in Chaps. 20 and 21, while devices in developmental stages are discussed in Chap. 90.

### 28.7.2 Indigent Patients

Some of the patients who attend my practice have difficulty affording physician fees, managed-care mandated copayments, and, most importantly, glaucoma medications. Some patients are unaware of medically related insurance programs for the indigent, such as Medicaid and local county assistance programs. We help them to apply for these programs when appropriate for their situations. Our billing department works out monthly payment plans that greatly assist some of these patients. For some patients who are elderly and poor we simply provide free care.

More challenging are the patients who cannot afford their glaucoma medications on a continuing or intermittent basis. Almost all patients, well-to-do or less fortunate economically, request sample bottles of eyedrops – some patients on every office visit. The pharmaceutical companies supply us with only a limited number of what they euphemistically refer to as "starter" bottles of drops. We try to limit the distribution of these samples to those patients who appear to us to be truly in difficult economic circumstances. Additionally, the pharmaceutical companies have fairly generous programs to provide free glaucoma medications to those patients who can demonstrate true financial need. It does place a resource burden on our staff to help patients fill out multiple forms, for us to receive shipments of drops designated for patients, and to distribute them to patients. Nonetheless, we do enroll patients in these programs for free medications as part of our ethical responsibility as a medical practice even though it is costly to us in resources used.

### 28.7.3 Refill Requests and Physician Phone Calls

Phone calls and facsimile requests for refill prescriptions are reviewed and acted upon by one of my ophthalmic assistants. They compare the request to the medications prescribed in the patient's chart, and also check to see that the patient has been seen by me or one of the group's physicians within the past 6 months. If they have a question about the appropriateness of a refill request, they defer action until they confer with me. Patients who have not been seen in 6 months are called and told that we will provide one refill only on emergent basis, but that in order to receive subsequent refills they must make an appointment to be seen by me or another physician in our group.

Patient phone calls about medication irritation or allergies or other glaucoma-related issues are first reviewed by an assistant, and anything other than simple questions are passed to me. I return patient phone calls at lunch time and at the end of the clinical day (or sooner if the concern is urgent). Telephone calls from physicians are taken immediately (I excuse myself from the examination lane if I am with a patient) or in some cases returned in between patient examinations.

### *28.7.4 Consultation Reports and Dictations*

All physicians referring patients to my practice for glaucoma consultation are sent written reports. For ophthalmologists and optometrists, I dictate a formal, personalized, consultation report describing my findings and treatment recommendations. I do this in between patient examinations, when the information is fresh in my mind and the chart is in front of me. For primary care physicians, and for the managed-care insurance companies that require a report of the patient's visit, I generally use a simple form to report this information. An example of this form may be seen as Appendix 9. I complete this form while I am still in the examination lane with the patient.

## 28.8 Conclusion

The comprehensive examination of the patient for glaucoma will continue to evolve both as we learn more about the disease process and as newer diagnostic technologies become available. Genetic testing for glaucoma variants, more objective and reliable structural optic nerve analyzers with progression analysis capabilities, and compliance monitoring devices will all aid us in the future to perform the best examinations we can. No instruments, however, can surpass the diagnostic acumen of the experienced and prepared physician who makes careful observations and who is aware of the signs and symptoms corresponding to glaucoma and other ophthalmic diseases.

## 28.1 Appendix 1: Medical History Questionnaire (MHQ)

Appendix A – Medical History Questionnaire

**MEDICAL HISTORY QUESTIONNAIRE**

Name _____ Date _____

Date of **birth** _____ Date of **last eye exam** _____

List any **medications** you currently take (prescription and over-the-counter):
_____
_____

Do you have **allergies** to any medications?  ☐ YES  ☐ NO
If YES, list the medications:
_____

List all **major illnesses** (glaucoma, diabetes, high blood pressure, heart attack, etc.) or **injuries** (concussion, etc.):
_____
_____

List any **surgeries** you have had (cataract, tonsillectomy, appendectomy):
_____
_____

Do you *currently* have any problems in the following areas? If "YES", please provide information.

| | YES | NO | Explanation of Problem |
|---|---|---|---|
| **EYES** (Glaucoma, cataract, retinal disease, etc.) | | | |
| Loss of vision | | | |
| Blurred vision | | | |
| Fluctuating vision | | | |
| Distorted vision (halos) | | | |
| Loss of side vision | | | |
| Double vision | | | |
| Dryness | | | |
| Mucous discharge | | | |
| Redness | | | |
| Sandy or gritty feeling | | | |
| Itching | | | |
| Burning | | | |
| Foreign body sensation | | | |
| Excess tearing/watering | | | |
| Glare/light sensitivity | | | |
| Eye pain or soreness | | | |
| Infection of eye or lid (blepharitis, stye) | | | |
| Tired eyes | | | |
| Crossed eyes, lazy eye | | | |
| Drooping eyelid | | | |
| **GENERAL/CONSTITUTIONAL** | | | |
| Fever | | | |
| Weight loss | | | |
| Other | | | |
| **EARS, NOSE, THROAT** (Sinus, ear infection, chronic cough, dry mouth, etc.) | | | |
| **CARDIOVASCULAR** (Heart, vessels, etc.) | | | |

| | | | |
|---|---|---|---|
| **CARDIOVASCULAR** (Heart, vessels, etc.) | | | |
| **RESPIRATORY** (Asthma, emphysema, etc.) | | | |
| **GASTROINTESTINAL** (Stomach ulcers, intestinal disease, etc.) | | | |
| **GENITAL, KIDNEY, BLADDER** | | | |
| **MUSCLES, BONES, JOINTS** (Arthritis, etc.) | | | |
| **SKIN** (Acne, warts, skin cancer, etc.) | | | |
| **NEUROLOGICAL** (Multiple sclerosis, etc.) | | | |
| **PSYCHIATRIC** (Anxiety, depression, insomnia) | | | |
| **ENDOCRINE** (Diabetes, hypothyroid, etc.) | | | |
| **BLOOD/LYMPH** (cholesterolemia, anemia, etc.) | | | |
| **ALLERGIC/IMMUNOLOGIC** (Hay fever, lupus, Sjogrens, etc.) | | | |

## FAMILY HISTORY

M=mother   F=father   S=sibling
GP=grandparent

| DISEASE | YES | NO | RELATIONSHIP TO PATIENT |
|---|---|---|---|
| Blindness | | | |
| Glaucoma | | | |
| Arthritis | | | |
| Cancer | | | |
| Diabetes | | | |
| Heart disease or high blood pressure | | | |
| Kidney disease | | | |
| Lupus | | | |
| Stroke | | | |
| Thyroid disease | | | |
| Other | | | |

## SOCIAL HISTORY

Current occupation: _____
Education (high school, vocational school, college degree): _____
Marital Status (married, divorced, single, widowed): _____
Living Arrangements: _____

Do you drive? ☐ YES ☐ NO
Do you have visual difficulty when driving? ☐ YES ☐ NO
Do you have problems with night vision? ☐ YES ☐ NO
Have you ever tried to wear contact lenses? ☐ YES ☐ NO
Do you currently wear contact lenses? ☐ YES ☐ NO
If YES, how long have you worn contact lenses? _____
Do you currently wear glasses? ☐ YES ☐ NO
If YES, how long have you had the current prescription? _____
Do you drink alcohol? ☐ YES ☐ NO    If YES:   occasional    1 per day    2-3 /day    4+ /day
Do you smoke?       ☐ YES ☐ NO    If YES:   occasional    ½ pack/day   1 pack/day   1+ pack
Have you ever had a blood transfusion? ☐ YES ☐ NO
History reviewed.    ☐ No Changes.    ☐ Additions as noted above.

Patent's Signature: _____ Date: _____

Physician's Signature: _____ Date: _____

## 28.2 Appendix 2: New Patient Welcome Letter

**GOOD MAN, MD**
Chief of Glaucoma Services

> **Appendix B**
>
> New Patient Welcome Letter

Dear New Patient:

Thank you very much for making an appointment to see me in consultation for glaucoma. I and my staff welcome you to our office. Let me tell you some of the things we will be doing during your visit here.

Your *glaucoma evaluation* may include several tests. For example, you may have your "field of vision" tested, a procedure which takes about 10 minutes for each eye. For scheduling reasons, this test may have been done before your visit with me today. My ophthalmic assistants will check your eyesight and measure the internal pressure of each eye (tonometry). They may measure the thickness of the cornea of each eye (central pachymetry). I will examine the structure of each eye under magnification through a slit-lamp biomicroscope. Then I will inspect the internal drainage system of each eye with a special lens (gonioscopy). Finally, we may use eye drops to dilate (enlarge) your pupils. This will allow me to look at your optic nerves and retinas. Often we take photographs or digital images of the optic nerves to compare with observations at future visits. The examination and tests are painless, but after I dilate your pupils, you will be sensitive to bright lights for several hours. Family members are welcome to observe the examination and to participate in our discussion about your eye problems.

Follow up glaucoma examinations for stable patients are usually done every three to four months. Patients usually have visual field examinations every six to eight months. Photography or digital imaging, and gonioscopy, are generally repeated at yearly intervals. Additional testing may be performed as indicated by your clinical condition.

The physicians at Visual Health want to provide you with the best possible eye care at the most reasonable cost. Fees for your *glaucoma evaluation* will vary with the services provided and the type of your medical insurance. I won't need to repeat any tests completed by your primary eye-care doctor, if I can obtain these results as part of your medical records. (My staff will provide you with forms to request your medical records from previous physicians.) Many patients now participate in "managed-care" insurance plans including HMOs that do not require "out of pocket" expenses for ophthalmology examinations, except perhaps for a small co-payment due at the time of your visit. However, these plans often do **require** some form of *"written approval"* or *"referral authorization,"* from your primary care physician. It is most important that you obtain and bring these referral forms with you to our office *or your examination may need to be rescheduled.*

We know that medical expenses are a major part of a family's budget. We will work with you to obtain the maximum allowable benefits for you under your medical insurance. If you have no insurance, or only limited insurance, we can set up a plan to help you pay your medical bills. Please ask your registration counselor for assistance. For your convenience, payment for services may be made with cash, check or major credit card.

**Your *glaucoma evaluation* will take about 90 minutes**. Please allow sufficient time in your schedule. I promise to answer all your questions and to do my best to teach you about your eye condition. I look forward to meeting you. Working together we can help to safeguard the precious gift of sight.

Good Man, M.D.

## GLAUCOMA - THE SNEAK THIEF OF VISION
Good Man, M.D.,

Glaucoma is the second most important cause of permanent blindness among the entire population of the United States (just behind macular degeneration) and the single most important cause of irreversible blindness among African Americans. Glaucoma is associated with a family history of the disease, being over 40 years old, nearsightedness, diabetes and migraine headaches.

What causes glaucoma? The eye is filled with a clear, watery fluid called aqueous humor. This fluid provides nourishment for the eye and helps it to maintain its round shape. The fluid must be drained from the eye as rapidly as it is produced. If the drainage system becomes clogged or blocked, excessive fluid pressure builds up within the eye. This pressure may damage the delicate optic nerve fibers found at the back of the eye, resulting in glaucoma, and loss of side vision at first. If untreated, eventually the entire optic nerve will be destroyed causing total blindness. Vascular factors (blood circulation) may also play a role in glaucoma. Research is ongoing to better understand glaucoma and to develop new therapies.

There are many different forms of glaucoma. Most kinds of glaucoma usually lack early symptoms. Thus, glaucoma is truly *"The Sneak Thief of Vision."* Vision lost from glaucoma is never regained. Fortunately, this devastating loss of sight is largely preventable through early diagnosis and treatment. The tests for glaucoma are simple and painless.

Glaucoma may usually be controlled with eye drops (and sometimes pills) taken every day throughout the patient's entire life. These medications act to decrease eye pressure either by helping the flow of fluid out of the eye or by decreasing the amount of fluid entering the eye. For some patients medications are poorly tolerated or not effective in controlling their glaucoma. For many of these individuals, a brief outpatient treatment with the ophthalmic lasers may help to reduce their eye pressure. In some cases, traditional glaucoma microsurgery may become necessary to form a new drainage pathway within the eye.

**Patients with all types of glaucoma need periodic eye examinations, generally 3 to 4 times a year, after their glaucoma has stabilized with treatment. Glaucoma sometimes gets worse without the patient being aware of it, requiring a change in treatment. As a rule, the optic nerve damage caused by glaucoma is permanent.** Drops, pills and surgery may prevent further eye damage from occurring, helping to preserve vision.

**Control of glaucoma by drugs can only be effective if patients take their medications on the treatment schedule prescribed by their doctor. Don't stop medication without first consulting your eye doctor. If you experience side effects, call and let us know. If your prescription glaucoma medications are running low, please call my office or have your pharmacy call my office to request refill authorization. You should NOT wait until your next scheduled appointment before obtaining refill prescriptions, nor do you have to make a "special" trip to my office. Do not run out of your medications; just call my office when you get low on your current supply.** Also, it is important to tell all of your physicians about your eye medications. Remember, to save *your* vision, *you* must help your eye care practitioner.

PLEASE READ THE INFORMATION BELOW AND SIGN WHERE INDICATED *AFTER* YOUR EXAMINATON

I acknowledge that I have read the information on both sides of this brochure and that I have been given a copy of it to take home. I acknowledge that I understand all the information presented in this brochure and that Dr. Schacknow has personally answered all my questions regarding my diagnosis and all recommended medical and/or surgical treatments for my eye conditions or diseases. I fully understand that it is *my* obligation to make sure that I see Dr. Good Man or any ophthalmologist of my choosing for follow-up glaucoma examinations every three to four months (or more often if so directed), for visual field examinations every six to eight months, and for optic nerve photography and gonioscopy at yearly intervals. I understand that glaucoma is a chronic, life-long condition that can result in permanent blindness. <u>I understand that my glaucoma may get worse without producing any symptoms such as pain or decreased vision, and that the only way to check on the stability of my glaucoma is by periodic visits with a qualified ophthalmologist.</u>

Patient (or representative): _____ Medical record # _____ Date: __/__/__

Family Member: _____ Witness: _____ Translator: _____

(French, Spanish, _____)

## 28.3 Appendix 3: Consent for Dilation

> Appendix C – Consent for Dilation

## Consent for Dilating Eye Drops
## Important Notice About Driving After Dilation

Dilating eye drops are used to dilate or enlarge the pupils of the eye to allow the ophthalmologist to get a better view of the inside of your eye. This will allow your ophthalmologist to better examine your retina and optic nerves.

Dilating drops frequently blur vision for a length of time that varies from person to person. During this time period you may find bright lights bothersome. You should wear your sunglasses if possible. "Disposable" sunglasses are available at the appointment checkout area. Please ask the clerk for a pair of them if you did not bring your own sunglasses with you.

It is not possible for your ophthalmologist to predict how much your vision will be affected or exactly how long the blurring effect or diminished vision will last after your examination. Because driving may be difficult immediately after an examination, it's best if you make arrangements not to drive yourself from the office. You should come to the office with a driver. If your vision is blurred, please do not attempt to drive. You should wait in our office until your vision returns to normal. This may take two to three hours. If necessary our office staff can assist you in arranging for alternative transportation.

*I hereby authorize Dr. GOOD MAN and/or such assistants as may be designated by him to administer dilating eye drops to me as part of my eye examination today and as part of future eye examinations should he feel that they are needed to diagnosis and treat my eye conditions. I am not aware of any allergies that I may have to dilating eye drops. I will not attempt to drive a motor vehicle from Dr. Good Man's office until my eyesight is no longer blurry from dilating drops, or, I will have someone else drive me from his office, now and on future visits when I am to be dilated.*

Patient's name (PLEASE PRINT) _____  Date: _____

Patient's signature: _____  CHART # _____

Witness: _____

## 28.4 Appendix 4: Consent for Medical Photography

> Appendix D – Consent for Medical Photography

### CONSENT FOR MEDICAL PHOTOGRAPHY

In connection with the ophthalmologic services that I am receiving from my physician, Dr. GOOD MAN, I consent that photographs may be taken of me or parts of my body, under the following conditions:

1. The photographs may be taken only with the consent of my physician and under such conditions and at such times as may be approved by him.

2. The photographs shall be taken by my physician or by a photographer approved by my physician.

3. The photographs shall be used for medical records and if, in the judgment of my physician, medical research, education or science will be benefited by their use, such photographs and information relating to my case may be published and republished, either separately or in connection with each other, in professional journals or medical books, or used for any other purpose which he may deem proper in the interest of medical education, knowledge, or research; provided, however, that it is specifically understood that in any such publication or use I shall not be identified by name.

4. The aforementioned photographs may be modified or retouched in any way that my physician, in his discretion, may consider desirable.

Patient's name (PLEASE PRINT) _____    Date: _____

Patient's signature: _____    Chart # _____

Witness: _____

## 28.5 Appendix 5: Physician's Practice Brochure

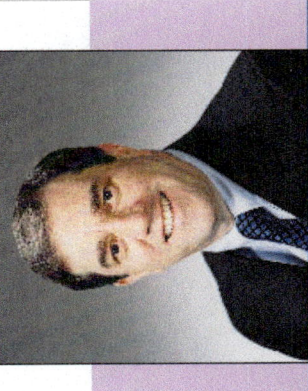

# VISUAL HEALTH
SPECIALISTS IN SIGHT

Paul N. Schacknow M.D., Ph.D., ophthalmologist is Chief of Glaucoma Services at Visual Health. He is a specialist in the medical, laser and surgical treatment of glaucoma patients. Dr. Schacknow, a native of Brooklyn, New York, did not take the typical career path to become a physician. He finished his undergraduate degree in psychology with honors at Brooklyn College and then completed his Ph.D. in auditory and visual psychophysics at the City University of New York. He was a college professor for the next seven years, teaching and doing research in the Division of Natural Sciences, State University at Purchase, New York. Seven years into his professorial career, he decided to undertake medical studies.

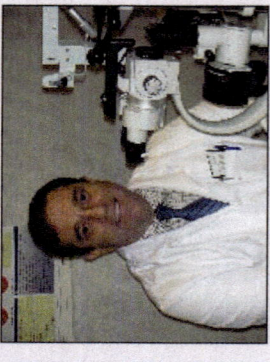

He entered the unique, accelerated, curriculum of the Ph.D. to M.D. Program at the University of Miami, receiving the Doctor of Medicine degree in 1983 after 23 months of study and training. He followed his medical and surgical internship at Framingham-Union Hospital in Massachusetts, with an ophthalmology residency at Harvard Medical School, at the world renowned Massachusetts Eye and Ear Infirmary. His formal ophthalmology training concluded in San Francisco at California Pacific Medical Center, with a fellowship in glaucoma management.

Dr. Schacknow is certified by the American Board of Ophthalmology. He is a Fellow of the American Academy of Ophthalmology and he has been elected to membership in the American Glaucoma Society. He currently holds an appointment as a Clinical Associate Professor in the Department of Surgery, Division of Ophthalmology, Nova Southeastern University, Fort Lauderdale, Florida.

He joined Visual Health in January 1992, after serving as the regional glaucoma specialist in Mobile, Alabama for three years. Dr. Schacknow's excellent academic training and extensive practice experience give him advanced skills and clinical insight to bring to the care of our glaucoma patients. He is an expert in the use of sophisticated computerized visual field and optic nerve-head analyzers for monitoring the progression of a patient's glaucoma. He has performed thousands of glaucoma surgical operations, employing state-of-the-art laser and microsurgical techniques, in patients who otherwise might have gone blind from advanced glaucoma. Dr. Schacknow is Medical Director of the Palm Beach Eye Foundation. He and his highly trained medical staff work with numerous pharmaceutical companies in ongoing clinical research projects to evaluate promising new medications for the treatment of glaucoma.

Dr. Schacknow participates in many additional activities in the professional eyecare community. He was President of the Palm Beach County Ophthalmology Society in 2001. He has published articles in peer-reviewed scientific journals and written book chapters on glaucoma diagnostic and surgical techniques. He is the senior editor of "The Glaucoma Book," to be published by Springer Scientific in 2008. He frequently is invited to lecture nationally and internationally at professional meetings of ophthalmologists, optometrists and vision research scientists.

He and his wife, Sharma, share their Palm Beach Gardens home with their son, Jeffrey Michael and an Australian terrier named "Spike." Dr. Schacknow enjoys gourmet cooking, fine dining and travel. He is addicted to playing with his home computer and surfing the Internet. Mrs. Schacknow is an attorney and tennis buff. Jeffrey, a high-school student, loves sports, science and Spike. (And of course his parents, too!) Our patients will enjoy Dr. Schacknow's outgoing personality, his caring attitude and his great sense of humor.

Dr. Schacknow works closely with his patients and their primary eyecare physicians for the diagnosis and management of their glaucoma. He is available to see new patients in our Lake Worth (561-964-0707) and Jupiter (561-747-1111) offices in Palm Beach County. His WebSite may be found at: http://www.glaucoma.eyemd.org

# 28.6 Appendix 6: Consultation Report Form

**Appendix E - Consultation Report Form**

**Glaucoma Consultation Report - New Patient**
**Your Practice Name**
**Good Man, MD**

Version 12.21.08

Patient:_____ Male – Female  [Box 1]
Chart #_____ Date:_____
Consult requested by: _____ (____ << report dictated)
Office: LW  JUP   Age: ___  Race: White Black Hispanic Asian Other
Primary language spoken is *English* unless next line is completed:
Spanish  French  Italian _____   Translator:_____

**Chief Complaint:**  [Box 2]
Sent by referring physician because of : _____
___high-IOP  ___narrow or closed angle(s)  ___uncontrolled GL
___suspicious optic nerves  ___family hx of GL  ___VF abnormality
___medication problem

Pt's comments: ___ pain  ___irritation  ___decreased vision  ___"bloodshot"
___itching  ___dermatitis  ___allergic reaction  ___feeling of increased eye pressure
___medication intolerance  ___fatigue  ___GI upset  ___dizziness  ___headache
___2nd opinion  ___change of insur. or new to local area (Hx of GL)
___out of meds  **DETAILS & COMMENTS:**

**Medical and Surgical History: GLAUCOMA**  [Box 3]
Date glaucoma first diagnosed or suspected: _____
Details:

**Previous Glaucoma & Other Ocular Medications:** ___ None
Medication/Dosage   Eye(s)   Dates (Mo/Yr)

**Ocular Medical & Surgical Hx (excluding glaucoma)**
(Please circle & then describe below. Include which eyes & dates of any surgeries)

Cataract Present  OD / OS     Cataract Surgery  OD / OS     Lens Implant  OD / OS
Lid Surgery  OD / OS   Diabetic Retinopathy  OD / OS   Diabetic Laser (PRP)  OD / OS
Retinal Detachment  OD / OS     LASIK - Refractive Surgery  OD / OS
Strabismus/Surgery  OD / OS    Trauma  OD / OS    Corneal Ulcer  OD / OS
Corneal Transplant  OD / OS    **DETAILS, OTHER CONDITIONS & COMMENTS:**

[Box 4]

**Glaucoma Laser & Surgical Treatments:** ___ None
Procedure        Eye        Date/ Name of Doctor

**Family Ocular History**

**Current Ocular Medications:** ___ None  [Box 5]
(Name and strength, eye(s), # of times per day, time of last dose)

**Current Systemic Medications:** ___ None  [Box 6]
(Name and strength, # of times per day, time of last dose)

**MEDICATION ALLERGIES:** ___ NONE  [Box 7]

V sc cc  OD _____ OS _____   [Box 8]
Far / Near              Pinhole

V sc cc  OD _____ OS _____   [Box 9]

**Current eyeglasses:**   [Box 10]
OD ____sphere ____cylinder ____axis ____near add
OS ____sphere ____cylinder ____axis ____near add

**Central Corneal Thickness (CCT):**  [Box 11]
OD: #1 _____ #2 _____   OS: #1 _____ #2 _____
Comments:

**Visual Fields**  HVF 24-2  GVF  Date_____ Done by:____
Previous VF (date) _____ at VH or by Dr. _____

OD Fixation/Reliability> Poor Fair Good   Cooperation> Poor Good
Interpretation by Dr. PNS: Normal   Gen-Depression   Central-Defect
NFB  Neuro  Non-Specific  Stable  Progression  **COMMENTS:**

OS Fixation/Reliability> Poor Fair Good   Cooperation> Poor Good
Interpretation by Dr. PNS: Normal   Gen-Depression
Central-Defect  NFB  Neuro  Non-Specific  Stable
Progression   **COMMENTS:**

[Box 12]

Patient's <u>Medical Hx</u>, <u>Review of Systems</u>, <u>Family Medical Hx</u> & pt's <u>Social History</u> are documented separately on form entitled "***Medical History Questionnaire***" completed on (date): _____  [Box 14]
This document was reviewed with the patient by Dr. GM _____

**Confrontation Visual Fields**   Notes by Dr. GM
Right Eye    Left Eye

[Box 13]

[Box 15]

| GLAUCOMA CONSULTATION REPORT   Page 2 | Patient: _____  Date: _____ |
|---|---|
| **Gonioscopy:** With Posner goniolens or _____<br>**OD** __ Angle open 360°, no pathology; Grade> Slit I II III IV __PAS<br>**OS** __ Angle open 360°, no pathology; Grade> Slit I II III IV __PAS<br>*Comments:*                                                    **Box 16** | **Tonometry:** By Goldmann applanation   or   Tonopen<br>T ____OD ____OS  Time: _____ AM / PM, by:<br>                                                         **Box 17**<br>Recheck: T ____OD ____OS, by _____ or Dr. GM |
| **RIGHT EYE** | **LEFT EYE** |
| Confrontation or Formal Visual Field: (see reverse side of page) | Confrontation or Formal Visual Field: (see reverse side of page) |
| **EOMS:** __NL in primary gaze __ NL sensory function _____ | **EOMS:** __NL in primary gaze __ NL sensory function _____ |
| **Adnexae**<br>**Lids:** __NL __Blepharitis __ Ptosis __Trichiasis _____<br>**Orbit**__NL  **Lacrimal Gland**__NL  **Lacrimal Drainage**__NL<br>**Preauricular Nodes**__NL | **Adnexae**<br>**Lids:** __NL __Blepharitis __ Ptosis __Trichiasis _____<br>**Orbit**__NL  **Lacrimal Gland**__NL  **Lacrimal Drainage**__NL<br>**Preauricular Nodes**__NL |
| **Pupil:** __PERRLA __APD ____Non-reactive   **Box 18**<br>Size > NL, Miotic, Dilated _____ Shape> NL or ____ | **Pupil:** __ __APD ____Non-reactive   **Box 19**<br>Size > NL, Miotic, Dilated _____ Shape> NL or ____ |
| **Iris:** __NL __Iridotomy __ Rubeosis ___Transill. Defects | **Iris:** __NL __Iridotomy __ Rubeosis ___Transill. Defects |
| **Conjunctiva:** __NL-> bulbar/palpebral __hyperemia<br>__ Ping/ Ptery ____subconj-heme | **Conjunctiva:** __NL-> bulbar/palpebral __hyperemia<br>__ Ping/ Ptery ____subconj-heme |
| **Cornea:** Epithelium__NL   Stroma__NL   Tear-film__NL<br>Endothelium__NL   __K'berg spindle __ guttatae _____<br>__PKP clear & compact | **Cornea:** Epithelium__NL   Stroma__NL   Tear-film__NL<br>Endothelium__NL   __K'berg spindle __ guttatae _____<br>__PKP clear & compact |
| **Anterior Chamber:** __NL depth & without inflammation<br>___cells ___flare ___hyphema ___hypopyon ___shallow | **Anterior Chamber:** __NL depth & without inflammation<br>___cells ___flare ___hyphema ___hypopyon ___shallow |
| Right eye was **NOT** dilated.  Right eye **WAS** dilated at ___<br>(phenylephrine 2.5% & tropicamide 1%) | Left eye was **NOT** dilated.  Left eye **WAS** dilated at ___<br>(phenylephrine 2.5% & tropicamide 1%) |
| **Lens:** __NL (no cataract, no pathology) __ Post.-synech.<br>__Aphakic __AC-IOL __PC-IOL __IRIS-IOL __PXF<br>Cataract >> ___Cortical ___Nuclear ___PSC _____<br>Posterior-capsule > __clear __hazy/wrinkled __open | **Lens:** __NL (no cataract, no pathology) __ Post.-synech.<br>__Aphakic __AC-IOL __PC-IOL __IRIS-IOL __PXF<br>Cataract >> ___Cortical ___Nuclear ___PSC _____<br>Posterior-capsule > __clear __hazy/wrinkled __open |
| **Posterior Segment (Vitreous & Fundus):**<br>**Vitreous:** __NL __floaters __PVD __asteroid hyalosis __ heme<br>**Retina:** (good-fair-poor view) direct-indirect 'scope  Volk 78 lens<br>**Macula:** __NL __ARMD-dry __ARMD-wet __hole/ERM<br>  __BDR __PDR  Other_____<br>Comments:_____<br>**Vessels:** __NL _____<br>**Periphery:** ___ NL _____<br>**Optic Nerve** (direct visualization by Dr. GM ): ___ stable<br>C/D ____V C/D ____H __Notch-INF / SUP __Pallor ____<br>*Fundus (Disc) photography* (date_____) by:_____<br>Interpretation by Dr. GM __ Consistent with direct visualization or<br>_____<br>Notes:<br><br>Previous disc photos (date) _____ | **Posterior Segment (Vitreous & Fundus):**<br>**Vitreous:** __NL __floaters __PVD __asteroid hyalosis __ heme<br>**Retina:** (good-fair-poor view) direct-indirect 'scope  Volk 78 lens<br>**Macula:** __NL __ARMD-dry __ARMD-wet __hole/ERM<br>  __BDR __PDR  Other_____<br>Comments:_____<br>**Vessels:** __NL _____<br>**Periphery:** ___ NL _____<br>**Optic Nerve** (direct visualization by Dr. GM ): ___ stable<br>C/D ____V C/D ____H __Notch-INF / SUP __Pallor ____<br><br>Interpretation by Dr. GM __ Consistent with direct visualization or<br>_____<br>Notes: |
| **Mental Status:** __Pt. is oriented to person, place & time.<br>__ Mood & affect are appropriate for office visit. | **Diagnoses & Clinical Impressions:**                    **Box 20** |
| **Discussion:** Diagnoses, clinical impressions and recommendations were discussed with the patient and all family members present. All questions were addressed and answered to their satisfaction. _____ GOOD MAN, MD | |
| Literature was given to the patient about:<br>__Glaucoma   ___Visual Fields   ___GDx / OCT<br>__Glauc. meds & side effects   ___Glauc. microsurgery<br>__Laser trabeculoplasty   ___Laser iridotomy | ____Refills & all new prescriptions given to pt. & reviewed with pt. and family members present |
| Schedule return visit in: ___ days, ___ weeks, ___ months<br>On next visit with Dr. GM ><br>___Refraction by optometrist   __HVF __GDx __OCT __CCT | **Recommendations:** __ continue current glaucoma medications, except:<br>                                                    **Box 21** |
| $T_a$, NO dilation  <or>  $T_a$, then dilate O__  ___ Disc photos after exam<br>___ Gonioscopy by Dr. GM _____       **Box 22** | |
| **TODAY:** __ Disc photos ___ Refract ___HVF ___GDx ___OCT ___CCT | Good Man, MD ____ |

## 28.7 Appendix 7: Consultation Report Form: Without Annotations

Appendix F - Consultation Report Form – without annotations

**Glaucoma Consultation Report - New Patient**
*Your Practice Name*
Good Man, MD

Version 12.21.08

Patient:_____ Male – Female
Chart #_____ Date:_____
Consult requested by: _____ (____ << report dictated)
Office: LW  JUP  Age:____ Race: White Black Hispanic Asian Other
Primary language spoken is *English* unless next line is completed:
Spanish  French  Italian _____  Translator:_____

**Chief Complaint:**
Sent by referring physician because of : _____
___high-IOP  __narrow or closed angle(s)  ___uncontrolled GL
__suspicious optic nerves  __family hx of GL  __VF abnormality
__medication problem

Pt's comments: ___ pain ___irritation ___decreased vision ___"bloodshot" __itching __dermatitis ___allergic reaction __feeling of increased eye pressure __medication intolerance __fatigue __GI upset ___dizziness ___headache

__2nd opinion ___change of insur. or new to local area (Hx of GL) ___out of meds  **DETAILS & COMMENTS:**

**Medical and Surgical History: GLAUCOMA**
Date glaucoma first diagnosed or suspected: _____
Details:

**Previous Glaucoma & Other Ocular Medications:** ___ None
Medication/Dosage    Eye(s)    Dates (Mo/Yr)

**Ocular Medical & Surgical Hx (excluding glaucoma)**
(Please circle & then describe below. Include which eyes & dates of any surgeries)

Cataract Present  OD / OS    Cataract Surgery  OD / OS    Lens Implant  OD / OS
Lid Surgery  OD / OS    Diabetic Retinopathy  OD / OS    Diabetic Laser (PRP)  OD / OS
Retinal Detachment  OD / OS    LASIK - Refractive Surgery  OD / OS
Strabismus/Surgery  OD / OS    Trauma  OD / OS    Corneal Ulcer  OD / OS
Corneal Transplant  OD / OS    **DETAILS, OTHER CONDITIONS & COMMENTS:**

**Glaucoma Laser & Surgical Treatments:** ___ None
Procedure    Eye    Date/ Name of Doctor

**Family Ocular History**

**Current Ocular Medications:** ___ None
(Name and strength, eye(s), # of times per day, time of last dose)

**Current Systemic Medications:** ___None
(Name and strength, # of times per day, time of last dose)

**MEDICATION ALLERGIES:** ____ NONE

**V** sc cc  OD    OS
Far / Near

**V** sc cc  OD    OS
Pinhole

**Current eyeglasses:**

OD ____sphere _____cylinder _____axis _____ near add

OS ____sphere _____cylinder _____axis _____ near add

**Central Corneal Thickness (CCT):**
OD: #1 _____ #2 _____    OS: #1 _____ #2_____
Comments:

56

**Visual Fields**  HVF$_{24-2}$  GVF  Date_____  Done by:____

Previous VF (date) _____ at VH or by Dr. _____

OD Fixation/Reliability> Poor Fair Good   Cooperation> Poor Good
Interpretation by Dr. PNS: Normal  Gen-Depression  Central-Defect
NFB  Neuro  Non-Specific  Stable  Progression    **COMMENTS:**

OS Fixation/Reliability> Poor Fair Good   Cooperation> Poor Good
Interpretation by Dr. PNS: Normal  Gen-Depression  Central-Defect  NFB  Neuro  Non-Specific  Stable  Progression
**COMMENTS:**

Patient's <u>Medical Hx</u>, <u>Review of Systems</u>, <u>Family Medical Hx</u> & pt's <u>Social History</u> are documented separately on form entitled "***Medical History Questionnaire***" completed on (date): _____

This document was reviewed with the patient by Dr. PNS _____

**Confrontation Visual Fields**
Right Eye    Left Eye

**Notes by Dr. PNS**

| **GLAUCOMA CONSULTATION REPORT** Page 2 | Patient: _____ Date: _____ |
|---|---|
| **Gonioscopy:** With Posner goniolens or _____<br>OD __ Angle open 360°, no pathology; Grade> Slit I II III IV __PAS<br>OS __ Angle open 360°, no pathology; Grade> Slit I II III IV __PAS<br>*Comments:* | **Tonometry:** By Goldmann applanation   or   Tonopen<br>T ____OD ____OS Time: _____ AM / PM, by: _____<br><br>Recheck: T ____ OD ____ OS, by _____ or Dr. PNS |

| **RIGHT EYE** | **LEFT EYE** |
|---|---|
| Confrontation or Formal Visual Field: (see reverse side of page) | Confrontation or Formal Visual Field: (see reverse side of page) |
| **EOMS:** __NL in primary gaze  __ NL sensory function _____ | **EOMS:** __NL in primary gaze  __ NL sensory function _____ |
| **Adnexae**<br>Lids: __NL __Blepharitis __ Ptosis __Trichiasis _____<br>Orbit__NL   **Lacrimal Gland** __NL   **Lacrimal Drainage** __NL<br>**Preauricular Nodes** __NL _____ | **Adnexae**<br>Lids: __NL __Blepharitis __ Ptosis __Trichiasis _____<br>Orbit__NL   **Lacrimal Gland** __NL   **Lacrimal Drainage** __NL<br>**Preauricular Nodes** __NL _____ |
| **Pupil:** __PERRLA __APD __Non-reactive<br>Size > NL, Miotic, Dilated _____ Shape> NL or _____<br>**Iris:** __NL __Iridotomy __Rubeosis __Transill. Defects | **Pupil:** __PERRLA __APD __Non-reactive<br>Size > NL, Miotic, Dilated _____ Shape> NL or _____<br>**Iris:** __NL __Iridotomy __Rubeosis __Transill. Defects |
| **Conjunctiva:** __NL-> bulbar/palpebral __hyperemia<br>__Ping/ Ptery _____subconj-heme<br>**Cornea:** Epithelium__NL   Stroma__NL   Tear-film__NL<br>Endothelium__NL __K'berg spindle __ guttatae _____<br>__PKP clear & compact _____ | **Conjunctiva:** __NL-> bulbar/palpebral __hyperemia<br>__Ping/ Ptery _____subconj-heme<br>**Cornea:** Epithelium__NL   Stroma__NL   Tear-film__NL<br>Endothelium__NL __K'berg spindle __ guttatae _____<br>__PKP clear & compact _____ |
| **Anterior Chamber:** __NL depth & without inflammation<br>___cells ___flare ___hyphema ___hypopyon ___shallow | **Anterior Chamber:** __NL depth & without inflammation<br>___cells ___flare ___hyphema ___hypopyon ___shallow |
| Right eye was **NOT** dilated.  Right eye **WAS** dilated at _____<br>(phenylephrine 2.5% & tropicamide 1%)<br>**Lens:** __NL (no cataract, no pathology) __ Post.-synech.<br>__Aphakic __AC-IOL __PC-IOL __IRIS-IOL __PXF<br>Cataract >> ____Cortical ____Nuclear ____PSC<br>Posterior-capsule > __clear __hazy/wrinkled __open | Left eye was **NOT** dilated.  Left eye **WAS** dilated at _____<br>(phenylephrine 2.5% & tropicamide 1%)<br>**Lens:** __NL (no cataract, no pathology) __ Post.-synech.<br>__Aphakic __AC-IOL __PC-IOL __IRIS-IOL __PXF<br>Cataract >> ____Cortical ____Nuclear ____PSC<br>Posterior-capsule > __clear __hazy/wrinkled __open |
| **Posterior Segment (Vitreous & Fundus):**<br>**Vitreous:** __NL __floaters __PVD __asteroid hyalosis __heme<br>Retina: (good-fair-poor view) direct-indirect 'scope  Volk 78 lens<br>Macula: __NL __ARMD-dry __ARMD-wet __hole/ERM<br>__BDR __PDR Other_____<br>Comments:_____<br>**Vessels:** __NL _____<br>**Periphery:** ___ NL _____<br>**Optic Nerve** (direct visualization by Dr. PNS):  ___ stable<br>C/D ___V C/D ___H ___Notch-INF / SUP __Pallor _____<br>*Fundus (Disc) photography* (date_____) by:_____<br>Interpretation by Dr. PNS __ Consistent with direct visualization or _____<br><br>Notes:<br><br><br>Previous disc photos (date) _____ | **Posterior Segment (Vitreous & Fundus):**<br>**Vitreous:** __NL __floaters __PVD __asteroid hyalosis __heme<br>Retina: (good-fair-poor view) direct-indirect 'scope  Volk 78 lens<br>Macula: __NL __ARMD-dry __ARMD-wet __hole/ERM<br>__BDR __PDR Other_____<br>Comments:_____<br>**Vessels:** __NL _____<br>**Periphery:** ___ NL _____<br>**Optic Nerve** (direct visualization by Dr. PNS):  ___ stable<br>C/D ___V C/D ___H ___Notch-INF / SUP __Pallor _____<br>Interpretation by Dr. PNS __ Consistent with direct visualization or _____<br><br>Notes: |
| **Mental Status:** __Pt. is oriented to person, place & time.<br>__ Mood & affect are appropriate for office visit. | **Diagnoses & Clinical Impressions:** |
| **Discussion:**  Diagnoses, clinical impressions and recommendations were discussed with the patient and all family members present.  All questions were addressed and answered to their satisfaction.    _____ **P. Schacknow, MD, PhD** | |
| Literature was given to the patient about:<br>__Glaucoma  ___Visual Fields  ___GDx / OCT<br>__Glauc. meds & side effects  ___Glauc. microsurgery<br>__Laser trabeculoplasty  ___Laser iridotomy | ___Refills & all new prescriptions given to pt. & reviewed with pt. and family members present |
| Schedule return visit in: ___ days, ___ weeks, ___ months<br>On next visit with Dr. PNS ><br>__Refraction by optometrist ___HVF ___GDx ___OCT___CCT<br><br>T$_a$, NO dilation  <or>  T$_a$, then dilate O__ ___ Disc photos after exam<br><br>___ Gonioscopy by Dr. PNS _____<br><br>**TODAY:** __ Disc photos ___ Refract ___HVF ___GDx ___OCT ___CCT | **Recommendations:** __ continue current glaucoma medications, except:<br><br><br><br><br><br>Good Man, MD ___ |

## 28.8 Appendix 8: Glaucoma Examination Report

Appendix G – Glaucoma Examination Report

**Glaucoma Examination Report**
**Established Patient**
*Your Practice Name*
**Good Man, MD**

Patient:_____ Male – Female
Chart #_____ Date:_____
Consult requested by: _____ (____ << report dictated)
Office: LW JUP    Age: ___   Race: White Black Hispanic Asian Other
Primary language spoken is *English* unless next line is completed:
Spanish  French  Italian _____    Translator:_____

**Chief Complaint:**
Sent by referring physician because of : _____
___high-IOP  __narrow or closed angle(s)   __uncontrolled GL
__suspicious optic nerves  __family hx of GL   __VF abnormality
___medication problem

Pt's comments: ___pain  ___irritation  ___decreased vision ___"bloodshot"
__itching  ___dermatitis  ___allergic reaction ___feeling of increased eye pressure  __medication intolerance   __fatigue  ___GI upset  ___dizziness
___headache

__2nd opinion  ___change of insur. or new to local area (Hx of GL)   ___out of meds  **DETAILS & COMMENTS:**

___Exam for monitoring of glaucoma progression and the following parameters: IOP DISCS HVF GDx compliance side-effects post-op

Date of last exam with Dr. GM _____

**History of Present Illness: GLAUCOMA**

Patient's <u>Medical Hx</u>, <u>Review of Systems</u>, <u>Family Medical Hx</u> & pt's <u>Social History</u> are documented separately on form entitled **"Medical History Questionnaire** (**MHQ***)"* completed on (date):_____
*Interim* changes to **MHQ** (Reviewed by Dr. PNS):  ___ No change

**Current Ocular Medications:** ___ None
(Name and strength, eye(s), # of times per day, time of last dose)

**Current Systemic Medications:** ___None
(Name and strength, # of times per day, time of last dose)

**MEDICATION ALLERGIES: ____ NONE**

**V** $_{sc}$ $_{cc}$ OD        OS
Far / Near

**V** $_{sc}$ $_{cc}$ OD        OS
Pinhole

**Current eyeglasses:**

OD _____sphere _____cylinder _____axis _____ near add

OS _____sphere _____cylinder _____axis _____ near add

**Refraction** (Vision with new refraction: OD 20/___ OS 20/___)

OD _____sphere _____cylinder _____axis _____ near add

OS _____sphere _____cylinder _____axis _____ near add

___ Rx given for new glasses  _____ Refer to optometrist

**Visual Fields** HVF$_{24-2}$  GVF    Date_____ Done by:____

Previous VF (date) _____ at VH or by Dr._____

OD Fixation/Reliability> Poor Fair Good   Cooperation> Poor Good
Interpretation by Dr. PNS: Normal   Gen-Depression   Central-Defect
NFB  Neuro  Non-Specific  Stable   Progression
**COMMENTS:**

OS Fixation/Reliability> Poor Fair Good   Cooperation> Poor Good
Interpretation by Dr. PNS: Normal  Gen-Depression  Central-Defect  NFB  Neuro  Non-Specific  Stable  Progression
**COMMENTS:**

**Scanning Laser Polarimetry** (GDx VCC):

Date_____ Done by:____ Previous GDx (date) _____ at VH

OD: Image Quality (Q) _____  NFI: _____  **Interpretation:**
Consistent with> DISC  VF  NL  OAG SUSPECT  OAG
Comments: Baseline  Stable  Progression

OS: Image Quality (Q) _____  NFI: _____  **Interpretation:**
Consistent with> DISC  VF  NL  OAG SUSPECT  OAG
Comments: Baseline  Stable  Progression

**ALSO SEE NARRATIVE REPORT WITH IMAGES & DATA ANALYSIS**

**Confrontation Visual Fields**
    Right        Left

**Notes by staff**

**Notes by Dr. Good Man**

| **GLAUCOMA EXAMINATION REPORT** Page 2 | Patient: _____ Date: _____ |
|---|---|
| **Gonioscopy:** Posner / 3-Mirror Goniolens<br>OD __ Angle open 360°, no pathology; Grade> Slit I II III IV __PAS<br>OS __ Angle open 360°, no pathology; Grade> Slit I II III IV __PAS<br>*Comments:* | **Tonometry:** By Goldmann Applanation or Tonopen Tactile<br>T ____OD ____OS Time: _____ AM / PM, by: _____<br><br>Recheck: T ____OD ____OS, by Dr. Good Man |

| **RIGHT EYE** | **LEFT EYE** |
|---|---|
| Confrontation or Formal Visual Field: (see reverse side of page) | Confrontation or Formal Visual Field: (see reverse side of page) |
| **EOMS:** __NL in primary gaze __ NL sensory function _____ | **EOMS:** __NL in primary gaze __ NL sensory function _____ |
| **Adnexae**<br>Lids: __NL __Blepharitis __Ptosis __Trichiasis _____<br>Orbit__NL  **Lacrimal Gland** __NL  **Lacrimal Drainage**__NL<br>**Preauricular Nodes**__NL | **Adnexae**<br>Lids: __NL __Blepharitis __Ptosis __Trichiasis _____<br>Orbit__NL  **Lacrimal Gland** __NL  **Lacrimal Drainage**__NL<br>**Preauricular Nodes**__NL |
| **Pupil:** __PERRLA ___APD ____Non-reactive<br>Size > NL, Miotic, Dilated     Shape> NL or _____ | **Pupil:** ___APD ____Non-reactive<br>Size > NL, Miotic, Dilated     Shape> NL or _____ |
| **Iris:** __NL __Iridotomy __Rubeosis ___Transill. Defects | **Iris:** __NL __Iridotomy __Rubeosis ___Transill. Defects |
| **Conjunctiva:** __NL-> bulbar/palpebral __hyperemia<br>   Ping/ Ptery _____ subconj-heme | **Conjunctiva:** __NL-> bulbar/palpebral __hyperemia<br>   Ping/ Ptery _____ subconj-heme |
| **Cornea:** Epithelium__NL   Stroma__NL   Tear-film__NL<br>Endothelium__NL   K'berg spindle __ guttatae _____<br>__PKP clear & compact _____ | **Cornea:** Epithelium__NL   Stroma__NL   Tear-film__NL<br>Endothelium__NL   K'berg spindle __ guttatae _____<br>__PKP clear & compact _____ |
| **Anterior Chamber:** __NL depth & without inflammation<br>___cells ___flare ___hyphema ____hypopyon ___shallow | **Anterior Chamber:** __NL depth & without inflammation<br>___cells ___flare ___hyphema ____hypopyon ___shallow |
| Right eye was **NOT** dilated. Right eye **WAS** dilated at _____<br>(phenylephrine 2.5% & tropicamide 1%) | Left eye was **NOT** dilated. Left eye **WAS** dilated at _____<br>(phenylephrine 2.5% & tropicamide 1%) |
| **Lens:** __NL (no cataract, no pathology) __ Post.-synech.<br>__Aphakic ___AC-IOL ___PC-IOL ___IRIS-IOL ___PXF<br>Cataract >> ____Cortical _____ Nuclear ___PSC _____<br>Posterior-capsule > __clear __hazy/wrinkled __open | **Lens:** __NL (no cataract, no pathology) __ Post.-synech.<br>__Aphakic ___AC-IOL ___PC-IOL ___IRIS-IOL ___PXF<br>Cataract >> ____Cortical _____ Nuclear ___PSC _____<br>Posterior-capsule > __clear __hazy/wrinkled __open |
| **Posterior Segment (Vitreous & Fundus):**<br>**Vitreous:** __NL __floaters __PVD __asteroid hyalosis __ heme<br>Retina: (good-fair-poor view) direct-indirect 'scope Volk 78 lens<br>Macula: __NL __ARMD-dry __ARMD-wet ___hole/ERM<br>          ___BDR __PDR  Other_____<br>Comments:_____<br>**Vessels:** __NL _____<br>**Periphery:** ___NL _____<br>**Optic Nerve** (direct visualization by Dr. PNS): ___ stable<br>C/D ____V C/D ____H ___Notch-INF / SUP ___Pallor _____<br>*Fundus (Disc) photography* (date_____) by:_____<br>Interpretation by Dr. GM __ Consistent with direct visualization or<br>_____<br>Notes:<br><br><br><br>Previous disc photos (date) _____ | **Posterior Segment (Vitreous & Fundus):**<br>**Vitreous:** __NL __floaters __PVD __asteroid hyalosis __ heme<br>Retina: (good-fair-poor view) direct-indirect 'scope Volk 78 lens<br>Macula: __NL __ARMD-dry __ARMD-wet ___hole/ERM<br>          ___BDR __PDR  Other_____<br>Comments:_____<br>**Vessels:** __NL _____<br>**Periphery:** ___NL _____<br>**Optic Nerve** (direct visualization by Dr. PNS): ___ stable<br>C/D ____V C/D ____H ___Notch-INF / SUP ___Pallor _____<br><br>Interpretation by Dr. GM __ Consistent with direct visualization or<br>_____<br>Notes: |
| **Mental Status:** __Pt. is oriented to person, place & time.<br>          __ Mood & affect are appropriate for office visit. | **Diagnoses & Clinical Impressions:** |
| **Discussion:** Diagnoses, clinical impressions and recommendations were discussed with the patient and all family members present. All questions were addressed and answered to their satisfaction.        _____ **G. Man, MD** | |
| Literature was given to the patient about:<br>__Glaucoma   ___Visual Fields   ___GDx-NFA<br>__Glauc. meds & side effects   ___Glauc. microsurgery<br>__Laser trabeculoplasty        ___Laser iridotomy | ___Refills & all new prescriptions given to pt. & reviewed with pt. |
| Schedule return visit in: ___ days, ___ weeks, ___ months<br>On next visit with Dr. GM ><br>___Refraction by optometrist ___HVF ___GVF ___GDx ___CCT<br><br>$T_a$, NO dilation <or> $T_a$, then dilate O__ ___ Disc photos after exam<br><br>___ Gonioscopy by Dr. GM _____<br><br>**TODAY:** __ Disc photos ___Refraction ___HVF ___GDx ___CCT | **Recommendations:**___ continue current glaucoma medications, except:<br><br><br><br><br><br><br><br>Good Man, MD ___ |

## 28.9 Appendix 9: Glaucoma Consult Examination Report to Referring Physician

Appendix H – Glaucoma Consult Examination Report to Referring Physician

**GLAUCOMA CONSULTATION EXAMINATION REPORT TO REFERRING PHYSICIAN**

To: Dr. _____  Date of Service: ___/___/_____

Exam Location: ___ Somewhere, NY (Voice phone 561-XXX-0707)   ___ Elsewhere, NY (Voice phone 561-XXX-8700)
FAX: Somewhere, NY (561-XXX-3181)    FAX: Elsewhere, NY (561-XXX - 6682)

Regarding: Patient _____  Date of Birth: ___/___/____

Practice Medical Record # _____  Health Plan / Insurance Type _____

| PRIMARY GLAUCOMA DIAGNOSIS | ADDITIONAL EYE DIAGNOSES |
|---|---|
| ___ Open Angle Glaucoma 365.11 | ___ Cataract (Nuclear 366.16) (Subcapsular 366.14) |
| ___ Anatomically Narrow Angles 365.02 | ___ Pseudophakia (intraocular lens implant) V43.1 |
| ___ Status/Post Acute Angle Closure Glaucoma 365.22 | ___ Dry Eye Syndrome 375.15 |
| ___ Pseudoexfoliation Glaucoma 365.52 | ___ Macular Degeneration (Dry 362.51) (Wet 362.52) |
| ___ Pigmentary Glaucoma 365.13 | ___ Diabetic Retinopathy Bckgrnd/362.01 Prolifer/362.02 |
| ___ Glaucoma Suspect 365.0 | ___ Blepharitis (Eyelid Inflammation) 373.0 |
| ___ Glaucoma, Neovascular 365.63 | ___ Conjunctivitis 077.9 (Viral) |
| ___ Glaucoma, Associated with Trauma 365.65 | ___ Uveitis 364.00 |
| ___ Low Tension Glaucoma 365.12 | |
| ___ Glaucoma Associated with Inflammation 365.62 | |

Best Corrected Vision: RIGHT 20/____  LEFT 20/____    Intraocular Pressure: RIGHT ____ LEFT _____ (mm Hg)

My examination reveals the patient
___ is clinically stable with adequate intraocular pressures. No glaucoma therapy indicated. Follow-up examination as below.
___ is newly diagnosed (as above) and requires treatment. Begin glaucoma therapy. *See list of medications below.*
___ is clinically stable with adequate intraocular pressures. Continue present therapy. *See list of medications below.*
___ is clinically stable but with borderline/high intraocular pressures. No change in therapy. Re-examine as indicated below.
___ is clinically stable but with borderline/high intraocular pressures. Change therapy. *See list of medications below.*

___ has intraocular pressure too high for health of optic nerve(s). Patient is on maximum medical therapy. **This patient requires laser trabeculoplasty (CPT 65855)** in RIGHT EYE, LEFT EYE, BOTH EYES. The laser procedure(s) should be performed in: < one week, < two weeks, < one month.
___ has anatomically narrow anterior chamber angles that are potentially occludable. This could lead to an emergent attack of acute angle closure glaucoma. **This patient requires laser iridotomy (CPT 66761)** in RIGHT EYE, LEFT EYE, BOTH EYES. The laser procedure(s) should be performed in: < one week, < two weeks, < one month.
___ has intraocular pressure too high for health of optic nerve(s). Patient is on maximum tolerated medical therapy. **This patient requires surgical trabeculectomy (CPT 66170)** in RIGHT EYE, LEFT EYE. The surgical procedure should be performed in: < one week, < two weeks, < one month.

**During this patient's next visit to my office I will perform an ophthalmic examination and the following procedures:**

___ Visual Field/92083    ___ Optic Nerve Photos/92250    ___ GDx or OCT Imaging/92135    ___ Pachymetry/76514
=================================================================================

___ Follow-up appointment with Dr. GOOD MAN in _____ days - weeks - months

___ Request consultation with Dr. _____ Purpose _____

___ Transfer of glaucoma eye care to Dr. _____

___ Co-management appointment with referring optometrist / ophthalmologist in ____ weeks -- months

| OPTHALMIC DROPS AND OINTMENTS | OPHTHALMIC ORAL MEDICATIONS |
|---|---|
|  |  |
|  |  |
|  |  |

_____ *Good Man, M.D.*, Chief of Glaucoma Services, Your Practice Name

# References

1. Jacobs EA. Patient centeredness in medical encounters requiring an interpreter. *Am J Med.* 2000;109(6):515.
2. Rivadeneyra R, Elderkin-Thompson V, Silver RC, Waitzkin H. Patient centeredness in medical encounters requiring an interpreter. *Am J Med.* 2000;108(6):470–474.
3. Takemura Y, Sakurai Y, Yokoya S, et al. Open-ended questions: are they really beneficial for gathering medical information from patients? *Tohoku J Exp Med.* 2005;206(2):151–154.
4. Sleath B, Roter D, Chewning B, Svarstad B. Asking questions about medication: analysis of physician-patient interactions and physician perceptions. *Med Care.* 1999;37(11):1169–1173.
5. Kaimbo DK, Buntinx F, Missotten L. Risk factors for open-angle glaucoma: a case-control study. *J Clin Epidemiol.* 2001;54(2):166–171.
6. Wilson MR, Hertzmark E, Walker AM, Childs-Shaw K, Epstein DL. A case-control study of risk factors in open angle glaucoma. *Arch Ophthalmol.* 1987;105(8):1066–1071.
7. Coleman AL, Miglior S. Risk factors for glaucoma onset and progression. *Surv Ophthalmol.* 2008;53(6 Suppl):S3–S10.
8. Deva NC, Insull E, Gamble G, Danesh-Meyer HV. Risk factors for first presentation of glaucoma with significant visual field loss. *Clin Experiment Ophthalmol.* 2008;36(3):217–221.
9. Rivera JL, Bell NP, Feldman RM. Risk factors for primary open angle glaucoma progression: what we know and what we need to know. *Curr Opin Ophthalmol.* 2008;19(2):102–106.
10. Boland MV, Quigley HA. Risk factors and open-angle glaucoma: classification and application. *J Glaucoma.* 2007;16(4):406–418.
11. Sommer A. Glaucoma risk factors observed in the Baltimore Eye Survey. *Curr Opin Ophthalmol.* 1996;7(2):93–98.
12. Brandt JD, Beiser JA, Gordon MO, Kass MA. Central corneal thickness and measured IOP response to topical ocular hypotensive medication in the Ocular Hypertension Treatment Study. *Am J Ophthalmol.* 2004;138(5):717–722.
13. Gordon MO, Beiser JA, Brandt JD, et al. The Ocular Hypertension Treatment Study: baseline factors that predict the onset of primary open-angle glaucoma. *Arch Ophthalmol.* 2002;120(6):714–720; discussion 829–730.
14. Brandt JD, Beiser JA, Kass MA, Gordon MO. Central corneal thickness in the Ocular Hypertension Treatment Study (OHTS). *Ophthalmology.* 2001;108(10):1779–1788.
15. Herndon L. Rethinking pachymetry and intraocular pressure. *Rev Ophthalmol.* 2002;9:07(7/15/02). <http://www.revophth.com/index.asp?page=1_144.htm>.
16. Brandt JD. Central corneal thickness, tonometry, and glaucoma risk–a guide for the perplexed. *Can J Ophthalmol.* 2007;42(4):562–566.
17. Bickley LS, Szilagyi PG. *Bates' Guide to Physical Examination and History Taking.* 8th ed. Philadelphia: Lippincott Williams & Wilkins; 2003.
18. Bobak SP, Goodwin JA, Guevara RA, Arya A, Grover S. Predictors of visual acuity and the relative afferent pupillary defect in optic neuropathy. *Doc Ophthalmol.* 1998;97(1):81–95.
19. Annette H, Kristina L, Bernd S, Mark-Oliver F, Wolfgang W. Effect of central corneal thickness and corneal hysteresis on tonometry as measured by dynamic contour tonometry, ocular response analyzer, and Goldmann tonometry in glaucomatous eyes. *J Glaucoma.* 2008;17(5):361–365.
20. Detry-Morel M. Currents on target intraocular pressure and intraocular pressure fluctuations in glaucoma management. *Bull Soc Belge Ophtalmol.* 2008;308:35–43.
21. Damji KF, Behki R, Wang L. Canadian perspectives in glaucoma management: setting target intraocular pressure range. *Can J Ophthalmol.* 2003;38(3):189–197.
22. Weinreb RN, Liu JH. Nocturnal rhythms of intraocular pressure. *Arch Ophthalmol.* 2006;124(2):269–270.
23. Liu JH, Gokhale PA, Loving RT, Kripke DF, Weinreb RN. Laboratory assessment of diurnal and nocturnal ocular perfusion pressures in humans. *J Ocul Pharmacol Ther.* 2003;19(4):291–297.
24. Liu JH, Kripke DF, Hoffman RE, et al. Nocturnal elevation of intraocular pressure in young adults. *Invest Ophthalmol Vis Sci.* 1998;39(13):2707–2712.
25. Mosaed S, Liu JH, Weinreb RN. Correlation between office and peak nocturnal intraocular pressures in healthy subjects and glaucoma patients. *Am J Ophthalmol.* 2005;139(2):320–324.
26. Nakakura S, Nomura Y, Ataka S, Shiraki K. Relation between office intraocular pressure and 24-hour intraocular pressure in patients with primary open-angle glaucoma treated with a combination of topical antiglaucoma eye drops. *J Glaucoma.* 2007;16(2):201–204.
27. Dev S, Damji KF, DeBacker CM, Cox TA, Dutton JJ, Allingham RR. Decrease in intraocular pressure after orbital decompression for thyroid orbitopathy. *Can J Ophthalmol.* 1998;33(6):314–319.
28. Johnstone MA, Albert DM. Prostaglandin-induced hair growth. *Surv Ophthalmol.* 2002;47(Suppl 1):S185–202.
29. Galloway GD, Eke T, Broadway DC. Periocular cutaneous pigmentary changes associated with bimatoprost use. *Arch Ophthalmol.* 2005;123(11):1609–1610.
30. Lagreze WD, Kardon RH. Correlation of relative afferent pupillary defect and estimated retinal ganglion cell loss. *Graefes Arch Clin Exp Ophthalmol.* 1998;236(6):401–404.
31. Martin TJ. Horner's syndrome, Pseudo-Horner's syndrome, and simple anisocoria. *Curr Neurol Neurosci Rep.* 2007;7(5):397–406.
32. Adie WJ. Complete and incomplete forms of the benign disorder characterised by tonic pupils and absent tendon reflexes. *Br J Ophthalmol.* 1932;16(8):449–461.
33. Lam DS, Tham CC, Lai JS, Leung DY. Current approaches to the management of acute primary angle closure. *Curr Opin Ophthalmol.* 2007;18(2):146–151.
34. La Hey E, Baarsma GS, De Vries J, Kijlstra A. Clinical analysis of Fuchs' heterochromic cyclitis. *Doc Ophthalmol.* 1991;78(3–4):225–235.
35. O'Connor GR. Doyne lecture. Heterochromic iridocyclitis. *Trans Ophthalmol Soc UK.* 1985;104(Pt 3):219–231.
36. Barr CC, Vine AK, Martonyi CL. Unexplained heterochromia. Intraocular foreign body demonstrated by computed tomography. *Surv Ophthalmol.* 1984;28(5):409–411.
37. Weinstein JM, Zweifel TJ, Thompson HS. Congenital Horner's syndrome. *Arch Ophthalmol.* 1980;98(6):1074–1078.
38. Gartner S, Henkind P. Neovascularization of the iris (rubeosis iridis). *Surv Ophthalmol.* 1978;22(5):291–312.
39. Ritch R. A unification hypothesis of pigment dispersion syndrome. *Trans Am Ophthalmol Soc.* 1996;94:381-405; discussion 405–389.
40. Wishart PK, Spaeth GL, Poryzees EM. Anterior chamber angle in the exfoliation syndrome. *Br J Ophthalmol.* 1985;69(2):103–107.
41. Laganowski HC, Kerr Muir MG, Hitchings RA. Glaucoma and the iridocorneal endothelial syndrome. *Arch Ophthalmol.* 1992;110(3):346–350.
42. Bonfioli AA, Orefice F. Sarcoidosis. *Semin Ophthalmol.* 2005;20(3):177–182.
43. Miki A, Saishin Y, Kuwamura R, Ohguro N, Tano Y. Anterior segment optical coherence tomography assessment of iris bombe before and after laser iridotomy in patients with uveitic secondary glaucoma. *Acta Ophthalmol.* 2008 October 24 [epub ahead of print].
44. Bruno CA, Alward WL. Gonioscopy in primary angle closure glaucoma. *Semin Ophthalmol.* 2002;17(2):59–68.
45. Spencer NA, Hall AJ, Stawell RJ. Nd:YAG laser iridotomy in uveitic glaucoma. *Clin Experiment Ophthalmol.* 2001;29(4):217–219.
46. Nichols JJ, Nichols KK, Puent B, Saracino M, Mitchell GL. Evaluation of tear film interference patterns and measures of tear break-up time. *Optom Vis Sci.* 2002;79(6):363–369.

47. Paschides CA, Kitsios G, Karakostas KX, Psillas C, Moutsopoulos HM. Evaluation of tear break-up time, Schirmer's-I test and rose bengal staining as confirmatory tests for keratoconjunctivitis sicca. *Clin Exp Rheumatol.* 1989;7(2):155–157.
48. Noecker R. Effects of common ophthalmic preservatives on ocular health. *Adv Ther.* 2001;18(5):205–215.
49. Leung EW, Medeiros FA, Weinreb RN. Prevalence of ocular surface disease in glaucoma patients. *J Glaucoma.* 2008;17(5):350–355.
50. Korb DR, Herman JP, Finnemore VM, Exford JM, Blackie CA. An evaluation of the efficacy of fluorescein, rose bengal, lissamine green, and a new dye mixture for ocular surface staining. *Eye Contact Lens.* 2008;34(1):61–64.
51. Feenstra RP, Tseng SC. What is actually stained by rose bengal? *Arch Ophthalmol.* 1992;110(7):984–993.
52. Calhoun FP Jr. Pigmentary glaucoma and its relation to Krukenberg's spindles. *Am J Ophthalmol.* 1953;36(10):1398–1415.
53. Posner A, Schlossman A. Syndrome of unilateral recurrent attacks of glaucoma with cyclitic symptoms. *Arch Ophthal.* 1948;39(4):517–535.
54. Pillai CT, Dua HS, Azuara-Blanco A, Sarhan AR. Evaluation of corneal endothelium and keratic precipitates by specular microscopy in anterior uveitis. *Br J Ophthalmol.* 2000;84(12):1367–1371.
55. Jones NP. Fuchs' heterochromic uveitis: a reappraisal of the clinical spectrum. *Eye.* 1991;5(Pt 6):649–661.
56. Moorthy RS, Mermoud A, Baerveldt G, Minckler DS, Lee PP, Rao NA. Glaucoma associated with uveitis. *Surv Ophthalmol.* 1997;41(5):361–394.
57. Adamis AP, Filatov V, Tripathi BJ, Tripathi RC. Fuchs' endothelial dystrophy of the cornea. *Surv Ophthalmol.* 1993;38(2):149–168.
58. Brooks AM, Grant G, Gillies WE. A comparison of corneal endothelial morphology in cornea guttata, Fuchs' dystrophy and bullous keratopathy. *Aust NZ J Ophthalmol.* 1988;16(2):93–100.
59. Kayes J, Holmberg A. The fine structure of the cornea in Fuchs' endothelial dystrophy. *Invest Ophthalmol.* 1964;3:47–67.
60. Jakus MA. Further observations on the fine structure of the cornea. *Invest Ophthalmol.* 1962;1:202–225.
61. Shields MB, ed. Glaucomas associated with intraocular hemorrhage and glaucomas associated with ocular trauma. In: *Textbook of Glaucoma.* Baltimore, MD: Williams and Wilkins; 1992:381–399.
62. Kloek C, Brauner S, Chen TC. Corneal blood staining after traumatic hyphema. *J Pediatr Ophthalmol Strabismus.* 2007;44(4):256.
63. Aonuma H, Matsushita H, Nakajima K, Watase M, Tsushima K, Watanabe I. Uveitis-glaucoma-hyphema syndrome after posterior chamber intraocular lens implantation. *Jpn J Ophthalmol.* 1997;41(2):98–100.
64. Ellingson FT. The uveitis-glaucoma-hyphema syndrome associated with the Mark VIII anterior chamber lens implant. *J Am Intraocul Implant Soc.* 1978;4(2):50–53.
65. Campbell DG, Simmons RJ, Grant WM. Ghost cells as a cause of glaucoma. *Am J Ophthalmol.* 1976;81(4):441–450.
66. Au Eong KG, Chua EC, Yip CC, Tun Y, Lim AS. Hypopyon – an unusual sign in acute angle-closure glaucoma. *Int Ophthalmol.* 1993;17(3):127–129.
67. Yi DH, Rashid S, Cibas ES, Arrigg PG, Dana MR. Acute unilateral leukemic hypopyon in an adult with relapsing acute lymphoblastic leukemia. *Am J Ophthalmol.* 2005;139(4):719–721.
68. Lobo A, Larkin G, Clark BJ, Towler HM, Lightman S. Pseudohypopyon as the presenting feature in B-cell and T-cell intraocular lymphoma. *Clin Experiment Ophthalmol.* 2003;31(2):155–158.
69. Jalali S, Das T, Gupta S. Presumed noninfectious endophthalmitis after cataract surgery. *J Cataract Refract Surg.* 1996;22(10):1492–1497.
70. Sari I, Akkoc N. Hypopyon uveitis. *J Rheumatol.* 2006;33(10):2097–2098.
71. Chang JH, McCluskey PJ, Grigg JR. Recurrent hypopyon in chronic anterior uveitis of pauciarticular juvenile idiopathic arthritis. *Br J Ophthalmol.* 2006;90(10):1327–1328.
72. Pearce A, Sugar A. Anterior uveitis and hypopyon. *Am J Ophthalmol.* 1992;113(4):471–472.
73. Zimmerman TJ, Kooner KS. *Clinical Pathways in Glaucoma.* New York: Thieme; 2001.
74. Casser L, Fingeret M, Woodcome HT. *Atlas of Primary Eyecare Procedures.* 2nd ed. Stamford, CT: Appleton & Lange; 1997.
75. Kaufman JH, Tolpin DW. Glaucoma after traumatic angle recession. A ten-year prospective study. *Am J Ophthalmol.* 1974;78(4):648–654.
76. Lehto I, Vesti E. Diagnosis and management of pigmentary glaucoma. *Curr Opin Ophthalmol.* 1998;9(2):61–64.
77. Naumann GO, Schlotzer-Schrehardt U, Kuchle M. Pseudoexfoliation syndrome for the comprehensive ophthalmologist. Intraocular and systemic manifestations. *Ophthalmology.* 1998;105(6):951–968.
78. Sampaolesi R, Zarate J, Croxato O. The chamber angle in exfoliation syndrome. Clinical and pathological findings. *Acta Ophthalmol Suppl.* 1988;184:48–53.
79. Browning DJ, Scott AQ, Peterson CB, Warnock J, Zhang Z. The risk of missing angle neovascularization by omitting screening gonioscopy in acute central retinal vein occlusion. *Ophthalmology.* 1998;105(5):776–784.
80. Becker B, Shaffer RN, Hoskins HD, Kass MA. *Becker-Shaffer's Diagnosis and Therapy of the Glaucomas.* 6th ed. St. Louis: Mosby; 1989.
81. Huang D, Swanson EA, Lin CP, et al. Optical coherence tomography. *Science.* 1991;254(5035):1178–1181.
82. Pavlin CJ, Harasiewicz K, Foster FS. Ultrasound biomicroscopy of anterior segment structures in normal and glaucomatous eyes. *Am J Ophthalmol.* 1992;113(4):381–389.
83. Pavlin CJ, Harasiewicz K, Sherar MD, Foster FS. Clinical use of ultrasound biomicroscopy. *Ophthalmology.* 1991;98(3):287–295.
84. Nolan WP, See JL, Chew PT, et al. Detection of primary angle closure using anterior segment optical coherence tomography in Asian eyes. *Ophthalmology.* 2007;114(1):33–39.
85. Pavlin CJ, Vasquez LM, Lee R, Simpson ER, Ahmed II. Anterior segment optical coherence tomography and ultrasound biomicroscopy in the imaging of anterior segment tumors. *Am J Ophthalmol.* 2009;147(2):214–219.
86. Pavlin CJ, McWhae JA, McGowan HD, Foster FS. Ultrasound biomicroscopy of anterior segment tumors. *Ophthalmology.* 1992;99(8):1220–1228.
87. Garcia JP Jr, Rosen RB. Anterior segment imaging: optical coherence tomography versus ultrasound biomicroscopy. *Ophthalmic Surg Lasers Imaging.* 2008;39(6):476–484.
88. Pavlin CJ, Ritch R, Foster FS. Ultrasound biomicroscopy in plateau iris syndrome. *Am J Ophthalmol.* 1992;113(4):390–395.
89. Radhakrishnan S, Goldsmith J, Huang D, et al. Comparison of optical coherence tomography and ultrasound biomicroscopy for detection of narrow anterior chamber angles. *Arch Ophthalmol.* 2005;123(8):1053–1059.
90. Kashiwagi K, Shinbayashi E, Tsukahara S. Development of a fully automated peripheral anterior chamber depth analyzer and evaluation of its accuracy. *J Glaucoma.* 2006;15(5):388–393.
91. Crick RP, Khaw PT. *A Textbook of Clinical Ophthalmology: A Practical Guide to Disorders of the Eyes and Their Management.* 3rd ed. River Edge, NJ: World Scientific; 2003.
92. Jonas JB, Gusek GC, Naumann GO. Optic disc, cup and neuroretinal rim size, configuration and correlations in normal eyes. *Invest Ophthalmol Vis Sci.* 1988;29(7):1151–1158.
93. Harizman N, Oliveira C, Chiang A, et al. The ISNT rule and differentiation of normal from glaucomatous eyes. *Arch Ophthalmol.* 2006;124(11):1579–1583.
94. Vilser W, Nagel E, Seifert BU, Riemer T, Weisensee J, Hammer M. Quantitative assessment of optic nerve head pallor. *Physiol Meas.* 2008;29(4):451–457.

# Chapter 29
# Glaucoma and Driving

Odette Callender

Many areas of the country do not have public transportation, making the ability to drive an essential part of maintaining one's independence. A July 2003 report issued by the Brookings Institution entitled "The Mobility Needs of Older Americans" found that increasing numbers of the elderly population are concentrated in suburban areas with no transportation options other than driving. According to the report, 56% of seniors live in suburban and rural areas, the number of miles driven by seniors increased from 12.7 miles a day in 1995 to 15.3 miles in 2001, and also seniors tend to be more receptive to transportation alternatives such as voucher and ride-sharing programs than to traditional means of public transportation.[1] The 2000 US Census counted approximately 35 million people were aged 65 years and over with approximately 4 million of them being over 85 years.[2] It is estimated that by 2050 the 85 years and older population will quadruple to more than 19.3 million.[3]

Per mile driven, crash rates increase starting at age 75 and markedly increase after age 80.[4] Between April 2001 and March 2002, the rate of fatal crashes per 100 million miles traveled was higher for drivers 80 and older than for drivers of any other age group except teenagers. Drivers 85 and older had the highest rate of fatal motor vehicle accidents. In 2006, 81% of fatal accidents involving older drivers happened during the day – 72% involved another vehicle. The Insurance Institute for Highway Safety (IIHS) released a study in March 2007 that indicated 40% of the fatal collisions of people aged 70 and older involving other vehicles occurred at intersections, compared with 23% for drivers aged 35–54, and the most common reason for intersection crashes for the oldest drivers was failure to yield.[1] The increased fatality rate is largely due to their increased susceptibility to injury.[4]

Many older Americans suffer from vision-threatening diseases such as macular degeneration and glaucoma that will increase driving difficulties. According to the 2000 US Census data, approximately 2.2 million US citizens have glaucoma. That number is projected to increase by 50% in 2020 to 3.36 million.[5] The number of office visits for glaucoma as the primary diagnosis among the elderly more than doubled from 1981 to 1991. It is projected that in 2050 those visits will increase to more than 16 million in patients 75 years and older.[6] With diseases such as macular degeneration that so noticeably affect central vision, it is easy for both patient and doctor to identify those who should not be driving. The situation is not always so obvious for patients with glaucoma. When compared to controls, glaucoma patients tend to avoid driving at night, in fog, in rain, during rush hour, on the highway, and in high-density traffic situations.[7] However with central vision maintained in glaucoma, even with very advanced disease, it tends to be harder for these patients to accept driving limitations.

Multiple studies have demonstrated an association of glaucoma with an increased risk of motor vehicle accidents (MVAs).[8] In an Alabama study, glaucoma patients were 3.6 times more likely to be involved in an injurious crash over a 5-year period.[9] A 5-year study in Halifax, Canada revealed that glaucoma patients were more than five times as likely to have been involved in a self-reported motor vehicle crash and over ten times more likely to have been at fault.[8] Glaucoma patients self-reported significantly more accidents and had three times the rate of simulator accidents in a study conducted by Szlyk et al in Chicago. Individuals with binocular peripheral field loss had accident rates twice as high as a normal control group in a California study.[10]

In the Szlyk et al study, glaucoma patients with less than 170 degrees of combined horizontal extent or less than 100 degrees of horizontal extent in the *better* eye with Goldmann visual field testing (III-4e target) were at greater risk for simulator accidents. The Goldmann horizontal extent in the *worse* eye was *not* significantly associated with driving performance. Humphrey visual field measures showed no significant correlation with driving performance.[10] An Australian study found that many patients with severe field defects on conventional, monocular automated perimetry, met driving standards when reevaluated with binocular Goldmann fields using the IV4e target[11] (IV4e is the standard used in Australia versus III4e in the United States[10]). Binocular Esterman testing, available on the Humphrey Visual Analyzer II perimeter, can be used as a substitute for Goldmann visual field to assess peripheral vision and may provide a more sensitive screening measure for peripheral visual field loss related to driving performance than threshold tests within the central visual field.[10] In the Esterman test, targets are presented at fixed brightness over the whole visual field, utilizing a 10 dB intensity stimulus with a Goldmann equivalent size of III-4-e. The test is typically done without the patient wearing glasses, so the field of vision is not limited by the frames. The monocular version tests a 100 point grid from 75 degrees temporally to 60 degrees nasally; the binocular version uses a 120-point grid to test 150 degrees bitemporally. In both the monocular and binocular versions the inferior field is tested more than the superior field (~50 degrees inferiorly vs. ~30 degrees superiorly).[12]

By applying the Advance Glaucoma Intervention Study (AGIS)-scoring system, McGwin et al correlated visual field defects in the central 24 degrees using the Humphrey Field Analyzer with police reported motor vehicle accidents in glaucoma patients over a 5½-year period. In the *better* eye, minor field defects (AGIS score 1–5) or moderate defects (AGIS score 6–11) were *not* associated with risk of involvement in a crash. Severe defects (AGIS score 12–20) were associated with an increased risk of a crash, but this was not statistically significant. Minor defects (AGIS score 1–5) in the *worse* eye did *not* increase the risk of a motor vehicle accident, but both moderate defects (score 6–11) and severe defects (score 12–20) significantly increased the risk. These findings are contrary to the conventional notion that the eye with better function dictates visual performance. In this study, the worse eye's visual field characteristics were significantly associated with crash involvement, whereas those of the better eye were not.[13]

It would appear that either a Binocular Esterman or the AGIS-scoring system applied to Humphrey visual field testing can assist in determining which glaucoma patients are more at risk for motor vehicle collisions. The Binocular Esterman is easy to administer and also easy to review the results with patients (dark areas show where lights were not seen in the periphery). The AGIS-scoring system is somewhat cumbersome, meant primarily for research,[14] and is a little harder to explain to patients (because it is just a number).

Driving is a very complex activity for which the following functional abilities have been identified as important for safe driving[15]:

- *High- and low-contrast visual acuity* – to read signs, detect hazards, and guide the vehicle properly under high and low visibility conditions.
- *Leg strength and stamina* – to use the gas and brake pedals effectively and timely in emergent situations.
- *Head/neck flexibility* – to rapidly check in both directions for cross-traffic, and to look over the shoulder before backing, merging, or changing lanes.
- *Short-term and working memory* – to remember and apply all rules and regulations for safe driving, sign messages, route directions, and other trip information while simultaneously attending to traffic.
- *Visualization of missing information* – to recognize a whole object when only part is in view, helping a driver anticipate and respond earlier to emerging safety threats.
- *Visual search with divided attention* – to rapidly scan the roadway environment for traffic control information, navigational cues, and conflicts with other vehicles or pedestrians, especially at intersections.

While intact central and peripheral vision are probably the most important criteria for safe driving, they are also the criteria easiest to test in the physician's office. There are vast differences among states regarding central and peripheral vision requirements for a driver's license.[16,17] While some states have strict vision requirements, others have no minimum standard for peripheral vision. Some require in-person license renewal allowing for at least a minimal assessment of cognitive function by the licensing counter personnel, but other states allow mail-in renewal so an older driver may go decades without being seen or tested by a department of motor vehicles representative.[17] As eye care professionals, we will often play a vital role in evaluating whether or not our patients are still capable of driving. Consider performing the binocular Esterman test (or AGIS scoring of Humphrey 24-2 fields) in patients with ocular diseases that can affect peripheral vision, especially when you are asked to complete drivers' license forms.

## References

1. Insurance Information Institute. Older drivers. <http://www.iii.org/media/hottopics/insurance/olderdrivers/> Accessed 08.03.08.
2. nationalatlas.gov. The 65 years and over population: 2000. <http://nationalatlas.gov/articles/people/a_age65pop.html> Accessed 08.03.08.
3. US Census Bureau. Projections of the total resident population by 5-year age groups, and sex with special age categories: middle series, 2050 to 2070. <http://www.census.gov/population/projections/nation/summary/np-t3-g.txt>; 2000 Accessed 08.03.08.
4. Insurance Institute for Highway Safety. Fatality facts 2006. <http://www.iihs.org/research/fatality_facts_2006/olderpeople.html> Accessed 08.03.08.
5. The Eye Diseases Prevalence Research Group – Friedman DS, Wolfs RCW, O'Colmain BJ, et al. Prevalence of open-angle glaucoma among adults in the United States. *Arch Ophthalmol.* 2004;122:532–538.
6. Friedman DS, Jampel HD, Muñoz B, West SK. The prevalence of open-angle glaucoma among blacks and whites 73 years and older. The Salisbury Eye Evaluation Glaucoma Study. *Arch Ophthalmol.* 2006;124:1625–1630.
7. McGwin G, Mays A, Joiner W, DeCarlo DK, et al. Is Glaucoma Associated with Motor Vehicle Collision Involvement and Driving Avoidance? *Invest Ophthalmol Vis Sci.* 2004;45:3934–3939.

8. Haymes SA, LeBlanc RP, Nicolela MT, et al. Risk of falls and motor vehicle collisions in glaucoma. *Invest Ophthalmol Vis Sci.* 2007;48:1149–1155.
9. Owsley C, McGwin G, Ball K. Vision impairment, eye disease, and injurious motor vehicle crashes in the elderly. *Ophthalmic Epidemiol.* 1998;5(2):101–113.
10. Szlyk J, Mahler CL, Seiple W, et al. Driving performance of glaucoma patients correlates with peripheral visual field loss. *J Glaucoma.* 2005;14(2):145–150.
11. McLean IM, Mueller E, Buttery RG, Mackey DA. Visual field assessment and the Austroads driving standard. *Clin Exp Ophthalmol.* 2002;30(1):3–7. <http://www3.interscience.wiley.com/journal/118962598/abstract> Accessed 08.10.08.
12. Eyetec.net. Module 15: visual fields, advanced concepts. http://www.eyetec.net/group3/M15S1.htm#Esterman%20Functional%20Tests Accessed 07.27.08.
13. McGwin G, Xie A, Mays A, Joiner W, et al. Visual field defects and the risk of motor vehicle collisions among patients with glaucoma. *Invest Ophthalmol Vis Sci.* 2005;46:4437-4441. <http://www.iovs.org/cgi/content/abstract/46/12/4437> Accessed 08.10.08.
14. Brusini P, Johnson CA. Staging Functional Damage in Glaucoma: Review of Different Classification Methods. *Surv Ophthalmol.* 2007;52(2):56–179.
15. Drivinghealth.com. DrivingHealth inventory – including UFOV. <http://www.drivinghealth.com/screening.htm> Accessed 08.12.08.
16. MD Support. State vision screening and standards for license to drive. <http://www.mdsupport.org/library/drivingrequirements.html> Accessed 08.03.08.
17. Getting Around. The role of the DMV. <http://www.getting-around.org/tools/dmv.cfm> Accessed 08.12.08.

# Chapter 30
# Electronic Medical Records in the Glaucoma Practice

Mildred M.G. Olivier and Linda Hay

Electronic health record (EHR) systems are an expanding technology with the potential to boost the efficiency of medical offices while improving patient safety and enhancing communication among healthcare providers. Although only an estimated 20% of US medical offices currently use EHRs,[1] this number is sure to grow substantially in the years to come. A survey conducted by the Medical Group Management Association (MGMA), published in 2008, looked at 135 ophthalmology practices. Of these, 86% had paper charts in files, and only 12% had EHRs. Fifty-three percent, however, were poised to adopt some form of EHRs within the next 24 months.[2] This chapter offers advice on selecting and implementing an EHR system as well as the legal aspects that should be considered as we come into this new era of electronic medical records. Support for EHRs stretches beyond the immediate medical community. In 2004, President Bush set a goal requiring all medical offices to have some form of operative EHRs by 2014.[3] President Obama's administration is fully committed to this concept as well.

At first glance, choosing an EHR system and incorporating it into a practice may appear time-consuming and expensive. Every practice is different in its staff size, patient numbers, and specialty and technology knowledge. In the long run a properly selected and operated EHR system may save practice time and money,[4] as well as increase patients' feelings of ease with their care. Patients are healthier, more engaged and more satisfied with the healthcare system, and doctors get the support and incentives necessary to help drive better outcomes.[5] An EHR system can also boost your staff's morale. Once installed, the system can cut down on the quantity of phone calls they must handle; decrease the amount of time they spend locating, pulling, and replacing patients' medical records and laboratory results; and maximize the efficiency of internal communications. In an era of pay-for-performance policies, EHRs may help provide the documentation needed for obtaining greater reimbursement and more malpractice-free credits, while also reducing medical errors. One also can draw on the database of codes and diagnoses of an EHR system to support clinical research by defining and fulfilling search parameters.

## 30.1 Initial Task Force

Put together a committee of personnel from various areas in your office – front desk staff, administrator, lead physician, technicians, and billing staff – to review available EHR systems. The group can determine what is needed to meet the requirements and preferences of each department, and build a consensus about what would be best for the office as a whole. Be sure to include on the committee both the person in the office who is the most enthusiastic about adopting an EHR system and the person who is the most reluctant. Their contrasting viewpoints will provide balance to the meetings. The committee should list the hardware, software, and budgetary costs required for your office. Do not forget to check with the local Medicare and other insurance providers to see if they have some specific requirements for electronic medical record and billing systems, as well as some suggestions for commercial systems that meet these requirements.

## 30.2 Find the Right EHR System

Currently, more than 400 companies sell a wide variety of EHR systems. The upside is that you have a lot of options. The downside is that choosing among them is a daunting process. An ophthalmic practice has specific requirements different from other medical specialties, which necessitates a system specifically designed or more adaptable to your practice needs, so it is imperative to conduct extensive research before buying an EHR system. Develop a request for proposals to help you distinguish the individual vendors. In fact, talking to other ophthalmologists in the neighborhood or when you attend professional conferences, especially if you are a subspecialist (glaucoma, retina, pediatric ophthalmology, etc.), can give you excellent insight into potential EHR systems to investigate and those to avoid.

In the twenty-first century, Internet searches are de rigueur before making any major purchase, and EHR systems are no exception.[6] A Web site worth a visit is the Commission for

Healthcare Information Technology (CHIT),[7] which certifies and endorses systems but does not measure how usable they are. The Web can also help you to determine the look of the EMR system you might choose. Appearance is important for the people who use any system. Your task force and others in the office can review appointment screens and the individual EMR pages. You may also want to ask how telephone calls, messages, and new documents can be identified in a chart by the physicians or other personnel.[7]

When assessing an EHR system, take into account its practicality. Does it mesh with your current technology, or are you going to have to replace or upgrade some components? Also, consider costs. These will be both initial and recurring. Costs include provider support, ongoing management and upgrades, privacy/security measures, and backup systems (both on- and off-site). Creating a spreadsheet of the different companies and the features of their systems can help you make a comparison.

If you and your staff lack the time or training to conduct your own Internet research, consider hiring a qualified consultant. A good consultant can help limit the number of companies to be reviewed and act as a liaison between your office and the representatives of EHR companies. When choosing a consultant, ensure that the individual you select has no biases or conflicts of interest (i.e., ties to one EHR company or another).[8]

After establishing the needs of your office, select vendors that seem to be the best match, preferably just three or four. Try to choose companies that have strong track records (have been around for 5–10 years and have more than 100 systems installed), accessible technical support teams (try calling and asking for some advice), and products that are HIPAA-compliant (ask to see documentation). In this instance, it may not be good to be an early adopter. Request a list from each vendor of local practices using their systems. Then call each practice to get their input regarding how pleased they are with the EHR system. If you can find some ophthalmology practitioners who are near your office, and if they like their specific system and vendor, try to arrange to visit them with one or two of your key personnel.

For those "references" you will speak with only by telephone, make sure you ask them how long they have had the system, what are its pluses and minuses, and how responsive the vendor is when problems occur or customization is needed. If possible, try to get a complete list from the vendor of all installations, do not have them cherry-pick and provide you with a list of just their most satisfied customers. Call a few at random and see if they offer differing perspectives on the system and service of the vendor. Most importantly, ask about costs for hardware, staff training, software, upgrades (and frequency) and service contracts (and hours of operation for technical support).

Have the three or four vendors that are the most promising companies, based on your research, come to your office with equipment and provide a demonstration. Ask if some of the hardware can be left for a week or so for various staff members to use and to become more familiar with its operation. Ask the vendors to leave copies of the operating manuals for your perusal. In order to allow the maximum number of physicians and key staff to view the vendor demonstrations, one can use lunchtime or after office hours time slots for visits by the different vendors.

Patient flow and intake time should be evaluated with various vendors to understand better how the system will be integrated into practice (and if possible correlate or at least coexist with your electronic billing systems). It is also important to consider the variety of intake documents that are now on paper in the office, and ask the vendor specifically where that information would be stored. This process will help to determine better how many papers may need to be scanned into the system. Do not forget to inquire whether the system comes with scanning software. Asking many of these questions early may decrease backend headaches for you and the staff.

Does the system provide a convenient means of dictation of office notes and consult letters? Is this done manually by typing or is voice recognition capability part of the system (and how well does it to work)? What kind of networking capabilities does the system have? Can EHRs be accessed from any computer via the Internet, by a physician at home who is responding to an "on call" request from a patient? Can the system be accessed remotely for troubleshooting, upgrading, and debugging by technicians from the vendors company? Does the EHR system physically reside on computer servers at your offices, or are the data sent to central servers over the Internet or virtual private networks that are owned by the vendor, or are they sent to a licensee?

### 30.2.1 Record-Keeping Methods

In medical offices across the country, an immense amount of time, energy, and space are consumed by the management of patient records. An effective EHR system can greatly reduce the hours and dollars dedicated to this process. Admittedly, the time investment may increase initially upon the adoption of EHRs. This happens because staff must enter old documents into the new system. Offices with a huge amount of data to upload may benefit from the hiring of high school students to come in on weekends, holidays, summers, or in the evenings to scan old information onto the EHR system. Some systems are set up for voice activation; others require typing. Choose the one that best suits your needs and existing hardware. Training for staff can be written off from your income taxes for the first year.

Some data may be entered by front office staff by either scannning or typing, but more complex aspect of the glaucoma examination will need to be input by technicians or physicians. Is there a fixed desk top computer in each exam room connected via Ethernet cabling to the servers? Do physicians and technicians perhaps employ portable laptops connected wirelessly to the servers? Do ophthalmic instruments (e.g., visual field machines, lensometers, and imaging devices) electronically transfer their information to the EHR or must their reports be transferred-scanned into the system?

### 30.2.2 Plan on Upgrades

As technology changes, your system will occasionally require updating. Negotiate the fees and terms of such upgrades in advance and be sure that they include training time for your staff. The cost ranges from $5,000 to $15,000.[9]

### 30.2.3 Consider Implementation

Decide whether you want the system to go live all at once or over time (e.g., over the course of 1 week, 1 month, or 1 year). The initial cost for an office has been estimated at $30,000–$50,000 per physician.[10,11]

### 30.2.4 Expect the Unexpected

Understand ahead of time who is/will be the legal owner of the records stored on the system (they should belong to your practice). Establish what kind of disaster recovery plan the EHR provider offers. Make sure that the system provides remote access to patients' charts, both from satellite locations and during off hours.

### 30.2.5 Additional Considerations

Other things to discuss with system manufacturers include:

#### 30.2.5.1 Records

Well-delineated folders need to be chosen to allow easy access to data such as visual fields, lab results, and operative reports.

#### 30.2.5.2 Format

The templates and screens provided by the vendor may need to be customized for the unique demands of your ophthalmology practice. Multispecialty ophthalmology practices may have different requirements from subspecialty practices. One of us writing this sidebar essay is an ophthalmologist in solo practice as a glaucoma subspecialist. The primary requirement needed to implement an EHR system into such a practice. My primary requirement was the ability to integrate existing patient photographs, visual fields, imaging studies, drawings, and gonioscopic details into the new electronic system and to make sure the system was flexible enough to work with any future upgrades to the existing office technology. Cost was a major consideration. A larger practice might have been able to divide the upfront costs and price of hardware more easily than can a solo office practitioner. Consider reducing cost be trying to integrate existing computers and other office hardware into the new EHR, not every vendor will be compatible with this option. Most EHR providers have pricing programs, including rental options, for smaller practices. Integrating the new technology into an EMR system has also brought new demands. At times separate software must be purchased in order to transfer information into an individual's chart into the new electronic health record.

Many ophthalmologists are technologically savvy as they have used computers and digital instruments in many ways both personally and professionally over the past two decades. Thus, in some practices, the ophthalmologists themselves can make suggestions to the vendor to purchase hardware, which is both cost-effective and easy to maintain. But be aware that committing your office to using a specific vendor and their hardware and software is akin to a marriage and should be approached with the same caution that one chooses a spouse. It is helpful to identify a technician or an individual in the office to be the in-house IT person who will both locally troubleshoot the system and interface with the technical support department of the vendor as needed. Having someone at hand who can do some troubleshooting for a variety of problems that may arise can save greatly on costs. Computer hardware itself is constantly becoming less expensive and computer capabilities and capacities (faster processors, increasing hard drive size) are increasing. Make sure your system, both hardware and software, is capable of growing with your practice. Implementing an effective EHR system is likely to be an expensive and somewhat painful process, and may be no longer optional as government mandates come into effect. But in the long run, you, your practice, and your patients will benefit from this twenty-first century way to practice ophthalmology.

## 30.3 Legal Aspects of Electronic Health Records

There are great benefits to the purchase and implementation of updated systems and technology. In the evaluation and assessment of new technology to enhance both performance and efficiency in the practice, however, the prudent practitioner must always consider potential legal risks and exposures that may arise as a result of and may be unique to any such updated systems or processes. The benefits to new systems and technologies that form the EHR, as described above, can be far more apparent than the risks by virtue of the fact that developers of new technologies focus on and market the care related benefits, but often analysis of related legal exposures is not typically part of the design and marketing process.

Given the cost of purchasing and implementing new technologies, the practitioner should investigate not only the cost, performance, and implementation issues, but should also investigate any potential legal related risks prior to purchase. Such an analysis will help provide a complete assessment of the risks and benefits of any product. The following provides guidelines to issues that the practitioner and the committee should assess.

### 30.3.1 Understand the Vital Role of Documentation in the Legal Process

The medical record is the best witness in any potential claim for malpractice. It is made contemporaneous to events, and it is made without bias or knowledge that anything bad has occurred. It does not suffer from forgetfulness over time. It is the proof that the practitioner provided proper, reasonable, and appropriate care. Years later, when memories fade, witnesses move on, and the details of the appropriateness of care become critically important, the record serves as the pivotal piece of evidence in a lawsuit. In a medical malpractice lawsuit, a plaintiff must prove his or her case by testimony of an expert critical of the care. The defendant must defend against those criticisms through supportive opinions of an expert as well as the defendant practitioner. It is far easier for a plaintiff's expert to criticize care when the records lack sufficient detail. Without adequate documentation, the plaintiff's expert often claims that if the care was not documented in the records, then the care did not occur. Reliance on the actual record as proof of the care provides stronger, objective evidence than simple reliance on sworn testimony years later.

### 30.3.2 Accurately Assess the Installation Time

The actual time needed to install new technologies can be quick or slow. Transition time is a critical period since there may be difficulties in access to that technology or system, and other modalities may be needed to maintain contemporaneous records. Methods for maintaining the consistency and integrity of records for care rendered during the installation process should be assessed by the committee and implemented prior to the actual installation so that any records prepared during this down time will be clear and contemporaneous if called into question years later. If the installation process is such that down time is lengthy, or the process is so different than the usual record keeping process, then the interim process should be detailed in a written document and kept in a file to help detail and explain how or why records were kept in such a manner so that the detail of this change in process can be explained at a later date if the need arises.

### 30.3.3 Predict the Changes in the Process of Recordkeeping

The time it takes to implement new technology in the office can mean a change in regular documentation practices. If there is a change in hardware or software, there is a change in process. A change in process means a change in the way records are kept, whether it is an issue of the nature of the procedure performed, or a change in the forms used. Any change in the processes of the practice will likely have some impact on the type or way a medical record is kept. Changes in the process mean less consistency, and the chance that important information may be lost in the translation. It is critical to know what changes will occur before they are implemented. If assessed, there may be steps that can be taken in the new process to help account for these changes. For example, if a new testing machine is acquired and the use of this new machine requires that a patient provide a critical piece of health history information to properly perform the testing, but the health history form in use does not require this piece of information, steps must be taken to change the process of recordkeeping to develop a new health history form. As part of the purchase assessment of this machine, there should be an accounting for a change in the health history process.

### 30.3.4 Know the Training Time Required

If issues in litigation arise concerning the appropriateness of care with new technologies, the issue of whether the practitioner and staff were properly trained in its use may be a basis for criticism, if that failure caused or contributed to an injury. As with any new process or technology, training is critical to appropriate use. Without accurate input of information needed to run the technology, later proof of the proper use may be difficult to assess. During this critical training period, understand that problems may occur, and know how to deal with them quickly and proactively. Be aware of the scope of the impact of any new technologies on the office processes and the medical record. The broader the scope of the impact, the more is the time that should be devoted to training. Having the committee available in the purchase process to focus on and assess these issues so they are handled in a timely and consistent manner is helpful. Ongoing assessment as to whether training is complete, and whether additional training is needed beyond the initial phase is also beneficial and should be documented to establish proper training and use.

### 30.3.5 Deal with Issues Related to Accurate Input of Information

Accurate input of information can be critical not only to substantive care issues, but also to recordkeeping issues. As such, typing accuracy can be critical not only to the substantive use of a technology or system, but also to the flow and clarity of the medical record itself. As technologies provide greater efficiencies such that actual typing is not needed (such as point and click or drag and drop methods), it becomes more imperative to have checks and balances in place to assess this accuracy. Methods that can be used in this regard are: ability and ease of use of spell check; regular auditing of records to assess accuracy of information; cross checks within systems to catch accuracy errors early; ability and understanding of the use of correction features; and limited access to the correction of errors after information has been downloaded or processed. Make sure that the system permits you to enter corrections to wrongly recorded information and that it provides some mechanisms for signing and dating any changes to the medical record (an audit trail for corrections.) It is imperative that a medical record that appears in court must never appear to have been altered after it was first recorded unless such changes are documented by signature and date they were made into the chart.

### 30.3.6 Be Aware of the Printed Format

Unlike old recordkeeping systems that were manual, new systems and documentation related to new technologies produce far different formats of medical records. Moreover, the use of electronic programs, systems or technologies may all have differing formats for both what the user sees onscreen as information is input or accessed, versus what the printed final form "record" shows. All users should be aware of how all versions appear on screen and on paper. The actual record used for legal purposes is that of the printed version. Because of this, it is critically important to view what the printed record looks like as this is what will be produced when records are requested. Certain types of printed records may appear confusing, or difficult to follow chronologically. Input or typographical errors that may not be apparent onscreen can be glaring in a printed version. Part of the regular audit process should include review of the printed record.

### 30.3.7 Beware the Lack of Narrative Information

From an efficiency perspective, technologies can, and are marketed to, decrease the time spent on actual input of narrative information. Use of menus, drop downs, and customization for particular processes or patients provide a clear benefit for both practitioner and staff. From a legal perspective, however, lack of narrative makes it far more difficult to determine what really transpired with this particular patient. Years later, when trying to reconstruct the care that took place, and to prove that the care was proper, the lack of any individual detail beyond pure demographics makes it harder to defend a claim. For example, a common defense in malpractice cases is that the patient failed to follow the doctor's advice as to follow up care. While a program for scheduling may have the benefit of automatically generating reminders to patients who have failed to return for care, there may not be easy access to input individualized issues in that failure to follow up that could strongly bolster a defense, or help witnesses remember what happened with this patient years before. In a lawsuit, for example, while it is good to have a printout showing that two reminder calls and two phone calls for follow-up were done, it is far better to have additional narrative notes from the office manager stating that there was a 10 min discussion with the patient in which the patient assured that he or she was off to work and so would absolutely call the next morning and schedule an appointment, and a subsequent 5 min phone call made the next week in which the patient said he or she could not then find a ride to the office, and the staff person advised that the office would arrange for transportation on the specified date. So make sure that the EHR system you purchase allows for free form text input in all important fields, including allowing for notes about missed and rescheduled appointments as well as notes on any phone conversations with the patients.

### 30.3.8 Know What Information Is Available

Electronic software systems and other technologies store far more data than does a written record. Electronic data may be embedded in documents and systems that are not apparent to the casual user. Records of keystrokes may be maintained in systems or backup systems and never truly deleted. Be aware that in a lawsuit, requests are being made to produce not only the written record, but embedded information inherent in the system or its backup data. Purchasers of systems should know what information is retained so that they can assure that anyone inputting information or using the technology knows what is retained, and so that, at a later point, if necessary, information can be recovered and produced.

### 30.3.9 Address Confidentiality Issues

With such an emphasis on the privacy and security of electronic medical records, including HIPAA, it is incumbent on the practitioner to know what privacy and security issues are a part of the system or program itself, and to assess the use of the technology in their own practice setting. Beyond basic requirements such as password use, accessibility by staff on a need-to-know basis, encryptions, and log-off times, the prudent practitioner should also consider those issues that relate to the personal nature of communication between the patient and the provider. While the EHR, as indicated above, can provide benefits to the patient, be aware that the use of electronic systems has the capability to lend an impersonal nature to the relationship with the patient. Laundry lists of symptoms or history as dictated by the programmer of a system might not cover every aspect critical to the care. It is imperative that the practitioner and the committee work to personalize the process for the patient, even if the technology helps streamline the process, and the confidentiality concerns create other issues. Disgruntled, unhappy patients are more likely to pursue a lawsuit if there is a bad result. Maintaining the personal touch with the patient will always serve the practitioner well in the event a problem occurs later.

Also be aware of the ever-expanding release of information electronically to physical locations outside the physical office such as home computers, blackberries, emails, billing services, etc. Care must be taken to assure that these outside sites maintain this personal information appropriately as well.

### 30.3.10 Policies Based on New Technologies

If new technologies require ongoing changes in process, new policies may help clarify the process and maintain consistency. If policies are adopted, they must be followed. Be aware that policies should be written as guidelines, not requirements that mandate the standard of care.

### 30.3.11 Use and Investigation of Resources

There are many resources available to the practitioner to help understand and assess the issues related to risk management with new technologies. Physician associations, office management associations, nurse and assistant organizations, risk management organizations, healthcare organizations, and insurance organizations or carriers, all may have resources available to address these concerns, and provide guidance for actual practice-related risks. As indicated previously, contacting references from the vendor (other users of the systems or technologies) can be a very helpful resource to investigate risk issues, assess practical risk problems and potential solutions, and may help to shape or develop policies. Inquiries to the vendor can be telling as well. If a vendor has never heard the term risk management, the practitioner and his or her committee may have to do more investigation.

### 30.3.12 Downtime for Updates, Maintenance, and Possible System Failure

Be aware of the requisite maintenance schedule, the need to update, time to download, repair or update new systems or technologies. Again, the seller and references from the seller can help to provide this information. Knowing what will occur when the system or technology is down periodically will help shape the course of care and recordkeeping during those times. If the down time will be significant or will require significant changes in the process or recordkeeping, know or have a clear policy on what to do in the interim. Be prepared also for what to do in the event of a system or technology failure. Depending on the nature and scope of the impact that such a failure may have on care or record keeping, it may be necessary to have a formal policy on what to do in the event of a failure. For example, if there is a scheduling program that not only sets all appointments but generates the entire new patient file record, forms, history and consents, and that system fails, there must be a consistent manual process followed for the opening of new records, to be sure that all proper information is covered and provided on that first visit and thereafter until the system is backup and running. It is during these times that potential legal exposures can occur. The importance of backup systems for electronic health systems cannot be overemphasized. A regular daily (onsite) or more often backup of all records/servers should be done with transfer occasionally of the physical media used for backup to offsite (safebox?) locations and perhaps multiple backups to several different physical media to several locations.

## 30.4 Conclusion

Choosing an EHR system is much like selecting a partner or a spouse. There are a lot of positive aspects in having an EMR system such as remote access from home, another office, or surgery suite. Patient access to information can be at the tip of your fingers. Everyone authorized can obtain information from the chart. Billing is not delayed by the disappearance of an individual's chart for key insurance information. One can customize the EHR so that documentation is consistent with the Physician Quality Reporting Initiative (PQRI) requirements, etc. This can lead to increased revenue and decreased practice liability for required documentation. The EHR system should provide the physician and staff with prompts as to what tests and procedures should be performed during the current office visit, helping to ensure that the best possible examination is done.

Making the correct choice on an EMR System can save a lot of pain and aggravation. If things do not work out, a painful (and costly) separation may occur. In 2004, the AMA stated that online communication may be the wave of the future. Prepare yourself with an EHR system.

## References

1. Fonkych K, Taylor R. The state and pattern of health information technology adoption [Internet]. 2005 [cited 2008 Sep 26]; Santa Monica (CA): Rand Corporation; 68 p. Available at: http://rand.org/pubs/monographs/2005/RAND_MG409.pdf.
2. Summary of AOA membership survey on electronic health records [Internet]. 2007 Sep [cited 2008 Sep 26]. Englewood (CO): Medical Group Management Association; Available at: http://www.aao.org/education/upload/09070_QOC_Survey_Rev1.pdf.
3. U.S. Department of Health & Human Services. HHS announces project to help 3.6 million consumers reap benefits of electronic health records [news release on the Internet]. 2007 Oct 30 [cited 2008 Sep 24]. Washington, DC: Available at: http://www.hhs.gov/news/press/2007pres/10/pr20071030a.html.
4. Rosenberg R. The automated glaucoma office. Glaucoma Today [Internet]. 2007 Dec [cited 2008 Sep 27]; Available at: http://www.glaucomatoday.com/articles/1107/GT1107_11.php.
5. Pope J. Implementing EHRs requires a shift in thinking. Health Manag Technol [Internet]. 2006 Jun [cited 2008 Sep 27]; Nelson Publishing, Inc. Available at: http://archive.healthmgttech.com/archives/0606/0606implementing_ehrs.htm.
6. Lynn J. Medscape today: choosing an EMR. Medscape Business Med [Internet]. 2008 April 11 [cited 2008 Sep 24]; New York: WebMD. Available at: http://www.medscape.com/viewarticle/571849.
7. Certification Commission for Healthcare Information Technology [Internet]. 2005–2008 [cited 2008 Sep 24]; Chicago (IL): Available at: http://www.cchit.org/index.asp.
8. Mastering patient flow [monograph on the Internet]. 2007 [cited 2008 Sep 24];3. Englewood (CO). Medical Group Management Association. 498 p. Available at: https://secure3.aao.org/store/common/index.cfm?mode=kilwwvgz&subsystem=ORD&primary_id=012181.
9. Adler K. Why it's time to purchase an electronic records system. Fam Pract Manag [Internet]. 2004 Nov/Dec [cited 2008 Sep 27]; American Academy of Family Physicians. Available at: http://www.aafp.org/fpm/20041100/43whyi.pdf.
10. Lohr S. Most doctors aren't using electronic health records. New York Times [Internet]. 2008 Jun 19 [cited 2008 Sep 24]; Available at: http://www.glaucomatoday.com/articles/1107/GT1107_11.php.

# Chapter 31
# Advanced Glaucoma and Low Vision: Evaluation and Treatment

Scott Robison

The hallmark of glaucoma is progressive vision loss, albeit in the early stages the vision loss is peripheral and often not discernible to the patient. Patients with advanced glaucoma may have significant vision loss, both peripheral and central, possibly with devastating impact on the patient's ability to perform their activities of daily living. Advanced glaucoma can be one of the most challenging and difficult conditions for the vision rehabilitation specialist to treat. The degree of success with the rehabilitation therapies currently available is limited, and rehabilitation itself does not protect against further vision loss that may continue to worsen even with the best medical and surgical care available to the patient. When the patient incurs vision loss that is functionally disabling, it is incumbent on the eye care provider, either ophthalmologist or optometrist, to have a strategy for vision rehabilitation (low vision) in place. Some rehabilitation services are easily provided in the office setting, while others must be referred out of office to provide the services the patient needs.

At initial diagnosis, patients with glaucoma may have little functional loss. These patients will only need general eye care to take care of their visual needs for routine daily activities. Glaucomatous optic neuropathy does not normally cause debilitating functional loss in its early stages, but educating the patient to potential rehabilitation services early in the disease process will make later transitions easier. Some patients at their initial diagnosis, or patients with longstanding recalcitrant glaucoma, may have significant functional vision loss. Those patients with significant loss of vision will need more extensive evaluation, and the therapeutic strategies may be more elaborate and complicated. When patients begin to experience vision loss that cannot be remediated by standard spectacle prescriptions, the patient should be entered into the vision rehabilitation system, either in-house or through referral to a vision rehabilitation specialist.

Functional loss frequently starts with mobility and ambulation problems. In a recent study, patients with peripheral field loss related to glaucoma demonstrated decreased traffic gap judgment in crossing the street, leading to increased risk of injury. As a group, they made 23% more errors in identifying a gap as crossable when it was too short.[2] Compared with control subjects, patients with glaucoma and reduced visual field were over three times more likely to have fallen in the last year and six times more likely to have been involved in a motor vehicle collision in the previous 5 years.[3] Noe et al. found that 25% of subjects with relatively minor visual field loss in both eyes reported a moderate to severe restriction in mobility activities.[4] According to McKean-Cowdin et al., greater severity of visual field loss related to glaucoma results in lower vision-related quality-of-life scores. In summary, people with glaucoma and reduced visual field experience more falls, more motor vehicle collisions, greater difficulty with mobility activities, increased risk of being hit by a car while crossing the street, and reduced quality of life.[5]

Some patients may have glaucoma as their primary and only ocular dysfunction, but many patients with glaucoma, who are often elderly, have other systemic or ocular health disorders as well. The low vision specialist needs to consider all eye and medical diseases even if the patient is referred for rehabilitation related to glaucoma. Patients with glaucoma and macular degeneration will have central acuity loss coupled with peripheral field loss, making the rehabilitation process more difficult. Cataract will reduce acuity and contrast sensitivity compounding the patient's functional loss. Diseases affecting the cornea may contribute to the patient's loss of function through glare sensitivity and decreased acuity.

## 31.1 Difficulties Experienced by Patients with Glaucoma

### 31.1.1 Visual Field Loss

The hallmark of moderate glaucoma is visual field loss. Paracentral scotomas coalesce into arcuate scotomas, ultimately forming double arcuate (ring) scotomas extending to the peripheral limits in all directions except temporally.[1,6] As the visual field loss increases with advanced glaucoma, only central and temporal islands of vision remain. At end stage, this results in visual fields with only remaining central and temporal islands of vision in advanced glaucoma. If the glaucoma is not controlled, the central island will diminish and eventually extinguish followed by the temporal island. Legal blindness is defined in most jurisdictions as 20° or less of total visual field in the horizontal meridian of the better-seeing eye. (Patients may also be described as legally blind based on acuity criteria alone, for example, less than 20/200 vision in the best-seeing eye.) Approximately 5% of patients with glaucoma go on to total blindness.[7] Early glaucomatous field loss will probably go unnoticed by the patient. As the field loss increases, patients may notice increased functional impairment. Mobility is often the first function affected. Peripheral field loss, without central acuity loss, will affect automobile driving skills first, then ambulation. Patients may complain of bumping into objects or people suddenly appearing as they enter from the patient's scotomas. The small visual field may cause difficulty keeping place while reading. Inferior arcuate defects also may affect reading, causing the patient to complain that their bifocals are no longer effective. As the central island starts to diminish, the central acuity will diminish as well. This decreases the patient's ability to spot distant objects, see faces, and discern print and near objects.

### 31.1.2 Visual Acuity

Central vision reduction usually occurs late in glaucoma, but studies have shown mild central and diffuse reduction in fields in the early stages.[1,8–13] Patients with glaucoma are more likely to reach the legal blindness standard for visual field than the standard of 20/200 in the better-seeing eye for acuity. Therefore, visual acuity may vary over a great range for different degrees of optic nerve head loss in glaucoma. Early acuity will often be normal even with progressing visual field defects. Visual acuity may be affected by concurrent eye disease. As the glaucoma progresses, there can be central field defects with significant central acuity loss. These patients are difficult to rehabilitate due to the small working field impeding the amount of magnification that will work for the patient.

### 31.1.3 Glare

As visual field and acuity decrease, patients will often complain of glare sensitivity. Glare sensitivity and photophobia are common problems in patients with glaucoma because of reduced contrast sensitivity, slower response times to light and dark adaptation, and decreased light absorption.[14] Glare can be compounded by cataract, dry eye, macular degeneration, or other ocular maladies. Glare may run the gamut from mildly annoying to debilitating. Glare is divided into two categories: discomfort glare and disability glare. Some glare can be alleviated with tints and anti-reflective coatings.

## 31.2 Definition of Vision Rehabilitation

*Vision rehabilitation*, or *low vision*, is the branch of eye care that takes care of patients with significant vision loss. The need for referral to a vision rehabilitation specialist depends upon the patient's needs and desires as well as the willingness of their eye care physician to provide low vision services. Some comprehensive practitioners do include vision rehabilitation as part of their practices and will only need to make referrals when the patient's vision loss exceeds their abilities and equipment. Much of vision rehabilitation can be done in the comprehensive ophthalmology or optometry office. The goal of vision rehabilitation is to increase the patient's ability to function with their vision loss, not to restore the vision that has been lost. By increasing patients' ability to function, they are better able to maintain their independence and are less likely to depend on others for help with their daily needs. This will help create greater confidence, self-esteem, self-reliability, and better quality of life. In patients with advanced glaucoma, the goals are to maintain their acuity with appropriate spectacles, maintain their reading and near-point functioning, offer help for any peripheral field loss, mitigate any glare the patient experiences, and be a conduit to networking the patient to any other services they require.

Referrals to vision rehabilitation usually occur after the patient has decreased vision loss of 20/40 or worse, or visual field defects that impact activities of daily living. By the time the patient has arrived at the legal blindness standard of a horizontal field of 20° or less in the better-seeing eye, they will be experiencing significant mobility problems. By then, the patient usually has gone through all recommended medical and surgical interventions. The most important determinant for referral is the impact the field or acuity loss is having on the patient. Glare may hasten the vision rehabilitation referral. The vision rehabilitation specialist will have a greater range of devices for rehabilitation to explore with the patient than the average primary care eye provider. Further, eye care practitioners specializing in low vision are committed to spending more "chair time" with the patient than is generally available to the comprehensive ophthalmologist, optometrist, or glaucoma specialist. Office records, including visual field exams, should accompany the patient who is seeing the low vision specialist in consultation.

The goals of vision rehabilitation are to maximize independence in the patient's activities of daily living. The problems most frequently experienced by patients with advanced glaucoma are those of ambulation, reading, spotting, and glare. For ambulation, there are optical devices to expand the visual field and prisms to displace the field to a more usable area. For reading, there are magnification and tracking strategies. For glare, there are tints and photochromic lenses as well as lighting strategies. And for other activities of daily living, there are a host of optical and non-optical strategies.

In all, there are many options that are available for the patient and the role of the vision rehabilitation specialist is to advise patients of these strategies and services. Finally, it is important that the patient and the referring physician have realistic expectations of the vision rehabilitation process. Patients who believe they are going to be cured or returned to their pre-glaucoma visual functioning will need to be educated to avoid severe disappointment. Patients need to move through the psychological stages of grief over their loss of vision before they are fully ready to engage in the vision rehabilitation process. It is also important that family members and other caretakers understand and participate in the vision rehabilitation process.

## 31.3 The Examination Sequence

### 31.3.1 Observation

Observe the patient when he or she approaches and enters the room. Patients with severe field loss may have someone leading them, or they may misjudge obstacles and walk into them while navigating. They may be using a cane or walker more for navigation than stability. Observe how they look at you when you call their name. Do they look directly at you or do they fixate you eccentrically? Observe if, and what, they are reading in the waiting area. Is it standard print or large print? Observe if they attempt to fill out a history form or other forms or if their caretakers complete them. Pay attention to the type of pen they use and the size of their writing. Observe interactions among the patient and accompanying friends or family members. These discreet observations may be clues to the level of the patient's functional disability.

### 31.3.2 History

Prior to the office visit, send the patient a health and social history questionnaire and a checklist of rehabilitation priorities. This should be in large print to facilitate the patient's ability to complete the form without the help of others. Included in the history should be the patient's general health history, ocular history, social history, their functional problems, and priorities for rehabilitation. The formal office examination starts with a review of these forms and the informal observations described previously. Ask accompanying friends or family members to participate in the historical review and to watch the examination if possible. These persons may help to obtain a more complete history and may describe patient daily needs that the patient may fail to articulate. There is some risk that the accompanying friends or family members will dominate the process and so this interview must be structured by the examiner.

#### 31.3.2.1 Health History

This is standard for all patients, but for the vision rehabilitation patient use large-print forms. Pay attention to any conditions or medications that could potentially further impair the patient's vision. Obtain a complete review of symptoms, full medication list, allergies, and history of general surgeries as these may help disclose something that the patient does not consider important but that might impact their ability to benefit from certain optical aids. Documentation of this information is also important for billing purposes, especially if using evaluation and management (E&M) codes.

#### 31.3.2.2 Ocular History

Ocular history includes any ocular surgeries, ocular medications, ocular problems identified in the past, and the natural history of current problems. Questions to ask include:

- Are there any other ocular conditions that will impact their vision?
- How and when does the patient take their glaucoma medications? What eye surgical procedures have they had, and what post-op regimen, short and long term, are they following?
- Particularly, have they had any previous vision rehabilitation services?
- Have any optical aid devices been prescribed before?
- Are they using the devices?
- Did they have training?
- Do they have spectacles?
- Do they use them?
- Or do they feel that they are not useful?

The patient's chief complaint will often be very general, for example, "I can't see distance objects" or "I run into things." If they are more specific, take special note of the complaints they enumerate, making use of a six-point history of present illness described as follows. The patient should be encouraged to elaborate on the problems they are having. It is important to elicit the functional challenges the patient is experiencing.

The six-point history should include:

1. Location – overall, central, peripheral, one eye, both eyes
2. Severity – rated from mild to disabling
3. Duration and onset – from recent to longstanding
4. Timing – constant or fluctuating

5. Modifying factors – what helps or hurts
6. Associated signs and symptoms – glare, contrast, etc.

The patient should then be asked to prioritize the goals he or she described on the pre-visit questionnaire. Have the family members present involved in this discussion. Have the patient rate which of his or her functional difficulties are most important to him or her. Those designated as most important will be addressed at the first visit. Generally, we start with the three goals and evaluate the success of achieving these goals at the first visit. Sometimes a single optical device can accomplish several of the goals. Once these goals are achieved, additional goals can be addressed.

### 31.3.2.3 Social History

It is important, with patients who have visual impairment, to understand their living situation and to elicit the functional challenges the patient is experiencing. First, try to identify the patient's support system – who helps him or her and if he or she lives alone or with family or other caregivers.

Next try to determine the patient's functional challenges by asking questions such as:

- What are their tasks at home?
- Do they cook?
- Do they clean?
- Do they do the laundry?
- Do they bathe themselves?
- Do they dress themselves?
- Do they ride the bus or take cabs?
- Do they drive?
- Who facilitates their transport?
- Do they use a wheelchair, walker, or cane?
- What is their level of education?
- Do they have a job?
- Do they want a job?
- What are their hobbies?
- Can they participate in them?
- Are there household tasks that they cannot perform?
- Do they have a social worker?
- Do they have a counselor or psychologist?
- Are they in assisted living?
- Are meals provided?
- What are the particulars of their living arrangements with regard to lighting, kitchen, bath, television size, radio, tape player, and computer?
- Do they live in a house or an apartment?
- Are there stairs, elevators, or long hallways?
- Do they wear spectacles?
- Have they obtained magnifiers on their own?
- What devices have they obtained that make things better – doorway peepholes, telescopes, software, etc.

## 31.4 Visual Acuity Measurement

During vision rehabilitation sessions, visual acuity measurements are typically done with high-contrast charts using bright lighting. Projection charts, typically used in general eye care, are not appropriate for most visually impaired patients due to low contrast, smaller optotype sizes, and few increments of acuity. Projection charts also tend to be presented in darkened rooms. This may give inaccurate acuity measurements as it can bring cataract, glare, pupil size, and other ocular anomalies into play. Testing should be done if possible at levels similar to what the patient will encounter at home or at work to simulate a "real world" experience. One good option is to use a brightly lit Sloan chart placed at 10 ft. Other practitioners may prefer the Early Treatment Diabetic Retinopathy Study (ETDRS) chart. However, the EDTRS chart does not have some of the larger letter sizes and must be repositioned frequently. The "Designs for Vision Distance Test Chart for the Partially Sighted," because of its larger available optotypes, is effective for patients with more severe acuity loss (Fig. 31.1).

Visual acuity measurement should be as accurate as possible so that calculations made will yield the best prescriptions for

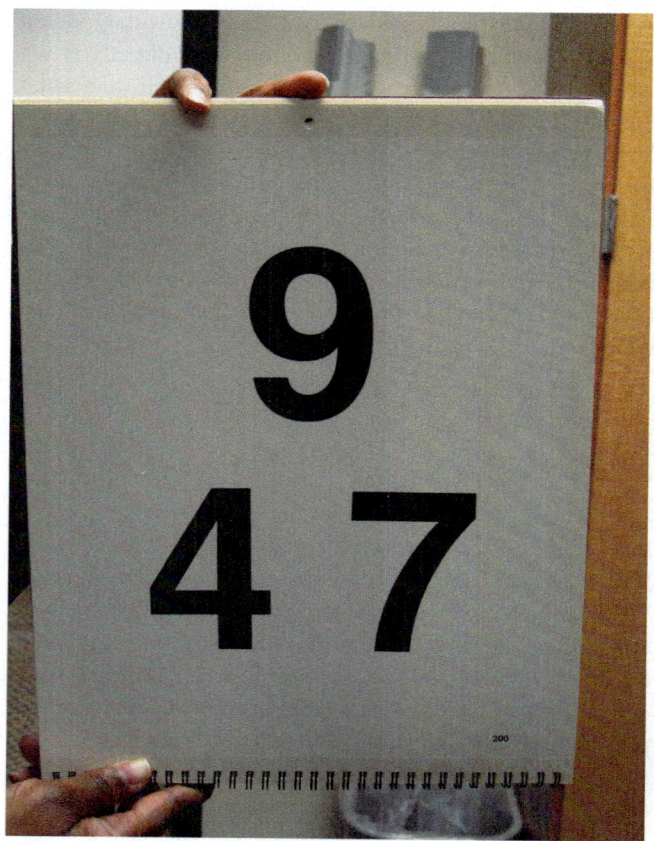

**Fig. 31.1** The designs for vision distance test chart for the partially sighted is effective for patients with more severe acuity loss

spectacles and devices. The patient is strongly encouraged to read the smallest characters that they can. Patients will often stop short of their true acuity and only with friendly but firm insistence will they push themselves to the limits of their true acuity. Encourage them to fixate eccentrically if necessary to improve performance. You may find that they already have a preferred locus of fixation. Some patients will not know how to properly find the optimum fixation point for best vision. They may know that there is a position that they occasionally find that yields best sight after shifting their gaze or moving their head. Encourage them to do so in your office. This will give you some idea of how well the patient will fair with eccentric fixation training. Patients that are reticent to try to read the acuity chart or quit easily may be depressed over their condition and lack motivation toward accepting functional help. These patients may not have fully accepted their vision loss. They may not be good candidates for vision rehabilitation until they have more fully worked through the process of grieving and acceptance.

### 31.4.1 Near Acuities

Near acuities should be done at the patient's most comfortable position with the spectacles or devices that they currently use. For example, if the patient has had an add of +4.00 prescribed in the past, they should read at a distance of 25 cm (10 in.) and reflexively move any near acuity card to that distance. The Bailey–Lovie Near Reading Card can be used for near acuities (Fig. 31.2). It does not test single letter acuity, but it is useful in gauging a patient's performance initially and can be used to make comparisons when evaluating the patient for near adds or magnifiers.

### 31.4.2 Visual Field Assessment

Evaluating the visual field is an important part of the low vision evaluation. If fields are not available, try to obtain them at the initial low vision visit. Use whatever form of perimetry available, be it automated perimetry, Goldmann perimetry, or the tangent screen. It is important to have an understanding of the size of the patient's remaining field when trying to rehabilitate a patient with advanced glaucoma. The Goldmann perimeter is probably the best option as it allows an easier assessment of the visual field using large stimuli. The Humphrey Automated 10-2 field may also help understand the remaining central field size of the patient with advanced glaucoma.

### 31.4.3 Refraction

All vision rehabilitation patients need a meticulous refraction. Patients often will arrive without any refractive correction, or corrections that are very old and ineffective. They may have only kept their vision care up-to-date in regard to their glaucoma and may have ignored getting new spectacles for some time. The refraction is the starting point upon which all optical devices are based. Use of a lensometer to determine the patient's current prescription will assist you in accurately

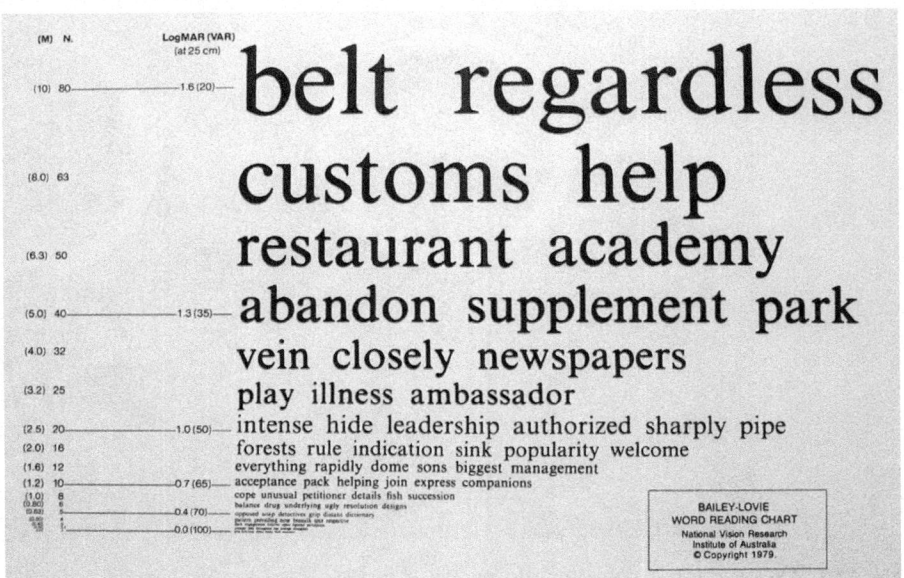

**Fig. 31.2** The Bailey–Lovie word reading card is effective for assessments of reading adds and near magnification

refracting the patient. Autorefractors will give one a starting point, especially with patients who are difficult to retinoscope, although the same reasons that make a patient difficult to retinoscope will give the auto refractor problems. Retinoscopy is still the mainstay of refraction for patients who have severe decreases in acuity. Older patients will tax your retinoscopy skills because they often have small pupils or media opacities in the visual axes. To increase the intensity of the reflex, radical retinoscopy can be used, which is retinoscopy done at shorter working distances than the usual 20–26 in. It is important to remember that the compensating power will be increased as the scoping distance decreases.[15] If your reflex is obtained at 25 cm, then you must compensate with 4 diopters of minus power for the net finding. Consider a dilated retinoscopy and bringing the patient back for device assessment if you have difficulty assessing the retinoscopic reflex. Keratometry or corneal topography can also be helpful in determining starting points for refraction, as they will help you determine corneal astigmatism.

Patients with vision loss often respond better to refractions done without a phoropter. The phoropter may inhibit their ability to eccentrically fixate. If there is a larger refractive error, the vertex distance of the phoropter as compared to the spectacles may be problematic. If you use the phoropter in these cases, measure the vertex distance and note it for use with the spectacle prescription. Prescriptions of greater than ± 4.00 diopters will be sensitive to vertex changes. If you use the phoropter, consider a ±0.50 or ±1.00 Jackson cross cylinder for cylinder assessment. Even when using the phoropter for determining the patient's distance prescription, the patient should have his or her add determination performed in a trial frame.

Trial frame refractions are a more effective way to refract patients with subnormal vision because they allow greater amounts of light to reach the eye, the doctor can view the patient's eye, the vertex distance can be regulated more easily, and the patient has a better understanding of the examination process. Trial frame refractions can be performed in several ways. Use of a standard trial frame is easiest because it usually allows four wells for trial lens insertion. Trial frames differ in their construction. Some trial frames are significantly lighter and easier to use, such as the "Universal," made by Oculus (Fig. 31.3). If the patient's retinoscopy and autorefraction indicate that the refraction is close to his or her current spectacles, Halberg clips may be used over the patient's glasses (Fig. 31.4). Halberg clips also allow for multiple wells for trial frame insertion. These clip onto the front of the patient's spectacles and function as a modified trial frame. Alternatively, lenses can even be dipped directly over a patient's spectacles.

Trial frame refractions are performed identically to those that are done in the phoropter. Start with retinoscopy findings, and also use information from lensometry, keratometry, and auto refractor readings. Add spherical lenses until you obtain the patient's best acuity, then use your ±0.50 or ±1.00D handheld

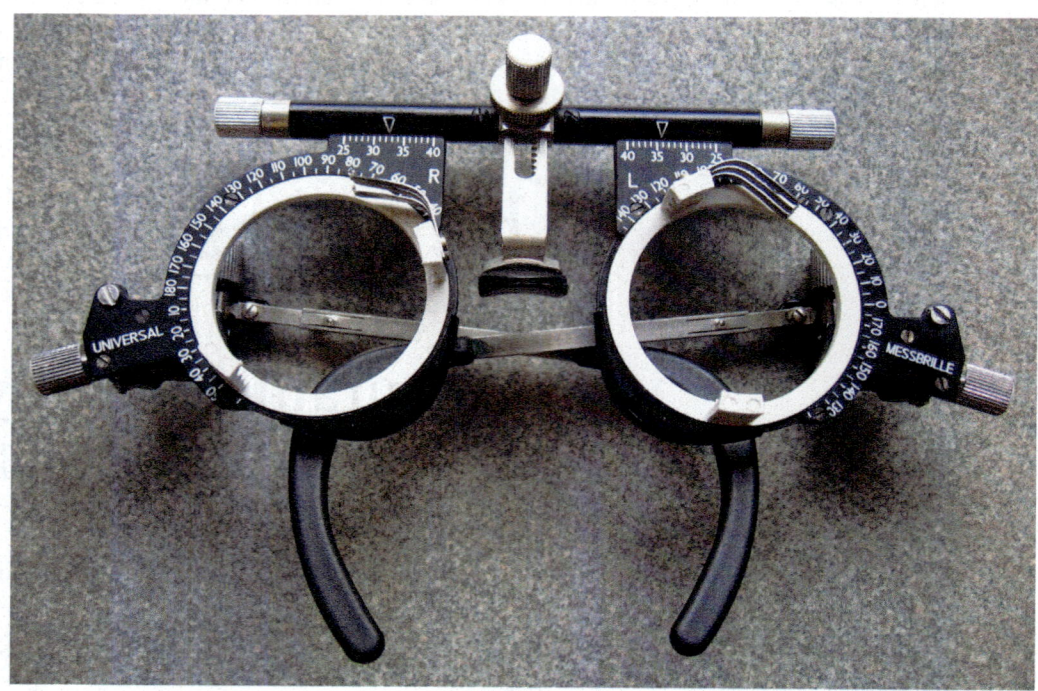

**Fig. 31.3** The universal trial frame from Oculus is an example of a lighter weight trial frame appropriate for trial frame refractions

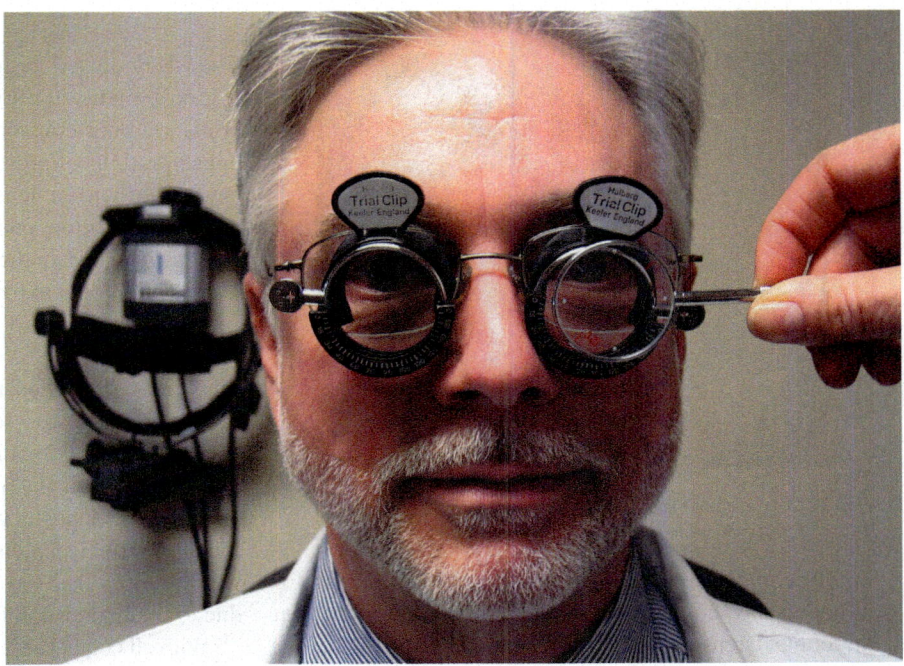

**Fig. 31.4** Halberg clips clip onto the patient's spectacles for trial frame refractions. The handheld Jackson Cross Cylinder is invaluable for trial frame refractions

Jackson cross cylinder to refine first the power, then the axis of cylinder. Then refine the sphere power if significant changes were made in the cylinder correction. You may have the patient self-refine the axis of the cylinder if you are having difficulty. Have them reach up and turn the axis knob of the trial frame, instructing the patient that they should be fine-tuning like they would the dial of a radio to bring in the station most clearly. See Sidebar 31.1 for discussion of contact lenses.

---

**SIDEBAR 31.1 Contact lenses and the glaucoma patient**

Jane Bachman Groth

The utilization of contact lenses in the glaucoma surgical population has been controversial. Significant risks have been associated with filtration blebs and contact lens wear. Thin-walled, avascular blebs with adjunctive antimetabolites have been shown to have a higher risk of endophthalmitis. With chronic trauma or daily placement of a contact lens, breakdown or bacterial infection of the bleb may be more likely. In certain cases, however, contact lenses are required for optimal visual correction. Whenever possible, it is imperative to carefully select the most appropriate candidates. Patient education is also critical to success and monitoring of potential side effects. Fitting philosophies are typically altered with the goal of decreasing risk in these patients.

A review of eight patients with filtering blebs who were fitted with contact lenses at Wills Eye Hospital was evaluated over a 9-year period. Patients were fitted with both soft and rigid gas-permeable contact lens modalities. Over an average follow-up period of 64.6 months, there were no significant complications noted. This study is significant as it shows that the risk of complications is lower than previously thought.

**Lens fit philosophy**

Optimal patient selection consists of characteristics of acceptable motivation, adequate agility with handling of the contact lenses, and good hygiene. Willingness to comply with careful follow-up is a must. Age is not a disqualifying factor.

History of a bleb leak, contact lens wear, contaminated eye drops, eyelid disease (such as blepharitis or rosacea), and conjunctivitis all may increase the risk of infection and endophthalmitis. Corneal health can be monitored with endothelial cell counts if necessary. Therefore, the most important requirement is the understanding of untoward symptoms signifying possible serious complications and the need to return for immediate follow-up if necessary.

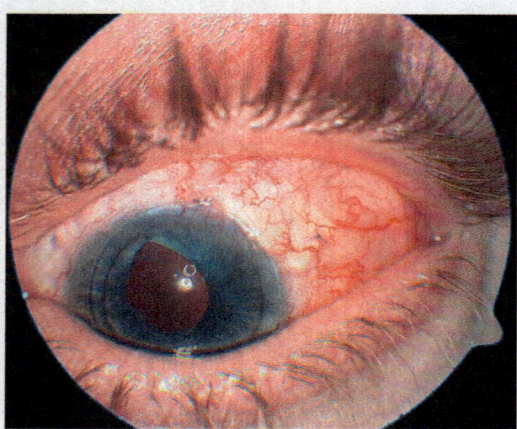

**Fig. 31.1-1** Contact lens used after surgery

Poorly compliant patients are at a much higher risk for infection and should not be fitted. It is recommended that the contact lens fit is not initiated until at least a year from the formation of the filtration bleb. A thicker-walled bleb is optimal so as to avoid leaks. The assurance of a Seidel negative bleb is essential to low-risk fitting.

Optimal fitting characteristics consist of several important factors. The first is lens type. Whenever possible, rigid gas-permeable lenses are recommended in order to provide the best oxygen transmission. In addition, custom design of the lens allows for the best fit for each patient. The relatively smaller diameter of a rigid lens (8.0–9.0 mm) may allow less physical contact with the bleb, thereby decreasing potential irritation (Fig. 31.1-1). Standard center thickness and tri-curve edge design exhibits less edge interaction with the bleb. However, the anterior surface of the bleb should be regularly observed for interface interaction. Careful documentation and anterior segment photography of the lens/bleb fit interaction aids in achieving the best fit relationship over time. A central fit with normal lens movement of 1–2 mm is desired. Superior fits are not advised. Soft lenses may decenter or ride over the top of the filtration bleb, which may cause undesirable movement. Smaller diameter soft, disposable daily wear lenses may be necessary if rigid fitting is not possible. Ultraviolet-absorbing rigid lenses should be used in aphakic patients. Extended wear regimens are discouraged due to higher risk of infection.

Fitting philosophy includes the flattest possible lens to allow good tear exchange and minimize corneal and bleb trauma. Corneal topographic analyses, including keratometry measurements, are essential to successful fitting.

It is not recommended that patients wear their contact lenses while instilling glaucoma medications. This is true whether the patient has had filtration surgery or not. The US Food and Drug Administration (FDA) considers it a contraindication to use glaucoma drops of any kind while wearing contact lenses – soft or rigid. Increased concentrations of preservatives and solution vehicle may cause the contact lens to become coated and degrade vision. In addition, increased contact time of the drug with the lens may irritate the corneal epithelium and may even lead to conjunctival toxicity.

While there is no clear recommendation regarding lens removal time for instillation of glaucoma medications, it is suggested that the lenses are kept out for a minimum of 15 min following administration of drops. A typical soft lens should be worn on a daily wear schedule and replaced at no later than 2 week intervals. As a result, any possible deposits will be discarded with the old lens. Ideally, daily wear disposable (discarded daily) lenses would be optimal. Overnight wear is not recommended due to the higher risk for infection.

With all contact lens types, a stringent cleaning regimen with careful compliance should be stressed. Hydrogen peroxide systems are very effective cleaners and are very well tolerated. Daily cleaners may be helpful as well if the lenses deposit frequently.

## Complications

Corneal physiologic changes that should be monitored in contact lens users include: superficial punctuate epitheliopathy, neovascularization, abrasions, and ulcers.

Bleb trauma and infection are very serious complications that can occur after filtering surgery. Both the patient and the physician should be aware of the signs and symptoms of these bleb-threatening occurrences. Increasing bleb vascularity is an ominous sign in the patient wearing contact lenses. If this is noted, altering the fit to include a smaller lens diameter, as well as a higher oxygen permeable lens is recommended. If this does not alleviate the increasing bleb vascularity, discontinuation of lens wear is necessary to avoid inflammatory bleb failure.

Direct bleb trauma may be commented on by the patient as increasing or new onset irritation. Sodium fluorescein staining at the bleb junction, or direct pain at the site, indicates an undesirable fit. Refitting should resolve this problem.

## Additional uses of contact lenses

Contact lenses are sometimes used with glaucoma patients not for refractive correction, but for therapeutic purposes. Opaque contact lens occlusion for enlarged

YAG laser iridotomy can be very helpful for chronic diplopia and/or glare. These are typically soft lenses, which can be custom colored to match the contralateral eye. The back portion of the lens is made opaque to shield out extraneous light, thereby decreasing bothersome glare and diplopia.

Contact lenses in glaucoma patients may be used as large diameter bandage lenses for management of leaking filtration blebs, particularly in those enhanced with antimetabolites. A 17.5 mm soft lens typically allows adequate coverage of the leaking bleb and may aid in sealing of the leak, hopefully avoiding more surgery.

Bandage lenses have also been utilized to alleviate corneal toxicity and erosions, irritation, and discomfort associated with antimetabolite 5-fluorouracil (5-FU) injections. This allows extending the periods of 5-FU administration with decreased toxicity to the patient and enhanced bleb longevity and success long term. Long-term bandage contact lenses have not been associated with corneal complications. Careful observation is recommended.

Contact lenses have also been shown to be useful for performing visual field examinations in glaucoma patients. High refractive error and aphakia exhibit better total field size, better blind spot size and plotting, and also less distortion secondary to prismatic effects when using contact lenses. There is also less chance of a "lens artifact" ring scotoma so long as the optic zone of the contact lens covers the pupil. Both soft and rigid lenses may be used for obtaining visual fields.

In the past, contact lenses had been used to enhance the delivery of glaucoma medications. Pilocarpine was studied for this purpose to retain the drug on the ocular surface for longer periods of time via a soft contact lens. Some use of Pilocarpine with a soft contact lens drug delivery system has been documented for acute angle closure glaucoma in India. Generally, contact lenses are not commonly used in this manner any more.

## Conclusion

Contact lenses may be an excellent alternative visual correction option for glaucoma patients. Care should be taken to optimize the fit to minimize the risks to the bleb and overall eye health. Patient selection and education regarding risks and need for follow-up are critical to success.

## Bibliography

Beckman RJ, Sofinski SJ, Greff LJ, et al. Bandage contact lens augmentation of 5-fluorouracil treatment in glaucoma filtration surgery. *Ophthalmic Surg.* 1991;22:563–564.

Bellows AR, McCulley JP. Endophthalmitis in aphakic patients with unplanned filtration blebs wearing contact lenses. *Ophthalmology.* 1981;88:839–844.

Blok MD, KOK JH, van Mil C, et al. Use of the megasoft bandage lens for treatment of complications after trabeculectomy. *Am J Ophthalmol.* 1990;110:264–268.

Dada VK, Acharjee SC. Soft lenses as therapeutic device. *Indian J Ophthalmol.* 1982;30:201–203.

Fresco BB, Trope GR. Opaque contact lenses for YAG laser iridotomy occlusion. *Optom Vis Sci.* 1992;69:656–657.

Grohe RM, Wyse TB. Fitting contact lenses in eyes with filtering blebs. *J Glaucoma.* 1998;7:439–445.

Gupta N, Weinreb RN. Filtering bleb infection as a complication of orthokeratology. *Arch Ophthalmol.* 1997;115:1076.

Hillman JS, Marsters JB, Broad A. Pilocarpine delivery by hydrophilic lens in the management of acute glaucoma. *Trans Ophthalmol Soc UK.* 1975;95:79–84.

Krohn DL. Enhancement of the sensitivity of the peripheral visual field of aphakic eyes by a soft contact lens correction. *Trans Am Ophthalmol Soc.* 1979;127:309–317.

Lois N, Dias JL, Cohen EJ. Use of contact lenses in patients with filtration blebs. *CLAO J.* 1997;23:100–102.

Mandelbaum S, Forster RK, Gelender H, et al. Late onset endophthalmitis associated with filtering blebs. *Ophthalmology.* 1985;92:964–972.

Marmion VJ, Jain MR. Role of soft contact lenses and delivery of drugs. *Trans Ophthalmol Soc UK.* 1976;96:319–321.

Samples JR, Andre M, MacRae SM. Use of gas permeable contact lenses following trabeculectomy. *CLAO J.* 1990;16:282–284.

Shoham A, Tessler Z, Finkelman Y, et al. Large soft contact lenses in the management of leaking blebs. *CLAO J.* 2000;26:37–39.

## 31.5 Vision Rehabilitation

### 31.5.1 Evaluation of Near Magnification

After completing the best distance refraction, next determine the proper amount of near magnification. Determination of near magnification for the low-vision patient may be very different from simply computing the "add" for a normally sighted patient with just age-related presbyopia and no visual disease like glaucoma. Near magnification may take the form of a near add, spectacle-mounted microscopes, handheld and stand magnifiers, telemicroscopes and/or electronic magnifiers, all of which are interchangeable when the equivalent power of each device is similar. There are several methods used as starting points for determining the near magnification. Kestenbaum's rule inverts the best corrected distance visual acuity to determine the starting near add for a 20/50 target (newspaper print) in diopters. For example, a patient with the best distance visual acuity of 20/140 will need

+7.00D lens to read newspaper print. Lebensohn's reciprocal of vision rule also uses best corrected distance visual acuity and the desired near acuity. The denominator of the distance acuity is divided by the denominator of the desired near acuity determining the amount of magnification needed. Using the previous example, the patient with best corrected distance visual acuity of 20/140 who wants to read 20/50 will need 140/50 or 2.8× magnification. Converting to diopters by the formula:

$$\text{Magnification} = \text{Diopters}/4$$

This is roughly +11.00D needed by Lebensohn's rule to read 20/50 print. Note the difference in the outcomes of each rule. At best, these rules are just starting points for determining near magnification, and distance acuity should probably not be used for determining near magnification due to the variables in correlating near and distance acuities.

A better method of determining near magnification is to find the patient's best near acuity (BNA), recording the optotype and the testing distance (TD). Determine the target near acuity (TNA) of what the patient would like to see or read. Using the three values, the new near target distance can be determined and the reciprocal of this value – the power of the near magnification – by the formula:

$$\text{BNA}/\text{TNA} = \text{TD}/n_{TD}$$

For example, a patient reads 3.0 M at 30 cm and they want to read newspaper print (1.0 M). The new target distance will be 10 cm and the reciprocal will be a +10.00 D lens. This would be the starting point for near magnification determination. The goal of near magnification determination is to find an add that will allow the patient to comfortably read their text size of choice or perform near tasks of choice. Generally 1.0 M is the target near acuity, as most newspapers and magazines are printed in that size print. If the patient's goal is reading the newspaper, determine the add that will allow them to read 1.0 M print. Then have the patient practice with a newspaper. If the patient desires a smaller sized near target, the magnification will need to be increased. After the starting point is determined, the near magnification should be adjusted using high contrast charts and finally refined using normal news or magazine print. Use a trial frame to adjust the power by dipping lenses over the starting point until the patient is comfortable with the power and acuity. Once the low-vision practitioner has determined the near magnification needed by the patient for a specific task (say reading the newspaper), then other devices of the same equivalent power can be substituted to meet the patient's other visual activity needs.[16]

Microscopes are spectacle-mounted convex lenses and come in four basic styles: full-field, half-eye, bifocal, and loupe. Standard bifocal reading adds can be obtained up to +8.00 D in a flat top bifocal style. Above +8.00 D, the bifocal must be specially constructed at a higher cost. Higher adds may be more practical for the patient if written as a reading-only prescription or if constructed as a spectacle-mounted magnifier (microscope). An alternative is to use a single vision lens such as a full-field or half-eye microscope.

The problems encountered with higher near powers are related to the short working distance (1/dioptic power). The power of the prescribed magnification will determine the focal length of the device. This is equal to the reading distance. Patients will quite often reject shorter working distances. There often seems to be an invisible wall, a psychological barrier that will not allow them to bring their material very close. Often this is the signal that this patient will work better with a stand or handheld minifier of equivalent power rather than spectacle magnification. High myopes will often remove their glasses to increase their magnification at near. Take advantage of the benefit their myopia affords them and add magnification on top of that. Patients with advanced glaucoma may reject the higher-powered adds due to a very small central field. These patients may even respond to a lesser add with a greater working distance and using larger print. Another problem encountered with patients having advanced glaucoma is that they have trouble finding their "add" because of their limited central field. In these patients, the options are to raise the add segment height significantly, go to a reading-only prescription, or to try to raise the remaining central field with prism in the add.

Although many patients with advanced glaucoma have good central acuities even as their visual fields diminish, some will indeed suffer loss of central vision as well as have severely restricted fields. The visual acuity loss may be glaucomatous or related to concurrent disease such as macular degeneration. Increasing magnification will increase their ability to resolve near printed materials and objects. An alternative to using a spectacle-mounted, high-powered near magnification is the use of a handheld, stand, or electronic minifier of equivalent power. These typically are used with a normal add between +2.00 to +4.00. The add will determine the distance of the reading material. Handheld minifiers are placed within the focal distance of the add, and the reading material is positioned at the focal distance of the magnifier. Magnification can be problematic for patients with advanced glaucoma because the magnified image can be greater than the usable field of the patient. The idea is to increase the size of the object to the point that it can be comfortably discerned without increasing the size beyond the available visual field.

Traditionally, the classic add that was used with handheld or stand magnifiers was a +4.00 diopter addition because of a presupposed working distance of 25 cm. Frequently, a +3.50 diopter add is more satisfactory. Using this lower power allows for an increased working distance. Also, this tends to be the highest power that can be obtained in a progressive

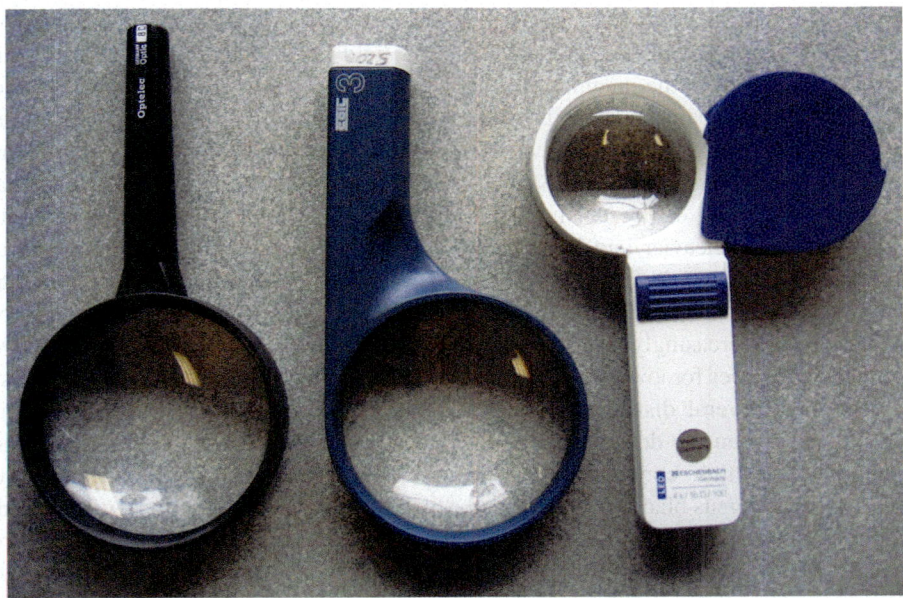

**Fig. 31.5** Handheld magnifiers come in a variety of sizes, shapes, and powers. Some have a light source. Many lighted handheld magnifiers use LCD illumination to conserve battery life

no-line bifocal and still maintain comfortable use of the bifocal. Progressive no-line bifocals do come in a +4.00 add, but they tend not to be as useful to the patients. Patients with advanced glaucoma will often prefer an add that is less powerful to increase the working distance, while forgoing some resolution.

Handheld magnifiers can be used without a bifocal add. The total magnification delivered to the patient will be less than when using an add. It is best to show the patient both options and let the patient pick the one they prefer. Handheld magnifiers are convex lenses that come in powers from less than one diopter to around 55 diopters (Fig. 31.5). They come in various sizes and styles, with or without illumination. Some have swing arms that allow the patient to use both hands. The advantages of using a handheld magnifier are that they are portable, light, often have an attached illumination device, and are relatively inexpensive. The disadvantages are that they do not have variable magnification and if the magnification becomes no longer adequate for the patient, they need to be replaced with a handheld magnifier with stronger magnification. All patients should be trained in the use of the magnifier with samples of material they will view when they return home.

Stand magnifiers require the use of an add or accommodation secondary to the fact that the material is set at a shorter distance than the focal point of the magnifier. This creates divergent waves leaving the magnifier, that require accommodation or an add to properly converge the rays onto retina. Stand magnifiers also are available in a variety of styles, with and without illumination (Fig. 31.6). Some have open stands,

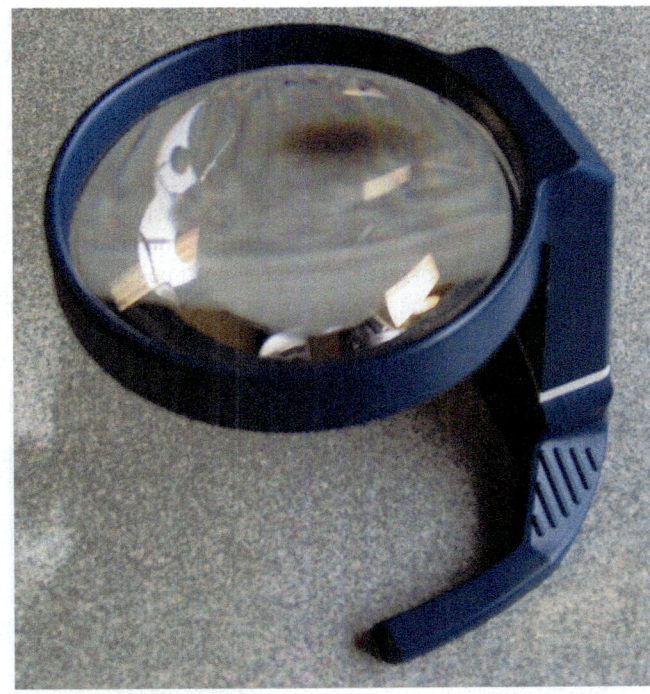

**Fig. 31.6** Stand magnifiers with lower power allow enough room to write under the lens. The greater the lens power the closer the lens must be to the object

for space to write, underneath the lens. Stand magnifiers are available in powers up to 100 diopters. The higher the power, the more likely the magnifier has illumination because of the difficulty of maintaining ambient illumination on the object.

One advantage of stand magnifiers compared to hand magnifiers is that they allow patients to use the device "hands-free." Further, because the distance from the magnifier to the material is fixed, there is less confusion manipulating the focal length for a clear image. Lower powers also allow writing beneath the lens. These devices do have the disadvantages of often requiring either an illuminating device or significant illumination. They also tend to be heavier and larger than hand-held magnifiers. As with handheld devices, they do not have the ability to vary magnification for different tasks.

Electronic magnification is increasingly becoming the gold standard of magnification devices for low vision patients. These expensive devices have several distinct advantages compared to simpler and less expensive devices. They can provide variable magnification, high contrast, reversible polarity – that is, white on black versus black on white – and very importantly, they can allow the patient to see objects at normal working distances. The disadvantage, especially of the closed-circuit televisions, is that they are not very portable and they are much more expensive than handheld or stand magnifiers. The inline closed-circuit television (CCTV) is the standard of the electronic magnifiers (Fig. 31.7). It is comprised of a monitor, a camera, and an XY table. The term "inline" refers to the fact that the patient, the material, and the monitor are all in a straight line. An XY table is a platform for the material that allows the patient to move the material forward and backward, as well as left and right, without actually touching the material. The CCTV works essentially by taking a real time picture of the material on the XY table and bringing it to the monitor for the patient to see. As the magnification increases, less of the material will be viewed on the monitor and the material must be moved using the XY table under the camera. Thus the patient can direct their gaze at one point and move the magnified print across the field of their gaze. They have variable magnification ranging from about 3× to about 75×. Increasing the size of the monitor will increase the total magnification of the unit. They come in color as well as black and white units. The color units can be manipulated so that there are different color combinations and polarities that allow for patient comfort in reading. They also come in true color for viewing photographs, objects, and color materials. Some units are available with auto-focusing while others are focused manually. Most have enough room between the camera and the XY table to perform writing tasks such as filling out a check. There is also enough space to view objects such as medicine bottles, canned goods, and dry goods. Some patients will also use them for creative tasks, such as needlework, painting, and drawing, instead of just reading. Newer designs digitally read the print on the page and are able to change the way the print is displayed. Full text, horizontal line, or word-by-word displays are available after the text has been read by the machine.

Patients with advanced glaucoma tend to do much better with the inline CCTV than optical magnification due to the greater working distance to the screen and their ability to manipulate the magnification. Patients with advanced glaucoma almost never use the unit at its highest level of magnification because the magnification of the material is greater than the extent of their visual field and the information at extended magnification is lost to them. While the closed-circuit TV system is the standard for the electronic magnifiers, there are many variations on this theme. Some electronic magnifiers move the camera into a unit very much like a computer mouse that is run across the material, then displaying the image on a monitor. The disadvantage of this system is that the monitor and mouse are not in line, but it does allow some portability from monitor to monitor. Other electronic monitors have the camera mounted on a swing arm (Fig. 31.8). This allows tasks that require significant amount of space to be performed underneath the camera. Reading tasks may not be as easy with this style of electronic magnifier, but the performance of arts-and-crafts may be easier. This system will also not be in-line, making it a less intuitive learning experience. With recent advances in microelectronics, many of these electronic magnifiers have been reduced in size and are now available as portable, handheld units (Fig. 31.9). These devices have smaller magnification capabilities than CCTVs but are extremely portable and user friendly. They function for several hours on a single battery charge and have the other advantages of color contrast and polarity manipulation. The portability and other features permit the patient to put them to good use for tasks outside the home, including shopping and banking.

Electronic magnifiers and computers require a spectacle add to maintain focus at the distance of the monitors.

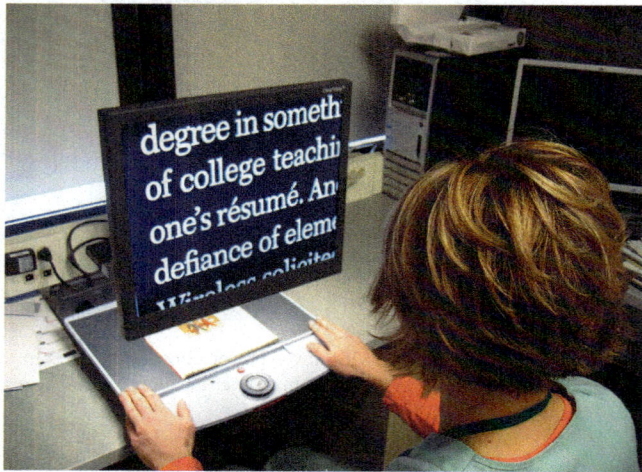

**Fig. 31.7** In-line Closed Circuit Televisions (CCTV) can deliver up to 60–80× magnification of reading material placed on their XY table. Often there is enough room between the camera and the table to view canned goods and health supplies or to perform craft activities

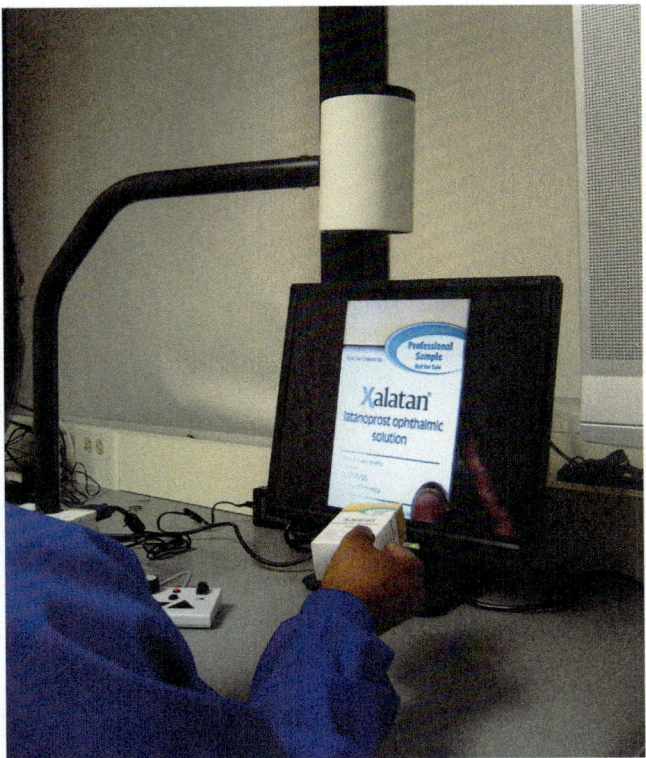

**Fig. 31.8** Optron is a swing-arm electronic magnifier. It is sturdier than other similar devices on the market. It uses an auto-focus camera to display color images up to 70× magnification. It is portable and has a clamp to secure the swing arm to a table. There is significant room between the camera and the base, which allows the undertaking of crafts or other tasks requiring more space

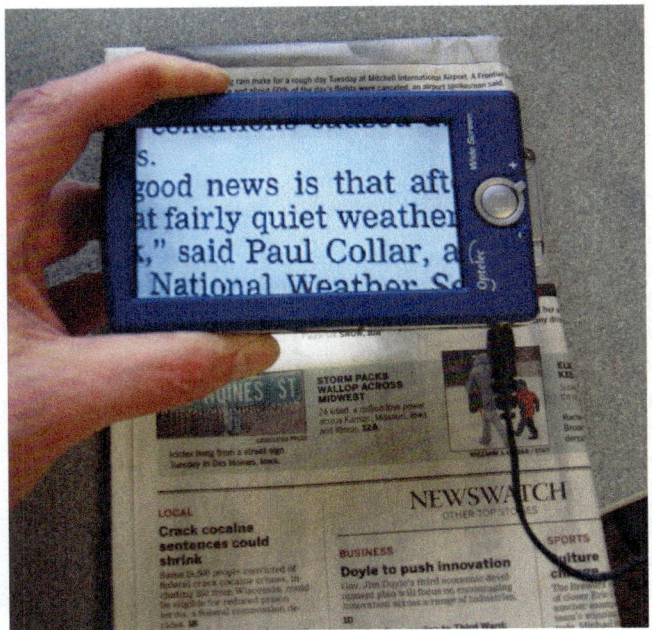

**Fig. 31.9** The compact is an example of the new generation of portable lightweight handheld electronic magnifiers. It has a 4.3 in. color LCD screen and magnification up to 10×. It runs about 3 h on a charge

Patients will often forgo the use of an add with these devices because they feel that the magnification is adequate. Conversely, they may also complain of asthenopia when using the monitor without an add; however, a quick demonstration of the usefulness of an "add" in the office will often change their minds. If the patient sits at a distance of 13 in. (33 cm) from the monitor, a spectacle add of +3.00 D should be prescribed to maintain the patient's focus at the plane of the monitor. The add will be less if the working distance is greater and more if the working distance is shorter.

Computer systems with specialized software can exceed the capabilities of straightforward CCTV systems. Of course, to fully benefit from sophisticated computer systems, the patient usually needs to have some pre-disability familiarity and comfort with using modern digital computers. While the current generation of Medicare age-plus patients is often computer-savvy, the present younger age group becomes senior citizens and it is likely that increasingly sophisticated hardware/software will benefit even more the next generation of glaucoma and other visually disabled patients. Many local associations for the blind offer computer training courses and more are likely to do so in the future. Ultimately, computer-based low-vision systems will offer the most capabilities of manipulating both text and pictorial information for the visually impaired patient. It is hoped that increasingly sophisticated software may actually be able to simplify the operation of these systems for patients. Systems that can read books and magazines, information from the Internet, perform online banking and shopping services, etc. are increasingly becoming available technologically and are generally within the financial resources of most low-vision patients. Some of the currently available computer/software packages are described as follows.

### 31.5.2 Computer Screen Magnification Programs

A screen magnifier is a type of assistive technology, usually in the form of software that interfaces with a computer's graphical output to present enlarged screen content (Fig. 31.10). Commonly used screen magnifiers include: ZoomText Magnifier (variable to 36× magnification), SeeIt Magnifier (up to 32× magnification), and The Magnifier, which provides 2–10× magnification. Computer manufacturers now include magnification programs standard in their operating systems. Most people with relatively normal sight will not look for these programs, but they are available to all persons with minor changes in display choices. A basic magnifier application has been included within the Microsoft Windows operating system since Windows XP, which has nine levels of magnification. Apple also provides a basic magnifier application.

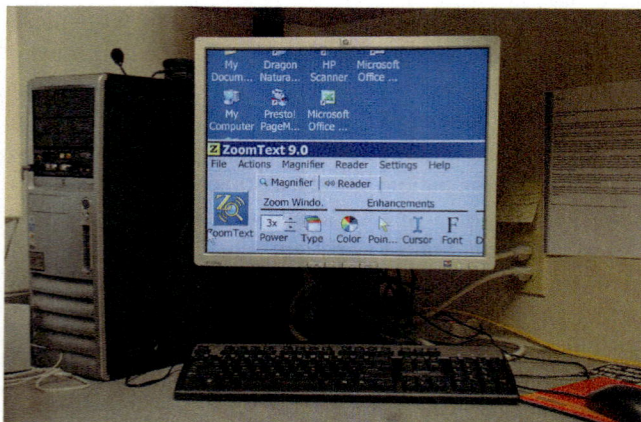

**Fig. 31.10** Zoomtext is a combination computer screen magnifier and screen reader. In this example, the monitor is 17 in. diagonal and the text magnification is at 3×. Zoomtext has the capability to magnify up to 36×

Magnification can also be obtained by increasing the size of the computer's monitor. For example, changing a monitor from 15 to 21 in. will increase the magnification by a factor of 1.4×.

### 31.5.3 Computer Screen Readers

Many of the programs that magnify the digital media on a computer will also read the contents of the screen. A screen reader is also a form of assistive technology. It is a software application that identifies and interprets what is displayed on the screen and then converts it to speech or Braille output. Once the material is recognized, the speed of speech, tone of speech, and type of voice can be manipulated. As the speech technology improves, these voices will be more lifelike in their sound. Commonly used screen magnifiers include: ZoomText Reader, Window-Eyes, JAWS, and Hal Screen Reader.

An extensive review of screen magnifiers and screen readers, often including free downloads, is available on the following websites: www.magnifiers.org and www.enablemart.com.

### 31.5.4 Reading Machines

Reading machines are stand-alone units that scan the material to be read, digitize the material, and then read it back audibly (Fig. 31.11). The units use optical character recognition programs, so handwritten text cannot be recognized. Newer units have built-in memory so that the material can be saved on compact discs and other material can be imported.

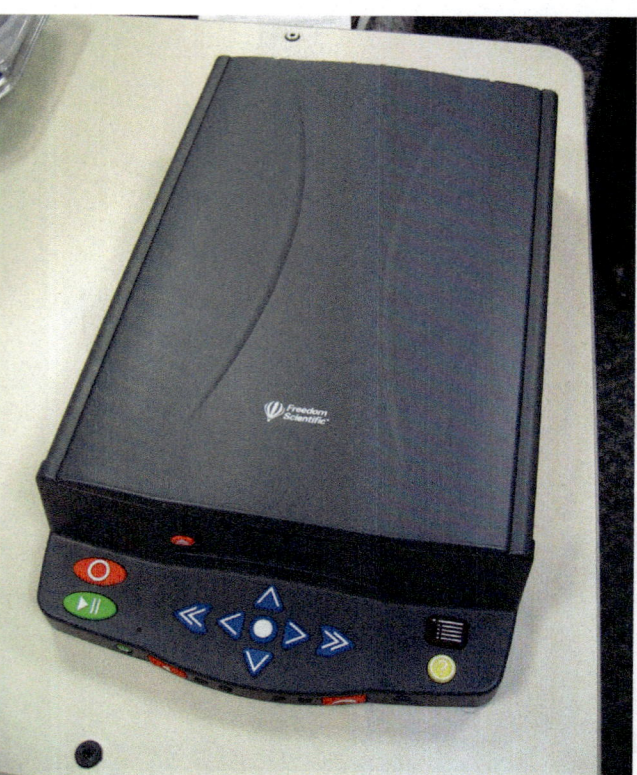

**Fig. 31.11** Sara is a stand-alone document reader made by Freedom Scientific that scans documents and reads the material back to the user

These newer units have monitors for following along with the text. An example of a stand-alone reading machine is the Sara manufactured by Freedom Scientific.

### 31.5.5 Handheld Scanner/Reader

The Kurzweil-National Federation of the Blind Reader is a handheld device housing a combination of digital camera and personal data assistant (PDA) (Fig. 31.12). The device takes a digital photograph of the material to be read, the PDA uses character recognition software to digitize the image to text, and then uses text-to-speech conversion technology to read the text to the user. Headphones can be used for privacy and the material can be digitally stored in the PDA for later use. The newest version released in spring 2008 uses cell phone technology essentially housing the entire package in a Nokia cell phone shell. This version has a 5 megapixel camera for photographing the material to be read, optical character recognition software, a money reader, global positioning system software, a screen reader, and a cell phone all in the shell of a normal cell phone. This device is exciting because it combines multiple devices that were often bulky

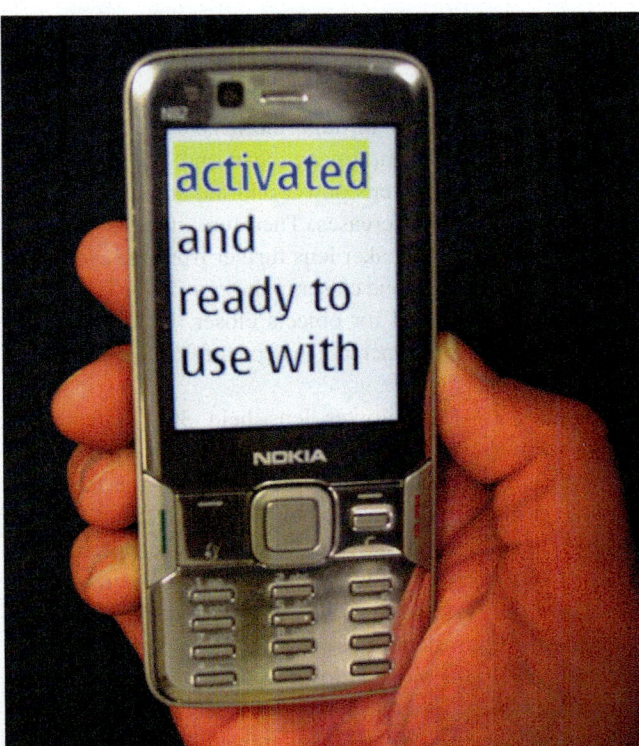

**Fig. 31.12** The knfb reader is a multifunctional phone with camera, optical character recognition, screen reading, money recognition, and GPS software housed in a Nokia cell phone shell. This exciting technology is the result of collaboration between Kurzweil Technologies and the National Foundation for the Blind

in the past and allows the visually impaired patient to be much more independent and mobile.

## 31.6 Evaluation of Field Enhancement Devices

Patients with advanced glaucoma may not complain of field loss until they have experienced significant loss of function. The larger their central field, the less likely it will impact their mobility and other daily living skills and the less likely they will be responsive to field enhancement. The challenge will be greater when the patient has significant problems, but the patient will be more motivated because of the loss of function.[17] Quite frequently, patients will not have functional loss until their central field reaches 10° or less. There are several strategies that can be applied when trying to manipulate visual fields for patients with advanced glaucoma. These strategies often differ significantly from each other, but the goal is to increase the usable visual field.

### 31.6.1 Scanning

Patients with constricted central fields sample their environment differently than people with full fields. When ambulating, they fixate over a larger area than normally sighted individuals, directing their gaze to objects to the side, the layout of wall and floor boundaries, or downward.[18] Because glaucomatous field loss is non-acute, some patients develop scanning techniques with time that allow them to navigate through their environment more efficiently. They will use head swings, eye sweeps, and a slower approach speed that they have developed over the course of their vision loss. All of these adaptations allow the patient to build a larger picture from the many small views they sample from their environment. Efficient scanning of the environment will significantly increase the functional field compared to the patient's demonstrable static visual field. The result is a patient who navigates their environment much more efficiently than one would expect.[22] These patients may not fare well with field enhancement devices due to their previously established scanning strategies – they may reject the new devices. Orientation and mobility instructors can improve the patient's scanning by helping the patient increase their awareness of the areas that need to be processed and by developing a systemic plan for search patterns.[17]

### 31.6.2 Field Expanders

Field expanders are devices used to attempt to increase the patient's usable field. They include optical minifiers, reverse telescopes, and prisms. The concept is to transfer the peripheral field into the usable remaining central field of the patient in two ways:

- By increasing the patient's working distance; and
- Through magnifications of the viewing area.

Increasing the patient's working distance is not always practical as objects can be too small to resolve or the needed distances are not available. Patients will perform better on a CCTV, not just because of the magnification but also because of the increased working distance. Patients will often spontaneously discover that they can push reading material farther away from them to increase their field of view.

Field expanders using optical magnification will increase the field of view, but they also decrease visual acuity proportionally. For example, a −3× device will increase a 10° field to 30°, but the corresponding decrease in acuity through the device may be from 20/20 to 20/60. Although the device is producing the desired increase in field, the patient may reject the device because of poor acuity.[17]

These devices also can disrupt the patient's usual scanning patterns. Low-vision patients use a dynamic scanning pattern of eye and head movements that effectively expands their range of functional field many times over their static visual field. Thus a patient may have a dynamic field four to five times the size of their static visual field with objects of normal size. When viewing through a field-expanding device, the patient is unable to engage in their usual low-vision scanning movements. Their field becomes limited to the field of the device with a corresponding decrease in object size. Any gain in the static field through the device may be counterbalanced by losses to the dynamic functional field.[17] These devices tend to be accepted for use in static situations, such as spotting objects or viewing through a window (Fig. 31.13), and not for dynamic use, such as ambulating. Even with the problems encountered with field expanders, some patients will use the devices effectively and with satisfaction. The more training the patient undergoes with the devices, the greater the likelihood of success with and continued use of the device.

### 31.6.3 Handheld Minus Lenses

Minus lenses minify and expand the field of view, acting as reverse telescopes with the minus lens acting as the objective and the patient's accommodation acting as the ocular. Patients hold the minus lens at arm's length, which gives a minified view of objects in front of them, allowing them to see more field as they view through the lens. The patient must accommodate to keep the image clear, and, as the eye-lens distance increases, the lens power and the amount of necessary accommodation decreases. Therefore, it is preferable to use a larger diameter weaker lens further from the eye than a smaller more powerful one closer to the eye. There is minimal accommodation needed for objects closer than infinity and there is a corresponding increase in depth of field for decreasing accommodation.[19]

Consider a −5.00 diopter lens held 30 cm from the patient's eye to view an object at optical infinity. The image through the lens will be at the focal point of the lens; i.e., 20 cm in front of the minus lens or 50 cm in front of the eye. The patient will have to accommodate or use a spectacle add to focus this image on the retina. The effective telescopic power for this system is 2/5 or 0.4× magnification. This would be the equivalent to using a 2.5× telescope in reverse. If the minus lens is moved closer to the eye, the magnification will decrease and the demand for accommodation will increase. Conversely, if the lens is moved farther away from the eye, magnification will be greater and the demand to accommodate will be less.[17]

The commercially developed minus lenses are inexpensive, lightweight, and very portable. Some are attached to a chain that can be worn around the neck, which is convenient for maintaining the proper distance from the eye. Others are constructed with a handle, similar to a handheld magnifier. Even easier is to dispense a minus lens blank from your optical dispensary. A hole can be drilled in the periphery of the lens and attached to a cord to wear around the neck. Fresnel lenses are another inexpensive option. They are extremely lightweight and easy to conceal. Cohen and Waiss suggested using large Fresnel lenses, the type that are affixed to the rear windows of vans, for viewing large fixed areas such as doorways, yards, or porches. They can be mounted on doors or windows in order to view those areas. They are available through auto and science supply retailers.[17]

Evaluate the usefulness of the lens by having the patient hold the lens at arm's length to view objects in the exam room or through the window of the exam room. Start with a −4.00 or −5.00 diopter lens and have the patient move the lens toward and away from them to see the changes in magnification. If the patient expresses further interest in this optical aid, train the patient to "spot" through the lens. They must move the head and lens as one unit, as if they were actually using (moving) a telescope. Test various lens powers to determine which is most effective for the patient.[17] Follow up this initial trial with further training.

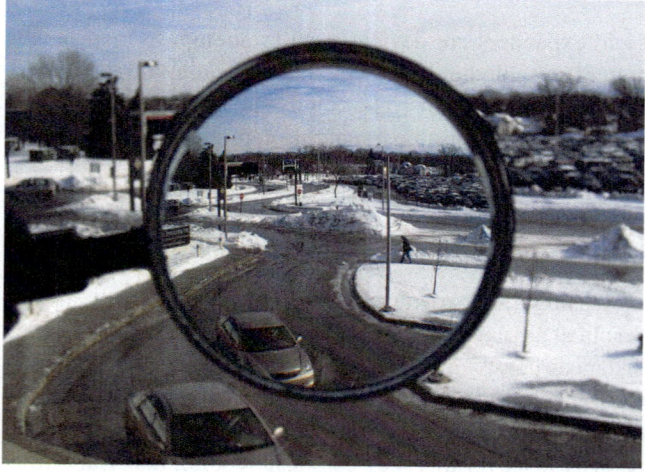

**Fig. 31.13** Distance view through a −4.00 diopter lens. Minus lenses increase the field of view through the lens while decreasing the acuity

## 31.6.4 Prisms

### 31.6.4.1 Fresnel Prisms

Fresnel prisms are thin prisms made of polyvinyl chloride. They are constructed of multiple individual prisms aligned together in series. This helps eliminate the thickness inherent with ophthalmic glass or plastic prisms. They are cut and easily applied to the patient's spectacle lenses (Fig. 31.14). They are available in powers up to 40 prism diopters. Most often, Fresnel prisms are thought of as temporary, but, because of their thin profile, patients often opt to continue with the Fresnel prism rather than grinding an ophthalmic prism into their lens. Fresnel prisms are easily removed and cleaned with warm soapy water, then reapplied, smoothing any air bubbles between their surface and the surface of the lens. They do tend to degrade and get brittle over time, so they need to be replaced periodically. Fresnel prisms degrade the visual acuity, decrease contrast, and have chromatic aberrations when viewing through them.[15]

Fresnel prisms can be used to "increase" the patient's field by applying them to the peripheral sides of the lens. The patient must look through the prism to gain any benefit. All other times they are looking through the carrier lens. Fresnel prisms are placed on the back side of the lens with the base away from the center. The concept is to have the patient look into the prism, which shifts the image of the view toward the center, reducing the distance the patient has to move their eyes to locate an object.[20]

There are several techniques using Fresnel prisms. The first is to apply base out only to the temporal side, also commonly used for hemianopia. This brings objects centrally from the periphery approximately 1° for every 2 prism diopters of Fresnel prism. For example, wearing a 40 prism diopter lens would expand a field by 20°. The patient's scanning movement is therefore reduced by an equal amount. In addition to a temporal prism, prisms can be applied nasally, superiorly, and inferiorly forming a ring around the central viewing area. Remember that all the prisms must be placed base away from center or base toward the scotoma. Thus the nasal prism will be base in, the temporal prism base out, the inferior prism base down, and the superior prism base up.[17] Decisions for the use of each will be determined by the specific needs of the patient. These spectacles will often only be used for ambulation and not for any near or reading tasks. If a patient has good scanning techniques, prisms may interfere and cause confusion.

### 31.6.4.2 Evaluation of the Prisms

Have the patient view a distant object. Introduce an opaque index card into the temporal side of the field until the patient can first detect it. This indicates where the central edge of the prism should be applied. Apply the prism base out. Repeat the procedure for nasal field, then the inferior and the superior fields. Have the patient scan the room and adjust the prisms to give the patient a comfortable central corridor. The patient should be encouraged to make eye movements into the prism to experience the change in field position and then return to the central corridor of the lens. The process is then repeated on the second eye as needed and adjusted accordingly to resolve any binocular conflicts. Have the patient then stand and walk, scanning into the prism and then back to the central corridor. If the response is still positive, train the patient to use the prisms while performing both near and distance tasks. A home trial is the next step, with adjustments made at follow-up after a week or two of wear. Training and wearing time are considered good predictors of continued use and satisfaction. Problems contributing to the discontinuation of Fresnel prisms are the inappropriate placement within the remaining field of the patient, visual acuity loss through the prism, glare through the prism, and difficulty in keeping the prisms clean.[21]

A second strategy for the prisms is Trifield glasses (Fig. 31.15). The spectacles are constructed by abutting the

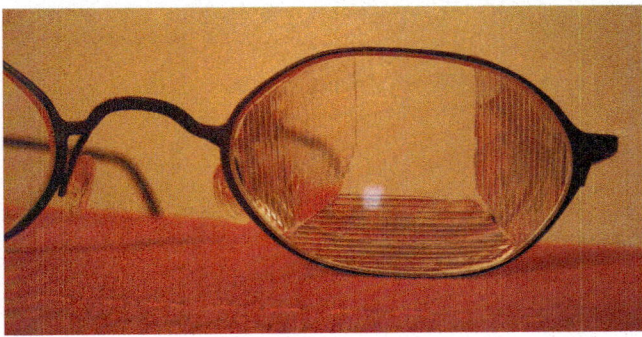

**Fig. 31.14** Fresnel prisms can be utilized to construct a channel lens in the office. The use of these prisms is quick, efficient, and inexpensive for evaluating the patient's response to channel lenses

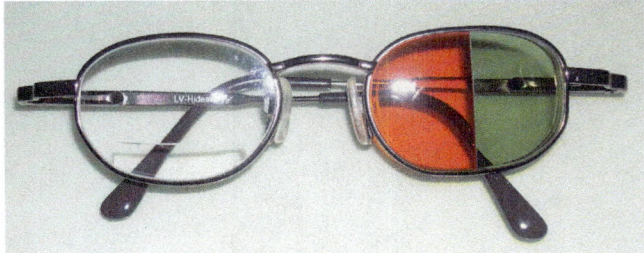

**Fig. 31.15** Trifield glasses have a spectacle lens with no prism on one side and a lens split with base in and base out prism. Each prism is tinted either *red* or *green* to heighten the patient's awareness of which field they are viewing (Courtesy of Eli Peli, Shepens Eye Research Institute, Harvard Medical School)

apices of two prisms at the center of the lens, each covering one half of the lens over the nondominant eye. The amount of prism must be greater than the remaining field to avoid diplopia. For help in determining the real direction of the objects, the right prism can be tinted red and the left prism green. The dominant eye has a normal prescription lens. This has been shown to increase field width, but patients can have problems determining the real direction of objects. The patient will have his or her view influenced by the prism in all directions on the nondominant side. These lenses can be constructed with Fresnel prisms or constructed using CR-39 plastic.

### 31.6.5 Inwave Channel Lenses

Channel lenses are the constructed version of multiple Fresnel prisms in one spectacle correction (Fig. 31.16). The original example of this is the Inwave lens that has multiple sections of base away from center prism within a single lens that shifts all the images toward the center. With this arrangement, the patient should only have to shift their eyes slightly to get into each of the prisms. The lens will have a center non-prismatic channel bordered by a temporal area 12 prism diopters base-out prism, with an identical area of nasal 12 prism diopters base-in prism, and an inferior area of 8 prism diopters base-down prism. The channel width ranges from 6 to 14 mm and the patients' refractive error can be ground into the lens. The patient's add can be incorporated into the lens up to +4.00 D and the segment line is generally at the level of the apex of the inferior prism.[22] It is important to keep the eye size of the spectacle frame as small as possible. Each one of these prisms will shift the image toward the center line, allowing the patient to use a smaller saccade to pick up objects in the field. The benefits of constructing the lens instead of using Fresnel prisms include better acuity, less chromatic aberration, better contrast, less distortion, and cosmetic attractiveness. Clip-on glare control lenses also can be made for the constructed version. The downside is that these lenses are expensive. Although no longer manufactured by the company that originally developed these lenses, there are labs that will custom make an Inwave style of lens such as Chadwick Optical Inc.[23]

### 31.6.6 Reverse Telescopes

Reverse telescopes are telescopes that have been turned around, with the patient looking through the objective lens and the ocular lens pointed at the object of regard (Fig. 31.17). Objects viewed through a reverse telescope appear smaller and the field of view is wider. The field of view is expanded by a factor that is equal to the magnification of the telescope when used for its original design. Therefore, the field viewed through a 3× telescope in the reverse direction will be three times wider. Because the angle subtended by the image is smaller, the visual acuity will be reduced with a reverse telescope.[20] The 3× reverse telescope will compress detail by three times and, therefore, decrease acuity by a factor of 0.33. A patient with 20/30 acuity will have approximately 20/100 acuity through the device. Reverse telescopes can be either Keplarian or Galilean and can be handheld, worn around the neck, or mounted in a spectacle frame. The patient's ability to use the device with a handheld telescope can be evaluated. If the patient desires the reverse telescope to be mounted in spectacles, it can be positioned either in the bioptic position or centrally. If the reverse telescope is

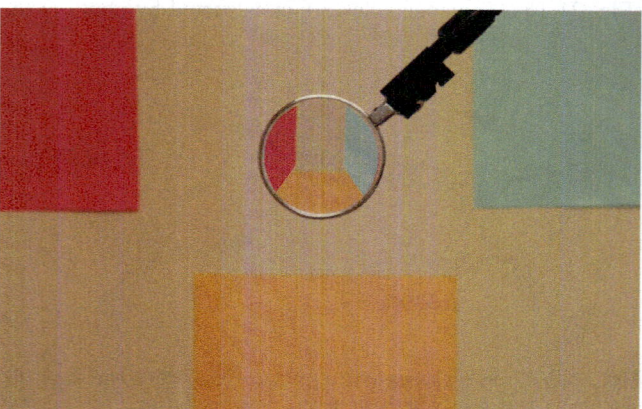

**Fig. 31.16** An Inwave trial channel lens positioned to demonstrate the prism nasally, temporally, and inferiorly. The central channel has no prism

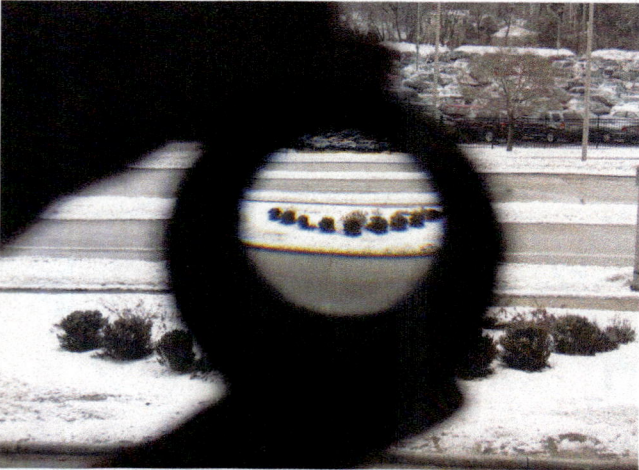

**Fig. 31.17** The view through a 2.5× telescope in reverse. Note the significant increase in field of view. This is accompanied by a proportional decrease in acuity

mounted in the bioptic position, the patient must tilt their head downward and look up through the objective when viewing the expanded field. When looking directly ahead, the patient will be viewing through the carrier lens of their spectacles. Patients function better using these telescopes in the bioptic position for mobility.

The handheld reverse telescope is positioned in front of the eye and all movements of the head must be matched by compensatory movements of the reverse telescope. Therefore, it is difficult to ambulate with the reverse telescope. It is normally used as a spotting device. This is also true of a mounted reverse telescope in the central full diameter position.

#### 31.6.6.1 Evaluating the Patient for a Reverse Telescope

Have the patient sit stationary and view a distant object. Start with a 2.5 or 2.8× Galilean telescope and have the patient view the same object looking through the objective lens of the telescope. If the patient responds positively, test telescopes of various powers until the preferred power is selected. The patient should get a sense of the viewing field and the acuity through the telescope. Encourage them to scan their surroundings for landmarks and hazards. Have the patient stand and move to another room, again scanning for potential hazards and landmarks. The patient will need to change the way they scan when using the telescope, using head and body rotation instead of eye scanning. Encourage the use of these rotations. If the response is still positive, consider the patient's anticipated use for the device to decide whether to dispense as handheld, bioptic, or centrally mounted. The patient will need continued training with the device, which is best done with orientation and mobility instructors.[17]

In the same vein, the most common field expander that patients purchase themselves is an apartment door "peephole." The common apartment door peephole is a reverse Galilean telescope in a plastic housing. It is approximately a 0.2× minifier and will decrease acuity. Kennedy et al., in a study of patients with retinitis pigmentosa, noted that the device was most helpful when used in scanning to locate people and objects when adequate illumination was available.[24] The device was more helpful in static rather than dynamic situations. Visual acuity was a limiting factor after 20/100. These apartment door peepholes are readily available to patients, are inexpensive and easily transportable, and patients are familiar with their function.

The Ocutech Image Minifier and the Multilens Optical Solutions Miniwider are two lightweight reverse telescopes specifically designed to reduce the barrel distortion characteristic of reverse telescopes. They are focusable and handheld or mounted.

### 31.6.7 Amorphic Lens

The amorphic lens was developed by William Feinbloom as a field expander consisting of cylinder lenses assembled in parallel axes creating an anamorphic system with one meridian unmagnified and the other magnified. Although no longer commercially available, there is historical value to awareness of this approach. When reversed, the amorphic lens gave the patient horizontal minification while the vertical remained unchanged. The resultant lens gave the patient a wider field of view when viewing through the lens. This lens was marketed by Designs for Vision in New York under the name New Horizons and came in minifying powers from 1.2× to −2.0× in increments of 0.2. The patient had to maintain the head in an upright position to keep vertical alignment. If the patient tilted their head toward their shoulder, there was loss of the vertical alignment leading to distortion of objects and patient disorientation. This reverse telescope was designed to be mounted centrally, but was more likely to be accepted if mounted bioptically.[20,25] Hoeft et al. found that one-third of the patients with retinitis pigmentosa in their study had improved mobility after 2 weeks of lens wear.[26] Szlyk et al. found 86% of their patients were satisfied with the devices and were able to be trained to perform functional tasks beyond peripheral awareness.[27] The differences in the studies may have been the placement in the bioptic position and a 3-month training period. Both studies were done with patients with retinitis pigmentosa, but since the peripheral field loss can be similar, patients with advanced glaucoma could experience similar benefits to training. The need for training is great for all the field expanding devices. When patients faired poorly with this device, it was due to the field distortion, the weight, and the poor cosmesis. There also could have been some disorientation, especially when used for dynamic scanning.

### 31.6.8 Electronic Field Enhancement

There is some work being done with electronic field manipulation by the Shepens Eye Research Institute in Massachusetts that may provide some benefit to patients with advanced glaucoma. Their device consists of a camera with a wide field of view mounted on one temple of a headset, a portable video processor to derive the edge images, and a display headset the size and shape of a pair of spectacles (Fig. 31.18). The Head Mounted Display (HMD) can provide 5× expanded field by superimposing minified edge images of a wider field over the wearer's see-through natural vision. These edge pixels in the display only occupy a small portion of field and would not interfere with the wearer's see-through vision. Shepens indicates that the resolution of the see-through view is as good as without. The visual information is coarse, but

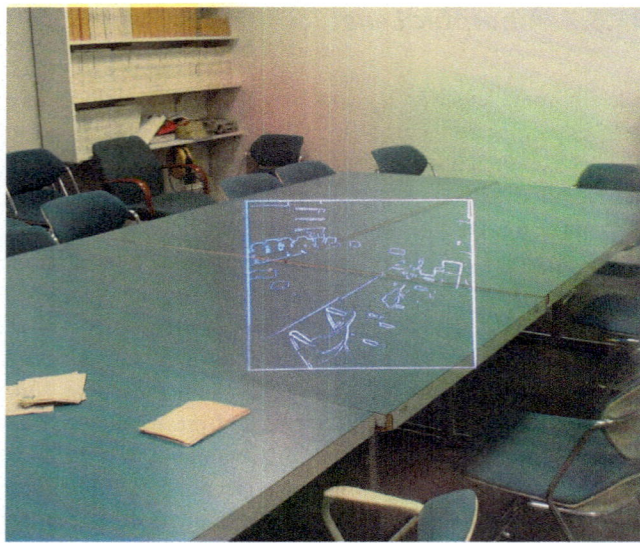
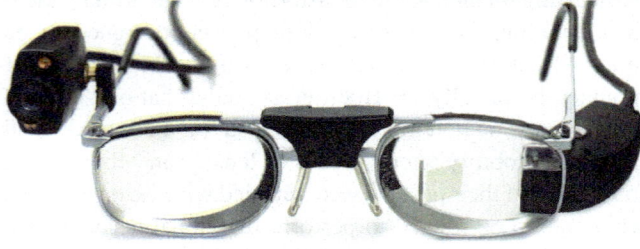

**Fig. 31.18** The HMD (head mounted display) developed at Shepens Eye Research Institute allows the patient to view through the lens while a leading edge image of the greater field of view is superimposed over the lens (Courtesy of Eli Peli, Shepens Eye Research Institute, Harvard Medical School)

may help the user detect obstacles that they would otherwise miss. The device is still in development and research stages and, at this time, is not commercially available.[28]

Patients with advanced glaucoma and significant field loss do not typically do well with optical expansion of fields. The field enhancement devices have some effectiveness if used appropriately, but are by no means a panacea for the constricted fields. Patients are much more likely to use and express satisfaction with the devices if they undergo extensive training. This extensive training requires commitment of considerable time on the part of the practitioner as well as the patient. They can work well for spotting tasks and some patients find them to be very helpful. Nonetheless, they have significant visual side effects and will not be a match for many patients.

### 31.6.9 Glare Control

Glare, photophobia, poor contrast sensitivity, and light adaption are problematic for patients with advancing glaucoma. Coincident ocular conditions may also contribute to the patient's difficulty. Glare is any light in the eye that does not contribute to the formation of the desired retinal image. There are two types of glare: discomfort glare and disability glare. Discomfort glare is light conditions that produce discomfort and reduce efficiency in performing visual tasks but do not interfere with visual resolution or identification of visual stimuli. Discomfort glare may be present when there is excessive light in the visual field. Discomfort glare can be lessened by reducing the excessive amount of light in the environment. If the lighting is under the patient's control, simply turning down the lights or adjusting the angle of the incoming light will help. When the illumination is not under the patient's control, indoors or outdoors, the use of absorptive lenses will help reduce discomfort glare. Discomfort may also be connected to excessive light contrasts, like unshaded windows or reflected light. The degree of discomfort will be greater the closer to the visual axis. Solutions to luminance contrast difficulties are to shade the windows, move lighting out of the visual axis, and turn to avoid reflections. Work spaces should be designed so that lighting is from above and behind the patient. Also, patients should position their back to windows when performing visual tasks. Disability glare is light conditions that reduce the resolution or ability to identify visual stimuli. Disability glare occurs when veiling luminances cause the observer to be unable to resolve the task at hand. An example of this is viewing through a dirty windshield while driving toward the sun. Solutions to disability glare are to try to adjust the source of the veiling luminances so that the glare is not direct or to remove the offending illumination source. Polarizing lenses can be effective. Anti-reflective coatings also can provide some benefit, but the lenses must be clean and free of scratches. Shorter wavelengths of light (bluer) scatter more than longer wavelengths (redder). Patients with glare issues will report intolerance to fluorescent lighting due to higher blue profile and feel more comfortable under incandescent lighting, which is richer in long wavelengths. Light absorptive lenses that block shorter wavelengths tend to give more comfort to patients experiencing glare. Yellow, amber, and browns selectively reduce shorter wavelengths and often will increase contrast and comfort.[29,30]

Tinted lenses are used for glare control. Patient preference often drives the choice of glare control lens. Yellow lenses reduce blue light, which is implicated in light scatter. Amber lenses have significant blue reduction but increased reduction of the total amount of light. The darker the tint, the more light will be blocked. Grey lenses can be used to reduce light intensity. There becomes a trade-off between reducing glare and reducing the amount of light. For example, the use of sunglasses in the daytime reduces glare to acceptable levels, but their use at night might reduce the light to levels that are not adequate for visual functioning. Patients should be evaluated under both indoor and outdoor conditions. Tints for outdoor sunlight conditions should include side and top shields to restrict extraneous light. Anti-reflection coatings can be considered for patients who are only mildly affected by glare.

Studies indicate that no single filter is beneficial for any particular disease.[31,32] Gormenzano and Stelmack designed a regimen to evaluate and prescribe filters. First, determine the best spectacle prescription. Then, occlude the eye with lesser acuity, or, if equal, the less dominant eye, to determine the hue and transmission that allows the best acuity and comfort for the better eye. This helps prevent prescribing filters that are too extreme or too dark. Use tint samples of known transmission to systematically evaluate the patient (Fig. 31.19). Quite often, 15–20% absorption is preferred because it is usually not too dark for indoor settings. Start with apricot and gray filters. Gray is neutral density and does not cast a hue. Apricot has blue-blocker qualities. Patients usually clearly prefer one tint to another. If they select gray, compare to brown, green, and blue. If they continue to prefer gray, try different transmission levels of gray. If the patient selects apricot, then have the patient make choices in the blue-blocker colors and then the different transmission levels. Make sure the filter is acceptable to the nondominant eye or the eye with lower acuity and then verify binocularly. Have the patient evaluate these tinted lenses under different light types and levels, such as fluorescent, incandescent, and sunlight. Cup hands around the sides of the trial frames to determine the need for side shields and visors. While patient acceptance is of paramount importance, the practitioner should also evaluate the patient performing their preferred near tasks and under different levels of illumination. Different filters may be needed for different levels of illumination.[32] There are many companies that produce filters of known transmissions. Corning photochromic filters (CPF) change transmission levels with changing levels of light. The patient's prescription can be ground into the CPF lens. There are also companies that will produce frames with tinted side shields. Tinted clip-ons or slip over sunshields are other options for providing the proper tinted lens to the patient.

Instructions on use of these filters will be invaluable to the patient. Educate the patient to the need for appropriate light transmission and teach them that one filter may not meet all their needs. When patients move from one light environment to another there will need to be an adjustment period. When moving from outdoors to indoors, they should change their filters at the threshold to facilitate the adjustment. Remove the darker filter and replace it with a filter that will work indoors. The opposite is true when moving from indoors to out. Patients will note improvement in their adaptation times when using filters in this manner.[33]

NoIR Medical Technologies at www.noir-medical.com has an extensive selection of glare-control glasses, clip-ons,

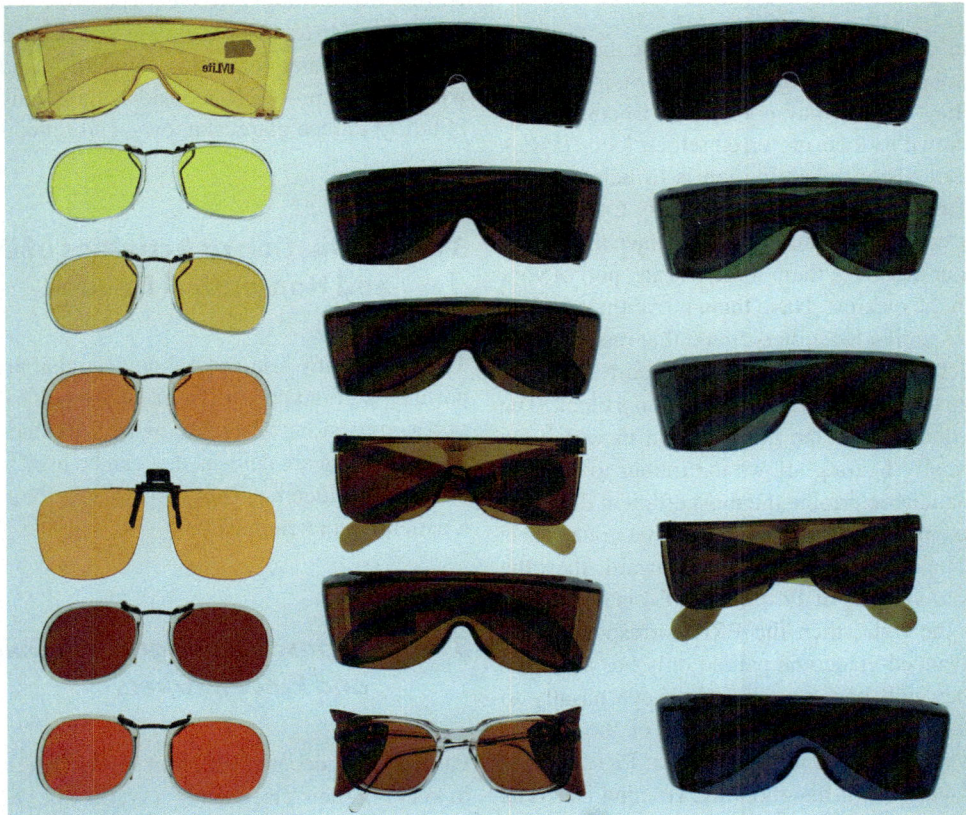

**Fig. 31.19** Examples of glare control filters including clip-ons, wrap around, side shields, and photochromic filters

and fit-overs. Technical-gear.com carries a selection of glare control glasses as well, including fit-overs and clip-ons.[34]

## 31.7 Training for Devices

Patients often find solutions that help by chance or by research. The solutions and devices that are used for patients with advanced glaucoma are often not intuitive and complicated. The likelihood of success with the devices if dispensed to patients that are not trained is significantly lower than if the time is spent working on the techniques and with the devices. Patients want easy solutions and, in the case of these devices, that is not likely. Emphasize the need for training and create an expectation that the patient will need to put some time and effort into the devices for them to work. Training and practice may be the difference between success and failure. Because of the time required to help ensure success with low vision devices, only highly motivated practitioners are likely to work successfully with low vision patients.

### 31.7.1 Preferred Retinal Locus and Eccentric Fixation Training

Some patients with advanced glaucoma may lose their central visual field but have a small island of preserved vision in their temporal field. They may or may not be able to control this preserved area, known as their preferred retinal locus (PRL). One of the goals of vision rehabilitation is to help patients locate their PRL and train them to eccentrically fixate to use the PRL. To determine the location of a PRL, have the patient look directly at your face. Ask them if there is any part of your face that comes in the clearest. Have them move their eyes in different directions until a location is found that results in the most complete picture of your face. The field corresponding to the PRL is often described in terms of time on a clock. The use of the clock dial to describe the direction in which the patient is eccentrically fixating allows the trainer to systematically help the patient determine the most efficient direction for viewing. For example, if the patient finds that your face is most clear when he or she looks slightly upward, then the PRL corresponds to viewing at 12 o'clock. If it is most clear when looking to the right, then the PRL corresponds to 3 o'clock. If the advanced glaucoma patient only has a temporal island then they will have to move their eye nasally to bring the island into play. Once the location of the PRL is established, work with the patient on using their PRL for near tasks, activities of daily living, and mobility. Training materials for eccentric fixation compiled by Gregory Goodrich can be found in *The Art and Practice of Low Vision*.[35]

## 31.8 Lighting

Lighting is very important to patients with advanced glaucoma. Difficulties involved with glare have been previously discussed, but there is need for significant lighting for the patient to function. Too much lighting will cause shadows, glare, and reflections. Too little lighting will not allow the patient to resolve objects in their environment for their required tasks. Consider the ambient or overall lighting of the patient's environs. Room lighting that is even, casts no shadow, and is adequate for mobility and activities of daily living is the first concern. Ambient lighting can take the form of fluorescent, incandescent, or halogen. Adequate light fixtures are needed to maintain the light evenly. Consider torchieres for bouncing the light off the ceiling to maintain a shadowless illumination. In addition to ambient lighting, it is desirable to have lighting that can be directed by hand for near visual tasks like reading. Gooseneck lamps are a particularly good source for this type of light so that reflections and glare can be minimized by changing the angle of the light. The light source for "directable" lamps can be fluorescent, incandescent, halogen, or light emitting diodes (LED). A gooseneck lamp can be moved close to the material taking advantage of the inverse square law of light intensity. This law states that when you move a light source closer to an object, the light intensity will be exponentially greater. Therefore a lamp that is positioned at four feet from an object will have a light intensity four times greater when moved in to 2 ft, and 16 times greater when moved in to 1 ft. Consider the layout of windows and blinds to reduce glare, shadows, and reflections.

## 31.9 Evaluation of Activities of Daily Living and Non-optical Devices

There are many non-optical devices that are valuable to the partially sighted patient. Some are meant to be used visually, others rely more on tactile or audible cues to be effective. The following are devices that can be used with patients with advanced glaucoma. They will vary in their effectiveness on a patient-to-patient basis.

### 31.9.1 Typoscopes, Signature Guides, and Place Markers

Patients with decent acuity but severe field loss will find help in keeping their place using a typoscope (Fig. 31.20). These are pocket-sized and convenient to use away from home. Patients will use the slot in the typoscope to track across

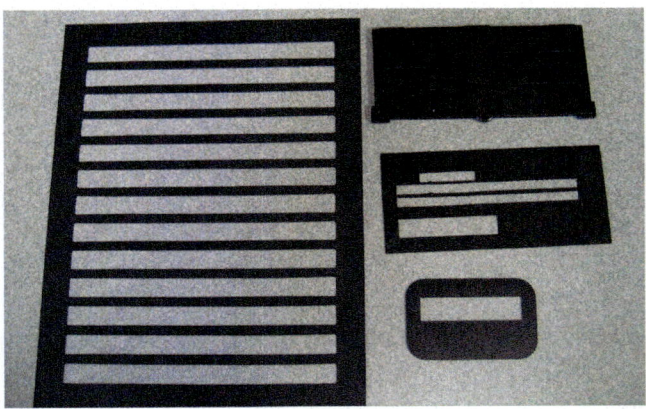

**Fig. 31.20** A variety of typoscopes. On the left is a full-page typoscope. On the right from top are an enclosing check template, lay-over check template, and a signature guide

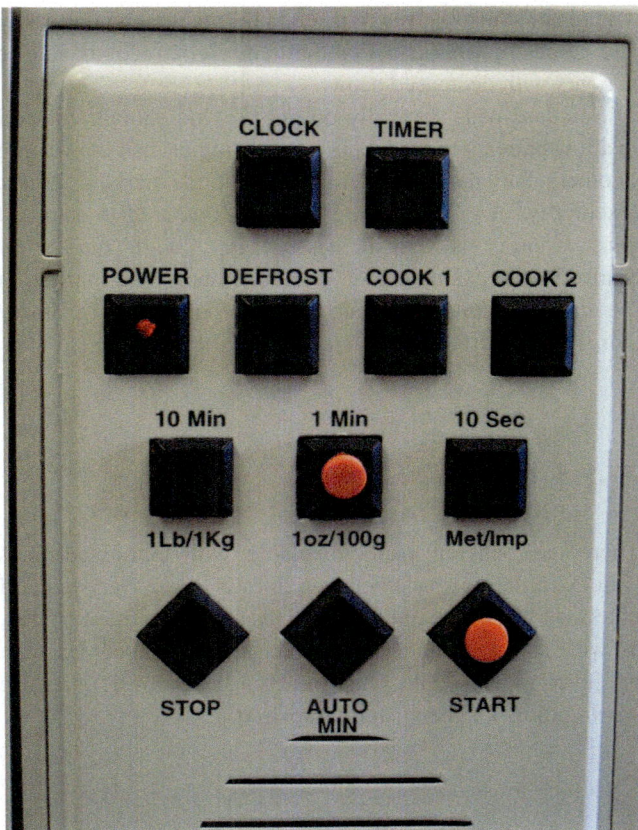

**Fig. 31.21** Tactile dots can be placed on appliance buttons to aid in the recognition of specific buttons. They are typically placed on the buttons that are used most frequently or the central button to help the patient navigate the keypad

lines of print or just the straight edge of the typoscope. Any straight edge, like a ruler or construction paper, can be used to help keep place on a line of print. These devices not only allow tracking from left to right along the flow of print but also assist in locating the beginning of the next line of print. The patient will follow the line that was just read back to the beginning then move down one line. Contrast may be increased and glare may also be reduced by the dark typoscope. Cues may not be limited to the straight edge itself, but the tactile response of holding the straight edge. Patients may also read and track print better by using their finger to move from word to word or by holding the beginning of the line of print as a tactile marker to indicate where to return to start the next line. Depending on their remaining field, the patient may also benefit from turning the page away from the horizontal, possibly even to a full 90°. This will be effective if the patient's vertical field is larger than their horizontal field.

Signature guides have a slot in the template to place over the area needed to be signed, allowing the patient to keep in a straight line. There are templates for placing over checks that have a slot for each field on the check. There are also writing guides for placement over 8.5 × 11-in. sheets of paper.

### 31.9.2 Tactile Dots, Plasticized Marking Pens, and Bold Line Markers

Tactile dots are inexpensive, raised, adhesive-backed dots about ¼-in. round that can be used to mark spots on appliances or any other place of importance to the patient (Fig. 31.21). Tactile dots can be used to give tactile input to locate frequently used buttons on items like the microwave oven or telephone. They can also be used to mark appliance dials on washing machines and stoves. For example, patients

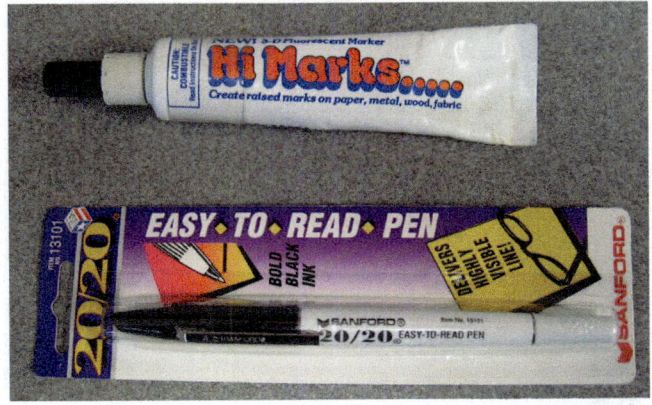

**Fig. 31.22** Top-Hi Marks fluorescent plasticized marker uses "plastic" ink to leave a raised mark for marking appliances and other commonly used dials. *Bottom* – The 20/20 marker made by Sanford is an example of a bold line marker

will place a dot at the 350° mark on their oven and place another dot on the dial mark. They then know that they are on the correct temperature when the dots are aligned. Plasticized marking pens are used similarly (Fig. 31.22).

The plastic "ink" leaves a raised mark that can be felt easily and comes in vibrant colors that tend to be recognizable to patients with decreased acuity.

Standard pens generally do not provide enough contrast to allow patients to read their own writing or read the writing of others. Patients will benefit from bold line markers, which, essentially, magnify the line of print compared to standard pens. Contrast is also increased. The "20/20" marker by Sanford is an example of a specialized bold line marker on the market, but most standard markers found in office supply stores will be effective.

### 31.9.3 Embossed Paper

There are pads of paper available with embossed lines (Fig. 31.23). The space between lines is larger than standard notebook lines. The lines themselves are noticeable to touch, as well as larger and bolder than normal paper. Used in conjunction with bold line markers, these can be effective writing tools for the visually impaired.

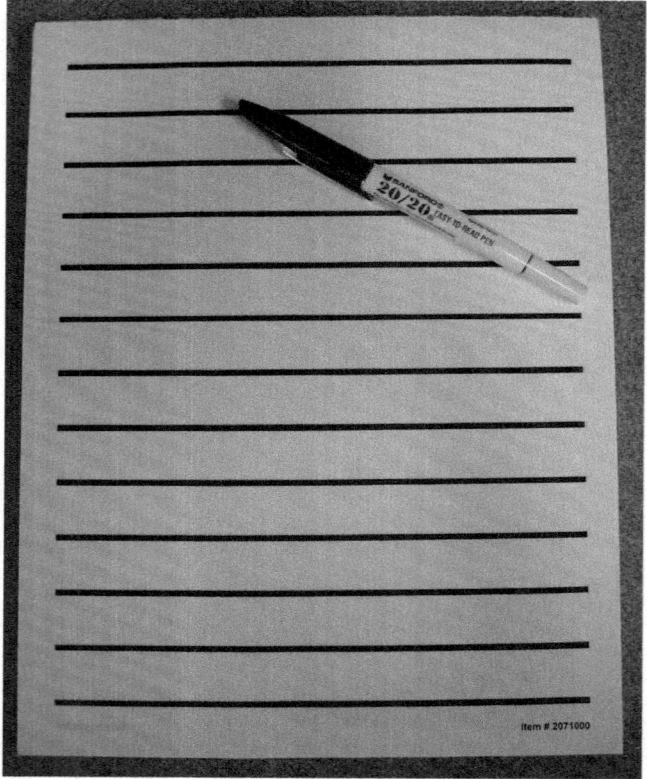

**Fig. 31.23** Embossed paper has darker embossed lines to improve contrast for writing tasks

### 31.9.4 Large-Print Checks

Checks can be ordered in larger sizes with larger print and embossed lines. These are readily available through most banks or can be obtained through check-making companies. As discussed earlier, there are signature templates that fit standard checks as well.

### 31.9.5 Adaptive Devices

There are many adaptive devices that are available on the market. They can be found by searching the World Wide Web, through catalogs, or through specialty stores. The hallmarks of adaptive devices typically are large print, large details, talking devices, or high contrast. The list of adaptive devices is actually pretty overwhelming. Many are very simple techniques using ordinary household items and easy to suggest to a patient. Others require specific devices that have to be obtained. Either way, there is a plethora of ideas and devices to be used in the public domain with a little searching. A few are mentioned as follows.

Large-print books, magazines, and other materials are available commercially and through libraries. Most libraries have a wide section of large-print books. Some major magazines like *Reader's Digest* produce a large-print edition, and there are large-print crosswords, word search, and other types of word games. Large-print playing cards come with large characters and suits. Some are printed with each suit in a different color to help identify the suit. Similarly, there are also large-print bingo cards and many large-print board games for patients who are visually impaired. Some of these games also incorporate tactile aspects, such as dominoes with raised dots.

Other adaptive devices are available with large details such as television remotes with keys that have numerals 3–10 times larger than the average remote (Fig. 31.24), large-faced telephones (Fig. 31.25), calculators, clocks, and kitchen timers. Alphabet and symbol stickers can be applied to computer keys. All of these items increase the magnification to the patient just by making the item larger.

### 31.9.6 Talking Devices

As their vision decreases and it becomes increasingly more difficult to identify objects and detail, some patients begin to use talking devices. These devices allow them to receive information auditorily rather than visually. Items in this category include talking watches, talking clocks, talking calculators, talking phones, and global positioning devices that talk.

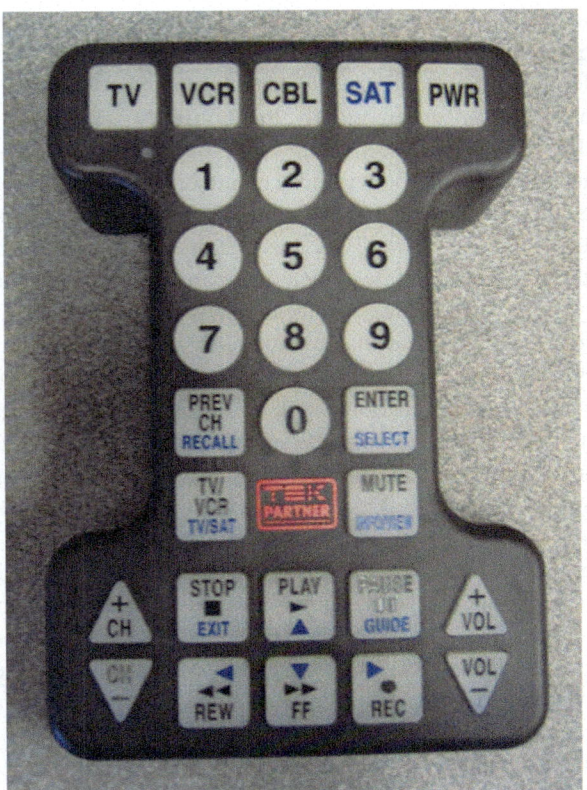

**Fig. 31.24** A universal remote with large buttons is an example of the adaptive technologies available in the marketplace that provide relative magnification through larger than normal sized numbers

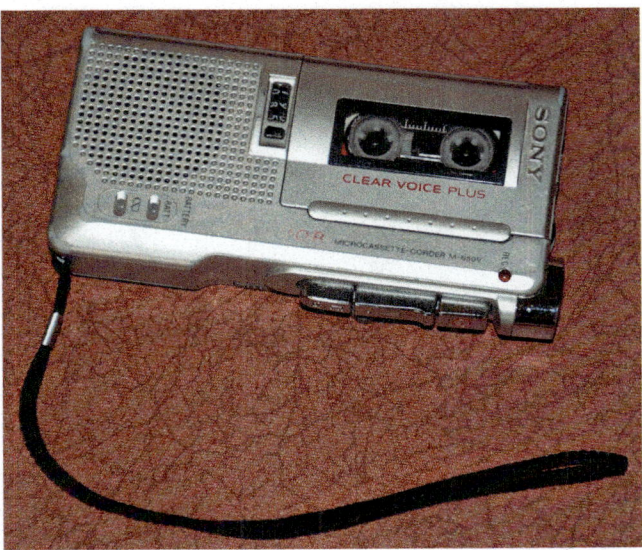

**Fig. 31.26** Cassette recorders or digital recorders are convenient tools for taking notes, creating grocery lists, and recording reminders

There are several talking devices available that enable patients to independently manage their healthcare needs including talking scales, blood pressure cuffs, thermometers, and glucometers.

Similarly, talking devices are available to manage meal preparation, including stoves, microwaves, and coffee makers. Some visually impaired patients will use handheld cassette or digital recorders to record their grocery lists and to record reminders for themselves (Fig. 31.26). It is an interesting scenario when a vision rehabilitationist dictates notes into a handheld recorder, and then the patient dictates instructions given to them into their own handheld recorder for reminding them later.

### 31.9.7 Labeling

Talking labels are another means of providing information aurally. They allow patients to record and store a voice message that can be played back with the push of a button. These systems allow speech patterns to be embedded on the label and affixed to an object. When the label is scanned with a handheld device, it will repeat what was recorded to the label. This is especially useful for people who take a variety of prescribed medications in order to avoid making a mistake. For patients who have a difficult time distinguishing color, color identifiers are available. These are small devices that, when held up to an object, announces the color. Labeling systems also come in tactile or Braille.

Labeling systems can be very simple (Fig. 31.27), such as sock holders that allow both socks to be put through one

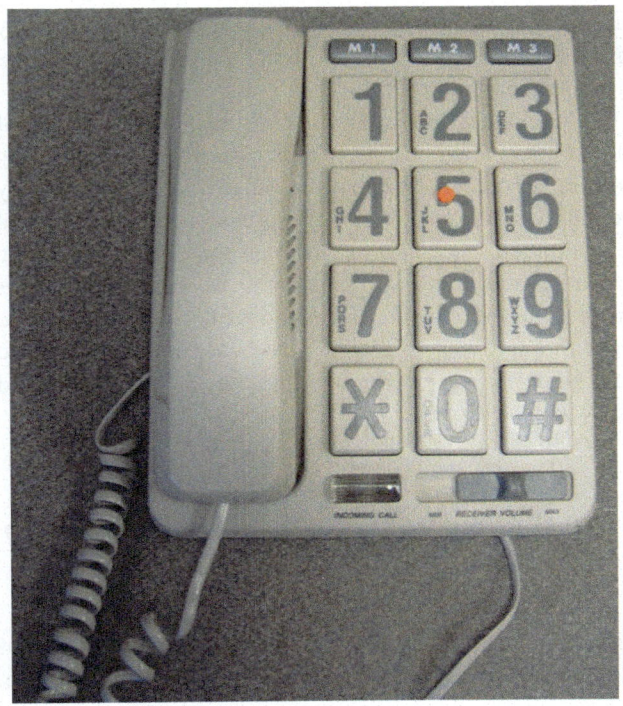

**Fig. 31.25** A large button telephone

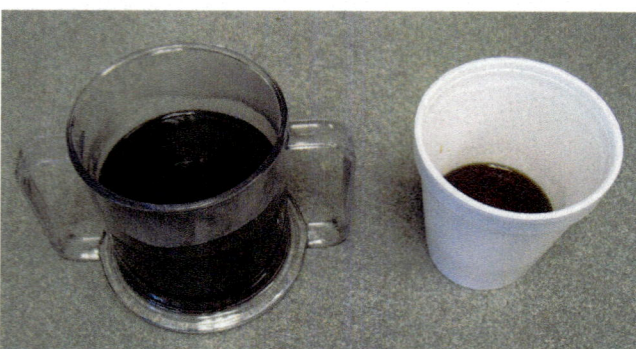

**Fig. 31.27** Cups that contrast the color of the liquid being poured assist patients in seeing when the cup is full and reduce the chance of over pouring

holder so that they do not become separated in the laundry, eliminating the need for matching. Another simple system is writing with a bold marker on note paper the name of a canned good and attaching the note with a rubber band to the can. After using the canned good, visually impaired patients can then remove the note and place it into a folder as part of their grocery list. Label makers provide labels with embossed print, enabling the patient a means of tactile identification.

### 31.9.8 Talking Books

Talking books are produced by the National Library Service for the Blind and Physically Handicapped (NLS), a division of the Library of Congress. NLS distributes talking books and playback equipment through a national network of cooperating libraries. The equipment and talking books are distributed free of charge to those who need them. The NLS is converting from cassette to digital media from 2008 to 2012 and both formats will be produced through the transition and for several years afterward. Patients can choose the books they want to hear or have them selected for them by choosing a category. Any healthcare provider can authorize talking books for their patient. Contact your state library for the necessary forms.

## 31.10 Networking

Because patients with advanced glaucoma have profound vision loss and, in some cases, total blindness, it is important to use a networked approach involving several health professionals supporting the low-vision practitioner. The team concept here is to work with the patient and the patient's family to create a support system to allow the patient to function in their home environment and in some cases work environment. The team includes other medical physicians, healthcare professionals, psychologists, social workers, rehabilitation teachers, occupational therapists, orientation and mobility instructors, adaptive technology specialists, private and state agencies for funding and benefits and, most importantly, the family.

First and foremost, it is important to educate the patient's family and friends about the true nature of the patient's visual disability and engage and encourage their willingness to provide a support system. They may not understand the degree or the significance of the patient's impairment, often because they see no external reasons for the patient's difficulties. The patient's eyes look normal and the family cannot understand why they are having such a hard time coping with activities of daily living. Education and demonstration of the patient's condition to the family will be very helpful in solidifying the family to support the patient. The family is often the first resource in psychological, financial, and material support. Try to include them in the examination process as well as some of the decision making. In the perfect world, family members will always rally around the visually impaired, but there are some families that do not fit that mold. Pay attention to those families that may make the process more difficult for the patient, and try to direct those patients to counseling services that will help counteract the negative impact of some detrimental family members.

Social workers are often the best resource to lead the team. They are well trained in counseling, educated in the team concept, and knowledgeable about funding and benefits through private and state agencies. Their training in counseling allows them to help the patient through the grieving process of their vision loss and keep them directed toward being functional in their environment. Often they will be the primary intake for the patient and will direct the patient through the vision rehabilitation process.

Psychologists and/or psychiatrists also may be needed if the patient is not adjusting to their vision loss. The grieving process for vision loss may be lengthy. The patient may exhibit symptoms of psychological dysfunction. As a visual rehabilitation specialist, you may have problems motivating the patient to work toward functioning or adapt the strategies that you are introducing if the patient has not been able to work through their grief. The psychologist will be able to help guide the patient through these levels of grieving and allow them to move forward.

### 31.10.1 Primary Service Providers in Low Vision Through "The Blindness System"

"The blindness system" is a well-developed network of libraries; state and federal agencies; and private, local, state, and national organizations serving the blind and visually impaired. "The blindness system" has been in existence for more than 100 years, with comprehensive services beginning after

World War II. Services in "the blindness system" are usually described as educational or rehabilitative programs. Certified vision rehabilitation therapists, certified orientation and mobility specialists, certified low vision therapists, teachers of children with visual impairment, and guide dog trainers are service providers through "the blindness system."[36]

A Certified Vision Rehabilitation Therapist (CVRT) (formerly Rehabilitation Teacher) has a bachelor's or master's degree in vision rehabilitation therapy or a related profession and is certified by the Academy for Certification of Vision Rehabilitation and Education Professionals (ACVREP). They instruct people with vision impairments in the use of compensatory skills and assistive technology. Specific areas of instruction include:

- Communication systems including Braille and computer access technology;
- Personal management including grooming, clothing organization, and medication management;
- Home management including organization and labeling, repairs, budgeting, and record-keeping;
- Activities of daily living including cooking, cleaning, and shopping;
- Leisure and recreation including hobbies, crafts, and sports;
- Psychosocial aspects of blindness; and
- Basic orientation and mobility skills such as sighted guide technique.

A CVRT can help enable the visually impaired live safe, productive, and independent lives.[31]

Certified Orientation and Mobility Specialists (COMS) hold a bachelor's or master's degree in orientation and mobility (O&M). They are certified by ACVREP. They provide instruction to individuals with visual impairment in the use of their remaining senses to determine their position within the environment and in techniques for safe movement from one place to another. Specific skills include:

- Residual vision stimulation and training
- Sighted guide techniques
- Locating dropped objects
- Cane techniques
- Soliciting/declining assistance
- Route planning
- Analysis and identification of intersections and traffic patterns
- Techniques for crossing the street
- Techniques for indoor travel, and
- Use of public transportation.[31]

Guide dogs are specifically trained dogs that act as a mobility tool to aid blind and visually impaired individuals. They begin formal training at 18 months and spend 4–6 months with a trainer prior to being matched with their blind person. They then spend 4 weeks training with their blind person and the trainer at a training center prior to returning home.[37,38]

Most established guide dog training centers require the following qualifications for their trainers: excellent physical health, stamina, a background in animal training, a college degree, the ability to teach or coach, and good interpersonal skills. Trainers serve an apprenticeship that varies between 2½ and 4 years.[37,38]

Certified Low Vision Therapists (CLVT) must have at least a bachelor's or master's degree in low vision or another field to apply to take the certification examination given by ACVREP. If the degree is in a field other than low vision, the applicant must possess verification of competency in specific areas of low vision and have 350 h of practice in low vision supervised by an OD or MD. The CLVT must complete a functional low vision evaluation that identifies visual impairments related to:

- Performance of activities of daily living including grooming, dressing, medication management, meal preparation, home management, shopping, and safety awareness training;
- Performance of educational pursuits;
- Performance of vocational pursuits; and
- Performance of leisure and social activities.

The CLVT trains patients in the use of optical devices prescribed by their eye doctor including handheld and stand magnifiers, spectacle-mounted magnifiers, telescopes, and field-enhancing devices. They train patients in the use of specific visual motor skills, such as identification and use of preferred retinal locus (PRL) for fixation, and address compensatory strategies for reduced visual field. The CLVT also provides instruction in the use of non-optical devices to maximize the use of other senses such as tactile or auditory strategies.[31]

Teachers of Children with Visual Impairment (TCVI) (formerly Vision Teachers) have a special education degree and additional certification in vision. They instruct and provide support services to enable children who are blind and visually impaired to participate in the least restrictive environment in which they are capable of learning – often mainstream classrooms. They work closely with the regular classroom teacher to assure that the student with impaired vision can access the regular curriculum. Duties may include transcribing materials into Braille or large print; teaching adaptive computer technology; and addressing daily living skills, social skills, and recreation and leisure activities.[31]

### 31.10.2 Reimbursement Sources

Services provided by the professionals within "the blindness system" are not reimbursed by insurance companies, including Medicare and Medicaid; however, funding is available through charitable organizations. The Center for Medicare and Medicaid Services (CMS) has a 5-year outpatient vision rehabilitation demonstration project in place in selected areas throughout the United States until March 31, 2011. The purpose of the project is to examine the impact of standardized Medicare coverage for vision rehabilitation services and to extend coverage under Part B for the same services to provide vision rehabilitation that would otherwise be payable when provided by an occupational or physical therapist if they are now provided by a vision rehabilitation professional under the general supervision of a qualified physician. This project covers services provided by certified low vision therapists (CLVT), certified orientation and mobility specialists (COMS), and certified vision rehabilitation therapists (CVRT).[39]

Following World War II, the US Veteran's Administration (VA) played a pivotal role in the development of vision rehabilitation services. The VA has its own network of comprehensive services for the blind and visually impaired, but services are restricted to veterans.

The alternative to "the blindness system" is the provision of low vision services through the healthcare system. Primary service providers are optometrists, ophthalmologists, and occupational therapists. Service delivery is not yet as comprehensive as "the blindness system," but services are reimbursed through medical insurance companies, including Medicare and Medicaid. Rehabilitation codes are the most reliable way to describe the services provided and for the patient to receive reimbursement. Evaluation and Management (E&M) codes are also used for reimbursement.

Occupational therapists have always treated patients with visual impairment, but formally reentered the field of low vision in 1991. This coincided with the Center for Medicare and Medicaid Services (CMS) acknowledging visual impairment as a physical impairment requiring rehabilitation. As of 2007, all occupational therapy program graduates have at least a master's degree, with a few programs offering entry-level doctoral degrees. Six months of supervised fieldwork, as well as passing national and state examinations, are required in order to practice. The American Occupational Therapy Association (AOTA) offers a specialty certification in low vision that provides formal recognition for those who have engaged in a voluntary process of ongoing, focused, and targeted professional development. This certification is not required for practice.

In general, occupational therapists work in a variety of settings to help patients improve their ability to perform tasks relevant to their living and work environments. Treatment focuses remediation of lost function or teaching strategies to compensate for loss of function. Related to low vision, in some settings, the occupational therapist may complete the low vision examination, although this is typically done by the eye care physician. Areas assessed include acuity, contrast sensitivity, visual field integrity, color vision, dark/light adaptation, and sensitivity to glare. The occupational therapist evaluates how the patient's visual deficits impair their ability to perform their daily tasks and life roles. The goals of treatment are to maximize independence either by instruction in the use of the patient's remaining vision or to instruct in compensatory strategies using magnification or other senses.[40]

Typical skills that an occupational therapist may teach in a low vision setting include:

- Identifying and using a preferred retinal locus (PRL) for reading and other activities of daily living;
- Use of magnification, including enlarging print, handheld and stand magnifiers, spectacle-mounted magnifiers, telescopes, and electronic magnification systems;
- Use of screen reader/screen magnifier computer software;
- Selection of proper lighting;
- Use of non-optical devices such as large-print checks, tactile markers for identifying appliance dials, bold-lined paper or templates for writing, talking watches, and talking glucometers;
- Methods to improve contrast for daily tasks; and
- Strategies to modify the home environment for improved organization and work simplification to reduce visual demand.

Adaptive technology specialists are able to evaluate, recommend, deliver, and train patients with severe vision loss on the use of adaptive technologies. These specialists will be the lead in setting up adaptive technologies for the patient in their home. They work with computer technologies that use magnification, auditory output and tactile outputs, as well as voice-activated technologies for those patients with severe visual impairment. At the most severe level, devices such as voice-activated computers and household equipment are used. Adaptive technology specialists are often contracted vendors, but can also be agents of the state.

### 31.10.3 Organizations and Resources for the Blind and Visually Impaired

Approximately 5% of patients with advanced glaucoma will become completely blind. These patients will need additional services to continue to be independent or partially independent. There are many organizations that offer services and information to blind and visually impaired patients and their families (Table 31.1). These organizations are available at the national level as well as the state and local levels. They range from private organizations to government agencies. There is a comprehensive directory of organizations and services available from the American Foundation for the Blind.[41]

Most communities have local resources that can be utilized by patients with blindness or visual impairment. The eye physician's office can contact local organizations and create

**Table 31.1** National organizations for the visually impaired

| Organization | Address | Telephone | Website |
| --- | --- | --- | --- |
| American Council of the Blind | 1155 15th St NW, Suite 1004, Washington, DC 20005 | (202) 467-5081<br>(800) 424-8666 | www.acb.org/ |
| American Foundation for the Blind | 11 Penn Plaza, Suite 300, New York, NY 10001 | (212) 502-7600<br>(800) 223-1839 | www.afb.org |
| American Printing House for the Blind | 1839 Frankfort Ave, P.O. Box 6085, Louisville, KY 40206-0085 | (502)895-2405 | www.aph.org |
| Associated Services for the Blind | 919 Walnut St, Philadelphia, PA 19107 | (215) 627-0600 | www.asb.org |
| Association for the Education and Rehabilitation of the Blind and Visually Impaired | 1703 N. Beauregard St, Suite 440, Alexandria, VA 22311 | (877)-492-2708 | www.aerbvi.org |
| Blinded Veterans Association | 477 H Street NW, Washington, DC 20001-2694 | (202) 371-8880 | www.bva.org |
| The Glaucoma Foundation | 80 Maiden Lane, Suite 700, New York, NY 10038 | (212)285-0080 | www.glaucomafoundation.org |
| Glaucoma Research Foundation | 251 Post Street, Suite 600, San Francisco, CA 4108 | (415)986-3162<br>(800)826-6693 | www.glaucoma.org |
| Lighthouse International | The Sol and Lillian Goldman, Building, 111 East 59th St, New York, NY 10022-1202 | (212) 821-9200<br>(800) 829-0500 | www.lighthouse.org |
| National Association for the Visually Handicapped | 22 West 21st St 6th Floor, New York, NY 10010 | (212) 889-3141<br>(212) 255-2804 | www.navh.org |
| National Association for Parents of Children with Visual Impairments | P.O. Box 317, Watertown, MA 02471 | (800) 562-6265<br>(617) 972-7441 | www.spedex.com/naprvil |
| National Federation of the Blind | 1800 Johnson St, Baltimore, MD 21230 | (410)659-9314 | www.nfb.org/ |
| National Industries for the Blind | 1310 Braddock Place, Alexandria, Virginia 22314-1691 | (703)310-0500 | www.nib.org/ |
| The National Library Service for the Blind and Physically Handicapped | Library of Congress, Washington, DC 20542 | (202) 707-5100 | www.loc.gov/nls/ |
| Prevent Blindness America | 211 West Wacker Dr. Suite 1700, Chicago, IL 60606 | (800) 331-2020 | www.preventblindness.org |
| Rehabilitation ServicesAdministration | 400 Maryland Ave. S.W., Washington, DC 20202-2800 | (202) 245-7488 | www.ed.gov/about/offices/list/osers/rsa |
| Research to Prevent Blindness | 645 Madison Ave Floor 21, New York, NY 10022-1010 | (800) 621-0026<br>(212) 752-4333 | www.rpbusa.org |

a resource list that can be distributed to their patients with visual impairment. These organizations include:

- *Libraries:* Most libraries have large-print publications and talking books available. They may also have programs to help people with special needs.
- *Banks:* Many banks offer large-print embossed checks, large-print bank statements, and some may deliver statements verbally on audio media.
- *Media outlets:* Some newspapers may have large-print versions, most have Web versions that can be read with screen readers, and newspapers are read over the radio or telephone by the staff or volunteers.
- *Transportation:* Many communities offer transportation at greatly reduced rates for people with visual impairment. Private organizations may provide transportation as well.
- *Taxes:* There are tax exemptions for the visually impaired.
- *Meals on wheels*: Meals can be delivered free-of-charge.
- *Utilities:* Many offer large-print billing. Telephone companies offer free directory service.
- *Support groups:* There may be support groups at the local level in many communities.
- *Lions Club International*: This international organization has chapters at the local level. They have many community-based eye health education programs and can be a local source of funding for vision-related projects.

There are also local and state: schools for the blind; foundations for the blind and visually impaired; homes for the blind and visually impaired; councils for the blind and visually impaired; and departments of rehabilitation services.

## 31.11 Conclusion

Advanced glaucoma presents with varied vision loss and function, from mild peripheral field defects and minimal functional loss to complete blindness. The advanced glaucoma patient will present a significant challenge to the eye care practitioner. There are many strategies to help these patients with varied results. The patient's functional problems should guide the choices of strategy. Some patients will have found appropriate strategies and remedies for their functional problems due to the slow course of vision loss, while others will need significant help visually, financially, and psychologically, as well as other forms of support. Networking of families, doctors, rehabilitation specialists, and organizations to the vision rehabilitation goals of patients will ease some of the problems the patient will experience with their declining vision. There are many organizations available at the community, state, national, and international level that will offer substantial help for patients.

The adaptive devices that are chosen for patients with advanced glaucoma will have results that differ from patient to patient. Finding help for the patient's complaints of field loss, glare, reading difficulties, and problems with activities of daily living will often be a daunting task. Some patients will reject the offered solutions and strategies immediately, but many will benefit from the strategies you have to offer. Remember that training will often be the most important aspect of whether a patient will have success with a particular device and show satisfaction.

The dedication and resources required to be a true vision rehabilitation specialist are outside the time and interest of most ophthalmologists and optometrists. As the patient with advanced glaucoma progress, their needs will be greater than the ability of the comprehensive eye care doctor to meet them. Referrals to the vision rehabilitation specialist may be the most appropriate course of action. To this end, the goals of discussing the devices and techniques in this chapter are not to serve strictly as an instructional or tutorial manual, but rather to educate the general eye care physician to the nuances of vision rehabilitation and aid them in setting patient expectations.

- Use the least magnification needed to perform the desired task for patients with advanced glaucoma. The trick is to not magnify greater than the patient's remaining field of vision.
- Computers are the ultimate in vision rehabilitation devices. They are able to manipulate any digital print. With the appropriate programs, they can recognize characters from print, recognize speech and translate to print, read from print audibly, and magnify print.
- The knfb Reader is a PDA, money reader, optical character recognition device, GPS, screen reader, camera, and phone all wrapped into a cell phone. The condensation of these devices into one manageable unit makes this device one of the most exciting new innovations in vision rehabilitation.
- Training will significantly increase the patient's chances of success with field enhancement devices. The more training the patient receives, the better the patient's chances of success. This is also true of other vision rehabilitation devices and techniques.
- There are many non-optical devices available that can enhance the quality of life for a patient with advanced glaucoma. Have some available in the office. For those items not available in the office, consider creating a fact sheet with websites and catalogs for patients with glaucoma.
- Talking books and the talking book player are free to the patient with a recommendation from their optometrist or ophthalmologist. Have forms available in the office to sign for the patient.
- Help the patient create as big a support network as possible. Include family members, other healthcare professionals, and funding sources.

**Acknowledgments** Many thanks to Jane Bachman Groth, Joseph Beringer, John Conto, David Deuker, Tricia Fekete, Serena Lynn, Laura Mazzie, Dennis Siemsen and Deb Wahlers for their contributions.

### 31.11.1 Clinical Pearls

- Observation of the patient's ability to move through the waiting room and exam room environment will help the clinician's assessment of the patient's functional status.
- A thorough history of the patient's visual difficulties in performing their activities of daily living is the key to directing the clinician to the most effective interventions.
- Using a near reading card with text instead of single letter acuity will allow the clinician to better assess the patient's near reading abilities and better assess magnification at near.
- Trial frame refractions are more effective than phoropter refractions for patients with visual impairment. They are more natural in terms of lighting and vertex distance and the patient will easily understand the prescription.

## References

1. Allingham RR, Damjii K, Freedman S, et al. *Shields' Textbook of Glaucoma.* 5th ed. Philadelphia, PA: Lippincott Williams & Wilkins; 2005:702.
2. Cheong AM, Geruschat DR, Congdon N. Traffic gap judgment in people with significant peripheral field loss. *Optom Vis Sci.* 2008; 85(1):26–36.
3. Haymes SA, Leblanc RP, Nicolela MT, et al. Risk of falls and motor vehicle collisions in glaucoma. *Invest Ophthalmol Vis Sci.* 2007;48: 1149–1155.
4. Noe G, Ferraro J, Lamoureux E, et al. Associations between glaucomatous visual field loss and participation in activities of daily living. *Clin Experiment Ophthalmol.* 2003;31(6):482–486.
5. McKean-Cowdin R, Wang Y, Wu J, et al. Impact of visual field loss on health-related quality of life in glaucoma: The Los Angeles Latino Eye Study. *Ophthalmology.* 2008;115(6):941–948.
6. Allingham RR, Damjii K, Freedman S, et al. Assessment of visual fields. In: *Shields' Textbook of Glaucoma.* 5th ed. Philadelphia, PA: Lippincott Williams & Wilkins; 2005.

7. Hattenhauer M, Johnson D, Ing H, et al. The probability of blindness from open-angle glaucoma. *Ophthalmology.* 1998;105:2099–2104.
8. Anctil J, Anderson D. Early foveal involvement and generalized depression of the visual field in glaucoma. *Arch Ophthalmol.* 1984;102:363.
9. Stamper RL. The effect of glaucoma on central visual function. *Trans Am Ophthalmol Soc.* 1984;82:792.
10. Drance SM. Diffuse visual field loss in open-angle glaucoma. *Ophthalmology.* 1991;98:1533.
11. Lachenmayr BJ, Drance SM, Chauhan BC, et al. Diffuse and localized glaucomatous field loss in light-sense, flicker and resolution perimetry. *Graefes Arch Clin Exp Ophthalmol.* 1991;229:267.
12. Lachenmayr BJ, Drance SM, Airaksinen PJ. Diffuse field loss and diffuse retinal nerve-fiber loss in glaucoma. *Ger J Ophthalmol.* 1992;1:22.
13. Polo V, Larrosa JM, Pinilla I, et al. Glaucomatous damage patterns by short-wavelength automated perimetry (SWAP) in glaucomatous suspects. *Eur J Ophthalmol.* 2002;12:49.
14. Brilliant RL, Ginsburg LH. *Rehabilitation of Peripheral Field Defects.* Boston, MA: Butterworth-Heinemann; 1999.
15. Ray JS. Visual rehabilitation and low vision therapy for the patient with glaucomatous vision loss. In: Sassani JW II, ed. *Ophthalmic Fundamentals: Glaucoma.* Thorofare, NJ: Slack, Inc; 1999.
16. Matchinski T, Brilliant R, Bednarksi M. Low vision near systems I: microscopes and magnifiers. In: Brilliant RL, ed. *Essentials of Low Vision Practice.* Boston, MA: Butterworth Heinemann; 1999.
17. Waiss B, Cohen JM. Visual impairment and visual efficiency training. In: Cold RG, Rosenthal BP, eds. *Remediation and Management of Low Vision.* St. Louis, MO: Mosby; 1996.
18. Turano K, Geruschat D, Baker F, et al. Direction of gaze while walking a simple route: persons with normal vision and persons with retinitis pigmentosa. *Optom Vis Sci.* 2001;78(9):667–675.
19. Kozlowski JM, Mainster M, Avila M. Negative-lens field expander for patients with concentric field constriction. *Arch Ophthalmol.* 1984;102(8):1182–1184.
20. Faye EE. *Clinical Low Vision.* 2nd ed. Boston, MA: Little, Brown and Company; 1984:529.
21. Hoppe E, Perlin R. The effectivity of fresnel prisms for visual field enhancement. *J Am Optom Assoc.* 1993;64(1):46–53.
22. Ray JR. *Visual Rehabilitation and Low Vision Therapy for the Patient with Glaucomatous Vision Loss.* Thorofare, NJ: Slack Incorporated; 1999.
23. Chadwick Optical Inc. 1763 Old River Rd. PO Box 485 White River JCT., Vermont, 05001, chadwickoptical@aol.com.
24. Kennedy W, Rosten J, Young L, et al. A field expander for patients with retinitis pigmentosa: a clinical study. *Am J Optom Physiol Opt.* 1977;11:744–755.
25. Herse P. Retinitis Pigmentosa: visual function and multidisciplinary management. *Clin Exp Optom.* 2005;88(5):335–350.
26. Hoeft W, Feinbloom W, Brilliant R, et al. Amorphic lenses: a mobility aid for patients with retinitis pigmentosa. *Am J Optom Physiol Opt.* 1984;62:142–148.
27. Szlyk J, Seiple W, Laderman D, et al. Use of bioptic amorphic lenses to expand the visual field in patients with peripheral loss. *Optom Vis Sci.* 1998;75:518–524.
28. Luo G, Lichtenstein L, Peli E. Collision judgment when viewing minified images through a HMD visual field expander. *Proceedings of SPIE, Ophthalmic Technologies XVII* 2007; 6426:64261Z.
29. Rosenberg R. Glare. In: Steun C, Arditi A, Horowitz A, et al., eds. *Vision Rehabilitation: Assessment, Intervention, and Outcomes.* New York, NY: Swerts & Zeitlinger; 2000.
30. Wolffsohn A, Cochrane H, Yoshimitsue S. Contrast is enhanced by yellow lenses because of selective reduction of short-wave-length light. *Optom Vis Sci.* 2000;77(2):73–81.
31. Nguyen TV, Hoeft WW. A study of corning blue blocker filters and related pathologies. *J Vis Rehabil.* 1994;8(3):15–21.
32. Gormezano S, Stelmack J. Efficient, effective clinical protocols for prescription of selective absorption filters. In: AA SC, Horowitz A, Lang M, et al., eds. *Vision Rehabilitation: Assessment, Intervention, and Outcomes.* New York, NY: Swerts & Zeitlinger; 2000.
33. Freedman PB, Jose RT. *The Art and Practice of Low Vision.* Newton, MA: Butterworth-Heinemann; 1997:320.
34. NoIR Medical Technologies, South Lyon, MI, http://www.noir-medical.com, 1-800-521-9746.
35. Goodrich GL. Low vision training. In: Freeman PB, Jose RT, eds. *The Art and Practice of Low Vision.* 2nd ed. Boston, MA: Butterworth-Heinemann; 1997.
36. AFB. An Introduction to Blindness Services in the United States. http://www.afb.org/Section.asp?Documentid=930.
37. http://www.guidedogsofamerica.org/. Last accessed August 10, 2008.
38. http://www.thepuppyplace.org. Last accessed August 10, 2008.
39. Medicare Learning Network. MLN Matters Number: MM3816. http://www.cms.hhs.gov/mlnmattersarticles/downloads/mm3816.pdf. Last accessed February 4, 2010
40. http://wmich.edu/hhs/blvs/rehabilitation-teaching.htm. Last accessed August 10, 2008.
41. *AFB Directory of Services for Blind and Visually Impaired Persons in the United States and Canada.* 25 ed. New York, NY: AFB Press; 1998.

# Chapter 32
# Glaucoma and Medical Insurance: Billing and Coding Issues

Cynthia Mattox

Accurate billing and coding allows you to practice medicine by providing you with the optimal and appropriate financial reimbursement for your work. Forgive the comparison, but even the most skillful car mechanic would quickly fail in business if he routinely neglected to charge for replacement parts or continually underestimated his labor time. Accurate billing ensures that you, your patient, and most likely the third-party payer are all receiving the ethically and legally appropriate charges and payments for services rendered.

Most ophthalmologists would rather spend their time treating patients in the clinic or the operating room (OR) than pore over a reimbursement report from the top three health plans for their practice. In this chapter, I hope to provide an overview of the tools you need to successfully code for the typical work done to treat glaucoma patients in the United States. Year by year, and sometimes suddenly, the rules for ophthalmology coding change. By knowing how to keep abreast of the rules, your practice will wither those changes promptly, minimizing any losses.

## 32.1 The Infrastructure

Most ophthalmology practices accept insurance payments and most accept Medicare. Most practices agree to submit insurance claims on behalf of their patients and receive payment directly from the insurer after submitting the bill, rather than from the patient at the time of service. For US Medicare patients, this requires a form signed by the patient to assign benefits to the practice. It must be in the chart, or available for review in the event of an audit. Medicare Part B coverage provides 80% of the full payment allowed by Medicare for a given service. Many, but not all, Medicare patients have a separate policy to cover the additional 20%, while patients covered by "Medicare Advantage" plans have the full cost of the ophthalmic service covered. Medicare, many Medicare Advantage, plans and private plans have a yearly deductible amount that must be paid out of pocket by the patient before insurance payments begin. Many private insurers require a co-pay from the patient at the time of service, and this amount varies by insurance product. This co-pay represents a portion of the full payment for the given service.

The complexity of insurance reimbursement requires that you have a "billing department." This department encompasses front-end work, which may include collecting insurance information from every patient at every visit, collecting co-pays, requesting signatures on beneficiary notices or insurance waivers, verifying addresses, recording primary care physician names, etc. This frontline information is crucial to efficient reimbursement. Depending on the practice, this information may be collected by the reception desk personnel, or by trained billing department employees.

The billing department again comes into play after the medical service in the office or operating room is rendered. An encounter form is generated either on paper or electronically, and codes describing the service and diagnosis must be entered correctly in the proper electronic format for the particular insurer. This demands the use of (often expensive) billing software. Time limits for claim submissions vary, with some private insurers allowing as little as 45 days, and Medicare allowing up to 1 year. Once the insurance claim is submitted, all or portions of it will be paid or rejected (or sometimes upon further inquiry said to be "lost" by the carrier). Rejections require additional work to evaluate, correct, resubmit, appeal, or bill to the patient. Most practices have experienced, well-trained coders who work with the physicians and administrators to deal with claims and rejections. The American Academy of Ophthalmic Executives offers courses, training programs, and certification for the highly complex and specific needs of ophthalmology coding.

Please keep in mind that the information in this chapter most often refers to the most common Medicare rules. At the time of this writing, there are numerous Medicare Carriers responsible for different states or regions of the country. The Medicare Carrier must abide by National Coverage policies, but where those do not exist, are free to create Local Medical policies, and may also interpret the rules slightly different. And so, some coverage policies will differ from state to state.

Many, but certainly not all, private payers use the basic Medicare rules for reimbursement, but often have variations. This is what makes coding and reimbursement practices so complex. It is important for you and your billing staff to remain current with the various rules from your Medicare carrier and from private payers that pertain to your practice.

### 32.1.1 Imperative Infrastructure Items

1. An appropriate fee schedule: Make sure your fee schedule is higher than the highest reimbursement from any payer with whom you have a contractual relationship.
2. A complete, easy-to-use office encounter form or software program. It should include:
   (a) all of the most common Current Procedural Terminology (CPT) codes used by the physicians in the practice (and a designated person who can research the less common procedure codes)
   (b) a way to indicate right/left/bilateral for those codes that require them
   (c) an indicator of specific global periods for all listed procedures
   (d) specific, yet abbreviated, list of diagnosis codes (and again a designee who can help look up the uncommon ones)
   (e) a list of modifiers to be used with exam codes
   (f) a list of modifiers to be used with procedure codes
   (g) a list of the patients' insurers
3. A separate surgical encounter form
   (a) Include all usual CPT codes used by your practice
   (b) Diagnosis codes – make sure all CPT codes have corresponding International Classification of Diseases, 9th Revision (ICD-9) diagnosis codes
   (c) Modifiers for procedure codes
   (d) List the patient's insurer
4. A separate form or section for inpatient coding
5. Billing software
6. Experienced coding personnel or special software to help check claims going out, and help work rejections

## 32.2 Coding and the Ophthalmologist

Unfortunately, there are few times the physician can delegate the responsibility of coding for services to a staff member. The ultimate responsibility for correct coding rests with the physician, both ethically and legally in terms of fraud and abuse issues. And familiarity with correct coding will actually increase revenue, either by appropriately billing for services with higher reimbursement, or by decreasing expenses by avoiding claim rejections and additional office staff time. There are, however, ways to streamline coding and have your staff assist you in the task throughout your clinic day.

Glaucoma patients undergo a multitude of tests usually performed by technicians and presented to you for interpretation and evaluation of the patient: pachymetry, visual field testing, optic nerve and retinal nerve fiber layer (RNFL) imaging, and optic disc photography. Having the technician check off the CPT code on the encounter form or electronic record for you is a good way to make sure the test is billed and you do not forget. However, there are a few caveats that only you as the physician-coder may be aware. For example, pachymetry is considered included in the payment for the exam by some payers, but not others. If you know which payers have refused to pay separately, you might not want to bill for pachymetry on the day of an exam to avoid having a rejected claim. On the other hand, one may deliberately decide to forego billing for pachymetry on a separate day because the cost of reimbursement may exceed the actual cost of processing a claim. Optic nerve photography 92250 and RNFL imaging 92135 are usually not paid for by Medicare or other payers if performed on the same date of service. This is a result of being bundled by Correct Coding Initiative (CCI). Some Medicare carriers and private payers have allowed the use of modifier -59 to "unbundle" these codes when medical necessity for both is present. Again, your knowledge will help you code correctly.

These examples may be causing you to throw up your hands and say, "I don't have time for this. I'm trying to take care of patients." A little bit of basic training, and then some routine maintenance of your knowledge base, along with help from your billing staff will quickly get you up to speed. Here are the basics:

### 32.2.1 Coding for Office Services

#### 32.2.1.1 Step One

First, determine if the patient is new to the practice. The definition of "new" is that the patient must not have been seen by *any* ophthalmologist in the practice over the prior 3 years. If they were seen within 3 years, that patient is an "Established Patient" of the practice. You and your fellow office ophthalmologists "share" the aspects of the coding experience, so that your reimbursement is somewhat dependent upon how other doctors have interacted with the patient.

Documentation: The chart or electronic data will indicate past visits to the practice. The physician should have access to the information, or the billing/technical staff should indicate the last visit date in the office note.

## 32.2.1.2 Step Two

The next step in coding for an office visit is to determine the level of service for the exam itself. Ophthalmologists are able to use either the "Eye Codes" (92002, 92004, 92012, and 92014) or the "Evaluation and Management Codes" (99202-5, 99212-5) or Consultation Codes (99242-5). Eye Codes consist of "intermediate" or "comprehensive" services; while the EM and Consultation Codes use Levels II, III, IV, and V. (Level I is reserved for nonMD services ordered by a physician, for example an IOP check performed by a technician or nurse – but not in conjunction with a special test or in the post-op period of a procedure). The various EM levels depend not only on the extent of exam provided, but also on the degree of medical complexity. A more complex problem along with a more extensive history and examination qualifies for a higher EM Level. Please read the CPT book for more detail. (Yes, it is confusing and probably the best source for understanding the intricacies of this somewhat arbitrary system.)

Documentation: Documentation requirements for the codes vary and are quite complex. Remember, the perspective of insurance companies, the federal government, and even attorneys is that if something is not documented in the chart, it never took place. The EM and Consult codes require a numerical counting of "elements" in the history and exam portions of the service that then need to be appropriate for the degree of medical complexity. The Eye Codes also list specifics to be included in both Intermediate and Comprehensive levels of service. The choice between using EM and Eye Codes should depend on the clinical situation because sometimes one over the other will be obvious. But many times, we have our choice, and although the EM and Eye Codes are similar in reimbursement for the similar level of work, one or the other may reimburse at a slightly higher amount. The ophthalmology practice that keeps abreast of the yearly changes in the Medicare fee schedule will be able to reap a small increase based on using the code that pays higher.

Consultation Codes are unique and in that they require documentation of a request for the consultation from the referring physician, and require a letter or indication of communication back to the referring physician regarding the patient's assessment and care program. A Consultation Code is only used for initial involvement in the problem for which the patient was referred. Subsequent services provided by the consultant for the same problem are coded as established patient exams. Consultants, however, may initiate treatment then return the patient to the physician who requested the consultation. If a written report is not sent to the referring physician, the consultation codes should not be used. Subspecialty practices that perform many consultations may get audited, and there must be copies of the written consultation reports in the patients' charts.

## 32.2.1.3 Step Three

Code for any Special Testing Services performed on the same date of exam, or on the date of service.

Remember that some tests are paid whether the test is performed unilaterally or bilaterally and do not take modifiers; e.g., gonioscopy, visual fields, and disc photography. Other test procedures require the presence of pathology in the eye(s) tested, and the use of a Right/Left/Bilateral modifier; e.g., RNFL imaging, ultrasound biomicroscope imaging, A-scan measurements, etc. By using modifiers to indicate that both eyes were tested, the reimbursement for the tests should be 100% payment for each eye.

Documentation: All Special Tests require a written order of the physician and an indication for the test, including which eye(s). Then an "interpretation and report" must be documented in the chart, either on the test printout or in the exam record. Other than right/left/bilateral for some of the tests, there are no other modifiers appended to Special Tests.

## 32.2.1.4 Step Four

Determine if any modifiers need to be appended to the Exam code based on all the services provided at the visit. The most commonly used modifiers for exams include the following:

- *57* indicates to the payer that based on the exam and clinical decision-making, a major surgical or laser procedure was indicated and performed on either the same date of service or the day after the exam.
- *24* indicates that an unrelated exam service was performed during the postoperative period of a procedure; i.e., not related to procedure or postoperative care.
- *25* indicates one of three things: (1) separately identifiable exam service above and beyond the usual service required for the minor procedure that is performed on the same day as the exam (some private payers require two separate diagnoses); (2) unbundles CCI edits involving special testing services – rarely applies to ophthalmology services; or (3) differentiates between two unrelated office visits on the same day by the same provider, or by more than one provider in a group.

## 32.2.1.5 Step Five: Office Procedures

A note on Global Periods: Remember that "minor" procedures have either a 0- or 10-day global period (some private payers have different number of days), while a "major" procedure has a 90-day global period. Global periods indicate that all postoperative care for that procedure is included in the payment for the procedure and cannot be billed separately.

Some minor procedures in glaucoma include: laser trabeculoplasty (10 days) (but not laser iridectomies); injection of air, fluid, medication into anterior chamber (10 days); therapeutic release of aqueous through paracentesis 0 days; subconjunctival or subTenon's injection 0 days; retrobulbar alcohol injection 0 days. Post-op visits within these time limits are not reimbursed; those outside of the limits are reimbursed as appropriately coded.

Major procedures include all other laser and operating room surgeries.

A typical glaucoma practice performs a number of office procedures. Depending on the situation, the coding will vary. Here are some typical examples:

1. If a patient is found to have a serious condition that requires urgent laser treatment or other major procedure on the same day as an exam, the exam code will require the use of a -57 modifier in order to be paid for the assessment as well as the major procedure.
2. If a procedure or laser is planned and scheduled for a later date, only the procedure or laser should be coded on the day it is performed. Any technician or physician work-up on the day of the laser/procedure is considered included in the laser/procedure payment.
3. Office procedures performed in the postoperative period as a result of a complication or as part of the usual postoperative care are considered part of the global payment for the original procedure. For example, reforming the anterior chamber at the slit lamp with a viscoelastic in the postoperative period of a filtration surgery is not separately billable. Why? Because the shallow anterior chamber would not have occurred except as a consequence of the surgery, and therefore is considered a complication of the original surgery, and included in the global payment. Now, if the patient needed to return to the operating room for choroidal drainage and anterior chamber reformation during the postoperative period, that is a different story and there is a modifier that will allow partial payment for the additional procedure (see coding modifier list that follows).
4. Another example is performing a "bleb needling revision." If this is necessary during the 90-day global period of the original filtration surgery, it would not be paid separately. However, if after the 90 days, or even years later, the bleb needling is performed to revive a failing bleb, it would be considered a new procedure with its own global period.
5. Modifiers for office procedures. The procedure modifiers are the same whether a procedure is performed in the office or operating room. The most common are:
    - *-50 Bilateral.* It is occasionally necessary or convenient to perform a procedure in both eyes on the same day. Medicare allows this with the use of the -50 bilateral modifier, but will pay only 50% for the procedure in the second eye (remember Special Tests performed bilaterally are paid at 100% each). Some private insurers may not pay at all for the second eye if done on the same day, so it is important to know their rules.
    - *-51 Multiple Procedures.* This is used to indicate that more than one procedure was performed in the same eye on the same day. Medicare will pay only 50% for the second procedure, so you should list the procedure with the highest reimbursement first. An example might be a laser iridotomy and laser iridoplasty performed together. There are some procedures and tests that are "bundled" with another one under CCI, and the higher paying code will be denied in favor of payment for the lower reimbursed code. An example is that gonioscopy is considered bundled on the day of a laser trabeculoplasty.
    - *-58 Staged* or more extensive procedure performed during the post-op period. Examples might include performing iridoplasty during the postoperative period of a laser iridotomy. Or cyclophotocoagulation during the postoperative period of a panretinal photocoagulation (PRP) performed for neovascular glaucoma. (Even if the PRP was performed by a retinal colleague in your group, assuming they were billing under the same tax ID number, this modifier is required). -58 begins a new global period of another 90 days.
    - *-79 Unrelated Procedure* during the postoperative period. The most common use of this is for the fellow eye's procedure. But a myriad of unrelated procedures could be envisioned and would use this modifier.

### 32.2.1.6 Step Six

Select the proper Diagnosis Codes for the examination, tests, and/or procedure. Keep in mind that many Coverage Policies for Special Tests and procedures require an appropriate diagnosis. For example, in order to be paid for doing a visual field test, there needs to be a diagnosis of glaucoma, glaucoma suspect, or a neurologic condition. If the special test or procedure is not linked to an appropriate diagnosis, it will likely be denied.

Most billing systems have a limited number of fields for listing diagnoses. And some payers accept only a certain number of fields. There is a possibility that health care systems in the future will prefer an exhaustive list of all diagnoses associated with a patient in order to better track outcomes of care and allow for more accurate profiling of patients, physicians, and costs of care. Currently, the best strategy is to list and link the codes that you know will allow for payment of the work you have done. In addition, you may want to list diagnosis codes that reflect the complexity of the patient encounter, or that increase the risk for future outcomes.

For example, if I see a patient with pseudoexfoliation (PXF), but following his or her as a glaucoma suspect with a visual field that particular visit, and also monitoring his or her cataract, I will code (1) glaucoma suspect, (2) cataract, and (3) pseudoexfoliation (PXF) syndrome. It is also important to code as specifically as possible, avoiding the generic codes that have "unspecified" in their description, if there is a more accurate code. So in the above example, I would use "cataract, nuclear sclerotic." If the patient at his or her next visit develops worsening of symptoms related to cataract, the decision is to perform surgery, and an A-scan/intraocular lens (IOL) calculation is performed that day, my list will be: (1) cataract, nuclear sclerotic, (2) PXF syndrome, and (3) glaucoma suspect, with special care to link the A-scan/IOL CPT code to diagnosis #1.

Again, there are at least yearly changes to the Diagnosis Codes, referred to as ICD codes, and updates to your forms and software are necessary.

### 32.2.2 Surgical Procedures

In selecting the appropriate surgical code, you must choose the most accurate and closely related category I or category III code from CPT. (Please also see the previous section on Office Procedures.) Surgeries performed in the operating room generally have a 90-day global period, with all postoperative care included in the payment for the procedure. Again, it is important to code an appropriate diagnosis for the given procedure. Modifiers play a large role in coding for glaucoma surgeries.

The -50 bilateral modifier is rarely used for intraocular glaucoma surgeries.

*-51 Multiple Procedure* applies if there is more than one procedure performed. The most common procedure probably being combined cataract and trabeculectomy surgery. For physician coding for the procedure, the most highly paid procedure is trabeculectomy and should be listed first. The second procedure would be the cataract/IOL surgery, and simply by listing it as a second procedure, it would be paid at 50% of its usual reimbursement. The -51 modifier is assumed. For the ASC or hospital reimbursement, however, the more highly paid procedure is the cataract/IOL (more supplies, etc.), and the facility will list it first on their claims.

*-58 Staged* or more extensive procedure performed during the post-op period. Examples might include performing a glaucoma drainage implant during the postoperative period of a rapidly failing trabeculectomy. Or glaucoma drainage implant during the postoperative period of a PRP performed for neovascular glaucoma (even if the PRP was performed by a retinal colleague in your group, assuming they were billing under the same tax ID number, this modifier is required). -58 begins a new global period of another 90 days, and allows payment of 100% for the procedure.

*-79 Unrelated Procedure* during the postoperative period. The most common use of this is for the procedure of the fellow eye. But a myriad of unrelated procedures could be envisioned and would use this modifier.

*-78 Related Procedure* during postoperative period requires unplanned return to the OR or Laser suite. This is used to code a procedure that is required due to a complication from the original procedure. This would be the modifier to use for choroidal drainage surgery to correct a flat anterior chamber that occurred as a result of a filtration surgery, for example. Another example would be to code for resuturing of a dehisced wound in a trabeculectomy that required a return to the OR. Using -78 allows payment of 80% of the usual reimbursement and does not start a new global period. The original global period is still in effect.

*-62* is used to indicate that two surgeons were involved with two or more distinct surgical procedures performed at the same time. An example might be a vitreoretinal surgeon performing a vitrectomy when the glaucoma surgeon performs a drainage implant with pars plana tube placement. Each surgeon codes their procedure along with the modifier, and dictates an operative note detailing their part of the procedure.

*-53* is used to describe a discontinued procedure after anesthesia or surgical prepping has been initiated. The most likely scenario would be in the case of a surgical cancellation due to a retrobulbar hemorrhage from the block.

*-80 Assistant Surgeon.* Some glaucoma surgeries allow the use of an assistant surgeon and some payers allow reimbursement to that assistant by billing the surgical CPT code with modifier -80 using the billing numbers of the assistant surgeon.

### 32.2.3 The Postoperative Period

The most common difficulties in coding correctly involve services provided during the postoperative period or global period. First, you must know the global period for the procedure and the payer. Remember that, with current reimbursement policy, all the physicians of your ophthalmology group who bill under the same tax ID number are considered the "same physician," because Medicare and other payers do not recognize a difference among ophthalmologists who are comprehensive ophthalmologists or subspecialists in ophthalmology. Second, the clinical situation and setting determines your ability to code and be reimbursed for a service during the global period.

If the clinical problem or reason for the visit is directly related to the original surgery, then the visit or service will be considered included in the global payment, even if there is a new diagnosis. A rule of thumb is to ask yourself, "Would the patient be having the current problem if the surgery had not been performed?" If the answer is most likely "no," then usually the service would be considered included as part of the post-op care.

If the answer is that the current problem is not likely to have been a consequence of the original surgery, then you can code for the service along with a modifier: a -24 appended to the exam code, and/or a -79 with a procedure code.

## 32.3 Coding and Billing Reconciliation

Once claims have been submitted to insurers, inevitably rejections will occur. It is important to review the rejected claims and evaluate the reasons for rejection. Scrutiny of your rejections will often lead to a better understanding of proper coding, but may also point to deficiencies in the billing system of your practice. For example, process errors such as failure to record primary care referral numbers or identification numbers can cause claim rejections that are irreversible. Some insurers will not pay claims if these items are not collected and recorded on the date of service. Sometimes the time it takes to correct a claim will cause it to go over the filing limits. Meticulous attention to data details upfront by your staff will reward the practice with prompt payment and less work to correct claims later.

Coding rejections will provide insight into some private payers coding rules. Many times these rules are not published and only after scrutinizing rejections will patterns become clear. Once a series of rejections occurs, it is easier to get answers from private payers as to the reason for the coding rejection, and either you can alter your behavior in coding or scheduling tests and procedures, or you can appeal the decision of the insurer. Having at least one physician in the practice who is familiar with coding rules and who can review these claim rejections periodically will help the billing staff form a strategy to avoid rejections in the future. A physician can also more easily translate to other physicians and help encourage "clean claims" with proper coding.

## 32.4 Other Resources and Suggestions

- Keep ahead of the time to file claims – billing personnel should know this for every payer your practice deals with.
- Consider software that "scrubs" your claims before sending them out, pointing out potential errors in coding that may cause rejections.
- Have someone in your office review every newsletter, email, or announcement from the health plans for items that might pertain to ophthalmology (remember it can pertain to imaging, multiple CPT code issues, optometrists versus MD distinctions in codes, routine versus medical/surgical care, claim filing methods or limits).
- Read the CPT book. Understand how to correctly select ICD diagnosis codes. Understand what CCI edits pertain to your procedures.
- Take a coding and reimbursement course as you begin your practice, and periodically thereafter.
- Understand what National Coverage Determinations and Local Coverage Determinations are in place for your Medicare carrier. Re-review them periodically.
- Review the Medicare fee schedule every time it changes (usually yearly, but in 2008 it was likely to be two times in the year).
- Review private health plan fee schedules whenever it is updated.
- Make sure your charges are above the reimbursement rate for every carrier you interact with.
- Hire knowledgeable people to deal with reimbursement and coding. But do not leave them in a vacuum without physician interaction and feedback.
  - Every large practice needs a physician liaison to the billing staff to translate issues back to the MDs.
- Periodically review reasons for claim denials – physician and billing personnel together.
- Consider an annual or biannual audit – either internally or by an outside consulting firm to learn where you may be under- or over-coding.
- Use American Academy of Ophthalmology (AAO) resources. Become a member of the American Academy of Ophthalmology Executives (AAOE). Take courses on billing and coding.
- Use state society resources. Most have a committee to deal with reimbursement issues.

Coding and billing properly takes time and attention to detail. Understanding the rules yourself and working with your staff to optimize your billing practices will be financially rewarding in the long run.

## Physician Quality Reporting Initiative

The Physician Quality Reporting Initiative (PQRI) was launched in the second half of 2007 as voluntary Centers for Medicare and Medicaid Services (CMS) program with the promise of a 1.5% bonus on all your Medicare payments for participating and reaching reporting criteria in those 6 months. Thanks to a huge AAO effort to develop measures, the bonus was and continues to be available to ophthalmologists by properly reporting on at least three measures. The program was expanded in 2008, and the bonus was increased to 2% beginning in 2009. Although the program is slated to continue, there is no Congressional funding beyond 2010. Currently, ophthalmology measures are available for diagnosis of primary open angle glaucoma, age-related macular degeneration, diabetic retinopathy, and cataract surgery. The AAO continues to develop additional measures in conjunction with the AMA Physician Consortium and through a rigorous vetting process with stakeholder organizations. Up to date information on participation can be found at the AAOE website: http://www.aao.org/advocacy/reimbursement/pqri/ and

CMS: http://www.cms.hhs.gov/pqri/.

## Electronic Prescribing

As part of the Medicare Improvements for Patients and Providers Act of 2008, the CMS has initiated a bonus program for physicians who qualify, adopt, and successfully report on electronic prescribing use. Beginning in 2009–2010, there is an opportunity for a 2% bonus on all your Medicare payments by successfully adopting e-prescribing. The bonus is reduced to 1.5% in 2011, 1% in 2012, and 0.5% in 2013. Importantly, beginning in 2012, there will be an automatic 1% reduction penalty to all your Medicare payments if you are not using e-prescribing by a yet-to-be announced date sometime after the beginning of 2010.

To receive the bonus, (1) you must receive at least 10% of your Medicare payments from office visits, (2) adopt a "qualified" e-prescribing program, and (3) then code on at least 50% of your Medicare office visits (not including postoperative visits). You are expected to code on every encounter whether or not prescriptions were filed electronically or not, with a choice of three separate codes. One is when you use e-prescribing, another for having access to e-prescribing but not for using it because no prescriptions were required, and the third code for not using e-prescribing either because state law did not allow it (in the case of some controlled substances) or because a patient requested paper prescriptions.

E-prescribing systems are available with or without an electronic medical record system. Several allow for the use of handheld personal digital assistants (PDAs) that have Internet access. Of course there is a cost for these systems. However, by most reports, e-prescribing has been shown to increase office efficiencies by reducing office staff time and effort in fielding phone calls from patients and pharmacists, creating documentation for prescriptions and refills, and allowing proper prescribing for a patient's insurance plan formulary. One feature of some systems that is of interest to glaucoma specialists is the ability to monitor the refill rates of patients and infer their adherence to therapy. Health policy experts are hopeful that the systems will encourage the use of less expensive medication choices or generics. And certainly there is the potential for reducing medication errors or harmful drug interactions.

For more information: http://www.cms.hhs.gov/EPrescribing/

# Chapter 33
# Medical Legal Considerations When Treating Glaucoma Patients

J. Wesley Samples and John R. Samples

The unique aspects of glaucoma care, due to its lifelong nature, represent specific medical-legal challenges. This is at least in part due to the fact that while loss of sight is infrequently life threatening, it is almost always devastating. Thus, patients who have suffered loss of sight are often well enough to personally pursue litigation. While glaucoma does not generate the most litigation in ophthalmology (cataract surgery lawsuits are more common),[1] civil suits claiming "failure to diagnose" glaucoma are relatively common. On average, 300 ophthalmologists per year were sued between 1985 and 2007, of which roughly one-quarter resulted in judgments against the ophthalmologists.[1] Side effects of glaucoma medications and the need to adequately warn the patient, and/or the patient's caregiver, about these side effects represent central challenges that must be addressed to ensure the high quality of care while also minimizing legal liability.

An initial diagnosis of glaucoma can be devastating. Patients often need time to digest the news, so it is always prudent to schedule a second visit within a few weeks after the diagnosis. This will give the patient a chance to ask questions about the disease and its treatment, and to understand that, they must be an active partner in any treatment plan.

Glaucoma patients are typically elderly and frightened by their increasingly poor vision. They are generally reluctant to accept the diagnosis of glaucoma, are often stressed, and also may be unable to fully understand the diagnosis. A perceived lack of empathy or concern on the doctor's part may make the patient angry and less receptive to listening to the physician. Because early, chronic open-angle glaucoma is symptomless, many patients may not fully believe the physician's diagnosis or understand that untreated glaucoma can cause irreversible blindness. Elderly patients may feel that they are "doing just fine" and feel no need for lifelong medical therapy. Additionally, many elderly glaucoma patients want to remain self-sufficient and not depend upon family members to drive them or help them with the activities of daily living. Such patients may continue to drive even after the glaucoma doctor tells them it is no longer safe for them to do so.

The need to inform the patients without alarming them, soliciting their cooperation in treatment, and keeping them informed about their status (even when we sometimes do not know the precise status of their optic nerve and visual field loss) can be a delicate balancing act.

While the primary reason glaucoma patients sue is for improper performance of a procedure, followed by errors in diagnosis,[2] a patient seeking out a glaucoma specialist may harbor unrealistic expectations, and this can ultimately lead to litigation too. Unrealistic expectations are considered among the greatest contributing factors to lawsuits. Patients with glaucoma will become blind without proper treatment. With proper treatment, most patients will avoid blindness, but in some patients the optic nerve damage may progress anyway, or they may have progressive visual field loss, or both. It is important to convey to patients that their medical compliance is the single greatest thing they can do to reduce their risk of vision loss. On the other hand, no matter how comforting the clinician wishes to be, he cannot guarantee the patient that treatment will completely eliminate any risk of blindness since a small percentage of even fully compliant patients will still lose their sight.

The prognosis for glaucoma, left untreated, is uniformly poor, but with treatment in most cases the disease can be controlled. Put another way, glaucoma is an optic neuropathy in which retinal ganglion cell loss is accelerated. As a result, the failure of treatment to be effective, since not every treatment is effective in every patient, might be something that a jury would find to be understandable and even acceptable. This is the reason that litigation regarding glaucoma may be more focused on other issues such as failure to make a correct diagnosis and the side effects of medications, rather than failure of treatment to be effective in a poor prognosis disease per se.

While the physician has a medical (and legal) duty to inform the patient about their prognosis, this has to be clinically tempered and the message delivered in such a way as to achieve the best possible outcome. Informing the patient of a poor prognosis requires empathy and a sense of timing. There are instances in glaucoma care where a measure of medical legal protection is achieved by documenting that the patient has a poor prognosis in the chart. In some instances, it may be accompanied by a letter to the patient.

## 33.1 Triage in the Office

All office staff needs to know how to handle triage at both the diagnosis and treatment stages. In glaucoma, there is a concern that the diagnosis of angle closure glaucoma may be missed. Diagnosis is addressed at length in its own chapter, but an example of a confounding diagnosis is given here for illustrative purposes. Halos are the classic manifestation of angle closure glaucoma, but nausea alone can be a presenting finding. When one of the coauthors (JRS) was a resident, one of his very first patients was hospitalized and had already undergone a barium enema and an upper gastrointestinal series for unexplained nausea before ultimately being diagnosed with angle closure glaucoma.

Another red flag for attention is red eye after surgery. With the increased recent use of mitomycin C in glaucoma surgery, bleb infections can be missed. Patients who call in with redness, irritation, or diminished vision in eyes that have undergone trabeculectomy may have a bleb infection. When a postsurgical patient calls in with red eye, "the sooner the better" is always the rule; the standard of care is to see such patients within a few hours and never more than 12 h later. If for whatever reason they cannot be seen within a few hours, they should be referred to an appropriate clinician, or, if it is after hours, they may be required to go to an emergency room.

In some instances, patients may travel to locations where there is no ophthalmologist. Recently one of the coauthors (JRS) was contacted by a patient with an obviously infected bleb who was traveling in rural Tahiti where there was no eye care available. When patients plan on traveling to remote locations, it is good to educate them about the signs and symptoms of infection prior to their travel and to provide an "emergency antibiotic" to carry with them. Since patients may not be accurate in detecting an infection, they are always advised to contact an ophthalmologist before starting the medication.

## 33.2 Compliance

When patients are relaxed and less stressed they are more likely to admit their noncompliance with physician instructions. When one of the coauthors (JWS) worked as an ophthalmic technician, he found that patients would often admit noncompliance to him because they perceived him as "just a kid checking the vision before the patient sees the ophthalmologist" and would often remark that "I tell your dad, the ophthalmologist, I am using the drops because that is what he wants to hear and it makes him happy." Compliance problems in glaucoma care are legendary and discussed in Chap. 55. The clinician has a medical and legal duty to inform the patients about the consequences of noncompliance. The discussion, which is mandatory for all glaucoma patients who are on topical medications, needs to be adjusted to the age, educational level, and ability to absorb and understand the information. "You have to be a broken record, or an MP3 player on repeat, informing the patient that glaucoma is a problem that does not go away and is not cured – and that they must return for regular monitoring."[2] Because of its chronic nature, glaucoma requires recruitment of family members and other care givers into the overall care plan, if for no other reason than to remind the patient to use their medications.

### 33.2.1 Drug Side Effects

Glaucoma medications may have serious systemic side effects that must be explained to the patient. Even when prescribed with verbal informed consent by the patient and even if the patient is given literature accompanying medication prescriptions, patients may sue if untoward events occur. Or, a patient's failure to follow daily medical regimens and postoperative instructions may lead to poor vision outcomes and therefore pose additional areas of potential legal concern.

There are specific duties when giving the patient a drug. One is medical and makes it incumbent upon the clinician to determine the presence of drug interactions and contraindications. Patients need to be instructed to contact the office whenever they experience side effects (see Chaps. 59 and 60). For example, since 2006 it has been recognized that African-Americans receiving beta-blockers as treatment for glaucoma are at increased risk for cardiovascular death. There have been very rare cases in which a patient died with a single use of a beta-blocker due to either reactive airway disease or heart block. It is common knowledge to not use beta-blockers when there is reactive airway disease or heart block. Treatment for other health conditions can be more nebulous. For example, beta-blockers used to be avoided for patients with congestive heart failure, but as we have learned that the failing heart has abnormal adrenergic tone, an increasing number of clinicians now use beta-blockers to treat congestive heart failure[3] (see Chap. 60).

In glaucoma, another similar question arises regarding when to use topical carbonic anhydrase inhibitors, which have a sulfa moiety. If the patient has a definite history of sulfa reaction such as erythema multiforme (or Stevens–Johnson syndrome), then carbonic anhydrase inhibitors should not be used. However, if the history is nebulous, such as the patient had a possible rash from a sulfa drug used to cure a urinary tract infection many years ago, then the treatment may proceed. The clinician has to take into account the quality of the history. However, there is a duty to warn the patient that should a rash and irritation develop around the eye then they should stop using the medication and contact the physician.

Physicians should also be aware that patients may undertake self-treatment with medications such as "natural" or herbal preparations. These unapproved therapies may lead to worsening of the visual outcome, especially if the patient ignores medically recognized therapies prescribed by the ophthalmologist. Patients on their own initiative occasionally smoke marijuana to control their glaucoma, or in some states marijuana may legally be prescribed.

## 33.3 Patient Expectations

Before a patient is seen in consultation, it is desirable to explain what they may expect at the time of consultation. This includes attention to duration of appointment, the effects of dilating drops, and therefore the need to bring a driver. If the patient has a caretaker, it may be useful for the caretaker to be present during the exam and subsequent discussion. Anecdotally, it appears that the presence of a caretaker during exams increases the likelihood of patient understanding and compliance.

Postsurgical recovery expectations may be a source of consternation between glaucoma doctors and their patients. When patients undergo trabeculectomy they need to be educated clearly about the rhythm of a normal postsurgical recovery, including stern warnings to avoid bending, lifting, or straining to minimize the risk of choroidal effusion or hemorrhage. Other procedures such as Ahmed tube implantation, Glaukos shunts, and Neomedix trabecutome may not create as much postoperative hypotony, and thus diminish the postoperative risk and need for activity restrictions. Patient education to manage expectations and enforce compliance need to be multi-pronged and should include education of the patient, education of caregivers, and handouts addressing the postoperative experience. The patient needs to be engaged in a dialogue, and encouraged to ask questions. A handout describing critical information for the three- to four-week period leading up to surgery is also useful. Another handout that has been very popular with patients is a list of the stages of recovery, starting with the patient being restricted to complete inactivity and building up to a full recovery (Table 33.1). While not comprehensive, such a device encourages patients to recognize that recovery takes place in steps.

**Table 33.1** Stages of postsurgical recovery for patients undergoing classic trabeculectomy or other glaucoma procedures where a low postoperative pressure is anticipated

| Stages of postsurgical recovery for trabeculectomy | | |
|---|---|---|
| Activity restrictions | | |
| Stages | Yes | No |
| Stage 1: Quiet, quiet, and more quiet. Especially important: no lifting, no bending, and no straining of any kind | • Bed rest only<br>• It is okay to be up for the bathroom and for meals, but otherwise lie flat with your head on the pillow<br>• Out for trips to the doctor only | • No activity whatsoever during stage 1<br>• Not even reading<br>• No TV (when one eye moves so does the other)<br>• No bending over to tie shoes<br>• No straining in the bathroom (use stool softeners) |
| Stage 2: A little, very light activity. Balanced with a lot of rest | • Same as stage 1, plus several short walks daily. Walking is okay<br>• TV is okay from about 10–15 feet | • Still no lifting, bending, or straining<br>• No bending over to tie shoes<br>• No straining in the bathroom |
| Stage 3: A little more activity, but start slow | • Same as stage 2, plus relative inactivity<br>• Plenty of bed rest<br>• Walking is okay<br>• TV and reading<br>• Riding in a car other than just to doctors office | • Still no lifting, bending, or straining |
| Stage 4 | • You can add washing hair at salon from Day 5 on; no soap in eyes!!!! (But of course, this was not a good idea even before surgery) | • No lifting over 5 lbs |
| Stage 5 | • Bending over is now okay<br>• Sex is okay<br>• Driving is okay if vision permits | • No lifting over 10 lbs |
| Stage 6 | • Continually build up physical activity<br>• Avoid any activity that distends the veins in the neck | • No heavy straining<br>• Avoid prolonged coughing<br>• Do not move heavy furniture<br>• No deep water diving |
| Stage 7 | • Unlimited activity | • No restrictions |

Important note: A "*stage*" does not mean a "*day*." Every eye recovery is different. Ask your doctor about the timing of each stage.

The glaucoma-treating physician may feel trapped between two diametrically opposed positions in the postoperative period: the need to approach the patient in a kind and gentle manner in the first few days after surgery and the need to adamantly enforce inactivity to avoid complications. A patient with a perception that a physician or a staff member lacks sympathy may lead to a legal claim. On the other hand, some patients need to be firmly guided to follow postoperative instructions, otherwise they may find it difficult to take physician instructions regarding inactivity and eye drops seriously.

### 33.3.1 Patient Complaints

If a patient complains, one should always respond quickly and effectively. While it is acknowledged that the "patient is not always right," even if the clinician is not in agreement, voicing empathy and understanding are important techniques in fielding a complaint, which often arises out of either high expectations or too little education about the disease. In some instances there may be an element of denial, and for that reason documentation is very important. When there is a complaint, it may be useful to point out that glaucoma is a difficult and chronic disease in contrast to other ophthalmic diseases where an improvement in acuity may be expected with surgical treatment. Of course, it is always best if the patient is aware of this prior to surgery. In some instances when there is a complaint, it may be useful to recruit family members into helping the patient to understand the situation and the disease process. In other instances, it may be best to refer the patient to a trusted colleague.

Psychologically, it is better to suggest a referral to a discontented patient rather than have the patient request one. Referral of an unhappy patient should always be prefaced with a phone call to the colleague. Choice of the doctor to whom one refers is exceedingly important. Although it may be difficult, it is usually best to give the doctor receiving the referral a free hand in treating the unhappy patient; explicit permission to treat or return the patient as appropriate will likely lead to a better encounter for both the patient and the doctor. Not every physician specialist recognizes that, with human nature and a chronic disease, some patients will always be unhappy and some will want to go from physician to physician until they either establish a good rapport or hear the positive message that they are seeking. The physician's own ego and compulsive nature may sometimes get in the way of effectively processing and acting upon a complaint.

It is useful to make others in the office aware of the complaint in case they come into contact with the patient. Front-desk and office personnel who would be expected to interface with the patient should be given a sense of how the complaint is to be handled. Finally, after a complaint is processed, practice personnel should always assess what happened and conduct introspection to see if the matter could have been handled better so that a similar complaint does not arise again. Realize that not all complaints are avoidable, whether they are related to wait time or poor outcome, but with good management, they will likely not proceed to a legal claim.

## 33.4 Clinical Guidelines and Evidence-Based Medicine

There has been a proliferation of glaucoma guidelines from a variety of sources in the last few years. Courts have recognized the need to depart from such guidelines in a number of instances. Clinical practice guidelines have played a large role in medical malpractice cases, in part because medical malpractice cases, by their very nature, focus on standard of care. Practice guidelines are supposed to provide a standard of care based on an evidence-based consensus in a particular area of medicine. An evidence-based approach to arguments concerning standard of care allows attorneys to litigate their cases according to a perceived standardized measure.

It has been suggested that attorneys have used clinical practice guidelines more frequently for "inculpatory than exculpatory purposes."[4,5] Although physician adherence to guidelines has been used as a shield in medical malpractice cases, the opposite has also been true. Maine (among other states) has created medical practice guidelines that, if adhered to by physicians, could be used as an affirmative defense in malpractice cases.[6] Recupero cites a Mississippi case in which departure from the guidelines was deemed medically necessary (Vede v. Delta Regional Medical Center 2006).[7] The plaintiff in this case developed a decubitus ulcer and asserted that he had not been turned every 2 h (in keeping with hospital policy and national guidelines). The hospital had departed from the policy because turning the patient caused airway obstruction and consequent drops in oxygen saturation. However, when practitioners depart from guidelines and there is a negative outcome, the deviation may bolster the case for the opposing side. The degree to which an ophthalmologist is held to the implementation of specific guidelines in glaucoma may depend upon the severity of the disease as evidenced by the status of the optic nerve. This is of particular concern in those cases in which guidelines with conflicting recommendations are introduced into the same malpractice case. Courts have permitted the juxtaposition of conflicting practice guidelines, allowing the jury to determine which evidence is most compelling.[4]

### 33.4.1 Standards of Glaucoma Treatment

There is a widespread perception in the medical community that providing a patient with the "gold standard" of care will protect physicians from malpractice litigation. Part of the dilemma is the nebulous definition of "gold standard." Arguably, physicians define it as the standard therapy that is in common practice on a national basis. However, the field of ophthalmology in particular has demonstrated that adhering to "the gold standard" may not always be sufficient to preclude a medical malpractice lawsuit based on negligence. In evaluating negligence, courts often look to the so-called "calculus" of Judge Learned Hand (United States v. Carroll Towing Co. 1947)[8]:

$$\text{Negligence} = (\text{Benefit} < \text{Probability of Injury} \times L)$$

where L = the cost of injury.

In the 1974 case *Helling v. Carey,* the court decided that this valuation suggested that an ophthalmologist had committed malpractice by failing to use noncontract tonometry to screen for glaucoma in a patient over the age of 40.[9,10] In many respects, it was a classic case of failure to diagnose. The decision was upheld by the Washington Supreme Court. The great irony of the case is that local and national standards of practice at the time did not mandate screening patients under the age of 40 for glaucoma. Furthermore, the lawsuit predated the widespread use of noncontact tonometry. It was the plaintiff's lawyers who sought out the inventor of the technology, and presented it to the court. The court was impressed by the simplicity and ease of the new noncontact tonometry technology, and was intent on demonstrating that malpractice is not excused just because a particular technology has not been adopted in common practice – especially when the burden on the practitioner is low in relation to the potentially great benefit for the patient."

The court reasoned that:

> "Under the facts of this case reasonable prudence required the timely giving of the pressure test to this plaintiff. The precaution of giving this test to detect the incidence of glaucoma to patients under 40 years of age is so imperative that irrespective of its disregard by the standards of the ophthalmology profession, it is the duty of the courts to say what is required to protect patients under 40 from the damaging results of glaucoma."[9]

This principal – the notion that adhering to custom might not always be reasonable – dates back to the 1932 negligence case of the sinking of *The T.J. Hooper* tugboat. Justice Hand, who presided over the case, stated that:

> "Indeed in most cases reasonable prudence is in fact common prudence, but strictly it is never a measure; a whole calling may have unduly lagged in the adoption of new and available devices…Courts must in the end say what is required; there are precautions so imperative that even their universal disregard will not excuse omission."[11]

Thus, where new potential treatment is cheap and risk free and the injury, though rare, is devastating, the doctor who fails to use the new treatment may be negligent in the eyes of a court, and a court may find a physician negligent, despite the physician's adherence to prevailing treatment practices.

In response to the ruling in *Helling*, the State of Washington passed a statute (RCW 4.24.290) that provided in part that:

> "In any civil action for damages based on professional negligence against…a member of the healing arts…the plaintiff in order to prevail shall be required to prove by a preponderance of the evidence that the defendant or defendants failed to exercise that degree of skill, care and learning possessed by other persons in the same profession…"[12]

A subsequent court confronted with a similar failure to diagnose a glaucoma scenario declined to apply the rule of *Helling* because of unique facts, but found that the standard embodied in the statute "allows ample scope for the application of the limited Helling rule."[12] Even more recent case law[12] from Washington makes special note of language in the statute (RCW 4.24.290) that "requires proof in a professional negligence action of failure to exercise the skill, care, and learning 'possessed' by others in the profession rather than that actually 'practiced'."[13] Thus, where a fact-intensive analysis finds application of the rule from *Helling* to be appropriate, negligence may be found in a case where the physician has simply provided treatment in line with that which is in common practice on a national basis. Under the Learned Hand calculus, this will be especially true when the other therapies and diagnostic methods possessed by others, but not part of the gold standard, are cheap relative to the cost of injury.

When considering a difficult patient, and hedging against a potential medical malpractice lawsuit by adhering to the gold standard, it is important to keep in mind that the gold standard itself may not provide much protection against a medical malpractice lawsuit. Rather, it is best to weigh the customary standard in light of recent advances. Ultimately, it may be that the best protection a physician has against malpractice litigation, with respect to all patients, even the "difficult" ones, is to keep abreast of advancements, read current journals and texts, and strive to apply them wherever they are needed.

## 33.5 Conclusion

As with all cases of diseases in which the prognosis without treatment is poor, physicians need to carefully document their conversations and interactions with the patient in the record, and in some rare instances in writing to the patient as well. Glaucoma is a chronic disease in most individuals and the need for treatment to prevent poor outcomes is something that all patients need to know. Vigilance and appropriate management of side effects of medications is key in patient management.

## References

1. Kirkner RM. How to manage your malpractice risks. *Rev Ophthalmol.* Jan 1, 2009. http://www.revophth.com/index.asp?page=1_14128.htm. Accessed May 2, 2009.
2. Craven ER. Malpractice costs rise as glaucoma surgery evolves. *Rev Ophthalmol.* August 1, 2007. http://www.revophth.com/index.asp?page=1_13470.htm. Accessed May 2, 2009.
3. Lama PJ. Topical β-adrenergic blockers and glaucoma: a heart-stopping association? *Ophthalmology* 2006;113(7):1067-1068.
4. Recupero PR. Clinical practice guidelines as learned treatises: understanding their use as evidence in the courtroom. September 2008. http://www.jaapl.org/cgi/content/full/36/3/290. Accessed May 17, 2009.
5. Hyams AL, Brandenburg JA, Lipsitz SR, Shapiro DW, Brennan TA. Practice guidelines and malpractice litigation: a two-way street. *Ann Intern Med.* March 15, 1995. http://www.annals.org/cgi/content/full/122/6/450. Accessed May 17, 2009.
6. Trail WR, Allen BA. Government created medical practice guidelines: the opening of Pandora's box. *J Law Health* 10 (1995/1996):231-258.
7. *Vede v. Delta Regional Medical Center.* 933 So.2d 31 (Miss. Ct. App., 2006).
8. *United States v. Carroll Towing Co.* 159 F.2d 169, 173 (2d Cir., 1947).
9. *Helling v. Carey.* 83 Wash.2d 514, 516, 519 P.2d 981, 982 (Sup. Ct. Wash., 1974).
10. *The T.J. Hooper.* 60 F.2d 737, 740 (Cir. Ct. App. 2d, 1932).
11. *Gates v. Jensen.* 924, 92 Wash.2d 246, 253, 595 P.2d 919 (Sup. Ct. Wash., 1979).
12. *Harris v. Groth.* 116, 99 Wash.2d 438, 443, 663 P.2d 113 (Sup. Ct. Wash., 1983).

# Part III
# The Glaucomas

# Chapter 34
# Primary Open Angle Glaucoma

Matthew G. McMenemy

Glaucoma is a significant global health problem. As of the year 2000, 67 million people worldwide were affected with "primary" glaucoma. Of these patients, 6.7 million were bilaterally blind.[1] Glaucoma is second only to cataracts as a cause of blindness worldwide. In the United States, where glaucoma accounts for 11% of all cases of blindness, it is the number two cause of blindness behind macular degeneration.[1-3] Among African-Americans, primary open angle glaucoma (POAG) is the leading cause of blindness[4-6] and POAG is also more prevalent in Hispanics relative to Caucasians.[7] More than two million Americans are affected with one variety or another of glaucoma, with most patients in the USA having POAG.[8]

Prevalence rates of glaucoma in various studies range from 0.5% to almost 9%.[9-27] In many population-based studies, POAG is the most common type of glaucoma.[9-11,13-18] While angle closure glaucoma is less common than POAG in Western nations with European-derived inhabitants, Asian populations tend to have higher rates of angle closure glaucoma (narrow angle glaucoma or NAG).[5,28] This finding may be real, or, in some instances, might be an artifact of health care availability in poorer countries. That is because POAG is relatively asymptomatic until late in the disease, while NAG may cause acute symptoms including visual loss and pain; therefore, NAG is more readily diagnosed as poorer patients may only avail themselves of emergency medical care. The incidence of POAG increases with age, and thus a population with a shorter average life span may also skew incidences of various glaucomas. There is no definite predilection for one sex over the other. POAG may be slightly more common in men,[10,29] although most studies show no sexual predilection,[11,18,24,25] and one study showed a higher prevalence among women.[23]

Patients with glaucoma have a significant risk of blindness. One twenty-year study that described predominately Caucasian patients with newly diagnosed and subsequently treated glaucoma found the risk of blindness in one eye was 27% and the risk of bilateral blindness was 9%.[30] In the Temba Glaucoma Study conducted in urban South Africa, 58% of patients were blind in at least one eye.[31] The Chen study found that 14.6% of patients were blind in one eye and 6.4% were blind in both eyes at 15 years.[32] These findings are summarized in Table 34.1.

In African-Americans, the incidence of glaucoma is up to six times higher in certain age groups compared to whites. POAG in blacks is more likely to lead to irreversible blindness. Glaucoma occurs 10 years earlier and progresses more rapidly in black compared to white patients. Historically, blacks tend to be less aware that they may have glaucoma with its sight-threatening consequences, and they respond more poorly to therapy, whether medical or surgical.[33]

Glaucoma patients are frequently unaware of their disease. Indeed, glaucoma is often referred to as the "sneak thief of sight." In most industrial societies, more than 50% of those affected are unaware of their condition.[1,34] The percentage of undiagnosed glaucoma may exceed this value in third world nations. Fifty-seven percent of POAG was previously undiagnosed in the Thessaloniki Eye Study, with a lack of regular visitation to an ophthalmologist being a major reason for the underdiagnosis.[35] In the Melbourne Visual Impairment Project, 50% were previously undiagnosed.[18] Seventy-four percent were undiagnosed in the Blue Mountain Study,[23] and 55% lacked an awareness of their glaucoma in the Baltimore Eye Study.[20] In the aforementioned Temba Glaucoma Study, 87% of patients were previously undiagnosed,[31] while an even greater 93% went undiagnosed in a rural South India study.[36] In the 9-year Barbados Eye Studies, over one-half of the participants with POAG were unaware of their diagnosis. Lack of knowledge of their disease was four times more likely when opticians or optometrists were the regular eye care providers compared with ophthalmologists.[37,38] Because open angle glaucoma has no early symptoms, periodic eye exams are an important component of the battle against glaucoma. These exams should become more frequent with age, perhaps every year for patients over 60 years of age. The overwhelming patient unawareness of their glaucoma is highlighted in Table 34.2.

Table 34.1 Risk of monocular or binocular blindness

| Study | Monocular blindness | Bilateral blindness |
|---|---|---|
| Primarily Caucasian Study[30] | 27% | 9% |
| Temba Glaucoma Study[31] | 58% | |
| Chen Study[32] | 14.6% | 6.4% |

Table 34.2 Patient's lack of awareness of glaucoma

| Study | Percent unaware of diagnosis |
|---|---|
| Framingham Study[12] | >50 |
| Thessaloniki Eye Study[35] | 57 |
| Melbourne Visual Impairment Project[18] | 50 |
| Blue Mountain Study[23] | 74 |
| Baltimore Eye Study[20] | 50 |
| Temba Glaucoma Study[31] | 87 |
| South India Study[36] | 93 |
| Barbados Eye Studies[38] | >50 |

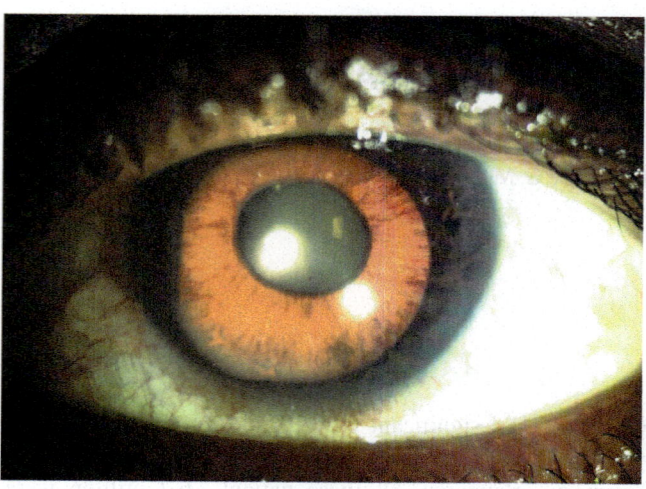

Fig. 34.1 African-American diabetic male with neovascularization of iris, ectropion uvea, and angle closure glaucoma

## 34.1 Definition

Glaucoma is an optic neuropathy with characteristic, usually progressive visual field loss and optic nerve cupping, often associated with elevated intraocular pressure (IOP). As we have seen above in the population-based studies, elevated IOP is not necessary to make the diagnosis of POAG. There are many varieties of glaucoma, so glaucoma classification systems are important in terms of treatment and prognosis. Accepted classification systems divide glaucoma into broad categories, including open versus closed angle glaucomas, and primary versus secondary glaucomas. Many of these varieties of glaucoma are discussed in detail in other chapters in this book. Here, we discuss POAG, or glaucoma with a visually open anterior chamber angle or "drain" (by gonioscopy) (see Figs. 34.1–34.4.) and without underlying, secondary ocular disease. If the angle formed by the iris plane, the ciliary body face, and the posterior cornea is greater than 20°, it is considered open. Otherwise, angles are described as either narrow or closed. POAG is the most common of the glaucomas, accounting for up to 75% of all glaucomas.

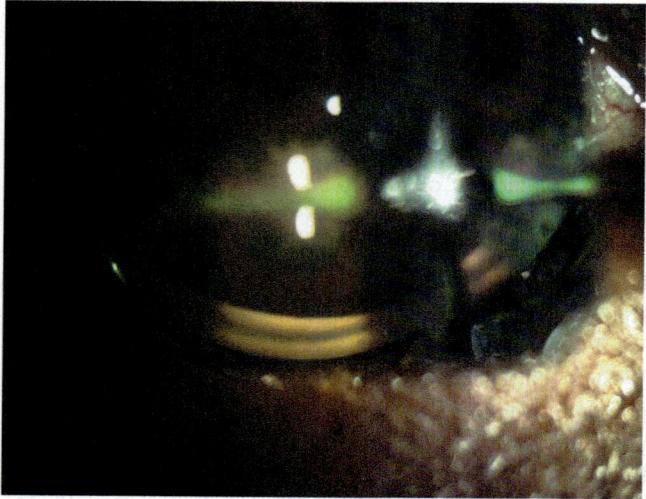

Fig. 34.2 Zeiss-style 4 mirror lens on the eye of the patient in Fig. 34.1. The angle is closed with no angle structures visible

## 34.2 Genetics

Von Graefe first recognized clusters of glaucoma patients within a family in 1869.[39] Duke-Elder subsequently described an autosomal dominant form of glaucoma.[40] Over the years, several modes of inheritance have been proposed, including gender-linked recessive, autosomal recessive, autosomal dominant, and multifactorial.[41] Referencing the Finnish Cohort Study, Teikari, in 1987, estimated the heritability of POAG at 13%.[42] Chang and coworkers studied the heritability of IOP and cup-to-disc ratio in an older population, and

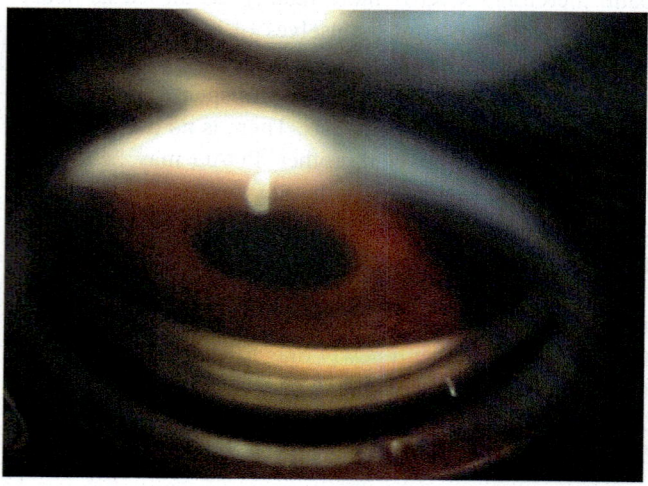

Fig. 34.3 Gonio lens on the eye of a patient with an open angle and visible angle structures

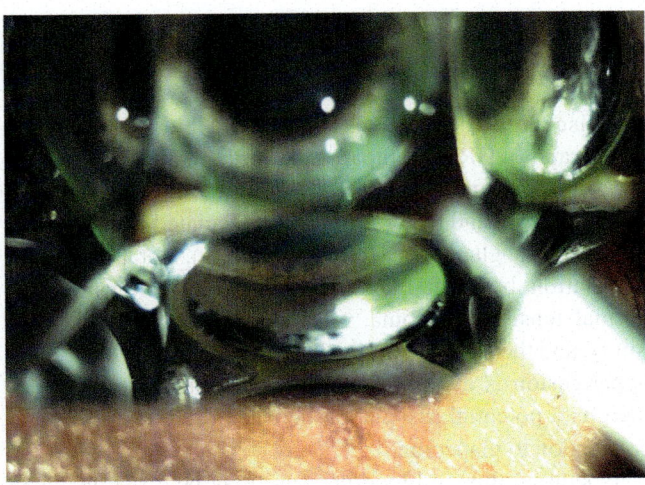

**Fig. 34.4** Gonio lens on the eye of a patient with narrow angles

concluded that C/D ratios are highly heritable, while IOP is moderately heritable.[43] Working with patients, their family members, and ophthalmologists, genetic researchers have identified 70 genes, loci, and alleles that cause glaucoma or syndromes associated with glaucoma. The distinct possibility exists that there are susceptibility genes for glaucoma. The glaucomas occurring as a result of these genes include infantile glaucoma, juvenile glaucoma, syndromic glaucoma, and some normal pressure and high pressure glaucomas. These glaucomas are the tip of the iceberg, as they may represent only a small portion of all glaucomas – although estimates of their actual frequency vary considerably.[44] It is believed that development of genomic testing panels will allow earlier detection of (1) patients at risk for glaucoma, (2) aggressive forms of glaucoma, and (3) patients responsive to a particular treatment. Armed with this knowledge, clinicians may tailor treatment of glaucoma on a personal or customized level.

## 34.3 Risk Factors

Of the many risk factors associated with open angle glaucoma, elevated IOP is the leading risk factor, and the only currently modifiable one. Upward of six million people in the United States have elevated IOP without demonstrable perimetric visual field damage.[45–47] It is important to understand that while no degree or level of IOP is diagnostic of glaucoma, glaucomatous optic disc damage may occur at almost any IOP but is more prevalent as IOP increases. Furthermore, as we will show, lowering IOP – regardless of the level at which disc and field damage originally occurred – seems to be beneficial in slowing or halting progression.

Prediction of which ocular hypertensives are most likely to develop glaucoma could allow a reduction of the prevalence and severity of POAG via the institution of earlier therapy. The Ocular Hypertension Treatment Study (OHTS) showed that reducing IOP a modest 20% in ocular hypertensive patients lowered the 5-year incidence of glaucoma from 9.5% in the control or untreated group to 4.4% – a 60% drop.[48] Treating all ocular hypertensives would subject many patients to unnecessary treatment, as well as the associated costs, side effects, and inconvenience. A more reasoned approach identifies those patients at high risk, and either initiates early treatment or pigeonholes those patients into closer monitoring. The European Glaucoma Prevention Study Group (EGPS) validated the results of the OHTS. In the OHTS observation group, the 5-year cumulative probability of developing open angle glaucoma was 9.5%, while in the EGPS observation group, the 5-year cumulative probability was higher at 16.8%. In the OHTS control group (no treatment), baseline older age, higher IOP, larger vertical cup/disc ratio, thinner central corneal thickness (CCT) measurement, and greater pattern standard deviation (PSD) were predictive factors for the development of POAG.[49] Interestingly, in the initial OHTS analysis, self-reported diabetes was protective with respect to the future development of glaucoma.[49] Subsequent publication did not support the protective association between diabetes and POAG, and suggested further study to clarify the association between diabetes and POAG.[50] The EGPS validated these same predictive factors.[51] Hazard ratios were the same among the OHTS and the EGPS, as well as pooled data from two other studies.[51–53] Additional risk factors were uncovered during follow-up of the trials, including IOP reduction,[54] IOP fluctuation,[55] optic disc hemorrhages,[56] and use of antihypertensive medications.[57]

Mean IOP reduction, mean IOP, presence of optic disc hemorrhages, and use of systemic diuretics are all predictors for the development of open angle glaucoma. These associations have been supported by the OHTS,[58] the Early Manifest Glaucoma Trial (EMGT),[59,60] and the EGPS studies. The greater the decrease in IOP, the lower is the mean IOP, and the smaller the area under the curve of IOP, the less is the risk of glaucoma. In the EGPS, for each 1 mmHg higher IOP per 12-month period, the increase in risk of developing OAG is 9% for a 5-year period.[61] Analysis of the EMGT data showed there was a 10–13% protection for each 1 mmHg lower IOP observed during a 5-year follow-up of POAG patients.

Controversy exists with respect to diurnal fluctuation and intervisit fluctuation of IOP as risk factors for the development and/or progression of glaucoma. The EGPS showed that intervisit IOP fluctuation over follow-up was not a risk factor for the development of glaucoma. In contrast, the Advanced Glaucoma Intervention Study (AGIS)[62] and other studies reported that intervisit fluctuation was a risk factor for the progression of POAG glaucoma.[63–66] In ocular hypertensives, Bengtsson et al showed that there was no association between diurnal fluctuation repeatedly measured over a 10-year follow-up with conversion to POAG.[67]

In the EMGT, he reported no association between diurnal fluctuation and progression of OAG in patients.[68]

Medeiros and Weinreb have reported that long-term fluctuations do not appear to be significantly associated with the risk of developing glaucoma in untreated ocular hypertensive subjects. Their study included 252 eyes of 126 patients with ocular hypertension. Forty eyes of 31 subjects developed glaucoma. The mean IOP in converters was 25.4 mmHg, compared to 24.1 mmHg in eyes that did not convert. IOP fluctuations were 3.16 mmHg in converters and 2.77 mmHg in nonconverters.[69]

According to a study by Leske and Heijl et al, treatment and follow-up IOP had a marked influence on progression, regardless of baseline IOP. Other significant factors were age, bilaterality, exfoliation, and disc hemorrhages. Optic disc hemorrhages are a well-known risk factor for the development and/or progression of glaucoma.[70–75] Meanwhile, lower systolic perfusion pressure, lower systolic blood pressure (BP), and cardiovascular disease history emerged as new predictors, suggesting a vascular role in progression. Another new factor was CCT.[76] In the EGPS, use of diuretics was associated with conversion to open-angle glaucoma, but the presence of systemic hypertension was not.[77] This effect may be due to a lower perfusion pressure, as low diastolic perfusion pressure has been associated with POAG.[78,79]

Treatment or overtreatment of systemic hypertension may cause a marked decrease in systemic blood pressure. This, in turn, may cause a chronic decrease of ocular blood flow (OBF), and ultimately loss of retinal ganglion cells (RGCs). In the Egna–Neumarkt Study,[80] a positive correlation was discovered between systemic blood pressure and IOP, and an association was found between POAG and systemic hypertension. Lower diastolic perfusion pressure is associated with a marked, progressive increase in the frequency of hypertensive glaucoma. The study found no relationship between systemic diseases of vascular origin and glaucoma. Poor perfusion of tissues can occur in the context of either hypertension or hypotension. Hypertension works by increasing peripheral vascular resistance in small vessels, while hypotension works by producing insufficient perfusion pressure of the optic disc. Low diastolic blood pressure, in the below 70 mmHg range, increased the incidence of glaucoma. In a Baltimore study, this association began at diastolic perfusion pressures less than 50 mmHg[78] while 23% of the Egna–Neumarkt glaucoma cases had ocular perfusion pressures (OPPs) less than 50 mmHg. It should be noted that this is not the most important mechanism of glaucoma in terms of frequency. Additionally, no link was found between glaucoma and the presence of diseases of other vascular tissues – angina, infarct, stroke, transient ischemic attack (TIA), and intermittent claudication. These findings were similar to those of Armaly, Drance, and Klein.[81–83] However, the findings were in disagreement with other authors.[84–90]

In the Thessaloniki Eye Study, nonglaucomatous individuals with systemic hypertension, whose medical treatment had induced a low diastolic pressure, had larger cup areas and cup/disc area ratios as assessed by Heidelberg retinal tomography (HRT) compared to individuals with higher diastolic pressures.[91] Dielemans et al found that systemic blood pressure and hypertension are associated with IOP and high tension glaucoma (IOP > 21 mmHg), but there is no association between blood pressure or hypertension and normal tension glaucoma.[92] The EGPS, Thessaloniki Eye Study, and the Punjabi report all confirmed that either treated hypertension is a risk factor for glaucoma progression, or there is a potential association between diuretics usage and conversion to glaucoma.[91,93,94]

Nocturnal dips in blood pressure may be a risk factor in glaucoma. Nocturnal pressure parameters, except pulse pressure, have been found to be lower in the patients with progressive field defects.[95] Graham and Drance reported that nocturnal dips in blood pressure were lower in patients with progressive field loss compared to patients with stable fields. This occurred in the context of good IOP control.[96]

Piltz–Seymour et al showed that laser Doppler flowmetry detected circulatory abnormalities in POAG suspects without manifest visual field changes. Decreases in flow in glaucoma suspects paralleled those of patients with POAG. The data suggested that compromised optic nerve blood flow (see Chap. 11) occurs early in glaucoma development and does not develop solely as a result of glaucoma damage.[97]

Thinner CCT is a risk factor for glaucoma and may correlate with disease severity.[98,99] In patients with open angle glaucoma, more significant field loss tends to occur in the eye with the thinner cornea.[100] Dueker et al have concluded that CCT is a risk factor for progression from ocular hypertension to POAG. Measurement of CCT is an important component of a complete eye exam, particularly if assessing patients with a risk of developing POAG. Evidence supporting the necessity of measuring CCT as part of screening for POAG or as a risk factor for glaucoma progression is not as strong.[101] See Chap. 8 for further discussion of the cornea.

Family history has long been known as a risk factor for glaucoma. In the Rotterdam Study, the lifetime absolute risk of glaucoma at age 80 was 10 times higher for individuals having relatives with glaucoma.[102] The Barbados Family Study of open-angle glaucoma, looking at inheritance of glaucoma in black families, found family history (see Chap. 9) to be a significant risk factor for the development of glaucoma.[103]

Martus and Stroux et al looked at predictive factors for progressive optic nerve damage in glaucoma. In patients with elevated IOP, significant predictive factors for eventual progression were older age, advanced perimetric damage, smaller neuroretinal rim, and larger area of beta zone peripapillary atrophy.[104] Budde has also studied zone beta peripapillary atrophy in glaucoma patients, and has concluded that it enlarges during follow-up in relatively few glaucoma patients. In refractive ranges above minus 3 diopters, enlargement of the beta zone occurs more frequently in progressive glaucoma than in nonprogressive glaucoma. He concluded that in view of its low frequency, enlargement of the beta zone may not be a useful marker for glaucoma progression. Enlargement of peripapillary beta zone was seen in 2.7% of glaucomatous eyes over 1.5 years. Enlargement of beta zone was observed in 4.4% of progressive glaucoma eyes versus 2.2% of stable glaucoma eyes. Finally, excluding eyes over minus 3 diopters, enlargement of beta zone occurred in 6.2% of progressive eyes versus 0.8% of stable eyes.[105] In the Beijing Eye Study, the beta zone of peripapillary atrophy (see Chap. 15, Sidebar 15.1) was significantly larger and occurred more frequently in glaucomatous eyes than in normal eyes of Chinese adults. No marked difference was noted between chronic open-angle glaucoma and primary angle closure glaucoma.[106]

Additional reported risk factors have included hypothyroidism and *Helicobacter pylori*. A study by Girkin at the Veterans Affairs Medical Center in Birmingham, Alabama found a greater risk of patients with a prior diagnosis of hypothyroidism developing glaucoma.[107] Kountouras et al identified a relationship between *H. pylori* and glaucoma.[108] However, these results were refuted by Galloway et al who found seropositivity for *H. pylori* was higher in patients with glaucoma (26%) than in controls (20.2%), but this difference was not statistically significant.[109]

Sleep apnea has been associated with glaucoma (see Chap. 12). In one study, 114 white patients were consecutively referred for polysomnographic evaluation of suspected sleep apnea syndrome (SAS). Sixty-nine of 114 patients had SAS. Three patients had POAG, while two had normal tension glaucoma. The incidence of glaucoma was 5 of 69, or 7.2%, which was significantly higher than the expected 2% incidence in the white population.[110] Geyer and Cohen et al found no difference in incidence of glaucoma in SAS (2%) and the general Caucasian population (1.7%).[111] POAG was present in 5 of 228 study patients. Although several studies suggest an association between SAS and glaucoma, many are case studies[112-115] and others have low sample size.[116-118] A large population report found a higher incidence of glaucoma in sleep disturbed patients with breathing disorders compared with normal sleeping individuals, although the study was based on a questionnaire rather than polysomnographic data.[119]

The recent Canadian Glaucoma Study (CGS) focused on systemic risk factors important to the progression of OAG. Investigators followed 258 patients for 5 years, and they identified four independent risk factors that were associated with glaucomatous visual field progression. Despite attempts to minimize the importance of IOP, it was identified as a significant risk factor for visual field progression. Other risk factors included baseline age, female sex, and abnormal baseline anticardiolipin antibody (ACA). The latter was associated with an almost fourfold increase in glaucoma progression as opposed to normal baseline ACA levels. Patients with diabetes, hypertension, cardiovascular disease, and migraine did not have an increased progression rate.[120] The risk factors are summarized in Table 34.3.

An evidence-based assessment of glaucoma risk factors by Friedman et al has concluded that although many risk factors have been reported, the risk factors most strongly supported by the literature include *higher IOP, greater cup-to-disc ratio, thinner central corneas*, and *older age*. Black race does not appear to be an independent risk factor, although black individuals tend to have thinner corneas, larger cup-to-disc ratios, and higher IOP, which do have strong associations with POAG.[121] The various risk factors are summarized in Table 34.4. When assessing these risk factors in a particular patient, it is important to remember that the risk models should not replace clinical judgment. The clinician must take into account life expectancy, patient health, costs, side effects of treatment, and patient preference when deciding to initiate or change glaucoma therapy.

**Table 34.3** Risk factors for the progression of OAG in the Canadian Glaucoma Study

| Risk factor | Hazard ratio |
| --- | --- |
| Abnormal baseline anticardiolipin levels | 3.86 |
| Higher baseline age | 1.04 per year |
| Female sex | 1.94 |
| Higher mean follow up IOP | 1.19 per 1 mmHg |

**Table 34.4** Summary of risk factors for diagnosis or progression of glaucoma

| Glaucoma risk factors |
| --- |
| **Increased IOP** |
| **Older age** |
| **Greater cup-to-disc ratio** |
| **Thin CCT** |
| **IOP reduction** |
| Optic disc hemorrhages |
| Antihypertensive use |
| Diurnal fluctuation[a] |
| Intervisit fluctuation[a] |
| Decrease systolic perfusion pressure |
| Lower systolic blood pressure |
| Vascular and/or cardiac disease[a] |
| Nocturnal blood pressure dip |
| Family history of glaucoma |
| Peripapillary atrophy |
| Hypothyroidism[a] |
| *H. pylori*[a] |
| Sleep apnea[a] |
| Anticardiolipin antibody |

Widely accepted and supported risk factors shown in bold.
[a]Controversial risk factors.

## 34.4 Clinical Assessment

POAG is indeed the "sneak thief of sight," because it is almost always insidious, slowly progressive, and pain free. Patients are typically unaware that they have the disease, as central vision is impacted only late in the course of the disease. It is typically bilateral, but can be asymmetric. Progressive loss of peripheral, paracentral, and central visual fields can lead to blindness. While normal patients have diurnal fluctuations in pressures of 2–6 mmHg, glaucoma patients can have much wider swings in pressure. The highest pressures in most patients are either in the early AM hours or upon awakening. However, some patients have their highest pressure in the afternoon. Some patients are able to tolerate high pressures without sustaining optic nerve damage. Others develop optic nerve injury despite apparently normal IOPs. Further, because an office visit is just one moment in time, it is a poor representation of the maximum IOP that may occur outside the office time frame. Thus, IOP alone cannot be used to make the diagnosis of POAG. The physician should also meticulously inspect the optic nerve head and associated retinal nerve fiber layer (RNFL). Imaging analysis devices (such as HRT, GDx, and OCT) may be useful to supplement direct visualization of the retinal by the examiner. Visual field testing should be obtained as well to determine functional loss of vision.

Gonioscopy is essential in the evaluation of all glaucoma suspects and patients (see Figs. 34.5–34.7). A nongonioscopy, slit-lamp angle grading system was devised by van Herick.[122] The angle between the observation system and the slit beam of the slit-lamp is set at 60°. The slit beam is oriented vertically and positioned at the corneal limbus. The peripheral anterior chamber depth is then compared to corneal thickness to estimate the depth of the anterior chamber. Angles are graded one through four, with grade 1 (shallow) consisting of an anterior chamber depth less than ¼ of the corneal thickness, and grade 4 (deep) being an anterior chamber depth greater than or equal to the corneal thickness. The van Herick grading system is good for suspecting narrow angles, but is not a substitute for gonioscopy (see Chap. 26), which should be performed during the initial assessment of all glaucoma suspects and patients. Periodic reevaluation should be performed as well, especially when confronted with a sudden elevation of pressure, shallowing of the anterior chamber, use of miotics, older hyperopes, cataract progression, or retinal vascular disease. Various angle grading systems exist for describing gonioscopic findings. In some systems where angles are graded 0–4, a grade 4 angle is wide open, while in other grading scales, a "4" may be a closed angle. The Shaffer gonioscopic classification system graded angles from Grade 0 representing a closed angle to Grade 3–4, consistent with a wide open, 20–45° angle where closure is impossible.[123] The Scheie classification system also graded angles as Grade 0–IV. In Grade 0, all structures of the angle are visible. In Grade I, it is difficult to see over the iris root and into the angle recess. With Grade II, the ciliary body is obscured. Grade III has an obscured posterior trabeculum, and finally Grade IV allows only visualization of Schwalbe's

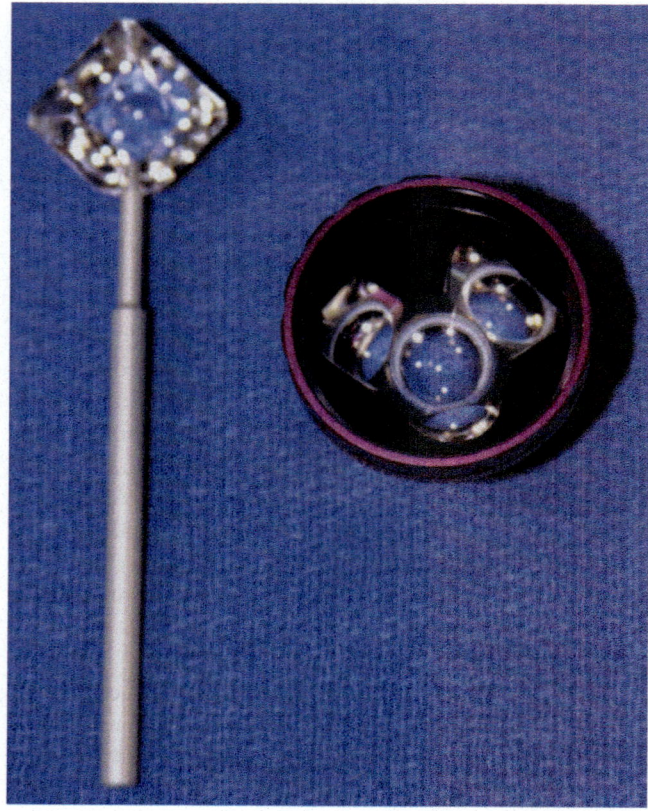

**Fig. 34.5** Two of several available gonioscopy lenses. (left) A Zeiss-style 4 mirror lens that couples to the eye with the patient's own tear film and (right) a Goldmann-style 3 mirror lens that requires goniosol to couple with the patient's eye

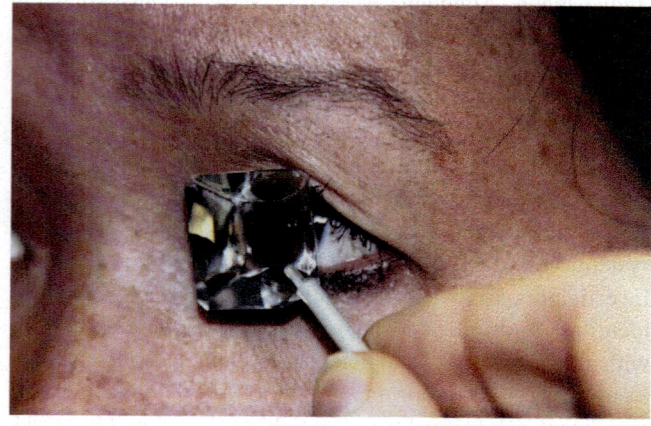

**Fig. 34.6** Zeiss-style 4 mirror lens on the eye of a patient

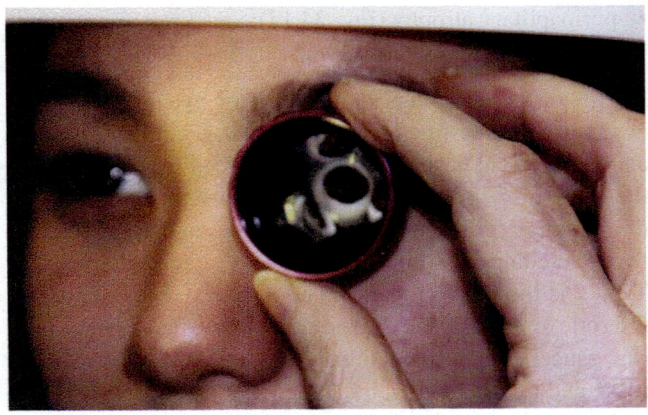

**Fig. 34.7** Goldmann-style 3 mirror lens on the eye of a patient

line.[124] This latter method eliminates the potential confusion of numerical grading systems.

The American Academy of Ophthalmology (AAO) has established Preferred Practice Pattern (PPP) guidelines.[125] Each recommendation is written on the basis of three principles: (1) each guideline is clinically relevant and detailed such that is it useful to eye care providers, (2) each guideline is given a rating relative to its importance in the care of the patient, and (3) each guideline is given a rating with respect to the strength of supporting evidence. It should be emphasized that the PPP guidelines provide a template for the general practice of eye care, but are not guidelines for the care of all individual patients. The initial exam history should contain an ocular history, a general medical history, a family history, a prior records review, and as assessment of the impact of the patient's visual function in relation to hobbies, employment, and daily living.

The primary ocular examination should include visual acuity, papillary evaluation, slit-lamp examination, IOP measurement, pachymetry, gonioscopy, stereoscopic evaluation of the optic nerve head and RNFL, color stereophotography or computer-generated image analysis, preferably dilated fundus examination, and visual field testing (see Chap. 28).

When therapy is needed, the PPP recommendation is to set a target pressure 20% less than the mean of multiple IOP measurements and less than or equal to 24 mmHg. I initially shoot for a drop of 30% from untreated baseline and IOP less than or equal to 21 mmHg. The treatment regimen should not only lower the IOP to the target pressure, but should be based on maximal effectiveness and tolerance. Follow-up exam histories should include the ocular history and medical history, with any updates since the last exam. Side effects of treatment medications should be noted. When appropriate, glaucoma medications, including frequency and time of last instillation, should be recorded. Compliance, or adherence, information should be obtained. Although it is frequently misleading, many patients will honestly volunteer that they missed their last dose or they miss multiple instillations during exam intervals. For example, a patient with IOP higher than the target pressure who admits to not using their glaucoma medications the prior evening or that morning, may not require a medication change or addition, but simply counseling to improve compliance.

PPP follow-up eye exams include visual acuity, slit-lamp exam, IOP measurement including time of the day, and gonioscopy when indicated. Patient education is an important component of treatment. This would include discussion of the following: risk factors, long-term prognosis, therapy as well as the need for long-term treatment, therapeutic alternatives including risks and benefits, training on drop instillation including punctal occlusion, and potential side effects of medications.

Frequency of examinations and testing is included in the AAO's PPP. Suspects may be followed as little as every 12–24 months. At the other extreme, the follow-up interval for uncontrolled glaucoma patients (i.e., target IOP not achieved) with high risk of damage are seen at intervals of 4 months or less. My approach has been to follow suspects annually, well-controlled patients every 6 months, and high-risk patients every 3 months. The PPP for testing of the optic nerve and visual field is every 3–24 months depending on treatment, whether target IOP is achieved, and risk of damage. In most instances, I get this testing once a year. However, if changes are noted, such as increased cupping, I may get visual field testing and documenting photos more often.

Quigley has studied practice patterns, and found that physicians varied dramatically in their adherence to PPPs, performing IOP measurements, disc evaluations and imaging, and visual field tests on 90% of OAG patients. These same ophthalmologists carried out gonioscopy, CCT measurement, and setting of target IOP in only half of their patients.[126]

Another recent study by Fremont et al assessed conformance of patterns of care for primary open-angle glaucoma with the AAO's PPPs.[127] Most elements of care during initial evaluations of POAG and follow-up visits were performed, including visual acuity examination, IOP check, slit-lamp examination, evaluation of the optic nerve head or nerve fiber layer, and fundus evaluation. However, frequency of other recommended processes fell woefully short. Gonioscopy was performed less than 50% of the time, optic nerve head drawing or photograph took place just over 50% of the time, and target pressures were documented 1.3% of the time. Failure to set a target pressure is worrisome, as future therapy is dependent on whether the IOP is above or below this target. Intervals between visits followed the PPPs. An increase in therapy was implemented in less than half the visits where IOP exceeded 25 mmHg. Intervals between visual fields were often surprisingly long. The study concluded that POAG is often undertreated.

Glaucoma should be considered in any patient undergoing an eye exam who has a family history of glaucoma. Glaucoma is more likely when a first-degree relative is affected and it is inherited more strongly through the female line. Clinically, glaucoma should be suspected if the IOP is elevated above 21 mmHg (although as we have seen, glaucoma may occur both above and below statistically average IOPs), if the cup-to-disc ratios are greater than 0.5, or if the cup-to-disc ratios are asymmetrical by 0.2 or more.

The ophthalmologist should carefully examine the optic nerve head, looking for:

- increased or progressive cupping (Figs. 34.8–34.10);
- vertical elongation of the cup (Figs. 34.11–34.18);
- nerve fiber layer (NFL) hemorrhages (Figs. 34.12, 34.19, and 34.20);
- nerve fiber layer thinning (Figs. 34.15 and 34.21);
- peripapillary atrophy (Fig. 34.17); and
- baring of the optic disc vessels.

Any of these findings should alert the eye doctor to initiate appropriate testing and, if indicated, therapy. Broadway and Drance et al have thoroughly described the evaluation of the optic disc in glaucoma, coming up with four types of discs. Type 1 is the focal glaucomatous disc, with polar or focal notching as well as progressive notch enlargement. Type 2 is the myopic glaucomatous disc. Type 3, or senile, sclerotic optic discs may show a moth-eaten neuroretinal rim, saucerization, peripapillary atrophy and choroidal sclerosis, and pallor. Finally, the Type 4 glaucoma disc has generalized enlargement of the optic disc cups. Findings may include concentric atrophy, temporal unfolding, extensive notching, or RNFL atrophy. Other features of the optic disc in glaucoma include cup deepening, neuroretinal rim slope

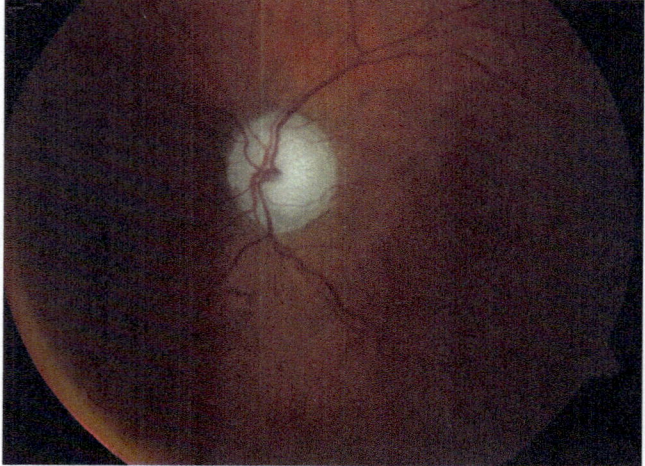

**Fig. 34.8** Generalized enlargement of the cup in a patient with advanced glaucoma

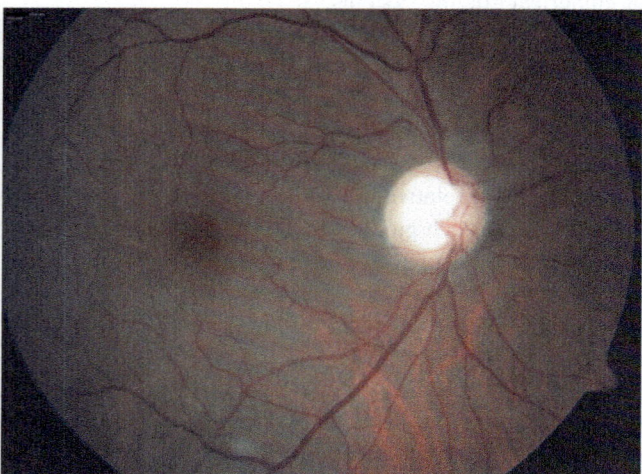

**Fig. 34.10** Generalized enlargement of the cup in a patient with advanced glaucoma

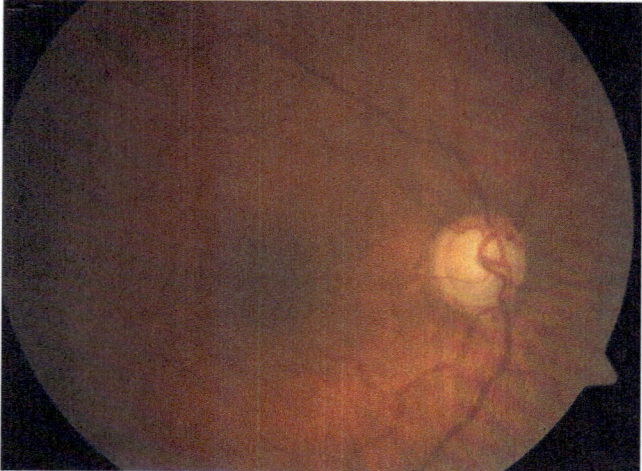

**Fig. 34.9** Generalized enlargement of the cup in a patient with glaucoma

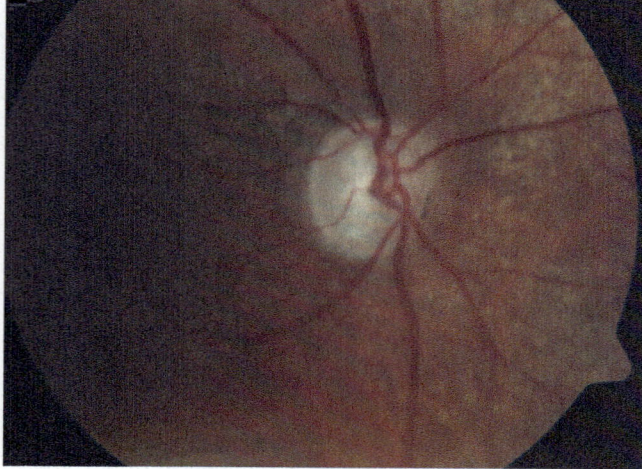

**Fig. 34.11** Vertical elongation of cup with thin rim superiorly and inferiorly in advanced glaucoma

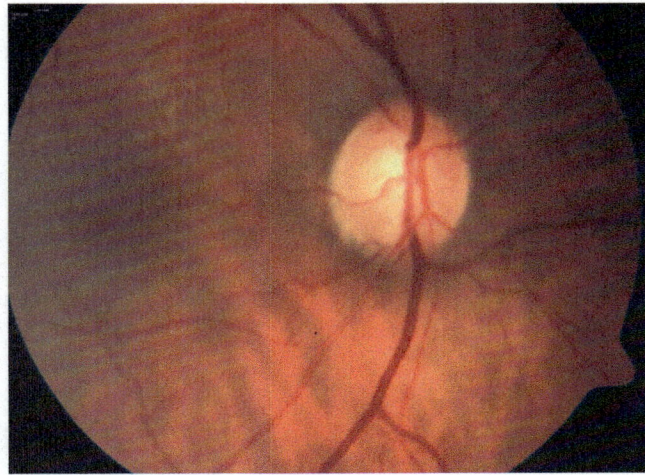

**Fig. 34.12** Vertical elongation of cup with thin rim inferiorly and a small nerve fiber layer hemorrhage inferiorly

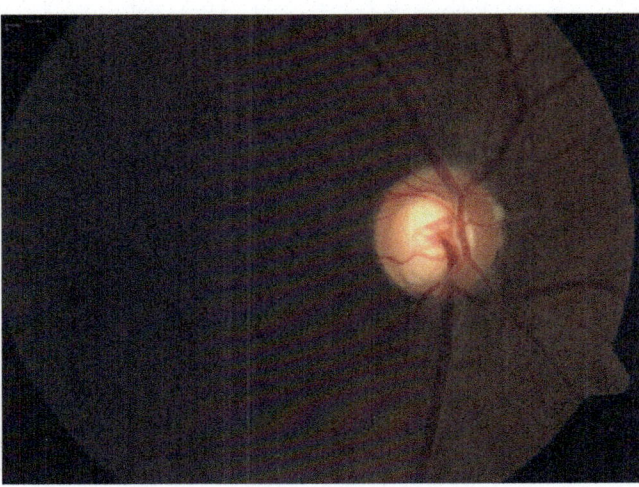

**Fig. 34.15** Vertical elongation of cup with thin rim inferiorly and inferior temporal nerve fiber layer loss

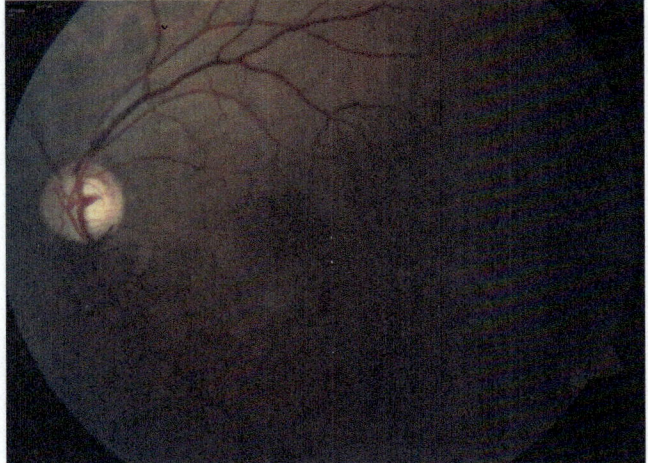

**Fig. 34.13** Vertical elongation of cup with thin rim inferiorly

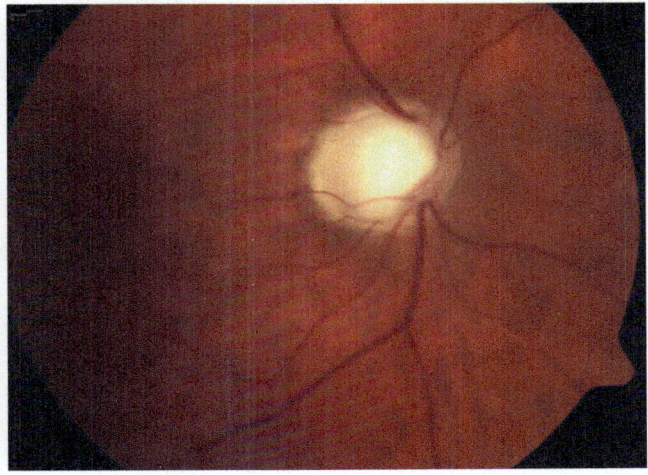

**Fig. 34.16** Vertical elongation of cup with thin rim inferiorly in Caucasian patient with advanced open angle glaucoma

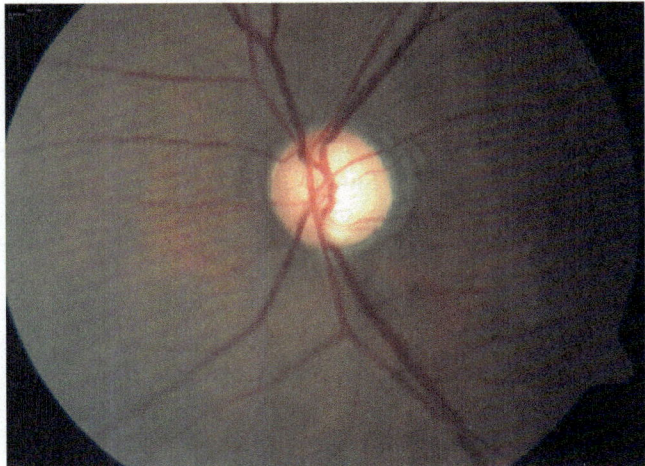

**Fig. 34.14** Vertical elongation of cup with thin rim inferiorly

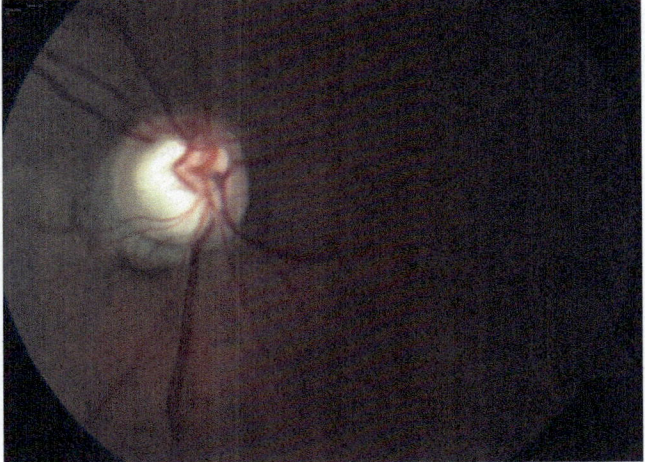

**Fig. 34.17** Vertical elongation of cup with thin rim inferiorly in patient with advanced glaucoma. Peripapillary atrophy is present as well

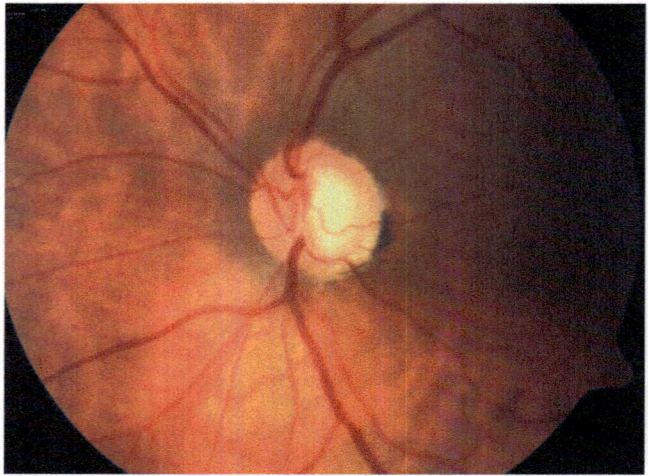

**Fig. 34.18** Vertical elongation of cup with thin rim inferiorly

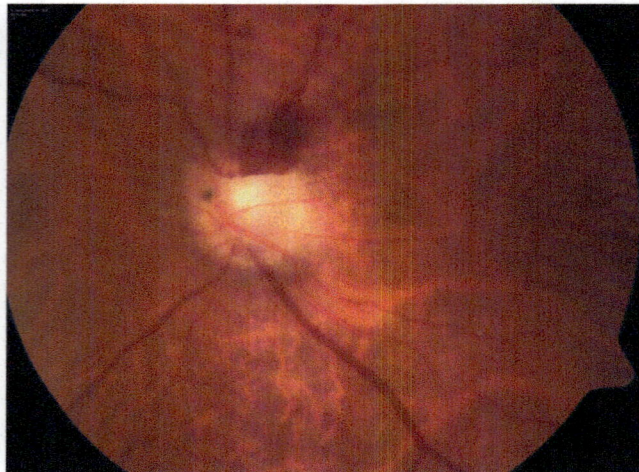

**Fig. 34.20** Superior nerve fiber layer hemorrhage

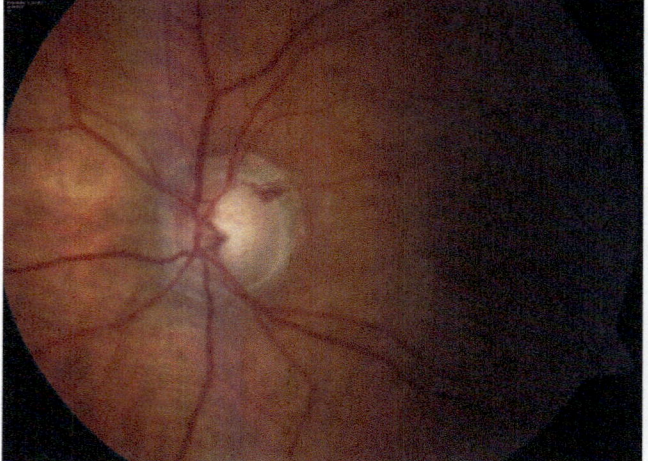

**Fig. 34.19** Nerve fiber layer hemorrhage with thin rim superiorly

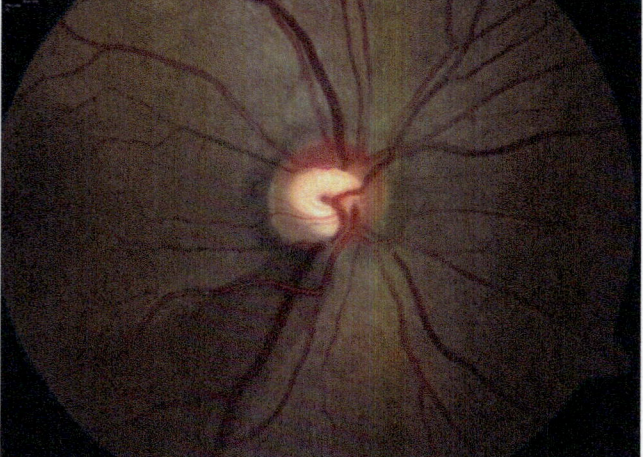

**Fig. 34.21** Thin rim inferiorly with nerve fiber layer loss inferior temporally

steepening, optic disc margin hemorrhages, pallor/cupping discrepancy, baring of a circumlinear vessel, RNFL defects, and peripapillary atrophy.[128] See Chap. 15 for discussion of the clinical examination of the optic nerve.

Bayer and Spaeth et al have developed a disk damage likelihood scale (DDLS) that correlates with visual field damage in patients with glaucoma.[129] DDLS classifies glaucomatous optic nerve damage based upon the narrowest radial width of rim and vertical disc diameter.

*Stereo disc photos or detailed drawings of the optic nerve, visual field testing, and IOP measurements should be standard and frequent components of the exam.* IOP measurements should take place at each glaucoma examination. Disc photos should be obtained early in the course of treatment anytime glaucoma is suspected. Photos may be repeated on an annual basis. Visual field testing should be obtained at least annually in capable patients, and may be repeated more often if progression is suspected. Kwan and Kim et al looked at the rate of visual field loss, as well as the long-term visual outcome in POAG. They found the average visual field decrease to be −1.5% per year. In those showing significant decrease, the rate was −2.1% per year. The cumulative rate of blindness was 19% at 22 years. This study was based on Goldmann perimetry.[130] Similar findings were obtained by Rasker and associates using automated perimetry.[131] Additional testing may include color perimetry, frequency doubling perimetry (FDP), optical coherence tomography (OCT), Glaucoma Diagnosis Device (GDx VCC), and Heidelberg retinal tomography (HRT). In one study, FDT had a 55.6% sensitivity and 92.7% specificity for detecting glaucoma.[132]

Technology may help us identify those ocular hypertensives more likely to develop glaucoma. The role of Doppler flowmetry in detecting early circulatory changes in OHT patients mimicking changes in frank OAG patients was described earlier in this chapter. Thinner OCT RNFL measurements at baseline have been associated with the development of glaucomatous change in glaucoma suspect eyes.[133] When compared with the GDx VCC, the Stratus OCT, and RNFL photography (structural exams), the Humphrey Matrix perimeter (a functional exam) was the best for detecting early glaucoma, with a specificity of 92.5% and a sensitivity of 90%. Combining the Humphrey Matrix perimeter and GDx VCC, specificity was 100% and sensitivity 90%.[134] Short wave-length automated perimetry (SWAP) and FDP showed similar ability to detect visual dysfunction in patients with preperimetric glaucoma.[135] Macular NFL thickness is reduced in glaucoma. Peripapillary NFL thickness outperformed both total macular and macular NFL thickness in terms of glaucoma detection and visual function correlation.[136] SWAP (at 79.6%), frequency doubling technology perimetry (FDP) (at 74.1%), and pattern electroretinography (PERG) (at 64.8%) have all been successful in detecting glaucomatous eyes prior to development of defects with standard white-on-white perimetry. A combination of SWAP and PERG was able to detect 88.9% of eyes before a prediction of field loss on standard automated perimetry (SAP).[137]

A panel led by Lin and Singh reviewed 159 articles dealing with optic nerve head and RNFL analysis. Eighty-two of the articles were determined to be useful based upon quality of scientific evidence. No studies were classified as having the highest level of evidence. The panel concluded that ONH and RNFL imaging devices provide quantitative information for the physician. No single imaging device outperforms others in distinguishing OAG from controls. The information from tests was useful when analyzed in conjunction with other relevant parameters.[138]

In the absence of frank optic nerve damage, the ophthalmologist should assess the patient's risk for developing glaucoma. Low-risk patients may be merely monitored without treatment. However, this decision should be made with the patient's understanding and verbally provided informed consent. It is useful to document this discussion in the medical chart. Some patients will be more comfortable treating their suspect status to prevent or delay glaucoma. After collaborative discussion with the patient, those perceived with high risk may be treated. Treatment should be undertaken within the clinical context of the patient's overall health and age. An elderly patient with minimal disc damage, who is in poor general health, and/or with limited life expectancy may be treated more conservatively than a younger patient with moderately advanced disease. Glaucoma risk calculators have been developed to help the clinician and patient with decision-making regarding treatment of the glaucoma suspect situation (see Sidebar 34.1). To date, there is no literature on how commonly these calculators are used in clinical practice.

Many ophthalmologists institute therapy in the absence of demonstrable visual field loss if the measured IOP is above a certain threshold, with consideration for the effect of any marked variation from "normal" CCT in the 540–560 µm range. For some doctors, treatment is started in all patients with a pressure above 21 mmHg, while for others the "magic number" is 25 mmHg, and still others treat IOPs above 30. Clearly this involves experience and clinical judgment given there is no universally accepted evidence-based standard of reference.

Normal pressure glaucoma or normal tension glaucoma is usually defined as POAG with pressures of 21 mmHg or less. Some physicians feel that both POAG and NTG are found along a continuous IOP spectrum related to a single disease entity, while others feel these may be two forms of glaucoma with different pathophysiologies. Nonetheless, serial tonometry is important in the diagnosis of these individuals, as often the higher pressures will be discovered at different times of the day, or may occur outside of normal office hours. Pachymetry is helpful in making this diagnosis, as many of these patients have thin corneas with their true IOPs higher than measured by Goldmann applanation tonometry. Splinter hemorrhages at the disc margin are common in normal pressure glaucoma and help to make the diagnosis in patients with low measured IOPs. Differential diagnosis of NTG includes POAG with large diurnal fluctuations, open angle glaucoma with thin CCT, systemic beta blockers masking the "true" elevated IOP, intermittent angle closure glaucoma, or prior corticosteroid-induced glaucoma. Other pathologies can mimic the visual field defects of glaucoma, including optic nerve head drusen or pits, retinal vascular disease or scarring, and ischemic optic neuropathy.

In many cases of apparent normal tension glaucoma, other causes of optic neuropathy are responsible. Some patients may have had an episodic event (e.g., cardiogenic shock or other one time vascular insufficiency) that caused optic nerve head cupping and is nonprogressive. This must be distinguished from progressive NTG that would require ongoing therapy. Carotid occlusive disease should be ruled out, as should cardiac disease. Auscultation and palpation of the carotid arteries is important. Carotid Doppler studies should be performed if indicated. Optic neuropathy can be seen following general anesthesia, hypotension, anemia, myocardial infarction, and shock. Vascular disorders such as syphilis, temporal arteritis, and systemic vasculitis should be considered. In many ways, NTG is a diagnosis of exclusion.

Therapy of normal tension glaucoma is more difficult than many other forms of glaucoma, because patients already have relatively low IOPs. Lowering of the pressure is beneficial in many patients (Normal Tension Glaucoma Treatment Study: NTGTS).[139] Further discussion of the diagnosis and treatment of NTG is elaborated in Chap. 35.

### Sidebar 34.1 Glaucoma suspects: When to treat, when to observe

Sophio Liao and Alan Robin

Multiple factors have been cited as risks for the development of primary open-angle glaucoma (POAG), including age, elevated intraocular pressure (IOP), African or Hispanic ancestry, a thin cornea, and family history of glaucoma. Deciding who is truly at increased risk and deserves closer monitoring can be difficult. The Ocular Hypertension Treatment Study (OHTS) group and the European Glaucoma Prevention Study (EGPS) provided some insight.

The OHTS group found that baseline age, vertical and horizontal C/D ratio, pattern standard deviation (PSD), central corneal thickness (CCT), and IOP were strong predictors of future development of POAG. African-American origin was not found to be an independent predictor of POAG; the increased incidence of POAG in these patients is likely attributable to their propensity for thinner CCT and larger C/D ratio. The study found that lowering IOP by 20% by use of topical medications in a group of patients with elevated IOP, and no evidence of glaucomatous damage was successful in delaying or preventing the onset of POAG.

At 5 years, only 4.4% of the treatment group developed POAG, compared with 9.5% of the observation group. The EGPS found that age, vertical C/D ratio, vertical C/D ratio asymmetry, thinner CCT, and PSD measurements on visual field testing were good predictors of the onset POAG. Although cardiovascular disease was not found to be a significant risk factor, the studies may not have powered to detect its true impact. A glaucoma suspect, as defined by the AAO, is a patient who demonstrates one of the three following findings in at least one eye:

1. optic nerve or nerve fiber layer defect such as an enlarged cup/disc ratio, asymmetric cup/disc ratios, notching/narrowing of the neural rim, or disc hemorrhage
2. visual field abnormality consistent with glaucoma
3. elevated IOP over 22 mmHg

All patients meeting at least one of these criteria should be routinely monitored with measurements of IOP, assessment of pupillary function, slit-lamp examination of the anterior segment, CCT measurement, gonioscopy, dilated fundus examination of the optic nerve head, RNFL, and fundus with documentation of any changes by photography and HRT or OCT, and evaluation of the visual field.

Treatment of high-risk glaucoma suspects should be initiated when the combination of known risk factors and the clinical picture indicate it is warranted. Of course, patients who develop optic nerve changes such as progressive disc cupping, RNFL loss, or glaucomatous visual field changes are considered to have progressed to POAG and treated as such.

The so-called risk calculators are available, but not widely used. For instance, a risk calculator based on the findings of the OHTS study was published to estimate the risk of developing POAG over 5 years. It incorporates diabetes mellitus as a risk-reducing factor, a finding from the OHTS study under much dispute, and is limited in applicability to those patients who fit the demographics and characteristics of the OHTS patient group. Furthermore, there are likely to be other, as yet undiscovered factors linked to increased or decreased risk of POAG development that are not incorporated into such risk calculators. For now, it is best to use clinical judgment, in conjunction with adjunctive testing and in the context of known risk factors, to decide who should be started on therapy and who should be observed. In particular, the strength of the OHTS study in finding that IOP lowering is strongly linked to a decreased risk of POAG, as well as the fact that the only modifiable risk factor known thus far is IOP, supports treating glaucoma suspects who have consistently elevated IOP. Treatment options should therefore begin with topical IOP-lowering medications with the goal of lowering IOP 20–30% and below 24 mmHg, typically with topical medications first.

## Bibliography

American Academy of Ophthalmology Glaucoma Panel. Primary Open-Angle Glaucoma Suspect. AAO Preferred Practice Patterns 2005;1–30.

Gordon MO, Beiser JA, Brandt JD, Heuer DK, Higginbotham EJ, Johnson CA, Keltner JL, Miller JP, Parrish RK 2nd, Wilson MR, Kass MA. The Ocular Hypertension Treatment Study: baseline factors that predict the onset of primary open-angle glaucoma. *Arch Ophthalmol.* 2002;120(6):714–720.

Johnson CA, Keltner JL, Cello KE, Edwards M, Kass MA, Gordon MO, Budenz DL, Gaasterland DE, Werner E. Ocular Hypertension Study Group. Baseline visual field characteristics in the ocular hypertension treatment study. *Ophthalmology* 2002;109(3):432–437.

Levine RA, Demirel S, Fan J, Keltner JL, Johnson CA, Kass MA; Ocular Hypertension Treatment Study Group. Asymmetries and visual field summaries as predictors of glaucoma in the ocular hypertension treatment study. Invest Ophthalmol Vis Sci. 2006;47(9):3896–3903.

Medeiros FA, Weinreb RN, Sample PA, Gomi CF, Bowd C, Crowston JG, Zangwill LM. Validation of a predictive model to estimate the risk of conversion from ocular hypertension to glaucoma. Arch Ophthalmol. 2005;123(10):1351–60.

Miglior S, Pfeiffer N, Torri V, Zeyen T, Cunha-Vaz J, Adamsons I (European Glaucoma Prevention Study Group). Predictive factors for open-angle glaucoma among patients with ocular hypertension in the European Glaucoma Prevention Study. Ophthalmology. 2007;114(1):3–9.

Miglior S, Torri V, Zeyen T, Pfeiffer N, Vaz JC, Adamsons I; EGPS Group. Intercurrent factors associated with the development of open-angle glaucoma in the European glaucoma prevention study. Am J Ophthalmol. 2007;144(2):266–275.

Miglior S, Zeyen T, Pfeiffer N, Cunha-Vaz J, Torri V, Adamsons I; European Glaucoma Prevention Study (EGPS) Group. Results of the European Glaucoma Prevention Study. Ophthalmology. 2005;112(3):366–375.

Ocular Hypertension Treatment Study Group and the European Glaucoma Prevention Study Group. The accuracy and clinical application of predictive models for primary open-angle glaucoma in ocular hypertensive individuals. Ophthalmology. 2008;115(11):2030–2036.

Tielsch JM, Katz J, Sommer A, Quigley HA, Javitt JC. Family history and risk of POAG. The Baltimore Eye Survey. Arch Ophthalmol. 1994;112(1):69–73.

## 34.5 Pathogenesis

Aqueous humor is produced by the nonpigmented epithelium of the ciliary body at a rate of 2.5 ml per min. Aqueous provides nutrition to the avascular tissues of the eye, including the lens, cornea, and vitreous. After being produced in the ciliary body, aqueous travels through the pupil into the anterior chamber. It exits the eye through two routes, the trabecular meshwork (so-called conventional outflow pathway or pressure-independent pathway) and uveoscleral pathway (so-called accessory outflow pathway or pressure-independent pathway). Resistance to aqueous outflow is within the structure of the trabecular meshwork, and the venous outflow system (see Sidebar 34.2). Eighty-five percent of the aqueous passes through the trabecular meshwork, while the other 15% exits via the uveoscleral venous system.

Although hypersecretion of aqueous is a possible mechanism of POAG, it either does not appear to be a real clinical entity or is certainly rare. Raised IOP leading to POAG occurs secondary to structural deficiencies in the trabecular meshwork. Pathologies include loss of the trabecular meshwork cells, plaques in the cribriform layer, and hyalinization of the trabecular beams. Narrowing of the collector channels can lead to an increased outflow resistance, with a subsequent rise in IOP.

A strong association exists between glaucoma and IOP. The higher the pressure, the greater is the likelihood of glaucoma. One study of a 5-year follow-up of ocular hypertensive patients without demonstrable glaucoma damage and with IOP of 22–30 mmHg revealed that 42% developed glaucoma.[140] Another study showed that the risk of developing glaucoma increases 10.5-fold when the pressure exceeds 24 mmHg compared to patients with lower pressures (sub-16 mmHg).[141] There may be a direct effect of increased IOP on the RGCs. The lamina cribrosa contains 10 lamellar sheets with pores through which pass bundles of RGC axons. It provides both structural support for the axons and contains the vascular supply for the optic nerve. High pressures distort and collapse the lamina cribrosa, resulting in mechanical and/or vascular damage to the optic nerve head.

Although there exists much evidence to support a pressure mechanism of glaucoma damage, it does not explain why some patients with normal pressures develop glaucoma and others with elevated pressure never develop glaucoma. There is an increased prevalence of glaucoma in patients with diabetes, hypertension, migraines, carotid occlusive disease, and cardiac disease. Glaucoma in these patients is likely due to a vascular etiology – decreased optic nerve head perfusion. There exists an ever-growing body of evidence suggesting that vascular factors, including OBF and OPP play a role in the pathogenesis and progression of glaucomatous optic neuropathy. This is summed up in the equation:

$$BP - IOP = Ocular\ Perfusion\ Pressure (OPP)$$

Four studies that support that low OPPs lead to increased glaucoma progression are summarized in Table 34.5. Several recent studies investigated OPP and glaucoma progression.

**Table 34.5** Population studies of OPP and glaucoma progression

| OPP and glaucoma progression: population studies |
|---|
| Baltimore Eye Survey (African–American and Caucasian)[78] |
| 6× excess of POAG in subjects with lowest category of Ocular Perfusion Pressure (OPP) |
| Egna-Neumarkt Study (Caucasian)[80] |
| Lower Diastolic Ocular Perfusion Pressure (DOPP) associated with marked, progressive increase in frequency of POAG |
| Barbados 4-Year Eye Study (African-Caribbean)[79] |
| 4-year risk of developing glaucoma increase dramatically at lower perfusion pressure |
| Projecto Ver (Hispanic)[16] |
| Found lower Diastolic Perfusion Pressure (DPP) associated with increased risk of POAG |

**Table 34.6** Panel assessment of glaucoma management

Consensus treatment preferences
- Medication is preferred over surgery as the initial therapy
- IOP lowering is the only effective treatment for POAG
- Prostaglandin analogs are the preferred medications
- Prostaglandins are the most effective agents
- Decreasing frequency of drop administration improves compliance
- Laser is used as second or third line
- Surgery should be performed when medications are ineffective, not available, or not complied with
- Trabeculectomy is the surgery of choice in eyes with no prior surgery
- Disc photos are needed
- Gonioscopy should be performed at least every 5 years

In the Barbados Eye 9-year Risk Factor Study – which studied a cohort of African–Caribbeans living in Barbados, West Indies – low mean perfusion pressure was the biggest risk factor associated with glaucoma progression, surpassing age, family history of glaucoma, IOP, and thinner CCT.[142] The EMGT was a randomized clinical trial comparing no treatment to treatment in initially diagnosed glaucoma. Following patients with higher baseline IOP revealed that patients with lower systolic blood pressure had an increased risk of glaucoma progression. Furthermore, in patients with lower baseline IOP, higher systolic blood pressure was associated with decreased risk of glaucoma progression.[76] In the Thessaloniki Eye Study, HRT testing was performed in 263 subjects. After excluding those who subsequently were identified with glaucoma, the study found that patients with diastolic blood pressure less than 90 mmHg as a result of systemic antihypertensive therapy had larger cup-to-disc ratios and cup areas on HRT compared to normal patients with diastolic blood pressure less than 90 mmHg and hypertensive patients with blood pressure of 90 mmHg or greater.[91]

There exists a relationship between nocturnal hypotension and OPP. Lowered blood pressure at night, coupled with the higher IOP in the supine position, compromises OPP. It is recommended that systemic blood pressure medications be taken in the morning as opposed to bedtime to minimize nocturnal hypotension. When treating glaucoma, use IOP lowering medications that lower IOP in both the day and night. Also, avoid glaucoma medications that lower systemic blood pressure at night; i.e., beta-blockers and alpha agonists.[96,143,144]

Low OPP is an important risk factor for glaucoma. Remembering the equation, BP−IOP=Ocular Perfusion Pressure, OPP is modifiable by lowering intraocular and improving perfusion pressure. New glaucoma strategies need to take advantage of this modifiable risk factor (see Chap. 11).

---

**SIDEBAR 34.2 Proteoglycan biosynthesis and degradation: What really causes glaucoma?**

Ted Acott, Kate Keller, Mary Kelley, and John Samples

Since the 1950s, glycosaminoglycans (GAGs), then known as mucopolysaccharides, have been the prime candidates for the outflow resistance molecules. Studies since then in a variety of species have supported a central role for these large, highly charged, extracellular matrix (ECM) components in providing the outflow resistance. Although establishing the exact role of GAGs in the outflow resistance of higher primates, particularly humans, has created controversy in the past, their direct involvement is generally accepted. With the exception of hyaluronan, which exists primarily as long chains or aggregate cables within the ECM, other GAGs are found as covalent side chains on proteoglycan core proteins.

Ongoing ECM turnover, mediated by a family of matrix metalloproteinases (MMPs), has been shown to be necessary for the day-to-day maintenance of the outflow resistance. The MMPs are zinc-dependent endopeptidases; collectively they degrade all types of ECM proteins, but they are heavily involved in processing a number of cytokines and other molecules. They are known to be involved in the cleavage of cell surface receptors, and chemokine in/activation. MMPs are also thought to play a major role on cell behaviors such as cell proliferation, adhesion, and migration. There are 22 members of the class in humans, and many of them have been found in the aqueous humor.

ECM turnover, initiated by MMPs in response to mechanical stretch or distortion of the juxtacanalicular ECM, is key to intraocular pressure (IOP) homeostasis. The initiation of ECM turnover involves ECM degradation at highly controlled and very dynamic focal areas at the cell surface, called podosome- or invadopodia-like structures (PILS), where MMP-2 and MMP-14 colocalize. Conceptually it is important to recognize that biosynthesis and degradation are taking place simultaneously in the outflow structures. In close concert with this ECM degradation is an extensive two-phase process of ECM biosynthetic replacement. In the first phase, matricellular and similar multidomain binding proteins are produced to hold and retain the ECM organization while the degraded ECM components are removed. In the second phase, replacement ECM components are produced and reintegrated into the ECM. The exact composition and amounts of the various components are adjusted slightly to increase or decrease the outflow resistance, depending on the direction of adjustment in IOP that is needed.

Recent studies of the ECM components produced by processes that modify the outflow resistance, such as mechanical stretch or IOP changes, TNFα (alpha), IL-1α (alpha) or TGFα (alpha), all implicate an interaction of the GAG, hyaluronan, and the proteoglycan, versican, as probably sources of the actual outflow resistance. Versican is a large aggregating proteoglycan with between 0 and 23 long and highly charged GAG sidechains (Fig. 34.2-1). In addition to the GAG sites, it has a variety of modular protein-binding domains that interact with a number of ECM proteins and with specific sites on hyaluronan. These manipulations of the outflow resistance change versican levels and produce alternative versican mRNA splicing, which modify the number of GAG chain attachment sites within the core protein. Additional recent studies provide further support for the idea that versican, acting in conjunction with hyaluronan, is a key component of the outflow resistance. It is likely that the highly charged side chains have a direct role in regulating the passage of aqueous through their "bottle brush" like structures. However, it should be noted that this idea remains tentative; but our belief, at the moment, is that versican is the major component in regulating outflow. Elsewhere in the text, the importance of cytokines modulating the response to laser has been discussed. It is likely that these cytokines change versican through MMPs. New methodologies that allow direct access to Schlemm's canal on a routine basis may provide a route by which versican may be directly altered to enhance outflow.

## Bibliography

Acott TS, Kelley MJ. Extracellular matrix in the trabecular meshwork (Review). *Exp Eye Res*. 2008;86:543–561.

Aga M, Bradley J, Keller K, Kelley M, Acott T. Specialized Podosome- or Invadopodia-like Structures (PILS) for Focal Trabecular Meshwork Extracellular Matrix Turnover. *Invest Ophthalmol Vis Sci*. 2008;49:5353–5365.

Bárány EH, Scotchbrook S. Influence of testicular hyaluronidase on the resistance to flow through the angle of the anterior chamber. *Acta Physiol Scand*. 1954;30:240–248.

Bradley JMB, Anderssohn AM, Colvis CM, et al. Mediation of laser trabeculoplasty-induced matrix metalloproteinase expression by IL-1β and TNFα. *Invest Ophthalmol Vis Sci*. 2000;41:422–430.

Bradley JMB, Kelley MJ, Zhu XH, Anderssohn AM, Alexander JP, Acott TS. Effects of mechanical stretching on trabecular matrix metalloproteinases. *Invest Ophthalmol Vis Sci*. 2001;42:1505–1513.

Bradley JMB, Vranka JA, Colvis CM, et al. Effects of matrix metalloproteinase activity on outflow in perfused human organ culture. *Invest Ophthalmol Vis Sci*. 1998;39:2649–2658.

Chen Y, Kelley MJ, Acott TS. DNA microarray analysis of gene expression in trabecular meshwork cells in response to TNFα and IL-1α. *Invest Ophthalmol Vis Sci*. 2005;46 (Abstract):#1349.

Hubbard W, Johnson M, Gong H, et al. Intraocular pressure and outflow facility are unchanged following acute and chronic intracameral chondroitinase ABC and hyaluronidase in monkeys. *Exp Eye Res*. 1997;65:177–190.

Keller K, Aga M, Bradley J, Kelley M, Acott T. Extracellular matrix turnover and outflow resistance. *Exp Eye Res*. 2009;88:676–682.

Keller KE, Bradley JM, Kelley MJ, Acott TS. Effects of modifiers of glycosaminoglycan biosynthesis on outflow facillity in perfusion culture. *Invest Ophthalmol Vis Sci*. 2008;49:2495–2505.

Keller KE, Kelley MJ, Acott TS. Extracellular matrix gene alternative splicing by trabecular meshwork cells in response to mechanical stretching. *Invest Ophthalmol Vis Sci*. 2007;48:1164–1172.

Kelley MJ, Rose AY, Song K, et al. Synergism of TNF and IL-1 in the induction of matrix metalloproteinase-3 in trabecular meshwork. *Invest Ophthalmol Vis Sci*. 2007;48:2634–2643.

Vittal V, Rose A, Gregory KE, Kelley MJ, Acott TS. Changes in gene expression by trabecular meshwork cells in response to mechanical stretching. *Invest Ophthalmol Vis Sci*. 2005;46:2857–2868.

Wight TN. Versican: a versatile extracellular matrix proteoglycan in cell biology. *Curr Opin Cell Biol*. 2002;14:617–623.

Wu YJ, La Pierre DP, Wu J, Yee AJ, Yang BB. The interaction of versican with its binding partners. *Cell Res*. 2005;15:483–494.

Zhao X, Russell P. Versican splice variants in human trabecular meshwork and ciliary muscle. *Mol Vis*. 2005;11:603–608.

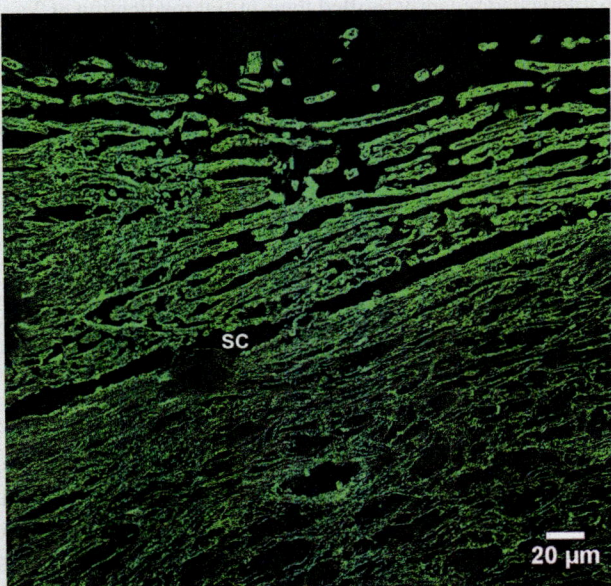

**Fig. 34.2-1** Versican localization in trabecular meshwork. Confocal image of versican immunostaining of 5μm section of human trabecular meshwork. Bar showing the scale and Schlemm's canal (SC) are labeled as indicated

## 34.6 Cost

The diagnosis and management of glaucoma are associated with considerable cost. Lee et al looked at insurance claims, finding the mean POAG costs to be $1,570 US in the first year, and $1,458 US in following years. Most of these dollar amounts were not pharmacy related. They accounted for about 10% of the patients' total health care costs.[145] A retrospective study in Sweden and the United States calculated the mean total POAG costs over 2 years were $1,972 US and $2,188 US.[146] In another US chart review study, mean POAG cost per year ranged from $623 US per patient to $2,511 US per patient for end stage disease.[147]

Kymes et al performed a cost utility analysis of the OHTS therapy. The OHTS concluded that treatment of ocular hypertension greater than or equal to 24 reduces the risk of POAG by 60% at 5 years. Treatment of patients with an annual risk greater than or equal to 5% is highly cost-effective. Treatment of patients with an annual risk greater than or equal to 2% is cost-effective. This may be one-third of patients with IOP greater than or equal to 24 mmHg.[148]

Stewart has calculated the cost-effectiveness of treating ocular hypertension. The incremental cost-effectiveness ratio (ICER) for all OHT patients to prevent one case from progressing to POAG over 5 years was $89,072. Using OHTS data and risk factors, the ICER could be reduced to less than $50,000.[149]

Pasquale et al found that patients with POAG had significantly higher adjusted total and condition-related health care charges during the first year of follow-up than patients with OHT using a multivariate analysis ($2,070 vs. $1,990, and $556 vs. $322). Females and older patients had higher charges than males and younger patients. Patients with comorbid conditions – including cataracts, cataract surgery, diabetic retinopathy, and blindness – had higher total and condition-related charges.[150]

## 34.7 Treatment and Compliance

POAG cannot be cured, and the damage done prior to diagnosis and initiation of therapy cannot be reversed. Slowing and rarely stopping progressive damage to the optic nerves requires lifelong treatment. Some patients are reluctant to start treatment, because they erroneously believe that treatment, once started, cannot be stopped upon reevaluation. These patients require appropriate education about their glaucoma as a disease process and about treatment options. They must be made to understand that optic nerve damage that is allowed to occur and perhaps progress is typically irreversible. Nevertheless, some patients will see an improvement in their visual field testing following IOP reduction.

While there are general principles regarding glaucoma management, there is not any treatment algorithm that is suitable for all patients. It is important to tailor treatment to the individual person. Most patients prefer medication to surgery as the initial treatment modality. Therapy typically begins with topical agents, but some ophthalmologists and patients prefer laser as the first option. Adherence to therapy diminishes with polypharmacology. Robin and Covert studied adherence to initial latanoprost primary therapy following adjunctive glaucoma therapy, and they found a significant decrease in refill interval of the primary drug. They recommended that the doctor, when adding a second adjunctive medication, needs to be cognizant of a possibility of decreased adherence to the first medication, as well as the possibility of poorer pressure control.[151] The fact that glaucoma is an asymptomatic long-term disease contributes to noncompliance with therapy. Other factors enhancing noncompliance or nonadherence include forgetfulness, complex treatment regimens, chronic use of medication, frequent administration, lack of noticeable benefit, side effects, financial burden, lack of understanding of their disease, and difficulty with administration. Reports of medication noncompliance range up to 80%.[152] Using Pilocarpine and an electronic monitoring device, Kass et al found that 15.2% of patients omitted at least 50% of doses and 6% of patients omitted at least 75% of doses. Patients took a mean of 76% of their drops, but reported 97% compliance.[153] In another study, one-half of patients who filled a glaucoma prescription discontinued all topical ocular hypotensive therapy within 6 months. Just 37% of these patients had recently refilled their initial medication at 3 years after the initial dispensing. Prostaglandins were associated with better persistence than other classes of medications.[154]

Many patients simply do not return to the eye doctor. A Yale study found that many African-Americans failed to access free eye care after glaucoma screening. Reasons for lack of follow-up included smoking, lack of access to transportation, and living alone.[155]

Patient knowledge and dose frequency can be used as starting points to improve compliance. A combination of patient education and prevention of forgetfulness seems to be successful in enhancing patient compliance. There are at present no determinants sensitive and specific enough to identify the potential noncompliers accurately.

Noncompliance is common (see Chap. 55). Field progression despite apparently good IOPs should alert the clinician to the possibility of noncompliance. To measure compliance, consider medication monitoring devices, (e.g., the Travatan Dosing Aid [TDA]) or inspection of pharmacy refill records. It is important for the physician and staff to educate patients and their families about glaucoma. Written materials may also be helpful. If the clinician suspects noncompliance, simplify dosing schedules (e.g., no more than two times per day) and consider medication compliance devices like the Travatan

Dosing Aid. The physician or staff should not only train the patient on how to instill eye drops but should watch the patient do so, perhaps using samples of artificial tear preparations. Training in digital punctal occlusion methods helps ensure proper use of eye drops and minimizes systemic absorption. Also, have the patient or family member wipe the eyelids to minimize local side effects. Tie drop instillation to daily activities, such as brushing one's teeth. Consider instillation devices for patients with manual dexterity issues. Personalize therapy for each patient, and choose therapy in the context of the patient's overall medical condition. The nerve fiber layer, cups, and pressures must be continually monitored with adjustments in treatment as necessary. Unfortunately, many physicians do not alter therapy based on reexamination of the patient. It is important to note that to date there are no objective studies linking noncompliance to progression.[156]

## 34.8 Conclusion

There is not a "magic pressure" above which all patients get glaucomatous loss, and below which damage does not occur (although glaucoma prevalence does increase with increasing IOP). Rather, the level at which glaucomatous damage occurs or progresses is particular to each individual patient. Therapy is usually instituted when loss seems likely to occur or has occurred. "Target IOP has come to represent our best clinical estimate of the IOP at which the pressure-related component of glaucomatous damage will be sufficiently slowed or arrested."[157] It is important to note that this "target pressure" is a dynamic concept, and not a static, one-time established value. Once a target has been set by the doctor based upon an initial evaluation of clinical parameters, it should be reevaluated at each office visit in light of the then existing clinical situation. If further optic nerve damage occurs or visual field loss worsens despite consistently achieving the target pressure, then a new lower target pressure must be set and obtained.

The only current treatment we have for POAG is lowering the patient's IOP. This goal can be achieved medically, or with laser or incisional surgeries. Most ophthalmologists and patients in the USA prefer starting with medical therapy. Initial laser and incisional surgery is more common in Europe. A meta-analysis of 11 different 24-h IOP studies evaluating the efficacy of glaucoma medicines by Stewart et al found that bimatoprost (29%) and travoprost (27%) were the most effective monotherapy treatments.[158] Argon laser trabeculoplasty was shown to be as effective as medical therapy at 2 years in the Glaucoma Laser Trial.[159] However, this study was conducted in the preprostaglandin analog era. A recent 5-year study found selective laser trabeculoplasty to be as effective as argon laser trabeculoplasty in eyes receiving maximum medical therapy.[160] Migdal and Hitchings compared long-term outcomes after early surgery versus laser and medicine in open angle glaucoma patients. Patients were followed a minimum of 5 years. Surgery resulted in the lowest IOPs. Visual fields worsened most in the medication group, and to a lesser extent in the laser group, but did not worsen in the surgery group.[161] These findings spurred the Collaborative Initial Glaucoma Treatment Study (CIGTS),[162] which randomized more than 600 patients to either trabeculectomy or medical treatment. At 5 years, the pressures were lower in the surgery group. Visual field deterioration was the same in both groups. Based on the results, the authors concluded that a switch to a "surgery-first" approach to glaucoma was not warranted. The results of large, multicenter, randomized clinical trials, as well as clinical experience, influence glaucoma therapy. A recently convened panel by Singh et al,[163] using principles of RAND-like methodology, tried to reach a consensus with respect to glaucoma diagnosis and management. Medical therapy was the preferred initial treatment of both OHT and POAG. Lowering IOP was the only effective therapy of POAG, with prostaglandin analogs being the agents of choice for initial treatment. If a glaucoma medication did not lower the pressure by at least 10%, another agent should be tried. Prostaglandin analogs were judged to be the systemically safest medications, while topical beta-blockers were the best in terms of ocular tolerance. Drugs that required fewer instillations per day were associated with better compliance. Therapy should be initiated with a one-eyed trial. The panel agreed that adjunctive therapy should be limited to one medication from each class, and therapy should be increased in the face of glaucoma progression, regardless of the pressure. Topical carbonic anhydrase inhibitors were felt to be of value when added to initial prostaglandin analog therapy. The panel supported second- or third-line use of laser trabeculoplasty. They also agreed that argon laser trabeculoplasty and selective laser trabeculoplasty are equal in terms of IOP lowering. Surgery should be entertained as an option when medications are not available, compliance is poor, or when the pressure on medications is unacceptably high. Trabeculectomy was scored as the initial surgery of choice for glaucoma patients, and the surgery should be enhanced with antifibrotic agents. The panel concurred that lower IOP is likely to occur with mitomycin C trabeculectomy than with glaucoma shunts and nonpenetrating glaucoma surgeries. The panel agreed that initial treatment should lower the IOP by 30%.

With respect to diagnostic testing, the panel agreed that disc photographs are needed, with stereo disc photography being the preferred method. Visual field testing should be obtained on all patients undergoing active glaucoma treatment, and FDP and SWAP can detect glaucoma earlier than standard visual field testing.

Agreed-upon consensus treatment preferences of glaucoma are listed in Table 34.6.

# References

1. Quigley HA. Number of people with glaucoma worldwide. *Br J Ophthalmol*. 1996;80:389–393.
2. Quigley HA, Vitale S. Models of open-angle glaucoma prevalence and incidence in the United States. *Invest Ophthalmol Vis Sci*. 1997;38:83–91.
3. Lighthouse International. New approach to assessing glaucoma risk may help physicians decide who needs treatment. Available at: http://www.lighthouse.org/education-services/profes0sional-education/patient-management/patient-management-disease-management/glaucoma/new-approach/Last accessed 9.03.08.
4. Sommer A, Tielsch JM, Katz J, et al. Racial differences in the cause-specific prevalence of blindness in east Baltimore. *N Engl J Med*. 1991;325:1412–1417.
5. Condon N, Wang F, Tielsch JM. Issues in the epidemiology and population based screening of POAG. *Surv Ophthalmol*. 1992;36:411–423.
6. Tielsch JM, Sommer A, Katz J, et al. Racial variations in the prevalence of primary open-angle glaucoma. The Baltimore Eye Survey. *JAMA*. 1991;266:369–374.
7. Varma R, Ying-Lai M, Francis BA, et al. Prevalence of open-angle glaucoma and ocular hypertension in Latinos: The Los Angeles Latino Eye Study. *Ophthalmology*. 2004;111(8):1439–1448.
8. The Eye Diseases Prevalence Research Group. Prevalence of open-angle glaucoma among adults in the United States. Last modified in December 2006. Available at http://www/nei/nih.gov/eyedata/pbd5.aspLast accessed 9.03.08.
9. Shiose Y, Kitazawa U, Tsukahara S, et al. Epidemiology of glaucoma in Japan. A nationwide survey. *Jpn J Ophthalmol*. 1991;35:133–155.
10. Leske MC, Connell AM, Schachat AP, Hyman L. The Barbados Eye Study. Prevalence of open-angle glaucoma. *Arch Ophthalmol*. 1994;112:821-829.
11. Bonomi L, Marchini G, Marraffa M, et al. Prevalence of glaucoma and intraocular pressure distribution in a defined population. The Egna-Neumarkt Study. *Ophthalmology*. 1998;105:209–215.
12. Leibowitz HM, Krueger DE, Maunder LR, et al. The Framingham Eye Study monograph; an ophthalmological and epidemiological study of cataract, glaucoma, diabetic retinopathy, macular degeneration, and visual acuity in a general population of 2631 adults, 1973–1975. *Surv Ophthalmol*. 1980; 24(supplement):335–610.
13. Foster PJ, Oen FTS, Machin D, et al. The prevalence of glaucoma in Chinese residents of Singapore. A cross-sectional population survey of the Tanjong Pagar district. *Arch Ophthalmol*. 2000;118:1105–1111.
14. Buhrmann RR, Quigley HA, Barron Y, et al. Prevalence of glaucoma in a rural East African population. *Invest Ophthalmol Vis Sci*. 2000;41:40–48.
15. Cedrone C, Culasso F, Cesareo M, et al. Prevalence of glaucoma in Ponza, Italy: A comparison of other studies. *Ophthalmic Epidemiol*. 1997;4:59–72.
16. Quigley HA, West SK, Rodriguez J, et al. The prevalence of glaucoma in a population-based study of Hispanic subjects. Proyecto VER. *Arch Ophthalmol*. 2001;119:1819–1826.
17. Rotchford AP, Johnson GJ. Glaucoma in Zulus. A population based cross-sectional surgery in a rural district in South Africa. *Arch Ophthalmol*. 2002;120:471–478.
18. Wensor MD, McCarty CA, Stanislavsky YL, et al. The prevalence of glaucoma in the Melbourne Visual Impairment Project. *Ophthalmology*. 1998;105:733–739.
19. Mason RP, Kosoko O, Wilson MR, et al. National survey of the prevalence and risk factors of glaucoma in St. Lucia, West Indies. Part 1. Prevalence findings. *Ophthalmology*. 1989;96:1363–1368.
20. Sommer A, Tielsch JM, Katz J, et al. Relationship between intraocular pressure and primary open angle glaucoma among white and black Americans. The Baltimore Eye Survey. *Arch Ophthalmol*. 1991;109:1090–1095.
21. Dandona L, Dandona R, Srinivas M, et al. Open-angle glaucoma in an urban population in southern India. The Andhra Pradesh Eye Disease Study. *Ophthalmology*. 2000;107:1702–1709.
22. Foster PJ, Baasanhu J, Alsbirk PH, et al. Glaucoma in Mongolia. A population-based survey in Hovsgol Province, Northern Mongolia. *Arch Ophthalmol*. 1996;68:626–629.
23. Mitchell P, Smith W, Attebo K, Healey PR. Prevalence of open-angle glaucoma in Australia. The Blue Mountains Eye Study. *Ophthalmology*. 1996;103:1661–1669.
24. Klein BEK, Klein R, Sponsel WE, et al. Prevalence of glaucoma. The Beaver Dam Eye Study. *Ophthalmology*. 1992;99:1499–1504.
25. Dielemans I, Vingerling JR, Wolfs RC, et al. The prevalence of primary open-angle glaucoma in a population-based study in the Netherlands. The Rotterdam Study. *Ophthalmology*. 1994;101:1851–1855.
26. Wolfs RC, Borger PH, Ramrattan RS, et al. Changing views on open-angle glaucoma: definitions and prevalences. The Rotterdam Study. *Invest Ophthalmol Vis Sci*. 2000;41:3309–3321.
27. Iwase A, Suzuki Y, Araie M, et al. The prevalence of primary open-angle glaucoma in Japanese. The Tajimi Study. *Ophthalmology*. 111;9:1641–1648.
28. Salmon JF, Mermoud A, Ivey A, et al. The prevalence of primary angle closure glaucoma and open angle glaucoma in Mamre, Western Cape, South Africa. *Arch Ophthalmol*. 1993;111:1623–1629.
29. Leske MC, Warheit-Roberts L, Wu SY. Open-angle glaucoma and ocular hypertension: the Long Island Glaucoma Case-Control Study. *Ophthalmic Epidemiol*. 1996;3:85–96.
30. Hattenhauer MG, Johnson DH, Ing HH, et al. The probability of blindness from open-angle glaucoma. *Ophthalmology*. 1998;105(11):2099–2104.
31. Rotchford A, Kirwin J, Muller M, et al. Temba Glaucoma Study: A population based cross-sectional survey in Urban South Africa. *Ophthalmology*. 2003;110(2):376–382.
32. Chen PP. Blindness in patients with treated open-angle glaucoma. *Ophthalmology*. 2003;110(4):726–733.
33. Racette L, Wilson MR, Zangwill LM, et al. Primary open-angle glaucoma in blacks: a review. *Surv Ophthalmol*. 2003;48(3):295–313.
34. The Eye Disease Research Group. Prevalence of open-angle glaucoma among adults in the United States. *Arch Ophthalmol*. 2004;122:532–538.
35. Topouzis F, Wilson MR, Harris A, Anastasopoulos E, et al. Prevalence of open-angle glaucoma in Greece: The Thessaloniki Eye Study. *Am J Ophthalmol*. 2007;1(4):511–519e1.
36. Ramakrishnan R, Nirmalan PK, Krishnadas R, et al. Glaucoma in a rural population of Southern India. The Aravind comprehensive eye survey. *Ophthalmology*. 2003;110(8):1484–1490.
37. Hennis A, Wu S-Y, Nemesure B, et al. Awareness of incident open-angle glaucoma in a population study. The Barbados Eye Studies. *Ophthalmology*. 2007;114(10):1816–1821.
38. Leske MC, Wu SY, Honkanen R, et al. Nine-year indidence of open-angle glaucoma in the Barbados Eye Studies. *Ophthalmology*. 2007;114(6):1058–1064.
39. Wolfs RC, Klaver CC, et al. Genetic risk of primary open-angle glaucoma (population based familial aggregation study). *Arch Ophthalmol*. 1998;116:1640–1645.
40. Duke-Elder S. *Disease of the Inner Eye. Text Book of Ophthalmology*. Vol 3. St. Louis: C V Mosby; 1945.
41. Chang TC, Congdon NG, Wojciechowski R, Munoz B, et al. Determinants of heritability of intraocular pressure and cup-to-disc ratio in a defined older population. *Ophthalmology*. 2005;112(7):1186–1191.
42. Teikari JM. Genetic factors in open-angle (simple and capsular) glaucoma. A population based twin study. *Acta Ophthalmol*. 1987;(65):715–720.
43. Chang TC, Congdon NG, Wojciechowski R, et al. Determinants and heritability of intraocular pressure and cup-to-disc ratio in a defined older population. *Ophthalmology*. 2005;112(7):1186-1191.
44. Moroi SE, Richards JE. Glaucoma and genomic medicine. *Glaucoma Today*. January/February 2008;6(1):16–24.

45. Leibowitz HM, Krueger DE, Maunder LR, et al. The Framingham Eye Study monograph: an ophthalmological and epidemiological study of cataract, glaucoma, diabetic retinopathy, macular degeneration, and visual acuity in a general population of 2631 adults, 1973–1975. *Surv Ophthalmology.* 1980;24(supplement):335–610.
46. Armaly MG, Kreuger DE, Maunder LR, et al. Biostatistical analysis of the Collaborative Glaucoma Study. I. Summary report of the risk factors for glaucomatous visual field defects. *Arch Ophthalmol.* 1980;98:2163–2171.
47. Quigley HA, Enger C, Katz J, et al. Risk factors for the development of glaucomatous visual field loss in ocular hypertension. *Arch Ophthalmol.* 1994;112:644–649.
48. Kass MA, Heuer DK, Higginbotham EF, et al. The Ocular Hypertension Treatment Study: a randomized trial determines that topical ocular hypotensive medication delays or prevents the onset of primary open angle glaucoma. *Arch Ophthalmol.* 2002;120: 701–713.
49. Gordon MO, Beiser JA, Brandt JD, et al. The Ocular Hypertension Treatment Study. Baseline factors that predict the onset of primary open angle glaucoma. *Arch Ophthalmol.* 2002;120:714–720.
50. Gordon MO, Beiser JA, Kass MA. Ocular Hypertension Treatment Study Group. Is a history of diabetes mellitus protective against developing primary open-angle glaucoma? *Arch Ophthalmol.* 2008:126(2):280–281.
51. The European Glaucoma Prevention Study Group. Predictive factors for open angle glaucoma among patients with ocular hypertension in the European Glaucoma Prevention Study. *Ophthalmology.* 2007;114:3–9.
52. Gordon MO, Torri V, Miglior S, et al. Validated model for the development of primary open-angle glaucoma in individuals with ocular hypertension. *Ophthalmology.* 2007;114(1):10–19.
53. Medeiros FA, Weinreb RN, Sample PA, et al. Validation of a predictive model to estimate the risk of conversion from ocular hypertension to glaucoma. *Arch Ophthalmol.* 2005;123:1351–1360.
54. Kass MA, Heuer DK, Higginbotham EJ, et al. The Ocular Hypertension Treatment Study. A randomized trial determines that topical hypotensive medication delays or prevents the onset of primary open angle glaucoma. *Arch Ophthalmol.* 2002;120:701–713.
55. Nouri-Mahdavi K, Hoffman D, Coleman AL, et al. Predictive factors for glaucomatous visual field progression in the Advanced Glaucoma Intervention Study. *Ophthalmology.* 2004;111:1627–1635.
56. Budenz DL, Anderson DR, Feuer WF, et al. Detection and prognostic significance of optic disc hemorrhages during the OHTS. *Ophthalmology.* 2006;116:2137–2143.
57. Langham MJ, Lancashire RJ, Cheng KK, et al. Systemic hypertension and glaucoma: mechanisms in common and co-occurrence. *Br J Ophthalmol.* 2005;89:960–963.
58. Kass MA, Heuer DK, Higginbotham EF, et al. The Ocular Hypertension Treatment Study. A randomized trial determines that topical hypotensive medication delays or prevents the onset of POAG. *Arch Ophthalmol.* 2002;120:701–713.
59. Heijl A, Leske MC, Bengtsson B, et al. Reduction of intraocular pressure and glaucoma progression. Results from the Early Manifest Glaucoma Trial. *Arch Ophthalmol.* 2002;120:1268–1279.
60. Leske MC, Heijl A, Hessein M, et al. Factors for glaucoma progression and the effect of treatment. The Early Manifest Glaucoma Trial. *Arch Ophthalmol.* 2003;121:48–56.
61. Miglior S, Torri V, et al. Intercurrent factors associated with the development of open angle glaucoma in the European Glaucoma Prevention Study. *Am J Opthalmol.* 2007;144(2):266–275.
62. Caprioli J, Coleman AL. Intraocular pressure fluctuation: a risk factor for visual field progression at low intraocular pressures in the Advance Glaucoma Intervention Study. *Ophthalmology.* 2008; 115(7):1123–1129.e3.
63. Stewart WC, Kolker AE, Sharpe ED, et al. Factors associated with long term progression or stability in primary open angle glaucoma. *Am J Ophthalmol.* 2000;130:274–279.
64. Niesel P, Flammer J. Correlations between intraocular pressure, visual field and visual acuity, based on 11 years of observations of treated chronic glaucomas. *Int Ophthalmol.* 1980;3:31–35.
65. Bergea B, Bodin L, Svedbergh B. Impact of intraocular pressure regulation on visual fields in open angle glaucoma. *Ophthalmology.* 1999;106:176–181.
66. Asrani S, Zeimer R, Wilensky J, et al. Large diurnal fluctuations in intraocular pressure are an independent risk factor in patients with glaucoma. *J Glaucoma.* 2000;9:134–142.
67. Bengtsson B, Heigl A. Diurnal IOP fluctuation: not an independent risk factor for glaucomatous visual field loss in high risk ocular hypertension. *Graefes Arch Clin Exp Ophthalmol.* 2005;243:513–518.
68. Bengtsson B, Leske MC, Hyman L. et al and the Early Manifest Glaucoma Trial. *Ophthalmology.* 2007;114:205–209.
69. Medeiros FA, Weinreb RN, et al. Long-term intraocular pressure fluctuations and risk of conversion from OHT to glaucoma. *Ophthalmology.* 2008;115(6):934–940.
70. Leske MC, Heijl A, Hussein M, et al. Factors for glaucoma progression and the effect of treatment. The Early Manifest Glaucoma Trial. *Arch Ophthalmol.* 2003;121:48–56.
71. Collaborative Normal Tension Glaucoma Study Group. The effectiveness of intraocular pressure reduction in the treatment of normal tension glaucoma. *Am J. Ophthalmology.* 1998;126:498–505.
72. AGIS Investigators. The Advanced Glaucoma Intervention Study (AGIS); 7. The relationship between control of intraocular pressure and visual field deterioration. *Am J Ophthalmology.* 2000;130:429–440.
73. Lichter PR, Musch DC, Gillespie BW, et al. CIGTS Study Group. Interim clinical outcome in the Collaborative Initial Glaucoma Treatment Study comparing initial treatment randomized to medication or surgery. Ophthalmology. 2001;108:1943–1953.
74. Drance S. Anderson DR, Schulzer M. and the Collaborative Normal Tension Glaucoma Study Group. Risk factors for progression of visual field abnormalities in normal tension glaucoma. *Am J Opthalmol.* 2001;131:699–708.
75. Budenz DL, Anderson DR, Feuer WJ, et al. Detection and prognostic significance of optic disc hemorrhages during the Ocular Hypertension Treatment Study. Ophthalmology. 2006;113: 2137–2143.
76. Leske MC, Heijl A, Hyman L, et al. Predictors of long-term progression in the early manifest glaucoma trial. Ophthalmology. 2007;114(11):1965–1972.
77. Miglior S, Torri V, et al. Intercurrent factors associated with the development of OAG in the EGPS. *Am J Opthalmol.* 144(2):266–275.
78. Tielsch JM, Katz J, Sommer A, et al. Hypertension, perfusion pressure, and POAG. A population based assessment. Arch Ophthalmol. 1995;113:216–221.
79. Leske MC, Wu S-Y, Nemesure B, et al. Incident OAG and blood pressure. Arch Ophthalmol. 2002;120:954–959.
80. Bonomi L, Marchini G, Marraffa M, et al. Vascular risk factors for primary open angle glaucoma: the Egna-Neumarkt Study. Ophthalmology. 2000;107:1287–1293.
81. Armaly MF. Glaucoma (review). Arch Ophthalmol. 1972;88: 439–460.
82. Drance SM. Some factors in the production of low tension glaucoma. Br J Ophthalmol. 1972;56:229–242.
83. Klein BE, Klein R. Intraocular pressure and cardiovascular risk variables. Arch Ophthalmol. 1981;99:837–839.
84. Wilson MR, Hertzmark E, Walker AM, et al. A case-control of risk factors in open-angle glaucoma. Arch Ophthalmol. 1987;105: 1066–1071.
85. Goldberg I, Hollow FC, Kass MA, Becker B. Systemic factors in patients with low-tension glaucoma. Br J Ophthalmol. 1981;65: 56–62.
86. Drance SM. The concept of chronic open-angle glaucoma: a personal view (review). *Ophthalmologica.* 1996;210:251–256.

87. Schulzer M, Drance SM, Carter CJ, et al. Biostatistical evidence for two distinct chronic open angle glaucoma populations. *Br J Ophthalmol*. 1990;74:196–200.
88. Flammer J, Orgul S, et al. The impact of ocular blood flow in glaucoma. *Prog Retin Eye Res*. 2002;21:359–393.
89. Fuschsjager-Maryl G, Wally B, Georgopoulos M, et al. Ocular blood flow and systemic blood pressure in patients with POAG and OHT. *Invest Ophthalmol Vis Sci*. 2004;45:834–839.
90. Hayreh SS, Zimmerman MB, Podhajsky P, et al. Nocturnal arterial hypotension and its role in optic nerve head and ocular ischemic disorders. *Am J Opthalmol*. 1994;117:603–604.
91. Topouzis F, Coleman AL, Harris A, et al. Association of blood pressure status with the optic disc structure in non-glaucoma subjects: the Thessaloniki Eye Study. *Am J Opthalmol*. 2006;142:60–67.
92. Dielemans I, Vingerling JR, Hofman A, Grobbee DE, de Jong PT. Primary open angle glaucoma, intraocular pressure, and systemic blood pressure in the general elderly population. The Rotterdam Study. *Ophthalmology*. 1995;102(1):54–60.
93. Miglior S, Torri V, Zeyen T, et al. The European Glaucoma Prevention Study (EGPS) Group. Intercurrent factors associated with the development of open angle glaucoma in the European Glaucoma Prevention Study. *Am J Opthalmol*. 2007;144:266–275.
94. Punjabi OS, Stamper RL, Bostrom AG, et al. Does treated systemic hypertension affect progression of optic nerve damage in glaucoma subjects? *Curr Eye Res*. 2007;32:153–160.
95. Drance SL, Drance SM, Wijsman K, et al. Ambulatory blood pressure monitoring in glaucoma. The nocturnal dip. *Ophthalmology*. 102(1):61–69.
96. Graham SL, Drance SM. Nocturnal hypotension: role in glaucoma progression. *Surv Ophthalmology*. 1999;43(1):S10–S16.
97. Piltz-Seymour JR, Grunwald, JE, Hariprasad, SM, et al. Optic nerve blood flow is diminished in eyes of POAG suspects. *Am J Opthalmol*. 2001;132(1):63–69.
98. Gordon MO, Beiser JA, Brandt JD, et al. The Ocular Hypertension Treatment Study: baseline factors that predict the onset of POAG. *Arch Ophthalmol*. 2002;120:714–720.
99. Herndon LW, Weizer JS, Stinnett SS. Central corneal thickness as a risk factor for advanced glaucoma damage. *Arch Ophthalmol*. 2004;122:17–21.
100. Rogers DL, Cantor RN, Catoira Y, et al. Central corneal thickness and visual field loss in fellow eyes of patients with open angle glaucoma. *Am J Ophthalmol*. 2007;143(1):159–161.
101. Dueker DK, Singh K, Lin SC, et al. Corneal thickness measurement in the management of POAG. A report by the American Academy of Ophthalmology. *Ophthalmology*. 2007;114(9):1779–1787.
102. Wolfs RCW, Klaver CCW, Ramrattan RS, et al. Genetic risk of primary open angle glaucoma. Population-based familial aggregation study. *Arch Ophthalmol*. 1998;116:1640–1645.
103. Leske MC, Nemesure B, He Q, Wu S-Y, et al. Patterns of open angle glaucoma in the Barbados Family Study. *Ophthalmology*. 2001;108:1015–1022.
104. Martus P, Stroux A, Budde WM, et al. Predictive factors for progressive optic nerve damage in various types of chronic open-angle glaucoma. *Am J Opthalmol*. 2005;139(6):999–1009.
105. Budde WN, Jonas JB. Enlargement of parapapillary atrophy in follow up of chronic open–angle glaucoma. *Am J Opthalmol*. 2004;137(4):646–654.
106. Xu L, Wang Y, et al. Differences in parapapillary atrophy between glaucomatous and normal eyes: The Beijing Eye Study. *Am J Opthalmol*. 2007;144(4):541–546.
107. Girkin CA, McGwin G, McNeal SF, et al. Hypothyroidism and the development of open-angle glaucoma in a male population. *Ophthalmology*. 2004;111(9):1649–1652.
108. Kountouras J, Mylopoulos N, Boura P, et al. Relationship between Helicobacter pylori infection and glaucoma. *Ophthalmology*. 2001;108:599–604.
109. Galloway PH, Warner SJ, Morshed MG, et al. Helicobacter pylori infection and the risk for open-angle glaucoma. *Ophthalmology*. 2003;110(5):922–925.
110. Mojon DS, Hess CW, Goldblum D, et al. High prevalence of glaucoma in patients with sleep apnea syndrome. *Ophthalmology*. 1999;106(5):1009–1012.
111. Geyer O, Cohen N, Segev E, et al. The prevalence of glaucoma in patients with sleep apnea syndrome: same as in the general population. *Am J Opthalmol*. 136(6):1093–1096.
112. Robert PY, Adenis JP, Tapie P, et al. Eyelid hyperlaxity and obstructive sleep apnea (OSA) syndrome. *Eur J Ophthalmol*. 1997;7:211–215.
113. McNab AA. Floppy eyelid syndrome and obstructive sleep apnea. *Ophthal Plast Reconstr Surg*. 1997;13:98–114.
114. Kremmer S, Selbach JM, Ayertey HD, Steuhl KP. Normal tension glaucoma, sleep apnea syndrome and nasal continuous positive airway pressure therapy: case report with a review of literature. *Klin Monatsbl Augenheilkd*. 2001;218(4):263–268.
115. Costarides MDM, AP GP, et al. Sleep disorders: a risk factor for normal-tension glaucoma? *J Glaucoma*. 2001;10:177–183.
116. Goldblum D, Mathis J, Bohnke M, et al. Nocturnal measurements of intraocular pressure in patients with normal-tension glaucoma and sleep apnea syndrome. *Klin Monatsbl Augenheilkd*. 2000;216:246–249.
117. Walsh JT, Montplaisir J. Familial glaucoma with sleep apnea: a new syndrome? *Thorax*. 1982;37:845–849.
118. Mojon DS, Hess CW, Goldblum D, Bohnke M, et al. Primary open-angle glaucoma is associated with sleep apnea syndrome. *Ophthalmologica*. 2000;214:115–118.
119. Onen SH, Mouriaux F, Berrandane L, et al. High prevalence of sleep-disordered breathing in patients with primary open angle glaucoma. *Acta Ophthalmol Scand*. 2000;78:638–641.
120. Chauhan BC, Mikelberg FS, Balaszi AG, LeBlanc RP, et al. Canadian Glaucoma Study: 2. Risk factors for the progression of open-angle glaucoma. *Arch Ophthalmol*. 2008;126(8):1030–1036.
121. Friedman DS, Wilson MR, Liebmann, JM, et al. An evidence-based assessment of risk factors for the progression of ocular hypertension and glaucoma. *Am J Opthalmol*. 2004;138(3):S19–S31.
122. van Herick W, Shaffer RN, Schwarts A. Estimation of width of angle of anterior chamber. Incidence and significance of the narrow angle. *Am J Ophthalmol*. 1969;68:626–629.
123. Hoskins HD Jr, Kass MA. *Becker-Shaffer's Diagnosis and Therapy of the Glaucomas*. 6th ed. St. Louis: Mosby; 1989:106–116.
124. Scheie HG. Width and pigmentation of the angle of the anterior chamber. A system of grading by gonioscopy. *Arch Ophthalmol*. 1957;58:510–512.
125. American Academy of Ophthalmology. *Primary Open Angle Glaucoma, Preferred Practice Pattern*. San Francisco: American Academy of Ophthalmology, 2005. Available at www.aao.org/ppp.
126. Quigley HA, Friedman DS, Hahn SR. Evaluation of practice patterns for the care of open-angle glaucoma compared with claims data. The Glaucoma Adherence and Persistency Study. *Ophthalmology*. 2007;114(9):1599–1606.
127. Fremont AM, Lee PP, Mangione CM, Kapur K, et al. *Arch Ophthalmol*. 2003;121:777–783
128. Broadway DC, Nicolela MT, Drance SM. Optic disc appearances in POAG. *Surv Ophthalmol*. 1999;43(Suppl 1):S223–S243.
129. Bayer A, Harasymowycz P, Henderer JD, Steinmann WG, Spaeth GL. Validity of a new disk grading scale for estimating glaucomatous damage: correlation with visual field damage. *Am J Ophthalmol*. 133(6):758–763.
130. Kwon YH, Kim C-S, Zimmerman MB, Alward WL, Hayreh SS. Rate of visual field loss and long term visual outcome in POAG. *Am J Opthalmol*. 2001;132:47–56.
131. Rasker MT, van den Enden A, Bakker D, Hoyng PF. Rate of visual field loss in progressive glaucoma. *Arch Ophthal*. 2000;118:481–488.

132. Iwase A, Tomidokoro A, Araie M, et al. Performance of frequency doubling technology perimetry in a population based prevalence survey of glaucoma. The Tajimi Study. *Ophthalmology*. 2007; 114(1):27–32.
133. Lalezary M, Medeiros FA, Weinreb RN, et al. Baseline optical coherence tomography predicts the development of glaucomatous change in glaucoma suspects. *Am J Opthalmol*. 2006;142(4): 576e1–576e8.
134. Hong S, Ahn H, Ha SJ, et al. Early glaucoma detection using the Humphrey Matrix Perimeter, GDx VCC, Stratus OCT, and Retinal Nerve Fiber Layer Photography. *Ophthalmology*. 2007;114(2): 210–215.
135. Leeprechanon N, Giaconi JA, Manassakorn A, et al. Frequency doubling perimetry and short-wavelength automated perimetry to detect early glaucoma. *Ophthalmology*. 2007;114(5):931–937.
136. Leung CKS, Chan W-M, Yung W-H, et al. Comparison of macular and peripapillary measurements for the detection of glaucoma. An Optical Coherence Tomography Study. *Ophthalmology*. 2005; 112(3):391–400.
137. Bayer AU, Erb C. Short wavelength automated perimetry, frequency doubling technology perimetry, and pattern electroretinography for prediction of progressive glaucomatous standard visual field defects. *Ophthalmology*. 2002;109(5):1009–1017.
138. Lin SC, Singh K, Jampel HD, et al. Optic Nerve Head and Retinal Nerve Fiber Layer Analysis, A Report by the American Academy of Ophthalmology. Ophthalmology 2007;114(10):1937–1949
139. Collaborative Normal-Tension Glaucoma Study Group. The effectiveness of intraocular pressure reduction in the treatment of normal-tension glaucoma. *Am J Ophthalmol*. 1998;126:498–505.
140. Schappert-Kimmijser J. A five year follow up of subjects with intraocular pressure of 22–30 mmHg without anomalies of the optic nerve and visual field typical for glaucoma at first investigation. *Ophthalmologica*. 1971;162(4):289–295.
141. Armaly MF, Krueger DE, Maunder L. Becker B, Hetherington J, et al. Biostatistical analysis of the collaborative glaucoma study. I. Summary report of the risk factors for glaucomatous visual-field defects. *Arch Ophthalmol*. 1980;98:2163–71.
142. Leske MC, Wu S-Y, Hennis A, Honkanen R, Nemesure B, Barbados Eye Studies Group. *Ophthalmology*. 2008;115(1):85–93.
143. Hayreh SS, Zimmerman MB, Podhajsky P, Alward WL. Nocturnal arterial hypotension and its role in optic nerve head and ocular ischemic disorders. *Am J Ophthalmol*. 1994;117(5):603–624.
144. Collignon N, Dewe W, Guillame S, Collignon-Brach. Ambulatory blood pressure monitoring in glaucoma patients. The nocturnal systolic dip and its relationship with disease progression. *Int Ophthalmol*. 1998;22(1):19–25.
145. Lee P, Levin L, Walt J, et al. Cost of patients with POAG. A retrospective study of commercial insurance claims data. *Ophthalmology*. 2007;114(7):1241–1247.
146. Gerdtham K-NG, UG AA. Costs of treating primary open angle glaucoma and ocular hypertension: a retrospective, observational two year chart review of newly diagnosed patients in Sweden and the United States. *J Glaucoma*. 1998;7:95–104.
147. Lee PP, Walt JG, et al. A multicenter, retrospective pilot study of resource use and costs associated with severity of disease in glaucoma. *Arch Ophthalmol*. 2006;124:12–19.
148. Kymes SM, Kass MA, Anderson DR, et al. Management of ocular hypertension: a cost-effectiveness approach from the OHTS. *Am J Opthalmol*. 2006;1(6):997–1008.
149. Stewart WC, Stewart JA, Nassar, Q et al. Cost-effectiveness of treating ocular hypertension. *Ophthalmology*. 2008;115(1):94–98.
150. Pasquale LR, Dolgitser M, Wentzloff JN, et al. Health Care Charges for Patients with Ocular Hypertension or POAG. Presented in part at: American Glaucoma Society meeting, March 2006, Charleston, South Carolina, and Association for Research and Vision in Ophthalmology meeting, May 2006, Fort Lauderdale, Florida. Opthalmology. Received 8 February 2007; received in revised for 10 April 2007; accepted 16 April 2007. Published online 22 August 2007.
151. Robin AL, Cover, D. Does adjunctive glaucoma therapy affect adherence to the initial primary therapy? *Ophthalmology*. 2005; 112(5):863–868.
152. Amon M, Menapace R, et al. Aspekte der Betreuung von Glaukompatienten und deren Auswirkung auf die Compliance. *Spektrum Augenheilkd*. 1990;4:5–8.
153. Kass MA, Meltzer DW, Gordon M, et al. Compliance with topical pilocarpine treatment. *Am J Opthalmol*. 1986;101:515–523.
154. Nordstrom BL, Friedman DS, et al. Persistence and adherence with topical glaucoma therapy. *Am J Opthalmol*. 2005;140(4): 598e1–598e11.
155. Gwira JA, Vistamehr S, Shelsta H, et al. Factors associated with failure to follow up after glaucoma screening. A study in an African American population. *Ophthalmology*. 2006;113(8):1315–1319.
156. Olthoff CMG, Schouten JSAG, et al. Noncompliance with ocular hypotensive treatment in patients with glaucoma or ocular hypertension. An evidence-based review. *Ophthalmology*. 2005; 112(6):953–961.
157. Fecthner RD, Singh K. Maximal glaucoma therapy. *J Glaucoma*. 2001;10(Suppl. 1):S73–S75.
158. Stewart WC, Konstas AGP, et al. Meta-analysis of 24 hour intraocular pressure studies evaluating the efficacy of glaucoma medicines. Ophthalmology. 2007. Received 8 March 2007; received in revised for 7 September 2007; accepted 2 October 2007; published online 17 December 2007.
159. The Glaucoma Laser Trial (GLT) 2. Results of Alt VS topical medicines. The Glaucoma Laser Trial Group. *Ophthalmology*. 1990;97(11):1403–1413.
160. Juzych MS, Chopra V, Banitt MR, et al. Comparison of long-term outcomes of selective laser trabeculoplasty versus argon laser trabeculoplasty in open-angle glaucoma. *Ophthalmology*. 2004; 111(10):1853–1859.
161. Migdal C, Gregory W, Hitchings R. Long-term functional outcome after early surgery compared with laser and medicine in open angle glaucoma. *Ophthalmology*. 1994;101(10):1651–1656.
162. Lichter PR, Musch DC, Gillespie BW, et al. Interim clinical outcomes in the Collaborative Initial Glaucoma Treatment Study comparing initial treatment randomized to medications or surgery. *Ophthalmology*. 2001;108:1943–1953.
163. Singh K, Lee BL, Wilson R, Glaucoma Modified RAND-Like Methodology Group. A panel assessment of glaucoma management: modification of existing RAND-like methodology for consensus in ophthalmology. Part II: Results and interpretation. *Am J Ophthalmol*. 2008;145(3):575–581.

# Chapter 35
# Normal Pressure Glaucoma

Bruce E. Prum

In 1857, the German ophthalmologist von Graefe described glaucomatous optic disc excavation with a "normal" intraocular pressure (IOP) by digital palpation. He called this "amaurosis and nerve head excavation."[1,2] At that time and for many decades following, open-angle glaucoma with a "normal" IOP was considered a rarity. In 1980, Levene, in a landmark paper, reviewed the definitions and known literature about this entity, which he called "low-tension glaucoma" (LTG).[3] He outlined six historical definitions for LTG – one descriptive only and five both causal and descriptive. He concluded that because of the uncertainty in causation of this glaucoma entity, the best definition of LTG was a descriptive one and included:

1. acquired cupping of the optic nerve,
2. corresponding visual field defects,
3. open anterior chamber angles, and
4. intraocular pressures ≤24 mmHg.

Our current understanding of primary open-angle glaucoma (POAG) is that it constitutes an optic neuropathy with characteristic structural optic nerve damage and functional visual field loss, without regarding the level of IOP.

With the advent of tonometric techniques for measuring IOP more accurately (in particular Goldmann applanation tonometry (GAT) in the 1950s), large, population-based, epidemiologic studies were conducted in the 1960s and 1970s to better determine the range of IOP seen in normal and glaucomatous eyes. It became clear that glaucomatous optic neuropathy with a normal IOP <22 mmHg (the statistical upper limit of normal range) was more common than previously believed, comprising as high as 30–50% of patients with POAG (see Sect. 35.2). Terminology for glaucomatous optic nerve disease with a normal IOP has evolved, even as its pathogenesis remains controversial. Many clinicians have traditionally thought of NTG as separate from HTG, and there is merit to consider these forms of glaucoma as distinct clinical entities. For our purposes, we call this form of glaucoma "normal-tension glaucoma" (NTG), but it has also variously been named low-pressure glaucoma, normal-pressure glaucoma, or low-tension glaucoma.

## 35.1 Definition

NTG, as discussed throughout this chapter, is a primary optic neuropathy of unknown cause characterized by:

1. *statistically normal range IOP <22 mmHg* on diurnal or multiple day measurements (some studies allow one IOP ≥22 and ≤24 mmHg)
2. *optic disc cupping and associated retinal nerve fiber layer loss*, often with flame-shaped, nerve fiber layer hemorrhages, similar to primary open-angle glaucoma with elevated intraocular pressures (so-called "high-tension" or "high-pressure" glaucoma, HTG)
3. *visual field defects consistent with the appearance of the optic nerve damage*, typically nerve fiber bundle defects such as arcuate scotomas, nasal steps, or paracentral scotomas
4. *an open anterior chamber angle without evidence of other causes of possible previously elevated IOP*, such as peripheral anterior synechiae from prior uveitis or angle closure, or angle recession from trauma
5. *absence of other causes of visual field loss or optic nerve damage that could mimic glaucoma*, such as congenital disc anomalies, a myopic tilted disc, optic nerve or pituitary/chiasmal tumors, previous ischemic optic neuropathy, cardiogenic shock or other nonrecurring vascular insult, where disc damage is typically nonprogressive.

## 35.2 Epidemiology

### 35.2.1 Population Studies

The IOP level at which the diagnosis of glaucomatous optic neuropathy has been made varies from the single digits to more than 50 mmHg. This modern understanding of the importance of IOP reduction for the treatment of all glaucomas is supported by many multicenter, randomized, prospective trials.[4–10]

Many studies of NTG have concluded that the prevalence of NTG among glaucoma patients is high but variable, depending on the population studied. These wide variations in observed prevalence are undoubtedly due to varying definitions of NTG based on optic nerve and visual field criteria without regard to diurnal IOP fluctuations or masqueraders of NTG.

## 35.2.2 Clinical Studies

In a large population-based study of almost 33,000 individuals in Malmo, Sweden, NTG was identified as the most frequent glaucoma diagnosis (52.9%) in newly diagnosed patients.[11] The detection of NTG was four times more common among unselected screened individuals (62% of whom had previously seen an ophthalmologist) compared with self-selected patients identified from routine clinical practice. The authors concluded that NTG is easily overlooked.

NTG prevalence varies widely among different ethnic populations. In the Baltimore Eye Survey (1991), the prevalence of POAG ranged from 1.3% with IOP 16–18 mmHg and 1.8% with IOP 19–21 mmHg up to as high as 26% for IOPs ≥35 mmHg.[12] Half of white and black patients with POAG had a screening IOP less than 21 mmHg, decreasing to 25% after one follow-up IOP and 15% after multiple follow-up IOPs. The incidence of POAG increased steadily with IOP elevation in both groups, but 16.7% of patients were ultimately diagnosed with NTG. In the recent Barbados Eye Study (2007) among Caribbean blacks of African ancestry, incident POAG was diagnosed in 4.4% of all followed-up patients and incident NTG was seen in one-third of all newly diagnosed cases over a 9-year period.[13]

In the Rotterdam Eye Study in Holland (1994) among whites, POAG prevalence was 1.1% overall with 38.9% of these diagnosed with NTG.[14] In the Egna–Neumarkt Study (1998) of mainly white individuals in northern Italy, the prevalence of POAG was 1.4% and NTG was 0.6%.[15] In the Blue Mountains Eye Study (1996) in Australia among white individuals, the prevalence of POAG increased from 0.9% with IOP 12–13 mmHg to 5.7% with IOP 22–23 mmHg, rising to 39% for IOP ≥28 mmHg.[16] In the recent Thessaloniki Eye Study in Greece (2007) among all white individuals, the prevalence of POAG varied from 2.7% to 3.8% depending upon the definition, but NTG with IOP ≤21 mmHg represented 59% of those identified.[17]

In the Los Angeles Latino Eye Study (2004) among Latinos of Mexican ancestry, the incidence of POAG was 4.4%.[18] IOP ≤21 mmHg was seen in 82% of these individuals. In the Tajimi Study in Japan (2004), overall POAG prevalence was 3.9%, comprised of NTG with IOP ≤21 mmHg in 3.6% and POAG with IOP ≥21 mmHg in 0.3%.[19] In rural India (2005), prevalence of POAG was 1.6% with NTG diagnosed in 67% of identified patients.[20] Clearly, NTG is a very common condition worldwide.

## 35.3 Risk Factors for NTG

### 35.3.1 IOP-Related

#### 35.3.1.1 Diurnal–Nocturnal Variation and Fluctuation of IOP

The Collaborative Normal Tension Glaucoma Study (CNTGS) (1998) was a randomized trial of treatment comparing reduction of IOP by 30% with observation in progressive NTG patients. It showed that aggressive IOP reduction could reduce progression of glaucomatous disease from 35% to 12% during approximately 5 years of follow-up.[5] Also, we know that IOP fluctuates during the waking day (diurnal variation) and while asleep at night (nocturnal variation), and from one office visit to another (usually between 8 AM to 5 PM). So, is it possible that some patients with "apparent" NTG may have IOPs that are much higher outside clinic exam hours or have increased IOP in the supine position during sleep? These "high" IOPs that occur outside the office visit time frame need to be considered when deciding a patient meets the criteria for NTG versus traditional HTG.

Several studies have demonstrated that IOP may peak when measured at times other than the usual time of office visits. Yamagami et al showed that in NTG patients mean diurnal IOP variation was 4.9 mmHg and peak IOPs most often occurred at 10 AM, but that 55% of peak IOPs occurred between 6 PM and 8 AM, outside usual clinic hours.[21] In another study, however, these researchers found that peak 24-h IOPs could be predicted from an average of six clinic IOPs.[22] A third 24-h IOP study concluded that IOP variation in NTG patients was similar to normal subjects and that sleep had little influence on 24-h IOP variation.[23] Sequential, day-long, office IOP measurements have recently been shown useful to help identify selected NTG patients demonstrating visual field deterioration with supposedly "controlled" IOP.[24] IOPs were all highest in the early morning hours in NTG, POAG, and glaucoma-suspect patients. IOP variations >5 mmHg were seen in 35% of subjects, and in the NTG group, there was a significant correlation between visual field deterioration and IOP peak and range, suggesting the importance of these factors to predict progression in NTG.

Diurnal IOPs in NTG patients ≤15 mmHg have been more frequently associated with retinal nerve fiber layer (RNFL) defects closer to fixation than in eyes with diurnal IOPs >15 mmHg.[25] The width of RNFL defects seen in this study, however, was not different between the two groups. These findings were interpreted by the authors to indirectly support an alternative pathogenesis for optic nerve damage other than direct IOP-related causation in NTG, such as optic nerve ischemia due to sectoral vascular insufficiency from small branches of the short posterior ciliary arteries supplying the laminar and prelaminar optic nerve.

Diurnal 24-h IOPs in NTG patients have also been observed to show a general decline over time or in relation to patient age. In one prospective Japanese study, one-ninth of patients with NTG were observed to have declining untreated IOPs over 3 years.[26] Yet, in another cross-sectional study of NTG patients after 4 weeks of medication washout, the mean, maximum, minimum, and IOP variation over 24 h did not differ between two patient groups divided by age <60 years versus >60 years. But 24-h IOP in this study correlated negatively with patient age >60 years.[27]

### 35.3.1.2 Asymmetry of Disease and IOP

A number of studies during the past 25 years have demonstrated asymmetric optic nerve and visual field damage in some NTG patients, that is, the most-affected eye has a higher IOP.[28-31] Note, however, that 24-h IOP in HTG eyes showed striking concordance of IOP variation between fellow eyes of 1.6–2.0 mmHg, and the estimated probability of a 2 mmHg difference was 68–90% and a 3 mmHg difference was 78–95% for all time intervals studied.[32] More recently, these same researchers looked at the diurnal IOP fluctuation in untreated glaucoma suspect (GS) and NTG eyes.[33] They took six IOP measurements from 7 AM to 10 PM to evaluate the concordance of IOP between fellow eyes. The mean absolute IOP difference between eyes was 1.4–1.9 mmHg in the GS eyes and 1.3–1.5 mmHg for the NTG eyes (correlation between fellow NTG eyes, $r=0.81$). The probability that the difference in IOP between fellow NTG eyes ranged within 3 mmHg was 86–93%. These more recent studies bring into question the likelihood that true 24-h IOP asymmetry, which was not measured in the early studies, was the cause of the observed intereye disease asymmetry. As a result, one might postulate non-IOP-related factors, which were incorrectly attributed to the difference in measured daytime IOPs, explain the observed asymmetry between fellow eyes of those NTG patients studied earlier.

Nocturnal, supine IOP rise may play a significant role in optic nerve damage seen clinically as "daytime" NTG. Even though we may never practically know how much our individual patients' IOPs may rise during sleep, nevertheless we can and should lower their daytime office IOPs with the most effective agents or interventions. We now know that prostaglandin analogs, laser trabeculoplasty (LTP) and surgical IOP lowering are the most effective interventions to lower daytime IOP and reduce 24-h fluctuations in IOP measured in the laboratory setting (see sections on medical, laser, and surgical therapy for details). Therefore, we should choose the best IOP-lowering therapy for each patient individually, based on the stage of disease, demonstrated rate of progression, life expectancy and willingness of the patient to engage in joint management of his or her own disease.

A number of studies have confirmed a thinner CCT (measured in μm by ultrasonic pachymetry) in NTG eyes vs. normal eyes vs. HTG eyes vs. OHT eyes, respectively. African-American patients have similarly been found with relatively thin CCTs in other population studies. For example, investigators found a similar CCT in normal eyes of Caucasians, Asians, and Hispanics (~550 μm), but thinner corneas in African-Americans (535 μm).[34] A recent study of 1,699 normal Latino eyes in Los Angeles found a normal CCT of 547 μm, in the same range as normal Caucasian, Chinese, Hispanic, and Filipino eyes studied elsewhere.[35]

Thin CCT was associated with localized retinal nerve fiber defects in NTG eyes,[36] with increased visual field defects (VFDs) at initial diagnosis but not with progression in POAG eyes,[37] with visual field progression in POAG eyes (529 vs. 547 μm for progressing vs. nonprogressing eyes),[38] and with a smaller IOP reduction in response to topical ocular hypotensive medications in OHT eyes.[39] From all evidence, consideration of CCT and its role in the diagnosis and progression of glaucoma is very important, with a thin CCT definitely associated with glaucomatous optic nerve and visual field damage and even response to IOP-lowering therapy.

In summary, in my practice I measure CCT in all glaucoma suspects and patients. If CCT is very thin (e.g., less than 500 μm), with an IOP <22 mmHg after multiple office-hour IOP measurements, and I suspect or diagnose NTG based on disc damage and/or VFDs, then I typically aim for a goal of at least a 30% IOP lowering (as supported by the CNTGS findings) with perhaps 5–10% more lowering tacked on as a clinical "safety-factor" for the unknown underestimation of true IOP.

Although this relationship of a thin CCT and NTG appears clear from multiple studies worldwide, new findings further confuse this seemingly simple association. In 2005, engineers modeled the biomechanics of the cornea and its relationship to IOP measured by GAT.[40] "Young's modulus of elasticity" sums all the elements that make up the biomechanical properties of corneal tissue; e.g., a cornea may be thick but soft, or thin and stiff in relation to applanation tonometry, and hence may affect IOP measurement unpredictably based on these multiple factors unrelated to CCT. They determined that Young's modulus was a more important determinant of error introduced into GAT (potentially affecting measurements of IOP by up to ~17 mmHg) than CCT or corneal curvature (which according to their model potentially affect IOP measurements by only 2.87 and 1.76 mmHg, respectively).

Iliev et al in 2007 attempted to overcome the limitations of our current knowledge about CCT and IOP as measured by GAT.[41] They proposed the "pressure-to-cornea index" ($PCI = IOP/CCT^3$, with IOP being the highest recorded IOP without treatment in mmHg and CCT measured in mm to integrate the combined risks of IOP and CCT for developing glaucoma). They found the PCI of normal eyes = 92, NTG eyes = 129, OHT eyes = 134, and HTG eyes = 174. Examining eyes with IOPs of 16–29 mmHg, they looked at the ability of the PCI to discriminate glaucoma eyes (NTG and HTG) from nonglaucoma eyes (controls and OHT) compared with three published formulas to correct IOP for CCT. They concluded that a PCI = 120–140 is the upper limit for "normality," with 120 as the cutoff for eyes with IOP ≤21 mmHg (i.e., NTG) and 140 the cutoff for eyes with IOP ≥22 mmHg (i.e., HTG). They even suggested that a treatment goal should be to lower the PCI to <100, the measured level for most normal eyes. However, the prognostic value of this index has not yet been proven in longitudinal studies. Much more work needs to be done to sort out the actual contribution of corneal factors as represented by CCT or eye tissue biomechanics to IOP estimation and optic nerve susceptibility to glaucoma damage.

To summarize the above studies:

1. CCT does appear to be significantly reduced in many eyes with NTG, and
2. A thin CCT is a risk factor for the diagnosis and progression of glaucomatous disc and visual field damage.

Eyes with a thin CCT may have higher IOPs than presumed by GAT and not be true NTG eyes (but HTG eyes). It is also logically possible that a thin CCT represents an inherent structural abnormality associated with the damage seen in glaucomatous optic discs and reflects an underlying structural weakness of the supportive collagen in the lamina cribrosa. Thus an inherent susceptibility to IOP-related damage occurs, even at normal IOP levels, which leads to loss of retinal ganglion cell axons over time. This of course then results in classic glaucomatous optic nerve cupping and visual field loss as seen in NTG.[42,43]

### 35.3.1.3 Different Measurement Techniques for a More "Accurate" IOP

A number of devices have been developed as alternatives to the GAT to attempt to measure IOP in settings of abnormal, irregular, scarred, pathologic, and postsurgical corneas (e.g., nystagmus, corneal edema, posttraumatic, keratoconus, Fuchs endothelial dystrophy, after corneal transplant, post-PRK, or post-LASIK). A more detailed discussion of these newer IOP measuring devices is found elsewhere in this book. Briefly, DCT has generally been found to be less affected by CCT than GAT, although not in all studies, and tends to measure IOP slightly higher than GAT. IOP measurements by pneumatonometer, TonoPen, and NCT all appear to be dependent on CCT, with the NCT most dependent and the TonoPen least dependent on CCT. The ORA seems to measure IOP independent of the effect of CCT and higher than GAT, while RBT measurements correlate with GAT and appear to be affected by CCT. The pressure phosphene tonometer has a wide variability in its ability to measure IOP accurately because of its very subjective end point in IOP determination. For the time being, the GAT still remains the IOP measurement device standard; it remains to be seen if future work may replace it with a newer device. As a practical matter, clinicians should check and calibrate their Goldmann tonometers monthly to avoid introducing additional measurement variability into inherent physiological variability of IOP.[44,45]

### 35.3.1.4 Effect of LASIK/PRK on IOP

The recent popularity of corneal refractive surgery such as photorefractive keratectomy (PRK) and laser assisted in situ keratomileusis (LASIK) has impacted the ophthalmologist caring for glaucoma patients. The corneal thinning resulting from these procedures results in underestimates of true, manometric IOP when using GAT. This may result in a generation of the overdiagnosis of NTG or underdiagnosis of true HTG in many patients if the examiner is either unaware of the corneal surgery or does not account for it when measuring IOP. Even when the physician is concerned about the effect of such corneal thinning, it is not clear as to which IOP measurement devices are most suitable for accurate measurement of true intraocular pressure. Generally, IOP measurements by GAT and NCT[46] are 2–5 mmHg lower after PRK/LASIK, depending on the amount of refractive correction achieved.[47–49] IOPs measured by the TonoPen[50] and pneumatonometer[51,52] appear less affected by refractive thinning. Measurement of IOP on the nasal, nonaffected cornea has been advocated to lessen the measurement inaccuracy.[53] Recent studies have suggested that IOP readings by the Pascal DCT are not affected by PRK/LASIK corneal thinning.[54–56] However, IOP measurements by the ORA are significantly reduced, with associated decreases in corneal hysteresis and corneal resistance factor, suggesting that LASIK permanently alters the viscoelastic properties of the cornea.[56] Finally, several correction algorithms for IOP following LASIK have been derived. These formulas may be considered when preoperative information about an individual patient is missing.[57–61]

In summary, the best and most pragmatic advice at this time is to obtain good baseline, office-hour IOP measurements before anticipated refractive surgery and then again, several months after surgery, when the patient is off all topical steroids. The difference in the average pre- and postoperative IOPs would be the patient's individual IOP correction factor. In the absence of preoperative data, perhaps one of the previously cited correction algorithms could be utilized.

### 35.3.2 Optic-Nerve Related

#### 35.3.2.1 Optic Disc Size

The optic nerve transmits to the brain the retinal ganglion cell axons gathered from a total retinal area of more than 1,000 mm$^2$, concentrated down into an area of 2–3 mm$^2$. Although anatomically small in size, the optic disc is the key intraocular structure we study to help discriminate normal from abnormal with respect to diagnosing and following glaucoma patients[62] (Fig. 35.1). The normal optic nerve has about 970,000 ± 240,000 axons, with a normal rate of age-related loss of about 4,900 axons per year.[63] The number of axons in the optic nerve is fairly constant from person to person, despite varying sizes of the scleral canal outlet. There is no significant correlation between axon count and size of the scleral canal, which ranges from 1.6 to 2.9 mm$^2$ in pathology specimens of normal eyes.[64] Clinically, optic disc area can range in extremes from 0.8 to 6 mm$^2$.[65] Some have suggested that a larger optic disc is more susceptible to IOP-induced damage.

Are myopia and optic disc size associated with NTG? In 1972, Tomlinson and Leighton compared the eyes of 11 NTG patients matched with respect to sex, age, and refractive with nonglaucomatous persons and HTG patients.[66] They found NTG eyes to have a longer overall axial length, with an increased cup-to-disc ratio (C/D), compared with normal and HTG eyes, although axial lengths and C/Ds did not differ between groups. Tomita et al used computerized image analysis to study the optic nerves in 26 NTG patients.[67] They found a larger optic disc area and a higher mean IOP, associated with greater visual field loss, in 8 of 22 patients with disc size and IOP asymmetry, suggesting a greater vulnerability to IOP in eyes with larger discs. However, in 1995, Jonas et al did not find any association between disc size, measured by morphometry, and visual field loss in NTG patients, but noted more cupping and visual field loss in eyes with the smaller disc, suggesting a selection bias in the earlier studies.[68]

#### 35.3.2.2 Comparisons of High- and Normal-Tension Glaucoma Discs

In his comprehensive article on NTG in 1980, Levene reviewed a total of 767 NTG cases.[3] He concluded that certain characteristics were more common in NTG than HTG. These features were:

1. Early, dense visual field defects extending to within 5° of fixation
2. Sudden visual field loss

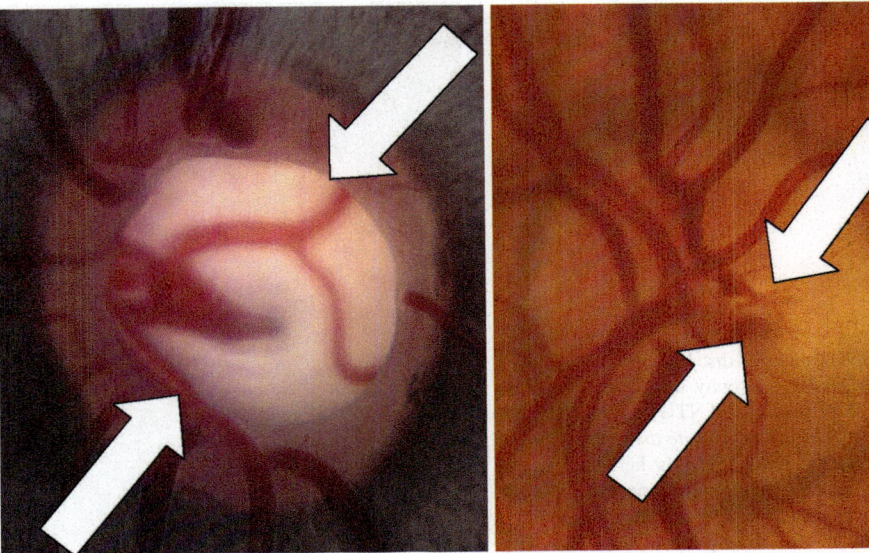

**Fig. 35.1** Two normal but differently sized optic discs with different cup/disc ratios (between the *white arrows* in figure 35.2). Note the large disc on the left with C/D ~0.6 in a 14-year-old African-American male, and the small disc with C/D ~0.2 in a 47-year-old Caucasian female. Both patients had normal RNFL thicknesses by OCT and normal visual fields

3. Early involvement of fixation
4. Slow progression of the field defect
5. A disproportion between the marked disc cupping noted and the limited, but centrally located, detectable visual field defects
6. High frequency of monocular cases
7. Female preponderance
8. Limited "sensitivity" of the field defect to even a marked reduction in IOP

Have these findings held up in studies subsequent to Levene's review? The finding of greater disc cupping associated with less generalized loss of visual field mean sensitivity, but a deeper central visual field loss, was confirmed by Gramer et al[69] but not by Lewis et al.[70] Caprioli and Spaeth examined eyes with early to moderate visual field loss and found the optic disc rim in NTG eyes to be significantly thinner inferiorly and infero-temporally than in HTG eyes with an average IOP 15 mmHg higher than the NTG eyes.[71] But they did not find comparative differences in disc pallor, peripapillary atrophy (PPA), disc hemorrhage, nasal cupping vessel overpass, and baring of the circumlinear vessels between groups. Cup contour was judged to be more gradually sloped toward the rim in NTG than HTG eyes, but HTG eyes had a steeper cup wall farther from the disc edge than in NTG. They also found initial VFDs to be closer to fixation in NTG and more peripheral, but progressing centrally, in HTG. They felt that their findings implied a different pathogenesis of optic nerve damage in these two groups, with NTG eyes more susceptible to vascular optic nerve injury and HTG eyes more susceptible to barotrauma, rather than vascular injury. These findings were confirmed by Heidelberg Retinal Tomography (HRT) in a study by Eid et al, who found larger cup areas and C/D ratios, smaller inferior neuroretinal rim (NRR) area, and a greater mean deviation of the superior rather than inferior arcuate visual field zone in NTG eyes, compared with HTG eyes.[72] They felt this indicated more vulnerability of the optic nerve to focal damage in NTG eyes. By contrast, Iester and Mikelberg[73] and Iester[74] did not find any differences in the optic nerve parameters measured by HRT between NTG and HTG eyes.

Others have compared the optic nerves of NTG and HTG patients. Tezel et al found only increased disc hemorrhages and arteriolar narrowing in NTG eyes.[75] Wang et al[76] found only an increase in PPA in NTG eyes with IOP ≤15 mmHg, while Miller and Quigley[77] found no differences between the two groups, except that an "hourglass appearance" of connective tissue bundles within the scleral lamina cribrosa was less common in NTG eyes. Miller and Quigley proposed that inherent, underlying differences in optic nerve head architecture of the lamina cribrosa that they observed might explain the variable sensitivity to IOP between HTG and NTG eyes.

### 35.3.2.3 Patterns of Optic Nerve Damage Observed in NTG Eyes

Attempts have been made to discriminate NTG from HTG based on observed patterns of optic disc cupping (focal vs. diffuse enlargement), disc hemorrhage occurrence, pattern of loss of the NRR, amount of PPA, amount and appearance of RNFL atrophy (localized vs. diffuse), and myopic tilting of the nerve (Figs. 35.2–35.6). Spaeth has written that "LTG is not a valid clinical entity, just as HTG is not a valid clinical

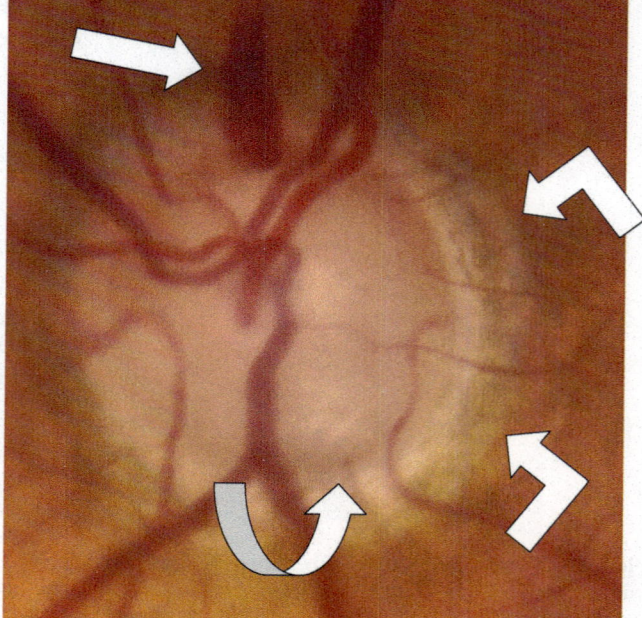

**Fig. 35.2** Color disc photograph of an optic disc hemorrhage, acquired pit of the optic nerve, and peripapillary atrophy in the left eye of an 84-year-old Caucasian male with very advanced NTG. A typical, flame-shaped, optic disc hemorrhage (ODH, *straight white arrow*) seen at the 12 o'clock position in the left eye. Note that this hemorrhage has occurred in an area of thinned, but relatively retained, neural rim at the superior pole of the disc (vertical cup/disc=0.9). By contrast, note the loss of the inferior neural rim at the 5–6 o'clock position, with focal deep excavation (an acquired pit of the optic nerve, APON, *curved white arrow*), associated focal pallor and visible lamina cribrosa pores deep in the cup. Note also typical, mild, β-zone peripapillary atrophy (*angled white arrows*) temporally and inferiorly beyond the disc margin

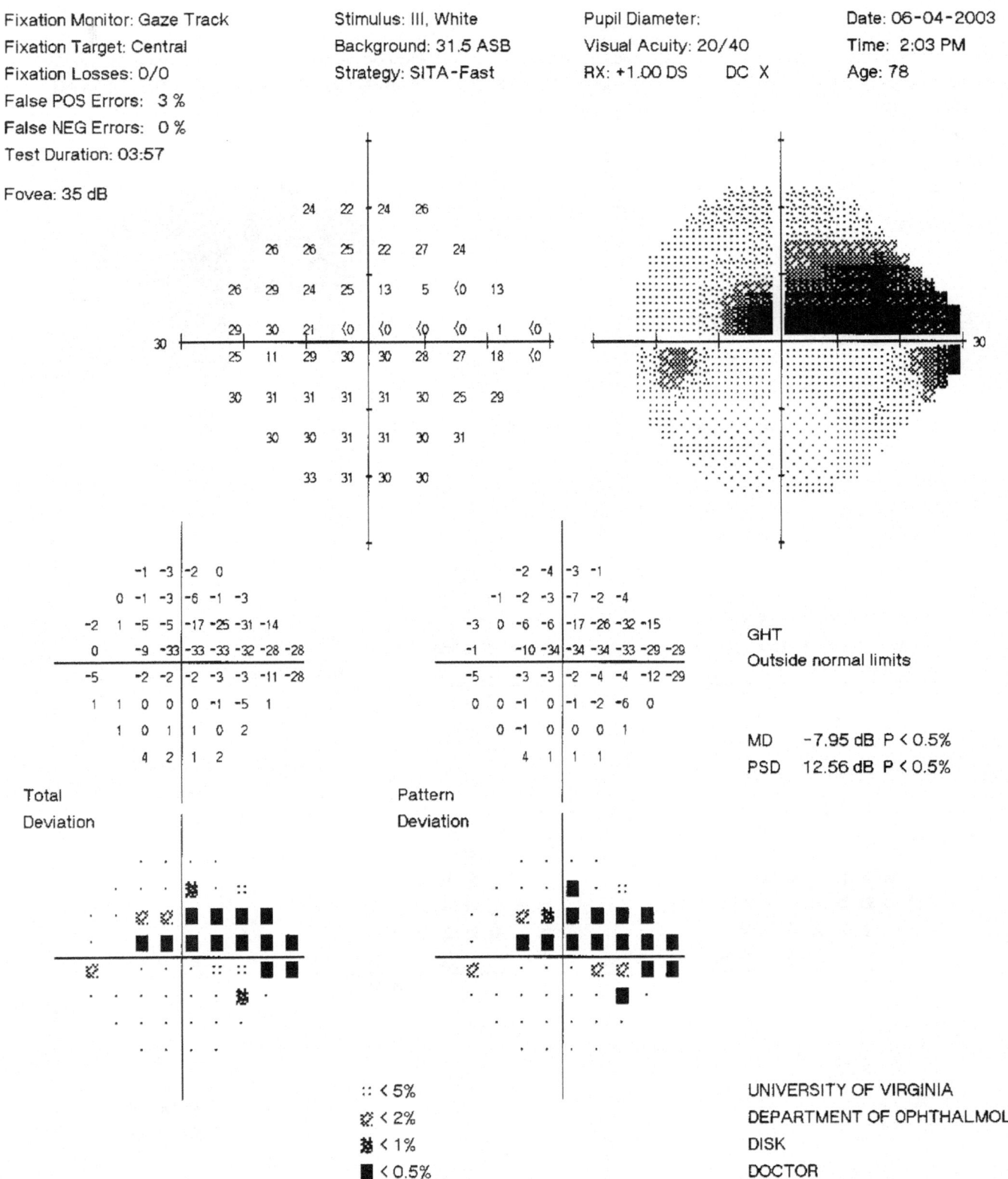

**Fig. 35.3** SITA standard 24-2 visual field of the NTG patient in Fig. 35.2. Note the dense superior arcuate scotoma (overall MD= −7.95), encroaching on the point 3° superonasal to fixation (−34 db), in this 24-2 visual field with 6° spacing of test points. This defect corresponds to the extensive loss of the inferior nerve rim. Note also that, despite the significant cupping of the optic disc seen in Figure 35.2, the inferior visual field only has an inferonasal scotoma, corresponding to the thin superior neural rim area where the dense ODH is located. Future follow-up will need to look carefully for changes in this region. The single, dense paracentral defect is expanded in the 10-2 field, with 2° spacing of test points, shown in Figure #4

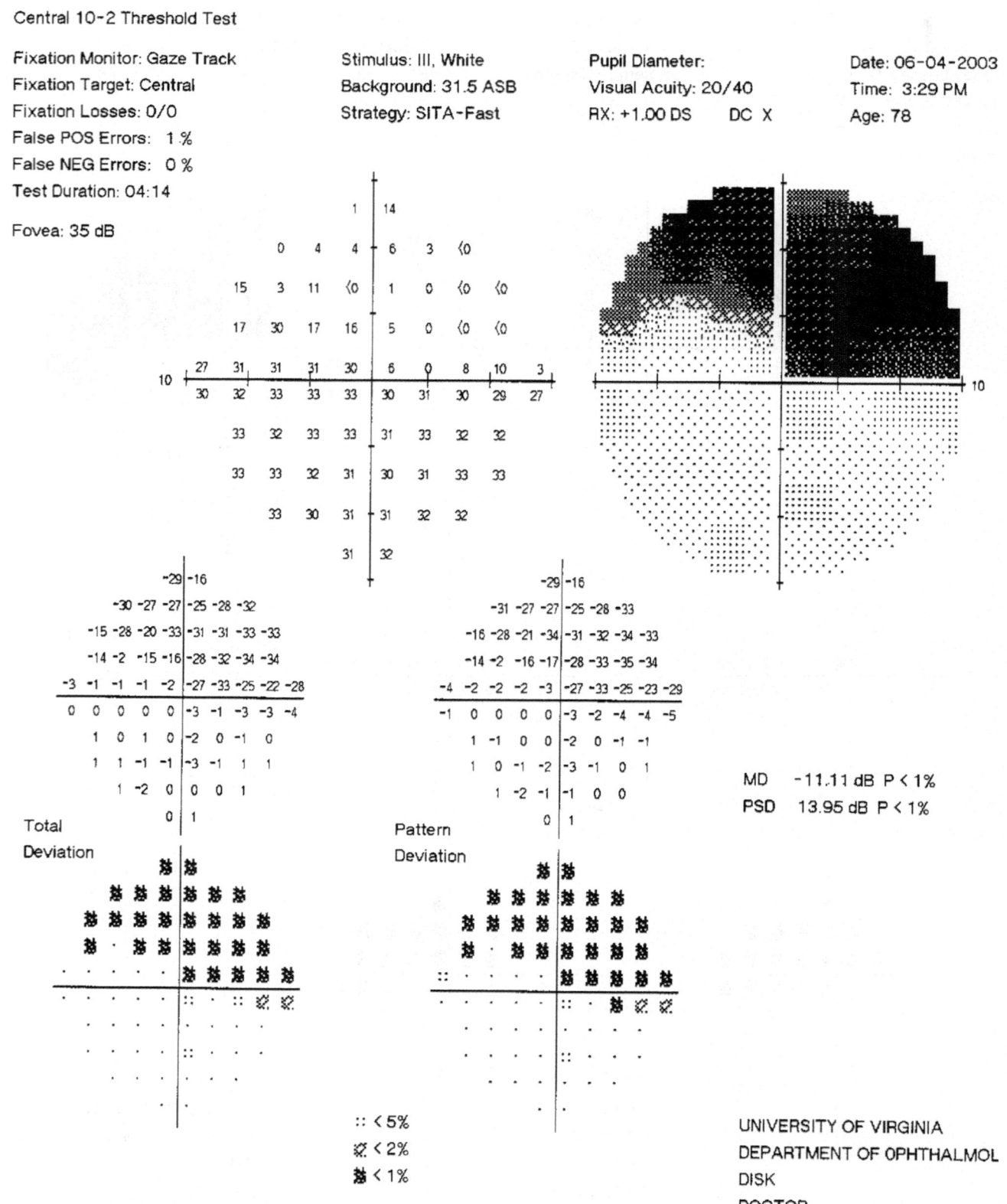

**Fig. 35.4** SITA standard 10-2 visual field of the NTG patient in Fig. 35.2. Note the dense superior visual field loss (MD= −11.11) to within 1° of fixation, associated with the deep APON seen in the disc photo in Fig. 35.2

| | OD (N=3) | OS (N=3) | OD-OS |
|---|---|---|---|
| Imax/Smax | 0.60 | 0.61 | -0.02 |
| Smax/Imax | 1.68 | 1.63 | 0.05 |
| Smax/Tavg | 1.63 | 2.03 | -0.40 |
| Imax/Tavg | 0.97 | 1.25 | -0.27 |
| Smax/Navg | 1.96 | 1.88 | 0.08 |
| Max-Min | 79.00 | 61.00 | 18.00 |
| Smax | 115.00 | 95.00 | 20.00 |
| Imax | 69.00 | 58.00 | 11.00 |
| Savg | 64.00 | 71.00 | -7.00 |
| Iavg | 56.00 | 49.00 | 7.00 |
| Avg.Thickness | 62.27 | 54.41 | 7.86 |

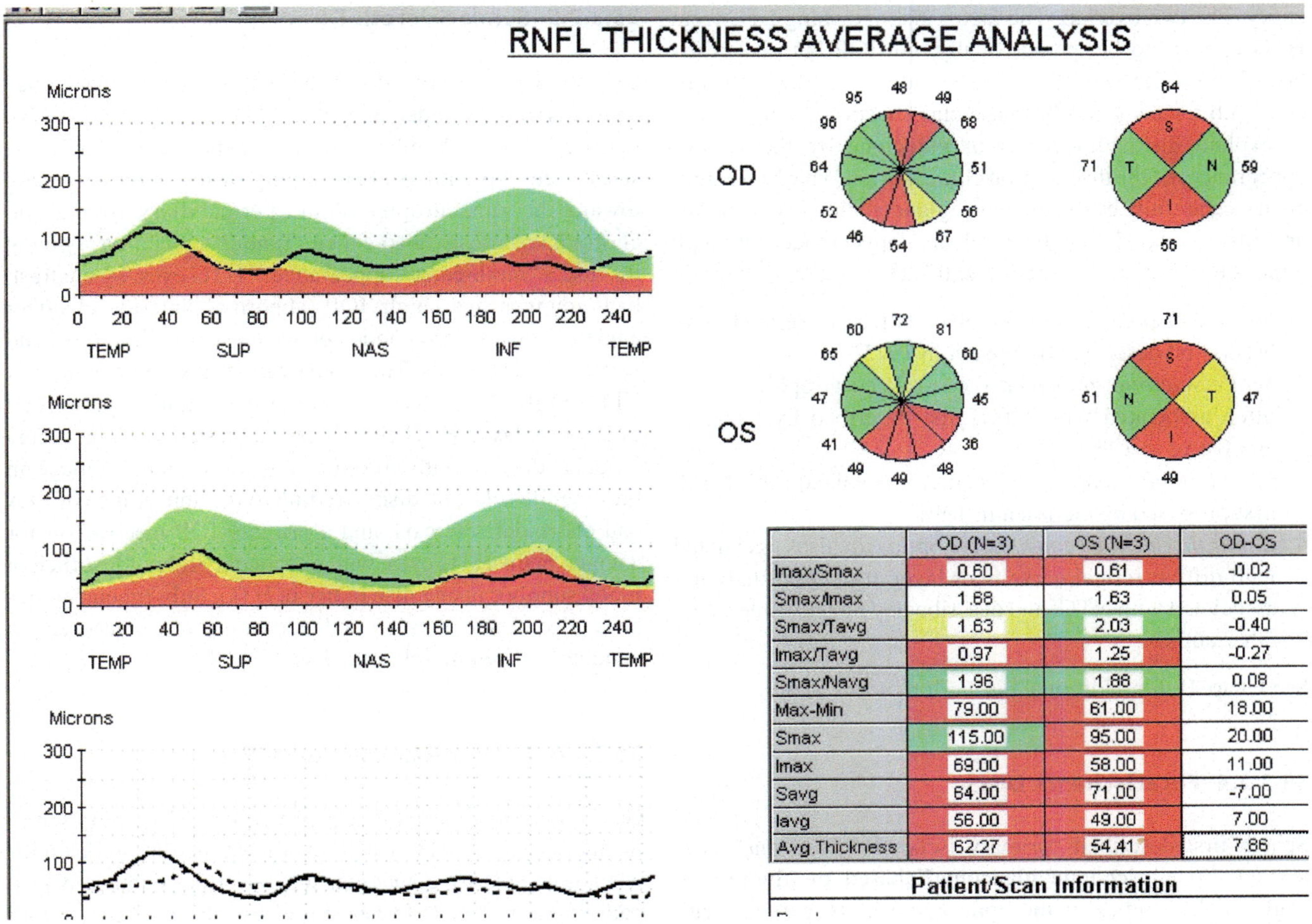

**Fig. 35.5** Optical coherence tomography of the peripapillary RNFL of the NTG patient in Figs. 35.2–35.5. The 12 o'clock sector OCT NFL thickness OS is still normal at 72 μm, compared to a markedly thinned NFL of 49 μm at the 6 o'clock sector OS (seen in the 12-clock-hour, pie pictograph, second from the top in the middle of the OCT printout). The patient's superior OCT NFL thickness OS (represented by the *black line* in the second TSNIT graph on the *center left*) is still in the green normal zone at 12 o'clock, but dips into the borderline yellow zone in the neighboring 11 and 1 o'clock sectors (seen in both the TSNIT graph and the pie pictograph). OCT here appears to detect early NFL loss in the two sectors flanking the 12 o'clock ODH and suggests the need for careful follow-up for future progressive thinning of the NFL in this region

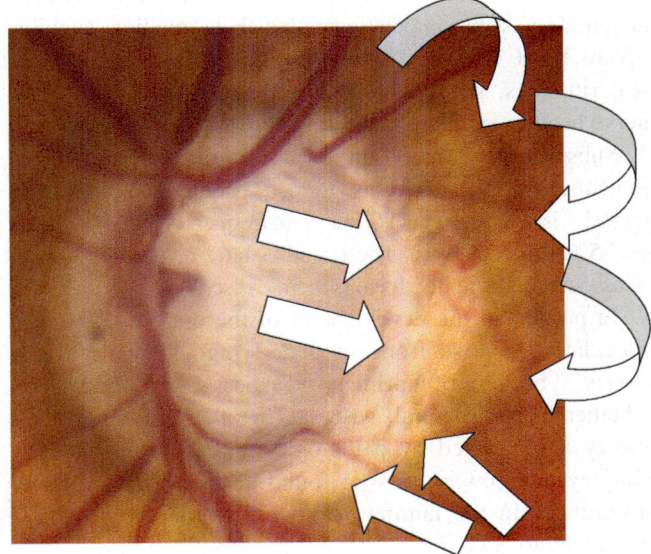

**Fig. 35.6** Color disc photograph of typical β-zone (white crescent of atrophy adjacent to the temporal edge of the disc, *straight arrows*) and α-zone (mottled area outside the area of alpha atrophy, *curved arrows*) peripapillary atrophy in the left eye of an 88-year-old female patient with extremely advanced NTG (C/D 0.95+). Note also the marked disc cupping, laminar pores visible in the depth of the cup, and loss of both superior and inferior disc neural rims

entity. The two overlap. The factor distinguishing LTG from HTG appears to be, paradoxically, not IOP but disk resistance."[78] Yet, he and others have studied the glaucomatous disc with a view toward disease classification, in an attempt to explain the pathogenesis of glaucoma by the various appearances of the disc seen on clinical exam. These researchers have carefully evaluated many glaucomatous optic nerves and discriminated four types of disc appearance, although none is exclusively associated with NTG:

1. *Focal ischemic glaucoma* discs often associated with NTG, first described by Spaeth in 1975[78]
2. *Senile sclerotic glaucoma* ("age-related atrophic") discs often associated with NTG, first described by Geijssen and Greve in 1987[79]
3. *Myopic glaucomatous* discs often associated with NTG, first proposed by Geijssen in 1991[80]
4. *Generalized enlargement of the optic cup* discs associated with diffuse retinal nerve fiber layer atrophy, usually not associated with NTG, and described by Spaeth[78] and many other authors.

See Chap. 18 for additional discussion of this topic.

### 35.3.2.4 Focal Ischemic Discs

Spaeth first described "primary ischemic glaucoma," later termed "focal ischemic glaucoma," based on fluorescein angiography studies of the optic nerve in 16 patients with clinical NTG.[78] These eyes were characterized by inferotemporal disc hypofluorescence; shallow and eccentric disc cupping with more pallor than expected; associated disc hemorrhages; and dense, often absolute, superior, paracentral scotomas, frequently noted by the patient. He did not comment on the amount of cupping compared to the visual field. In the NTG patients with this focally damaged disc appearance, he found a possible association with diabetes mellitus, syphilis, severe heart disease, "hemodynamic crises," and platelet abnormalities, suggesting localized ischemia of the optic nerve head to explain the disc injury.

Subsequent studies[81-87] have all confirmed that the focal ischemic disc appearance, also termed "acquired pit of the optic nerve,"[83] is seen also in HTG but more frequently in NTG (~15% vs. 75%, respectively[83]). These studies have revealed a number of associations with the focal ischemic disc.

In particular, the development of the optic pit has been speculated to arise from an underlying "laminar insufficiency"[83] because of a primary weakness of the optic nerve, whether from structural, vascular, or other etiologies. This theory is supported by pathologic findings from work by Quigley and coworkers who found a number of structural differences in the lamina cribrosa of patients with NTG compared to HTG.[88,89]

### 35.3.2.5 Senile Sclerotic Discs

Geijssen and Greve first described "senile sclerotic glaucoma" characterized by older age, relatively low IOP (or NTG), normal anterior chamber angles, "senile excavation" or a saucerized cup with gradual sloping of the optic nerve cup toward the rim, atrophy of the peripapillary retina, and choroidal sclerosis (also called "fundus tesselation") giving the disc a "moth-eaten" appearance.[79] HTG eyes, by contrast, had younger age, high IOP, abnormal anterior chamber angles, deep and steep optic nerve excavation, little PPA, and no choroidal sclerosis. They found larger superior than inferior VFDs in the NTG eyes, compared with equal superior and inferior VFDs in HTG eyes. They suggested a primary local vascular disease with chronic ischemia causing damage in these senile sclerotic discs, leading to the appearance of PPA and choroidal sclerosis, and a primary IOP mechanism for damage in the HTG eyes, with a secondary role of insufficient blood supply causing disc injury in HTG. Subsequent studies have also found similar and additional characteristics in patients with senile sclerotic discs.[81,85,90,91]

### 35.3.2.6 Myopic Glaucomatous Discs

Geijssen first proposed that myopic eyes might represent a distinct group of NTG with a characteristic disc appearance when damaged by glaucoma, separate from damage due to pathologic myopia.[80] In her study, she observed disc tilting with oblique insertion, shallow cupping, temporal crescents or PPA, and typical glaucomatous thinning and excavation of the superior and inferior poles of the NRR. Subsequent studies have confirmed these and other findings in this type of myopic glaucomatous disc damage.[81,85,92,93]

### 35.3.2.7 Generalized Enlargement of the Optic Cup Discs

Spaeth first called this type of optic nerve damage "primary hyperbaric glaucoma," characterized by elevated IOP; a normal disc fluorescein pattern; more symmetric, round enlargement of the optic cup; and visual field loss more often peripheral than central.[78] He proposed that disc damage in this group of eyes was purely mechanical in etiology from the chronic effects of elevated IOP. Other studies have also found a number of characteristics in patients with generalized optic cup enlargement.[81,85,92,93]

In summary, while these four types of disc cupping are often typical of eyes with NTG, they are not generally predominant in this disease entity. However, their identification may help target disease management from an ocular (e.g., degree of necessary IOP-lowering) and systemic (e.g., treatment of cardiovascular risk factors) point of view.

### 35.3.2.8 Neuroretinal Rim Loss

Jonas et al examined the pressure-dependence of NRR in patients with NTG.[94] They found that optic disc size actually decreased with decreasing maximal IOP in eyes with the focal ischemic disc appearance, suggesting a vasogenic reason for the nerve fiber loss. This finding was also suggested by another study that found an abnormal retrobulbar circulation in NTG eyes.[95] Yet, Jonas et al also found a correlation between a smaller NRR area in eyes with a relatively higher IOP compared with eyes with a lower IOP in all three of the focal ischemic, senile sclerotic, and myopic glaucomatous disc types seen in the NTG eyes he studied.[94] This suggests a baro-traumatic mechanism for damage in all these disc types characteristic of NTG.

Tan et al utilized the HRT to study NRR loss in OHT, OHT converters, NTG suspects, and NTG eyes.[97] These researchers found reproducible loss of NRR primarily at the superior and inferior poles of the OHT groups, especially inferiorly, consistent with prior studies showing vertical cup elongation in early glaucoma. NRR loss was detected in 11% of OHT suspects and in 90% of OHT eyes converting to glaucoma. NRR loss was detected in 58% of NTG suspects but in only 54% of NTG eyes, and in 3 of 5 NTG converters in whom VFDs developed. Temporal rim loss in these eyes correlated with dense paracentral VFDs, as seen in other studies previously mentioned.

### 35.3.2.9 Optic Disc Hemorrhage

Optic disc hemorrhages (ODHs) are a hallmark of progressive glaucomatous optic nerve damage. ODHs were characterized by Drance et al in the 1970s as localized ischemic optic neuropathy, and they noted a 20% prevalence in NTG patients.[96–99] Since then, many studies have examined patients with NTG and ODHs to elucidate their characteristics and associations and to correlate ODHs with disease state.

ODHs may be linear, flame-shaped, splinter-shaped, or occasionally blot-type and rounded. They usually are found in the prelaminar area of the optic nerve and peripapillary retina, and rarely in the depth of the optic disc cup. They have a much higher frequency (~3:1) of ODHs in the inferior versus the superior disc pole of the disc. ODHs in NTG eyes have recently been found to be associated with branch retinal vein occlusions in the contralateral eye, suggesting a possible common microvascular thrombotic mechanism.[100,101]

Jonas and Budde investigated glaucomatous eyes with very high IOP (juvenile open-angle glaucoma) and very low IOP (NTG), in order to increase the possibility to detect differences in optic nerve appearance between the groups.[102] In contrast to earlier studies, these authors found that the optic nerves in these two groups were similar in number of detectable localized retinal nerve fiber layer defects (RNFLDs), size of PPA, optic cup depth, steepness of disc cupping, rim/disc area ratio, retinal arteriole diameter, and degree of focal arteriolar narrowing. However, NTG eyes did have broader localized RNFLDs, more frequent NRR notches, and more frequent and larger ODHs.[102] They speculated that the lower frequency of detected ODH and NRR notches in high-pressure JOAG eyes resulted directly from the larger transmural pressure gradient across the small vessels of the optic disc in NTG eyes. Therefore, a small vessel rupture on the optic nerve in eyes with NTG would lead to a larger disc hemorrhage that reabsorbed more slowly, and hence have a higher chance to be detected in disc photos than in eyes with HTG. An ODH due to a similar vessel rupture in an HTG eye would be smaller, more easily reabsorbed, more easily missed in a disc photo, and lead to a smaller resulting RNFLD seen on subsequent clinical exam. Thus, the relative paucity of ODH in HTG vs. NTG may be an artifact of the examination that may not reflect the true frequency of occurrence.

Based on their findings, these researchers further speculated that the pathogenic mechanisms of disc damage in NTG and HTG may rather be more similar than different. This conclusion also agrees with:

1. The *clinical findings* of some similarities in disc damage appearance between NTG and HTG eyes by Caprioli and Spaeth,[71]
2. The *pathologic findings* by Miller and Quigley of abnormal laminar architecture in NTG eyes making them potentially more susceptible to IOP damage,[77] and
3. The *beneficial response to IOP-lowering* in a large subset of NTG eyes seen in the CNTGS.[4,5]

For all the apparent differences observed when comparing NTG and HTG eyes, these findings imply a shared element of IOP-mediated damage for both NTG and HTG eyes.

In summary, ODHs serve as an easily identifiable sign of disease progression and should always be carefully searched for on clinical exam and review of disc photos. Their occurrence should prompt more investigation within 2–6 weeks into the status of a patient's disease state such as:

1. optic disc photos and computerized disc imaging at current visit to document the ODH,
2. VF testing with 24-2 or even central 10-2 programs, if a paracentral defect is suspected based on the ODH location, to look for change in or new VFDs,
3. more frequent IOP monitoring at various times throughout the day to detect unsuspected IOP spikes,
4. usually more aggressive IOP control to reduce IOP an additional 15–20% from established current baseline,
5. repeat optic nerve evaluation with dilation to look for ODH resolution, new and/or recurrent ODHs, and
6. subsequent careful disease state monitoring with VF testing and optic nerve exam to establish future stability.

### 35.3.2.10 Peripapillary Atrophy

PPA is separated into two zones: zone alpha ($\alpha$) – a peripheral zone with irregular hyper- and hypopigmentation from loss of the RPE; and zone beta ($\beta$) – a central, whitish zone with visible choroidal vessels and sclera because of loss of both RPE and photoreceptors (Figs. 35.6–35.8). This atrophy is felt to develop due to loss of the peripapillary choroidal branches from the short posterior ciliary arteries, which penetrate centripetally into the prelaminar portion of the optic nerve head in a sectoral fashion. These branches supply the optic nerve axons and collagenous laminar beams with blood. Absence or dysfunction of these branches would cause segmental ischemia and damage to the optic nerve head leading to axonal loss, focal disc notching, cupping, and acquired pits of the optic nerve with associated PPA.

Anderson first suggested that peripapillary halos or atrophy were more common in NTG than HTG eyes.[103] Geijssen and Greve in 1987 first described the association of PPA with larger superior than inferior VFDs in the NTG senile sclerotic disc, compared to little PPA and equal VFDs in the superior and inferior regions in HTG discs.[79] They concluded that primary local optic disc microvascular insufficiency could explain the pathogenesis of disc damage in NTG eyes, while in HTG eyes elevated IOP played a primary role and vascular insufficiency a secondary role in the pathogenesis of disc damage. Their findings are similar to those by Kawano et al in 2006, who found that only the inferior half of zone-beta ($\beta$) PPA correlated with glaucomatous VF damage.[104] Further, inferior PPA also correlated with axial length, while superior PPA correlated only with axial length but not VF damage. They felt these findings suggested that the inferior region of the ONH is more vulnerable to damage in NTG than the superior region, and therefore inferior PPA is more clinically significant in NTG than superior PPA.

Similarly, Buus and Anderson found the incidence of PPA to be 64% in NTG discs and only 34% in OHT discs.[105] This difference persisted even after exclusion of eyes with myopia greater than −4 diopters. Araie et al also found that the extent of PPA in untreated NTG eyes correlated with VF progression.[106] But, Tezel et al found that zone beta ($\beta$) PPA was detected more often in NTG than HTG eyes, presumably because the NTG eyes were seen at a more advanced stage of disease.[75] They felt that the final appearance of the optic nerve damage was similar in NTG and HTG eyes for the same degree of damage, regardless of the possible different mechanisms for the optic neuropathy observed in the two groups. This was con-

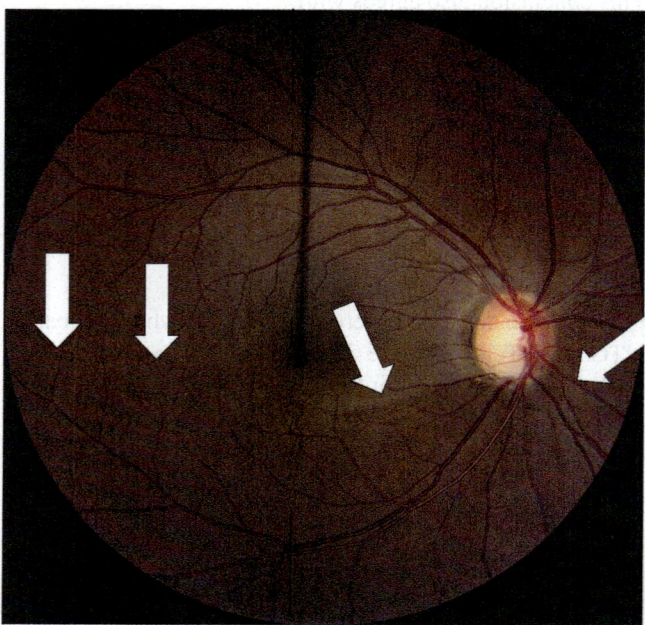

**Fig. 35.7** Color disc photograph showing loss of the inferior NFL with focal cupping in the right eye of a 41-year-old Hispanic female with moderately advanced NTG, OD>OS. Classical, deep, inferior excavation/cupping and focal pallor of the right eye optic nerve rim with marked loss of the associated inferior arcuate NFL (vertical cup/disc = 0.75–0.8). Note the distinct loss of inferior NFL striations with absence of typical high NFL reflectance inferiorly and a resulting dull, dark, wedge-shaped defect from 4 to 8 o'clock, with clear and sharp visibility of the blood vessels and their margins in this region, as a result of the loss of the surrounding NFL (between *white arrows*). By contrast, these brightly reflected NFL striations are seen easily at the superior pole of the disc where the neural rim is well retained, with blurring of the blood vessel margins due to the normally thick NFL surrounding the vessels in this area

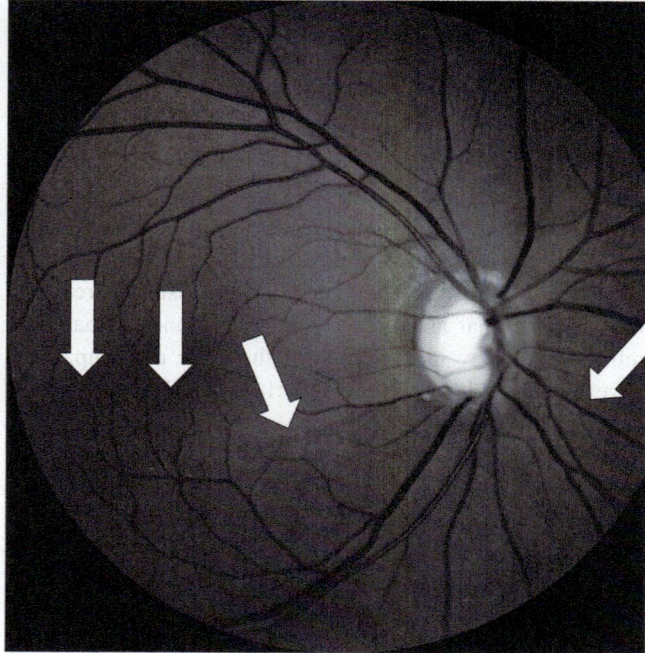

**Fig. 35.8** Red-free NFL photograph of the right eye of the NTG patient in Fig. 35.7. Note the very dense loss of inferior NFL seen in the dark, wedge-shaped, extensive defect, radiating out from approximately the 4 o'clock to the 7:30–8 o'clock position on the nerve rim (between *white arrows*), seen also in Fig. 35.7

firmed by Jonas and Xu, who did not find larger areas of zone alpha (α) or beta (β) PPA in NTG eyes compared with HTG eyes, after exclusion of eyes with myopia greater than −8 diopters, when eyes were matched for stage of disease by the amount of remaining NRR area and visual field loss.[107]

In summary, beta (β) PPA is a sign associated with advancing glaucomatous optic neuropathy. Its presence should lead the clinician to look for other signs of related disc damage such as associated disc notching or rim thinning, disc hemorrhages, RNFL loss, and prompt VF testing to detect possible early disease, where NTG has not necessarily been suspected previously.

## 35.4 Visual Field Defects

### 35.4.1 Patterns of Loss

#### 35.4.1.1 Dense, Focal, and Central vs. Peripheral and Diffuse

As documented from review of the early classical literature on NTG and from his own retrospective case series, Levene[3] concluded that VFDs in NTG eyes tend to:

1. Involve fixation early
2. Be dense and to within 5° of fixation
3. Occur suddenly
4. Be disproportionately less extensive than expected from the advanced optic nerve damage observed
5. Be monocular
6. Progress slowly

In a retrospective review of NTG patients in 1976, Chumbley and Brubaker noted a nerve fiber bundle pattern of Goldmann visual field defects (VFDs) in all eyes that could be evaluated.[108] Superior arcuate scotomas were seen in 84% and inferior arcuate scotomas in 58%, and both defects in 41% of eyes (Figs. 35.9–35.13). Interestingly, VFDs involved the macula in 25% of eyes either at initial exam or progressed to involve the macula on follow-up in their study group.

In NTG/VF studies during the 1980s:

1. Motolko et al found no difference between the two glaucoma groups.[109]
2. Hitchings and Anderton found "steeper sided" VFDs in NTG.[110]
3. Caprioli and Spaeth found VFDs with a steeper slope, closer to fixation, and greater depth in NTG.[111]
4. King et al found a slightly greater mean eccentricity from fixation of 4.86° vs. 2.96°, but no difference in slope or depth, of VFDs in NTG.[112]

In eyes with a classic, localized VFD in one hemifield only, Drance et al found the spared hemifield of HTG eyes to have twice as much diffuse loss as NTG eyes, supporting the hypothesis that elevated IOP affects visual function diffusely, while localized VFDs are less influenced by IOP-mediated damage.[113] This same group studied NTG and HTG eyes matched for extent of VF damage, pupil size, and visual acuity and found that the NTG eyes had greater areas of normal sensitivity, hence more localized damage, than HTG eyes.[114] But these researchers did not feel that this study proved a differential mechanism of damage between the two groups, because both groups also showed localized VFD, hypothesized to arise from ischemic, pressure-independent mechanisms. Asymmetric IOP in NTG patients, however, has been demonstrated in other studies to be associated with greater VFDs in the eye with the higher IOP.[115-118] Other studies have concluded that "the effect of IOP on the type of visual field damage in glaucoma patients with relatively low IOP is not clearly apparent in our study."[119]

Further comparisons of visual fields in NTG and HTG eyes have shown a greater amount of localized VFDs in the *inferior* hemifield of NTG eyes from one US study,[120] but a more depressed area of sensitivity in the *superior* hemifield in NTG eyes compared with more diffuse damage in HTG eyes from another Japanese study.[121] Again, comparing VFDs in the central 10° in NTG versus HTG eyes from Japan, Koseki et al found a greater amount of VFDs in the superior arcuate area extending down to the horizontal meridian, nasal to fixation, in NTG eyes compared with a more diffuse pattern of damage seen in HTG eyes.[121] In a large comparative study from Britain, the frequency of unilateral VFDs in over 700 patients was similar in NTG (25%) and HTG (31%) eyes.[122] However, patients with unilateral field loss were younger, and in NTG patients, the left eye was 2.1 times more likely to be affected, whereas in HTG patients, both eyes had an equal chance to be affected. Additional studies utilizing SLP in NTG eyes with localized VFDs in one hemifield have determined that the RNFL is thinner in areas with the normal hemifield in these NTG eyes, compared with normal eyes.[123,124] This is a hopeful finding of probable subclinical RNFL damage now detectable by this new technology at an early stage of disease, just as seen with OCT discussed earlier, that might have been too subtle to identify previously, except with the most expert of red-free photographic techniques. This gives us encouragement that the new imaging technology can now do a much better job of picking up early NTG damage so clinicians can diagnose NTG earlier, to treat it earlier and perhaps more effectively.

Interestingly also, in a recent Japanese study of 94 consecutive NTG patients younger than 61 years, MRI scans detected ischemic changes in the brain in 34% of patients, whose VFDs were relatively deeper in the inferior, nasal to pericentral region than in patients without such MRI findings.[125] The implications for these findings are unclear, because MRI scanning is too expensive for routine use in otherwise apparently straight-forward NTG patients. MRI

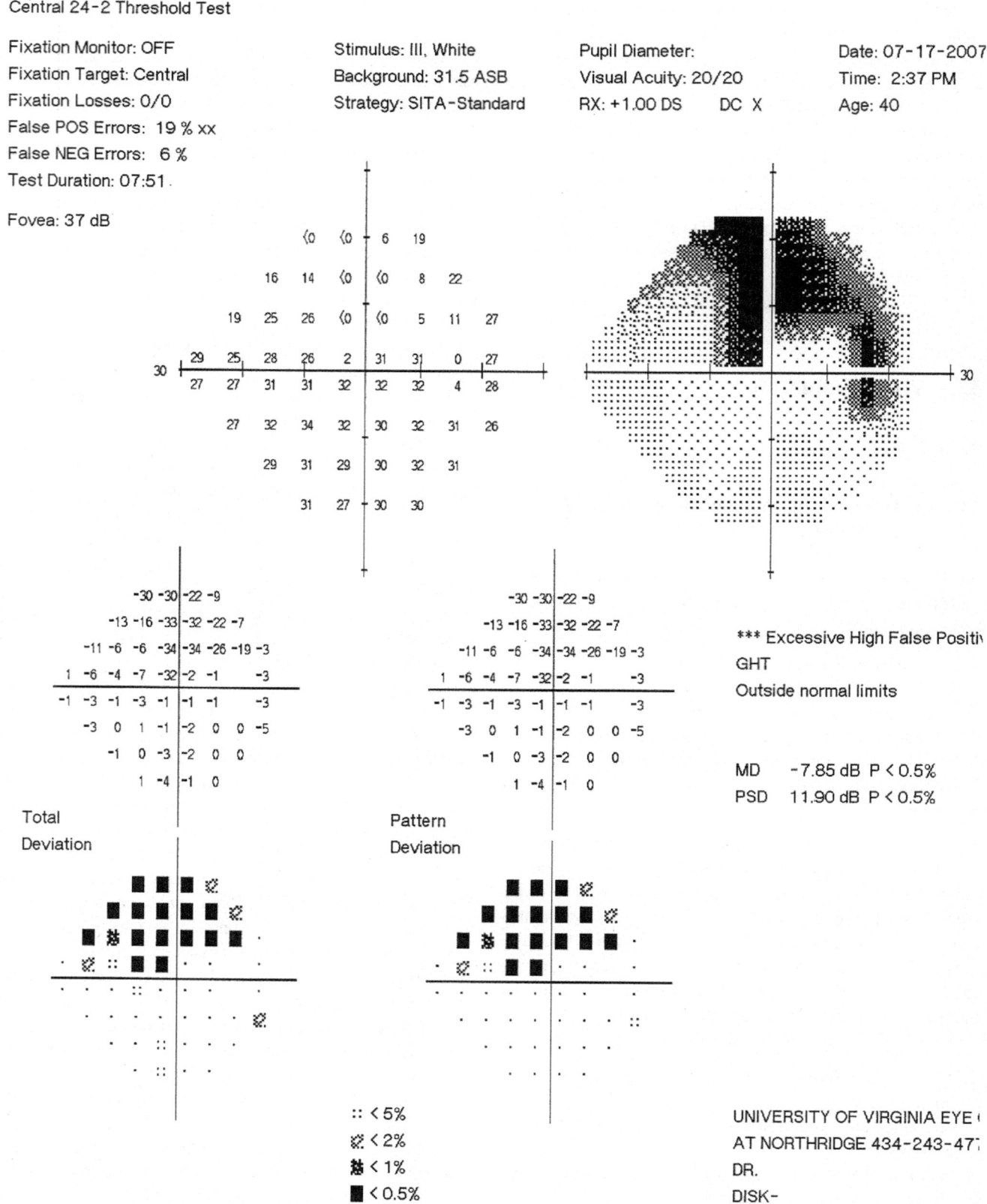

**Fig. 35.9** SITA standard 24-2 visual field of the NTG patient in Figs. 35.7 and 35.8. Note the dense superior arcuate scotoma (overall MD=−7.85) and the dense superonasal paracentral defect (−32 dB) in the single point near fixation on this 24-2 field, with 6° spacing of test points. This single point defect is expanded in the 10-2 field, with 2° spacing of test points, shown in Fig. 35.10

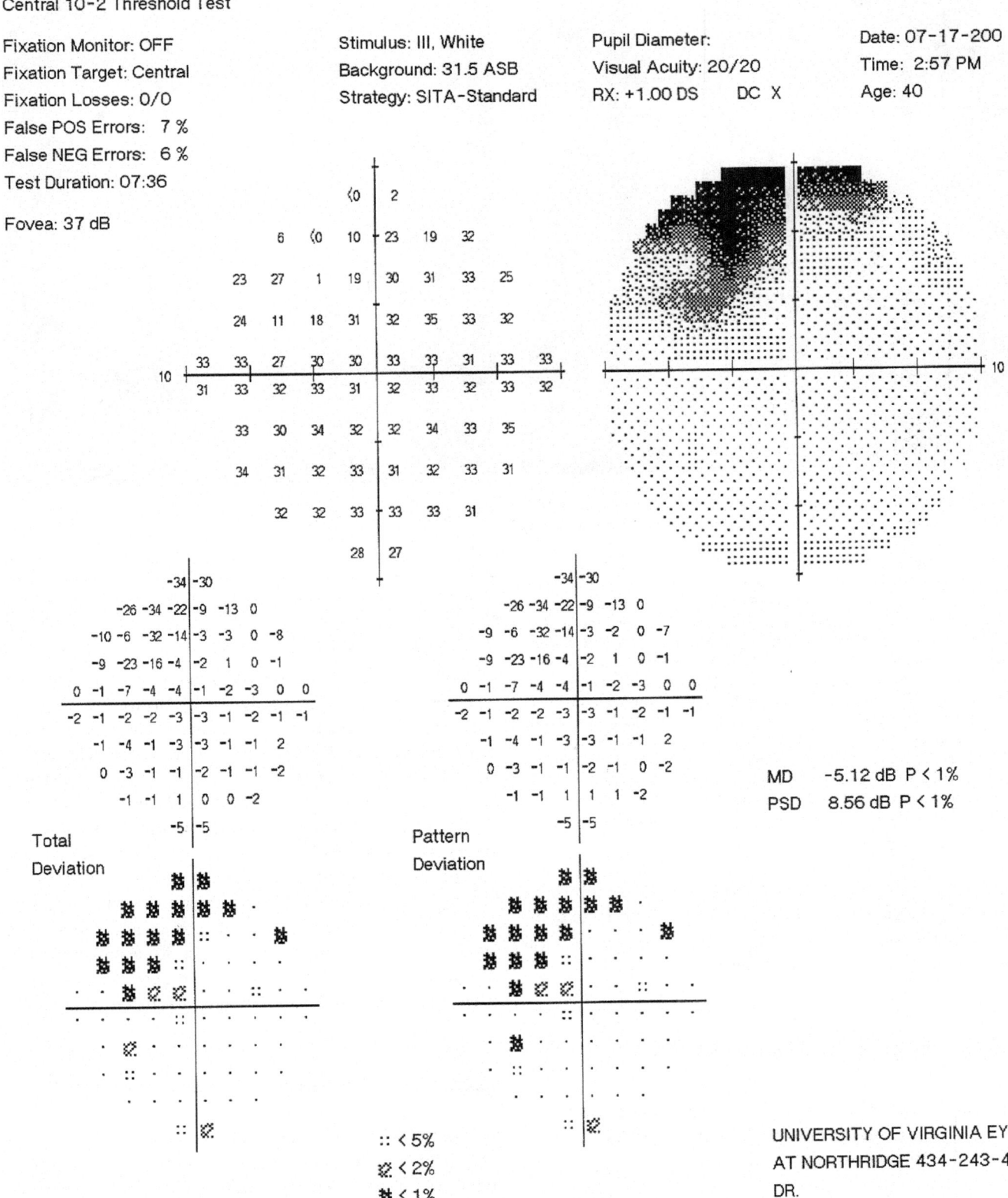

**Fig. 35.10** SITA standard 10-2 visual field of the NTG patient in Figs. 35.7 and 35.8. Note the moderately dense superior arcuate scotoma extending to within 3° of fixation superonasally, with points of depression in this superonasal area ranging from −14 to −34 dB. This fairly extensive area of significant visual field involvement (overall MD=−5.12, involving 16 test points) is represented by only the single paracentral point with a MD=−32 in the 24-2 field in Fig. 35.9. Use of the 10-2 program can enhance detection of early paracentral visual field loss and can be used to effectively follow progression that might easily be missed on the 24-2 program

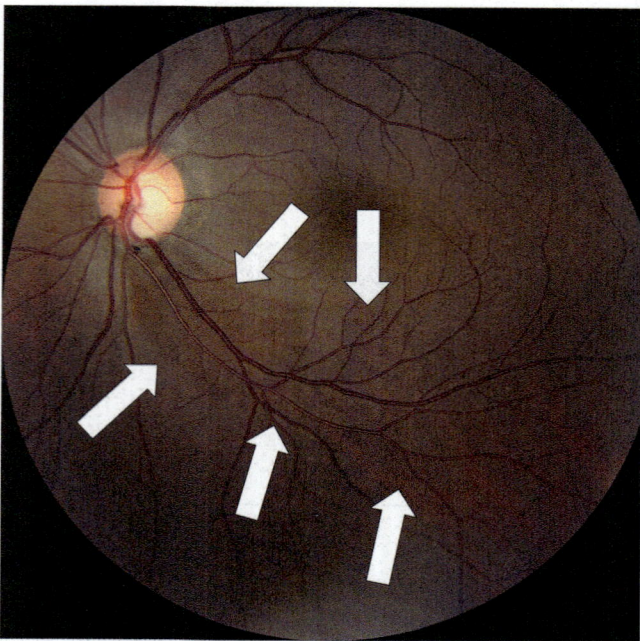
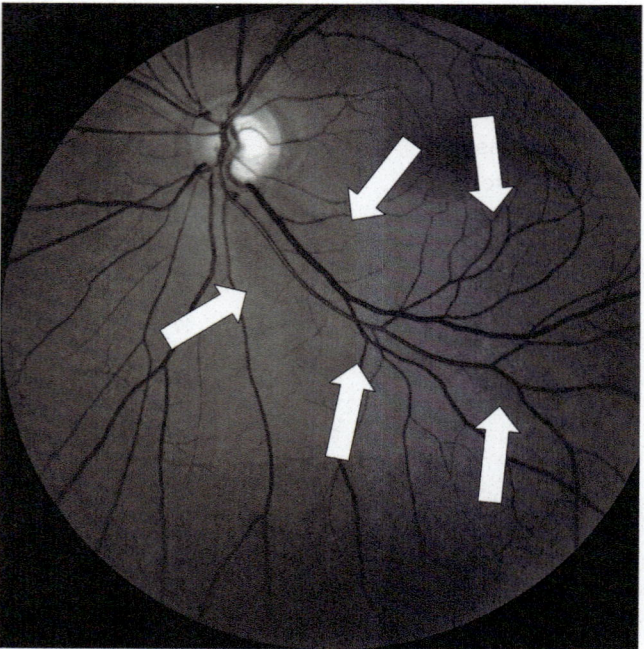

**Fig. 35.11** Color disc photograph showing loss of the inferior NFL with focal cupping in the left eye of the 41-year-old Hispanic female with moderately advanced NTG, OD>OS, seen in Figs. 35.7–35.10. Classical, deep, inferior excavation/cupping and focal pallor of the left eye optic nerve rim with marked loss of the associated inferior arcuate NFL (vertical cup/disc = 0.75–0.8). Note the smaller, wedge-shaped, NFL defect radiating out from approximately the 4:30–5 o'clock to the 6 o'clock position on the nerve rim (between *white arrows*), compared with the defect OD seen in Figs. 35.7 and 35.8. Note again the distinct loss of inferior NFL striations with absence of typical high NFL reflectance inferiorly and a resulting dull, dark, wedge-shaped defect from 4:30–5 o'clock to 6 o'clock. The blood vessels and their margins in this inferior region are clear and sharp, as a result of the loss of the surrounding NFL. By contrast, the brightly reflected NFL striations are seen easily at the superior pole of the disc, where the neural rim is well retained, resulting in blurring of the blood vessel margins due to the normally thick NFL surrounding the vessels in this superior area

**Fig. 35.12** Red-free NFL photograph of the left eye of the NTG patient in Fig. 35.10. Note the dense loss of the inferior NFL shown by the dark, wedge-shaped, defect radiating out from approximately the 4:30–5 o'clock to the 6 o'clock position on the nerve rim (between *white arrows*). This defect is but less extensive than the NFL defect OD seen in Figs. 35.7 and 35.8

exams might be indicated for those NTG patients in whom there is a clinical or historical suspicion of neurologic damage, or perhaps an unusual pattern of VFD suggestive of a hemianopia crossing the horizontal meridian.

### 35.4.2 Progression Characteristics

#### 35.4.2.1 How Often Do NTG Patients Need to Have a VF Test to Detect Glaucomatous VF Progression?

This question was examined in a British study of six untreated NTG eyes with 119 retinal locations deteriorating by ≥1 dB/year, all of whom had three VFs per year for 4 years.[126] When the tests were "thinned" to the more usual one test/year and compared with the actually completed three tests/year, only 45% of deteriorated eyes were detected over the same 4-year time span. Testing only yearly led to an average delay of 1.1 years in the detection of progression. The lesson here is that more frequent VF testing results in better detection of visual field progression (Figs. 35.14 and 35.15). To detect stability or progression in eyes with very advanced or end-stage damage, it is recommended to use the central 10° VF test program with 2° spacing of test points in eyes with dense paracentral defects, such as often may be seen in NTG. Alternatively, for advanced disease, using the size V stimulus combined with the central 10° visual field test, has been advocated when visual sensitivity on the standard 24° or 30° test with the size III stimulus at 6° spacing of test points is greatly reduced, such as when the overall mean deviation is less than −25 dB.[127]

#### 35.4.2.2 How Often Does VF Damage Progress in NTG?

Similar to the Chumbley and Brubaker study cited earlier,[108] a 1985 British study found VF progression by Goldmann testing in 40% of untreated NTG patients followed for a mean of 10.5 years[128] (Fig. 35.16). Visual field loss more often progressed in an already damaged hemifield (1:2 chance) than developed de novo (1:4 chance) in an uninvolved hemifield. It took an average of 4.4 years to see progression, with an average of 1.5 VF tests per year (Figs. 35.17 and 35.18).

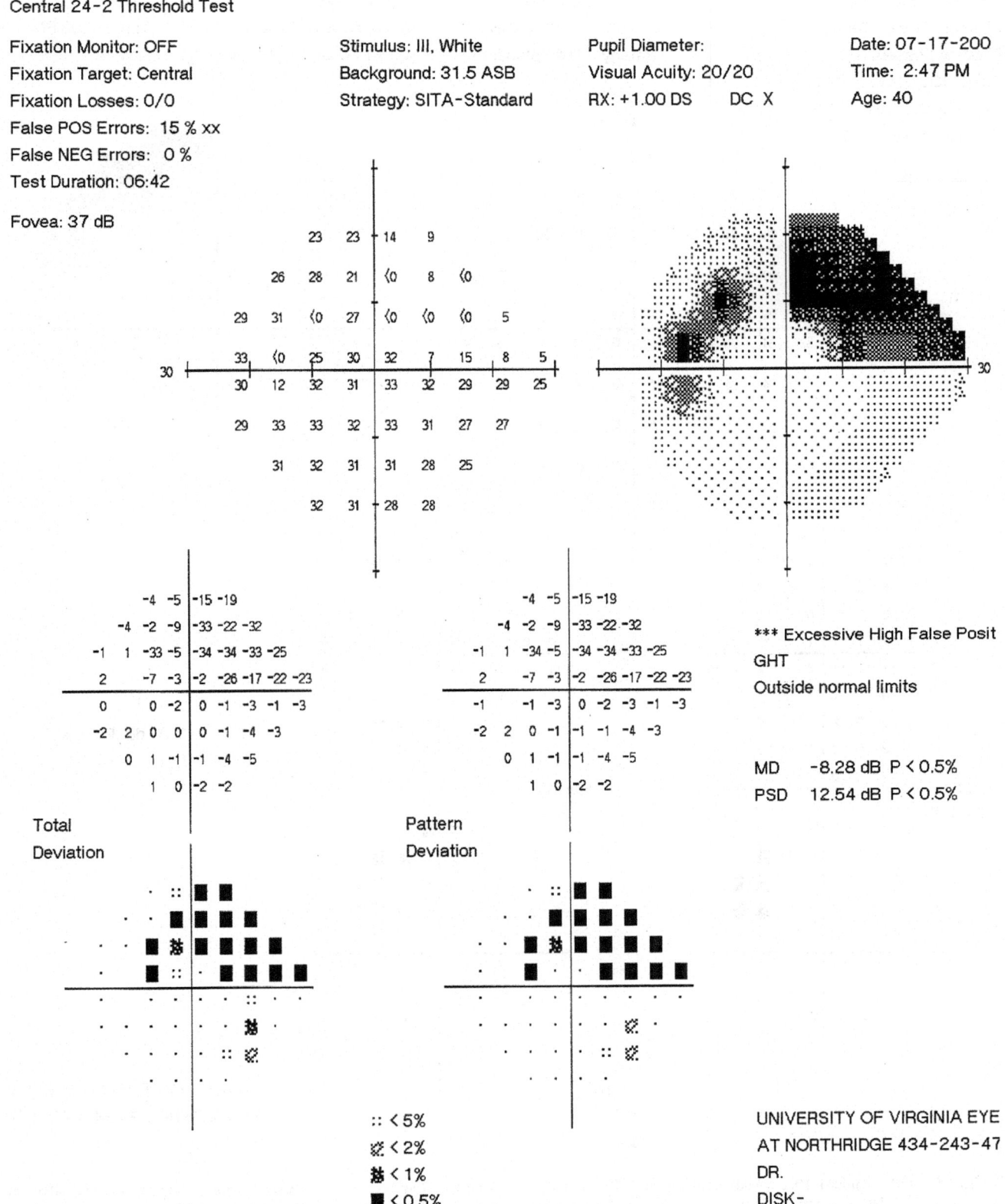

**Fig. 35.13** SITA standard 24-2 visual field of the NTG patient in Figs. 35.11 and 35.12. Note the dense superior arcuate scotoma (overall MD=−8.28) here OS, similar to that seen in the OD, but with the absence of a dense superior paracentral defect near fixation, as seen in the OD in Fig. 35.9. On the 10-2 field shown in Fig. 35.14, a central defect is found, however, although it is less extensive than in the defect OD in seen Fig. 35.10

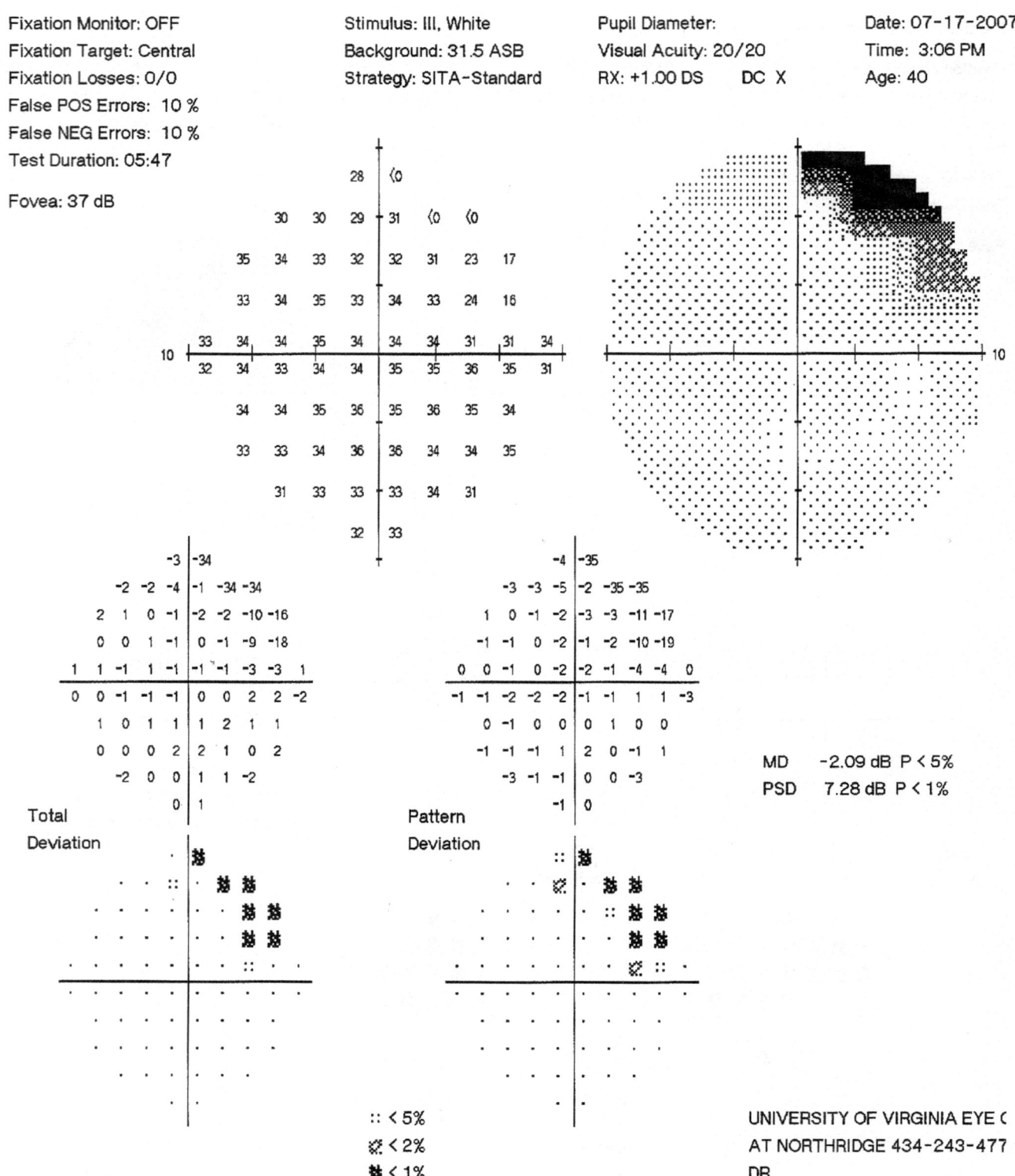

**Fig. 35.14** SITA standard 10-2 visual field of the NTG patient in Figs. 35.9 and 35.10. Note the mild superior arcuate scotoma (overall MD = −2.09, involving six test points) extending to within 5° of fixation superonasally. This subtle defect is not seen in the superonasal paracentral point (−2 dB) in the 24-2 field in Fig. 35.13 and is not as extensive as the defect OD seen in Fig. 35.10. This finding indicates that a patient can have significant paracentral visual field loss that is not well represented on the 24-2 program. Consequently, the author would advocate for more frequent assessment of the central 10-2 visual field in patients felt to be at risk for paracentral visual field loss, based on the appearance of their optic nerve or computerized imaging of the peripapillary NFL, or even based on patient complaints of "blind spots" or defects near the center of their vision that might be mistakenly ascribed to macular edema from diabetes or from macular degeneration changes

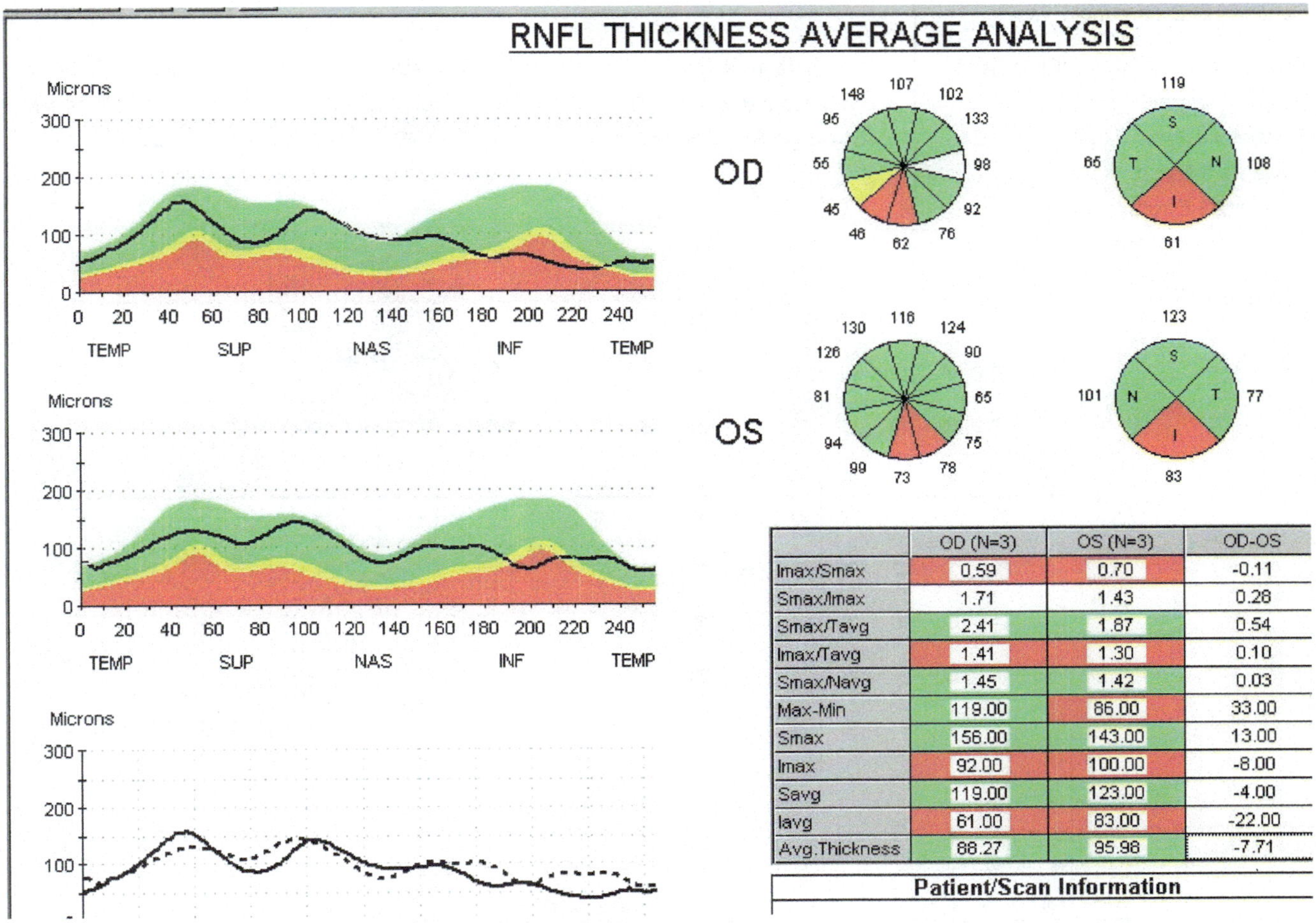

# 35 Normal Pressure Glaucoma

**Fig. 35.15** Optical coherence tomography of the peripapillary RNFL of the patient in Figs. 35.7–35.14. Note the markedly thinned inferior and inferotemporal OCT NFL sectors in both eyes of the NTG patient seen in Figs. 35.7–35.14. NFL sector thicknesses are 62, 46, and 45 μm OD (red 6 and 7 o'clock and yellow 8 o'clock sectors, respectively, in *upper center* pie pictograph) and are much thinner than the 78, 73, and 75 μm measured in the mirror image sectors OS (red 5 and 6 o'clock and green 4 o'clock sectors, respectively, in the *middle center* pie pictograph). By contrast, note the well-preserved superior NFL thicknesses OU (all superior sectors have normal NFL thicknesses denoted by the *green color* in the pie pictographs), which correspond with the normal, superior, optic disc neural rims seen clinically in the color disc photos in Figs. 35.7 and 35.11

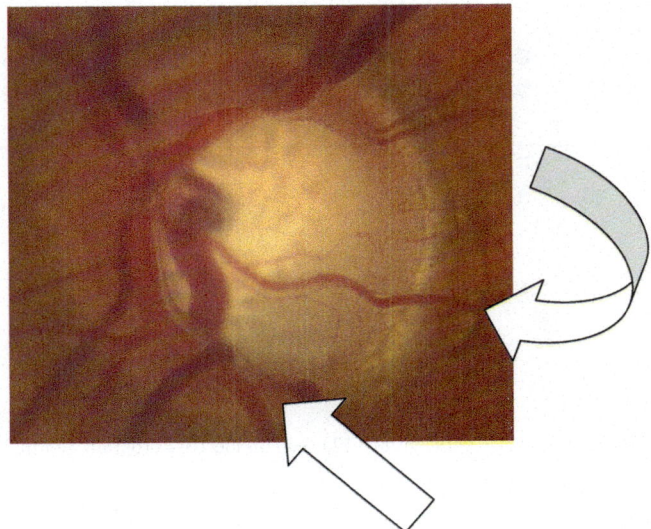

**Fig. 35.16** Color disc photograph OS of a 58-year-old, Caucasian, female patient with early NTG. Note loss of the inferotemporal nerve rim and associated notch of the rim at the 5–6 o'clock position (*straight white arrow*) and mild adjacent PPA (*curved white arrow*)

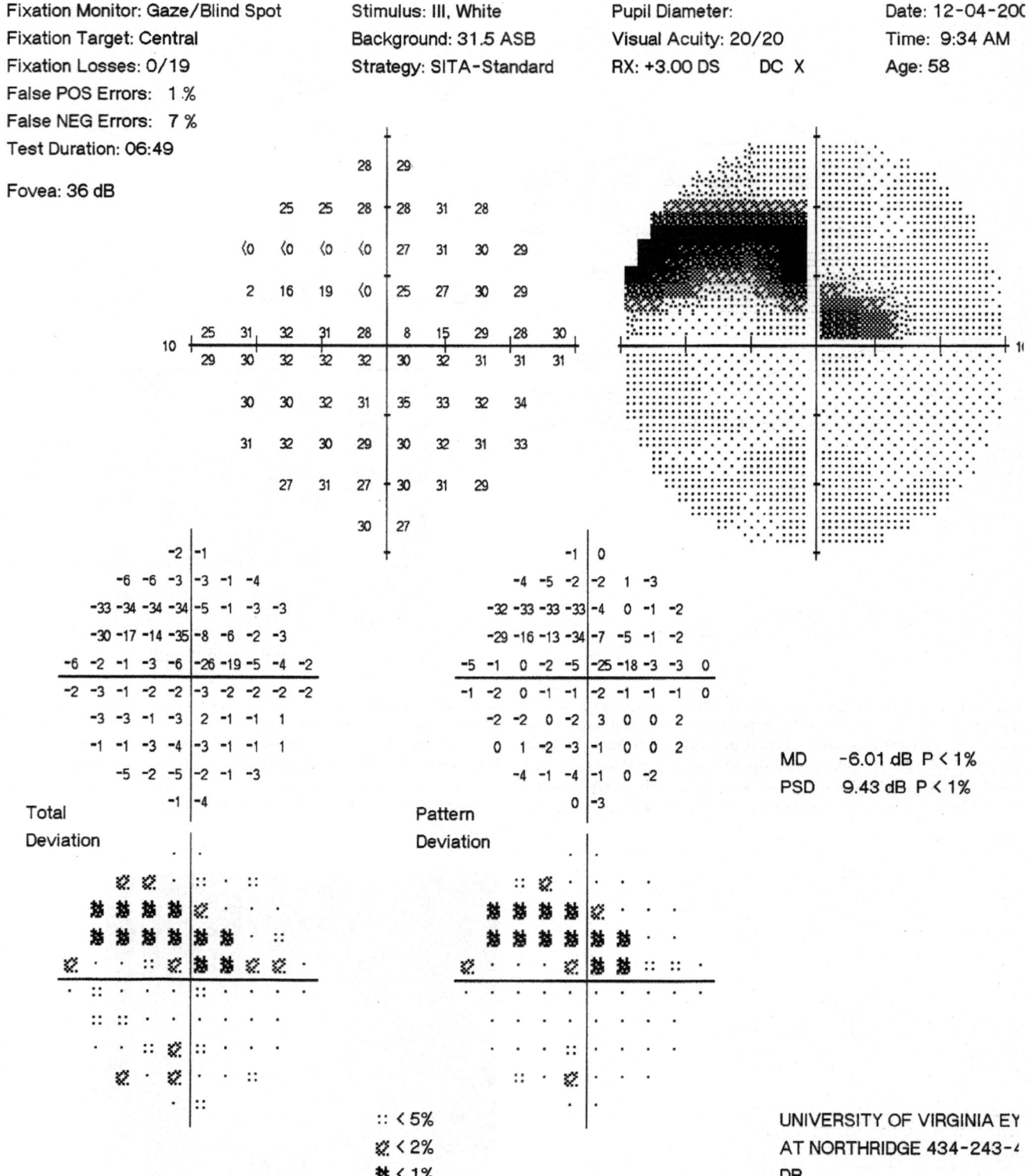

**Fig. 35.17** Dense paracentral VFD seen on the 10-2 program first in 2006 and stable here in 2008

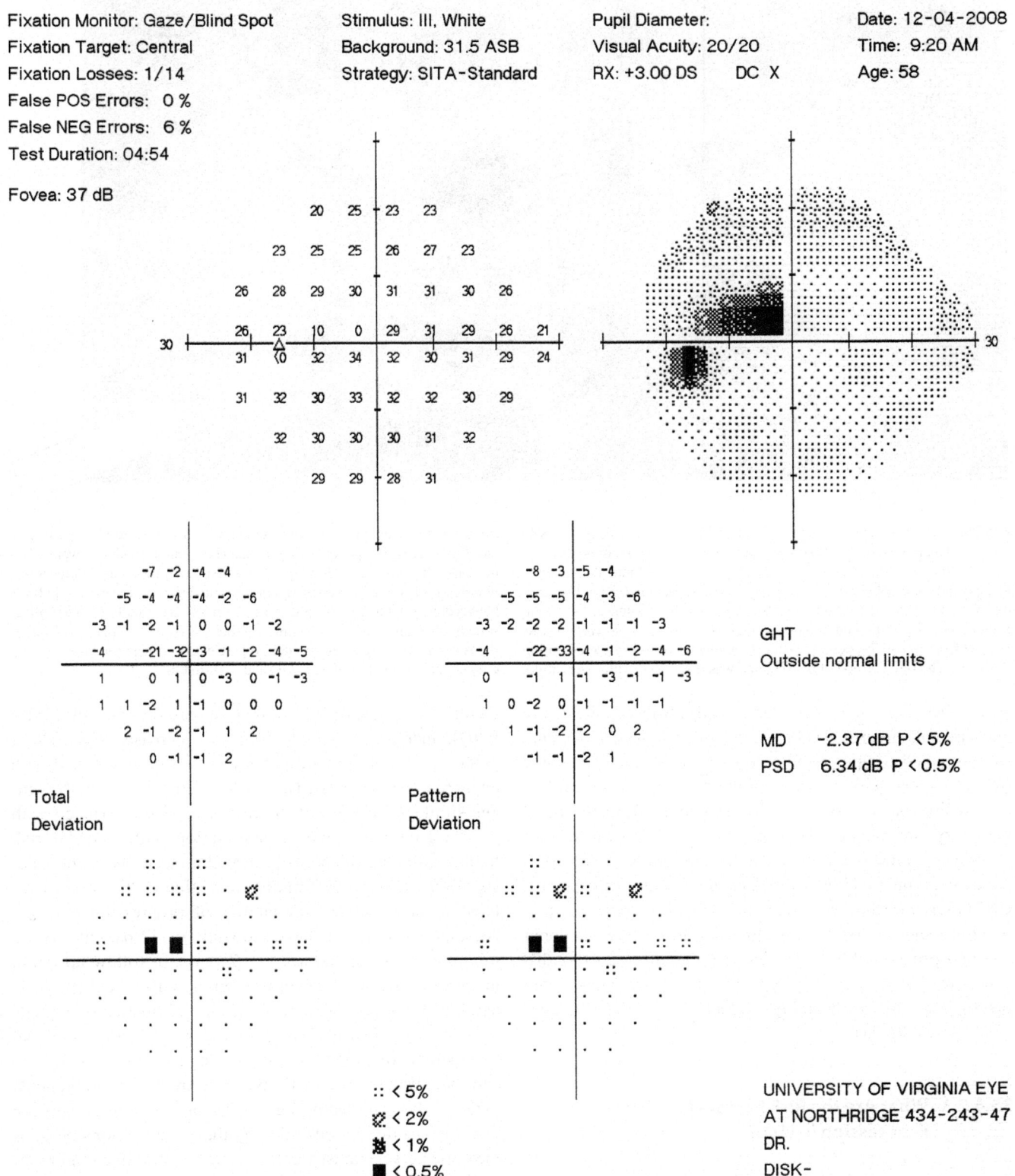

**Fig. 35.18** Dense paracentral VFD seen here on the 24-2 program first in 2008 but missed in 2004–2007

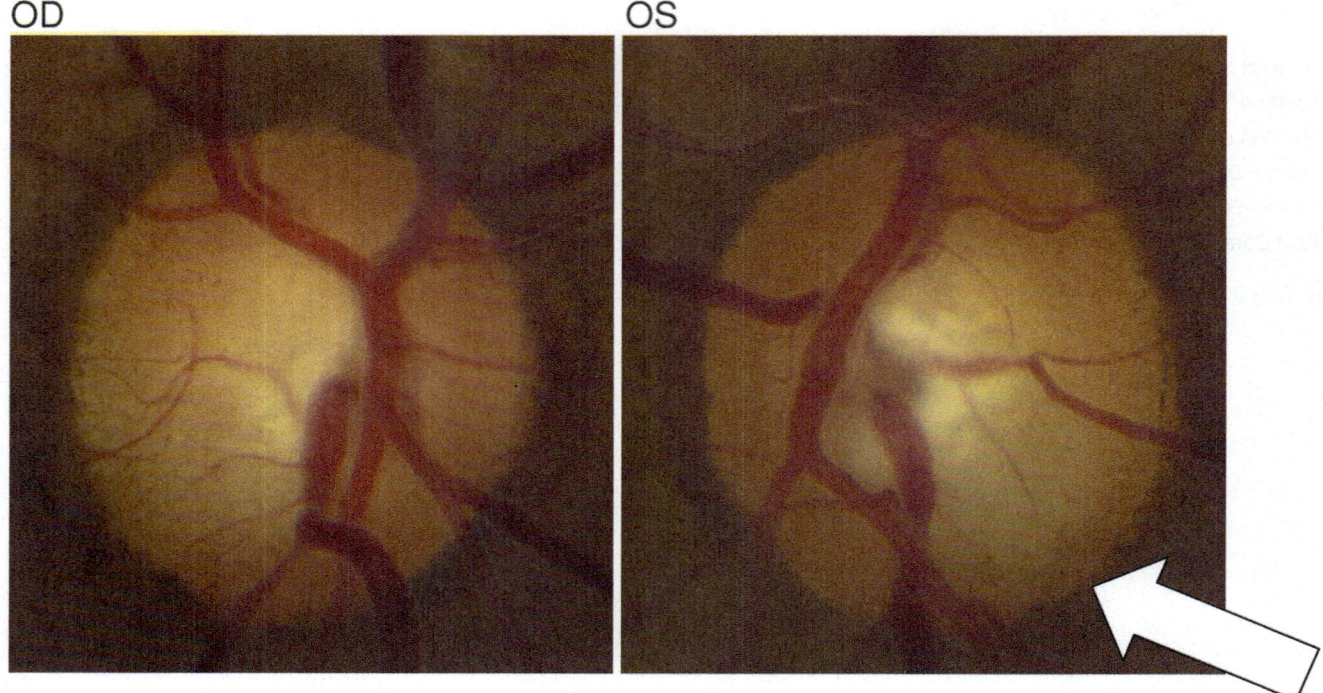

**Fig. 35.19** Color disc photographs of early NTG, OS>OD, in a 64-year-old African-American female. (*left*) Note the central, even, round optic disc cup OD (C/D=0.3–0.4), which was normal and stable without documented change and a normal visual field over 9 years of follow-up. (*right*) The optic disc OS, however, showed documented, progressive thinning of the neural rim and developed a notch at the 5 o'clock position (*straight white arrow*, vertical C/D=0.6–0.7) over 5–7 years. An ODH was never observed during this time. The inferotemporal disc change was associated with a very mild, superonasal visual field change on standard white-on-white SITA perimetry (see Fig. 35.20). The patient's mother had HTG, but the patient never had an untreated IOP above 21 mmHg over 9 years of follow-up. Interestingly, despite the clear disc asymmetry, there was no observed asymmetry in IOPs between eyes. Untreated IOPs during this time were usually 15–19 mmHg, sometimes higher OD or sometimes higher OS by 2–4 mmHg, and sometimes equal OU over a full diurnal cycle. Central corneal thicknesses were only slightly thinned at 503 μm OD and 519 μm OS

In another US study of moderate and advanced, medically and surgically treated NTG eyes, VF progression was detected by automated computerized perimetry in 53% at 3 years and 62% at 5 years, with the most common VFD (76%) identified as a dense, paracentral scotoma, extending from the nasal periphery toward a point 8° from fixation.[129] This rate of progression was much higher than the 42% rate seen in a comparative group of HTG eyes. The multicenter, prospective CNTGS found that in untreated NTG eyes approximately one-third showed localized progression in 3 years and about one-half progressed in 5–7 years, at a rate of −0.2 to −2 dB/year, but that change was typically small and slow, often insufficient to measurably affect the MD index[130] (Figs. 35.19–35.24).

### 35.4.2.3 What Are the Risk Factors for Visual Field Progression in NTG?

A retrospective study of untreated, early NTG patients (initial MD ≥ −5 dB) from Japan found definite VF progression in 48% of them over a mean follow-up of 42 months, with a calculated rate of progression of 80% at 65 months.[131] Risk factors for progression included increased cup-to-disc ratio (C/D), increased area of PPA, and increased IOP. These authors felt that the risk of VF progression associated with an increased C/D implied a pressure-dependence to ON damage similar to HTG; but the increased risk associated with greater PPA suggested an association with vascular risk factors affecting the peripapillary choroid in the pathogenesis of ON damage. A 3 mmHg reduction in IOP was calculated to decrease the probability of progression to 37%. Another retrospective Japanese study of 47 patients with a minimum 5 years, and average 7 years, of follow-up found nonuse of calcium channel blockers (CCBs), beta (β) PPA, and ODH, but not mean, peak or diurnal fluctuation of IOP, to be associated with VF progression.[132] They concluded that risk factors other than IOP play a role in progression of NTG and that systemic use of CCBs (used by half of the patients in the study) is protective against VF progression, suggesting that the vasodilation afforded by these medications protects the optic nerve against vascular insufficiency, that might otherwise lead to progressive ON and VF damage.

A role for vascular insufficiency in NTG was suggested by the results of several studies examining retrobulbar circulation in NTG eyes with visual field progression. Yamazaki

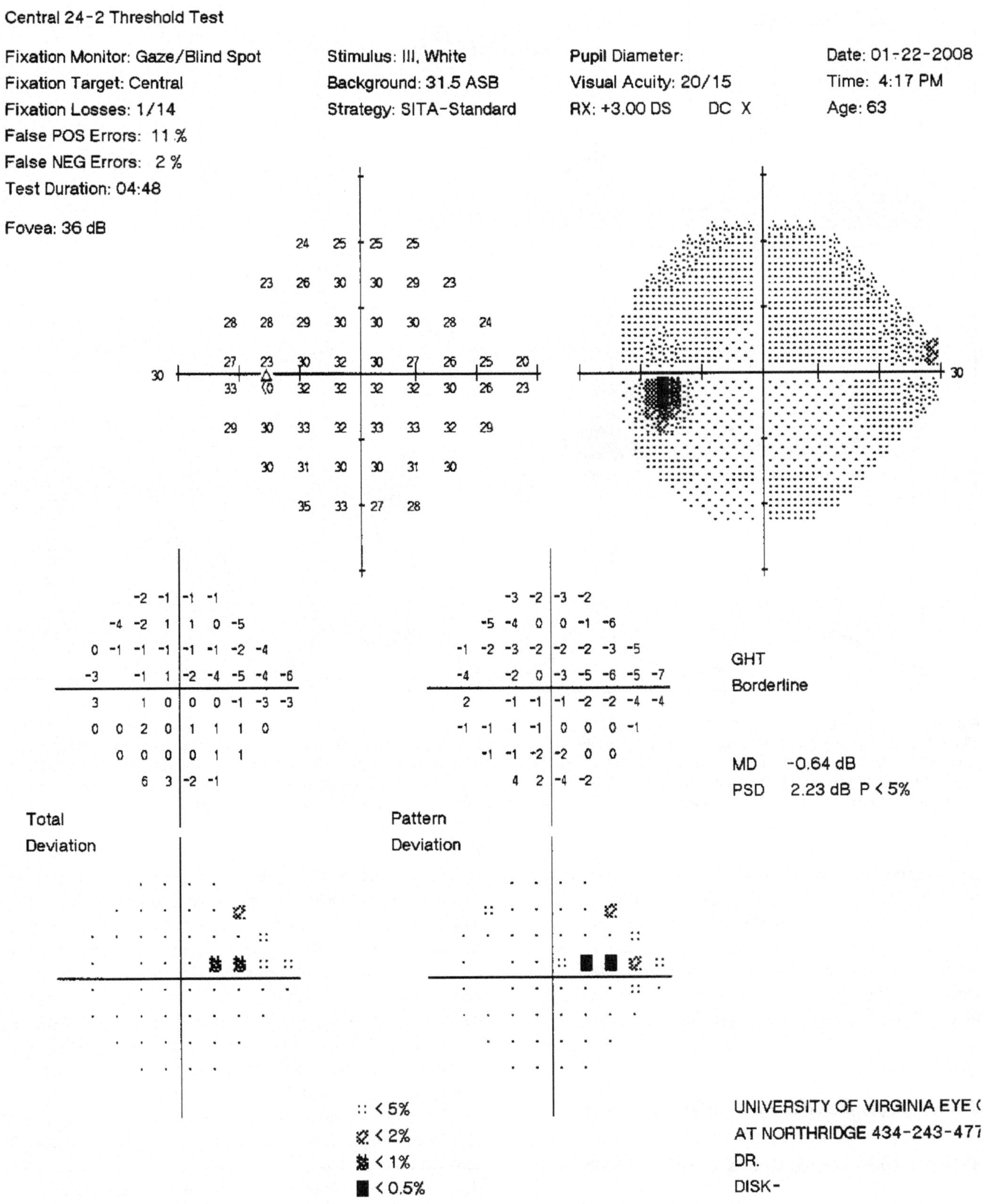

## 35 Normal Pressure Glaucoma

**Central 24-2 Threshold Test**

Fixation Monitor: Gaze/Blind Spot
Fixation Target: Central
Fixation Losses: 1/14
False POS Errors: 11 %
False NEG Errors: 2 %
Test Duration: 04:48

Fovea: 36 dB

Stimulus: III, White
Background: 31.5 ASB
Strategy: SITA-Standard

Pupil Diameter:
Visual Acuity: 20/15
RX: +3.00 DS     DC  X

Date: 01-22-2008
Time: 4:17 PM
Age: 63

GHT
Borderline

MD    -0.64 dB
PSD   2.23 dB  P < 5%

Total Deviation

Pattern Deviation

:: < 5%
▨ < 2%
▩ < 1%
■ < 0.5%

UNIVERSITY OF VIRGINIA EYE (
AT NORTHRIDGE 434-243-477
DR.
DISK-

**Fig. 35.20** SITA standard 24-2 visual field OS of the NTG patient in Fig. 35.16. Note the very mild superior arcuate scotoma and superior nasal depression on this visual field OS, with a mean deviation of only −0.64 dB, corresponding to the early notch in the optic nerve rim seen in Fig. 35.19. Standard SITA perimetry on the 10-2 program OS was normal, however. The standard SITA 24-2 and 10-2 visual fields OD were also completely normal

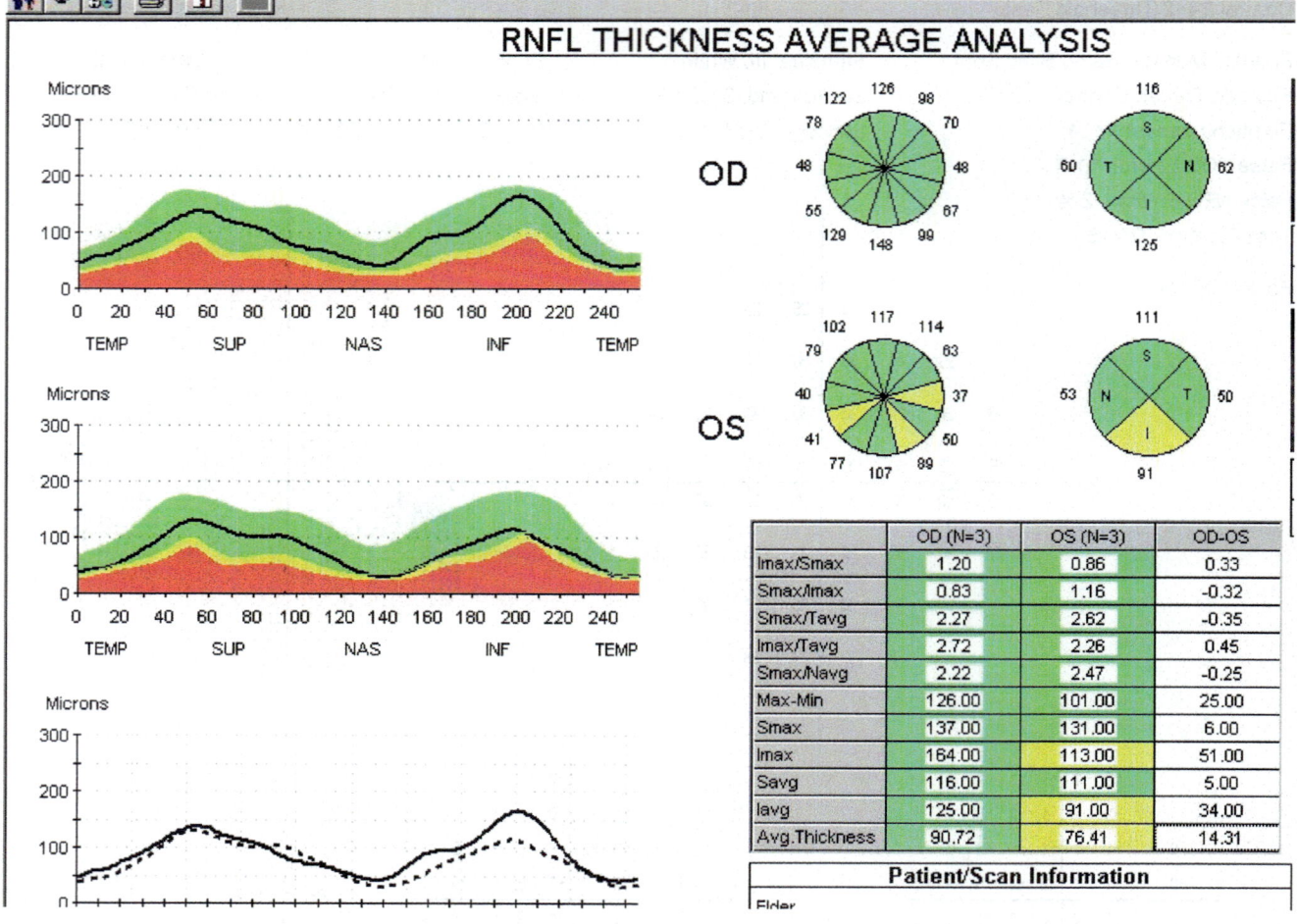

**Fig. 35.21** OCT NFL thickness of the NTG patient in Figs. 35.19 and 35.20. Note the asymmetric thinning of the inferior NFL thickness OS, seen on both the TSNIT graph on the *left* and on the *lower center* pictograph of this OCT printout. Average inferior quadrant NFL thickness is 125-μm OD and 91-μm OS (seen in the quadrant pictographs on the *top right*). There is definite 5 o'clock sector thinning of 89 μm OS (a *borderline yellow color* in the sector pie pictograph in the *center*), corresponding to the clinical notch of the optic nerve seen in Fig. 35.19. By comparison, the mirror image NFL thickness in the 8 o'clock sector OD is a normal 129 μm (a *green color* in the *top center* sector pie pictograph)

and Drance found NTG eyes with VF progression to have decreased blood flow velocities and increased resistive indices in their retrobulbar arteries compared with nonprogressing eyes with NTG or eyes with HTG.[133] Tanaka et al found minimum flow velocity of the central retinal artery and elevated cholesterol level to be associated with VF progression in 48 NTG eyes followed for more than 5 years.[134]

### 35.4.3 Age, Gender and Refractive Error

#### 35.4.3.1 Old > Young, Unless Myopic; Female > Male

The association of myopia and glaucoma is well established. Perkins and Phelps found an incidence of myopia of 27.4% in HTG and 22.4% in NTG eyes compared to 6.9% in the normal population.[137] Geijssen in 1991 was the first to describe the association of the myopic glaucomatous disc and NTG, later confirmed by other studies.[80] Araie et al found a significant positive association with degree of myopia and VF loss in the inferior, cecocentral area in both NTG and HTG; but, surprisingly, in NTG eyes only there was a negative association between high myopia and superior, cecocentral VF loss.[135] These authors concluded that myopic NTG eyes, especially with high myopia, are more likely to lose central vision, and therefore visual field tests of the central 10° may be critical to evaluate progression. But a later study from this same group found high myopia to be associated with more VF damage in a point just temporal and inferior to fixation in HTG eyes, but with less damage at these points in NTG.[136] However, they found high myopia to be associated with more VF damage at points nasal and inferior to fixation in the NTG eyes.

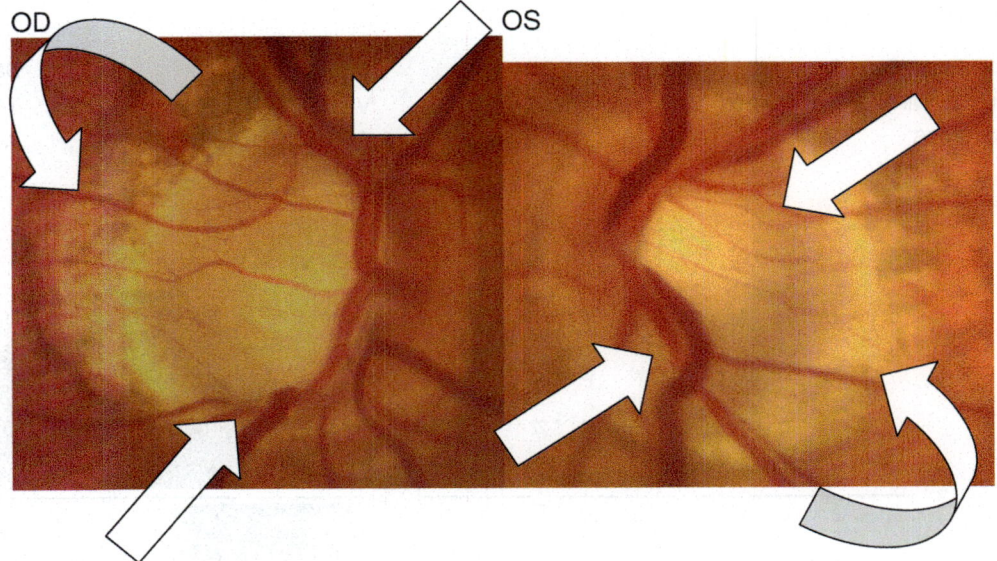

**Fig. 35.22** Color disc photographs of very advanced, but asymmetric, NTG, OD>>OS, in a 62-year-old Caucasian female with moderate myopia (−3.00 diopters). Note asymmetric loss of the OD rim inferiorly with focal notch (*inferior straight white arrow*, and vertical C/D ~0.9–0.95, between *straight white arrows*, *left photo*) and PPA (*curved white arrow*, *left photo*) and much less cupping OS (vertical C/D ~0.6–0.7 with even rim, between *straight white arrows*, *right photo*) but some mild PPA inferotemporally (*curved white arrow*, *right photo*). The visual field OD was very damaged, with probable early progression on both the 24-2 and 10-2 programs (see Figs. 35.23 and 35.24), but the VF OS showed only mild superior arcuate depression on the 24-2 program (MD=−0.09 to −1.74, during this time, not shown) and was essentially normal on the 10-2 program (not shown)

## 35.5 Systemic Factors

Migraine, vasospasm, cardiovascular disease, nocturnal hypotension, vascular dysregulation, autoimmunity, anemias, and diabetes, along with other systemic conditions and genetic factors, have all been associated with NTG. However, their significance in HTG and NTG will be discussed in detail in other chapters in this book. See Table 35.1 for systemic factors to consider when approaching evaluation of the NTG patient. Specifically, two interesting systemic associations with NTG are discussed in detail below.

**Table 35.1** Systemic factors that may play a role in NTG

| |
|---|
| Migraine headache and Raynaud's phenomenon |
| Vasospasm |
|     Endothelins |
|     C reactive protein |
|     Platelet aggregation, etc. |
|   Vascular disease – carotid disease, ASCVD, MI, blood vessel, cholesterol, inflammation |
| Nocturnal hypotension |
| Vascular dysregulation |
| Autoimmunity |
| Shock syndromes/hypotension |
| Anemias? |
| Diabetes mellitus |
| Obstructive sleep apnea syndrome |

### 35.5.1 Migraine Headache and Raynaud's Phenomenon

Supporting the concept of ischemia and vasospasm as a cause of optic nerve damage in glaucoma, US researchers found a higher prevalence of headache, and specifically migraine headache, in NTG patients (86%) than normals (64%),[138,139] but this association was found to be significant in Japanese NTG (17%) versus HTG (11%) versus normal (12%) patients.[140] Conversely, many migraine patients without the diagnosis of glaucoma have been found to have VFDs, often defined as "glaucomatous-like," in up to 35–62% of patients with normal IOPs.[141,142] Finally, as mentioned previously, the multicenter, prospective CNTGS recently found a 2.58 increased relative risk of VF progression in untreated NTG patients with migraine versus without migraine headache, even when controlling for patient sex.[143]

In summary, a preponderance of evidence thus supports an association between the vasospastic element of migraine and the pathogenesis of glaucomatous optic neuropathy in NTG, although the pathophysiology of this damage is unknown. Whether treatment of vasospasm with vasodilating drugs may be beneficial in NTG is discussed later (see Sect. 35.12).

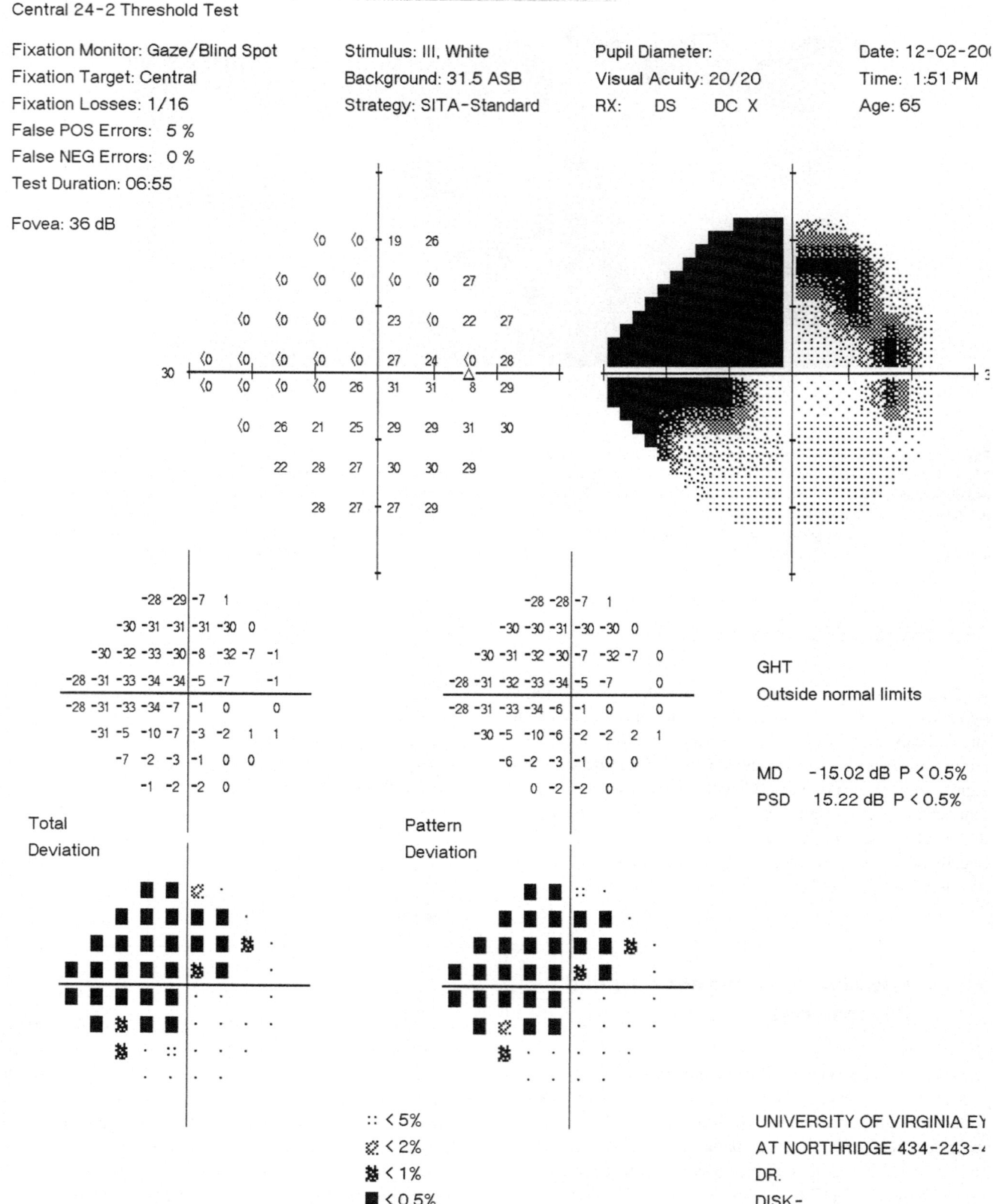

**Fig. 35.23** SITA standard 24-2 visual field OD of patient in Fig. 35.22. MD progressed from between −12.2 and −13.7 dB in 2006 and 2007 to −15.02 dB in 2008, shown here

# 35 Normal Pressure Glaucoma

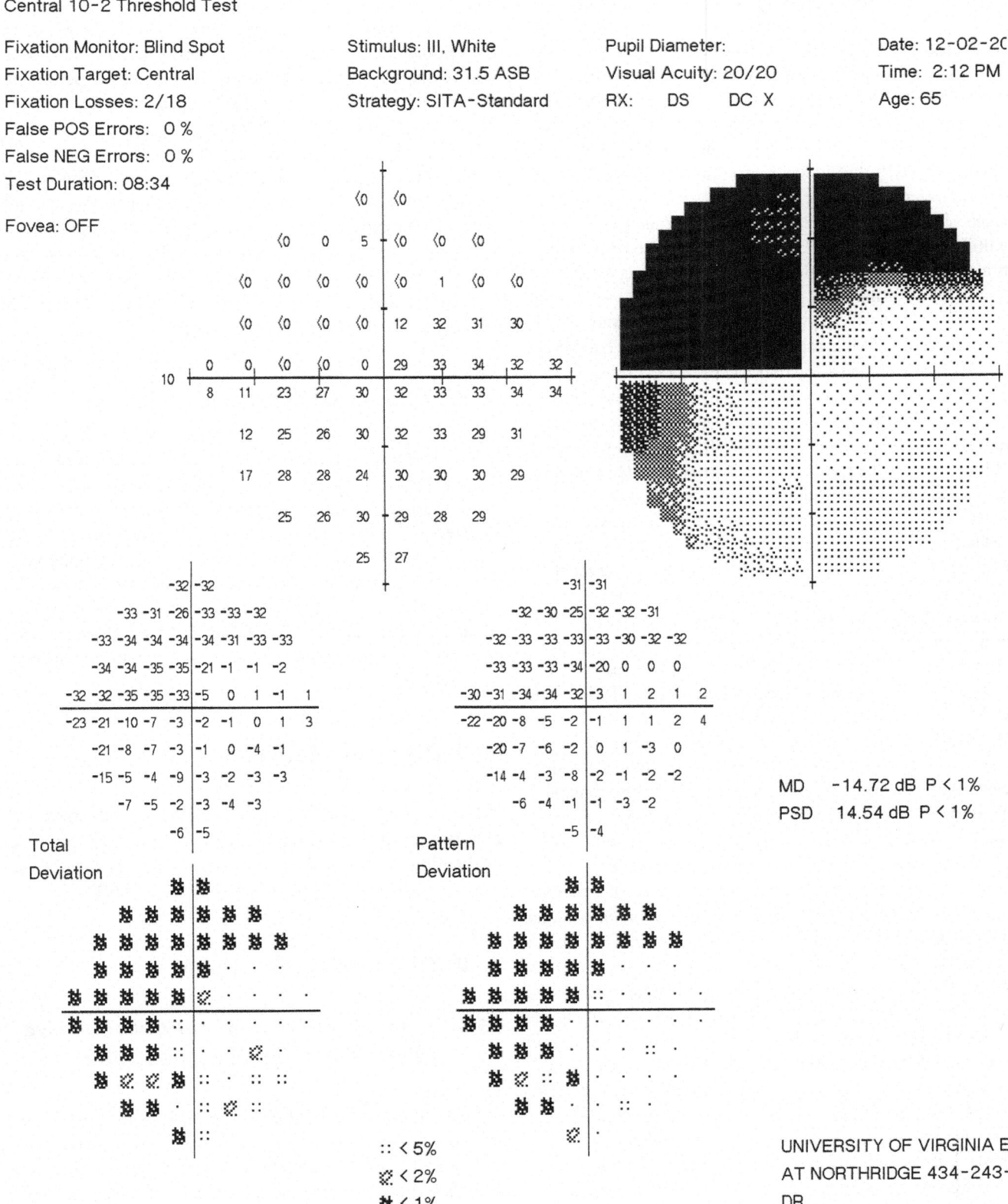

Fig. 35.24 SITA standard 10-2 visual field OD of patient in Figs. 35.22 and 35.23. MD progressed from −10.6 in 2005 to −14.7 dB in 2008, shown here. Note dense, superior arcuate scotoma to 1° of fixation superonasally with MD=−32 dB in this position

### 35.5.2 Obstructive Sleep Apnea Syndrome

The intriguing association of obstructive sleep apnea syndrome (OSAS) and glaucoma was first reported in a 1982 case series of five affected persons in two generations of the same family.[144] VF defects associated with OSAS have stabilized or reversed with treatment by continuous positive airway pressure (CPAP) during sleep at night.[145] In a study of 114 consecutive patients sent for a sleep study in one clinic, 3 patients had POAG, 2 had NTG, and all patients with glaucoma in this group had OSAS.[146] IOP was not elevated during sleep in a group of OSAS patients in one study, suggesting that repetitive nocturnal hypoxia may cause the optic nerve damage observed in some patients.[147] In another study of the association of OSAS and NTG, 5/9 NTG patients had OSAS, 2/9 NTG patients had sleep hypopnea, 2/4 NTG suspects had OSAS, 1/4 NTG suspects had sleep hypopnea, and 1/4 NTG suspects had upper airway resistance syndrome by polysomnography.[148] By contrast, only 1/30 comparison patients without NTG had a positive sleep history and also had upper airway resistance syndrome by polysomnography.

One NTG patient with OSAS and documented progressive VFDs over 5 years, despite successful medical and surgical treatment to lower IOP, was stabilized for the subsequent 3½ years after institution of CPAP.[149] Polysomnography in 16 consecutive NTG patients showed a high prevalence of OSAS in 50% of patients 45–64 years old and in 63% of patients >64 years old, suggesting the value of sleep studies and treatment in this group.[150] A study of 66 patients from Turkey with OSAS found significantly decreased RNFL by SLP, correlated with the degree of measured hypoxia, compared to 20 controls, suggesting chronic, decreased ocular perfusion-related hypoxia and vasospasm as a possible cause to explain this finding, which might precede clinically detectable glaucoma.[151] Another Chinese study of 41 patients with OSAS found that moderate and severe OSAS is associated with a higher incidence of VFDs and glaucomatous ON changes four times higher than in controls.[152] However, in a larger study from Israel, the prevalence of glaucoma in OSAS patients (2% of 228 patients) was found to be similar to the general Caucasian population.[153] And, still another very large nested case-control study of more than 7,000 patients in the US Veterans Administration hospital system did not find an association between OSAS and the diagnosis of glaucoma.[154]

A recent Italian study of 51 consecutive patients with OSAS, however, found an incidence of unsuspected NTG of 5.9%, but no patient in the control group had OSAS or NTG.[155] These authors underscored the importance of obtaining a sleep history in patients with NTG to refer for appropriate polysomnography and treatment, when indicated. Finally, a very recent study of ocular blood flow in 31 OSAS patients compared with 25 controls found a 12.9% prevalence of glaucoma in the OSAS patients, all of whom had severe OSAS, and suggested that VFDs may be due to ON perfusion defects, which appear to increase as the resistivity index increases in the ophthalmic and central retinal arteries.[156] Indeed, these new findings will need to be further investigated to determine if the optic neuropathy seen in some patients with OSAS is true NTG and treatable by IOP-lowering or simply another glaucoma mimic that is IOP-independent.

Perhaps, with all this new evidence to suggest a possible association between OSAS, decreased ocular perfusion and optic nerve hypoxia, and glaucoma or glaucoma-like damage of the optic nerve, it is indeed wise to refer patients who are suspects for NTG or HTG with a positive sleep history for sleep studies to determine if they have unsuspected OSAS and might benefit from CPAP therapy.

## 35.6 Differential Diagnosis

The differential diagnosis of NTG has been discussed many times at length. It includes congenital or acquired optic nerve anomalies, ON damage associated with prior intermittent/undetected or prior known elevated IOP now normalized, compressive lesions of the optic nerve, ischemic optic neuropathies, myopia with tilted discs, shock-induced optic neuropathy, hereditary optic neuropathies, and nutritional or toxic optic neuropathies. See Table 35.2 for other diagnoses to consider when examining the patient whom you suspect may have NTG.

## 35.7 Diagnostic Evaluation

Table 35.3 outlines the appropriate elements of the medical/ophthalmic history, ophthalmic exam, ocular and systemic testing options, medical exam considerations, and follow-up strategy for a patient with known or suspected NTG.

## 35.8 IOP-Lowering Treatment

### 35.8.1 Guidelines Based on the Collaborative Normal Tension Glaucoma Study

The findings of the CNTGS have become the most important evidence to date that lowering of IOP is beneficial in patients with NTG. This 10 year study, begun in 1988, tested the hypothesis that lowering of IOP in patients with NTG has long-term benefit. Two hundred and thirty patients with unilateral or bilateral NTG documented by glaucomatous optic nerve cupping were enrolled at 24 centers. Patients had documented VF loss, and a median IOP of 20 mmHg or less.

**Table 35.2** Differential diagnostic possibilities for NTG

Prior or intermittently elevated IOP
  Angle Closure – old AACG, CACG, Intermittent ACG
  Old Uveitis, Glaucomatocyclitic crisis
  Old trauma
  Residual steroid-induced
  Burned out pigmentary glaucoma
  Use of systemic medications, e.g., beta blockers, which might lower IOP
  Undetected, wide diurnal IOP fluctuation
  Nocturnal elevation of IOP in supine position only
Congenital optic nerve anomalies
  Optic nerve pits
  Optic nerve drusen
  Optic nerve coloboma
  Morning glory syndrome
  Optic nerve hypoplasia
Ocular disorders
  Degenerative myopia
  Retinal degenerations
  Myelinated nerve fibers
  Branch retinal vein occlusions
  Choroidal nevus or melanoma
  Retinoschisis
  Chorioretinal disease or scarring
Myopia with tilted disc syndrome
  Especially in young, Chinese males?
Compressive lesions
  Optic nerve – tumors, dolichoectatic carotid artery
  Pituitary/chiasm – tumors, aneurysms, cysts, chiasmatic arachnoiditis
Ischemic optic neuropathy
  Nonarteritic vs. arteritic/temporal arteritis
Shock-induced
  Hypotension/hypovolemia
Inherited optic nerve degenerative disorders
  Leber's hereditary optic neuropathy,
  Autosomal dominant optic neuropathy of Kjer
Nutritional/toxic optic neuropathies
  Tobacco/alcohol-related
  Vitamin B12 and folate deficiency
  Methanol induced
Tonometric error
  Thin CCT and underestimated IOP
  Low scleral rigidity

**Table 35.3** Elements of the medical and ocular exam for NTG

Medical/ocular history
  Migraine, Raynaud's syndrome, cold hands and feet, Prinzmetal's angina
  Patient age and associated morbidity/longevity
  Systemic nocturnal hypotension – overtreatment of HBP
Visual acuity
  Snellen acuity
  Color vision testing
Refractive error
Intraocular pressure
  Techniques – GAT, DCT, ORA, pneumatonometer, TonoPen

**Table 35.3** (continued)

  Confounding of CCT
  Positional changes – supine and yoga head stands in Sirsasana
  Diurnal and multiple day measurements, nocturnal?
Pachymetry for CCT
Gonioscopy to R/O uveitis/PAS, trauma/angle recession, PG/pigment
Iris/lens appearance to R/O PG, trauma, pseudoexfoliation
Optic nerve appearance
  Size
  Cupping patterns – APON/focal ischemic, senile sclerotic/age-related atrophic, myopic glaucomatous, notching, sloping, excavation, laminar dots/pore visibility, pallor, vessel patterns
  Hemorrhages
  RNFL
  PPA
  Tilting
  Document appearance – stereo photos, Stratus OCT, GDx VCC, HRT3
  Assess ON blood flow? – Color Doppler, velocimetry, flowmetry, FA
Risk factors for progression of ON damage – IOP fluctuation, ODH, migraine, female sex, age?
Visual field
  SITA SAP – size III vs. V stimulus, 24-2/30-2 vs. 10-2 pattern
    establish a good baseline
    frequent follow-up, q 3–6 months.
    use 10-2 program if VFD close to fixation
    use 10-2/size V program if very advanced damage
  SITA SWAP
  FDT Matrix
  Assess risk factors for progression of VF damage
MRI/CT ± contrast – indications
  Loss of central acuity not explained by clinical exam
  Disc pallor out of proportion to disc cupping
  Young age
    Hemianopic VFD not respecting the horizontal meridian, but respecting the vertical midline, particularly in the contralateral eye
  Unilateral progression despite equal IOPS in both eyes
  Unilateral or asymmetrical dyschromotopsia
Other possible tests, as indicated
  Cold challenge – nailbed capillaroscopy for vasospasm assessment
  24 h BP monitoring
    Blood tests – CBC, VDRL, FTA, ANA, ESR, Chem 12, Viscosity, CRP, complement C3 and 4, cholesterol, platelet aggregation, endothelins?, B12?, Folate?
    Carotid artery studies – Doppler U/S, MRA, angiogram
General systemic medical examination for:
  Monoclonal gammopathy of undetermined significance
  Autoimmune disease
  Blood pressure regulation to avoid nocturnal hypotension
  Treatment of cardiovascular disease
  Treatment of anemia
  Treatment of arrhythmia
  Treatment of congestive heart failure
  Systemic immunosuppression therapy in selected individuals?
Follow-up
  Risk factor assessment
  Diurnal vs. repeated IOP measurements for baseline IOP and fluctuation
  Role of 24-h IOPs?
  Good VF baseline

(continued)

**Table 35.3** (continued)

Frequent disc exams for ODH

Baseline ON photos and computerized imaging with periodic reimaging

Target IOP determination derived from studies with periodic reassessment

**Table 35.4** Summary of results from the CNTGS reports[4,5,129]

1. 1992: 30% IOP reduction from a mean of 16.9 mmHg was achieved in 57% of NTG patients without surgery
2. 1994: Early errors occurred in diagnosis of VF progression in NTG – more testing to confirm progression (in 4/5 repeated VF tests) reduced false positive rate from 57% to 2%
3. 1998: Comparison of VF progression between groups – reduction in rate for treated (12%) versus untreated (35%) NTG patients, when corrected for cataract (mostly seen in trabeculectomy eyes, 16/34)
4. 1998: Effectiveness of IOP reduction in NTG – VF progression seen in 20% of treated patients vs. 60% of untreated patients
5. 2001: Natural history of untreated NTG – 30% show small, localized progression by 3 years and 50% show small, localized progression by 7 years, not affecting the MD, but some progress faster
6. 2001: Factors increasing relative risk for progression of VFDs in NTG – migraine = 2.58, disc hemorrhage = 2.72, female gender = 1.85, Asians < Whites
7. 2003: Factors that predict the benefit of IOP lowering in NTG – no ODH, female gender, family history of glaucoma, no family history of stroke, no personal history of CVD, mild disc excavation, females (but not all) with migraine

Patients were randomized immediately if the VFD threatened fixation or they had previous documented VF progression; or randomized to observation and then to treatment later if the VF progressed, ON cupping progressed, or a new ODH developed. Treatment required a 30% reduction in IOP by medical therapy (excluding beta blockers and alpha adrenergic agents), LTP, or trabeculectomy. The findings of this study were published in seven reports from 1992 to 2003 and conclusively demonstrated the benefit of IOP-lowering to many, but not all, patients with NTG (see Table 35.4 for summary).

Glaucoma medical therapy developed since the initiation of the CNTGS (e.g., prostaglandin analog drops) may achieve lower IOPs without the need for laser or incisional surgeries. It is therefore possible that more NTG patients will achieve adequate target IOPs with medical therapy.

## 35.9 Medications: Many Classes Available

Discussion of all the classes of ocular hypotensive medications and their specific effects in patients with NTG is beyond the scope of this section but is found in several reviews.[157-160] Here, we highlight a number of pertinent studies on medical IOP-lowering therapy in NTG. To achieve effective IOP-lowering as in the CNTGS, it is suggested that clinicians aim for a 30% lowering of IOP in all patients with NTG. Whether this can be achieved with monotherapy or not is usually decided on a case-by-case basis in the clinic, which likely can only partially be answered by review of the studies to be presented.

### 35.9.1 Compliance Issues in NTG

A recent, retrospective study of noncompliance with clinic follow-up and visual field testing was conducted in 203 NTG suspects from Seattle, Washington.[161] Researchers found a 46% noncompliance rate. Noncompliance was associated with younger age (50 vs. 55 years), English-speaking patients, and lack of health insurance. Not surprisingly, lack of health insurance had the strongest association for noncompliance with follow-up visits. The question of why noncompliance is higher in NTG remains.

## 35.10 Laser Trabeculoplasty

In the CNTGS, use of argon laser trabeculoplasty (ALT) alone was effective to reduce IOP by 30% in 7% of patients, and in 23% of patients when combined with pilocarpine.[157,162] Another early, prospective French study found no effect of ALT to reduce IOP in a group of 29 eyes followed for 4 years.[163] However, in medically treated NTG eyes undergoing ALT in other studies:

1. Nakayama[164] reported a 2–3 mmHg lowering of IOP,
2. de Jong et al[165] found a 13% IOP lowering,
3. Ticho and Nesher[162] showed a 2.2–9.9 mmHg reduction in IOP (average 34.4%),
4. Schwartz et al reported a 73% success rate with a 4.9 mmHg IOP reduction in diurnal IOP at 12 months in those successful eyes. However, they described a decreasing IOP effect over the 22 months of follow-up.[166]

A recent prospective study of the nocturnal IOP-lowering effect of LTP in medically treated HTG patients found that the mean, peak, and range of nocturnal supine IOPs were decreased more consistently than during the diurnal period.[167] Hence, perhaps LTP is reasonable also to help reduce nocturnal supine IOPs in NTG patients, even if it does not seem to have much effect during daytime IOP measurements.

Selective laser trabeculoplasty is a new laser procedure felt to work by targeting pigmented cells in the trabecular meshwork and does not seem to cause thermal damage as in standard LTP. No studies of its use in NTG exist. However, several studies of HTG and OHT patients have shown a significant correlation between initial IOP and IOP-lowering effect. One study found that eyes with IOP ≤21 mmHg had an average IOP reduction of only 4.8% (0.74 mmHg) compared with a 20.4% (5.8 mmHg) reduction in eyes with IOP ≥21 mmHg.[168] This suggests that the effectiveness of SLT in NTG patients may be minimal, if any at all.

## 35.11 Filtering Surgery

### 35.11.1 Trabeculectomy

In the CNTGS, 43% of patients required a trabeculectomy in order to achieve a 30% lowering of IOP.[168a] The benefit to preservation of VF from this amount of IOP lowering, however, could not be ascertained until correction for the development of cataract, which occurred more frequently in the surgery group (16/34) than medically treated group (7/34) or the control group (11/34).[4]

This represented 14% of the control patients, 11% of the medically treated patients, and 26% of the surgically treated patients, a near doubling of risk with surgery. Clearly, surgical control of IOP comes at the cost of producing visually significant cataracts. One might argue that modern, clear corneal, small incision cataract surgery techniques with foldable intraocular lenses are minimally invasive, and that the cost of generating this reversible impairment to visual function, therefore, is relatively small in light of the long-term, permanent risk of irreversible loss of VF with uncontrolled IOP in NTG. But, even so, the risk of trabeculectomy failure following clear corneal cataract surgery is also not small.[169–171] As expected for this challenging disease to treat, a number of studies of the surgical management of NTG exist.

Abedin et al found that IOP lowering by full thickness sclerostomy achieved an IOP of ≤12 mmHg or less and preserved VF in 13 eyes with progressive NTG.[172] De Jong et al found that filtering surgery reduced IOP by 20% or more in 21/26 NTG eyes with progressive VF loss and lowered IOP by 6.8 mmHg (37%), compared with the contralateral nonoperated eye at 1 year, with a significant decrease in diurnal IOP variation from 4.3 to 2.1 mmHg.[173] Hitchings and coworkers showed a reduced rate of VF loss with surgery in 18 NTG patients with bilaterally progressive disease, undergoing unilateral trabeculectomy, over a follow-up of 2–7 years, with average preoperative IOPs of 17.2 mmHg decreased by 31%.[174] Yamamoto et al found IOP lowering from 13.9 to 7.9 mmHg in 42 eyes with NTG undergoing trabeculectomy.[175] Cataract progressed in 19%, hypotony maculopathy occurred in 12%, and VF deteriorated in two patients despite IOPs of 8 and 9 mmHg.

Koseki and colleagues showed prospectively that IOP lowering from 16 to 9.2 mmHg at 2 years by trabeculectomy with antimetabolites in 21 NTG patients with progressive VF loss could retard subsequent VF loss, as measured by an increase in MD slope from −1.48 to +0.13 dB/year.[176] Similarly, Bhandari et al showed that IOP lowering by trabeculectomy slowed the loss of VF in 17 NTG eyes with progressive disease.[177]

### 35.11.2 Trabeculectomy with 5-Fluorouracil and Mitomycin C

Hagiwara and coworkers prospectively demonstrated an IOP lowering from 14.8 to 9.6 mmHg by trabeculectomy with mitomycin C (MMC) in 21 NTG eyes over 2–7 years, with a reduction in MD slope to −0.37 dB/year in operated eyes versus −0.71 dB/year in the contralateral nonoperated eyes.[178] Visual acuity decreased in six operated and five nonoperated eyes, with cataract developing in 29% of the 21 operated eyes and 19% of the 21 nonoperated eyes. Visual field loss was also slowed or halted with surgical lowering of IOP by 20–30% in a study by Membrey et al in 61 NTG eyes, when VF loss was measured by pointwise linear regression analysis.[179] However, use of MMC was associated with a greater risk of VF deterioration compared with no antimetabolite or 5-fluorouracil (5FU) use. These researchers concluded that 5FU was preferable to MMC for this reason.

Shigeeda and colleagues also used antimetabolite-augmented trabeculectomy in 23 progressive NTG patients and found IOP reduction from 16.2 to 11 mmHg, over at least 5 years with a mean of 6 years of follow-up, associated with an increase in MD slope from −1.05 to −0.44 dB/year.[180] Jongsareejit et al found trabeculectomy with MMC to lower IOP significantly from 15.9 mmHg to 8–11 mmHg in 39 eyes throughout follow-up of 3 or more years (mean 4.2 years), with cumulative survival of VF of 39% and 41% at 4 years achieved with an IOP lowering of 20% and 30%, respectively.[181] However, they observed shallow anterior chambers (6), choroidal detachments (9), hypotony maculopathy (7), bleb leak (1), cataract (3), and blebitis (2), but no endophthalmitis postoperatively. Recently, Miyake et al retrospectively demonstrated that the reduction of IOP by trabeculectomy with MMC in 50 NTG eyes from 15.3 to 11.3 mmHg also decreased the rate of ODH from 42% to 8.8% following surgery.[182] In a group of 99 HTG eyes followed in the same study, the reduction in IOP from 19.6 to 11.1 mmHg was associated with a reduction in ODH from 33% to 5.5%. These researchers speculated that the reason for the decrease in ODH associated with surgical lowering of IOP was due to one or both of (1) a direct action of the postoperatively lowered IOP or (2) amelioration of blood circulation around the optic nerve head secondary to the decreased IOP.

If, as we believe, ODHs are:

1. an expression of pathological damage at the level of the microvasculature of the optic nerve head,
2. a harbinger of subsequent damage to the retinal ganglion cells and the nerve fiber layer, and
3. a precursor to future irreversible VF loss associated with glaucoma,

then certainly aggressive lowering of IOP by surgical means seems to be a reasonable course for NTG patients experiencing

**Table 35.5** Possible surgical procedures to consider in NTG eyes

Trabeculectomy with or without 5FU or MMC
  Trabeculectomy with express shunt
  Glaucoma drainage implants
  Nonpenetrating surgery
    Viscocanalostomy
    Nonpenetrating deep sclerectomy with collagen implant
  Trabeculotomy
  Trabectome?
  Canaloplasty/trabecular tightening?
  I-stent trabecular microbypass stent?
  SOLX suprachoroidal shunt?
  Cyclophotocoagulation
    Noncontact
    Contact – Diode G Probe
    Endocyclophotocoagulation with phaco
  Cataract surgery alone with potential postop IOP decline

progressive optic nerve and VF damage, especially if associated with an ODH.

Lastly, aggressive surgical intervention always brings the possibility of feared loss of remaining central visual function, often termed "snuff-out" of the optic nerve, particularly in patients with advanced glaucomatous disease. A recent retrospective review of 117 patients with severe glaucoma undergoing trabeculectomy over a 7-year period found only seven eyes to lose central vision postoperatively – three from hypotony maculopathy, two from uncontrolled IOP, and one from inflammatory reaction.[183] Patients losing central vision had higher preoperative IOPs (27 mmHg) and complication rates (43%) compared to those who did not lose central vision (19.7 mmHg and 4%, respectively). Therefore, with modern surgical trabeculectomy techniques employing judicious use of antimetabolites, coupled with selective postoperative suture release to enhance aqueous outflow while avoiding profound and early hypotony, we can be confident that loss of central acuity is rare due to the effect of trabeculectomy in NTG eyes (see Table 35.5 for a list of alternative surgical techniques for IOP lowering).

## 35.12 Non-IOP-Lowering Therapy (Neuroprotection?)

### 35.12.1 Calcium Channel Blockers and Optic Nerve Blood Flow

With the awareness of, and evidence for, the possible role of vasospasm and vascular insufficiency in the pathogenesis of NTG, researchers have tried to target this element of the disease to see if systemic vasodilation therapy might have a beneficial effect to slow or halt disease progression. In an effort to see if alternative treatments might address the special subgroup of NTG patients who have migraine headache, Raynaud's syndrome, vasospastic tendencies (as demonstrated by slow recovery from constriction of capillaries in the hand in response to cold water immersion), and focal ischemic damage to the optic disc, researchers have studied a number of compounds and their local vasodilatory effects in the optic nerve. A few small studies have looked at the long-term effect of vasodilators to protect against VF loss in NTG patients. This effort to find drugs that could possibly enhance blood flow to the optic nerve might loosely be termed a search for "neuroprotection" of the optic nerve – a relatively new concept in glaucoma therapy. Attention has been directed mostly to the class of drugs known as calcium channel blockers.

#### 35.12.1.1 Nifedipine

A prospective, 6-month, Japanese study of nifedipine in 25 NTG patients showed a benefit in six patients with continual VF improvement over the short course of the study, especially in younger patients with a higher initial mean sensitivity, lower IOP, and better recovery from cold exposure.[184] A Finnish study of nifedipine and acetazolamide in NTG patients found no effect of either therapy to prevent progressive loss of NRR, even in patients with demonstrated cold hands and feet and a positive response to cold challenge.[185] A retrospective US survey of HTG and NTG patients on concurrent therapy with several different CCBs, however, suggested that in NTG patients taking these medications only 2/18 (11%) eyes progressed by VF analysis compared to 10/18 (56%) that progressed while not on CCB therapy, with 0/18 that progressed by ON criteria while on CCBs compared to 8/18 (44%) not on CCB treatment.[186] By contrast, CCB therapy in HTG had no effect on rate of VF or ON progression. Another US study examined the serial course of VFs and optic nerve damage in a group of 43 OAG patients taking various CCBs for nonocular disease and compared them to a control group with the same ocular diagnoses but no systemic CCB treatment.[187] These investigators, however, could not find any difference in IOP and stability or change in VFs and ONs between groups, even among the NTG subset in their study population.

Gaspar et al studied short-term treatment with nifedipine in 59 patients with VF defects and saw an average improvement in VF MD of 1.2 dB after treatment.[188] Improvement was better in younger patients but worse in patients with optic nerve excavation, and no improvement was seen with anterior ischemic optic neuropathy. Six months of treatment with nifedipine improved contrast sensitivity at six cycles per degree in 16/21 NTG patients who could tolerate the medication, but nifedipine did not alter average retrobulbar blood flow in these subjects.[189] However, patients experiencing the most improvement in retrobulbar blood flow also experienced the most improvement in visual function.

### 35.12.1.2 Brovincamine

Brovincamine, a selective cerebral vasodilating CCB at one time available in Japan, was shown to improve or stabilize visual fields in NTG patients in two independent, prospective, randomized trials. The first trial by Sawada et al showed VF improvement in a subset of 6/14 patients compared to 0/14 in the placebo group over a mean of 3.2 years with a minimum of 2.5 years of follow-up.[190] Patients with better recovery from cold exposure and higher systolic BP showed the most benefit. A second 2-year study of 48 patients by Koseki et al showed progressive VF deterioration in six VF test points (in the superior arcuate and superior nasal step region) in the control group compared to no deteriorating points in the brovincamine group.[191] The authors of both studies felt that their results suggested the distinct potential for brovincamine to stabilize or improve VFs in NTG patients and suggested the need for further large-scale trials.

### 35.12.1.3 Nilvadipine

Several short-term studies examining the vascular effects of nilvadipine by color Doppler imaging and scanning laser Doppler flowmetry have been performed in animals and humans. This CCB has been shown to:

1. Decrease vascular resistance in distal retro-orbital vessels,[192]
2. Reduce orbital vascular resistance and increase optic disc blood flow,[193]
3. Increase blood velocity, and probably blood flow, in the optic nerve, choroid and retina of rabbits and also increase blood velocity in the human optic nerve head,[194] and
4. Reduce the resistance index of orbital vessels, similar to $CO_2$ inhalation.[195]

### 35.12.1.4 Nimodipine

Nimodipine, FDA-approved in the US, is a centrally acting CCB like brovincamine. Its effect on visual function and ocular blood flow assessed by laser Doppler flowmetry has been investigated in a number of very short-term studies. Results of these studies have shown:

1. Improved contrast sensitivity in NTG patients and controls after a single dose,[196]
2. Improved VF performance in NTG patients and improved color vision in both NTG and normal patients, without change in macular hemodynamics, after a single dose in NTG,[197]
3. Significant increase in contrast sensitivity in healthy subjects without a change in optic nerve blood flow over 3 days,[198]
4. Normalization of retinal capillary blood flow in NTG patients with vasospastic hyperreactivity after a single dose,[199]
5. Increased optic nerve head and choroidal blood flow and improved color contrast sensitivity in NTG patients, but no correlation between the improved contrast sensitivity and ocular blood flow.[200]

### 35.12.1.5 Caution on CCBs and Development of OAG

Despite these potential demonstrated benefits of CCBs, as in all areas of medicine, research in larger groups of patients often sheds new light on previous evidence of a therapeutic benefit from a drug that may only have been tested in a few individuals. The case with oral CCBs and their potential benefit in NTG is not an exception. A recent, large, population-based study of over 3,800 individuals, in Rotterdam, the Netherlands prospectively examined the association between the use of antihypertensive medications and incident open-angle glaucoma over an average follow-up of 6.5 years.[201] During this period, 87 cases of open-angle glaucoma developed, and use of CCBs *increased* the relative risk of incident OAG by 1.8-fold, while use of beta blockers *did not increase* the risk of developing OAG. No other antihypertensive drug class was associated with incident OAG.

These investigators speculated that the increased risk of OAG associated with CCBs may be due to a reduction in BP without a reduction in IOP, leading to a decrease in OPP, despite the demonstrated potential for dilation of ophthalmic and posterior ciliary blood vessels by this class of drug. They further felt that, based on the results of their study, the hypothesis of increased resistance in optic nerve perfusion caused by beta blockers seems unlikely on theoretical grounds, giving no cause for stopping beta blockers in glaucoma patients. Contrary to previous suggestions of the benefit from CCBs and potential harm from beta blockers in some NTG patients seen in earlier small studies, these investigators felt that the strong association of CCBs with incident OAG and lack of such an association with beta blockers was enough to advise that use of

CCBs or discontinuation of beta blockers in NTG patients *could not be recommended.*

In summary, there is evidence on the benefit of systemic CCBs in NTG patients with vasospastic tendencies. However, this evidence is still very preliminary, is based on only a few studies with small numbers of patients, and it seems to conflict with new epidemiologic studies linking use of CCBs to an increased incidence of OAG. Hence, use of CCBs to protect the optic nerve by theoretically increasing blood flow in NTG cannot be advised at this time.

### 35.12.1.6 Memantine and Excitotoxicity

Memantine, an NMDA antagonist, has shown mild success in slowing the progression of symptoms of Alzheimer's disease and demonstrated bench research potential to be useful for neuroprotection in glaucoma.[202] However, a recent prospective, randomized, multicenter trial of memantine in medically treated NTG patients was stopped because of lack of efficacy endpoints reached. The search for neuroprotective medications for glaucoma will likely continue, despite this setback.

## 35.13 Conclusion

1. True NTG is most often a slowly progressive disease if untreated.
2. True NTG must be distinguished from "pseudo NTG" or POAG/HTG (e.g., with a thin CCT, increased supine/nocturnal IOP) and other congenital or acquired disc damage (e.g., AION, myopia, etc.)
3. True NTG is not rare in all racial groups worldwide.
4. True IOP is a misnomer, as newer techniques evolve to measure this ocular parameter and POAG (whether NTG or HTG) occurs at all levels of IOP.
5. Characteristic ON and VF findings are often seen in true NTG eyes (e.g., four types of discs and associated VFD).
6. Eyes with discs suspicious for NTG should lead to VF testing, computerized and photographic ON imaging, and close follow-up for change and diurnal/ nocturnal IOP assessment.
7. While risk factors for NTG exist, none are truly treatable to slow the disease progression except for IOP.
8. The CNTGS has clearly shown that a 30% lowering of IOP is the best available therapy for progressing NTG.
9. Medications, laser, and filtering surgery can achieve a 30% IOP reduction to stabilize NTG damage.
10. Future studies will help to elucidate if non-IOP-lowering (neuroprotective?) strategies or treatment will also help to slow progression in NTG. None are currently available or well-proven.

## References

1. von Graefe A. Amaurose mit Sehnervenexcavation. *Archiv für Ophthalmol.* 1857;3:484-487.
2. von Graefe A. Die iridectomie bei amauros mit sehnervenexcavation. *Archiv für Ophthalmol.* 1857;3:546.
3. Levene RZ. Low-tension glaucoma: a critical review and new material. *Surv Ophthalmol.* 1980;24:621-663.
4. The Collaborative Normal-Tension Glaucoma Treatment Study Group. Comparison of glaucomatous progression between untreated patients with normal-tension glaucoma and patients with therapeutically reduced intraocular pressure. *Am J Ophthalmol.* 1998;126:487-497.
5. The Collaborative Normal-Tension Glaucoma Treatment Study Group. The effectiveness of intraocular pressure reduction in the treatment of normal-tension glaucoma. *Am J Ophthalmol.* 1998; 126:498-505.
6. The Advanced Glaucoma Intervention Study (AGIS) 4: Comparison of treatment outcomes within race. Seven-year results. *Ophthalmology.* 1998;105:1146-1164.
7. The Advanced Glaucoma Intervention Study (AGIS) 7: The relationship between control of intraocular pressure and visual field deterioration. *Am J Ophthalmol.* 2000;130:429-440.
8. Lichter PR, Musch DC, Gillespie BW, et al. Interim clinical outcomes in the Collaborative Initial Glaucoma Treatment Study comparing initial treatment randomized to medications or surgery. *Ophthalmology.* 2001;108:1943-1953.
9. Heijl A, Leske MC, Bengtsson B, et al, for the Early Manifest Glaucoma Trial Group. Reduction in intraocular pressure and glaucoma progression: results from the Early Manifest Glaucoma Trial. *Arch Ophthalmol.* 2002;120:1268-1279, discussion 1371-1372.
10. Kass MA, Heuer DK, Higginbotham EJ, et al. The Ocular Hypertension Treatment Study: a randomized trial determines that topical ocular hypotensive medications delays or prevents the onset of primary open angle glaucoma. *Arch Ophthalmol.* 2002;120:701-713, discussion 829-830.
11. Grodum K, Heijl A, Bengtsson B. A comparison of glaucoma patients identified through mass screening and in routine clinical practice. *Acta Ophthalmol Scand.* 2002;80:627-631.
12. Sommer A, Tielsch JM, Katz J, et al. Relationship between intraocular pressure and primary open angle glaucoma among white and black Americans. The Baltimore eye survey. *Arch Ophthalmol.* 1991;109:1090-1095.
13. Leske MC, Wu SY, Honkanen R, et al. Nine-year incidence of open-angle glaucoma in the Barbados eye study. *Ophthalmology.* 2007;114:1058-1064.
14. Dielemans I, Vingerling JR, Wolfs RC, et al. The prevalence of primary open-angle glaucoma in a population-based study in the Netherlands. The Rotterdam study. *Ophthalmology.* 1994;101:1851-1855.
15. Bonomi L, Marchini G, Marraffa M, et al. Prevalence of glaucoma and intraocular pressure distribution in a defined population. The Egna-Neumarkt study. *Ophthalmology.* 1998;105:209-215.
16. Mitchell P, Smith W, Attebo K, et al. Prevalence of open-angle glaucoma in Australia. *Ophthalmology.* 1996;103:1661-1669.
17. Toupozis F, Wilson MR, Harris A, et al. Prevalence of open-angle glaucoma in Greece: the Thessaloniki eye study. *Am J Ophthalmol.* 2007;144:511-519.
18. Varma R, Ying-Lai M, Francis BA, et al. Prevalence of open-angle glaucoma and ocular hypertension in Latinos: the Los Angeles Latino eye study. *Ophthalmology.* 2004;111:1439-1448.

19. Iwase A, Suzuki Y, Araie M, et al. The prevalence of primary open-angle glaucoma in Japanese. The Tajimi study. *Ophthalmology.* 2004;111:1641-1648.
20. Vijaya L, George R, Paul PG, et al. Prevalence of open-angle glaucoma in a rural south Indian population. *Invest Ophthalmol Vis Sci.* 2005;46:2261-4467.
21. Yamagami J, Araie M, Shirato S, et al. [Diurnal variation of intraocular pressure in low tension glaucoma]. *Nippon Ganka Gakkai Zasshi.* 1991;95:495-499.
22. Yamagami J, Araie M, Aihara M, et al. Diurnal variation in intraocular pressure of normal-tension glaucoma eyes. *Ophthalmology.* 1993;100:643-650.
23. Ido T, Tomita G, Kitazawa Y. Diurnal variation of intraocular pressure in normal-tension glaucoma. Influence of sleep and arousal. *Ophthalmology.* 1991;98:296-300.
24. Collaer N, Zeyen T, Caprioli J. Sequential office pressure measurements in the management of glaucoma. *J Glaucoma.* 2005;14:196-200.
25. Kim DM, Seo JH, Kim SH, et al. Comparison of localized retinal nerve fiber layer defects between low-teen intraocular pressure group and a high-teen intraocular pressure group in normal-tension glaucoma. *J Glaucoma.* 2007;16:293-296.
26. Oguri A, Yamamoto T, Kitazawa Y. Spontaneous intraocular pressure reduction in normal-tension glaucoma and associated clinical factors. *Jpn J Ophthalmol.* 2000;44:263-267.
27. Okada K, Tsumamoto Y, Yamaski M, et al. The negative correlation between age and intraocular pressures measured nytohemerally in elderly normal-tension glaucoma patients. *Graefes Arch Clin Exp Ophthalmol.* 2003;241:19-23.
28. Cartwright MJ, Anderson DR. Correlation of asymmetric damage and asymmetric intraocular pressure in normal-tension glaucoma (low-tension glaucoma). *Arch Ophthalmol.* 1988;106:898-900.
29. Crichton A, Drance SM, Douglas GR, et al. Unequal intraocular pressure and its relation to asymmetric visual field defects in low-tension glaucoma. *Ophthalmology.* 1989;96:1312-1314.
30. Haefliger IO, Hitchings RA. Relationship between asymmetry in visual field defects and intraocular pressure difference in an untreated normal (low) tension glaucoma population. *Acta Ophthalmol (Copenh).* 1990;68:564-567.
31. Yamagami J, Shirato S, Araie M. The influence of the intraocular pressure on the visual field of low-tension glaucoma. *Acta Soc Ophthalmol Jpn.* 1990;94:514-518.
32. Dinn RB, Zimmerman MB, Shuba LM, et al. Concordance of diurnal intraocular pressure between fellow eyes in primary open-angle glaucoma. *Ophthalmology.* 2007;114:915-920.
33. Shuba LM, Doan AP, Maley MK, et al. Diurnal fluctuation and concordance of intraocular pressure in glaucoma suspects and normal tension glaucoma patients. *J Glaucoma.* 2007;16:307-312.
34. Shimmyo M, Ross AJ, Moy A, et al. Intraocular pressure, Goldmann applanation tension, corneal thickness, and corneal curvature in Caucasians, Asians, Hispanics, and African Americans. *Am J Ophthalmol.* 2003;136:603-613.
35. Hahn S, Azen S, Ying-Lai M, et al. Central corneal thickness in Latinos. *Invest Ophthalmol Vis Sci.* 2003;44:1508-1512.
36. Choi HJ, Kim DM, Hwang SS. Relationship between central corneal thickness and localized retinal nerve fiber layer defect in normal-tension glaucoma. *J Glaucoma.* 2006;15:120-123.
37. Shah H, Kniestedt C, Bostrom A, et al. Role of central corneal thickness on baseline parameters and progression of visual fields in open angle glaucoma. *Eur J Ophthalmol.* 2007;17:545-549.
38. Kim JW, Chen PP. Central corneal pachymetry and visual field progression in patients with open-angle glaucoma. *Ophthalmology.* 2004;111:2126-2132.
39. Brandt JD, Beiser JA, Gordon MO, et al. Central corneal thickness and measured high IOP response to topical ocular hypotensive medication in the Ocular Hypertension Treatment Study. *Am J Ophthalmol.* 2004;138:717-722.
40. Liu J, Roberts CJ. Influence of corneal biomechanical properties on intraocular pressure measurement: quantitative analysis. *J Cataract Refrac Surg.* 2005;31:146-155.
41. Iliev ME, Meyenberg A, Buerki E, et al. Novel pressure-to cornea index in glaucoma. *Br J Ophthalmol.* 2007;91:1364-1368.
42. Brandt JD. Central corneal thickness, tonometry, and glaucoma – a guide for the perplexed. *Can J Ophthalmol.* 2007;42:562-563.
43. Brandt JD. Central corneal thickness – tonometry artifact, or something more? *Ophthalmology.* 2007;114:1963-1964.
44. Chuo JY, Mikelberg FS. Calibration errors of Goldmann tonometers in a tertiary eye care centre. *Can J Ophthalmol.* 2007;42:712-714.
45. Kumar N, Jivan S. Goldmann applanation tonometer calibration checks: current practice in the UK. *Eye.* 2007;21:733-734.
46. Gerzozi HJ, Chung HS, Lang Y, et al. Intraocular pressure and photorefractive keratectomy: a comparison of three different tonometers. *Cornea.* 2001;20:33-36.
47. Chatterjee A, Shah S, Bessant DA, et al. Reduction in intraocular pressure after excimer laser photorefractive keratectomy. Correlation with pretreatment myopia. *Ophthalmology.* 1997;104:355-359.
48. Mardelli PG, Piebenga LW, Whitacre MM, et al. The effect of excimer laser photorefractive keratectomy on intraocular pressure measurements using the Goldmann applanation tonometer. *Ophthalmology.* 1997;104:945-948, discussion 949.
49. Munger R, Hodge WG, Mintsioulis G, et al. Correction of intraocular pressure for changes in central corneal thickness following photorefractive keratectomy. *Can J Ophthalmol.* 1998;33:159-165.
50. Levy Y, Zadok D, Glovinsky Y, et al. Tono-pen versus Goldmann tonometry after excimer laser photorefractive keratectomy. *J Cataract Refract Surg.* 1999;25:486-491.
51. Zadok D, Tran DB, Twa M, et al. Pneumotonometry versus Goldmann applantion tonometry after laser in situ keratomileusis for myopia. *J Cataract Refract Surg.* 1999;25:1344-1348.
52. Duch S, Serra A, Castenera J, et al. Tonometry after laser in situ keratomileusis. *J Glaucoma.* 2001;10:261-265.
53. Park HJ, Uhm KB, Hong C. Reduction in intraocular pressure after laser in situ keratomileusis. *J Cataract Refract Surg.* 2001;27:303-309.
54. Siaganos DS, Papastergiou GI, Moedas C. Assessment of the Pascal dynamic contour tonometer in monitoring intraocular pressure in unoperated eyes and eyes after LASIK. *J Cataract Refract Surg.* 2004;30:746-751.
55. Liu L, Lei C, Li X, et al. Measurement of intraocular pressure after LASIK by dynamic contour tonometry. *J Huazhong Univ Sci Technolog Med Sci.* 2006;26:372-373.
56. Pepose JS, Feigenbaum SK, Qazi MA, et al. Changes in corneal biomechanics and intraocular pressure following LASIK using static, dynamic and noncontact tonometry. *Am J Ophthalmol.* 2007;143:39-47.
57. Kierstein EM, Hüsler A. Evaluation of the Orssengo-Pye IOP corrective algorithm in LASIK patients with thick corneas. *Optometry.* 2005;76:536-543.
58. Chang DH, Stulting RD. Change in intraocular pressure measurements after LASIK the effect of the refractive correction and the lamellar flap. *Ophthalmology.* 2005;112:1009-1016.
59. Kohlhaas M, Spörl E, Böhm AG, et al. Applanation tonometry in "normal" patients and patients after LASIK. *Klin Monatsbl Augenhilkd.* 2005;222:823-826.
60. Yang CC, Wang IJ, Chang YC, et al. A predictive model for postoperative intraocular pressure among patients undergoing laser in situ keratomileusis (LASIK). *Am J Ophthalmol.* 2006;141:530-536.
61. Kohlhaas M, Spoerl E, Boehm AG, et al. A correction formula for the real intraocular pressure after LASIK for the correction of myopic astigmatism. *J Refract Surg.* 2006;22:263-267.

62. Jonas JB, Papastathopoulos KI. Optic disc shape in glaucoma. *Graefes Arch Clin Exp Ophthalmol.* 1996;234:S167-S173.
63. Mikelberg FS, Drance SM, Schulzer M, et al. The normal human optic nerve. Axon count and axon diameter distribution. *Ophthalmology.* 1989;96:1325-1328.
64. Mikelberg FS, Yidegiligne HM, White VA, et al. Relation between optic nerve axon number and axon diameter to scleral canal area. *Ophthalmology.* 1991;98:60-63.
65. Jonas JB, Budde WM, Panda-Jonas S. Ophthalmoscopic evaluation of the optic nerve head. *Surv Ophthalmol.* 1999;43:293-320.
66. Tomlinson A, Leighton DA. Ocular dimensions in low tension glaucoma compared with open-angle glaucoma and the normal. *Br J Ophthalmol.* 1972;56(2):97-105.
67. Tomita G, Nyman K, Raitta C, et al. Interocular asymmetry of optic disc size and its relevance to visual field loss in normal-tension glaucoma. Graefes Arch Clin Exp Ophthalmol. 1994;232: 290-296.
68. Jonas JB, Stürmer J, Papastathopoulos KI, et al. Optic disc size and optic nerve damage in normal pressure glaucoma. Br J Ophthalmol. 1995;79:1102-1105.
69. Gramer E, Althaus G, Leydhecker W. Site and depth of glaucomatous visual field defects in relation to sized of the neuroretinal edge zone of the optic disk in glaucoma without hypertension, simple glaucoma, pigmentary glaucoma. A clinical study with the Octopus perimeter 201 and the optic nerve analyzer. Klin Monatsbl Augenheilkd. 1986;189:190-198.
70. Lewis RA, Hayreh SS, Phelps CD. Optic disk and visual field correlations in primary open-angle glaucoma and low-tension glaucoma. Am J Ophthalmol. 1983;96:148-152.
71. Caprioli J, Spaeth GL. Comparison of the optic nerve head in high- and low-tension glaucoma. Arch Ophthalmol. 1985;103:1145-1149.
72. Eid TE, Spaeth GL, Moster MR, et al. Quantitative differences between the optic nerve head and peripapillary retina in low-tension and high-tension primary open-angle glaucoma. Am J Ophthalmol. 1997;124:805-813.
73. Iester M, Mikelberg FS. Optic nerve head morphologic characteristics in high-tension and normal-tension glaucoma. Arch Ophthalmol. 1999;117:1010-1013.
74. Iester M. Comparison of optic disc parameters between normal-tension glaucoma and visual-field-matched high tension glaucoma. In: Wall M, Mills RP, eds. Perimetry Update 2000/2001. The Hague, The Netherlands: Kugler Publications; 2001:323-329.
75. Tezel G, Kass MA, Kolker AE, et al. Comparative optic disc analysis in normal pressure glaucoma, primary open-angle glaucoma, and ocular hypertension. Ophthalmology. 1996;103:2105-2113.
76. Wang XH, Stewart WC, Jackson GJ. Differences in optic discs in low-tension glaucoma patients with relatively low or high pressures. Acta Ophthalmol Scand. 1996;74:364-367.
77. Miller KM, Quigley HA. Comparison of optic disc features in low-tension and typical open-angle glaucoma. Ophthalmic Surg. 1987;18:882-889.
78. Spaeth GL. Fluorescein angiography: its contribution towards understanding the mechanisms of visual loss in glaucoma. Trans Am Ophthalmol Soc. 1975;89:457-465.
79. Geijssen HC, Greve EL. The spectrum of primary open angle glaucoma. I: senile sclerotic glaucoma versus high tension glaucoma. Ophthalmic Surg. 1987;18:207-213.
80. Geijssen HC. Studies on Normal Pressure Glaucoma. Amsterdam, The Netherlands: Kugler Publications; 1991:1-178.
81. Geijssen HC, Greve GL. Focal ischaemic normal pressure glaucoma versus high pressure glaucoma. Doc Ophthalmol. 1990;75: 291-301.
82. Javitt JC, Spaeth GL, Katz LJ, et al. Acquired pits of the optic nerve. Increased prevalence in patients with low-tension glaucoma. *Ophthalmology.* 1990;97:1038-1043, discussion 1043-1044.
83. Spaeth GL. A new classification of glaucoma including focal glaucoma. Surv Ophthalmol. 1994;38:S9-S17.
84. Yamazaki Y, Hayamizu F, Miyamoto S, et al. Optic disc findings in normal tension glaucoma. Jpn J Ophthalmol. 1997;41:260-267.
85. Ugurlu S, Weitzmann M, Nduaguba C, et al. Acquired pit of the optic nerve: a risk factor for progression of glaucoma. Am J Ophthalmol. 1998;125:457-464.
86. Nduaguba C, Ugurlu S, Caprioli J. Acquired pits of the optic nerve in glaucoma: prevalence and associated visual field loss. Acta Ophthalmol Scand. 1998;76:273-277.
87. Jonas JB, Budde WM. Optic cup deepening correlated with optic nerve damage in focal normal-pressure glaucoma. J Glaucoma. 1999;8:227-231.
88. Quigley HA, Addicks EM. Regional differences in the structure of the lamina cribrosa and their relation to glaucomatous optic nerve damage. Arch Ophthalmol. 1981;99:137-143.
89. Quigley HA, Green WR. The histology of human glaucoma cupping and optic nerve damage: clinicopathologic correlation in 21 eyes. *Ophthalmology.* 1979;86:1803-1830.
90. Jonas JB, Gründler A. Optic disc morphology in "age-related atrophic glaucoma". *Graefes Arch Clin Exp Ophthalmol.* 1996;234: 744-749.
91. Nicolela MT, McCormick TA, Drance SM, et al. Visual field and optic disc progression in patients with different types of optic disc damage: a longitudinal prospective study. *Ophthalmology.* 2003;110:2178-2184.
92. Broadway DC, Nicolela MT, Drance SM. Optic disk appearances in primary open angle glaucoma. Surv Ophthalmol. 1999; 43:S223-S243.
93. Pederson JE, Anderson DR. The mode of progressive disc cupping in ocular hypertension and glaucoma. Arch Ophthalmol. 1980; 98:490-495.
94. Jonas JB, Gründler AE, Gonzales-Cortés J. Pressure-dependent neuroretinal rim loss in normal-pressure glaucoma. Am J Ophthalmol. 1998;125:137-144.
95. Nicolela MT, Walman BE, Buckley AR, et al. Various glaucomatous optic nerve appearances: a color Doppler imaging study of retrobulbar circulation. *Ophthalmology.* 1996;103:1670-1679.
96. Drance SM, Begg IS. Sector hemorrhage – a probable acute ischemic disc change in chronic simple glaucoma. Can J Ophthalmol. 1970;5:137-141.
97. Tan JCH, Poinoosawmy D, Hitchings RA. Tomographic identification of neuroretinal rim loss in high-pressure, normal pressure and suspected glaucoma. Invest Ophthal Vis Sci 2004;45:2279-2285.
97a. Begg IS, Drance SM, Sweeney VP. Ischaemic optic neuropathy in chronic simple glaucoma. Br J Ophthalmol. 1971;55:73-90.
98. Drance SM. Some factors in the production of low tension glaucoma. Br J Ophthalmol. 1972;56:229-242.
99. Drance SM. Disc hemorrhage in the glaucomas. Surv Ophthalmol. 1989;33:331-337.
100. Kim SJ, Park KH. Four cases of normal-tension glaucoma with disk hemorrhage combined with branch vein occlusion in the contralateral eye. Am J Ophthalmol. 2004;137:357-359.
101. Yoo YC, Park KH. Disc hemorrhage in patients with both normal-tension glaucoma and branch vein occlusion in different eyes. *Korean J Ophthalmol.* 2007;21:222-227.
102. Jonas JB, Budde WM. Optic nerve head appearance in juvenile-onset chronic high-pressure glaucoma and normal-pressure glaucoma. *Ophthalmology.* 2000;107:704-711.
103. Anderson DR. Correlation of peripapillary anatomy with the disc damage and field abnormalities in glaucoma. In: Greve EL, Heijl A, eds. Fifth International Visual Field Symposium. 1982. The Hague: Dr. W. Junk; 1983:1-10. (Doc Ophthalmol Proc Ser; 35).
104. Kawano J, Tomidokoro A, Mayama C, et al. Correlation between hemifield visual field damage and corresponding parapapillary

105. Buus DR, Anderson DR. Peripapillary crescents and halos in normal-tension glaucoma and ocular hypertension. *Ophthalmology*. 1989;96:16-19.
106. Araie M, Sekine M, Suzuki Y, et al. Factors contributing to the progression of visual field damage in eyes with normal-tension glaucoma. *Ophthalmology*. 1994;101:1440-1444.
107. Jonas JB, Xu L. Parapapillary chorioretinal atrophy in normal-pressure glaucoma. *Am J Ophthalmol*. 1993;115:501-505.
108. Chumbley LC, Brubaker RF. Low-tension glaucoma. *Am J Ophthalmol*. 1976;81:761-767.
109. Motolko M, Drance SM, Douglas GR. Visual field defects in low-tension glaucoma. Comparison of defects in low-tension glaucoma and chronic open angle glaucoma. *Arch Ophthalmol*. 1982;100:1074-1077.
110. Hitchings RA, Anderton SA. A comparative study of visual field defects seen in patients with low-tension glaucoma and chronic simple glaucoma. *Br J Ophthalmol*. 1983;67:818-821.
111. Caprioli J, Spaeth GL. Comparison of visual field defects in the low-tension glaucomas with those in the high-tension glaucomas. *Am J Ophthalmol*. 1984;97:730-737.
112. King D, Drance SM, Douglas G, et al. Comparison of visual field defects in normal-tension glaucoma and high-tension glaucoma. *Am J Ophthalmol*. 1986;101:204-207.
113. Drance SM, Douglas GR, Airaksinen JP, et al. Diffuse visual field loss in chronic open-angle and low-tension glaucoma. *Am J Ophthalmol*. 1987;104:577-580.
114. Chauhan BC, Drance SM, Douglas GR, et al. Visual field damage in normal-tension glaucoma and high-tension glaucoma. *Am J Ophthalmol*. 1989;108:636-642.
115. Crichton A, Drance SM, Douglas GR, et al. Unequal intraocular pressure and its relation to asymmetric visual field defects in low-tension glaucoma. *Ophthalmology*. 1989;96:1312-1314.
116. Haefliger IO, Hitchings RA. Relationship between asymmetry of visual field and intraocular pressure difference in an untreated normal (low) tension glaucoma population. *Acta Ophthalmol (Copenh)*. 1990;68:564-567.
117. Araie M, Kitazawa M, Koseki N. Intraocular pressure and central visual field of normal tension glaucoma. *Br J Ophthalmol*. 1997;81:852-856.
118. Chauhan BC, Drance SM. The influence of intraocular pressure on visual field damage in patients with norml-tension and high-tension glaucoma. *Invest Ophthalmol Vis Sci*. 1990;31:2367-2372.
119. Zeiter JH, Shin DH, Juzych MS, et al. Visual field defects in patients with normal-tension glaucoma and patients with high-tension glaucoma. *Am J Ophthalmol*. 1992;114:758-763.
120. Araie M, Yamagami J, Suziki Y. Visual field defects in normal-tension and high-tension glaucoma. *Ophthalmology*. 1993;100:1808-1814.
121. Koseki N, Araie M, Suzuki Y, et al. Visual field damage proximal to fixation in normal- and high-tension glaucoma eyes. *Jpn J Ophthalmol*. 1995;39:274-283.
122. Poinoosawmy D, Fontana L, Wu JX, et al. Frequency of asymmetric visual field defects in normal-tension glaucoma and high-tension glaucoma. *Ophthalmology*. 1998;105:988-991.
123. Reyes TD, Tomita G, Kitazawa Y. Retinal nerve fiber layer thickness within the area of apparently normal visual field in normal-tension glaucoma with hemifield defect. *J Glaucoma*. 1998;7:329-335.
124. Choi J, Cho HS, Lee CH, et al. Scanning laser polarimetry with variable corneal compensation in the area of apparently normal hemifield in eyes with normal-tension glaucoma. *Ophthalmology*. 2006;113:1954-1960.
125. Suzuki J, Tomidokoro A, Araie M, et al. Visual field damage in normal-tension glaucoma patients with or without ischemic changes in cerebral magnetic resonance imageing. *Jpn J Ophthalmol*. 2004;48:340-344.
126. Viswanathan AC, Hitchings RA, Fitzke FW. How often do patients need visual field tests? *Graefes Arch Clin Exp Ophthalmol*. 1997;235:563-568.
127. Zalta AH. Use of the central 10° field and size V stimulus to evaluate and monitor small central islands of vision in end stage glaucoma. *Br J Ophthalmol*. 1991;75:151-154.
128. Anderton SA, Coakes RC, Poisoowanamy S, et al. The nature of visual loss in low tension glaucoma. In: Heijl A, Greve EL, eds. *Proceedings of the 6th International Visual Field Symposium*. Dordrecht, The Netherlands: Dr W Junk Publishers; 1985:393-386.
129. Gliklich RE, Steinemann WC, Spaeth GL. Visual field change in low-tension glaucoma over a five-year follow-up. *Ophthalmology*. 1989;96:316-320.
130. Collaborative Normal-Tension Glaucoma Study Group. Natural history of normal-tension glaucoma. *Ophthalmology*. 2001;108:247-253.
131. Araie M, Sekine M, Suzuki Y, et al. Factors contributing to the progression of visual field damage in eyes with normal-tension glaucoma. *Ophthalmology*. 1994;101:1440-1444.
132. Daugeliene L, Yamamoto T, Kitazawa Y. Risk factors for visual field damage progression in normal-tension glaucoma. *Graefes Arch Clin Exp Ophthalmol*. 1999;237:105-108.
133. Yamazaki Y, Drance S. The relationship between progression of visual field defects and retrobulbar circulation in patients with glaucoma. *Am J Ophthalmol*. 1997;124(3):287–295.
134. Tanaka C, Yamazaki Y, Yokoyama H. [Study on the progression of visual field defect and clinical factors in normal-tension glaucoma]. *Nippon Ganka Gakkai Zasshi*. 2000;104:590-595.
135. Araie M, Arai M, Koseki N, et al. Influence of myopic refraction on visual field defects in normal tension and primary open angle glaucoma. *Jpn J Ophthalmol*. 1995;39:60-64.
136. Mayama C, Suzuki Y, Araie M, et al. Myopia and advanced-stage open-angle glaucoma. *Ophthalmology*. 2002;109:2072-2077.
137. Perkins ES, Phelps CD. Open angle glaucoma, ocular hypertension, low-tension glaucoma and refraction. *Arch Ophthalmol*. 1982;100:1464-1467.
138. Corbett JJ, Phelps CD, Eslinger P, et al. The neurologic evaluation of patients with low-tension glaucoma. *Invest Ophthalmol Vis Sci*. 1985;26:11011104.
139. Phelps CD, Corbett JJ. Migraine and low-tension glaucoma. A case-control study. *Invest Ophthalmol Vis Sci*. 1985;26:1105-1108.
140. Usui T, Iwata K, Motohiro S, et al. Prevalence of migraine in low-tension glaucoma and primary open-angle glaucoma. *Br J Ophthalmol*. 1991;75:224-226.
141. Lewis RA, Vijayan N, Watson CW, et al. Visual field loss in migraine. *Ophthalmology*. 1989;96:321-326.
142. Comoǧlu S, Yarangümeli A, Köz OG, et al. Glaucomatous visual field defects in patients with migraine. *J Neurol*. 2003;250:201-206.
143. Drance S, Anderson DR, Schulzer M, et al. Risk factors for progression of visual field abnormalities in normal-tension glaucoma. *Am J Ophthalmol*. 2001;131:699-708.
144. Walsh JT, Montplaisir J. Familial glaucoma with sleep apnoea: a new syndrome? *Thorax*. 1982;37:845-849.
145. Mojon DS, Mathis J, Zulauf M, et al. Optic neuropathy associated with sleep apnea syndrome. *Ophthalmology*. 1998;105:874-877.
146. Mojon DS, Hess CW, Goldblum D, et al. High prevalence of glaucoma in patients with sleep apnea syndrome. *Ophthalmology*. 1999;106:1009-1012.
147. Goldblum D, Mathis J, Böhnke M, et al. [Nocturnal measurements of intraocular pressure in patients with normal-tension glaucoma and sleep apnea syndrome]. *Klin Monatsbl Augenheilkd*. 2000;216:246-249.

148. Marcus DM, Costarides AP, Gokhale P, et al. Sleep disorders: a risk factor for normal-tension glaucoma? *J Glaucoma*. 2001;10: 177-183.
149. Kremmer S, Selbach JM, Ayertey HD, et al. [Normal tension glaucoma, sleep apnea syndrome and nasal continuous positive airway pressure therapy – case report with a review of the literature]. *Klin Monatsbl Augenheilkd*. 2001;218:263-268.
150. Mojon DS, Hess CW, Goldblum D, et al. Normal-tension glaucoma is associated with sleep apnea syndrome. *Ophthalmologica*. 2002;216:180-184.
151. Kargi SH, Altin R, Koksai M, et al. Retinal nerve fibre layer measurements are reduced in patients with obstructive sleep apnoea syndrome. *Eye*. 2005;19:575-579.
152. Tsang CS, Chong SL, Ho DK, et al. Moderate to severe obstructive sleep apnoea patients is associated with a higher incidence of visual field defect. *Eye*. 2006;20:38-42.
153. Geyer O, Cohen N, Segev E, et al. The prevalence of glaucoma in patients with sleep apnea syndrome: same as in the general population. *Am J Ophthalmol*. 2003;136:1093-1096.
154. Girkin CA, McGwin G Jr, McNeal SF, et al. Is there an association between pre-existing sleep apnoea and the development of glaucoma? *Br J Ophthalmol*. 2006;90:679-681.
155. Sergi M, Salerno DE, Rizzi M, et al. Prevalence of normal tension glaucoma in obstructive sleep apnea syndrome patients. *J Glaucoma*. 2007;16:42-46.
156. Karakucuk S, Goktas S, Aksu M, et al. Ocular blood flow in patients with obstructive sleep apnea syndrome (OSAS). *Graefes Arch Clin Exp Ophthalmol*. 2008;246:129-134.
157. Kass M. The treatment of normal-tension glaucoma. In Peril to the nerve – glaucoma and clinical neuro-ophthalmology. In: Leader BJ, Calkwood JC, eds. *Proceedings of the 45th annual symposium of the New Orleans academy of ophthalmology*. The Hague, The Netherlands: Kugler Publications; 1998:61-72.
158. Hoyng PFJ, Kitazawa Y. Medical treatment of normal-tension glaucoma. *Surv Ophthalmol*. 2002;47(suppl 1):S116-S124.
159. Kitazawa Y, Yamamoto T. Contemporary treatment of normal-tension glaucoma. *Ophthalmol Clin N Am*. 1991;4:889-895.
160. Cantor L. Achieving low target pressures with today's glaucoma medications. *Surv Ophthalmol*. 2003;48(suppl 1):S8-S16.
161. Ngan R, Lam DL, Mudumbai RC, et al. Risk factors for noncompliance with follow-up among normal-tension glaucoma suspects. *Am J Ophthalmol*. 2007;144:310-311.
162. Ticho U, Nesher R. Laser trabeculoplasty in glaucoma. Ten-year evaluation. *Arch Ophthalmol*. 1989;107:844-846.
163. Demailly P, Lehrer M, Kretz G. [Argon laser trabeculoretraction in chronic open-angle glaucoma with normal pressure. A prospective study on the tonometric and perimetric effect]. *J Fr Ophtalmol*. 1989;12:183-189.
164. Nakayama T. An analysis of progressive LTG at our clinic. *Folia Ophthalmol Jpn*. 1987;38:1895-1901.
165. de Jong N, Greve EL, Hoyng PFJ, et al. Results of a filtering procedure in low tension glaucoma. *Int Ophthalmol*. 1989;13: 131-138.
166. Schwartz AL, Perman KI, Whitten M. Argon laser trabeculoplasty in progressive low-tension glaucoma. *Ann Ophthalmol*. 1984;16: 560-562.
167. Lee AC, Mosaed S, Weinreb RN, et al. Effect of laser trabeculoplasty on nocturnal intraocular pressure in medically treated glaucoma patients. *Ophthalmology*. 2007;114:666-670.
168. Johnson PB, Katz LJ, Rhee DJ. Selective laser trabeculoplasty: predictive value of early intraocular pressure measurements for success at 3 months. *Br J Ophthalmol*. 2006;90:741-743.
168a. Schulzer MD. The Normal Tension Glaucoma Study Group. Intraocular pressure reduction in normal-tension glaucoma patients. *Opthalmology*. 1992;99:1468-1470.
169. Ehrnrooth P, Lehto I, Puska P, et al. Phacoemulsification in trabeculectomized eyes. *Acta Ophthalmol Scand*. 2005;83:561-566.
170. Inal A, Bayraktar S, Inal B, et al. Intraocular pressure control after clear corneal phacoemulsification in eyes with previous trabeculectomy: a controlled study. *Acta Ophthalmol Scand*. 2005;83:554-560.
171. Rebolleda G, Muñoz-Negrete FJ. Phacoemulsification in eyes with functioning filtering blebs: a prospective study. *Ophthalmology*. 2002;109:2248-2255.
172. Abedin S, Simmons RJ, Grant WM. Progressive low-tension glaucoma: treatment to stop glaucomatous cupping and field loss when these progress despite normal intraocular pressure. *Ophthalmology*. 1982;89:1-6.
173. de Jong N, Greve EL, Hoyng PF, et al. Results of a filtering procedure in low tension glaucoma. *Int Ophthalmol*. 1989;13:131-138.
174. Hitchings RA, Wu J, Poinoosawmy D, et al. Surgery for normal tension glaucoma. *Br J Ophthalmol*. 1995;79:402-406.
175. Yamamoto T, Ichien M, Suemori-Matushita H, et al. [Trabeculectomy for normal-tension glaucoma]. *Nippon Ganka Gakkai Zasshi*. 1994;98:579-583.
176. Koseki N, Araie M, Shirato S, et al. Effect of trabeculectomy on visual field performance in central 30 degrees field in progressive normal-tension glaucoma. *Ophthalmology*. 1997;104:197-201.
177. Bhandari A, Crabb DP, Poinoosawmy D, et al. Effect of surgery on visual field progression in normal-tension glaucoma. *Ophthalmology*. 1997;104:1131-1137.
178. Hagiwara Y, Yamamoto T, Kitazawa Y. The effect of mitomycin C trabeculectomy on the progression of visual field defect in normal-tension glaucoma. *Graefes Arch Clin Exp Ophthalmol*. 2000;238:232-236.
179. Membrey WL, Bunce C, Poinoosawmy DP, et al. Glaucoma surgery with or without adjunctive antiproliferaties in normal tension glaucoma: 2 Visual field progression. *Br J Ophthalmol*. 2001;85:696-701.
180. Shigeeda T, Tomidokoro A, Araie M, et al. Long-term follow-up of visual field progression after trabeculectomy in progressive normal-tension glaucoma. *Ophthalmology*. 2002;109:766-770.
181. Jongsareejit B, Tomidokoro A, Mimura T, et al. Efficacy and complications after trabeculectomy with mitomycin C in normal-tension glaucoma. *Jpn J Ophthalmol*. 2005;49:223-227.
182. Miyake T, Sawada A, Yamamoto T, et al. Incidence of disc hemorrhages in open-angle glaucoma before and after trabeculectomy. *J Glaucoma*. 2006;15:164-171.
183. Law SK, Nguyen AM, Coleman AL, et al. Severe loss of central vision in patients with advanced glaucoma undergoing trabeculectomy. *Arch Ophthalmol*. 2007;125:1044-1050.
184. Kitazawa Y, Shirai H, Go FJ. The effect of Ca2(+)-antagonist on visual field in low-tension glaucoma. *Graefes Arch Clin Exp Ophthalmol*. 1989;227:408-412.
185. Lumme P, Tuulonen A. Neuroretinal rim area in low tension glaucoma: effect of nifedipine and acetazolamide compared to no treatment. *Acta Ophthalmol*. 1991;69:293-298.
186. Netland PA, Chaturvedi N, Dreyer EB. Calcium channel blockers in the management of low-tension and open-angle glaucoma. *Am J Ophthalmol*. 1993;115:608-613.
187. Liu S, Araujo SV, Spaeth GL, et al. Lack of effect of calcium channel blockers on open-angle glaucoma. *J Glaucoma*. 1996;5:187-190.
188. Gaspar AZ, Flammer J, Hendrickson P. Influence of nifedipine on the visual fields of patients with optic-nerve-head disease. *Eur J Ophthalmol*. 1994;4:24-28.
189. Harris A, Evans DW, Cantor LB, et al. Hemodynamic and visual function effects of oral nifedipine in patients with normal-tension glaucoma. *Am J Ophthalmol*. 1997;124:296-302.
190. Sawada A, Kitazawa Y, Yamamoto T, et al. Prevention of visual field defect progression with brovincamine in eyes normal-tension. *Ophthalmology*. 1996;103:283-288.

191. Koseki N, Araie M, Yamagami J, et al. Effects of brovincamine on visual field damage in patients with normal-tension glaucoma with low-normal intraocular pressure. *J Glaucoma*. 1999;8:117-123.
192. Yamamoto T, Niwa Y, Kawakami H, et al. The effect of nilvadipine, a calcium-channel blocker, on the hemodynamics of retrobulbar vessels in normal-tension glaucoma. *J Glaucoma*. 1998;7:301-305.
193. Tomita G, Niwa Y, Shinohara H, et al. Changes in optic nerve head blood flow and retrobulbar hemodynamics following calcium-channel blocker treatment normal-tension glaucoma. *Int Ophthalmol*. 1999;23:3-10.
194. Tomita K, Araie M, Tamaki Y, et al. Effects of nilvadipine, a calcium antagonist, on rabbit ocular circulation and optic nerve head circulation in NTG subjects. *Invest Ophthalmol Vis Sci*. 1999;40:1144-1151.
195. Niwa Y, Yamamoto T, Harris A, et al. Relationship between the effect of carbon dioxide inhalation or nilvadipine on orbital blood flow in normal-tension glaucoma. *J Glaucoma*. 2000;9:262-267.
196. Bose S, Piltz J, Breton ME. Nimodipine, a centrally active calcium channel antagonist, exerts a beneficial effect on contrast sensitivity in patients with normal-tension glaucoma and in control subjects. *Ophthalmology*. 1995;102:1236-1241.
197. Piltz J, Bose S, Lanchoney D. The effect of nimodipine, a centrally active calcium channel antagonist, on visual function and macular blood flow in patients with normal-tension glaucoma and control subjects. *J Glaucoma*. 1998;7:336-340.
198. Boehm AG, Breidenbach KA, Pillunat LE, et al. Visual function and perfusion of the optic nerve head after application of centrally acting calcium-channel blockers. *Graefes Arch Clin Exp Ophthalmol*. 2003;241:34-38.
199. Michalk F, Michelson G, Harazny J, et al. Single-dose nimodipine normalizes impaired retinal circulation in normal tension glaucoma. *J Glaucoma*. 2004;13:158-162.
200. Luksch A, Rainer G, Koyuncu D, et al. Effect of nimodipine on ocular blood flow and colour contrast sensitivity in patients with normal tension glaucoma. *Br J Ophthalmol*. 2005;89:21-25.
201. Müskens RPHM, de Voogd S, Wolfs RCW, et al. Systemic antihypertensive medication and incident open-angle glaucoma. *Ophthalmology*. 2007;114:2221-2226.
202. Lipton SA. Pathologically-activated therapeutics for neuroprotection: mechanism of NMDA receptor block by memantine and S-nitrosylation. *Curr Drug Targets*. 2007;8:621-632.

# Chapter 36
# Primary and Secondary Angle-Closure Glaucomas

Marshall N. Cyrlin

Almost 70 million cases of glaucoma have been diagnosed worldwide, approximately half of which are classified as angle-closure glaucoma (ACG).[1] Lowe, in 1955, emphasized the study of the anterior chamber angle facilitating the early classification of angle-closure glaucoma.[2] Among patients with angle closure, primary angle-closure glaucoma (PACG) is the most common diagnosis. PACG is more common in Asians than in any other ethnic group.[3] PACG, primary open angle glaucoma (POAG), and chronic angle-closure glaucoma (CACG) are collectively a major cause of bilateral blindness worldwide, and responsible for more than 90% of the bilateral blindness in China.[4] It is estimated that by the year 2020, there will be approximately 21 million of cases of PACG, with more than 5.3 million bilaterally blind individuals as a result of angle closure.[5]

## 36.1 Definitions and Classification

Angle closure results from apposition of the peripheral iris to the trabecular meshwork (iridotrabecular contact – ITC). This can sufficiently obstruct the outflow of aqueous and result in glaucoma. The best method of classifying the various types of angle-closure glaucoma continues to be debated, as each has various strengths for different circumstances, but all are sound approaches based on etiology that guide the clinician to the correct and effective therapy.[6] Four current methods for diagnosing the classification of angle-closure glaucoma are summarized in Table 36.1, with additional discussion following.

### 36.1.1 International Society of Geography and Epidemiology of Ophthalmology Classification

Foster and associates have published a classification of angle closure that has been widely used in prevalence studies and epidemiological research.[7] It specifies three stages (PACS, PAC and PACG) in the progression of angle closure from ITC, and from signs of disease, such as elevated intraocular pressure and peripheral anterior synechia, to frank optic nerve damage as the result of chronically elevated pressure.

#### 36.1.1.1 Primary Angle-Closure Suspect

The individual with an anatomically narrow angle can be classified as a primary angle-closure suspect (PACS) when gonioscopy reveals a shallow peripheral angle recess with the iris close to the trabecular meshwork. The PACS has iridotrabecular contact (ITC) in three or more quadrants, no peripheral anterior synechiae, and normal intraocular pressure (IOP), optic nerve and visual field.[3]

Even without a history of sub-acute or acute angle closure attacks, this patient is at risk for future angle closure. If it is not deemed necessary to treat the eyes at the time of initial diagnosis, the patient should, however, be educated as to the potential for acute angle closure and the need for immediate care should symptoms occur. It may be wise to advise the patient to have an examination before any travel, and/or against extended travel to locations where eye care is not readily available.

#### 36.1.1.2 Primary Angle Closure

In an acute primary angle closure attack, there is a sudden obstruction of the anterior chamber (AC) angle with an acute elevation of the intraocular pressure to very high levels. This results in characteristic symptoms and ultimately blindness if left untreated. In PAC, the individual has iridotrabecular contact (ITC) in three or more quadrants, either elevated IOP and/or primary peripheral anterior synechiae (PAS), with normal optic nerve and normal visual field.[3]

**Table 36.1** Four methods for diagnosing angle-closure glaucoma.

Current diagnostic approaches

| Symptoms-based | Mechanism-based | Angle-closure configuration-based | International Society of Geography and Epidemiology of Ophthalmology (ISGEO) |
|---|---|---|---|
| Acute angle-closure | Pupillary block | Pure pupillary block | Primary angle closure suspect (PACS) |
| Angle closes suddenly with high intraocular pressure (IOP), symptoms & rapid optic nerve damage | Restriction of aqueous flow from posterior to anterior chamber | Shallow anterior chamber (AC), more anterior lens position, strong pupillary block tendency | Angle occludable, no peripheral anterior synechiae (PAS) Nl IOP, optic nerve, VF |
| Sub-acute angle-closure | Plateau iris | Non-pupillary block | Primary angle closure (PAC) |
| Milder, self limiting acute angle closure, may be intermittent | Anteriorly positioned ciliary processes push iris forward | Deeper AC, more posterior lens position, anterior positioned ciliary body (plateau), iris crowding | Angle occludable, increased IOP and/or PASNl optic nerve, VF |
| Chronic angle-closure | Lens induced angle-closure | Multiple mechanisms | Primary angle-closure glaucoma (PACG) |
| Partially closed angle, increased IOP, symptoms mild or absent until very late | Block results from swollen or mobile lens | | |
| Latent angle-closure | Retrolenticular mechanisms | Features of both pupillary block and non-pupillary block, difficult to distinguish prior to laser iridotomy | |
| Shallow AC, narrow angle, at risk for closure, nl IOP, nl optic nerve | Increased retrolenticular pressure, from ciliary block, posterior aqueous diversion | | Primary angle closureAbnormal optic nerve, VF |
| | | Note: The angle closure approach is limited to primary angle-closure glaucoma; it does not consider degree of angle obstruction or abnormal optic nerve | |
| Note: Symptom-based classification does not describe degree of angle obstruction or presence of nerve damage | Note: Mechanism-based classification is easy to understand and aids in determining the choice of treatment | | Note: The ISGEO classification defines three stages in the natural history, glaucoma is defined by abnormal optic nerve, visual field |

#### 36.1.1.3 Primary Angle-Closure Glaucoma

In PACG, the individual has ITC in three or more quadrants, with evidence of glaucomatous damage to the optic nerve or visual field.[3]

In chronic PACG, the angle usually closes gradually over time. Sustained ITC may result in a pathophysiologic cascade of trabecular dysfunction, PAS, increased IOP, optic nerve damage and visual field loss. Because the pressure rises gradually, the patient may have no symptoms until there is advanced glaucomatous visual loss. In this regard, the natural history of asymptomatic progression to blindness may be analogous to POAG.

### 36.1.2 Mechanistic (Pathophysiologic) Classification

Ritch and Lowe[8] proposed a classification based on the angle anatomy and mechanisms of outflow obstruction. Primary and secondary angle closures can also be classified mechanistically by the presence or absence of pupillary block and whether the iris is anatomically "pushed forward" or "pulled forward" to the trabecular meshwork (Table 36.2). Four successive levels of anatomic levels of angle closure have been described: iris (pupillary block), ciliary body (plateau iris), the lens (phacomorphic glaucoma), and vectors posterior to the lens (malignant glaucoma). Angle closure may result from blockage of outflow with one or more of these anatomical changes, with one or more mechanisms involved. Pupillary block may occur to some degree in other forms of glaucoma and must be ruled out. A consensus statement from the 3rd Global Association of International Glaucoma Societies (AIGS) Consensus Meeting on Angle-Closure Glaucoma concluded the following: "Although the amount of pupillary block may vary among eyes with angle closure, all eyes with angle closure require treatment with iridotomy."[3]

The possibility to visualize the anterior segment structures with imaging techniques such as ultrasound biomicroscopy (UBM) and optical coherence tomography (OCT) has enhanced our ability to better anatomically classify the angle-closure glaucoma, determine the mechanisms involved and institute proper therapy. Imaging can often clarify nebulous situations, particularly if one clinician has found the angle to be open when another has not. Further discussion of imaging is given in Chap. 27.

**Table 36.2** Mechanisms of angle-closure glaucoma.

Underlying mechanisms of angle-closure glaucoma
*Posterior mechanisms – Iris pushed forward*
With pupillary block
 Pupillary block glaucoma (primary angle closure)
  Lens-related mechanisms
   Subluxation of lens (partial zonular dehiscence)
   Mobile lens syndrome (weakened or lax zonules)
   Intumescent lens (phacomorphic)
   Implantable contact lens (ICL)
  Posterior synechiae
  Crystalline lens
  Pseudophakia
  Iris-vitreous block in aphakia
  Uveitis
Without pupillary block
 Plateau iris configuration/syndrome (anteriorly located ciliary processes)
 Pseudoplateau iris (iris ciliary body cysts, tumors)
 Malignant Glaucoma (aqueous misdirection syndrome, ciliary block)
 Lens-related mechanisms
  Subluxation of lens (partial zonular dehiscence)
  Mobile lens syndrome (weakened or lax zonules)
  Intumescent lens (phacomorphic)
 After cataract extraction (vitreous displaced forward)
 Uveal edema (after central retinal vein occlusion, after extensive panretinal photocoagulation (PRP), after scleral buckling procedures)
 Tumors
  Retinoblastoma
  Malignant melanoma
 Cysts
  Iris
  Ciliary body
 Retrolenticular tissue
  Persistent hyperplastic primary vitreous (PHPV)
  Retinopathy of prematurity (ROP)
*Anterior mechanisms – Iris pulled forward*
Membrane contraction
 Iridocorneal endothelial syndrome (ICE) – migration of corneal endothelium
 Posterior polymorphous dystrophy (PPMD)
 Penetrating and nonpenetrating trauma
 Neovascular glaucoma (NVG)
Inflammatory precipitate contraction
Inflammatory membrane
 Fuch's heterochromic iridocyclitis
 Syphilitic interstitial keratitis

## 36.1.3 Plateau Iris Configuration and Plateau Iris Syndrome

Plateau Iris Configuration and Plateau Iris Syndrome are conditions that are often confused with pupillary block and PAC. Plateau iris configuration is an anatomically abnormal anterior segment configuration that has the potential to result in angle closure. On gonioscopy in plateau iris, the root of the iris may be short and inserted more anteriorly on the ciliary face. This results in a plateau configuration with a shallow peripheral angle and a sharp drop-off of the peripheral iris. The anterior chamber may be of normal depth centrally and the iris only slightly convex.

Plateau iris syndrome may develop spontaneously or after pupillary dilation and may present with symptoms identical to an acute angle closure (pupillary block) attack. In some cases, there may also be an additional element of relative pupillary block. Ultrasound biomicroscopy (UBM), when available, is especially useful in the assessment and differentiation of pupillary block and plateau iris configurations. Imaging under both light and dark conditions is helpful. In a recent study, Filho and associates compared the UBM findings between plateau iris configuration (PIC) and primary open angle glaucoma with narrow angles (POAGNA).[9] They found that PIC eyes are characterized by a more crowded anterior segment compared with POAGNA eyes. However, when the same parameters were evaluated between light and dark circumstances, no changes occurred.

The etiology of a glaucoma attack may not be appreciated without imaging. The episode is therefore often treated with laser iridotomy. An iridotomy may not open the angle or may only open it partially. An eye with an open laser iridotomy and plateau iris configuration may ultimately undergo an acute attack, confirming the diagnosis.

Laser peripheral iridoplasty can open the angle in plateau iris syndrome.[10] This technique is not readily embraced by all ophthalmologists – some voicing discomfort over the inflammatory changes created by the application of the laser to the iris. This technique employs argon laser burns of low power and large spot size to the peripheral iris adjacent to the angle to physically pull open the angle. The eye is pretreated with apraclonidine or brimonidine. The argon laser treatment parameters are set to produce contraction burns (500 µm spot, 0.5–0.7 s, 80–100 mW). The Abraham lens is used to place the burns as peripherally as possible. The laser power should be adjusted accordingly so that the spots produce contraction – not penetration. Failure to see any contraction is an indication of too low power or PAS holding the iris to the sclera and preventing contraction. A full treatment requires from 20 to 24 spots over 360°. Overtreatment should be avoided. Approximately two spot diameters should be left between each spot and radial iris vessels should be avoided. Postoperatively, the patient is treated with topical steroid drops with the pressure monitored as with any other glaucoma laser procedure.[11] A primary treatment of combined peripheral iridoplasty and laser iridotomy performed sequentially has also been proposed.[12] A patient with plateau iris configuration is susceptible to undergoing further shallowing of the anterior chamber with aging and may also develop pupillary block (see Chap. 62 for further discussion of plateau iris syndrome).

## 36.2 Primary Angle-Closure Glaucoma Versus Secondary Angle-Closure Glaucoma

Angle-closure glaucoma has two pathophysiologic etiologies. The final common mechanism of each type is appositional obstruction of the trabecular meshwork by peripheral iris. This results in an impairment of aqueous outflow accompanied by a sudden (acute) or gradual (chronic) increase in intraocular pressure. Raised IOP and subsequent glaucomatous damage to the optic nerve result either from mechanisms that push the iris forward from behind, or from mechanisms that pull the iris forward into contact with the trabecular meshwork. Degrees of closure range from iridotrabecular contact (ITC) with normal intraocular pressure to total trabecular outflow occlusion with elevated pressure and eventual peripheral anterior synechiae (PAS).

Primary angle closure is caused by pupillary block that results in appositional and/or synechial closure of the anterior chamber angle. Conditions that were previously classified as primary angle-closure glaucoma, such as plateau iris, are generally associated with anatomic abnormalities of the anterior chamber. Conditions classified as secondary angle-closure glaucoma are associated with other ocular or systemic abnormalities.

In cases of primary acute angle closure attack or an acute secondary angle closure, the intraocular pressure can rapidly elevate to a dangerous level. Prompt diagnosis and treatment are paramount as blindness may ensue quickly.

## 36.3 Gonioscopy

Gonioscopy is essential to identifying the underlying anatomy and pathophysiology of angle closure in order to properly classify the type of glaucoma and initiate treatment.

Gonioscopy as a technique to visualize the anterior chamber angle was devised by Trantas in the1880s.[13] His method employed indenting the sclera and viewing with a direct ophthalmoscope. Koeppe gonioscopy, a method rarely used today both because of the elaborate setup it requires and because it is time-consuming to perform, is an excellent method of "direct" gonioscopy. A dome-shaped Koeppe lens is applied to each eye with the patient in the exam chair in the recumbent position and the angle is viewed directly through the lens with a handheld source of magnification and illumination (Fig. 36.1a, b). The advantages of this method are that there is no distortion of the anatomy and that corresponding area of the angle in each eye can easily be compared by placing a lens on each eye and then viewing back and forth. The disadvantages of Koeppe lenses are that they require extra diagnostic equipment, cannot be used at the slit lamp and do not allow for compression gonioscopy that would allow dynamic manipulation of the anterior chamber angle. Because the lens remains on the eye without any pressure from the examiner's hands, there is no possibility that the act of holding the lens on the eye can deform the angle. Deformation of the angle is a common problem by novice gonioscopists.

Current commonly employed methods of gonioscopy are termed "indirect" because the lenses are mirrored and the portion of the angle viewed is 180° away, as seen through the mirror. The widespread use of gonioscopy following the introduction of the Goldmann lens in 1938 greatly improved the understanding of anterior chamber anatomy and the pathogenesis of the angle-closure glaucoma. The three mirror Goldmann lens (Fig. 36.2) is the most versatile Goldmann type lens because in addition to the mirror for examining the angle, the other portions of the lens can also be used to view the posterior pole and more peripheral retina. The two mirror Goldmann and single mirror Goldmann lenses are smaller and easier to manipulate at the slit lamp. The advantage of the Goldmann type of lens is that it does not distort the appearance

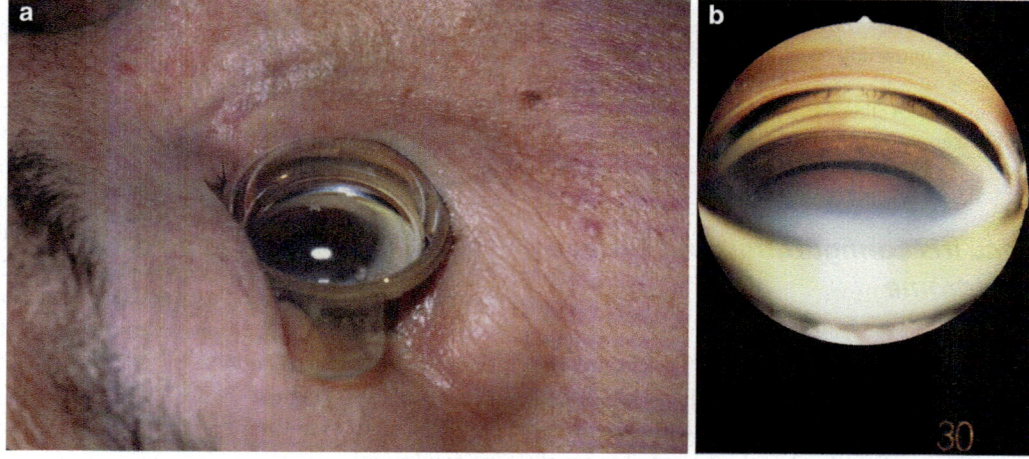

**Fig. 36.1** (a) Keoppe lens placed on eye in the recumbent position for direct gonioscopy (b) View through Koeppe lens of open, heavily pigmented angle

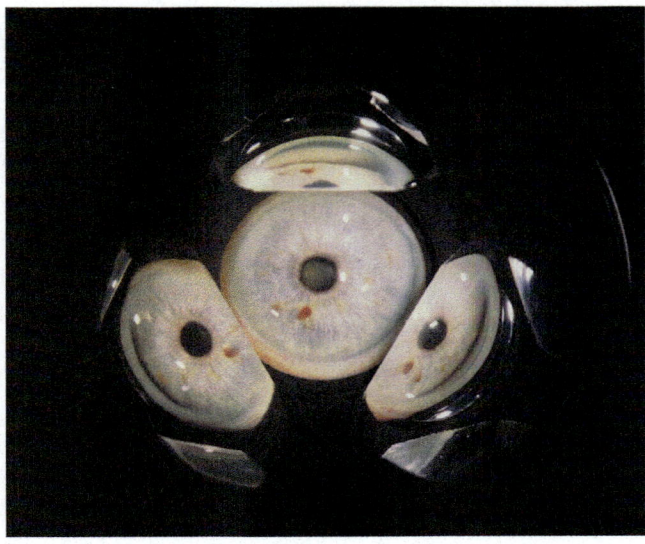

**Fig. 36.2** View through Goldmann three-mirror lens. The top mirror (*angle mirror*) shows an open angle

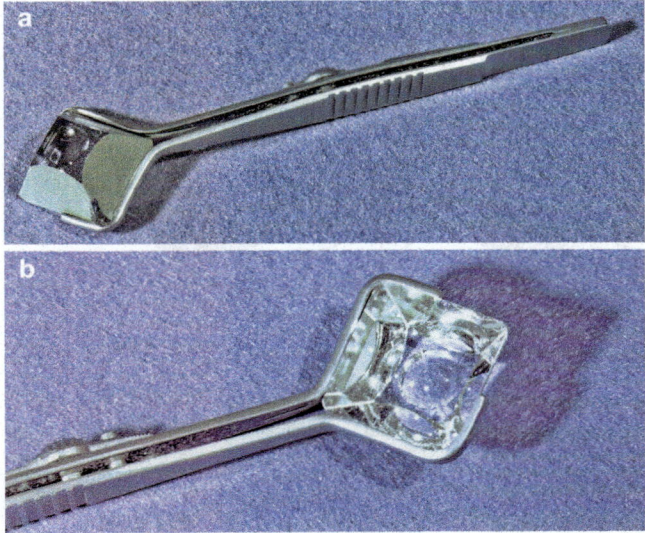

**Fig. 36.3** Zeiss lens. (**a**) Undersurface of Zeiss four-mirror lens shows the concave face of the lens which is applied to the tear film of the cornea. (**b**) Closeup of the clinician's (*slit lamp*) view of the four mirrors

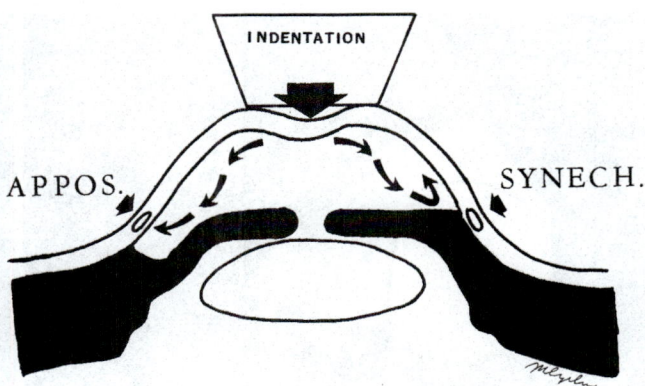

**Fig. 36.4** Compression gonioscopy. Compression with the four-mirror lens is employed to indent the cornea and force fluid into the peripheral angle. When the angle closure is appositional (iridotrabecular contact) the iris is pushed away allowing access of aqueous to the trabecular meshwork. When the angle closure is synechial the angle cannot be opened by compression.

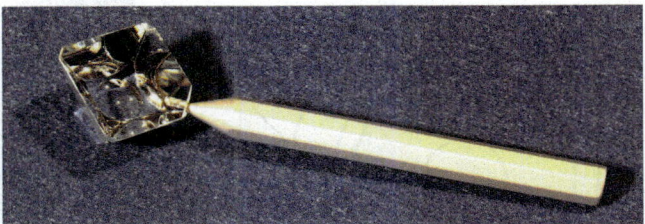

**Fig. 36.5** Posner four-mirror indirect gonioscopy lens

of the angle. The disadvantage is that viscous gonio solution must be employed as a coupling agent between the lens and the patient's corneal surface.

The original Zeiss lens is a pyramidal, silvered glass, four mirror lens with a shallow corneal curvature on its ocular surface. Nonsilvered versions with high-index glass, which afford an excellent view, are now available. The traditional lens is clipped into a retaining fork on a metal handle that is held in the clinician's fingertips (Fig. 36.3a, b). One advantage of this lens is that it is convenient to use during a routine slit lamp examination, as it is placed directly on the tear film and does not require a sticky gonio solution. At the conclusion of the gonio exam, the cornea remains clean and there is nothing to rinse off from the eye. Another major advantage is that the Zeiss lens may be employed to perform "compression gonioscopy." Compression gonioscopy is the intentional depression of the cornea with the gonioscopy lens to force fluid into the peripheral angle open in an attempt to widen or open it (Fig. 36.4). This technique is useful to determine if the narrow angle has appositional closure, synechial closure, or both.[14] The findings from this "dynamic gonioscopy" can aid the clinician in determining whether the patient would best benefit from laser iridotomy, trabeculectomy, or other glaucoma procedure. The disadvantage of the Zeiss lens is that the clinician must be wary not to unintentionally compress the cornea when initially viewing the angle structures, and thus erroneously overestimate the depth of the angle or its susceptibility for closure. The Zeiss lens (and its derivatives) requires more skill by the examiner, than does the Goldmann lens, to get an adequate view of angle structures.

The Posner lens (Fig. 36.5) is a variation of the Zeiss type lens with the four mirror lens mounted on a wand

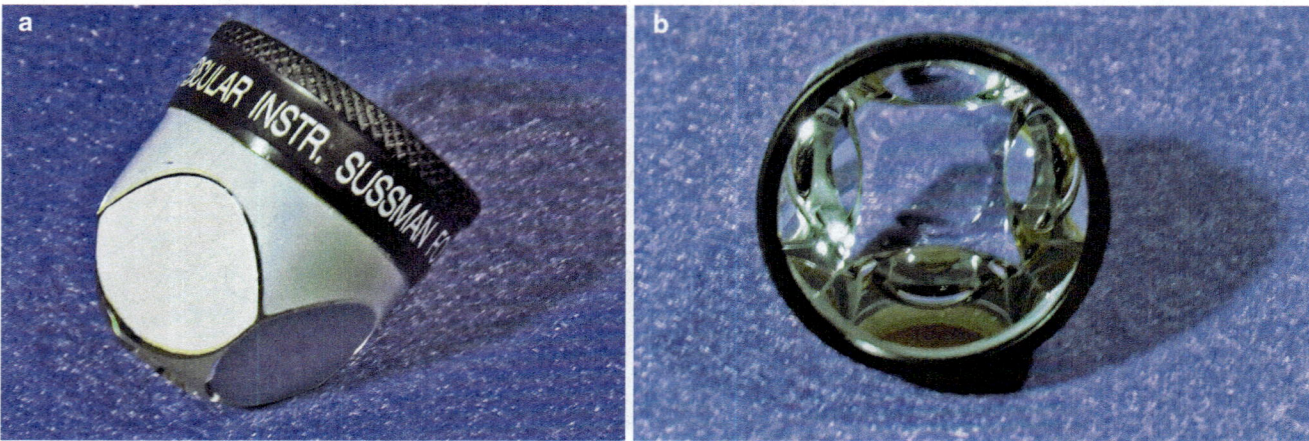

**Fig. 36.6** (**a**) Sussman four-mirror indirect gonioscopy lens side view. (**b**) Sussman four-mirror indirect gonioscopy lens mirror view. The central concave surface is applied to the tear film of the cornea and the angle is viewed through each of the mirrors

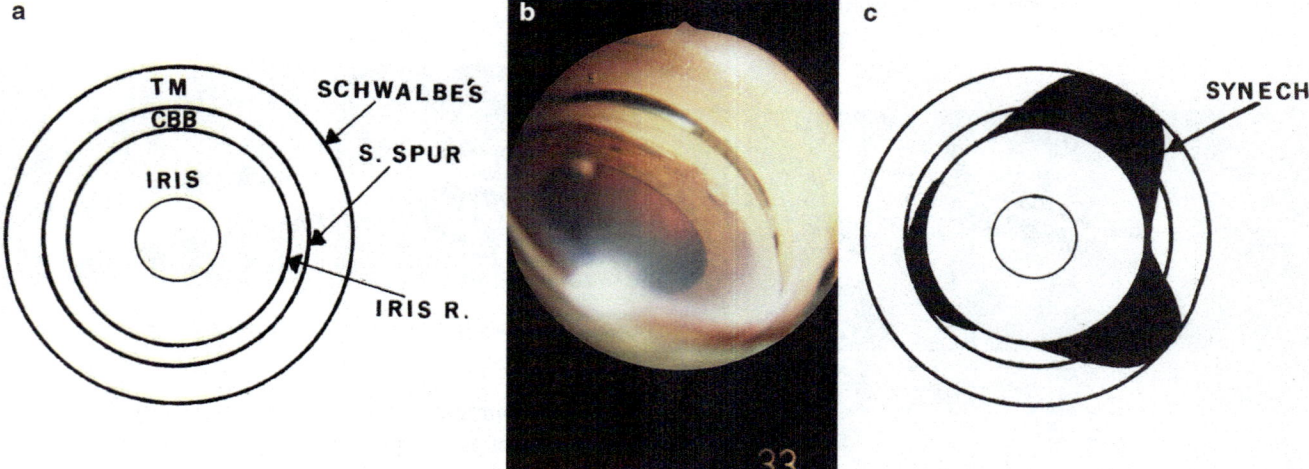

**Fig. 36.7** Diagramming the angle (**a**) Blank chart for diagramming the angle with the landmarks of Schwalbe's line, scleral spur and iris root indicated by lines and trabecular meshwork (TM), ciliary body band (CBB) and iris indicated by concentric rings. (**b**) Gonioscopic photographic (through Koeppe lens) of synechial angle closure. (**c**) Angle diagram of synechial angle closure depicting synechia completely covering the TM band and lower synechia up to the inferior border of the TM

shaped handle. The Sussman lens (Fig. 36.6a, b) is a similar four mirror lens mounted in a retaining ring and is directly held in the fingertips as is the Goldmann lens. The Posner and Sussman lenses are used in a similar fashion as the Zeiss lens to view the anterior chamber angle and to perform compression. In some patients, the corneal ocular surface curvature of these types of lenses does not well match that of the patient's cornea, and it is difficult to get the tear film to fill the interface appropriately. In these instances, a single drop of a thick artificial tear solution can often remedy this problem. With experience, most ophthalmologists easily master the technique of using these gonio lenses that use only tears as a coupling medium.

Various grading systems have been proposed to describe the appearance of the AC angle and its probability of closure.[15]

- The Scheie system grades the angle from "0 wide open" to "4 closed."
- The Shaffer system, the most widely used, grades the angle from "0 closed" to grade "4 wide open." A grade 1 angle would be considered possibly to probably occludable.
- The Spaeth system is more descriptive and specifies the iris insertion, amount of pigment, and the configuration of the iris.

The findings of the gonioscopy exam may be diagramed on a chart of concentric rings (Fig. 36.7a) with pathology such as closure or synechiae charted (Fig. 36.7b, c).

Gonioscopy lenses have therapeutic as well as diagnostic uses. In cases of acute angle closure attacks, dynamic gonioscopy (with Zeiss, Posner, or Sussman lenses) can sometimes

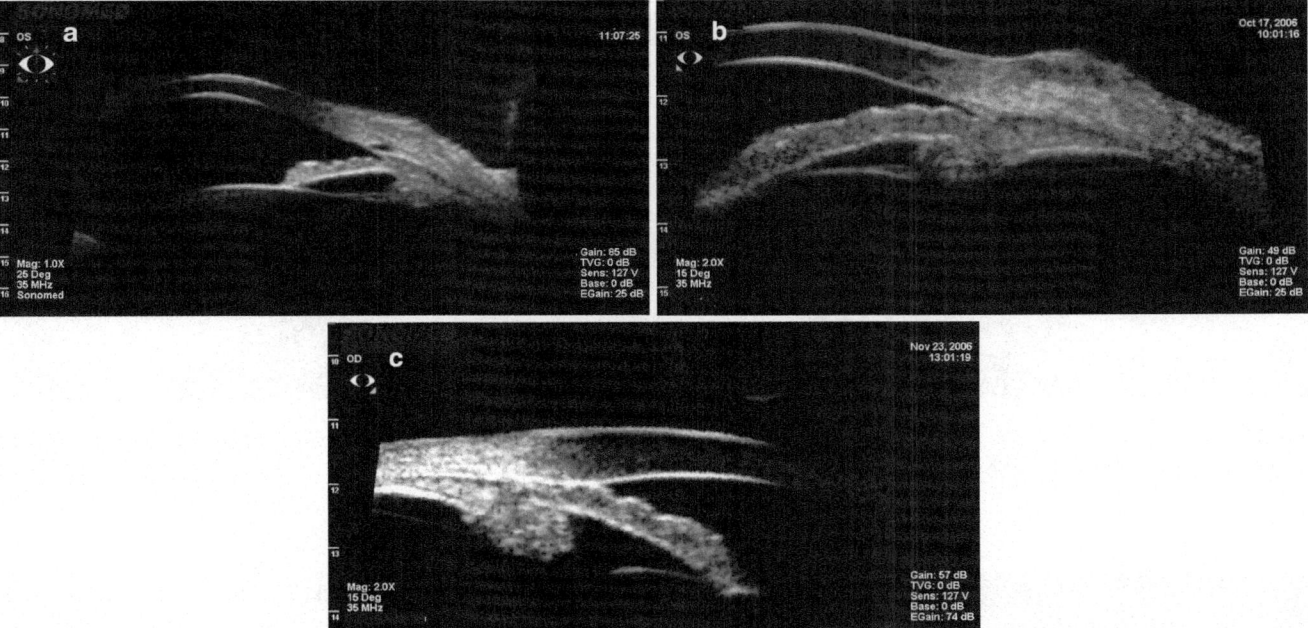

**Fig. 36.8** (a) UBM open angle. The anterior chamber is deep with the iris well away from the TM. The lucency internal to the TM is Schlem's canal. The ciliary sulcus is imaged as the larger lucent area posterior to the iris. (b) UBM narrow angle. The iris is convex and the peripheral anterior chamber is shallow but the angle is not closed. (c) UBM closed angle. The angle is closed with iridotrabecular contact. (Images courtesy of Sonomed, Inc., Lake Success, NY)

be used to interrupt the attack by compressing the cornea to relieve apposition and forcibly opening the peripheral angle after medical therapy has been initiated. The flat, nonsilvered portion of these lenses (between the mirrors) may also be applied to a filtering bleb after trabeculectomy surgery to compress the conjunctiva and visualize the underlying sutures to perform laser suture lysis when a lens dedicated for this purpose is not available. Gonioscopy is discussed in greater detail in Chap. 26.

## 36.4 Anterior Segment Imaging

### 36.4.1 Ultrasound Biomicroscopy, Optical Coherence Tomography, Scanning Peripheral Anterior Chamber Depth Analyzer, Dark-Room Infrared Gonioscopy

Imaging techniques such as ultrasound biomicroscopy (UBM) and optical coherence tomography (OCT), although not usually available to the community-based physician, have proven to be a useful adjunct to gonioscopy. Compared to gonioscopy, they are more objective, not as dependent on patient cooperation, and more precise in determining the anterior segment anatomy.[16-18] The role of UBM in the differential diagnosis of angle-closure glaucoma has been extensively reviewed by Tello et al[19] The standard UBM images the anterior segment with ultrasound in the low frequency range. It is useful to view the angle, iris, lens, postlenticular space, and ciliary body (Fig. 36.8a–c). The newer higher-frequency UBM can visualize Schlemm's canal and the angle, and can be used for imaging in the operating room. UBM can be used to elucidate pathophysiologic mechanisms in narrow angle and angle closure eyes. It is especially helpful in the assessment of pupillary block (Fig. 36.9a, b) and plateau iris configurations (Fig. 36.10). UBM is valuable in evaluating the persistence of appositional angle closure after laser iridotomy in the fellow eyes after acute primary angle closure.[20]

Optical coherence tomography images the anterior segment with light rather than ultrasound (Fig. 36.11a, b). It does not require direct ocular contact and is more comfortable for the patient. OCT is excellent at imaging structures anterior to the iris, but is not good at penetrating the pigmentation of the iris. Refer to Chap. 27 for further discussion of imaging.

The Scanning Peripheral Anterior Chamber depth analyzer (SPAC) obtains rapid slit photographs of the central and peripheral anterior chamber and creates an anterior iris surface contour. This measure can be compared to sample databases.[21]

A new imaging method for evaluating the angle is Dark-room Infrared Gonioscopy (DIG). Gonioscopy is performed

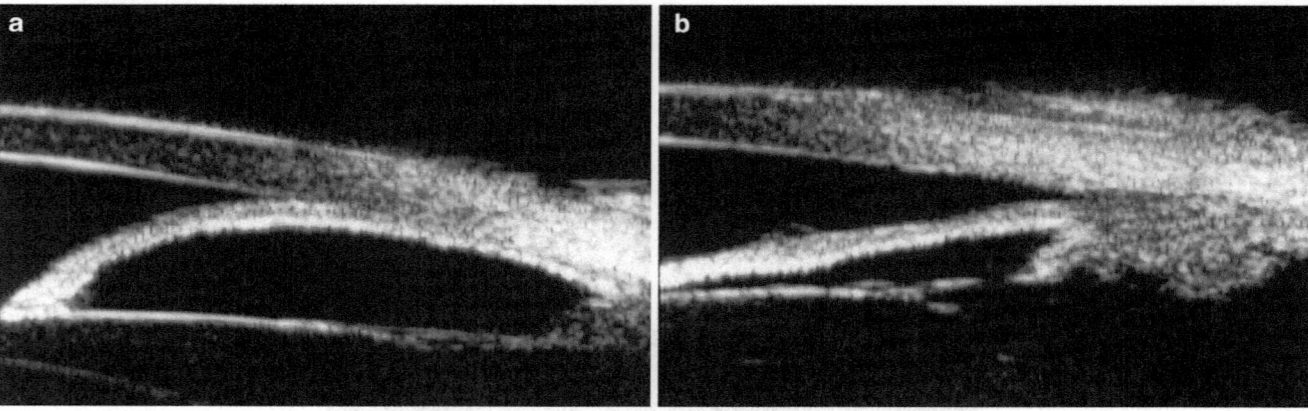

**Fig. 36.9** (a) Pupillary block. The convex iris is bowed forward occluding the angle. (b) Pupillary block broken with angle opened by laser iridotomy. (Images courtesy of Fred Kapetansky, M.D.)

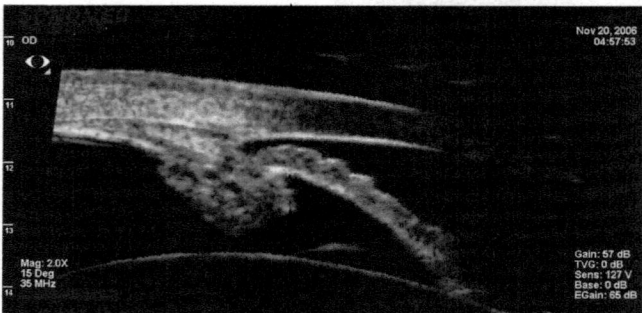

**Fig. 36.10** Plateau iris. There is a shallow peripheral angle with a sharp drop off of the peripheral iris. (Image courtesy of Sonomed, Inc., Lake Success, NY)

with infrared light eliminating the bright light of the slit lamp. This makes it possible to view the dynamics of the angle in the dark as well as light or accommodative stimulation. Although there is no commercially available instrument available at present, by modifying currently available video instruments DIG can be performed.[22]

## 36.5 Pathogenesis and Pathophysiology of the Angle-Closure Glaucoma

Angle-closure results from appositional obstruction of the trabecular meshwork by the peripheral iris. This can be a consequence of an abnormal relationship between the size and position of the structures of the anterior segment and the relative pressure differential between the anterior and posterior chambers. Blockage of the meshwork may occur by forces acting at four successive anatomic levels, as proposed by Ritch et al[8] The first anatomic level described is at the iris. Mechanistically, this is the site of pupillary block. The next anatomic level is at the ciliary body, the level at which plateau iris syndrome occurs. The third level is the lens, which is involved in phacogenic mechanisms. The fourth anatomic level relates to forces posterior to the lens. This level has therefore been described as retinovitreal or uveal. Mechanistically this level is the site of malignant glaucoma and secondary angle closure syndromes. Furthermore, each level of block can have some component of block of the level preceding it, creating a situation in which multiple mechanisms should be considered and treated. Anterior segment abnormalities – such as inflammatory, fibrotic, or fibrovascular conditions – can pull the peripheral iris forward to cause appositional and eventual synechial closure of the angle. Pupillary block, plateau iris, aqueous misdirection, or posterior segment abnormalities – such as choroidal swelling, choroidal hemorrhage, choroidal detachment, tumor, or space occupying lesions – can push the iris forward from behind to cause appositional and eventual synechial closure of the angle. (Table 36.2) Of these various mechanisms, pupillary block is by far the most common. Further, the mechanisms are not mutually exclusive and relative pupillary block may be present.

### 36.5.1 Pupillary Block Mechanism

Pupillary block is the most frequent etiology of angle closure[23,24] and the underlying mechanism of most cases of PACG. Flow through the pupil is compromised and the peripheral iris bows forward against the trabecular meshwork. Pupillary block is maximum at the point of mid-dilation (Fig. 36.12). Outflow is impeded and the pressure gradient between the posterior and anterior chambers increases until eventually there is no outflow. Eyes with preexisting

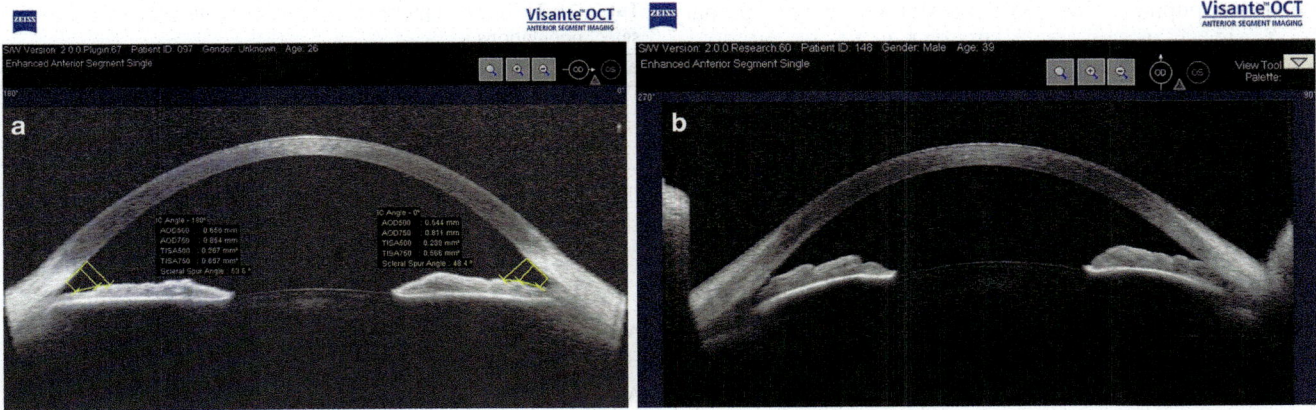

**Fig. 36.11** (a) Anterior segment OCT. OCT of open angle with anterior segment measurements. (b) OCT of narrow angle with convex iris. (Images courtesy of Zeiss-Humphrey Meditec)

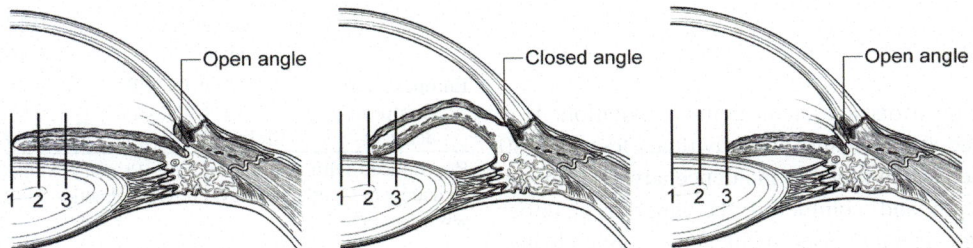

**Fig. 36.12** Pupillary Block mechanism. (**1**) The pupil is constricted and the angle is open. (**2**) The pupil is in the mid-dilated position. Pupillary block is maximal in this position and as a result the iris is bowed anteriorly and the angle narrows. (**3**) The pupil is more completely dilated and the relative pupillary block is diminished, with a return to a flatter iris configuration. If full-blown angle closure occurs, the iris may stay in the mid-dilated position until the angle closure attack is broken

shallow anterior chambers are predisposed to pupillary block. (This is why gonioscopy should be performed on *all* patients with eyes that appear to have shallow anterior chambers by slit lamp examination.) Apposition of the pupil to anterior lens capsule is the greatest in the mid-dilated position. This apposition can be relieved by constriction of the iris or dilation of the pupil away from the mid position. Surgical iridectomy or laser iridotomy will permanently eliminate angle closure from pupillary block (but not cure plateau iris configuration as described later).

Another form of a more chronic pupillary block can occur when the pupil is completely adherent to the lens capsule (secluded) by posterior synechia. This is often the result of an inflammatory process. The pressure gradient balloons the iris forward resulting in iris bombé (Fig. 36.13).

It is essential that all cases of pupillary block be interrupted in order that anatomic appositional closure does not result in permanent synechial closure. If that occurs, relieving the pupillary block may not restore normal intraocular pressure, because access to the trabecular meshwork is prevented, and additional surgical measures may become necessary to lower IOP to safe levels.

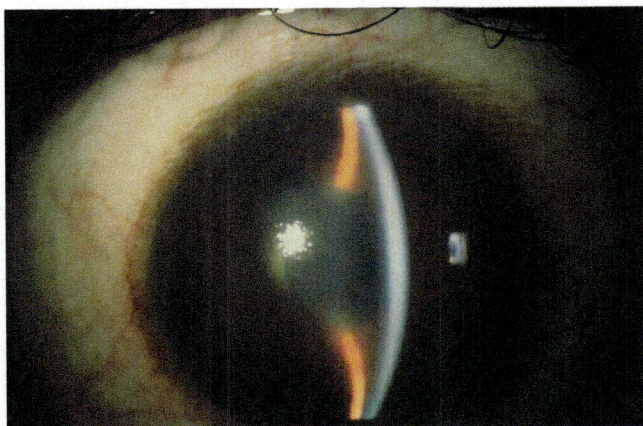

**Fig. 36.13** Iris bombe with secluded pupil secondary to inflammatory glaucoma

## 36.6 Primary Angle-Closure

Primary angle-closure glaucoma is associated with relative pupillary block in most of the cases.[23,24] It must be differentiated from plateau iris configuration and lens induced secondary pupillary block. Risk factors for developing primary angle-closure glaucoma are well established and are discussed in the following sections.

## 36.6.1 Risk Factors for Developing Primary Angle-Closure

The major risk factors for angle closure are advancing age, female gender, and Asian ethnicity.[25-31] Women have shallower anterior chambers than men. The anterior chamber shallows with age.[32,33] Biometric risk factors include small anterior segment dimensions and refractive error with axial and limbal anterior chamber depth the most strongly correlated to PAC and PACG.[34,35]

### 36.6.1.1 Age

PACG is generally a disease of an aging population. It is uncommon to see angle closure in individuals less than 40 years of age, after which time the incidence advances by the decade. The depth and volume of the anterior chamber decrease with age. The increased incidence of angle closure with age can be attributed to the normal increase in thickness of the lens with age, akin to the increasing rings and thickness of a tree trunk with age. As cataracts mature, the preexisting shallow anterior chamber and forward movement of the lens can result in increasing pupillary block. In young patients, PACG is typically associated with other anatomical abnormalities.[36] In a young angle closure patient, consideration should be given to plateau iris mechanism.

### 36.6.1.2 Gender

Independent of race, primary angle closure has a two to four times greater prevalence for women than men. This increase cannot be accounted for by women's somewhat smaller anterior chamber depth (ACD) and axial lengths.[37]

### 36.6.1.3 Race

The prevalence of PACG in patients older than age 40 varies greatly depending on race (Table 36.3). The difference in some of the biometric parameters (anterior chamber depth, axial length, which will be discussed) accounts for some of the variation in white and Inuit populations. However, biometric findings alone cannot justify the increased incidence in the Chinese and East Asian populations. In addition, acute forms are more prevalent in whites, whereas Africans and Asians are more likely to suffer from asymptomatic chronic disease. The burden

**Table 36.3** Reported prevalence of angle-closure glaucoma among select populations.

| Population | Location or sub-population | Reported prevalence (%) |
|---|---|---|
| Inuit | Alaskan Inuit[38,39] | 2.65–3.8 (age >40) |
| | East Greenlandic Inuit[40] | 2.5 (age ≥40) |
| | Taiwan[41] | 3.0 (age ≥40) |
| | Mongolia[42] | 1.4 (age ≥40) |
| | Singapore Chinese[43] | 1.25 (age ≥60) |
| | Southern India[44] | 1.08 (age ≥40) |
| Asian | Japan[26] | 0.34 (age ≥40) |
| Hispanic | Arizona, U.S.[45] | 0.1 (age >40) |
| African and African-derived | Baltimore, U.S.[46] | 0.9 (age ≥40) |
| | Tanzania, East Africa[47] | 0.58 (age ≥40) |
| | South African Zulus[48] | 0.5 (age ≥40) |
| | Italy[49] | 0.6 (age >40) |
| | Baltimore, U.S.[46] | 0.4 (age ≥40) |
| | Bedford, United Kingdom[50] | 0.17 (age >40) |
| | Sweden[51] | 0.1 (age 55–69) |
| European and European-derived | United Kingdom[52] | 0.09 (age ≥40) |
| | Beaver Dam, U.S.[53] | 0.04 (age ≥43) |
| | Ireland[54] | 0.009 (age >50) |

Reproduced with permission from Primary Angle Closure, American Academy of Ophthalmology, Preferred Practice Patterns (PPP), 2008, p 6, www.aao.org

of angle-closure glaucoma is greater in Asian countries. There has been controversy regarding the explanation the greater rate of angle closure in this demographic.[37,44,48,55-60]

### 36.6.1.4 Genetic Predisposition

It has been reported that angle-closure glaucoma patients and their siblings, but not their offspring, have axial lengths less than normal.[61] In population studies, first-degree relatives (parents, siblings, and offspring) of primary angle-closure glaucoma patients are found to be at greater risk. Indeed, it may be prudent to examine the first-degree relatives of a patient who presents with angle-closure glaucoma. In whites, the prevalence increases 1–12%. In the Inuit population, the risk is 3.5-fold and in the Chinese, the risk is sixfold greater than in the general population.[37] Nanophthalmos, a secondary angle closure has been associated with chromosomal abnormalities.

### 36.6.1.5 Biometrics

Anterior chamber dimensions may be measured by optical pachymetry, OCT, UBM, Scheimpflug photography, and SPAC. The OCT can measure central anterior chamber depth, corneal curvature, and axial length by a combination of infrared partial coherence biometry and optical method. The Pentacam uses other methods to measure central ACD by rotating Scheimpflug photography to yield more insight into angle structures. Small anterior segments and short axial lengths are typical in patients who develop primary angle closure. The primary findings predisposing to angle closure are a shallow anterior chamber depth, a thicker lens, increased anterior curvature of the lens, a shorter axial length, a small corneal diameter, and radius of corneal curvature. An anterior chamber depth (ACD) of less than 2.5 mm increases the chances of primary angle closure, whereas most patients with primary angle closure have an ACD of less than 2.1 mm. Advances in biometry techniques have demonstrated a definite association between ACD and peripheral anterior synechia (PAS). An ACD of greater than 2.4 mm is not typically associated with primary PAS. There is, however, a strong correlation of increasing PAS formation with an ACD shallower than 2.4 mm. The previous notwithstanding, angle closure still occurs with deep anterior chambers in some cases.[35,37,60,62,63]

### 36.6.1.6 Iris Cross-Sectional Area

Quigley and associates recently studied the change of iris cross-sectional (CS) area with pupillary dilation as a risk factor in angle closure. They employed anterior segment OCT in angle-closure and open angle glaucoma eyes and evaluated the change in CS with pupil dilation. In addition to iris CS area, they considered iris CS area/mm of pupil diameter change. They found that the iris loses almost half of its volume as the pupil increases from 3 to 7 mm in diameter. This was presumed to be due to loss of extracellular fluid. Smaller iris CS area change with physiologic pupil dilation was considered to be a possible risk factor for angle closure. It was postulated that dynamic iris change deserves testing as a prospective indicator of angle closure.[64]

### 36.6.1.7 Refractive Error

Primary angle closure has an increased incidence in hyperopic individuals independent of race. Hyperopic eyes have smaller depth and volume.[65] Angle closure in myopic patients should arouse suspicion of another underlying mechanism for pupillary block.

## 36.6.2 Acute Primary Angle-Closure and Sub-acute Primary Angle-Closure

### 36.6.2.1 Symptoms

Acute primary angle-closure, an "acute glaucoma attack," results from sudden pupillary block causing a typical symptom complex. In a matter of minutes, the patient may go from a state of good vision, with a white and comfortable eye, to blurred vision with a red and painful eye. The blurred vision may be accompanied by halos or rainbows around lights as a result of light scattering caused by corneal edema. (The pumping action of the corneal endothelium is compromised by the acutely raised IOP.) Ocular pain and or headache are typical. The elevated pressure may induce nausea and or vomiting. The latter symptoms may rarely be prominent enough to cause some individuals to go to the emergency room for evaluation of an acute abdominal disorder.

Upon careful ocular history taking, some patients report that under the appropriate circumstances, they may suffer symptoms consistent with what is termed as a sub-acute, intermittent, or prodromal angle closure attack. Pupillary block is initiated and patient relates having had one or several episodes of altered vision and or discomfort. The symptoms can abate if the pupillary block spontaneously resolves when circumstances initiating the attack reverse. This may happen when miosis results from the patient going into brightly lit environment or by going to sleep. The diagnosis of sub-acute angle closure is made by the clinical history and the physical findings of an anatomically narrow, occludable angle. Performing gonioscopy in these patients, preferably with compression using a Zeiss or similar lens, is absolutely essential in determining if the symptomology is a prodrome to acute angle closure.

### 36.6.2.2 Signs

Patients suffering from an acute primary angle closure attack typically manifest hyperemic conjunctiva and episclera, tearing, corneal edema, elevated intraocular pressure, a shallow anterior chamber, minimal cell or flare, and a fixed or sluggish mid-dilated or irregular pupil (Fig. 36.14). The corneal

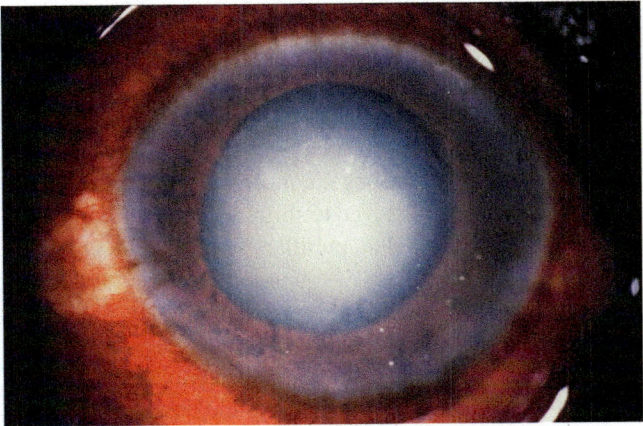

**Fig. 36.14** Acute angle-closure attack. The eye is hyperemic with corneal edema, elevated intraocular pressure, shallow anterior chamber and dilated irregular pupil

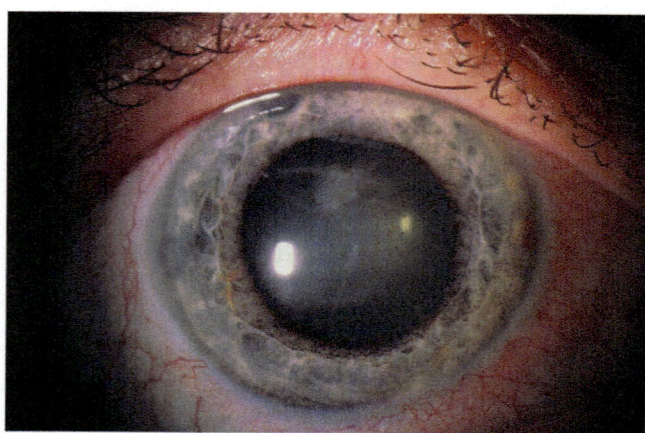
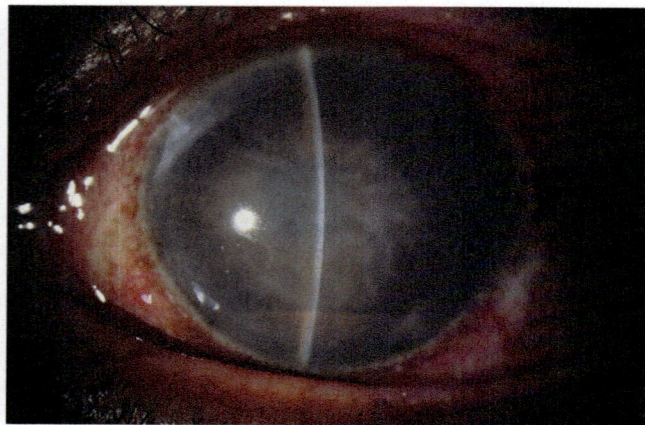

**Fig. 36.15** Sequellae of severe acute angle-closure glaucoma attack include glaukomflecken (white superficial lens opacities), iris atrophy with pigment release from elevated IOP (note surgical iridectomy which was necessary to break attack)

**Fig. 36.16** Acute angle closure treated with strong miotic resulting in sterile hypopyon

edema may be so dense as to obscure the view of the anterior chamber and angle until the intraocular pressure is reduced. The markedly elevated intraocular pressure can result in focal glaucoma induced lens opacities that are localized infarctions (glaukomflecken) (Fig. 36.15), iris atrophy, and decreased pupillary reactivity. Inflammation with appositional touch of the peripheral iris to sclera leads to PAS.

### 36.6.2.3 Medical Treatment of Acute PACG

The initial treatment for an acute attack of PACG is to lower the intraocular pressure and relieve the pupillary block. Fortunately in PACG, the attack is generally monocular, and acute attention is initially directed toward the "attack eye."

Medical treatment is initiated with topical miotic drops, beta blockers, alpha-adrenergic agents, and carbonic anhydrase inhibitors. If the patient is not nauseated, then oral carbonic anhydrase may be administered. In some instances, it may also be helpful to treat the nausea directly. It is best to use intermediate strength miotic drops (pilocarpine hydrochloride 2%) and not to repeat more than approximately three times in an hour. Stronger concentrations of pilocarpine (e.g., 4%) have been observed to shift the lens–iris diaphragm forward, exaggerating the pupillary block. The pupillary response (constriction) may be blunted until the intraocular pressure drops below 40 mmHg, because at very high pressures, the iris is ischemic and the muscles therefore cannot respond to the cholinergic stimulation. Multiple doses of pilocarpine eye drops may cause systemic cholinergic symptoms exacerbating those of the attack itself. Stronger miotics, in addition to further narrowing of the peripheral angle, also can increase inflammation (Fig. 36.16).

In those cases in which there is no substantial intraocular pressure reduction to the previous regimen, or in which the level of the intraocular pressure threatens optic nerve perfusion, oral osmotic (50% glycerin or isosorbide) or intravenous mannitol solutions (1–2 gm/kg) may be required. System concerns in very elderly or frail individuals, and the use of oral glycerin in diabetics, tempers the use of the agents for some patients.

If the pupil does not constrict and the pupillary block is not abated, the Zeiss-type gonio-lens may be employed to attempt to force aqueous into the peripheral angle, open it, and possibly break the attack.[66] In the absence of an appropriate lens, the tip of the Goldmann applanation tonometer can be removed from the slit lamp mount and manually used to compress the central cornea. If there is substantial corneal edema, care must be taken not to abrade the cornea by these methods. These approaches are most successful after an initial medical lowering of the intraocular pressure. The status of the optic nerve and the lens should be documented, if possible, at the time of presentation. Glaukomflecken, opacities in the anterior lens caused by infarcts secondary to acutely high IOP, should be recorded if present.

### 36.6.2.4 Laser and Surgical Treatment of Acute PACG

In cases of markedly elevated IOP threatening the optic nerve, emergency paracentesis may be necessary.[67] Paracentesis can be done as an initial treatment or in conjunction with medical therapy. This may be performed at the slit lamp or under the microscope following adequate topical anesthesia (proparacaine or tetracaine) and surgical prep (povidone iodine). A paracentesis blade or 26-gauge needle on a syringe with the plunger removed may be used to release aqueous. This procedure, when undertaken in patients with markedly shallow anterior chambers and dilated pupils, must be performed with extreme care so as not to injure the lens. A risk to the lens is present due to the shallow chamber. It is best to pass the needle horizontally across the anterior chamber, angling it away from the lens of the eye. This procedure, when successful, does have the advantages of rapidly reducing the IOP, interrupting the acute attack, and reducing pain. By reducing corneal edema it facilitates the performance of laser iridotomy. Currently, laser iridotomy (Yttrium-Aluminum-Garnet [YAG] or argon laser) is the primary initial treatment for PACG. Once the attack has been broken and the corneal edema has cleared sufficiently, laser iridotomy should be performed. Sometimes, the attack cannot be aborted medically and the cornea remains edematous. Topical glycerin is often helpful to clear the cornea long enough to provide a view for laser treatment to create a peripheral iridotomy. The iris tends to be swollen and boggy during the acute phase of the attack, making performing a laser peripheral iridotomy more difficult than in a quiet eye with a narrow but open angle. It is sometimes impossible to create an iridotomy due to edema in the iris (see Chap. 61, Sidebar 61.3).

YAG laser iridotomy tends to be easier to do than argon laser in very lightly and very heavily pigmented eyes, as it is not dependent upon pigment for absorption of the energy. Argon laser iridotomy is the most easily performed in patients with light brown or hazel colored irides (Fig. 36.17). With all laser modalities it is generally best to treat in the base of an iris crypt (thinner total iris tissue to penetrate) in one of the superior quadrants (less likelihood of glare symptoms if a truly peripheral iridectomy [PI] is done "under the lid"). The physician should use a specifically designed laser iridotomy lens that has a convex lens button to disperse the beam at the corneal plane and concentrate it at the iris surface. If the iris is treated at the 12 o'clock position, rising vapor bubbles may obscure the iridotomy before it can be completed. For this reason, 11 or 1 o'clock may be preferable. Placing iridotomies high and under the lid can avoid the rare side effect of the patient being troubled by incident light striking an iridotomy. Patients on anticoagulants or those with bleeding tendencies or iris neovascularization are more likely to bleed with YAG than with argon iridotomy, which cauterizes as it penetrates. Bleeding can be avoided by pretreating the iridotomy site with large spot, low-power argon laser before using the YAG to create the opening. Sometimes, this technique of first treating with large diameter argon laser spots and then "blasting" through with a few final YAG bursts of energy is also helpful to penetrate very thick brown irides.[1] Usually it is also necessary to perform laser on the fellow eye as soon as possible to protect it from future angle closure. Occasionally the eyes are asymmetric – with respect to the depths of the anterior chamber angles. Mild miotics may be used prophylactically to prevent angle closure in the contralateral eye until laser iridotomy can be performed.

Another approach to relieving ITC is to perform laser peripheral iridoplasty.[68-71] This may be effective in breaking the acute attack of angle closure. It is performed as was described for plateau iris syndrome. The peripheral iris may be difficult to treat secondary to the shallow peripheral anterior chamber and the proximity to the corneal endothelium with the potential of subsequent corneal decompensation.

In rare instances where the attack cannot be broken and the cornea cleared for laser, surgical iridectomy is required. The angle must be opened expediently to avoid synechia formation and permanent partial or complete angle closure. In cases of prolonged angle closure attacks, surgical iridectomy may break the pupillary block, but there may not be sufficient remaining functional angle for maintaining intraocular pressure control. Trabeculectomy, although initially successful, has a poor prognosis for long-term function in acutely inflamed eyes.[72] On the other hand, if angle closure has been present for a long time, peripheral anterior synechia will have formed and an iridectomy may no longer be curative, making trabeculectomy or a similar outflow procedure desirable even if it will eventually be doomed to failure.

### 36.6.2.5 Narrow or Occludable Anterior Chamber Angle

At times the clinician will identify patients who have shallow peripheral anterior chambers during a routine slit lamp examination with no history to support a diagnosis of sub-acute angle closure (Fig. 36.18). The Van Herick classification system for limbal anterior chamber depth (LACD) can be used

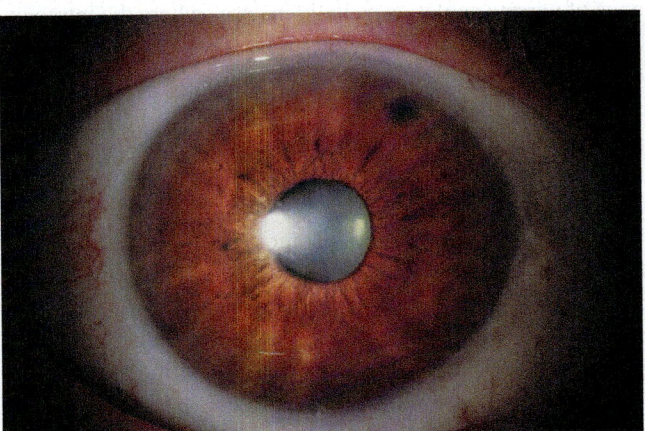

**Fig. 36.17** Argon laser iridotomy. Light to medium brown or hazel eyes are the easiest to treat

---

[1] This two-stage laser technique was described in a personal communication with Paul N. Schacknow, MD, PhD.

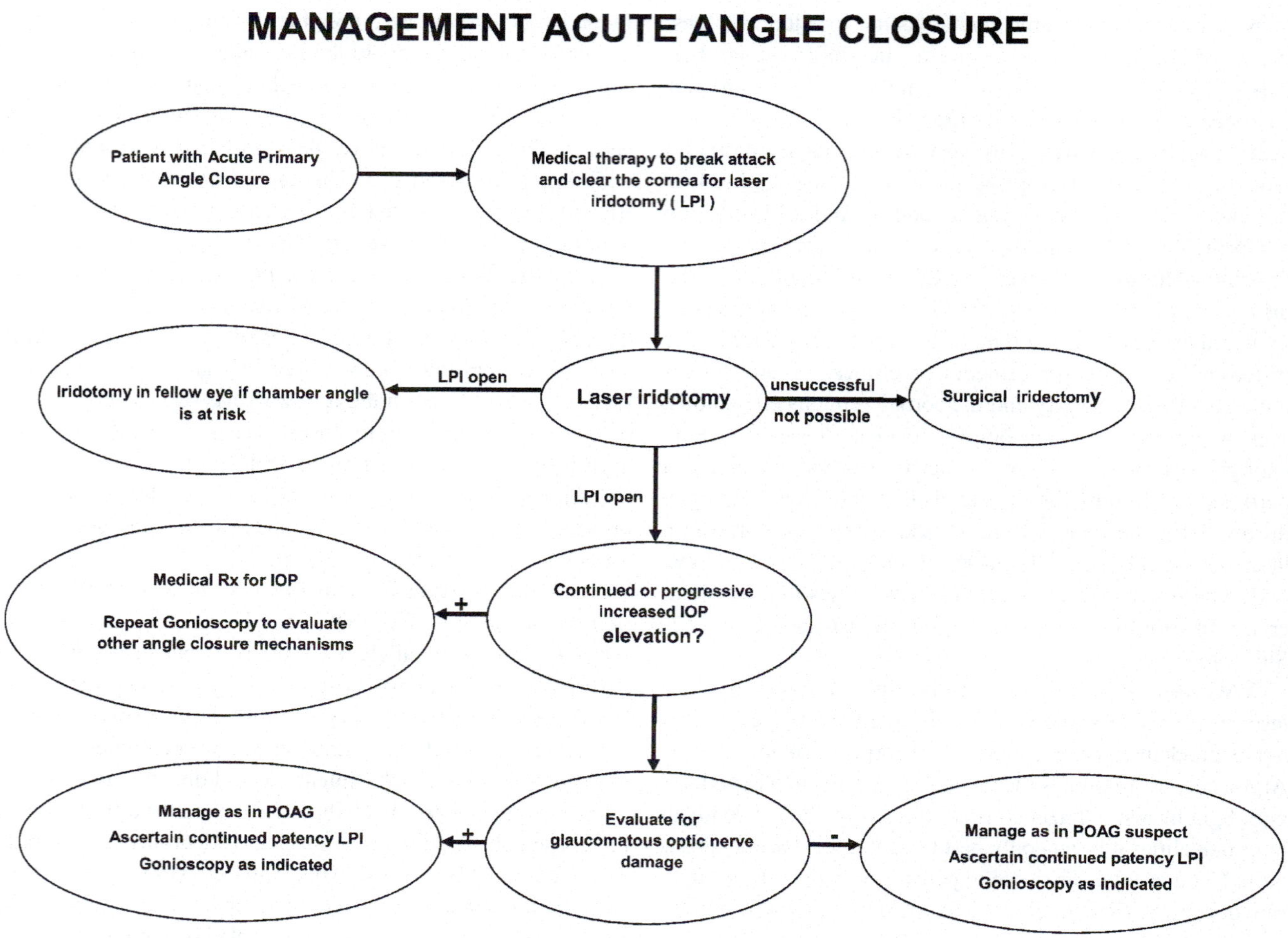

## MANAGEMENT ACUTE ANGLE CLOSURE

**Fig. 36.18** Management of acute angle closure

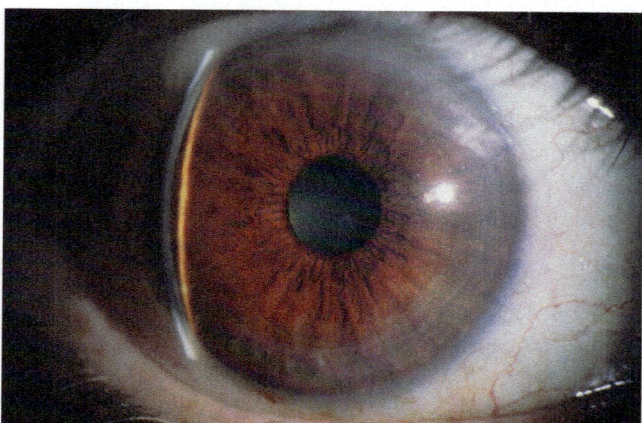

**Fig. 36.19** Limbal anterior chamber depth. Shallow peripheral anterior chamber as estimated by Van Herick classification for limbal anterior chamber depth (LACD)

for evaluation and documentation[75] (Fig. 36.19). If available, chamber depth can also be recorded by optical pachymetry[73,74] or by contemporary quantitative imaging methods.[75,76]

Gonioscopy is mandatory in addition to the slit lamp exam. With the ease of examination afforded by the Zeiss and similar lenses, gonioscopy should be included in all initial anterior segment exams regardless of slit lamp appearance. Compression gonioscopy should be performed in the presence of narrow angles, especially in cases where the intraocular pressure is elevated, to determine whether any synechial closure has occurred. Charting of the width of the angle should be documented by the Shaffer or the Spaeth grading system. If there is significantly elevated intraocular pressure, and especially if there is synechial closure, then prophylactic laser iridotomy may be indicated.

In eyes with normal intraocular pressure and slit to ITC angles, the value of prophylactic laser iridotomy has not been well established.[73,74] The generally favorable risk to benefit ratio has allowed for the widespread performance for many patients. It should especially be considered in patients with narrow angles who have symptoms consistent with angle closure, those who must undergo repeated dilation, who need anticholinergics or similar medication, and those who do not have immediate access to emergency ophthalmologic care.

It should also be considered when a previously normal IOP is elevated or when the angle has been observed to become progressively narrower or develops PAS.

In patients with normal intraocular pressures and angles, which are considered to be occludable, a discussion of the potential for acute angle closure should be undertaken in terms suitable for a layperson. Although generally safe, laser iridotomy has the theoretical potential for cataract,[77] endothelial cell dysfunction,[78] and corneal decompensation.[79] All patients with narrow angles should be made aware of conditions and medications, such as anti-cholinergics, antihistamines, sedatives, and any over the counter drugs with "glaucoma warnings" that may precipitate an acute angle closure attack. In particular, many elderly patients take chronic anticholinergic medications for bladder control. If symptoms occur, they must be counseled to seek immediate medical treatment by an eye care physician.

Prior to the advent of safe, easy to perform laser iridotomy, there was a greater need to better predict those patients at risk for acute angle closure. Dark room prone and pharmacological provocative tests were employed to assist in deciding which patients were candidates for prophylactic surgical iridectomies, which clearly have a poorer risk to benefit ratio than the modern laser iridotomy. An elevation of 8 mmHg of intraocular pressure, in the presence of gonioscopic angle closure, was considered a positive provocative test, suggesting the risk of future acute angle closure, although this is not always certain. A negative provocative test does not rule out the possibility of angle closure.[80] Despite the fact that provocative tests are not routinely performed in the twenty-first century, any narrow angle patient who is dilated should have the intraocular pressure checked and gonioscopy repeated if IOP is elevated. If the pupils are to be dilated with a weak agent such as tropicamide 0.5 or 1% and angle closure occurs, it can usually be reversed with pilocarpine drops. If a patient with well open iridectomies or iridotomies goes into angle closure after dilation, a diagnosis of plateau iris should be entertained.

## 36.7 Chronic Angle-Closure

Chronic angle closure is a term used for eyes in which the angle gradually narrows without precipitating an acute attack. With time, synechia develop and the intraocular pressure rises gradually. Early on this condition should be treated with laser iridotomy. Patients with chronic angle closure and significantly elevated IOP develop glaucomatous optic neuropathy and visual field loss similar to primary open angle glaucoma. These patients may have more extensive disc and field damage, and it may be difficult to establish a target IOP. Their corneas are usually clear, nonedematous, as the endothelium has had time to adapt to the slowly rising IOPs and still functions adequately as a pump to prevent aqueous from entering the stroma. These patients should be treated medically in a similar fashion to POAG, but miotics – especially strong miotics – should be avoided. Prostaglandin analogue therapy can be particularly effective. These patients are not good candidates for laser trabeculoplasty but can benefit from trabeculectomy or combined phacotrabeculectomy.

## 36.8 Combined Mechanism Glaucoma (Mixed Mechanism Glaucoma)

An open angle glaucoma patient may narrow, then deepen after laser iridotomy, but with the pressure remaining elevated, with or without peripheral anterior synechial formation. This condition is termed "combined mechanism" glaucoma or "mixed mechanism" glaucoma. Combined mechanism glaucoma may also occur in a patient who is initially diagnosed as narrow angle and despite open iridotomy, manifests reduced outflow and increased intraocular pressure. These eyes are treated as chronic angle closure. Patients may also have glaucoma with more than one pathophysiologic etiology. The causes enumerated above are not mutually exclusive. When two or more processes, though not necessarily chronic angle closure, occur simultaneously the term mixed-mechanism glaucoma may be used. The patients are treated with the modalities appropriate to each of the underlying etiologies of the mixed mechanisms of their glaucomas.

## 36.9 Secondary Angle Closure with Pupillary Block

### 36.9.1 Lens Induced

Various forms of lens-induced "secondary angle closure" with pupillary block have been described. Tarongoy et al have recently reviewed the role of the lens in the pathogenesis, prevention, and treatment of angle-closure glaucoma.[81]

Phacomorphic glaucoma occurs secondary to a large anteriorly displaced lens (Fig. 36.20). The lens may become acutely intumescent because of imbibing water from the aqueous. Laser peripheral iridoplasty may be performed urgently to open the peripheral angle. Dilation followed by cataract extraction is curative. Penetrating trauma to the anterior segment can result in delayed swelling of the lens (Fig. 36.21) requiring surgical removal.

In Weill–Marchesani syndrome (microspherophakia), patients are characteristically of short stature with spade-like

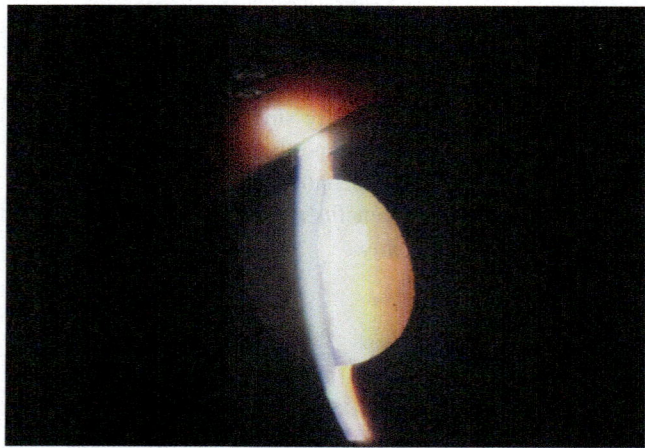

**Fig. 36.20** Phacomorphic glaucoma. Large swollen lens results in secondary angle closure

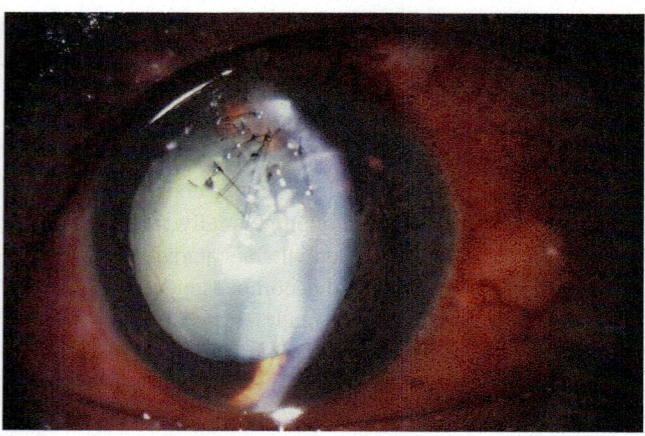

**Fig. 36.21** Traumatic cataract. Swollen lens secondary to penetrating trauma results in secondary angle closure following repair of corneal laceration

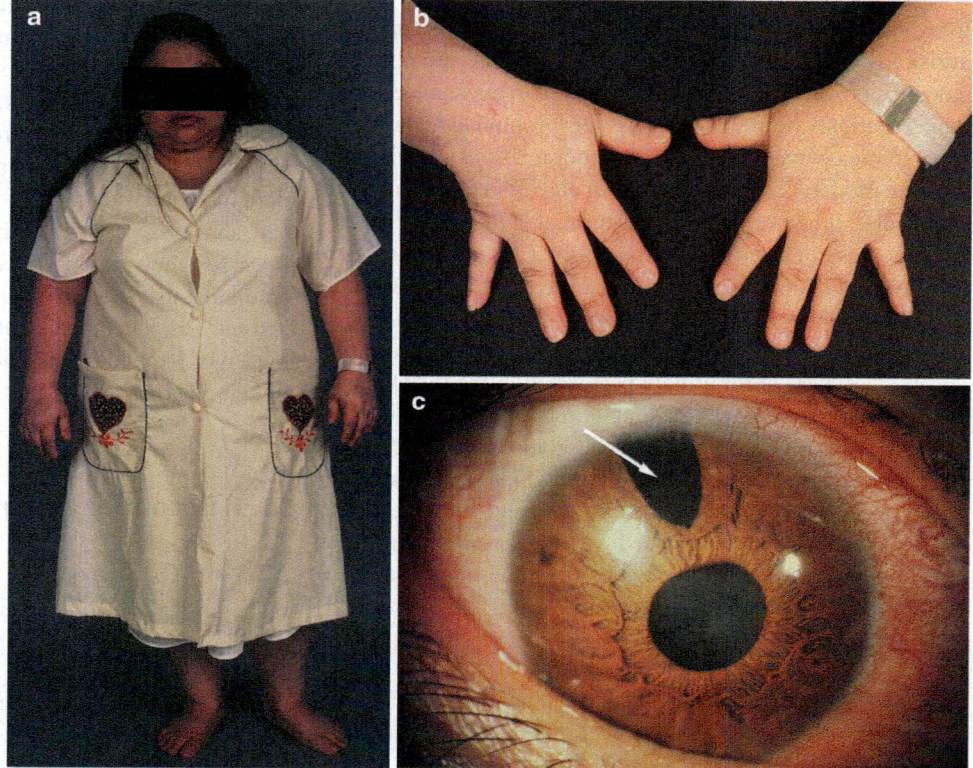

**Fig. 36.22** (**a**) Weill–Marchesani body habitus. (**b**) Brachydactyly. (**c**) Shallow anterior chamber due to forward movement of the microspherophakic lens (edge of lens – *arrow*) after pupillary block relieved by iridectomy

hands (brachydactyly) (Fig. 36.22a–c). The lens is small and there is a laxity of the zonules. Glaucoma is common. The lens can displace forward resulting in pupillary block with markedly elevated intraocular pressure (Fig. 36.23a). In these cases, pilocarpine increases the pupillary block. Dilation and laser iridotomy may relieve the pupillary block (Fig. 36.23b, c).

Partially or completely dislocated lenses in numerous conditions associated with ectopia lentis[82] can result in secondary angle-closure. Marfan syndrome is an autosomal dominant condition with a physical appearance the opposite of Weill–Marchasani. Marfan syndrome patients are tall, with long slender fingers and toes (arachnodactyly) (Fig. 36.24a, b). They are subject to frequent cardiovascular disease, scleral stretching, and retinal detachment.[83] Ectopia lentis usually occurs in the fourth to fifth decade of life with the lens commonly subluxing upward (Fig. 36.24c). Surgical removal of the lens is often necessary.

Homocystinuria is an autosomal recessive disease manifesting in a disorder of homocysteine metabolism.

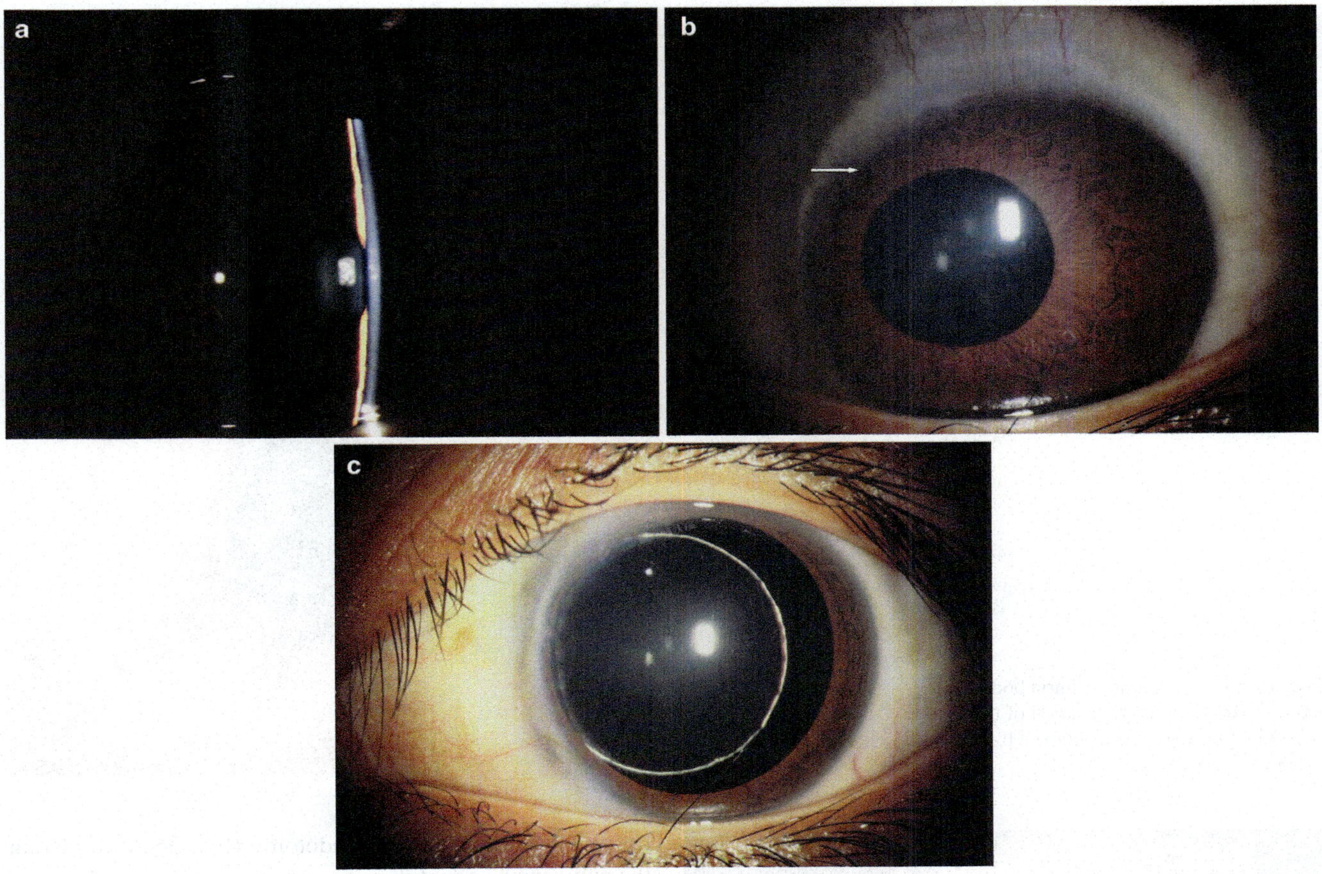

**Fig. 36.23** (a) Weill–Marchesani shallow AC, with pupillary block. (b) Pupillary block relieved with laser iridotomy and dilating. (c) Microspherophakia well visualized with pupil widely dilated

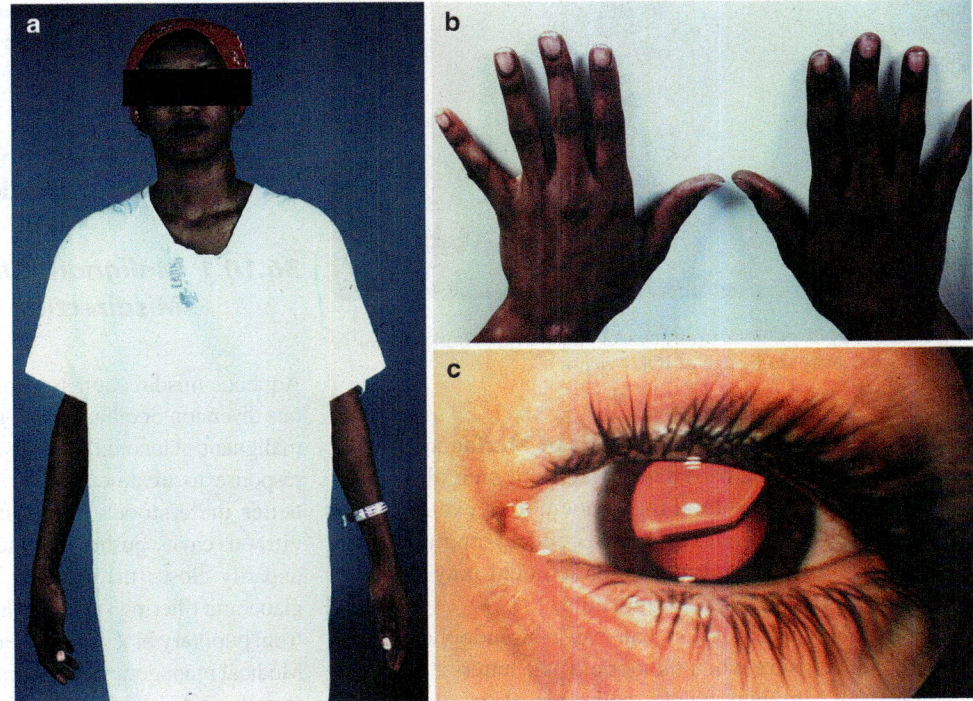

**Fig. 36.24** (a) Marfan syndrome body habitus. (b) Arachnodactyly. (c) Upward dislocation of abnormally shaped lens

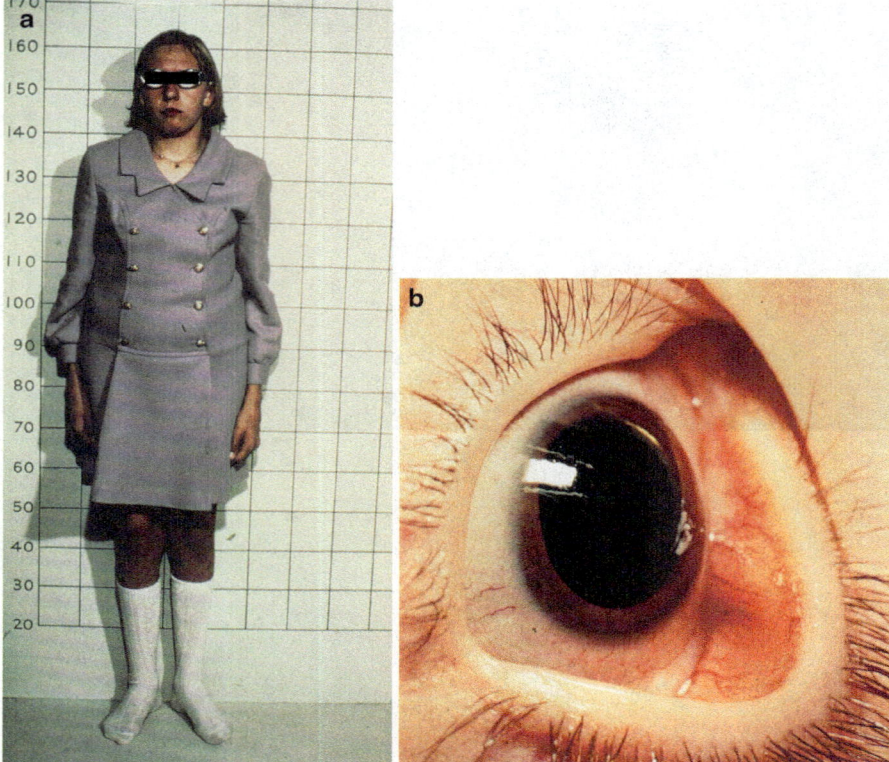

**Fig. 36.25** (a) Homocystinuria body habitus. (b) Anterior dislocation of the lens with pupillary block relieved by dilating

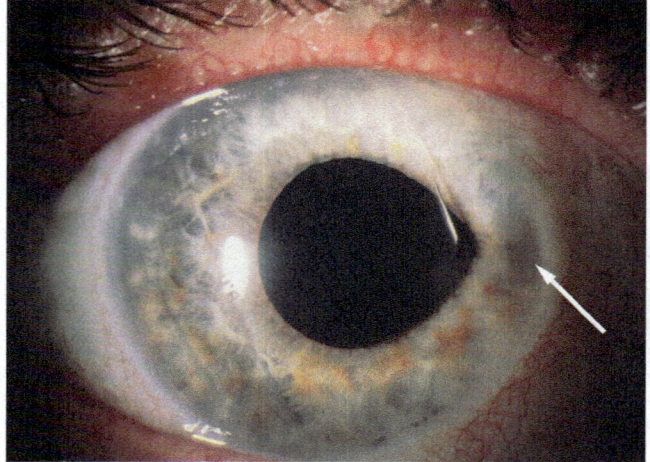

**Fig. 36.26** Pupillary block from anterior chamber IOL broken by laser (iris retracted away from edge of IOL – *arrow*)

Their body habitus is similar to that of Marfan syndrome patients (Fig. 36.25a, b). They suffer from mental retardation and are subject to fatal thromboembolic events, especially under general anesthesia. Secondary angle closure due to ectopia lentis and retinal detachment may occur as in individuals with Marfan syndrome.

Intraocular lenses (IOLs) can cause pseudophakic secondary angle closure when the optic of the anterior chamber lens (ACIOL) implant blocks communication of aqueous between the posterior and anterior chambers. Emergency treatment consists of laser iridotomy (Fig. 36.26). Dilating the pupil can be effective as a temporizing measure. All anterior chamber intraocular lens implantations should be accompanied by prophylactic iridectomies. Phakic lens implants for refractive surgery can cause pupillary block and angle closure. This may be avoided in many cases[84] by proper sizing of the lens and prophylactic laser iridotomies.

## 36.10 Secondary Angle-Closure Without Pupillary Block

### 36.10.1 Malignant Glaucoma-Aqueous Misdirection Syndrome

Aqueous misdirection syndrome is also termed posterior aqueous diversion or ciliary block glaucoma. It was originally named malignant glaucoma[85] because of its relentless course and poor response to treatment, until its physiologic mechanisms were better understood. The posterior flow of aqueous into the vitreous cavity pushes the anterior hyaloid face forward and secondarily closes the angle. It may occur following cataract or glaucoma filtering surgery. The diagnosis must be differentiated from pupillary block and suprachoroidal effusion or hemorrhage. Medical management includes hypotensive agents, atropine, and steroids. YAG laser destruction of the anterior hyaloid face or argon laser to the ciliary processes can sometimes be helpful.

Pars plana vitrectomy with incision of the anterior hyaloid face is usually curative. See Chap. 37 for further discussion of malignant glaucoma.

## 36.11 Neovascular Glaucoma

Neovascular glaucoma results from the occlusion of the trabecular meshwork and secondary closure of the angle by fibrovascular membrane formation. New vessels may originate at the pupillary margin and extend peripherally (rubeosis iridis, Fig. 36.27) or originate at the root of the iris and extend anteriorly to the trabecular meshwork, closing the angle. The neovascularization is typically associated with ischemic ocular conditions, most notably proliferative diabetic retinopathy and ischemic central vein occlusion. The intraocular pressure rises slowly, and there may not be any symptoms until the disease advances. At this point the disease results in a red, painful eye with marked corneal edema and little or no vision.

Primary treatment is directed at the underlying etiology and includes retinal photocoagulation[86] and anti-VEGF (vascular endothelial growth factor) drugs such as Avastin[87] and Lucentis. The glaucoma may be managed with standard pharmacologic therapy, but prostaglandin agents and miotics should be avoided so as not to increase inflammation. Once the ischemia has been stabilized, surgical treatment for the glaucoma consists of trabeculectomy with antifibrotic agents (5-fluorouracil, mitomycin-C) or aqueous tube shunt implantation. Advanced cases may require topical atropine 1% and steroid drops to quiet the inflammatory response. There are patients who respond poorly to surgery and are candidates for laser cyclodestructive procedures (transcleral diode laser or endophotocyclocoagulation [ECP]). Cyclocryocoagulation therapy causes marked pain and inflammation and should be avoided. Refer to Chap. 40 for further discussion of neovascular glaucoma.

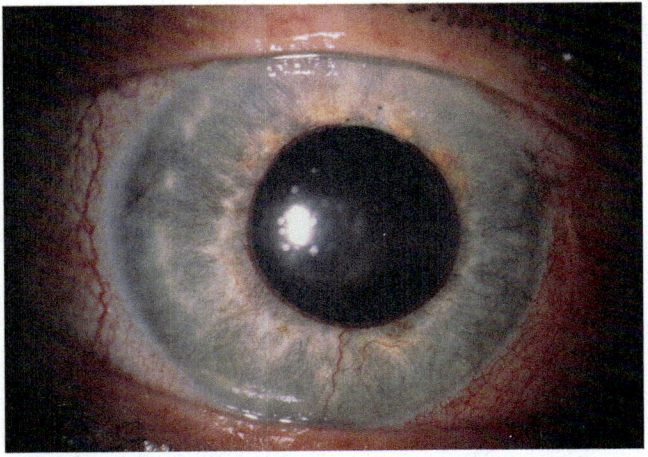

**Fig. 36.27** Neovascular glaucoma with rubeotic vessels from the pupillary margin with ectropion to the angle with secondary closure from fibrovascular membrane

## 36.12 Iridocorneal Endothelial Syndrome

Iridocorneal endothelial (ICE) syndrome was termed to encompass a spectrum of abnormalities that share a disorder of the corneal endothelium.[88,89] The major clinical presentations are:

- Progressive Iris Atrophy in which iris pathologies (atrophy, stretching and melting holes and corectopia) are progressive and predominate (Fig. 36.28a, b).

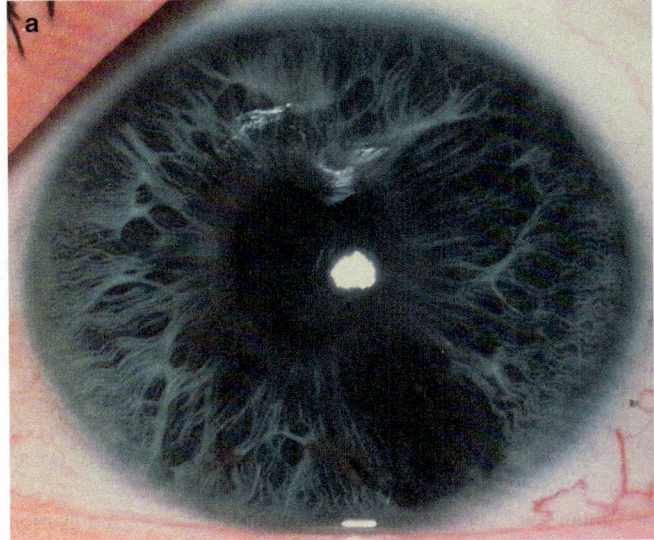 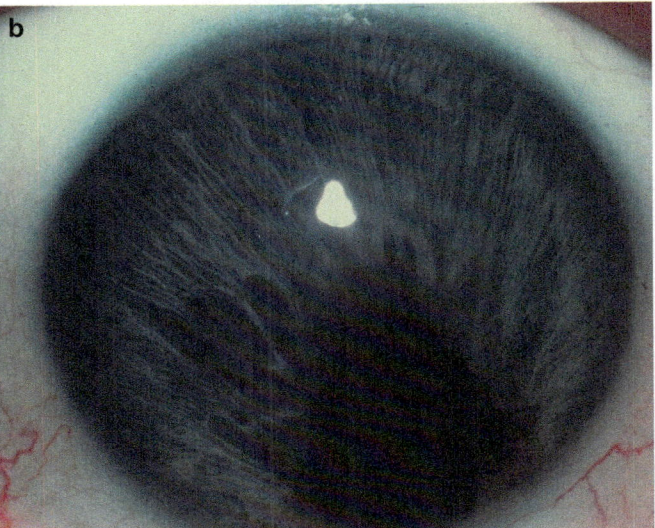

**Fig. 36.28** Progressive iris atrophy with atrophy, stretching and melting holes, correctopia. (**a**) Early stage. (**b**) Late stage.

- Chandler Syndrome in which iris pathologies are mild and corneal edema, even at low IOP predominates.
- Cogan–Reese Syndrome in which nodular pigmented lesions of the iris surface predominate.

Angle-closure results from a form of migratory corneal endothelium extending across the angle and later across the iris. A secondary glaucoma subsequently develops. Advanced disease results in diffuse corneal edema with elevated intraocular pressure. Standard medical therapy is helpful early on but the disease may eventually become refractory. Surgical success is limited and the long term prognosis is poor. Refer to Chap. 46 for a further discussion of ICE syndrome.

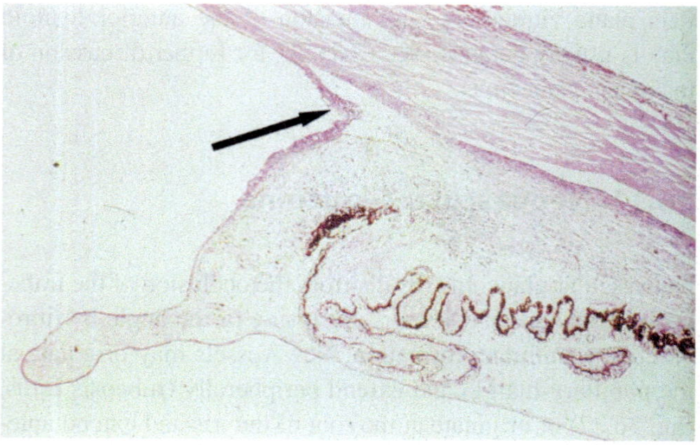

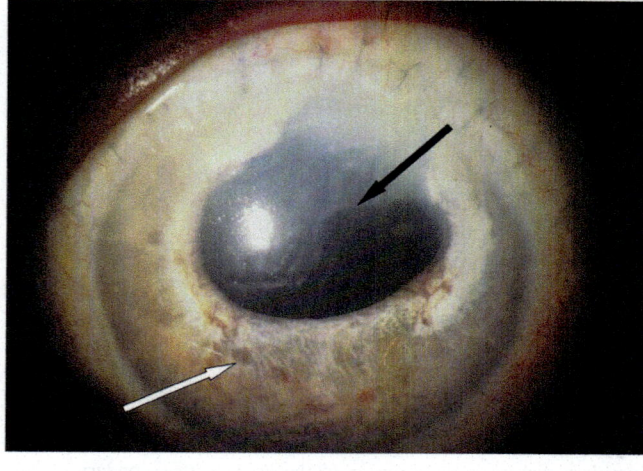

**Fig. 36.30** Epithelial downgrowth (ingrowth) photomicrograph with abnormal tissue growing across the angle and onto the iris (*arrow*)

## 36.13 Epithelial and Fibrous Downgrowth

Epithelial (Figs. 36.29 and 36.30) and fibrous downgrowth (Fig. 36.31) are rare surgical complications resulting in secondary angle closure. Inciting factors include fistula and hypotony. The abnormal tissue grows across the angle and onto the iris. Epithelial ingrowth (downgrowth) has a graver prognosis (see Chap. 74). It can be differentiated from fibrous tissue by treating suspected tissue with low-energy argon laser. Epithelial tissue characteristically reacts with a whitish fluffy reaction termed "popcorning," while uninvolved iris turns brownish black.[90] Standard glaucoma medical therapy and surgical therapy are generally ineffective. Surgical removal or destruction of the pathologic tissue can be helpful in the early stages.

**Fig. 36.31** Fibrous downgrowth. Retrocorneal membrane (*black arrow*), absence of whitish "popcorning" lesions from diagnostic argon laser, brown laser burns indicate uninvolved iris tissue (*white arrow*)

## 36.14 Inflammation

Inflammation associated with a variety of ocular and systemic conditions can cause trabeculitis or synechia formation with secondary angle closure. Medical treatment should avoid the use of miotics and may include cycloplegic agents and topical or systemic steroids. Surgical treatment includes trabeculectomy with antifibrotic agents or aqueous tube shunt surgery.

Posterior scleritis (Fig. 36.32) may result in large uveal effusions resulting in secondary angle closure. The incidence of glaucoma over an 11-year period has been reported as high

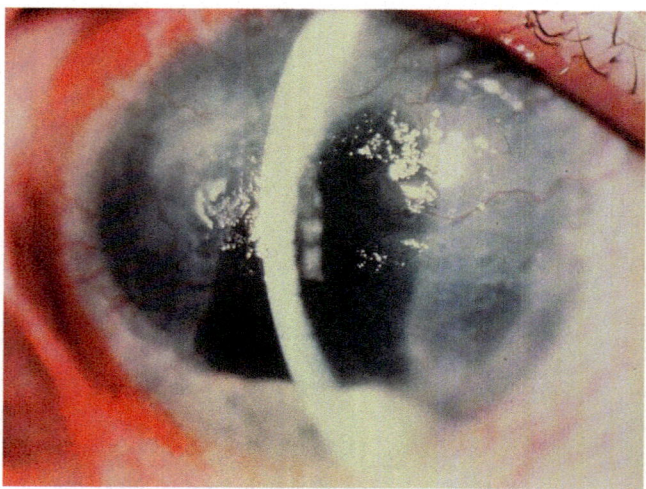

**Fig. 36.29** Epithelial downgrowth (ingrowth)

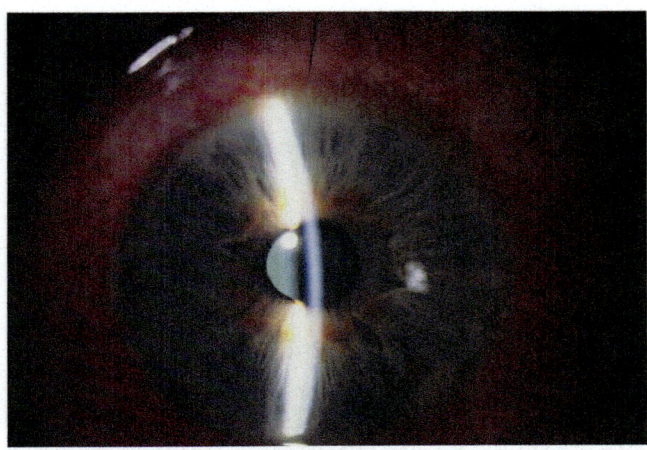

**Fig. 36.32** Posterior scleritis with choroidal effusion, shallow anterior chamber and secondary angle closure

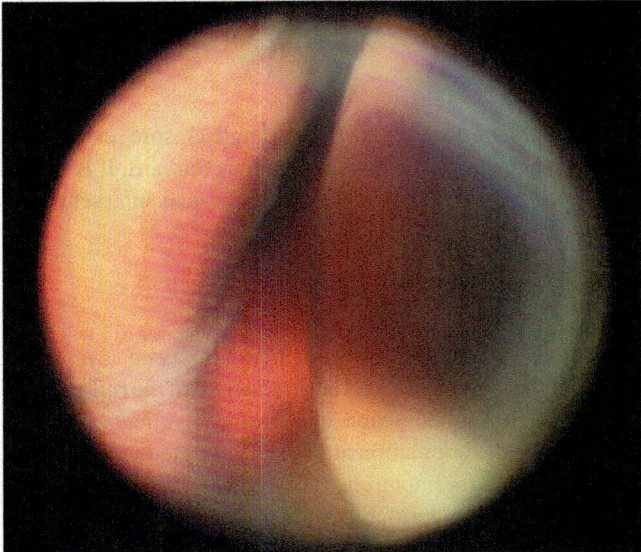

**Fig. 36.33** Massive choroidal effusion with secondary angle closure

as 13% in patients with scleritis. An acute angle-closure glaucoma is usually the result of ciliary body rotation rather than pupil block, and therefore will not respond to peripheral iridotomy. It may completely resolve with medical therapy when the inflammation subsides. Chronic angle closure may result in widespread peripheral anterior synechiae and permanent angle closure requiring surgical intervention.[91] For further discussion of uveitis and glaucoma, see Chap. 41.

## 36.15 Retinal Disorders and Posterior Segment Disorders

Various retinal disorders and treatments can result in secondary angle-closure glaucoma. Primary or secondary uveal effusions (Fig. 36.33) can cause a forward displacement of the iris. Central retinal vein occlusion (CRVO) can cause choroidal swelling with secondary closure[92] as can extensive retinal photocoagulation for CRVO or proliferative diabetic retinopathy.

Treatment consists of topical ocular hypotensive and anti-inflammatory agents. Laser iridotomy is not indicated. This form of closure usually occurs within the first 30 days after the CRVO and is not related to the neovascular glaucoma that typically occurs 90 days later. Mechanical secondary angle closure can result from scleral buckling procedures[93] or expansion of a gas bubble placed in the eye during vitrectomy. If medical therapy is unsuccessful, removal (Fig. 36.34a, b) or repositioning of the buckling material or some of the gas bubble may be necessary. Retinopathy can cause mixed mechanism disease because of retro-lental mass, inflammation, rubeosis, and secondary angle-closure (Fig. 36.35). Tumors such as malignant melanoma can push the lens forward causing angle closure (Fig. 36.36). Refer to Chap. 80 for discussion of retinal surgery and glaucoma.

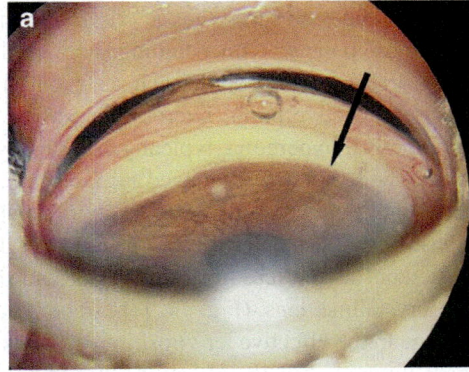
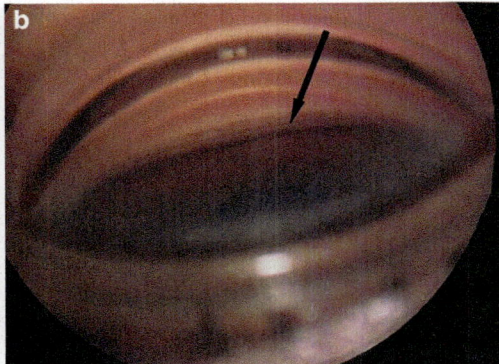

**Fig. 36.34** Angle closure secondary to anteriorly displaced scleral buckle encircling band "indenting" the angle (*arrow*) and causing increased IOP. (**a**) Gonioscopic view of compressed angle (*arrow*) prior to removal of encircling band. (**b**) Gonioscopic view of open angle (*arrow*) following removal of encircling band

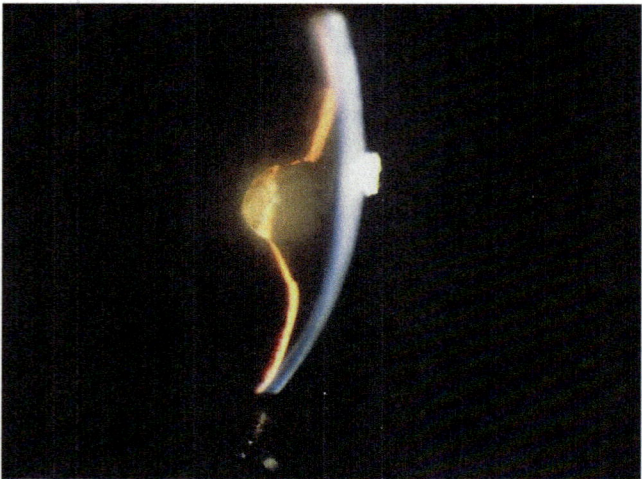

**Fig. 36.35** Endstage retinopathy of prematurity (ROP) with retro-lental mass, inflammation, rubeosis, secondary angle closure, and iris bombé

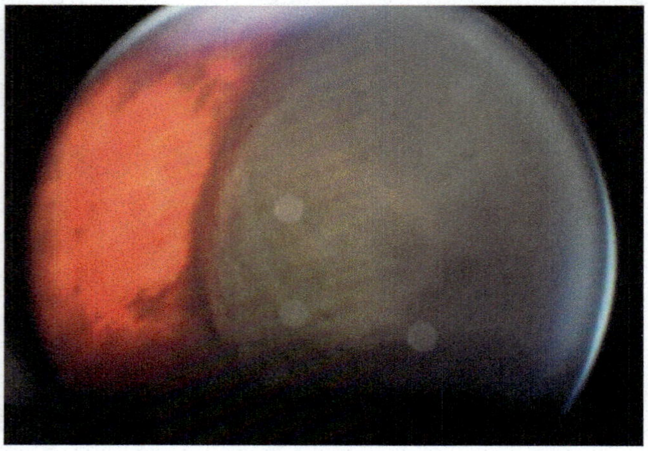

**Fig. 36.36** Malignant melanoma of the choroid acting as a posterior mass pushing forward resulting in secondary angle closure

## 36.16 Drug-Induced Secondary Angle-Closure Glaucoma

Topiramate (Topamax) systemic medical therapy for epilepsy, migraine, and other neurological conditions is well documented to cause acute bilateral secondary angle-closure glaucoma[94] (see Sidebar 36.1). The angle closure results from a sudden uveal effusion pushing the lens forward. It is treated medically until it resolves. Laser or surgical intervention is rarely required.

---

**SIDEBAR 36.1. Topiramate, uveal effusion, and secondary angle-closure glaucoma**

Theodoros Filippopoulos and Cynthia L. Grosskreutz

Topiramate (Topamax, Ortho-McNeil Neurogics Inc, Titusville, New Jersey) is a relatively new antiepileptic drug currently FDA-approved for migraine prophylaxis as well. Topiramate is a sulfamate substituted monosaccharide that has also been used off label for depression, neuropathic pain, pseudotumor cerebri, bipolar disorder, to treat alcohol dependence, and as a weight reduction agent. Since its introduction in 1995 (1996 in the US), several cases of transient myopia, uveal effusions, and bilateral angle-closure glaucoma have been published that established a direct causal relationship between the use of this medication and the observed ocular side effects. This has resulted in a specific postmarketing warning in topiramate's US labeling in 2001.

Topiramate can cause acute secondary angle-closure glaucoma without pupillary block. Typically, affected patients (85%) present within 2 weeks after the introduction of topiramate to their treatment regimen with blurry vision in both eyes as the first symptom secondary to a myopic refractive shift. Very infrequently only one eye is involved. Any age group can be affected, with the reported average age of 34–37 years. This group of patients probably reflects the population at risk being treated with topiramate for the aforementioned indications. With slit lamp examination, the anterior chamber is seen to be uniformly shallow, while the iris assumes a planar configuration as a result of the anterior displacement of the lens–iris diaphragm. Gonioscopy reveals bilateral appositional angle closure in eyes that were previously thought not to be at risk for angle closure. Classic iris bombé is not found with these patients. Other findings commonly associated with acute angle closure, such as a middilated and/or sluggish reactive pupil, microcystic corneal edema, and conjunctival hyperemia, typically accompany the clinical picture with topiramate induced angle closure. Ophthalmic ultrasonography reveals 360° of choroidal (uveal) effusions, a shallow anterior chamber due to forward displacement of the lens–iris diaphragm, and thickening of the crystalline lens (Fig. 36.1-1). The thickening and change in the effective lens position accounts for the transient myopic shift in refraction. In addition, ultrasound biomicroscopy of the affected angles has demonstrated ciliary body thickening and an annular ciliochoroidal

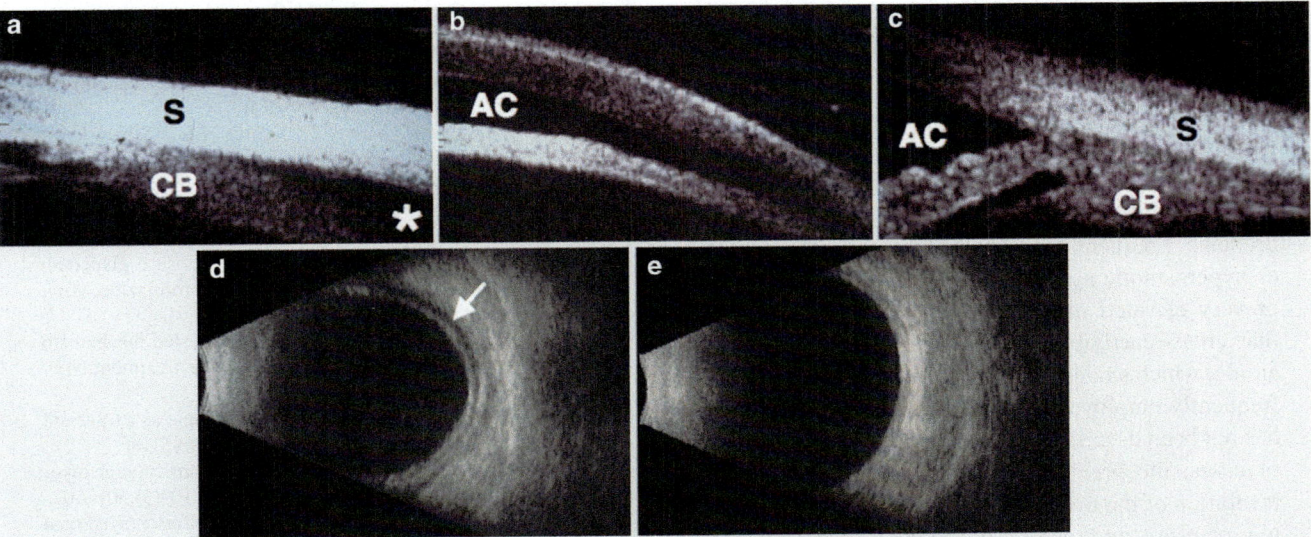

**Fig. 36.1-1** Ultrasound biomicroscopy images (UBM) and ophthalmic ultrasound images (b-scan) before (**a, b, d**) and after (**c, e**) resolution of secondary angle closure due to topiramate. The UBM shows a supraciliary effusion (*), demonstrated in A, which causes anterior rotation of the lens–iris diaphragm and a significant decrease of the anterior chamber depth (**b**). The normal anatomy of a deep chamber with a well-defined ciliary sulcus is restored a few days later after the discontinuation of the offending drug (**c**). Ophthalmic ultrasound demonstrates a choroidal effusion at presentation (**d**) that has resolved a few days later. (Reprinted with permission from Sankar PS, Pasquale LR, Grosskreutz CL. Uveal effusion and secondary angle-closure glaucoma associated with topiramate use. *Arch Ophthalmol* 2001;119(8):1210-1211. American Medical Association, © 2001. All rights reserved.)

(supraciliary) effusion. Both the ciliary body swelling and the ciliochoroidal (supraciliary) effusion allow for relaxation of the zonules and explain the thickening of the lens and the forward displacement of the lens–iris diaphragm. Depending on the degree and rate of intraocular pressure, elevation headache, nausea/vomiting, and periocular pain can confuse the clinical picture. This may lead to late recognition of the diagnosis, frequently after unnecessary central nervous system (CNS) imaging studies have been obtained in the emergency room.

The clinical constellation of bilateral angle closure, especially if encountered in younger patients where angle closure is extremely rare, narrows the differential diagnosis significantly. Once suspected, the presence of uveal effusions should be confirmed with ultrasonography or ultrasound biomicroscopy if available, and the patient's medication list should be reviewed. Other uncommon reasons of ciliochoroidal effusions, such as systemic diseases, orbital/ocular inflammatory, neoplastic, traumatic processes, surgery, or venous, can be usually be ruled out by the patient's history.

Topiramate exerts its anticonvulsant effect by multiple mechanisms including a state-dependent sodium channel blockade, augmentation of GABA activity, and antagonization of excitatory amino acid receptors. It also possesses a weak carbonic anhydrase activity. The propensity of sulfa-related compounds to produce transient myopia and/or secondary angle closure has been described in the past in association with acetazolamide, sulfamethoxazole, indapamide, and hydrochlorothiazide. The exact mechanism resulting in uveal effusions is unknown. The working hypothesis about the pathogenesis of the uveal effusions is an idiosyncratic breakdown in the blood–ocular barrier allowing net fluid accumulation within the suprachoroidal space that extends anteriorly. The above theory is further supported by the finding of a high protein concentration in the cerebrospinal fluid (CSF) of patients who received a lumbar puncture as part of their work-up before the diagnosis was established. High CSF protein levels suggest a concurrent breakdown in the blood–brain barrier. In addition, the reported faster resolution of the secondary angle closure in patients treated with a combination of mannitol and high-dose intravenous steroids further supports this hypothesis. There is also evidence supporting a dose-dependent response because at least five cases occurred within hours after doubling the dose of topiramate and because rechallenging of one patient with a lower dose of topiramate failed to reproduce the initially observed induced myopia.

Treatment requires immediate discontinuation of the offending agent along with administration of aqueous suppressants and topical steroids. A peripheral iridotomy is not necessary or useful because the mechanism of angle closure is not relative pupillary block in this case.

Pilocarpine is contraindicated because it can aggravate the angle closure by relaxing the zonules and allowing further anterior displacement of the lens–iris diaphragm. In contrast, cycloplegics have a role as they tighten the zonules and displace the lens–iris diaphragm posteriorly, making trabecular meshwork available for aqueous drainage. Frequently, oral carbonic anhydrase inhibitors or hyperosmotic agents are required in the acute setting of very elevated intraocular pressures. It is interesting that cross-reactivity between topiramate and acetazolamide, which shares a similar sulfonamide moiety and is frequently employed in the treatment of this glaucoma, has not been described to our knowledge. In the majority of cases, the previously mentioned approach leads to resolution of the uveal effusion, improvement in intraocular pressure, and reversal of the induced myopia within a few days. Recently, a more rapid resolution of the uveal effusion and secondary angle-closure glaucoma has been documented with a combination of intravenous mannitol and methylprednisolone. Surgical intervention is seldom necessary. When needed, one can consider drainage of the suprachoroidal effusion, if conservative management fails and the risk of corneal decompensation is imminent due to lenticular–corneal touch.

## Bibliography

Banta JT, Hoffman K, Budenz DL, et al. Presumed topiramate-induced bilateral acute angle-closure glaucoma. *Am J Ophthalmol* 2001;132(1):112–114.

Beasley FJ. Transient myopia and retinal edema during hydrochlorothiazide (hydrodiuril) therapy. *Arch Ophthalmol* 1961;65:212-213.

Beasley FJ. Transient myopia and retinal edema during ethoxzolamide (cardrase) therapy. *Arch Ophthalmol* 1962;68:490–491.

Bovino JA, Marcus DF. The mechanism of transient myopia induced by sulfonamide therapy. *Am J Ophthalmol* 1982;94(1):99–102.

Chen TC, Chao CW, Sorkin JA. Topiramate induced myopic shift and angle closure glaucoma. *Br J Ophthalmol* 2003;87(5):648–649.

Craig JE, Ong TJ, Louis DL, Wells JM. Mechanism of topiramate-induced acute-onset myopia and angle closure glaucoma. *Am J Ophthalmol* 2004;137(1):193–195.

Fan JT, Johnson DH, Burk RR. Transient myopia, angle-closure glaucoma, and choroidal detachment after oral acetazolamide. *Am J Ophthalmol* 1993;115(6):813–814.

Fraunfelder FW, Fraunfelder FT, Keates EU. Topiramate-associated acute, bilateral, secondary angle-closure glaucoma. *Ophthalmology* 2004;111(1):109–111.

Garland MA, Sholk A, Guenter KE. Acetazolamide-induced myopia. *Am J Obstet Gynecol* 1962;84:69–71.

Geanon JD, Perkins TW. Bilateral acute angle-closure glaucoma associated with drug sensitivity to hydrochlorothiazide. *Arch Ophthalmol* 1995;113(10):1231–1232.

Grinbaum A, Ashkenazi I, Gutman I, et al. Suggested mechanism for acute transient myopia after sulfonamide treatment. *Ann Ophthalmol* 1993;25(6):224–226.

Gubbay SS. The occurrence of drug-induced myopia as a transient side effect of topiramate. *Epilepsia* 1998;39(4):451.

Ikeda N, Ikeda T, Nagata M, et al. Pathogenesis of transient high myopia after blunt eye trauma. *Ophthalmology* 2002;109(3):501–507.

Ikeda N, Ikeda T, Nagata M, et al. Ciliochoroidal effusion syndrome induced by sulfa derivatives. *Arch Ophthalmol* 2002;120(12):1775.

Kaniecki R. Neuromodulators for migraine prevention. *Headache* 2008;48(4):586–600.

Lachkar Y, Bouassida W. Drug-induced acute angle closure glaucoma. *Curr Opin Ophthalmol* 2007;18(2):129–133.

Liebmann JM, Weinreb RN, Ritch R. Angle-closure glaucoma associated with occult annular ciliary body detachment. *Arch Ophthalmol* 1998;116(6):731–735.

Medeiros FA, Zhang XY, Bernd AS, Weinreb RN. Angle-closure glaucoma associated with ciliary body detachment in patients using topiramate. *Arch Ophthalmol* 2003;121(2):282–285.

Parikh R, Parikh S, Das S, et al. Choroidal drainage in the management of acute angle closure after topiramate toxicity. *J Glaucoma* 2007;16(8):691–693.

Postel EA, Assalian A, Epstein DL. Drug-induced transient myopia and angle-closure glaucoma associated with supraciliary choroidal effusion. *Am J Ophthalmol* 1996;122(1):110–112.

Rhee DJ, Goldberg MJ, Parrish RK. Bilateral angle-closure glaucoma and ciliary body swelling from topiramate. *Arch Ophthalmol* 2001;119(11):1721–1723.

Rhee DJ, Ramos-Esteban JC, Nipper KS. Rapid resolution of topiramate-induced angle-closure glaucoma with methylprednisolone and mannitol. *Am J Ophthalmol* 2006;141(6):1133–1134.

Ritch R, Chang BM, Liebmann JM. Angle closure in younger patients. *Ophthalmology* 2003;110(10):1880–1889.

Sankar PS, Pasquale LR, Grosskreutz CL. Uveal effusion and secondary angle-closure glaucoma associated with topiramate use. *Arch Ophthalmol* 2001;119(8):1210–1211.

Thambi L, Kapcala LP, Chambers W, et al. Topiramate-associated secondary angle-closure glaucoma: a case series. *Arch Ophthalmol* 2002;120(8):1108.

Viet Tran H, Ravinet E, Schnyder C, et al. Blood-brain barrier disruption associated with topiramate-induced angle-closure glaucoma of acute onset. *Klin Monatsbl Augenheilkd* 2006;223(5):425–457.

## 36.17 Nanophthalmos

Nanophthalmos is characterized by a short, less than 20 mm axial length eye with a small corneal diameter, large lens, and thick sclera. It has been associated with one recessive gene (MFRP, 11q23) and two autosomal dominant genes (NNO1, 11p and locus VMD2, 11q12).[95] The patients are susceptible to angle closure at an earlier age than PAC. These patients are at high risk for choroidal effusion and nonrhegmatogenous retinal detachment. They are at high risk for complications during surgery, and prophylactic posterior sclerotomies should be considered if intraocular surgery is necessary.

## 36.18 Conclusion

Angle-closure glaucoma is a major cause of blindness worldwide. Many individuals remain as suspects at risk for future disease while others present as acute emergencies or are subject to chronic asymptomatic loss of vision. It is essential for the clinician to be able to identify and classify those at risk and those with disease in order to initiate an effective follow-up or treatment plan. Patients do not always fall neatly into textbook classifications, particularly with angle-closure glaucoma, and consideration should always be given to mixed-mechanism disease We are fortunate to have an improved understanding of the risk factors, inheritance, and pathophysiology of the spectrum of angle-closure glaucoma. Continued advances in diagnostics, imaging systems, and therapeutics have revolutionized the management of angle-closure glaucoma. Particularly noteworthy is the development and widespread availability of laser iridotomy for the prevention and treatment of pupillary block.

## References

1. Hyams S. *Angle-closure glaucoma, a comprehensive review of primary and secondary angle-closure glaucoma*. Amsterdam: Kugler & Ghedini; 1990, p 1.
2. Lowe RF. A history of primary angle closure glaucoma. *Surv Ophthalmol*. 1995;40:163–170.
3. Foster PJ. Epidemiology, classification and mechanism. In: Weinreb, RN, Friedman, DS, eds. *Angle closure and angle closure glaucoma*. The Hague, The Netherlands: Kuegler; 2006:1–20
4. Foster PJ, Johnson GJ. Glaucoma in China: how big is the problem? *Br J Ophthalmol*. 2001;85:1277–1282.
5. Quigley HA, Broman AT. The number of people with glaucoma worldwide in 2010 and 2020. *Br J Ophthalmol*. 2006;90:262–267.
6. Wang N, Li S, Liang Y. Classification. In: Hong C, Yamamoto T, eds. *Angle closure glaucoma*. Amsterdam, The Netherlands: Kuegler; 2007:41–55.
7. Foster PJ, Buhrman RR, Quigley HA, Johnson GJ. The definition and classification of glaucoma in prevalence surveys. *Br J Ophthalmol*. 2002;86:238–242.
8. Ritch R, Lowe RF. Angle-Closure Glaucoma - Clinical Types. In: Ritch R, Shields MB, Krupin T, eds. *The glaucomas*. 2nd ed. St. Louis: Mosby; 1996:801–840.
9. Filho AD, Cronemberger S, Mérula RV, Calixto N. Comparative study between plateau iris configuration and primary open angle glaucoma with narrow angle using ultrasound biomicroscopy. *Invest Ophthalmol Vis Sci* 2009;43:ARVO E-Abstract 3363
10. Ritch R, Tham CCY, et al. Argon laser peripheral iridoplasty in the management of plateau iris syndrome: long-term follow-up. *Ophthalmology*. 2004;111:104–108.
11. Ritch R. Laser and medical treatment of primary angle closure glaucoma. In: Weinreb RN, Friedman DS, eds. *Angle closure and angle closure glaucoma*. The Hague, The Netherlands: Kuegler; 2006:37–54
12. Peng D, Zhang X, Yu K. Argon laser peripheral iridoplasty and laser iridectomy for plateau iris glaucoma. *Zhonghua Yan Ke Za Zhi*. 1997;33:165–168.
13. Dellaporta A. Historical notes on gonioscopy. *Surv Ophthalmol*. 1975;20:137–149.
14. Forbes M. Gonioscopy with corneal indentation: a method for distinguishing between appositional closure and synechial closure. *Arch Opthalmol*. 1966;76:488–497.
15. Friedman DS, Mingguang H. Anterior chamber angle assessment techniques. *Surv Ophthalmol*. 2008;53:250–273.
16. Ritch R, Liebman J, Tello C. A construct for understanding angle closure glaucoma: the role of ultrasound biomicroscopy. *Ophthalmol Clin North Am*. 1995;8:281–293.
17. Lieberman J. Ultrasound biomicroscopy. In: Weinreb RN, Friedman DS, eds. *Angle closure and angle closure glaucoma*. The Hague, The Netherlands: Kuegler; 2006:71
18. Baskaran M. Devices for screening for angle closure. In: Weinreb RN, Friedman DS, eds. *Angle closure and angle closure glaucoma*. The Hague, The Netherlands: Kuegler; 2006:73–74.
19. Tello C, Rothman R, Ishikawa H, Ritch R. Differential diagnosis of the angle closure glaucomas. *Ophthalmol Clin North Am*. 2000;13:443–453.
20. Yao B, Wu L, Zhang C, Wang X. Ultrasound biometric features associated with angle closure in fellow eyes of acute primary angle closure after laser iridotomy. *Ophthalmology*. 2009;116:444–448.
21. Kashiwagi K, Kashiwagi F, Toda Y, et al. A newly developed peripheral anterior chamber depth analysis system: principle, accuracy and reproducibility. *Br J Ophthalmol*. 2004;88:1036–1041.
22. Asawaphureekorn S. New approaches to visualize the anterior chamber angle. In: Hong C, Yamamoto T, eds. *Angle closure glaucoma*. Amsterdam, The Netherlands: Kuegler; 2007:101–113.
23. Nolan WP, Foster PJ, Devereux JG, Uranchimeg D, Johnson GJ, Baasanhu J. YAG laser iridotomy treatment for primary angle-closure in east Asian eyes. *Br J Ophthalmol*. 2000;84:1255–1259.
24. Gazzard G, Friedman DS, Devereux JG, Chew PT, Seah SK. A prospective ultrasound biomicroscopy evaluation of changes in anterior segment morphology after laser iridotomy in Asian eyes. *Ophthalmology*. 2003;110:630–638.
25. Ramakrishnan R, Nirmalan PK, Krishnadas R, et al. Glaucoma in a rural population of southern India: the Aravind comprehensive eye survey. *Ophthalmology*. 2003;110:1484–1490.
26. Shiose Y, Kitazawa Y, Tsukuhara S, et al. Epidermiology of glaucoma in Japan – a nationwide glaucoma survey. *Jpn J Ophthalmol*. 1991;35:133–153.
27. Foster PJ, Gaasanhu J, Alsbirk PH, Munkhbayar D, Uranchimeg D, Johnson GJ. Glaucoma in Mongolia – a population-based survey in Hövsgöl Province, Northern Mongolia. *Arch Ophthalmol*. 1996; 114:1235–1241.
28. Yamamoto T, Iwase A, Araie M, et al. The Tajimi Study report 2: prevalence of primary angle closure and secondary glaucoma in a Japanese population. *Ophthalmology*. 2005;112:1661–1669.
29. Bourne RRA, Sukudom P, Foster PJ, et al. Prevalence of glaucoma in Thailand: a population based survey in Rom Klao District, Bangkok. *Br J Ophthalmol*. 2003;87:1069–1074.
30. Salmon JF, Mermoud A, Ivey A, Swanevelder SA, Hoffman M. The prevalence of primary angle-closure glaucoma and open angle glaucoma in Mamre, Western Cape, South Africa. *Arch Ophthalmol*. 1993;111:1263–1269.
31. Seah SKL, Foster PJ, Chew PT, et al. Incidence of acute primary angle-closure glaucoma in Singapore. An island-wide survey. *Arch Ophthalmol*. 1997;115:1436–1440.
32. Alsbirk PH. Anterior chamber depth in Greenland Eskimos. I. A population study of variation with age and sex. *Acta Ophthalmol*. 1974;52:551–564.
33. Foster PJ, Alsbirk PH, Baasanhu J, Munkhbayar D, Uranchimeg D, Johnson GJ. Anterior chamber depth in Mogolians. Vatiation with age, sex and method of measurement. *Am J Ophthalmol*. 1997;124:53–60.

34. Foster PJ, Devereux JG, Alsbirk PH, et al. Detection of gonioscopically occludable angles and primary angle closure glaucoma by estimation of limbal chamber depth in Asians: modified grading scheme. *Br J Ophthalmol.* 2000;84:186–192.
35. Devereux JG, Foster PJ, Baasanhu J, et al. Anterior chamber depth measurement as a screening tool for primary angle-closure glaucoma in an East Asian population. *Arch Ophthalmol.* 2000;118:257–263.
36. Chang BM, Liebman JM, Ritch R. Angle closure in younger patients. *Trans Am Ophthalmol Soc.* 2002;100:201–214.
37. Angle Closure Glaucoma. Coffi, G.A., Durcan, F.J. Girkin, C. A. et al Chapter 5 in Section 10 of Basic and Clinical Science Course 2008-2009. publisher American Academy of Ophthalmology; 2008; 5:126–128.
38. Van Rens GH, Arkell SM, Charlton W, Doesburg W. Primary angle-closure glaucoma among Alaskan Eskimos. *Doc Ophthalmol.* 1988;70:265–276.
39. Arkell SM, Lightman DA, Sommer A, et al. The prevalence of glaucoma among Eskimos of northwest Alaska. *Arch Ophthalmol.* 1987;105:482–485.
40. Bourne RR, Sorensen KE, Klauber A, et al. Glaucoma in east greenlandic inuit – a population survey in Ittoqqortoonmiit (Scoresbysund). *Acta Ophthalmol Scand.* 2001;79:462–467.
41. Congdon NG, Quigley HA, Hung PT, et al. Screening techniques for angle-closure glaucoma in rural Taiwan. *Acta Ophthalmol Scand.* 1996;74:113–119.
42. Foster PJ, Baasanhu J, Alsbirk PH, et al. Glaucoma in Mongolia. Apopulation-based survey in Hovsgol province, northern Mongolia. *Arch Ophthalmol* 1996;114:1235–1241
43. Sim DH, Goh LG, Ho T. Glaucoma pattern amongst the elderly Chinese in Singapore. *Ann Acad Med Singapore.* 1998;27(6):819–823.
44. Dandona L, Dandona R, Mandal P, et al. Angle-closure glaucoma in an urban population in southern India: the Andhra Pradesh Eye Disease Study. *Ophthalmology.* 2000;107:1710–1716.
45. Quigley HA, West SK, Rodriguez J, et al. The prevalence of glaucoma in a population-based study of Hispanic Subjects: Proyecto VER. *Arch Ophthalmol* 2001;119(12):1819–1826.
46. Tielsch JM, Katz J, Singh K, et al. A population-based evaluation of glaucoma screening: the Baltimore Eye Survey. *Am J Epidemiol* 1991;134:1102–1110.
47. Buhrmann RR, Quigley HA, Barron Y, et al. Prevalence of glaucoma in a rural East African population. *Invest Ophthalmol Vis Sci* 2000;41:40–48.
48. Rotchford AP, Johnson GJ. Glaucoma in Zulus: a population-based cross-sectional survey in a rural district in South Africa. *Arch Ophthalmol.* 2002;120:471–478.
49. Bonomi L, Marchini G, Marraffa M, et al. Prevalence of glaucoma and intraocular pressure distribution in a defined population. The Egna-Neumarkt Study. *Ophthalmology.* 1998;105:209–215.
50. Bankes JL, Perkins ES, Tsolakis S, Wright JE. Bedford glaucoma survey. *Br Med J.* 1968;1:791–796.
51. Bengtsson B. The prevalence of glaucoma. *Br J Ophthalmol* 1981;65:46–49.
52. Hollows FC, Graham PA. Intra-ocular pressure, glaucoma, and glaucoma suspects in a defined population. *Br J Ophthalmol* 1966;50:570–586.
53. Klein BE, Klein R, Sponsel WE, et al. Prevalence of glaucoma. The Beaver Dam Eye Study. *Ophthalmology.* 1992;99:1499–1504.
54. Coffey M, Reidy A, Wormald R, et al. Prevalence of glaucoma in the west of Ireland. *Br J Ophthalmol* 1993;77:17–21.
55. Bonomi L, Marchini G, Marraffa M, et al. Epidemiology of angle-closure glaucoma: prevalence, clinical types, and association with peripheral anterior chamber depth in the Egna-Neumarket Glaucoma Study. *Ophthalmology.* 2000;107:998–1003.
56. Congdon N, Wang F, Tielsch JM. Issues in the epidemiology and population-based screening of primary angle-closure glaucoma. *Surv Ophthalmol.* 1992;36:411–423.
57. Erie JC, Hodge DO, Gray DT. The incidence of primary angle-closure glaucoma in Olmstead County, Minnesota. *Arch Ophthalmol.* 1997;115: 177–181.
58. Foster PJ, Oen FT, Machin D, et al. The prevalence of glaucoma in Chinese residents of Singapore: a cross-sectional population survey of the Tanjong Pagar district. *Arch Ophthalmol.* 2000;118:1105–1111.
59. Congdon NG, Qi Y, Quigley HA, et al. Biometry and primary angle-closure glaucoma among Chinese, White and Black populations. *Ophthalmology.* 1997;104:1489–1495.
60. Aung T, Nolan WP, Machin D, et al. Anterior chamber depth and the risk of primary angle closure in 2 East Asian populations. *Arch Ophthalmol.* 2005;123:527–532.
61. Stanley H. Biometry. In: Stanley H, ed. *Angle closure glaucoma.* Amsterdam: Kugler & Ghedini; 1990.
62. Congdon NG, Youlin Q, Quigley H, et al. Biometry and primary angle-closure glaucoma among Chinese, white, and black populations. *Ophthalmology.* 1997;104:1489–1495.
63. Marchini G, Pagliarusco A, Toscano A, Tosi R, Brunelli C, Bonomi L. Ultrasound biomicroscopic and conventional ultrasonographic study of ocular dimensions in primary angle closure glaucoma. *Ophthalmology.* 1998;105:2091–2098.
64. Quigley HA, Silver DM, Friedman DS, et al. Iris cross-sectional area decreases with pupil dilation and its dynamic behavior is a risk factor in angle closure. *J Glaucoma.* 2009;18:173–183.
65. Fontana SC, Brubaker RF. Volume and depth of the anterior chamber in the normal aging human eye. *Arch Ophthalmol.* 1980;98: 1803–1808.
66. Forbes M. Indentation gonioscopy and efficacy of iridectomy in angle-closure glaucoma. *Trans Am Ophthalmol Soc.* 1974;72:488–515.
67. Lam DS, Chua JK, Tham CC, Lai JS. Efficacy and safety of immediate anterior chamber paracentesis in the treatment of acute primary angle-closure glaucoma: a pilot study. *Ophthalmology.* 2002;109:64–70.
68. Lam DS, Lai JS, Tham CC, Chua JK, Poon AS. Argon laser peripheral iridoplasty versus conventional systemic medical therapy in treatment of acute primary angle-closure glaucoma: a prospective, randomized, controlled trial. *Ophthalmology.* 2002;109:1591–1596.
69. Lai JS, Tham CC, Chua JK, et al. To compare argon laser peripheral iridoplasty (ALPI) against systemic medications in treatment of acute primary angle-closure: mid-term results. *Eye.* 2006;20:309–314.
70. Lai JS, Tham CC, Chua JK, et al. To compare argon laser peripheral iridoplasty (ALPI) against systemic medications in treatment of acute primary angle-closure: mid-term results. *Eye* 2006;20:309–314.
71. Quaranta L, Bettelli S, et al. Argon laser iridoplasty as primary treatment for acute angle closure glaucoma: a prospective clinical study. *Acta Ophthalmol Scand Suppl.* 2002;236:16–17.
72. Aung T, Tow SL, Yap EY, et al. Trabeculectomy for acute primary angle closure. *Ophthalmology.* 2000;107:1298–1302.
73. Alsbirk PH. Anatomical risk factors in primary angle-closure glaucoma. A ten-year follow-up survey based on limbal and axial anterior chamber depths in a high risk population. *Int Ophthalmol.* 1992;16:265–272.
74. Wilensky JT, Kaufman PI, Frohlichstein D, et al. Follow-up angle-closure glaucoma suspects. *Am J Ophthalmol* 1993;115:338–346.
75. Ritch R, Stegman Z, Liebmann J. Mapstone's hypothesis confirmed. *Br J Ophthalmol.* 1995;79:300.
76. Gazzard G, Foster PJ, Friedman DS, Khaw PT, Seah SK. Light to dark physiological variation in irido-trabecular angle width [videotape]. *Br J Ophthalmol* 2004;88:1357–1482.
77. Lim LS, Husain R, Gazzard G, Seah SK, Aung T. Cataract progression after prophylactic laser peripheral iridotomy: potential implications for the prevention of glaucoma blindness. *Ophthalmology.* 2005;112:1355–1359.
78. Robin AL, Pollack IP. A comparison of neodymium:YAG and argon laser iridotomies. *Ophthalmology.* 1984;91:1011–1016.

79. Schwartz GF, Steinmann WC, Spaeth GL, Wilson RP. Surgical and medical management of patients with narrow anterior chamber angles: comparative results. *Ophthalmic Surg.* 1992;23:108–112.
80. Friedman DS, Thomas R, Alsbirk PH, Gazzard G. Detection of primary angle closure glaucoma. In: Weinreb RN, Friedman DS, eds. *Angle closure and angle closure glaucoma.* The Hague, The Netherlands: Kuegler; 2006:55–63.
81. Tarongoy P, Ho CL, Walton DS. Angle-closure glaucoma: the role of the lens in the pathogenesis, prevention and treatment. *Surv Ophthalmol.* 2009;54:211–225.
82. Nelson L, Maumenee IH. Ectopia lentis. *Surv Ophthalmol.* 1982;27:143–157.
83. Nemet AY, Assia EI, Apple DJ, Barequet IS. Current concepts of ocular manifestations in Marfan syndrome. *Surv Ophthalmol.* 2006;51:561–575.
84. Lovisolo CF, Reinstein DZ. Phakic intraocular lenses. *Surv Ophthalmol.* 2005;50:549–587.
85. von Graefe A. Beitrage zur Palhologie und Therapie des Glaukoms. *Arch Ophthalmol* 1869;15:108.
86. Klein R. Prevention of visual loss from diabetic retinopathy. *Surv Ophthalmol.* 2002;47:S246–S252.
87. Gunther JB, Altaweel MM. Bevacizumab (Avastin) for the treatment of. *Surv Ophthalmol.* 2009;54:372–400.
88. Yanoff M. Iridocorneal endothelial syndrome: unification of a disease spectrum. *Surv Ophthalmol.* 1979;24:1–20.
89. Hemady RK, Patel A, Blum S, Nirankari VS. Bilateral iridocorneal endothelial syndrome case report and review of the literature. *Cornea.* 1994;13:368–372.
90. Vargas LG, Vroman DT, Soloman KD, Holzer MP, et al. Epithelial downgrowth after clear cornea phacoemulsification. *Ophthalmology* 2002;12:2331–2335.
91. Okhravi N, Odufuwa B, McCluskey P, Lightman S. Scleritis. *Surv Ophthalmol* 2005;50:351–363
92. Mendelsohn AD, Jampol LM, Schoch D. Secondary angle-closure after central retinal vein occlusion. *Am J Ophthalmol.* 1985;100:581–585.
93. Sodhi A, Leung L, Do DV, Gower EW, Schein OD, Handa JT. Recent trends in the Management of Rhegmatogenous Retinal Detachment. *Surv Ophthalmol* 2008;53:50–67
94. Levy J, Yagev R, Petrova A, Lifshiz T. Topiramate-induced bilateral angle-closure glaucoma. *Can J Ophthalmol.* 2006;41:221–225.
95. Wiggs JL. Genetic etiologies of glaucoma. *Arch Ophthalmol* 2007;125(1):30–37.

# Chapter 37
# Malignant Glaucoma (Posterior Aqueous Diversion Syndrome)

Marshall N. Cyrlin

Von Graefe[1] first used the term *malignant glaucoma* to describe a devastating and unusual form of glaucoma that occurred following ocular surgery. This sequelae was associated with increased intraocular pressure (IOP) and flattening or shallowing of the anterior chamber. The word *malignant* was used to characterize the uniformly grave visual prognosis, but because of its relationship to cancer, many have objected to its use, preferring the term *misdirection of aqueous*. The current definition has been expanded to include *classic malignant glaucoma* and *nonphakic malignant glaucoma* as well as disorders occurring in other clinical situations. Classic malignant glaucoma is usually associated with a specific clinical scenario that occurs after incisional surgery (iridectomy or filtration) for primary angle-closure glaucoma, secondary or chronic angle-closure glaucoma, or at times open-angle glaucoma in phakic patients (Table 37.1). The occurrence of malignant glaucoma after cataract surgery and the persistence of malignant glaucoma following cataract surgery in the classic form have been termed as *aphakic malignant glaucoma*. The diagnosis *nonphakic malignant glaucoma* has been suggested for both aphakic and pseudophakic types[2] and may also be applied to the development of malignant glaucoma after combined cataract and filtration surgery. The term *malignant-like glaucoma* has been proposed for instances with similar clinical presentations but where different underlying pathophysiology may be present.[2]

The term *malignant glaucoma* is unacceptable to some clinicians because to patients it may suggest cancer and it is not related to the underlying pathophysiology of the disease. Instead, various other descriptions such as *aqueous misdirection syndrome, ciliary block glaucoma*,[3,4] and *direct lens block glaucoma*[5] have been proposed. Nonetheless, the term *malignant glaucoma* is still used often because it is readily understood by most clinicians to define the classic phakic and nonphakic forms and is based on actual pathophysiologic mechanisms (Table 37.2).

## 37.1 Classic Malignant Glaucoma

The pathognomonic findings of classic malignant glaucoma are increased IOP or unexpected normal IOP following glaucoma surgery, central (axial) shortening of the anterior chamber, open iridotomy or iridectomy, and no evidence for choroidal effusion or hemorrhage. Historically, it has an occurrence between 0.6 and 4% of eyes that are diagnosed with acute angle-closure glaucoma.[6–8] The chance of the onset of malignant glaucoma following surgery for angle-closure glaucoma is the greatest when the angle is not completely opened at the time of surgery, regardless of whether or not the IOP has been reduced prior to the procedure.[9] In one study, a relationship between chronic angle-closure and malignant glaucoma was reported in 10 of 14 eyes.[10] Classic malignant glaucoma typically develops after surgical peripheral iridectomy or filtering (full-thickness sclerectomy or trabeculectomy) surgery in phakic patients (Figs. 37.1 and 37.2). Elevated IOP and shallowing of the chamber can occur during the surgery, immediately afterward, after the discontinuation of cycloplegics,[9] after the initiation of miotics,[9,11] or quite some time later.[11–15] If one eye develops malignant glaucoma after surgery, the contralateral eye will probably do likewise. Although the IOP may in some cases be in the teens to low 20s following filtration surgery, it may at times be 40–60 mmHg or greater. Miotics are ineffective in lowering IOP and instead may further increase the pressure. Conventional filtering surgery in patients who have had previous peripheral iridectomy does not reverse the problem.

## 37.2 Non-phakic Malignant Glaucoma

*Malignant glaucoma in aphakia* is a term for eyes with persistence of preexisting malignant glaucoma after cataract surgery as well as in patients with malignant glaucoma

**Table 37.1** Classic malignant glaucoma

*Diagnostic criteria for classic malignant glaucoma*

Flattening or shallowing of the axial (central anterior chamber with peripheral flattening

Increased or greater than expected IOP after filtering surgery

Absence of pupillary block following iridotomy or iridectomy

*Anticipated response to treatment*

No reduction of IOP following miotic therapy

Reduction of IOP or reversal with aqueous suppressant, mydriatic-cycloplegic and/or osmotic therapy

Generally resolved by disruption of the anterior hyaloid by laser or surgery

**Table 37.2** Clinical manifestations of malignant glaucoma

Classic malignant glaucoma
Non-phakic malignant glaucoma
   Aphakic
   Pseudophakic
Malignant-like glaucoma

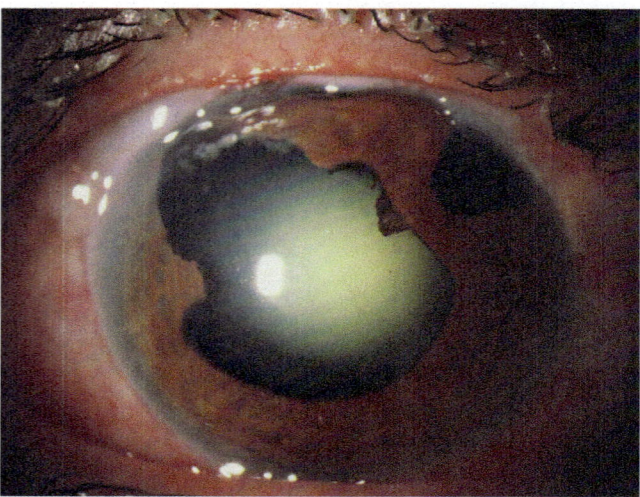

**Fig. 37.2** Classic malignant glaucoma with central and peripheral flat chambers after sector iridectomy and subsequent trabeculectomy. Reproduced with permission from Cyrlin M. Malignant glaucoma. In: Albert DM, Jakobiec FA, eds. *Principles and Practice of Ophthalmology*, 2nd edition. WB Saunders, 2000:2834–2846

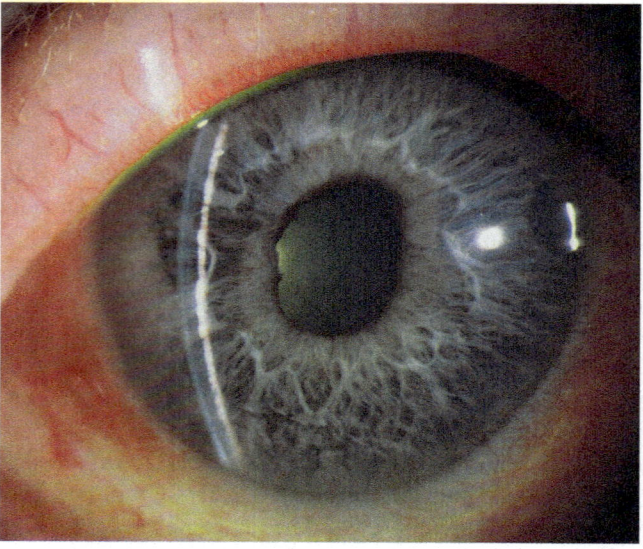

**Fig. 37.1** Classic malignant glaucoma with central and peripheral flat chambers after a surgical peripheral iridectomy. Reproduced with permission from Cyrlin M. Malignant glaucoma. In: Albert DM, Jakobiec FA, eds. *Principles and Practice of Ophthalmology*, 2nd edition. WB Saunders, 2000:2834-2846

occurring following routine cataract surgery. Reports of non-phakic malignant glaucoma have increased during the past few decades. It has been noted after cataract surgery in eyes with[16] or without[7,16] preexisting glaucoma. It has been described in eyes undergoing anterior chamber intraocular lens implantation at the time of cataract extraction.[17] Pseudophakic malignant glaucoma should be considered after surgery in patients with axial shallowing of the anterior chamber and in eyes with a shallow chamber and pressures in the teens or higher after a combined phacotrabeculectomy with lens implant.[18] Malignant glaucoma has also been reported following Nd:YAG laser capsulotomy,[19] diode laser cyclocoagulation,[20] and aqueous tube shunt surgery.[21]

## 37.3 Other Malignant Glaucoma Syndromes

Numerous clinical entities share some or all the findings of classic phakic and nonphakic malignant glaucoma. Malignant glaucoma, malignant-like glaucoma,[2] and other entities defined by their presumed pathophysiologic mechanisms have been described by various authors. An extensive review of case reports in the literature has been presented by Luntz and Rosenblatt.[22]

Table 37.3 lists the circumstances when a clinical picture consistent with classic malignant glaucoma, but not necessarily occurring after typical incisional surgery, has been reported.

The presence of diagnostic criteria and the response to treatment as described earlier distinguish between malignant glaucoma and malignant-like glaucoma. The need for a patent iridectomy or iridotomy before the diagnosis is made cannot be emphasized enough.

## 37.4 Pathogenesis

The clinical findings in malignant glaucoma and its various presentations previously have been thought to be primarily the end result of aqueous misdirection or posterior aqueous diversion (Fig. 37.3a, b). Shaffer recognized early the effects of aqueous accumulation in the vitreous and its possible function in the pathogenesis of classic malignant glaucoma.[33] By definition, malignant glaucoma does not result from pupillary block and is not relieved by laser iridotomy or surgical iridectomy. Mechanisms that involve various contributions of the lens or zonules, ciliary processes, anterior hyaloid face, or vitreous body have been proposed.

The term *ciliary block* has been used by some clinicians to emphasize the presumed role of the ciliary processes in blocking the forward flow of aqueous in many cases.[3,4] Swollen, anteriorly displaced ciliary processes may be pressed up against the lens or against abnormally forward vitreous in phakic patients, or the ciliary processes may be touching or adherent to vitreous in aphakic patients.[8] Anterior displacement of the lens has also been attributed to ciliary muscle contraction[5] and loose zonules.[38,39] Swelling, spasm, or displacement of the ciliary processes could then be enhanced by miotics or inflammation. Direct lens block, as described by Levene,[3] would result from anterior displacement of the lens with shallowing of both the peripheral and the central anterior chamber. Emphasizing posterior aqueous diversion, ciliary block, or direct lens block as the primary mechanisms in malignant glaucoma underestimates the role of the anterior hyaloid and vitreous, which are probably of greater significance.

One of the great puzzles about malignant glaucoma is that laboratory studies suggest that at physiological rates of aqueous production, malignant glaucoma should not occur. Epstein and colleagues have proposed that resistance to the forward flow of aqueous could be further exacerbated by a diminution of anterior hyaloid surface area resulting from apposition to the peripheral lens or ciliary body. Malignant glaucoma would result from a persistent expansion of the vitreous volume in an eye with a relatively impermeable and diminished anterior hyaloid surface rather than from isolated pools of trapped aqueous in the vitreous cavity (Fig. 37.4).[40,41] Quigley has hypothesized a vicious circle of elevated pressure, vitreous compaction and dehydration, resulting in a further reduction in fluid conductivity, and shallowing of the chamber.[42]

The final common pathway of the various contributing mechanisms in malignant glaucoma is a self-perpetuating

**Table 37.3** Clinical picture consistent with classic malignant glaucoma

*After laser treatment for glaucoma*
After laser iridectomy:
   Narrow angle[2]
   Acute angle closure[23]
   Chronic angle closure[24,25]
After laser suture lysis following trabeculectomy[24,26,27]
After Nd:YAG laser cyclophotocoagulation[28]
*After miotics*
With prior glaucoma surgery:
Iridectomy[29]
Filtration[11]
Without prior surgery[30]
*After trauma*[5]
*Associated with retinal disease*
Retinopathy of prematurity[31,32]
After retinal detachment surgery[33]
After central vein occlusion[34]
*Associated With Inflammation*[5]
*Associated With Infection*
Fungal keratomycosis[35]
Nocardia asteroidis[36]
*Spontaneously*[37,38]

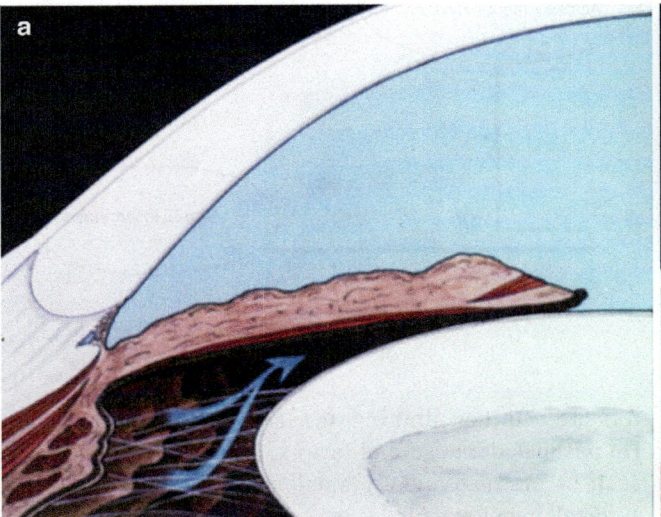 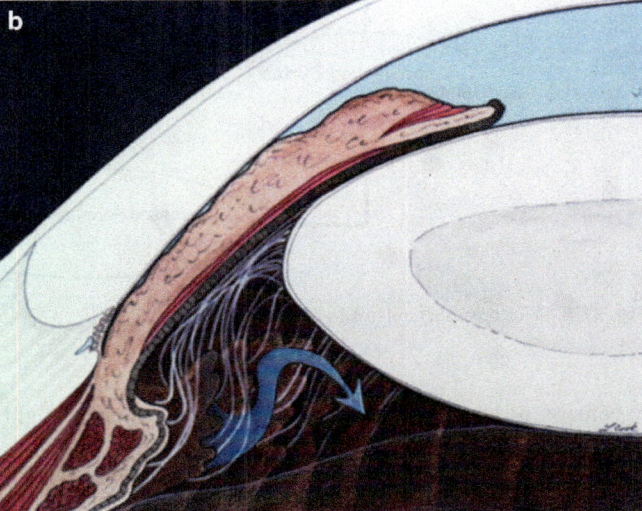

**Fig. 37.3** (a) Normal pathway of aqueous passage from the posterior to anterior chamber (*arrows*). (b) Aqueous misdirection posteriorly to the vitreous (*arrows*) in malignant glaucoma. Illustrations courtesy of B. Thomas Hutchinson, MD. Reproduced with permission from Cyrlin M. Malignant Glaucoma. In: Albert DM, Jakobiec FA (eds). Principles and Practice of Ophthalmology, 2nd edition. WB Saunders, 2000; 2834–2846

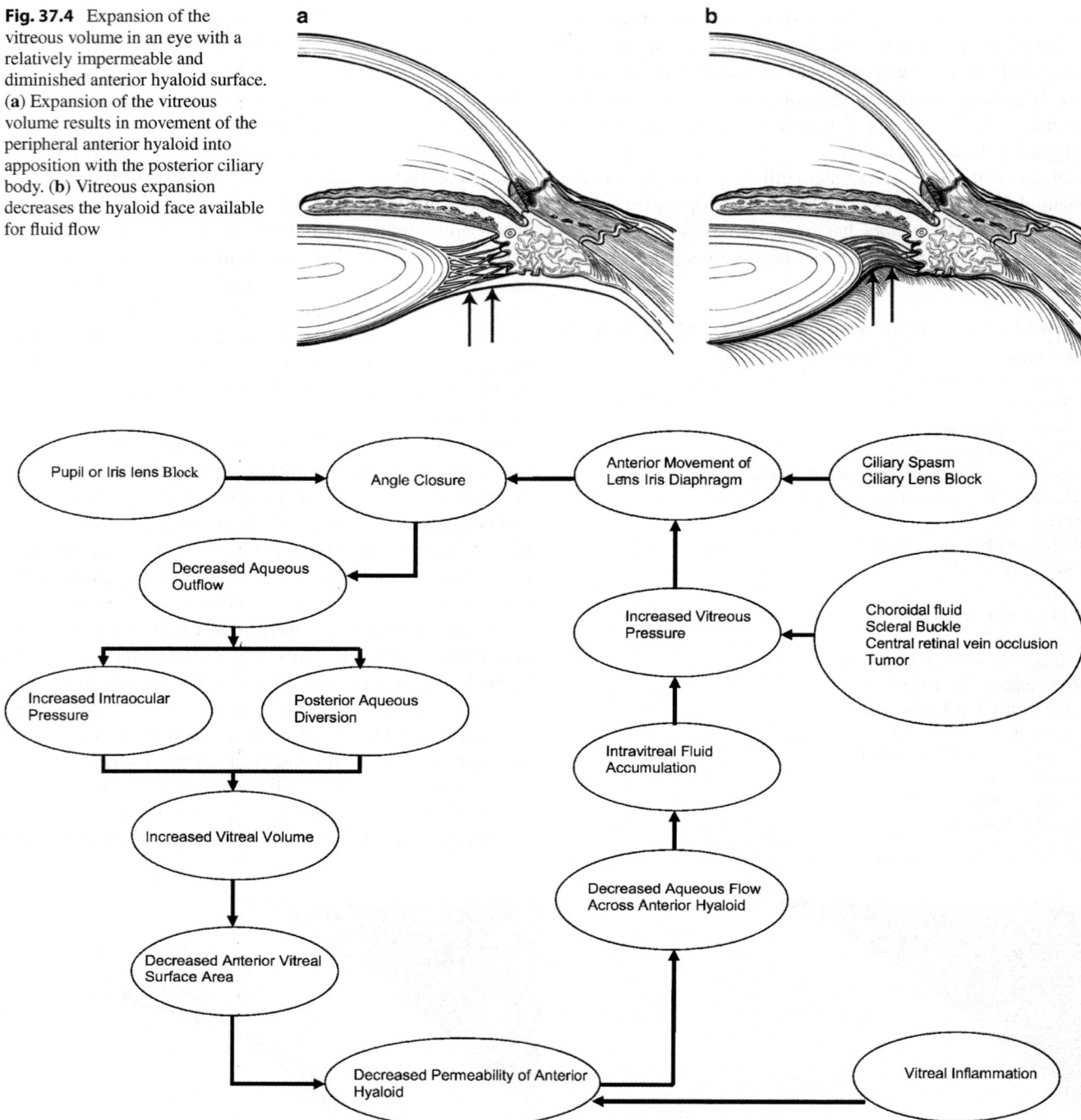

**Fig. 37.4** Expansion of the vitreous volume in an eye with a relatively impermeable and diminished anterior hyaloid surface. (**a**) Expansion of the vitreous volume results in movement of the peripheral anterior hyaloid into apposition with the posterior ciliary body. (**b**) Vitreous expansion decreases the hyaloid face available for fluid flow

**Fig. 37.5** Vitreous mechanisms in malignant glaucoma

expansion of the vitreous (Fig. 37.5).[22] Epstein has brought these mechanisms together into what he terms "unifying concepts in malignant glaucoma."[43,44] He stressed the presence of retrolenticular block that involves the anterior hyaloid face. Of highest significance is the relationship of the hyaloid face to the ciliary body. The hyaloid represents an impermeable barrier that pools aqueous posteriorly. It then expands forward, further limiting the area for fluid exchange. He postulated that several factors, alone or in combination, such as an anatomically small middle segment, sudden surgical hypotony of the eye, inflammation with hyaloid condensation, other causes of hyaloid abnormalities, or any sudden blockage of the posterior to anterior flow of aqueous, may initiate a malignant glaucoma condition.

Quigley and associates suggest that both primary angle closure and malignant glaucoma may be related to concurrence of several contributing factors that include a small eye, susceptibility for choroidal expansion, and decreased fluid conductivity of the vitreous.[45] Regardless of the underlying factor, disruption of the anterior hyaloid face with the Nd:YAG laser can cure classic phakic, aphakic, and pseudophakic malignant glaucoma.[46–48]

## 37.5 Differential Diagnosis

Malignant glaucoma usually presents as a postoperative flat central anterior chamber in an eye with normal or elevated IOP. The diagnoses that it is most commonly confused with are pupillary block, choroidal effusion, and suprachoroidal hemorrhage (Table 37.4). Ultrasound biomicroscopy, where available, may be useful in the differential diagnosis of malignant glaucoma and malignant glaucoma-like syndromes.

### 37.5.1 Pupillary Block

Pupillary-block glaucoma is often the most difficult condition to differentiate from malignant glaucoma. In pupillary-block glaucoma, the pressure is usually high and the anterior chamber is shallow to flat. In most cases, the anterior chamber in pupillary-block glaucoma remains deeper centrally than peripherally, whereas in malignant glaucoma, axial shallowing is much more typical. This difference in axial depth cannot be relied upon, however, and marked axial shallowing may be observed in some patients receiving strong miotics. One must ascertain the patency of an iridotomy or iridectomy. This can usually be done by careful slitlamp examination. Previously made iridectomies should be fully patent and not occluded by ciliary processes, inflammatory debris, the anterior hyaloid face, vitreous, retained lens material, or intraocular lenses. If communication between the posterior and anterior chambers cannot be determined with absolute certainty, another opening should be created, preferably with the argon or Nd:YAG laser. In most cases of pure pupillary-block glaucoma, the anterior chamber deepens after laser treatment. In rare cases where papillary-block has been present for a long time, deepening may not occur.

### 37.5.2 Choroidal Effusion

Choroidal effusion is associated with a shallow or flat anterior chamber after filtering surgery. The IOP is usually low. On funduscopic examination, light brown peripheral choroidal elevations that contain a straw-colored fluid are generally visible. If visibility is poor or choroidal effusion cannot be discerned, B-scan ultrasonography may be needed.[49] However, conventional B-scan ultrasonography is often not capable of detecting small or annular supraciliary effusions, and ultrasound biomicroscopy (UBM) may be helpful to rule out peripheral effusions. When choroidal effusion is causative, one or more posterior sclerotomies with drainage of the choroidal fluid and anterior chamber reformation through a paracentesis is curative. With rare exceptions, fluid is not present in the suprachoroidal space in patients with malignant glaucoma.[6]

### 37.5.3 Suprachoroidal Hemorrhage

Suprachoroidal hemorrhage presents with a shallow or flat chamber at the time of surgery or usually within 1 week postoperatively. Typically, the IOP is high when the hemorrhage occurs and then it drops. The sudden onset of ocular pain – at

**Table 37.4** Differential diagnosis of malignant glaucoma

| Pupillary block | Choroidal effusion | Suprachoroidal hemorrhage | Malignant glaucoma |
|---|---|---|---|
| Anterior chamber (AC) flat or shallow | AC flat or shallow | AC flat or shallow | AC flat or shallow |
| Intraocular pressure (IOP) normal or elevated | IOP subnormal or low | IOP normal or elevated | IOP normal or elevated |
| Fundus appears normal | Large, smooth, light brown choroidal elevations | Dark brown or dark red choroidal elevations | No choroidal elevation |
| No suprachoroidal fluid | Straw-colored fluid present | Light red or dark red blood | No suprachoroidal fluid |
| Choroidal drainage does not cure | Drainage does cure | Drainage does cure | Does not cure |
| Iridotomy/iridectomy does cure | Does not cure | Does not cure | Does not cure |
| Does not have patent Iridotomy/iridectomy | Has patent Iridotomy/iridectomy | Has patent Iridotomy/iridectomy | Has patent Iridotomy/iridectomy |
| Onset early or late postoperatively | Onset first 5 days postoperatively, occasionally later | Onset at surgery or first 5 days postoperatively, rarely later | At surgery or first 5 days postoperatively, but sometimes weeks to months postoperatively |

times severe – and increased inflammation are characteristic. Fundus findings on examination are similar to those with choroidal effusion except for a darker brown or dark red appearance of the choroidal elevations. When posterior sclerotomies and drainage are performed, bright or dark red blood, rather than straw-colored fluid is obtained. If the blood is not drained acutely it may be clotted and may not flow freely. Eventually, the blood will liquefy and can be removed.

### 37.5.4 Overfiltration and Wound Leakage

Overfiltration and wound leakage are also associated with shallow or flat postoperative anterior chambers with low intraocular pressures and are usually not confused with malignant glaucoma. They may, however, by resulting in an acute decompression of the anterior chamber, allow anterior movement of the peripheral hyaloid into apposition with the ciliary body. This could secondarily lead to expansion of the vitreous volume and the initiation of malignant glaucoma.[44]

### 37.5.5 Ultrasound Biomicroscopy

High-frequency ultrasound biomicroscopy (UBM) provides detailed imaging of the anterior and middle segment structures of the eye. It is possible to accurately elucidate the relationship of the anatomic positions of the cornea, iris, angle, lens or intraocular lens, ciliary body, and hyaloid face. The relative depths of the anterior and posterior chambers can be determined. Thus, UBM where available is a valuable tool in the differential diagnosis of pupillary block, secondary angle closures, suprachoroidal effusion, suprachoroidal hemorrhage, and the malignant glaucoma-like syndromes. Liebmann and coworkers reported a series of six patients with presentations clinically indistinguishable from that of malignant glaucoma by thorough examination as well as by standard B-scan ultrasonography. In these cases, the correct diagnosis of annular supraciliary effusion resulting in secondary angle-closure glaucoma was determined only by ultrasound biomicroscopy[50] (Fig. 37.6).

## 37.6 Management

The medical and surgical management of malignant glaucoma has greatly improved with advances in our understanding of the pathophysiologic mechanisms of this disease and current treatment options. Cataract extraction alone as an early treatment for phakic malignant glaucoma did not prove

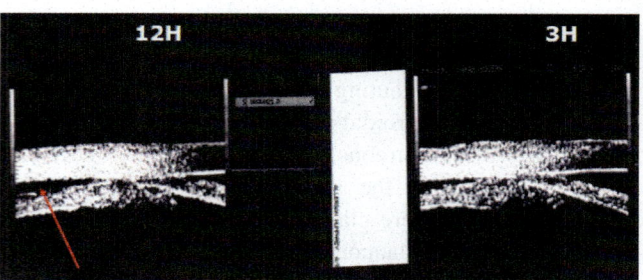

**Fig. 37.6** Annular choroidal on UMB rules out malignant glaucoma. Effusion at the 12 o'clock position (12H) arrow is greater than the shallower area effusion at the 3 o'clock (3H) position. Courtesy of Jeffrey Liebmann M.D. and Tiago Prata, M.D

successful unless vitreous loss with disruption of the anterior hyaloid face occurred at the time of the procedure.[33,51] Early attempts at treatment with miotics actually worsened the situation and can even precipitate malignant glaucoma.[6] In 1962, Chandler and Grant advocated the effective use of cycloplegic-mydriatic drugs.[39] The following year, Weiss and colleagues suggested treatment with intravenous hyperosmotic agents.[52] Oral and topical aqueous suppressants have added to our pharmacologic armamentarium.

### 37.6.1 Medical Treatment

Current medical treatment consists of atropine (1% drops up to q.i.d.), phenylephrine (2.5–10% drops up to q.i.d.), a topical p-blocker (b.i.d.), and an oral carbonic anhydrase inhibitor (acetazolamide, 250 mg q.i.d. or 500 mg sequel b.i.d., or methazolamide, 50 mg b.i.d.) or topical carbonic anhydrase inhibitor (dorzolamide or brinzolamide t.i.d.). Cyclopentolate (1%) may be better as an initial cycloplegic agent, with the atropine used for longer-term administration. It is absolutely essential to warn patients of the side effects of anticholinergics when using cyclogyl or atropine. Punctal occlusion may be recommended. The addition of α-agonists (apraclonidine or brimonidine t.i.d.) may also be helpful. In phakic patients, the atropine or cyclopentolate relaxes the sphincter muscle of the ciliary body. The phenylephrine stimulates the α-adrenergic receptors of the longitudinal muscle of the ciliary muscle. This combination tightens the zonules and helps to pull the anteriorly displaced lens back. This would help to increase the surface area of the anterior hyaloid. The $a_2$-agonists, β-blockers, and carbonic anhydrase inhibitors lower IOP by decreasing aqueous secretion and secondarily preventing further expansion of the vitreous. An oral osmotic agent (50% glycerol or isosorbide) or intravenous 20% mannitol in a dosage of 1–2 g/kg can be administered, with caution, every 12–24 h. The osmotic agents further reduce vitreous volume, deepen the anterior chamber, and possibly increase vitreous permeability.

Topical steroids may also be helpful in reducing inflammation and, based upon the pathophysiology may have a role in reducing ciliary body edema.[41] Oral steroids have been recommended for some cases of malignant-like (pseudomalignant) glaucoma.[53] Medical therapy has been reported to be curative in 50% of patients within 5 days.[6,7,10] Intensive medical therapy should be initiated immediately and continued for at least 5 days along with laser treatment, if visibility for laser treatment is good, and there is not excessive inflammation. After resolution, administration of at least one drop of atropine daily may be required indefinitely to prevent relapse[9] unless laser treatment or surgery proves curative.

## 37.7 Argon Laser Treatment and Nd:YAG Anterior Hyaloidotomy and Capsulotomy

Argon laser treatment of the ciliary processes, with or without adjunctive medical therapy, has been advocated for phakic and aphakic malignant glaucoma.[54,55] Nd:YAG laser treatment to open the anterior hyaloid face or posterior lens capsule, in cases of aphakia has been used more successfully.[46–48,56] Tello and colleagues documented the anatomic changes in the positions of the iris, intraocular lens, and ciliary body and the chamber depth with ultrasound biomicroscopy before and after the resolution of pseudophakic malignant glaucoma by Nd:YAG laser treatment of the anterior hyaloid face.[57] Nd:YAG treatment may be cautiously delivered through a preexisting laser iridotomy, or through a newly made one, to the anterior hyaloid in phakic patients. This should not be attempted unless visualization and focusing are excellent so as not to injure the crystalline lens, zonules, or ciliary body.

In pseudophakic patients it is necessary to create an open communication between the posterior and anterior segment with laser treatment to the lens capsule and residual lens material, if necessary, in addition to the vitreous face. Although it is not currently recommended, cyclocryotherapy has also been reported in the past as a treatment for malignant glaucoma.[58]

## 37.8 Surgical Therapy

When medical or laser therapy is not successful in relieving malignant glaucoma, vitreous surgery is indicated. Historically, Simmons and coworkers advocated a "surgical confirmation procedure" in which other diagnostic possibilities such as pupillary block or choroidal effusion are ruled out in the operating room before proceeding with vitreous surgery. They emphasized that the success of Chandler's manual deep vitreous surgery method, which was originated prior to the widespread availability of automated pars plana vitrectomy, is dependent on exacting attention to all the details as recommended.[7,8] Luntz and colleagues, to the contrary, have described cases in which suprachoroidal effusion and vitreous pooling of aqueous have occurred simultaneously, necessitating drainage of both the suprachoroidal space and vitreous cavities.[59] Automated mechanical vitrectomy through a posterior sclerotomy in phakic eyes or through a limbal approach in nonphakic eyes is currently a preferred alternative to the manual method and is often curative.[57,60–66] Disruption of an impermeable anterior hyaloid face at the time of vitrectomy is essential to the treatment of this disease in addition to reduction of vitreous volume, and deepening of the anterior chamber (Fig. 37.7a, b). Lois and associates have described a new surgical approach, zonulo-hyaloido-vitrectomy,

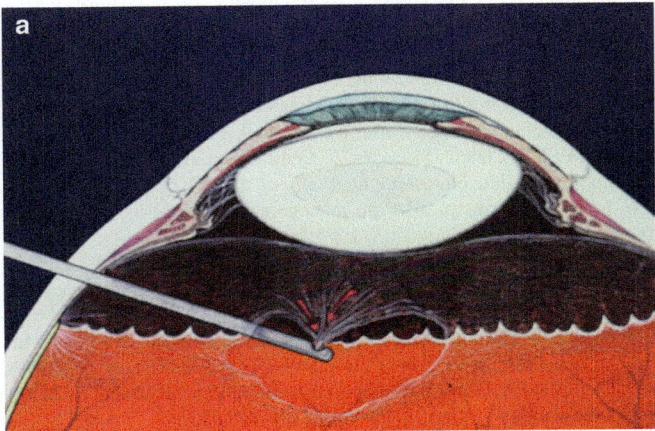 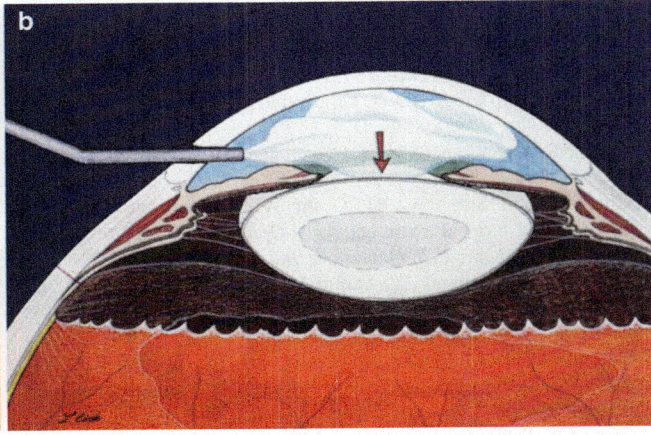

**Fig. 37.7** (a) Posterior sclerotomy with disruption of the anterior hyaloid face and automated mechanical vitrectomy for malignant glaucoma. (b) Deepening of the anterior chamber with a viscoelastic agent (arrow through a paracentesis after vitrectomy. Illustrations courtesy of B. Thomas Hutchinson, M.D. Reproduced with permission from Cyrlin M. Malignant Glaucoma. In: Albert DM, Jakobiec FA, eds. *Principles and Practice of Ophthalmology*, 2nd edition. WB Saunders, 2000; 2834–2846

in the management of pseudophakic malignant glaucoma. This procedure involves the performance of zonulectomy, hyaloidectomy, and anterior vitrectomy through a peripheral iridectomy or iridotomy via the anterior chamber.[67]

## 37.9 Management of the Contralateral Eye

After an episode of malignant glaucoma in one eye, the risk of malignant glaucoma in the contralateral eye is significant if surgery is needed after an acute angle-closure attack.[68] It may be advisable to create a laser iridectomy in the fellow eye, without pretreatment with miotics, before surgical intervention on the involved eye.[8]

## 37.10 Conclusion

At the time the term malignant glaucoma was proposed, it was truly a disease with a malignant course, resulting in a blind and often painful eye. Over the years, our better understanding of the pathophysiology coupled with improvements in our diagnostic, medical, and surgical armamentarium have allowed clinicians to make an accurate diagnosis and promptly institute effective treatment.

## References

1. von Graefe A. Beitrage zur Palhologie und Therapie des Glaukoms. *Arch Ophthalmol.* 1869;15:108.
2. Levene R. Malignant glaucoma: Proposed definition and classification. In: Shields MB, Pollack I, Kolker A, eds. *Perspectives in Glaucoma. Transactions of the First Scientific Meeting of the American Glaucoma Society.* Thorofare, NJ: Slack; 1988:243-350.
3. Weiss DI, Shaffer RN. Ciliary block (malignant glaucoma). *Trans Am Acad Ophthalmol Otol.* 1972;76:450.
4. Shaffer RN, Hoskins HD Jr. Ciliary block (malignant glaucoma). *Ophthalmology.* 1978;85:215.
5. Levene R. A new concept of malignant glaucoma. *Arch Ophthalmol.* 1972;87:497.
6. Chandler PA, Simmons RJ, Grant WM. Malignant glaucoma: Medical and surgical treatment. *Am J Ophthalmol.* 1968;66:495.
7. Simmons RJ. Malignant glaucoma. *Br J Ophthalmol.* 1972;56:263.
8. Simmons RJ, Thomas IV, Yaqub MK. Malignant glaucoma. In: Ritch R, Shields MB, Krupin T, eds. *The Glaucomas.* CV Mosby: St. Louis; 1989:1251–1263.
9. Simmons RJ. Malignant glaucoma. III In: Epstein DL, ed. *Chandler and Grant's Glaucoma.* Philadelphia, PA: Lea & Febiger; 1986:264–278.
10. Trope GE, Pavlin CJ, Bau A, et al. Malignant glaucoma: Clinical and ultrasound biomicroscopic features. *Ophthalmology.* 1994;101:1030.
11. Merritt JC. Malignant glaucoma induced by miotics postoperatively in open-angle glaucoma. *Arch Ophthalmol.* 1977;95:1988.
12. Hoshiwara I. Case report of simultaneous malignant glaucoma occurring 3 years after glaucoma surgery. *Arch Ophthalmol.* 1964;72:601.
13. Gorin G. Angle-closure glaucoma induced by miotics. *Am J Ophthalmol.* 1966;62:1063.
14. Jafar MS, Tomey KF. Malignant glaucoma manifesting bilaterally 15 months after peripheral iridectomy. *Glaucoma.* 1982;4:177.
15. Ellis PP. Malignant glaucoma occurring 16 years after successful filtering surgery. *Ann Ophthalmol.* 1984;16:177.
16. Wollensak I, Pham DT, Anders N. Ciliolenticular block as a late complication in pseudophakia. *Ophthalmologe.* 1995;92:280.
17. Hanish SJ, Lamberg RL, Gordon JM. Malignant glaucoma following cataract extraction and intraocular lens implant. *Ophthalmic Surg.* 1982;13:713.
18. Epstein DL. Pseudophakic malignant glaucoma-Is it really pseudomalignant? *Am J Ophthalmol.* 1987;103:231.
19. Arya SK, Sonika S, Kochhar S. Malignant glaucoma as a complication of Nd:YAG laser posterior capsulotomy. *Ophthalmic Surg Lasers Imaging.* 2004;35:248–250.
20. Azuara-Blanco A, Dua HS. Malignant glaucoma after diode laser cyclophotocoagulation. *Am J Ophthalmol.* 1999;127:467–469.
21. Greenfield DS, Tello C, Budenz DL, Liebman JM, Ritch R. Aqueous misdirection after glaucoma drainage device implantation. *Ophthalmology.* 1999;106:1035–1040.
22. Luntz MH, Rosenblatt M. Malignant glaucoma. *Surv Ophthalmol.* 1987;32:73.
23. Brooks AM, Halper CA, Gillies WE. Occurrence of malignant glaucoma after laser iridotomy. *Br J Ophthalmol.* 1989;73:617.
24. Robinson A, Plialnic M, Deutsch D, et al. The onset of malignant glaucoma after prophylactic laser iridotomy. *Am J Ophthalmol.* 1990;110:95.
25. Aminlati A, Sassani JW. Simultaneous bilateral malignant glaucoma following laser iridotomy. *Graefes Arch Clin Exp Opbthalmol.* 1993;231:12.
26. Di Sclafani M, Liebmann JM, Ritch R. Malignant glaucoma following argon laser release of scleral flap sutures after trabeculectomy. *Am J Ophthalmol.* 1989;108:597.
27. Macken P, Buys Y, Trope GE. Glaucoma laser suture lysis. *Br J Ophthalmol.* 1996;80:398.
28. Hardten DR, Brown JD. Malignant glaucoma after Nd:YAG cyclophotocoagulation. *Am J Ophthalmol.* 1991;111:245.
29. Pecora JL. Malignant glaucoma worsened by miotics in a postoperative angle-closure glaucoma patient. *Ann Ophthalmol.* 1979;11:1412.
30. Rieser JC, Schwartz B. Miotic-induced malignant glaucoma. *Arch Ophthalmol.* 1972;87:706.
31. Pollard AF. Secondary angle closure glaucoma in cicatricial retrolental fibroplasia. *Am J Ophthalmol.* 1980;89:651.
32. Kushner BJ. Ciliary block in retinopathy of prematurity. *Arch Ophthalmol.* 1982;100:1078.
33. Lowe RF. Malignant glaucoma related to primary angle closure glaucoma. *Aust N Z J Ophthalmol.* 1979;7:11.
34. Weiss IS, Deiter PO. Malignant glaucoma syndrome following retinal detachment surgery. *Ann Ophthalmol.* 1974;6:1099.
35. Weber PA, Cohen JS, Baker O. Central retinal vein occlusion and malignant glaucoma. *Arch Ophthalmol.* 1987;105:635.
36. Jones BR. Principles in the management of oculomycosis. *Trans Am Acad Ophthalmol Otol.* 1975;79:15.
37. Lass JH, Thoft RA, Bellows AR, et al. Exogenous Nocardia asteroides endophthalmitis associated with malignant glaucoma. *Ann Ophthalmol.* 1981;13:317.
38. Schwartz AL, Anderson DR. "Malignant glaucoma" in an eye with no antecedent operation or miotics. *Arch Ophthalmol.* 1975;93:379.
39. Chandler PA, Grant WM. Mydriatic-cycloplegic treatment in malignant glaucoma. *Arch Ophthalmol.* 1962;68:353.
40. Epstein DL, Hashimoto JM, Anderson PJ, Grant WM. Experimental perfusions through the anterior and vitreous chambers with possible relationships to malignant glaucoma. *Am J Ophthalmol.* 1979;88:1078.
41. Epstein DL. Malignant glaucoma. In: Jakobiec FA, Sigelman J, eds. *Advanced Techniques in Ocular Surgery.* WB Saunders: Philadelphia, PA; 1984:158–168.

42. Quigley HA. Malignant glaucoma and fluid flow rate. [Editorial]. *Am J Ophthalmol.* 1980;89:879.
43. Epstein DL. Unifying concepts in malignant glaucoma. *Glaucoma Under Pressure 1997 Symposium. American Academy of Ophthalmology Specialty Day.* San Francisco, October 1997.
44. Epstein DL. The malignant glaucoma syndromes. In: Epstein DL, Allingham RR, Schuman JS, eds. *Chandler and Grant's Glaucoma.* Media, PA: Williams & Wilkins; 1997:285–303.
45. Quigley HA, Friedman DS, Congdon NG. Possible mechanisms of primary angle-closure and malignant glaucoma. *J Glaucoma.* 2003;12:167–180.
46. Epstein DL, Steinert RF, Puliafito CA. Neodymium-YAG laser therapy to the anterior hyaloid in aphakic malignant (ciliovitreal block glaucoma). *Am J Ophthalmol.* 1984;98:137.
47. Little BC, Hitchings RA. Pseudophakic malignant glaucoma: Nd:YAG capsulotomy as a primary treatment. *Eye.* 1993;7:102.
48. Little BC. Treatment of aphakic malignant glaucoma using Nd:YAG laser posterior capsulotomy. *Br J Ophthalmol.* 1994;78:499.
49. Dugel PR, Heuer OK, Thach AB, et al. Annular peripheral choroidal detachment simulating aqueous misdirection after glaucoma surgery. *Ophthalmology.* 1997;104:439.
50. Liebmann JM, Weinreb RN, Ritch R. Angle-closure glaucoma associated with occult annular ciliary body detachment. *Arch Ophthalmol.* 1998;16:731.
51. Rheindorf O. Uber Glaukom. *Klin Monatsbl Augenheilkd.* 1877;25:148.
52. Weiss DI, Shaffer RN, Harrington DO. Treatment of malignant glaucoma with intravenous mannitol infusion: Medical reformation of the anterior chamber by means of an osmotic agent: A preliminary report. *Arch Ophthalmol.* 1963;69:154.
53. Beckman H, Blau RP. Oral steroid therapy for ciliary (pseudomalignant glaucoma). *Glaucoma.* 1981;3:169.
54. Herschler J. Laser shrinkage of the ciliary processes: A treatment for malignant (ciliary block) glaucoma. *Ophthalmology.* 1980;87:1155.
55. Weber PA, Henry MA, Kapetansky FM, et al. Argon laser treatment of the ciliary processes in aphakic glaucoma with flat anterior chamber. *Am J Ophthalmol.* 1984;97:82.
56. Risco JM, Tomey KF, Perkins TW. Laser capsulotomy through intraocular lens positioning holes in anterior aqueous misdirection. *Arch Ophthalmol.* 1989;107:1569.
57. Momeda S, Hayashi H, Oshima K. Anterior pars plana vitrectomy for phakic malignant glaucoma. *Jpn J Ophthalmol.* 1983;27:73.
58. Benedikt O. A new operative method for the treatment of malignant glaucoma. *Klin Monatsbl Augenheilkd.* 1977;170:665.
59. Luntz MH, Harrison R, Schenker H. Management of secondary glaucoma. In: Luntz MH, Harrison R, Schencker HI, eds. *Glaucoma Surgery.* Baltimore: Williams & Wilkins; 1984:107–116.
60. Boke W, Teichmann KDS, Junge W. Experiences with ciliary block ("malignant") glaucoma. *Klin Monatsbl Augenheilkd.* 1980;177:407.
61. Koerner FH. Anterior pars plana vitrectomy in ciliary and iris block glaucoma. *Graefs Arch Clin Exp Ophthalmol.* 1980;214:119.
62. Weiss H, Shin DH, Kollarits CR. Vitrectomy for malignant (ciliary block) glaucomas. *Int Ophthalmol Clin.* 1981;21:113.
63. Lynch MG, Brown RH, Michels RG, et al. Surgical vitrectomy for pseudophakic malignant glaucoma. *AM J Ophthalmol.* 1986;102:148.
64. Byrnes GA, Leen MM, Wong TP, et al. Vitrectomy for ciliary block (malignant) glaucoma. *Ophthalmology.* 1995;102:1308.
65. Harbour JW, Rubsamen PE, Palmberg P. Pars plana vitrectomy in the management of phakic and pseudophakic malignant glaucoma. *Arch Ophthalmol.* 1996;114:1073.
66. Tsai JC, Barton KA, Miller MH, et al. Surgical results in malignant glaucoma refractory to medical or laser therapy. *Eye.* 1997;11:677.
67. Lois N, Wong D, Groenwald C. New surgical approach in the management of pseudophakic malignant glaucoma. *Ophthalmology.* 2001;108:780–783.
68. Shields MB. Glaucomas following ocular surgery. In: Shields MD, ed. *Textbook of Glaucoma.* Baltimore: Williams & Wilkins; 1998:345–3500.

# Chapter 38
# Pigmentary Dispersion Syndrome and Glaucoma

Celso Tello, Nathan Radcliffe, and Robert Ritch

Pigment dispersion syndrome (PDS) and pigmentary glaucoma (PG) are two successive stages of the same disease process characterized by disruption of the iris pigment epithelium and deposition of the dispersed pigment granules throughout the anterior segment. The classic diagnostic triad that characterizes the pigment dispersion syndrome consists of corneal endothelial pigmentation (Krukenberg spindle, Fig. 38.1); slit-like, radial, mid-peripheral iris transillumination defects (Fig. 38.2); and dense homogeneous pigmentation of the trabecular meshwork (Fig. 38.3). In PDS, the anterior chamber is often deeper than normal both centrally and peripherally. The iridocorneal angle is typically wide open, the iris is inserted posteriorly into the ciliary body, and the configuration of the peripheral iris is concave[1] (Fig. 38.4). Pigmentary glaucoma is defined as glaucomatous optic neuropathy attributable to elevated intraocular pressure (IOP) from PDS.

## 38.1 Pathophysiology of Pigment Dispersion Syndrome

The underlying mechanism responsible for PDS is a concave iris contour that allows apposition of its posterior surface to the zonular bundles. The iris is also larger in patients with PDS, contributing to its concavity. Campbell hypothesized that friction between zonules and the peripheral iris in predisposed eyes is the cause of the pigment liberation in pigmentary dispersion syndrome.[2] Furthermore, a reverse pupillary block mechanism may exist, in which the iris drapes over the lens and acts as a "flap valve," preventing aqueous in the anterior chamber from returning to the posterior chamber.[3] The pressure in the anterior chamber then exceeds that of the posterior chamber, pushing the iris posteriorly, creating a concave configuration, and forcing the iris pigment epithelium into contact with the zonular bundles. Mechanical rubbing during pupillary movement disrupts the iris pigment epithelium, releasing pigment granules into the aqueous humor. Greater iridozonular contact will cause greater pigment dispersion.[4] The accumulation of pigment granules in the intertrabecular meshwork increases the resistance of aqueous egress through this structure, elevating IOP.

The act of blinking generates reverse pupillary block by compressing the anterior chamber and pushing the iris and aqueous humor posteriorly.[5] When ultrasound biomicroscopy is performed on normal patients and on patients with untreated PDS, the iris configuration is initially concave. After an eyelid speculum is placed, inhibiting blinking, the iris gradually becomes less concave. Pressure builds in the posterior chamber pushing the iris forward. Once blinking is restored, the original concave configuration is reestablished.

Exercise (jogging, playing basketball, and bouncing during dancing) can cause the release of pigment as a result of pupillary movement in young PDS patients. We have seen pigment liberation and elevated IOP after exercise in a patient with PDS that was high enough to produce corneal edema. The type of exercise that induces pigment liberation may differ between patients. For example, we recall one patient who was a soccer player with pigmentary glaucoma. We asked him to return to our office after a workout that included running and kicking, and his pressures were normal after this exercise. However, when he returned to our office after a soccer match, his pressures were elevated. We concluded that the act of "heading" the ball (unique to the soccer match) was responsible for pigment liberation in his particular case. The phenomenon of exercise-induced IOP elevation in PDS can be prevented completely by miotic-induced relative pupillary block.[6] The use of laser iridotomy (discussed later) to eliminate reverse pupillary block inhibits exercise-induced pigment release incompletely.[7]

Pharmacologic pupillary dilation in PDS may result in significant pigment liberation into the anterior chamber.[8] This pigment liberation may be accompanied by IOP elevation because of acute obstruction of the aqueous outflow pathway by pigment granules. The fact that delayed IOP elevation follows dilation in PDS is not well recognized, however, the astute clinician will

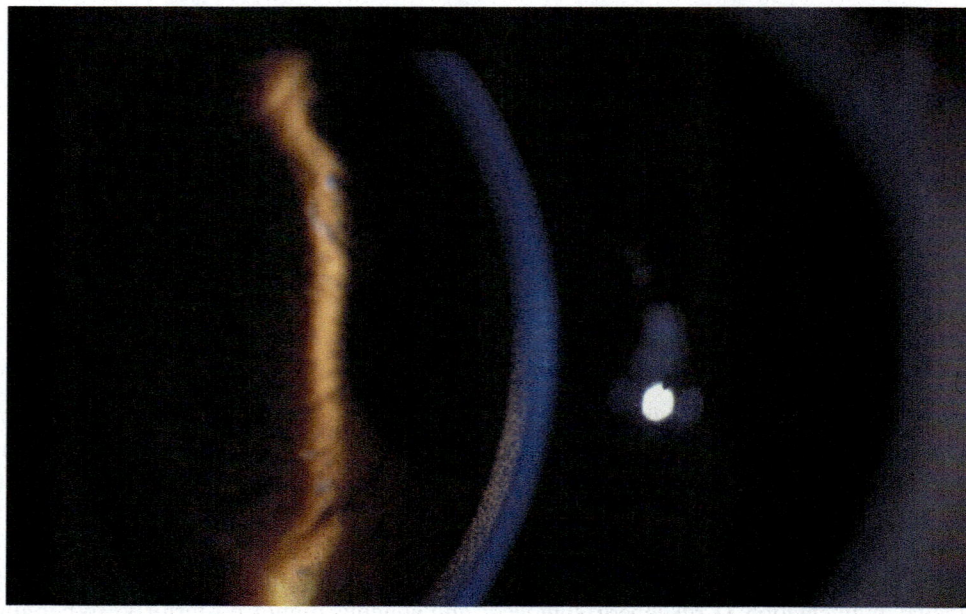

**Fig. 38.1** Pigment dispersion syndrome with Krukenberg spindle

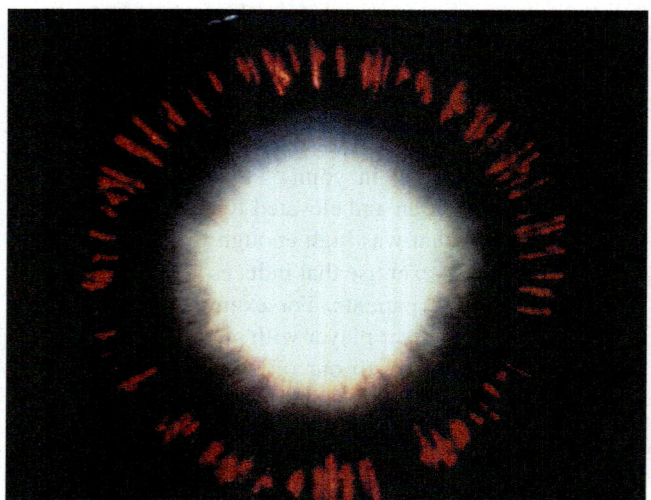

**Fig. 38.2** Midperipheral, radial, slit-like pattern transillumination defects are seen most commonly inferonasally in young PDS/PG patients

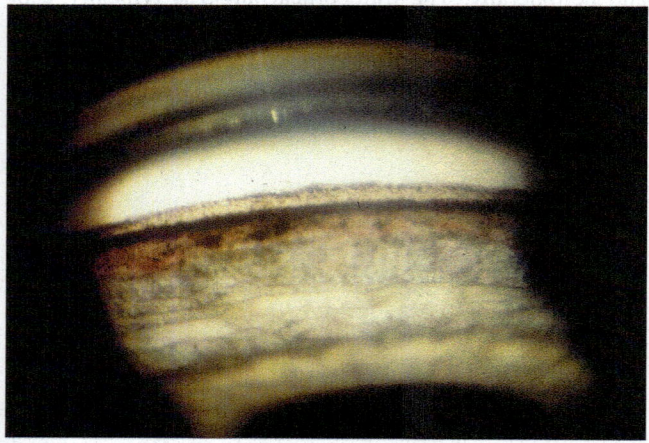

**Fig. 38.3** In PDS, the angle is characteristically wide open, with a homogeneous, dense hyperpigmented band on the trabecular meshwork. The iris insertion is posterior and the peripheral iris approach is often concave

measure IOP after dilation in all patients. In PDS, the maximal anterior chamber pigment dispersion may occur shortly after dilation, while the maximal elevation in IOP may occur several hours after dilation, when anterior chamber pigment is decreasing. This lag probably reflects the time necessary for pigment to obstruct the trabecular meshwork, reduce aqueous humor outflow, and for pressure to build within the eye.

## 38.2 Presentation

Patients with PDS are usually myopic, so fortunately they often seek eye care for spectacle or contact lens correction. Upon examination, they may be noted to have elevated IOP or pigment dispersion. Pigment dispersion syndrome itself may present symptomatically. The classic presentation is that of a young

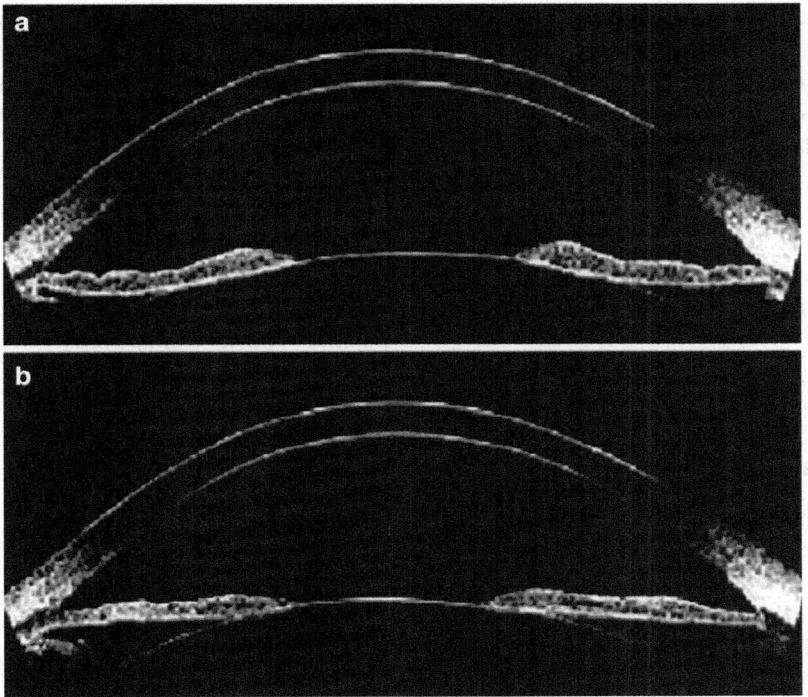

**Fig. 38.4** Slit-lamp optical coherence tomography demonstrates iris concavity in a young PDS patient

(20- to 40-year-old) myopic male who experiences blurry vision or eye pain after exercise.[9] Occasionally, trauma followed by eye pain may be the heralding event, and furthermore trauma may exacerbate preexisting pigmentary glaucoma.

## 38.3 Examination

The key to making the diagnosis of PDS lies in performing a thorough exam with an appropriately high index of suspicion. With respect to refractive error, most patients with PDS will be myopic, some will be emmetropic, and very few will be hyperopic.[10,11] On pupillary examination, hyperplasia of the iris dilator muscle in PDS can cause deformation of the pupil in the direction of maximal iris transillumination. These changes may also result in anisocoria, with the less involved pupil being smaller.[12,13] In severe cases, an efferent pupillary defect may be present.

Slit-lamp examination should be performed with high magnification and in complete darkness with all room lights and computer monitors turned off to aid in the detection of anterior chamber pigment and iris transillumination defects. Corneal endothelial pigment appears as a central, vertical, brown band (Krukenberg spindle, with a "pine tree" shape), the pattern of pigmentation resulting from aqueous convection currents.[14] While the Krukenberg spindle may appear dense on slit lamp biomicroscopy, this pigment almost never interferes with visual acuity, and, in fact, most of our younger patients with PDS (including those with dense Krukenberg spindles) usually have 20/15 corrected visual acuity. When the Krukenberg spindle is less dense, the endothelial pigment granules have the appearance of an extremely fine cinnamon powder and may be difficult to detect, particularly in patients who have passed the active liberation stage. Clinically, loss of iris pigment appears as a midperipheral, radial, slit-like pattern of transillumination defects seen most easily by retroillumination.[15] These defects are most often present inferonasally and are more apparent in lighter irides. The presence, amount, and distribution of iris transillumination defects should be noted as this information is useful for grading, for staging, and for following the disease.

On gonioscopy, the angle is typically Shaffer grade IV ("wide open"), the iris is inserted posteriorly into the ciliary body, and the configuration of the peripheral iris is concave. The amount of trabecular meshwork pigmentation should be graded and documented separately in the superior and inferior angles of both eyes. Pigment may also be deposited on Schwalbe's line, on the zonules, on the posterior capsule of the lens, at the level of the insertion of the posterior zonular fibers (Zentmayer ring) and on the posterior lens central to Weigert's ligament (Scheie's stripe).

After pupillary dilation, the anterior chamber should be evaluated in complete darkness for pigment and the IOP should be monitored. Ideally, the pressure is checked at least 1 h after dilation is complete. Treatment with a single drop of brimonidine is usually effective in treating pigment-related IOP spikes in the office. The peripheral retina must be carefully examined, as lattice degeneration may be present in up to 20% of patients.[16] Furthermore, retinal breaks are present in up to 11.7%, and rhegmatogenous retinal detachments requiring surgery may occur in 3.3% of patients.[16] Optic nerve examination with careful drawing or stereophotography should be performed as for any patient, noting the size of the optic nerve, the presence or absence of peripapillary atrophy, nerve fiber layer defects, disc hemorrhages, or neuroretinal rim thinning.

## 38.4 Diagnosis and Differential Diagnosis of PDS

To make the diagnosis of PDS, we require the presence of Krukenberg spindles, dense homogenous trabecular meshwork pigmentation and a posterior iris insertion, with the presence of iris transillumination defects being confirmatory but not necessary. Many conditions other than PDS will cause the dispersion of pigment or of pigmented cells throughout the anterior chamber. The ophthalmologist must use all of the available information, age, history of presenting illness, past ocular history, refractive error, and examination findings to distinguish these conditions from true PDS.

Other disorders that have been reported to cause anterior segment pigment dispersion include exfoliation syndrome (XFS), diabetes, herpetic eye disease, iris pigment epithelitis, radiation, trauma, iris pigment epithelial cysts, ciliary body cysts, iris nevus, and melanoma or melanocytoma of the anterior and posterior segment. Exfoliation syndrome can be detected by the presence of exfoliation material on the pupillary border or by the presence of exfoliation material on the anterior capsule after pupillary dilation. Melanomas and melanocytomas can produce unilateral pigment dispersion; however, other signs of intraocular tumor should be present such as iris or ciliary body mass, focal angle closure (atypical for a patient with true PDS), inflammation, or a sentinel scleral vessel. None of these conditions will have the radial, midperipheral transillumination defects usually seen in PDS.

It is important to remember that the presence of PDS does not preclude other eye conditions in which pigment dispersion may be present. In fact, XFS may be more common in PDS than it is in the general population. The onset of newly elevated IOPs in a patient in his or her sixth decade who has a prior diagnosis of PDS or PG is suggestive of exfoliation syndrome. Patients who may have both PDS and XFS have been described as having the "overlap syndrome."[17]

Pigmented Long Anterior Zonules (PLAZ), also known as pigmented lens striae, occur when abnormally long and anteriorly inserted zonules are present on the face of the anterior lens capsule, usually bilaterally. This iridozonular apposition creates a special type of pigment dispersion as the zonules rub against the posterior surface of the iris, liberating pigment into the anterior chamber. Krukenberg spindles, densely pigmented trabecular meshwork, and pigmented zonules may be seen on examination. Iris transillumination defects are not typically found in PLAZ, nor is there reverse pupillary block. Unlike PDS, PLAZ is common in black patients, and its incidence increases with hyperopia, age, and female gender.[18] Finally, PLAZ is in some cases associated with a CTRP5 genetic mutation and late-onset macular degeneration.[19]

## 38.5 Asymmetric or Unilateral PDS

In general, PDS is bilateral. In all cases of PDS where asymmetric pigment dispersion is present there is either increased relative pupillary block in the less-involved eye (reducing peripheral iridozonular contact) or greater iridozonular contact in the more-involved eye. Patients will rarely present with heterochromia because of deposition of pigment particles on the iris surface when the involvement is asymmetric. We have observed asymmetric PDS caused by anisometropia, with the less myopic eye being less involved. Unilateral cataract, anisometropia, trauma, angle recession, and Marfan's syndrome have been reported in unilateral or highly asymmetric PDS. Two pupillary disorders – Horner's syndrome and Adie's pupil – can result in asymmetric PDS, with the involved eye being less pigmented in Horner's syndrome and more pigmented in Adie's pupil. In patients in whom no clear cause for asymmetric PDS is found, a more posterior iris insertion and greater iridolenticular contact will be present in the eye with the greater PDS.[4] PDS may resolve as a result of cataract extraction, lens subluxation, chronic treatment with pilocarpine, or iridotomy.

## 38.6 Inheritance/Epidemiology

PDS shows autosomal dominant heritability with incomplete penetrance.[20] The most significant risk factors for the development of the phenotypic expressions of PDS are young age, male gender, myopia, European ancestry, and a positive family history. Although men and women are equally affected, men are more likely to develop glaucoma in a ratio of approximately 3:1.[21] Men are more likely to develop PG from PDS, are diagnosed with PG at an earlier age, and are more likely to require filtering surgery.[11]

As a result of obstruction of the intertrabecular meshwork by pigment granules and possible failure or breakdown of normal phagocytic function of trabecular endothelial cells, the IOP elevates in many PDS patients. Pigment dispersion syndrome may be present in up to 2.45% of the Caucasian population.[22] PDS is rare in blacks, and has an estimated prevalence of about 15 cases per 10,000.[23] In black patients, whose irides may not display classic transillumination defects, infrared pupillography may be helpful. Signs of pigment liberation in blacks (particularly middle-aged black women) may also suggest the PDS-like findings of PLAZ, previously discussed.

The frequency with which PDS converts to PG has probably been greatly overestimated. The three studies that have examined patients longitudinally suggest that up to 50% will eventually develop PG.[24-26] However, the true rate of PDS in the general population may be an order of magnitude greater than has previously been suspected, and we estimate that the true rate of progression from PDS to PG is around 10%.

## 38.7 Temporal Evolution of PDS

Active release of pigment usually occurs during the second to fourth decade of life, when accommodation may play a significant role in the mechanism of the disease. The fact that accommodation increases iris concavity not only in PDS patients but also in myopes without PDS and normal eyes suggests that the iris in PDS, in addition to being morphologically larger and concave, could be naturally predisposed to release its pigment.[27] After the cessation of the pigment liberation phase, however, the IOP may or may not normalize.

The regression phase typically begins in the middle age. During middle age, there is a loss of accommodation with the onset of presbyopia and development of relative pupillary block secondary to increased lens thickness. These two changes presumably both contribute to the cessation of pupillary block and decrease the severity of pigment liberation. Once the eye has reached the regression phase, the transillumination defects may disappear, the IOP may return to normal, and the trabecular meshwork pigmentation may decrease. The only remaining sign may be the "pigment reversal sign," where the trabecular meshwork is found to be darker superiorly compared with inferiorly. This finding alone may distinguish patients with "burned out" pigmentary glaucoma who are now in the regression phase. Older patients presenting with PG may only have very subtle manifestations, if any, of PDS, and they may be misdiagnosed as primary open-angle glaucoma or normal-tension glaucoma.[28]

## 38.8 Treatment

In deciding whether to treat the patient with PDS, the ophthalmologist should initially approach the patient in a similar manner to any other glaucoma suspect. In our practice, we make use of the concept of the pigment dispersion syndrome suspect (PDSS) to help follow patients who are at risk for PDS or who may have had it in the past. For example, consider a 50-year-old myopic male with an IOP of 12 OU, an inferior notch in the optic nerve OS, and a superior arcuate defect in the left visual field. On gonioscopy OS, the trabecular meshwork has 2+ pigmentation superiorly and 1+ pigmentation inferiorly (a reversal sign). This patient is a strong pigment dispersion syndrome suspect and is also a normal tension glaucoma suspect, and in either case, he has open angle glaucoma.

We also use the term exfoliation suspect (XFSS). At times it may be difficult to distinguish exfoliation syndrome and PDS, as some patients may have both (overlap syndrome).[17] Generally, PDSS refers to a patient with pigmentation only on the corneal endothelium or in the angle who does not have typical iris transillumination defects. This may occur with patients who are at early or late stages of the disease. XFSS refers to patients who have light pigment dispersion, a Sampaolesi's line or peripupillary iris ruff transillumination defects but in whom exfoliative material is not directly visible. For patients in whom the IOP elevates along with the presence of pigment liberation in the anterior chamber, the diagnosis of PDS or exfoliation syndrome is more likely.

The treatment of PDS/PG is aimed at reversing the iris concavity, preventing pigment release, and therefore lowering IOP. Theoretically, miotics are ideal drugs to treat PDS/PG. Pupillary constriction reverses the iris concavity and eliminates iridozonular contact (inhibiting pigment release). By creating tension over the scleral spur, miotics increase aqueous outflow through the trabecular meshwork (lowering IOP) and enhance the clearance of pigment through the trabecular meshwork (increasing outflow facility). In patients with iris concavity and active release of pigment, low-concentration pilocarpine can be used as tolerated. Pilocarpine Ocuserts were in many respects the best available type of miotic therapy, and in the past, we had excellent success with them. Ocuserts immobilized the pupil to approximately 3 mm without causing extreme miosis or accommodative spasm, allowing normal functioning. Unfortunately, they are no longer manufactured and alternative miotic formulations require frequent dosing in order to be effective. The peripheral retina should be examined carefully prior to treatment with miotics, both because lattice degeneration is commonly found in patients with PDS and because the incidence of retinal detachment is higher than average in these patients.

Because miotics are poorly tolerated and have a less favorable risk profile in the younger population, once the IOP is elevated, we prefer to treat with prostaglandin analogues that produce an excellent IOP response by increasing uveoscleral outflow. We have found prostaglandin analogues to be effective as monotherapy, and their IOP-lowering effects are also additive in patients already on miotic therapy.[29] Agents that lower IOP by reducing aqueous production hypothetically may diminish the rate of clearance of the pigment from the trabecular meshwork, possibly exacerbating the disease process. Furthermore, these agents may inhibit relative pupillary block, which is therapeutic in PDS.

Argon laser trabeculoplasty and selective laser trabeculoplasty are alternative treatments to lower IOP, mostly in young pigmentary glaucoma patients. The success rate of argon laser trabeculoplasty (ALT) in PG is greater in younger patients than in older ones and decreases with age.[30] Selective laser trabeculoplasty may result in marked rises of IOP secondary to pigment release. In patients with PDS, any laser surgery should be performed with low laser power to avoid release of pigment and IOP elevation.

Laser iridotomy (LI) equalizes pressures between the anterior and posterior chambers, flattens the iris, eliminates iridozonular contact, and occasionally decreases further liberation of pigment. Theoretically, by preventing pigment liberation from the iris, the meshwork should be able to clear itself of previously deposited pigment. Proper patient selection for laser iridotomy is important and somewhat controversial. Ideally, patients should still be in the pigment liberation stage. This may be determined by the presence of pigment liberation into the anterior chamber with resulting IOP elevation after pupillary dilation. We also perform this procedure on young patients (under 40) who have visual symptoms or elevated IOP with exercise.

Patients who have uncontrolled glaucoma possibly requiring filtering surgery are suboptimal candidates for laser iridotomy, because years may be required to achieve resolution of trabecular meshwork dysfunction. Although the benefits of LI in PDS are inconclusive, in young patients with iris concavity, active release of pigment and ocular hypertension, LI may be of benefit for years. If laser peripheral iridotomy is to be performed, we prefer argon laser to YAG. The YAG laser causes significant pigment liberation and inflammation, and may overwhelm the already compromised trabecular meshwork, resulting in IOP elevation.

## 38.9 Future Directions

With the elucidation iridozonular contact and reverse pupillary block as the underlying mechanism for PDS, new questions are raised. What factors make one patient with reverse pupillary block more likely to liberate pigment than another? Why will one patient with pigment liberation and heavily pigmented trabecular meshwork develop elevated IOP while another will not? Finally, are some patients with PDS and elevated IOP more susceptible to optic nerve damage than others? These questions may be answered when the genetic etiologies for PDS, a condition with autosomal dominant inheritance and variable penetrance, are discovered.

## 38.10 Clinical Pearls

1. The fact that delayed IOP elevation follows dilation in PDS is not well recognized, however, the astute clinician will measure IOP after dilation in all patients.
2. While Krukenberg spindles may appear dense at the slit lamp, these almost never interfere with visual acuity.
3. Treatment with a single drop of brimonidine is usually effective in treating pigment-related IOP spikes after pupillary dilation.
4. The peripheral retina must be carefully examined in patients with pigment dispersion syndrome, as lattice degeneration may be present in up to 20% of patients.
5. Exfoliation syndrome may be more common in pigment dispersion syndrome than it is in the general population. The onset of newly elevated IOPs in a patient in his or her sixth decade who has a prior diagnosis of PDS or PG is suggestive of exfoliation syndrome.[5]
6. Later in life, the only remaining sign of PDS may be the "pigment reversal sign," where the trabecular meshwork is found to be darker superiorly when compared with inferiorly. This finding alone may distinguish patients with "burned out" pigmentary glaucoma from those with normal tension glaucoma.
7. For patients in whom the IOP elevates along with the presence of pigment, the diagnosis of PDS or XFS is more likely.
8. In young patients with iris concavity, active release of pigment, and ocular hypertension, LI may be of benefit for years.
9. In patients with iris concavity and active release of pigment, low-concentration pilocarpine can be used as tolerated.
10. Treatment with aqueous suppressants may diminish the rate of clearance of the pigment from the trabecular meshwork, possibly exacerbating the disease process. Furthermore, these agents may inhibit relative pupillary block, which is therapeutic in PDS.
11. Prostaglandin analogues are often effective as monotherapy in these patients.
12. Elevated IOP induced by exercise can be inhibited by the use of pilocarpine 0.5% drops immediately before the activity.
13. The peripheral retina should be examined carefully prior to treatment with miotics since lattice degeneration is commonly found in patients with PDS, and the incidence of retinal detachment is higher than average.

14. In patients undergoing laser iridotomy to relieve reverse papillary block, argon laser peripheral iridotomy is preferred to YAG laser iridotomy. The YAG laser causes significant pigment liberation and inflammation, and may overwhelm the already compromised trabecular meshwork, resulting in IOP elevation.

The authors do not have any financial interest in any technique or device described in this chapter.

## References

1. Sokol J, Stegman Z, Liebmann JM, et al. Location of the iris insertion in pigment dispersion syndrome. *Ophthalmology*. 1996;103(2):289–293.
2. Campbell DG. Pigmentary dispersion and glaucoma: a new theory. *Arch Ophthalmol*. 1979;97:1667–1672.
3. Karickhoff JR. Reverse pupillary block in pigmentary glaucoma: follow up and new developments. *Ophthalmic Surg*. 1993;24: 562–563.
4. Kanadani FN, Dorairaj S, Langlieb AM, et al. Ultrasound biomicroscopy in asymmetric pigment dispersion syndrome and pigmentary glaucoma. *Arch Ophthalmol*. 2006;124(11):1573–1576.
5. Liebmann JM, Tello C, Chew SJ, et al. Prevention of blinking alters iris configuration in pigment dispersion syndrome and in normal eyes. *Ophthalmology*. 1995;102(3):446–455.
6. Schenker HI, Luntz MH, Kels B, et al. Exercise-induced increase of intraocular pressure in the pigmentary dispersion syndrome. *Am J Ophthalmol*. 1980;89(4):598–600.
7. Haynes WL, Alward WL, Tello C, et al. Incomplete elimination of exercise-induced pigment dispersion by laser iridotomy in pigment dispersion syndrome. *Ophthalmic Surg Lasers*. 1995;26(5): 484–486.
8. Kristensen P. Mydriasis-induced pigment liberation in the anterior chamber associated with acute rise in intraocular pressure in open-angle glaucoma. *Acta Ophthalmol*. 1965;43:714–724.
9. Farrar SM, Shields MB, Miller KN, Stoup CM. Risk factors for the development and severity of glaucoma in the pigment dispersion syndrome. *Am J Ophthalmol*. 1989;108(3):223–229.
10. Sugar HS. Pigmentary glaucoma: a 25-year review. *Am J Ophthalmol*. 1966;62:499–507.
11. Scheie HG, Cameron JD. Pigment dispersion syndrome: a clinical study. *Br J Ophthalmol*. 1981;65:264–269.
12. Alward WL, Haynes WL. Pupillometric and videographic evaluation of anisocoria in patients with the pigment dispersion syndrome. *Invest Ophthalmol Vis Sci*. 1991;32(suppl):1109.
13. Feibel RM, Perlmutter JC. Anisocoria in the pigmentary dispersion syndrome. *Am J Ophthalmol*. 1990;110:657–660.
14. Krukenberg F. Beiderseitige angeborene Melanose der Hornhaut. *Klin Monatsbl Augenheilkd*. 1899;37:254–258.
15. Scheie HG, Fleischhauer HW. Idiopathic atrophy of the epithelial layers of the iris and ciliary body: a clinical study. *Arch Ophthalmol*. 1958;59:216–228.
16. Weseley P, Liebmann J, Walsh JB, et al. Lattice degeneration of the retina and the pigment dispersion syndrome. *Am J Ophthalmol*. 1992;114(5):539–543.
17. Ritch R, Mudumbai R, Liebmann JM. Combined exfoliation and pigment dispersion: paradigm of an overlap syndrome. *Ophthalmology*, 2000;107(5):1004–1008.
18. Roberts DK, Lo PS, Winters JE, et al. Prevalence of pigmented lens striae in a black population: a potential indicator of age-related pigment dispersal in the anterior segment. *Optom Vis Sci*. 2002;79(11): 681–687.
19. Ayyagari R, Mandal MN, Karoukis AJ, et al. Late-onset macular degeneration and long anterior lens zonules result from a CTRP5 gene mutation. *Invest Ophthalmol Vis Sci*. 2005;46(9):3363–3371.
20. Andersen JS, Pralea AM, DelBono EA, et al. A gene responsible for the pigment dispersion syndrome maps to chromosome 7q35-q36. *Arch Ophthalmol*. 1997;115(3):384–388.
21. Bick MW. Sex differences in pigmentary glaucoma. *Am J Ophthalmol*. 1962;54:831–837.
22. Ritch R, Steinberger D, Liebmann JM. Prevalence of pigment dispersion syndrome in a population undergoing glaucoma screening. *Am J Ophthalmol*. 1993;115:707–710.
23. Roberts DK, Chaglasian MA, Meetz RE. Clinical signs of the pigment dispersion syndrome in blacks. *Optom Vis Sci*. 1997;74(12): 993–1006.
24. Migliazzo CV, Shaffer RN, Nykin R, et al. Long-term analysis of pigmentary dispersion syndrome and pigmentary glaucoma. *Ophthalmology*. 1986;93:1528–1536.
25. Farrar SM, Shields MB, Miller KN, et al. Risk factors for the development and severity of glaucoma in the pigment dispersion syndrome. *Am J Ophthalmol*. 1989;108:223–229.
26. Richter CU, Richardson TM, Grant WM. Pigmentary dispersion syndrome and pigmentary glaucoma. A prospective study of the natural history. *Arch Ophthalmol*. 1986;104:211–215.
27. Pavlin CJ, Harasiewicz K, Foster FS. Posterior iris bowing in pigmentary dispersion syndrome caused by accommodation. *Am J Ophthalmol*. 1994;118(1):114–116.
28. Ritch R. Nonprogressive low-tension glaucoma with pigmentary dispersion. *Am J Ophthalmol*. 1982;94:190–196.
29. Toris CB, Zhan GL, Zhao J, et al. Potential mechanism for the additivity of pilocarpine and latanoprost. *Am J Ophthalmol*. 2001;131(6): 722–728.
30. Ritch R, Liebmann J, Robin A, et al. Argon laser trabeculoplasty in pigmentary glaucoma. *Ophthalmology*. 1993;100(6):909–913.

# Chapter 39
# Exfoliation Syndrome and Glaucoma

Anastasios G. P. Konstas, Gábor Holló, and Robert Ritch

## 39.1 Definition, Terminology, and Prevalence

Exfoliative glaucoma (XFG) is the most common type of secondary open-angle glaucoma.[1] Its worldwide prevalence makes it critical for ophthalmologists to be familiar with the full clinical spectrum of the disease.[1-3] Exfoliation syndrome (XFS) and XFG were initially described in 1917 by the Finnish ophthalmologist John Lindberg. In 1924, it was determined that XFG develops from XFS. Both conditions currently affect 60–70 million people worldwide. Of these, 15–17 million people have increased intraocular pressure (IOP) and 5–6 million are estimated to suffer from XFG.[3] Both XFS and XFG are characterized by the systemic synthesis and accumulation of an abnormal fibrillar material, called exfoliation material. Originally it was believed that the sole source of this abnormal material is the lens. The terms exfoliation material, XFS, XFG, and capsular glaucoma were introduced based on this early theory. True exfoliation of the lens capsule is a different and an exceedingly rare entity, which occurs as a consequence of thermal damage of the lens. Exfoliation syndrome and XFG – the term used in this chapter – and pseudoexfoliation (the term preferred by other investigators) are different names for the same condition.

> Exfoliative glaucoma (XFG) is the most common type of secondary open angle glaucoma worldwide.

Exfoliative glaucoma is common in several parts of the world, but prevalence figures show a wide variation between 0.2% and 27% for XFS, and between 0.07% and 14.2% for XFG,[2] depending on the region. In Europe, XFS and XFG are very common in the Nordic countries, Greece and Turkey, and less common in Central Europe, Germany, and Spain. The condition is present in America and Africa, and has been detected also in Central and East Asia. Based on current findings, XFS appears to be very common in Australia among the aboriginal people, though XFG is rare in this population.[1-3]

No proper evaluative scale has been developed as yet to facilitate research and clinical characterization of the condition. Such a scale will provide a better understanding of the exfoliation process as it relates to the progression of glaucoma and also to the new genetic findings. A new scheme is currently under consideration.

## 39.2 Genetics, Histology, Biochemistry, and Pathophysiology

The genetic background of XFS and XFG remained unclear until 2007, when the Reykjavik study identified specific single nucleotide polymorphisms associated with exfoliation.[4] Historically, autonomic dominant inheritance, mitochondrial transmission, and environmental influences were proposed as potential sources for XFG and XFS.[1] However, the 2007 discovery of the role played by lysyl oxidase-like protein 1 (LOXL1) gene polymorphism in the development of the condition has shed light on its genetic background.[4] LOXL1 is a member of a gene family that plays an important role in elastin metabolism. Synthesis of exfoliation material has always been attributed to disturbed elastin metabolism, leading XFS to be considered a systemic elastin fibrillopathy disease. This may explain the histological findings and several XFS-related intraocular and extraocular complications. It is hypothesized that dysfunction of the LOXL1 gene may lead to the progressive accumulation of exfoliation material. In the general populations of Iceland and Sweden, the high-risk haplotype of LOXL1 is very common; it is found in approximately 50% in the general population, and 25% of the population is homozygous for this mutation. For these individuals, the risk for development of XFG is approximately 2.47 times higher than that for the general population and 700 times higher than the risk for people carrying the low-risk haplotype. The importance of LOXL1 gene polymorphism in the development of the disorder has recently been confirmed in a Midwest American population cohort[5] and in the German and Italian populations.[6] Intensive worldwide genetic

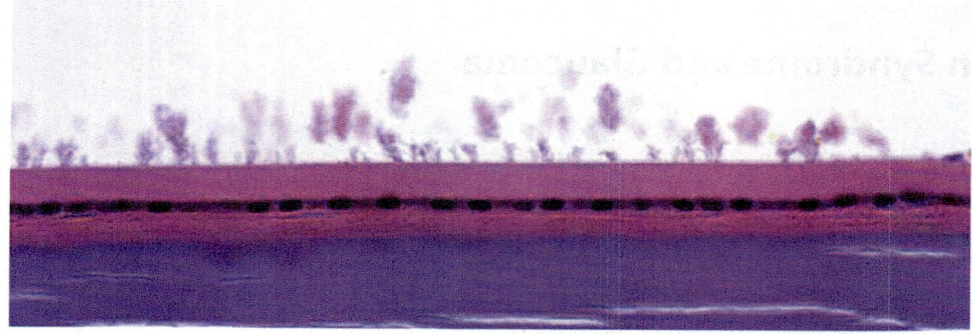

**Fig. 39.1** Light microscopic appearance of exfoliation material deposition on the lens surface. Courtesy of Ursula Schloetzer-Schrehardt

research is currently being carried out to clarify the precise role of LOXL1 mutations worldwide. In the Japanese population, XFS and XFG seem to be associated with different LOXL1 polymorphisms compared to the white populations.[7,8] A commercial test is currently available for the two single nucleotide polymorphisms found on this gene. While its importance for research is unquestionable, the clinical value of using it to predict who is going to get exfoliation remains to be determined.

> Exfoliation material synthesis may be related to disturbed elastin metabolism. Specific mutations of the LOXL1 gene, a member of the lysyl oxidase gene family which plays a key role in elastin metabolism, are strongly associated with the development of XFS and XFG.

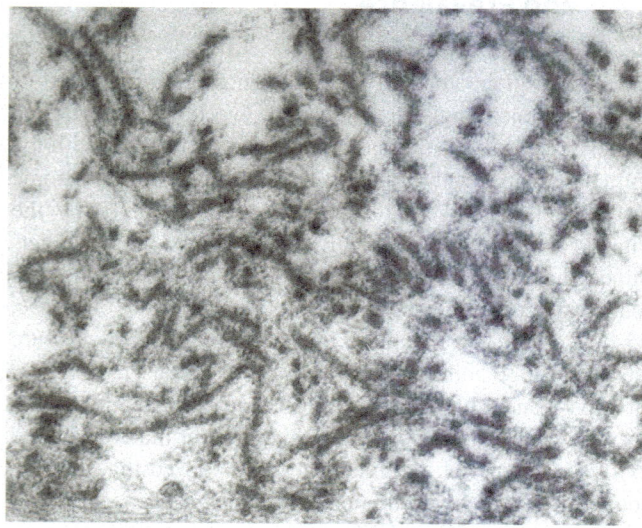

**Fig. 39.2** Electron microscopic appearance of exfoliation material aggregates. Courtesy of Ursula Schloetzer-Schrehardt

XFS is an age-dependent, generalized disorder of the extracellular matrix metabolism, which is rarely manifested clinically before the age of 60 years. Nevertheless, before XFS and XFG become clinically detectable, exfoliation material aggregates can be identified by transmission electron microscopy within ocular tissues.[9,10] Ultrastructurally, exfoliation deposits are electron dense, elastotic material that appears fibrillar in structure (Fig. 39.1–39.3). Histochemical studies reported that exfoliation material consists of a core protein surrounded by glycoconjugates, giving it a glycoprotein/proteoglycan structure. Generally, exfoliation aggregates can be seen both intracellularly while being synthesized and extracellularly where they are deposited. Though intraocular and extraocular exfoliation material are not morphologically, or biochemically identical, they both represent the same type of abnormal fibrillopathy.[10] Recent research data suggest that the exfoliation-related biochemical changes are influenced by increased oxidative stress, which, as a part of a vicious circle, is enhanced by the exfoliation-induced tissue damage.[11] Development of nuclear cataract is more common in patients with XFS/XFG and may probably be related to increased oxidative stress in the anterior segment of the eye.[11]

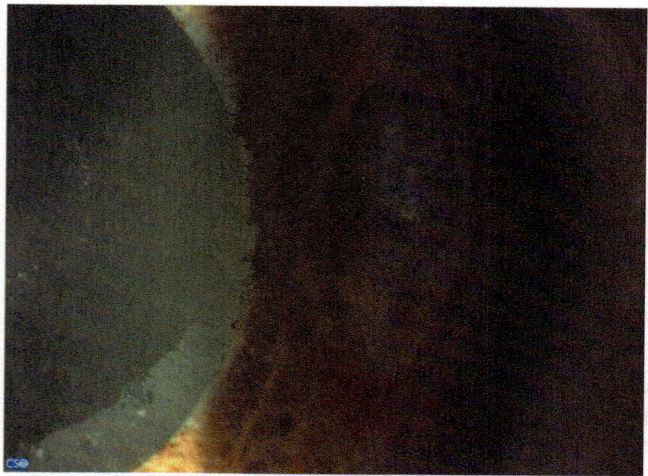

**Fig. 39.3** Classic slit-lamp appearance of exfoliation material deposition on the lens. The central disc and peripheral granular zone are evident together with marked pupillary ruff atrophy

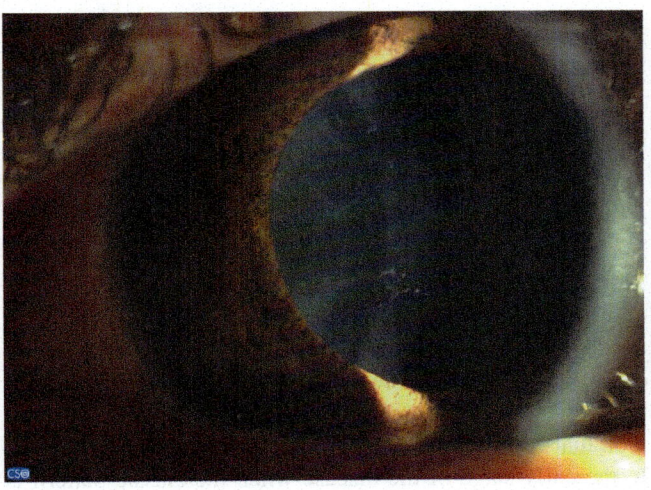

**Fig. 39.4** Biomicroscopic appearance of an eye with exfoliation syndrome. A subtle bridge connects the central disc with the peripheral granular zone

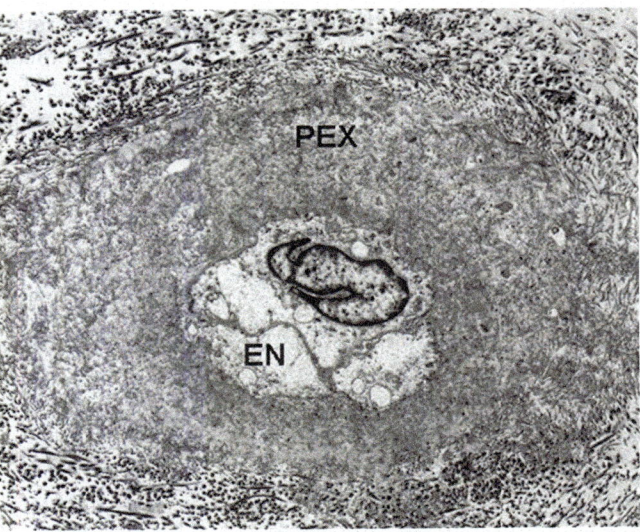

**Fig. 39.5** Ultrastructural appearance of an iris ghost vessel. Exfoliation material (PEX) completely surrounds the obliterated lumen of the vessel. EN=endothelium of the vessel. Courtesy of Ursula Schloetzer-Schrehardt

Intraocular synthesis and accumulation of exfoliation material predominantly involve the anterior segment of the eye; exfoliation aggregates are synthesized by the non-pigmented ciliary epithelial cells, trabecular endothelial cells, vascular endothelial cells in the iris, and pre-equatorial lens epithelium cells. After reaching the extracellular space, exfoliation aggregates are deposited around the cells of origin, but may also be passively transported by the aqueous humor and be deposited upon the zonular apparatus, anterior lens surface, pupillary margin, and within the outflow system. In the trabecular meshwork (together with the pigment granules liberated from the pupillary margin and the posterior layer of the iris), the accumulated exfoliation material can reduce aqueous humor outflow leading to a gradual increase of intraocular pressure (IOP) and subsequent development of XFG with optic nerve head damage. Exfoliation aggregates have been identified in many different systemic organs, such as connective tissues, skin, heart muscle cells, striated muscle cells, and large vessel walls.[10]

Exfoliation material is not only synthesized and accumulated in different tissues, but, more importantly by disturbing extracellular matrix metabolism it can induce alterations in function.[1,2,12] These XFS-related degenerative changes are clinically important and must be known by all ophthalmologists (Fig. 39.4). First, XFS causes zonular fragility and disruption that subsequently may lead to lens subluxation, which results in surgical complications during phacoemulsification cataract surgery, and in extreme cases may lead to pupillary block or secondary angle-closure glaucoma. The zonular fragility, thinning of the equatorial lens capsule, and reduced dilatation of the pupil are thought to be responsible for the increased complication rate during cataract surgery, as well as the postoperative decentration of intraocular lenses even years after uncomplicated cataract surgery. In some cases, exfoliation-induced corneal degenerative changes may impact the number and shape of corneal endothelial cells, which may lead to corneal decompensation even after uncomplicated phacoemulsification cataract surgery or following marked elevation of IOP.[3]

The degenerative changes induced by XFS and XFG in the iris result in the reduced pupillary dilatation in these patients. Further, degenerative changes and exfoliation deposits around the wall of iris vessels lead to micro-occlusions, formation of ghost vessels (Fig. 39.5), and secondary micro-neovascularization. These changes are important clinically since they result in increased vascular permeability and impairment of the blood-aqueous barrier function, which can lead to increased incidence of posterior synechiae formation and more severe inflammation after intraocular surgery. Retrobulbar perfusion may also be impaired in XFS and XFG.

Though rarely appreciated by ophthalmologists, XFS patients may also exhibit systemic vascular involvement. There are reports of impaired regulation of heart function and reduced precapillary perfusion.[12] In the large vessels, rigidity increases and elasticity decreases compared to the age-matched elderly population.[13] Plasma homocysteine level is also increased in XFS and XFG, and homocysteine level increases with the duration of XFS.[13] Since disturbed homocysteine metabolism and the consequent increase of the plasma homocysteine level are responsible for several serious vascular diseases including ocular vascular occlusions (e.g., retinal vein occlusion), XFS/XFG patients with a positive vascular history can benefit from a consultation with an internist or a cardiologist. These systemic alterations can explain why XFS is frequently associated with systemic vascular diseases.[14] At present, however, we do not recommend performing homocysteine level testing routinely in these patients.

> XFS and XFG are systemic disorders with several ocular and extraocular sequelae.

## 39.3 Evolution of XFG from XFS

Both XFS and XFG may present clinically as unilateral disease. In clinically apparent unilateral disease, ultrastructural investigation of the clinically unaffected fellow eye can often

> In 10 years, one-third of the clinically unilateral exfoliation cases convert to bilateral disease, whereas 30% of the XFS eyes without IOP elevation convert to XFG.

document the morphological presence of exfoliation material. Thus, unilateral XFS may only be a cross-sectional clinical category, and not a true biological entity. This issue is of practical importance, since clinically detectable XFS or XFG often develops in the fellow eye over time.[15,16] Statistically, over a period of 10 years, approximately one in three cases of clinically unilateral exfoliation cases convert to bilateral exfoliation.[16] The implication is that careful slitlamp examination is required at each follow-up visit, and re-consideration of the classification of the fellow eye may be necessary if exfoliation material or elevated pressure occur.

The cumulative risk for XFG development in eyes with manifest XFS but without IOP elevation is approximately 30% in 10 years and most of these cases convert within the first 5 years.[15] Pressure elevation is an important indicator of the conversion process. It is thought that IOP elevation in XFS and XFG is caused by blockage within the trabecular meshwork by exfoliation material and pigment granules released from the posterior iris layer and pupillary margin. It seems likely that the meshwork becomes overwhelmed with a loss of functional reserve for handling the exfoliation and pigment deposits, and it may be that the macrophage response of trabecular cells is no longer able to deal with the abnormal material. Subsequent development of IOP elevation and exaggerated 24-h IOP fluctuation lead to optic nerve head damage, and from this point the condition is classified as XFG. The presence of exfoliation in ocular hypertension doubles the risk of glaucoma development.

## 39.4 Clinical Diagnosis of XFG

The clinical diagnosis of XFG relies upon the clinical detection of exfoliation material.[1] In the fully developed form of XFS, exfoliation material is visible on the anterior lens surface in a typical configuration. The relatively homogenous central disc corresponds to the size of the undilated pupil. The central disc is surrounded by a clear intermediate zone. The peripheral zone is a granular, often layered ring of exfoliation material deposits. This classic presentation, however, is not always evident and there are subtle signs of the condition years before the classic appearance. It is important to recognize that even when it is typically present it is common that XFS cannot be visualized without pupil dilatation. In the early stage of the disease when the classic pattern is often not yet fully developed, exfoliation material may only be seen on the peripheral part of the anterior lens capsule. Detection of the early exfoliation signs can be facilitated using low intensity slitlamp illumination. The beam should be positioned at approximately 45° from the axis of observation. Fine exfoliation aggregates can often be visible upon the pupillary margin, and less frequently on the iris, corneal endothelium, and sometimes may be seen with gonioscopy upon the trabecular meshwork. Due to the degenerative changes associated with the condition, the iris is atrophic, with transillumination defects, and the pupillary margin can demonstrate a moth-eaten appearance due to loss of pigment. Nuclear cataract is more common in XFS and XFG. In some cases, phacodonesis, subluxation, or even luxation of the lens can occur as consequence of zonular damage. Iris pigment liberation and deposition are early and typical signs in the condition. Pigment granules are frequently seen deposited on the anterior lens surface after pupil dilatation. Fine pigment deposits are commonly seen on the iris surface and less frequently upon the corneal endothelium. Pigment accumulation in the angle is pathognomonic of the condition and is seen as a wavy pigment deposition above Schwalbe's line (called Sampaolesi's line) and as dense, dark pigment accumulated unevenly within the trabecular meshwork (Fig. 39.6). The amount of pigment granules varies considerably and correlates well with the severity of the disease.

In XFG, all characteristics of XFS are present (Fig. 39.7), accompanied by elevated IOP and an optic nerve head showing typical glaucomatous neuroretinal rim loss.[17-19] This is usually diffuse, and in many cases very advanced when the diagnosis is made. The diffuse optic nerve head damage is due to the high pressure characteristics of XFG where IOP can in some instances be as high as 60 mmHg at diagnosis.[18] XFG is characterized by worse 24-h characteristics than primary open-angle glaucoma (POAG).[17] Despite the high pressure characteristics, XFG is usually asymptomatic and not associated with pain or discomfort. Due to its unilateral presentation or the different degree of severity between the two

# 39 Exfoliation Syndrome and Glaucoma

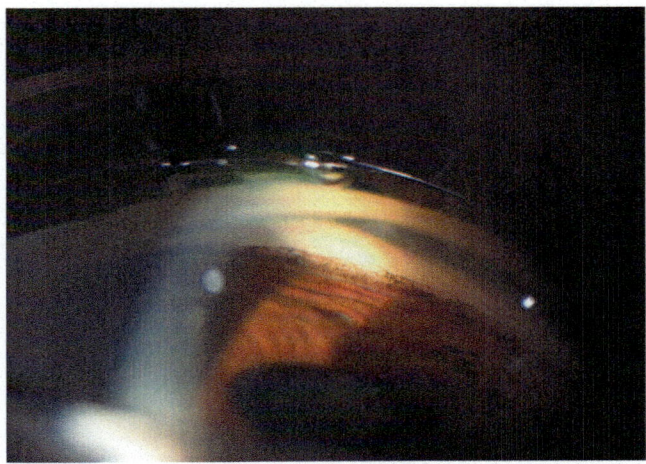

**Fig. 39.6** Typical gonioscopic appearance of an eye with exfoliative glaucoma (XFG). Dense, uneven pigmentation can be seen below Sampaolesi's line

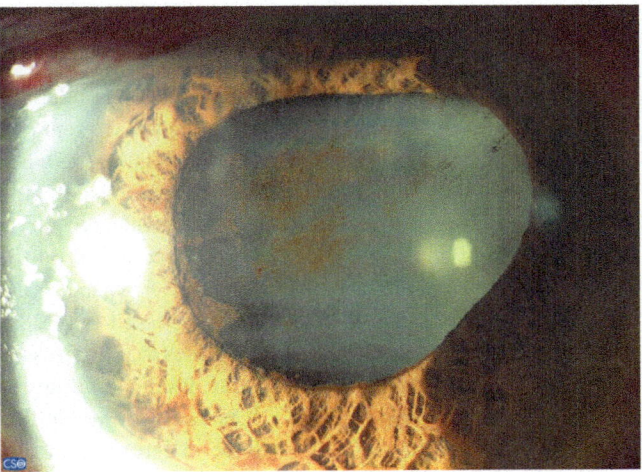

**Fig. 39.7** Dense deposition of pigment on the surface of the lens together with posterior synechiae following intense dilatation of the pupil in an eye with XFG

eyes, the patient's realization of visual loss can be delayed. Owing to the large 24-h IOP fluctuation in XFG, IOP assessment should not rely on a single pressure reading; ideally a 24-h IOP curve should be carried out, or at least a daytime pressure curve with three IOP readings (morning, afternoon, and evening).

It is necessary to establish the correct diagnosis and identify the IOP peaks in XFG management. An IOP curve is also valuable in evaluating the true magnitude of IOP reduction in XFG. Practitioners are often reluctant to perform diurnal curve studies as part of their routine evaluation of their glaucoma patients, but it is important to realize that in XFG, proper diagnosis and management cannot be obtained on the basis of a single IOP measurement.

When the pupil is pharmacologically dilated in XFS and XFG (which is vital to establish the diagnosis), pigment is frequently released from the posterior iris layer. This may result in acute pressure elevation. In order to prevent acute damage due to this IOP spike, the pressure should ideally be measured 2–3 h after dilatation and if necessary, additional IOP lowering medication should be employed.

> XFG is characterized by worse 24-h IOP characteristics than POAG. A single IOP measurement is often insufficient to evaluate the real IOP in this glaucoma. A pressure curve may better delineate pressure characteristics and facilitate diagnosis and management.

## 39.5 Differential Diagnosis of XFG

In order to provide tailor-made management, XFG must be differentiated from other glaucoma types.[1,19] In POAG, there is no clinical evidence of exfoliation material and the IOP characteristics (e.g., IOP fluctuation) are better, the disease is typically bilateral, there are no pigmentary signs, and optic nerve head damage is generally less severe. Though IOP in juvenile open-angle glaucoma is usually high, the patients are much younger that XFG patients. Young age is also a key differential with pigmentary glaucoma where pigmentary signs and IOP characteristics resemble those of XFG. Further, in pigmentary glaucoma, the extent of pigment liberation is greater, iris transillumination defects are typically radial, pigment deposits upon the cornea endothelium form a central vertical spindle (Krukenberg's spindle), and the trabecular pigmentation is dense and homogeneous.

Occasionally, exfoliation and pigment deposits on the corneal endothelium are incorrectly ascribed inflammatory precipitates. Thus, XFG should also be differentiated from uveitic glaucoma. Since narrow angle, high IOP, and anterior movement of the lens due to zonular weakness can be seen in XFG just like in angle-closure glaucoma, these two glaucomas are sometimes difficult to differentiate. They often can be distinguished by their different natural course and history and via indentation gonioscopy. Finally, exfoliation keratopathy should be distinguished from Fuchs's dystrophy (which starts in the center and spreads to the periphery later) as well as pseudophakic or aphakic bullous keratopathy (which starts on the periphery and progresses to the central cornea).

> XFG should be differentiated from POAG, juvenile open-angle glaucoma, pigmentary glaucoma, uveitic glaucoma, and primary angle-closure glaucoma

There is a higher incidence of cataract (especially nuclear cataract) in XFS and XFG, thus, cataract surgery is often required. Importantly, the rate of surgical complications is higher in eyes with exfoliation than in eyes without.[20] The cataract surgeon needs to anticipate surgical problems, and should use gentle movements and minimal pressure, especially when performing capsulorhexis and nucleus fragmentation. Due to inadequate pupil dilation and zonular fragility, complications may occur in XFS/XFG. With phacoemulsification the complication rate has diminished compared with extracapsular cataract surgery. Nevertheless, the rate of posterior capsular breaks, vitreous loss, and even drop of the nucleus into the vitreous cavity are thought to be more frequent in XFG, but there is insufficient controlled data with adequately powered studies to elucidate this. The use of a capsular tension ring may be required more often.[20] In the early postoperative period, the pre-existent breakdown of blood-aqueous barrier increases the chances for inflammation or fibrinoid reaction. Postoperatively, anterior capsular contraction and phimosis are more common in XFG. Decentration, dislocation, or even luxation of the capsular bag–IOL complex may occur many years after uncomplicated cataract surgery (Fig. 39.8).

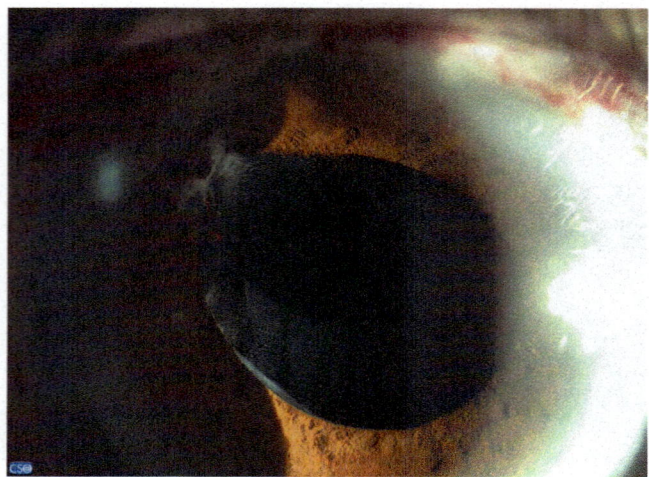

**Fig. 39.8** Atypical, gradual accumulation of exfoliation material on the surface of an intraocular lens 4 years after complicated phaco cataract surgery

> An increased rate of surgical complications can occur with cataract surgery in patients with XFS/XFG. The presence of exfoliation material should be carefully monitored prior to cataract surgery. In eyes with exfoliation, atraumatic surgical techniques and careful postoperative monitoring are required.

## 39.6 Medical Therapy for XFG

Exfoliative glaucoma is a leading cause of visual loss in the elderly and can carry a poor prognosis in some instances. It is thought to be a more severe glaucoma with faster progression than POAG.[1,2,21] This is due to several clinical characteristics including older age, higher mean and peak IOP, wider 24-h IOP fluctuation and more visual field damage at diagnosis. It has never been elucidated to date whether the worse prognosis in XFG is due to the difference in age, the worse 24-h IOP characteristics of XFG, or to a poorer response of XFG to medical therapy.[22-24] Although published literature suggests that XFG generally responds less well to medical therapy than POAG, this may simply reflect the worse IOP characteristics in XFG.[24] Previous studies suggest that absolute IOP reduction and the percentage fall of pressure with medical therapy in XFG are often higher than in POAG. Nevertheless, in many XFG cases, it is more difficult to reach the predetermined target IOP with monotherapy.[23] Therefore in XFG, more medication becomes necessary to control the pressure and laser or surgical intervention are more often required.

In patients with XFG, there is a dose–response relationship between levels of IOP lowering and the subsequent rate of progression.[22] There is a strong linear correlation between untreated 24-h IOP characteristics and mean visual field defect at diagnosis.[17] In the first study that evaluated target pressure in XFG and the influence of IOP reduction on the long-term stability or progression within 5 years, XFG patients with a mean IOP ≤ 17 mmHg progressed only 28% of the time compared with 70% of XFG cases that progressed with a mean IOP ≥ 20 mmHg.[23] Stepwise, medical therapy in XFG is currently similar to POAG. It is likely, however, that future medical therapy in XFG will be different from that employed in POAG. Medical therapy includes beta-adrenergic antagonists, alpha-adrenergic agonists, miotics, carbonic anhydrase inhibitors, and prostaglandin analogues. Despite the arrival of new classes of topical medications, which have significantly reduced the rate of surgery in XFG (just like in POAG), the trend remains for XFG to respond less well to monotherapy, to require more often adjunctive therapy, maximal medical therapy, and, finally, to require sooner and more often surgical intervention. At the present time, the impact of new medications on the long-term prognosis of XFG remains unknown.[24]

In XFG, response to timolol has been reported to be less favorable than in POAG.[22,25-27] In a 24-h study, despite a greater mean 24-h IOP reduction with timolol, XFG patients still exhibited worse 24-h IOP characteristics and greater fluctuation of IOP than age-matched patients with POAG.[27] However, the short-term as well as the long-term success rates of IOP control with timolol therapy are low. Indeed, only 8% of XFG patients versus 33% of POAG patients were successfully controlled with timolol monotherapy after 3 years.[26] Dorzolamide was documented to be efficacious as monotherapy in XFG.[28] In another study[29], dorzolamide was additive to timolol over 24 h but it did not alter the worse IOP characteristics compared with POAG.

In a parallel study in 50 XFG patients, the fixed combination of dorzolamide/timolol was found to provide significantly greater diurnal IOP reduction (45%) compared with either latanoprost (34%) or travoprost (36%) monotherapy.[30] This means diurnal reduction was greater than that reported for POAG patients with these drugs. The dorzolamide/timolol fixed combination has also been evaluated as initial therapy in XFG and was found to be a viable option.[31] In a crossover study, Konstas and associates[31] employed this fixed combination as initial therapy in 65 newly diagnosed patients with XFG with a mean pretreatment IOP of 31.2 mmHg. After 2 months of therapy, the fixed combination provided a mean reduction of 13.1 mmHg (42%) at peak.

To date there is limited information for the response and success rate with the prostaglandin analogues in XFG. In a recent prospective parallel diurnal study, latanoprost was slightly more effective than timolol monotherapy in lowering IOP in eyes with XFG.[32] There was a trend for better diurnal IOP control and significantly less diurnal IOP fluctuation with latanoprost therapy.

In a parallel study[30], travoprost was found to obtain similar reduction in diurnal IOP (36%) in patients with XFG compared with latanoprost (34%). In a more recent crossover study, however,[33] in 42 XFG patients mean 24-h IOP with travoprost (17.3 mmHg) was significantly better than that with latanoprost (17.8 mmHg) and this difference was attributed to significantly better IOP control with travoprost at 18:00 (16.7 mmHg versus 17.9 mmHg). A recently published study investigated the efficacy of bimatoprost compared with latanoprost in XFG.[34] This multicenter, crossover, 3-month study investigated the diurnal IOP control obtained with bimatoprost versus latanoprost in 129 consecutive XFG patients. Bimatoprost obtained significantly lower diurnal IOP than latanoprost (17.6 mmHg versus 18.6 mmHg) after 3 months of chronic therapy. In a recent meta-analysis of 24-h studies, the results of prostaglandin monotherapy for patients with XFG demonstrated in general that both untreated baseline and treatment arms were higher in XFG and the 24-h IOP reductions from baseline were greater than observed in the POAG patients.[35]

Adjunctive latanoprost therapy is safe and well tolerated for the long-term treatment of patients with XFG.[24,36] One study reported that latanoprost is more effective as adjunctive therapy with timolol than dorzolamide.[36] The role of fixed combinations (e.g., dorzolamide/timolol, latanoprost/timolol, travoprost/timolol, bimatoprost/timolol, and brimonidine/timolol fixed combinations) in the medical therapy of XFG requires further elucidation. In certain XFG patients with high baseline IOP and advanced damage, fixed combinations may be the best initial choice for therapy. It is conceivable that these XFG patients will benefit from initial medical therapy with fixed combinations. In medicine, initial therapy with fixed combinations was found to provide improved clinical outcome in real life practice. Fixed combinations obtain better IOP control than concomitant unfixed therapies and reduce the incidence of adverse events. In XFG, fixed combinations should be used earlier and more frequently in the stepwise therapy of XFG because of the worse 24-h IOP characteristics, the faster progression, and worse prognosis.

Future research on the efficacy of new medications specifically in XFG may determine the best initial and stepwise therapy in this secondary glaucoma. The target 24-h IOP that will ensure stability in all XFG patients remains to be determined. Such information is especially important, because XFG is a severe form of open-angle glaucoma, more often associated with vision loss than POAG. The future focus on therapy in XFG should not only be IOP reduction and will probably include innovative approaches that may slow the progression from XFS to XFG, or even prevent the development of XFG.

> Medical therapy is more difficult in XFG. Although the IOP reduction may be initially greater, the worse 24-h IOP characteristics in this condition make it more difficult to obtain the desired target pressure. Therefore, adjunctive therapy is often needed. Fixed combination drugs should be used earlier in XFG.

## 39.7 Argon Laser Trabeculoplasty in XFG

Argon laser trabeculoplasty (ALT) is a successful and well-established photocoagulative procedure for lowering IOP in XFG.[37] Most studies show a better response to ALT in XFG than in POAG; nevertheless, late failure may be more common in XFG.[37-41] Traditionally, ALT has been recommended when IOP is not satisfactorily controlled with maximum tolerated medical therapy, as an option before filtering surgery. However, when medical treatment is contraindicated and in elderly or non-compliant patients, ALT may also be a valuable option as first choice of treatment.[38,42] XFG is characterized by dense trabecular pigmentation, therefore XFG eyes with open anterior chamber angles are particularly suitable for ALT. Since the amount of pigmentation of the meshwork directly influences the outcome, and in XFG the meshwork is generally more heavily pigmented, the power selected should be less than that selected with POAG. The optimal power setting is determined by the heat-induced reaction of the trabecular meshwork, which determines if the power setting is appropriate. Ideally, the IOP should be checked during the first 6 h postoperatively. If it is not possible, pre-treatment with topical apraclonidine and the use of oral acetazolamide postoperatively is recommended to prevent an ALT-induced IOP-spike. Topical steroids or topical nonsteroidal anti-inflammatory drops are to be used four times daily for 7 days. Close monitoring is suggested in cases of advanced glaucoma, one-eye patient, high pre-laser IOP, and repeated trabeculoplasty. The result of ALT cannot be evaluated before 4–6 weeks. ALT has very few complications – the commonest is a transient elevation of IOP, which is more common in XFG than in POAG. In some eyes, there is a formation of small peripheral anterior synechiae (especially after posteriorly placed burns or in patients with narrow angles). Late gradual IOP elevation due to loss of ALT effect is common. Although conceivably ALT may decrease the success of subsequent filtration surgery, there is no controlled evidence to support this hypothesis.

In most studies, the initial pressure lowering effect of ALT was greater in XFG than in POAG, at least during the first 12–24 months.[39-42] On an average, an IOP decrease of about 30% can be expected in XFG with ALT. Though the success criteria vary among studies, the success rate reported after one year ranges between 70% and 90%. However, the laser effect declines over time, and the subsequent failure rate is higher in XFG (approximately 10% per year) than that seen in POAG.[37] The higher rate of failure is not surprising, since exfoliation material and pigment granules are continuously accumulating in XFG, leading to a functional blockage of the trabecular meshwork. Nevertheless, a number of studies report success rates close to 50% after 5 years of follow-up. Despite the poorer long-term success, ALT is a valuable treatment option in XFG, since success of medical therapy and filtration surgery are also worse in XFG compared with POAG.

Since topical medication may cause local or systemic adverse effects and may influence the quality of life, primary ALT may be considered in XFG.[38] Evidence from Scandinavia[37] suggests that initial ALT treatment is particularly successful in XFG and at least as good as initial medical therapy. In a long-term study,[38] the probability of success (defined as no medication required) after primary ALT was 80% after 2 years, 54% after 5 years, and 36% after 8 years in XFG.

Selective laser trabeculoplasty (SLT) is a relatively new technique, similar in principle to ALT, that utilizes a Q-switched 532 nm Nd:YAG laser, which selectively targets the intracellular melanin granules in the trabecular meshwork cells.[43] Using short exposition time, very low power, and wide area of laser application, thermal damage and disruption of the trabecular meshwork is reduced. Because of its non-destructive nature, repeated treatments with SLT are theoretically possible, and SLT in theory can be employed in eyes where ALT has failed. Similarly to ALT, topical alpha-agonists or systemic carbonic anhydrase inhibitors should be given since temporary IOP elevation can also be encountered after SLT. Little information on the specific effectiveness of SLT in XFG is available at present.[37,44] Most published studies were performed on eyes with POAG or on a mixed population of POAG and XFG cases. It is logical that in XFG the SLT energy settings should be significantly lower to avoid pressure spikes after therapy. In XFG, the IOP reduction reported in the first post-treatment year seems to be similar (approximately 30%) to that detected in POAG. The IOP reduction is more pronounced if the pre-treatment pressure is higher; i.e., around 30 mmHg. Early IOP spikes is the commonest complication of the procedure and have been repeatedly detected in eyes with XFG after SLT.

## 39.8 Surgery in XFG

Surgery is usually considered the final step in the management of XFG. It is indicated when medical and laser therapy has failed to obtain the predetermined target pressure, or when visual field loss and/or optic disc damage progress despite conservative treatment. The decision on filtering surgery should be made on an individual basis, carefully considering the risk/benefit ratio.[45] Increased rate of surgical complications is well documented in XFG, but at the same time, the need for surgery is more frequent in XFG compared to POAG. Trabeculectomy is still recognized as the standard surgical procedure in progressive or uncontrolled XFG.[46-48] Furthermore, some new surgical modalities (e.g., trabecular aspiration and goniocurettage) have been proposed for XFG surgery.[49-53] The surgical technique in trabeculectomy does not differ from that used in other types of glaucoma. Importantly, there is no controlled study to date examining the long-term success of trabeculectomy in XFG compared with POAG.

Following trabeculectomy, patients with XFG may progress less frequently than those with POAG.[47] Mean postoperative IOP has been reported lower after 6 months of follow-up in XFG compared to POAG.[48] Trabeculectomy in XFG is thought to be more successful with the concomitant use of antimetabolites (mitomycin C or 5-fluorouracil), but their influence on the long-term success in XFG remains to be determined. When XFG coexists with advanced lens opacities, combined surgery may be considered. This procedure may be effective in reducing IOP as well as the number of glaucoma medications needed, but the long-term success of IOP reduction again needs to be determined in controlled trials.

Trabeculectomy and combined surgery may be associated with several intraoperative and postoperative complications in XFG. Phacodonesis due to zonular fragility may lead to intraoperative zonular rupture and subsequent lens subluxation. The incidence of vitreous loss or late incarceration of vitreous into the internal ostium of the filtration site is higher than in non-XFG eyes.[45] Iris vasculopathy can result in the development of intraoperative or early postoperative hyphema. Cataract formation after trabeculectomy is frequent in XFG. Like in other types of glaucoma, overfiltration and wound leakage lead to reduced anterior chamber depth and postoperative hypotony. In patients with XFG, surgery may exacerbate the preexisting blood-aqueous barrier breakdown, which may lead to marked postoperative inflammation, fibrinoid reaction, and posterior synechia formation.[3] In some cases, the size of Schlemm's canal may decrease after surgery, which can lead to difficulties of IOP control if the filtering procedure later fails. The success of long-term IOP control can be compromised if capsular rupture and vitreous loss occurs in combined phaco-trabeculectomy due to poor pupil dilation and underlying zonular fragility. It is not known if long-term success in XFG is worse than with POAG due to an increased rate of scarring in eyes with XFG resulting from higher levels of transforming growth factor beta 1 (TGFβ1)[1,3] and the breakdown of the blood aqueous barrier. Furthermore, because of the higher IOP and the older age of XFG patients, complications such as choroidal detachment and suprachoroidal hemorrhage may occur more frequently.

New surgical modalities (deep sclerectomy and viscocanalostomy) that are supposed to bypass the functional blockage of the trabecular meshwork have also been tried in XFG.[49-52] These techniques may avoid some unfavorable consequences of trabeculectomy; i.e., increased probability for postoperative inflammation, hypotony, and cataract formation. Limited information is available on the effectiveness of deep sclerectomy in XFG. Drolsum et al[49] investigated the success of deep sclerectomy using two different implants in XFG versus POAG, and suggested that deep sclerectomy may be more successful in XFG (61% versus 38% complete success after 1.5 years follow-up). In both POAG and XFG patients, IOP reduction found after deep sclerectomy with mitomycin C was significantly lower than that obtained without mitomycin C. No controlled comparative data are available between deep sclerectomy and trabeculectomy specifically in XFG. Trabecular aspiration is another new, non-filtering glaucoma procedure in XFG.[53] It is designed to increase trabecular outflow in XFG patients. In this procedure, trabecular debris and pigment are aspirated with a suction force of 100–200 mmHg under light tissue-instrument contact, using a modified intraocular aspiration probe. As a primary procedure in XFG, trabecular aspiration resulted in a mean IOP reduction of 49% at almost 15 months after surgery. When aspiration was combined with phacoemulsification, it was significantly more effective in IOP lowering than cataract surgery alone and reduced the need for adjunctive medical therapy, although less than phaco-trabeculectomy.

Since XFG is a difficult form of glaucoma with worse IOP characteristics than POAG, if a low target pressure is required, trabeculectomy should be considered as the surgery of choice.[54] Non-penetrating procedures can be considered in XFG despite the high cost of the implants in XFG cases with less damage when less IOP reduction is needed due to a favorable side effect profile.

**Acknowledgments** Supported in part by a Pythagoras grant (Dr. Konstas); a Hungarian National Health Grant (ETT 001/2009), (Dr. Holló); and a Horizon Award, Allergan, Inc., and Edith C. Blum Foundation, New York, NY (Dr. Ritch).

## References

1. Ritch R, Schlötzer-Schrehardt U. Exfoliation syndrome. *Surv Ophthalmol*. 2001;45:265–315.
2. Ringvold A. Epidemiology of the pseudoexfoliation syndrome. A review. *Acta Ophthalmol Scand*. 1999;77:371–375.
3. Ritch R, Schlotzer-Schrehardt U, Konstas AG. Why is glaucoma associated with exfoliation syndrome? *Prog Retin Eye Res*. 2003;22:253–275.
4. Thorleifsson G, Magnusson KP, Sulem P, et al. Common sequence variants in the LOXL1 gene confer susceptibility to exfoliation glaucoma. *Science*. 2007;317:1397–1400.
5. Fingert JH, Alward WA, Kwon YH, Wang K, Streb LM. LOXL1 mutations are associated with exfoliation syndrome in patients from the Midwestern United States. *Am J Ophthalmol*. 2007;144:974–975.
6. Pasutto F, Krumbiegel M, Marin CY, et al. Associations of LOXL1 common sequence variants in German and Italian patients with pseudoexfoliation syndrome and pseudoexfoliation glaucoma. *Invest Ophthalmol Vis Sci*. 2008;49:1459–1463.
7. Ozaki M, Lee KYC, Vithana FN, et al. Association of LOXL1 gene polymorphism with pseudoexfoliation in the Japanese. *Invest Ophthalmol Vis Sci*. 2008;49:3976–3980.
8. Hayashi H, Gotoh N, Ueda Y, Nakanishi H, Yoshimura N. Lysyl oxidase-like 1 polymorphism and exfoliation syndrome in the Japanese population. *Am J Ophthalmol*. 2008;145:582–585.
9. Schlötzer-Schrehardt U, Naumann GOH. Trabecular meshwork in pseudoexfoliation syndrome with and without open-angle glaucoma. *Invest Ophthalmol Vis Sci*. 1995;36:1750–1764.
10. Naumann GOH, Shclötzer-Schrehardt U, Kühle M. Pseudoexfoliation syndrome for the comprehensive ophthalmologist. *Ophthalmology*. 1998;105:951–968.
11. Koliakos GG, Konstas AGP, Schrehardt-Schloetzer U, Bufidis T, Georgiadis N, Ringvold A. Ascorbic acid concentration is reduced in the aqueous humor of patients with exfoliation syndrome. *Am J Ophthalmol*. 2002;134:879–883.
12. Visontai ZS, Horváth T, Kollai M, Holló G. Decreased cardiovagal regulation in exfoliation syndrome. *J Glaucoma*. 2008;17:133–138.
13. Visontai Z, Merisch B, Kollai M, Holló G. Increase of carotid artery stiffness and decrease of baroreflex sensitivity in exfoliation syndrome and glaucoma. *Br J Ophthalmol*. 2006;90:563–567.
14. Mitchell P, Wang JJ, Smith W. Association of pseudoexfoliation syndrome with increased vascular risk. *Am J Ophthalmol*. 1997;124:85–687.
15. Tarkkanen A, Kivelä T. Cumulative incidence of converting from clinically unilateral to bilateral exfoliation syndrome. *J Glaucoma*. 2004;13:181–184.
16. Puska P. Unilateral exfoliation syndrome: conversion to bilateral exfoliation and to glaucoma. A prospective 10-year follow-up study. *J Glaucoma*. 2002;11:517–524.
17. Konstas AGP, Matziris DA, Stewart WC. Diurnal intraocular pressure in untreated exfoliation and primary open-angle glaucoma. *Arch Ophthalmol*. 1997;28:111–117.

18. Konstas AGP, Holló G, Astakhov YS, et al. Presentation and long-term follow-up of exfoliation glaucoma in Greece, Spain, Russia and Hungary. *Eur J Ophthalmol.* 2006;16:60–66.
19. Thygesen J. Ocular clinical findings in exfoliation syndrome. In: Holló G, Konstas AGP, eds. *Exfoliation Syndrome and Exfoliative Glaucoma.* Savona, Italy: Dogma S.r.l; 2008:105–112.
20. Teus MA, de Benito-Llopis L. Update on cataract surgery in exfoliation syndrome. In: Holló G, Konstas AGP, eds. *Exfoliation Syndrome and Exfoliative Glaucoma.* Savona, Italy: Dogma S.r.l; 2007:127–132.
21. Vesti E, Kivel AT. Exfoliation syndrome and exfoliation glaucoma. *Prog Retin Eye Res.* 2000;19:268–345.
22. Konstas AGP, Tsironi S, Kozobolis VP. Medical therapy of exfoliative glaucoma. In: Holló G, Konstas AGP, eds. *Exfoliation Syndrome and Exfoliative Glaucoma.* Savona, Italy: Dogma S.r.l; 2008:137–144.
23. Konstas AGP, Holló G, Akopov EL, et al. Factors associated with long-term progression or stability in exfoliation glaucoma. *Arch Ophthalmol.* 2004;122:29–33.
24. Konstas AGP, Tsironi S, Ritch R. Current concepts in the pathogenesis and management of exfoliation syndrome and exfoliative glaucoma. *Compr Ophthalmol Update.* 2006;7:131–141.
25. Takki KK, Klemetti A, Valle O. The IOP-lowering effect of timolol in simple and capsular glaucoma. A multicenter study in Finland. *Graefes Arch Clin Exp Ophthalmol.* 1982;218:83–87.
26. Blika S, Saunte E. Timolol maleate in the treatment of glaucoma simplex and glaucoma capsulare. A three-year follow up study. *Acta Ophthalmol (Copenh).* 1982;60:967–976.
27. Konstas AG, Matziris DA, Gate EA, Stewart WC. Effect of timolol on the diurnal intraocular pressure in exfoliation and primary open-angle glaucoma. *Arch Ophthalmol.* 1997;115:975–979.
28. Heijl A, Strahlman E, Sverrisson T, et al. A comparison of dorzolamide and timolol in patients with pseudoexfoliation and glaucoma or ocular hypertension. *Ophthalmology.* 1997;104:137–142.
29. Konstas AGP, Maltezos A, Bufidis T, Hudgins AG, Stewart WC. Twenty-four hour control of intraocular pressure with dorzolamide and timolol maleate in exfoliation and primary open-angle glaucoma. *Eye.* 2000;14:73–77.
30. Parmaksiz S, Yuksel N, Karabas VL, Ozkan B, Demirci G, Caglar Y. A comparison of travoprost, latanoprost, and the fixed combination of dorzolamide and timolol in patients with pseudoexfoliation glaucoma. *Eur J Ophthalmol.* 2006;16:73–80.
31. Konstas AG, Kozobolis VP, Tersis I, Leech J, Stewart WC. The efficacy and safety of the timolol/dorzolamide fixed combination vs latanoprost in exfoliation glaucoma. *Eye.* 2003;17:41–46.
32. Konstas AG, Mylopoulos N, Karabatsas CH, et al. Diurnal intraocular pressure reduction with latanoprost 0.005% compared to timolol maleate 0.5% as monotherapy in subjects with exfoliation glaucoma. *Eye.* 2004;18:893–899.
33. Konstas AGP, Kozobolis VP, Katsimpris IE, et al. Efficacy and safety of latanoprost versus travoprost in exfoliative glaucoma patients. *Ophthalmology.* 2007;114:653–657.
34. Konstas AGP, Holló G, Irkec M, et al. Diurnal IOP control with bimatoprost vs latanoprost in exfoliative glaucoma: a crossover observer-masked 3-center study. *Br J Ophthalmol.* 2007;91:757–760.
35. Stewart WC, Konstas AGP, Nelson LA, Kruft B. Meta-analysis of 24-hour intraocular pressure studies evaluating efficacy of glaucoma medicines. *Ophthalmology.* 2008;115:1117–1122.
36. Petounis A, Mylopoulos N, Kandarakis A, Andreanos D, Dimitrakoulias N. Comparison of additive intraocular pressure-lowering effect of latanoprost and dorzolamide when added to timolol in patients with open-angle glaucoma or ocular hypertension: a randomized open-label, multicenter study in Greece. *J Glaucoma.* 2001;10:316–324.
37. Odberg T. Laser therapy of exfoliative glaucoma. In: Holló G, Konstas AGP, eds. *Exfoliation Syndrome and Exfoliative Glaucoma.* Savona, Italy: Dogma S.r.l; 2008:149–153.
38. Odberg T, Sandvik L. The medium and long-term efficacy of primary argon laser trabeculoplasty in avoiding topical medication in open angle glaucoma. *Acta Ophthalmol Scand.* 1999;77:176–181.
39. Threlkeld A, Hertzmark E, Sturm RT, et al. Comparative study of the efficacy of argon laser trabeculoplasty for exfoliation and primary open-angle glaucoma. *J Glaucoma.* 1996;5:311–316.
40. Higginbotham EJ, Richardson TM. Response of exfoliation glaucoma to laser trabeculoplasty. *Br J Ophthalmol.* 1986;70:837–839.
41. Psilas P, Prevezas D, Petroutsos G, et al. Comparative study of argon laser trabeculoplasty in primary open-angle and pseudoexfoliation glaucoma. *Ophthalmologica.* 1989;198:57–63.
42. Tuulonen A, Niva A-K, Alanko HI. A controlled five-year follow-up study of laser trabeculoplasty as primary therapy for open-angle glaucoma. *Am J Ophthalmol.* 1987;104:334–338.
43. Hodge WG, Damji KF, Rock W, Buhrmann R, Bowel AM, Pan Y. Baseline IOP predicts selective laser trabeculoplasty success at 1 year post-treatment: results from a randomised clinical trial. *Br J Ophthalmol.* 2005;89:1157–1160.
44. Melamed S, Ben Simon GJ, Levkovitch-Verbin H. Selective laser trabeculoplasty as primary treatment for open-angle glaucoma. *Arch Ophthalmol.* 2003;121:957–960.
45. Kozobolis VP, Konstas AGP. Filtering surgery in exfoliative glaucoma. In: Holló G, Konstas AGP, eds. *Exfoliation Syndrome and Exfoliative Glaucoma.* Savona, Italy: Dogma S.r.l; 2008:157–161.
46. Tørnqvist G, Drolsum L. Trabeculectomies. A long-term study. *Acta Ophthalmol (Copenh).* 1991;69:450–454.
47. Popovic V, Sjostrand J. Course of exfoliation and simplex glaucoma after primary trabeculectomy. *Br J Ophthalmol.* 1999;83:305–310.
48. Konstas AGP, Jay JL, Marshall GE, Lee WR. Prevalence, diagnostic features and the response to trabeculectomy in exfoliation glaucoma. *Ophthalmology.* 1993;100:619–627.
49. Drolsum L. Deep sclerectomy in patients with capsular glaucoma. *Acta Ophthalmol Scand.* 2003;81:567–572.
50. Kozobolis VP, Christodoulakis EV, Tzanakis N, Zacharopoulos I, Pallikaris IG. Primary deep sclerectomy versus primary deep sclerectomy with the use of mitomycin C in primary open-angle glaucoma. *J Glaucoma.* 2002;11:287–293.
51. Shaarawy T, Nguyen C, Schnyder C, Mermoud A. Five year results of viscocanalostomy. *Br J Ophthalmol.* 2003;87:441–445.
52. Wishart PK, Wishart MS, Porooshani H. Viscocanalostomy and deep sclerectomy for the surgical treatment of glaucoma: a long-term follow-up. *Acta Ophthalmol Scand.* 2003;81:343–348.
53. Jacobi PC, Dietlein TS, Krieglstein GK. Comparative study of trabecular aspiration vs trabeculectomy in glaucoma triple procedure to treat pseudoexfoliation glaucoma. *Arch Ophthalmol.* 1999;117:1311–1318.
54. Ritch R, Konstas AGP, Schlötzer-Schrehardt U: Exfoliation syndrome and exfoliative glaucoma. In Glaucoma: Medical diagnosis and therapy, Shaarawy TM, Sherwood MB, Hitchings RA, Crowston JG, eds, *Saunders* 2009;1:339–348.

# Chapter 40
# Neovascular Glaucoma

Donald Minckler

Neovascular glaucoma (NVG) is an apt generic term originally proposed by Weiss and colleagues in 1963 for the secondary glaucoma due to proliferation of fibrovascular tissue with progressive closure of the anterior chamber angle.[1,2] Simply defined, neovascularization (NV) in any organ system implies growth of vessels into or onto tissues not normally vascularized, such as cornea, vitreous, sub-retinal space, and the iris and meshwork surfaces and interstices.

Although still among the most complicated and difficult types of glaucoma to manage, clarification of the association of NVG with elaboration of vascular endothelial growth factor (VEGF) by ischemic retina has recently led to a new therapy option, anti-VEGF intravitreal injection, and new hope for an improving treatment algorithm.[3,4]

## 40.1 Pathophysiology

NV and NVG have been associated with a remarkable number of clinical disorders, the common denominator of which is retinal ischemia.[2–4] The most common systemic correlate, accounting for over one-third of NVG cases, is long-standing diabetes, which after a decade or more may lead to retinal capillary compromise triggering VEGF production by under-perfused retinal tissues. The second major association of ocular importance, accounting for approximately another third of NVG cases, is central retinal vein occlusion (CRVO), specifically those variations that are accompanied by areas of retinal capillary non-perfusion and ischemia (see Sidebar 40.1). A third group of associations includes orbital ischemia from carotid occlusive disease and dozens of other disorders that individually are also capable of provoking NVG. Entities in this "other" category include central or branch artery occlusions, retinal detachment, tumors (especially retinoblastoma), radiation retinopathy, sickle cell disease, and many others including numerous infectious and inflammatory diseases – many of unknown etiology such as Eales disease.[2]

## 40.2 Differential Diagnosis

The term "pseudo neovascularization" has been used to describe prominent iris and/or angle vessels that are abnormally leaky, occurring in Fuch's heterochromic iridocyclitis and pseudoexfoliation syndrome. Abnormally prominent iris vasculature can accompany acute angle-closure glaucoma and ocular trauma. Neovascularization (rete mirabile) occasionally noted gonioscopically around anterior segment wounds, including cataract incisions and trabeculectomy fistulas, is more appropriately considered aberrant wound healing than secondary to tissue ischemia.

Neovascularization of the iris may rarely be present in adults with retinopathy of prematurity (ROP) who can present with progressive angle-closure. However, the pathophysiology of angle-closure in such patients may also involve retrolental fibrosis and cataract. Neovascularization of the iris has been demonstrated experimentally in kittens with ROP.[5]

In diabetes, the sequence of capillary compromise and regional retinal ischemia is more likely and accelerated with type I diabetes and insulin-dependence compared to type II disease. Proliferative retinopathy, while physiologically understandable as an attempt to improve blood flow locally, unfortunately leads to substantial collateral damage. Untreated, intra-retinal, and extra-retinal proliferation of new vessels associated with diabetes eventually leads to extension of fragile immature vasculature from the retina and optic disc into the vitreous, with high risk of vitreous hemorrhage and the long-term consequence of fibrous organization and retinal detachment. Retinal complications include microaneurysms, intra-retinal hemorrhages and exudates, and macular edema. Besides stimulating local

> **SIDEBAR 40.1. Open angle glaucoma and central retinal vein occlusion**
>
> Meena Beri
>
> The association of Central Retinal Vein Occlusion (CRVO) and glaucoma/elevated intraocular pressure (IOP) has long been observed. The first person to note the role of glaucoma in the development of CRVO seems to have been Verhoeff in 1913.
>
> CRVO is a multifactorial disease with several risk factors; i.e., age, systemic arterial hypertension, diabetes, dysproteinemia, and hyperviscosity disorders predisposing an eye to have CRVO develop and other factors precipitating it. Hemi-CRVO is a variant of CRVO. In this condition, the eyes have a congenital abnormality of two trunks of central retinal vein in the optic nerve instead of one.
>
> While CRVO and HCVRO share same clinical and pathogenetic features, they should be differentiated from major branch retinal vein occlusion. CRVO/HCRVO consist of two distinct varieties: ischemic and non-ischemic.
>
> Earlier observations of association of CRVO and glaucoma were based on histopathologic evidence. Subsequent studies based on non-randomized comparative case series of 674 consecutive patients reported overall prevalence of glaucoma 9.9% and of ocular hypertension 16.2%.
>
> **Elevated Intraocular Pressure in Pathogenesis of CRVO/HCRVO** Verhoeff postulated that probably the increased IOP compresses and collapses the wall of the central retinal vein (CRV) leading to intimal/endothelial proliferation, which he found in his histopathologic studies to be the primary cause. This further leads to stasis of circulation and subsequent thrombosis of the central retinal vein. Others have reported a significant prevalence of exfoliation syndrome with in CRVO compared with control eyes, thought likely due to the high pressures seen in exfoliation. Stasis of circulation caused by elevated IOP might be one of the contributing factors in Virchow's triad for development of thrombosis.
>
> **Ocular Hypotension with CRVO/HCRVO** The association of ocular hypotony in eyes with CRVO is well established since reported for the first time by Moore in 1922. The pathogenesis still remains an enigma. Theoretically, retinal hypoxia and liberation of hypotensive factor by the hypoxic retina leads to fall of IOP. This may be a self-limited problem. However, patients with an ischemic CRVO/HCRVO may develop NVG.
>
> **The Take-Home Messages**
>
> 1. Patients with CRVO/HCRVO have higher than normal prevalence of glaucoma/OHT.
> 2. Presence of hypotony in the affected eye with CRVO/HCRVO can be misleading. Such eyes may still develop NV if they have ischemia.
> 3. The author recommends that the fellow eye with elevated pressure/OHT should be treated with ocular hypotensive agents in order to avoid its progression into glaucoma and to prevent development of CRVO/HCRVO.
> 4. The eye with CRVO/HCVO with hypotony needs no further lowering of IOP by ocular hypotensive agents. However, the eye should be monitored periodically for future consideration of glaucoma therapy as IOP tends to equalize over time.
>
> **Bibliography**
>
> Cursiefen C, Kuchle M, et al. Pseudoexfoliation syndromein eye with ischemic central retinal vein occlusion: a histopathologic and electron microscopic study. *Acta Ophthalmol Scand.* 2001;79:476–478.
>
> Hayreh SS. Central retinal vein occlusion. *Ophthalmol Clin North Am.* 1998;11:559–590.
>
> Hayreh SS, et al. Hemi-central retinal vein occlusion. Pathogenesis, clinical features and natural history. *Arch Opthalmol.* 1980;98:1600–1609.
>
> Hayreh SS, et al. IOP abnormalities associated with central and hemicentral retinal vein occlusion. *Ophthalmology.* 2004;111(1):133–141.
>
> Hayreh SS, et al. Systemic diseases associates with various type of retinal vein occlusion. *Am J Ophthalmol.* 2001;131:61–77.
>
> Moore RF. Some observation on intraocular tension in cases of thrombosis of retinal veins. *Trans Ophthalmol Soc UK.* 1922;42:115–126.
>
> Saatci OA, Ferliel ST, et al. Pseudoexfoliation and glaucoma in eyes with retinal vein occlusion. *Int Ophthalmol.* 1999;23:75–78.
>
> Verhoeff FH. The effect of chronic glaucoma on the central retinal vessels. *Arch Opthalmol.* 1913;42:145–152.

fibrovascular proliferation, VEGF diffuses throughout the vitreous anteriorly and where concentrated at the disc, pupil, and in the angle can provoke neovascular budding from adjacent capillaries.

### 40.2.1 Clinical Presentations

The first clinically apparent manifestations of anterior segment NV (pre-NVG) associated with diabetic retinopathy are often tiny red nubbins or non-radial, irregular surface capillaries adjacent to the pupil or iris defects. Early on, these may not become visible at the slit lamp until irritation during examination and gonioscopy or after topical drugs for pupil dilation. They may also become obvious during fluorescein iris angiography (Fig. 40.1). Under the continued influence of VEGF, a fibrovascular membrane erupts onto and covers the iris surface usually emanating from peripupillary capillaries, eventually spreading to and vaulting the scleral spur to arborize anteriorly across the meshwork (Fig. 40.2). Contraction within the growing membrane, which can occur before IOP elevates, often rolls the pupillary edge anteriorly, producing characteristic ectropion uvea (Fig. 40.3). During the intermediate and later phases of evolving NVG, contraction of the angle membrane produces progressive up-ratcheting of the peripheral iris into contact with the meshwork that progresses from the iris recess in a posterior to anterior direction to complete angle closure via peripheral anterior synechia (PAS) formation (Fig. 40.4). Outflow through the meshwork progressively decreases,

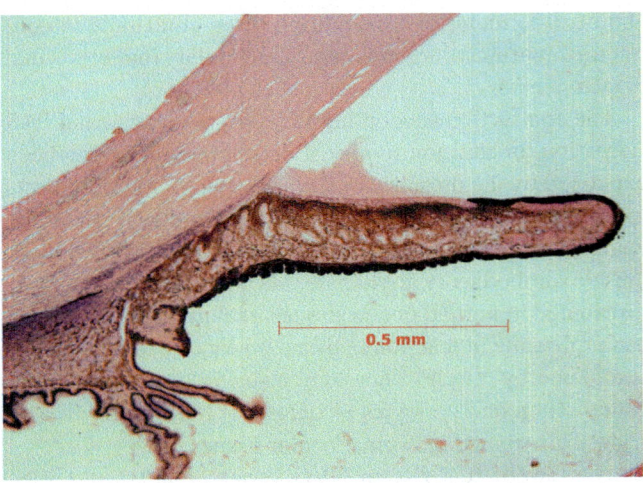

**Fig. 40.3** Photomicrograph illustrating ectropion uvea as a consequence of neovascularization (NV) associated with advanced diabetic vitreoretinopathy and retinal detachment. The pupil is everted bending the sphincter anteriorly due to contraction of a fibrovascular membrane on the iris surface continuous with the same process that has closed the angle by pulling the iris anteriorly (photomicrograph; hematoxylin and eosin; celloidin embedding, original ×10)

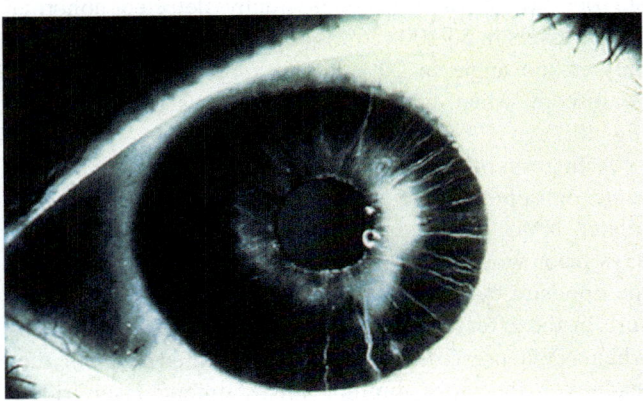

**Fig. 40.1** Iris angiogram illustrating early leak from new vessels at pupil margin

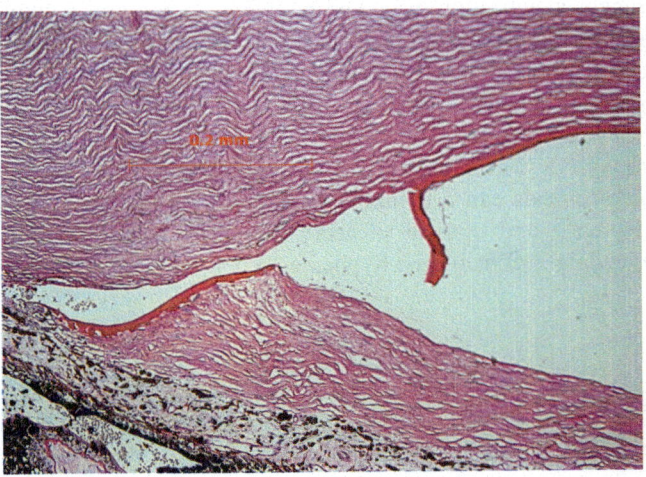

**Fig. 40.4** Massive end-stage fibrosis along the anterior iris surface. An artifactually fractured Descemet's membrane indicates where the "false" angle formed anterior to complete angle-closure in diabetes related neovascular glaucoma (photomicrograph; periodic-acid Schiff; original ×100)

eventually overwhelming compensatory mechanisms, possibly including decreased aqueous production, and marked elevation of IOP ensues. After angle closure, continuing high IOP with corneal edema and bullous keratopathy provoke cycles of pain and inflammation with eventual resolution by fibrovascular resurfacing of the cornea and ingrowth into the corneal stroma. Eyes that survive until very late stages may develop thick iris membranes with variable obliteration of the anterior chamber by fibrosis. Vascularization along the lens capsule or lens remnants

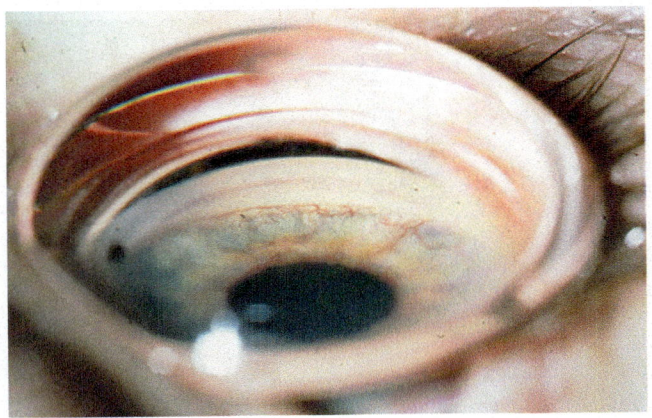

**Fig. 40.2** Clinical gonioscopy via Köeppe lens of fully developed rubeosis and angle-closure in diabetes

and cyclitic membrane formation often contribute to contracting vitreous organization, and total funnel retinal detachment.

The contraction accounting for ectropion uveae and PAS formation, in addition to retinal detachment, has long been explained by the presence of a population of myofibroblasts in the fibrovascular membranes, the cytoplasm of which contains arrays of contractile fibrils that react with smooth muscle antibodies (Fig. 40.5).[6,7] Myofibroblasts are widely distributed in normal ocular tissues, including the uvea, and can proliferate in reaction to tissue injury or when indirectly stimulated by VEGF. They may also evolve from vascular endothelium and pericytes or quiescent fibroblasts, all also widely distributed in normal ocular tissues.

The rate of IOP rise in NVG varies greatly but can be abrupt, leading to a presentation confused with acute primary angle-closure and often to laser peripheral iridectomy, seldom indicated as pupillary block is rarely present. Headache and corneal edema with vision decrease are common if IOP rises rapidly. Typical clinical signs of NVG in cases presenting with acute IOP elevation usually include ocular pain, ciliary flush, corneal bedewing, often obvious rubeosis, ectropion uvea, and hyphema. When gonioscopy is possible, variable angle closure with broad peripheral anterior synechiae (PAS) is typical. If gonioscopy is not possible due to corneal opacity, anterior segment imaging with high resolution ultrasound or optical coherence tomography (OCT) can establish the diagnosis of angle-closure. Paracentesis can accomplish rapid, usually transient, IOP decrease and corneal clearing, but may provoke angle bleeding and increased hyphema. When IOP is elevated in NVG, abnormal vessels are always present in the angle, usually in several quadrants or circumferentially in diabetes and CRVO (see Sidebar 40.2). Neovascularization of the angle may be segmental and limited to a few clock hours anterior to a branch vein occlusion (BVO).

## 40.2.2 Diabetes

The likelihood of NVG developing in diabetic patients is correlated with glucose control. In the Diabetes Control and Complications Trial (DCCT), 24% of standard treatment group patients developed NVG over 9 years compared to 8% in the intensively treated group.[8]

A unique and landmark study conducted between 1984 and 1990 in diabetic eyes found that 31 of 100 nonconsecutive diabetic patients (59 males, 41 females) without previous laser therapy had IOPs greater than 21 mmHg in one or both eyes. Standard gonioscopy revealed angle vessels in 30/100 (30%), but gonioangiography detected abnormal angle vessels in 56/100 (56%). Importantly, NV was present only in the angle in 20%, reinforcing the importance of gonioscopy when evaluating diabetic eyes (Fig. 40.6 and Fig. 40.7).[9]

A history of diabetes and typical retinopathy in the same or opposite eye would strongly support diabetic-related NVG. Painless sudden decrease in vision 60–90 days prior would be typical of CRVO. An open angle in the opposite eye essentially rules out primary angle-closure in the affected eye, the most common misdiagnosis when NVG presents with acutely elevated IOP, in turn leading to the most common mistreatment: laser iridectomy. The most florid examples of rubeosis follow CRVO

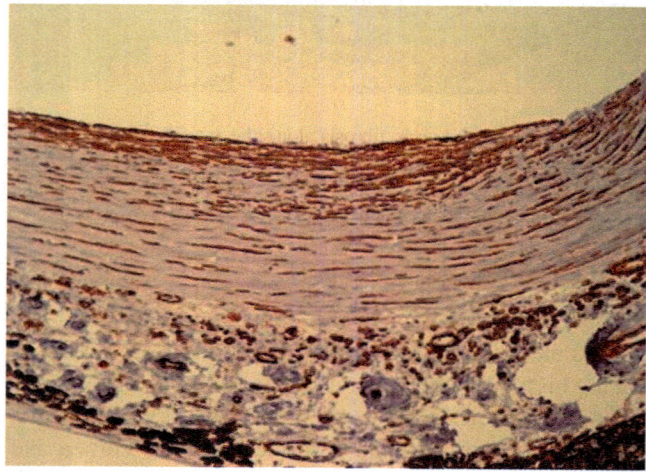

**Fig. 40.5** SMA (smooth muscle antigen) immunostaining positive cells are reddish brown within the membrane and along the anterior iris, from same case as in Fig. 40.4. (photomicrograph; original ×200; SMA [smooth muscle actin] immunostain)

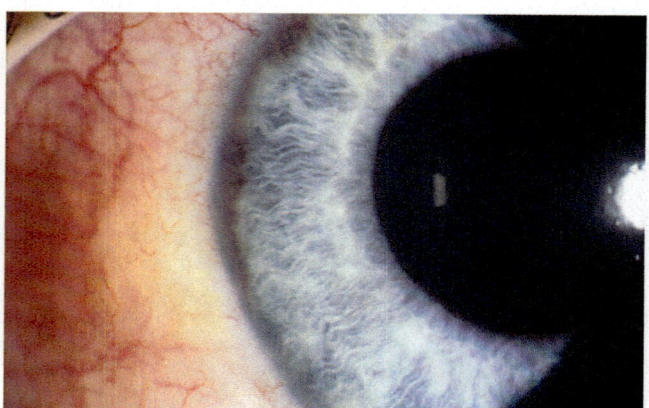

**Fig. 40.6** Clinically obvious angle neovascularization in type I diabetes without pupillary neovascularization being evident.

## SIDEBAR 40.2. Central retinal vein occlusion and monitoring risk of neovascular glaucoma

John Hyatt, Sarwat Salim, and Peter A. Netland

Central retinal vein occlusion (CRVO) is a well-known cause of vision loss, not only due to characteristic acute retinal changes, but also due to its sequelae, such as neovascular glaucoma (NVG) and macular edema. In an effort to improve outcomes, there has been much discussion regarding identification of patients with CRVO who are at greatest risk of developing NVG for timely intervention.

CRVO accounts for about one-third of cases of NVG. Not only can CRVO lead to NVG, but elevated intraocular pressure may play a role in its etiology. Neovascularization (NV) of the iris or angle after CRVO is a critical clinical finding that can result in NVG if not recognized and treated promptly. In the Central Vein Occlusion Study (CVOS), 16% of the eyes developed NV. Hayreh et al found that approximately 10% of eyes with CRVO developed NV, while the incidence increased to 45% in eyes with prominent retinal ischemia. The amount of retinal ischemia seen on fluorescein angiography (FA) has been shown to correlate with development of anterior segment NV. This link is explained by the elaboration of VEGFs by ischemic retina, coinciding with formation of NV. Quantifying retinal ischemia by FA to assess risk of anterior segment NV at times can be problematic because transmission blockage secondary to acute hemorrhage can limit accurate delineation of ischemic retina. There also is controversy in the literature surrounding what terminology and threshold to use for classifying a patient as having an "ischemic" or "non-perfused" CRVO. Though the Central Retinal Vein Occlusion Study (CVOS) used ten or more disc areas of retinal non-perfusion as a cut-off, a significant percentage of patients initially classified as perfused later developed NV. Subsequently, 30 disc areas of non-perfusion at presentation emerged as a more accurate predictor of development of NV. Of the eyes in the CVOS where retinal hemorrhages initially precluded adequate classification of retinal ischemia on presentation, 83% eventually demonstrated evidence of significant ischemia.

Visual acuity also predicts the likelihood of developing NV. Overall, the CVOS showed a linear correlation between decreasing Snellen visual acuity and risk for NV. In the subset of patients who presented within 1 month after the initial insult, 56% of the eyes with visual acuity less than 20/200 manifested NV during the study. This finding proved more predictive than any other variable, including nonperfusion on FA.

Neovascularization and associated glaucoma are usually seen within the first few months after the occlusion, giving rise to the commonly used term "90 day glaucoma." In the CVOS population, the steepest rise in NV formation was during the first 4 months. While analyzing the rate of NV occurring in patients with ischemic CRVO, Hayreh et al noted a similar precipitous rise in the first few months. In both of these studies, the risk of NV formation stabilized after about 8 months, with a very slow increase in the following years. The rapid development of anterior segment NV in some patients with CRVO makes the first few months after onset a critical time for monitoring and intervention.

At the conclusion of the CVOS, the investigators recommended frequent follow-up in the first 6 months after onset with attention paid to recognizing NV in the anterior segment by meticulously examining the undilated pupillary border and performing gonioscopy, since NV might develop in the anterior chamber angle first. Their schedule was approximately monthly, with potentially longer spacing between appointments for stable or improving eyes with visual acuity better than 20/200 on presentation. Notably, they found that prophylactic panretinal photocoagulation (PRP) did not prevent formation of NV in susceptible eyes. However, they conducted PRP at the earliest signs of NV in an effort to prevent development of NVG, resulting in regression of NV in the first month in 56% of previously untreated eyes. The mechanism by which PRP works is unclear. It is believed to reduce retinal oxygen demand, reducing hypoxic stimulus and subsequent release of VEGF.

Recently, newer anti-VEGF agents have been used in CRVO eyes to specifically evaluate their effect on macular edema and visual acuity over fairly short follow-up times. Two small retrospective studies using Avastin showed improvement of varying levels in visual acuity and macular edema and a lower incidence of NV than one might expect from the percentages quoted in the CVOS. A recent prospective, non-comparative trial of Avastin used in 46 patients with CRVO present for anywhere up to 150 weeks showed that injections during the first 6 months resulted in significant improvement in visual acuity. Individuals who presented within 3 months had better final visual acuity outcomes than those who presented greater than 3 months after onset of symptoms. The ongoing Rubeosis Anti-VEGF (RAVE) trial will utilize a longer follow-up time and specifically investigate whether use of an anti-VEGF agent soon after onset of ischemic CRVO will prevent NVG and reduce the need for PRP.

## Bibliography

Aiello LP, Avery RL, Arrigg PG, et al. VEGF in ocular fluid of patients with diabetic retinopathy and other retinal disorders. *N Engl J Med*. 1994;331:1519–1520.

A randomized clinical trial of early panretinal photocoagulation for ischemic central vein occlusion. The Central Vein Occlusion Study Group N report. *Ophthalmology*. 1995;102:1434–1444.

Boyd SR, Zachary I, Chakravarthy U, et al. Correlation of increased VEGF with NV and permeability in ischemic central vein occlusion. *Arch Ophthalmol*. 2002;120:1644–1650.

Ferrara DC, Koizumi H, Spaide RF. Early bevacizumab treatment of central retinal vein occlusion. *Am J Ophthalmol*. 2007;144:864–871.

Hayreh SS. Neovascular Glaucoma. *Prog Retin Eye Res*. 2007;26(5):470–485.

Hayreh SS, Rojas P, Podhajsky P, et al. Ocular NV with retinal vascular occlusion – III. Incidence of ocular NV with retinal vein occlusion. *Ophthalmology*. 1983;90:488–506.

Hsu J, Kaiser RS, Sivalingam A, et al. Intravitreal bevacizumab (Avastin) in central retinal vein occlusion. *Retina*. 2007;27:1013–1019.

Pe'er J, Folberg R, Itin A, et al. VEGF upregulation in human central retinal vein occlusion. *Ophthalmology*. 1998;105:412–416.

Priluck IA, Robertson DM, Hollenhorst RW. Long-term follow-up of occlusion of the central retinal vein in young adults. *Am J Ophthalmol*. 1980;90:190–202.

Prilinger SG, Wolf AH, Kreutzer TC, et al. Intravitreal bevacizumab injections for treatment of central retinal vein occlusion: 6-month results of a prospective trial. *Retina*. 2007;27:1004–1012.

Rubeosis Anti-VEGF (RAVE) Trial for Ischemic Central Retinal Vein Occlusion. http://clinicaltrials.gov/ct2/show/nct00406471. Accessed August 30, 2008.

The Central Vein Occlusion Study Group. Baseline and early natural history report. *Arch Ophthalmol*. 1993;111:1087–1095.

The Central Vein Occlusion Study Group: Natural history and clinical management of central retinal vein occlusion. *Arch Ophthalmol*. 1997;115:486–491.

Tripathi RC, Li J, Tripathi BJ, et al. Increased level of VEGF in aqueous humor of patients with NVG. *Ophthalmology*. 1998;105:232–237.

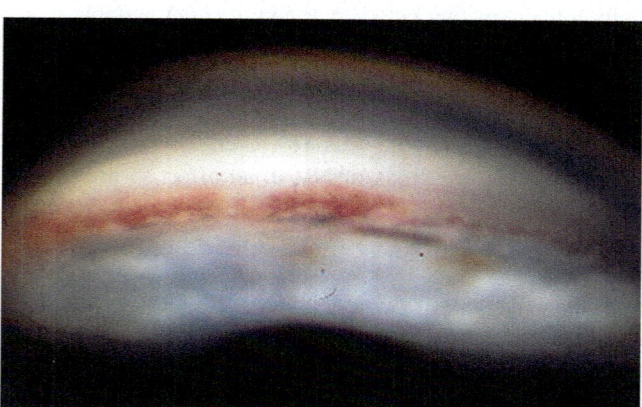

**Fig. 40.7** Clinically obvious angle NV in type I diabetes without pupillary NV being clinically evident

in which relatively huge vessels can course irregularly across the iris surface.

## 40.3 Treatment of Neovascular Glaucoma

Early recognition of NVG in at-risk eyes is crucial to favorable long-term outcome. If the patient presents in crisis, the immediate goal is to lower IOP and clear the cornea to permit assessment of anterior and posterior involvement. Recognition of retinal ischemia should prompt urgent intravitreal anti-VEGF injection and subsequent pan-retinal photocoagulation (PRP) with follow-on medication as necessary to control IOP and allow time (2–6 weeks) for vessel remission. If NV goes into remission but IOP remains unacceptable in spite of maximal medication, then filtering surgery (trabeculectomy or aqueous shunt) is indicated. In the face of persistent rubeosis and high IOP, an aqueous shunt is probably preferable but will likely provide only transient benefit. With unclear media (persisting corneal edema, cataract) ultrasound evaluation is often necessary to evaluate the potential for an anterior chamber shunt for temporary relief of IOP, hoping for corneal clearing. In cases with advanced cataract, cataract extraction or pars plana vitrectomy, lensectomy, endolaser, and shunt-tube repositioning via the pars plana may be indicated. With an opaque cornea but useful vision potential, a keratoprosthesis-pars plana vitrectomy, lensectomy, endolaser, shunt installation, and penetrating keratoplasty may still be possible.

### 40.3.1 PRP

Following numerous publications on treatment of diabetic retinopathy by photocoagulation in 1976, pan-retinal photocoagulation (PRP) has remained the "gold standard" treatment for diabetic retinopathy.[10] Rubeosis will often regress within 3–6 weeks of adequate PRP and in many cases remain quiescent thereafter. Recurrence of proliferative retinopathy after complete PRP may respond to additional PRP, traditionally the first-choice additional intervention. Meshwork vessels noted gonioscopically prior to PRP with open or only partially closed angles, often become invisible over several subsequent weeks with stabilization of angle-closure and improvement in IOP control.

## 40.3.2 Anti-VEGF

Vascular endothelial growth factor is a key regulator of angiogenesis; stimulates proliferation, migration, and survival of endothelial cells; promotes vascular permeability; and induces endothelial vasodilatation. VEGF-A, commonly known as VEGF, is the only member of the VEGF gene family induced by hypoxia.[11] Recent and ongoing clinical studies have clearly documented the clinical benefits of intravitreal injections – of bevacizumab (Avastin), ranibizumab (Lucentis), and pegaptanib (Macugen) – in some types of macular degeneration and have generated great hope for improved therapy in other retinal bleeding disorders including diabetic retinopathy.[12] Several recent case reports, albeit with only days to a few weeks follow-up, provide incentive for continued study of these new therapies.[13-18] At present, bevacizumab intravitreal injections are widely used as the initial therapy for NVG, prior to PRP, which is seemingly logical, especially if the angle is still at least partially open. Remarkable remission of iris and angle vessels, as with disc or retinal NV, may be seen over a few days; and clinically the duration of effect (suppression) of iris and angle NV after an intravitreal injection of bevacizumab without additional therapy lasts approximately 3–6 weeks. Pharmacokinetic studies in rabbits comparing 0.5 mg intravitreal ranibizumab (Lucentis) to 1.25 mg bevacizumab (Avastin) indicated that the vitreous half-life of ranibizumab is 2.28 days compared to 4.32 days for bevacizumab.[19] Cross-over to the uninjected opposite rabbit eye was found only with bevacizumab.[19]

## 40.3.3 Medical Therapy of Neovascular Glaucoma

The rationale for specific topical agents in neovascular glaucoma depends on the stage of the disease when discovered. If the angle is sufficiently closed to explain high IOP, aqueous suppressants (beta-blockers, alpha-agonists, systemic carbonic anhydrase inhibitors) are the most likely to be beneficial. Miotic agents may only add irritation and are usually ineffective in lowering IOP. Prostaglandins may be helpful but also prove irritating. If photophobia is present, steroids and cycloplegics may be useful. Paracentesis may precipitate bleeding from iris or angle vessels but can provide a jump start for medical therapy, temporarily lowering IOP with instant relief of pain and corneal edema. Atropine and topical steroids have been widely recommended for chronic use in otherwise intractable NVG in poor vision eyes and can mitigate discomfort, usually from corneal edema, long-term. Over months in some blind painful eyes with NVG, the corneal surface may vascularize and pain may disappear.

## 40.3.4 Surgical Therapy of Neovascular Glaucoma

### 40.3.4.1 Trabeculectomy

Generally, substantial benefit to long-term outcome in NVG will result from pre-surgical control of IOP via anti-VEGF intravitreal injection and PRP. Venting aqueous via filtering surgery when ischemic retinal tissues are still generating VEGF just transfers the stimulus for fibrovascular proliferation to extraocular tissues, leading to high risk of surgical failure. Filtering surgery or shunt installations in the face of florid NV will often be complicated by excessive bleeding, either extra- or intraocular. While aqueous shunts have the advantage of not requiring an iridectomy when placed in the anterior chamber, they have the disadvantage of requiring substantial space between the cornea and iris for anterior chamber tube insertion. They can be successfully placed through peripheral iris (PAS) into the posterior chamber in pseudophakic eyes or via the pars plana in vitrectomized eyes.

Pre-PRP trabeculectomy for NVG in the older literature was reported as having relatively poor success, approximately 50–60% at 1-year with improvement after anti-fibrotic use began.[20] Tsai et al reported follow-up out to 5 years in a retrospective case series after 5-flurouracil (5-FU) use in 34 eyes undergoing filtering surgery for NVG, 85% of which had prior retinal ablation. Success at 1 year (IOP<21 with/without medications) was poor among patients <50 years of age (23%), mostly type I diabetics, but far better (95%) among those >50 years of age, mostly type II diabetics.[21] In a prospective randomized trial comparing 5-FU to mitomycin-C (MMC) in non-NVG filtering surgery, Kitazawa et al found MMC superior (88% vs. 47% success defined as IOP≤20 mmHg).[22] However, in a recent randomized prospective study of filtering surgery in NVGs comparing 5-FU to MMC, there was no difference in IOP outcomes (IOP<21 mmHg) at 35 months between the two agents.[23] Although there is ongoing experimentation, no reports have yet appeared regarding the benefits, if any, of the new anti-VEGF agents to long-term outcome after filtering surgery in NVG.

### 40.3.4.2 Aqueous Shunts

Aqueous shunts are preferred by many for NVG not responding to PRP and maximal medications. Advantages of shunts include no necessity for an iridectomy during anterior chamber installation, decreasing the risk of bleeding. In any case, a shunt is likely to better tolerate intraoperative and postoperative bleeding or massive fibrin reaction than trabeculectomy with an increased likelihood of continued function. Non-valved shunts (Baerveldt, Molteno) are probably less likely to be obstructed by hemorrhage or fibrin than valved shunts (Ahmed, Krupin). Shunts are technically easier to place in inflamed eyes than standard filters and may be the best option for rapid IOP control when hyphema, inflammation, and corneal edema preclude PRP. Tissue plasminogen activator (tPA) may be useful to clear fibrin or blood after trabeculectomy or shunt installations.[24] No studies have yet been published as to the additional benefits, if any, of anti-VEGF prior to or after aqueous shunt installations in NVG. Long-term outcome of Molteno implants in NVG has been recently updated by Every et al who found IOPs < 21 mmHg with success rates at 1, 2, and 5 years respectively of 72, 60, and 40% with double-plate Molteno implants.[25] In an earlier report by Broadway et al, a small series of double-plate Molteno implants in NVG cases were only 40% successful at 2 years.[26]

In a quasi-randomized prospective trial, Susanna et al did not find partial excision of Tenon's with MMC during Ahmed shunt installations helpful in refractory NVG.[27] Costa et al also found MMC not useful in Ahmed shunt installations in a mixed group of neovascular and non-neovascular refractory glaucomas.[28] Cantor et al also found no benefit of MMC with double-plate Molteno implants in a small study of mixed neovascular and non-neovascular cases.[29] Among published prospective randomized trials, only Duan et al found benefit of MMC including ultrasound evidence of larger blebs.[30] Lima et al found no difference in outcomes in a series of mixed neovascular and non-neovascular refractory cases between endocyclophotocoagulation and Ahmed shunts.[31]

### 40.3.4.3 Cyclophotocoagulation

Most glaucoma specialists prefer filtering surgery or aqueous shunts to cyclophotocoagulation in eyes with vision better than 20/400, based on the presumption that the latter is more destructive, only temporizing, and more likely to provoke phthisis. Transscleral diode, probably the most generally available method of cyclodestruction present in the United States, is effective and less likely to result in phthisis than earlier methods such as cyclocryotherapy (Fig. 40.8).[32,33] Endoscopic cyclophotocoagulation (ECP) has become increasingly popular, but for maximal effect requires two-site intraocular surgery and may be more appropriate as the glaucoma part of combined cataract and glaucoma procedures in relatively healthy non-neovascular eyes than for IOP control in NVG.[34]

## 40.4 Conclusion

Our understanding of the pathophysiology and therapy of NVG has come a long way in a relatively short time. Quoting Duke-Elder (1969) "…the only practical treatment, if a

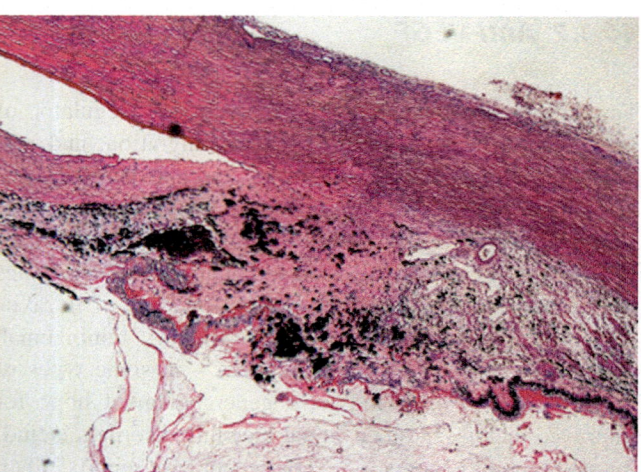

**Fig. 40.8** Relatively discrete anterior and mid-ciliary body injury after cyclodiode treatment many months before enucleation. Disruption of ciliary muscle and pigment dispersion, some in macrophages, is apparent. The anterior-most ciliary processes appear to have been spared (hematoxylin and eosin, original magnification ×50)

retrobulbar injection of alcohol or cyclodiathermy fails to relieve the pain, is enucleation."[35] Surely the most fundamentally important advances in therapy since Duke-Elders' time have included the realization that PRP could in most cases stabilize the disease and that tight glucose control greatly decreased its incidence. Perhaps we are now on the threshold of vastly improved adjunctive treatment with the new anti-VEFG agents.

## References

1. Weiss DI, Shaffer RN, Nehrenberg TR. Neovascular glaucoma complicating carotid-cavernous fistula. *Arch Ophthalmol.* 1963; 69:304–307.
2. Wand M. Neovascular glaucoma. In: Ritch R, Shields MB, Krupin T, eds. *The Glaucomas – Clinical Science.* 2nd ed. St. Louis: Mosby; 1996:1073–1129. Ch 51.
3. Sivak-Callcott JA, O'Day DM, Gass JD, et al. Evidence-based recommendations for the diagnosis and treatment of neovascular glaucoma. *Ophthalmology.* 2001;108:1767–1776.
4. Hayreh SS. Neovascular glaucoma. *Prog Retin Eye Res.* 2007; 26(5):470–485.
5. Yoneya S, Numaga T, Yamazaki S, et al. Neovascularization of iris demonstrated in kittens with ROP. *Nippon Ganka Gakkai Zasshi.* 1982;86(9):1251–1261.
6. Bron AJ, Tripathi RC, Tripathi BJ. *Wolff's Anatomy of the Eye and Orbit.* London: Chapman and Hall Medical; 1993:377. Ch 11.
7. Sassani JT, Eagle RC. The myofibroblastic component of rubeosis iridis. *Ophthalmology.* 1983;90:721–728.
8. Diabetes control and complications trial research group. Progression of retinopathy with intensive versus conventional treatment in the Diabetes Control and Complications Trial. *Ophthalmology.* 1995;102:647–661.
9. Ohnishi Y, et al. Fluorescein gonioangiography in diabetic neovascularization. *Graefes Arch Clin Exp Ophthalmol.* 1994;232:199–204.

10. Diabetic retinopathy study group. Preliminary report on effects of photocoagulation therapy. *Am J Ophthalmol.* 1976;81:383–396.
11. Ferrara N. Vascular endothelial growth factor: basic science and clinical progress. *Endocr Rev.* 2004;25:581–611.
12. Andreoli CM, Miller JW. Anti-vascular endothelial growth factor therapy for ocular neovascular disease. *Curr Opin Ophthalmol.* 2007;18:502–508.
13. Avery RL. Regression of retinal and iris neovascularization after intravitreal bevacizumab (Avastin) treatment. *Retina.* 2006;26:354–356.
14. Davidorf FH, Mouser JG, Derick RJ. Rapid improvement of rubeosis iridis from a single bevacizumab (Avastin) injection. *Retina.* 2006;26:354–356.
15. Kahook MY, Schuman JS, Noecker RJ. Intravitreal bevacizumab in a patient with neovascular glaucoma. *Ophthalmic Surg Lasers Imaging.* 2006;37:144–146.
16. Paula JS, Jorge R, Costa RA, et al. Short-term results of intravitreal bevacizumab (Avastin) on anterior segment neovascularization in neovascular glaucoma. *Acta Ophthalmol Scand.* 2006;84:556–557.
17. Grisanti S, Bieter S, Peters S, et al. The Tuebingen bevacizumab study group. Intravitreal bevacizumab (Avastin) in the treatment of neovascular glaucoma. *Am J Ophthalmol.* 2006;142:158–160.
18. Yazdani S, Hendi K, Pakravan M. Intravitreal bevacizumab (Avastin) injection for neovascular glaucoma. *J Glaucoma.* 2007;16:437–439.
19. Bakri SJ, Snyder R, Reid JM, et al. Pharamoacokinetics of intravitreal ranibizumab (Lucentis). *Ophthalmology.* 2007;114:2179–2182.
20. Katz LJ, Costa VP, Spaeth GL. Filtration surgery. In: Ritch R, Shields MB, Krupin T, eds. *The Glaucomas.* 2nd ed. St. Louis: Mosby; 1996:1682. Ch 83.
21. Tsai JC, Feuer WJ, Parrish RK 2nd, et al. 5-Flurouracil filtering surgery and neovascular glaucoma – long-term follow-up of the original pilot study. *Ophthalmology.* 1995;102:887–892.
22. Kitazawa Y, Kawase K, Matsushita H, et al. Trabeculectomy with mitomycin. A comparative study with fluorouracil. *Arch Ophthalmol.* 1991;109:1693–1698.
23. Sisto D, Vetrugno M, Trabucco T, et al. The role of antimetabolites in filtration surgery for neovascular glaucoma: intermediate-term follow-up. *Acta Ophthalmol Scand.* 2007;85:267–271.
24. Sidoti PA, Morinelli EN, Heuer DK, et al. Tissue plasminogen activator and glaucoma drainage implants. *J Glaucoma.* 1995;4:258–262.
25. Every SG, Molteno AC, Bevin TH, et al. Long-term results of Molteno implant insertion in cases of neovascular glaucoma. *Arch Ophthalmol.* 2006;124:355–360.
26. Broadway DC, Tester M, Schulzer M, et al. Survival analysis for success of Molteno tube implants. *Br J Ophthalmol.* 2001;85:689–695.
27. Susanna R Jr, Latin American Glaucoma Society. Partial Tenon's capsule resection with adjunctive MMC in Ahmed glaucoma valve implant surgery. *Br J Ophthalmol.* 2003;87:994–998.
28. Costa VP, Azuara-Blanco A, Netland PA, et al. Efficacy and safety of adjunctive mitomycin-C during Ahmed glaucoma valve implantation: a prospective randomized clinical trial. *Ophthalmology.* 2004;111:1071–1076.
29. Cantor L, Burgoyne J, Sanders S, et al. The effect of mitomycin C on Molteno implant surgery: a 1-year randomized masked, prospective study. *J Glaucoma.* 1998;7:240–246.
30. Duan X, Jiang Y, Qing G. Long-term follow-up study on Hunan aqueous drainage implantation combined with mitomycin-C for refractory glaucoma. *Yan Ke Xue Bao Bian Ji Bu.* 2003;19(2):81–85.
31. Lima FE, Magacho L, Carvalho DM, et al. A prospective, comparative study between endoscopic cyclophotocoagulation and the Ahmed drainage implant in refractory glaucoma. *J Glaucoma.* 2004;13:233–237.
32. Callens C, D'Hondt K, Zeyen T. The long-term effect of diode laser cyclodestruction on intraocular pressure. *Bull Soc Belge Ophthalmol.* 2003;289:81–86.
33. Hamard P, Gayraud JM, Kopel J, et al. Treatment of refractory glaucomas by transscleral cyclophotocoagulation using semiconductor diode laser. Analysis of 50 patients followed-up over 19 months. *J Fr Ophthalmol.* 1997;20:125–133.
34. Kahook MY, Lathrop KL, Noecker RJ. One-site versus two-site cyclophotocoagulation. *J Glaucoma.* 2007;16:527–530.
35. Duke-Elder S, Jay B. System of ophthalmology. *Haemorrhagic Glaucoma*, vol. XI. London: Henry Kimpton; 1969:667.

# Chapter 41
# Inflammatory Disease and Glaucoma

Sunita Radhakrishnan, Emmett T. Cunningham Jr, and Andrew Iwach

## 41.1 Introduction

Elevated intraocular pressure (IOP) is a common, but challenging complication of ocular inflammation. When IOP elevation in the setting of uveitis is temporary and does not damage the optic nerve, the term uveitis-related ocular hypertension is most appropriate. Uveitic "glaucoma" must be reserved for cases of uveitis in which elevated IOP is associated with optic nerve damage, which manifests as changes in the optic nerve structure and/or the presence of visual field defects.

The overall prevalence of secondary glaucoma in all forms of uveitis has been reported to be between 5 and 19% in adults and from 5 to 13.5% in children.[1] Anterior uveitis, older age at presentation, and chronic inflammation are all related to a higher prevalence of uveitic glaucoma. Certain types of uveitis, such as herpetic keratouveitis and anterior uveitis, associated with Juvenile Idiopathic Arthritis are also associated with a higher prevalence of secondary glaucoma.

## 41.2 Mechanisms of Elevated IOP in Patients with Uveitis

### 41.2.1 How Does Inflammation Affect the IOP?

Inflammation in the eye results in multiple cellular, biochemical, and morphological alterations that can affect IOP. In general, acute inflammation tends to cause a decrease in IOP, initially due to a combination of decreased aqueous production and increased aqueous outflow. This change in aqueous dynamics is offset in two ways. First, the appearance of inflammatory cells and proteins in the aqueous renders it more viscous or "plastic." Second, the trabecular meshwork itself can be altered by the direct involvement in the inflammatory response or via inflammatory mediators (trabeculitis). Thus, the initial IOP can be increased, normal, or decreased. Moreover, the relative contributions of decreased inflow and increased outflow resistance can vary throughout the course of the inflammatory process. Morphologic changes in the anterior chamber angle can also result in elevated IOP, by either pupillary block or non-pupillary block mechanisms. The treatment of uveitis with corticosteroids can result in elevated outflow resistance and thereby increase the IOP. Finally, chronic, progressive morphological changes in the ciliary body can result in chronic hypotony and eventually phthisis.

### 41.2.2 Clinical Classification of Uveitis-Related Elevation in IOP

For clinical purposes, it is useful to consider the status of the anterior chamber angle as well as the timing of the rise in IOP relative to the onset of inflammation. Based on these factors, uveitic ocular hypertension or glaucoma can be classified as follows (see Fig. 41.1):

1. Inflammatory Ocular Hypertension Syndromes (IOHS)
2. Acute Uveitic Angle Closure
3. Corticosteroid-Induced Ocular Hypertension/Glaucoma
4. Chronic, Mixed-Mechanism Ocular Hypertension/Glaucoma

#### 41.2.2.1 Inflammatory Ocular Hypertension Syndromes

Elevated IOP in patients with IOHS is believed to result from direct inflammation of the trabecular meshwork or trabeculitis. The IOP elevation in these syndromes parallels the course of the inflammation. The most common condition causing IOHS is herpetic anterior uveitis caused by either herpes simplex or herpes zoster infection. Other well-recognized causes of IOHS include cytomegalovirus infection, sarcoidosis, toxoplasmosis, syphilis, and Posner Schlossman syndrome.[2,3]

Traditionally, herpetic anterior uveitis can be caused by either herpes simplex virus (HSV) or varicella zoster virus (VZV), and nearly 30% of patients with anterior uveitis caused by either of these viruses develop secondary ocular

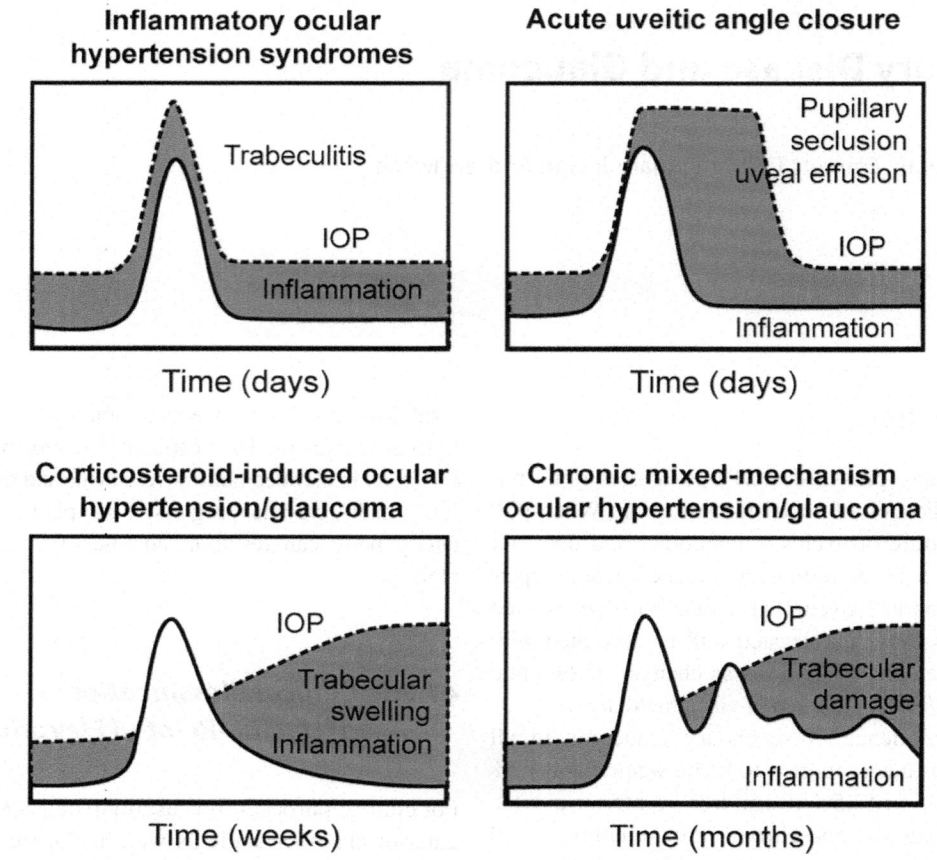

**Fig. 41.1** Classification scheme for elevated IOP in uveitis based on underlying mechanism and timing of IOP rise with respect to the onset of inflammation.

hypertension. Corneal epithelial or stromal involvement is common in such cases and should be looked for to support the diagnosis. Iris stromal atrophy, either patchy or sectoral (see Fig. 41.2), is caused by virus-induced ischemia and is a unique finding that differentiates herpetic anterior uveitis from other causes of IOHS, but may not be present in all cases.

In Posner Schlossman syndrome, or glaucomatocyclitic crisis, there is unilateral, episodic and acute, severe elevation of IOP. Patients are generally young and present with pain and blurred vision. The inflammation seen in this syndrome is characteristically mild and appears out of proportion to the rise in IOP. A number of authors have reported herpes virus DNA in patients diagnosed clinically as having Posner Schlossman syndrome, suggesting that at least some patients with this condition have what might be considered *form fruste* herpetic anterior uveitis.

IOHS may be confused with clinical entities in which noninflammatory material blocks the trabecular pores causing a rise in IOP. Thus, lens material in phacolytic glaucoma, red blood cells in microhyphema, and photoreceptor outer segments in Schwartz – Matsuo syndrome may all mimic inflammatory cells and result in misdiagnosis as IOHS.

The importance of identifying IOHS lies in the fact that most causes of this rather unique presentation are infectious in nature. Once IOHS is accurately diagnosed, an appropriate workup to identify and treat the causative microbial agent can be initiated. In general, co-management of these cases with a specialist in ocular inflammation is desirable.

#### 41.2.2.2 Acute Uveitic Angle Closure

In this category, elevation in IOP occurs with or soon after the onset of inflammation but may take longer to resolve than the inflammation. Acute uveitic angle closure can be caused by two mechanisms:

1. Pupillary block: Seclusion of the pupil by extensive posterior synechiae or an inflammatory pupillary membrane can result in iris bombe and angle closure (see Fig. 41.3). This mechanism can occur even in patients with open angles prior to the onset of uveitis.

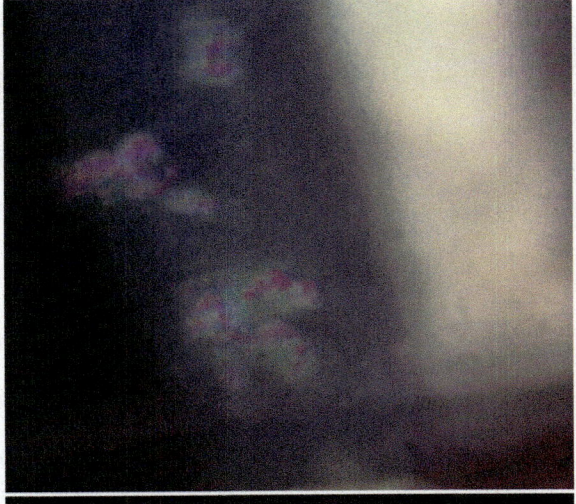

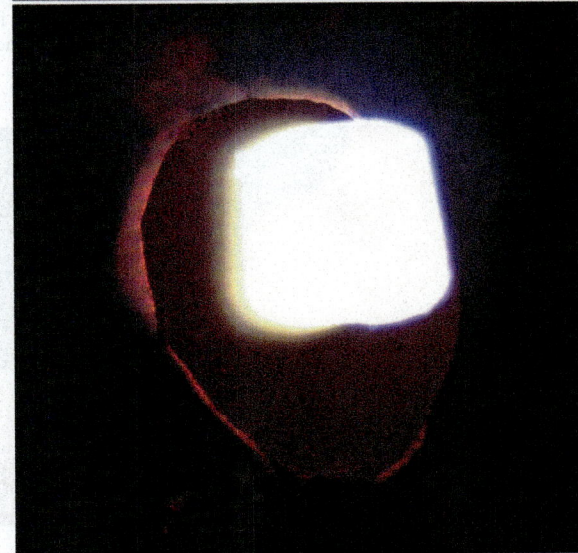

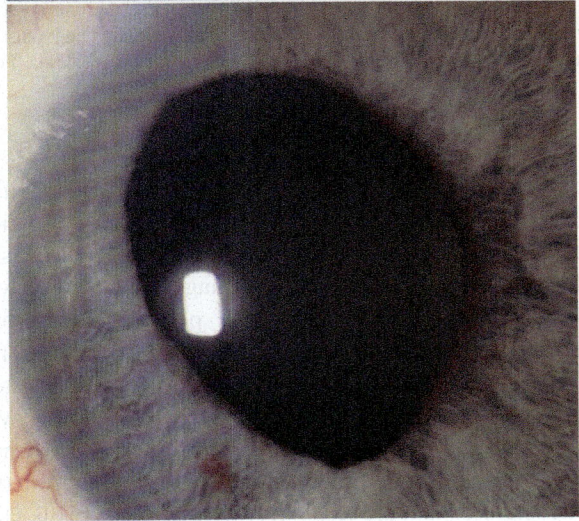

**Fig. 41.2** A patient with herpes zoster keratouveitis. Top panel shows multiple pseudodentrites stained centrally with Rose Bengal and outlined in green by pooled fluorescein. Middle and bottom panels show correctopia with areas of atrophy at the pupillary margin visualized using transillumination. Iris atrophy can be observed in the setting of both herpes simplex and herpes zoster infection

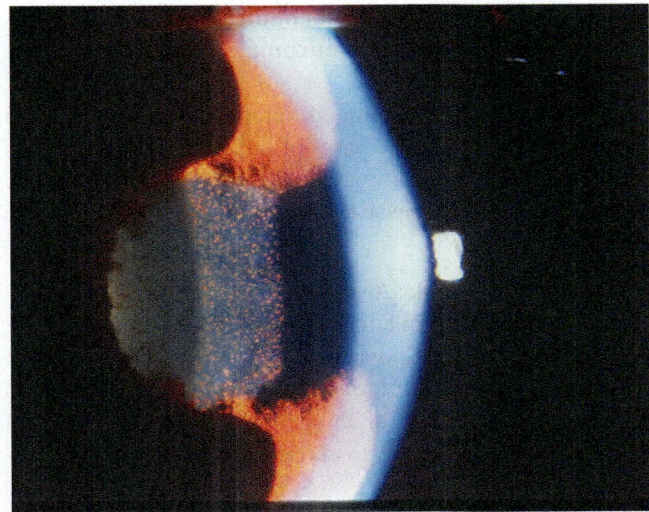

**Fig. 41.3** Iris bombe in a patient with seclusion following a severe episode of HLA-B27 associated anterior uveitis

2. Non-pupillary block: A forward movement of the lens-iris diaphragm due to ciliochoroidal effusion can also result in angle closure by a "pushing" mechanism. Iris bombe is not seen with this mechanism.

Detailed slit lamp examination can usually help differentiate the two mechanisms; however, in some cases, imaging of the posterior chamber with ultrasound biomicroscopy may be required. Identifying the mechanism of angle closure in this category is important because treatment differs significantly between the two. In pupillary-block angle closure, the recommended treatment is a laser peripheral iridotomy, whereas in non-pupillary block angle closure due to a ciliochoroidal effusion, cycloplegia, and systemic corticosteroids are the mainstay of treatment. Understanding the mechanism of angle closure also helps in establishing the diagnosis, as ciliochoroidal effusions are more common in certain uveitic conditions such as Vogt-Koyanagi-Harada disease, scleritis, and sympathetic ophthalmia.

### 41.2.2.3 Corticosteroid-Induced Ocular Hypertension/Glaucoma

Corticosteroid-induced IOP elevation tends to occur days to weeks after the onset of uveitis and initiation of treatment with corticosteroids. The mechanism is believed to be related to a reduction in aqueous outflow mediated by wide-ranging effects on the trabecular meshwork at the cellular and biochemical levels. All routes of corticosteroid administration can be associated with elevated IOP, including topical, periocular intraocular, systemic, and intranasal (see Chap. 57 Intravitreal Steroids).

### 41.2.2.4 Chronic, Mixed-Mechanism Ocular Hypertension/Glaucoma

Many patients with uveitis develop ocular hypertension months to years after the onset of inflammation for reasons unrelated to IOHS, acute angle closure, or corticosteroids. Mechanisms of IOP elevation in this group of patients can be classified as follows:

1. Chronic closed angle: Angle closure by the "pulling" mechanism occurs via formation of peripheral anterior synechiae or of vascular membranes such as in Fuchs heterochromic iridocyclitis and other forms of chronic uveitis.
2. Open angle: In spite of an open angle, there is increased outflow resistance due to chronic damage to the trabecular meshwork.

Juvenile Idiopathic Arthritis, sarcoidosis, and Fuchs heterochromic iridocyclitis are commonly associated with chronic mixed-mechanism IOP elevation. In Fuchs iridocyclitis, there is chronic, usually unilateral, low-grade iridocyclitis characterized by diffusely distributed stellate keratic precipitates and iris heterochromia (see Fig. 41.4), often accompanied by whitish vitreous cellular infiltrates. Unlike many types of uveitis, the inflammation in this entity is often asymptomatic and posterior synechiae are uncommon despite the presence of persistent inflammation. Nearly all patients develop posterior subcapsular cataract and up to 60% develop secondary glaucoma.

In sarcoidosis-related anterior uveitis, the incidence of glaucoma ranges from 11 to 26%. The inflammation in sarcoidosis tends to be "fibrin-rich" with the formation of iris nodules (see Fig. 41.5) and keratic precipitates on the trabecular meshwork resulting in the development of posterior and anterior peripheral synechiae, respectively. The uveitis also tends to be chronic with morphological changes in the angle being common in the later stages.

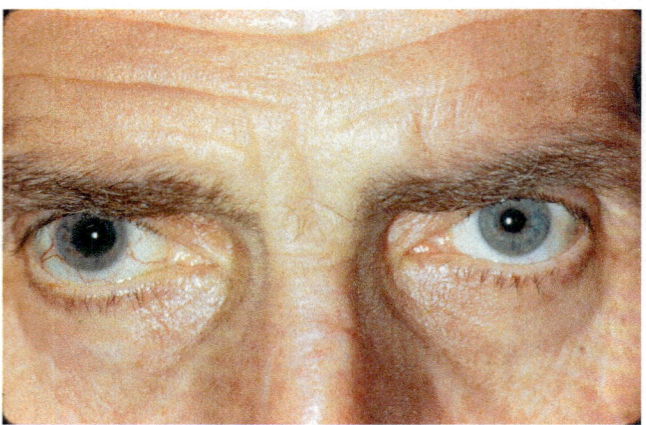

**Fig. 41.4** Iris heterochromia in a patient with Fuchs heterochromic iridocyclitis. Note that the affected, right eye is darker in appearance in this patient with lightly pigmented irides, whereas the affected iris in a patient with darkly pigmented irides is typically lighter in appearance

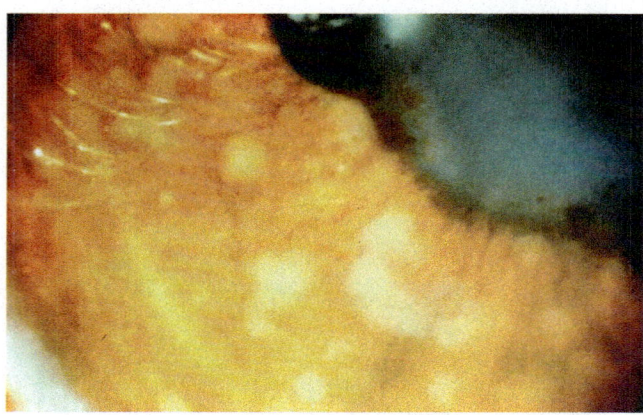

**Fig. 41.5** Busacca nodules on the iris in a patient with sarcoidosis. Reproduced with permission from Cunningham ET Jr. Diagnosis and management of acute anterior uveitis. *Am Acad Ophthalmol*, Focal Points 2002

## 41.3 Managing Elevated IOP in Patients with Uveitis

### 41.3.1 General Principles

Co-management with a uveitis specialist is ideal, but not always feasible. In general, the underlying inflammation must be treated as necessary. Under-treating uveitis with corticosteroids in order to minimize IOP elevation is a short-sighted strategy because the long-term risks of chronic inflammation far outweigh the benefits of short-term IOP control. Treatment of IOP elevation must be undertaken with the optic nerve status in mind. In many patients with uveitis, the optic disc is not severely damaged and the target IOP does not need to be very low. The timing of IOP elevation can also help in management – a patient with acute rises in IOP observed only during episodes of inflammation can probably be managed adequately with medical therapy alone, whereas a patient with chronic mixed mechanism glaucoma is more likely to require surgical intervention. In patients who develop ocular hypertension in response to corticosteroids, alternative therapy with weaker corticosteroids or immunosuppressive therapy may be considered, although it should be remembered that corticosteroids that are less likely to raise IOP are also less likely to control moderate to severe inflammation. Use of long-acting depot corticosteroid preparations in these patients must be undertaken with particular caution, and preferably only after a sustained trial of either topical or systemic corticosteroid therapy has shown that the risk of corticosteroid induced ocular hypertension is low.

## 41.3.2 The Therapeutic Armamentarium

Treatment options available in the management of uveitic glaucoma are as follows:

Topical hypotensive therapy for raised IOP in uveitis is similar to treatment for primary open angle glaucoma (POAG) with a few caveats. Prostaglandin analogs, which have replaced beta-blockers as first line of therapy for POAG in many practices, must be used with caution in patients with uveitis because they may have a proinflammatory effect. Although no clear cause-effect relationship has been demonstrated, a number of case reports have suggested that these drugs may exacerbate preexisting iridocyclitis, promote recurrences of herpetic keratitis or keratouveitis, and promote the formation of cystoid macular edema.[4,5] It seems most prudent, therefore, that these agents be used as second- or third-line therapy in patients with uveitis and that when they are used, the treating physician remains mindful of the possibility for inflammatory side effects. It must be noted, however, that prostaglandin analogs are not contraindicated in uveitic ocular hypertension/glaucoma and that they can be very useful in many patients, especially when controlling the IOP would otherwise require surgery. Medications that are definitely proinflammatory and must be avoided in patients with active uveitis include pilocarpine, epinephrine, and epinephrine prodrugs. For these reasons, beta-blockers are usually the first line of management for raised IOP in uveitis, followed by carbonic anhydrase inhibitors (topical and/or systemic) and alpha agonists.

### 41.3.2.1 Laser Procedures

*Laser peripheral iridotomy* is the treatment of choice for acute angle closure due to pupillary block. The inflammatory response following laser iridotomy in patients with uveitis tends to be more severe and prolonged than in patients with primary angle closure, hence the need for aggressive treatment with corticosteroids must be anticipated. In addition, there is a higher rate of closure of the iridotomy[6] and hence performing at least two iridotomies is recommended.

*Laser trabeculoplasty*: Laser trabeculoplasty does not play a significant role in the management of elevated IOP related to uveitis.

*Cyclophotocoagulation* must be used with extreme caution in uveitic glaucoma for two reasons. First, the procedure can exacerbate inflammation and second, there is a greater risk of atrophy in a ciliary body that has already sustained damage from recurrent inflammation; this can eventually lead to hypotony and/or phthisis.

### 41.3.2.2 Surgery

The decision to perform surgery depends on the IOP, the degree of nerve damage, and response as well as tolerance to medical therapy. It is beneficial to have the inflammation controlled prior to surgery, but in many patients with uveitis-associated increase in IOP, surgery is performed on an emergent rather than elective basis. These patients are for the most part already on some form of corticosteroid therapy and it is worthwhile to consider the use of systemic, periocular, and/or intraocular corticosteroids in the perioperative period. Many uveitis specialists recommend IV Solumedrol 250–1,000 mg given intraoperatively followed by a quickly tapered dose of oral prednisone, 0.5–1.5 mg/kg/day, in the postoperative period.

Both trabeculectomy with antimetabolites and aqueous drainage devices have been successfully used in the management of uveitic glaucoma. The choice depends on the likelihood of failure of trabeculectomy and surgeon preference. Active uveitis, inflammation that is difficult to control, younger age, and history of prior trabeculectomy are all associated with high risk for failure of filtering surgery and an aqueous drainage device is preferable in these patients. Patients with uveitis have a greater risk of developing hypotony following either type of surgery and modifications to the surgical technique are performed to safeguard against it. In recent years, intravitreal drug delivery devices, such as the Retisert implant,[7] are being used with increasing frequency in patients with uveitis. It is important to communicate with the surgeon that the inferotemporal quadrant may be the best position for the placement of such sustained release devices so that a superior trabeculectomy or placement of a drainage device in the superotemporal or inferonasal quadrants may be performed in the future as indicated.

*Trabeculectomy*: Trabeculectomy without antifibrosis agents has a relatively low (30–50%) chance of survival in patients with uveitis,[8,9] therefore use of either 5-fluorouracil (5-FU) or mitomycin-C (MMC) is recommended. Success rates of 75–90% with mitomycin-C[10,11] and 50–90% with 5-fluorouracil[9,12-14] have been reported depending on the definition of success, lens status, and level of risk for failure. There is no direct comparative study to support the use of one agent over the other, and the choice depends mainly on surgeon preference. Many surgeons also use 5-FU injections postoperatively.

Uveitic eyes are particularly at risk for postoperative hypotony, therefore the scleral flap must be sutured tightly. If hypotony does develop and is accompanied by shallowing of the anterior chamber, cycloplegia can help move the lens-iris diaphragm posteriorly. The frequency of postoperative corticosteroid therapy is determined based on the balance between the need to control active inflammation and the need to accelerate healing (thereby decreasing overfiltration). Topical corticosteroids are generally used for 6–8 weeks postoperatively and may need to be tapered slowly.

*Aqueous Drainage Devices*: In recent years, the indications for aqueous drainage implantation have expanded considerably. For many surgeons, aqueous drainage devices are the procedure of choice in uveitic glaucoma. Both the valved Ahmed and the non-valved Baerveldt implant have been used for IOP control in such patients. When using the Baerveldt implant, the choice between the 250 mm$^2$ or the 350 mm$^2$ device should theoretically be based on the balance between the opposing risks of hypotony and postoperative encapsulation. In practice, however, the 350 mm$^2$ device tends to be used most commonly. There are a relatively small number of studies that have reported outcomes of aqueous drainage device implantation specifically in uveitic patients. Of these, the longest follow-up with Ahmed implants was reported by Papadaki and associates[15] and the largest series of uveitic patients with Baerveldt implants was reported by Ceballos and associates.[16]

Success rates in the study by Papadaki and associates were 77% and 57% at 1 and 4 years, respectively, with the definition of success being IOP of 5–21 mmHg plus 25% lowering from preoperative levels. At 4 years follow-up, 74% of patients required topical medication for IOP control. The overall complication rate was 12% per person-years with corneal edema or graft failure being the most common (3.2% per person-years). The occurrence of severe hypotony defined as flat anterior chamber, choroidal effusion, hypotony maculopathy, or any combination thereof was 1.2% per person-years. In the study by Ceballos and colleagues,[16] the success rate was 92% at 2 years with the definition of success being IOP of 5–21 mmHg without need for further glaucoma surgery, loss of light perception, or phthisis. The most common complications were choroidal effusions (4 of 24 eyes), hypotony, and cystoid macular edema (3 of 24 eyes for both).

*Other Surgical Procedures*: Goniotomy,[17] viscocanalostomy,[18] and trabeculodialysis[19,20] have all been reported for the treatment of uveitic glaucoma with success rates varying from 50 to 71%. Trabeculodialysis is a modified goniotomy procedure in which the trabecular meshwork is further released via wing incisions to maximize direct aqueous access into Schlemm's canal. In our experience, this procedure is especially useful in children with uveitis and elevated IOP. A newer device, called the Trabectome[21] has recently been developed for ab-interno trabeculectomy. Although, there is no data yet on its efficacy in patients with uveitic glaucoma, it may be an attractive option in patients with well-controlled inflammation and mild optic nerve damage.

### 41.3.3 Specific Treatment Strategies

Management can be tailored to the individual patient based on the mechanism of IOP elevation:

#### 41.3.3.1 Management of IOHS

A complete history and directed uveitis workup should be performed for all patients with uveitis, regardless of whether the IOP is elevated, low, or normal (see Sidebar 41.1). In patients with IOHS and no clear evidence of herpetic infection, most would recommend testing for sarcoidosis with a chest X-ray and serum angiotensin converting enzyme (ACE) or lysozyme level and for syphilis with an FTA-ABS and a VDRL or RPR. The fundus should also be examined carefully for any evidence of toxoplasmic retinochoroiditis. Patients with Posner-Schlossman syndrome can be especially challenging to diagnose as the inflammatory response can be very subtle and the eye examination is typically normal between attacks. The IOP elevation in patients with IOHS typically reverses with treatment of the underlying inflammatory/infectious condition with topical corticosteroids and/or antimicrobial therapy as indicated. Patients with herpetic keratouveitis can develop a chronic relapsing-remitting course and may eventually require surgical intervention.

#### 41.3.3.2 Management of Uveitic Angle Closure

For pupillary-block acute angle closure, laser peripheral iridotomy is the treatment of choice. At least two iridotomies are recommended due to the possibility of aqueous in the posterior chamber being loculated as well as the high rate of closure. Patients require close monitoring of IOP as well as inflammation following the laser procedure.

In angle closure due to a ciliochoroidal effusion or serous retinal detachment, systemic corticosteroids are indicated. Cycloplegia helps in shifting the lens-iris diaphragm posteriorly and long-acting cycloplegics such as atropine, homatropine, or scopolamine are preferred. A retina or uveitis specialist must be consulted in these cases as the underlying etiologies commonly involve the posterior segment and may have a systemic component as well.

#### 41.3.3.3 Management of Corticosteroid-Induced Ocular Hypertension/Glaucoma

In these patients, treatment of inflammation must be considered primary with IOP elevation managed secondarily by any means necessary. The choice of IOP-lowering treatment depends on the state of the inflammation and the extent of optic nerve damage. For example, a patient with active uveitis, moderate to advanced optic nerve damage, and pressure in the 40s is likely to do better with an aqueous drainage device. On the other hand, a patient with corticosteroid-induced hypertension in an eye that is now quiet may do very well with topical medications alone. In selected cases, removal of a periocular or intraocular depot of corticosteroid may result in successful resolution of the IOP elevation. In patients who require chronic corticosteroid therapy, "soft" corticosteroids such as loteprednol and rimexolone may be considered, but only once the inflammation has been largely controlled. Lowering the dose of corticosteroid can also be effective, for example using Pred-mild (0.12% prednisolone acetate) instead of Pred Forte (1% prednisolone acetate), but again should not be considered unless the inflammation is largely controlled. Nonsteroidal immunosuppressive therapy is usually considered for patients requiring long-term use of oral corticosteroids to control inflammation. It is important to note that it takes several weeks to produce an effective anti-inflammatory effect with immunosuppressive agents, and patients must be maintained on corticosteroids until then. Most patients with corticosteroid-induced ocular hypertension can be managed with topical medications, the exception being patients with IOP elevation due to the intravitreal fluocinolone implant (FA). Goldstein and associates reported that 37% of patients with the FA implant required IOP lowering surgery.[28]

### 41.3.3.4 Management of Chronic Mixed-Mechanism Ocular Hypertension/Glaucoma

Management is similar to any chronic mixed-mechanism glaucoma, with both medications and surgery being effective.

---

**SIDEBAR 41.1. Laboratory testing for uveitis in the glaucoma patient**

Omar Chaudhary and Sandra M. Johnson

Once the clinical diagnosis of uveitis has been determined in a patient, the next step is the work-up to discover its possible etiology. A wide variety of ocular and systemic diseases have been associated with uveitis. Thus, it is prudent to have a systematic manner to approach the diagnosis. If an underlying diagnosis is found, it can aid in appropriate treatment and management while contributing to the overall health of the patient.

Most clinicians have recommended avoiding blanket laboratory testing for each patient diagnosed with uveitis, because this has a low diagnostic yield with frequent false positives. It is also very expensive to do a large number of laboratory tests. Instead, it is more appropriate to use the history and physical exam to suggest a differential diagnosis that can be explored with a smaller number of laboratory tests and imaging procedures to confirm the etiology of the uveitis.

Clues from the uveitis history such as onset, duration, severity, and monocular vs. binocular involvement can help characterize the illness. Family history can also help uncover genetic disorders with uveitis components such as HLA-B27 related diseases. A thorough review of systems is often most helpful, as patients may exhibit signs and symptoms of an underlying systemic disorder that causes uveitis, at the time of presentation (see Table 41.1).

The workup of uveitis begins with narrowing the differential based on the location of inflammation. While some overlap occurs, some diseases mainly present with anterior segment inflammation (iritis or iridocyclitis) while others cause intermediate segment (pars planitis or peripheral retinitis) or posterior segment inflammation (choroiditis or choreoretinitis).

**Anterior Uveitis**

Anterior uveitis accounts for the vast majority of uveitis cases and can be divided into two broad groups based on the presence or absence of granulomatous inflammation (see Table 41.2). The presence of inflammatory nodules on the surface of the iris or mutton-fat keratic precipitates (large greasy, yellowish-white accumulations of inflammatory cells) indicates granulomatous inflammation.

All patients should have a work-up with the first case of anterior granulomatous uveitis. Lab work-up may not need to be extensive, because the past medical history, review of systems, and physical exam may point to a causative etiology. For example, herpes zoster can be suspected when interstitial corneal inflammation and iris atrophy accompanies the uveitis.

Basic laboratory work-up for all cases of *granulomatous* uveitis includes complete blood count (CBC) with differential, angiotensin converting enzyme (ACE) level, and chest X-ray to evaluate for sarcoidosis or tuberculosis, and RPR or VDRL. Even though syphilis accounts for less than 1% of uveitis cases, it should be routinely tested for because it is easily treated and syphilis may have serious neurological consequences if untreated.

**Table 41.1** Review of systems

| | |
|---|---|
| Headache | Sarcoidosis, Behçet disease, CNS lymphoma, VKH, polyarteritis nodosa, Lyme disease, toxoplasmosis, CMV |
| Neuropathy | Lyme disease, syphilis, multiple sclerosis, herpes zoster, CMV, Behçet disease |
| Cough/shortness of breath | Wegener's granulomatosis, tuberculosis, sarcoidosis |
| Diarrhea | Inflammatory bowel disease, reactive arthritis |
| Arthritis | Lyme disease, ankylosis spondylitis, reactive arthritis, inflammatory bowel disease, psoriatic arthritis, syphilis, SLE, Behçet disease, Juvenile Idiopathic Arthritis, sarcoidosis |
| Rash | Herpes zoster, Lyme disease, syphilis, psoriatic arthritis, Behçet disease, SLE, leprosy, inflammatory bowel disease, reactive arthritis |
| Oral ulcers | Behçet disease, SLE, inflammatory bowel disease, herpes zoster |
| Hematuria | Wegener's granulomatosis, SLE, polyarteritis nodosa, TINU |
| Eye Trauma | Sympathetic ophthalmia |
| Genital ulcers | Syphilis, Behçet disease, reactive arthritis |
| Ethnicity | Behçet disease – Mediterranean, Middle Eastern, Asian |

*VKH*, Vogt-Koyanagi-Harada syndrome; *CMV*, Cytomegalovirus; *SLE*, systemic lupus erythematosus; *TINU*, Tubulointerstitial Nephritis and Uveitis syndrome

**Table 41.2** Causes of anterior uveitis

| Granulomatous | Non-granulomatous |
|---|---|
| Idiopathic Sarcoidosis | HLA-B27 related |
| Auto-immune | Ankylosis spondylitis |
|   Multiple sclerosis | Psoriatic arthritis |
|   Vogt-Koyanagi-Harada syndrome | Inflammatory bowel disease |
| | Reactive arthritis |
|   Sympathetic ophthalmia | Infectious |
| Infectious | Syphilis |
|   Syphilis | Lyme disease |
|   Lyme disease | Herpes zoster |
|   Tuberculosis | Other |
|   Herpes zoster | Sarcoidosis |
|   Coccidiomycosis | Juvenile Idiopathic Arthritis |
|   Leprosy | Tubulointerstitial Nephritis and Uveitis syndrome |
|   Toxoplasmosis | |
|   Brucellosis | Fuchs heterochromic iridocyclitis |

Further work-up depends on the remaining differential. Lyme disease and toxoplasmosis serologies and a PPD may be performed. If sarcoidosis is still suspected, a chest computed tomorgraph (CT) is warranted, as 10% of patients may not have hilar lymphadenopathy seen on a chest X-ray. In addition, an enlarged lacrimal gland or conjunctival nodules may be biopsied to assess for sarcoidosis.

For nongranulomatous uveitis, further workup is usually not recommended, until after the first episode if the past medical history and review of systems are negative. However, with recurrent episodes or with severe attacks, testing for HLA-B27 is recommended, as its associated diseases have been found in up to half of cases of anterior uveitis. An ACE level and CXR should also be ordered to evaluate for sarcoidosis as well as an RPR or VDRL for syphilis. Lyme serologies and serum creatinine to evaluate for tubulointerstital nephritis associated uveitisTINU are also recommended. More in-depth workup can include a chest CT, ANA, rheumatoid factor (RF), and sacroiliac X-rays.

Physical exam findings can also aid with diagnosis. Keratic precipitates can still be seen in nongranulomatous uveitis, however they usually accumulate over the inferior half of the cornea, occasionally forming a hypopyon as seen in HLA-B27 associated uveitis. The presence of heterochromia is seen in Fuchs heterochromic iridocyclitis.

### Intermediate Uveitis

The majority of intermediate uveitis cases are idiopathic, however each patient should be evaluated for systemic diseases that can present in this manner. Again, a history and detailed review of systems will aid in diagnosis. Sarcoidosis, syphilis, and Lyme disease can cause intermediate uveitis and a CBC, ACE level, chest X-ray (CXR), VDRL or RPR, and Lyme serologies should be routinely ordered. If the patient also has neurologic findings, a diagnosis of multiple sclerosis may be considered.

### Posterior Uveitis

There are a wide variety of causes of chorioretinitis including both systemic diseases and those that are confined to the eye. A thorough history can help tailor the work-up, however if the review of systems are unremarkable, additional laboratory testing will likely not aid with diagnosis.

Systemic diseases such as sarcoidosis, Behçet disease, Sjogren's syndrome, Wegeners granulomatosis, systemic lupus erythematosis (SLE), multiple sclerosis, and polyarteritis nodosa should be considered. Infectious diseases such as syphilis, toxoplasmosis, tuberculosis, West Nile virus, Lyme, herpes zoster (ARN) also cause posterior uveitis. Cytomegalovirus (CMV) should also be considered in immunocompromised hosts.

Each patient should receive a CBC, ACE level, RPR or VDRL, and a CXR as a part of the initial work-up. A fluorescein angiography or retinal biopsy should be considered if retinal vasculitis is present. An evaluation by a retinal specialist is very helpful.

While a substantial portion of uveitis cases are idiopathic, other causes of ocular symptoms such as intraocular malignancies should be considered. They can be misdiagnosed as uveitis and should be considered if the symptoms are not responsive to steroid therapy. Primary CNS lymphoma is the most common malignancy to present similarly to uveitis and can be evaluated with an MRI of the head, vitreous biopsy, or lumbar puncture.

## Bibliography

Jabs DA, Nussenblatt RB, Rosenbaum JT. Standardization of uveitis nomenclature for reporting clinical data. Results of the First International Workshop. *Am J Ophthalmol*. Sep 2005;140(3):509-516.

McCannel CA, Holland GN, Helm CJ et al. Causes of uveitis in the general practice of ophthalmology. *Am J Ophthalmol*. 1996;121:35-46.

Rothova A, Buitenhuis HJ, Meenken C et al. Uveitis and systemic disease.

Tay-kearney M, Schwam BL, Lowder C et al. Clinical features and associated systemic diseases of HLA-B27 uveitis. *Am J Ophthalmol*. 1996;121:47-56.

Weiner A, BenEstra D. Clinical patterns and associated conditions in chronic uveitis. *Am J Ophthalmol*. 1991;112:151-158.

## Corticosteroid-Induced Ocular Hypertension/Glaucoma

Elevated intraocular pressure (IOP) can occur as a result of systemic (oral, intravenous, or inhaled) or ocular (topical, periocular, or intravitreal) administration of corticosteroids. The mechanism of increased IOP is increased resistance to aqueous outflow. Risk factors associated with corticosteroid-induced IOP rise[22] include primary open angle glaucoma (POAG), glaucoma suspect status, and a family history of glaucoma. Children as a group tend to be at greater risk of developing corticosteroid-induced ocular hypertension, for reasons that are not entirely clear. Patients with connective tissue disease, high myopia, and type 1 diabetes mellitus have also shown to be at increased risk for developing a corticosteroid-induced elevation in IOP.

The extent of IOP elevation depends on the potency of the corticosteroid, the dose and duration of treatment, the route of administration, and the patient's susceptibility to corticosteroid-induced ocular hypertension.[23] Intraocular administration is most frequently associated with IOP elevation and the most rapid rise is also seen with this mode of corticosteroid delivery. When treated with topical corticosteroids for 4–6 weeks, 5% of the population demonstrates a rise in IOP > 16 mmHg, and 30% have a rise of 6–15 mmHg.[24,25] With intraocular administration, a higher prevalence of IOP elevation has been reported; 40–50% with intravitreal triamcinolone (IVTA) injection[26,27] and 71% with the fluocinolone acetonide (FA) intravitreal implant.[28] Most patients with IVTA-induced IOP elevation require only topical medications for IOP control whereas in the FA implant study[28] ,37% required IOP lowering surgery.

## 41.4 Conclusion

The mechanism of elevated IOP in uveitis is multifactorial. Management can be especially challenging in patients with corticosteroid-induced ocular hypertension; however, adequate control of inflammation must be the primary goal. Understanding the mechanism of IOP elevation can help in establishing a diagnosis as well as in directing therapy, which differs in many aspects from treatment of non-uveitic glaucomas. Finally, the expertise of a uveitis specialist can be very helpful in the management of this complex condition.

## 41.5 Clinical Pearls

1. Adequate control of inflammation is the primary goal in patients with uveitis and elevated intraocular pressure.
2. Aqueous suppressants are the first line of therapy, followed by carbonic anhydrase inhibitors, alpha agonists, and finally, prostaglandin analogs, which must be used with caution.
3. Laser trabeculoplasty is contraindicated in uveitis-related elevated IOP.
4. With the increasing use of intravitreal corticosteroids, more patients with uveitis will require medical and surgical management of corticosteroid-induced elevated intraocular pressure.

5. Trabeculectomy performed without antimetabolites has a high chance of failure in patients with uveitic glaucoma.
6. Patients with uveitis are at greater risk for hypotony after any IOP lowering surgery.
7. Ciliodestructive procedures must be avoided in uveitic glaucoma due to the potential of causing hypotony and eventual phthisis.

## References

1. Moorthy RS, Mermoud A, Baerveldt G, et al. Glaucoma associated with uveitis. *Surv Ophthalmol*. 1997;41:361-394.
2. Reddy S, Cubillan LDP, Havakimyan A, Cunningham ET. Inflammatory ocular hypertension syndrome (IOHS) in patients with syphilitic uveitis. *Br J Ophthalmol*. 2007;91:1610–1612.
3. Westfall AC, Lauer AK, Suhler EB, Rosenbaum JT. Toxoplasmosis retinochoroiditis and elevated intraocular pressure. *J Glaucoma*. 2005;14:3–10.
4. Warwar RE, Bullock JD, Ballal D. Cystoid macular edema and anterior uveitis associated with Latanoprost use: experience and incidence in a retrospective review of 94 patients. *Ophthalmology*. 1998;105:263–268.
5. Wand M, Gilbert CM, Liesegang TJ. Latanoprost and herpes simplex keratitis. *Am J Ophthalmol*. 1999;127:602-604.
6. Spencer NA, Hall AJ, Stawell RJ. Nd:Yag laser iridotomy in uveitic glaucoma. *Clin Experiment Ophthalmol*. 2001;29:217–219.
7. Retisert (Bausch & Lomb/Control Delivery Systems). Lim LL, Smith JR, Rosenbaum JT. Curr Opin Invest Drugs. 2005;6:1159–1167
8. Stavrou P, Murray PI. Long-term follow-up of trabeculectomy without antimetabolites in patients with uveitis. *Am J Ophthalmol*. 1999;128:434–439.
9. Towler HMA, Bates AK, Broadway DC, et al. Primary trabeculectomy with 5-fluorouracil for glaucoma secondary to uveitis. *Ocul Immunol Inflamm*. 1995;3:163–170.
10. Prata JA, Neves RA, Minckler DS, et al. Trabeculectomy with mitomycin C in glaucoma associated with uveitis. *Ophthalmic Surg Lasers*. 1994;25:616–620.
11. Noble J, Derzko-Dzulynsky L, Rabinovitch T, Birt C. Outcome of trabeculectomy with intraoperatieve mitomycin C for uveitic glaucoma. *Can J Ophthalmol*. 2007;42:89–94.
12. Towler HM, McCluskey P, Shaer B, et al. Long-term follow-up of trabeculectomy with intraoperative 5-fluorouracil for uveitis-related glaucoma. *Ophthalmology*. 2000;107:1822–1828.
13. Jampel HD, Jabs DA, Quigley HA. Trabeculectomy with 5-fluorouracil for adult inflammatory glaucoma. *Am J Ophthalmol*. 1990;109:168–173.
14. Patitsas CJ, Rockwood EJ, Meisler DM, et al. Glaucoma filtering surgery with postoperative 5-Fluorouracil in patients with intraocular inflammatory disease. *Ophthalmology*. 1992;99:594–599.
15. Papadaki TG, Zacharopoulos IP, Pasquale LR, et al. Long-term results of Ahmed glaucoma implantation for uveitic glaucoma. *Am J Ophthalmol*. 2007;144:62–69.
16. Ceballos EM, Parrish RK II, Schiffman JC. Outcome of Baerveldt glaucoma drainage implants for the treatment of uveitic glaucoma. *Ophthalmology*. 2002;109:2256–2260.
17. Freedman SF, Rodriguez-Rosa RE, Rojas MC, Enyedi LB. Goniotomy for glaucoma secondary to chronic childhood uveitis. *Am J Ophthalmol*. 2002;133:617–621.
18. Miserocchi E, Carassa RG, Bettin P, Brancato R. Viscocanalostomy in patients with glaucoma secondary to uveitis: preliminary report. *J Cataract Refract Surg*. 2004;30:566–570.
19. Williams RD, Hoskins HD, Shaffer RN. Trabeculodialysis for inflammatory glaucoma: a review of 25 cases. *Ophthalmic Surg*. 1992;23:36–37.
20. Kanski JJ, McAllister JA. Trabeculodialysis for inflammatory glaucoma in children and young adults. *Ophthalmology*. 1985;92:927–930.
21. Minckler D, Baerveldt G, Ramirez MA, et al. Clinical results with the Trabectome, a novel surgical device for treatment of open-angle glaucoma. *Trans Am Ophthalmol Soc*. 2006;104:40–50.
22. Jones R, Rhee DJ. Corticosteroid-induced ocular hypertension and glaucoma: a brief review and update of the literature. *Curr Opin Ophthalmol*. 2006;17:163–167.
23. Clark A. Steroids, ocular hypertension, and glaucoma. *J Glaucoma*. 1995;4:354–369.
24. Armaly MF. Statistical attributes of the steroid hypertensive response in the clinically normal eye. I. The demonstration of three levels of response. Invest Ophthalmol. 1965;4:187–197
25. Becker B. Intraocular pressure response to topical corticosteroids. *Invest Ophthalmol*. 1965;26:198–205.
26. Jonas JB, Degenrigh RF, Kreissig I, et al. Intraocular pressure elevation after intravitreal triamcinolone acetonide injection. *Ophthalmology*. 2005;112:593–598.
27. Rhee DJ, Peck RE, Belmont J, et al. Intraocular pressure alterations following intravitreal triamcinolone acetonide. *Br J Ophthalmol*. 2006;90:999–1003.
28. Goldstein DA, Godfrey DG, Hall A, et al. Intraocular pressure in patients with uveitis treated with fluocinolone acetonide implants. *Arch Ophthalmol*. 2007;125:1478–1485.

# Chapter 42
# Posner–Schlossman Syndrome

Raghu C. Mudumbai and Sarwat Salim

Posner–Schlossman Syndrome (PSS), otherwise known as glaucomatocyclitic crisis, is an uncommon form of open angle glaucoma. This unilateral condition typically affects young to middle-aged individuals and is characterized by recurrent episodes of mild, nongranulomatous anterior uveitis with markedly elevated intraocular pressure (IOP).[1] Some patients may have associated systemic disorders, mostly of allergic and gastrointestinal origin.[2] A possible role of herpes simplex virus infection has also been postulated.[3]

During an acute attack, a patient presents with minimal symptoms of ocular discomfort and blurred vision, often of short duration. On clinical examination, mild iridocyclitis is noted with slight ciliary flush, corneal edema, small to mid-sized nonpigmented keratic precipitates on the central and inferior cornea. Usually, there is a trace cell and flare in the anterior chamber. Of note, posterior synechiae and peripheral anterior synechiae are characteristically absent. In some cases, iris hypochromia, which may lead to confusion with Fuchs' heterochromic iridocyclitis, may be present.[1] The associated rise in IOP is usually out of proportion to the inflammatory process and reaches levels in the range of 40–60 mmHg. Gonioscopy reveals an open angle, and occasionally, keratic precipitates may be present on the trabecular meshwork. Between attacks, both the anterior chamber and IOP return to normal, requiring no long-term treatment.

Although PSS is usually a self-limited condition, some cases with advanced optic nerve cupping and associated visual field loss have been described. Jap et al.[4] reported that patients with diagnosis of PSS for 10 or more years were three times more likely to develop glaucomatous optic neuropathy when compared with patients with less than 10 years of disease. Reduction in aqueous outflow facility due to inflammatory changes in the trabecular meshwork and increased aqueous humor production secondary to augmented levels of prostaglandins have been implicated in IOP spikes and subsequent glaucoma.[5,6] Although initially described as a distinct entity from primary open angle glaucoma, some studies have suggested an association with primary open angle glaucoma.[7,8]

Treatment of PSS is directed at controlling the inflammation and associated IOP elevation. Inflammation responds well to topical corticosteroids. Usually, elevated IOP normalizes with the control of inflammation or may necessitate glaucoma medical therapy. Aqueous suppressants are usually effective in controlling IOP. Efficacy of prostaglandin analogs in PSS is not well established. Prophylactic therapy for glaucoma or uveitis does not prevent recurrences and is not recommended between attacks. In rare, uncontrolled cases, glaucoma filtration surgery may be required.

Other differential diagnoses to consider in the setting of mild anterior chamber inflammation include Fuchs' heterochromic iridocyclitis (FHI) and herpetic uveitis. FHI is usually asymptomatic and presents as chronic inflammation with the eventual formation of a posterior subcapsular cataract and significant secondary glaucoma. Unlike PSS, the uveitis of FHI does not respond well to topical steroids. Herpetic uveitis typically has more pronounced intraocular inflammation, lasts longer, and requires more aggressive treatment.

Recognizing PSS is invaluable for counseling patients and providing appropriate care. Once identified as PSS, patients can be educated to the relatively good prognosis and need to seek medical care during acute attacks. Recently, PSS has been linked to NAION during acute elevation in IOP in patients with susceptible small cup-disc ratios.[9] Careful follow-up can prevent such problems and avoid unnecessary surgical intervention.

## References

1. Posner A, Schlossman A. Syndrome of unilateral recurrent attacks of glaucoma with cyclitic symptoms. *Arch Ophthalmol*. 1948;39:517–535.
2. Knox DL. Glaucomatocyclitic crises and systemic disease: peptic ulcer, other gastrointestinal disorders, allergy and stress. *Trans Am Ophthalmol Soc*. 1988;86:473–495.
3. Yamamoto S, Pavan-Langston D, Tada R, et al. Possible role of herpes simplex virus in the origin of Posner-Schlossman syndrome. *Am J Ophthalmol*. 1995;119:796–798.
4. Jap A, Sivakumar M, Med M, et al. Is Posner Schlossman syndrome benign? *Ophthalmology*. 2001;108:913–918.
5. Spivey BE, Armaly MF. Tonographic studies in glaucomatocyclitic crisis. *Am J Ophthalmol*. 1963;55:47–51.
6. Nagataki S, Mishima S. Aqueous humor dynamics in glaucomatocyclitic crisis. *Invest Ophthalmol*. 1976;15:365.
7. Kass MA, Becker B, Kolker AE. Glaucomatocyclitic crisis and primary open angle glaucoma. *Am J Ophthalmol*. 1973;75:668.
8. Raitta C, Vannas A. Glaucomatocyclitic crisis. *Arch Ophthalmol*. 1977;95:608–612.
9. Irak I, Katz BJ, Zabriskie NA, et al. Posner-Schlossman syndrome and nonarteritic anterior ischemic optic neuropathy. *J Neuroophthalmol*. 2003;4:264–267.

# Chapter 43
# Fuchs' Uveitis Syndrome and Glaucoma

Edney R. Moura Filho and Thomas J. Liesegang

## 43.1 History and Clinical Features

Lawrence[1] first described Fuchs' uveitis syndrome (FUS) in 1843. In 1906, in a series of 38 patients, Ernst Fuchs'[2] described a condition called complicated heterochromia, which was characterized by heterochromia, inflammation, and cataract. This disorder has also been called Fuchs' heterochromic uveitis and Fuchs' heterochromic cyclitis. However, vitreous opacities and chorioretinal scars are common, and therefore the frequently used term cyclitis is not entirely accurate.[3]

In 1955, Franceschetti[4] reported on 62 patients with FUS, and Kimura[5] later described 23 patients with the syndrome. In 1973, Lowenfield and Thompson[6,7] described other characteristics, such as cataracts, glaucoma, and vitreous opacities, which are associated with the disease.

FUS counts for 2–11% of all cases of anterior uveitis[8] and is currently considered an unusual form of uveitis that has a variable clinical appearance. Clinical criteria for establishing the diagnosis of FUS have not yet been internationally accepted.

According to the guidelines of the International Uveitis Study Group,[9] the classic features of FUS include a chronic unilateral nongranulomatous inflammation mainly involving the anterior uvea, insidious onset, low grade in activity, affecting of both genders equally, a preponderance in those between 20 and 45 years old, unresponsiveness to corticosteroid therapy, absence of systemic disorders, and generally a good prognosis except for the development of cataract and glaucoma.

The disease has no racial or sexual predilection and can involve either eye in patients of all ages.[10] About 7.8–10% of patients have bilateral disease which requires an astute clinician to recognize.[11] If the disease is unilateral at presentation, it usually remains a unilateral disease.[12]

The presence of heterochromia has been an over emphasized feature of FUS. The heterochromia can show wide variation and is an inconsistent feature of the disease. Some patients remain unaware of it, and in others, it remains very subtle to the observer. Others describe the heterochromia or iris changes since youth.[10,13,14] Daylight examination is usually best for detecting subtle heterochromia. A heterochromia is usually most evident in blue-eyed patients (Figs. 43.1. and 43.2.). In brown irides (in whites,[5] blacks,[15] or Asians[16]), the heterochromia can be subtle or absent because both layers of the iris (anterior and posterior) are of the same color and texture.[17] In some individuals, there is more atrophy of the anterior iris layer such that the iris can appear darker in the affected eye (reversed heterochromia) from the pigmentation of the posterior iris layer. If both eyes are involved, there is also an absence of heterochromia. In some patients, heterochromia never develops although the anterior iris stroma maintains a washed out appearance in comparison with the normal eye.[10] In each of these situations, there are other features present which establish the diagnosis.[18,19]

Heterochromia being absent,[20] and the various clinical signs[20] not always being present at the same time, FUS can be difficult to diagnose. Incorrect diagnosis may lead to unnecessary corticosteroid therapy and to misleading expectations for the course of the disease.

Iris changes often precede heterochromia. They include iris stromal smoothing with loss of the normal corrugated texture. Quantitative analysis of scattered light from iris and ocular structures has also been used but remains a research tool.[21]

Iris nodules are common, occurring in more than 30% of cases.[4,11,21] They are typically small and translucent and can be on the pupil margin (Koeppe nodules) or iris surface (Busacca nodules). Small, refractile iris crystals are typical of FUS.[22,23] These crystals represent Russell bodies and can occur in other chronic uveitidies.[23,24]

There is minimal and variable cell and flare.[12] Keratic precipitates are not always stellate and generalized, and all distributions and types of keratic precipitates, including "mutton fat," have been described (Fig. 43.3.).

Gonioscopy may disclose several abnormalities. Vessels can be seen in the angle of the anterior chamber (possibly related to atrophy of the iris and better visualization).[10] These fine vessels, present in the angle, probably are susceptible to the frequent filiform hemorrhages noted in association with

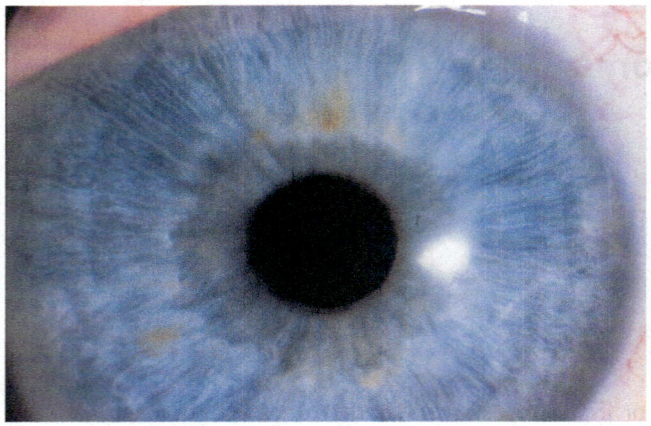

**Fig 43.1** The right eye of patient with Fuchs' uveitis demonstrating lack of crisp iris detail, indistinct washed out appearance, and slight heterochromia in comparison with normal left eye (Fig. 43.2.). This eye also demonstrated fine iris neovascularization and cholesterol crystals in the anterior chamber

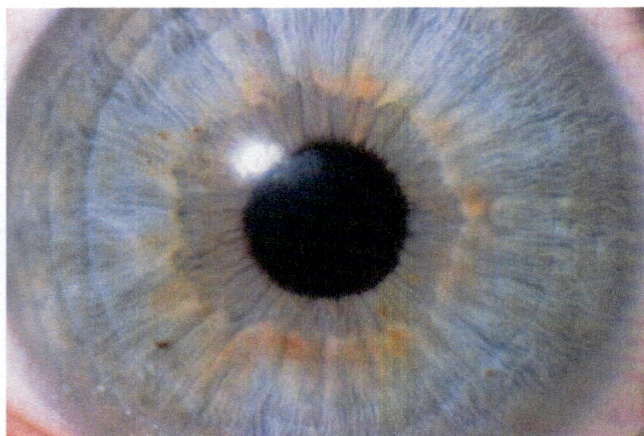

**Fig. 43.2** The normal left eye of patient in Fig. 43.1. for comparison

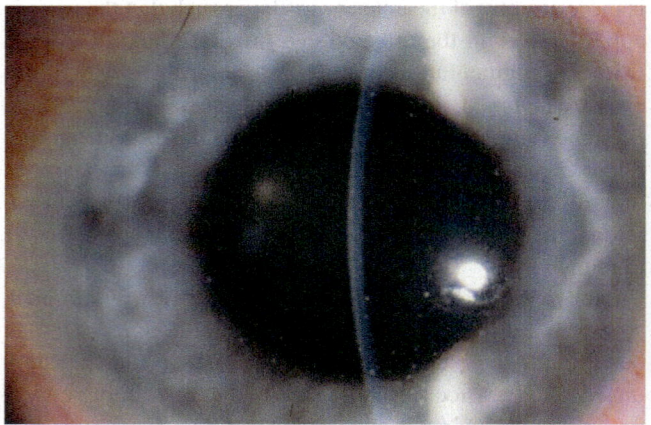

**Fig. 43.3** Slit beam through cornea of patient with Fuchs' uveitis demonstrating fine keratic precipitates (KP) on the back of the cornea, even extending to the superior cornea. The extension of KP the upper cornea is almost diagnostic of Fuchs' uveitis. There are fine filaments between the KP throughout the back of the cornea

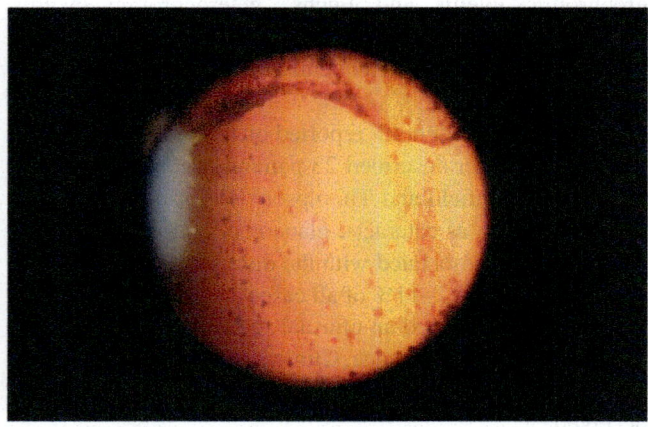

**Fig. 43.4** Retroillumination view of anterior segment in patient demonstrating the KP on the superior and inferior cornea and the vitreous cells and debris characteristic of Fuchs' uveitis

paracentesis of the anterior chamber and may be responsible for some of the flare seen in the syndrome.[25] The angle can have a dirty dullness or filmy appearance, but there is no increased pigmentation.[10]

A hyphema may also occur in association with trivial trauma, gonioscopy, applanation tonometry, or mydriasis spontaneously.[11,13,26] The occurrence of hyphema does not necessarily correlate with the clinical signs of iris neovascularization or with the presence of abnormal vessels in the iridocorneal angle.[10,11]

Vitreous cells are present in almost all patients with FUS. The cells may remain dustlike or progress to heavy and stringy veils as they cling to a degenerative vitreous framework (Fig. 43.4.). They can interfere with vision and/or become an annoyance. The vitreous debris can vary in density over time. With cataract surgery (especially intracapsular cataract surgery), dense vitreous veils can form, possibly related to bleeding from a ciliary body blood cyst. Vitrectomy is occasionally necessary to eliminate the heavy vitreous veils.[10,11,27]

Cataracts are an invariable feature after prolonged follow-up of FUS. They originate as posterior subcapsular cataracts and have a tendency to progress rapidly to maturity. They may progress to shrunken hypermature lenses and the iris heterochromia may become more prominent as the cataract matures.[10] The prognosis for cataract surgery varies in the literature probably related to the variability and severity of the overall disease process in the individual eye.[12]

Studies have documented clinically evident corneal edema after cataract surgery.[10,28] The corneal edema can be central or peripheral with the latter similar to that described by Brown and McLean.[57] Peripheral corneal edema may occur prior to cataract surgery.

Patients with FUS usually do not present as emergencies.[12] IOP elevation is not as common as with glaucomatocyclitic crisis but may occur as a late, serious complication. Glaucoma, usually chronic open-angle glaucoma, has been associated with FUS in 9–59% of cases,[13,14] with the higher figures seen in series with a long-term follow-up. It is the most common cause of permanent visual loss in patients with FUS.[10] The glaucoma typically persists after the uveitis has subsided.

## 43.2 Etiology and Pathogenesis

Different explanations for the pathomechanism have been proposed in FUS. Some findings support a genetic basis for the disease,[14] but data on HLA typing has been either contradictory or very weak. Because chorioretinal scarring is found in some FUS patients, the association of ocular toxoplasmosis with FUS has also been suggested.[29,30] Melamed et al.[31] suggested that the neural changes may be the initial abnormality in FUS and that adrenergic denervation may also be involved. Unilateral heterochromia has also been associated with sympathetic paralysis and the assumed "trophic" function of the sympathetic nervous system.[21,32] Ocular trauma has been cited as precipitating uveitis, but hypotheses suggesting that trauma can lead to FUS have not established a pathogenic connection.[33]

In 2004, Quentin and Reiber[34] provided two compelling lines of evidence to suggest that most cases of FUS in a European population were associated with chronic rubella infection. Birnbaum et al.[35] also reported on the decreasing prevalence of FUS in a single tertiary ophthalmologic center since the introduction of mass vaccination against the rubella virus. The vaccination occurs with a live pathogen vaccine and was reported to cause temporary uveitis and conjunctivitis that demonstrated positive results for rubella virus by PCR.[36,37]

Several factors have been reported in the etiology of glaucoma in FUS. Secondary glaucoma is not a result of a steroid-responsive trabeculitis, the drainage angle is usually open, and although peripheral anterior synechiae can occur, they are not a regular or marked feature.[10,38] Huber[39] considered the main cause of ocular hypertension to be an increase of the outflow resistance located in the trabeculum. Chandler and Grant[40] stated that rubeosis of the iris in the anterior chamber angle induces the development of chronic secondary glaucoma. Peripheral anterior synechiae, trabecular sclerosis, lens induced glaucoma, an abnormal felt-like membrane in the angle, trabecular spaces filled with plasma cells, and steroid induction have also been reported as possible causes.[6,13,17,39,41–46] Glaucoma is more common in patients with progressive iris atrophy.[12] Most patients, however, have no apparent cause.

## 43.3 Management

No anti-inflammatory treatment is known to change the course of FUS; therefore, treatment should be mostly reserved to the sight-threatening complications: cataract, glaucoma, and vitreous opacification.

Part of the cells and flare seen in FUS may be a consequence of blood aqueous barrier breakdown and leakage rather than active inflammation. They also show limited response to topical steroids.[25] While of questionable benefit, topical and periocular steroids may promote cataract formation and glaucoma. Although there are no randomized controlled trials addressing the use of steroids in FUS, occasional and short time use of corticosteroids may be indicated if a symptomatic exacerbation in the uveitis occurs. Long-term steroids should be avoided in FUS.

A short trial of topical steroids may also be helpful to differentiate FUS from conditions such as glaucomatocyclitic crisis and idiopathic anterior uveitis with trabeculitis, in which the initial appearance can be similar, but the response to steroids is markedly different.

Glaucoma is one of the most problematic complications of FUS. There is no general agreement on the prognosis of glaucoma in FUS, and most authors report their conclusions on cases with a short control period. Some workers[13,47] claimed a favorable outlook when the glaucoma was treated early. Other studies[5,17] suggest that glaucoma usually becomes refractory to medical treatment. In the series reported by Liesegang,[10] the prognosis was poorer than previously reported, although the author demonstrated success in controlling IOP by combined medical and surgical therapy in 21 of 32 patients.

In the early stages, the elevated intraocular pressure may be intermittent and associated with increased intraocular inflammation.[48] This may respond to topical corticosteroids. Topical and systemic glaucoma medications are later required with a variable longterm effect. Argon laser trabeculoplasty is usually not successful and may be contraindicated in view of the inflammatory nature of the condition and the presence of peripheral anterior synechiae, fine vessels in the angle, or a felt-like membrane in the angle. Glaucoma filtration surgery is frequently necessary but has all the attendant risks associated with glaucoma surgery in a patient with uveitis, including bleb failure.[12,13] The role of wound modulators (5-fluorouracil, mitomycin) has not been extensively evaluated. Use of light cryotherapy prior to filtration surgery may reduce complications related to neovascularization.[17] Patients who do not respond to filtration surgery may need a shunt implantation. Some patients require enucleation because of absolute or rubeotic glaucoma.[10,13,45,49]

A high index of suspicion and regular follow-up in patients with FUS are warranted to detect glaucoma early. Medical and surgical treatment for reducing IOP should be especially aggressive in these patients. They can have wide fluctuations of IOP and baseline investigations, including optic disk photography, Heidelberg retinal tomography imaging or OCT, and visual fields can help detect progression. Patients with FUS and glaucoma are often less responsive to medical therapy. In his series of patients with FUS, Liesegang[10] reported 66% of patients with secondary glaucoma requiring surgery. La Hey et al.[50] reported failed medical therapy in 73% of cases. Despite surgery (trabeculectomy with 5-fluorouracil), only 72% of these patients achieved IOP less than 21 mmHg even with additional medication. Jones[13] described 27 patients with FUS and glaucoma, only 63% of whom remained controlled on topical medication. Half the patients undergoing trabeculectomy failed to respond to treatment, and four eyes ultimately required enucleation with end-stage glaucoma. Merayo–Lloves et al.,[51] in a retrospective study, found that FUS accounted for 19% of the cases of secondary glaucoma in patients with uveitis. Despite aggressive medical and surgical therapy, progressive visual field loss and optic nerve damage occurred in a third of patients. The authors concluded that glaucoma was an under-appreciated, vision-threatening complication in patients with uveitis.

With newer topical ocular hypotensive medications, it is hoped that fewer patients will require surgical intervention. The highest reported success rate for trabeculectomy without adjuvant anti-metabolites in uveitic glaucoma (from different etiologies) is 54% after 5 years.[52] With additional intraoperative 5-fluorouracil, a success rate of 67% at 5 years was reported.[53] Mitomycin-C did not show any obvious advantages over 5-fluorouracil, but there may be a bias in case selection.[54–56] Molteno et al.[57] reported 87% of patients with uveitic glaucoma controlled at 5 years.

## References

1. Lawrence W. Changes in colour in the iris. In: Hays I, ed. *A Treatise on Diseases of the Eye*. Philadelphia: Lea & Blauchard; 1853:411–416.
2. Fuchs E. Ueber komplikationen der Heterochromie. *Z Augenheilkd*. 1906;15:191–212.
3. Mohamed Q, Zamir E. Update on Fuchs' uveitis syndrome. *Curr Opin Ophthalmol*. 2005;16:356–363.
4. Franceschetti A. Heterochromic cyclitis (Fuchs' syndrome). *Am J Ophthalmol*.. 1955;39:50–58.
5. Kimura SJ. Fuchs' syndrome of heterochromic cyclitis in brown-eyed patients. *Trans Am Ophthalmol Soc*. 1978;76:76–89.
6. Lowenfield IE, Thompsom S. Fuchs' heterochromic cyclitis. A critical review of the literature. I. Clinical characteristics of the syndrome. *Surv Ophthalmol*. 1973;17:394–457.
7. Lowenfield IE, Thompsom S. Fuchs' heterochromic cyclitis. A critical review of the literature. I. Etiology and mechanisms. *Surv Ophthalmol*. 1973;18:2–61.
8. Tran VT, Auer C, Guex-Crosier Y, Pittet N, Herbort CP. Epidemiological characteristics of uveitis in Switzerland. *Int Ophthalmol*. 1994;18:293–298.
9. Bloch-Michel E, Nussenblatt RB. International Uveitis Study Group recommendations for the evaluation of intraocular inflammatory disease. *Am J Ophthalmol*. 1987;103:234–235.
10. Liesegang TJ. Clinical features and prognosis in Fuchs' uveitis syndrome. *Arch Ophthalmol*. 1982;100:1622–1626.
11. Jones NP. Fuchs' heterochromic uveitis: a reappraisal of the clinical spectrum. *Eye*. 1991;5:649–661.
12. Liesegang TJ. Fuchs uveitis syndrome. In: Pepose JS, Holland GN, Wilhelmus KR, eds. *Ocular Infection & Immunity*. St Louis: Mosby; 1996:495–506.
13. Jones NP. Glaucoma in Fuchs' heterochromic uveitis: aetiology, management and outcome. *Eye*. 1991;5:662–667.
14. Jones NP. Fuchs' heterochromic uveitis: an update. *Surv Ophthalmol*. 1993;37:253–272.
15. Tabbut BR, Tessler HH, Williams D. Fuchs' heterochromic iridocyclitis in blacks. *Arch Ophthalmol*. 1988;106:1688–1690.
16. Jain IS, Gupta A, Gangwar DN, Dhir SP. Fuchs' heterochromic cyclitis: some observations on clinical picture and on cataract surgery. *Ann Ophthalmol*. 1983;15:640–642.
17. O'Connor GR. Heterocromic iridocyclitis. Doyne lecture. *Trans Ophthalmol Soc UK*. 1985;104:219–231.
18. Donoso LA, Eigerman RA, Magargal LE. Fuchs' heterochromic cyclitis associated with subclavian steal syndrome. *Ann Ophthalmol*. 1981;13:1153–1155.
19. Clarnella-Cantani A. and Leonardi E. Bilateral Fuchs's syndrome of heterochromic cyclitis. *Clin Oculist Patol Oculare*. 1982;3:91–94.
20. La Hey E, Baarsma GS, de Vries J, Kijlstra A. Clinical analysis of Fuchs' heterochromic cyclitis. *Documenta Ophtalmologica*. 1991;78:225–235.
21. La Hey E, Ijspeert JK, van den Berg TJ, Kijlstra A. Quantitative analysis of iris translucency in Fuchs' heterochromic cyclitis. *Invest Ophthalmol Vis Sci*. 1993;34:2931–2942.
22. Zamir E, Margalit E, Chowers I. Iris crystals in Fuchs' heterochromic iridocyclitis. *Arch Ophthalmol*. 1998;116:1394.
23. Callear AB, Reynolds A, Harry J, Murray PI. Iris crystals in chronic uveitis. *Br J Ophthalmol*. 1999;83:703.
24. Lam S, Tessler HH, Winchester K, et al. Iris crystals in chronic iridocyclitis. *Br J Ophthalmol*. 1993;77:181–182.
25. Norrsell K, Holmer AK, Jacobson H. Aqueous flare in patients with monocular iris atrophy and uveitis: a laser flare and iris angiography study. *Acta Ophthalmol Scand*. 1998;76(4):405–412.
26. Feldman ST, Deutsch TA. Hyphema following Honan balloon use in Fuchs' heterochromic iridocyclitis. *Arch Ophthalmol*. 1986;104:967.
27. Ward DM, Hart CT. Complicated cataract extraction in Fuchs's heterochromic uveitis. *Br J Ophthalmol*. 1967;51:530–538.
28. Kimura SJ, Hogan MJ, Thygeson P. Fuchs' Syndrome of Heterochromic cyclitis. *Arch Ophthalmol*. 1955;54:179–186.
29. De Abreu MT, Belfort R, Hirata PS. Fuchs' heterochromic cyclitis and ocular toxoplasmosis. *Am J Ophthalmol*. 1982;93:739–742.
30. La Hey E, Rothova A, Baarsma GS, de Vries J, van Knapen F, Kijlstra A. Fuchs' heterochromic iridocyclitis is not associated with ocular toxoplasmosis. *Arch Ophthalmol*. 1992;110(6):806–811.
31. Melamed S, Lahav M, Sandbank U, et al. Fuchs' heterochromic iridocyclitis, an electron microscopic study of the iris. *Invest Ophthalmol Vis Sci*. 1978;17:1193–1198.
32. Aggarwal RK, Luck J, Coster DJ. Horner's syndrome and Fuchs' heterochromic uveitis. *Br J Ophthalmol*. 1994;78(12):949.
33. La Hey E, Baarsma GS, Rothova A, et al. High incidence of corneal epithelium antibodies in Fuchs' heterochromic cyclitis. *Br J Ophthalmol*. 1988;72:921–925.

34. Quentin CD, Reiber H. Fuchs heterochromic cyclitis: rubella virus antibodies and genome in aqueous humor. *Am J Ophthalmol.* 2004;138:46–54.
35. Birnbaum AD, Tessler HH, Schultz KA, et al. Epidemiological relationship between Fuchs heterochromic iridocyclitis and the United States rubella vaccination program. *Am J Ophthalmol.* 2007;144:424–428.
36. Kitaichi N, Ariga T, Ohno S, Shimizu T. Acute unilateral conjunctivitis after rubella vaccination: the detection of the rubella genome in the inflamed conjunctiva by reverse transcriptase-polymerase-chain reaction. *Br J Ophthalmol.* 2006;90:1436–1437.
37. Islam SM, El-Sheikh HF, Tabbara KF. Anterior uveitis following combined vaccination for measles, mumps, and rubella (MMR): a report of two cases. *Acta Ophthalmol Scand.* 2000;78:590–592.
38. Amsler M, Verrey F. Heterochromie de Fuchs et fragilite vasculaire. *Ophthalmologica.* 1946;111:177.
39. Huber A. Das Glaucom bei komplizierten Hetcrochromie Fuchs. *Ophthalmologica.* 1961;142:66–115.
40. Chandler PA, Grant WM. *Lectures on Glaucoma.* Philadelphia: Lea and Febiger; 1965.
41. Benedikt O, Roll P, Zirm M. The glaucoma in heterochromic cyclitis of Fuchs. Gonioscopic studies and electron microscopic investigations of the trabecular meshwork. *Klin Monatsbl Augenheilkd.* 1978;173:523–533.
42. Berger BB, Tessler HH, Kottow MH. Anterior segment ischaemia in Fuchs' heterochromic cyclitis. *Arch Ophthalmol.* 1980;98:499–501.
43. Hart CT. The IOP in Fuch's heterochromic cyclitis. *Trans Ophthalmol Soc UK.* 1971;91:771–775.
44. Hart CT, Ward DM. Intraocular pressure in Fuchs's heterochromic uveitis. *Br J Ophthalmol.* 1967;51:739–743.
45. Lerman S, Levy C. Heterochromic iritis and secondary neovascular glaucoma. *Am J Ophthalmol.* 1964;57:479–481.
46. Perry HD, Yanoff M, Scheie HG. Rubeosis in Fuchs heterochromic iridocyclitis. *Arch Ophthalmol.* 1975;93:337–339.
47. Lemke L. Das Glaucoma bei Heterochromiecyclitis. *Ophthalmologica.* 1966;151:457–464.
48. Pietruschka G, Priesz G. Secondary glaucoma with heterochromia cyclitis according to Fuchs. *Klin Monatsbl Augenheilkd.* 1974;164:609–615.
49. Norn MS. Cataract extraction in Fuchs' heterochromia: follow-up of 19 cases. *Acta Ophthalmologica.* 1968;46:685–699.
50. La Hey E, de Vries J, Langerhorst CT, et al. Treatment and prognosis of secondary glaucoma in Fuchs' heterochromic iridocyclitis. *Am J Ophthalmol.* 1993;116:327–340.
51. Merayo-Lloves J, Power WJ, Rodriguez A, et al. Secondary glaucoma in patients with uveitis. *Ophthalmologica.* 1999;213:300–304.
52. Stavrou P, Murray PI. Long-term follow-up of trabeculectomy without antimetabolites in patients with uveitis. *Am J Ophthalmol.* 1999;128:434–439.
53. Towler HMA, Bates AK, Broadway DC, et al. Primary trabeculectomy with 5 fluorouracil for glaucoma secondary to uveitis. *Ocul Immunol Inflamm.* 1995;3:163–170.
54. Towler HM, McCluskey P, Shaer B, et al. Long-term follow-up of trabeculectomy with intraoperative 5-fluorouracil for uveitis-related glaucoma. *Ophthalmology.* 2000;107:1822–1828.
55. Jampel HD, Jabs DA, Quigley HA. Trabeculectomy with 5-fluorouracil for adult inflammatory glaucoma. *Am J Ophthalmol.* 1990;109:168–173.
56. Sung VC, Barton K. Management of inflammatory glaucomas. *Curr Opin Ophthalmol.* 2004;15:136–140.
57. Molteno, AC, Sayawat N, Herbison, P. Otago glaucoma surgery outcome study: long-term results of uveitis with secondary glaucoma drained by Molteno implants. *Ophthalmology.* 2001;108:605–613.

# Chapter 44
# Herpes Simplex Related Glaucoma

Edney R. Moura Filho and Thomas J. Liesegang

The word "herpes" derives from the Greek verb meaning "to creep or crawl" and was used to describe spreading cutaneous lesions in the writings of Hippocrates some 25 centuries ago.[1] There are now eight recognized human herpes viruses: herpes simplex virus type 1 (HSV-1), HSV-2, varicella–zoster virus (VZV), cytomegalovirus, Epstein–Barr virus, human herpes virus 6 (associated with roseola infantum), human herpes virus 7 (associated with roseola infantum and febrile convulsions), and human herpes virus 8 (associated with Kaposi sarcoma and lymphomas).[2]

HSV is endemic in virtually every human society throughout the world, from urban to remote native tribes. There are two distinct serotypes of HSV: HSV type 1 (HSV-1) and type 2 (HSV-2). They are transmitted by direct skin or mucous membrane contact, by venereal routes, or by maternal genital infection to the newborn. HSV-1 classically causes infections above the waist, for example, the eye, nares, or mouth (cold sores); HSV-2 usually causes infections below the waist, for example, the genitals. In recent years, however, HSV-1 is increasingly frequent in genital infections.

## 44.1 Ocular HSV and Glaucoma

In the ocular area, HSV causes disease of the lids (eyelid vesicles), conjunctiva (inflammation and vesicles), sclera (scleritis), cornea (keratitis), the anterior part within the eye (anterior uveitis), the retina (retinitis), or, less commonly, in the choroid (choroiditis) or optic nerve (optic neuritis)[3] (Figs. 44.1 and 44.2). Although many of the manifestations begin as the result of the HSV viral infection itself, many manifestations are the aftermath of the body's response to the infection in terms of mounting an inflammatory response, an immune response, vascular leakage, scarring, and nerve damage. Actual virus particles have been identified in the human iris,[4] aqueous,[5,6] and cornea.[7] HSV has also been implicated as a secondary cause of high intraocular pressure (IOP) and glaucoma.

In a study at Mayo Clinic in Rochester, Minnesota, 121 patients with their first recognized clinical episode of ocular HSV were followed for up to 33 years.[8] The initial episodes of ocular HSV involved the lids or conjunctiva in 54%, the superficial cornea in 63%, the deep cornea in 6%, and the uvea in 4%. The disease was bilateral in 12%, and the predominant form of recurrent disease was dendritic corneal involvement, although 20% had only recurrent lid involvement. Significant stromal disease developed in 20% of patients. Patients tended to get a recurrence of the same type of ocular disease that they had previously, that is, patients with epithelial disease tended to get recurrent epithelial disease; this was similar for conjunctival disease and stromal disease. Seventy percent of eyes maintained 20/20 vision; only three of 130 eyes had final vision that was worse than 20/100.

In a retrospective study by Falcon and Williams,[9] 50 patients who developed high IOP in association with HSV keratouveitis were studied. These patients had suffered from recurrent HSV disease from a few weeks to 30 years before presenting with high IOP. The authors reported that glaucoma could be overlooked in a disease process that occurs in an acute, chronic, and intermittent fashion. Moreover, increased IOP as a consequence of prior damage to the trabecular meshwork by HSV keratouveitis could also be overlooked. The authors also reported that the nature of the first attack of ocular herpes differed from that occurring in association with increased IOP. Patients who presented with their first episode of ocular herpes had either a dendritic or amoeboid ulcer (40%) or stromal disease (60%). Patients with ocular herpes who presented with increased IOP had stromal keratitis (96–100%) or a metaherpetic ulcer (4%). Most of the patients with stromal keratitis also had an anterior chamber inflammatory reaction. Another feature noted by the authors was the preponderance of patients with uveitis in the group who developed increased IOP compared with the group who did not. The frequency of ocular hypertension was greater (2.4 episodes) among patients with irregular stromal keratitis as compared to patients with disciform keratitis (1.8 episodes).

Van der Lelij et al[10] reported on a large cohort of patients who were initially seen with unilateral anterior uveitis in association with sectoral iris atrophy, but no evidence of prior or concurrent epithelial or stromal keratitis. Evidence for either HSV or VZV infection was found in every patient with

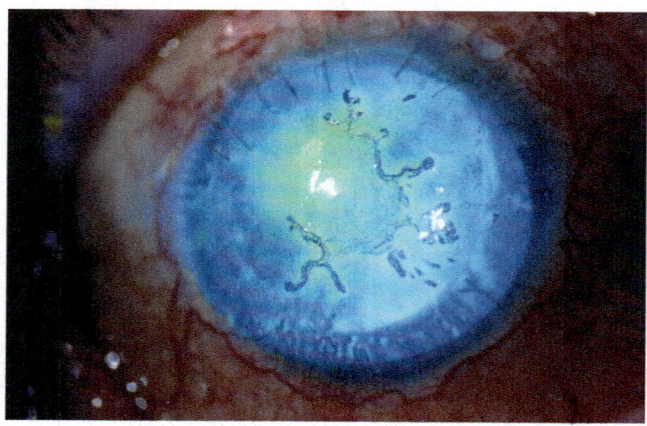

**Fig. 44.1** Herpes simplex epithelial keratitis. Multiple and extensive corneal dendrites stained with fluorescein and highlighted with a cobalt blue filter in HIV+ patient with herpes simplex epithelial keratitis

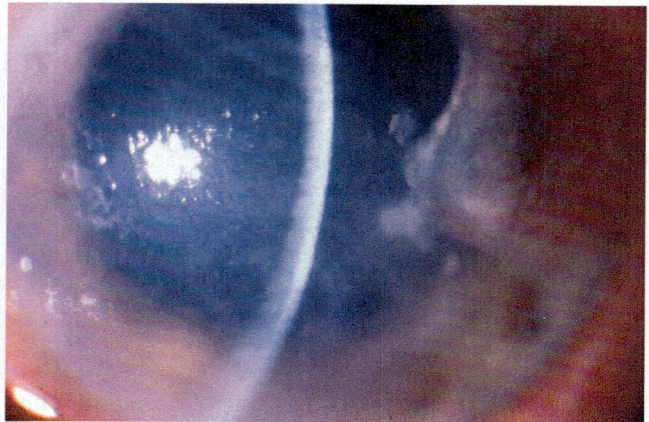

**Fig. 44.3** HSV stromal keratouveitis and glaucoma. Chronic HSV keratitis now demonstrating stromal edema, corneal folds, keratic precipitates, uveitis, increased intraocular pressure, as well as superficial peripheral lipid deposition, anterior stromal scarring, and corneal vascularization

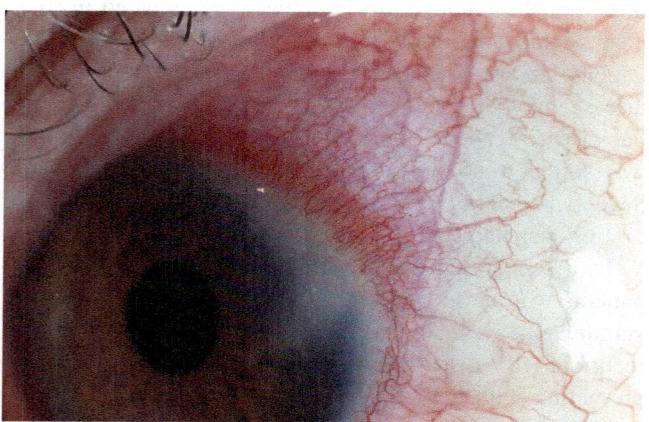

**Fig. 44.2** HSV episcleritis and peripheral stromal keratitis. Patient demonstrates mild scleritis with purplish hue and associated mild peripheral keratitis. Patient had increased intraocular pressure

active uveitis. HSV accounted for more than 80% of cases. VZV-induced iritis was, however, more common in patients over 50 years of age, accounting for approximately 60% of cases in this age group. Both VZV- and HSV-associated anterior uveitis tended to recur on average once per year. Additional findings in their cohort that supported the diagnosis of herpetic anterior uveitis included acutely elevated intraocular pressure, pupillary distortion, recurrent fever blisters, punctate keratopathy, and decreased corneal sensation.

### 44.1.1 Pathogenesis of Glaucoma Associated with HSV

The pathogenesis of HSV keratouveitic glaucoma is controversial. Some authors suggested that increased IOP is not secondary to inflammation, but a result of steroid therapy.[11]

Hogan et al[12] reported severe and widespread alterations in the anterior segment in a pathologic study of whole, enucleated eyes with absolute glaucoma and herpetic keratouveitis. The trabecular bands were thick and edematous and a mix of fibrin and chronic inflammatory cells obstructed the outflow channels between the bands. Posterior synechia were extensive, and the anterior lens showed signs of cataractous change. The anterior ciliary body also showed signs of chronic inflammation.

Another study by Tiwari et al[13] demonstrated evidence that human trabecular meshwork cells are susceptible to HSV-1 entry and are capable of supporting viral replication. The authors believe that damage to cells forming the trabeculum of the eye by HSV-1 infection could contribute to the development of glaucoma. Primary cultures of human trabecular meshwork cells were used as an in vitro model to demonstrate the ability of HSV-1 to enter into and establish a productive infection of the trabeculum.

Townsend and Kaufman[14] reported that 13 of 36 HSV infected rabbits (36%) developed increased IOP during the observation period. The IOP began to rise 4–8 days after infection and coincided with peaks in anterior chamber reaction. A diffuse mononuclear cell infiltration of the iris root and trabecular meshwork with disruption of the lamellar arrangement was present on histologic examination of the eyes. All animals with persistent pressure elevations had anterior synechia and 50% of these animals had retrocorneal membranes covering 180° of the angle circumference.

These findings suggest that increased IOP in HSV keratouveitic glaucoma is related to trabecular blockade or trabeculitis (Figs. 44.3–44.5). Inflammatory cells, fibrin, and plasma proteins may produce a physical blockade of the trabecular meshwork.[12] Retrocorneal membrane obstruction

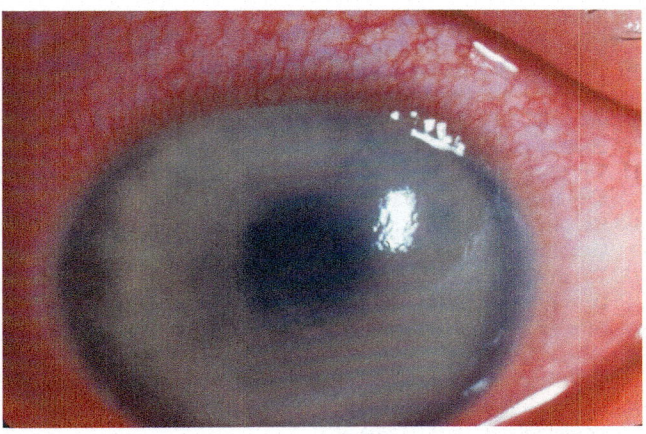

**Fig. 44.4** Acute HSV keratouveitis and edema. Patient with acute recurrence of HSV demonstrating episcleritis, corneal edema, keratic precipitates, uveitis, and increased intraocular pressure

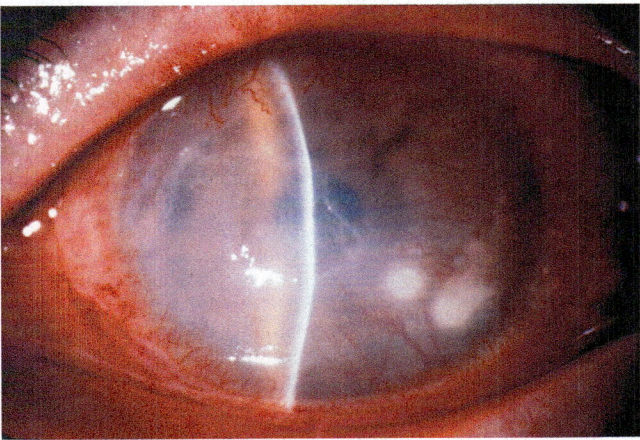

**Fig. 44.5** Chronic HSV stromal keratitis and uveitis. Patient with long standing chronic HSV keratitis demonstrating multifocal stromal infiltrates, shallow sterile epithelial ulceration, stromal neovascularization, keratic precipitates, uveitis, and increased intraocular pressure

of the angle may also contribute to rises in IOP.[14] Thick and edematous trabecular bands, which may present clinically as limbitis, appear to obstruct trabecular outflow.[12] Posterior synechia formation could cause pupillary blockade and secondary angle-closure glaucoma. However, angle closure was not implicated as a cause of increased IOP in any of the 50 patients studied by Falcon and Williams.[9]

The treatment of HSV keratouveitis with topical steroids may increase IOP, as suggested by Thygeson.[11] In contradiction, all patients in another study[6] were noted to have increased IOP before steroid therapy was commenced. The final possibility is preexisting ocular hypertension or glaucoma, which stresses the importance of an awareness of dual mechanisms of disease.

## 44.1.2 Management of Glaucoma Associated with HSV

The management of glaucoma occurring secondary to HSV keratouveitis starts with the treatment of the viral disease itself. The historical treatment of epithelial HSV has been with topical antiviral agents.[15] There have been three topical antiviral eye medications (idoxuridine, vidarabine, trifluridine) for HSV in the United States, but only trifluridine is presently available at this time. Acyclovir ophthalmic ointment is not available in the United States. These are all effective and nearly equivalent.[15] Adding topical interferon speeds epithelial healing but it remains a research drug. These antivirals are used to treat epithelial disease, but also as prophylaxis for recurrent epithelial HSV in high-risk situations such as with the concomitant use of topical corticosteroids or after corneal transplant surgery.[15]

The stromal disease and anterior segment inflammation (anterior uveitis, trabeculitis, endotheliitis) requires the addition of anti-inflammatory agents; NSAIDs have not been found to be effective in this disease. Patients usually require continual topical corticosteroid with a very careful, prolonged reduction schedule, using different techniques (i.e., dose reduction or frequency reduction) varying with the patient or disease process. Disciform endotheliitis and trabeculitis are usually exquisitely sensitive to topical corticosteroids, and early intervention leads to complete resolution.

With long-term steroid use, the possibility of steroid-induced ocular hypertension should be kept in mind. However, a drop in IOP from steroid suppression of the trabeculitis will likely precede any steroid-induced pressure rise.[11]

Antiglaucoma medications may need to be added to adequately control the ocular hypertension with attention being paid to the status of the optic nerve. If medications are used, it may be advisable to avoid the use of miotics. Opinions vary on whether or not it is helpful to avoid prostaglandins in the presence of intraocular inflammation. The IOP tends to return to normal as the intraocular inflammation resolves, although, patients may develop persistent IOP elevation requiring chronic therapy. Filtration surgery may be required in a few cases.[10]

The role of steroids and antiviral medications in the treatment and prevention of ocular HSV disease was evaluated in the Herpetic Eye Disease Study,[16–20] although it did not address the specific question of glaucoma associated with HSV. Summary of the results are as follows: Oral acyclovir can reduce the recurrences of stromal keratitis, during the period the agent is administered.[16] Topical trifluridine eye drops did not add to the use of oral acyclovir in preventing stromal keratitis and iridocyclitis.[17] Although topical steroids hasten healing times, they do not make a significant difference in the visual outcome.[17] There was no additive effect of oral acyclovir to patients with stromal keratitis already receiving trifluridine and topical steroids.[18] There is only marginal benefit to adding oral acyclovir to patients with HSV iridocyclitis already receiving trifluridine and topical steroids.[19] Long-term suppressive oral acyclovir therapy reduces the rate of recurrent HSV epithelial keratitis and stromal keratitis during the period of time the agent is taken.[20]

Other studies prior to the HEDS reported that oral acyclovir was effective in prophylaxis of recurrent epithelial HSV, following a prior episode provided the acyclovir is continued.[21] Because of the high incidence of HSV epithelial keratitis following corneal transplantation, prophylactic oral acyclovir is routinely administered for several months after transplantation with reduction in the rate and duration of recurrences of HSV.[22]

The use of some glaucoma medications is controversial in HSV infection. Topical b-blockers (timolol),[23,24] prostaglandin F2a analogs (latanoprost),[24-26] and prostamide analogs (bimatoprost)[27] have been implicated in the reactivation of HSV ocular disease in anecdotal human reports. On the other hand, other authors believe that the prevalence of ocular HSV in patients treated with ocular hypotensive therapy is no different than that found in the general population[28] and that a true scientifically proven causal relationship has not been confirmed.[29] They suggest that case reports lack statistical validity to suggest causation, but may be valuable for signaling potential adverse drug reactions.

## References

1. Pepose JS, Leib DA, Stuart PM, Easty DL. Herpes simplex virus diseases anterior segment of the eye. In: Pepose JS, Holland GR, Wilhelmus KR, eds. *Ocular Infection and Immunity*. St Louis: Mosby-Year Book; 1996:905–932.
2. Miyagawa H, Yamanishi K. The epidemiology and pathogenesis of infections caused by the high numbered human herpesviruses in children: HHV-6, HHV-7 and HHV-8. *Curr Opin Infect Dis*. 1999;12:251–255.
3. Kimura SJ. Herpes simplex uveitis: a clinical and experimental study. *Trans Am Ophthalmol Soc*. 1962;60:440–470.
4. Witmer R, Iwamoto T. Electron microscope observation of herpes-like particles in the iris. *Arch Ophthalmol*. 1968;79:331–337.
5. Sundmacher R, Neumann-Haefelin D. Herpes simplex virus isolations from the aqueous of patients suffering from focal iritis, endotheliitis, and prolonged disciform keratitis with glaucoma. *Klin Monatsbl Augenheilkd*. 1979;175:488–501.
6. Pavan-Langston D, Brockhurst RJ. Herpes simplex panuveitis. *Arch Ophthalmol*. 1969;81:783–787.
7. Pavan-Langston D. Viral disease of the ocular anterior segment: basic science and clinical disease. In: Foster S, Azar D, Dohlman C, eds. *Smolin and Thoft's the Cornea: Scientific Foundations and Clinical Practice*. 4th ed. Philadelphia, PA: Lippincott Williams & Wilkins; 2005:297–397.
8. Liesegang TJ, Melton LJ III, Daly PJ, Ilstrup DM. Epidemiology of ocular herpes simplex. Incidence in Rochester, Minn, 1950 through 1982. *Arch Ophthalmol*. 1989;107:1155–1159.
9. Falcon MG, Williams HP. Herpes simplex keratouveitis and glaucoma. *Trans Ophthalmol Soc UK*. 1978;98:101–104.
10. Van der Lelij A, Ooijman FM, Kijlstra A, Rothova A. Anterior uveitis with sectoral iris atrophy in the absence of keratitis: a distinct clinical entity among herpetic eye diseases. *Ophthalmology*. 2000;107:1164–1170.
11. Thygeson P. Chronic herpetic keratouveitis. *Trans Am Ophthalmol Soc*. 1967;65:211–226.
12. Hogan MJ, Kimura SJ, Thygeson P. Pathology of herpes simplex keratouveitis. *Trans Am Ophthalmol Soc*. 1963;61:75–99.
13. Tiwari V, Clement C, Scanlan PM, Kowlessur D, Yue BYJT, Shukl D. A role for herpesvirus entry mediator as the receptor for herpes simplex virus 1 entry into primary human trabecular meshwork cells. *J Virol*. 2005;79:13173–13179.
14. Townsend WM, Kaufman HE. Pathogenesis of glaucoma and endothelial changes in herpetic keratouveitis in rabbits. *Am J Ophthalmol*. 1971;71:904–910.
15. Liesegang TJ. Herpes simplex viruses ocular disease. In: Studahl M, Cinque P, Bergstrom T, eds. *Herpes Simplex Viruses*. Vol. 36. Boca Raton: Taylor & Francis; 2006:239–274. Infectious Disease and Therapy, Chapter 10.
16. Herpetic Eye Disease Study Group. Acyclovir for the prevention of recurrent herpes simplex virus eye disease. *N Engl J Med*. 1998;339:300–306.
17. The Herpetic Eye Disease Study Group. A controlled trial of oral acyclovir for the prevention of stromal keratitis or iritis in patients with herpes simplex virus epithelial keratitis. The Epithelial Keratitis trial. *Arch Ophthalmol*. 1997;115:703–712.
18. Barron BA, Gee L, Hauck WW, et al. Herpetic Eye Disease Study. A controlled trial of oral acyclovir for herpes simplex stromal keratitis. *Ophthalmology*. 1994;101:1871–1882.
19. The Herpetic Eye Disease Study Group. A controlled trial of oral acyclovir for iridocyclitis caused by herpes simplex virus. *Arch Ophthalmol*. 1996;114:1065–1072.
20. The Herpetic Eye Disease Study Group. Oral acyclovir for herpes simplex virus eye disease: effect of prevention of epithelial keratitis and stromal keratitis. *Arch Ophthalmol*. 2000;118:1030–1036.
21. Simon AL, Pavan-Langston D. Long-term oral acyclovir therapy. Effect on recurrent infectious herpes simplex keratitis in patients with and without grafts. *Ophthalmology*. 1996;103:1399–1404. discussion 1404–1405.
22. Barney NP, Foster CS. A prospective randomized trial of oral acyclovir after penetrating keratoplasty for herpes simplex keratitis. *Cornea*. 1994;13:232–236.
23. Hill JM, Shimomura Y, Dudley JB, et al. Timolol induces HSV-1 ocular shedding in the latently infected rabbit. *Invest Ophthalmol Vis Sci*. 1987;28:585–590.
24. Deai T, Fukuda M, Hibino T, et al. Herpes simplex virus genome quantification in two patients who developed herpetic epithelial keratitis during treatment with antiglaucoma medications. *Cornea*. 2004;23:125–128.
25. Wand M, Gilbert CM, Liesegang TJ. Latanoprost and herpes simplex keratitis. *J Ophthalmol*. 1999;127:602–604.
26. Ekatomatis P. Herpes simplex dendritic keratitis after treatment with latanoprost for primary open angle glaucoma. *Br J Ophthalmol*. 2001;85:1008–1009.
27. Kroll DM, Schuman JS. Reactivation of herpes simplex virus keratitis after initiating bimatoprost treatment for glaucoma. *Am J Ophthalmol*. 2002;133:401–403.
28. Bean G, Reardon G, Zimmerman TJ. Association between ocular herpes simplex virus and topical ocular hypotensive therapy. *J Glaucoma*. 2004;13:361–364.
29. Camras CB. Latanoprost increase the severity and recurrence of herpetic keratitis in the rabbit: latanoprost and herpes simplex keratitis. *Am J Ophthalmol*. 2000;129:271–272.

# Chapter 45
# Herpes Zoster Related Glaucoma

Edney R. Moura Filho and Thomas J. Liesegang

Varicella–zoster virus causes two distinct syndromes. Primary infection presents as varicella (or chickenpox), a contagious and usually benign childhood illness that occurs in epidemics among susceptible children. The reactivation of the virus, usually associated with decline in cell-mediated immunity, occurs as herpes zoster (HZ) (shingles). Varicella is spread through droplet infection with an initial viremia, and subsequent viral spread to the skin and the eye. It is easily disseminated to susceptible individuals. Ninety-five percent of the population has serological evidence of prior VZV infection with or without symptomatic varicella. The incidence of varicella has diminished 70% after implementation of the varicella vaccine in 1995.

Herpes zoster ophthalmicus (HZO) is defined as HZ involvement of the ophthalmic division of the fifth cranial nerve. The ophthalmic division further divides into the nasociliary, frontal, and lacrimal branches, of which the frontal nerve is most commonly involved with HZO.[1] Without the use of antiviral therapy, approximately 50% of HZ patients develop ocular involvement.[2,3] There is a long list of complications from HZ, including those that involve the optic nerve and retina in HZO, but the most frequent and debilitating complication of HZ regardless of dermatomal distribution is post-herpetic neuralgia (PHN), a neuropathic pain syndrome that persists or develops after the zoster rash has resolved.

## 45.1 Herpes Zoster Ophthalmicus and Glaucoma

Herpes zoster presents as an acute, painful, vesicular eruption distributed along a single dermatome. Most cases of HZO have a prodromal period before skin eruptions that may include fever, malaise, headache, and pain in the eye.[4]

Hutchinson's sign is defined as skin lesions at the tip, side, or root of the nose and is a strong predictor of ocular inflammation and corneal denervation in HZO, especially if both branches of the nasociliary nerve are involved.[5,6]

A study by Thean et al.[7] identified the clinical features of uveitis secondary to HZO. Most patients were immunocompetent. The course of the uveitis was generally uniphasic in nature and of a relatively short duration. There was a high incidence of secondary glaucoma, with 15% of all patients requiring surgical intervention. The visual loss in several patients was not directly related to the uveitis and secondary glaucoma but to other complications associated with HZO. The authors report that the secondary glaucoma may be the result of several mechanisms: (1) plugging of the trabecular meshwork due to the presence of cellular debris and iris pigment; (2) trabeculitis; (3) pupillary-block glaucoma secondary to posterior synechiae, with resultant iris bombé; (4) peripheral anterior synechiae; or (5) chronic open-angle glaucoma presumably due to damage to the trabecular meshwork or as a result of the use of topical steroids (Figs. 45.1– 45.3).

Van der Lelij et al.[8] reported on a large cohort of patients who were initially seen with unilateral anterior uveitis in association with sectoral iris atrophy but no evidence of prior or concurrent epithelial or stromal keratitis (Fig. 45.4). Evidence for either HSV or VZV infection was found in every patient with active uveitis. HSV accounted for more than 80% of cases. VZV-induced iritis was, however, more common in patients over 50 years of age, accounting for approximately 60% of cases in this age group. Both VZV- and HSV-associated anterior uveitis tended to recur on average once per year. Additional findings in their cohort that supported the diagnosis of herpetic anterior uveitis included acutely elevated intraocular pressure, pupillary distortion, recurrent fever blisters, punctate keratopathy, and decreased corneal sensation.

## 45.2 Management of HZO

A course of systemic antiviral agents (acyclovir, valacyclovir, or famciclovir) is advised for all patients with defects of cell-mediated immunity. Controversy lingers regarding the use of antivirals for localized zoster in the normal host although they are recommended for all patients with HZO. Although any of the three systemic antivirals may lessen the complications of ocular zoster, there does not appear to be

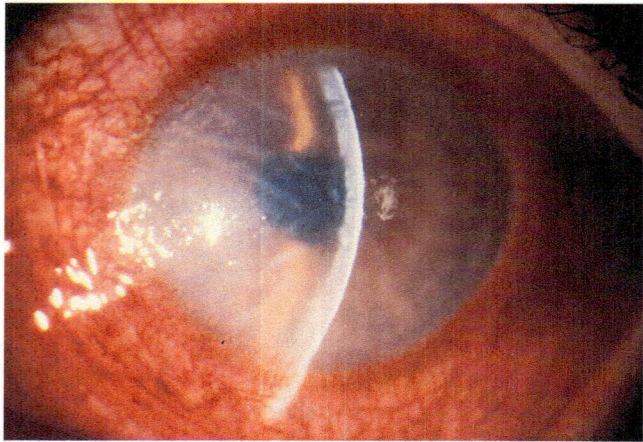

**Fig. 45.1** Acute severe keratouveitis and glaucoma in patient with herpes zoster ophthalmicus. Patient demonstrates episcleritis, corneal folds, keratic precipitates, uveitis, and increased intraocular pressure. Responded to topical steroids and temporary glaucoma medication

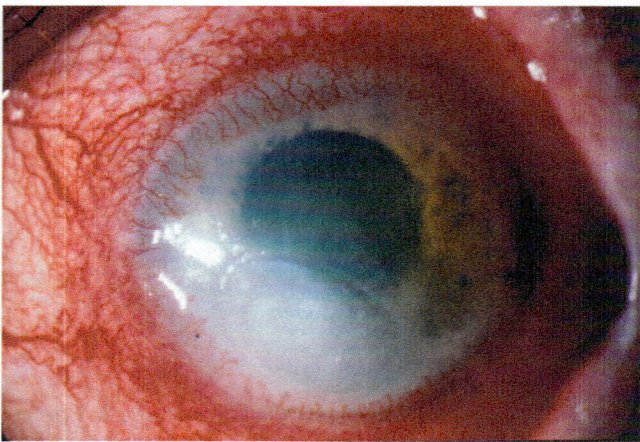

**Fig. 45.3** Chronic keratouveitis, sterile neurotrophic ulcer, and glaucoma in patient with prior herpes zoster ophthalmicus. Patient demonstrates episcleritis, corneal epithelial ulcer with dense stromal infiltrate, uveitis, and increased intraocular pressure

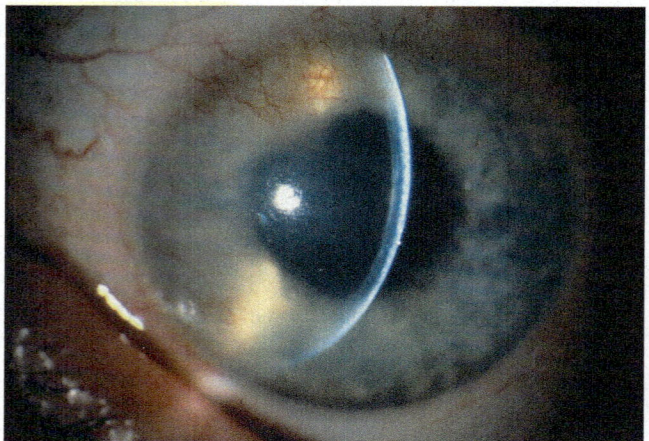

**Fig. 45.2** Chronic keratouveitis and glaucoma in patient with prior herpes zoster ophthalmicus. Patient demonstrates anterior corneal scarring, dense superior pannus and intrastromal vessels, keratic precipitates, uveitis, and increased intraocular pressure

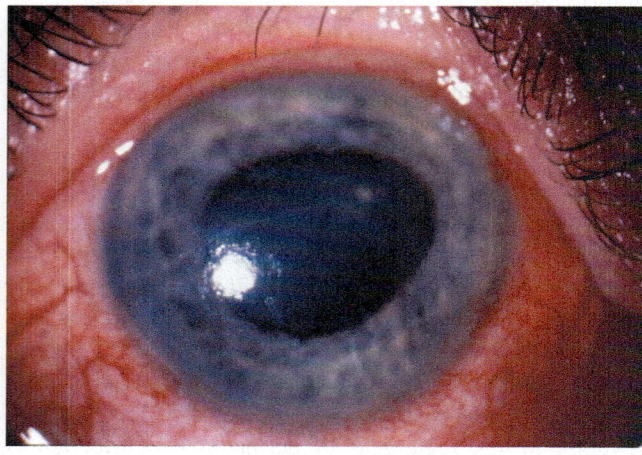

**Fig. 45.4** Chronic neurotrophic keratitis, sector iris atrophy in patient with prior herpes zoster ophthalmicus. Patient had irregular corneal surface, lack of corneal sensation, slightly irregular pupil with a sector of iris atrophy and increased intraocular pressure

convincing or consistent evidence of the benefit of the systemic antivirals in preventing or treating the most severe complications of HZO. The drugs should be administered within 72 h of the onset of the rash. Patients receiving combined corticosteroids and antivirals have acceleration in cutaneous healing rates and a better quality of life, decreased use of analgesics, a decrease in the time to uninterrupted sleep, and a decrease in time to resumption of normal activities of daily living compared to those with antiviral alone. Steroids should not be used in those with depressed cell-mediated immunity. Acyclovir-resistant VZV have been reported in patients with advanced AIDS, requiring therapy with alternative drugs (e.g., foscarnet). There is no role for topical antiviral drugs in the management of herpes zoster (as opposed to HSV keratouveitis).

Most treatment plans for PHN have anecdotal reports rather than controlled trials, so effectiveness is both complex and difficult to evaluate. Early antiviral appears to modify later PHN only marginally. For persistent cases, management in conjunction with a pain expert and a multifaceted approach is recommended. A variety of pharmacologic therapies exist for those who are not helped by mild analgesia. Clinical trials have shown that opioids, tricyclic antidepressants, and gabapentin reduce the severity or duration of post herpetic neuralgia, either as single agents or in combination.

Topical steroids are recommended for chronic episcleritis and keratitis and for all cases of iritis. Careful monitoring of the use of topical steroids with very slow reduction and withdrawal prevents rebound effects and helps to detect steroid responders. Complications from severe neurotrophic keratopathy or exposure keratitis can require surgical intervention such as a partial tarsorrhaphy. Occasionally corneal surgery may be required in cases of perforation from neurotrophic corneas. Following a penetrating keratoplasty, HZO patients require close monitoring and therapy with lubrication and possibly lateral tarsorrhaphies. Cataract and glaucoma operations are generally uncomplicated, but topical steroids must be used postoperatively. Systemic steroids are indicated for markedly hemorrhagic rashes, proptosis with external ophthalmoplegia, optic neuritis, and contralateral hemiplegia.

The management of increased IOP and glaucoma occurring secondary to HZO is directed initially at halting or preventing reactivation of viral disease. Supplemental antiglaucoma medications may need to be added to adequately control the ocular hypertension. Suggested options include b-blockers, a-agonist, and carbonic anhydrase inhibitors (oral and topical). The IOP usually returns to normal as the intraocular inflammation resolves. Although the majority of patients who develop glaucoma are controlled with topical medication, some patients may require the temporary use of systemic carbonic anhydrase inhibitors. For those with persistent high IOP and controlled inflammation, trabeculectomy with antifibrotic agents should be considered. Glaucoma drainage devices have been proposed as useful alternatives[9-12] especially for those with active inflammation.

Although there have been anecdotal case reports suggesting an association between prostaglandins (PG) analogues and the development of anterior uveitis or cystoid macular edema (CME), there is scant evidence from controlled clinical trials and experimental studies to support these associations.[13-17] A study by Chang et al.[18] shows that PG analogues are potent drugs that lower raised IOP in patients with uveitis. This study was unable to demonstrate any major increase in the frequency of either anterior uveitis or CME. Based on the results of this study, the benefit of improved IOP control may outweigh the potential increased risks of anterior uveitis or CME in these patients, particularly given that there is more visual loss with glaucoma in patients with uveitis.[19] However, the study was in patients with secondary IOP elevation due to multiple causes of uveitis and not HZO related.

If coexisting lid, IOP, tear film, and corneal sensation deficits are addressed properly and ocular inflammation is controlled, then other types of ocular surgeries have a high success rate.[20] Marsh and Cooper[21] found that the surgical results for corneal scars, glaucoma, and cataracts were no different between HZO patients and routine cases, except that they noted a tendency for prolonged inflammation after surgery in HZO patients.

# References

1. Edgerton A. Herpes zoster ophthalmicus: report of cases and a review of the literature. *Trans Am Ophthalmol Soc.* 1942;40:390-439.
2. Harding SP. Management of ophthalmic zoster. *J Med Virol.* 1993;(Suppl 1):97-101.
3. Harding SP, Lipton JR, Wells JC. Natural history of herpes zoster ophthalmicus: predictors of postherpetic neuralgia and ocular involvement. *Br J Ophthalmol.* 1987;71:353-358.
4. Liesegang TJ. Herpes zoster ophthalmicus natural history, risk factors, clinical presentation, and morbidity. *Ophthalmology.* 2008;115:S3-S12.
5. Hutchinson J. A clinical report on herpes zoster ophthalmicus (shingles affecting the forehead and nose). *R Lond Ophthalmic Hosp Rep.* 1865;5:191-215.
6. Zaal MJ, Volker-Dieben HJ, D'Amaro J. Prognostic value of Hutchinson's sign in acute herpes zoster ophthalmicus. *Graefes Arch Clin Exp Ophthalmol.* 2003;241:187-191.
7. Thean JH, Hall AJ, Stawell RJ. Uveitis in Herpes zoster ophthalmicus. *Clin Experiment Ophthalmol.* 2001;29:406-410.
8. Van der Lelij A, Ooijman FM, Kijlstra A, Rothova A. Anterior uveitis with sectoral iris atrophy in the absence of keratitis: a distinct clinical entity among herpetic eye diseases. *Ophthalmology.* 2000;107:1164-1170.
9. Da Mata A, Burk SE, Netland PA, et al. Management of uveitic glaucoma with Ahmed glaucoma valve implantation. *Ophthalmology.* 1999;106:2168-2172.
10. Molteno AC, Sayawat N, Herbison P. Otago glaucoma surgery outcome study: long-term results of uveitis with secondary glaucoma drained by Molteno implants. *Ophthalmology.* 2001;108:605-613.
11. Ceballos EM, Parrish RK 2nd, Schiffman JC. Outcome of Baerveldt glaucoma drainage implants for the treatment of uveitic glaucoma. *Ophthalmology.* 2002;109:2256-2260.
12. Kok H, Barton K. Uveitic glaucoma. *Ophthalmol Clin North Am.* 2002;15:375-387.
13. Stjernschantz JW. From PGF(2alpha)-isopropyl ester to latanoprost: a review of the development of xalatan: the Proctor Lecture. *Invest Ophthalmol Vis Sci.* 2001;42:1134-1145.
14. Wand M, Shields BM. Cystoid macular edema in the era of ocular hypotensive lipids. *Am J Ophthalmol.* 2002;133:393-397.
15. Schumer RA, Camras CB, Mandahl AK. Latanoprost and cystoid macular edema: is there a causal relation? *Curr Opin Ophthalmol.* 2000;11:94-100.
16. Hoyng PF, Rulo AH, Greve EL, et al. Fluorescein angiographic evaluation of the effect of latanoprost treatment on blood-retinal barrier integrity: a review of studies conducted on pseudophakic glaucoma patients and on phakic and aphakic monkeys. *Surv Ophthalmol.* 1997;41(Suppl 2):S83-S88.
17. Furuichi M, Chiba T, Abe K, et al. Cystoid macular edema associated with topical latanoprost in glaucomatous eyes with a normally functioning blood-ocular barrier. *J Glaucoma.* 2001;10:233-236.
18. Chang JH, McCluskey P, Missotten T, Ferrante P, Jalaludin B, Lightman S. Use of ocular hypotensive prostaglandin analogues in patients with uveitis: does their use increase anterior uveitis and cystoid macular oedema? *Br J Ophthalmol.* 2008;92:916-921.
19. Neri P, Azuara-Blanco A, Forrester JV. Incidence of glaucoma in patients with uveitis. *J Glaucoma.* 2004;13:461-465.
20. Pavan-Langston D, Yamamoto S, Dunkel EC. Delayed herpes zoster pseudodendrites. Polymerase chain reaction detection of viral DNA and a role for antiviral therapy. *Arch Ophthalmol.* 1995;113:1381-1385.
21. Marsh RJ, Cooper M. Ophthalmic zoster: mucous plaque keratitis. *Br J Ophthalmol.* 1987;71:725-728.

# Chapter 46
# Iridocorneal Endothelial Syndrome and Glaucoma

Sarwat Salim and Peter A. Netland

Iridocorneal endothelial (ICE) syndrome represents a spectrum of disease, encompassing three clinical variations: Chandler's syndrome, progressive iris atrophy, and Cogan-Reese syndrome. This acquired, unilateral disorder typically manifests in young to middle adulthood and predominantly affects women, although bilateral involvement and occurrence in a child have been reported.[1,2] A high percentage of patients with ICE syndrome develop secondary glaucoma.

The underlying mechanism linking all three variants is an abnormality of the corneal endothelium. Clinically, a fine "hammered-silver" appearance of the Descemet's membrane is noted, which may be associated with corneal edema in moderate to advanced cases. On specular microscopy, the endothelial cells are reduced in number and appear pleomorphic with dark–light reversal (the cell boundaries appear bright with dark cell surfaces). These cells acquire characteristics of epithelial cells, such as presence of desmosomes, intracytoplasmic filaments, and microvilli.

The abnormal endothelial cells can migrate as a membrane over adjacent structures, including the iris and the trabecular meshwork.[3] These cells also have been shown to secrete an abnormal basement membrane, similar to Descemet's.[4] Contraction of this membrane leads to associated iris changes, iridotrabecular synechiae, and secondary glaucoma. A viral etiology has been proposed for this corneal endotheliopathy based on a history of inflammation in some affected eyes and the presence of inflammatory cells observed in corneal specimens.[5] Herpes simplex virus DNA has been demonstrated with polymerase chain reaction in corneal specimens obtained from patients with ICE syndrome.[6]

The three entities in their purest form may be easily recognized clinically; however, clear categorization can be difficult at times since patients may exhibit different clinical manifestations at various stages of the disease. In general, the extent of iris involvement is a differentiating factor among the three variants. Chandler's syndrome usually presents with corneal edema and minimal iris alterations, and is often not recognized initially by the clinician. Progressive iris atrophy is characterized by extensive iris stromal atrophy associated with corectopia and ectropion uveae. These latter findings are usually seen in the quadrant with peripheral anterior synechiae, with formation of stretch holes in the opposite quadrant. In Cogan-Reese syndrome, any degree of iris atrophy may be present, but the predominant feature is the presence of multiple, pigmented, pedunculated iris nodules (Fig. 46.1a, b). These nodules are composed of tissue resembling iris stroma and are often surrounded by endothelial tissue.

The prevalence of glaucoma in ICE syndrome has been reported to be as high as 82%.[3] Glaucoma appears to be more frequent and severe in patients with progressive iris atrophy and Cogan-Reese syndrome as compared with Chandler's syndrome. The anterior chamber angle is usually open early in the disease process, and some patients may develop glaucoma at this stage. Often, broad peripheral anterior synechiae are present in the drainage angle, resulting from contraction of the abnormal basement membrane (Fig. 46.2a, b). These often extend to Schwalbe's line, leading to aqueous outflow obstruction and culminating in secondary angle closure glaucoma.[7]

Management of patients with ICE syndrome requires treatment for corneal edema, glaucoma, or both. Mild cases of corneal edema are often managed with soft contact lenses and hypertonic saline solutions. In advanced cases, penetrating or endothelial keratoplasty may be required, although the failure rate is high with need for repeat corneal grafts. In some cases, the corneal edema may be improved with reduction in intraocular pressure. Medical therapy for glaucoma is usually initiated with aqueous suppressants, but often fails. Laser trabeculoplasty is ineffective due to the structural alterations in the angle recess.

Surgical intervention is eventually required in a high percentage of patients with ICE syndrome and glaucoma. The most commonly performed surgical procedure is trabeculectomy, with variable success rates reported. Shields et al[8] reported a success rate of 69% in 33 cases with trabeculectomy. Doe et al[9] demonstrated improved outcomes with concomitant use of antifibrosis agents. In general, the higher failure rate is attributed to a younger patient population with excessive scarring. Endothelialization of the fistula in the bleb cavity can lead to obstruction of aqueous flow.[10] Aqueous drainage implants have shown favorable outcomes in a small number of cases, but further studies are warranted to validate these results in a large series.[11]

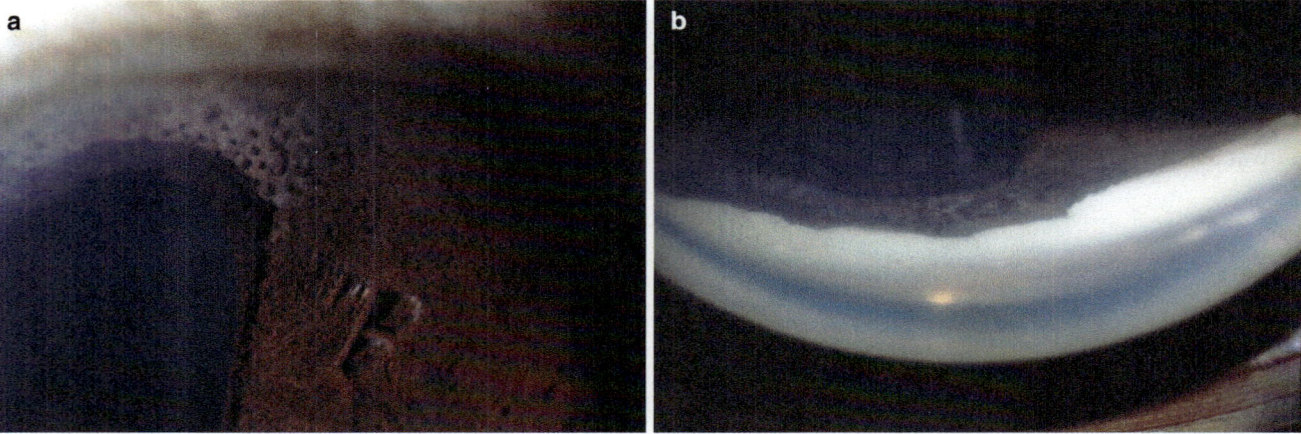

**Fig. 46.1** A 39-year-old African-American woman with Cogan-Reese syndrome. (**a**) Multiple, pigmented, pedunculated nodules and ectropion uvea (*left*) are located adjacent to relatively normal-appearing iris (*right*). (**b**) Peripheral anterior synechia observed by gonioscopy in the anterior chamber angle adjacent to the abnormal iris

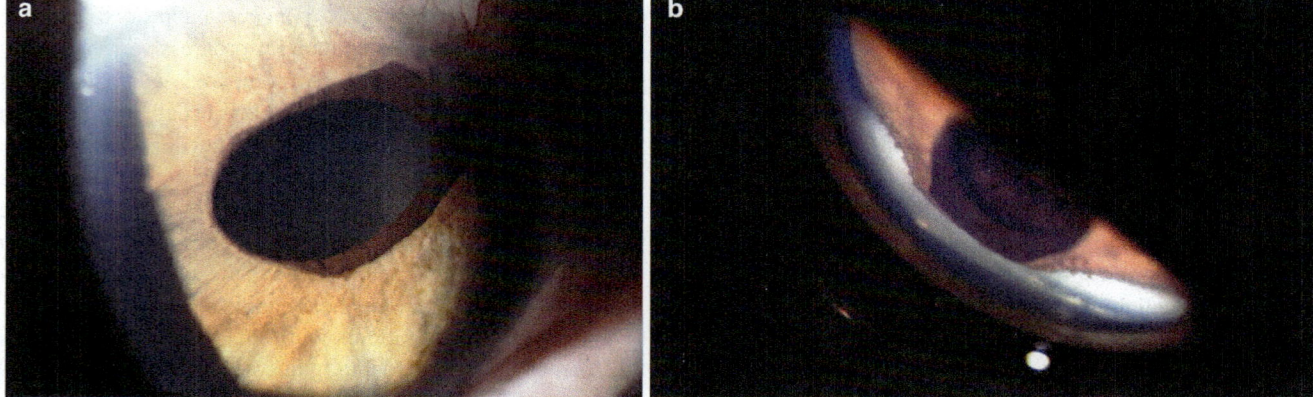

**Fig. 46.2** A 47-year-old Caucasian woman with Cogan-Reese syndrome. (**a**) Corectopia and ectropion uvea are present. (**b**) Gonioscopy shows broad peripheral anterior synechia in the anterior chamber angle

# References

1. Des Marchais B, Simmons RB, Simmons RJ, Shields MB. Bilateral Chandler syndrome. *J Glaucoma*. 1999;8(4):276–277.
2. Salim S, Shields MB, Walton D. Iridocorneal endothelial syndrome in a child. *J Pediatr Ophthalmol Strabismus*. 2006;43(5):308-310.
3. Hirst LW, Quigley HA, Stark W, et al. Specular microscopy of iridocorneal endothelial syndrome. *Am J Ophthalmol*. 1980;89: 11–21.
4. Campbell DG, Shields MB, Smith TR. The corneal endothelium and the spectrum of essential iris atrophy. *Am J Ophthalmol*. 1978;86:317–324.
5. Alvarado JA, Murphy CG, Maglio M, et al. Pathogenesis of Chandler's syndrome, essential iris atrophy, and the Cogan-Reese syndrome. Alterations of the corneal endothelium. *Invest Ophthalmol Vis Sci*. 1986;27:873–882.
6. Alvarado JA, Underwood JL, Green WR, et al. Detection of herpes simplex viral DNA in the iridocorneal endothelial syndrome. *Arch Ophthalmol*. 1994;112:1601–1609.
7. Salim S, Shields MB. Pretrabecular mechanisms of intraocular pressure elevation. In: Tombran-Tink J, Barnstable CJ, Shields MB, eds. *Mechanisms of the glaucomas*. New Jersey: Humana; 2008:83–97.
8. Shields MB, Campbell DG, Simmons RJ. The essential iris atrophies. *Am J Ophthalmol*. 1978;85:749–759.
9. Doe EA, Budenz DL, Gedde SJ, et al. Long-term surgical outcomes of patients with glaucoma secondary to the iridocorneal endothelial syndrome. *Ophthalmology*. 2001;108:1789–1795.
10. Yanoff M, Scheie H, Allman M. Endothelialization of filtering bleb in iris nevus syndrome. *Arch Ophthalmol*. 1976;94:1933–1936.
11. Kim DK, Aslanides IM, Schmidt CM, et al. Long-term outcome of aqueous shunt surgery in ten patients with iridocorneal endothelial syndrome. *Ophthalmology*. 1999;106:1030–1034.

# Chapter 47
# Ghost Cell Glaucoma

Dinorah P. Engel Castro and Cynthia Mattox

Ghost cell glaucoma was first described in 1976 by Campbell[1] and coworkers as a transient secondary open angle glaucoma in which the trabecular meshwork is obstructed by degenerated red blood cells called "ghost cells." Ghost cells may develop in any remaining red blood cells 7–10 days following vitreous hemorrhage from any etiology. The erythrocytes become spherical, less pliable, and partially lose their intracellular hemoglobin, causing them to appear tan-colored. The denaturized hemoglobin left in the cytoplasm binds to the internal surface of the cell membrane forming granules (Heinz bodies). Ghost cells, once formed, may remain for months in the vitreous cavity after hemorrhage. These vitreous ghost cells can gain access to the anterior chamber through a disrupted anterior hyaloid face, or an open posterior capsule from previous surgery,[2] after traumatic injury[3] or spontaneously.[4] Ghost cells are less pliable than fresh cells; thus, once in the anterior chamber, they may obstruct the trabecular meshwork and markedly increase intraocular pressure.

Ghost cell glaucoma has rarely been associated with complicated intracapsular or extracapsular cataract surgeries in which hyphema or vitreous hemorrhage developed. Ghost cell glaucoma has been more commonly described when a vitreous hemorrhage was not completely removed during vitrectomy[2] or as a consequence of vitreous hemorrhage caused by trauma,[3] or after hemorrhage from a retina disorder such as proliferative diabetic retinopathy.[4] A single case report describes ghost cell glaucoma after a vitreous hemorrhage from a snake bite.[5]

Diagnosis of this condition can be made clinically given a history of previous vitreous hemorrhage following trauma or surgery, or associated with a preexisting disease. In biomicroscopy, the anterior chamber is filled with small tan-colored cells that may become layered in the inferior anterior chamber angle (candy-stripe sign). The anterior chamber cellular reaction appears out of proportion compared to the aqueous flare or conjunctival injection. IOP can be markedly increased, resulting in corneal edema. Gonioscopically, the angle appears normal except for the ghost cells layered over the trabecular meshwork inferiorly.[6] In questionable situations, an anterior chamber aspirate can be obtained and ghost cells may be observed on microscopic examination[7,8] (See Fig. 47.1).

Differential diagnosis of ghost cell glaucoma includes the less common hemolytic and hemosiderotic glaucomas, uveitic glaucoma, and endophthalmitis. Neovascular glaucoma, which may present with anterior chamber and vitreous hemorrhage, should also be ruled out by carefully evaluating the iris and the angle.

IOP reduction is the goal of treatment for ghost cell glaucoma. Although ghost cell glaucoma is not a permanent condition, it may take months until the degenerated cells are completely removed from the anterior chamber and vitreous. Management needs to be titrated, as with all glaucomas, to what is known about the status of the optic nerve. If medical management fails, irrigation of the anterior chamber along with a posterior vitrectomy may be necessary to clear the blood and ghost cells.[9]

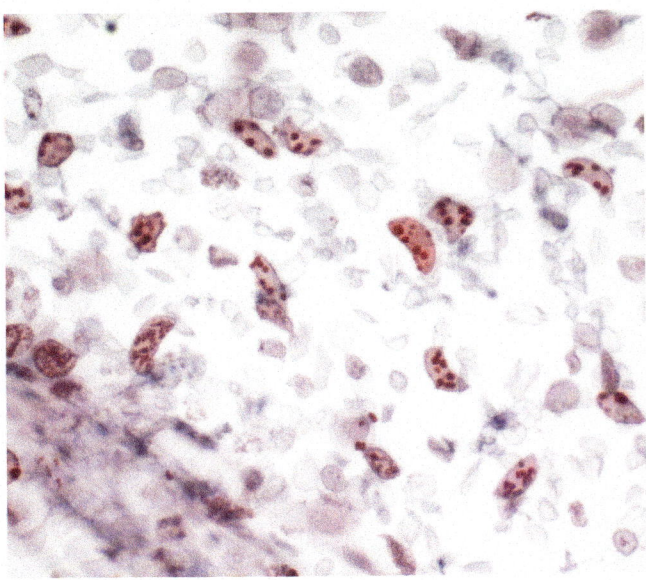

**Fig. 47.1** Anterior chamber aspirate stained with hematoxilin-eosin, showing a spherical erythrocyte with denaturized hemoglobin granule bound to the internal surface of the cell membrane (Heinz body)

# References

1. Campbell DG, Simmons RJ, Grant WM. Ghost cells as a cause of glaucoma. *Am J Ophthalmol*. 1976;81:441-450.
2. Campbell DG, Simmons RJ, Tolentino FI, McMeel JW. Glaucoma occurring after closed vitrectomy. *Am J Ophthalmol*. 1977;83:63-69.
3. Campbell DG. Ghost cell glaucoma following trauma. *Ophthalmology*. 1981;88:1151-1158.
4. Mansour AM, Chess J, Starita R. Nontraumatic ghost cell glaucoma – a case report. *Ophthalmic Surg*. 1986;17:34-36.
5. Rojas L, Ortiz G, Gutiérrez M, Corredor S. Ghost cell glaucoma related to snake poisoning. *Arch Ophthalmol*. 2001;119:1212-1213.
6. Campbell DG, Schertzer R. Ghost cell glaucoma. In: Ritch R, Shields MB, Krupin T, eds. *The Glaucomas*. 2nd ed. St Louis: Mosby-Year Book; 1996.
7. Cameron JD, Havener VR. Histologic confirmation of ghost cell glaucoma by routine light microscopy. *Am J Ophthalmol*. 1983;96:251-252.
8. Summers CG, Lindstrom RL, Cameron JD. Phase contrast microscopy. Diagnosis of ghost cell glaucoma following cataract extraction. Surv Ophthalmol. 1984;28:342-344.
9. Abu el-Asrar AM, al-Obeidan SA. Pars plana vitrectomy in the management of ghost cell glaucoma. *Int Ophthalmol*. 1995;19:121-124.
10. Campbell DG, Essigmann EM. Hemolytic ghost cell glaucoma. Further studies. *Arch Ophthalmol*. 1979;1997:2141-2146.
11. Summers CG, Lindstrom RL. Ghost cell glaucoma following lens implantation. *J Am Intraocul Implant Soc*. 1983;9:429-433.

# Chapter 48
# Fuchs' Endothelial Dystrophy and Glaucoma

Blair Boehmer and Clark Springs

Fuchs' Endothelial Dystrophy (FED) is a common disorder of the cornea that causes slow progressive endothelial degeneration with subsequent corneal edema and loss of vision in late stages. It is characterized by a thickened Descemet's membrane (DM) from the aberrant deposition of widespaced collagen and the development of guttae, or posterior excrescences that represent projections of abnormal extracellular matrix between DM and endothelial cells.[1,2] The bilateral, though asymmetric, condition often presents clinically between the fourth and seventh decades of life and is reported to have a female predominance as high as 3.5:1.[3] Pedigree analysis reveals an autosomal dominant inheritance pattern with variable expressivity, although sporadic cases are also reported.[4] While several hypotheses exist, the primary etiology of FED is unknown. Multiple studies have proposed an association between FED and glaucoma including primary open angle, angle closure, and other glaucomas. The relationships remain unclear.

## 48.1 Primary Open Angle Glaucoma

Abnormal aqueous outflow and elevated IOP has been demonstrated in patients with corneal guttata in several studies. Buxton et al. report that tonography in patients with guttata revealed a facility of outflow less than normal in 82% of eyes and an elevated IOP/outflow facility ratio in 70%, implying involvement of the trabecular meshwork (TM).[5] These data were used to support Kolker and Hetherington's position that 10–15% of patients with FED had concomitant primary open angle glaucoma as well as the suggestion that "glaucoma should be suspected in all patients who have endothelial dystrophy."[6] Specular microscopy was subsequently used in a recreation of Buxom's protocol that showed no correlation of aqueous outflow with the presence or severity of guttata.[7] A study by Burns et al. actually demonstrated a negative correlation between IOP and guttata, although increased corneal thickness may have confounded tonometry in this case.[8] Abnormal composition of aqueous humor has been found in FED patients with respect to the level of fibrinogen-related molecules. This has been thought to theoretically predispose the TM to dysfunction.[9] However, no differences in fibrinogen-related metabolites, glucose, $CO_2$, $HCO_3$, or pH were noted when aqueous was compared to normal controls in an analysis by Wilson et al.[10] Krachmer studied 71 patients with FED in 64 families and found only one case of POAG.[11] Similarly, no correlation between the conditions was found on a pedigree analysis by Magovern.[12]

## 48.2 Angle Closure Glaucoma

FED has also been associated with an increased incidence of angle closure glaucoma. A study by Bigar and Witmer reported bilateral endothelial dystrophy in 35% of patients with angle closure glaucoma, while Rice claims that FED patients typically have shallower anterior chambers.[13,14] The implications of these statements, if accurate, are weighty and would affect differential diagnosis and treatment in both conditions. Based on these studies and Fuchs' own refractions that yielded an average spherical equivalent of +2.45D in a subset of his patients, Pitts and Jay confirmed through clinical measurements of 24 FED patients that Fuchs' dystrophy is associated with axial hypermetropia and shallow anterior chamber.[15] A similar refractive error of +2.48D was reported with mean values for axial length and anterior chamber depth significantly less than in controls.[14] Initially, the correlation with angle closure was attributed to corneal edema crowding the anterior chamber, but angle closure is frequently seen before progression to endothelial decompensation. In 73% of FED patients with angle closure, an acute attack occurred prior to clinically significant corneal disease.[16] In contrast, Brooks et al. observed no association between the conditions and showed significantly shallower anterior chambers in patients with isolated angle closure glaucomas than FED. Also, within the angle closure group, only one of 88 participants had changes consistent with FED, much less than Bigar's estimate of 35%.[17] Unfortunately, increased pressure negatively affects the corneal endothelium as evidenced by reduced endothelial cell densities in patients with acute or chronic angle closure, thus obscuring the correlation.[18] Although the conditions may exacerbate each other, several authors conclude that a causal relationship is improbable in either direction, but an association may exist through genetic linkage.[15] While FED does not manifest clinically until later in life, this is a reasonable assumption as the TM and corneal endothelium share a neural crest origin, and microscopy shows alterations in DM, specifically a thickened posterior banded layer and a thin or absent posterior nonbanded layer that suggest dysfunction from a very early age.[1,19]

## 48.3 Oxidative Stress and Apoptosis

High levels of oxidative damage and apoptosis have been implicated in the disease process of both glaucoma and FED. Through molecular analysis, recent research shows that apoptosis is the cause of endothelial cell death in FED with evidence pointing to oxidative stress as catalyst.[20-22] Clusterin, a protein that acts as a cytoprotector or proapoptic depending on posttranslational modification, is upregulated, and both forms are overexpressed in Fuch's endothelial cells.[23] Jurkunas et al. also reveal significantly decreased expression of peroxiredoxins, a novel class of antioxidants, in FED endothelium when compared to controls.[24] Epithelial cells in the disease also show abnormal levels of apoptosis regulator proteins, Bax, cathepsin, survivin, and p27 suggesting excessive apoptosis.[25] In relation to glaucoma, aerobic reactions, superoxide anions, and $H_2O_2$ in the anterior chamber expose the TM to high levels of oxidative stress. Such chronic insult is suggested to play a role in TM dysfunction.[26,27] In addition, studies indicate that retinal ganglion cells in glaucomatous eyes die by apoptosis through increases in several activation signals.[28] DeLaPaz and Epskin have shown decreased activity of human TM superoxide dismutase in the aging eye, and a threefold increase in TM 8-OHdg, a marker of oxidative stress, is seen in POAG patients. Certain products of lipid peroxidation are also elevated in the serum of glaucoma patients.[26,29] In addition, null mutations in a glutathione transferase are associated with development of POAG.[26] These putative alterations in mechanisms designed to protect cells from oxidative stress may play a role in pathogenesis of FED and glaucoma.

## 48.4 Other Considerations

Genetic studies point to involvement of collagen VIII gene COL8A2 or, more recently, sodium borate transporter SLC4A11 as a cause of FED.[30] While SLC4A11 products are not expressed in the TM, collagen VIII is produced and forms porous hexagonal lattice structures that may provide support and protection from compressive forces.[31] Therefore, abnormal collagen VIII could be a factor in both diseases. Fluid balance is integral to glaucoma and FED disease processes. Aquaporins, a class of transmembrane proteins that regulate cellular water flux, are expressed in TM, ciliary body, and corneal endothelial tissues.[32] Analysis by Kenney et al. reveals a significant decrease in AQP1 in FED corneas, likely contributing to development of edema.[33] AQP1 expression in the TM is also shown to affect the outflow facility. AQP1 and AQP4 are both expressed in nonpigmented ciliary body cells and likely modulate aqueous humor production. Certain glaucoma treatments are aimed at their regulation.[34,35] Hormonal influences are suggested in FED, as a female predominance exists; however, there is no consensus on a similar epidemiology in glaucoma.[1]

## 48.5 Conclusion

Currently, the association between glaucoma and FED is unclear, but the evidence is slightly more convincing in relation to angle closure glaucoma. Increased IOP and duration of elevation both exacerbate corneal endothelial damage, but neither in a consistent nor predictable fashion. Some recommend closer monitoring of IOP in FED patients and possibly performing a combined cataract extraction with penetrating keratoplasty to prevent occurrence of angle closure.[15] Analysis of the literature, however, does not strongly support any specific treatment or evaluation of FED or glaucoma in relation to the other. Each patient should be managed individually on a case-by-case basis. Further research on these subjects will hopefully elucidate any association that may exist between the two relatively common diseases.

## References

1. Adamis AP, Filatov V, Tripathi BJ, Tripathi RC. Fuchs' endothelial dystrophy of the cornea. *Surv Ophthalmol*. 1993;38(2):149-167.
2. Gottsch JD, Zhang C, Sundin OH, Bell WR, Stark WJ, et al. Fuchs corneal dystrophy: aberrant collagen distribution in an L450W mutant of the COL8A2 gene. *Invest Ophthalmol Vis Sci*. 2005;46(12):4504-4511.
3. Afshari NA, Pittard AB, Siddiqui A, Klintworth GK. Clinical study of Fuchs corneal endothelial dystrophy leading to penetrating keratoplasty. *Arch Ophthalmol*. 2006;124(6):777-780.
4. Rosenblum P, Stark WJ, Maumenee IH, Hirst LW, Maumenee AE. Hereditary Fuchs' dystrophy. *Am J Ophthalmol*. 1980;90(4):455-462.
5. Buxton JN, Preston RW, Riechers R, Guibault N. Tonography in cornea guttata. *Arch Ophthalmol*. 1967;77(5):602-603.
6. Kolker AE, Hetherington J. *Becker-Shaffer's Diagnosis and Therapy of the Glaucomas*. 4th ed. St. Louis: Mosby; 1976.

7. Roberts CW, Steinert RF, Thomas JV, Boruchoff SA. Endothelial guttata and facility of aqueous outflow. *Cornea*. 1984;3(1):5-9.
8. Burns RR, Bourne WM, Brubaker RF. Endothelial function in patients with cornea guttata. *Invest Ophthalmol Vis Sci*. 1981;20(1):77-85.
9. Bramson T, Stenbjerg S. Fibrinolytic factors in aqueous humor and serum from patients with Fuchs' dystrophy and patients with cataract. *Acta Ophthalmol*. 1979;57(3):470-476.
10. Wilson SE, Bourne WM, Maguire LJ, Rahhal FM, Ribaudo RK, et al. Aqueous humor composition in Fuchs' dystrophy. *Invest Ophthalmol Vis Sci*. 1989;30(3):449-453.
11. Krachmer JH, Purcell JJ, Young CW, Bucher KD. Corneal endothelial dystrophy: a study of 64 families. *Arch Ophthalmol*. 1978;96(11):2036-2039.
12. Magovern M, Beauchamp GR, McTigue JW, Fine BS, Baumiller RC. Inheritance of Fuchs' combined dystrophy. *Ophthalmology*. 1979;86(10):1897-1923.
13. Bigar F, Witmar R. Corneal endothelial changes in primary acute angle-closure glaucoma. *Ophthalmology*. 1982;89(6):596-599.
14. Pitts JF, Jay JL. The association of Fuchs's corneal endothelial dystrophy with axial hypermetropia, shallow anterior chamber, and angle closure glaucoma. *Br J Ophthalmol*. 1990;74(10):601-604.
15. Fuchs E. Dystrophia epithelialis corneae. *Graefes Arch Clin Exp Ophthalmol*. 1910;76(3):478-508.
16. Lowenstein A, Geyer O, Hourvitz D, Lazar M. The association of Fuchs's corneal endothelial dystrophy with angle closure glaucoma. *Br J Ophthalmol*. 1991;75(8):510.
17. Brooks AM, Grant G, Gillies WE. The significance of anterior chamber depth in Fuch's corneal dystrophy and cornea guttata. *Cornea*. 1994;13(2):131-135.
18. Sihota R, Lakshmaia C, Titiyal JS, Dada T, Agarwal HS. Corneal endothelial status in the subtypes of primary angle closure glaucoma. *Clin Exp Ophthalmol*. 2003;31:492-495.
19. Wilson SE, Bourne WM. Fuchs' dystrophy. *Cornea*. 1988;7(1):2-18.
20. Borderie VM, Baudrimont M, Vallee A, Ereau TL, Gray F, et al. Corneal endothelial cell apoptosis in patients with Fuchs' dystrophy. *Invest Ophthalmol Vis Sci*. 2000;41(9):2501-2505.
21. Li QJ, Ashraf FM, Shen D, Green RW, Satrk WJ, et al. The role of apoptosis in the pathogenesis of Fuchs endothelial dystrophy of the cornea. *Arch Ophthalmol*. 2001;119(11):1597-1604.
22. Wang Z, Handa JT, Green WR, Stark WJ, Weinberg RS, et al. Advanced glycation end products and receptors in Fuchs' dystrophy corneas undergoing Decemet's stripping with endothelial keratoplasty. *Ophthalmology*. 2007;114(8):1453-1460.
23. Jurkunas UV, Bitar MS, Rawe I, Harris DL, Colby K, et al. Increased clusterin expression in Fuchs' endothelial dystrophy. *Invest Ophthalmol Vis Sci*. 2008;49(7):2946-2955.
24. Jurkunas UV, Rawe I, Bitar M, Zhu C, Harris DL, et al. Decreased expression of peroxiredoxins in Fuchs' endothelial dystrophy. *Invest Ophthalmol Vis Sci*. 2008;49(7):2956-2963.
25. Szentmary N, Szende B, Suveges I. P53, CD95, cathepsin and survivin pathways in Fuchs' dystrophy and pseudophakic bullous keratopathy corneas. *Histol Histopathol*. 2008;23:911-916.
26. Chen JZ, Kadlubar FF. A new clue to glaucoma pathogenesis. *Am J Med*.2003; 697-698.
27. Green K. Free radicals and aging of anterior segment tissues of the eye: a hypothesis. *Ophthalmic Res*. 1995;27(suppl 1):143-149.
28. Kumarasamy NA, Lam FS, Wang AL, Theoharides TC. Glaucoma: current and developing concepts for inflammation, pathogenesis and treatment. *Eur J Inflamm*. 2006;4(3):129-137.
29. Yildirim O, Ates NA, Ercan B, Muslu N, Unlu A, et al. Role of oxidative stress enzymes in open angle glaucoma. *Eye*. 2005;19:580-583.
30. Vithana EN, Morgan PE, Ramprasad V, Tan DT, Yong VH, et al. SLC4A11 mutations in Fuchs endothelial corneal dystrophy. *Hum Mol Genet*. 2008;17(5):656-666.
31. Acott TS, Kelley MJ. Extracellular matrix in the trabecular meshwork. *Exp Eye Res*. 2008;86:543-561.
32. Stamer DW, Snyder RW, Smith BL, Agre P, Regan JW. Localization of aquaporin CHIP in the human eye: implications in the pathogenesis of glaucoma and other disorders of ocular fluid balance. *Invest Ophthalmol Vis Sci*. 1994;35(11):3867-3872.
33. Kenney CM, Atilano SR, Zorapapel N, Holguin B, Gaster RN, et al. Altered expression of aquaporins in bullous keratopathy and Fuchs' dystrophy corneas. *J Histochem Cytochem*. 2004;52(10):1341-1351.
34. Stamer WD, Peppel K, O'Donnell ME, Roberts BC, Wu F, et al. Expression of aquaporin-1 in human trabecular meshwork cells: role in resting cell volume. *Invest Ophthalmol Vis Sci*. 2001;42(8):1803-1811.
35. Chatterton JE. RNAi-mediated inhibition of aquaporin 1 for treatment of IOP-related conditions; Patent No. 20080214486. United States, 2008.

# Chapter 49
# Ocular Trauma and Glaucoma

Helen Tseng and Kenneth Mitchell

## 49.1 Introduction

Blunt or penetrating ocular trauma can result in an elevated intraocular pressure (IOP). This elevation in IOP can cause early or late glaucoma, depending on the nature of the injury. Although glaucoma associated with trauma is a multifactorial disease process, the main underlying feature is reduced aqueous humor outflow through the trabecular meshwork channels.

## 49.2 Epidemiology and Pathogenesis

Blunt ocular trauma commonly causes anterior segment damage as the cornea and sclera are displaced posteriorly. This compressive deformation causes posterior displacement of the iris–lens diaphragm with subsequent expansion at the equator of the eye. Such damage may cause various anterior and posterior ocular tissues to tear, as illustrated in Fig. 49.1. The most common injuries following blunt ocular trauma are angle recession (52–80.5%), hyphema (49%), and iris injury (37.3%).[1,2] Development of glaucoma after ocular contusion is 3.39% after 6 months with independent risk factors including hyphema, baseline visual acuity <20/200, lens injury, angle recession, and advancing age, in decreasing order.[3]

Penetrating ocular trauma can also cause an elevated IOP from intraocular inflammation, secondary angle closure, intraocular hemorrhage, lens injury, or epithelial downgrowth.[4] There is a 2.67% risk of developing glaucoma after penetrating ocular injury,[5] and the most common anterior segment injuries are iridodialysis (50%) and corneal injury (41%).[2]

Globes that have suffered penetrating injuries are usually first examined in the emergency room setting. The management of open globes is beyond the purview of this chapter. Here, we will discuss the diagnosis and treatment of glaucoma in traumatized eyes that are stable with respect to globe integrity.

## 49.3 Diagnosis

A complete history of the nature and timing of the current injury, past ocular injury, any preexisting glaucoma, and past medical history, including sickle cell disease, coagulation defects, tetanus vaccination status, and use of anticoagulants needs to be obtained. Next, a complete ophthalmologic exam including visual acuity, pupil exam, IOP measurement, slit-lamp exam, and fundus exam (if possible) should be performed. Special attention should be taken to check for any lens damage, zonular injury, and peripheral retinal lesion. During the initial exam, careful gonioscopy can be performed; however, there is a risk that this exam may increase any intraocular bleeding. Therefore, it may be prudent to postpone this exam until 4 weeks after initial injury. Gonioscopy may reveal shallow anterior chamber depth, iris tears, trabecular meshwork tears, or angle recession as manifested by a white distinct scleral spur or a broad ciliary body band. Examination of the atraumatic eye should be done for comparison.

Elevated IOP secondary to trauma can cause early or late onset glaucoma depending on the damage and independent risk factors for glaucoma. Early onset glaucoma can occur with intraocular inflammation, trabecular meshwork damage, hyphema, and chemical trauma. Late onset glaucoma is more common with angle recession, ghost cells, lens injury, secondary angle closure, cyclodialysis cleft closure, epithelial downgrowth, retinal detachment,[6] and retained intraocular foreign body.

## 49.4 Early Onset Glaucoma After Trauma

### 49.4.1 Intraocular Inflammation After Trauma

Anterior segment inflammation may be present after blunt or penetrating trauma. This inflammation may result in ocular hypotension with decreased aqueous production.

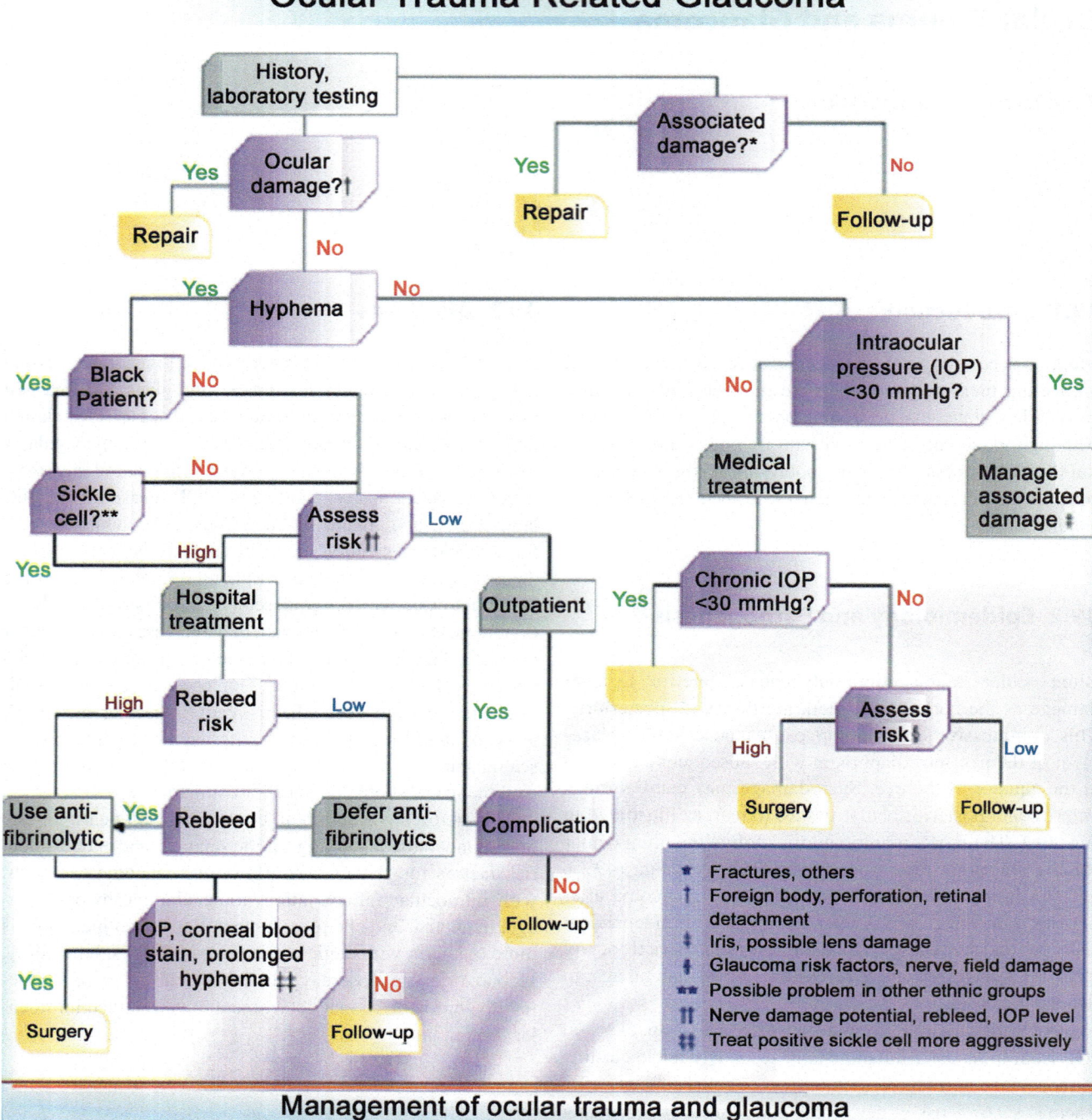

**Fig. 49.1** Ocular trauma glaucomas and their management. Reproduced with permission from Yanoff M, Duker JS, eds: Ophthalmology, 3rd ed. 2008 Mosby

However, it can also cause a rise in IOP with trabecular blockade with inflammatory cells and particulate debris (blood, iris pigment, lens particles, vitreous). Trabeculitis, the notion that the meshwork becomes inflamed and obstructed, may explain an elevated IOP when the level of anterior chamber inflammation is low and there is no lens material or blood seen in the anterior chamber. With penetrating injuries, Girkin et al. found that baseline intraocular inflammation was highly associated with the future development of glaucoma in a multivariate analysis.[5]

## 49.4.2 Trabecular Meshwork Injury

Direct damage to the trabecular meshwork outflow channels can cause an early rise in IOP. Gonioscopy findings include focal hemorrhage in Schlemm's canal, full-thickness rupture of trabecular meshwork, a trabecular flap, or cyclodialysis.[7]

## 49.4.3 Hyphema

Traumatic hyphemas generally result from a tear in the ciliary body or iris (Fig. 49.2).

The amount of blood in the anterior chamber determines the grade:

- Grade 1: blood fills less than one-third of the anterior chamber.
- Grade 2: blood fills one-third to one-half of the anterior chamber.
- Grade 3: blood fills one-half to less than 100% of the anterior chamber.
- Grade 4 or Eight-ball hyphema: blood or clot fills entire anterior chamber.

Red blood cells clog the trabecular meshwork, which, in combination with any concurrent ocular injury, can elevate the IOP. These patients need to be monitored for rebleeding, which is usually a higher grade than the initial bleed. Rebleeding is thought to be secondary to clot lysis and retraction from traumatized vessels. Risk factors for rebleeding include young age, African descent, larger initial hyphema, ocular hypotony or hypertension, and aspirin use.[4] Frequent exams are necessary to monitor IOP and for corneal bloodstaining.

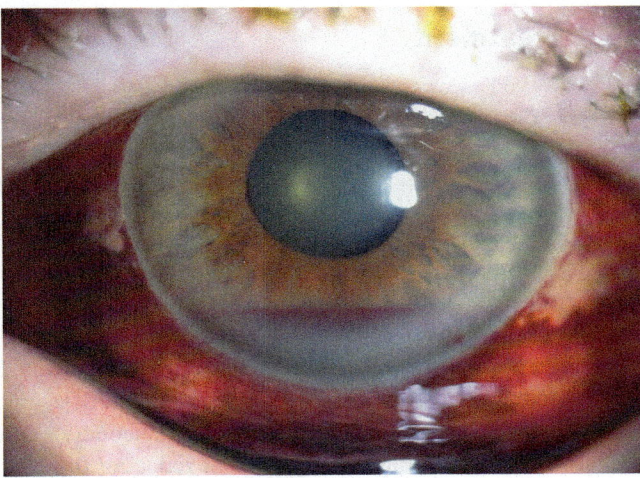

**Fig. 49.2** Hyphema. Layered blood in the anterior chamber, which may cause elevated IOP as the red blood cells clog the trabecular meshwork. Courtesy of Department of Ophthalmology, University of South Carolina

The cornea can develop a yellow/brown discoloration as hemoglobin and hemosiderin penetrate the corneal stroma. The risk of glaucoma must be assessed in each individual patient. Patients with preexisting glaucoma and sickle-cell disease are especially at risk. A sickle cell test and hemoglobin electrophoresis should be performed on patients of African and Hispanic ethnicity. Sickle-cell patients are more sensitive to IOP spikes as their optic nerves exist in a chronic relatively hypoxic state with their decreased blood flow.

## 49.4.4 Chemical Injuries

Alkaline injury is more likely to cause ocular hypertension and subsequent glaucoma than acid injury. Alkaline exposure causes an almost immediate shrinkage of the scleral collagen, which can elevate IOP to 40–50 mmHg. Next, a second elevation of IOP is noted within a few hours as prostaglandins are released.[6] This type of injury may also cause late onset glaucoma as peripheral anterior synechiae develop with possible trabecular meshwork scarring and pupillary block.

## 49.5 Late Onset Glaucoma After Trauma

### 49.5.1 Angle Recession

Angle recession is the result of a tear between the longitudinal and circular muscles of the ciliary body. Gonioscopy may reveal a broad ciliary band or very white scleral spur in comparison to the nontraumatic eye. Fifty to eighty-one percent of posttraumatic eyes develop angle recession and 6–20% of these eyes develop glaucoma. There is a higher risk of developing ocular hypertension if greater than 240° of the angle is affected. This elevation can occur months to years after the initial trauma. The underlying pathology of this late ocular hypertension is thought to be an extension of Descemet's membrane, which covers the trabecular meshwork and blocks outflow.

### 49.5.2 Ghost Cell Glaucoma

The red blood cells of a vitreous hemorrhage can lose their pliable biconcave disc shape and hemoglobin, and degenerate into tan/khaki spherical ghost cells. These ghost cells can fill the anterior chamber and form a tan hypopyon. Given their rigid spherical shape, it is difficult to traverse through the trabecular meshwork so they clog the outflow pathway.

On gonioscopy, the angle may appear normal with a tan layer coating the trabeculum, especially inferiorly. The subsequent IOP rise is proportional to the amount of ghost cells. This elevated IOP tends to occur 3–4 weeks after the development of a vitreous hemorrhage.[8]

### 49.5.3 Secondary Angle Closure

Intraocular inflammation and blood secondary to trauma are common. Persistent inflammation can lead to the formation of peripheral anterior synechiae. If extensive enough, the patient may develop angle closure glaucoma. Penetrating trauma commonly results in peripheral anterior synechiae formation and the angle should be swept at the time of primary closure to minimize the risk.

### 49.5.4 Lens Injury

There are four main types of traumatic lens injury that can lead to secondary glaucoma: lens subluxation, lens swelling, and a phacolytic or phacoanaphylactic process. Lens subluxation or dislocation from traumatic zonular damage can cause anterior or posterior displacement. This lens instability can lead to pupillary block and eventual creeping angle closure. Lens swelling/hydration from trauma can cause phacomorphic glaucoma with associated pupillary block. Phacolytic glaucoma results from the release of lens proteins through an intact capsule. Macrophages in the anterior chamber engulf these proteins and clog the trabecular meshwork. Phacoanaphylactic glaucoma is a granulomatous inflammatory reaction to lens particles released from a disrupted lens capsule.[7]

### 49.5.5 Cyclodialysis Cleft Closure

Cyclodialysis is the separation of the ciliary body from the scleral spur. This creates a direct pathway for aqueous fluid to the suprachoroidal space and can result in temporary or chronic hypotony. This cleft can close months to years later and result in a precipitous rise in IOP, presumably from the initial trauma's effect on outflow channels.

### 49.5.6 Epithelial Downgrowth

Epithelial downgrowth is a potential complication of penetrating ocular injury and less commonly occurs as a complication of elective microsurgery. The traumatic wound creates a pathway for epithelium to enter the anterior chamber. The creeping membrane creates a classic scalloped edge on the corneal endothelium and can extend to the iris and angles structures. Iris involvement can be confirmed if the membrane whitens with argon laser application. This topic is explored in greater depth in Chap. 74.

### 49.5.7 Retained Intraocular Foreign Body

Rarely, an iron-containing retained intraocular foreign body can cause siderosis bulbi. The iron exposure can cause iris heterochromia and ocular hypertension as the toxic iron coats the trabecular meshwork. Less frequently, copper-containing foreign bodies cause chalcosis with subsequent glaucoma. Both siderosis and chalcosis can also cause retinal dysfunction, which mimics glaucomatous visual field changes.

### 49.5.8 Rhegmatogenous Retinal Detachment

Ocular trauma may result in retinal dialysis, tears, and detachment. Rhegmatogenous retinal detachment is more commonly associated with ocular hypotension with decreased ciliary body aqueous production. However, 5–10% of these patients may develop Schwartz-Matsuo syndrome. In these cases, the retinal detachment causes the release of rod outer segments that can migrate into the anterior segment. There, these proteins can clog the outflow pathway with subsequent ocular hypertension. A thorough exam of the peripheral retina is imperative to make this diagnosis, which is often mistaken for inflammatory glaucoma. Repair of the retinal detachment usually results in rapid improvement of IOP.[6]

## 49.6 Treatment

### 49.6.1 General Principles of Medical and Surgical Management

Each patient must be assessed for their individual risk of developing posttraumatic glaucoma to guide treatment. In contrast, patients with preexisting glaucoma should be managed more aggressively and may require expeditious surgical management. As always, management needs to be dictated by the status of the optic nerve. The management of ocular hypertension and subsequent posttraumatic glaucoma should focus on the underlying etiology and at reducing the IOP. Any inflammation should be treated with topical steroids. As these patients may require a prolonged course of steroids, they should be carefully monitored for any IOP steroid response. The mainstay for IOP treatment is aqueous suppressants, including beta blockers, alpha agonists, and carbonic anhydrase inhibitors (if not contraindicated). Cycloplegics should be considered to increase uveoscleral outflow and to control ciliary spasm. Generally, miotics are avoided as they may worsen inflammation. Prostaglandin analogues can be tried in the absence of cystoid macular edema as a "last resort" before recommending surgical management. If medical management fails and there is progression of optic nerve damage, then surgical intervention must be considered. Current filtration surgery options include trabeculectomy, with or without adjunctive antimetabolite use, tube shunt implantation, and cilioablative procedures. More specific medical and surgical treatment plans are usually necessary for certain cases, including hyphema, angle recession, and ghost cell glaucoma.

### 49.6.2 Hyphema Treatment

The two main goals in the treatment of traumatic hyphemas are IOP control and prevention of rebleeding. This can usually be achieved in an outpatient setting unless there is concern for noncompliance, other high risk ocular injuries, or the patient is at high risk for a rebleed. All patients should be restricted to bed rest/limited activity. An eye shield should be worn at all times; a patch should be avoided as this may prevent recognition of decreased vision. The head of the bed should be elevated and treatment with atropine and topical steroids are used. Both aspirin and nonsteroidal anti-inflammatory drugs should be avoided. IOP control should consist of topical beta-blockers and alpha agonists. Carbonic anhydrase inhibitors can be used topically and systemically in nonsickle cell disease/trait patients. They should be avoided in these patients as the associated increased systemic acidity may induce a crisis. Methazolamide causes less acidosis and, if necessary, may be considered with adequate hydration. Indications for surgical intervention are IOP>50 mmHg for 5 days, IOP>35 mmHg for 7 days, unresolved total hyphema for 9 days, or corneal blood staining.[9] Surgical interventions include paracentesis, anterior chamber washout, and clot expression, which may necessitate the utilization of a vitrectomy instrument.

Traumatic hyphemas have a 0.4–35% rate of rebleed, usually within 2–5 days. For prevention of rebleeding, one can consider aminocaproic acid or systemic steroids. Aminocaproic acid inhibits fibrinolysis and therefore decreases the rate of clot hemolysis. A randomized clinical trial found the same 7.1% rate of rebleed when patients were treated with oral aminocaproic acid 50 mg/kg every 4 h for 5 days versus oral prednisone 40 mg/day divided dose.[10] Use of aminocaproic acid has also resulted in longer duration of clot and its cessation may cause an IOP spike as the clot begins to lyse. The use of topical aminocaproic acid is currently under debate.

### 49.6.3 Angle Recession Glaucoma Treatment

Angle recession glaucoma is often refractory to aqueous suppressant therapy. Miotics should be avoided since the subsequent decrease in uveoscleral outflow will compound the decreased conventional outflow. If medical therapy fails, the surgical options include trabeculectomy with or without antimetabolite and tube shunt implantation. Laser trabeculoplasty is not effective. A retrospective study by Mermoud et al. found that trabeculectomy with adjunctive antimetabolite had a statistically significant greater reduction in IOP than trabeculectomy without antimetabolite and Molteno tube implantation after 6 months. This group also required less postoperative glaucoma medication. However, 3/20 of these patients developed late bleb infection.[11]

### 49.6.4 Ghost Cell Glaucoma Treatment

If medical management of IOP is inadequate, then surgical treatment options include anterior chamber wash-out or vitrectomy to remove as many red blood cells as possible.

## References

1. Canavan YM, Archer DB. Anterior segment consequences of blunt ocular injury. *Br J Ophthalmol.* 1982;66:549–555.
2. Ozer PA, Yalvac IS, Satana B, Eksioglu U, Duman S. Incidence and risk factors in secondary glaucomas after blunt and penetrating ocular trauma. *J Glaucoma.* 2007;16:685–690.
3. Girkin CA, McGwin G Jr, Long C, Morris R, Kuhn F. Glaucoma after ocular contusion: a cohort study of the United States Eye Injury Registry. *J Glaucoma.* 2005;14:470–473.
4. Schmidt C. Glaucoma Associated with Trauma. In: Eid T, Spaeth G, eds. *The Glaucomas.* Philadelphia, PA:Lippincott Williams&Wilkins; 2000:18 1–189.
5. Girkin CA, McGwin G Jr, Morris R, Kuhn F. Glaucoma following penetrating ocular trauma: a cohort study of the United States Eye Injury Registry. *Am J Ophthalmol.* 2005;139:100–105.
6. Shingleton B. Glaucoma due to trauma. In: Epstein D, ed. *Chandler and Grant's Glaucoma.* 4th ed. Baltimore, MD: Williams&Wilkins; 1997:395–403.
7. Kuhn F, Pieramici D. *Ocular Trauma: Principles and Practice.* New York, NY: Thieme; 2002.
8. Epstein D. Hemolytic or ghost-cell glaucoma. In Epstein D, ed. *Chandler and Grant's Glaucoma.* 4th ed. Baltimore, MD: Wiliiams&Wilkins; 1997:412–415.
9. Berke S. Post-traumatic glaucoma. In: Yanoff M, Duker J, eds. *Ophthalmology.* 2nd ed. St Louis, MO:Mosby; 2004: 1518-1521.
10. Farber MD, Fiscella R, Goldberg M. Aminocaproic acid versus prednisone for the treatment of traumatic hyphema. *Ophthalmology.* 1991;98:279–286.
11. Mermoud A, Salmon JF, Barron A, Straker C, Murray AD. Surgical management of post-traumatic angle recession glaucoma. *Ophthalmology.* 1993;100:634–642.

# Chapter 50
# Infantile, Childhood, and Juvenile Glaucomas

David S. Walton

The childhood glaucomas are a clinically diverse group of ocular disorders. On examination many different potential primary and secondary etiologies of the glaucoma must be considered. The systemic conditions associated with the pediatric glaucomas also need to be recognized. The profound and common anterior segment abnormalities secondary to the increased intraocular pressure (IOP) seen in these children makes their conditions seem more similar than is necessarily true. The purpose of this chapter is to provide information to assist with the examination of children with glaucomas to enable physicians to recognize them more accurately, so that more appropriate and optimum glaucoma treatment decisions will be made.

Infantile primary congenital glaucoma (PCG) is the most common primary glaucoma seen in infants and older children. It is a hereditary childhood glaucoma secondary to abnormal development of the filtration angle. Other less frequent infantile glaucoma conditions must be differentiated from this type. Glaucoma surgery has dramatically improved the visual prognosis for children affected with these glaucomas. The optimum selection of glaucoma surgery/glaucoma therapy depends on many factors, including an accurate diagnosis of the presence, severity, and type of glaucoma. Late recognition and delayed IOP control can result in permanent and severe visual morbidity. Associated secondary amblyopia and refractive errors are common. Clinical monitoring of these young glaucoma patients is demanding, requires specialized instrumentation and skills, and is often carried out for uncooperative young patients. This care is best managed by ophthalmologists who possess the motivation and clinical experience with childhood glaucoma and the necessary specialized surgical and examination skills. Successful infantile glaucoma control is a lifelong goal requiring perseverance by patients, by their parents, and by their caregivers.

The primary developmental glaucomas are subclassified according to the presence or absence of systemic or other ocular anomalies, and the secondary childhood glaucomas are classified according to their etiologies.

*Developmental glaucoma* is a term used to broadly encompass all glaucomas resulting from abnormal development of the aqueous outflow system, which may or may not be associated with a systemic anomaly. In 1984, Hoskins and Shaffer classified the developmental glaucomas anatomically related to anomalies of the trabecular meshwork alone (*isolated trabeculodysgenesis*), in combination with the iris (*iridotrabeculodysgenesis*), or with the cornea (*corneotrabeculodysgenesis*).[1]

*Congenital glaucoma* is a term also broadly used when responsible developmental anomalies are suspected. *Primary congenital glaucoma* (PCG) is the term now recommended for all three clinical age-of-diagnosis related subdivisions of PCG with the clinical features, gonioscopic abnormalities, and genetics of isolated trabeculodysgenesis or iridotrabeculodysgenesis. The designation *juvenile glaucoma* is best reserved for patients with primary *juvenile open-angle glaucoma* (JOAG) who have normal gonioscopic findings, frequent myopia, and *acquired* glaucoma associated with autosomal dominant inheritance.

Most primary childhood glaucomas are genetically determined. When the genetic basis for childhood glaucoma can be identified, it becomes possible to reclassify and associate patients more meaningfully. The clinical examination reveals the severity of the disease and provides the most reliable and available information to determine the diagnosis and clinical management of the glaucoma patient. This clinical information is necessary also to direct genetic testing, which in the future may become more important for more specific disease-related genetic therapy.

## 50.1 Terminology Problems

The nomenclature for childhood glaucoma is plagued with confusing terminology. The childhood glaucomas are classified into *primary* and *secondary* groups (Table 50.1).

## 50.2 Pathophysiology of Infantile Glaucoma

Very little information is known pertaining to the causes of the impaired outflow in each of the primary childhood glaucomas. The secondary glaucomas can be understood related

**Table 50.1** The primary and secondary pediatric glaucomas

I. *Developmental glaucomas*
  A. Primary congenital glaucoma (PCG)
    1. Newborn primary congenital glaucoma
    2. Infantile primary congenital glaucoma
    3. Late-recognized primary congenital glaucoma
  B. Juvenile open-angle glaucoma (JOAG)
  C. Primary glaucomas associated with systemic diseases
    1. Sturge–Weber syndrome
    2. Neurofibromatosis (NF-1)
    3. Stickler syndrome
    4. Oculocerebrorenal syndrome (Lowe)
    5. Rieger syndrome
    6. SHORT syndrome
    7. Hepatocerebrorenal syndrome (Zellweger)
    8. Marfan syndrome
    9. Rubinstein–Taybi syndrome hepatic fibrosis, hypothyroidism
    10. Infantile glaucoma with retardation and paralysis
    11. Oculodentodigital dysplasia
    12. Glaucoma with microcornea and absent sinuses
    13. Mucopolysaccharidosis
    14. Trisomy 13
    15. Caudal regression syndrome
    16. Trisomy 21 (Down syndrome)
    17. Cutis marmorata telangiectatica congenita
    18. Warburg syndrome
    19. Kniest syndrome (skeletal dysplasia)
    20. Michel's syndrome
    21. Nonprogressive hemiatrophy
    22. PHACE syndrome
    23. Soto syndrome
    24. Linear scleroderma
    25. GAPO syndrome
    26. Roberts' pseudothalidomide syndrome
    27. Wolf–Hirschhorn (4p-) syndrome
    28. Robinow syndrome
    29. Fetal hydantoin syndrome
    30. Nail–patella syndrome
    31. Proteus syndrome
    32. Cranio–cerebello–cardiac (3C) syndrome
    33. Brachmann–deLange syndrome
    34. Rothmund–Thomson syndrome
    35. 9p deletion syndrome
    36. Phakomatosis pigmentovascularis (PPV)
    37. Nevoid basal cell carcinoma S. (Gorlin S)
    38. Epidermal Nevus syndrome (Solomon S)
    39. Androgen insensitivity, pyloric stenosis
    40. Diabetes mellitus, polycystic kidneys
  D. Primary glaucomas with associated ocular anomalies
    1. Aniridia
      a. congenital aniridic glaucoma
      b. acquired aniridic glaucoma
    2. Congenital ocular melanosis
    3. Sclerocornea
    4. Congenital iris ectropion syndrome
    5. Peters' syndrome
    6. Iridotrabecular dysgenesis (iris hypoplasia)
    7. Posterior polymorphous dystrophy
    8. Idiopathic or familial elevated venous pressure
    9. Congenital anterior (corneal) staphyloma
    10. Congenital microcoria
    11. Congenital hereditary endothelial dystrophy
    12. Axenfeld–Rieger anomaly

II. *Secondary (acquired) glaucomas*
  A. Traumatic glaucoma
    1. Acute glaucoma
      a. Angle concussion
      b. Hyphema
      c. Ghost cell glaucoma
    2. Glaucoma related to angle-recession
    3. Arteriovenous fistula
  B. Glaucoma with intraocular neoplasms
    1. Retinoblastoma
    2. Juvenile xanthogranuloma (JXG)
    3. Leukemia
    4. Melanoma of ciliary body
    5. Melanocytoma
    6. Iris rhabdomyosarcoma
    7. Aggressive iris nevi
    8. Medulloepithelioma
    9. Mucogenic glaucoma with iris stromal cyst
  C. Glaucoma related to chronic uveitis
    1. Open-angle glaucoma
    2. Angle-blockage mechanisms
      a. Synechial angle closure
      b. Iris bombe with pupillary block
    3. Trabecular meshwork endothelialization
  D. Lens-related glaucoma
    1. Subluxation-dislocation with pupillary block
      a. Marfan syndrome
      b. Homocystinuria
      c. Weill–Marchesani syndrome
      d. Axial-subluxation high myopia syndrome
      e. Ectopia lentis et papillae
    2. Spherophakia with pupillary block
    3. Phacolytic glaucoma
  E. Glaucoma following lensectomy for congenital cataracts
    1. Pupillary-block glaucoma
    2. Infantile aphakic open angle glaucoma
  F. Glaucoma related to corticosteroids
  G. Glaucoma secondary to rubeosis
    1. Retinoblastoma
    2. Coats' disease
    3. Medulloepithelioma
    4. Familial exudative vitreoretinopathy
    5. Subacute/chronic retinal detachment

to the primary ocular disease complicated by glaucoma, e.g., neoplasm or uveitis. Some information is available, however, from studies of PCG.

PCG is felt to result from an abnormality of the trabecular meshwork that may represent a developmental arrest or relative immaturity of the trabecular tissue causing increased resistance to aqueous outflow.[2,3] Initially, the defect was thought to be an imperforate membrane lining the anterior chamber angle based on its gonioscopic appearance suggesting a "clothed membrane with a shagreened surface".[4,5] Evidence of this membrane has not been found.[6]

The histopathology of PCG is characterized by an anterior insertion of the iris and ciliary body with variable exposure of the trabecular meshwork to the anterior chamber.[6] The anterior iris insertion may cover a variable amount of ciliary body band and trabecular meshwork. The anterior portion of the ciliary body overlaps the posterior portion of the trabecular meshwork with underdevelopment of the angle recess. The longitudinal fibers of the ciliary muscle insert directly into the corneoscleral meshwork passing in front of the internal tip of an underdeveloped scleral spur. In one study (77.8%), eyes with PCG had either an invisible or narrow ciliary body band compared to only 13.8% of control eyes.[7]

Anderson showed that the trabecular meshwork is porous and that the intertrabecular beam spaces are present, but also that the trabecular beams in between these spaces are abnormally thickened.[6] Maul et al. found an increased amount of collagen fibrils in the core of the trabecular beams.[8] The juxtacanalicular meshwork in eyes with PCG had been found to be thicker than in normal eyes.[6,8,9] Unlike the corneoscleral meshwork, this external layer of the meshwork is normally compact with a lack of intertrabecular spaces.[9] The cells in the juxtacanalicular layer are normally round with short cytoplasmic processes and are surrounded by extracellular materials comprising of collagen, elastic fibers, and amorphous substances, giving it a compact appearance.[8,9]

Enucleated eyes of premature infants reveal that the trabecular sheets first appear on the anterior chamber side of the trabeculum and gradually progress with fetal age toward Schlemm's canal.[3] The trabecular meshwork at 42 weeks of gestation shows intertrabecular spaces similar to that seen in adult eyes, with only a few layers of cells in the juxtacanalicular area. Hence, it has been postulated that the thicker-compact juxtacanalicular meshwork seen in PCG is perhaps the result of delayed differentiation.[3]

The absence of Schlemm's canal has also been described in PCG, but this is an exception and indicates more severe maldevelopment.[10,11] Both immaturity of the juxtacanalicular meshwork and/or underdevelopment of Schlemm's canal or collector channels could explain the failure of goniotomy.[11]

Similarity of the angle histopathology in PCG, glaucoma with the Sturge–Weber syndrome, and in the maternal rubella syndrome with glaucoma[12] suggests that a common pathway for angle development is affected in these diverse conditions. The underlying mechanism of trabecular dysgenesis is still unknown even though the genetic basis for PCG has been determined in many cases.[13,14] The most probable mechanism is offered by Anderson who reported that excessive formation of collagen in the trabecular tissue results in thickened and taut trabecular beams that prevent posterior sliding of the peripheral iris and ciliary body along the inner eye surface, resulting in the anterior location of the uveal tract and underdevelopment of the angle recess.[6] The success of goniotomy in PCG may be explained by the relief of tension on the thickened and compact trabecular meshwork, with resultant decreased resistance to the outflow of aqueous.[6]

## 50.3 Epidemiology and Genetics

PCG, which accounts for approximately 55% of primary pediatric glaucomas and is the most common type, is hereditary with a variable incidence in different populations, but with an overall occurrence of 1 in 10,000 births.[15,16] The majority (about 75%) of PCG cases are bilateral, and asymmetric expression should be suspected in clinically apparent unilateral cases.[12] More than 80% present within the first year of life, with 25% diagnosed in the neonatal period, and 60% within the first 6 months of life.[12]

The majority of PCG cases are sporadic, but 10–40% are familial with frequent related consanguinity.[17] In most familial cases, transmission is autosomal recessive with variable expression and penetrance of 40–100%.[17] Three loci for PCG have been found.[17-19] The initial locus on chromosome 2p21 (GLC3A) was described in 1995 by Sarfarazi et al who identified significant genetic linkage to this region in 11 of 17 Turkish families.[13,17] Although three chromosomal loci have been linked to PCG, only the gene CYP1B1 in locus GLC3A has been identified.[14] Mutations in the CYP1B1 gene were found responsible for 87% of familial cases, but present only in 27% of sporadic cases of PCG.[17] Approximately, 45 mutations of this gene have been identified and include deletion, insertion, point mutation, missense, nonsense, frameshift, and terminator mutations.[20] Genotype–phenotype correlation was described related to the success of glaucoma management and abnormalities secondary to elevated IOP; the most severe phenotype was associated with frameshift mutations.[20] In cases of parent–child transmission, molecular analysis invariably found homozygosity or compound heterozygosity for the mutant alleles in the affected parent and gene carrier status in the normal parent.[21] These are examples of pseudodominance involving an autosomal recessive trait.

PCG is genetically distinct from conditions classified as an anterior segment dysgenesis or Axenfeld–Rieger syndrome/anomaly, which is transmitted by autosomal dominant inheritance resulting from mutations in the transcription factor genes PITX2 or FOXC1.[22,23] PCG is also unrelated to JOAG in which the MYOC (TIGR) gene has been identified at locus GLC1A on chromosome 1q25.[24] Glaucoma associated with a facial nevus flammeus (Schirmer–Sturge–Weber Syndrome) is the most common nonhereditary primary glaucoma seen in infancy.

Importantly, in the evaluation of a child with a primary childhood glaucoma it is frequently informative to exam all other family members for evidence of related disease. This especially includes younger and future siblings and parents. The penetrance and expressivity of PCG is highly variable.[17] Complete examination of siblings is essential to rule out the presence of glaucoma, which could be easily missed if the clinical presentations are quite different and less severe than present in the affected sibling. When autosomal dominant inheritance is responsible for anterior segment dysgenesis, highly variable expressivity is frequent and the examination of parents and other family members of suspected cases is frequently informative and always indicated.

## 50.4 Clinical Features

The signs and symptoms of glaucoma in infancy are variable dependent on the child's age, the severity of glaucoma, the presence of associated ocular anomalies, and the development of secondary corneal IOP related abnormalities (Table 50.2). Very few children are asymptomatic and show minimal evidence of glaucoma.

Infants are most likely to present with subtle corneal enlargement and diffuse corneal opacification, which is often recognized promptly by physicians or parents. The classic symptoms of epiphora, photophobia, and blepharospasm are secondary to corneal edema and opacification, and breaks in Descemet's membrane. Infants may exhibit irritable behavior, which may be mistakenly attributed to colic or formula intolerance. The epiphora may be misinterpreted as evidence of a congenital nasolacrimal duct obstruction, or a "red eye" mimicking conjunctivitis, leading to further delayed diagnosis. The corneas are often diffusely thick due to stromal edema and later become thin with pathologic corneal enlargement. Alternatively, focal stromal thickening and opacification occur in association with breaks (Haab's striae) in Descemet's membrane. These defects are typically horizontal, curvilinear, and parallel to the limbus in the peripheral cornea. Progressive corneal enlargement secondary to the IOP ceases by 3–4 years of age. Both parents and physicians may accept corneal enlargement as a normal variation, even when more exaggerated unilaterally. The etiologic differential diagnosis of the classical signs of infantile glaucoma is tabulated for reference in Table 50.3.

In older children, astigmatism and progressive axial myopia cause symptomatic decreased uncorrected visual acuity and refractive amblyopia. These children with a late-recognized infantile glaucoma may be asymptomatic and discovered to have elevated IOP or optic nerve cupping on routine ocular examination or when examined for unrelated ocular conditions. While cupping of the optic nerve in glaucoma is generally a gradual process in older children and adults, it can occur rapidly in infants. Reversibility of the cupping with normalization of IOP in young children occurs due to suspected increased elasticity of the lamina cribrosa.

**Table 50.2** Signs and symptoms of glaucoma in infancy

| Symptoms | Signs |
| --- | --- |
| Photophobia | Buphthalmos |
| Epiphora | Corneal enlargement |
| Blepharospasm | Corneal edema |
| Red eye | Corneal size asymmetry |
| Irritability | Breaks in Descemet's membrane |
| Cloudy cornea | Iris and pupillary abns. |
| Enlarged cornea/eye | Elevated IOP |
| Poor vision | Visual impairment |
| Asymptomatic | Myopia/astigmatism |
| Irritability | Optic nerve cupping |

**Table 50.3** Differential diagnoses of the classical signs and symptoms of PCG

1. *Corneal edema or opacity*
   Ocular
       Birth trauma
       Sclerocornea
       Keratitis
       Limbal dermoid
       Congenital hereditary endothelial dystrophy
       Posterior polymorphous corneal dystrophy
       Anterior staphyloma
       Peters' anomaly
   Systemic
       Mucopolysaccharidoses I, II, III
       Mucolipidoses IV
       Cystinosis
       Generalized gangliosidosis I
       Infantile Niemann–Pick disease
       De Barsy syndrome
       Familial dysautonomia
2. *Corneal enlargement*
       Axial myopia
       Hereditary megalocornea
       Keratoglobus
3. *Epiphora and "red eye"*
       Conjunctivitis
       Corneal abrasion
       Congenital nasolacrimal duct obstruction
       Uveitis
       Keratitis
4. *Photophobia*
   Ocular
       Keratitis
       Aniridia
       Iritis
       Cataract
       Achromatopsia
       Posterior polymorphous dystrophy
   Systemic
       Albinism
       Meningitis
       Posterior fossa tumor[37]

## 50.5 The Examination

The clinical examination (Table 50.4) of a child with glaucoma requires patience, time, and skill. A detailed examination utilizing a table-mounted slit-lamp for tonometry and biomicroscopy of the anterior segment and optic nerve head is not possible in most children under 5 years of age, but an informative office evaluation can still be obtained.

An appropriate *medical and family history* and examination of family members is essential due to the genetic basis of some types of childhood glaucoma. *A general physical examination* is also indicated when evidence of a systemic and/or ocular developmental defect suggests diagnoses other than isolated glaucoma, or when general anesthesia is planned. Because children resist being held down or touched in the eye region, clinical information must be gained by careful inspection before laying hands on them. The presence of glaucoma may be obvious on inspection alone by observing the presence of hazy, enlarged or asymmetrical corneas, light sensitivity, and abnormal visual behavior.

Vision assessment includes observing the child's behavior, interest in toys, willingness to follow objects, presence of nystagmus, and pupillary reactivity. The relative function of the two eyes should be compared when clinically appropriate.

The inspection and *examination of the anterior segment* is facilitated by the use of a penlight and a handheld slit-lamp, which allow maneuverability regardless of the child's position. Magnification obtained with loupes or with the oculars present on handheld slit-lamps is useful. The corneal size and clarity should be studied. Asymmetry in cornea size is usually more obvious on inspection than by measurement. Breaks in Descemet's membrane must be identified and differentiated from other abnormalities such as the more vertically oriented defects seen after forceps-induced birth trauma, or the irregular-scattered defects seen with posterior polymorphous dystrophy.

The *iris and pupil* should be carefully studied for abnormalities such as iris stromal hypoplasia, pupillary ectopia, and pupillary enlargement and irregularity as seen with newborn PCG, Axenfeld–Rieger anomaly, and aniridia. The *anterior chambers* are typically deep, and the lenses are clear in most PCG patients.

*Tonometry* is an essential component of the examination and can be the most difficult part with an uncooperative child. The best IOP measurements are taken with a sleeping or relaxed child using topical anesthesia. IOP readings are variably altered by sedation and general anesthesia, and falsely elevated with a struggling patient. Time and patience are the most important requirements for success. Repeated measurements during the same or return office visits may be necessary. Parents can help by holding the child to provide reassurance and to distract the patient with a toy or a bottle. Tonometry efforts should be initially directed to the more normal eye as IOP measurements are more critical in determining if this eye has glaucoma. Various instruments have been used in the measurement of IOP in children. The Perkins applanation tonometer probably ranks highest in terms of accuracy and the Tono-Pen (Medtronic Solan, Jacksonville, Florida, USA) highest in ease of use. The corneal thickness should be measured when possible to improve the interpretation of the eye pressure measurements. The Schiotz tonometer is still useful to give an indication of the IOP in the young or struggling child examined in the supine position, although its accuracy is most affected by corneal thickness and curvature, and scleral rigidity. In older cooperative children the familiar slit-lamp mounted Goldman tonometer may be used more confidently.

*Gonioscopy* is indispensable for determining the type of childhood glaucoma and the choice of surgery. When corneal clarity permits, simultaneous bilateral examination of the angles may be performed with Koeppe lenses. A handheld microscope and a customized illuminator for gonioscopy are recommended. Direct gonioscopy by this method can often be performed in the office with a sleeping/feeding infant or a cooperative child lying supine after topical anesthesia. An older child may permit indirect gonioscopy at the slit-lamp. However, a detailed gonioscopic examination of a young child most often requires general anesthesia. Epithelial removal can be performed to obtain a clear view when the cornea is cloudy due to epithelial edema.

The angle appearance in primary infantile glaucoma can vary according to the severity of angle anomalies. Typically, the iris inserts more anteriorly than normal with variable obscuration of the ciliary body band. There is an altered translucency of the angle face causing indistinct definition of the different angle structures (ciliary body band, scleral spur, and trabecular meshwork). The peripheral iris often appears hypoplastic with scalloping at its insertion and with visibility of the peripheral iris pigment epithelium. In more severe angle presentations, the angle may be so underdeveloped that minimal visible angle structures anterior to the iris insertion can be identified, with complete absence of the scleral spur

**Table 50.4** Examination for infantile glaucoma

History and systemic examination
Examination of relatives
General inspection (for photophobia, corneal size and asymmetry, and systemic defects)
Vision assessment
Tonometry
Anterior segment examination (cornea, anterior chamber, iris, and pupil)
Gonioscopy
Fundoscopy and optic nerve head evaluation
Ultrasonography
Retinoscopy

and ciliary body band. The presence of multiple abnormal iris processes, iridocorneal pillars, and excessive thickening of Schwalbe's line should suggest the diagnosis of anterior segment dysgenesis related to an Axenfeld–Rieger anomaly.

*Optic nerve head examination* may be performed with a direct or indirect ophthalmoscope. Examination with an indirect ophthalmoscope allows three-dimensional assessment of the optic disc as well as detection of posterior segment abnormalities. An A-scan ultrasound examination is useful to obtain the axial length of each eye, which increases abnormally with the severity and duration of the glaucoma. B-scan ultrasound of the posterior segment may yield useful information when cloudy corneas preclude a good view of the fundus; advanced cupping can be recognized and unexpected retinal defects ruled out.

A complete office examination is usually sufficient to either exclude glaucoma, or to diagnose suspected glaucoma and justify general anesthesia for a more detailed examination before probable surgery. The role of the examination-under-anesthesia (EUA) is to add to rather than replace the office examination. It should follow the office examination and precede any planned glaucoma surgery. Essential information that can be obtained during the EUA is listed in Table 50.5. Operating room preparation for this examination is often helpful given the extensive amount of necessary equipment that is required.

## 50.6 Principles of Treatment

The management of an infant or child with glaucoma is challenging. It is a chronic disease affecting infants and young children with normal life expectancies. The IOP-reducing benefit of each treatment modality may not persist. Treatments should be carefully tailored with the goal of long-term control of the IOP with minimum risk to the eye to enable meaningful preservation of vision for life.

Surgery constitutes the mainstay of therapy for childhood glaucoma. Medications alone in young children with glaucoma are rarely completely effective, but play an important secondary role as adjunctive treatment. Because angle surgery enjoys striking success rates for infantile PCG, it should be considered

**Table 50.5** Information to be obtained under EUA

| |
|---|
| Intraocular pressures |
| Corneal diameters |
| Anterior segment assessment |
| Gonioscopic observations |
| Retinoscopy measurements |
| Optic nerve head assessment |
| Photographic documentation |

first and will often be the initial procedure of choice. Other surgical procedures must be considered when appropriate angle surgery has failed or is unlikely to succeed because of gonioscopic evidence of a severe filtration angle anomaly.

### 50.6.1 Medical Treatment

Infants with glaucoma typically respond poorly to medical therapy alone. Medications are important when used before surgery as a temporizing measure in infants unfit for surgery or anesthesia, to prepare a patient for goniosurgery by clearing the cornea, and for adjunctive therapy in complicated cases unsuitable or only partially controlled by surgical therapy. Medications will have different risk factors and benefit profiles in children compared to adults, and ophthalmologists ordering them for infants and children should be aware of these differences. Ocular surface toxicity and allergy are also real problems complicating continuous topical treatment when started at a young age. Children are also often unable to communicate adverse effects of drugs, which gives importance to the observations of parents and physicians who need to assess the appearance of the eye; look for systemic signs; and note changes in behavior, appetite, and growth.

#### 50.6.1.1 Oral Carbonic Anhydrase Inhibitors

Oral carbonic anhydrase inhibitors (CAIs) – acetazolamide or methazolamide – are the most effective and potent IOP lowering drugs for children with glaucoma. At acetazolamide dosages of 10–15 mg/kg/day by mouth, it is generally safe for use in the short term and often reduces IOP by a third.[25] It is useful to clear the cornea before goniosurgery and to improve IOP control after a failed surgical procedure prior to further glaucoma surgery.

#### 50.6.1.2 Beta-Adrenergic Antagonists

Beta-adrenergic antagonists (beta-blockers) have been used extensively for the treatment of glaucoma in infancy to adolescence. Studies have found IOP-lowering the efficacy of 20–30% in responsive cases of childhood glaucoma, but none has looked at its efficacy in PCG.[26,27] Severe systemic side effects from topical timolol are rare in infants and children but bronchospasm and bradycardia have been reported,[27-29] especially with the higher concentration of 0.5%. Apnea has been described in neonates and a toddler, although other factors such as coexistent congenital disorders could also have contributed to the apneic spells.[29,30]

### 50.6.1.3 Beta-Adrenergic Agonist

Brimonidine, a relatively selective alpha-agonist, reduces IOP by decreasing aqueous production and increasing uveoscleral outflow.[31] Brimonidine passes through the blood-brain barrier, potentially causing central nervous system (CNS) toxicity.[32] There are reports of bradycardia, hypotension, hypothermia, hypotonia, apnea, and unresponsiveness in infants after topical brimonidine.[33-36] A study on the safety and efficacy of brimonidine in older children 2.4–16.8 years of age reported somnolence and extreme fatigue following brimonidine administration and also showed a 6.7% average IOP reduction in the group, which is much less than that shown in adult studies.[37] Brimonidine should be avoided in infancy and toddlers and be used with caution in older children.

### 50.6.1.4 Prostaglandin Analogues

Latanoprost, travoprost, and bimatoprost have been shown to be very effective in the treatment of adult glaucoma, have similar chemical structures, and reduce IOP primarily by enhancing uveoscleral outflow.[38] They also have very similar side effects, the most prominent of which are conjunctival hyperemia, iris and skin pigmentation, and accelerated eyelash growth.[38] Their use and efficacy in children has not been widely reported. Disappointingly little IOP lowering and a high nonresponse rate in children has been reported, although they are safe systemically.[39,40] A significant IOP-lowering effect was found in some older children with primary juvenile glaucoma or Sturge–Weber related glaucoma.[39,40] The average age of nonresponders was 5 years versus 11 years for responders.[40]

### 50.6.1.5 Miotics

Miotics such as pilocarpine are ineffective for infantile glaucoma. Symptoms of ciliary spasm and visual blurring from the induced myopia occur in children.

## 50.6.2 Goniotomy

Barkan developed the goniotomy technique and described its successful use for infants with glaucoma.[41,42] This seminal accomplishment offered for the first time a successful therapy for infantile glaucoma heretofore considered a hopeless disease.

### 50.6.2.1 Indications

Goniotomy is the procedure of choice for children with this primary infantile congenital glaucoma (PCG). Preoperative gonioscopic evaluation is an essential preparation for goniosurgery. Inadequate pressure control after an initial goniotomy often indicates the need for repeat goniosurgery. Repeat goniotomy should also be considered with a reoccurrence of glaucoma irrespective of the patient's age even into adulthood. The severe angle anomaly with extreme forward insertion of the iris and minimal development of the trabeculum typically seen with *primary newborn glaucoma* decreases the potential for a successful goniotomy. The indication for goniotomy is also much less certain for other primary glaucomas, including glaucoma with a nevus flammeus (SWS), Axenfeld-Rieger syndrome, and neurofibromatosis. *Late-recognized PCG* can be difficult to distinguish from primary juvenile glaucoma, but fortunately goniotomy is indicated for both of these conditions. It is also the procedure of choice for glaucoma secondary to chronic anterior uveitis when the filtration angle is not complicated by synechia.[43]

### 50.6.2.2 Goniotomy Technique

Goniotomy is performed utilizing a light source, magnification instrument, fixation forceps, operating gonioscopic lens, and a suitable goniotomy needle or knife. Following the positioning of the globe and with the trabecular meshwork in view through an operating lens, the cutting instrument is entered into the anterior chamber through the peripheral cornea and brought into contact with the mid section of the trabeculum (Fig. 50.1). A

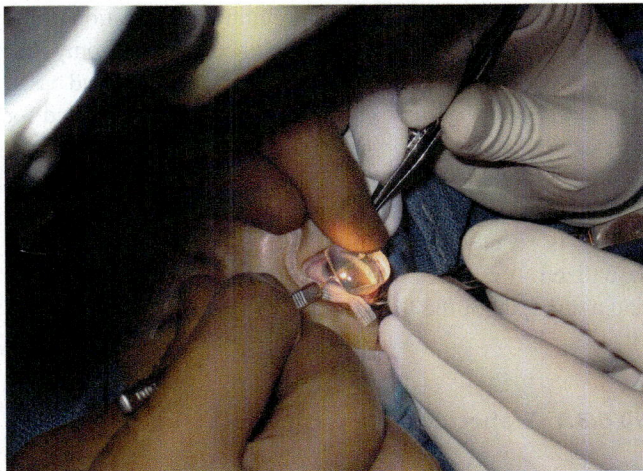

**Fig. 50.1** The goniotomy procedure is performed with simultaneous viewing of the trabecular meshwork in the filtration angle

circumferential incision is then made in the trabeculum and the instrument is removed without causing injury to the cornea or lens.[44]

### 50.6.2.3 Results

The outcome of goniotomy surgery for PCG overall is very favorable with a reported success rate over 80%.[45] Patients recognized to have glaucoma between birth and 2 months of age have a lower success rate with goniotomy,[46-48] which may correlate with their severe filtration angle anomaly. Goniotomy surgery was performed for 335 eyes and glaucoma control was achieved with single goniotomy in 71% (239) of eyes and by one or more goniotomies in 94% (313) of eyes.[49] Relapse following successful goniotomy is unusual.[48]

Surgical complications after goniotomy surgery are rare. A postoperative hyphema is a constant finding after goniosurgery and usually of no clinical significance. Occasionally, a significant amount of blood will reflux into the anterior chamber during the first 72 h after surgery; when this becomes complicated by an elevated IOP, washout of the blood should be considered.

## 50.6.3 Trabeculotomy

Trabeculotomy ab externo is an alternative procedure to goniotomy for PCG. Its successful use for infantile glaucoma was recognized early and favorable results were reported.[50,51] The efficacy of this newer operation compared favorably with goniotomy.[51] The results of trabeculotomy and goniotomy for infantile glaucoma were compared and found equally effective and safe, and the significant advantage of trabeculotomy for those cases with a cloudy cornea limiting visualization of the angle was described.[52] Primary combined trabeculotomy–trabeculectomy was performed for 144 eyes with PCG, and based on a success rate of over 90% at 6 months, recommended for cases with significant corneal edema.[53]

Trabeculotomy may be a more appropriate choice for surgeons not experienced with goniotomy, especially when the cornea is so cloudy that the angle cannot be comfortably visualized. It requires more operating time than goniotomy, and a quadrant of the limbus must be used for this surgery.

### 50.6.3.1 Trabeculotomy Technique

The operative technique of trabeculotomy has been modified very little.[54] The superior quadrants are best saved for alternative surgery. A limbus-based scleral flap is created to expose the sclerolimbal junction, followed by a radial incision centered over this landmark to unroof and expose Schlemm's canal. Trabeculotomy probes are then introduced into Schlemm's canal and rotated into the anterior chamber in a plane parallel to the iris to create a fistula between the canal and the anterior chamber.[55] The anterior chamber is then deepened and the scleral flap and conjunctiva repositioned.

An alternative and technically more difficult variation of this procedure, which has proven effective, is to thread a suture circumferentially through Schlemm's canal followed by its removal into and out of the anterior chamber, which creates a circumferential communication between these structures.[56]

### 50.6.3.2 Results

Study of the long-term effectiveness of trabeculotomy has confirmed its efficacy for PCG. Trabeculotomy in 99 eyes was reported with a probability of success after one or more surgeries at 5 and 10 years to be 92% and 82%, respectively.[57] Trabeculotomy for 46 children with PCG and a mean age of approximately 4 years (range 13–88 months) achieved success in 87% (68) eyes using custom probes for 102 procedures.[58] Complications after standard trabeculotomy are unusual.

## 50.6.4 Trabeculectomy

Before the use of goniosurgery for children, filtering surgery was performed with little expectation for success. Procedures done included limbo-scleral trephine and posterior lip sclerectomy. Beauchamp studied the use of trabeculectomy for seven children refractory to angle surgery; four patients were followed and three of the eight operated eyes were adequately controlled.[59] Introduction of trabeculectomy lessened the risks of filtration surgery in young children but did not significantly improve glaucoma control. The addition of antimetabolites administered during pediatric trabeculectomy surgery improved the surgical outcome.[60]

The indication for trabeculectomy surgery for childhood patients is persistence of an unacceptable eye pressure elevation following an appropriate number of angle incision operations. The condition of the superior conjunctiva related to previous surgery, patient age, potential for follow-up examinations, postoperative contact lens use, and the risk of postoperative infection – all must carefully be considered. Children under 1 year of age show a significantly lower success rate than older patients.[61] An explanation for this failure is not clear. The surgery is not more complicated with the use of an antimetabolite, but the postoperative care is difficult for these young patients. Their postoperative course is often characterized by decreasing evidence of external filtration even in patients who achieve improved initial IOP control and evidence of external filtration. Favorable outcome with combined trabeculotomy–trabeculectomy for PCG patients under 1 month of age has been described.[47]

### 50.6.4.1 Trabeculectomy Technique

The trabeculectomy surgical procedure for children does not vary significantly from the technique performed for adults. A fornix-based flap is manufactured that spares the surgeon the need to enter through the youthful conjunctiva and Tenon's layers, which are substantially thicker than those found in adult eyes (and vascularized Sturge–Weber patients). If used, mitomycin-C 0.2–0.4 mg/cc is applied to the scleral flap region and broadly more posteriorly.[62] A scleral flap is created with adequate extension anteriorly to facilitate entry into the anterior chamber in front of the abnormal anterior insertion of the iris. After a punch removal of a small section of trabeculum and peripheral cornea, the iridectomy is performed. The flap is closed with nylon or absorbable sutures and the conjunctiva is closed tightly. Absorbable 10–0 stitches allow tension on the scleral flap to be released at a time 3–4 weeks following the procedure.

### 50.6.4.2 Results

The results of trabeculectomy procedures are encouraging with 60–70% of patients successfully controlled during the first 2 years after surgery.[60,61,63] Complications after trabeculectomy with use of adjunctive antifibrosis agents are frequent.[60,61,63] After surgery, shallowing of the anterior chamber is frequent and choroidal expansion occurs variably in proportion to the degree and duration of hypotony. Chronic postoperative hypotony with maculopathy occurs infrequently. Non-progressive subcapsular lens opacities occur even after only a few weeks of hypotony. Failure is associated with decreasing evidence of subconjunctival filtration, often without evidence internally of blockage of the sclerostomy. Ciliary processes can be seen in the internal sclerostomy with both functioning and nonfunctioning results. Late-onset, bleb-related endophthalmitis occurs acutely with an expected occurrence rate of (7–17 %)[60,61,64] and typically occurs within a 3-year period following surgery.[64] Candidate patients remain at risk when thin-avascular blebs develop even in the absence of aqueous leakage. Following trabeculectomy for PCG, thin-avascular blebs were observed after 18 months in 33% and 67% of eyes following use of 0.2 mg/cc and 0.4 mg/cc of mitomycin-C, respectively.[65] Bleb excision followed by conjunctival advancement is necessary and becomes mandatory for blebs that become at risk for infection; it is a procedure that fortunately is associated with a low incidence of bleb failure.[66]

## 50.6.5 Glaucoma Drainage Devices

Glaucoma implant surgery is an important treatment alternative for children who are poor candidates for goniosurgery and trabeculectomy or who have proven to be refractory to these procedures. Molteno pioneered the contemporary translimbal glaucoma implant and now its use has been widely adopted and its efficacy and complications are better understood.[67,68] Introduction of the Baerveldt implant (Pharmacia & Upjohn, Inc., Kalamazoo, Michigan) in 1990 made available a silicone nonvalved implant and the Ahmed Glaucoma Valve implant (New World Medical, Inc., Rancho Cucamonga, California) was designed with a valve to lessen the occurrence of immediate postoperative hypotony.

The indications for childhood glaucoma implant surgery have expanded beyond being only an option to consider after other procedures have failed. Many patients with childhood glaucoma will have initial goniosurgery; and if unsuccessful or no longer indicated, trabeculectomy and Glaucoma Drainage Devices (GDD) surgery then must be considered. When preoperative gonioscopy in infancy reveals a severe angle anomaly, goniosurgery has only a small chance of success, and the outcome of trabeculectomy at this age even with antimetabolite augmentation is poor; hence, these infants are strong candidates for primary glaucoma implant surgery.[69] When the outcome of 32 patients with a mean age of 7 months treated with glaucoma implants and 19 patients with a mean age of 5 months treated with trabeculectomy were compared, the success probability at 77 months was 53% and 19%, respectively.[70]

### 50.6.5.1 Glaucoma Tube Insertion Technique

The surgical technique is similar for all types of glaucoma implants. The superior temporal quadrant is the preferred site to maximize the distance of the drainage plate from the optic nerve and to lessen the risk of postoperative eyelid deformity. Following a peritomy, the implant device is secured to the sclera with its anterior edge approximately 7 mm from the limbus. I recommend that the plate may be trimmed prior to insertion as necessary to facilitate its entry. The tube is shortened and beveled and placed into the anterior chamber parallel to the iris, taking into account the frequent anterior insertion of the iris especially in children with PCG. Peripheral contact between the iris and the tube will result in correctopia. The tube can be tied with a 7–0 absorbable suture to impede flow and decrease the risk of hypotony.

Finally, the tube is protected with sclera or pericardium and the limbal peritomy is closed.

### 50.6.5.2 Results

The results of glaucoma implant surgery for the pediatric glaucomas and for PCG are favorable.[71,72] In a cohort of 14 PCG eyes, including 9 eyes with a history of previous cycloablation, success was achieved in 93% (13) of eyes with the continued use of medications.[72] Importantly, the potential success of implant surgery for refractory PCG has greatly decreased the use of destructive cycloablative procedures. With use of the Ahmed implant for 60 pediatric glaucoma eyes – including 25 with PCG–IOP control was achieved in 73% (44 eyes) at last examination with continued use of medications in 77%; however, complications occurred in 50% (30 eyes).[73] The complications of pediatric glaucoma implant surgery are varied and frequent.[72,73] Early hypotony and tube-related problems are most common and often require intervention.[72] Glaucoma implant tube exposure puts an eye at significant risk for infection and postoperative endophthalmitis and must be corrected promptly by recovering the tube.[74]

## 50.6.6 Cyclodestruction

Cyclodestructive procedures are selectively used to improve aqueous outflow for childhood glaucoma that has proven refractory to medical therapy and to conventional surgical procedures, and work by decreasing aqueous production. The required ciliary epithelial ablation can be clinically produced by cyclocryotherapy, or by transscleral or endoscopic diode laser cyclophotocoagulation.

The indications for using any of these intentionally damaging procedures must also consider the long-term visual and anatomic prognosis and the parents' own expectations for their child's affected eye.

The ocular indications include a blind painful eye, a blind eye with a high pressure and rapidly deteriorating cornea, an eye proven to be refractory to all more conservative treatment alternatives, an eye with anatomic defects that preclude other glaucoma procedures, and a patient who is not a candidate for either prolonged general anesthesia or intraocular surgery.

### 50.6.6.1 Cycloablation Technique

The cycloablation surgical procedures differ, but have in common the direction of destructive energy targeted for the ciliary epithelium and the need for general anesthesia. The cyclocryotreatment and the transscleral laser probes are applied externally to the retrolimbal conjunctiva, while the laser endoscope is entered through the anterior chamber to approximate the ciliary processes.

### 50.6.6.2 Results

The reported results of cyclodestructive procedures for PCG patients are difficult to interpret – because of the limited number of reported cases and their use primarily for eyes with advanced disease – but are of value. The results of cyclocryotherapy for 37 PCG eyes with the history of previous eye surgery were compared to those for 12 eyes without prior procedures, and control was achieved in 31% and 30%, respectively.[75] Twenty-five PCG eyes were in a cohort of 64 eyes with pediatric glaucoma treated with cyclocryotreatment, which achieved success in 44% (28) at last examination (mean, 4.8 ± 3.3 years) with an average of 4.1 ± 4.0 treatments for each eye.[76] Twenty-six PCG eyes were in a series of 77 refractory pediatric glaucoma eyes treated with laser diode cyclophotocoagulation that collectively achieved a success rate of 30% after approximately 4 years.[77] Four eyes of 3 patients with PCG and a history of multiple previous conventional glaucoma procedures were treated with endoscopic diode laser photocoagulation and success was achieved in 1 eye.[78]

Cyclodestructive operations are followed by many complications, including phthisis,[76,77] retinal detachment,[76,77] and chronic hypotony and cataracts.[75] Not yet reported is the chronic postcyclodestruction anterior segment syndrome seen frequently in children successfully controlled by these procedures, and which is characterized by band keratopathy, corneal edema and endothelial cell drop out, chronic anterior chamber flare, posterior synechia and microcoria, and slowly progressive cataracts.

## 50.7 Clinical Pearls

1. There are many primary and secondary causes of childhood glaucoma; some are associated with systemic disease and are genetically determined. Following the initial clinical assessment, the findings should be reviewed using the table of known glaucoma causes and systemic associations as a guide.
2. Raised IOP in early childhood causes profound anterior segment abnormalities. Corneal enlargement, opacification, exaggerated anterior chamber depth, and Descemet's membrane breaks are important signs of glaucoma. The breaks remain permanently visible and become an important evidence of a raised IOP before 2 years of age.

3. Informative office and operating room tonometry is an essential information for the management of children with glaucoma. When children come to an office/clinic environment for testing, parents should assist with holding, distracting, or feeding the children to enable this test to be as reliable as possible. Frequent reexamination is often required to follow children satisfactorily.
4. Inspection of the irides of children with glaucoma will often be very helpful in determining the cause and severity of the anterior segment anomaly. In an infant, this is best done with a focal illuminator, hand-held slit beam, and a magnifying loupe. In some cases a Koeppe lens can also be utilized to obtain more magnification and to visualize the angle structures.
5. Medical treatments for childhood glaucoma have a limited usefulness in young children. Acetazolamide is effective and can safely be given at a dose of 10–15 mg/day PO. Patients should be monitored for loss of appetite, excessive fatigue, and other signs of metabolic acidosis. Brimonidine should be avoided.
6. Goniosurgery is always the first consideration for surgery for childhood glaucoma. Some conditions respond more favorably than others. Children in the first year of life with mild-to-moderate expression of infantile PCG respond very well with this type of surgery.
7. Trabeculectomy surgery has an important place in the treatment of the pediatric glaucomas. Patients must be followed indefinitely for evidence of bleb thinning, and parents need to remain vigilant for signs of infection.
8. Glaucoma drainage device surgery is important for children when other procedures have failed or are not indicated. The drainage plate may be trimmed to accommodate a smaller eye. After surgery, a hand slit beam is very helpful to assess the drainage tube in the anterior chamber and a Koeppe lens may be used to restudy the tube entry position in the angle or assess the patency of the tube.
9. Refractive and strabismus amblyopia are important causes of vision loss in children with glaucoma. Early optical and occlusion therapies are important for these children.

## References

1. Hoskins DH, Shaffer RN, Hetherington J. Anatomical classification of the developmental glaucomas. *Arch Ophthalmol*. 1984;102:1331-1336.
2. Anderson DR. Pathology of the glaucomas. *Br J Ophthalmol*. 1972;56:146-157.
3. Tawara A, Inomata H. Developmental immaturity of the trabecular meshwork in congenital glaucoma. *Am J Ophthalmol*. 1981;92: 508-525.
4. Barkan O. Pathogenesis of congenital glaucoma: gonioscopic and anatomic observation of the angle of the anterior chamber in the normal eye and in congenital glaucoma. *Am J Ophthalmol*. 1955;40:1-11.
5. Worst JGF. Congenital glaucoma: remarks on the aspect of chamber angle, ontogenetic and pathogenetic background, and mode of action of goniotomy. *Invest Ophthalmol*. 1968;7:127-134.
6. Anderson DR. The development of the trabecular meshwork and its abnormality in primary infantile glaucoma. *Trans Am Ophthalmol Soc*. 1981;79:458-485.
7. Tawara A, Inomata H, Tsukamoto S. Ciliary body band width as an indicator of goniodysgenesis. *Am J Ophthalmol*. 1996;122: 790-800.
8. Maul E, Strozzi L, Munoz C, et al. The outflow pathway in congenital glaucoma. *Am J Ophthalmol*. 1980;89:667-675.
9. Tawara A, Inomata H. Congenital abnormalities of the trabecular meshwork in primary glaucoma with open angle. *Glaucoma*. 1987;9:28-34.
10. Maumenee AE. The pathogenesis of congenital glaucoma: a new theory. *Trans Am Ophthalmol Soc*. 1958;56:507-570.
11. Wright JD, Robb RM, Deuker DK, et al. Congenital glaucoma unresponsive to conventional therapy: a clinicopathological case presentation. *J Pediatr Ophthalmol Strabismus*. 1983;20: 172-179.
12. Kolker AE, Hetherington J. Congenital glaucoma. In: *Becker-Shaffer's Diagnosis and Therapy of the Glaucomas*. 5th ed. St Louis: CV Mosby; 1983: 317 [Chapter 18].
13. Sarfarazi M, Arkarsu AN, Hossain A, et al. Assignment of a locus(GLC3A) for primary congenital glaucoma(buphthalmos) to 2p21 and evidence for genetic heterogeneity. *Genomics*. 1995;30: 171-178.
14. Stoilov I, Nurten A, Sarfarazi M. Identification of three different truncating mutations in cytochrome P4501B1 (CYP1B1) as the principal cause of primary congenital glaucoma in families linked to the GLC3A on chromosome 2p21. *Hum Mol Genet*. 1997;6: 641-647.
15. Miller SJH. Genetic aspects of glaucoma. *Trans Ophthalmol Soc UK*. 1966;86:425-434.
16. Taylor RH, Ainsworth JR, Evans AR, et al. The epidemiology of pediatric glaucoma: The Toronto experience. *J AAPOS*. 1999;3: 308-315.
17. Sarfarazi M, Stoilov I. Molecular genetics of primary congenital glaucoma. *Eye*. 2000;14:422-428.
18. Akarsu AN, Turacli ME, Aktan SG, et al. A second locus (GLC3B) for primary glaucoma (buphthalmos) maps to the 1p36 region. *Hum Mol Genet*. 1996;5:1199-1203.
19. Stoilov IR, Sarfarazzi M. The Third Genetic Locus(GLC3C) for Primary Congenital Glaucoma (PCG) Maps to Chromosome 14q24.3. Fort Lauderdale (FL): Association for Research in Vision and Ophthalmology; 2002.
20. Panicker SG, Mandal AN, Reddy ABM, et al. Correlations of genotype with phenotype in Indian patients with primary congenital glaucoma. *Invest Ophthalmol Vis Sci*. 2004;45:1149-1156.
21. Bejjani BA, Stockton DW, Lewis RA, et al. Multiple CYP1B1 mutations and incomplete penetrance in an inbred population segregating primary congenital glaucoma suggest frequent de novo events and a dominant modifier locus. *Hum Mol Genet*. 2000;9:367-374.
22. Alward WLM, Semina EV, Kalenak JW, et al. Autosomal dominant iris hypoplasia is caused by a mutation in Rieger syndrome (RIEG/PITX2) gene. *Am J Ophthalmol*. 1998;125:98-100.
23. Nishimura DY, Swiderski RE, Alward WLM, et al. The forkhead transcription factor gene FKHL7 is responsible for glaucoma phenotypes which map to 6p25. *Nat Genet*. 1998;19:140-147.
24. Alward WLM, Fingert JH, Coote MA, et al. Clinical features associated with mutations in the chromosome 1 open angle glaucoma gene (GLC1A). *N Engl J Med*. 1998;338:1022-1023.
25. Freedman SF. Primary congenital glaucoma. In: Albert DM, Jacobiec FA (aus): *Principles and Practice of Ophthalmology*. WB Saunders Company; 2000.

26. Zimmerman TJ, Kooner KS, Morgan KS. Safety and efficacy of timolol in pediatric glaucoma. *Surv Ophthalmol.* 1983;28:262.
27. Hoskins HDJ, Hetherington JJ, Magee SD, et al. Clinical experience with timolol in childhood glaucoma. *Arch Ophthalmol.* 1985;103:1163.
28. McMahon CD, Hetherington JJ, Hoskins HDJ, et al. Timolol and pediatric glaucomas. *Ophthalmology.* 1981;88:249.
29. Williams T, Ginther WH. Hazard of ophthalmic timolol. *N Eng J Med.* 1982;306:1485.
30. Olson RJ, Bromberg BB, Zimmerman TJ. Apneic spells associated with timolol therapy in a neonate. *Am J Ophthalmol.* 1979;88:120-121.
31. Toris CB, Gleason ML, Camras CB, et al. Effects of brimonidine on aqueous humor dynamics in human eyes. *Arch Ophthalmol.* 1995;113:1514-1517.
32. Juzych M, Robin A, Novack G. Alpha-2 agonists in glaucoma therapy. In: Zimmerman T, Kooner K, Sharir M, Fechtner R, eds. *Textbook Of Ocular Pharmacology.* Philadelphia: Lippincott-Raven; 1997: 247-54.
33. Carlsen JO, Zabriskie NA, Kwon YH, et al. Apparent central nervous system depression in infants after the use of topical brimonidine. *Am J Ophthalmol.* 1999;128:255-256.
34. Korsch E, Grote A, Seybold M, et al. Systemic adverse effects of topical treatment with brimonidine in an infant with secondary glaucoma. *Eur J Pediatr.* 1999;158:685.
35. Mungan NK, Wilson TW, Nischal KK, et al. Hypotension and bradycardia in infants after the use of topical brimonidine and beta-blockers. *J AAPOS.* 2003;7:69-70.
36. Berlin RJ, Lee UT, Samples JR, et al. Ophthalmic drops causing coma in an infant. *J Pediatr.* 2001;138:441-443.
37. Enyedi LB, Freedman SF. Safety and efficacy of brimonidine in children with glaucoma. *J AAPOS.* 2001;5:281-284.
38. Parrish RK, Palmberg P. Sheu WP; XLT Study Group. A comparison of latanoprost, bimatoprost, and travoprost in patients with elevated intraocular pressure: a 12-week, randomized, masked-evaluator multicenter study. *Am J Ophthalmol.* 2003;135:688-703.
39. Enyedi LB, Freedman SF. Latanoprost for the treatment of pediatric glaucoma. *Surv Ophthalmol.* 2002;47(Suppl 1):S129-S132.
40. Enyedi LB, Freedman SF, Buckley EG. The effectiveness of latanoprost for the treatment of pediatric glaucoma. *J AAPOS.* 1999;3:33-39.
41. Barkan O. Technic of goniotomy. *Arch Ophthalmol.* 1938;19:217-223.
42. Barkan O. Operation for congenital glaucoma. *Am J Ophthalmol.* 1942;25:552-568.
43. Ho CL, Walton DS. Goniosurgery for glaucoma secondary to chronic anterior uveitis. prognostic factors and surgical technique. *J Glaucoma.* 2004;13:445-449.
44. Walton DS. Goniotomy. In: JT, ed. *Glaucoma Surgery.* St Louis, MO: Mosby-Year-Book, Inc.; 1992:107-121.
45. de Luise VP, Anderson DR. Primary infantile glaucoma (congenital glaucoma). *Surv Ophthalmol.* 1983;28:1-19.
46. Boughton Wl, Parks MM. An analysis of treatment of congenital glaucoma by gonitomy. *Am J Ophthalmol.* 1981;91:566-572.
47. Mandal AK, Gothwal VK, Bagga H, et al. Outcome of surgery on infants younger than 1 month with congenital glaucoma. *Ophthalmology.* 2003;110:1909-1915.
48. Shaffer RN. Prognosis of goniotomy in primary infantile glaucoma (trabeculodysgenesis). *Tr Am Oph Soc..* 1982;80:321-325.
49. Russell-Eggitt IM, Rice NSC, Barrie J, et al. Relapse following goniotomy for congenital glaucoma due to trabecular dysgenesis. *Eye.* 1992;6:197-200.
50. McPherson SD Jr. Results of external trabeculotomy. *Trans Am Ophthalmol Soc.* 1973;71:163-170.
51. McPherson SD Jr, MacFarland D. External trabeculotomy for developmental glaucoma. *Ophthalmol.* 1980;87:302-305.
52. McPherson SD Jr, Berry DP. Goniotomy vs external trabeculotomy for developmental glaucoma. *Ophthalmol.* 1980;87:302-305.
53. Mandal A, Naduvilath TJ, Jayagandan DO. Surgical results of combined trabeculotomy-trabeculectomy for developmental glaucoma. *Ophthalmology.* 1998;105:974-982.
54. Harms H, Dannheim R. Epicritical consideration of 300 cases of trabeculotomy ab externo. *Trans Ophthalmol Soc UK.* 1969;89:491-499.
55. Shrader CE, Cibis GW. Trabeculotomy. In: J T, ed. *Glaucoma Surgery.* St Louis, MO: Mosby-Year Book, Inc.; 1992:123-131.
56. Mendicino ME, Lynch MG, Drack A, et al. Long-term surgical and visual outcomes in primary congenital glaucoma: 360 degrees trabeculotomy versus goniotomy. *J AAPOS.* 2000;4:205-210.
57. Akimoto M, Tamihara H, Negi A, et al. Surgical results of trabeculotomy ab externo for developmental glaucoma. *Arch Ophthalmol.* 1994;112:1540-1544.
58. Filous A, Brunova B. Results of the modified trabeculotomy in the treatment of primary congenital glaucoma. *J AAPOS.* 2002;6:182-186.
59. Beauchamp GR, Parks MM. Filtering surgery in children: barriers to success. *Ophthalmol.* 1979;86:170-180.
60. Beck AD, Wilson WR, Lynch MG, et al. Trabeculectomy with adjunctive mitomycin-C in pediatric glaucoma. *Am J Ophthalmol.* 1998;126:648-657.
61. Freedman S, McCormick K, Cox T. Mitomycin-C augmented trabeculectomy with postoperative wound modulation in pediatric glaucoma. *J AAPOS.* 1999;3:117-124.
62. Wells AP, Cordeiro MF, Bunce C, et al. Cystic bleb formation and related complications in limbus- versus fornix-based conjunctival flaps in pediatric and young adult trabeculectomy with mitomycin C. *Ophthalmology.* 2003;110:2192-2197.
63. Susanna R, Oltrogge EW, Carani JE, et al. Mitomycin as adjunct chemotherapy with trabeculectomy in congenital and developmental glaucomas. *J Glaucoma.* 1995;4:151-188.
64. Sidoti PA, Belmonte SJ, Liebmann JM, et al. Trabeculectomy with mitomycin-C in the treatment of pediatric glaucoma. *Ophthalmology.* 2000;107:422-429.
65. Agarwal HC, Sood NN, Sihota R, et al. Mitomycin-C in congenital glaucoma. *Ophthalmol Surg Lasers.* 1997;28:979-985.
66. Tannenbaum DP, Hoffman D, Greaney MJ, et al. Outcomes of bleb excision and conjunctival advancement for leaking or hypotonous eyes after glaucoma filtering surgery. *Br J Ophthalmol.* 2004;88:99-103.
67. Hill R, Heur D, Baerveldt G, et al. Molteno implantation for glaucoma in young patients. *Ophthalmology.* 1991;98:1042-1046.
68. Nesher R, Sherwood M, Kass M, et al. Molteno implants in children. *J Glaucoma* 1992;1:228-232.
69. Walton DS, Katsavounidou G. Newborn primary congenital glaucoma:2005 update. *J Pediatr Ophthalmol Strabismus.* 2005;42:333-341.
70. Beck AD, Freedman S, Kammer J, Jin J. Aqueous shunt devices compared with trabeculectomy with mitomycin-C for children in the first two years of life. *Am J Ophthalmol.* 2003;136:994-1000.
71. Coleman A, Smyth R, Wilson R, Tam M. Initial clinical experience with the ahmed glaucoma valve implant in pediatric patients. *Arch Ophthalmol.* 1997;115:186-191.
72. Englert J, Freedman S, Cox T. The ahmed valve in refractory pediatric glaucoma. *Am J Ophthalmol.* 1999;127:34-42.

73. Morod Y, Donaldson C, Kim Y, et al. The Ahmed drainage implant in the treatment of pediatric glaucoma. *Am J Ophthalmol*. 2003;135:821-829.
74. Al-Torbaq AA, Edward DP. Delayed endopthalmitis in a child following an Ahmed glaucoma valve implant. *J AAPOS*. 2002;6:123-125.
75. Al Faran MF, Tomey KF, Mutlaq FA. Cyclocryotherapy in selected cases of congenital glaucoma. *Ophthalmic Surg*. 1990;21:794-798.
76. Wagle NS, Freedman SF, Buckley EG, et al. Long-term outcome of cyclocryotherapy for refractory pediatric glaucoma. *Ophthalmology*. 1998;105:1921-6; discussion 1926-1927.
77. Kirwan JF, Shah P, Khaw PT. Diode laser cyclophotocoagulation: role in the management of refractory pediatric glaucomas. *Ophthalmology*. 2002;109:316-323.
78. Plager DA, Neely DE. Intermediate-term results of endoscopic diode laser cyclophotocoagulation for pediatric glaucoma. *J AAPOS*. 1999;3:131-137.

# Part IV
# The Medical Treatment

# Chapter 51
# Medications Used to Treat Glaucoma

Paul N. Schacknow and John R. Samples

## 51.1 Glaucoma Therapy

### 51.1.1 Treatment Goals

The goals of glaucoma therapy for the patient and the physician are ultimately the same ones, but they are often approached from very different perspectives. Most patients with glaucoma visit their ophthalmologist on a regular basis because they understand that they have a potentially blinding disease that requires compliance with examinations and therapy. The patient's goal is to preserve the vision manifested in his or her visual field. While the treating ophthalmologist's overriding goal also is to preserve visual function for the patient, the doctor's immediate goal is to preserve those physiological structures whose anatomy underlies the basis for the ability to see. In treating the patient, the ophthalmologist needs to take into account new understandings of risk factors as well as new concepts, such as those that suggest that aging is a major risk factor for glaucoma.

The attempt to stabilize or at least minimize the damage to both structure and function involves three therapeutic approaches:

1. The reduction of intraocular pressure to or below a presumed "safe" target pressure that arrests the disease process or slows it sufficiently that patients will have the preservation of visual acuity and visual field consistent with their activities of daily living and their expected life span. Different optic nerves demand different intraocular pressures in order not to sustain progression. The same pressure does not suit every optic nerve. Target intraocular pressure (IOP) gives us a means of tracking the patient from visit to visit, but one must realize that there are little data on how to actually set the target IOP.
2. Maintaining and theoretically increasing ocular perfusion pressure to the optic nerve and retina. Vascular factors play a significant role in maintaining the health of the optic nerve. This is addressed in Chap. 11.
3. Protecting the optic nerve head and retinal ganglion cells from chemical mediators and other damaging agents that may result from intraocular pressure, vascular insult, or other unknown factors. Thus, neuroprotection is the final goal of all glaucoma therapies, although the term itself considers treatment approaches separate from directly lowering intraocular pressure or raising ocular perfusion pressure.

Numerous well-controlled scientific studies have provided scientific evidence that reduction of intraocular pressure should be a cornerstone of glaucoma therapy. Medical therapy tends to be the first choice for most forms of open angle glaucoma (OAG) in the United States,[1] although in Europe surgical intervention is somewhat more common as first-line therapeutic intervention.[2] Laser trabeculoplasty[3-5] – selective laser trabeculoplasty (SLTP) in particular[6] – is an option being offered as initial therapy for OAG. However, narrow or closed angle glaucomas are more likely treated as surgical diseases.

The Collaborative Initial Glaucoma Treatment Study (CIGTS)[7] showed that visual field preservation was similar after 5 years for both medical and surgical treatment. Most North American physicians prefer medical therapy as initial treatment because of the potential risk of surgical misadventures, surgical side effects, and the chronic risk of infection. Both short- and long-term use of glaucoma medications are associated with cellular changes in the conjunctival tissue that may increase the risk of scarring and decrease the success of subsequent incisional glaucoma surgery.[8-10] Medical therapies for glaucoma are taking into consideration reducing or eliminating preservative components such as benzalkonium chloride (BAK), which is associated with damaging effects to the conjunctiva, cornea, and the interior cells of the eye such as the corneal endothelium and trabecular cells in some instances.[11]

### Defining Maximum Tolerated Medical Therapy

During the 1970s, 1980s, and 1990s, the Zeitgeist was such that most medical insurance carriers required that the patient should have exhausted "maximum tolerated medical therapy (MTMT)" before the insurance carrier would consider either laser trabeculoplasty or incisional glaucoma surgery. In many cases, patients were using three, four, or even five different topical medications and perhaps an oral carbonic anhydrase inhibitor. This common use of maximal therapy in all instances resulted in great expense for the patient, poor compliance with complicated and expensive dosing regimens, preservative overload, and symptoms of ocular irritation. MTMT offers little benefit in terms of further reduction of intraocular pressure over what could be accomplished with only one or two different drops. Sherwood and his colleagues at the University of Florida have more recently shown that compliance indeed decreases with the number of drops used, more so as time passes, and with little benefit in the reduction of intraocular pressure for the third or fourth medication.[12] We would like ophthalmologists to evolve from the concept of "maximum *tolerated* medical therapy" to the idea of "maximum *acceptable* medical therapy" or perhaps better "maximum *reasonable* medical therapy." The idea is that given all the problems, with using three or more topical medications and oral anti-glaucoma medications as well, it is more reasonable to try patients on a single topical glaucoma medication as a first-line agent. If this has only partial success in reaching target pressure, consider adding a second topical agent. If further pressure reduction is required, try substitution of one agent for another or perhaps add a second bottle if it is a combination product of two topical medications. The goal is to keep the number of topical medications at no more than three, and the number of bottles at no more than two. If this maximum reasonable medical therapy is unsuccessful, then laser trabeculoplasty, incisional surgery, or one of the new surgical methods would come next in the sequence of treatment.

## 51.2 Medical Therapy

### 51.2.1 Intraocular Pressure Control is the Mainstay of Treatment

#### 51.2.1.1 Medical Therapy to Control Intraocular Pressure

In the United States, the Food and Drug Administration (FDA) has granted approval for glaucoma medications based on their ability to lower intraocular pressure. Considerations of visual field preservation, vascular dysregulation, the toxic effects of preservatives, dosing regimens to optimize compliance, and neuroprotection have not played any role in the FDA drug approval process. Yet all these factors remain major concerns for clinicians in the day-to-day care of glaucoma patients.

The role of fluctuations in intraocular pressure, minute by minute, day to day, and month by month, with respect to the progression of optic nerve head damage and visual field loss, is a matter of interest and controversy.[13-17] Some studies have concluded that fluctuations in intraocular pressure make a significant and independent contribution to glaucoma progression separate from the magnitude of intraocular pressure. Other studies, generally those looking at earlier in the disease course of the patient, suggest that fluctuations in pressure play little role. It seems likely that fluctuation is more important among specific subpopulations of glaucoma patients.[15] Because of the possible role of fluctuations in the progression of glaucoma, it is important to consider the clinical characteristics of medications for treating glaucoma with respect to not only their ability to lower intraocular pressure but providing relatively flat 24-h circadian IOP curves and both diurnal and nocturnal IOP control (Sidebar 51.1).

---

### SIDEBAR 51.1 Circadian variation of aqueous humor dynamics: implications for glaucoma therapy

Arthur J. Sit

Intraocular pressure (IOP) varies dynamically throughout the circadian cycle. Diurnal variations in IOP were first described by Drance who found that daytime IOP tends to be highest in the morning and decreases over the course of the day. However, 24-h IOP profiles measured in the physiologic positions (upright while awake, supine while asleep) indicate that peak IOP occurs during the nocturnal period for most normal subjects as well as glaucoma patients. The reasons for this pattern are unclear, but may have significant implications for the management of glaucoma.

IOP varies with posture, and the elevation of IOP at night can be at least partially explained by the change from the sitting position to the supine position. When IOP measured in the supine-only position is considered, most of the nocturnal elevation of IOP is eliminated for normal subjects, while glaucoma patients show a slight decrease in nocturnal IOP. However, these findings present a paradox since numerous studies on aqueous humor flow indicate that aqueous humor production in the nocturnal period drops by at least 50% in normal and glaucomatous eyes. If all other factors remained equal, there should be a significant decline in nocturnal IOP, which is not seen in either the supine or physiologic positions.

A recent study examining the circadian variations in aqueous humor dynamics investigated other factors that could produce the observed circadian IOP pattern. Outflow facility measured with Schiotz tonography appeared to decrease slightly at night but not enough to compensate for the decrease in aqueous production. Mathematical modeling of aqueous humor outflow dynamics suggested that the most likely factor responsible for the nocturnal IOP pattern was a change in episcleral venous pressure. However, other factors may have contributed as well, including changes in uveoscleral flow. This research is ongoing, and the mechanisms responsible for the 24-h IOP pattern remain to be elucidated.

Consistent reduction of IOP over the 24-h period is a goal in glaucoma treatment even if the exact reasons for the circadian IOP pattern may be unclear. However, some common glaucoma medications demonstrate a circadian variation in efficacy. The reasons for this can be understood from their mechanisms of action and our current understanding of aqueous humor dynamics.

Beta-adrenergic blockers, such as timolol, appear to lower IOP during the daytime but have reduced or minimal effect during the nighttime. Orzalesi et al found that twice a day, timolol had no statistically significant IOP lowering effect when compared with baseline when IOP was measured in the supine position during the night. Liu et al confirmed this finding, demonstrating that timolol gel-forming solution lowered IOP once during the day, but had essentially no IOP lowering effect during the night when IOP was measured in physiologic positions (sitting during the day and supine at night). Quaranta et al did find a statistically significant IOP reduction with twice a day timolol when IOP was measured sitting during the day and supine at night, but of smaller magnitude than during the day. These results are not surprising when the mechanism of action of timolol is considered. Studies of aqueous humor flow using anterior segment fluorophotometry have repeatedly demonstrated that timolol is a potent aqueous suppressant during the day, but does not significantly reduce aqueous flow at night. This is likely related to the normal reduction in aqueous production at night that likely occurs because of a nocturnal decrease in circulating beta-adrenergic agonists. Interestingly, when IOP is measured in the sitting position during the nocturnal period, timolol does appear to maintain IOP lowering effect, although less than during the diurnal period. This suggests the possibility of different mechanisms of action for timolol in the sitting and supine positions. However, the clinical significance of this finding is unclear since most individuals will assume a supine position for sleep.

The prostaglandin analogs (PGs) have excellent IOP control throughout the 24-h period, although less at night than at the day. Reduction of IOP from PGs is considered to result from an increase of aqueous humor outflow, presumably from the enhanced uveoscleral outflow. The long-term effect is likely related to the remodeling of the extracellular matrix in the ciliary muscle bundles by matrix metalloproteinases, but other mechanisms such as an increase in conventional outflow facility also appear to be involved. The decrease in nocturnal efficacy may be related to the slight decrease in conventional outflow facility that occurs at night. As well, there appears to be a more rapid attenuation of the IOP lowering effect during the diurnal period than during the nocturnal period after stopping treatment with PGs. This suggests that improvement of conventional outflow facility may be more important during the day, but the effect is of shorter duration than the remodeling of the uveoscleral outflow pathway.

Alpha-2-adrenergic agonists appear to have variable IOP lowering effect with unclear nocturnal efficacy. Orzalesi et al found that brimonidine lowered IOP significantly during the day, but did not significantly lower IOP at night. In contrast, Quaranta et al found statistically significant IOP reduction throughout the 24-h period with brimonidine, but less than with latanoprost at all time points. The mechanism of action of brimonidine is also unclear. It appears to be an aqueous suppressant but may also have effects on the uveoscleral outflow pathways. The nocturnal effects of brimonidine on aqueous humor flow are currently unknown.

Carbonic anhydrase inhibitors (CAIs) are aqueous suppressants that reduce aqueous humor production. Since they act directly upon carbonic anhydrase in the ciliary body to reduce aqueous humor formation, they are not influenced by the circadian variation of circulation hormones like beta-blockers. As a result, CAIs reduce IOP during the day as well as at night, although less than with PGs.

The 24-h efficacy of cholinergic agonists like pilocarpine is unknown. However, these medications reduce IOP by improving conventional outflow facility. If outflow facility only changes minimally at night, we may speculate that cholinergic agonists will reduce IOP during the nocturnal period, but this remains to be demonstrated.

## Conclusion

Optimal therapy for glaucoma would involve IOP control throughout the 24-h period. However, not all therapies are equally efficacious at all times of the day and night. Understanding of the mechanisms of action of different therapies, along with the knowledge of the circadian changes in aqueous humor dynamics, allows us to predict the therapies that will provide the most consistent IOP reduction. As well, understanding of aqueous humor dynamics may help in the development of future therapies with consistent 24-h IOP control.

## Bibliography

Brubaker RF. Flow of aqueous humor in humans [The Friedenwald Lecture]. *Invest Ophthalmol Vis Sci.* 1991;32(13):3145-3166.

Dailey RA, Brubaker RF, Bourne WM. The effects of timolol maleate and acetazolamide on the rate of aqueous formation in normal human subjects. *Am J Ophthalmol.* 1982;93(2):232-7.

Drance SM. The significance of the diurnal tension variations in normal and glaucomatous eyes. *Arch Ophthalmol.* 1960;64: 494-501.

Dubiner HB, Sircy MD, Landry T, et al. Comparison of the diurnal ocular hypotensive efficacy of travoprost and latanoprost over a 44-hour period in patients with elevated intraocular pressure. *Clin Ther.* 2004;26(1):84-91.

Garcia-Feijoo J, Martinez-de-la-Casa JM, Castillo A, et al. Circadian IOP-lowering efficacy of travoprost 0.004% ophthalmic solution compared to latanoprost 0.005%. *Curr Med Res Opin.* 2006;22(9):1689-1697.

Ingram CJ, Brubaker RF. Effect of brinzolamide and dorzolamide on aqueous humor flow in human eyes. *Am J Ophthalmol.* 1999;128(3):292-296.

Kacere RD, Dolan JW, Brubaker RF. Intravenous epinephrine stimulates aqueous formation in the human eye. *Invest Ophthalmol Vis Sci.* 1992;33(10):2861-2865.

Kaufman PL, Barany EH. Loss of acute pilocarpine effect on outflow facility following surgical disinsertion and retrodisplacement of the ciliary muscle from the scleral spur in the cynomolgus monkey. *Invest Ophthalmol.* 1976;15(10):793-807.

Konstas AG, Boboridis K, Tzetzi D, et al. Twenty-four-hour control with latanoprost-timolol-fixed combination therapy vs latanoprost therapy. *Arch Ophthalmol.* 2005;123(7):898-902.

Konstas AG, Katsimbris JM, Lallos N, et al. Latanoprost 0.005% versus bimatoprost 0.03% in primary open-angle glaucoma patients. *Ophthalmology.* 2005;112(2):262-266.

Konstas AG, Lake S, Economou AI, et al. 24-Hour control with a latanoprost-timolol fixed combination vs timolol alone. *Arch Ophthalmol.* 2006;124(11):1553-1557.

Konstas AG, Maltezos AC, Gandi S, et al. Comparison of 24-hour intraocular pressure reduction with two dosing regimens of latanoprost and timolol maleate in patients with primary open-angle glaucoma. *Am J Ophthalmol.* 1999;128(1):15-20.

Konstas AG, Papapanos P, Tersis I, et al. Twenty-four-hour diurnal curve comparison of commercially available latanoprost 0.005% versus the timolol and dorzolamide fixed combination. *Ophthalmology.* 2003;110(7):1357-1360.

Larsson LI. Aqueous humor flow in normal human eyes treated with brimonidine and timolol, alone and in combination. *Arch Ophthalmol.* 2001;119(4):492-495.

Lim KS, Nau CB, O'Byrne MM, et al. Mechanism of action of bimatoprost, latanoprost, and travoprost in healthy subjects. A crossover study. *Ophthalmology.* 2008;115(5):790-795 e4.

Liu JH, Kripke DF, Hoffman RE, et al. Nocturnal elevation of intraocular pressure in young adults. *Invest Ophthalmol Vis Sci.* 1998;39(13):2707-2712.

Liu JH, Kripke DF, Twa MD, et al. Twenty-four-hour pattern of intraocular pressure in the aging population. *Invest Ophthalmol Vis Sci.* 1999;40(12):2912-2917.

Liu JH, Kripke DF, Weinreb RN. Comparison of the nocturnal effects of once-daily timolol and latanoprost on intraocular pressure. *Am J Ophthalmol.* 2004;138(3):389-395.

Liu JH, Zhang X, Kripke DF, Weinreb RN. Twenty-four-hour intraocular pressure pattern associated with early glaucomatous changes. *Invest Ophthalmol Vis Sci.* 2003;44(4):1586-1590.

Lutjen-Drecoll E, Wiendl H, Kaufman PL. Acute and chronic structural effects of pilocarpine on monkey outflow tissues. *Trans Am Ophthalmol Soc.* 1998;96:171-191; discussion 92-95.

McCannel CA, Heinrich SR, Brubaker RF. Acetazolamide but not timolol lowers aqueous humor flow in sleeping humans. *Graefes Arch Clin Exp Ophthalmol.* 1992;230(6):518-520.

Orzalesi N, Rossetti I, Bottoli A, et al. Comparison of latanoprost, brimonidine and a fixed combination of timolol and dorzolamide on circadian intraocular pressure in patients with primary open-angle glaucoma and ocular hypertension. *Acta Ophthalmol Scand Suppl.* 2002;236:55.

Orzalesi N, Rossetti L, Bottoli A, et al. The effect of latanoprost, brimonidine, and a fixed combination of timolol and dorzolamide on circadian intraocular pressure in patients with glaucoma or ocular hypertension. *Arch Ophthalmol.* 2003;121(4):453-457.

Orzalesi N, Rossetti L, Bottoli A, Fogagnolo P. Comparison of the effects of latanoprost, travoprost, and bimatoprost on circadian intraocular pressure in patients with glaucoma or ocular hypertension. *Ophthalmology.* 2006;113(2):239-246.

Orzalesi N, Rossetti L, Invernizzi T, et al. Effect of timolol, latanoprost, and dorzolamide on circadian IOP in glaucoma or ocular hypertension. *Invest Ophthalmol Vis Sci.* 2000;41(9): 2566-2573.

Ota T, Murata H, Sugimoto E, et al. Prostaglandin analogues and mouse intraocular pressure: effects of tafluprost, latanoprost, travoprost, and unoprostone, considering 24-hour variation. *Invest Ophthalmol Vis Sci.* 2005;46(6):2006-2011.

Quaranta L, Gandolfo F, Turano R, et al. Effects of topical hypotensive drugs on circadian IOP, blood pressure, and calculated diastolic ocular perfusion pressure in patients with glaucoma. *Invest Ophthalmol Vis Sci.* 2006;47(7):2917-2923.

Schadlu R, Maus TL, Nau CB, Brubaker RF. Comparison of the efficacy of apraclonidine and brimonidine as aqueous suppressants in humans. *Arch Ophthalmol.* 1998;116(11):1441-1444.

Sit AJ, Nau CB, McLaren JW, et al. Circadian variation of aqueous dynamics in young healthy adults. *Invest Ophthalmol Vis Sci.* 2008;49(4):1473-1479.

Sit AJ, Weinreb RN, Crowston JG, et al. Sustained effect of travoprost on diurnal and nocturnal intraocular pressure. *Am J Ophthalmol.* 2006;141(6):1131-1133.

Topper JE, Brubaker RF. Effects of timolol, epinephrine, and acetazolamide on aqueous flow during sleep. *Invest Ophthalmol Vis Sci.* 1985;26(10):1315-1319.

Toris CB, Gleason ML, Camras CB, Yablonski ME. Effects of brimonidine on aqueous dynamics in human eyes. *Arch Ophthalmol.* 1995;113(12):1514-1517.

Toris CB, Zhan G, Fan S, et al. Effects of travoprost on aqueous humor dynamics in patients with elevated intraocular pressure. *J Glaucoma.* 2007;16(2):189-195.

Toris CB, Zhan GL, Camras CB, McLaughlin MA. Effects of travoprost on aqueous humor dynamics in monkeys. *J Glaucoma.* 2005;14(1):70-73.

Tsukamoto H, Larsson LI. Aqueous humor flow in normal human eyes treated with brimonidine and dorzolamide, alone and in combination. *Arch Ophthalmol.* 2004;122(2):190-193.

Walters TR, DuBiner HB, Carpenter SP, et al. 24-Hour IOP control with once-daily bimatoprost, timolol gel-forming solution, or latanoprost: a 1-month, randomized, comparative clinical trial. *Surv Ophthalmol.* 2004;49 Suppl 1:S26-S35.

Weinreb RN, Toris CB, Gabelt BT, et al. Effects of prostaglandins on the aqueous humor outflow pathways. *Surv Ophthalmol.* 2002;47 Suppl 1:S53-S64.

## 51.3 The Decision to Treat

### 51.3.1 Risks and Benefits of Treatment

#### 51.3.1.1 Setting Target Pressure

The rationale for beginning medical treatment of glaucoma is based on the assumption that lowering intraocular pressure is the most important thing we presently offer the glaucoma patient. Many multicenter, randomized clinical trials have sustained the importance of lowering intraocular pressure.[18] Some of these studies are shown in Table 51.1.

There are, of course, many other non-IOP factors that influence the choice of medical therapy as initial treatment for any given patient. The decision really rests upon the clinician's accounting of risk factors for an individual patient. In addition to the ability of medications to lower intraocular pressure, we must also consider the natural course of the disease and the age of the patient, topical and systemic side effects of medications, preservative toxicities, dosing intervals, adherence to medical regimens and, of course, the possibility of no treatment at all for select patients.

As experienced clinicians, we must consider both the risks and benefits of starting medical therapy for a specific patient. The best predictor of the IOP that an eye will sustain in the future is the pressure that it has had in the past.[19] Before beginning medical therapy, the physician should set a "target-IOP" for the patient. The target-IOP is the clinician's best estimate of the maximum intraocular pressure the specific glaucoma patient can tolerate without further damage to their optic nerves and visual fields.[20] This IOP may, of course, differ between the two eyes of the patient. We emphasize that this target pressure is only a clinical estimate and must be updated periodically if progression is noted. It is unfortunate that many ophthalmologists do not reassess the IOP of the patient at each visit with respect to the clinical findings![21]

The target pressure may serve as a useful reminder for managing the patient, though very often, clinicians articulate the fear that writing such a number in the medical record will work against them in court. First, note that medical malpractice cases in glaucoma care are rare and commonly surround the issue of failure to diagnose.[22,23] Second, once the ophthalmologist perceives and acts upon the target pressure as an ever-evolving concept based on the current clinical condition of their patient, modified if necessary at each visit, the physician is unlikely to visit target pressure as a legal matter. As of this writing, we are unaware of any instance where target pressure has been invoked in a medical-legal case. Therapy may be adjusted in line with the setting of a new target pressure at each clinical visit as circumstances dictate.

**Table 51.1** Multicenter, randomized controlled clinical trials demonstrating importance of reduced intraocular pressure to slow or halt progression of glaucoma

| NEI-sponsored clinical trials | | | | |
|---|---|---|---|---|
| Trial | Number of patients/eyes | Diagnosis | Treatments | Follow-up |
| EMGT[1] | 255 patients | OAG | Therapy (argon laser trabeculoplasty and betaxolol) vs. Observation | 4–9 years |
| OHTS[2] | 1,636 patients | OHT | Medical therapy vs. observation | 5 years |
| CIGITS[3] | 607 patients | OAG | Medical therapy vs. surgery | 5 years |
| AGIS[4] | 738 eyes | OAG | Argon laser trabeculoplasty vs. surgery | 8 years |
| CNTGS[5] | 140 eyes | NTG | Medical therapy and/or surgery vs. observation | 7 years |

Rather than a single numerical value for an initial target pressure, most glaucoma specialists set a preliminary goal for target IOP as a *range* of percentage reduction from the initial presenting IOP in the office setting.[24,25] Expert panel recommendations for initial target pressure range from 25% reduction for patients with mild glaucoma to more than 35% initial reduction for patients with severe damage.[26] Factors to be considered in determining initial and subsequent target pressures include the IOP level at which the optic nerve damage occurred ("diagnostic" IOP), the extent of glaucomatous damage (cup-to-disc ratio, disc hemorrhage, visual fields, optic nerve head appearance, and retinal nerve fiber layer imaging), the rate of progression of glaucomatous damage if known, the presence of other known risk factors (age, race, CCT, family history/ genetic predisposition), expected lifespan, and finally the patient's medical history (systemic hypertension, diabetes, sleep apnea, age, systemic medications).

Some specialists feel that patients are ill-served by setting a target pressure or target-IOP range. One argument sometimes advanced against using a target range is that, theoretically, it seems likely there should be some absolute value of intraocular pressure below which the patient's glaucoma will not progress, and by using a range, we are simply admitting that we do not know how low to go for that individual patient. But setting a target-IOP range is useful when it is based on the clinician's experience and the many factors described previously, as long as it is reevaluated at each office visit based on clinical findings.

Intraocular pressure determinations are made in the ophthalmologist's office during clinic hours. Recent studies have suggested that a large proportion of patients' highest daily IOPs occur outside the usual office hours,[27,28] and may also be the highest during the portion of the night when the patient is supine and sleeping. Target-IOPs have traditionally been determined based on one or two measurements of the patient's IOP during usual daylight office hours, and thus may not be representative of the true IOPs when glaucomatous damage may occur, Patients who suffer from sleep apnea[29-34] or may have body builds with "thick" necks may pose additional problems when trying to determine their true IOPs and setting target-pressures. Most patients have their highest intraocular pressure upon awakening. This may mean that it is ideal to dose medication upon awakening rather than waiting until later in the morning. Occasional clinic visits early in the morning before the office normally would open and may reveal elevated intraocular pressures that would not otherwise be detected.

Patients should be involved in discussions about target-IOPs. Patients need to be apprised that simply determining how close their IOP is to "target" at each office visit is not sufficient to determine the stability or progression of their glaucoma. Changes in the optic nerve head, via ophthalmoscopy, photography or imaging devices, and functional visual field and acuity changes are the true measures of glaucoma status. IOP is an easily measured but poor surrogate for "defining" glaucoma.

## 51.4 Anatomy and Physiology of Aqueous Humor Production and Outflow

In the first section of this chapter, we have had a discussion of the rationale behind the medical therapy of glaucoma. Before beginning a discussion of the medications themselves, we will now describe the anatomical and physiological substrates related to the ingress and outflow of aqueous humor within the eye.

### 51.4.1 Anatomy of Aqueous Humor Production

The lens and cornea are avascular structures that are supplied nonetheless with nutrients and oxygen by the aqueous humor, which also serves to remove metabolic waste products as it is drained from the eye. Aqueous humor is produced within the 70–80 ciliary processes that are radial folds in the pars plicata of the ciliary body. Both active and passive mechanisms are involved in aqueous production. The two-layered epithelium covering the ciliary processes are sealed together by tight junctions (zonula occludens) forming the blood–aqueous barrier between the posterior chamber and blood vessels that pass through the ciliary body and its processes.[35,36]

Passive mechanisms of aqueous production include *diffusion* and *ultrafiltration*:

- *Diffusion* – lipid-soluble substances pass through the cell membrane in response to a concentration gradient across the membrane.
- *Ultrafiltration* – water and water-soluble molecules flow through micropores in the cell membrane based on an osmotic gradient, IOP, blood pressure in the ciliary vasculature, and the plasma oncotic pressure (from colloidal proteins).

Active mechanisms of aqueous production involve *secretion*:

- *Secretion* – large water-soluble molecules are actively moved across cell membranes. This requires and involves enzymes (e.g., Na-K ATPase and glycolytic) found in nonpigmented epithelial cells. The majority of aqueous production is mediated by active transport mechanisms.

Aqueous production starts in the blood with the final product eventually reaching the anterior chamber. The route is as follows (Fig. 51.1):

**Fig. 51.1** Route of aqueous humor production and outflow

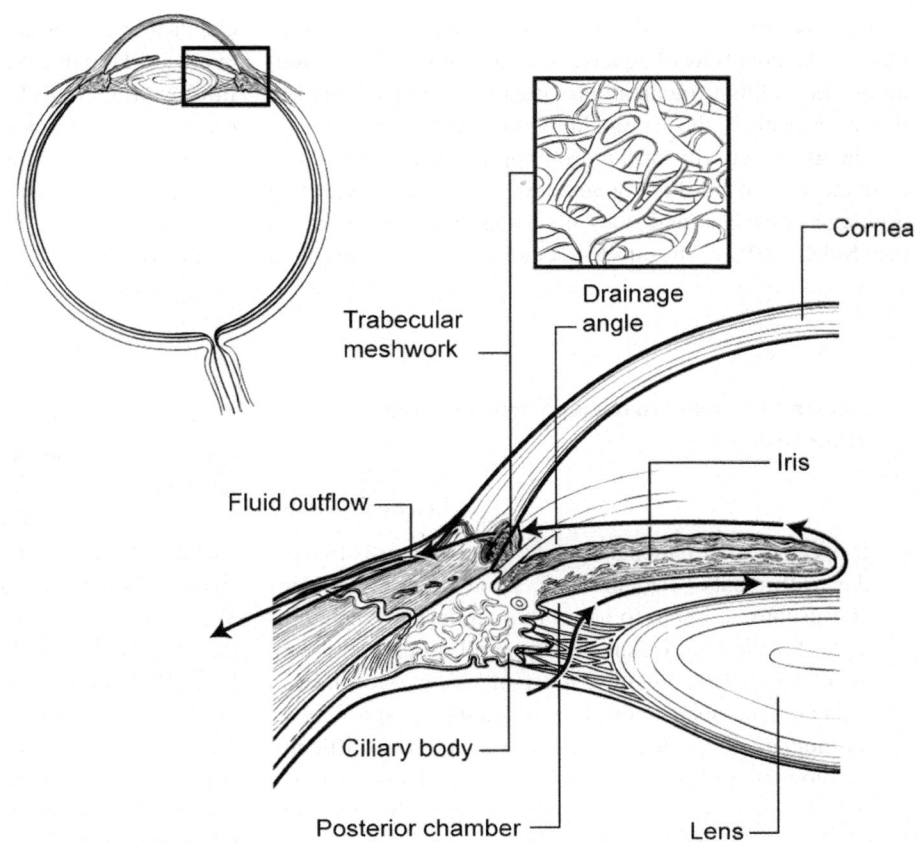

Blood plasma ultrafiltrate > capillary endothelial cells > ciliary process interstitial tissue > pigmented epithelium > nonpigmented epithelium (active transport) > posterior chamber > pupil > anterior chamber.

Aqueous humor is a "complex mixture of electrolytes, organic solutes, growth factors, and other proteins that supply nutrients to the nonvascularized tissues of the anterior chamber (i.e., trabecular meshwork (TM), lens, and corneal endothelium)."[37] Aqueous is produced at a rate of 2.0–3.0 μl/min. or 1.5% of anterior chamber volume/min. The anterior chamber holds approximately 250 μl of aqueous humor, the posterior chamber about 60 μl of aqueous humor. All the aqueous is replenished about every 1.5–2 h during the daytime hours. Relative to blood plasma, aqueous has approximately 15 times greater ascorbate and much less protein (0.02% in aqueous versus 7% in plasma). Aqueous humor formation decreases with sleep[38] (suppression of 45±20%) and advancing age[39] (decrease of 2.5% per decade). Men and women on average have the same rate of aqueous flow.[38]

After entering the anterior chamber and angle structures, there are two pathways for the outflow of aqueous humor from the eye.[40] The "conventional" or trabecular meshwork outflow path is said to be "pressure-dependent." This pathway is usually thought to account for about 80% of aqueous outflow. The route of aqueous outflow through the trabecular meshwork is:

Anterior chamber > trabecular meshwork > Schlemm's Canal > scleral collector channels > episcleral aqueous veins > anterior ciliary veins > superior ophthalmic veins > venous system.

The "unconventional" or uveoscleral outflow path is said to be "pressure-independent." This pathway accounts for the remaining 20% of aqueous outflow, although there is conjecture that the actual number is higher. The root of aqueous outflow through the uveoscleral pathway is:

Anterior chamber > iris root > ciliary body interstitial tissue > suprachoroidal space (negative pressure) > sclera? vortex veins? along the nerves? > posterior ciliary veins > venous system.

The majority of glaucoma medications are eyedrops that are placed on the surface of the eye. They enter through the conjunctiva and cornea, with the fornix serving as a reservoir. Usually drops are applied in great excess, and most of the medication does not enter the eye. The root of absorption into the eye from an eyedrop is from the conjunctival cul-de-sac, then becoming part of the tear film (mucin, water, and oil) that is 7–9 μm thick, then passively diffusing into cornea and conjunctiva and then becoming part of the aqueous humor. Peak concentration of drug in the aqueous humor takes from 30 to 60 min. Glaucoma drugs are generally not uniformly distributed throughout the eye, because of both physical barriers like iris, lens, and cillary body, as well as circulatory factors like bulk flow of aqueous humor and the blood circulation. In addition, medications often differentially bind to tissues, especially those containing melanin.[40]

The great majority of the drop applied to the eye (some estimate this to be 80% or greater) exits via the lacrimal drainage apparatus and does not enter into the eye at all (see Sidebar 51.2). The cul-de-sac holds at most 30 μL of an eye drop. Most of the drop drains from the cul-de-sac of the eye within the first 5 min. Blinking eliminates about 2 μL of fluid from the cul-de-sac.[41] The route of nasolacrimal duct drainage is: conjunctival cul-de-sac > inferior and superior nasal puncta > canaliculi > lacrimal sac > nasolacrimal duct > Valve of Hasner > inferior nasal turbinate > then absorption into the vascularized nasopharyngeal mucosa or swallowed.[40]

### Sidebar 51.2  How to use eye drops to treat glaucoma

*Odette Callender*

It is easy to tell patients to "take these two pills twice a day with meals." Patients understand these instructions and usually are able to adapt this regimen to their lifestyle. Swallowing is something we all do naturally and, even if currently healthy, most of us have swallowed pills at some point in our lives – vitamins, aspirin, acetaminophen, ibuprofen, etc. For those who have difficulty swallowing, pills can often be crushed and dissolved in a liquid or mixed with food. We can usually discretely swallow a pill even when in a public venue.

How about the doctor instead instructing the patient to "take these two drops twice a day?" This may be a tall order requiring much more than just adapting the schedule to the patient's lifestyle. Instilling drops in our eyes is not something we do naturally. In fact quite the opposite is true given the instinctive protective reflex of closing your eyes when something approaches them. Not only do our patient's have to overcome this natural reflex, but many of them are elderly and have difficulty handling the small bottles of eye drops because of arthritis or perhaps cognitive issues. Many people have never had to use eyedrops before the prescription you just gave to them. It's impossible to discretely instill an eyedrop at the dinner table. Using eyedrops requires a new skill set and social adjustments different from taking other kinds of medications prescribed by noneyecare physicians. Yet when writing a prescription or providing a sample, do you (or your staff) routinely ask patients if they have ever instilled drops in their eyes before? Does your practice routinely provide written or hands-on instruction on how to instill eye drops? Do you watch patients demonstrate instillation of drops with perhaps a sample bottle of artificial tears? With our incredibly busy office/clinic schedules, the answer to these questions is often NO.

A study by Winfield et al looking at the causes of patient noncompliance revealed a wide variety of problems patients have instilling their drops. The most important finding was that 69% of those patients in the study stated that they would *not* have reported compliance barriers to their physician even if specifically questioned. We cannot rely on patients to tell us spontaneously that they are having difficulty using their drops, but we as their physicians must instead take a proactive approach. One-on-one training between patients and physicians or staff, while ideal, is often not feasible. In office video, education is likely only available in a limited number of practices. Written material gives the patient something which they may refer and share with family and friends who may assist with drop instillation. Step by step instructions that include answers to "frequently asked questions" will benefit patients while saving you and your staff time. Any patients for whom we prescribe drops, not just our glaucoma patients, can benefit from such instructions.

It is instructive to occasional ask your long term patients to demonstrate drop instillation in the office. You may be in for a rude awakening when you find that more of the medication reaches their cheeks than their fornices! Such a situation provides an opportunity for reinstruction in instillation techniques. Do not let your patient leave the office until you feel comfortable that they or their accompanying care provider can accurately administer glaucoma drop medications. Provide instructions for both new and "experienced" patients and consider offering compliance and/or instillation aids. Although 78% of patients in the study by Winfield et al responded favorably to the suggestion of using compliance aids, none of them were aware that aids were available.

Many doctors instruct patients to perform punctual occlusion. However, despite instruction many patients do not perform proper punctual occlusion negating the benefits. "Nasolacrimal occlusion, a technique in which digital pressure on the periphery of the nasolacrimal drainage system, obstructs drainage to the nasopharyngeal mucosa, and has been shown to significantly decrease systemic absorption. Eyelid closure for 5 min following drug application also achieves the same purpose by inhibiting nasolacrimal pump action." This drop instruction sheet describes eyelid closure, that may be easily done by all patients without requiring digital dexterity. It is a reasonable alternative to punctual occlusion. If you prefer that patients perform punctual occlusion, they should also do so while closing their eyes. We personally demonstrate punctual occlusion on ourselves and then ask the patient to do so in front of us. We reinstruct them and guide their fingers as necessary to adequately perform this technique.

## Bibliography

Gerber SL, Cantor LB, Craig Brater D. Systemic drug interactions with topical glaucoma medications. *Surv Ophthalmol.* 1990;35(3):205-218.

Winfield AJ, Jessiman D, Williams A, Esakowitz L. A study of the causes of non-compliance by patients prescribed eyedrops. *Br J Ophthalmol.* 1990;74:477-480.

## 51.5 Corneal Penetration by Drugs

The multilayered cornea is not easily penetrated by drugs. The corneal structure may be described as a lipid–water–lipid sandwich[57] (Fig. 51.2). The zonula occludens (tight junctions) limit the passage of aqueous-based medications through the epithelium and into the stroma. Some preservatives, such as benzalkonium chloride (BAK), act as detergents and break up the tight junctions, greatly enhancing the entrance of water-soluble substances.

Unfortunately, BAK contributes greatly to symptoms of ocular surface disease experienced by many glaucoma patients, and its presence has been ubiquitous in glaucoma medications.[8,10,42-44] Newer drugs, such as brimonidine[45,46] with Purite and travoprost[47] with the preservative sofZia, and timolol in the single-use Occudose form do not contain BAK (see Sidebar 51.3 for more discussion on the role of preservatives in glaucoma medications and ocular surface disease.) Lipid-based molecules do easily penetrate the corneal epithelium, but have somewhat retarded passage through the stroma of the cornea. Hydrophilic drug molecules can be esterified to become lipophilic and function as "prodrugs," that easily pass through the corneal epithelium. The cornea is rich in esterases that in turn hydrolyze the ester bond as the drug passes through it. Glaucoma medications such as Propine (esterified epinephrine) and latanoprost and travoprost (esterifed derivatives of prostaglandin $F_{2\alpha}$ (F2 alpha) make use of the prodrug principle. As prodrugs, these compounds are about ten times[48] more soluble than their original molecules.

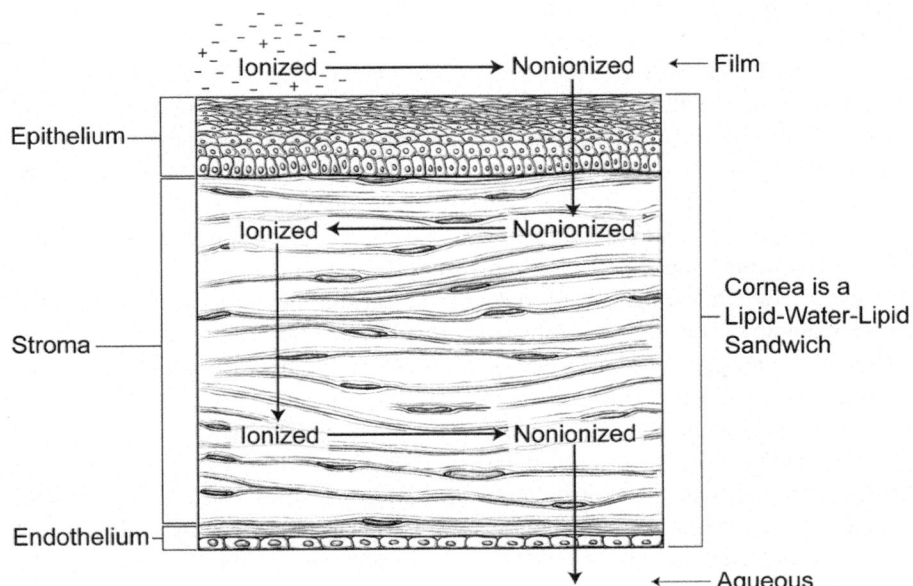

**Fig. 51.2** Anatomy of drug penetration into the eye

### Sidebar 51.3 Preservatives and glaucoma medications

Clark L. Springs

Ocular surface disease (OSD) in the glaucoma patient is a frequent cause of discomfort and visual degradation. It is often under-recognized, undertreated, and a frequent source of frustration for patient and physician, alike. OSD encompasses aqueous tear deficiency, lipid abnormalities (i.e., meibomian gland dysfunction, blepharitis), and mucin deficiencies due to decreased goblet cell function. These deficiencies can lead to increased tear osmolarity, an upregulation in inflammatory mediators, and, ultimately, ocular irritation. A variety of risk factors can contribute to this dysfunctional tear state such as age, systemic diseases and medications, as well as preservatives in topical ophthalmic medications. Climate and relative humidity are also a major factor.

Benzalkonium chloride (BAK), a quaternary ammonium compound with surfactant properties, is the most commonly used preservative in topical ophthalmic medications. It is a highly effective antimicrobial agent that prevents contamination. BAK can also enhance corneal penetration of some drugs by separating the epithelium. The mechanism of action of BAK is by irreversible binding of cell membranes altering cell permeability.

The effects of BAK are nonselective, which can adversely affect the health of various ocular tissues. On the ocular surface, BAK can decrease tear break-up time and compromise epithelial cell integrity, which can impair healing and exacerbate OSD. In the conjunctiva, BAK can induce chronic subclinical inflammation and fibroblastic transformation, which can negatively impact goblet cell density and accessory lacrimal gland function. The effects of BAK are dose dependent and cumulative. In cell culture systems, at a concentration of 0.0001%, cell arrest occurs; at 0.01% apoptosis occurs; and at 0.05–0.1% cell necrosis occurs. The concentration of BAK in commercially available glaucoma medications ranges from 0.05 to 0.2%.

In glaucoma, the use of chronic BAK may be a significant concern. Many patients are elderly, and use multiple ophthalmic medications on a chronic basis for the treatment of their glaucoma and other ophthalmic conditions (e.g., OSD). These factors can be responsible for poor tolerance of glaucoma eye drops, due to inflammation and toxicity. Further, patients undergoing glaucoma filtering have a higher rate of failure if they have been on topical medications preserved with BAK. BAK has also been implicated in the exacerbation of postoperative cystoid macular edema because of its ability to breakdown the blood–aqueous barrier. Between 8 and 15% of the US population have symptoms of ocular surface disease. However, in the glaucoma population, the prevalence of OSD symptoms is significantly higher, 40–58%. Further, the severity of ocular surface symptoms increased with the number of medications used.

Currently, ophthalmologists do not have a single practical, reproducible test that can help them diagnose and stage OSD. Physicians must therefore rely on their clinical judgment and formulate treatment plans based on a combination of objective testing and their assessment of individual patients' symptoms. Questionnaires such as the Ocular Surface Disease Index are well validated tools for detecting and staging ocular surface disease especially when they are used in conjunction with clinical testing. In 2007, the International Dry Eye Workshop published its guidelines for diagnosing and treating ocular surface disease. In addition to identifying critical clinical tests, this report recommended that physicians adhere to the following sequence when objectively assessing patients for OSD:

1. Measure tear breakup time with fluorescein staining
2. Perform vital staining with lissamine green or rose bengal
3. Evaluate the production of tears with Schirmer testing
4. Assess the morphology of the eyelids and meibomian glands
5. Test the function of the meibomian glands.

Performing these tests out of order may affect their integrity and provide inaccurate information.

The elimination of BAK from OTC lubricants is recognized as the single most critical advance in the treatment of OSD. Similarly, limitation of BAK load in glaucoma drops is a desirable goal and one that is being actively pursued by industry. Preservative-free preparations can be compounded extemporaneously and a topical preservative-free beta blocker is commercially available (Timoptic OcuDose; Merck, Whitehouse Station, New Jersey). The cost and inconvenience of preservative-free preparations is often prohibitive. Gentler oxidizing preservatives that dissipate on the ocular surface have recently been introduced in topical glaucoma medications. Brimonidine preserved with sodium chlorite (Alphagan-P; Allergan, Irvine, California) is the only alpha-agonist available in a BAK-free formulation. Travaprost preserved with a buffered solution of borate, zinc, and polyols (Travatan-Z; Alcon Laboratories, Ft. Worth, Texas) is currently the only commercially available prostaglandin analog without BAK. In an in vitro model of conjunctival epithelial cells, travoprost without BAK maintained cell viability is comparable to physiologic buffered saline, while BAK-preserved preparations demonstrated significant loss of cell viability and apoptotic activity. An in vivo rabbit model has shown a beneficial effect of the oxidizing preservatives sodium chlorite and Sofzia with preservation of microvilli and less conjunctival inflammation, in comparison to BAK containing glaucoma medications. Horsley and Kahook found that replacing latanoprost with 0.02% BAK with travoprost Sofzia for 8 weeks increased the mean tear breakup time of 20 consecutive patients (40 eyes) from $2.02 \pm 0.71$ to $6.34 \pm 1.31$ ($p < 0.001$). The patients also reported an improvement in their dry eye symptoms on the Ocular Surface Disease Index at the end of the study ($26.31 \pm 8.25$–$16.56 \pm 6.19$ ($p < 0.001$)). Further studies are underway to determine the significance of this preliminary report.

In summary, OSD is a serious and debilitating condition that is prevalent among the elderly. Further, OSD appears to be exacerbated by the use of topical ophthalmic medications preserved with BAK. Together, these factors increase the risk that elderly glaucoma patients will develop OSD.

Physicians can prevent or minimize OSD among their glaucoma patients by carefully evaluating clinical signs and symptoms. Minimizing or eliminating exposure to extrinsic factors such as the preservative BAK may reduce the incidence and severity of OSD among those who use glaucoma medications.

## Bibliography

Baudouin C, de Lunardo C. Short term comparative study of topical 2% carteolol with and without benzalkonium chloride in healthy volunteers. *Br J Ophthalmol*. 1998;82:39-42.

Baudouin C, Pisella PJ, Fillacier K, et al. Ocular surface inflammatory changes induced by topical antiglaucoma drugs *Ophthalmology*. 1999;106(3):556-563.

Baudouin C, Riancho L, Warnet J, et al. In vitro studies of antiglaucomatous prostaglandin analogues: travoprost with and without benzalkonium chloride and preserved latanoprost. *Invest Ophthalmol Vis Sci*. 2007;48:4123-4128.

Bourcier T, DeSaint Jean M, Brignole F, Goguel A, Baudouin C. Expression of CD40 and CD40 ligand in the human conjunctival epithelium. *Curr Eye Res*. 2000;20:85-94.

Broadway DC, Grierson I, O'Brien C, et al. Adverse effects of topical antiglaucoma medication. *Arch Ophthalmol*. 1994;112:1437-1445.

De Saint Jean M, Debbasch C, Brignole F, Warnet JM, Baudouin C. Relationship between in vitro toxicity of benzalkonium chloride (BAC) and preservative-induced dry eye. *Adv Exp Med Biol*. 2002;506(Pt A):697-702.

Fechtner R, Budenz, D, Godfrey D. Prevalence of ocular surface disease symptoms in glaucoma patients on IOP-lowering medications. Poster presented at: *The 18th Annual Meeting of the American Glaucoma Society*; March 8, 2006; Washington, DC.)

Horsley MB, Kahook MY. Changes in tear break-up time and ocular surface disease index after initiation of travoprost with Sofzia in patients previously using latanoprost with benzalkonium chloride. Poster presented at: *The 18th Annual Meeting of the American Glaucoma Society*; March 8, 2006; Washington, DC.

Kahook MY, Noecker RJ. Comparison of corneal and conjunctival changes after dosing of travoprost preserved with Sofzia, latanoprost with 0.02% benzalkonium chloride, and preservative-free artificial tears. *Cornea*. 2008;27(3):339-343.

Leung EW, Medeiros FA, Weinreb RN. Prevalence of ocular surface disease in glaucoma patients. *J Glaucoma*. 2008;17(5):350-355.

Management and therapy of dry eye disease: report of the management and therapy subcommittee of the international dry eye workshop (2007). *Ocul Surf*. 2007;5(2):163-178.

Miljanovic B. Dana R. Sullivan DA. Schaumberg DA. Impact of dry eye syndrome on vision-related quality of life. [Journal Article. Randomized Controlled Trial. Research Support, N.I.H., Extramural. Research Support] *Am J Ophthalmol*. 2007;143(3):409-415.

Miyake K, Ibaraki N, Goto Y, et al. ESCRS Binkhorst lecture 2002: pseudophakic preservative maculopathy. *J Cataract Refract Surg*. 2003;29:1800-1810.

Montes-Mico R. Role of the tear film in the optical quality of the human eye. *J Cataract Refract Surg*. 2007;33(9):1631-1635.

Noecker R. Effects of common ophthalmic preservatives on ocular health. *Adv Ther*. 2001;18:205-215.

Noecker RJ, Herrygers LA, Anwaruddin R. Corneal and conjunctival changes caused by commonly used glaucoma medications. *Cornea*. 2004;23(5):490-496.

Ocular Surface 2007 Report of the International Dry Eye Workshop. *Ocul Surf*. 2007;5(2):65-206.

Sasaki H, Nagano T, Yamamura K, Nishida K, Nakamura J. Ophthalmic preservatives as absorption promoters for ocular drug delivery. *J Pharm Pharmacol*. 1995;47(9):703-707.

Schiffman RM, Christianson MD, Jacobsen G, Hirsch JD, Reis BL. Reliability and validity of the ocular surface disease index. *Arch Ophthalmol*. 2000;118:615-621

Schiffman RM, Christianson MD, Jacobsen G, Hirsch JD, Reis BL. Reliability and validity of the ocular surface disease index [see comment]. [Journal Article Research Support, Non-U.S. Gov't] *Arch Ophthalmol*. 2000;118(5):615-621.

## 51.6 Prostaglandins vs. Prostamides

Allergan contends that bimatoprost, with an amide moiety rather than an ester group, does not function as a prodrug, but enters the eye through the sclera as an intact prostamide.[49] Several studies have shown, however, that amidases within the corneal epithelium cleave the amide group from the basic bimatoprost molecule. This hydrolyzed bimatoprost molecule has been shown to activate the same prostaglandin FP receptors as the hydrolyzed molecules of latanoprost and travoprost.[50,51] It is our opinion that most glaucoma specialists consider bimatoprost, latanoprost, and travoprost to likely work through the same set of receptors and have the same mechanism(s) of action.[50]

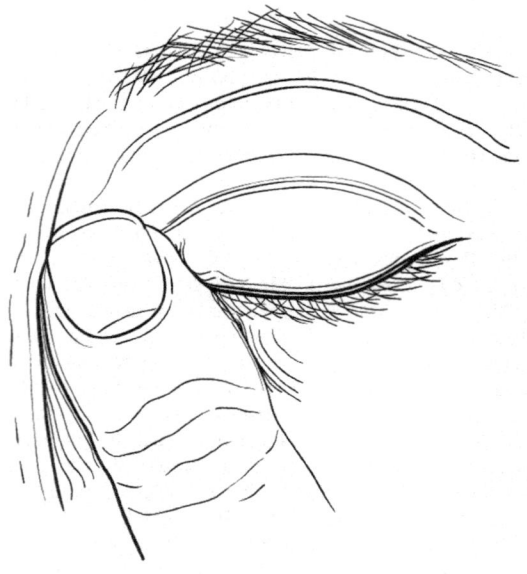

**Fig. 51.3** Nasolacrimal occlusion digital massage technique

Relatively high concentrations of active medications found in glaucoma drops can result in significant systemic side effects when these drops get into the body after exiting the eye through the nasolacrimal duct system. Occlusion of the nasolacrimal puncta near the medial canthus of both upper and lower eyelids of each eye after topical application of glaucoma drops may reduce systemic absorption up to 70%. The technique of nasolacrimal punctal obstruction (NLO) can be easily taught to patients (Fig. 51.3), but it is important to watch them personally demonstrate the technique in the office.[52,53] In many cases, patients incorrectly use digital pressure on the nasal bones or through the eyelid in the middle of the globe rather than over the anatomical area where the puncta are found. Patients should be asked to perform NLO for between 2 and 5 min, although this is often impractical 100% of the time. Hand washing and keeping the nails trimmed are often neglected but useful adjuncts for nasal lacrimal duct obstruction.

## 51.7 Pharmacological Basis of Drug Activity: The Autonomic Nervous System

Medications work by acting on receptors found on nerve cells and target end-organs. Drugs used to treat glaucoma, both eyedrops and oral agents, act as either agonists or antagonists after binding to receptors. What follows is a brief discussion of the organization of the nervous system, and the major receptor classes that are of interest to us regarding the biological activity of glaucoma drugs.

These sympathetic nerve ganglia start within the vertebral column found between the first thoracic segment and the third lumbar segments of the spinal cord. These ganglia contain not only the sympathetic trunks but also include the cervical ganglia that send sympathetic nerve fibers to the head and thorax organs and to the celiac and mesenteric ganglia, that in turn direct sympathetic fibers to the abdominal organs. The neurotransmitter secreted by the preganglionic cells is *acetylcholine* where they synapse with the postganglionic cell. The postganglionic cell soma is found in the ganglion – its nerve fiber distributed to target organs or glands.

*Norepinephrine* is found at the synapses of postganglionic cells where they join with the target site. Depolarization of the cell membrane causes the release of norepinephrine stored within granules. *Epinephrine* is the neurotransmitter secreted by the adrenal medulla directly into the blood where it circulates to reach target organs.

The adrenergic receptors are the major receptor subtypes found within the sympathetic nervous system. A landmark study by Ahlquist[54] in 1948 described two classes of adrenergic receptors – alpha and beta – based on the potency of response to neurotransmitters. When first proposed, this idea was considered radical, because at that time, most scientists thought it was the neurotransmitter itself that determined the response of the end organ, not the receptor that was activated.

There are two alpha receptor subtypes. The neurotransmitters *epinephrine* and *norepinephrine* stimulate both subtypes equally well. The alpha-$_1$ receptor is the more common, and it is found mostly in smooth muscles and some glands. The alpha$_2$ receptor is found at presynaptic terminals of the adrenergic nerves. It functions as an auto-receptor, which when activated decreases the subsequent release of neurotransmitter in a negative feedback loop.

Three subclasses of beta receptors have been identified. Beta$_1$ receptors are located in heart muscle and kidney. When stimulated, they increase heart rate and contractility and cause the release of renin from the kidney. Both epinephrine and norepinephrine are effective in stimulating beta-$_1$ receptors. Beta$_2$ receptors reside in smooth muscle that relaxes upon activation. Beta$_2$ agonists cause bronchodilation in the lungs and vasodilation in skeletal and cardiac muscle. Epinephrine is much more effective in stimulating these receptors than norepinephrine. The final beta$_3$ receptor class is found in fat cells. Activation promotes lipolysis, causing the release of fatty acids. Both epinephrine and norepinephrine work about equally well in activating these receptors.

Norepinephrine can be an agonist that affects both pre- and postsynaptic receptors. It can be removed by uptake into the presynaptic neuron or by uptake into the postsynaptic

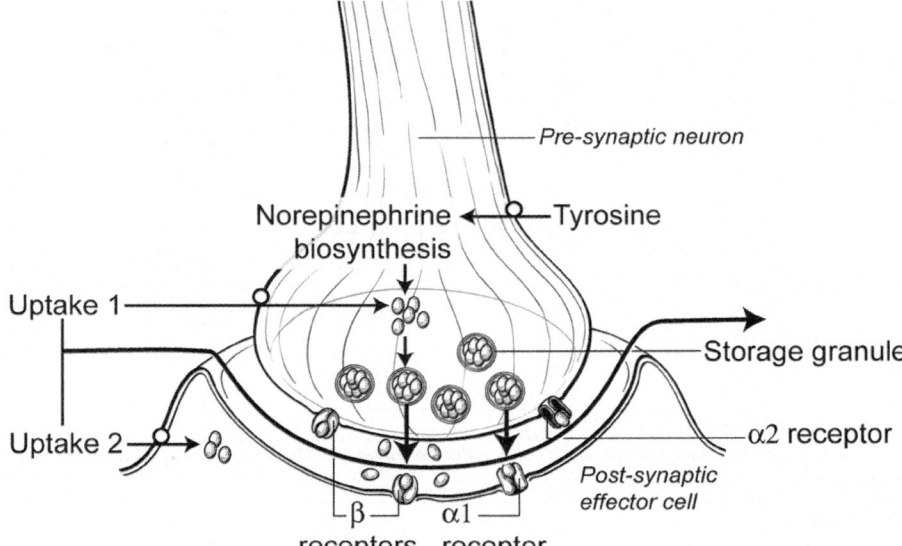

**Fig. 51.4** Stimulation and the activation of neurotransmitter

neuron (see Fig. 51.4). Some norepinephrine simply leaks out of the synapse into the general circulation.[55] Both epinephrine and norepinephrine are deactivated by catechol-O-methyltransferase (COMT), which is found on the postsynaptic cell membrane. They are also inactivated by monoamine oxidase-a (MOA-a),[56] which occurs after "uptake 1" as depicted in Fig. 51.4.

Some adrenergic agonists are said to be direct acting, that is, they bind directly to the receptor and cause a response through their intrinsic activity. Other adrenergic agonists act indirectly by binding to the receptor and causing the release of either epinephrine or norepinephrine. Some indirect agonists work by inhibiting the reuptake of norepinephrine into the synapse. Finally, some drugs work as "mixed-action agonists," that is, they have both direct agonist characteristics, but also cause the release of epinephrine and norepinephrine

Both adrenergic agonists and adrenergic antagonists (blocking agents) may demonstrate nonselectivity by activating several of the beta-receptor subtypes, or they may be relatively selective and have greater activity at a specific subtype. For example, beta-blockers such as timolol eye drops are nonselective, activating both $beta_1$ and $beta_2$ subtypes, while betaxolol eye drops have much greater activity at the $beta_1$, rather than the $beta_2$, subtype of receptor. Alpha-agonists such as apraclonidine eye drops are nonselective activating both $alpha_1$ and $alpha_2$ receptors, while brimonidine eye drops are relatively selective with greater activity for the $alpha_2$ receptor. These differences in relative selectivity result in variation in both drug potency and side effect profiles for these agents. For example, nonselective beta-blockers such as timolol lower intraocular pressure more than $beta_1$ selective agonists such as betaxolol, but betaxolol is less likely to have an adverse effect on the respiratory function than timolol. Similarly, apraclonidine causes more allergic dermatitis and hyperemia than brimonidine, likely due to it being less selective in its receptor class activation. "Original" versions of ophthalmic medications, both for glaucoma and other eye diseases, have often been improved upon in second- and third-generation varieties by making them more selective for the receptors they activate.

Some of the parasympathetic nerve ganglia begin inside the skull (cranial nerves CN III – oculomotor nerve; CN VII – facial nerve; CN IX – glossopharyngeal nerve; and CN X – vagus nerve). Other parasympathetic ganglia originate from the sacral region of the vertebral column (spinal nerves S2 and S4). About 75% of all parasympathetic nerve fibers belong to the vagus nerve.

Similar to the sympathetic nervous system, there are several receptor subtypes within the parasympathetic system (see Fig. 51.5). The parasympathetic nerves release acetylcholine as the neurotransmitter. *Nicotinic receptors* are found at the synapses between pre-and postganglionic neurons. *Muscarinic receptors* are found on all effector cells stimulated by postganglionic parasympathetic fibers. Five different types of muscarinic receptors have been described. All five receptor classes are found within the central nervous system, while receptors M1–M4 are found in various tissues[57]:

- M1 – Secretory glands
- M2 – Heart muscle
- M3 – Smooth muscles and glands. Pilocarpine acts here.
- M1, M3 and M5 receptors activate phospholipase C, generating two secondary messengers (IP3 and DAG), leading to increased intracellular calcium
- M2 and M4 inhibit adenylate cyclase, which decreases the production of the second messenger cAMP.
- M2 receptors in the heart are important for closing calcium channels, reducing heart contractility and rate.

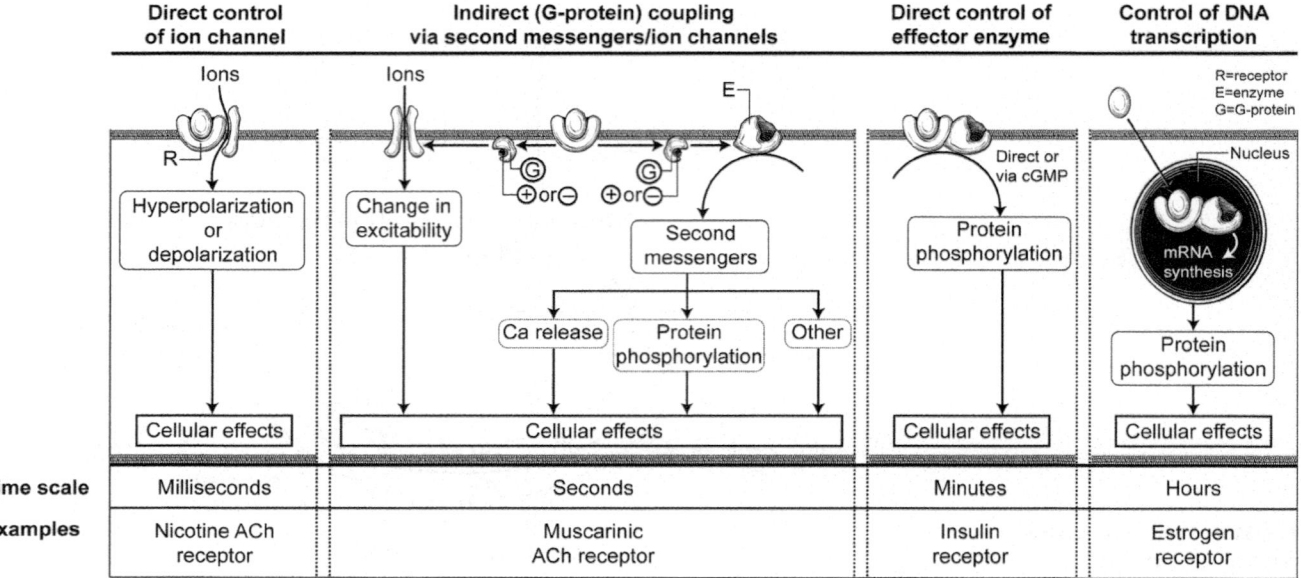

**Fig. 51.5** Parasympathetic receptors-subtypes

## 51.8 Medications for Glaucoma Therapy

*Pharmacodynamics* is the branch of medicinal chemistry that is concerned with how a drug works, its mechanisms of action, and the physiological and medically beneficial effects of the drug. Drugs work by binding to regulatory macromolecules, such as the receptors we have described in the previous section, or in some cases by attaching to and working with enzymes. Recall that drugs that bind to receptors may be agonists or antagonists (or in some cases have mixed action). *Pharmacokinetics*, however, is concerned with the "where" and "when" of drug functionality, the absorption, distribution, metabolism, and excretion of medications.

Glaucoma drugs come in many preparations. Topical medications for glaucoma are available as aqueous solutions, suspensions, ointments, inserts placed within the fornices of the eye, and gels. Punctal plugs may be used in the future to administer glaucoma medications.[58] Systemic medications used to treat glaucoma also have several routes of administration, oral, intravenous, intraocular injections, and periocular injections[59] (e.g., anecortave acetate,[59] still being studied in clinical trials). While the ophthalmologist is most concerned about the activity of the medication contained within the bottle, inactive ingredients in the container help adjust the pH, viscosity, and osmolarity (effective tonicity of dissolved concentrates) of the vehicle to facilitate delivery and stability of the medication. The normal pH of tears is 7.4; if the drug vehicle pH is much different than that then reflex tearing will occur. The addition of methylcellulose and polyvinyl alcohol enhances drug absorption by increasing corneal contact time.

The US Food and Drug Administration requires all multidose containers to have adequate protection from contaminating bacteria and yeasts, and as described earlier, the most common[60] of these in ophthalmic preparations is benzalkonium chloride (BAK).

### 51.8.1 Choosing a Drug for Primary Therapy of Glaucoma

What are the characteristics of an ideal drug for glaucoma therapy? Primarily, both the physician and the patient want a drug that is efficacious in preserving visual acuity and visual field, that is, they want a drug that works! They want drugs that will slow down or halt the progression of glaucoma, both structurally and functionally. Second, glaucoma medications ideally should be extremely "patient friendly," so that patients will be inclined to use them. The former US Surgeon General, C. Everett Koop, purportedly has commented "Drugs don't work in patients who don't take them," a succinct statement of the importance of *medication compliance*.

Tables 51.2 and 51.3 summarize both the efficacy and compliance-related factors desirable in glaucoma medications. Some of these attributes are present in the medications available today; some are on the horizon and some in the more distant future. As we look at the different classes of glaucoma medications and evaluate their pros and cons, keep in mind the various factors listed in these two tables.

Tolerability and safety also are important aspects for choosing and continuing glaucoma medications. While tolerability

**Table 51.2** Efficacy characteristics of an ideal glaucoma drug: "the drug works"

| | Available in current drugs | Future availability |
|---|---|---|
| Maximum IOP lowering as monotherapy | Prostaglandin class lowers IOP about 30%[211] | New classes of receptors and intraocular target sites undergoing research |
| High responder rates to desired target IOP | PGAs and beta-blockers have response rates (as monotherapies) of 50–70% | Genetic profiling may help select high response drugs for individual patients[427] |
| Flat 24 h IOP curves (low IOP fluctuation) and diurnal and nocturnal control of IOP | PGAs have fairly flat 24 h IOP curves; beta-blockers do not work at night[87] | Highest IOPs may be when supine[85,428,429] – drug research in the future will likely require 24 h studies |
| No tachyphylaxis (short-term) or long-term drift | PGAs have good long term track records; some controversy about beta-blocker "drift"[164,168,170,172,430] | New classes of receptors and intraocular target sites undergoing research |
| Increase ocular blood flow – ocular perfusion pressure | Some evidence that topical carbonic anhydrase inhibitors (TCAIs) may increase ocular[93,431-437] blood flow and that PGAs and TCAIs may increase ocular perfusion pressure[92] | This will be a major area of research. Vascular insufficiency has long been thought to be a major factor in glaucoma[438-440] |
| Disease modifying agents (e.g., "fix" the TM or other outflow pathways) | None at the moment | Cytochalasin B,[441,442] Ethacrynic acid[443,444] Rho-kinase inhibitors[445] |
| Neuroprotection by direct action on retinal ganglion cells | Controversy regarding role of topical brimonidine[374,376,377] as neuroprotective; oral memantine trials halted in early 2008 (failed to reach endpoint) | "Neuroprotection" has been the elusive holy grail of glaucoma, much searched for but to date not found. The hunt continues |

**Table 51.3** Compliance characteristics of a desirable glaucoma drug: "patients will adhere to its use"

| | Presently available | Future availability |
|---|---|---|
| Once a day or less frequent dosing intervals | PGAs, beta-blockers – Q Day | Look for better than once a day applications in the future (anecortave acetate?)[59] |
| Multiple medications in one container – better compliance, less total preservative dose | Combination products: Cosopt Combigan | In development PGA/beta-blocker combinations available outside USA |
| Long duration of action in case of missed doses | PGAs[180,199] | Ongoing research |
| No BAK or other detergent-type preservatives | Alphagan –P Travatan Z Timolol Ocudose | Many future glaucoma drugs will have newer, non-detergent, preservatives |
| Easy to hold/use bottle and or dosing aid | Yes – but patients vary in their preferences for containers Travatan Dosing Aid and Pfizer Xal-Ease device for Xalatan[446,447] | Improvements are possible in addressing issues such as pliability |
| No systemic side effects | Timolol – many PGAs – few Alpha-agonist – moderate TCAIs – few | Ongoing research |
| No topical side effects | Timolol – few PGAs – hyperemia, periorbital skin hyperpigmentation, lash growth Alpha-agonist – conjunctivitis, dermatitis – common TCAIs – stinging (dorzolamide), dermatitis | Ongoing research |
| Compliance monitoring readily available | No – efforts have been (e.g., Travatan Dosing Aid) made but no device is in widespread clinical use[446] | Yes – bottle communication with wireless bus at home or concept of a "Universal Medical Bus" for medications to communicate |
| Cost and insurance coverage | Generic drugs are available | More on the way |

is often evident based on patent symptoms (e.g., hyperemia, itching), potential safety issues may be substantially more subtle. Often new and established patients complete medical history questionnaires that also contain a "review of systems." These documents are helpful because they suggest to the treating physician areas of possible systemic side effects with potential glaucoma medications, but they cannot entirely substitute for a thorough interview with the patient by the eye doctor. The danger of increasingly high clinic volumes of patients and shorter patient interviews is that important systemic medical issues will be missed that may result in the patient sustaining side effects. As glaucoma consultants, we have too often seen referred patients who come into our offices on topical beta-blockers, started by their community ophthalmologists who had not inquired about any history of asthma or chronic obstructive pulmonary disease (COPD). While a detailed medical history questionnaire is very helpful, the personal interaction between the patient and the physician results in a better likelihood of uncovering potential medication/medical-history interactions and adverse effects.

### 51.8.1.1 Choice of the Initial Agent

As explained earlier in this chapter, the rationale for treatment of glaucoma is based on the assumption that lowering intraocular pressure *currently* is the most important thing we can do for the patient. At the present time, benefits such as improved blood flow or direct neuroprotection of retinal ganglion cells are secondary considerations when choosing primary monotherapy for patients with ocular hypertension or open angle glaucoma. Pilocarpine was introduced in the late nineteenth century to treat glaucoma. Figure 51.6 shows the timeline of development for glaucoma medications used in the USA.

Medications for the treatment of glaucoma may be divided into six classes (seven classes if we include fixed-combinations of products) as shown in Table 51.4. Table 51.5 depicts the relative potencies of glaucoma agents with respect to lowering intraocular pressure.

A meta-analysis of 28 randomized clinical trials[61] summarizing the relative effectiveness of the more commonly used glaucoma medications for lowering IOP is shown in Table 51.6.

### 51.8.1.2 Beta-Adrenergic Antagonists

As early as 1967 it was found that the nonselective beta-blocker propranolol reduced IOP when administered intravenously.[62] A paper by Katz et al in 1976 demonstrated that topical timolol reduced IOP in normal volunteers.[63] From the

**Table 51.4** Glaucoma drug treatment options

Beta-adrenergic antagonists
Hypotensive lipids
Carbonic anhydrase inhibitors
Topical, oral
Sympathomimetic agonists
Non-selective, selective
Parasympathomimetic agents
Miotics
Fixed combinations
Hyperosmotic agents

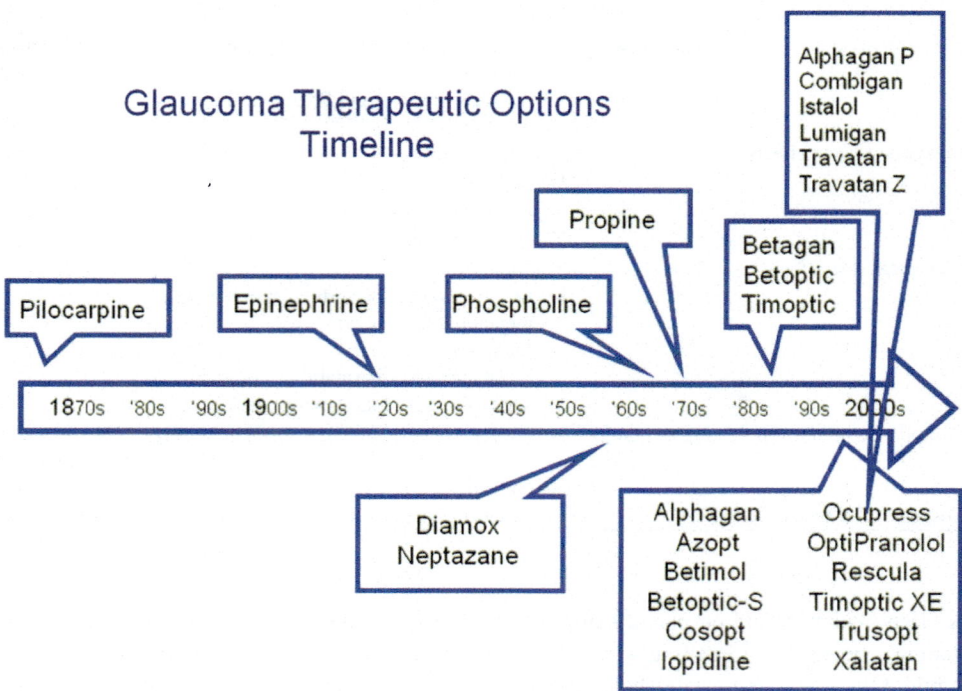

**Fig. 51.6** Glaucoma therapeutic options timeline

**Table 51.5** Maximum IOP lowering as monotherapy

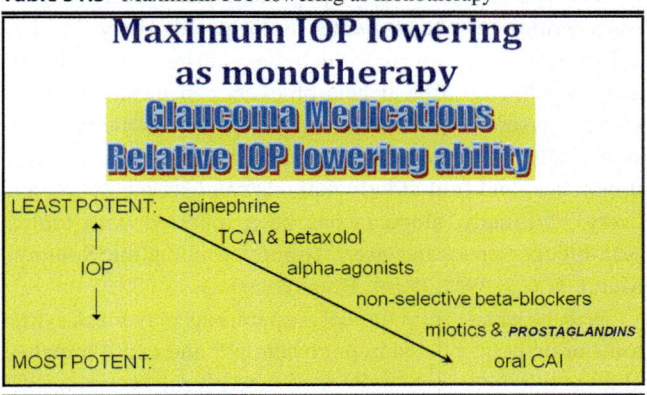

**Table 51.6** Intraocular pressure-lowering effects of glaucoma medications based on a meta-analysis of 28 randomized clinical trials through 2003

| IOP lowering effects of common glaucoma medications | | |
|---|---|---|
| | Peak IOP | Trough IOP |
| Betaxolol | −23% | −20% |
| Timolol | −27% | −26% |
| Dorzolamide | −22% | −17% |
| Brinzolamide | −17% | −17% |
| Brimonidine | −25% | −18% |
| Latanoprost | −31% | −28% |
| Travoprost | −31% | −29% |
| Bimatoprost | −33% | −28% |

late 1970s through the beginning of the twenty-first century, beta-adrenergic antagonists ("beta-blockers") became the mainstay of initial clinical treatment for lowering intraocular pressure in glaucoma patients. Timoptic was introduced by Merck in 1978. This and other nonselective beta-blockers reduce IOP by about 20–25% by suppression of aqueous humor formation. These drops inhibit cyclic adenosine monophosphate (cAMP) in ciliary epithelium. Carteolol has "intrinsic sympathomimetic activity" (ISA) and subsequently may have less effect on lipid profiles than other nonselected beta-blockers.[64-66] Only the generic version of carteolol is sold in the USA. There have been reports of anterior uveitis in patients using metipranolol, persisting even after its reformulation.[67-74] This drug has fallen out of favor in the United States.

Beta-blockers are available in solutions, gel forming solutions, and suspensions. In the United States, the following brands are available:

*Generic/brand names*
- *Nonselective* ($B_1$–$B_2$ blockade) – timolol maleate (Timoptic, Timoptic XE, Timoptic Ocudose, Timolol GFS, Istalol); timolol hemihydrate (Betimol), levobunolol (Betagan); metipranolol (Optipranolol 0.3%), carteolol HCl (Ocupress 1%)
- *Selective* (B1 ≫ B2 blockade) – Betoptic-S.25%

All are available in both 0.25 and 0.50% concentrations except as noted. Most of the pressure reduction activity of these drugs is mediated through their action on the beta-$_2$ receptors. Nonselective beta-blockers lower IOP on average 20–25%. Although most ophthalmologists prescribe the 0.50% concentration of the nonselective beta-blockers, adequate aqueous concentrations are achieved with lesser amounts of drug, and the 0.25% commercial preparations are close to the peak of the dose response curve.[75] These high aqueous concentrations of drug, even with the 0.25% dose, explain why betaxolol, which is highly selective for the beta-1 receptor, reaches a sufficient concentration to lower intraocular pressure, which is mediated through the beta-2 receptor.[76-79] Betaxolol lowers IOP 15–20%, but it does not lower pressure as much as the nonselective beta-blockers (20–25%).[80-83]

All of the listed medications use benzalkonium chloride as the preservative, except Timoptic-XE and Timolol GFS, which use benzododecinium bromide 0.012% (also a quaternary ammonium compound) and Timolol Ocudose, which is supplied in preservative-free unit-dose 0.2 ml containers. Approved dosing per the package inserts is every 12 h, except for once per day dosing (usually in the morning) for Timoptic XE and Timolol GFS, and for Istalol, which contains sorbic acid and is more lipophilic. The greatest activity of the medications occurs between 2 and 4 h after instillation.[84] Beta-blockers take about 4 weeks to fully leave the body.

Beta-blockers have little activity during the evening and night-time hours, when aqueous production by the ciliary body is reduced because of natural circadian factors.[38,85,86] Circulating catecholamine concentration (especially epinephrine) is lowest at night, resulting in a deceased sympathetic tone that appears necessary for the production of aqueous. It has been hypothesized that if there is a low sympathetic tone, little aqueous is being produced above a basal level, and thus there is little for the beta-antagonist drugs to "block."[87] Thus, beta-blockers do not provide effective 24-h control of intraocular pressure.[85] Therefore, drugs that affect aqueous *outflow* (e.g., hypotensive lipids), rather than aqueous *production*, may be more effective agents at reducing *nocturnal* intraocular pressure.

While many beta-blockers in solution form are approved for twice a day dosing, most of the benefit of this class of medication can be achieved by a single morning dose.[88-90] Because beta-blockers do not appear to work as well at night, the evening dose is superfluous and increases the risk of side effects. Also, there is some concern that nocturnal effects of beta-blockers may lower ocular perfusion pressure.[91-105] This would be especially worrisome in patients with normal tension glaucoma. There is some evidence that betaxolol may increase retinal and choroidal blood flow by acting on voltage-dependent calcium channels.[102,106-115] It may thus have some neuroprotective effect separate from its IOP lowering properties.[116,117] Levobunolol has an active metabolite (dihydrobunolol) that may contribute to its longer duration of activity when compared with timolol.[118,119]

Topical beta-blockers have few ocular side effects.[120,121] Istalol and Betimol sting more than other products Timoptic-XE and timolol gel forming solution (timolol – GFS) may blur vision upon installation. Betoptic-S comes as a suspension that helps minimize stinging.[122] All topical beta-blockers cause some corneal anesthesia and punctuate staining.[123] Although their ocular side effects may just be a nuisance, their systemic side effects may be dramatic and even life-threatening in some instances. As described earlier in this chapter, there are two major forms of beta agonist activity: $beta_1$, which largely affects cardiac muscle, and $beta_2$, which largely affects pulmonary function. Well-known systemic side effects of beta-blockers limit their use in glaucoma patients who suffer from respiratory ailments. Betaxolol is a relatively selective $beta_1$ antagonist and is thought to be safer than the nonselective beta-blockers for use in patients with pulmonary conditions. However, no beta-blocker is safe enough to use in patients with severe reactive airway disease. Fortunately, for these patients, we have a number of good alternative preparations for both primary and adjunctive glaucoma therapies.

Recently, congestive heart failure (CHF) has become only a relative contraindication to the use of oral beta-blockers systemically[124-128] and similarly for the use of beta-blocker eye drops. Nonetheless, it is prudent to check with the patient's family physician or cardiologist before instituting such therapy in patients with known CHF. Steps taken to limit the systemic side effects of beta-blockers include reduced concentrations (0.25% compared to 0.5%) and $beta_1$-selective preparations (e.g., betaxolol), along with nasolacrimal duct occlusion. Topical beta-blockers used to treat glaucoma are less effective at lowering IOP in patients already taking oral beta-blockers.[129,130] This "double dosing" by topical and oral routes significantly increases the risk of systemic side effects. In most cases, patients using oral beta-blockers should not receive topical beta-blockers as their initial glaucoma therapy.

Because of these scientific issues and medical-legal concerns, when prescribing beta-blocker eye drops, physicians must be acutely aware of their potential interaction with the patient's general medical problems. Before initiating therapy with a topical beta-blocker, the patient's pulse rate and systemic blood pressure should be checked and recorded in the medical record. This should be repeated at subsequent office visits. Ask about a history of heart block, CHF, bradycardia, and any incidences of fainting.[131] Patients also should be asked about smoking, asthma, and COPD.[131] Patients using topical beta-blockers may exhibit decreased exercise tolerance, less so with $beta_1$-selective agents.[132-137] As with oral beta-blockers, lipid profiles may be affected unfavorably with decreased high density lipoprotein (HDL) and increased triglycerides.[138] The patient's lipid profile may be less affected with Ocupress, which has intrinsic sympathetic activity (ISA).[64] Topical beta-blockers can produce central nervous system effects including depression, anxiety, confusion, hallucinations, drowsiness, weakness, memory loss, impotence, and frail elderly patients can become "weak and dizzy."[139] Finally, alopecia has been reported with topical beta-blockers (package insert, Timoptic Ophthalmic Solution, Merck & Co., West Point, Pennsylvania.)

Beta-blockade from topical preparations may mask symptoms of diabetic-related hypoglycemia[140] and cause impaired glucose tolerance (inhibit lipolysis and glycogenolysis).[141-149] Beta-blockade can mask symptoms of thyrotoxicosis and abrupt cessation may cause it.[150-154]

Patients with dark irises, including African–Americans, may have less intraocular lowering pressure effect from beta-blockers because of binding of the medication to melanin.[155-158] (This is also true for pilocarpine[159] and adrenergic agonists[160] used to treat glaucoma.)

Topical beta-blockers applied unilaterally may exhibit some "cross-over" of IOP lowering in the contralateral eye.[84,161-163] This makes a "one-eyed" trial of a beta-blocker somewhat difficult to evaluate.

These agents generally do not exhibit tachyphylaxis or short-term "escape," although one early report[164] suggests tachyphylaxis does occur. There is more controversy, however, about long-term drift of IOP with topical beta-blockers.[165-171] A recent well-designed study suggests that long-term drift of beta-blockers is an urban myth among ophthalmologists.[172]

### 51.8.1.3 Hypotensive Lipids

Hypotensive lipids (HLs) for treating OAG fall into three sub-categories. The prostaglandin analogues (PGAs) include latanoprost (Xalatan 0.005%) and travoprost (Travatan and Travatan Z, both 0.004%); there is one prostamide – bimatoprost (Lumigan 0.03%); and the deconsanoid class is represented by unoprostone isopropyl (Rescula 0.15%). They are all derivatives of prostaglandin $F_{2\alpha}$, based on pioneering work by Bito, Stjernschantz, and Camras.[173-176] This class of glaucoma medications increase both trabecular meshwork and uveoscleral outflow,[177-179] and are less affected by circadian variations in aqueous production than the beta-blockers.[180,181] Although these drugs have this dual mechanism of action, most of the increased outflow facility can be attributed to their effects on the pressure-independent uveo-scleral outflow pathway.[179]

Only bimatoprost and latanoprost are currently (as of December 2008) approved as first-line agents by the FDA in the USA. However, in clinical practice, travoprost and travoprost without BAK (Travatan Z) free are also used as first-line agents by the great majority of practicing ophthalmologists and optometric physicians. Unoprostone isopropyl is very infrequently used as either first-line or adjunctive therapy in the United States, although it is popular in Japan where it was developed. It requires twice per day dosing (the other hypotensive lipids are dosed once per day) and lowers IOP to a much lesser extent than the other products of this class. Unless noted otherwise, the phrase "hypotensive lipids" (HLs) subsequently used in this chapter shall refer only to bimatoprost, latanoprost, and travoprost (with or without BAK).

The hypotensive lipids have become accepted by ophthalmologists as first-line therapy in the USA, Europe, and South America for most forms of open angle glaucoma. Cost considerations and later introductions have limited their use in Asia and Africa, where beta-blockers and miotics are still popular.

Early drugs developed to control glaucoma either decreased aqueous production (beta-blockers) or increased conventional, trabecular-meshwork-mediated outflow (miotics). The major innovation of the HL medications is their ability to increase uveoscleral outflow (with a small to moderate affect on TM function as well). The prototype molecule, prostaglandin $F_{2\alpha}$ does itself lower IOP, but it was found to produce too much inflammation and ocular symptoms intolerable to patients and was thus never developed into a commercial product.[174] Molecular engineering has led to derivatives of this parent compound with acceptable efficacy and safety profiles.

Most scientists agree that the mechanism of action for increased uveoscleral outflow involves activation of the FP class of prostaglandin receptors found at the iris root and ciliary body. Stimulation of these receptors results in the up-regulation of matrix metalloproteinases (which are similar to collagenases) that in turn result in a remodeling of extracellular matrix and widening of intermuscular spaces in the ciliary body. Aqueous may then more easily exit the eye around the cellular structures.[182-185] A study in FP-receptor-deficient mice, with presumed functional uveoscleral outflow pathways, showed no affect of any of the four hypotensive lipids on reduction of intraocular pressure.[186]

How do the commercial preparations differ? As described earlier in this chapter, all of the HLs function as prodrugs. Latanoprost, travoprost, and unoprostone are esterified derivatives of prostaglandin $F_{2\alpha}$, while bimatoprost contains an amide group in the same position as the isopropyl ester of the other molecules. The chemical structures of the compounds are shown in Fig. 51.7.

The ester or amide portions of the molecules are cleaved by abundant corneal enzymes, with the free acid forms of the lipids entering into the anterior chamber in sufficient concentration to activate the FP prostaglandin receptors of the ciliary body that is bathed in aqueous. The ester moiety is easily cleaved, allowing the drugs to be manufactured at relatively low concentrations (latanoprost 0.005%, travoprost 0.004%; unoprostone has a higher concentration 0.15% but is a relatively ineffective drug – we will not consider it in subsequent discussion). The amide group on the bimatoprost molecule is not as easily separated from the free acid.[187] The clinical product used to treat glaucoma has a concentration (0.03%) six to eight times greater than the other HLs.

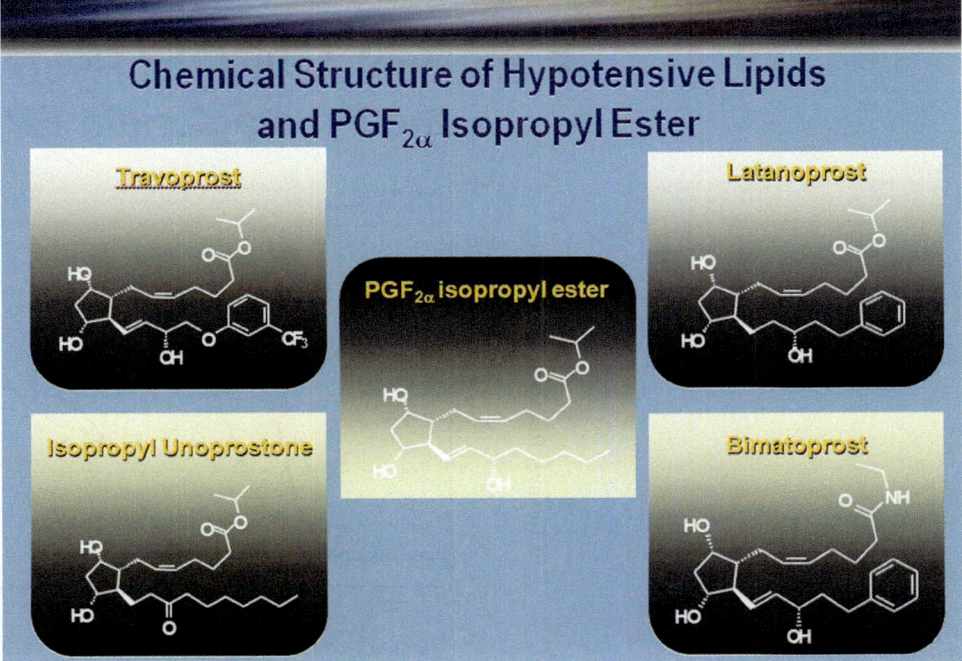

**Fig. 51.7** Structure of the hypotensive lipids. Courtesy of Alcon Labs, Fort Worth, Texas

This increased concentration allows sufficient free acid to enter the eye to effectively activate the FP receptors.[188] Thus, it would appear that bimatoprost lowers IOP by uveoscleral outflow in the same manner as the other HLs.[50,189] However, the manufacturer (Allergan, Irvine, California) has sponsored research suggesting that the entire bimatoprost molecule acts primarily by passing through intact sclera to activate "prostamide" receptors on the ciliary body with subsequent increase in uveoscleral outflow facility.[190] There is one study using a preparation of feline iris sphincter that demonstrates binding of the full bimatoprost molecule to receptors that appear to be distinct from prostaglandin FP receptors.[191] (And recall the murine study described above that showed no reduction in IOP when bimatoprost was applied to the eyes of FP receptor deficient mice.[186]) No published studies have found these receptors in the ciliary body nor has a prostamide receptor been "cloned" using standard biological techniques. Bimatoprost has been used clinically since 2001. While prostamide receptors may exist, clinically bimatoprost seems to function as a prostaglandin analogue, with both increased activity of the conventional and nonconventional outflow pathways. The authors look forward to a research that may demonstrate the presence of the receptors in the relevant tissues and their binding and activation by the nonhydrolyzed version of bimatoprost. From a clinical perspective, in our practices, we consider the three major HLs as belonging to the same class of medication.

Variations in the $PGF_{2\alpha}$ molecule result in changes in potency and side effects. Latanoprost was the first HL to be developed commercially (by Pharmacia, now Pfizer). It became available in the USA in 1996. In order to reduce the hyperemia associated with $PGF_{2\alpha}$, the unsaturated (double) bond between carbons 13 and 14 was saturated. This resulted in some loss of potency, but by reducing hyperemia made the drug acceptable to real world patients. Because there is no major clinical difference in IOP-lowering efficacy whether this class of drugs is dosed daytime or nighttime, it has become customary to prescribe the HLs at bedtime, so that the majority of the immediate hyperemia associated with drug dosing occurs while the patient is asleep. These drugs do have some "chronic" hyperemia that tends to subside over several months of use. Occasionally patients prefer morning dosing, which is acceptable from an efficacy perspective. Clinical IOP-lowering efficacy of the HLs is better with QD dosing (at the commercially available concentrations) rather than BID dosing.[192-194] Systemic half-life of the drugs are brief (e.g., latanoprost 17 min). The peak plasma concentration of latanoprost is about $10^{-10}$ M or less, and there is little if any effect of the drugs on the IOP of the contralateral eye when dosed unilaterally.[195]

Both bimatoprost and travoprost came to the US market in March 2001. To improve efficacy, Alcon Laboratories modified the $PGF_{2\alpha}$ molecule to create travoprost by adding a CF3 on the unsaturated benzene ring. This allows for a tighter bonding of the travoprost free acid to the FP receptors.[196,197] This results in a longer duration, clinically useful, IOP-lowering effect of both original travoprost and the BAK-free version.[180,198,199] This could be important in patients who occasionally miss doses. The functional activities of the HLs are shown in Fig. 51.8 using an in vitro technique employing phosphoinositide (PI) turnover and intracellular

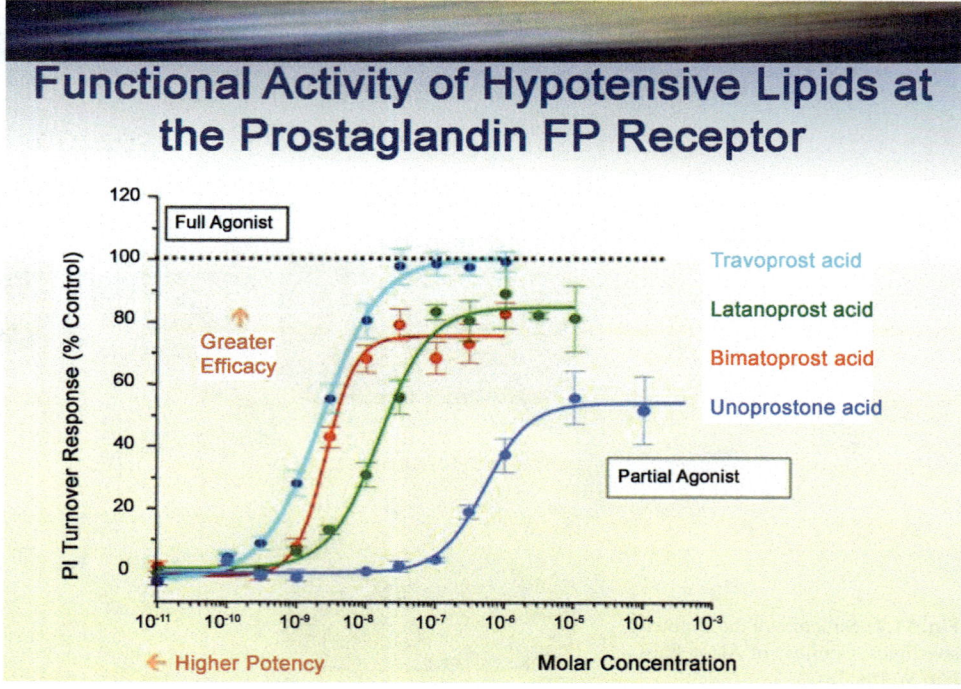

**Fig. 51.8** Functional activity of hypotensive lipids at PG FP receptor. Courtesy of Alcon Labs, Fort Worth, Texas

Ca² mobilization on cultured human trabecular meshwork cells of nonglaucomatous donor eyes.

Alcon kept the double bond between carbons 13 and 14, increasing efficacy but resulting in more hyperemia for travoprost than found in the commercial latanoprost preparation (the newer travoprost without BAK has slightly less hyperemia than the original product, but both versions produce more clinical hyperemia than latanoprost).[47,200] Most of the hyperemia associated with the HLs results from dilated conjunctival vessels in response to direct activation of FP receptors found in the vasculature muscle walls.[201] This is not a toxic or allergic response, but is, however, of cosmetic concern to the patient. Allergan, when designing bimatoprost, also kept the unsaturated double bond between carbons 13 and 14 and added the amide group, where the other products have the isopropyl ester. As discussed earlier, bimatoprost has a six- to eightfold greater concentration than the other HLs. This may be related to the clinical observation that bimatoprost causes more red eye than the other two products.[200,202,203] A newer version of bimatoprost is planned with decreased drug concentration and increased BAK resulting in less hyperemia (Latanoprost causes the least conjunctival hyperemia, a bit more with travoprost.)[204]

Additionally, the HLs activate more than just the FP class of prostaglandin receptors. The EP class of prostaglandin receptors mediates inflammatory byproducts. Funk in a recent (2001) review[205] of eicosanoid biology said, "Prostaglandins act both at peripheral sensory neurons and at central sites…to evoke hyperalgesia. Recent data support involvement of…EP$_1$ receptors in pain."[206-208] Table 51.7 shows the relative binding affinities for the HLs at both FP and EP$_1$ receptors. It is desirable for glaucoma drugs to have high binding affinities for the FP receptors (to lower IOP) and low binding affinities to the EP$_1$ receptors (to minimize inflammation). Here, we see that bimatoprost is a better agonist at the EP$_1$ receptor than the three other products. Thus, the increased hyperemia seen with bimatoprost may result both from its affinity for EP$_1$ receptors (inflammatory hyperemia) as well as its relatively higher concentration (vasodilatory hyperemia in response to FP receptor activation). From a clinical perspective, most patients find that the hyperemia of all the HLs decreases sufficiently over a month or two to become cosmetically acceptable.[209,210] We have found that prospectively discussing conjunctival hyperemia with patients before initiating HL therapy greatly decreases their emergent phone calls and "drop-in" office visits.

While conjunctival hyperemia is clinically apparent to the patients, their companions, and the treating physician, other aspects of ocular surface disorders may be less obvious but even more important to chronic disease management. As noted earlier in this chapter, the BAK found in most glaucoma medications may play an important role in causing the signs and symptoms of ocular surface disease and subclinical inflammation (see Sidebar 51.3). The newer formulation of travoprost without BAK, with the preservative sofZia, seems equally effective as the original product but with improved ocular surface health.[11,47] New glaucoma products without BAK are under development by the pharmaceutical industry.

The three hypotensive lipids lower intraocular pressure on average between 25 and 30%. This is greater than the nonselective beta-blockers, which lower IOP between 20 and 25%. The only randomized controlled clinical trial directly comparing the three agents found them to be on average about the same in IOP-lowering efficacy (with a slight, 0.5 mmHg, advantage to bimatoprost) and confirmed the clinical impression that latanoprost had the lowest rate of conjunctival hyperemia.[211] The previously mentioned meta-analysis by van der Valk of 28 clinical studies also shows the HLs to be roughly equivalent in their ability to lower intraocular pressure.[61] A more recent meta-analysis of nine studies that had to compare at least two prostaglandin analogues as monotherapy, found that travoprost and bimatoprost lowered IOP −0.98 mmHg (95% CI: −2.08; 0.13; $p=0.08$) and −1.04 mmHg (95% CI: −2.11; 0.04; $p=0.06$) respectively, when compared with latanoprost.[212]

The HLs have relatively flat IOP curves over 24 h, demonstrating both low circadian IOP fluctuation and, unlike the beta-blockers, effective diurnal and nocturnal IOP control.[85,180,181,199,203] They do not evidence short-term escape or long-term drift.[213-215]

HLs have few systemic side-effects. HLs should generally be avoided in women of child bearing age without adequate birth control or who are pregnant, because although plasma concentrations of topical HLs are low, there is a theoretical risk of abortion due to the action of prostaglandin molecules on uterine smooth muscle.[216-218] There are no references in the ophthalmic literature that this has ever happened

**Table 51.7** Binding affinity of hypotensive lipids at prostaglandin receptors. Used with permission of Alcon Labs, Fort Worth, Texas

### Binding Affinity of Hypotensive Lipids Prostaglandin Receptors

| Compound | Receptor Binding Affinity (Ki, nM) | |
|---|---|---|
| | FP | EP$_1$ |
| Travoprost (acid) | 52 ± 2 | 9,540 |
| Bimatoprost (acid) | 83 ± 2 | 95 |
| Latanoprost (acid) | 92 ± 14 | 2000 |
| PGF$_{2\alpha}$ | 129 ± 12 | 600 |
| Unoprostone (acid) | 5,649 ± 893 | 12,000 |

Note: Lower number implies higher affinity

Adapted from MR Hellberg, et al. 2001, J. Ocular Pharmacol. Therapeu. 17(5)421-432 and NA Sharif et al., 2001, Eur. J. Pharmacol. 432, 211-213 (see Chap. 58 for discussion of glaucoma therapy during pregnancy.) There are some reports of muscle aches, gastrointestinal upset and influenza-like symptoms with the use of topical HLs to treat glaucoma.[219,220]

There have been case reports of reactivation of clinically dormant herpes simplex virus (HSV) keratitis by patients who begin HLs, confirmed in some cases upon rechallenging the eyes involved. We generally avoid using HLs in patients with a history of HSV keratitis.[221-227]

The use of HLs has been associated with cystoid macular edema (CME) especially in patients who have undergone cataract surgery and intraocular lens implantation, more often if the posterior capsule is ruptured[228-230] (some researchers feel that post-cataract CME may be related to eye drop preservatives.[231]) Sometimes, this CME is clinically apparent with complaints of reduced visual acuity and contrast sensitivity, sometimes, this CME is picked up by fluorescein angiography or optical coherence tomography. In our experience, this HL-related CME almost always improves by withdrawal of the agent and treatment with topical steroids and nonsteroidal anti-inflammatory drugs (NSAIDs). In our practices, we generally try to discontinue HLs several weeks before cataract surgery and try to avoid reinstituting them for about 3 months after surgery. Fortunately, many open angle glaucoma patients undergoing phacoemulsification cataract surgery have a "honeymoon" period of reduced intraocular pressure lasting several months or more and may require less glaucoma medical therapy during that time.[232-234] Thus, they suffer no harm by temporarily suspending the HL postoperatively. If the posterior capsule is broken, we may avoid the further use of HLs at all. To attempt to prevent CME, many anterior segment surgeons pretreat all patients about to undergo cataract surgery with topical steroids and NSAIDs, especially if they have been using hypotensive lipids.[235] Some cataract surgeons continue to use previously prescribed HLs throughout the perioperative period.[236] The authors do not advise doing so unless IOP control is lost without the use of HLs in the immediate postoperative time frame.

There have been a several studies reporting an association of HLs with the development of anterior uveitis or the worsening of preexisting uveitis.[237-245] Because prostaglandins are proinflammatory compounds, most glaucoma experts do not recommend their use in patients with uveitis, uveitic glaucoma, or neovascular glaucoma. There appears to be little role for HLs in managing an attack of acute angle closure glaucoma, but these agents do appear useful for various forms of chronic angle closure glaucoma.[246,247] Finally, the three hypotensive lipids are not additive in their effects, that is, using (for example) bimatoprost in the AM and latanoprost in the PM will result in slightly worse lowering of IOP than using either drug alone.[248]

There are several ocular-related side effects of HLs that may be described as cosmetic. Hyperemia, discussed previously, may be intolerable to some patients. Proactive discussion of this issue may improve patient adherence with HLs. A small to moderate percentage of patients (<20%) using the HLs develop permanent, clinically noticeable changes in iris color, with increasing plumpness of melanocytes (stimulation of melanogenesis) perhaps through an effect on tyrosinase, but no increase in their number. This change in iris color reflects no mutagenesis, but is of cosmetic concern to some patients[249] (not unreasonably, many elderly glaucoma patients are unconcerned about eye color changes if the medications will help save their sight.) Purely blue eyes are rarely affected and fully darker brown eyes show no visibly detectable changes. It is the hazel and green eyes that may become noticeably browner. These color changes may occur with greater frequency than generally supposed, as Teus et al have shown in a 2002 study comparing patients who received latanoprost in only one eye.[250]

These color changes are more frequent with latanoprost than bimatoprost or travoprost (per the package inserts). Again, proactive conversation with the patient about this possibility before starting a hypotensive lipid will avoid unhappiness and potential medico-legal complications. Because of concerns about iris heterochromia (and possible lash growth described below) we almost never prescribe the use of HLs when glaucoma medication is needed only in one eye.[250] Figure 51.9 depicts a patient whose irides are different colors after using bimatoprost in only one eye.

Both hypertrichosis and periorbital skin hyperpigmentation are common side effects for patients who use the topical HLs.[251-261] The lashes may become thicker, longer, and increase in quantity (Fig. 51.10). They may become darker although poliosis has been reported.[262] Many women find the lash effects desirable,[263] and Allergan now has a commercial product (Latisse) for lash enhancement using bimatoprost 0.03% as the active ingredient. For those patients who are bothered by the changed lashes, there is good news. Lashes

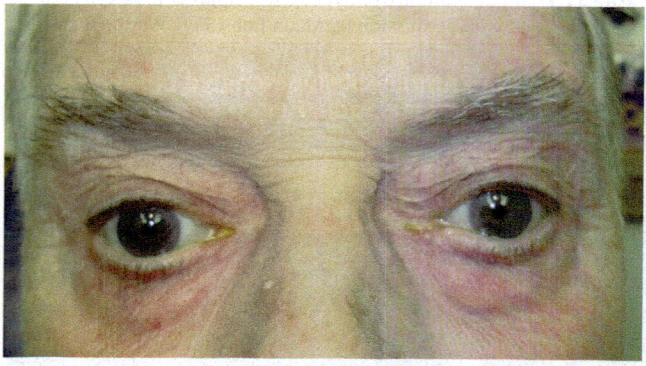

**Fig. 51.9** Only the right eye was treated with bimatoprost. The patient had similar hazel irides before treatment. The iris of the right eye is now much darker than the left one. Courtesy of Drs. Tarek Shazly and Mark Latina

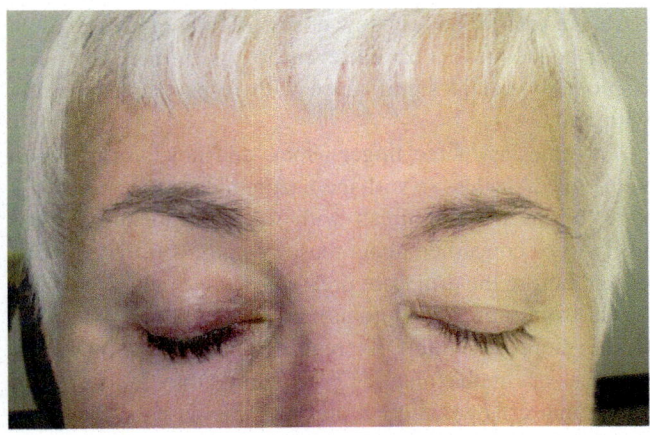

**Fig. 51.10** Lash changes with bimatoprost. Only the right eye was treated. Courtesy of Drs. Tarek Shazly and Mark Latina

naturally fall out and are replaced about every 12 weeks, so once the medication is stopped, the situation reverses itself.[264] (Recall that induced iris color changes are not reversible.) There is a report of hyperpigmentation and hypertrichosis of the vellus hair on the malar region after unilateral treatment with bimatoprost in a Hispanic patient. These phenomena reversed 2 months after the discontinuation of bimatoprost.[265] Hyperpigmentation of the lids and periorbital skin is more common in people with darker skin (Asian, Hispanics, and African-Americans) than very pale skin. The skin pigmentation changes appear to only affect the epidermis, which similar to eye lashes, is periodically renewed.[258] Most patients find that undesirable skin pigmentation reverses with cessation of the drug. In our clinical experience, bimatoprost is more likely to affect the lashes and periorbital skin than the other two HLs. Some patients find that using petroleum jelly to coat the lash margins and skin below the lower lids, just before taking their HL eye drops, helps reduce these side effects.

### 51.8.1.4 Carbonic Anhydrase Inhibitors

The zinc-enzymes classified as carbonic anhydrases (CAs) are widespread through the bacteria and plant and animal kingdoms. There are at least 14 known varieties of the alpha-CAs ($\alpha$-CA) whose main function is the hydration of $CO_2$ to bicarbonate ($HCO^-$). Two of these enzymes are important for the production of aqueous humor by the epithelium of the ciliary processes, cytoplasmic CA II and membrane-bound CA IV.[266,267] Part of aqueous production involving active secretion relies on the formation of bicarbonate by these enzymes to correct the imbalance caused by the ATPase-fueled transport of sodium into the space between the non-pigmented ciliary epithelial cells. More than 99% of the activity of these enzymes must be inhibited to successfully decrease aqueous production.[268]

In 1954, Becker demonstrated that acetazolamide, a sulfonamide-based carbonic anhydrase inhibitor (CAI), could lower intraocular pressure in human subjects.[269] The IOP-lowering affect of CAIs may be enhanced by the metabolic acidosis they can cause.[270] Acetazolamide is more likely to cause clinically relevant systemic acidosis than methazolamide at therapeutic doses.[271] This may be one of the reasons that acetazolamide at full doses lowers IOP better than full doses of methazolamide. CA isoenzymes are present in many tissues in addition to ciliary processes, including corneal endothelium, iris, retinal pigment epithelium, red blood cells, brain, and kidney. Oral CAIs, while extremely effective in lowering IOP, may have profound medicinal and side effects on the body.[268] For this reason, chronic use of oral CAIs is generally reserved as therapy of last resort for patients who have tried topical medications (and perhaps laser treatments) without adequate control, and who for one reason or another are not good candidates for glaucoma surgical intervention. Oral CAIs are also used on a temporary basis for emergent situations with acute rise of IOP. Examples of these situations include early postretinal and early postcataract surgeries and acute angle closure glaucoma until laser therapy becomes available.[272,273]

Before initiating treatment with oral or topical CAIs, the physician must inquire about sulfonamide allergies. Many patients have been treated with sulfonamide-based antibiotics for bladder infections and may consider any gastrointestinal insult caused by these antibiotics as allergic symptoms. Patients should be specifically asked about breathing difficulties and skin reactions,[274,275] which are the most common form of allergic manifestations to sulfonamide antibiotics. Stevens–Johnson syndrome (erythema multiforme major) has been reported with the oral CAIs.[276] This may be more common in Japanese and Korean patients.[277,278] Fortunately, there are significant structural differences between sulfonamide antibiotics and the CAIs used to treat glaucoma, but prudence suggests avoiding *oral* CAIs in any patients with true allergies to any sulfonamide medication.[279] On occasion we have cautiously used *topical* CAIs with patients who have an ambiguous history of sulfonamide allergy symptoms. We explain the possible risks, have them use the drops while in the office, keep them around for several hours, and tell them that in the rare event of an allergic reaction we will call for emergency medical services. In our practices, we have never had a patient who has had an acute event under these circumstances.

Oral CAIs are powerful agents for lowering IOP (between 25 and 30%)[280] and may do so very well when other medical therapies are unable to reach the target IOP in chronic glaucomas, or to temporarily bring IOP to safe levels in acute emergent situations. But their systemic side effects are legion and often serious, in addition to the allergic respiratory and skin problems discussed previously. The limited data available suggest that the topical CAIs (TCAIs), while theoretically capable of causing all the same systemic mischief as the oral agents, have mostly ocular and periorbital side effects.

The two common oral CAIs are acetazolamide (Diamox) and methazolamide (Neptazane). Dichlorphenamide (Daranide) is also available, but not popular. Diamox is available as "regular" tablets (62.5, 125, and 250 mg) and in timed-release, 500 mg "Sequels." Diamox regular is generally prescribed QID as 250-mg tablets for chronic use or better as Diamox Sequels 500 mg Q 12 h. The Sequels produce less GI symptoms and less fluctuation in IOP over 24 h, but are considerably more expensive than the standard tablets that are also generically available. Neptazane tablets are prescribed Q 12 h or TID in either 25 or 50-mg dosages. They do come in generic varieties as well.

In a situation that requires acute lowering of IOP, we often prescribe one regular 250 mg Diamox tablet, with relatively quicker onset of action, and at the same time, we have the patient take a Diamox Sequel for its sustained effect. Patients who may have nausea or vomiting from acutely high IOP, as in angle closure situations, may not tolerate the oral preparations. Acetazolamide is excreted unchanged by the renal system. Methazolamide undergoes first-pass metabolism by the liver. CAs in the kidney promote the absorption of bicarbonate through the renal tubules. CAIs cause alkalinization of the urine along with increased micturition, both day and night, and potassium excretion. Patients prescribed chronic oral CAIs should have their electrolytes monitored, perhaps with the assistance of their family physician, especially if taking other potassium-wasting drugs such as thiazide diuretics and oral corticosteroids.[281,282] This is especially important in patients taking cardiac glycosides, such as digitalis, because hypokalemia can be lethal in the presence of digitalis. Systemic side effects are generally dose-related *except* for the blood dyscrasias, which will be discussed later.[283] Kidney stone occurrence may be up 50 times greater in patients taking oral CAIs than prevalent in the general population.[284] Systemic CAIs cause the kidney to secrete less magnesium and citrate and an alkaline urine. This contributes to the formation of calcium phosphate and oxalate based stones.

Methazolamide at lower doses is less likely to cause urolithiasis because of less acidosis and no change in concentrations of urinary citrate.[271,285,286] If it is necessary to prescribe oral CAIs, methazolamide is preferred to acetazolamide in patients with a history of kidney stones.

Salicylates interact with oral CAIs. Patients taking high-dose aspirin can get tinnitus, increased respiratory rate, and even confusion and coma.[287-290] They should be warned of these symptoms and told to avoid high doses of aspirin if oral CAIs are prescribed. The low dose of 81 mg of aspirin often prescribed to prevent cardiac events by its antiplatelet effects is probably not of significance with respect to interacting with oral CAIs.

Paresthesias of the fingers, toes, and nose are common with oral CAIs, less so with methazolamide at lower doses.[291] Paresthesias may diminish with time.[271] Patients are less likely to be concerned about these symptoms if they are discussed before the drugs are prescribed.

Gastrointestinal symptoms are also common with oral CAIs, more so with QID regular Diamox than Diamox Sequels or methazolamide.[292] Patients may suffer from abdominal cramps, nausea, and in some cases severe diarrhea.[293] Symptoms may improve as time passes, but some patients must discontinue oral CAIs because of these difficulties. The oral CAIs cause a strange metallic taste with foods and carbonated beverages – patients should be warned this is likely to occur.[294] We have had more than one patient return a case of "bad" beer to the store after initiating acetazolamide therapy.[295] (We apologized to them for our lapse in not discussing this side effect of hypogeusia!) Also note that topical CAIs, when drained onto the tongue via the nasolacrimal duct, may produce "funny" taste sensations for a short time after contact. Lower doses of oral CAIs disrupt taste sensations to a lesser degree than do higher doses.

Patients taking oral CAIs, usually after several months, can have an unexpected onset of a malaise-syndrome complex involving – to varying degrees – tiredness, lack of appetite (that may be accompanied by weight loss), and even severe depression.[293] Generalized apathy may ensue. Patients with mild dementia may seem to get worse. Often, neither the patient nor family members attribute the slow onset of this malaise-syndrome to oral CAIs that may have been started several months earlier. The symptoms resolve, slowly, with reduced drug dosage or more often with discontinuation of the offending drug. Similarly, decreased libido and even impotency can result from oral CAIs, again often not attributed to the drugs.[296,297] Patients and physicians must be aware of these possibilities.

Blood dyscrasias from oral CAIs (none has been reported in the literature from topical CAIs as of mid-2009) are extremely serious events. They fall into two categories: one that is sudden and is irreversible, with a high mortality rate (about 50% for patients with aplastic anemia); and another that is drug-dose dependent and may be reversible with termination of the CAI. Fortunately, the incidence of aplastic anemia associated with oral CAIs is low. Keisu et al in 1990[298] estimated it is "approximately one in 18,000 patient years." Patients present with a constellation of symptoms, including fever, easily bruised skin, purpura, sore throat, paleness, nosebleeds, petechaie, and perhaps jaundice.[298,299] The use of blood tests to monitor for blood dyscrasias is controversial.[300] In an editorial in 2000,[301] Fraunfelder and Bagby weigh the pros and cons of doing routine, periodic blood tests on patients taking oral CAIs, hopefully to catch early any abnormalities and to be able to cease the drug and treat the reversible cases. Because of the serious nature of these dyscrasias, and the fact that only about half of the patients have an irreversible, potentially fatal variation, they recommend that "a standard CBC, consisting of white blood count with differential, hemoglobin, hematocrit, and platelet count, should be repeated every 1–2 months during the first 6-month period and then at 6-month intervals." In our experience, few ophthalmologists ever get diagnostic blood tests on patients beginning or continuing oral CAI therapy.[302] By custom we do not, but we are fortunate not to have had any patients so affected in our practices. Luckily the odds against this happening seem to have been in our favor. Physicians may feel the inconvenience and cost of these tests outweigh the probability of finding and successfully treating affected patients. Patients should be aware of the untoward symptoms and report them on an emergent basis. Given all of the above problems with oral CAIs, they should generally be used only temporarily in acute situations of very high IOP or when all other means of treatment have failed and surgery is not a good option.

The glaucoma community was pleased when, 41 years after Becker first used acetazolamide to treat glaucoma, effective TCAIs were introduced. Dorzolamide[303-306] (Trusopt 2%) first appeared in 1995, followed by brinzolamide[306-309] (Azopt 1%) in 1998. Generic versions of dorzolamide became available in November, 2008. The pH of dorzolamide is mildly acidic (5.6). This results in the drops stinging and burning on instillation, which is tolerated by most patients if they are warned about these side effects when the drops are first prescribed. Azopt is prepared as a micro-fine suspension at a pH (7.5) similar to tears, resulting in more comfortable application of the drop.[310] The suspension vehicle causes a short period of mild blurring of vision and a whitish residue to form on the eyelids. Most patients seem to prefer the relative comfort of Azopt compared to that of Trusopt (and presumably the recently introduced (November 2008) generic formulation of dorzolamide).[310,311] Most importantly, both dorzolamide and brinzolamide lower IOP to the same extent, about 20%.[312] The authors usually prescribe Azopt because of comfort, unless insurance and formulary issues otherwise dictate. Azopt may be very useful in pediatric applications where comfort is important to ensure compliance.[313,314]

Do these TCAIs lower intraocular pressure as well as the oral CAIs? In a word, "no," they do not. Dorzolamide decreases aqueous production by about 70% of the amount of a full dose of acetazolamide.[315] Dorzolamide is relatively selective for the $\alpha$-CAs II isoenzyme when compared with the $\alpha$-CA IV isoenzyme (38:1).[268] Acetazolamide can inhibit *both* isoenzymes to more fully suppress aqueous flow than the more selective TCAIs. We look forward to research that would yield topical carbonic anhydrase inhibitors that would suppress both forms of the ciliary process $\alpha$-CA isoenzymes. To review, the topical CAIs lower IOP about 20% (similar to betaxolol), the oral CAIs closer to 30%. Further, patients receiving a full dose of oral CAIs are unlikely to see any additional pressure lowering by also using topical dorzolamide or brinzolamide. This is true for the TCAI component in combination products of TCAIs and timolol (Cosopt with dorzolamide and Azarga with brinzolamide). Stated differently, the TCAI portion of these combination products is superfluous when patients are also taking oral CAIs.

There has been a question as to whether these topical CAIs inhibit CA isoenzymes in the corneal endothelium to a degree that causes clinical compromise. It would appear that healthy corneas can tolerate these drugs used as chronic glaucoma agents, but that corneas with borderline endothelial function, including transplants, may not.[316-318] We feel that corneas that do "decompensate" after TCAI therapy likely recover with cessation of such therapy.

One important feature of both topical[319,320] and oral[87,321] CAIs is that they work to suppress aqueous and lower IOP throughout the 24-h day, both in the diurnal and nocturnal time periods. Recall that Brubaker et al[38,87] have shown with fluorophotometry, and Liu et al[85] in clinical settings, that beta-antagonists do not work at night when sympathetic tone is minimal. Thus, TCAIs may be more useful agents than beta-blockers because, as we believe, glaucomatous damage may occur at any hour of the day. Nocturnal lowering of IOP is important to slow or halt progression of glaucoma.

Because they only lower IOP about 20%, when compared with HLs that lower IOP about 30%, they are more suitable as secondary and adjunctive agents than as primary monotherapy for glaucoma. Using TCAIs as adjunctive glaucoma therapy is more fully discussed in Chap. 52. Interestingly, with respect to the combination TCAI/timolol products, it is only the TCAI component that is helpful to lower IOP at night, as the beta-blocker is ineffective during the nocturnal period as previously mentioned.

The package inserts for both dorzolamide and brinzolamide indicate that they are approved for TID dosing. Clinicians have found that in the real world, patients rarely take these medications three times a day, but that in fact they usually skip the middle of the day dose. This of course results in a fluctuation in control of intraocular pressure. This is especially problematic if these drugs are prescribed as sole agents. (Some postapproval studies have shown equivalent clinical efficacy comparing TID and BID dosing.[322]) Because of compliance, twice per day dosing is more commonly prescribed when the TCAI drugs are used as adjunctive therapy to HLs or nonselective beta-blockers. Indeed, when these medications are added to beta-blockers (timolol) to form combination products, such as Cosopt and Azarga, they are in fact dosed twice per day (see Sidebar 51.4 and Chap. 52).

> **SIDEBAR 51.4 Carbonic anhydrase inhibitors**
>
> Sophio Liao and Alan Robin
>
> In managing primary open angle glaucoma, treatment should be tailored to the individual patient with the goal of stabilizing optic nerve fiber layer status, controlling intraocular pressure (IOP), and stabilizing visual fields in the context of optimizing quality of life. Although it is acceptable to treat first with laser trabeculoplasty, initial therapy most often comprises one or more topical eyedrops with the goal of decreasing intraocular pressure by 20–30%. When management by topical drops alone fails to lower IOP sufficiently, oral carbonic anhydrase inhibitors (CAI), first introduced to the treatment of glaucoma in 1954, are very useful adjuncts or substitutions. CAIs work by reducing the production of aqueous humor and have been shown to reduce IOP by 30% alone. Oral CAIs have even demonstrated an additive IOP-lowering effect when used in conjunction with topical CAIs in children with pediatric glaucoma, a result not consistently found in the adult population. CAIs include acetazolamide, methazolamide, and diclorphenamide. Acetazolamide is the most commonly used, and is supplied in 125 or 250-mg tablets, or 500-mg sustained-release capsules. It may be dosed up to 250 mg four times daily or 500-mg SR capsules twice a day. CAIs are not first-line choices for treatment, despite impressive IOP-lowering effects, due to their numerous adverse effects. These include malaise, depression, confusion, a metallic taste in the mouth, anorexia, diarrhea, decreased libido, paresthesias, kidney stones, metabolic acidosis, and blood dyscrasias. Use of oral CAIs is contraindicated in patients with a history of kidney stones or other renal disease, liver disease, cardiac disease, Addison's disease, severe chronic obstructive pulmonary disease, and in patients with sulfonamide allergy out of concern for sulfa cross-reactivity. In the acute setting, oral CAIs are also particularly useful. If aggressive topical therapy does not break an acute glaucoma attack, the next step is the use of oral CAIs.
>
> Concern about harmful effects of oral CAIs led to the development of topical formulations that are now widely used. There has been some concern amongst providers about the use of topical CAIs in patients with reported sulfonamide allergies. Despite decreased systemic absorption of topical versus oral medications, there remains concern about the theoretical cross-reactivity between even a small amount of CAI and sulfonamides. However, increased incidence of allergic reactions to topical CAI formulations has never been proven. Since the 1950s, five case reports have been published, and were recently reviewed by Johnson et al Three of those reports concerned patients who had no history of sulfa allergy; the other two reports were found not to demonstrate any true linkage between the patients' stated sulfa hypersensitivity and cross-reactivity with CAIs. Given this information, there is as yet no evidence for concern regarding the use of topical CAIs in patients with known sulfa allergies, whereas the use of oral CAIs in these patients is contraindicated. Of course, it is up to the individual ophthalmologist to take this information into account when making a clinical decision whether or not to utilize topical CAIs.
>
> **Bibliography**
>
> American Academy of Ophthalmology Glaucoma Panel. Primary Open-Angle Glaucoma. *AAO Preferred Practice Patterns* 2005; 1-30.
> Alward WL. Medical management of glaucoma. *N Engl J Med.* 1998;339(18):1298-1307.
> Friedland BR, Maren TH. The role of carbonic anhydrase in lens ion transport and metabolism. *Ann N Y Acad Sci.* 1984;429:582-586.
> Johnson KK, Green DL, Rife JP, Limon L. Sulfonamide cross-reactivity: fact or fiction? *Ann Pharmacother.* 2005;39:290-301.
> Kaur IP, Smitha R, Aggarwal D, Kapil M. Acetazolamide: future perspective in topical glaucoma therapeutics. *Int J Pharm.* 2002;248(1-2):1-14.
> Sabri K, Kevin AV. The additive effect of topical dorzolamide and systemic acetazolamide in pediatric glaucoma. *J AAPOS.* 2006;10(5):464-468.

#### 51.8.1.5 Sympathomimetic Agonists

The sympathomimetic agonists used to treat glaucoma may be divided into those that are nonselective and activate both alpha and beta receptors, and those that are selective for alpha receptors alone. The nonselective drugs are represented by epinephrine compounds and dipivefrin HCl, while the available selective sympathetic agonists consist of various preparations of apraclonidine and brimonidine.

Along with pilocarpine, epinephrine was one of the first agents used to treat glaucoma (see Table 51.5). It functions as a mixed alpha and beta agonist. Early after administration, it causes an increase in aqueous production by its action on the beta receptors on the ciliary processes. Alpha adrenergic stimulation reduces ultrafiltration because of vasoconstriction and decreased ciliary body blood flow. These early effects diminish in several hours. The predominant effect of epinephrine is an increase in both conventional (trabecular meshwork) and unconventional (uveoscleral) outflow facility for a net reduction in IOP. There may be long-term changes in the glycosamine biochemistry of the trabecular meshwork as well.[323] Epinephrine is available in both branded and generic versions in concentrations of 0.25, 0.50, 1.0, and 2.0%.

Epinephrine frequently causes ocular irritation (toxic rather than allergic reactions) with follicular conjunctivitis. Rebound conjunctival hyperemia occurs several hours after administration; first, the musculature lining the conjunctival blood vessel contracts causing blanching, then, the muscles relax past their "neutral" tone and fill with blood causing the hyperemic appearance.

Oculosympathetic innervation in the orbit includes Mueller's muscle, which when stimulated by epinephrine may cause eyelid retraction. Similarly, stimulation of the iris dilator muscles by epinephrine causes mydriasis. Epinephrine (and dipivefrin) should not be used to treat open angle glaucoma in patients who also have narrow anterior chamber angles because of the potential for papillary block with drug-induced iris dilation. Epinephrine has been associated with a significant percentage (up to 30%) of cystoid macular edema (CME) when used in aphakes[324] (not common anymore) or in pseudophakes with torn or opened posterior capsules (the Irvine–Gass Syndrome[325]). This CME is usually clinically apparent as reduced acuity and contrast sensitivity. Finally, chronic use of epinephrine to treat glaucoma has been associated with black adrenochrome deposits on the conjunctiva and contact lenses used by the patient.[326-333] Topical epinephrine also can raise systemic blood pressure, cause headaches and precipitate cardiac arrhythmias in susceptible individuals.[334,335]

To lessen the frequency and magnitude of some of the side effects of epinephrine eye drops, dipivefrin HCl (Propine) was created as a prodrug. Two pivaloyl groups were added to the basic epinephrine molecule, considerably enhancing its lipophilicity and its ability to penetrate the cornea and then enter into the aqueous. Dipivefrin is effective at a clinically available concentration of 0.1%, 10 to 20 times less concentrated than commercial epinephrine eye drops. While all of the ocular and systemic side effects of epinephrine eye drops can and do occur with Propine, they do so to a lesser extent.[48,334,336-344] Although neither drug currently is very popular for glaucoma treatment in the USA, we note that Propine has largely supplanted the use of epinephrine when nonselective sympathomimetic agents are used at all. Both forms of the medication reduce IOP about 18–21%.[345]

The selective alpha agonist agents used to treat glaucoma are modifications of the clonidine molecule (similar to the development of the HLs that were derived from $PGF_{2\alpha}$). Clonidine, developed to control systemic blood pressure, easily crosses the blood–brain barrier. When used topically, the raw clonidine molecule does lower IOP, but it also gets absorbed systemically in sufficient concentration to cause systemic hypotension.[346-348] Two topical alpha-adrenergic agonists are available for glaucoma therapy, apraclonidine (Iopidine) which is relatively nonselective for $alpha_1$ and $alpha_2$ receptors, and brimonidine (Alphagan and generic) that is more selective for $alpha_2$ than $alpha_1$ receptors. These drugs work by preventing the release of norepinephrine at presynaptic terminals. They both decrease aqueous production, and they may have some effect on episcleral venous pressure[349] as well as uveoscleral outflow.[349,350] Brimonidine may also affect conventional outflow in a positive manner.[351] These drugs lower intraocular pressure between 20 and 25%, about as well or just slightly less than the nonselective beta-blockers.

Iopidine (0.5 and 1.0%) received FDA approval in 1992. It is more polar than clonidine and thus less likely to cause systemic side effects. It is sometimes used to block postoperative rises in IOP after glaucoma laser surgery, including peripheral iridotomies (YAG and Argon), trabeculoplasties (both ALT and SLT), and YAG posterior capsulotomies.[352-355] The authors rarely, if ever, use it chronically to treat open angle glaucomas, because in our experience, and in the literature,[356] apraclonidine: (a) does not lower IOP in about 1/3 of patients, (b) has extreme tachyphylaxis (loss of effect) within about 90 days in about 1/3 of patients, and finally (c) causes blepharoconjunctivitis with red eyes, conjunctival follicles, pruritis, and periorbital dermatitis in about 1/3 of patients. Pupil dilation and lid retraction may also occur in a significant fraction of patients.[357]

Alphagan 0.2%, containing BAK as a preservative, was introduced in the USA in 1996.[358-361] It is now available generically (as brimonidine) in the same concentration. That branded product has been discontinued by Allergan and supplanted with Alphagan-P in both 0.15 and 0.10% concentrations, containing Purite as the preservative. Purite is reported to be "gentler to the cornea than benzalkonium chloride",[362] and its formulation allows enhanced penetration of brimonidine through the cornea allowing lower concentrations of the active medication.[43,363] Brimonidine has significantly fewer of the problems found with apraclonidine because of its increased selectivity for the $alpha_2$ receptor.[364] Brimonidine is suitable for chronic administration to treat glaucoma patients. Nonetheless, we have found that with the original version of Alphagan, and the current generic version of brimonidine in the 0.2% strength with BAK, about 25% of patients who use these drugs suffer from a severe conjunctival hyperemia and periorbital dermatitis in the first 18 months or so of use, necessitating discontinuing the medications. These symptoms clear up within days of stopping the offending medication.

The newer lower concentrations of Alphagan-P, which contain the preservative Purite instead of BAK, seem to be better tolerated, with a decreased incidence of allergy and almost as good intraocular pressure control as with the higher (0.2%) concentration of the original drug.[46,365] The concentration of brimonidine was reduced and the preservative was changed because of the high degree of clinical intolerance with the original formulation. But the incidence of this clinical intolerance to the alpha agonist medications, even with reduced concentrations, is still much higher, in our experience, than that of other topical glaucoma preparations. We might note that dorzolamide and brinzolamide, the TCAIs, have topical toxicities/allergies including periorbital dermatitis in the 5–15% range, but still less than the frequency seen with the alpha agonists. When choosing an alpha-adrenergic agonist, we prefer the 0.1% concentration of Alphagan-P, because of the reduced frequency of side effects.

The pharmacokinetics of topically administered brimonidine requires that it be dosed three times per day, similar to the TCAIs. As they do with the TCAIs, patients usually skip the middle dose when these drugs are used as monotherapeutic agents. The daily dose of the alpha agonist is given just twice a day when used as part of the product Combigan, which contains brimonidine and timolol (with BAK). The alpha agonist component wanes in its ability to lower IOP in the wee hours of the morning, as compared to TCAIs, thus perhaps giving some advantage to using Cosopt over Combigan.[366] Of course, the beta-blocker component of both of these combination products does not work during the nocturnal time period, reducing the overall utility of these products at night.

Brimonidine must be used with caution in two special populations: (a) neonates and young children, and (b) the frail and elderly. With very young patients, brimonidine has resulted in apnea and coma.[367-370] In our clinical experience with some elderly patients, lethargy and mental confusion have resulted from topical brimonidine dosing. In these groups of patients the drug seems to cross the blood brain barrier in sufficient concentration to cause these severe side effects. We refrain from using alpha-adrenergic agonists in children less than 12 years of age and also in slightly built elderly people over age 85. In those elderly patients for whom we do prescribe brimonidine, we question them about symptoms of fatigue, weakness, and dizziness on the first and occasional subsequent visits after beginning use of the medication. We note that sleepiness and fatigue may occur in patients of any age who use these topical medications.

These alpha-adrenergic agonists should not be used in patients taking monoamine oxidase inhibitors (MAOIs) because they may precipitate a hypertensive crisis. They are also contraindicated in patients taking tricyclic antidepressants because of an increased risk of central nervous system (CNS) mediated depression.[371]

While the TCAIs produce some taste perversion as we have previously described (especially with carbonated beverages), the alpha agonist class of drugs causes symptoms of dry mouth (and dry nose) when drained through the nasolacrimal duct into the throat.[359,360,372,373] Some patients hardly notice this issue, while some complain bitterly about it. This especially may be a problem for patients with Sjogren's syndrome. Instruction in digital nasolacrimal duct occlusion is helpful in reducing these symptoms.

Brimonidine's FDA-approved indication for use in the treatment of glaucoma is for the lowering of intraocular pressure. A number of studies suggest that brimonidine may have a direct role in providing neuroprotection for retinal ganglion cells (RGCs). In rodent models with laser-induced ocular hypertension[374] or optic nerve crush injury,[375] parenterally administered brimonidine promoted RGC survival when compared with animals who had received placebo treatments but not the alpha-adrenergic agonist. Studies by Kent[376,377] suggest that topical administration of brimonidine results in concentrations of the agent in the vitreous that should be sufficient to provide neuroprotection of retinal ganglion cells. Various mechanisms have been proposed for this possible neuroprotective action of these alpha-2 adrenergic agonists. These include up-regulation of neurotrophic factors such as "basic fibroblast growth factor,"[378] and attenuation of the release of glutamate, an excitatory toxic agent found in excess in the vitreous of patients with elevated IOP and glaucoma.[379,380] In our clinical experience, and based on discussions with many glaucoma specialists, we feel that brimonidine is almost always prescribed for patients solely with respect to its ability to lower intraocular pressure. Nonetheless, some physicians do add brimonidine for its presumed neuroprotective effect to their mix of "maximal medical therapy" for patients with glaucoma who have progressive optic nerve and visual field damage that does not seem to be sufficiently controlled by other medications and/or laser and surgical options. Currently, there are no published clinical studies indicating that using brimonidine in this manner has any beneficial effect on halting or slowing glaucoma progression independently from lowering of IOP.

### 51.8.1.6 Parasympathomimetic Agents

The parasympathomimetic medications are the oldest form of eye drops used to treat glaucoma (see Fig. 51.6). Because they all have the side effect of acting on the iris sphincter muscle to make the pupil smaller, we shall use the simpler name "miotics" when referring to these agents. The miotics are subdivided into two classes based on mechanism of action, the *direct* acting cholinergic agents, and the *indirect* acting anti-cholinesterase agents. The direct acting agents mimic the action of acetylcholine on the postganglionic parasympathetic receptor target sites (motor end plates) on the ciliary body. The indirect acting cholinergic agents disrupt the activity of acetylcholinesterase that works to degrade the neurotransmitter acetylcholine. This prolongs the action of acetylcholine at the synapse. Following the activation of these receptors, the longitudinal ciliary muscle contracts, pulls on the attached scleral spur, that in turn tightens the trabecular meshwork increasing the outflow of aqueous humor. This lowers intraocular pressure.

Miotic agents may *reduce* uveoscleral outflow.[381] However, there are reports of miotics being adjunctive to HLs.[382-384] We have found mixed results with our patients when using HLs and miotics concomitantly.

Pilocarpine, most commonly used in concentrations of 1–4%, is available both in branded (IsoptoCarpine, Pilocar) and generic preparations. It is used four times per day. Pilopine HS OPHTH Gel 4% is used once nightly. They are both direct acting agents. Carbachol (Isoptocarbachol) is available in concentrations of 1–3%, and has mixed activity, functioning as both direct and indirect acting agent. It is prescribed three times per day. Because these direct acting agents bind to melanin in the iris and ciliary body, the stronger concentrations are often required to adequately treat patients with brown irises as compared to patients with blue or hazel iris color. Indirect acting agents include echothiophate iodide (Phospholine iodide) and demecarium bromide (Humorsol) both supplied in 0.125 and 0.250% concentrations. These drugs irreversibly inhibit cholinesterase. They have long durations of action and can be dosed once or twice per day. Manufacturing problems have caused these drugs to be in limited supply and they are rarely used in the United States. Their use is also limited by their relatively common side effects.

Local side effects of these miotic agents include the previously mentioned miosis, increased lacrimation, induced accommodation, and brow ache.[385] We usually start patients on 1 or 2% pilocarpine and increase to the 4% concentration if necessary after several weeks. This allows them to tolerate what can be a severe brow ache with the higher strength. This discomfort subsides as the muscles adapt to chronic dosing of the medication. Induced near accommodation (myopia) is particularly troublesome to young, phakic patients, especially with the waxing and waning of accommodation every 4–6 h given the normal QID dosing of drugs like pilocarpine. Miotic agents, especially the strong indirect acting ones, promote the development of cataracts and are relatively contraindicated in phakic patients.[386] Patients with preexisting cataracts will find that the miosis induced by these agents results in a further blurring of vision and reduced amount of light getting to the retina. For all these reasons, we almost never prescribe miotic agents to phakic individuals. In fact, because of these side effects, coupled with the need for four times per day dosing, we hardly prescribe miotic agents at all, except for the rare pseudophakic or aphakic patient who has not responded to other medications, laser therapy, and for whom surgery is not indicated or has been ineffective.

We note that miotic agents can disrupt the blood brain barrier and should not be used chronically in patients with ocular inflammation. Nonetheless, in situations of acute rise in intraocular pressure to dangerous levels, such as after some retina surgeries or other intraocular procedures, we have found that short-term use of pilocarpine at 2 or 4% concentrations can sometimes provide temporary relief (for a day or two) of high IOP until a change in the clinical situation occurs. The increased tension on the trabecular meshwork may facilitate the egress of surgical debris from the anterior chamber. We often couple this with frequent dosing of topical steroids. This miotic/steroid therapy may allow a patient to go overnight or through the weekend without an urgent surgical procedure to lower intraocular pressure. It is important to warn the patient about potential brow ache.

These agents cause a forward shift of the lens–iris diaphragm and can precipitate pupillary block and angle closure glaucoma in predisposed eyes as the angle becomes compromised.[387] Although pilocarpine may be helpful for breaking an acute attack of angle closure glaucoma, by causing miosis and pulling the mid-dilated pupil away from the lens it is blocking, stronger concentrations of pilocarpine may aggravate rather than help papillary block. The 4% concentration of pilocarpine may move the lens–iris diaphragm too far forward. We confine ourselves to using no more than 2% pilocarpine when treating a patient with acute angle closure and pupillary block. Further, if intraocular pressure is over about 40 mmHg, the blood supply to the iris sphincter muscle is compromised. The ischemic muscle cannot contract in response to pilocarpine. Thus, there is little benefit of this agent until the pressure can be reduced by topical beta-blockers, brimonidine, TCAIs, oral CAIs, oral osmotic agents, or emergent paracentesis.

Chronic use of any of the miotics may lead to the formation of posterior synechiae,[388] leading in rare cases to an occluded pupil. The indirect acting miotics and higher concentrations of pilocarpine may cause iris pigment cysts[385] and pseudopemphigoid.[389,390] Highly myopic patients may suffer retinal tears or detachments with the stronger concentrations of miotic agents.[391] All myopic patients, and those with a previous history of retinal detachments, should undergo a peripheral retina examination before commencing miotic therapy. This should be repeated yearly in the absence of any symptoms. We find that it is often difficult to dilate and examine well the posterior segment of patients on prolonged miotic therapy. B-scan retinal ultrasound may prove helpful, although it is a less desirable substitute for a dilated peripheral retinal examination.

Systemic side effects of the parasympathomimetic agents include crampy gastrointestinal upset, diarrhea, increased salivation,[392] and increased secretion of stomach acid.[385] Because cholinesterase activity is suppressed by the indirect acting miotics, succinylcholine should not be administered to patients undergoing anesthesia until at least 6 weeks after ceasing these glaucoma drugs.[393]

Today, miotic agents for glaucoma are used more as the exception in Western countries rather than as the rule. They may be helpful in select patients when no other combination of medications can bring the patients' disease under control. Globally, they are still widely prescribed for patients who cannot afford, or who do not have access to, the more recently developed glaucoma medications.

### 51.8.1.7 Hyperosmotics

Hyperosmotic agents are never used for the chronic control of glaucoma. They are used in acute situations where it is desired to temporarily bring down high intraocular pressure that cannot easily be done so by other means. Examples include acute angle closure glaucoma and preoperatively before incisions are made into the anterior chamber during cataract or cornea surgeries. These agents increase the osmolality of the blood, creating a high osmotic gradient between the systemic circulation and the vitreous. Water is "sucked" from the vitreous cavity and enters the general circulation, thereby reducing intraocular pressure. Large, rapid doses of these agents cause a greater osmotic difference, a greater removal of water from the vitreous, and a greater reduction of intraocular pressure. Their effects wear off quickly as there is a rapid re-equalization of the osmotic gradient between the blood and the vitreous cavity. Thus, it is important that some more definitive means of lowering intraocular pressure be achieved within several hours of administering these medications, as if nothing else is done, the intraocular pressure will again rise once the compartments have equilibrated.[394,395]

The hyperosmotic agent mannitol (Osmitrol, 20 and 50% solutions) is given parenterally (intravenously). There are two oral hyperosmotic agents, glycerin 50% (Osmoglyn) and isosorbide 40% solution (Ismotic). Oral glycerin should not be used in diabetic patients as it is metabolized to glucose. For these patients, isosorbide solution is preferred.[394] Any of these drugs can cause electrolyte disturbances and should be used with caution in frail or elderly people. They are contraindicated in patients with kidney failure or who undergo dialysis. The fluid shifts may cause congestive heart failure and expansion of blood volume. Generally speaking, these are medications of last resort and only to be used in emergent situations.[396]

Patients with acutely high intraocular pressures may be nauseated. Serving the oral solutions over ice helps palatability. They should be imbibed over about 30 min, several sips at a time. It is not uncommon for patients who take these oral preparations to engage in emesis. For patients who present with moderate to severe nausea, IV mannitol or IV acetazolamide may be better choices than the oral hyperosmotics. We employ both oral and parenteral versions of the hyperosmotics with great caution (see Sidebar 51.5). The availability of laser peripheral iridotomy has reduced the need for these medications for most patients with acute pupillary-block angle-closure glaucoma.

---

#### Sidebar 51.5 Hyperosmotic agents for the acute management of glaucoma

Kayoung Yi and Teresa C. Chen

Intravenous (IV) mannitol and oral glycerin (glycerol) are the most commonly used hyperosmotic agents. Because of their potentially life-threatening side effects, hyperosmotic agents or osmotics are usually reserved for emergency situations to lower intraocular pressure (IOP) when other medications have proven insufficient. Concern about side-effects has led some physicians to abandon their use completely. Hyperosmotics are also used to lower IOP preoperatively in order to decrease the risk of certain intra- and postoperative complications. Since hyperosmotics penetrate the blood–ocular barrier poorly, these agents work by creating a large osmotic gradient for water to leave the eye. Other osmotic agents, which are now seldom used, include isosorbide, alcohol, and urea.

Mannitol IV infusion: dosing and administration

Mannitol IV infusion is typically administered over 30–60 min using a 20% premixed solution (Fig. 51.5-1) at a dose of 1–2 g/kg of body weight. The authors prefer the lower dose of 1 g/kg, which works sufficiently and has less potential for side effects. It is important to note that too rapid an infusion of mannitol will cause a shift of intracellular water into the extracellular space resulting in cellular dehydration with a higher risk of hyponatremia, congestive heart failure, and pulmonary edema. Slow administration may decrease the risk of intracranial bleeding in predisposed patients. Doses in excess of 200-g IV mannitol per day have also been associated with acute renal failure. For these reasons, mannitol should be avoided or used with caution in patients with cardiac, pulmonary, and/or renal problems.

Mannitol IV push: dosing and administration

Although the indications are limited, mannitol may be administered IV push over 3–5 min as a 25% injection using 50 ml single dose vials (Fig. 51.5-2). Mannitol IV push may be used for cases where more conservative medical treatments do not lower extremely elevated eye pressures or when emergent laser or surgical treatment is not possible. In rare instances, their use may be appropriate when there is positive vitreous pressure during cataract surgery. Because of the significant general medical risks of IV push, the IV push route is preferably administered by a physician for the reasons noted above, but slow administration is always preferable. Because of mannitol's limited solubility, storage at room temperature (25°C) is recommended. If crystallization is seen (Fig. 51.5-3), the solution should be warmed prior to use since mannitol

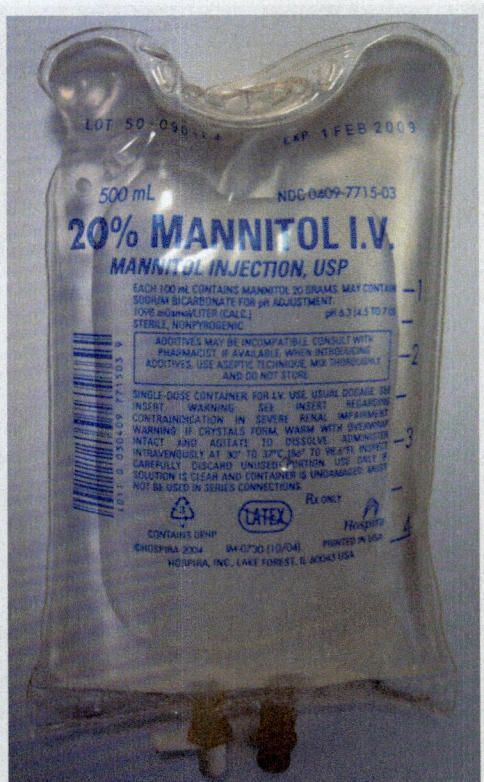

**Fig. 51.5-1** For IV infusion, 20% mannitol (200 mg/ml) can be purchased in 250 or 500-ml bags (Mannitol 20%, Hospira Worldwide Inc., Lake Forest, IL; Mannitol 20%, B. Braun Medical Inc., Sheffield, United Kingdom; Osmitrol 20%, Baxter Medication Delivery, Deerfield, IL)

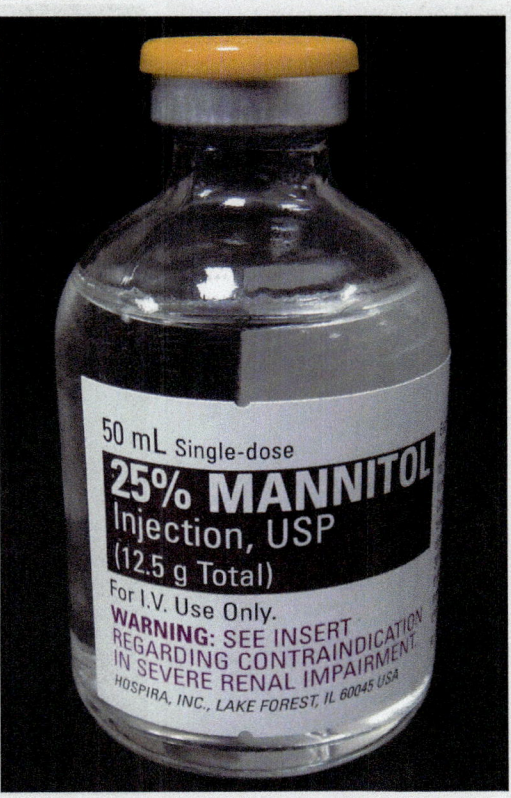

**Fig. 51.5-2** For IV push, 25% mannitol can be purchased as 50-ml single dose vials (Mannitol 25%, American Regent Inc., Shirley, NY)

should not be administered if crystals are present. Intraocular pressure reduction occurs within 45 min of administration and can last up to 6 h. Peak effect occurs 1–2 h after administration.

Oral glycerin: dosing and administration

Glycerin (or glycerol) is usually given as a 50% oral solution at a dose of 1–1.5 g/kg of body weight, or 2–3 ml of 50% glycerin solution per kg of body weight (approximately 4–6 oz per individual). Because of its unpleasantly sweet taste, it is often given with juice or over ice. Onset of action can occur within 10 min, with a peak effect at approximately 1 h, and duration of action up to 4–5 h.

Glycerin is metabolized to glucose and should not be used in diabetics. Glycerin solution may be used for the cardiovascular or severely dehydrated patient who may not be able to use mannitol.

Oral glycerin: Massachusetts Eye and Ear Infirmary Recipe

Glycerin had been sold as Osmoglyn (50% solution, 220-ml bottle by Alcon Laboratories Inc., Fort Worth, TX), however, it is no longer marketed in the United States. Isosorbide (Ismotic) had been used as an alternative to oral glycerin in patients with diabetes, but it is also no longer marketed in the United States. Because Osmoglyn and Ismotic are no longer commercially sold, we mix our own oral glycerin 50% solution (Fig. 51.5-4) using a recipe courtesy of the Massachusetts Eye and Ear Infirmary Department of Pharmacy (Table 51.5-1). The expected yield for this recipe is 900 ml using Crystal Light (a powdered sugar-free drink mix, Kraft Foods, Inc, Northfield, IL), sterile water for irrigation (900 ml), and Glycerin USP (450 ml, Humco, Texarkana, TX). This oral glycerin solution can be stored for up to 3 months in a refrigerator.

Side effects of the hyperosmotic agents

Despite their efficacy, hyperosmotics are not commonly used because of their potential for serious side effects. The typical dosages for mannitol and glycerin are for one time use and not for long-term pressure control. Repeat administration of osmotics without adequate fluid replacement may result in severe

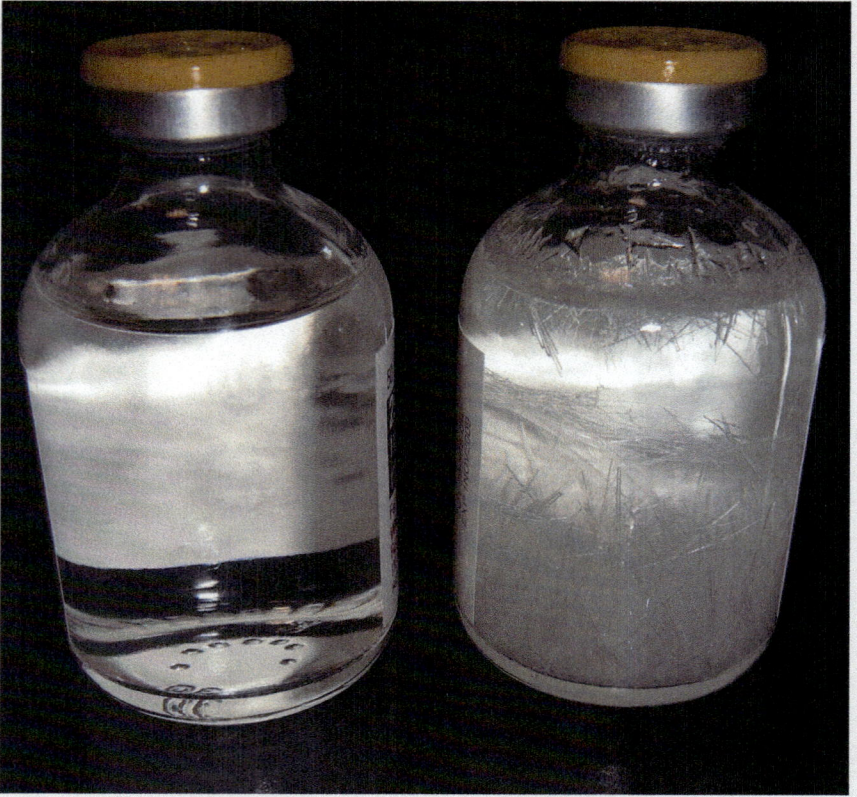

**Fig. 51.5-3** Two 25% mannitol single dose vials are shown in order to demonstrate the absence (*left bottle*) and presence (*right bottle*) of crystals. Before administering the mannitol, the crystals should be dissolved by warming and shaking

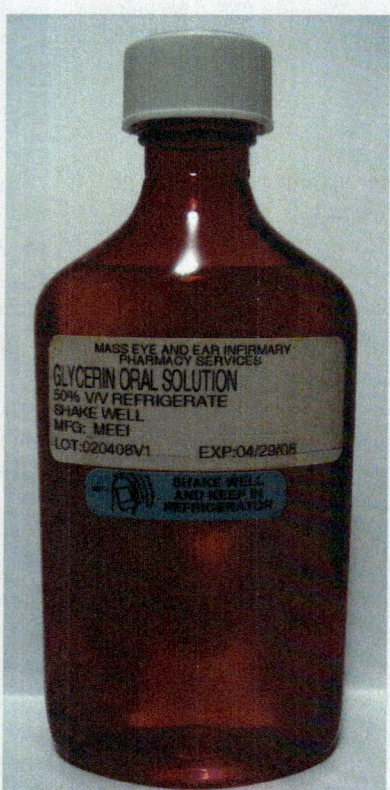

**Fig. 51.5-4** 50% glycerin oral solution from the Massachusetts Eye and Ear Infirmary, Harvard Medical School

headache, disorientation, and confusion from cerebral dehydration.

Although IV mannitol is preferred over glycerin for patients who are nauseated or diabetic, mannitol can be associated with side effects such as a chilly sensation, dizziness, urinary retention, pulmonary edema, congestive heart failure, renal failure, and intracranial hemorrhage. Intravenous mannitol should be used with caution in patients with cardiac, pulmonary, or renal dysfunction. Hyperosmotic agents, especially mannitol, are contraindicated in patients with renal failure, as they may induce diuresis and resultant electrolyte imbalance, which may then lead to seizures and coma.

Glycerin has been associated with nausea, vomiting, calories, and headaches. Glycerin should not be used in diabetic patients.

Use of pre-operative mannitol

Hyperosmotics may be used to reduce eye pressure before various types of intraocular surgery, especially prior to glaucoma surgery when the preoperative IOP is very high, i.e., around 50 mmHg. Preoperative lowering of IOP with hyperosmotics may decrease the risk of certain intraoperative and postoperative complications, such as suprachoroidal hemorrhages and decompression retinopathy. These complications are more commonly seen with a sudden drop of eye pressure from very

Table 51.5-1 Massachusetts Eye and Ear Infirmary Recipe for oral glycerin (glycerol) 50% solution

| Ingredients | Procedure |
|---|---|
| Crystal Light, lemon flavored | 1. Weigh out 2 g lemon flavored Crystal Light |
| | 2. Add the 2 g of Crystal Light to 900 ml of sterile water for irrigation and shake well |
| Sterile water for irrigation | 3. Measure 450 ml of glycerin |
| Glycerin USP | 4. Q.s. to 900 ml with Crystal Light diluting solution (1:1 ratio of 450 ml Glycerin with 450 ml of Crystal Light diluting solution) |
| | 5. Stir well to ensure even distribution of components |
| | 6. Transfer 225 ml of the solution each to four 240 ml amber plastic bottles, cap and label |
| | 7. Store in a refrigerator (for up to 3 months) |

q.s quantum sufficient (as much as is sufficient, enough).

high to zero, which can occur at the time of the initial surgical incision.

When using mannitol preoperatively, 20% mannitol may be given as a slow infusion over 60 min starting 1–1.5 h before surgery in order to achieve the maximum IOP reduction before surgery. Although 1 g/kg can be used, others have suggested using 100 ml of 20% mannitol (or a 20 g dose of mannitol). Mannitol can lower the IOP and increase the anterior chamber depth by dehydrating the vitreous. Preoperative ocular digital massage also helps lower the IOP and reduce positive pressure.

**Acknowledgments** Massachusetts Eye and Ear Infirmary Pharmacy Department: Judy Yee RPH, Ann Papadopoulos RPH, Christine Finn PharmD.

## Bibliography

Allingham RR, Damji K, Freedman S, et al. Hyperosmotics. In: Allingham RR, Damji KF, Freedman S, Moroi SE, eds. *Shields' Textbook of Glaucoma*. 5th ed. Philadelphia, PA: Lippincott Williams & Wilkins; 2005.

Awasthi P, Mathur SP, Srivastava MP. Oral glycerol in cataract surgery. *Br J Ophthalmol*. 1967;51:130-131.

de Ocampo G, Balolong ED, Bernardino V Jr. Pre-operative use of mannitol as ocular anti-hypertensive agent. *Eye Ear Nose Throat Mon*. 1965;44:75-82.

Dudley DF, Leen MM, Kinyoun JL, et al. Retinal hemorrhages associated with ocular decompression after glaucoma surgery. *Ophthalmic Surg Lasers*. 1996;27:147-150.

Feitl ME, Krupin T. Hyperosmotic agents. In: Ritch R, Shields MB, Krupin T, eds. *The Glaucomas*. 2nd ed. St. Louis, MO: Mosby-Year Book; 1996.

Hill K. Ocular osmotherapy with mannitol. *Am J Ophthalmol*. 1964;58:79-83.

Kolker AE. Hyperosmotic agents in glaucoma. *Invest Ophthalmol*. 1970;9:418-423.

Maris PJ Jr, Mandal AK, Netland PA. Medical therapy of pediatric glaucoma and glaucoma in pregnancy. *Ophthalmol Clin North Am*. 2005;18:461-468.

McCurdy DK, Schneider B, Scheie HG. Oral glycerol: the mechanism of intraocular hypotension. *Am J Ophthalmol*. 1966;61:1244-1249.

Miettinen R, Airaksinen PJ, Pihlajaniemi R, et al. Preoperative timolol and ocular compression in cataract surgery. *Acta Ophthalmol (Copenh)*. 1982;60:622-627.

O'Keeffe M, Nabil M. The use of mannitol in intraocular surgery. *Ophthalmic Surg*. 1983;14:55-56.

Singh A. Medical therapy of glaucoma. *Ophthalmol Clin North Am*. 2005;18:397-408.

Smith EW, Drance SM. Reduction of human intraocular pressure with intravenous mannitol. *Arch Ophthalmol*. 1962;68:734-737.

Speaker MG, Guerriero PN, Met JA, et.al. A case-control study of risk factors for intraoperative suprachoroidal expulsive hemorrhage. *Ophthalmology*. 1991;98:202-209.

Taylor DM. Expulsive hemorrhage; some observations and comments. *Trans Am Ophthalmol Soc*. 1974;72:157-169.

Tsai JC, Forbes M. Hyperosmotic agents used to control acute elevation of intraocular pressure in glaucoma. In: Tsai JC, Forbes M, eds. *Medical Management of Glaucoma*. 2nd ed. West Islip, NY: Professional Communications Inc; 2004.

## 51.9 Adjunctive Therapy and Combination Agents

A number of factors must be considered when selecting one or more adjunctive medications as either concomitant or combination therapies. While opinions among glaucoma specialists vary, it is estimated that between 30 and 50% of glaucoma patients will require more than one medical therapy to achieve adequate intraocular pressure control. Complex dosing schedules lead to poor compliance.[397,398] Multiple doses of medication increase preservative load and ocular surface disease.[10] Cost considerations limit compliance and refill rates.[398] Side effect rates, both local and systemic, increase as medications are added.[399]

Most ophthalmologists are choosing the hypotensive lipids – bimatoprost, latanoprost, and travoprost – as their drugs of first choice because they achieve maximum lowering of intraocular pressure as single agents, they only require once-per-day dosing, and have minimal ocular and virtually no systemic side effects. They have replaced the nonselective beta-blockers as initial agents of choice in many countries. Their major downside is that they are currently branded products in most parts of the world and their high cost is a major stumbling block for most patients, especially those with limited or no drug insurance plans. Single medication adjunctive agents to HLs may be chosen from the beta-blockers, the alpha agonists, and the topical carbonic anhydrase inhibitors. Miotic agents are generally not added to hypotensive lipids. They differ with respect to their ability to provide diurnal and nocturnal control, dosing schedules, side effect profiles, and additivity with respect to lowering intraocular pressure when added to the primary hypotensive lipid agents.

Combination products containing hypotensive lipids and beta-blockers are available in many parts of the world but not in the United States. These include DuoTrav (travoprost and timolol), Xalacom (latanoprost and timolol), and Ganfort (bimatoprost and timolol).[400-425] The FDA does not feel that the additional pressure lowering achieved by the combinations, as compared to the HLs alone, warrants any additional safety risk achieved by combining the medications. Yet, such medications minimize the preservative exposure to the eye and offer maximum efficacy for patients who are only wiling to use a single medication once a day. In the USA, we have had Cosopt (containing dorzolamide and timolol) for over 10 years (now also sold generically) and more recently Combigan (containing brimonidine and timolol) has become available. These products may be used as sole therapies, that is two drugs in one bottle and nothing else, or the combination product might be adjunctive to a third "primary" initial agent. A stepped approach to adjunctive medications for glaucoma is best. In many cases, we switch from one primary monotherapy to another before adding adjunctive therapy in requiring the use of two or more agents.

## 51.10 Pragmatic Considerations When Prescribing Medications for Glaucoma Patients

The authors of this chapter are glaucoma consultants who treat a wide spectrum of patients. Some are glaucoma suspects with ocular hypertension or optic nerves that appear at risk, some have early open angle glaucoma and some are tertiary care referrals with advanced disk and visual field damage. Choosing the appropriate medical therapy for patients at different stages along the glaucoma disease spectrum requires two factors: (1) an understanding of the drugs themselves as described in this chapter, and (2) a commitment by the physician to understand the unique personalities, social support mechanisms, and economic circumstances of his or her patients as individual human beings. Understanding the evidenced-based science of glaucoma medical therapy must be combined with a commitment to ensure patient adherence with prescribed medical regimens. This section of the chapter discusses some of the practical considerations for treating patients with glaucoma with adequate medical therapy.

Patients vary in their desire to actively participate in their care. In the twenty-first century, more and more patients are knowledgeable about the glaucoma disease process. They avidly surf the Internet to learn about the medications and their side effects. They read lay patient-centered books and pamphlets about glaucoma. Many of them are able to describe some of the subtypes of primary and secondary glaucomas. Some patients still rely on the traditional paternalistic model of the doctor being the expert and the patient being a relatively passive recipient of the physician's presumed wisdom about glaucoma diagnosis and treatment options. For all these patients, the modern physician must spend adequate "chair time" to understand the specifics of the patient's disease and the patient's ability to cope with chronic treatment requirements.

Many patients feel that glaucoma is a disease that is "embodied" in the absolute value of their intraocular pressure alone apart from other factors. They need to understand the reason doctors do functional and structural diagnostic testing in addition to measuring their IOPs. They need to understand the virtually symptomless early history of their disease. They need to comprehend that taking the eye drops every day is important, but that it will not make them see better or feel better. As physicians, we must encourage them not to skip doses. We must try to educate them, prospectively, to deal with side effects such as conjunctival hyperemia, in spite of the fact that these drops do not help them achieve better visual acuity or wider visual fields. We should try to use medications with less BAK preservative load, when appropriate, to minimize ocular surface disease signs and symptoms.

Interestingly, primary care physicians and internists are often unaware of the significant systemic absorption and plasma concentrations of topical ophthalmic medications. As mentioned previously, these topical drugs may have serious systemic side effects and interactions with oral medications used for nonophthalmic treatments. It is incumbent on the eye physician to interact, by telephone and or written communications, with the patient's other physicians and make them aware of the systemic pharmacological effects of the "drops in those little bottles." Internists are often surprised but gladdened by such prospective phone calls by ophthalmologists, before their patients suffer congestive heart failure or respiratory distress, or cardiac arrhythmias, or systemic hypotension or hypertension.

Some patients are unable to purchase the expensive newer medications. As physicians, we need to take the time to work with the pharmaceutical industry to participate in the indigent patient assistance programs they offer to ensure that our patients receive these valuable newer products. This requires expending expensive, nonreimbursable, time on the part of the physician and allied staff. But it is our ethical obligation to assist patients in this matter. We must learn some of the arrangements that different managed care pharmacies have regarding prescription drug copayments and dispensing different monthly quantities of drugs. Bottles holding larger quantities of drug generally result in better medication compliance because they require less frequent efforts on the part of the patient to obtain refill prescriptions.

Physicians need to occasionally watch patients administer eye drops to themselves. We have been amazed at how often patients, especially patients new to glaucoma treatment, place eyedrops on their cheeks or on their noses, rather than within the fornices of their eyes! Even with adequate placement, many patients dispense two or three or even more eyedrops every time they take their medications. This not only increases the risk of systemic and topical side effects, but it is one of the major reasons that the quantity of medication dispensed by the pharmacy does not last until the date that the patient's insurance company is willing to pay for a refill.

We find that *prospectively* discussing medication quantities, topical and systemic side effects, costs, generic availability, and office policies regarding refill request telephone calls result in much better patient compliance, fewer patient complaints, and fewer avoidable phone calls and drop-in office visits regarding problematic aspects of medication use. In our practices, we find that this prospective conversation best occurs between the physician and the patient, rather than between an ophthalmic assistant and the patient. This extra, prospectively offered "chair time," saves much postvisit "nuisance calls" from patients, including those that inevitably occur late at night and on weekends to the on-call physician. Patients are much less concerned about the continued use of medication that they are prospectively made aware may cause conjunctival hyperemia. They are more likely just to discontinue the use of such a medication, with or without a phone call to their physician, if the symptom happens without the patient having been made aware of its potential occurrence.

Physicians must teach ophthalmic assistants to ask open-ended questions when interviewing patients about their medication use during routinely scheduled office visits. If the assistant simply names the medications prescribed by the physician, and also suggests their dosing intervals, most patients will simply say "yes" to these prompts and agree that these suggested answers are indeed exactly what they do. If instead the assistant requires the patients to name their medications, and tell how often and when they are using them, a different set of answers may occur. Telling some patients to use their medication "four times each day" results in some patients using all their drops between 9 and 10 o'clock in the morning, some synchronizing the eye drops with the three meals and a bedtime dose, and some spacing their medicines almost exactly 6 h apart and waking up in the middle of the night to do so! The patient must be told in appropriate language exactly what it is that their ophthalmologist or optometrist would like them to do to comply properly with medical therapy. Brief or abbreviated conversations often result in patient misunderstanding. We usually ask our patients to repeat verbally the instructions we just gave them. We are amazed at how often they cannot do so even before they leave the office. In addition to verbal instructions about medication use, we provide written instructions on preprinted forms for each patient. We then have them read these instructions out loud and make sure that they understand what we have asked them to do.

We find that some patients would like to rely on samples or "starter" bottles of medication provided by their physician for the great majority of the bottles of medication that they use. Certainly we cannot do so both ethically and pragmatically in a busy practice with many, many patients and only a few bottles of samples. Indeed, we reserve such sample medications for patients who are new to glaucoma therapy, as well as for those who are truly indigent. We try to supply patients with prescriptions for generic versions of medication when appropriate. (We do acknowledge the academic controversy as to whether generic forms of medication are completely equivalent to their branded counterparts.[426])

## 51.11 Conclusion

Eliciting compliance is the key to successful glaucoma therapy. Selection of medications should be based on scientific concepts such as receptor binding, duration of action, and consideration of preservatives. Obviously, not every medication is good for every patient and what is a good first medication is not always a good second one. Future developments in glaucoma therapy will get us away from medications needed even just "once-a-day" and thereby increase compliance.

## References

1. Higginbotham EJ. Initial treatment for open-angle glaucoma-medical, laser or surgical? Medication is the treatment of choice for chronic open-angle glaucoma. *Arch Ophthalmol.* 1998;116(2): 239-240.
2. Hitchings R. Initial treatment for open-angle glaucoma-medical, laser, or surgical? Surgery is the treatment of choice for open-angle glaucoma. *Arch Ophthalmol.* 1998;116(2):241-242.
3. Jampel HD. Initial treatment for open-angle glaucoma-medical, laser, or surgical? Laser trabeculoplasty is the treatment of choice for chronic open-angle glaucoma. *Arch Ophthalmol.* 1998;116(2): 240-241.

4. The Glaucoma Laser Trial. I. Acute effects of argon laser trabeculoplasty on intraocular pressure. Glaucoma Laser Trial Research Group. *Arch Ophthalmol.* 1989;107(8):1135-1142.
5. The Glaucoma Laser Trial (GLT) and glaucoma laser trial follow-up study: 7. Results. Glaucoma Laser Trial Research Group. *Am J Ophthalmol.* 1995;120(6):718-731.
6. McIlraith I, Strasfeld M, Colev G, Hutnik CM. Selective laser trabeculoplasty as initial and adjunctive treatment for open-angle glaucoma. *J Glaucoma.* 2006;15(2):124-130.
7. Feiner L, Piltz-Seymour JR. Collaborative Initial Glaucoma Treatment Study: a summary of results to date. *Curr Opin Ophthalmol.* 2003;14(2):106-111.
8. Baudouin C. Side effects of antiglaucomatous drugs on the ocular surface. *Curr Opin Ophthalmol.* 1996;7(2):80-86.
9. Baudouin C. Mechanisms of failure in glaucoma filtering surgery: a consequence of antiglaucomatous drugs? *Int J Clin Pharmacol Res.* 1996;16(1):29-41.
10. Baudouin C, Pisella PJ, Fillacier K, et al. Ocular surface inflammatory changes induced by topical antiglaucoma drugs: human and animal studies. *Ophthalmology.* 1999;106(3):556-563.
11. Kahook MY, Noecker RJ. Comparison of corneal and conjunctival changes after dosing of travoprost preserved with sofZia, latanoprost with 0.02% benzalkonium chloride, and preservative-free artificial tears. *Cornea.* 2008;27(3):339-343.
12. Neelakantan A, Vaishnav HD, Iyer SA, Sherwood MB. Is addition of a third or fourth antiglaucoma medication effective? *J Glaucoma.* 2004;13(2):130-136.
13. Asrani S, Zeimer R, Wilensky J, Gieser D, Vitale S, Lindenmuth K. Large diurnal fluctuations in intraocular pressure are an independent risk factor in patients with glaucoma. *J Glaucoma.* 2000;9(2):134-142.
14. Bengtsson B, Leske MC, Hyman L, Heijl A. Fluctuation of intraocular pressure and glaucoma progression in the early manifest glaucoma trial. *Ophthalmology.* 2007;114(2):205-209.
15. Caprioli J, Coleman AL. Intraocular pressure fluctuation a risk factor for visual field progression at low intraocular pressures in the advanced glaucoma intervention study. *Ophthalmology.* 2008;115(7):1123-1129 e1123.
16. Hughes E, Spry P, Diamond J. 24-hour monitoring of intraocular pressure in glaucoma management: a retrospective review. *J Glaucoma.* 2003;12(3):232-236.
17. Medeiros FA, Weinreb RN, Zangwill LM, et al. Long-term intraocular pressure fluctuations and risk of conversion from ocular hypertension to glaucoma. *Ophthalmology.* 2008;115(6):934-940.
18. Wilson MR, Gaasterland D. Translating research into practice: controlled clinical trials and their influence on glaucoma management. *J Glaucoma.* 1996;5(2):139-146.
19. Anderson DR. Glaucoma: the damage caused by pressure. XLVI Edward Jackson memorial lecture. *Am J Ophthalmol.* 1989;108(5):485-495.
20. Weinreb RN. Lowering intraocular pressure to minimize glaucoma damage. *J Glaucoma.* 2001;10(5 Suppl 1):S76-S77.
21. Fremont AM, Lee PP, Mangione CM, et al. Patterns of care for open-angle glaucoma in managed care. *Arch Ophthalmol.* 2003;121(6):777-783.
22. Craven ER. Risk management issues in glaucoma: diagnosis and treatment. *Surv Ophthalmol.* 1996;40(6):459-462.
23. Classe JG. Glaucoma – a clinicolegal review. *J Am Optom Assoc.* 1997;68(6):389-394.
24. Palmberg P. Evidence-based target pressures: how to choose and achieve them. *Int Ophthalmol Clin.* 2004;44(2):1-14.
25. Palmberg P. How clinical trial results are changing our thinking about target pressures. *Curr Opin Ophthalmol.* 2002;13(2):85-88.
26. Coleman AL, Baerveldt G, Bournias TE, eds. Evidence-based management of glaucoma: recommendations of an expert panel. In: *Glaucoma Disease Management Guide.* Montvale, NJ: Thomson-PDR; 2003.
27. Nakakura S, Nomura Y, Ataka S, Shiraki K. Relation between office intraocular pressure and 24-hour intraocular pressure in patients with primary open-angle glaucoma treated with a combination of topical antiglaucoma eye drops. *J Glaucoma.* 2007;16(2):201-204.
28. Mosaed S, Liu JH, Weinreb RN. Correlation between office and peak nocturnal intraocular pressures in healthy subjects and glaucoma patients. *Am J Ophthalmol.* 2005;139(2):320-324.
29. Kremmer S, Niederdraing N, Ayertey HD, Steuhl KP, Selbach JM. Obstructive sleep apnea syndrome, normal tension glaucoma, and nCPAP therapy – a short note. *Sleep.* 2003;26(2):161-162.
30. Marcus DM, Costarides AP, Gokhale P, et al. Sleep disorders: a risk factor for normal-tension glaucoma? *J Glaucoma.* 2001;10(3):177-183.
31. Mojon DS, Hess CW, Goldblum D, et al. Normal-tension glaucoma is associated with sleep apnea syndrome. *Ophthalmologica.* 2002;216(3):180-184.
32. Mojon DS, Hess CW, Goldblum D, Bohnke M, Korner F, Mathis J. Primary open-angle glaucoma is associated with sleep apnea syndrome. *Ophthalmologica.* 2000;214(2):115-118.
33. Onen SH, Mouriaux F, Berramdane L, Dascotte JC, Kulik JF, Rouland JF. High prevalence of sleep-disordered breathing in patients with primary open-angle glaucoma. *Acta Ophthalmol Scand.* 2000;78(6):638-641.
34. Pearson J. Glaucoma in patients with sleep apnea. *Ophthalmology.* 2000;107(5):816-817.
35. Civan MM, Macknight AD. The ins and outs of aqueous humour secretion. *Exp Eye Res.* 2004;78(3):625-631.
36. Macknight AD, McLaughlin CW, Peart D, Purves RD, Carre DA, Civan MM. Formation of the aqueous humor. *Clin Exp Pharmacol Physiol.* 2000;27(1-2):100-106.
37. Fautsch MP, Johnson DH. Aqueous humor outflow: what do we know? Where will it lead us? *Invest Ophthalmol Vis Sci.* 2006;47(10):4181-4187.
38. Reiss GR, Lee DA, Topper JE, Brubaker RF. Aqueous humor flow during sleep. *Invest Ophthalmol Vis Sci.* 1984;25(6):776-778.
39. Diestelhorst M, Kriegistein GK. Does aqueous humor secretion decrease with age? *Int Ophthalmol.* 1992;16(4–5):305-309.
40. Lee PS, H and Lin, S. Medical Therapy of Glaucoma: Mechanisms of Action and Rational Selection of Therapies *American Academy of Ophthalmology, Annual Meeting;* 2007.
41. Netland PA, American Academy of Ophthalmology. *Glaucoma Medical Therapy : Principles and Management.* 2nd ed. New York: Oxford University Press In cooperation with the American Academy of Ophthalmology; 2008.
42. Leung EW, Medeiros FA, Weinreb RN. Prevalence of ocular surface disease in glaucoma patients. *J Glaucoma.* 2008;17(5):350-355.
43. Noecker R. Effects of common ophthalmic preservatives on ocular health. *Adv Ther.* 2001;18(5):205-215.
44. Baudouin C. The pathology of dry eye. *Surv Ophthalmol.* 2001;45(Suppl 2):S211-S220.
45. Mundorf T, Wilcox KA, Ousler GW 3rd, Welch D, Abelson MB. Evaluation of the comfort of Alphagan P compared with Alphagan in irritated eyes. *Adv Ther.* 2003;20(6):329-336.
46. Katz LJ. Twelve-month evaluation of brimonidine-purite versus brimonidine in patients with glaucoma or ocular hypertension. *J Glaucoma.* 2002;11(2):119-126.
47. Lewis RA, Katz GJ, Weiss MJ, et al. Travoprost 0.004% with and without benzalkonium chloride: a comparison of safety and efficacy. *J Glaucoma.* 2007;16(1):98-103.
48. Garzia R. An advance in ophthalmic pharmacology. The use of the epinephrine pro-drug dipivalyl epinephrine in the treatment of glaucoma. *J Am Optom Assoc.* 1982;53(9):727-730.

49. Krauss AH, Woodward DF. Update on the mechanism of action of bimatoprost: a review and discussion of new evidence. *Surv Ophthalmol.* 2004;49(Suppl 1):S5-S11.
50. Camras CB, Sharif NA, Wax MB, Stjernschantz J. Bimatoprost, the prodrug of a prostaglandin analogue. *Br J Ophthalmol.* 2008;92(6):862-863. Author reply 863-864.
51. Maxey KM, Johnson JL, LaBrecque J. The hydrolysis of bimatoprost in corneal tissue generates a potent prostanoid FP receptor agonist. *Surv Ophthalmol.* 2002;47(Suppl 1):S34-S40.
52. Zimmerman TJ, Kooner KS, Kandarakis AS, Ziegler LP. Improving the therapeutic index of topically applied ocular drugs. *Arch Ophthalmol.* 1984;102(4):551-553.
53. Ariturk N, Oge I, Erkan D, Sullu Y, Sahin M. The effects of nasolacrimal canal blockage on topical medications for glaucoma. *Acta Ophthalmol Scand.* 1996;74(4):411-413.
54. Ahlquist RP. A study of the adrenotropic receptors. *Am J Physiol.* 1948;153(3):586-600.
55. Esler M, Jennings G, Lambert G, Meredith I, Horne M, Eisenhofer G. Overflow of catecholamine neurotransmitters to the circulation: source, fate, and functions. *Physiol Rev.* 1990;70(4):963-985.
56. Goldstein DS. *The Autonomic Nervous System in Health and Disease.* New York: M. Dekker; 2001.
57. Eglen RM, Watson N. Selective muscarinic receptor agonists and antagonists. *Pharmacol Toxicol.* 1996;78(2):59-68.
58. QLT Plug Delivery I. A Safety Study of the Latanoprost Punctal Plug Delivery System (L-PPDS) in Subjects with Ocular Hypertension or Open Angle Glaucoma. http://clinicaltrials.gov/ct2/show/NCT00820300. Accessed 11 April 2009.
59. Robin AL, Clark AF, Covert DW, et al. Anterior juxtascleral delivery of anecortave acetate in eyes with primary open-angle glaucoma: a pilot investigation. *Am J Ophthalmol.* 2009;147(1):45-50.
60. Abelson M, Fink K. How to handle BAK. *Rev Ophthalmol.* 2002;9(12). Published Last Modified Date. Accessed Dated Accessed.
61. van der Valk R, Webers CA, Schouten JS, Zeegers MP, Hendrikse F, Prins MH. Intraocular pressure-lowering effects of all commonly used glaucoma drugs: a meta-analysis of randomized clinical trials. *Ophthalmology.* 2005;112(7):1177-1185.
62. Phillips CI, Howitt G, Rowlands DJ. Propranolol as ocular hypotensive agent. *Br J Ophthalmol.* 1967;51(4):222-226.
63. Katz IM, Hubbard WA, Getson AJ, Gould AL. Intraocular pressure decrease in normal volunteers following timolol ophthalmic solution. *Invest Ophthalmol.* 1976;15(6):489-492.
64. Stewart WC, Dubiner HB, Mundorf TK, et al. Effects of carteolol and timolol on plasma lipid profiles in older women with ocular hypertension or primary open-angle glaucoma. *Am J Ophthalmol.* 1999;127(2):142-147.
65. Chrisp P, Sorkin EM. Ocular carteolol. A review of its pharmacological properties, and therapeutic use in glaucoma and ocular hypertension. *Drugs Aging.* 1992;2(1):58-77.
66. Freedman SF, Freedman NJ, Shields MB, et al. Effects of ocular carteolol and timolol on plasma high-density lipoprotein cholesterol level. *Am J Ophthalmol.* 1993;116(5):600-611.
67. Kamalarajah S, Johnston PB. Bilateral anterior uveitis associated with 0.3% minims metipranolol. *Eye.* 1999;13(Pt 3a):380-381.
68. Fraunfelder FW, Rosenbaum JT. Drug-induced uveitis. Incidence, prevention and treatment. *Drug Saf.* 1997;17(3):197-207.
69. Patel NP, Patel KH, Moster MR, Spaeth GL. Metipranolol-associated nongranulomatous anterior uveitis. *Am J Ophthalmol.* 1997;123(6):843-844.
70. Watanabe TM, Hodes BL. Bilateral anterior uveitis associated with a brand of metipranolol. *Arch Ophthalmol.* 1997;115(3):421-422.
71. Beck RW, Moke P, Blair RC, Nissenbaum R. Uveitis associated with topical beta-blockers. *Arch Ophthalmol.* 1996;114(10):1181-1182.
72. Burvenich H. Metipranolol associated granulomatous anterior uveitis: not so uncommon as thought. *Bull Soc Belge Ophtalmol.* 1995;257:63-66. discussion 66-67.
73. O'Connor GR. Granulomatous uveitis and metipranolol. *Br J Ophthalmol.* 1993;77(8):536-538.
74. Akingbehin T, Villada JR. Metipranolol-associated granulomatous anterior uveitis. *Br J Ophthalmol.* 1991;75(9):519-523.
75. Mottow-Lippa LS, Lippa EA, Naidoff MA, Clementi R, Bjornsson T, Jones K. .008% timolol ophthalmic solution. A minimal-effect dose in a normal volunteer model. *Arch Ophthalmol.* 1990;108(1):61-64.
76. Vuori ML, Ali-Melkkila T, Kaila T, Iisalo E, Saari KM. Beta 1- and beta 2-antagonist activity of topically applied betaxolol and timolol in the systemic circulation. *Acta Ophthalmol (Copenh).* 1993;71(5):682-685.
77. Vuori ML, Kaila T, Iisalo E, Saari KM. Concentrations and antagonist activity of topically applied betaxolol in aqueous humour. *Acta Ophthalmol (Copenh).* 1993;71(5):677-681.
78. Vuori ML, Ali-Melkkila T. The effect of betaxolol and timolol on postoperative intraocular pressure. *Acta Ophthalmol (Copenh).* 1993;71(4):458-462.
79. Vuori ML, Ali-Melkkila T, Kaila T, Iisalo E, Saari KM. Plasma and aqueous humour concentrations and systemic effects of topical betaxolol and timolol in man. *Acta Ophthalmol (Copenh).* 1993;71(2):201-206.
80. Gaul GR, Will NJ, Brubaker RF. Comparison of a noncardioselective beta-adrenoceptor blocker and a cardioselective blocker in reducing aqueous flow in humans. *Arch Ophthalmol.* 1989;107(9):1308-1311.
81. Stewart RH, Kimbrough RL, Ward RL. Betaxolol vs timolol. A six-month double-blind comparison. *Arch Ophthalmol.* 1986;104(1):46-48.
82. Long DA, Johns GE, Mullen RS, et al. Levobunolol and betaxolol. A double-masked controlled comparison of efficacy and safety in patients with elevated intraocular pressure. *Ophthalmology.* 1988;95(6):735-741.
83. Feghali JG, Kaufman PL, Radius RL, Mandell AI. A comparison of betaxolol and timolol in open angle glaucoma and ocular hypertension. *Acta Ophthalmol (Copenh).* 1988;66(2):180-186.
84. Zimmerman TJ, Kaufman HE. Timolol, dose response and duration of action. *Arch Ophthalmol.* 1977;95(4):605-607.
85. Liu JH, Kripke DF, Weinreb RN. Comparison of the nocturnal effects of once-daily timolol and latanoprost on intraocular pressure. *Am J Ophthalmol.* 2004;138(3):389-395.
86. Ericson LA. Twenty-four hourly variations in the inflow of the aqueous humour. *Acta Ophthalmol (Copenh).* 1958;36(3):xxx.
87. Topper JE, Brubaker RF. Effects of timolol, epinephrine, and acetazolamide on aqueous flow during sleep. *Invest Ophthalmol Vis Sci.* 1985;26(10):1315-1319.
88. Letchinger SL, Frohlichstein D, Glieser DK, et al. Can the concentration of timolol or the frequency of its administration be reduced? *Ophthalmology.* 1993;100(8):1259-1262.
89. Wandel T, Charap AD, Lewis RA, et al. Glaucoma treatment with once-daily levobunolol. *Am J Ophthalmol.* 1986;10(3):298-304.
90. Soll DB. Evaluation of timolol in chronic open-angle glaucoma. Once a day vs twice a day. *Arch Ophthalmol.* 1980;98(12):2178-2181.
91. Costagliola C, Parmeggiani F, Virgili G, et al. Circadian changes of intraocular pressure and ocular perfusion pressure after timolol or latanoprost in Caucasians with normal-tension glaucoma. *Graefes Arch Clin Exp Ophthalmol.* 2008;246(3):389-396.
92. Quaranta L, Gandolfo F, Turano R, et al. Effects of topical hypotensive drugs on circadian IOP, blood pressure, and calculated diastolic ocular perfusion pressure in patients with glaucoma. *Invest Ophthalmol Vis Sci.* 2006;47(7):2917-2923.
93. Fuchsjager-Mayrl G, Wally B, Rainer G, et al. Effect of dorzolamide and timolol on ocular blood flow in patients with primary open angle glaucoma and ocular hypertension. *Br J Ophthalmol.* 2005;89(10):1293-1297.

94. Fuchsjager-Mayrl G, Wally B, Georgopoulos M, et al. Ocular blood flow and systemic blood pressure in patients with primary open-angle glaucoma and ocular hypertension. *Invest Ophthalmol Vis Sci.* 2004;45(3):834-839.
95. Arend O, Harris A, Wolter P, Remky A. Evaluation of retinal haemodynamics and retinal function after application of dorzolamide, timolol and latanoprost in newly diagnosed open-angle glaucoma patients. *Acta Ophthalmol Scand.* 2003;81(5):474-479.
96. Sato T, Muto T, Ishibashi Y, Roy S. Short-term effect of beta-adrenoreceptor blocking agents on ocular blood flow. *Curr Eye Res.* 2001;23(4):298-306.
97. Lubeck P, Orgul S, Gugleta K, Gherghel D, Gekkieva M, Flammer J. Effect of timolol on anterior optic nerve blood flow in patients with primary open-angle glaucoma as assessed by the Heidelberg retina flowmeter. *J Glaucoma.* 2001;10(1):13-17.
98. Sponsel WE, Mensah J, Kiel JW, et al. Effects of latanoprost and timolol-XE on hydrodynamics in the normal eye. *Am J Ophthalmol.* 2000;130(2):151-159.
99. Arend O, Harris A, Arend S, Remky A, Martin BJ. The acute effect of topical beta-adrenoreceptor blocking agents on retinal and optic nerve head circulation. *Acta Ophthalmol Scand.* 1998;76(1):43-49.
100. Greve EL, Rulo AH, Drance SM, Crichton AC, Mills RP, Hoyng PF. Reduced intraocular pressure and increased ocular perfusion pressure in normal tension glaucoma: a review of short-term studies with three dose regimens of latanoprost treatment. *Surv Ophthalmol.* 1997;41(Suppl 2):S89-S92.
101. Grunwald JE. Effect of timolol maleate on the retinal circulation of human eyes with ocular hypertension. *Invest Ophthalmol Vis Sci.* 1990;31(3):521-526.
102. Pillunat L, Stodtmeister R. Effect of different antiglaucomatous drugs on ocular perfusion pressures. *J Ocul Pharmacol.* 1988;4(3):231-242.
103. Pillunat LE, Stodtmeister R, Wilmanns I, Metzner D. Effect of timolol on optic nerve head autoregulation. *Ophthalmologica.* 1986;193(3):146-153.
104. Hayreh SS, Podhajsky P, Zimmerman MB. Beta-blocker eyedrops and nocturnal arterial hypotension. *Am J Ophthalmol.* 1999;128(3):301-309.
105. Hayreh SS, Podhajsky P, Zimmerman MB. Role of nocturnal arterial hypotension in optic nerve head ischemic disorders. *Ophthalmologica.* 1999;213(2):76-96.
106. Yarangumeli A, Kural G. Are there any benefits of Betoptic S (betaxolol HCl ophthalmic suspension) over other beta-blockers in the treatment of glaucoma? *Expert Opin Pharmacother.* 2004;5(5):1071-1081.
107. Dong Y, Ishikawa H, Wu Y, Shimizu K, Goseki T, Yoshitomi T. Effect and mechanism of betaxolol and timolol on vascular relaxation in isolated rabbit ciliary artery. *Jpn J Ophthalmol.* 2006;50(6):504-508.
108. Wood JP, Schmidt KG, Melena J, Chidlow G, Allmeier H, Osborne NN. The beta-adrenoceptor antagonists metipranolol and timolol are retinal neuroprotectants: comparison with betaxolol. *Exp Eye Res.* 2003;76(4):505-516.
109. Melena J, Stanton D, Osborne NN. Comparative effects of antiglaucoma drugs on voltage-dependent calcium channels. *Graefes Arch Clin Exp Ophthalmol.* 2001;239(7):522-530.
110. Hirooka K, Kelly ME, Baldridge WH, Barnes S. Suppressive actions of betaxolol on ionic currents in retinal ganglion cells may explain its neuroprotective effects. *Exp Eye Res.* 2000;70(5):611-621.
111. Melena J, Wood JP, Osborne NN. Betaxolol, a beta1-adrenoceptor antagonist, has an affinity for L-type Ca2+ channels. *Eur J Pharmacol.* 1999;378(3):317-322.
112. Yu DY, Su EN, Cringle SJ, Alder VA, Yu PK, DeSantis L. Systemic and ocular vascular roles of the antiglaucoma agents beta-adrenergic antagonists and Ca2+ entry blockers. *Surv Ophthalmol.* 1999;43(Suppl 1):S214-S222.
113. Gross RL, Hensley SH, Gao F, Wu SM. Retinal ganglion cell dysfunction induced by hypoxia and glutamate: potential neuroprotective effects of beta-blockers. *Surv Ophthalmol.* 1999;43(Suppl 1):S162-S170.
114. Setoguchi M, Ohya Y, Abe I, Fujishima M. Inhibitory action of betaxolol, a beta 1-selective adrenoceptor antagonist, on voltage-dependent calcium channels in guinea-pig artery and vein. *Br J Pharmacol.* 1995;115(1):198-202.
115. Bessho H, Suzuki J, Tobe A. Vascular effects of betaxolol, a cardioselective beta-adrenoceptor antagonist, in isolated rat arteries. *Jpn J Pharmacol.* 1991;55(3):351-358.
116. Osborne NN, Ugarte M, Chao M, et al. Neuroprotection in relation to retinal ischemia and relevance to glaucoma. *Surv Ophthalmol.* 1999;43(Suppl 1):S102-S128.
117. Osborne NN, Wood JP, Chidlow G. Invited review: neuroprotective properties of certain beta-adrenoceptor antagonists used for the treatment of glaucoma. *J Ocul Pharmacol Ther.* 2005;21(3):175-181.
118. Rakofsky SI, Melamed S, Cohen JS, et al. A comparison of the ocular hypotensive efficacy of once-daily and twice-daily levobunolol treatment. *Ophthalmology.* 1989;96(1):8-11.
119. Derick RJ, Robin AL, Tielsch J, et al. Once-daily versus twice-daily levobunolol (0.5%) therapy. A crossover study. *Ophthalmology.* 1992;99(3):424-429.
120. McMahon CD, Shaffer RN, Hoskins HD Jr, Hetherington J Jr. Adverse effects experienced by patients taking timolol. *Am J Ophthalmol.* 1979;88(4):736-738.
121. Van Buskirk EM. Adverse reactions from timolol administration. *Ophthalmology.* 1980;87(5):447-450.
122. Weinreb RN, Caldwell DR, Goode SM, et al. A double-masked three-month comparison between 0.25% betaxolol suspension and 0.5% betaxolol ophthalmic solution. *Am J Ophthalmol.* 1990;110(2):189-192.
123. Van Buskirk EM. Corneal anesthesia after timolol maleate therapy. *Am J Ophthalmol.* 1979;88(4):739-743.
124. Packer M, Colucci WS, Sackner-Bernstein JD, et al. Double-blind, placebo-controlled study of the effects of carvedilol in patients with moderate to severe heart failure. The PRECISE Trial. Prospective Randomized Evaluation of Carvedilol on Symptoms and Exercise. *Circulation.* 1996;94(11):2793-2799.
125. Packer M, Bristow MR, Cohn JN, et al. The effect of carvedilol on morbidity and mortality in patients with chronic heart failure. U.S. Carvedilol Heart Failure Study Group. *N Engl J Med.* 1996;334(21):1349-1355.
126. Packer M. New concepts in the pathophysiology of heart failure: beneficial and deleterious interaction of endogenous haemodynamic and neurohormonal mechanisms. *J Intern Med.* 1996;239(4):327-333.
127. Packer M. Beta-blockade in the management of chronic heart failure. Another step in the conceptual evolution of a neurohormonal model of the disease. *Eur Heart J.* 1996;17 Suppl B:21-23.
128. Effect of metoprolol CR/XL in chronic heart failure: Metoprolol CR/XL Randomised Intervention Trial in Congestive Heart Failure (MERIT-HF). *Lancet.* 1999;353(9169):2001-2007.
129. Goldberg I, Adena MA. Co-prescribing of topical and systemic beta-blockers in patients with glaucoma: a quality use of medicine issue in Australian practice. *Clin Experiment Ophthalmol.* 2007;35(8):700-705.
130. Schuman JS. Effects of systemic beta-blocker therapy on the efficacy and safety of topical brimonidine and timolol. Brimonidine Study Groups 1 and 2. *Ophthalmology.* 2000;107(6):1171-1177.
131. Nelson WL, Fraunfelder FT, Sills JM, Arrowsmith JB, Kuritsky JN. Adverse respiratory and cardiovascular events attributed to timolol ophthalmic solution, 1978-1985. *Am J Ophthalmol.* 1986;102(5):606-611.

132. Diggory P, Cassels-Brown A, Vail A, Abbey LM, Hillman JS. Avoiding unsuspected respiratory side-effects of topical timolol with cardioselective or sympathomimetic agents. *Lancet*. 1995;345(8965):1604-1606.
133. Gullestad L, Dolva LO, Soyland E, Kjekshus J. Difference between beta-1-selective and non-selective beta-blockade during continuous and intermittent exercise. *Clin Physiol*. 1988;8(5):487-499.
134. Nieminen T, Lehtimaki T, Maenpaa J, Ropo A, Uusitalo H, Kahonen M. Ophthalmic timolol: plasma concentration and systemic cardiopulmonary effects. *Scand J Clin Lab Invest*. 2007;67(2):237-245.
135. Stewart WC, Stewart JA, Jackson AL. Cardiovascular effects of timolol maleate, brimonidine or brimonidine/timolol maleate in concomitant therapy. *Acta Ophthalmol Scand*. 2002;80(3):277-281.
136. Stewart WC, Stewart JA, Crockett S, Kubilus C, Brown A, Shams N. Comparison of the cardiovascular effects of unoprostone 0.15%, timolol 0.5% and placebo in healthy adults during exercise using a treadmill test. *Acta Ophthalmol Scand*. 2002;80(3):272-276.
137. Dickstein K, Aarsland T. Comparison of the effects of aqueous and gellan ophthalmic timolol on peak exercise performance in middle-aged men. *Am J Ophthalmol*. 1996;121(4):367-371.
138. Bartlett JD, Olivier M, Richardson T, Whitaker R Jr, Pensyl D, Wilson MR. Central nervous system and plasma lipid profiles associated with carteolol and timolol in postmenopausal black women. *J Glaucoma*. 1999;8(6):388-395.
139. Zimmerman T. Medicinal therapy for glaucoma. In: SG ETM, ed. *The Glaucomas: Concepts and Fundamentals*. Philadelphia: Lippincott Williams and Wilkins; 2000:27-45.
140. Velde TM, Kaiser FE. Ophthalmic timolol treatment causing altered hypoglycemic response in a diabetic patient. *Arch Intern Med*. 1983;143(8):1627.
141. McGill JB, Bakris GL, Fonseca V, et al. beta-blocker use and diabetes symptom score: results from the GEMINI study. *Diabetes Obes Metab*. 2007;9(3):408-417.
142. Lama PJ. Systemic adverse effects of beta-adrenergic blockers: an evidence-based assessment. *Am J Ophthalmol*. 2002;134(5):749-760.
143. Hirsch IB, Boyle PJ, Craft S, Cryer PE. Higher glycemic thresholds for symptoms during beta-adrenergic blockade in IDDM. *Diabetes*. 1991;40(9):1177-1186.
144. Marker JC, Hirsch IB, Smith LJ, Parvin CA, Holloszy JO, Cryer PE. Catecholamines in prevention of hypoglycemia during exercise in humans. *Am J Physiol*. 1991;260(5 Pt 1):E705-E712.
145. Verschoor L, Wolffenbuttel BH, Weber RF. Beta-blockade and carbohydrate metabolism: theoretical aspects and clinical implications. *J Cardiovasc Pharmacol*. 1986;8(Suppl 11):S92-S95.
146. Mills GA, Horn JR. Beta-blockers and glucose control. *Drug Intell Clin Pharm*. 1985;19(4):246-251.
147. Ostman J. beta-adrenergic blockade and diabetes mellitus. A review. *Acta Med Scand Suppl*. 1983;672:69-77.
148. Lager I. Adrenergic blockade and hypoglycaemia. *Acta Med Scand Suppl*. 1983;672:63-67.
149. Schluter KJ, Kerp L. Beta-adrenoceptor blocking agents induce different counter-regulatory responses to insulin. *J Pharmacol*. 1983;14(Suppl 2):49-60.
150. Fraser T, Green D. Weathering the storm: beta-blockade and the potential for disaster in severe hyperthyroidism. *Emerg Med (Fremantle)*. 2001;13(3):376-380.
151. Strube PJ. Thyroid storm during beta blockade. *Anaesthesia*. 1984;39(4):343-346.
152. Shenkman L, Podrid P, Lowenstein J. Hyperthyroidism after propranolol withdrawal. *JAMA*. 1977;238(3):237-239.
153. Pimstone BL. Beta-adrenergic blockade in thyrotoxicosis. *S Afr Med J*. 1969:Suppl:27-30.
154. Schweitzer P, Pivonka M, Zeman R, Gregorova J, Merstenova E. The acute hemodynamic changes of beta-adrenergic blockade in patients with thyrotoxicosis. *Z Kreislaufforsch*. 1968;57(12):1212-1220.
155. Katz IM, Berger ET. Effects of iris pigmentation on response of ocular pressure to timolol. *Surv Ophthalmol*. 1979;23(6):395-398.
156. Olateju SO, Ajayi AA. The lack of efficacy of topical beta-blockers, timolol and betaxolol on intraocular pressure in Nigerian healthy volunteers. *Eye*. 1999;13(Pt 6):758-763.
157. Soltau JB, Zimmerman TJ. Changing paradigms in the medical treatment of glaucoma. *Surv Ophthalmol*. 2002;47(Suppl 1):S2-S5.
158. Araie M, Takase M, Sakai Y, Ishii Y, Yokoyama Y, Kitagawa M. Beta-adrenergic blockers: ocular penetration and binding to the uveal pigment. *Jpn J Ophthalmol*. 1982;26(3):248-263.
159. Lyons JS, Krohn DL. Pilocarpine uptake by pigmented uveal tissue. *Am J Ophthalmol*. 1973;75(5):885-888.
160. Patil PM, Jacobowitz D. Unequal accumulation of adrenergic drugs by pigmented and nonpigmented iris. *Am J Ophthalmol*. 1974;78(3):470-477.
161. Dunham CN, Spaide RF, Dunham G. The contralateral reduction of intraocular pressure by timolol. *Br J Ophthalmol*. 1994;78(1):38-40.
162. Zimmerman TJ, Kaufman HE. Timolol. A beta-adrenergic blocking agent for the treatment of glaucoma. *Arch Ophthalmol*. 1977;95(4):601-604.
163. Radius RL, Diamond GR, Pollack IP, Langham ME. Timolol. A new drug for management of chronic simple glaucoma. *Arch Ophthalmol*. 1978;96(6):1003-1008.
164. Boger WP 3rd. Shortterm "escape" and longterm "drift." The dissipation effects of the beta adrenergic blocking agents. *Surv Ophthalmol*. 1983;28 Suppl:235-242.
165. Lee PY, Podos SM, Serle JB, Camras CB, Severin CH. Intraocular pressure effects of multiple doses of drugs applied to glaucomatous monkey eyes. *Arch Ophthalmol*. 1987;105(2):249-252.
166. Zimmerman TJ, Canale P. Timolol – further observations. *Ophthalmology*. 1979;86(1):166-169.
167. Batterbury M, Harding SP, Wong D. Long-term drift and timolol therapy: possible role for pulsed therapy. *Int Ophthalmol*. 1992;16(4–5):321-324.
168. Gandolfi SA. Restoring sensitivity to timolol after long-term drift in primary open-angle glaucoma. *Invest Ophthalmol Vis Sci*. 1990;31(2):354-358.
169. Markowitz S, Morin JD. Timolol: a 4-year follow-up study. *Can J Ophthalmol*. 1983;18(6):278-280.
170. Steinert RF, Thomas JV, Boger WP 3rd. Long-term drift and continued efficacy after multiyear timolol therapy. *Arch Ophthalmol*. 1981;99(1):100-103.
171. Gandolfi SA, Vecchi M. Serial administration of adrenergic antagonist and agonist ("pulsatile therapy") reduces the incidence of long-term drift to timolol in humans. *Invest Ophthalmol Vis Sci*. 1996;37(4):684-688.
172. Bengtsson B, Heijl A. Lack of long-term drift in timolol's effectiveness in patients with ocular hypertension. *Invest Ophthalmol Vis Sci*. 2001;42(12):2839-2842.
173. Bito LZ. A new approach to the medical management of glaucoma, from the bench to the clinic, and beyond: the Proctor Lecture. *Invest Ophthalmol Vis Sci*. 2001;42(6):1126-1133.
174. Bito LZ, Stjernschantz J, Resul B, Miranda OC, Basu S. The ocular effects of prostaglandins and the therapeutic potential of a new PGF2 alpha analog, PhXA41 (latanoprost), for glaucoma management. *J Lipid Mediat*. 1993;6(1-3):535-543.
175. Camras CB, Siebold EC, Lustgarten JS, et al. Maintained reduction of intraocular pressure by prostaglandin F2 alpha-1-isopropyl ester applied in multiple doses in ocular hypertensive and glaucoma patients. *Ophthalmology*. 1989;96(9):1329-1336. Discussion 1336-1327.
176. Camras CB, Bito LZ. Reduction of intraocular pressure in normal and glaucomatous primate (Aotus trivirgatus) eyes by topically applied prostaglandin F2 alpha. *Curr Eye Res*. 1981;1(4):205-209.

177. Brubaker RF, Schoff EO, Nau CB, Carpenter SP, Chen K, Vandenburgh AM. Effects of AGN 192024, a new ocular hypotensive agent, on aqueous dynamics. *Am J Ophthalmol.* 2001;131(1):19-24.
178. Bahler CK, Howell KG, Hann CR, Fautsch MP, Johnson DH. Prostaglandins increase trabecular meshwork outflow facility in cultured human anterior segments. *Am J Ophthalmol.* 2008;145(1):114-119.
179. Lim KS, Nau CB, O'Byrne MM, et al. Mechanism of action of bimatoprost, latanoprost, and travoprost in healthy subjects. A crossover study. *Ophthalmology.* 2008;115(5):790-795 e794.
180. Dubiner HB, Sircy MD, Landry T, et al. Comparison of the diurnal ocular hypotensive efficacy of travoprost and latanoprost over a 44-hour period in patients with elevated intraocular pressure. *Clin Ther.* 2004;26(1):84-91.
181. Walters TR, DuBiner HB, Carpenter SP, Khan B, VanDenburgh AM. 24-Hour IOP control with once-daily bimatoprost, timolol gel-forming solution, or latanoprost: a 1-month, randomized, comparative clinical trial. *Surv Ophthalmol.* 2004;49(Suppl 1):S26-S35.
182. Lindsey JD, Kashiwagi K, Kashiwagi F, Weinreb RN. Prostaglandin action on ciliary smooth muscle extracellular matrix metabolism: implications for uveoscleral outflow. *Surv Ophthalmol.* 1997;41(Suppl 2):S53-S59.
183. Lutjen-Drecoll E, Tamm E. Morphological study of the anterior segment of cynomolgus monkey eyes following treatment with prostaglandin F2 alpha. *Exp Eye Res.* 1988;47(5):761-769.
184. Sagara T, Gaton DD, Lindsey JD, Gabelt BT, Kaufman PL, Weinreb RN. Topical prostaglandin F2alpha treatment reduces collagen types I, III, and IV in the monkey uveoscleral outflow pathway. *Arch Ophthalmol.* 1999;117(6):794-801.
185. Gaton DD, Sagara T, Lindsey JD, Weinreb RN. Matrix metalloproteinase-1 localization in the normal human uveoscleral outflow pathway. *Invest Ophthalmol Vis Sci.* 1999;40(2):363-369.
186. Ota T, Aihara M, Narumiya S, Araie M. The effects of prostaglandin analogues on IOP in prostanoid FP-receptor-deficient mice. *Invest Ophthalmol Vis Sci.* 2005;46(11):4159-4163.
187. Hellberg MR, Ke TL, Haggard K, Klimko PG, Dean TR, Graff G. The hydrolysis of the prostaglandin analog prodrug bimatoprost to 17-phenyl-trinor PGF2alpha by human and rabbit ocular tissue. *J Ocul Pharmacol Ther.* 2003;19(2):97-103.
188. Camras CB, Toris CB, Sjoquist B, et al. Detection of the free acid of bimatoprost in aqueous humor samples from human eyes treated with bimatoprost before cataract surgery. *Ophthalmology.* 2004;111(12):2193-2198.
189. Sharif NA, Williams GW, Kelly CR. Bimatoprost and its free acid are prostaglandin FP receptor agonists. *Eur J Pharmacol.* 2001;432(2-3):211-213.
190. Cantor LB, Hoop J, Wudunn D, et al. Levels of bimatoprost acid in the aqueous humour after bimatoprost treatment of patients with cataract. *Br J Ophthalmol.* 2007;91(5):629-632.
191. Spada CS, Krauss AH, Woodward DF, et al. Bimatoprost and prostaglandin F(2 alpha) selectively stimulate intracellular calcium signaling in different cat iris sphincter cells. *Exp Eye Res.* 2005;80(1):135-145.
192. Alm A, Stjernschantz J. Effects on intraocular pressure and side effects of 0.005% latanoprost applied once daily, evening or morning. A comparison with timolol. Scandinavian Latanoprost Study Group. *Ophthalmology.* 1995;102(12):1743-1752.
193. Alm A, Widengard I, Kjellgren D, et al. Latanoprost administered once daily caused a maintained reduction of intraocular pressure in glaucoma patients treated concomitantly with timolol. *Br J Ophthalmol.* 1995;79(1):12-16.
194. Linden C, Alm A. Latanoprost twice daily is less effective than once daily: indication of receptor subsensitivity? *Curr Eye Res.* 1998;17(6):567-572.
195. Sjoquist B, Stjernschantz J. Ocular and systemic pharmacokinetics of latanoprost in humans. *Surv Ophthalmol.* 2002;47(Suppl 1):S6-S12.
196. Hellberg MR, Sallee VL, McLaughlin MA, et al. Preclinical efficacy of travoprost, a potent and selective FP prostaglandin receptor agonist. *J Ocul Pharmacol Ther.* 2001;17(5):421-432.
197. Sharif NA, Kelly CR, Crider JY, Williams GW, Xu SX. Ocular hypotensive FP prostaglandin (PG) analogs: PG receptor subtype binding affinities and selectivities, and agonist potencies at FP and other PG receptors in cultured cells. *J Ocul Pharmacol Ther.* 2003;19(6):501-515.
198. Sit AJ, Weinreb RN, Crowston JG, Kripke DF, Liu JH. Sustained effect of travoprost on diurnal and nocturnal intraocular pressure. *Am J Ophthalmol.* 2006;141(6):1131-1133.
199. Gross RL, Peace JH, Smith SE, et al. Duration of IOP reduction with travoprost BAK-free solution. *J Glaucoma.* 2008;17(3):217-222.
200. Stewart WC, Kolker AE, Stewart JA, Leech J, Jackson AL. Conjunctival hyperemia in healthy subjects after short-term dosing with latanoprost, bimatoprost, and travoprost. *Am J Ophthalmol.* 2003;135(3):314-320.
201. Chen J, Woodward DF. Prostanoid FP receptor mediated, endothelium dependent vasodilatation and the ocular surface hyperemic response to PGF2 alpha and related compounds. *Adv Exp Med Biol.* 2002;507:331-336.
202. Gandolfi SA, Cimino L. Effect of bimatoprost on patients with primary open-angle glaucoma or ocular hypertension who are nonresponders to latanoprost. *Ophthalmology.* 2003;110(3):609-614.
203. Konstas AG, Katsimbris JM, Lallos N, Boukaras GP, Jenkins JN, Stewart WC. Latanoprost 0.005% versus bimatoprost 0.03% in primary open-angle glaucoma patients. *Ophthalmology.* 2005;112(2):262-266.
204. Honrubia F, Garcia-Sánchez J, Polo V, de la Casa JM, Soto J. Conjunctival hyperemia with the use of latanoprost versus other prostaglandin analogues in patients with ocular hypertension or glaucoma: a meta-analysis of randomized clinical trials. *Br J Ophthalmol.* http://bjo.bmj.com/cgi/content/abstract/bjo.2007.135111v1 ed: published online 19 Nov 2008; 2009.
205. Funk CD. Prostaglandins and leukotrienes: advances in eicosanoid biology. *Science.* 2001;294(5548):1871-1875.
206. Narumiya S, FitzGerald GA. Genetic and pharmacological analysis of prostanoid receptor function. *J Clin Invest.* 2001;108(1):25-30.
207. Tilley SL, Coffman TM, Koller BH. Mixed messages: modulation of inflammation and immune responses by prostaglandins and thromboxanes. *J Clin Invest.* 2001;108(1):15-23.
208. Sugimoto Y, Narumiya S, Ichikawa A. Distribution and function of prostanoid receptors: studies from knockout mice. *Prog Lipid Res.* 2000;39(4):289-314.
209. Abelson MB, Mroz M, Rosner SA, Dirks MS, Hirabayashi D. Multicenter, open-label evaluation of hyperemia associated with use of bimatoprost in adults with open-angle glaucoma or ocular hypertension. *Adv Ther.* 2003;20(1):1-13.
210. Trattler W, Noecker RJ, Earl ML. A multicentre evaluation of the effect of patient education on acceptance of hyperaemia associated with bimatoprost therapy for glaucoma or ocular hypertension. *Adv Ther.* 2008;25(3):179-189.
211. Parrish RK, Palmberg P, Sheu WP. A comparison of latanoprost, bimatoprost, and travoprost in patients with elevated intraocular pressure: a 12-week, randomized, masked-evaluator multicenter study. *Am J Ophthalmol.* 2003;135(5):688-703.
212. Denis P, Lafuma A, Khoshnood B, Mimaud V, Berdeaux G. A meta-analysis of topical prostaglandin analogues intra-ocular pressure lowering in glaucoma therapy. *Curr Med Res Opin.* 2007;23(3):601-608.
213. Goldberg I. Comparison of tropical travoprost eye drops given once daily and timolol 0.5% given twice daily in patients with open-angle glaucoma or ocular hypertension. *J Glaucoma.* 2001;10:414-422. *J Glaucoma.* 2002;11(3):275.

214. Cohen JS, Gross RL, Cheetham JK, VanDenburgh AM, Bernstein P, Whitcup SM. Two-year double-masked comparison of bimatoprost with timolol in patients with glaucoma or ocular hypertension. *Surv Ophthalmol*. 2004;49(Suppl 1):S45-S52.
215. Bayer A, Weiler W, Oeverhaus U, Skrotzki FE, Stewart WC. Two-year follow-up of latanoprost 0.005% monotherapy after changing from previous glaucoma therapies. *J Ocul Pharmacol Ther*. 2004;20(6):470-478.
216. Higginbotham EJ. Managing glaucoma during pregnancy. *JAMA*. 2006;296(10):1284-1285.
217. Maris PJ Jr, Mandal AK, Netland PA. Medical therapy of pediatric glaucoma and glaucoma in pregnancy. *Ophthalmol Clin North Am*. 2005;18(3):461-468, vii.
218. Johnson SM, Martinez M, Freedman S. Management of glaucoma in pregnancy and lactation. *Surv Ophthalmol*. 2001;45(5):449-454.
219. Lee YC. Abdominal cramp as an adverse effect of travoprost. *Am J Ophthalmol*. 2005;139(1):202-203.
220. Papachristou GC, Ritch R, Liebmann JM. Gastrointestinal adverse effects of prostaglandin analogues. *Arch Ophthalmol*. 2008;126(5):732-733.
221. Schumer RA, Camras CB, Mandahl AK. Putative side effects of prostaglandin analogs. *Surv Ophthalmol*. 2002;47 Suppl 1:S219.
222. Kroll DM, Schuman JS. Reactivation of herpes simplex virus keratitis after initiating bimatoprost treatment for glaucoma. *Am J Ophthalmol*. 2002;133(3):401-403.
223. Wand M, Gilbert CM, Liesegang TJ. Latanoprost and herpes simplex keratitis. *Am J Ophthalmol*. 1999;127(5):602-604.
224. Deai T, Fukuda M, Hibino T, Higaki S, Hayashi K, Shimomura Y. Herpes simplex virus genome quantification in two patients who developed herpetic epithelial keratitis during treatment with antiglaucoma medications. *Cornea*. 2004;23(2):125-128.
225. Gordon YJ, Yates KA, Mah FS, Romanowski EG. The effects of Xalatan on the recovery of ocular herpes simplex virus type 1 (HSV-1) in the induced reactivation and spontaneous shedding rabbit models. *J Ocul Pharmacol Ther*. 2003;19(3):233-245.
226. Kothari MT, Mehta BK, Asher NS, Kothari KJ. Recurrence of bilateral herpes simplex virus keratitis following bimatoprost use. *Indian J Ophthalmol*. 2006;54(1):47-48.
227. Ekatomatis P. Herpes simplex dendritic keratitis after treatment with latanoprost for primary open angle glaucoma. *Br J Ophthalmol*. 2001;85(8):1008-1009.
228. Halpern DL, Pasquale LR. Cystoid macular edema in aphakia and pseudophakia after use of prostaglandin analogs. *Semin Ophthalmol*. 2002;17(3-4):181-186.
229. Ahad MA, McKee HD. Stopping prostaglandin analogues in uneventful cataract surgery. *J Cataract Refract Surg*. 2004;30(12):2644-2645.
230. Altintas O, Yuksel N, Karabas VL, Demirci G. Cystoid macular edema associated with latanoprost after uncomplicated cataract surgery. *Eur J Ophthalmol*. 2005;15(1):158-161.
231. Miyake K, Ibaraki N. Prostaglandins and cystoid macular edema. *Surv Ophthalmol*. 2002;47(Suppl 1):S203-S218.
232. Yalvac I, Airaksinen PJ, Tuulonen A. Phacoemulsification with and without trabeculectomy in patients with glaucoma. *Ophthalmic Surg Lasers*. 1997;28(6):469-475.
233. McGuigan LJ, Gottsch J, Stark WJ, Maumenee AE, Quigley HA. Extracapsular cataract extraction and posterior chamber lens implantation in eyes with preexisting glaucoma. *Arch Ophthalmol*. 1986;104(9):1301-1308.
234. Steuhl KP, Marahrens P, Frohn C, Frohn A. Intraocular pressure and anterior chamber depth before and after extracapsular cataract extraction with posterior chamber lens implantation. *Ophthalmic Surg*. 1992;23(4):233-237.
235. Wittpenn JR, Silverstein S, Heier J, Kenyon KR, Hunkeler JD, Earl M. A randomized, masked comparison of topical ketorolac 0.4% plus steroid vs steroid alone in low-risk cataract surgery patients. *Am J Ophthalmol*. 2008;146(4):554-560.
236. Wand M, Shields BM. Cystoid macular edema in the era of ocular hypotensive lipids. *Am J Ophthalmol*. 2002;133(3):393-397.
237. Smith SL, Pruitt CA, Sine CS, Hudgins AC, Stewart WC. Latanoprost 0.005% and anterior segment uveitis. *Acta Ophthalmol Scand*. 1999;77(6):668-672.
238. Fechtner RD, Khouri AS, Zimmerman TJ, et al. Anterior uveitis associated with latanoprost. *Am J Ophthalmol*. 1998;126(1):37-41.
239. Warwar RE, Bullock JD, Ballal D. Cystoid macular edema and anterior uveitis associated with latanoprost use. Experience and incidence in a retrospective review of 94 patients. *Ophthalmology*. 1998;105(2):263-268.
240. Sacca S, Pascotto A, Siniscalchi C, Rolando M. Ocular complications of latanoprost in uveitic glaucoma: three case reports. *J Ocul Pharmacol Ther*. 2001;17(2):107-113.
241. Suominen S, Valimaki J. Bilateral anterior uveitis associated with travoprost. *Acta Ophthalmol Scand*. 2006;84(2):275-276.
242. Faulkner WJ, Burk SE. Acute anterior uveitis and corneal edema associated with travoprost. *Arch Ophthalmol*. 2003;121(7):1054-1055.
243. Packer M, Fine IH, Hoffman RS. Bilateral nongranulomatous anterior uveitis associated with bimatoprost. *J Cataract Refract Surg*. 2003;29(11):2242-2243.
244. Parentin F. Granulomatous anterior uveitis associated with bimatoprost: a case report. *Ocul Immunol Inflamm*. 2003;11(1):67-71.
245. Fortuna E, Castaneda-Cervantes RA, Bhat P, Doctor P, Foster CS. Flare-up rates with bimatoprost therapy in uveitic glaucoma. *Am J Ophthalmol*. 2008;146(6):876-882.
246. Aung T, Wong HT, Yip CC, Leong JY, Chan YH, Chew PT. Comparison of the intraocular pressure-lowering effect of latanoprost and timolol in patients with chronic angle closure glaucoma: a preliminary study. *Ophthalmology*. 2000;107(6):1178-1183.
247. Saw SM, Gazzard G, Friedman DS. Interventions for angle-closure glaucoma: an evidence-based update. *Ophthalmology*. 2003;110(10):1869-1878. quiz 1878-1869, 1930.
248. Doi LM, Melo LA Jr, Prata JA Jr. Effects of the combination of bimatoprost and latanoprost on intraocular pressure in primary open angle glaucoma: a randomised clinical trial. *Br J Ophthalmol*. 2005;89(5):547-549.
249. Stjernschantz JW, Albert DM, Hu DN, Drago F, Wistrand PJ. Mechanism and clinical significance of prostaglandin-induced iris pigmentation. *Surv Ophthalmol*. 2002;47(Suppl 1):S162-S175.
250. Teus MA, Arranz-Marquez E, Lucea-Suescun P. Incidence of iris colour change in latanoprost treated eyes. *Br J Ophthalmol*. 2002;86(10):1085-1088.
251. Johnstone MA. Hypertrichosis and increased pigmentation of eyelashes and adjacent hair in the region of the ipsilateral eyelids of patients treated with unilateral topical latanoprost. *Am J Ophthalmol*. 1997;124(4):544-547.
252. Tosti A, Pazzaglia M, Voudouris S, Tosti G. Hypertrichosis of the eyelashes caused by bimatoprost. *J Am Acad Dermatol*. 2004;51(5 Suppl):S149-S150.
253. Stecchi G, Saccucci S, Molinari S, De Gregorio F. Eyelash hypertrichosis induced by topical latanoprost: 6-month follow-up study. *Acta Ophthalmol Scand Suppl*. 2002;236:56-57.
254. Demitsu T, Manabe M, Harima N, Sugiyama T, Yoneda K, Yamada N. Hypertrichosis induced by latanoprost. *J Am Acad Dermatol*. 2001;44(4):721-723.
255. Strober BE, Potash S, Grossman ME. Eyelash hypertrichosis in a patient treated with topical latanoprost. *Cutis*. 2001;67(2):109-110.
256. Herane MI, Urbina F. Acquired trichomegaly of the eyelashes and hypertrichosis induced by bimatoprost. *J Eur Acad Dermatol Venereol*. 2004;18(5):644-645.

257. Wand M. Latanoprost and hyperpigmentation of eyelashes. *Arch Ophthalmol.* 1997;115(9):1206-1208.
258. Kapur R, Osmanovic S, Toyran S, Edward DP. Bimatoprost-induced periocular skin hyperpigmentation: histopathological study. *Arch Ophthalmol.* 2005;123(11):1541-1546.
259. Herndon LW, Robert DW, Wand M, Asrani S. Increased periocular pigmentation with ocular hypotensive lipid use in African Americans. *Am J Ophthalmol.* 2003;135(5):713-715.
260. Kook MS, Lee K. Increased eyelid pigmentation associated with use of latanoprost. *Am J Ophthalmol.* 2000;129(6):804-806.
261. Wand M, Ritch R, Isbey EK Jr, Zimmerman TJ. Latanoprost and periocular skin color changes. *Arch Ophthalmol.* 2001;119(4):614-615.
262. Chen CS, Wells J, Craig JE. Topical prostaglandin F(2alpha) analog induced poliosis. *Am J Ophthalmol.* 2004;137(5):965-966.
263. Shaikh MY, Bodla AA. Hypertrichosis of the eyelashes from prostaglandin analog use: a blessing or a bother to the patient? *J Ocul Pharmacol Ther.* 2006;22(1):76-77.
264. O'Toole L, Cahill M, O'Brien C. Eyelid hypertrichosis associated with latanoprost is reversible. *Eur J Ophthalmol.* 2001;11(4):377-379.
265. Hart J, Shafranov G. Hypertrichosis of vellus hairs of the malar region after unilateral treatment with bimatoprost. *Am J Ophthalmol.* 2004;137(4):756-757.
266. Wistrand PJ, Garg LC. Evidence of a high-activity C type of carbonic anhydrase in human ciliary processes. *Invest Ophthalmol Vis Sci.* 1979;18(8):802-806.
267. Matsui H, Murakami M, Wynns GC, et al. Membrane carbonic anhydrase (IV) and ciliary epithelium. Carbonic anhydrase activity is present in the basolateral membranes of the non-pigmented ciliary epithelium of rabbit eyes. *Exp Eye Res.* 1996;62(4):409-417.
268. Maren TH. Carbonic anhydrase: chemistry, physiology, and inhibition. *Physiol Rev.* 1967;47(4):595-781.
269. Becker B. Decrease in intraocular pressure in man by a carbonic anhydrase inhibitor, diamox; a preliminary report. *Am J Ophthalmol.* 1954;37(1):13-15.
270. Bietti G, Virno M, Pecori-Giraldi J. Acetazolamide, metabolic acidosis, and intraocular pressure. *Am J Ophthalmol.* 1975;80(3 Pt 1):360-369.
271. Maren TH, Haywood JR, Chapman SK, Zimmerman TJ. The pharmacology of methazolamide in relation to the treatment of glaucoma. *Invest Ophthalmol Vis Sci.* 1977;16(8):730-742.
272. Lam DS, Lai JS, Tham CC, Chua JK, Poon AS. Argon laser peripheral iridoplasty versus conventional systemic medical therapy in treatment of acute primary angle-closure glaucoma: a prospective, randomized, controlled trial. *Ophthalmology.* 2002;109(9):1591-1596.
273. Hoh ST, Aung T, Chew PT. Medical management of angle closure glaucoma. *Semin Ophthalmol.* 2002;17(2):79-83.
274. Turtz CA, Turtz AI. Toxicity due to acetazolamide (diamox). *AMA Arch Ophthalmol.* 1958;60(1):130-131.
275. Spring M. Skin eruptions following the use of diamox. *Ann Allergy.* 1956;14(1):41-43.
276. Sud RN, Grewal SS. Stevens-Johnson syndrome due to Diamox. *Indian J Ophthalmol.* 1981;29(2):101-103.
277. Shirato S, Kagaya F, Suzuki Y, Joukou S. Stevens-Johnson syndrome induced by methazolamide treatment. *Arch Ophthalmol.* 1997;115(4):550-553.
278. Flach AJ, Smith RE, Fraunfelder FT. Stevens-Johnson syndrome associated with methazolamide treatment reported in two Japanese-American women. *Ophthalmology.* 1995;102(11):1677-1680.
279. Strom BL, Schinnar R, Apter AJ, et al. Absence of cross-reactivity between sulfonamide antibiotics and sulfonamide nonantibiotics. *N Engl J Med.* 2003;349(17):1628-1635.
280. Friedland BR, Mallonee J, Anderson DR. Short-term dose response characteristics of acetazolamide in man. *Arch Ophthalmol.* 1977;95(10):1809-1812.
281. Bateson MC. Dietary potassium and diuretic therapy. *Am Heart J.* 1974;88(1):124-125.
282. Bateson MC, Lant AF. Dietary potassium and diuretic therapy. *Lancet.* 1973;2(7825):381-382.
283. Dahlen K, Epstein DL, Grant WM, Hutchinson BT, Prien EL Jr, Krall JM. A repeated dose-response study of methazolamide in glaucoma. *Arch Ophthalmol.* 1978;96(12):2214-2218.
284. Kass MA, Kolker AE, Gordon M, et al. Acetazolamide and urolithiasis. *Ophthalmology.* 1981;88(3):261-265.
285. Stone RA, Zimmerman TJ, Shin DH, Becker B, Kass MA. Low-dose methazolamide and intraocular pressure. *Am J Ophthalmol.* 1977;83(5):674-679.
286. Shields MB, Simmons RJ. Urinary calculus during methazolamide therapy. *Am J Ophthalmol.* 1976;81(5):622-624.
287. Anderson CJ, Kaufman PL, Sturm RJ. Toxicity of combined therapy with carbonic anhydrase inhibitors and aspirin. *Am J Ophthalmol.* 1978;86(4):516-519.
288. Rousseau P, Fuentevilla-Clifton A. Acetazolamide and salicylate interaction in the elderly: a case report. *J Am Geriatr Soc.* 1993;41(8):868-869.
289. Sweeney KR, Chapron DJ, Brandt JL, Gomolin IH, Feig PU, Kramer PA. Toxic interaction between acetazolamide and salicylate: case reports and a pharmacokinetic explanation. *Clin Pharmacol Ther.* 1986;40(5):518-524.
290. Liddell NE, Maren TH. CO2 retention as a basis for increased toxicity of salicylate with acetazolamide: avoidance of increased toxicity with benzolamide. *J Pharmacol Exp Ther.* 1975;195(1):1-7.
291. Becker B, Middleton WH. Long-term acetazoleamide (diamox) administration in therapy of glaucomas. *AMA Arch Ophthalmol.* 1955;54(2):187-192.
292. Epstein DL, Grant WM. Carbonic anhydrase inhibitor side effects. Serum chemical analysis. *Arch Ophthalmol.* 1977;95(8):1378-1382.
293. Alward WL. Medical management of glaucoma. *N Engl J Med.* 1998;339(18):1298-1307.
294. Miller LG, Miller SM. Altered taste secondary to acetazolamide therapy. *J Fam Pract.* 1990;31(2):199-200.
295. Graber M, Kelleher S. Side effects of acetazolamide: the champagne blues. *Am J Med.* 1988;84(5):979-980.
296. Wallace TR, Fraunfelder FT, Petursson GJ, Epstein DL. Decreased libido – a side effect of carbonic anhydrase inhibitor. *Ann Ophthalmol.* 1979;11(10):1563-1566.
297. Epstein RJ, Allen RC, Lunde MW. Organic impotence associated with carbonic anhydrase inhibitor therapy for glaucoma. *Ann Ophthalmol.* 1987;19(2):48-50.
298. Keisu M, Wiholm BE, Ost A, Mortimer O. Acetazolamide-associated aplastic anaemia. *J Intern Med.* 1990;228(6):627-632.
299. Lubeck MJ. Aplastic anemia following acetazolamide therapy. *Am J Ophthalmol.* 1970;69(4):684-685.
300. Zimran A, Beutler E. Can the risk of acetazolamide-induced aplastic anemia be decreased by periodic monitoring of blood cell counts? *Am J Ophthalmol.* 1987;104(6):654-658.
301. Fraunfelder FT, Bagby GC. Monitoring patients taking oral carbonic anhydrase inhibitors. *Am J Ophthalmol.* 2000;130(2):221-223.
302. Mogk LG, Cyrlin MN. Blood dyscrasias and carbonic anhydrase inhibitors. *Ophthalmology.* 1988;95(6):768-771.
303. Balfour JA, Wilde MI. Dorzolamide. A review of its pharmacology and therapeutic potential in the management of glaucoma and ocular hypertension. *Drugs Aging.* 1997;10(5):384-403.
304. Herkel U, Pfeiffer N. Update on topical carbonic anhydrase inhibitors. *Curr Opin Ophthalmol.* 2001;12(2):88-93.
305. Pfeiffer N. Dorzolamide: development and clinical application of a topical carbonic anhydrase inhibitor. *Surv Ophthalmol.* 1997;42(2):137-151.
306. Stewart WC. Perspectives in the medical treatment of glaucoma. *Curr Opin Ophthalmol.* 1999;10(2):99-108.

307. DeSantis L. Preclinical overview of brinzolamide. *Surv Ophthalmol.* 2000;44(Suppl 2):S119-S129.
308. March WF, Ochsner KI. The long-term safety and efficacy of brinzolamide 1.0% (azopt) in patients with primary open-angle glaucoma or ocular hypertension. The Brinzolamide Long-Term Therapy Study Group. *Am J Ophthalmol.* 2000;129(2):136-143.
309. Sugrue MF. Pharmacological and ocular hypotensive properties of topical carbonic anhydrase inhibitors. *Prog Retin Eye Res.* 2000;19(1):87-112.
310. Silver LH. Ocular comfort of brinzolamide 1.0% ophthalmic suspension compared with dorzolamide 2.0% ophthalmic solution: results from two multicenter comfort studies. Brinzolamide Comfort Study Group. *Surv Ophthalmol.* 2000;44 Suppl 2:S141-145.
311. Barnebey H, Kwok SY. Patients' acceptance of a switch from dorzolamide to brinzolamide for the treatment of glaucoma in a clinical practice setting. *Clin Ther.* 2000;22(10):1204-1212.
312. Ingram CJ, Brubaker RF. Effect of brinzolamide and dorzolamide on aqueous humor flow in human eyes. *Am J Ophthalmol.* 1999;128(3):292-296.
313. Moore W, Nischal KK. Pharmacologic management of glaucoma in childhood. *Paediatr Drugs.* 2007;9(2):71-79.
314. Terraciano AJ, Sidoti PA. Management of refractory glaucoma in childhood. *Curr Opin Ophthalmol.* 2002;13(2):97-102.
315. Maus TL, Larsson LI, McLaren JW, Brubaker RF. Comparison of dorzolamide and acetazolamide as suppressors of aqueous humor flow in humans. *Arch Ophthalmol.* 1997;115(1):45-49.
316. Kaminski S, Hommer A, Koyuncu D, Biowski R, Barisani T, Baumgartner I. Influence of dorzolamide on corneal thickness, endothelial cell count and corneal sensibility. *Acta Ophthalmol Scand.* 1998;76(1):78-79.
317. Giasson CJ, Nguyen TQ, Boisjoly HM, Lesk MR, Amyot M, Charest M. Dorzolamide and corneal recovery from edema in patients with glaucoma or ocular hypertension. *Am J Ophthalmol.* 2000;129(2):144-150.
318. Zhao JC, Chen T. Brinzolamide induced reversible corneal decompensation. *Br J Ophthalmol.* 2005;89(3):389-390.
319. Orzalesi N, Rossetti L, Invernizzi T, Bottoli A, Autelitano A. Effect of timolol, latanoprost, and dorzolamide on circadian IOP in glaucoma or ocular hypertension. *Am J Ophthalmol.* 2000;130(5):687.
320. Orzalesi N, Rossetti L, Invernizzi T, Bottoli A, Autelitano A. Effect of timolol, latanoprost, and dorzolamide on circadian IOP in glaucoma or ocular hypertension. *Invest Ophthalmol Vis Sci.* 2000;41(9):2566-2573.
321. McCannel CA, Heinrich SR, Brubaker RF. Acetazolamide but not timolol lowers aqueous humor flow in sleeping humans. *Graefes Arch Clin Exp Ophthalmol.* 1992;230(6):518-520.
322. Silver LH. Dose-response evaluation of the ocular hypotensive effect of brinzolamide ophthalmic suspension (Azopt). Brinzolamide Dose-Response Study Group. *Surv Ophthalmol.* 2000;44 Suppl 2:S147-S153.
323. Nordmann JP. Aqueous Suppressants. In: Weinreb R, Kitazawa Y, Krieglstein GK, eds. *Glaucoma in the 21st Century.* London: Mosby; 2000:109-116.
324. Mackool RJ, Muldoon T, Fortier A, Nelson D. Epinephrine-induced cystoid macular edema in aphakic eyes. *Arch Ophthalmol.* 1977;95(5):791-793.
325. Gass JD, Norton EW. Cystoid macular edema and papilledema following cataract extraction. A fluorescein fundoscopic and angiographic study. *Arch Ophthalmol.* 1966;76(5):646-661.
326. Fong DS, Frederick AR Jr, Richter CU, Jakobiec FA. Adrenochrome deposit. *Arch Ophthalmol.* 1993;111(8):1142-1143.
327. Kaiser PK, Pineda R, Albert DM, Shore JW. 'Black cornea' after long-term epinephrine use. *Arch Ophthalmol.* 1992;110(9):1273-1275.
328. Pardos GJ, Krachmer JH, Mannis MJ. Persistent corneal erosion secondary to tarsal adrenochrome deposit. *Am J Ophthalmol.* 1980;90(6):870-871.
329. McCarthy RW, LeBlanc R. A 'black cornea' secondary to topical epinephrine. *Can J Ophthalmol.* 1976;11(4):336-340.
330. Schmitt H, Remler O. Adrenochrome conjunctival inclusions following a local adrenaline therapy (author's transl). *Klin Monatsbl Augenheilkd.* 1974;165(2):332-336.
331. Sugar J. Adrenochrome pigmentation of hydrophilic lenses. *Arch Ophthalmol.* 1974;91(1):11-12.
332. Green WR, Kaufer GJ, Dubroff S. Black cornea: a complication of topical use of epinephrine. *Ophthalmologica.* 1967;154(2):88-95.
333. Reinecke RD, Kuwabara T. Corneal Deposits Secondary to Topical Epinephrine. *Arch Ophthalmol.* 1963;70:170-172.
334. Kerr CR, Hass I, Drance SM, Walters MB, Schulzer M. Cardiovascular effects of epinephrine and dipivalyl epinephrine applied topically to the eye in patients with glaucoma. *Br J Ophthalmol.* 1982;66(2):109-114.
335. Davidson SI. Systemic effects of eye drops. *Trans Ophthalmol Soc U K.* 1974;94(2):487-495.
336. Mills KB, Jacobs NA. A single-blind randomised trial comparing adrenaline 1.0% with dipivalyl epinephrine (propine) 0.1% in the treatment of open-angle glaucoma and ocular hypertension. *Br J Ophthalmol.* 1988;72(6):465-468.
337. Coleiro JA, Sigurdsson H, Lockyer JA. Follicular conjunctivitis on Dipivefrin therapy for glaucoma. *Eye.* 1988;2(Pt 4):440-442.
338. Cebon L, West RH, Gillies WE. Experience with dipivalyl epinephrine. Its effectiveness, alone or in combination, and its side effects. *Aust J Ophthalmol.* 1983;11(3):159-161.
339. Wandel T, Spinak M. Toxicity of dipivalyl epinephrine. *Ophthalmology.* 1981;88(3):259-260.
340. Podos SM, Ritch R. Epinephrine as the initial therapy in selected cases of ocular hypertension. *Surv Ophthalmol.* 1980;25(3):188-194.
341. Goldberg I, Kolker AE, Kass MA, Becker B. Dipivefrin: current concepts. *Aust J Ophthalmol.* 1980;8(2):147-150.
342. Kramer SG. Epinephrine distribution after topical administration to phakic and aphakic eyes. *Trans Am Ophthalmol Soc.* 1980;78:947-982.
343. Theodore J, Leibowitz HM. External ocular toxicity of dipivalyl epinephrine. *Am J Ophthalmol.* 1979;88(6):1013-1016.
344. Kohn AN, Moss AP, Hargett NA, Ritch R, Smith H Jr, Podos SM. Clinical comparison of dipivalyl epinephrine and epinephrine in the treatment of glaucoma. *Am J Ophthalmol.* 1979;87(2):196-201.
345. Kass MA, Mandell AI, Goldberg I, Paine JM, Becker B. Dipivefrin and epinephrine treatment of elevated intraocular pressure: a comparative study. *Arch Ophthalmol.* 1979;97(10):1865-1866.
346. Hodapp E, Kolker AE, Kass MA, Goldberg I, Becker B, Gordon M. The effect of topical clonidine on intraocular pressure. *Arch Ophthalmol.* 1981;99(7):1208-1211.
347. Harrison R, Kaufmann CS. Clonidine. Effects of a topically administered solution on intraocular pressure and blood pressure in open-angle glaucoma. *Arch Ophthalmol.* 1977;95(8):1368-1373.
348. Petursson G, Cole R, Hanna C. Treatment of glaucoma using minidrops of clonidine. *Arch Ophthalmol.* 1984;102(8):1180-1181.
349. Reitsamer HA, Posey M, Kiel JW. Effects of a topical alpha2 adrenergic agonist on ciliary blood flow and aqueous production in rabbits. *Exp Eye Res.* 2006;82(3):405-415.
350. Toris CB, Camras CB, Yablonski ME. Acute versus chronic effects of brimonidine on aqueous humor dynamics in ocular hypertensive patients. *Am J Ophthalmol.* 1999;128(1):8-14.
351. Benozzi J, Jaliffa CO, Firpo Lacoste F, Llomovatte DW, Keller Sarmiento MI, Rosenstein RE. Effect of brimonidine on rabbit tra-

351. becular meshwork hyaluronidase activity. *Invest Ophthalmol Vis Sci.* 2000;41(8):2268-2272.
352. Robin AL, Pollack IP, DeFaller JM. Effects of topical ALO 2145 (p-aminoclonidine hydrochloride) on the acute intraocular pressure rise after argon laser iridotomy. *Arch Ophthalmol.* 1987;105(9):1208-1211.
353. Pollack IP, Brown RH, Crandall AS, Robin AL, Stewart RH, White GL. Prevention of the rise in intraocular pressure following neodymium-YAG posterior capsulotomy using topical 1% apraclonidine. *Arch Ophthalmol.* 1988;106(6):754-757.
354. Brown RH, Stewart RH, Lynch MG, et al. ALO 2145 reduces the intraocular pressure elevation after anterior segment laser surgery. *Ophthalmology.* 1988;95(3):378-384.
355. Fourman S. Effects of topical ALO 2145 (p-aminoclonidine hydrochloride, aplonidine hydrochloride) on the acute intraocular pressure rise after argon laser iridotomy. *Arch Ophthalmol.* 1988;106(3):307-309.
356. Araujo SV, Bond JB, Wilson RP, Moster MR, Schmidt CM Jr, Spaeth GL. Long term effect of apraclonidine. *Br J Ophthalmol.* 1995;79(12):1098-1101.
357. Yuksel N, Guler C, Caglar Y, Elibol O. Apraclonidine and clonidine: a comparison of efficacy and side effects in normal and ocular hypertensive volunteers. *Int Ophthalmol.* 1992;16(4–5):337-342.
358. Greenfield DS, Liebmann JM, Ritch R. Brimonidine: a new alpha2-adrenoreceptor agonist for glaucoma treatment. *J Glaucoma.* 1997;6(4):250-258.
359. Schuman JS, Horwitz B, Choplin NT, David R, Albracht D, Chen K. A 1-year study of brimonidine twice daily in glaucoma and ocular hypertension. A controlled, randomized, multicenter clinical trial. Chronic Brimonidine Study Group. *Arch Ophthalmol.* 1997;115(7):847-852.
360. Derick RJ, Robin AL, Walters TR, et al. Brimonidine tartrate: a one-month dose response study. *Ophthalmology.* 1997;104(1):131-136.
361. Serle JB. A comparison of the safety and efficacy of twice daily brimonidine 0.2% versus betaxolol 0.25% in subjects with elevated intraocular pressure. The Brimonidine Study Group III. *Surv Ophthalmol.* 1996;41 Suppl 1:S39-S47.
362. Cantor LB, WuDunn D, Catoira-Boyle Y, Yung CW. Absorption of brimonidine 0.1% and 0.15% ophthalmic solutions in the aqueous humor of cataract patients. *J Glaucoma.* 2008;17(7):529-534.
363. Acheampong AA, Small D, Baumgarten V, Welty D, Tang-Liu D. Formulation effects on ocular absorption of brimonidine in rabbit eyes. *J Ocul Pharmacol Ther.* 2002;18(4):325-337.
364. Gordon RN, Liebmann JM, Greenfield DS, Lama P, Ritch R. Lack of cross-reactive allergic response to brimonidine in patients with known apraclonidine allergy. *Eye.* 1998;12(Pt 4):697-700.
365. Whitson JT, Ochsner KI, Moster MR, et al. The safety and intraocular pressure-lowering efficacy of brimonidine tartrate 0.15% preserved with polyquaternium-1. *Ophthalmology.* 2006;113(8):1333-1339.
366. Orzalesi N, Rossetti L, Bottoli A, Fumagalli E, Fogagnolo P. The effect of latanoprost, brimonidine, and a fixed combination of timolol and dorzolamide on circadian intraocular pressure in patients with glaucoma or ocular hypertension. *Arch Ophthalmol.* 2003;121(4):453-457.
367. Al-Shahwan S, Al-Torbak AA, Turkmani S, Al-Omran M, Al-Jadaan I, Edward DP. Side-effect profile of brimonidine tartrate in children. *Ophthalmology.* 2005;112(12):2143.
368. Bowman RJ, Cope J, Nischal KK. Ocular and systemic side effects of brimonidine 0.2% eye drops (Alphagan) in children. *Eye.* 2004;18(1):24-26.
369. Enyedi LB, Freedman SF. Safety and efficacy of brimonidine in children with glaucoma. *J AAPOS.* 2001;5(5):281-284.
370. Mungan NK, Wilson TW, Nischal KK, Koren G, Levin AV. Hypotension and bradycardia in infants after the use of topical brimonidine and beta-blockers. *J AAPOS.* 2003;7(1):69-70.
371. Schuman JS. Short- and long-term safety of glaucoma drugs. *Expert Opin Drug Saf.* 2002;1(2):181-194.
372. Simmons ST. Efficacy of brimonidine 0.2% and dorzolamide 2% as adjunctive therapy to beta-blockers in adult patients with glaucoma or ocular hypertension. *Clin Ther.* 2001;23(4):604-619.
373. Walters TR. Development and use of brimonidine in treating acute and chronic elevations of intraocular pressure: a review of safety, efficacy, dose response, and dosing studies. *Surv Ophthalmol.* 1996;41(Suppl 1):S19-S26.
374. WoldeMussie E, Ruiz G, Wijono M, Wheeler LA. Neuroprotection of retinal ganglion cells by brimonidine in rats with laser-induced chronic ocular hypertension. *Invest Ophthalmol Vis Sci.* 2001;42(12):2849-2855.
375. Wheeler LA, Lai R, Woldemussie E. From the lab to the clinic: activation of an alpha-2 agonist pathway is neuroprotective in models of retinal and optic nerve injury. *Eur J Ophthalmol.* 1999;9 Suppl 1:S17-S21.
376. Kent AR, King L, Bartholomew LR. Vitreous concentration of topically applied brimonidine-purite 0.15%. *J Ocul Pharmacol Ther.* 2006;22(4):242-246.
377. Kent AR, Nussdorf JD, David R, Tyson F, Small D, Fellows D. Vitreous concentration of topically applied brimonidine tartrate 0.2%. *Ophthalmology.* 2001;108(4):784-787.
378. Wen R, Cheng T, Li Y, Cao W, Steinberg RH. Alpha 2-adrenergic agonists induce basic fibroblast growth factor expression in photoreceptors in vivo and ameliorate light damage. *J Neurosci.* 1996;16(19):5986-5992.
379. Dreyer EB, Grosskreutz CL. Excitatory mechanisms in retinal ganglion cell death in primary open angle glaucoma (POAG). *Clin Neurosci.* 1997;4(5):270-273.
380. Donello JE, Padillo EU, Webster ML, Wheeler LA, Gil DW. alpha(2)-Adrenoceptor agonists inhibit vitreal glutamate and aspartate accumulation and preserve retinal function after transient ischemia. *J Pharmacol Exp Ther.* 2001;296(1):216-223.
381. Crawford K, Kaufman PL. Pilocarpine antagonizes prostaglandin F2 alpha-induced ocular hypotension in monkeys. Evidence for enhancement of Uveoscleral outflow by prostaglandin F2 alpha. *Arch Ophthalmol.* 1987;105(8):1112-1116.
382. Toris CB, Zhan GL, Zhao J, Camras CB, Yablonski ME. Potential mechanism for the additivity of pilocarpine and latanoprost. *Am J Ophthalmol.* 2001;131(6):722-728.
383. Zhong Y, Gao J, Ye W, Huang P, Cheng Y, Jiao Q. Effect of latanoprost acid and pilocarpine on cultured rabbit ciliary muscle cells. *Ophthalmic Res.* 2007;39(4):232-240.
384. Toris CB, Alm A, Camras CB. Latanoprost and cholinergic agonists in combination. *Surv Ophthalmol.* 2002;47(Suppl 1):S141-S147.
385. Zimmerman TJ, Wheeler TM. Miotics: side effects and ways to avoid them. *Ophthalmology.* 1982;89(1):76-80.
386. Abraham SV, Teller JJ. Influence of various miotics on cataract formation. *Br J Ophthalmol.* 1969;53(12):833-838.
387. Gorin G. Angle-closure glaucoma induced by miotics. *Am J Ophthalmol.* 1966;62(6):1063-1067.
388. Khaw PT, Shah P, Elkington AR. Glaucoma-2: treatment. *BMJ.* 2004;328(7432):156-158.
389. Ekong AS, Foster CS, Roque MR. Eye involvement in autoimmune blistering diseases. *Clin Dermatol.* 2001;19(6):742-749.
390. Bhol K, Mohimen A, Neumann R, et al. Differences in the anti-basement membrane zone antibodies in ocular and pseudo-ocular cicatricial pemphigoid. *Curr Eye Res.* 1996;15(5):521-532.
391. Pape LG, Forbes M. Retinal detachment and miotic therapy. *Am J Ophthalmol.* 1978;85(4):558-566.
392. Takakura AC, Moreira TS, Laitano SC, De Luca LA Jr, Renzi A, Menani JV. Central muscarinic receptors signal pilocarpine-induced salivation. *J Dent Res.* 2003;82(12):993-997.

393. Eilderton TE, Farmati O, Zsigmond EK. Reduction in plasma cholinesterase levels after prolonged administration of echothiophate iodide eyedrops. *Can Anaesth Soc J.* 1968;15(3):291-296.
394. Bruckner HL. Glycerol versus isosorbide. *Ann Ophthalmol.* 1972;4(8):629-633.
395. Mehra KS, Singh R, Char JN, Rajyashree K. Lowering of intraocular tension. Effects of isosorbide and glycerin. *Arch Ophthalmol.* 1971;85(2):167-168.
396. Fraunfelder FT, Fraunfelder FW, Randall JA. *Drug-Induced Ocular Side Effects.* 5th ed. Boston: Butterworth-Heinemann; 2001.
397. Katz LJ. Modern alchemy: fixed combinations of glaucoma drugs. *Am J Ophthalmol.* 2005;140(1):125-126.
398. Tsai JC, McClure CA, Ramos SE, Schlundt DG, Pichert JW. Compliance barriers in glaucoma: a systematic classification. *J Glaucoma.* 2003;12(5):393-398.
399. Robin AL, Covert D. Does adjunctive glaucoma therapy affect adherence to the initial primary therapy? *Ophthalmology.* 2005;112(5):863-868.
400. Larsson LI. Effect on intraocular pressure during 24 hours after repeated administration of the fixed combination of latanoprost 0.005% and timolol 0.5% in patients with ocular hypertension. *J Glaucoma.* 2001;10(2):109-114.
401. Larsson LI. The effect on diurnal intraocular pressure of the fixed combination of latanoprost 0.005% and timolol 0.5% in patients with ocular hypertension. *Acta Ophthalmol Scand.* 2001;79(2):125-128.
402. Lass JH, Eriksson GL, Osterling L, Simpson CV. Comparison of the corneal effects of latanoprost, fixed combination latanoprost-timolol, and timolol: a double-masked, randomized, one-year study. *Ophthalmology.* 2001;108(2):264-271.
403. Calissendorff B, Sjoquist B, Hogberg G, Grunge-Lowerud A. Bioavailability in the human eye of a fixed combination of latanoprost and timolol compared to monotherapy. *J Ocul Pharmacol Ther.* 2002;18(2):127-131.
404. Pfeiffer N. A comparison of the fixed combination of latanoprost and timolol with its individual components. *Graefes Arch Clin Exp Ophthalmol.* 2002;240(11):893-899.
405. Konstas AG, Kozobolis VP, Tersis I, Leech J, Stewart WC. The efficacy and safety of the timolol/dorzolamide fixed combination vs latanoprost in exfoliation glaucoma. *Eye.* 2003;17(1):41-46.
406. Diestelhorst M, Larsson LI. A 12 week study comparing the fixed combination of latanoprost and timolol with the concomitant use of the individual components in patients with open angle glaucoma and ocular hypertension. *Br J Ophthalmol.* 2004;88(2):199-203.
407. Hamacher T, Schinzel M, Scholzel-Klatt A, et al. Short term efficacy and safety in glaucoma patients changed to the latanoprost 0.005%/timolol maleate 0.5% fixed combination from monotherapies and adjunctive therapies. *Br J Ophthalmol.* 2004;88(10):1295-1298.
408. Olander K, Zimmerman TJ, Downes N, Schoenfelder J. Switching from latanoprost to fixed-combination latanoprost-timolol: a 21-day, randomized, double-masked, active-control study in patients with glaucoma and ocular hypertension. *Clin Ther.* 2004;26(10):1619-1629.
409. Konstas AG, Lake S, Economou AI, Kaltsos K, Jenkins JN, Stewart WC. 24-Hour control with a latanoprost-timolol fixed combination vs timolol alone. *Arch Ophthalmol.* 2006;124(11):1553-1557.
410. Martinez A, Sanchez M. A comparison of the safety and intraocular pressure lowering of bimatoprost/timolol fixed combination versus latanoprost/timolol fixed combination in patients with open-angle glaucoma. *Curr Med Res Opin.* 2007;23(5):1025-1032.
411. Rossetti L, Karabatsas CH, Topouzis F, et al. Comparison of the effects of bimatoprost and a fixed combination of latanoprost and timolol on circadian intraocular pressure. *Ophthalmology.* 2007;114(12):2244-2251.
412. Lazaridou MN, Montgomery DM, Ho WO, Jaberoo D. Changes in intraocular pressure following a switch from latanoprost monotherapy to latanoprost/timolol fixed combination therapy in patients with primary open-angle glaucoma or ocular hypertension: results from a clinical practice database. *Curr Med Res Opin.* 2008;24(10):2725-2728.
413. Martinez A, Sanchez M. Bimatoprost/timolol fixed combination vs latanoprost/timolol fixed combination in open-angle glaucoma patients. *Eye (Lond).* 2009;23(4):810-818.
414. Brandt JD, Cantor LB, Katz LJ, Batoosingh AL, Chou C, Bossowska I. Bimatoprost/timolol fixed combination: a 3-month double-masked, randomized parallel comparison to its individual components in patients with glaucoma or ocular hypertension. *J Glaucoma.* 2008;17(3):211-216.
415. Martinez A, Sanchez M. Efficacy and safety of bimatoprost/timolol fixed combination in the treatment of glaucoma or ocular hypertension. *Expert Opin Pharmacother.* 2008;9(1):137-143.
416. Robin AL. A double-masked, randomized, parallel comparison of a fixed combination of bimatoprost 0.03%/timolol 0.5% with non-fixed combination use in patients with glaucoma or ocular hypertension. *Eur J Ophthalmol.* 2007;17(4):685-686. author reply 686-687.
417. Hommer A. A double-masked, randomized, parallel comparison of a fixed combination of bimatoprost 0.03%/timolol 0.5% with non-fixed combination use in patients with glaucoma or ocular hypertension. *Eur J Ophthalmol.* 2007;17(1):53-62.
418. Day DG, Sharpe ED, Beischel CJ, Jenkins JN, Stewart JA, Stewart WC. Safety and efficacy of bimatoprost 0.03% versus timolol maleate 0.5%/dorzolamide 2% fixed combination. *Eur J Ophthalmol.* 2005;15(3):336-342.
419. Konstas AG, Mikropoulos D, Haidich AB, Ntampos KS, Stewart WC. Twenty-four-hour intraocular pressure control with the travoprost/timolol maleate fixed combination compared with travoprost when both are dosed in the evening in primary open-angle glaucoma. *Br J Ophthalmol.* 2009;93(4):481-485.
420. Arend KO, Raber T. Observational study results in glaucoma patients undergoing a regimen replacement to fixed combination travoprost 0.004%/timolol 0.5% in Germany. *J Ocul Pharmacol Ther.* 2008;24(4):414-420.
421. Hollo G, Kothy P. Intraocular pressure reduction with travoprost/timolol fixed combination, with and without adjunctive brinzolamide, in glaucoma. *Curr Med Res Opin.* 2008;24(6):1755-1761.
422. Herceg M, Noecker R. Travoprost/timolol fixed combination. *Expert Opin Pharmacother.* 2008;9(6):1059-1065.
423. Noecker RJ, Awadallah NS, Kahook MY. Travoprost 0.004%/timolol 0.5% fixed combination. *Drugs Today (Barc).* 2007;43(2):77-83.
424. Schuman JS, Katz GJ, Lewis RA, et al. Efficacy and safety of a fixed combination of travoprost 0.004%/timolol 0.5% ophthalmic solution once daily for open-angle glaucoma or ocular hypertension. *Am J Ophthalmol.* 2005;140(2):242-250.
425. Barnebey HS, Orengo-Nania S, Flowers BE, et al. The safety and efficacy of travoprost 0.004%/timolol 0.5% fixed combination ophthalmic solution. *Am J Ophthalmol.* 2005;140(1):1-7.
426. Cantor LB. Ophthalmic generic drug approval process: implications for efficacy and safety. *J Glaucoma.* 1997;6(5):344-349.
427. Wirtz MK, Acott TS, Samples JR, Morrison JC. Prospects for genetic intervention in primary open-angle glaucoma. *Drugs Aging.* 1998;13(5):333-340.
428. Liu JH, Bouligny RP, Kripke DF, Weinreb RN. Nocturnal elevation of intraocular pressure is detectable in the sitting position. *Invest Ophthalmol Vis Sci.* 2003;44(10):4439-4442.
429. Liu JH, Kripke DF, Hoffman RE, et al. Nocturnal elevation of intraocular pressure in young adults. *Invest Ophthalmol Vis Sci.* 1998;39(13):2707-2712.
430. Boger WP 3rd. Timolol: short term "escape" and long term "drift". *Ann Ophthalmol.* 1979;11(8):1239-1242.

431. Barnes GE, Li B, Dean T, Chandler ML. Increased optic nerve head blood flow after 1 week of twice daily topical brinzolamide treatment in Dutch-belted rabbits. *Surv Ophthalmol*. 2000;44(Suppl 2):S131-S140.
432. Bergstrand IC, Heijl A, Harris A. Dorzolamide and ocular blood flow in previously untreated glaucoma patients: a controlled double-masked study. *Acta Ophthalmol Scand*. 2002;80(2):176-182.
433. Costagliola C, Campa C, Parmeggiani F, et al. Effect of 2% dorzolamide on retinal blood flow: a study on juvenile primary open-angle glaucoma patients already receiving 0.5% timolol. *Br J Clin Pharmacol*. 2007;63(3):376-379.
434. Grunwald JE, Mathur S, DuPont J. Effects of dorzolamide hydrochloride 2% on the retinal circulation. *Acta Ophthalmol Scand*. 1997;75(3):236-238.
435. Harris A, Arend O, Arend S, Martin B. Effects of topical dorzolamide on retinal and retrobulbar hemodynamics. *Acta Ophthalmol Scand*. 1996;74(6):569-572.
436. Martinez A, Gonzalez F, Capeans C, Perez R, Sanchez-Salorio M. Dorzolamide effect on ocular blood flow. *Invest Ophthalmol Vis Sci*. 1999;40(6):1270-1275.
437. Pillunat LE, Bohm AG, Koller AU, Schmidt KG, Klemm M, Richard G. Effect of topical dorzolamide on optic nerve head blood flow. *Graefes Arch Clin Exp Ophthalmol*. 1999;237(6):495-500.
438. Hayreh SS. Pathogenesis of visual field defects. Role of the ciliary circulation. *Br J Ophthalmol*. 1970;54(5):289-311.
439. Hayreh SS. Pathogenesis of cupping of the optic disc. *Br J Ophthalmol*. 1974;58(10):863-876.
440. Hayreh SS, Revie IH, Edwards J. Vasogenic origin of visual field defects and optic nerve changes in glaucoma. *Br J Ophthalmol*. 1970;54(7):461-472.
441. Robinson JC, Kaufman PL. Phalloidin inhibits epinephrine's and cytochalasin B's facilitation of aqueous outflow. *Arch Ophthalmol*. 1994;112(12):1610-1613.
442. Robinson JC, Kaufman PL. Cytochalasin B potentiates epinephrine's outflow facility-increasing effect. *Invest Ophthalmol Vis Sci*. 1991;32(5):1614-1618.
443. Melamed S, Kotas-Neumann R, Barak A, Epstein DL. The effect of intracamerally injected ethacrynic acid on intraocular pressure in patients with glaucoma. *Am J Ophthalmol*. 1992;113(5):508-512.
444. Epstein DL. Open angle glaucoma. Why not a cure? *Arch Ophthalmol*. 1987;105(9):1187-1188.
445. Rao PV, Deng PF, Kumar J, Epstein DL. Modulation of aqueous humor outflow facility by the Rho kinase-specific inhibitor Y-27632. *Invest Ophthalmol Vis Sci*. 2001;42(5):1029-1037.
446. Friedman DS, Jampel HD, Congdon NG, Miller R, Quigley HA. The TRAVATAN Dosing Aid accurately records when drops are taken. *Am J Ophthalmol*. 2007;143(4):699-701.
447. Semes L, Shaikh AS. Evaluation of the Xal-Ease latanoprost delivery system. *Optometry*. 2007;78(1):30-33.

# Chapter 52
# Choosing Adjunctive Glaucoma Therapy

Jess T. Whitson

Glaucoma is a group of optic neuropathies characterized by retinal ganglion cell death, irreversible optic nerve damage, and vision loss. The treatment of glaucoma consists of reducing intraocular pressure (IOP) to a target level that is presumed to prevent further optic nerve deterioration.[1] This presumption of clinical stability should be reevaluated at each clinical encounter with the patient and a new lower target IOP level estimated if progression has occurred.

Typically treatment begins with the initiation of topical medical therapy. Currently, five classes of medications are commonly used for the reduction of IOP (Table 52.1). These include alpha-adrenergic agonists, beta-adrenergic antagonists (beta-blockers), carbonic anhydrase inhibitors (CAIs), cholinergics or miotics, and prostaglandin analogs (PGAs). Topical beta-blockers, which reduce IOP by decreasing aqueous humor production, were approved for clinical use in the late 1970s.[2] These agents are either nonselective (timolol, levobunolol, metipranolol, and carteolol), inhibiting both $\beta_1$- and $\beta_2$-adrenergic receptors, or selective (betaxolol), preferentially inhibiting $\beta_1$-receptors. Due to their IOP-lowering efficacy, local tolerability, and twice-daily dosing schedule, beta-blockers remained the initial agent of choice for glaucoma therapy for many years following their introduction. With the availability of generic versions of these products, cost considerations still contribute to their popularity as both monotherapeutic and adjunctive agents, even as more effective but more expensive classes of medications have come to the market.

In recent years, however, the PGAs have emerged as a popular class for monotherapy, and the leading initial agent of choice for most patients with glaucoma or ocular hypertension.[3] Latanoprost was the first PGA to be introduced for the treatment of glaucoma in the United States (1996) followed several years later by bimatoprost (2001) and travoprost (2001). The PGAs lower IOP primarily by increasing uveoscleral outflow of aqueous humor,[4-6] although there is some evidence of a dual mechanism of action for these drugs, with some effect on enhancing trabecular meshwork outflow.[5,7-9] The PGAs offer the glaucoma patient excellent IOP-lowering efficacy, typically reducing IOP by about 30% from baseline.[10]

The PGAs provide effective diurnal and circadian IOP control and minimize IOP fluctuation, a potential risk factor for glaucomatous progression.[11] Unlike beta-blockers, the PGAs show little, if any, evidence of tachyphylaxis.[12] Finally, they are prescribed with a simple once-daily dosing regimen and pose very few systemic safety concerns. This chapter will discuss various options and strategies for the selection and use of adjunctive agents in patients being treated with a PGA as first-line therapy for glaucoma, who fail to reach target pressures.

## 52.1 Need for Adjunctive Glaucoma Therapy

Provided adequate IOP reduction is achieved, treatment of glaucoma with a single agent –or monotherapy – is advantageous to both the treating physician as well as the patient. Treatment with a single agent eliminates the possibility of a "washout effect," which may occur when a second drop of medication is administered before the first drop is absorbed by the eye.[13] Furthermore, a patient is more likely to be compliant with a simple drug regimen than a more complex one.[14] Finally, monotherapy reduces the eye's exposure to the preservative benzalkonium chloride (BAK), which has been shown to cause dose-dependent toxic effects on the ocular surface and tear film.[15] As seen in the literature and clinical practice, however, many glaucoma patients will require an adjunctive agent for adequate reduction in IOP, even when treated first-line with a PGA. The Ocular Hypertension Treatment Study (OHTS) evaluated the ability of medical therapy to prevent or delay the development of glaucoma in patients with elevated IOP. Over 40% of the patients enrolled in the treatment arm of this study required two or more medications to achieve the relatively modest target pressure reduction goal of 20% or more from baseline.[16] The Collaborative Initial Glaucoma Treatment Study (CIGTS) is currently comparing medical therapy with trabeculectomy as the initial intervention in newly diagnosed glaucoma. Almost three-fourths of the patients randomized to the medication arm in the CIGTS required two or more agents to achieve a more aggressive

**Table 52.1** Classes of agents used for the treatment of glaucoma

Alpha-adrenergic agonists
Beta-blockers
Carbonic anhydrase inhibitors
   Oral
   Topical
Cholinergics (miotics)
Prostaglandin analogs

**Table 52.2** Mechanism of action of drugs used for the treatment of glaucoma

Decrease aqueous humor production
   Alpha-adrenergic agonists
   Beta-blockers
   Carbonic anhydrase inhibitors
Increase aqueous humor outflow
   Alpha-adrenergic agonists
   Cholinergics
   Prostaglandin analogs

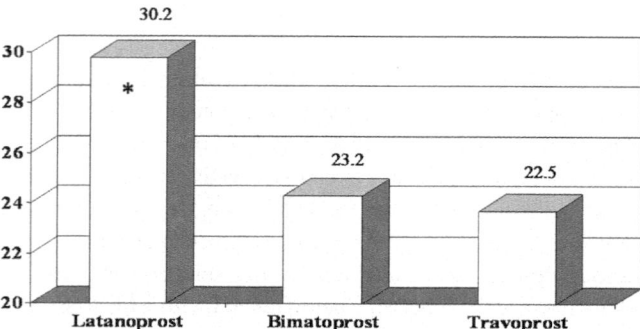

*$P < .0001$ versus bimatoprost or travoprost.
Adapted from [12]

**Fig. 52.1** Frequency of adjunctive medication use with prostaglandin analogs. Results from a review of a large prescription plan database of over 13,000 patients who were prescribed an adjunctive agent for glaucoma following initiation of PGA therapy with either latanoprost, bimatoprost, or travoprost. (Reproduced from Whitson, JT. "Glaucoma: a review of adjunctive therapy and new management strategies," Expert Opinion on Pharmacotherapy, 2007, Dec. 8(18):3237-3249, with kind permission of Informa UK Ltd.)

treatment reduction goal of about 35% from baseline.[17] Finally, a recent evaluation of prescription data from a large nationwide managed care plan demonstrated that almost 30% of patients treated first-line with a PGA will require an additional agent for IOP control within 1 year[18] (Fig. 52.1).

After initiation of PGA therapy, the patient should be evaluated 4–6 weeks later to allow adequate time for maximal IOP reduction to occur. Typically, one should expect a reduction in IOP of about 30% from baseline with PGA monotherapy.[10,19] If the patient demonstrates less than ideal IOP reduction with the initial agent, consider switching to a different PGA before adding another medication ("substitution monotherapy"). Unlike other classes of glaucoma drugs – such as beta-blockers or topical CAIs, which typically show a comparable IOP response between agents of the same class in a given patient – the PGAs can sometimes demonstrate more individual patient variability. The reason for this remains unclear. While responder rates for all three PGAs are quite high, a patient with an inadequate IOP response from one PGA may respond better to another one.[20] Once maximal IOP lowering from the PGA is achieved, adjunctive therapy should be considered should that patient require additional reduction in IOP in order to stabilize their disease.

The selection of appropriate adjunctive glaucoma therapy can be a difficult task. A recent article noted that if a physician considers all the different formulations and concentrations of agents on the market as of 2002, and no more than one medication is selected from each class, then there are currently more than 56,000 different combinations of medications that can be used for the treatment of glaucoma.[21] To simplify the selection process, four broad criteria may be used to evaluate the appropriate agent to use adjunctively with a PGA. These criteria include safety and tolerability, efficacy, mechanism of action, and convenience of the dosing regimen. Obviously, the safety and tolerability of any agent is important to consider, especially when selecting it for use on a long-term basis. Most ophthalmologists expect at least a 15% additional reduction in IOP from the second agent when added to a patient on monotherapy. Additionally, minimizing IOP fluctuation on a diurnal and nocturnal basis should be emphasized. Recent studies demonstrate that large fluctuations in IOP can lead to progression of glaucoma.[11,22,23] Selection of an adjunctive agent that lowers IOP by reducing aqueous humor production will complement the increased aqueous outflow produced by the PGA (Table 52.2). Finally, an adjunctive medication dosing regimen should be kept as simple as possible to maximize patient compliance.

Typically, the selection of an adjunctive agent for a PGA involves choosing from one of three classes of medications: alpha-adrenergic agonists, beta-blockers, and topical CAIs. Due to local tolerability issues and more frequent dosing requirements, the cholinergics, or miotics, are no longer commonly used in modern clinical practice except in a few special situations.

## 52.2 Classes of Medications Used for Adjunctive Therapy

### 52.2.1 Alpha-Adrenergic Agonists

The only alpha-adrenergic agonist commonly used today for chronic glaucoma therapy is the $\alpha_2$-selective agent, brimonidine. A dual mechanism of action, including reduction of aqueous humor production and increase of aqueous humor outflow, has been described for brimonidine.[24] This drug was originally formulated as a 0.2% solution, but due to a relatively high allergy rate was recently reformulated as both a 0.15% and a 0.1% solution preserved with stabilized oxychloro complex (Purite®) instead of BAK (brimonidine-P). The newer formulations have significantly lower rates of allergic conjunctivitis than the original solution.[25] Brimonidine is labeled for three-times-a-day dosing, although most clinicians use it twice daily, especially when used as an adjunctive agent. When added to latanoprost, brimonidine produced an additional reduction in IOP of 32.2%, or 5.9 mmHg ($p<0.001$), in a large, open-label, phase IV community trial.[26] Other postmarketing studies have shown both brimonidine 0.2% and brimonidine-P 0.15% to be effective adjunctive agents when used with a PGA, producing additional reductions in IOP ranging from 2.0 to 5.1 mmHg.[27,28]

### 52.2.2 Beta-Blockers

The nonselective beta-blockers include carteolol, levobunolol, metipranolol, and timolol. The cardioselective agent betaxolol is somewhat less effective at IOP reduction than the nonselective agents, but is also less likely to induce pulmonary side effects in patients with asthma or other types of airway disease. Beta-blockers lower IOP by decreasing production of aqueous humor during waking hours.[29] Recent reports indicate that these agents have minimal effect on aqueous humor production at night,[30] however, and thus are often less effective at reducing IOP during nighttime hours.[31]

Early experience using a beta-blocker as an adjunctive agent for a PGA seemed promising. Once-daily beta-blocker therapy and use of an aqueous inflow suppressant combined with the aqueous outflow enhancing properties of the PGA made sense clinically because of complementary mechanisms of action. Using a beta-blocker (an aqueous suppressant) in the morning and a PGA (outflow enhancer) at night is a simple regimen for the patient to follow. Furthermore, initial reports of a small number of patients showed additional reductions in IOP ranging from 14 to 21% when timolol 0.5% was added to latanoprost 0.005%.[32,33] More recent studies, however, have been less encouraging. Bucci[34] found a similar reduction in mean diurnal IOP using the combination of latanoprost and timolol when compared to latanoprost alone ($6.1 \pm 0.3$ mmHg vs. $5.5 \pm 0.3$ mmHg). More recently, Manni and colleagues[35] found no statistically significant difference in mean diurnal IOP in patients treated with either bimatoprost 0.03% versus latanoprost and timolol after 6 months of therapy. Higginbotham and coworkers[36] compared latanoprost monotherapy to fixed combination latanoprost/timolol and found that after 6 months of therapy, the fixed combination product produced a final mean diurnal IOP less than 1 mmHg lower than latanoprost alone ($19.9 \pm 3.4$ mmHg vs. $20.8 \pm 4.6$ mmHg). Due to the lack of additional IOP-lowering efficacy produced by the beta-blocker shown in this and other fixed combination products, at this time, the US Food and Drug Administration has not formally approved any PGA/beta-blocker combination agent for clinical use and it appears unlikely these PGA/beta-blocker products will ever come to market in the USA. Some PGA/beta-blocker combinations have been approved outside the United States. These include DuoTrav (travoprost/timolol), Ganfort (bimatoprost/timolol), and Xalacom (latanoprost/timolol).

### 52.2.3 Topical Carbonic Anhydrase Inhibitors

Like beta-blockers, topical CAIs, which include brinzolamide and dorzolamide, reduce IOP by decreasing aqueous humor production.[37,38] Although the topical CAIs are formally approved for three-times-a-day dosing, most clinicians use these agents twice a day, especially when used as adjunctive medications. Brinzolamide taken twice daily has been shown to be equally effective as either brinzolamide or dorzolamide taken three times daily in patients with open-angle glaucoma or ocular hypertension.[39] Studies evaluating the efficacy of dorzolamide when used adjunctively with latanoprost demonstrate additional IOP reduction of up to 3 mmHg and overall reduction in IOP of about 40% from baseline.[40,41] Brinzolamide has also been shown to be additive to the PGAs, producing an additional 4.2 mmHg (18.4%) reduction in IOP when used in patients with open-angle glaucoma or ocular hypertension treated with travoprost[42] and an additional 5.2 mmHg (24.6%) reduction in IOP when used adjunctively with latanoprost.[43] Moreover, the combination of a topical CAI and a PGA appears to be very effective at controlling IOP on a 24-h basis. A recent study by Nakamoto and Yasuda[44] revealed that both diurnal and nocturnal mean IOP were reduced significantly more with the combination of brinzolamide and latanoprost than with latanoprost alone in 22 patients with normal tension glaucoma after 8 weeks of therapy (diurnal mean IOP reduction: latanoprost and brinzolamide = 19.8%, latanoprost alone = 14.1%, $p<0.001$; nocturnal mean IOP reduction: latanoprost and brinzolamide = 13.4%, latanoprost = 10.0%, $p<0.05$).

## 52.3 Studies Comparing Adjunctive Agents for Glaucoma Therapy

Until recently, most comparative glaucoma drug studies found in the literature focused on head-to-head comparisons of single agents used as monotherapy. As medical therapy

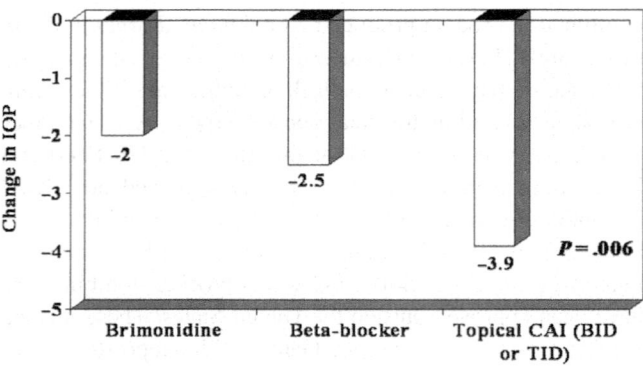

**Fig. 52.2** Agents used in combination with PGAs. Results from a retrospective comparison of additional reduction in IOP produced by various agents when used in combination with latanoprost in patients with glaucoma or ocular hypertension

for glaucoma has grown increasingly complex, however, the need has arisen to design trials that can help to determine the safest and most effective combination of agents for our patients. In 2002, O'Connor and colleagues[45] published one of the first studies to compare the efficacy of different medications used in combination with a PGA. This retrospective review compared the additional IOP reduction produced by timolol, brimonidine, or dorzolamide when added to latanoprost in 73 glaucoma patients with inadequately controlled IOP. After 1 year of therapy, dorzolamide, taken either two or three times daily, produced the greatest additional IOP reduction (3.9 mmHg), followed by timolol (2.5 mmHg) and brimonidine (2.0 mmHg) ($p=0.006$) (Fig. 52.2). More recently, Reis and colleagues[46] compared timolol, brinzolamide, or brimonidine used adjunctively with travoprost in a prospective, randomized, investigator-masked study. After 4 weeks of therapy, both timolol and brinzolamide produced significantly greater additional IOP reduction compared to brimonidine ($3.9 \pm 1.8$ mmHg vs. $4.0 \pm 2.1$ mmHg vs. $2.3 \pm 1.8$ mmHg, $p=0.01$). Following the publication of these two studies, other head-to-head comparisons of adjunctive agents used with a PGA for the treatment of glaucoma began to appear in the literature.

### 52.3.1 Brimonidine Versus Topical CAIs

In a prospective, double-masked, crossover comparison, Konstas and colleagues[47] found that brimonidine-P 0.15% and dorzolamide 2%, each used twice daily, produced equivalent final mean 24-h IOP when added to latanoprost in 31 patients with open-angle glaucoma or ocular hypertension after 6 months of therapy (brimonidine-P: $16.9 \pm 1.5$ mmHg, dorzolamide: $16.8 \pm 1.5$ mmHg, $p=0.66$). More recently, Noecker and colleagues[48] compared brimonidine-P 0.15% with dorzolamide 2% as adjunctive therapy to latanoprost in 70 patients with glaucoma or ocular hypertension in a prospective, randomized, double-masked clinical trial. After 3 months, the additional IOP reduction produced by each agent was statistically equivalent at both peak (brimonidine-P: 6.0 mmHg, dorzolamide: 4.6 mmHg, $p=0.167$) and trough (2.7 mmHg vs. 2.9 mmHg, $p=0.810$). In another study, however, Feldman and colleagues[49] found greater additional mean IOP reduction produced by the topical CAI compared to brimonidine-P when added to patients treated with travoprost. In this prospective, randomized, double-masked trial, final mean diurnal IOP was significantly lower in patients treated with adjunctive brinzolamide 1.0% than brimonidine-P 0.15% after 3 months of therapy ($18.6 \pm 0.25$ mmHg vs. $19.3 \pm 0.27$ mmHg, $p=0.035$).

### 52.3.2 Beta-Blockers Versus Topical CAIs

In a prospective, randomized, double-masked clinical trial, Hollo and colleagues[50] compared timolol to brinzolamide, each given twice daily as adjunctive therapy, to patients treated with travoprost. After 3 months, final mean diurnal IOP was statistically equivalent ($18.1 \pm 2.7$ mmHg vs. $18.1 \pm 3.0$ mmHg, $p=0.96$). Martinez-de-la-Casa and colleagues[51] found greater overall IOP reduction produced by concomitant travoprost and brinzolamide than with fixed combination latanoprost/timolol (Fig. 52.3). After 3 months of therapy, final mean diurnal IOP was $16.9 \pm 0.9$ mmHg for the concomitant therapy group versus $18.1 \pm 1.0$ mmHg for the fixed combination group ($p=0.015$).

### 52.3.3 Beta-Blockers Versus Brimonidine

Netland and colleagues[52] compared brimonidine-P and bimatoprost versus timolol and latanoprost in 28 patients with glaucoma or ocular hypertension in a prospective, multicenter trial. After 3 months of therapy, each treatment group achieved statistically equivalent reductions in IOP from baseline ranging from 8.5 to 9.0 mmHg for brimonidine-P/bimatoprost and 7.5 to 7.7 mmHg for timolol/latanoprost ($p=$NS). A significantly higher percentage of patients treated with brimonidine-P/bimatoprost in this study achieved a final IOP of 16 mmHg or lower (69.2% vs. 27.3%, $p=0.024$). More recently, Mundorf and colleagues[53] compared brimonidine-P 0.15% and timolol as adjunctive therapy with either latanoprost or bimatoprost in 77 patients

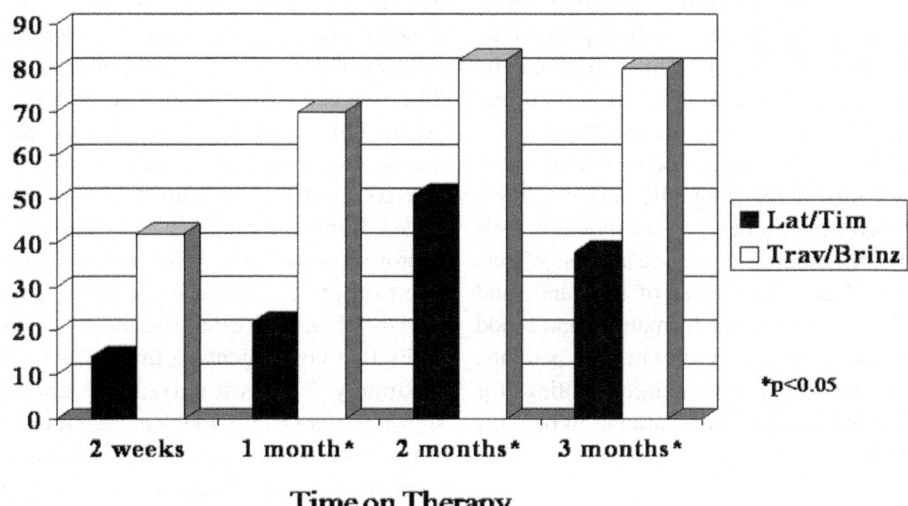

**Fig. 52.3** Concomitant travoprost/brinzolamide versus fixed combination latanoprost/timolol. Comparison of the percentages of patients achieving IOP of less than 18 mmHg following treatment with either concomitant travoprost/brinzolamide or fixed combination latanoprost/timolol. (Reproduced from Whitson, JT. "Glaucoma: a review of adjunctive therapy and new management strategies," Expert Opinion on Pharmacotherapy, 2007, Dec. 8(18):3237-3249, with kind permission of Informa UK Ltd.)

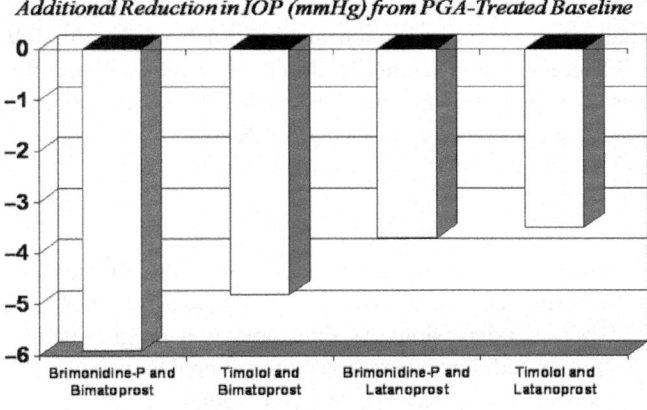

**Fig. 52.4** Brimonidine-P 0.15% versus timolol 0.5% adjunctive therapy with PGAs. Additional reduction in mean IOP produced by either timolol or brimonidine-P when added to either bimatoprost or latanoprost after 3 months of therapy. (Reproduced from Whitson, JT. "Glaucoma: a review of adjunctive therapy and new management strategies," Expert Opinion on Pharmacotherapy, 2007, Dec. 8(18):3237-3249, with kind permission of Informa UK Ltd.)

with glaucoma or ocular hypertension. After 3 months, brimonidine-P produced greater reduction in mean IOP than timolol when added to bimatoprost (5.9 mmHg vs. 4.8 mmHg). The two agents, however, were comparable when added to latanoprost (3.7 mmHg vs. 3.5 mmHg) (Fig. 52.4).

## 52.4 Other Options for Adjunctive Glaucoma Therapy

In modern clinical practice, the primary choices for adjunctive therapy for patients treated with a PGA typically include a beta-blocker, brimonidine, or a topical CAI. Two other options for adjunctive medical therapy may also be considered in some situations. These include the cholinergics and the oral CAIs.

The cholinergics, or miotics, include both direct-acting (pilocarpine) and indirect-acting (echothiophate iodide) agents. These medications reduce IOP by increasing aqueous humor outflow through the trabecular meshwork pathway.[54] They cause contraction of the ciliary muscle that stretches the trabecular meshwork, which is anchored at the scleral spur. Pilocarpine may work against the increased facilitation of uveoscleral outflow induced by PGAs, because of decreased interstitial space between muscle fiber bundles of the contracted ciliary body.[55] Studies have shown additional reduction in IOP of at least 15% when pilocarpine is added to ocular hypertensive patients treated with latanoprost.[56–61] Pilocarpine is available in concentrations ranging from 0.5 to 6.0%. Disadvantages of pilocarpine include its four-times-a-day dosing regimen, induced myopia and accommodative spasm in younger patients, and reduction of vision from pupillary miosis in patients with cataractous lens changes.

Older, pseudophakic patients, however, often tolerate this drug well. A once-daily 4% ophthalmic gel is also available, which is usually dosed at bedtime. When prescribing both pilocarpine gel and a PGA at bedtime, it is important to instruct the patient to use the gel at least 5 min after instillation of the PGA to ensure complete absorption of the eye drop.

The oral CAIs include acetazolamide and methazolamide. These drugs are very effective at reducing IOP, and have shown additivity to PGAs in clinical studies.[62] Unfortunately, their use is often limited by the numerous systemic adverse effects they produce, which include paresthesias of the hands and feet, nausea, weight loss, kidney stone formation, and blood dyscrasias.[63–73] Due to their poor tolerability in most patients, the oral CAIs are most commonly used in urgent settings for acute reduction in IOP or as short-term treatment in patients on maximal topical therapy.

## 52.5 Fixed Combination Agents

For those patients who require more than one glaucoma medication for adequate IOP control, fixed combination agents offer several practical advantages over concomitant therapy. By combining two drugs in one bottle, compliance may be enhanced through a simplified regimen. Also, less exposure to preservatives such as BAK occurs, and the potential for "washout effect" is eliminated. Finally, depending on the patient's insurance benefits, lower copayments may benefit the patient economically and, therefore, also contribute to better compliance.

Currently, two fixed combination glaucoma products are available for clinical use in the United States. Timolol 0.5%/dorzolamide 2.0% (Cosopt) was introduced in 1998. Cosopt reduces IOP by 27–33% from baseline and provides similar 24-h IOP control to latanoprost in patients with glaucoma or ocular hypertension.[74,75] A postmarketing open-label trial has demonstrated that Cosopt further lowers IOP by 29% ($p<0.001$) when used adjunctively with latanoprost.[76] Timolol 0.5%/ brimonidine 2.0% (Combigan) has recently been approved for use by the US Food and Drug Administration, and like Cosopt, it is dosed twice daily. Combigan reduces IOP by 4.4–7.6 mmHg from baseline and is equivalent in efficacy to its two components – timolol and brimonidine – taken separately.[77] Interestingly, large comparative trials have shown a significantly lower allergy rate with the fixed combination product Combigan when compared to brimonidine 0.2% alone.[77] Combigan is also a very effective adjunctive agent, further reducing IOP by 6.9 mmHg (29%) from a PGA-treated baseline.[78]

Fixed combination products have been developed for each of the PGAs (bimatoprost, latanoprost, and travoprost) with timolol. Both bimatoprost 0.03%/timolol 0.5% (Ganfort) and travoprost 0.004%/timolol 0.5% (DuoTrav) have been shown to produce comparable reductions in IOP when compared to their individual components taken concomitantly.[79,80] Moreover, latanoprost 0.005%/timolol 0.5% fixed combination (Xalacom) produces greater reduction in IOP than either latanoprost or timolol taken alone.[36] Each of the timolol/PGA combination agents is dosed once daily. Currently, none are approved for clinical use in the United States but are available in other parts of the world (Sidebar 52.1).

---

**Sidebar 52.1 Combination medical therapy for glaucoma**

Todd D. Severin

Medical therapy remains the mainstay for the first-line treatment of glaucoma. While medical monotherapy (the use of one topical medication for intraocular pressure control) is the preferred medical regimen, several limitations to successful monotherapy exist. Primarily, in a large number of patients being treated for glaucoma, monotherapy has the potential to lose its effectiveness over time. There may be several mechanisms for this loss of effectiveness, but two primary mechanisms have been discussed:

1. Tachyphylaxis: The GLT demonstrated the prevalence of tachyphylaxis to beta-blocker monotherapy. After 2 years of therapy, 50% of the beta-blocker treated patients lost effectiveness with initial therapy, requiring additional medications to maintain control.
2. Disease progression: As glaucoma is a progressive disease, additional therapy is often required to maintain adequate intraocular pressure (IOP) control to prevent glaucomatous disk damage. In the Collaborative Initial Glaucoma Treatment Study (CIGTS) trial, >75% of patients required ≥2 agents to reach target IOP after 2 years. The Ocular Hypertension Treatment Study (OHTS) demonstrated that 49% of patients required ≥2 agents to reach 20% IOP reduction at 5 years.

In all, pharmacy surveillance data has demonstrated that greater than 40% of all glaucoma patients require adjunctive therapy to maintain adequate IOP control.

Historically, when monotherapy fails to adequately control IOP, the clinician has two medical choices: switch therapy to a different monotherapeutic agent or add additional agents to the primary monotherapy. Switch therapy is a relatively new term in the glaucoma vernacular. Simply, it states that if one agent fails to adequately control IOP (i.e., a prostaglandin) successful monotherapy may still be achieved with the substitution of a different prostaglandin agent or another monotherapeutic agent, like a beta-blocker.

When switch therapy has failed to maintain adequate control with a monotherapeutic agent, additional agents must be added to the primary therapy. While often effective, this medical regimen, called adjunctive therapy, has several limitations:

1. Lack of efficacy of additional medications: A 2004 study by Neelakantan and colleagues found that adding a third or fourth antiglaucoma medication only produced a clinically significant reduction in IOP in 40–60% of patients. Based on Kaplan–Meier analysis, the cumulative probability of achieving success in lowering IOP when both efficacy and safety are considered was:

    - 27% for a third medication and 31% for a fourth medication at 6 months
    - 14% for both a third and fourth medication at 1 year

2. Medication washout: It is important for patients using multiple eyedrops to wait an appropriate amount of time after the instillation of the first drug before instilling the second medication to avoid "washing out" or diluting the first drug. Suggested time interval between drops by consensus is at least 5 min, a duration many patients find difficult to maintain, particularly when combined with the recommended eyelid closure or punctual occlusion.
3. Preservative load: Benzalkonium chloride (BAK), the main preservative used in ophthalmologic medications, has been shown to increase the incidence of ocular surface disease through damage to epithelial cells and epithelial cell tight junctions. As BAK is present in most antiglaucoma preparations, the use of multiple medications to control glaucoma may result in an increased exposure to BAK, putting the patient at risk of developing ocular surface disease.
4. Adherence with medical regimen: Adding medications to a patient's treatment regimen affects compliance or adherence to the prescribed regimen. In one study, nonadherence was documented in 67.7% of patients taking more than one medication. In another study by Robin and Covert, it was discovered that adding a second agent to a patient's regimen affected the patient's adherence to the first medication. Of 1,784 patients who used two different medications, the average refill interval for the first medication was 40.6 days before the addition of adjunctive therapy and 47.4 days after the addition of adjunctive therapy, demonstrating an increased lack of adherence to the prescribed medical regimen.

One solution to overcome these limitations of adjunctive therapy is the use of two or more medications combined in fixed concentrations into one bottle – a treatment option known as *combination therapy*. Theoretically, combination therapy offers several distinct advantages over the standard approach to adjunctive therapy:

- Fewer bottles
- Fewer daily drops
- Improved compliance
- Minimizes possible confusion
- Eliminates potential washout effect
- Possibly better efficacy than the two agents used separately
- Cost-effectiveness for patients by reducing number of co-pays for prescriptions
- Allows for simpler treatment regimens

Currently, there are several combination agents available for the treatment of glaucoma:

- Cosopt – dorzolamide/timolol
- Combigan – brimonidine/timolol
- E-pilo – epinephrine/timolol
- Timpilo – pilocarpine/timolol
- Ganfort – bimatoprost/timolol
- DuoTrav – travoprost/timolol
- Xalacom – latanoprost/timolol

Only two fixed combination agents from this list are currently available in the United States: dorzolamide/timolol and brimonidine/timolol. Both combination medications have been shown to be at least as effective at lowering IOP as the individual constituents within each combination. In one study, 74 glaucoma patients previously using dorzolamide plus a topical beta-blocker were switched to fixed combination dorzolamide/timolol in one eye. The previous dorzolamide and topical beta-blocker concomitant regimen was continued in the other eye as an internal control. The authors concluded that in a real-life clinical practice, the dorzolamide/timolol fixed combination provided significantly greater IOP lowering than its components taken separately. This benefit is felt to be related to the previously mentioned decrease in medication washout.

Two identical, multicenter, randomized, double-masked, 12-month clinical studies, with enrollment of greater than 1,000 patients have also demonstrated the fixed brimonidine/timolol combination to be safe, well-tolerated, and equally as effective as concomitant administration of the two separate components.

A systematic review of the literature on the efficacy of fixed combination therapy compared to their unfixed components in reducing intraocular pressure was performed by Cox et al. In this paper, the authors concluded that based on the evidence available up to May 2007 fixed combination therapies were equally safe and effective in reducing IOP as the nonfixed components administered concomitantly. The main side effects reported in these studies were hyperemia, ocular irritation, and keratitis.

Any usage of fixed combination products needs to be appropriate and accompanied by a clear understanding of the risk, side effects, and possible negatives of combination therapy. While generally shown to be safe, combination therapy:

1. Is associated with the combined side effects of the component medications used concomitantly.
2. Must be administered with a clear understanding of the contraindications to the usage of each of the component medications.
3. Reaction to one component of the combination would require the discontinuation of the entire combination product.
4. May be costlier than individual therapy, particularly with the usage of generic equivalents.

Fixed combinations, thereby, offer an attractive alternative to traditional adjunctive therapy. Employing these newer agents, patients may be able to effectively control their IOP with fewer bottles of medicine and potentially fewer side effects with easier adherence. Employing these agents, a stepwise approach to medical therapy would be:

1. Initiation of monotherapy agent, primarily a prostaglandin analog or beta-blocker.
2. If target pressure is not reached, consideration of switching therapy to another monotherapy agent.
3. If the switch is ineffective or not instituted, adjunctive therapy can be instituted with complementary mechanism to primary agent, such as a topical carbonic anhydrase inhibitor, alpha-agonist, or beta-blocker added to a prostaglandin.
4. Consideration can be given to changing a two-drug regimen (i.e., prostaglandin and beta-blocker) to appropriate combination if available.
5. If the first adjunct is not effective at reaching target pressure (i.e., prostaglandin and timolol), discontinue the first adjunct and institute combination therapy, resulting in a combination of prostaglandin analog and either timolol/dorzolamide fixed combo or timolol/brimonidine fixed combo.
6. Adjunctive therapy can be stepwise increased by adding the final complementary adjunctive agent, resulting in combinations of prostaglandin/fixed timolol–dorzolamide and brimonidine or prostaglandin/fixed timolol–brimonidine and dorzolamide.

As such, combination therapy may offer the clinician an effective alternative to the traditional concept of adjunctive therapy. By providing a fixed combination of more than one medication in each bottle, combination therapy may result in an easier, more effective medical regimen for glaucoma patients.

## Bibliography

Boger WP 3rd. Short-term "escape" and longterm "drift." The dissipation effects of the beta adrenergic blocking agents. *Surv Ophthalmol.* 1983;28(suppl):235-242.

Choudhri S, Wand M, Shields MB. A comparison of dorzolamide-timolol combination versus the concomitant drugs. *Am J Ophthalmol.* 2000;130:832-833.

Cox JA, Mollan SP, Bankart J, Robinson R. Efficacy of antiglaucoma fixed combination therapy versus unfixed components in reducing intraocular pressure: a systematic review. *Br J Ophthalmol.* 2008;92:729-734.

Lichter PR, Musch DC, Gillespie BW; the CIGTS Study Group. Interim clinical outcomes in the Collaborative Initial Glaucoma Treatment Study comparing initial treatment randomized to medications or surgery. *Ophthalmology.* 2001;108:1943-1953.

National Drug Code Data, July 2005. <http://www.fda.gov/cder/ndc/> Accessed 03.04.09.

Neelakantan A, Vaishnav HD, Iyer SA, Sherwood MB. Is addition of a third or fourth antiglaucoma medication effective? *J Glaucoma.* 2004;13:130-136.

Patel SC, Spaeth GL. Compliance in patients prescribed eyedrops for glaucoma. *Ophthalmic Surg.* 1995;26:233-235.

Pisella PJ, Pouliquen P, Baudouin C. Prevalence of ocular symptoms and signs with preserved and preservative free glaucoma medication. *Br J Ophthalmol.* 2002;86:418-423.

Robin AL, Covert D. Does adjunctive glaucoma therapy affect adherence to the initial primary therapy? *Ophthalmology.* 2005;112:863-868.

Sherwood, Craven ER, Chou C, et al. Twice-daily 0.2% brimonidine-0.5% timolol fixed combination therapy vs monotherapy with timolol or brimonidine in patients with glaucoma or ocular hypertension: a 12-month randomized trial. *Arch Ophthalmol.* 2006; 124(9):1230-1238.

## 52.6 Limitations/Other Treatment Options

While the traditional stepwise approach for adding medications is usually effective for control of IOP, adjunctive glaucoma therapy does have limitations. In particular, once two or three bottles of drugs are being used by the patient, the addition of more medication to that patient's regimen is often not successful at producing further reduction in IOP. Neelakantan and colleagues[81] have shown that adding a third or fourth bottle of medication to a patient's existing regimen results in a 20% or greater additional reduction in IOP only 14% of the time. Moreover, patients with more complex drug regimens are less likely to be compliant with therapy than those with simpler ones.[14]

For those patients on maximal-tolerated medical therapy who need further reduction in IOP, other options include laser trabeculoplasty and filtration surgery. Both argon laser trabeculoplasty (ALT) and selective laser trabeculoplasty (SLT) reduce IOP by increasing outflow of aqueous humor through the trabecular meshwork pathway.[82,83] ALT was described over 20 years ago and involves the placement of evenly spaced, nonpenetrating argon laser burns over the circumference of the trabecular meshwork. SLT employs a Q-switched, frequency-doubled Nd:YAG laser to selectively deliver energy to pigmented trabecular meshwork cells in a process termed photothermolysis. Comparable reductions in IOP between ALT and SLT have been reported.[84] Since SLT is thought to be less destructive to the architecture of the trabecular meshwork, it may be more repeatable than ALT. Eyes with previously failed ALT have been shown to respond better to SLT than to repeat ALT (reduction in IOP: $6.8 \pm 2.4$ mmHg with SLT vs. $3.6 \pm 1.8$ mmHg with repeat ALT, $p = 0.01$).[85] Like other treatment options for glaucoma, a more robust IOP response is typically seen with laser trabeculoplasty the earlier it is used in the treatment paradigm. Finally, filtration surgery, or trabeculectomy, may be used in those patients who are refractory to both medical and laser therapy. Trabeculectomy surgery involves the creation of a fistula into the anterior chamber and subsequent drainage of aqueous humor into the subconjunctival space, which results in the formation of a filtration "bleb." Antifibrotic agents, such as 5-fluorouracil or mitomycin-C, may reduce the postoperative subconjunctival scarring response and improve the success rate of trabeculectomy surgery.[86,87]

## 52.7 Beyond IOP: Diastolic Ocular Perfusion Pressure

While reduction of IOP remains the cornerstone for effective glaucoma therapy, several recent population-based, epidemiologic studies have demonstrated that low diastolic ocular perfusion pressure (DOPP) is an important and potentially modifiable risk factor for this disease. DOPP may be defined as:

$$DOPP = DBP - -IOP$$

where DBP stands for diastolic blood pressure. The proposed mechanism is that lower DOPP at the optic nerve head compromises ocular blood flow thus leading to glaucomatous damage.[88] The Baltimore Eye Survey,[89] the Egna-Neumarkt Study,[90] and the Proyecto Ver[91] each showed significantly higher prevalence rates for glaucoma among patients with lower DOPP. In the Barbados Eye Study,[92,93] low DOPP was a significant risk factor for the development of new cases of glaucoma in a large cohort of African-Caribbeans after both 4 and 9 years of follow-up.

A recent study by Quaranta and coworkers[94] has shown that topical glaucoma medications can affect DOPP in patients with glaucoma. In this prospective, double-masked, randomized study, 27 patients with newly diagnosed glaucoma were treated with timolol 0.5% at 8 A.M. and 8 P.M., brimonidine 0.2% at 8 A.M. and 8 P.M., dorzolamide 2% at 8 A.M., 2 P.M. and 8 P.M., and latanoprost 0.005% at 8 P.M. The duration of each treatment period was 6 weeks, with a 4-week washout period between each treatment. IOP and systemic blood pressure were measured around the clock at 2-h intervals at baseline and after each treatment period. Each medication lowered IOP significantly at all time points compared to baseline. Mean 24-h DOPPs were $50.7 \pm 5.9$ mmHg at baseline, $53 \pm 5.5$ mmHg with timolol, $46.2 \pm 5.4$ mmHg with brimonidine, $55.9 \pm 4.6$ mmHg with dorzolamide, and $56.4 \pm 4.9$ mmHg with latanoprost. Because of the significant reduction it induced in systemic blood pressure, mean 24-h DOPP was significantly lowered by brimonidine compared to baseline ($p < 0.0001$). Treatment with dorzolamide or latanoprost caused no reduction in systemic blood pressure, however, and as a result, each of these drugs produced a significant increase in 24-h DOPP ($p < 0.001$). While this is a relatively short-term study, it does raise some interesting questions on the effect that topical medications may have on DOPP with chronic treatment that require further investigation.

## 52.8 Conclusion: Making Sense of Adjunctive Glaucoma Therapy

The introduction of the PGAs for glaucoma therapy has had a dramatic impact on the medical treatment of this disease. These agents offer a number of advantages over other classes of medications, including robust reductions in IOP in most patients, effective pressure control on a 24-h basis, once-daily therapy, and very few systemic safety concerns. For these reasons and more, the PGAs have become a favored first-line choice for glaucoma therapy among many ophthalmologists.

It is clear from the literature review discussed in this chapter, however, that no single class of medication has emerged as the ideal adjunctive agent for a PGA. Each of the three commonly used classes of adjunctive agents – beta-blockers, brimonidine, and topical CAIs – offers distinct advantages and disadvantages for the patient. Beta-blockers were introduced for clinical use more than 25 years ago and were once a mainstay for first-line glaucoma therapy. Following the introduction of latanoprost in 1996, the use of a PGA/beta-blocker regimen became a popular combination for glaucoma therapy among many ophthalmologists. Advantages of beta-blockers include once-daily formulations and the availability of generics. However, recent studies have shown that beta-blockers may not be the most effective option for adjunctive therapy in many patients with glaucoma. Beta-blockers often provide minimal additional IOP reduction when added to a PGA.[34–36] Moreover, these agents have little effect on aqueous humor production during nighttime hours[30] and may result in poor nocturnal IOP control.[31]

Brimonidine-P (0.15 or 0.1%) has been shown to add effectively to a PGA.[26–28] It is also formulated with the preservative, Purite®, which is gentler on the ocular surface than other products preserved with BAK, especially in those patients with dry eye or ocular surface disease. Brimonidine-P also has a significantly lower allergy rate than the original 0.2% solution preserved with BAK.[25] Moreover, brimonidine-P is devoid of many of the systemic adverse effects associated with beta-blockers and can be used safely in patients with asthma or other types of restrictive airway disease. Disadvantages of brimonidine-P include less consistent 24-h IOP control compared with PGAs or topical CAIs.[75,95]

The topical CAIs also add effectively to a PGA.[40–44] This class of agents offers excellent 24-h IOP control and is safe and well-tolerated by most patients. While it is still unclear which adjunctive agent is best for a PGA, most of the comparative studies published to date favor the topical CAIs over the beta-blockers[45,51] or brimonidine.[45,46,49] Within the topical CAI class, most patients prefer brinzolamide to dorzolamide due to its more neutral pH and less likelihood to sting upon instillation.[96] Some patients, however, prefer the solution dorzolamide to the foreign body sensation produced by the particulate crystals in the suspension brinzolamide. Both of the topical CAIs may produce a transient metallic taste in some patients following instillation.[97,98] While the topical CAIs are devoid of many of the serious systemic effects seen with the oral CAIs, they should be avoided in patients with a known sulfa hypersensitivity.

The medical management of glaucoma has changed greatly in recent years. In particular, the introduction of the PGAs has had a dramatic impact on the way ophthalmologists manage their patients. Furthermore, safe and effective adjunctive agents, such as brimonidine and the topical CAIs, have given us new therapeutic options for those patients who need greater reduction in IOP than that provided by a PGA alone. Comparative studies are currently underway to help determine the most effective option for adjunctive therapy. While there is clearly no ideal drug, or combination of drugs, for each and every patient, we now have a variety of agents from which to choose to help us individualize our treatment strategies and better care for our patients with glaucoma.

This work was supported in part by an unrestricted educational grant from Research to Prevent Blindness, New York, New York.

## References

1. American Academy of Ophthalmology. *Primary open-angle glaucoma, preferred practice pattern*. San Francisco: American Academy of Ophthalmology. <http://one.aao.org/CE/Practice Guidelines/PPP_Content.aspx?cid=a5a59e02-450b-4d50-8091-b2d-d21ef1ff2>; 2005 Accessed 31.01.08.
2. Zimmerman TJ, Kaufman HE. Timolol. A beta-adrenergic blocking agent for the treatment of glaucoma. *Arch Ophthalmol*. 1977;95(4): 601–604.
3. Soltau JB, Zimmerman TJ. Changing paradigms in the medical treatment of glaucoma. *Surv Ophthalmol*. 2002;47(Suppl 1):S2–S5.
4. Lee PY, Podos SM, Severin C. Effect of prostaglandin F2 alpha on aqueous humor dynamics of rabbit, cat, and monkey. *Invest Ophthalmol Vis Sci*. 1984;25(9):1087–1093.
5. Brubaker RF, Schoff EO, Nau CB, et al. Effects of AGN 192024, a new ocular hypotensive agent, on aqueous dynamics. *Am J Ophthalmol*. 2001;131(1):19–24.
6. Toris CB, Camras CB, Yablonski ME. Effects of PhXA41, a new prostaglandin F2 alpha analog, on aqueous humor dynamics in human eyes. *Ophthalmology*. 1993;100(9):1297–1304.
7. Ziai N, Dolan JW, Kacere RD, Brubaker RF. The effects on aqueous dynamics of PhXA41, a new prostaglandin F2_ analogue, after topical application in normal and ocular hypertensive human eyes. *Arch Ophthalmol*. 1993;111:1351–1358.
8. Camras CB, Siebold EC, Lustgarten JS, et al. Maintained reduction of intraocular pressure by prostaglandin F2_-1- isopropyl ester applied in multiple doses in ocular hypertensive and glaucoma patients. *Ophthalmology*. 1989;96:1329–1337.
9. Christiansen GA, Nau CB, McLaren JW, Johnson DH. Mechanism of Ocular Hypotensive Action of Bimatoprost (Lumigan) in Patients with Ocular Hypertension or Glaucoma. *Ophthalmology*. 2004; 111:1658–1662.
10. Parrish RK, Palmberg P, Sheu WP. A comparison of latanoprost, bimatoprost, and travoprost in patients with elevated intraocular pressure: a 12-week, randomized, masked-evaluator, multicenter study. *Am J Ophthalmol*. 2003;135:688–703.
11. Asrani S, Zeimer R, Wilensky J, et al. Large diurnal fluctuations in intraocular pressure are an independent risk factor in patients with glaucoma. *J Glaucoma*. 2000;9(2):134–142.
12. Hedman K, Watson PG, Alm A. The effect of latanoprost on intraocular pressure during 2 years of treatment. *Surv Ophthalmol*. 2002;47(Suppl 1):S65–S76.

13. Chrai SS, Makoid MC, Eriksen SP, et al. Drop size and initial dosing frequency problems of topically applied ophthalmic drugs. *J Pharm Sci.* 1974;63(3):333–338.
14. Patel SC, Spaeth GL. Compliance in patients prescribed glaucoma medications. *Ophthalmic Surg.* 1995;26(3):233–236.
15. Broadway DC, Grierson I, O'Brien C, et al. Adverse effects of topical antiglaucoma medication. *Arch Ophthalmol.* 1994;112:1437-1445.
16. Kass MA, Heuer DK, Higginbotham EJ, et al. The ocular hypertension treatment study: a randomized trial determines that topical ocular hypotensive medication delays or prevents the onset of primary open-angle glaucoma. *Arch Ophthalmol.* 2002;120(6):701–713.
17. Lichter PR, Musch DC, Gillespie BW, et al. Interim clinical outcomes in the collaborative initial glaucoma treatment study comparing initial treatment randomized to medications or surgery. *Ophthalmology.* 2001;108(11):1943–1953.
18. Covert D, Robin AL. Adjunctive glaucoma therapy use associated with travoprost, bimatoprost, and latanoprost. *Curr Med Res Opin.* 2006;22(5):971–976.
19. Van der Valk R, Webers CA, Schouten JS, Zeegers MP, Hendrikse F, Prins MH. Intraocular pressure–lowering effects of all commonly used glaucoma drugs: a meta-analysis of randomized trials. *Ophthalmology.* 2005;112:1177–1185.
20. Gandolfi SA, Cimino L. Effect of bimatoprost on patients with primary open-angle glaucoma or ocular hypertension who are non-responders to latanoprost. *Ophthalmology.* 2003;110(3):609–614.
21. Realini T, Fechtner RD. 56, 000 ways to treat glaucoma. *Ophthalmology.* 2002;109(11):1955–1956.
22. Hughes E, Spry P, Diamond J. 24-hour monitoring of intraocular pressure in glaucoma management: a retrospective review. *J Glaucoma.* 2003;12(3):232–236.
23. Nouri-Mahdavi K, Hoffman D, Coleman AL, et al. Predictive factors for glaucomatous visual field progression in the Advanced Glaucoma Intervention Study. *Ophthalmology.* 2004;111(9):1627–1635.
24. Toris CB, Gleason ML, Camras CB, et al. Effects of brimonidine on aqueous humor dynamics in human eyes. *Arch Ophthalmol.* 1995;113: 1514–1517.
25. Katz LJ. Twelve-month evaluation of brimonidine-purite in patients with glaucoma or ocular hypertension. *J Glaucoma.* 2002;11:119–126.
26. Lee DA, Gornbein JA. Effectiveness and safety of brimonidine as adjunctive therapy for patients with elevated intraocular pressure in a large, open-label community trial. *J Glaucoma.* 2001;10(3): 220–226.
27. Erdogan H, Toker I, Arici MK, et al. A short-term study of the additive effect of latanoprost 0.005% and brimonidine 0.2%. *Jpn J Ophthalmol.* 2003;47(5):473–478.
28. Mundorf T, Noecker RJ, Earl M. Ocular hypotensive efficacy of brimonidine 0.15% as adjunctive therapy with latanoprost 0.005% in patients with open-angle glaucoma or ocular hypertension. *Adv Ther.* 2007;24:302–309.
29. Wilson RP, Kanal N, Spaeth GL. Timolol: its effectiveness in different types of glaucoma. *Ophthalmology.* 1979;86:43–50.
30. Rettig ES, Larsson LI, Brubaker RF. The effect of topical timolol on epinephrine-stimulated aqueous humor flow in sleeping humans. *Invest Ophthalmol Vis Sci.* 1994;35:554–559.
31. Liu JH, Kripke DF, Weinreb RN. Comparison of the nocturnal effects of once-daily timolol and latanoprost on intraocular pressure. *Am J Ophthalmol.* 2004;138:389–395.
32. Rulo AH, Greve EL, Hoyng PF. Additive effect of latanoprost, a prostaglandin F2 alpha analogue and timolol in patients with elevated intraocular pressure. *Br J Ophthalmol.* 1994;78(12):899–902.
33. Stewart WC, Day DG, Sharpe ED, et al. Efficacy and safety of timolol solution once daily vs. timolol gel added to latanoprost. *Am J Ophthalmol.* 1999;128(6):692–696.
34. Bucci MG. Intraocular pressure-lowering effects of latanoprost monotherapy versus latanoprost or pilocarpine in combination with timolol: a randomized, observer-masked multicenter study in patients with open-angle glaucoma. Italian Latanoprost Study Group. *J Glaucoma.* 1999;8(1):24–30.
35. Manni G, Centofanti M, Parravano M, et al. A 6-month randomized clinical trial of bimatoprost 0.03% versus the association of timolol 0.5% and latanoprost 0.005% in glaucomatous patients. *Graefe's Arch Clin Exp Ophthalmol.* 2004;242(9):767–770.
36. Higginbotham EJ, Feldman R, Stiles M, et al. Latanoprost and timolol combination therapy vs. monotherapy: one-year randomized trial. *Arch Ophthalmol.* 2002;120(7):915–922.
37. Wang R-F, Serle JB, Podos SM, et al. MK-507 (L-671, 152), a topically active carbonic anhydrase inhibitor, reduces aqueous humor production in monkeys. *Arch Ophthalmol.* 1991;109: 1297–1299.
38. DeSantis L. Preclinical overview of brinzolamide. *Surv Ophthalmol.* 2000;44(Suppl 2):S119–S129.
39. Silver LH. Clinical efficacy and safety of brinzolamide (Azopt), a new topical carbonic anhydrase inhibitor for primary open-angle glaucoma and ocular hypertension. Brinzolamide Primary Therapy Study Group. *Am J Ophthalmol.* 1998;126(3):400–408.
40. Arici MK, Topalkara A, Guler C. Additive effect of latanoprost and dorzolamide in patients with elevated intraocular pressure. *Int Ophthalmol.* 1998;22(1):37–42.
41. Chiselita D, Apatachioae I, Poiata I. The ocular hypotensive effect of the combination of latanoprost with dorzolamide. *Oftalmologia.* 1999;46(4):39–45.
42. Franks W; Brinzolamide Study Group. Ocular hypotensive efficacy and safety of brinzolamide ophthalmic suspension 1% added to travoprost ophthalmic solution 0.004% therapy in patients with open-angle glaucoma or ocular hypertension. *Curr Med Res Opin.* 2006;22(9):1643–1649.
43. Shoji N, Ogata H, Suyama H, et al. Intraocular pressure lowering effect of brinzolamide 1.0% as adjunctive therapy to latanoprost 0.005% in patients with open-angle glaucoma or ocular hypertension: an uncontrolled, open-label study. *Curr Med Res Opin.* 2005; 21(4):503–508.
44. Nakamoto K, Yasuda N. Effect of concomitant use of latanoprost and brinzolamide on 24-hour variation of IOP in normal-tension glaucoma. *J Glaucoma.* 2007;16(4):352–357.
45. O'Connor DJ, Martone JF, Mead A. Additive intraocular pressure lowering effect of various medications with latanoprost. *Am J Ophthalmol.* 2002;133(6):836–837.
46. Reis R, Queiroz CF, Santos LC, et al. A randomized, investigator-masked, 4-week study comparing timolol maleate 0.5%, brinzolamide 1%, and brimonidine tartrate 0.2% as adjunctive therapies to travoprost 0.004% in adults with open-angle glaucoma or ocular hypertension. *Clin Ther.* 2006;28(4):552–559.
47. Konstas AG, Karabatsas CH, Lallos N, et al. 24-hour intraocular pressures with brimonidine purite versus dorzolamide added to latanoprost in primary open-angle glaucoma subjects. *Ophthalmology.* 2005;112(4):603–608.
48. Noecker RJ. Brimonidine purite 0.15% versus dorzolamide 2% used as adjunctive therapy to latanoprost. *Presented at the annual meeting of the American Glaucoma Society*, San Francisco, CA, 2007 (poster).
49. Feldman RM, Tanna AP, Gross RL, et al. Comparison of the ocular hypotensive efficacy of adjunctive brimonidine 0.15% or brinzolamide 1% in combination with travoprost 0.004%. *Ophthalmology.* 2007;114(7):1248–1254.
50. Hollo G, Chiselita D, Petkova N, et al. The efficacy and safety of timolol maleate versus brinzolamide each given twice daily added to travoprost in patients with ocular hypertension or primary open-angle glaucoma. *Eur J Ophthalmol.* 2006;16(6):816–823.
51. Martinez-de-la-Casa JM, Castillo A, Garcia-Feijoo J, et al. Concomitant administration of travoprost and brinzolamide versus fixed latanoprost/timolol combined therapy: three-month

comparison of efficacy and safety. *Curr Med Res Opin.* 2004; 20(9):1333–1339.
52. Netland PA, Michael M, Rosner SA, et al. Brimonidine Purite and bimatoprost compared with timolol and latanoprost in patients with glaucoma and ocular hypertension. *Adv Ther.* 2003;20(1):20–30.
53. Mundorf T, Dirks M, Noecker RJ, et al. Brimonidine purite 0.15% versus timolol 0.5% as adjunctive therapy with lipids. *Presented at the annual meeting of the American Glaucoma Society*, Snowbird, UT, 2005.
54. Nietgen GW, Schmidt J, Hesse L, et al. Muscarinic receptor functioning and distribution in the eye: molecular basis and implications for clinical diagnosis and therapy (review). *Eye.* 1999;13(Pt 3a): 285–300.
55. Toris CB, Zhan G-L, Zhao J, Camras CB, Yablonski ME. Potential mechanism for the additivity of pilocarpine and latanoprost. *Am J Ophthalmol.* 2001;131:722–728.
56. Fristrom B, Nilsson SE. Interaction of PhXA41, a new prostaglandin analogue, with pilocarpine. A study on patients with elevated intraocular pressure. *Arch Ophthalmol.* 1993;111(5):662–665.
57. Camras CB, Wang R-F, Podos SM. Effect of pilocarpine applied before or after prostaglandin F2a on IOP in glaucomatous monkey eyes. *Invest Ophthalmol Vis Sci.* 1990;31:150.
58. Villumsen J, Alm A. Effect of the prostaglandin F2a analogue PhXA41 in eyes treated with pilocarpine and timolol. *Invest Ophthalmol Vis Sci.* 1992;33:1248.
59. Friström B, Nilsson SEG. Interaction of PhXA41, a new prostaglandin analogue, with pilocarpine. A study on patients with elevated intraocular pressure. *Arch Ophthalmol.* 1993;111:662–665.
60. Kent AR, Vroman DT, Thomas TJ, Herbert RL, Crosson CE. Interaction of pilocarpine with latanoprost in patientswith glaucoma and ocular hypertension. *J Glaucoma.* 1999;8:257–262.
61. Shin DH, McCracken MS, Bendel RE, et al. The additive effect of latanoprost to maximum-tolerated medications with low-dose, high-dose and no pilocarpine therapy. *Ophthalmology.* 1999;106:386–390.
62. Rulo AH, Greve EL, Hoyng PF. Additive ocular hypotensive effect of latanoprost and acetazolamide. A short-term study in patients with elevated intraocular pressure. *Ophthalmology.* 1997;104(9): 1503–1507.
63. Epstein DL, Grant WM. Carbonic anhydrase inhibitor side effects. *Arch Ophthalmol.* 1977;95:1378–1382.
64. Wallace TR, Fraunfelder FT, Petursson GJ, Epstein DL. Decreased libido – a side effect of carbonic anhydrase inhibitor. *Ann Ophthalmol.* 1979;11:1563–1566.
65. Epstein RJ, Allen RC, Lunde MW. Organic impotence associated with carbonic anhydrase inhibitor therapy for glaucoma. *Ann Ophthalmol.* 1987;19:48–50.
66. Heller I, Halevy J, Cohen S, Theodor E. Significant metabolic acidosis induced by acetazolamide: not a rare complication. *Arch Intern Med.* 1985;145:1815–1817.
67. Kass MA, Kolker AE, Gordon M, et al. Acetazolamide and urolithiasis. *Ophthalmology.* 1981;88:261–265.
68. Howlett SA. Renal failure associated with acetazolamide therapy for glaucoma. *South Med J.* 1975;68:504–506.
69. Higenbottam T, Ogg CS, Saxton HM. Acute renal failure from the use of acetazolamide (Diamox). *Postgrad Med J.* 1978;54:127–128.
70. Fraunfelder FT, Meyer SM, Bagby GC Jr, Dreis MW. Hematologic reactions to carbonic anhydrase inhibitors. *Am J Ophthalmol.* 1985;100:79–81.
71. Werblin TP, Pollack IP, Liss RA. Blood dyscrasias in patients using methazolamide (Neptazane) for glaucoma. *Ophthalmology.* 1980;87:350–354.
72. Weiss IS. Hirsutism after chronic administration of acetazolamide. *Am J Ophthalmol.* 1974;78:327–328.
73. Shirato S, Kagaya F, Suzuki Y, Joukou S. Stevens-Johnson syndrome induced by methazolamide treatment. *Arch Ophthalmol.* 1997;115:550–553.
74. Boyle JE, Ghosh K, Gieser DK, et al. A randomized trial comparing the dorzolamide-timolol combination given twice daily to monotherapy with timolol and dorzolamide. *Ophthalmology.* 1999; 106(12 Suppl):10–16.
75. Orzalesi N, Rossetti L, Bottoli A, et al. The effect of latanoprost, brimonidine, and a fixed combination of timolol and dorzolamide on circadian intraocular pressure in patients with glaucoma or ocular hypertension. *Arch Ophthalmol.* 2003;121(4):453–457.
76. Bastien N, Psaradellis F, Sampalis J, et al. Effect of dorzolamide-timolol (Cosopt(R)) co-administered with latanoprost™ or dorzolamide-timolol alone in patients with open angle glaucoma or ocular hypertension not adequately controlled on latanoprost. *Presented at the annual meeting of the Association for Research in Vision and Ophthalmology*, Fort Lauderdale, FL, 2006:441–B176.
77. Sherwood MB, Craven ER, Chou C, et al. Twice-daily 0.2% brimonidine-0.5% timolol fixed-combination therapy vs monotherapy with timolol or brimonidine in patients with glaucoma or ocular hypertension: a 12-month randomized trial. *Arch Ophthalmol.* 2006;124(9):1230–1238.
78. Nixon DR, Hollander DA. Comparison of the efficacy and tolerability of twice-daily Combigan™ vs. Cosopt(R) fixed-combination therapies. *Presented at the annual meeting of the American Academy of Ophthalmology*, New Orleans, LA, 2007.
79. Hommer A; Ganfort Investigators Group I. A double-masked, randomized, parallel comparison of a fixed combination of bimatoprost 0.03%/timolol 0.5% with non-fixed combination use in patients with glaucoma or ocular hypertension. *Eur J Ophthalmol.* 2007; 17(1):53–62.
80. Hughes BA, Bacharach J, Craven ER, et al. A three-month, multicenter, double-masked study of the safety and efficacy of travoprost 0.004%/timolol 0.5% ophthalmic solution compared to travoprost 0.004% ophthalmic solution and timolol 0.5% dosed concomitantly in subjects with open angle glaucoma or ocular hypertension. *J Glaucoma.* 2005;14(5):392–399.
81. Neelakantan A, Vaishnav HD, Iyer SA, et al. Is addition of a third or fourth antiglaucoma medication effective? *J Glaucoma.* 2004; 13(2):130–136.
82. Babizhayev MA, Brodskaya MW, Mamedov NG, et al. Clinical, structural and molecular phototherapy effects of laser irradiation on the trabecular meshwork of human glaucomatous eyes. *Graefes Arch Clin Exp Ophthalmol.* 1990;228(1):90–100.
83. Kramer TR, Noecker RJ. Comparison of the morphologic changes after selective laser trabeculoplasty and argon laser trabeculoplasty in human eye bank eyes. *Ophthalmology.* 2001;108(4): 773–779.
84. Damji KF, Bovell AM, Hodge WG, et al. Selective laser trabeculoplasty versus argon laser trabeculoplasty: results from a 1-year randomised clinical trial. *Br J Ophthalmol.* 2006;90(12): 1490–1494.
85. Damji KF, Shah KC, Rock WJ, et al. Selective laser trabeculoplasty versus argon laser trabeculoplasty: a prospective randomised clinical trial. *Br J Ophthalmol.* 1999;83(6):718–722.
86. Ruderman JM, Welch DB, Smith MF, et al. A randomized study of 5-fluorouracil and filtration surgery. *Am J Ophthalmol.* 1987; 104(3):218–224.
87. Palmer SS. Mitomycin as adjunct chemotherapy with trabeculectomy. *Ophthalmology.* 1991;98(3):317–321.
88. Hayreh SS. Anatomy and physiology of the optic nerve head. *Trans Am Acad Ophthalmol Otolaryngol.* 1974;78(2):OP240–OP254.
89. Tielsch JM, Katz J, Sommer A, Quigley HA, Javitt JC. Hypertension, perfusion pressure, and primary open-angle glaucoma. A population-based assessment. *Arch Ophthalmol.* 1995; 113(2):216–221.
90. Bonomi L, Marchini G, Marraffa M, Bernardi P, Morbio R, Varotto A. Vascular risk factors for primary open angle glaucoma: the Egna-Neumarkt Study. *Ophthalmology.* 2000;107(7):1287.

91. Quigley HA, West SK, Rodriguez J, Munoz B, Klein R, Snyder R. The prevalence of glaucoma in a population-based study of Hispanic subjects: Proyecto VER. *Arch Ophthalmol.* 2001;119(12):1819–1826.
92. Leske MC, Connell AM, Wu SY, et al. Incidence of open-angle glaucoma: the Barbados Eye Studies. The Barbados Eye Studies Group. *Arch Ophthalmol.* 2001;119(1):89–95.
93. Leske MC, Wu S-Y, Hennis A, Honkanen R, Nemesure B. Risk factors for incident open-angle glaucoma: the Barbados Eye Studies. The Barbados Eye Studies Group. *Ophthalmology.* 2008;115:85–93.
94. Quaranta L, Gandolfo F, Turano R, et al. Effects of topical hypotensive drugs on circadian IOP, blood pressure, and calculated diastolic ocular perfusion pressure in patients with glaucoma. *Invest Ophthalmol Vis Sci.* 2006;47:2917–2923.
95. Orzalesi N, Rossetti L, Invernizzi T, et al. Effect of timolol, latanoprost, and dorzolamide on circadian IOP in glaucoma or ocular hypertension. *Invest Ophthalmol Vis Sci.* 2000;41(9):2566–2573.
96. Barnebey H, Kwok SY. Patients' acceptance of a switch from dorzolamide to brinzolamide for the treatment of glaucoma in a clinical practice setting. *Clin Ther.* 2000;22(10):1204–1212.
97. Silver LH. Ocular comfort of brinzolamide 1.0% ophthalmic suspension compared with dorzolamide 2.0% ophthalmic solution: results from two multicenter comfort studies. Brinzolamide Comfort Study Group. *Surv Ophthalmol.* 2000;44(suppl 2):S141–S145.
98. Sall K. The efficacy and safety of brinzolamide 1% ophthalmic suspension (Azopt) as a primary therapy in patients with open-angle glaucoma or ocular hypertension. Brinzolamide Primary Therapy Study Group. *Surv Ophthalmol.* 2000;suppl 2:S155–S162.

# Chapter 53
# Monocular Drug Trials for Glaucoma Therapy in the Community Setting

Tony Realini

The clinical management of glaucoma would be far simpler if all patients responded equally well to therapy with IOP-lowering medication. Unfortunately, this is not the case. Consider that timolol offers median IOP reduction of approximately 5–6 mmHg. This does not mean that every patient will manifest a 5–6 mmHg IOP reduction. Rather, it means that half of the patients will enjoy an IOP reduction exceeding this median amount, while the other half will have a lesser IOP reduction. There is currently no way of identifying a priori how patients will respond to their medication; we are limited to a trial and error approach, a so-called n-of-one trial.

Therefore, when initiating medical therapy for IOP reduction in eyes with glaucoma, it is incumbent upon the clinician to confirm that the chosen therapy is efficacious in the individual patient. This task is less straightforward than it might seem. IOP is a dynamic parameter, much like systemic blood pressure or blood glucose levels. IOP varies spontaneously over time, and can be influenced by such varied factors as time of day, body position, hydration status, the season of the year, and even the tightness of a necktie, among others.[1] Of these, circadian IOP variation – the regular, cyclical rhythm of IOP that occurs every 24 h – is considered to be a key source of spontaneous IOP variation. The clinical consequence of spontaneous IOP variation is that a single measurement is not greatly informative of IOP behavior. To fully characterize long-term IOP variation requires multiple measurements over time, days, weeks, and months. Unlike blood pressure or blood glucose, which can be easily measured by patients at home, providing clinicians with a plethora of data to guide clinical management decisions, there is no easy way by which patients can measure their IOP at home. Thus, when managing IOP control, clinicians are limited to the data they collect during scheduled office visits. Consequently, characterizing long-term IOP variation can require multiple office visits over time, becoming both time-consuming and costly. And when initiating medical therapy for IOP reduction, IOP variation must be characterized both before and after the initiation of therapy, making the process doubly time-consuming and costly.

## 53.1 The Monocular Therapeutic Drug Trial

The monocular therapeutic drug trial was developed as a clinical tool to aid clinicians in distinguishing between the therapeutic and spontaneous components of IOP variation when initiating medical therapy. The monocular drug trial is elegant in its simplicity: measure IOP in both eyes, initiate treatment in one eye, then measure IOP in both eyes a few weeks later, at the same time of day as the initial measurement to minimize circadian IOP variation. The IOP change in the treated eye represents the sum of both a therapeutic IOP change and a spontaneous IOP change. The IOP change in the untreated eye represents purely spontaneous IOP change. Subtracting the IOP change in the untreated eye from the IOP change in the treated eye yields the true therapeutic IOP change attributable to treatment. As a clinical example, consider a patient whose IOP values are 25 mmHg in both eyes before treatment, and 18 and 23 mmHg in the right and left eyes, respectively, following a course of treatment in the right eye only. The 7-mmHg reduction in the right eye represents both therapeutic and spontaneous components of IOP change. The 2-mmHg reduction in the left eye represents purely spontaneous IOP change. The 5-mmHg difference represents the true therapeutic effect of the treatment.

The monocular trial's clinical utility requires that several key assumptions be true. In recent years, a growing body of research has called many of these assumptions – and the clinical value of the monocular trial itself – into question. It is useful to review each of these assumptions, their role in supporting the monocular trial, and the data supporting or challenging their validity.

### 53.1.1 Fellow Eyes Exhibit Symmetrical Spontaneous IOP Variation

The monocular trial is predicated on the assumption that the untreated eye tells us what the treated eye would have done had it not been treated, so that one eye can serve as a control for its fellow eye. This requires that spontaneous

IOP variation over time occurs symmetrically in fellow eyes. The existing data does not support this assumption. Katavisto compared diurnal IOP curve shapes between fellow eyes of 236 glaucoma patients, reporting that 45% of subjects had different IOP curve shapes in their fellow eyes.[2] Wilensky and colleagues confirmed this in their report demonstrating that 33% of ocular hypertensive patients and 36% of glaucoma patients exhibited different IOP curve shapes between fellow eyes.[3] Several years ago, we demonstrated that the majority of glaucoma patients – and half of normal subjects – experience periodic asymmetric IOP fluctuations in which the IOP in one eye changes by 3 mmHg or more relative to the change in the fellow eye from one visit to the next.[4] Other groups have recently reported low-to-moderate correlation of fellow-eye IOP in both normal subjects and glaucoma patients.[5,6] In contrast, another group has reported that the diurnal variation of intraocular pressure in glaucoma suspects and both high-tension and low-tension glaucoma patients is largely concordant between fellow eyes.[7,8]

## 53.1.2 There Is No Contralateral Crossover IOP Reduction Arising from Monocular Therapy

The monocular trial requires that the IOP change in the untreated eye be purely spontaneous and uninfluenced by therapy in the fellow eye. The validity of this assumption depends upon the medication chosen for the monocular trial. For beta-blockers in particular, this assumption is patently false, as a significant contralateral crossover effect has been well-described. The magnitude of this crossover effect for beta-blockers was recently established by the Ocular Hypertension Treatment Study, in which a mean 1.5 mmHg reduction in IOP was observed in fellow eyes during monocular trials with beta-blockers.[9] The potential contralateral effects of other IOP-lowering drug classes have not been fully characterized. It is generally assumed that prostaglandins, once systemically absorbed, are metabolized too quickly to manifest a significant contralateral IOP response. For example, the half-life of latanoprost acid in the aqueous humor was about 2.5 h, while its half-life in the systemic circulation – which might mediate crossover effects – was only 17 min.[10]

## 53.1.3 Circadian IOP Variation Follows a Sustained Daily Rhythm

Measuring pretreatment and on-treatment IOP at the same time of day theoretically eliminates the component of spontaneous IOP change attributable to diurnal variation. This practice assumes that there is a sustained and reproducible circadian IOP rhythm that a given eye follows day after day. Katavisto reported that 80% of glaucomatous eyes exhibited reproducible diurnal IOP curve shapes using Schiøtz tonometry more than 40 years ago.[2] In contrast, Wilensky and colleagues reported that only 28% of eyes with ocular hypertension and 34% of eyes with primary open-angle glaucoma (POAG) had reproducible curve shapes on retesting using a home applanation tonometer, operated by the patient, which was developed by one member of the research team.[3,11] The reproducibility of IOP rhythms in both normal and glaucomatous eyes over time, assessed using the clinical standard Goldmann tonometry, is the subject of an ongoing study in our lab, and data addressing this assumption of the monocular drug trial is soon forthcoming from us. In the meantime, there is little relevant data suggesting that the assumption is valid.

## 53.1.4 Fellow Eyes Respond Symmetrically to a Given IOP-Lowering Medication

The monocular trial does not require – and advocates of the monocular trial do not expressly recommend – that the second-treated eye should undergo formal evaluation of drug efficacy after a successful monocular trial. It is assumed that if the medication used for the monocular trial was effective in the first-treated eye, then the fellow eye will have a similar therapeutic response once bilateral treatment is initiated. Our group recently reported that fellow eyes do, in fact, respond symmetrically to a given IOP-lowering agent, with a coefficient of determination ($r^2$) of 0.7 (that is, 70% of the IOP reduction seen in one eye was determined by the IOP reduction in the fellow eye) based on a single pair of pretreatment and on-treatment measurements.[12] In contrast, Young and coworkers evaluated the bilateral IOP response to latanoprost monotherapy and reported significantly lower coefficients of determination for the correlation of IOP reduction between fellow eyes, ranging from 0.274 for daytime IOP measurements to 0.413 for 24-h circadian IOP measurements.[13] More research is required on this important point, but in the meantime, the assumption that fellow eyes respond symmetrically to a given IOP-lowering medication is far from established.

## 53.1.5 Patients Take Their Medications as Prescribed

The monocular trial, by definition, requires that patients use the drop in only one eye. If patients treat both eyes, or treat the wrong eye, the monocular trial provides no useful data. It is well-established that patients frequently misunderstand directions for medication use. This is particularly problematic when drug samples are given (as is often the case when first initiating therapy, when the monocular trial is utilized) because, unless we write down the directions for the trial for each patient, the patient does not have the directions printed on the bottle or box to refer back to in case of confusion. Even when the directions are clearly understood, a whole host of other barriers to compliance may prevent patients from following the directions. Particularly problematic is that noncompliant patients do not often confess to their behavior, nor are physicians easily able to identify the potentially noncompliant patients. It is essentially axiomatic in glaucoma that this assumption is invalid.

### 53.1.6 What Does This Mean for the Monocular Trial?

So if the assumptions underlying the monocular trial are not convincingly valid, what does this mean for the monocular trial itself? The monocular trial is designed to tell us if a drug is working or not, but does it really tell us anything about how well the drug might work in the fellow eye? We conducted a retrospective evaluation of our own experience with the monocular drug trial in order to determine the relationship between the IOP reduction seen during the monocular trial and the IOP reduction seen when the same drug was subsequently administered to the fellow eye.[14] In our 52-patient series, the coefficient of determination was 0.0174, demonstrating that there was no relationship between the IOP reduction in first-treated eyes verses second-treated eyes. Other groups have since investigated this important clinical issue. Dayanir and colleagues conducted a similar retrospective evaluation and found moderate correlation between first- and second-treated eyes among high-tension glaucoma patients (coefficient of determination = 0.293) but not low-tension glaucoma patients (coefficient of determination = 0.096).[15] In a thorough but complex retrospective analysis of their monocular trial data, Leffler and colleagues found a non-significant relationship between IOP in the first- and second-treated eyes after a monocular trial followed by bilateral therapy.[16] Takahashi and coworkers have conducted a prospective analysis of the monocular drug trial, oddly in normal subjects, and have found a similar lack of correlation between first-treated and second-treated IOP reduction (coefficient of determination = 0.097).[17]

Several of these groups have suggested modifications that improve the utility of the monocular trial. Sit and coworkers suggested that the monocular trial may be improved by using multiple IOP measurements obtained over the course of a day rather than a single measurement at both the pretreatment and on-treatment assessments.[6] This approach has not yet been evaluated prospectively, and if effective, such a modification might have value that outweighs the inconvenience to the patient. Interestingly, the analyses by both Leffler's[16] and Takahashi's[17] groups suggested that the monocular trial may offer little benefit over simultaneously initiating therapy in both eyes. Takahashi's team reported that when considering the correlation between first-treated and second-treated eyes, the coefficient of determination for fellow-eye IOP reductions was essentially equivalent whether or not the change in the untreated eye was subtracted from the change in the treated eye after the monocular trial (0.097 vs. 0.102, respectively).[17] Leffler's team compared the results of both monocular and binocular trials and found little difference in the correlation of IOP responses in fellow-eye pair whether medication was started in one or both eyes initially.[16]

If, as suggested by the data from both Takahashi's[17] and Leffler's[16] groups, there is no need for the "control" data provided by the untreated fellow eye during a monocular trial, then there is no compelling reason to utilize a monocular trial at all. Rather, if both eyes require treatment, then both eyes should be treated, and each eye should be assessed for treatment efficacy individually (but simultaneously). This has the added benefit of not delaying treatment in the fellow eye while awaiting the results of the monocular trial. The only reason left to consider a monocular trial is based on safety rather than efficacy: a monocular therapeutic trial exposes only one eye to the drug (and exposes the individual to one-half of the bilateral dose), thus potentially reducing the impact that might arise if a serious drug-related event were to occur. In some cases, such as the initiation of a topical carbonic anhydrase inhibitor in a patient with a known sulfa allergy, a monocular trial may be appropriate.

### 53.1.7 A New Clinical Approach to Assessment of Drug Efficacy

Ironically, the monocular drug trial was developed to minimize the impact of spontaneous IOP variation, but it fails precisely because of IOP variation: it assumes that spontaneous IOP variation is both predictable and symmetrical between fellow eyes, neither of which appears to be true.

So how should we assess the efficacy of newly initiated topical IOP-lowering therapy if not by the monocular drug trial? We strongly recommend obtaining multiple baseline IOP measurements before initiating therapy in order to more fully characterize an individual patient's inherent IOP variation. The American Academy of Ophthalmology recommends obtaining multiple baseline measurements.[18] Equally important is to obtain multiple on-treatment IOP measurements. Why are we in such a hurry to lower IOP that we feel we have to decide whether or not to continue a given medication based on a single on-treatment IOP? It is worth considering that glaucoma is a chronic and usually slowly progressive disease. Instances in which emergent IOP reduction is required are quite uncommon. We don't need to be in such a hurry to lower IOP that we sacrifice accuracy for rapidity. We can, and probably should, continue a medication beyond the first on-treatment visit even if it has only lowered IOP by 1–2 mmHg. Often in these cases, subsequent assessments at future visits will demonstrate significantly lower IOP measurements. Has the drug simply taken longer to take effect? Probably not. Rather, we undervalue the importance of reducing a patient's range of IOP. If a drug lowers a patient's IOP range from the neighborhood of 20–28 mmHg to the neighborhood of 15–20 mmHg, this may be therapeutically adequate for some people. And note that this patient's IOP can be 20 mmHg both before and after the initiation of therapy. With only a single pretreatment IOP and a single posttreatment IOP, you may not be able to discern the true therapeutic value of a newly initiated drug. We should stop asking "What is the patient's IOP?" and start asking "What is the patient's IOP range?", which can only be determined by obtaining multiple measurements over time.

In summary, the monocular trial is a creative, yet ultimately flawed, method of distinguishing between spontaneous and therapeutic IOP variation in the assessment of the efficacy of newly initiated IOP-lowering therapy. The assumptions required by the monocular trial simply are not supported by both old and emerging data. The monocular trial itself, in several reports, offers little if anything over simultaneous bilateral therapy. Its only legitimate role in glaucoma management is to assess the safety and tolerability of a given drug in a given patient before beginning long-term bilateral therapy. To best assess the long-term efficacy of a given drug in a given patient, multiple IOP measurements should be obtained both before and after initiating therapy. We should refrain from discarding a drug that fails to show a huge IOP drop at the very first on-treatment IOP assessment. Rather, we should acknowledge that glaucoma is a long-term disease, and we should give the drugs a chance to show us how well they work by measuring on-treatment IOP over several visits.

# References

1. Teng C, Gurses-Ozden R, Liebmann JM, Tello C, Ritch R. Effect of a tight necktie on IOP. *Br J Ophthalmology*. 2003;87:946–948.
2. Katavisto M. The diurnal variations of ocular tension in glaucoma. *Acta Ophthalmol Suppl*. 1964; Suppl 78:1–130.
3. Wilensky JT, Gieser DK, Dietsche ML, Mori MT, Zeimer R. Individual variability in the diurnal intraocular pressure curve. *Ophthalmology*. 1993;100:940–944.
4. Realini T, Barber L, Burton D. Frequency of asymmetric intraocular pressure fluctuations among patients with and without glaucoma. *Ophthalmology*. 2002;109:1367–1371.
5. Liu JH, Sit AJ, Weinreb RN. Variation of 24-hour intraocular pressure in healthy individuals: right eye versus left eye. *Ophthalmology*. 2005;112:1670–1675.
6. Sit AJ, Liu JH, Weinreb RN. Asymmetry of right versus left intraocular pressures over 24 hours in glaucoma patients. *Ophthalmology*. 2006;113:425–430.
7. Dinn RB, Zimmerman MB, Shuba LM, et al. Concordance of diurnal intraocular pressure between fellow eyes in primary open-angle glaucoma. *Ophthalmology*. 2007;114:915–920.
8. Shuba LM, Doan AP, Maley MK, et al. Diurnal fluctuation and concordance of intraocular pressure in glaucoma suspects and normal tension glaucoma patients. *J Glaucoma*. 2007;16:307–312.
9. Piltz J, Gross R, Shin DH, et al. Contralateral effect of topical beta-adrenergic antagonists in initial one-eyed trials in the ocular hypertension treatment study. *Am J Ophthalmol*. 2000;130:441–453.
10. Sjöquist B, Stjernschantz J. Ocular and systemic pharmacokinetics of latanoprost in humans. *Surv Ophthalmol*. 2002;47(Suppl 1):S6-S12.
11. Zeimer RC, Wilensky JT, Gieser DK, Mori MM, Baker JP. Evaluation of a self tonometer for home use. *Arch Ophthalmol*. 1983;101:1791–1793.
12. Realini T, Vickers WR. Symmetry of fellow-eye intraocular pressure responses to topical glaucoma medications. *Ophthalmology*. 2005;112:599–602.
13. Young A, Liu JHK, Weinreb RN. ARVO 2006. *Invest Ophthalmol Vis Sci*. 2006; E-Abstract 437. Available online at http://www.iovs.org
14. Realini T, Fechtner RD, Atreides SP, Gollance S. The uniocular drug trial and second-eye response to glaucoma medications. *Ophthalmology*. 2004;111:421–426.
15. Dayanir V, Cakmak H, Berkit I. The one-eye trial and fellow eye response to prostaglandin analogues. *Clin Experiment Ophthalmol*. 2008;36:136–141.
16. Leffler CT, Amini L. Interpretation of uniocular and binocular trials of glaucoma medications: an observational case series. *BMC Ophthalmol*. 2007;7:17.
17. Takahashi M, Higashide T, Sakurai M, Sugiyama K. Discrepancy of the intraocular pressure response between fellow eyes in one-eye trials versus bilateral treatment: verification with normal subjects. *J Glaucoma*. 2008;17:169–174.
18. American Academy of Ophthalmology. *Primary Open-Angle Glaucoma: Preferred Practice Pattern*. San Francisco: American Academy of Ophthalmology; 2005.

# Chapter 54
# Neuroprotection of Retinal Ganglion Cells

Alvaro P.C. Lupinacci, Howard Barnebey, and Peter A. Netland

Therapeutic efforts for treatment of glaucoma have focused on reduction of intraocular pressure as the main objective. In clinical practice, intraocular pressure (IOP) control has been expected to slow or arrest the glaucoma progression. However, clinicians have been confronted with significant glaucoma progression even when achieving control of intraocular pressure. In the Collaborative Normal-Tension Glaucoma Study, following medical or surgical treatment to achieve at least 30% reduction of intraocular pressure, 12% of patients experienced continued visual field loss secondary to optic nerve damage.[1]

In eyes with glaucoma, histologic studies have shown a selective loss of retinal ganglion cell bodies and their axons, which travel through the optic nerve toward the lateral geniculate nucleus in the brain. This neuronal death and loss of axons account for the characteristic optic nerve cupping and visual field loss observed in glaucoma patients.[2-8] In patients with glaucoma, permanent neural damage may occur in other areas of the visual pathway, including the lateral geniculate nucleus and the occipital cortex. Recent interest has focused on the mechanisms of damage of these neural cells, both with and without elevated intraocular pressure. There has also been interest in using new therapeutic strategies in glaucoma patients other than reducing the intraocular pressure. Neuroprotection is a strategy intended to prevent neuronal injury in glaucoma patients, thereby preventing optic nerve damage and vision loss.[9-15]

## 54.1 Mechanisms of Ganglion Cell Death in Glaucoma

Observations in humans and experimental animals indicate that cell death in glaucoma occurs principally by the apoptotic pathway. In apoptosis, cell death occurs when caspases and other enzymes condense cell organelles and fragment the cell's DNA. The compartmentalized cellular debris is then phagocytosed by adjacent cells, without an inflammatory response. The apoptotic pathway is not completely understood but several sites are subject to promising therapeutic strategies.[3,4,8,16-18] Apoptosis is often referred to as "programmed cell death."

Genes that control apoptosis are the subject of intensive research. Examples of the genetic regulation of apoptosis are the BCL-2 gene product and the BCL-X gene product (BAX protein). The BCL-2 protein blocks apoptosis, whereas the BAX protein stimulates apoptosis. Depending on the balance of these proteins, the cell either lives or becomes apoptotic. Gene therapy to inhibit the apoptotic pathway is one potential neuroprotective strategy separate from the lowering of IOP.[10,19]

Deprivation of metabolic substrates, such as glucose and oxygen, may trigger apoptosis. Disruption of the microcirculation could cause potentially damaging problems due to interruption of nutrient delivery or waste removal.[20-22] Autoimmune reactions, attributed to cytolytic T-lymphocytes or other immune system components, could cause ganglion cell death.[3,23-s27]

Neurons are dependent on growth factors for survival. These factors are small peptides classified as neurotrophins, cytokines, or growth factors. One neurotrophin required by ganglion cells is brain-derived neurotrophic factor (BDNF). Neurotrophins are taken up by ganglion cell axons from the brain and transmitted to the retina by retrograde axoplasmic transport. Axonal transport may be disrupted by either vascular ischemia or by mechanical compression, both of which could occur in glaucoma. Neurotrophin deprivation could lead to apoptosis of retinal ganglion cells.[2,3,5,10,28-31]

Another possible cause of apoptosis is excitotoxicity. The primary excitotoxin in the brain is glutamate. In the brain, high local concentrations of glutamate overstimulate ganglion cell surface receptors, including the $N$-methyl-D-aspartate (NMDA) receptor. This leads to massive calcium influx and death of the cell. Very high levels of glutamate may stimulate cell necrosis, but lower elevations of glutamate may initiate apoptosis. Glutamate release is a common response to cellular ischemia, so this mechanism is consistent with a primary ischemic injury in glaucoma.[32-34] Although initial studies showed increased glutamate levels in human glaucoma,[15,33] subsequent studies were unable to reproduce these findings.[35]

Nitric oxide synthase generates nitric oxide from l-arginine. High levels of nitric oxide may generate peroxynitrate, which can nitrosylate and fragment DNA and bind to tyrosine residues in cell proteins, thereby leading to cell death. Neufeld and coworkers have demonstrated increased levels of nitric oxide synthase isoforms (NOS-1,2,3) in the optic nerve head of patients with primary open-angle glaucoma. Interestingly, nitric oxide synthase in the vascular endothelium may cause vasodilation and increased volumetric blood flow.[3,20,21,36]

The apoptotic process may continue even after the initial insult has been withdrawn. In glaucoma patients, even after intraocular pressure control, optic nerve cupping and visual field loss may be observed. Schwartz and coworkers have found that when the optic nerve of a rat is partially crushed there is an initial or primary degeneration followed by a secondary degeneration that occurs over a few weeks. Drugs that block receptors for glutamate inhibit this secondary degeneration. It is possible that the initially injured cells released excitotoxins that caused adjacent cells to subsequently die, keeping the apoptotic process active even after the trigger stimulus had ceased.[25,37]

Thus, genetic regulation, retrograde axonal neurotrophin transportation, metabolic substrate and waste circulation, autoimmune regulation, excitotoxicity regulation, and nitric oxide synthase control are possible strategies for neuroprotection treatment in glaucoma.

## 54.2 Neuroprotection in Glaucoma

Neuroprotection in glaucoma is intended to prevent or inhibit the death of neurons in ganglion cells and other neuronal cells affected by the disease. Of course, lowering IOP is in this sense neuroprotective, but in the context of this chapter we are looking for other ways to prevent destructive cellular events or enhance the survival of cells exposed to injurious stimuli, reducing the irreversible loss of ganglion cells. Neuroprotection as a therapeutic strategy may be an adjunctive therapy, in combination with ocular hypotensive or vasoactive treatments. Neuroprotection may also be the primary or secondary intention of a therapy. Whenever nerve cell injury and death are involved in a pathologic condition such as glaucoma, neuroprotection may be attempted clinically, independent of the original cause of the condition.[10–14]

There are currently no drugs that are approved for use in glaucoma patients with an indication or a marketing claim for neuroprotection. However, currently available ocular hypotensive drugs have been tested for their neuroprotective properties, and other drugs are under investigation for treatment of glaucoma patients.

Gene therapy is one approach that may be tried in the future. For example, increasing the expression of bcl-2 or suppressing bcl-x may prevent ganglion cells from dying by apoptosis. Another approach would be to replace deficient neurotrophins. Injection of neurotrophins or other growth factors into the vitreous can reduce apoptosis after optic nerve transection. Although neurotrophins have systemic side effects and administration is difficult, analogues or alternative routes of drug administration may help with these problems. Aurintricarboxylic acid prevents activation of a nuclease that cleaves DNA during apoptosis and can block apoptosis of sympathetic neurons in culture after nerve growth factor withdrawal. These approaches are of interest, but are still far from clinical application.[2,3,10,28,31]

Drugs that may influence excitotoxicity and antioxidants are under active investigation. NMDA antagonists have been of interest in order to reduce both primary and secondary neuronal cell loss in glaucoma. Unfortunately, NMDA receptors may have multiple neurophysiological effects, and NMDA antagonists can have broad impact on neurological activity. Some NMDA antagonists have been developed with apparently less systemic side effects. The amantadine derivative Memantine, which is an NMDA antagonist that is directed at controlling glutamate-mediated excitotoxicity, showed promise in experimental research.[32,34,38] However, clinical trial results did not show a clear benefit of this drug.[35]

Brimonidine is a currently approved alpha-2-agonist that appears to have neuroprotective properties in experimental conditions.[19,34,39,40] Clinical trials are needed to establish the actual neuroprotective activity of brimonidine. Calcium channel antagonists may partially ameliorate NMDA receptor-mediated neurotoxicity of retinal ganglion cells in vitro, and they may have other vascular and neuroprotective properties.[10,41] Drugs that block nitric oxide synthase, such as arginine analogs, and drugs that block free radical lipid peroxidation, such as the 21-amino-steroid tirilazad mesylate, are of interest.[21,38,41] Estrogen and erythropoietin[42–44] also may have some activity as neuroprotectants.[45,46]

There is interest in neuroprotective effects of the immune system. Autoimmune T cells have been found to slow the rate of "secondary degeneration" in experimental studies, which has been termed "neuroprotective autoimmunity." Glatiramer acetate (copaxone) has been used as an antigen to cross react with myelin and stimulate a protective T-cell response. Whether or not a "glaucoma vaccine" is feasible will require further clinical trials.[24,25,27,47]

Many potential causes of ganglion cell death have been linked to ischemia. Ischemia may influence retrograde transport of brain-derived growth factors. Ischemia is also a well-known stimulus of glutamate release, and may be related to the excitotoxicity pathway.[17,48] Vasoprotection, improving optic nerve blood circulation, can be considered a form of neuroprotection.[22] Various systemic medications may influence the ocular circulation, and several anti-glaucoma medications have effects on intraocular pressure as well as effects on the ocular circulation. Ocular perfusion pressure, hypotension, and microcirculatory abnormalities are being actively investigated for a possible role in glaucoma, which may provide the basis for hemodynamic neuroprotective treatment strategies.

Some natural compounds such as *epigallocatechin gallate* (present in green tea), *Fructus lycii*, and *Ginkgo biloba* are being studied as possible neuroprotective and vasoactive drugs.[49-51] Stem cells are also being tested in experimental studies.[52] Bioenergetic studies are being performed on several neurodegenerative diseases, including glaucoma.[53] Bioenergetics is a quantum physics approach to biological systems, studying the influence of electromagnetic (light and other waves), electric, and chemical energies on organisms. Acupuncture and homeopathy are examples of the application of bioenergetic concepts in the medical field. Biophotonics, which uses pulses of light at different wave-lengths to improve health and organic functions, is another example of a bioenergetic application.

Retinal ganglion cell analysis is of great importance in neuroprotection research. Equipment using fluorescently labeled annexin 5 and confocal laser scanning ophthalmoscopy is able to visualize retinal ganglion cells undergoing the apoptotic process. Called "DARC" from Detection of Apoptotic Retinal Cells, this equipment may be an important step toward developing neuroprotective glaucoma therapies.[54]

Experimental models have provided evidence for benefits of neuroprotective treatments. These models have included ischemia-reperfusion models, optic nerve transsection and crush models, and excitotoxicity models. In experimental studies, a variety of drugs have shown benefits that appear to be non-IOP dependent. However, clinical studies in humans are needed to provide further evidence for the efficacy of neuroprotective treatments.

## 54.3 Conclusion

Glaucoma is a characteristic optic neuropathy with selective loss of retinal ganglion cells. The death of ganglion cells in glaucoma is primarily by apoptosis influenced by various factors that have been identified as genetic, neurotrophic, autoimmune, and excitotoxic. Neuroprotective drugs are under investigation. In the future, these drugs may be used by themselves, or in combination with other treatments for glaucoma that improve blood supply and/or reduce intraocular pressure.

## References

1. Anderson DR. Collaborative normal tension glaucoma study. *Curr Opin Ophthalmol*. 2003;14(2):86–90.
2. Weber AJ, Harman CD, Viswanathan S. Effects of optic nerve injury, glaucoma, and neuroprotection on the survival, structure, and function of ganglion cells in the mammalian retina. *J Physiol*. 2008;586(Pt 18):4393–4400.
3. Wax MB, Tezel G. Neurobiology of glaucomatous optic neuropathy: diverse cellular events in neurodegeneration and neuroprotection. *Mol Neurobiol*. 2002;26(1):45–55.
4. McKinnon SJ. Glaucoma, apoptosis, and neuroprotection. *Curr Opin Ophthalmol*. 1997;8(2):28–37.
5. Lipton SA. Retinal ganglion cells, glaucoma and neuroprotection. *Prog Brain Res*. 2001;131:712–718.
6. Levin LA. Neuroprotection and regeneration in glaucoma. *Ophthalmol Clin North Am* 2005;18(4):585–596, vii.
7. Levin LA. Mechanisms of optic neuropathy. *Curr Opin Ophthalmol*. 1997;8(6):9–15.
8. Farkas RH, Grosskreutz CL. Apoptosis, neuroprotection, and retinal ganglion cell death: an overview. *Int Ophthalmol Clin*. 2001;41(1):111–130.
9. Yoles E, Schwartz M. Potential neuroprotective therapy for glaucomatous optic neuropathy. *Surv Ophthalmol*. 1998;42(4):367–372.
10. Whitcup SM. Clinical trials in neuroprotection. *Prog Brain Res*. 2008;173:323–335.
11. Weinreb RN. Glaucoma neuroprotection: What is it? Why is it needed? *Can J Ophthalmol*. 2007;42(3):396–398.
12. Wein FB, Levin LA. Current understanding of neuroprotection in glaucoma. *Curr Opin Ophthalmol*. 2002;13(2):61–67.
13. Osborne NN, Chidlow G, Nash MS, Wood JP. The potential of neuroprotection in glaucoma treatment. *Curr Opin Ophthalmol*. 1999;10(2):82–92.
14. Osborne NN, Chidlow G, Layton CJ, Wood JP, Casson RJ, Melena J. Optic nerve and neuroprotection strategies. *Eye*. 2004;18(11):1075–1084.
15. Dreyer EB. The potential for neuroprotection in glaucoma. *Ophthalmol Clin North Am*. 1997;10:365–376.
16. Weinreb RN. Neuroprotection–possibilities in perspective. *Surv Ophthalmol*. 2001;45(Suppl 3):S241–S242.
17. Osborne NN. Pathogenesis of ganglion "cell death" in glaucoma and neuroprotection: focus on ganglion cell axonal mitochondria. *Prog Brain Res*. 2008;173:339–352.
18. Nickells RW. Retinal ganglion cell death in glaucoma: the how, the why, and the maybe. *J Glaucoma*. 1996;5(5):345–356.
19. Kalapesi FB, Coroneo MT, Hill MA. Human ganglion cells express the alpha-2 adrenergic receptor: relevance to neuroprotection. *Br J Ophthalmol*. 2005;89(6):758–763.
20. Rosa RH Jr, Hein TW, Yuan Z, et al. Brimonidine evokes heterogeneous vasomotor response of retinal arterioles: diminished nitric oxide-mediated vasodilation when size goes small. *Am J Physiol Heart Circ Physiol*. 2006;291(1):H231–H238.
21. Neufeld AH, Hernandez MR, Gonzalez M. Nitric oxide synthase in the human glaucomatous optic nerve head. *Arch Ophthalmol*. 1997;115(4):497–503.
22. Harris A, Ciulla TA, Kagemann L, Zarfati D, Martin B. Vasoprotection as neuroprotection for the optic nerve. *Eye* 2000;14(Pt 3B):473–475.
23. Schwartz M, London A. Glaucoma as a neuropathy amenable to neuroprotection and immune manipulation. *Prog Brain Res*. 2008;173:375–384.
24. Schwartz M. Harnessing the immune system for neuroprotection: therapeutic vaccines for acute and chronic neurodegenerative disorders. *Cell Mol Neurobiol*. 2001;21(6):617–627.
25. Schwartz M. Physiological approaches to neuroprotection. boosting of protective autoimmunity. *Surv Ophthalmol*. 2001;45(Suppl 3):S256–S260; discussion S273–S276.
26. Bakalash S, Kipnis J, Yoles E, Schwartz M. Resistance of retinal ganglion cells to an increase in intraocular pressure is immune-dependent. *Invest Ophthalmol Vis Sci*. 2002;43(8):2648–2653.
27. Bakalash S, Kessler A, Mizrahi T, Nussenblatt R, Schwartz M. Antigenic specificity of immunoprotective therapeutic vaccination for glaucoma. *Invest Ophthalmol Vis Sci*. 2003;44(8):3374–3381.
28. Neufeld AH, Liu B. Glaucomatous optic neuropathy: when glia misbehave. *Neuroscientist*. 2003;9(6):485–495.

29. Osborne NN, Ugarte M, Chao M, et al. Neuroprotection in relation to retinal ischemia and relevance to glaucoma. *Surv Ophthalmol*. 1999;43(Suppl 1):S102–S128.
30. Cordeiro MF, Erskine L. Back to basics – ephrins, axonal guidance, neuroprotection and glaucoma. *Br J Ophthalmol*. 2007;91(9):1106.
31. Tezel G. TNF-alpha signaling in glaucomatous neurodegeneration. *Prog Brain Res*. 2008;173:409–421.
32. Lipton SA. Pathologically-activated therapeutics for neuroprotection: mechanism of NMDA receptor block by memantine and S-nitrosylation. *Curr Drug Targets*. 2007;8(5):621–632.
33. Dreyer EB. A proposed role for excitotoxicity in glaucoma. *J Glaucoma*. 1998;7(1):62–67.
34. Dong CJ, Guo Y, Agey P, Wheeler L, Hare WA. Alpha2 adrenergic modulation of NMDA receptor function as a major mechanism of RGC protection in experimental glaucoma and retinal excitotoxicity. *Invest Ophthalmol Vis Sci*. 2008;49(10):4515–4522.
35. Osborne NN. Recent clinical findings with memantine should not mean that the idea of neuroprotection in glaucoma is abandoned. *Acta Ophthalmol* 2008.
36. Neufeld AH, Sawada A, Becker B. Inhibition of nitric-oxide synthase 2 by aminoguanidine provides neuroprotection of retinal ganglion cells in a rat model of chronic glaucoma. *Proc Natl Acad Sci U S A*. 1999;96(17):9944–9948.
37. Schwartz M. Neuroprotection as a treatment for glaucoma: pharmacological and immunological approaches. *Eur J Ophthalmol*. 2003;13(Suppl 3):S27–S31.
38. Kitaoka Y, Kumai T. Modulation of retinal dopaminergic cells by nitric oxide. A protective effect on NMDA-induced retinal injury. *In Vivo*. 2004;18(3):311–315.
39. Wheeler L, WoldeMussie E, Lai R. Role of alpha-2 agonists in neuroprotection. *Surv Ophthalmol*. 2003;48(Suppl 1):S47–S51.
40. Wheeler LA, Woldemussie E. Alpha-2 adrenergic receptor agonists are neuroprotective in experimental models of glaucoma. *Eur J Ophthalmol*. 2001;11(Suppl 2):S30–S35.
41. Chidlow G, Wood JP, Casson RJ. Pharmacological neuroprotection for glaucoma. *Drugs*. 2007;67(5):725–759.
42. Tsai JC, Song BJ, Wu L, Forbes M. Erythropoietin: a candidate neuroprotective agent in the treatment of glaucoma. *J Glaucoma*. 2007;16(6):567–571.
43. Zhong L, Bradley J, Schubert W, et al. Erythropoietin promotes survival of retinal ganglion cells in DBA/2J glaucoma mice. *Invest Ophthalmol Vis Sci*. 2007;48(3):1212–1218.
44. Weishaupt JH, Rohde G, Polking E, Siren AL, Ehrenreich H, Bahr M. Effect of erythropoietin axotomy-induced apoptosis in rat retinal ganglion cells. *Invest Ophthalmol Vis Sci*. 2004;45(5):1514–1522.
45. Kumar DM, Simpkins JW, Agarwal N. Estrogens and neuroprotection in retinal diseases. *Mol Vis*. 2008;14:1480–1486.
46. Zhou X, Li F, Ge J, et al. Retinal ganglion cell protection by 17-beta-estradiol in a mouse model of inherited glaucoma. *Dev Neurobiol*. 2007;67(5):603–616.
47. Schori H, Kipnis J, Yoles E, et al. Vaccination for protection of retinal ganglion cells against death from glutamate cytotoxicity and ocular hypertension: implications for glaucoma. *Proc Natl Acad Sci U S A*. 2001;98(6):3398–3403.
48. Lagreze WA, Muller-Velten R, Feuerstein TJ. The neuroprotective properties of gabapentin-lactam. *Graefes Arch Clin Exp Ophthalmol*. 2001;239(11):845–849.
49. Yu MS, Lai CS, Ho YS, et al. Characterization of the effects of anti-aging medicine Fructus lycii on beta-amyloid peptide neurotoxicity. *Int J Mol Med*. 2007;20(2):261–268.
50. Chung HS, Harris A, Kristinsson JK, Ciulla TA, Kagemann C, Ritch R. Ginkgo biloba extract increases ocular blood flow velocity. *J Ocul Pharmacol Ther*. 1999;15(3):233–240.
51. Zhang B, Rusciano D, Osborne NN. Orally administered epigallocatechin gallate attenuates retinal neuronal death in vivo and light-induced apoptosis in vitro. *Brain Res*. 2008;1198:141–152.
52. Bull ND, Johnson TV, Martin KR. Stem cells for neuroprotection in glaucoma. *Prog Brain Res*. 2008;173:511–519.
53. Schober MS, Chidlow G, Wood JP, Casson RJ. Bioenergetic-based neuroprotection and glaucoma. *Clin Experiment Ophthalmol*. 2008;36(4):377–385.
54. Guo L, Cordeiro MF. Assessment of neuroprotection in the retina with DARC. *Prog Brain Res*. 2008;173:437–450.

# Chapter 55
# Compliance and Adherence: Lifelong Therapy for Glaucoma

Alan Robin, Betsy Sleath, and David Covert

## 55.1 The Problem

The Early Manifest Glaucoma Trial randomized those with early diagnosed previously untreated glaucoma into two groups: no treatment or treatment with a combination of laser trabeculoplasty plus betaxolol ophthalmic solution. At a median follow-up of 8 years, 67% of all subjects progressed and treatment significantly decreased the rate of progression.[1] Despite the initially optimistic news, the results are not as encouraging as they might seem. As one might imagine, 76% of the control group progressed. However, despite apparent treatment, 59% of the treated glaucoma patients also progressed. One would like to know why more than 50% of those under treatment still experience additional glaucomatous progression.

Almost all of the government-sponsored multicentered trials in ophthalmology did not simultaneously evaluate compliance to therapy. Many studies, such as the Advanced Glaucoma Intervention Study,[2] find a direct correlation between lowering intraocular pressure (IOP) and successful therapy as measured by stable visual fields. The authors consider that this success is due in total to the degree of IOP lowering by either laser, surgery, medication, or a combination of these modalities. What these authors do not examine is why some patients achieve adequately low IOPs while others do not. While there may be fundamental biological differences among patients, the answer could also be in part related to patient adherence to prescribed medical therapy.

Does adherence matter? There is good evidence in the systemic literature that there is a direct relationship between adherence and successful outcomes. In many diseases, such as systemic hypertension, there is a direct correlation between adherence and outcome. There is also a direct correlation between intervention and the ability to improve patient disease outcomes. There has been a large void in our systematic research into adherence with glaucoma therapy from the mid 1980s to the first part of this century. During that period of time, the treatment of glaucoma has markedly changed: There has been the advent of three new classes of intraocular pressure-lowering medications (alpha agonists, topical carbonic anhydrase inhibitors, and prostaglandin analogs), the common use of antimetabolites in filtration surgery, the acceptance of laser trabeculoplasty as a commonly used initial glaucoma therapy, as well as the emergence of the acceptance of surgical shunts in glaucoma therapy. Over the last decade, there has been a renewed interest in adherence in glaucoma therapy.

In the United States, medical therapies are still the most common initial treatment used in glaucoma management. They have become easier for patients because much of the first-line treatment may be used just once daily (prostaglandin analogs and nonselective beta blockers) and the medication side effect profiles have improved compared to the older drugs available 10 or more years ago. The use of adjunctive therapy (such as a prostaglandin analog and topical carbonic anhydrase inhibitor) has become commonplace. Why then is adherence such an important issue for management of patients with glaucoma?

Medication adherence, or compliance, is the extent to which a patient acts in accordance with a prescribed interval, medication concentration, and dosing regimen. There are many ways of defining adherence, none of which is perfect. First one can look at *the percent of doses* taken. An example here would be a woman on a once-daily oral contraceptive. At the end of the month, to be totally adherent, one would expect that all her pills would be used. However, if a woman takes all 30 pills for the month on the first day, there would be 100% adherence, but the desired effects might not occur.

A second way of evaluating adherence is to evaluate *coverage*. Coverage is the proportion of time for which the interval between doses is no more than 2 h more than the nominal dosing interval. This makes no adjustment for overdosing. An example here would be for a once-daily medication used over 2 months: If a patient took 30 doses at 20-h intervals and 30 doses at 28-h intervals, the percent coverage would be 1,260/1,440 h (88%).

A third way of assessing adherence is to evaluate *dosing errors*. This allows one to evaluate both over- and under-adherence to a specific dosing regimen. If a patient was supposed to take a medication at 8 A.M. and 8 P.M., but instead took it at 8 A.M., noon, and 8 P.M., this would be considered one dosing error. Finally, one can look at the interdose interval, or the interval between doses. Here an individual who took a BID medication every 9 h half the time and 15 h half the time will have an average interdose interval of 12 h. Although each of these is a valid assessment of adherence, each only tells part of the total story.

Adherence to the treatment of chronic diseases is estimated to be 75%,[3] but may be actually lower with asymptomatic diseases like glaucoma. Kass et al used an electronic monitor in two tandem studies of patients using one medication and found that the mean percent of doses taken was 65% for pilocarpine taken four times daily and 73% for timolol taken twice daily.[4,5] Beyond just taking the appropriate dose at the correct time, adherence with eye drops can be far more complex for the patient compared to adherence with conventional medication regimens (pills and injections). When using eye drops, the patient must be able to place a single drop in the eye without missing the eye while avoiding touching the tip of the bottle to the eye. The patient may also need to apply multiple drops in the eye with an appropriate amount of time separating the drops. A study by Tsai et al found that 17% of patients relied on others for administration of drops due to poor vision and a lack of manual dexterity.[6] We have considered success of the proper administration of a single eye drop to the eye without eye drop bottle, eyelid, or eye contamination.[7] In 140 subjects, all of whom stated that they administered their own eye drops and had a minimum of 6 months experience on glaucoma medical therapy (95% treated for over 1 year), we found that only 83% of subjects actually were able to properly administer a medication to the eye. In addition, only 51% (72/140) were able to use the bottle without contamination, and only 44% (62/140) were able to squeeze a single drop from the bottle. Most eye physicians do not spend much time considering the difficulties of eye drop administration by the patient. One must not only persist with use of a medication, but also execute instillation correctly to achieve the therapeutic benefit. These medication administration difficulties with eye drops are analogous to the problems patients have with using inhalers for asthma, dermatologic creams, and insulin therapy for diabetes. No research has been done on the "best techniques" for eye drop administration and as such there are no standard methods to teach eye drop instillation.

Furthermore, we have no knowledge of how individuals with poorer central vision from retinal disease or advanced field loss from glaucoma are able to administer eye drops. Do they have more problems than people who are normal sighted? Is the use of eye drops more difficult for people with good sight in only one of their eyes as compared to patients who have good binocular visual capabilities? Finally, our knowledge of subjects actually being observed administering eye drops is limited to a few other studies with conflicting results.[8-11]

It is therefore important for us to actually observe our patients in the clinic using eye drops. We cannot assume *a priori* that patients know how to do this, or that they are good at administering eye drops without instruction and feedback after being observed in this process. Many elderly patients with glaucoma have minimal or no family support. They often live by themselves and may not be able to self-administer or have difficulty remembering to take their eye drops at prescribed intervals. In the future we may wish to strive for different types of medical therapies that are long-lasting and that do not require the skills needed for proper drop installation. These therapies, under development, may include long-acting injectable or peribulbar agents, drug eluting implantable devices, drug saturated punctal plugs, and as yet undetermined technologies.

More complex dosing regimens may affect adherence negatively. One drug is often not adequate to control IOP and additional glaucoma medications are required to meet the target pressure. The Ocular Hypertension Treatment Study (OHTS) found that in eyes without significant optic nerve damage at possible risk of developing glaucoma, to reach a modest reduction in IOP of 20% or more long-term, more than 40% of patients needed additional medication within 5 years after starting treatment.[12] The Advanced Glaucoma Intervention Study (AGIS) and the Collaborative Initial Glaucoma Treatment Study (CIGTS) found that in patients with glaucoma, the number of patients requiring more than one medication might be as high as 80% when the disease is more severe.[13,14] The addition of another eye drop medication can be both costly and confusing to the patient, especially with an asymptomatic disease like glaucoma. A study by Robin et al used electronic monitoring to capture the patient dosing experience and found that more complex dosing regimens resulted in poorer adherence and that it was the addition of the second medication that apparently caused the problem.[15] A survey by Sleath et al of patients who were taking two or more medications for glaucoma found that close to half of the patients reported having difficulties administering their drops and nearly a quarter of the patients waited less than 3 min between instillations of multiple glaucoma medications.[16]

## 55.2 Provider–Patient Communication About Glaucoma and Adherence

Additional factors that can create adherence problems for patients include the cost of treatment, side effects, the number and complexity of systemic medications, and a lack of understanding of the need for chronic therapy.[17-19] Approximately 50% of individuals who start on glaucoma medications discontinue them within 6 months.[20,21] Provider–patient communication about glaucoma can be a critical factor that impacts treatment adherence. For example, Tsai et al conducted structured interviews with 48 glaucoma patients and found that communication with providers was cited as an important barrier to medication adherence.[22] Similarly, Taylor et al found that poor provider–patient communication was cited as one of the main reasons for eye drop nonadherence among glaucoma patients.[17] Even more importantly, providers have been found to overestimate patient medication adherence and research has shown that the ability of providers to detect nonadherent patients is poor.[23] Patient demographic characteristics, such as socioeconomic status and level of education are poor predictors of patient adherence to medication regimen.

The following aspects of the provider–patient relationship have been found to be related to poor adherence: (a) inadequate communication, (b) poor rapport, and (c) inadequate provider monitoring of medication use.[24] Each of these areas will be discussed and strategies on how to improve the provider–patient relationship in these areas will be presented.

### 55.2.1 Inadequate Communication

Inadequate communication can negatively influence patient adherence. Research has shown that on average, patients recall and comprehend as little as 50% of what their providers tell them.[25,26] Several other studies have shown that patients have unmet needs for more information from their providers.[27-29] For example, Herndon et al reviewed the results of surveys returned by 4,310 subscribers to the Glaucoma Research Foundation newsletter.[30] Slightly more than half of the respondents reported that they had been told that glaucoma could lead to blindness; 11% reported that they were not told much at all about glaucoma. Only 69% identified intraocular pressure (IOP) as the most important factor impacting their risk of vision loss, and just 49% understood the importance of monitoring IOP. Another study found that 15% of glaucoma patients stated that no one gave them information about their glaucoma medications and 20% stated that no one showed how to use their eye drops.[31]

Educating patients about glaucoma and its treatment is especially important because of the uniqueness of the disease: It is a chronic illness that is symptomless until far advanced. The American Academy of Ophthalmology Guidelines for primary open-angle glaucoma suggests that eye care providers discuss the following at glaucoma visits[32]:

1. Side effects of glaucoma medications
2. Frequency and time of use of last glaucoma medication(s)
3. Review of medication use
4. Physical or emotional changes that occur when taking glaucoma medications (because glaucoma can impact quality of life)
5. Diagnosis, severity of the disease, prognosis and management plan, and likelihood of long-term therapy, and
6. Eyelid closure and nasolacrimal occlusion when applying topical medications in order to reduce systemic absorption[32]

It is important for eye care providers to use the "teach-back technique" with patients because it allows eye care providers a chance to assess patient comprehension and recall.[33] One study found that diabetic patients whose physicians assessed recall or comprehension were more likely to have adequate glycemic control than patients whose physicians did not assess recall or comprehension.[34] To use the "teach-back" technique, eye care providers just need to ask patients to repeat back how they will use a medication so that the provider can then correct any errors in understanding. The following dialog between an ophthalmologist and a glaucoma patient is a good example of how one can use the "teach-back technique":

> OPHTHALMOLOGIST: We are going to leave you on the steroid eye drop but change that to every 3 hours. ... So you're going to take the steroid eye drop how often?
>
> PATIENT: Every 3 hours.
>
> OPHTHALMOLOGIST: That was your test (laughing)
>
> PATIENT: Good. I finally passed a test (laughing)

It is also important to use as many senses as possible. Not only listening and repeating, but also putting instructions in writing. Preprinted forms that may be easily customized for each patient as they are sitting in your examination cubicle are helpful in reminding patients about medications and side effects. In this way, when a patient leaves your office, he will have an additional reminder of what has transpired. An important note is to not refer to medications by their top colors. Many medications' tops can be used on other classes of medications so that a patient may think he is taking the medications correctly but in actuality may be inadequately dosing or creating a potentially dangerous situation (e.g., substituting the tops of a nonselective beta-blocker and topical carbonic anhydrase inhibitor would result in taking the carbonic anhydrase inhibitor once daily – an inadequate amount – and the beta-blocker three times daily – an amount that could potentially cause serious adverse events).

### 55.2.2 Poor Rapport

Rapport issues can also impact the provider–patient relationship and subsequent medication adherence. For example, one study found that diabetic patients reported being less motivated to adhere when their providers scolded them.[35] Street et al found that diabetic patients had poorer metabolic control after interacting with providers who were more controlling and directive.[36]

Provider behavior is often viewed as being on a continuum that ranges from using a paternalistic style where the provider dominates and controls the decisions made during an encounter to using a patient-centered or collaborative goal-setting style where both the provider and patient are involved in making treatment decisions.[37] The term "compliance" is more in line with the paternalistic viewpoint. The term "adherence" suggests more of a partnership between the patient and the physician. An encounter that is patient-centered and focuses on collaborative goal setting is one in which the provider is (a) receptive to the patient's opinions and expectations and (b) involves the patient in decision-making about treatment.[38] Using a patient-centered style can potentially improve patient adherence because both the provider and the patient are part of the treatment decisions being made. The following excerpt from a glaucoma patient visit illustrates an ophthalmologist using a patient-centered interaction style:

> PATIENT: I don't like the Brand A prostaglandin because it does seem to make my eye sore. It's been that way since Dr. __ switched me to Brand A prostaglandin from Brand B prostaglandin. I had been on the Brand B prostaglandin for years.
>
> OPHTHALMOLOGIST: Would you like us to switch you to another medicine that may be a little better but has the same pressure effect?
>
> PATIENT: Well, curiously my right eye was always good with the Prostaglandin B or Prostaglandin A, but my left eye wasn't good with the Prostaglandin B—you know my left eye you just operated on. He switched me to the Prostaglandin A for both eyes 'cause that is easier.
>
> OPHTHALMOLOGIST: Would you like me to switch you back to the Prostaglandin B?
>
> PATIENT: Yes, I would.
>
> OPHTHALMOLOGIST: Okay, we will.

### 55.2.3 Inadequate Provider Monitoring

Inadequate provider monitoring of patient problems and concerns can also negatively impact patient adherence.[25] Sleath and colleagues analyzed 467 audiotapes of physician–patient encounters from 11 primary care settings.[39] All patients were on one or more prescription medications. Nearly half of all patients were not asked how their medications were helping and more than 66% were not asked about barriers or side effects. Prior work has found that glaucoma patient-reported problems in using eye drops were related to patient adherence.[16,40] This underscores the importance of eye care providers monitoring medication use through the use of open-ended questions. Eye care providers seeing glaucoma patients could ask open-ended questions such as:

- "How are you using your eye drops?"
- "How are your eye drops working?"
- "What problems or barriers do you have to using your eye drops?"
- "Many of my patients tell me they find it hard to take their eye drops every day. What makes it hard for you to take all your medicines?"

In summary, eye care provider–patient communication about glaucoma may be a critical factor that impacts treatment adherence.[17,22] Eye care providers should make sure to: (a) adequately educate patients about their medication regimens and use the "teach-back" technique to assess patient comprehension and recall, (b) establish rapport with patients and use a patient-centered or collaborative goal-setting interaction style, (c) adequately monitor patient medication use through the use of open-ended questions, and (d) use both written and verbal instructions. Staff members who establish excellent ongoing personal relationships with the patient may be able to help the physician in monitoring patient adherence.

## 55.3 The Economic Impact of Patient Nonadherence

Patient adherence when less than optimal can reduce therapeutic benefit. The relationship between adherence, clinical effectiveness, and disease progression is complex. However, the expectation from less-than-desired patient adherence is less-than-optimal therapeutic effect, which could lead to disease progression and visual field loss. The economic impact of poor adherence or persistence is difficult to quantify but could be significant. The economic implication of disease progression is increasing health-care costs. When a patient's glaucoma is getting worse, the physician must attempt to separate lack of adequate efficacy of the medical treatment versus poor adherence to that therapy. Changing from one eye drop that the patient is not using consistently to another eye drop that they will use equally nonconsistently will not solve the problem of slowing disease progression.

Studies have looked at the relationship between nonadherence, IOP control, and the progression of disease, but the results were not consistent. A study by Konstas et al[41] found higher IOPs and worse visual field loss in the nonadherent group; however, a study by Spaeth[42] found the opposite, showing good visual field maintenance with poor adherence. A review of these two studies and other studies by Olthoff et al[43] could not find an association between poor adherence, IOP control, and visual field loss. Although this relationship could not be established, a number of studies[12,14,44,45] have shown that IOP control slows or prevents the development of glaucoma. Therefore, the theoretical implication of poor adherence is uncontrolled IOP leading to disease progression over the long term.

This relationship between nonadherence, IOP control, and disease progression is further complicated by other factors such as patient nonresponse to treatment unrelated to adherence and "forgiveness" of the therapy regimen. Nonresponse to treatment could be related to genetic profile, pharmacokinetic and pharmacodynamic factors, and misdiagnosis. The "forgiveness" of a drug, that is the ability of a drug to maintain therapeutic activity despite nonadherence by the patient, is well documented in the area of glaucoma drugs, more specifically with prostaglandin analogs.[46] A number of studies have shown that the IOP lowering capabilities of prostaglandin analogs prescribed once a day can reach well beyond the 24-h dosing period interval, providing some measure of "forgiveness" to patients who are not adherent to their treatment regimen.[47-49] Therefore, loss of therapeutic activity is less likely to occur due to a late or missed dose. Physicians should consider using glaucoma medications with very long half-lives and infrequent dosing intervals given the natural tendency for patients to be less than perfectly adherent to their medication regimens.

Initially, poor adherence would result in lower drug acquisition costs for the health-care payer and the patient in terms of fewer copayments. However, lower than desired therapeutic response may result in additional costs due to unnecessary changes in medication regimen such as switching to another drug or addition of a second concomitant drug. The addition of a second drug could actually reduce adherence further due to a more complex dosing regimen. This may lead to the addition of a third or fourth drug, which would not solve the problem as these additional medications are also not taken appropriately.[50] The addition of more drugs increases the risk of side effects and preservative-related ocular surface inflammation.[51] Costs would increase significantly if unnecessary surgery is also performed to meet the therapeutic target. Quite often the practitioner will take the path of treatment escalation before determining whether nonadherence is the reason for the less-than-desired therapeutic response. If nonadherence is the reason, medication changes will lead to further therapeutic failure and unnecessary costs. The eventual use of surgery to meet the therapeutic target for IOP control will eliminate the adherence issue, but a successful outcome comes at a high cost to the health-care payer and the patient.

While patient nonadherence may initially result in lower drug therapy acquisition costs, overall health-care resource utilization and costs in the long term would be higher as disease progression leads to visual field loss and decreased patient functioning.[52] A study of health-care resource use at different stages of disease for primary open-angle glaucoma (POAG) showed a dramatic increase in direct costs going from $623 per patient for POAG suspects or early stage disease to $2,511 per patient for end-stage disease.[53] Medication costs represented the largest portion of health-care costs at each stage of disease, but the cost of surgery approached the level of drug cost as the average number of surgeries increased with worsening disease severity. For those patients reaching end-stage disease and eventually blindness, it has been estimated that the costs for benefits, health care, and reduced tax revenues total $1.5 billion annually.[54] Loss of visual field also leads to indirect costs from the decreased ability of a patient to complete daily activities and the increased risk of falls and car accidents.[55,56]

## References

1. Leske CM, Heijl A, Hyman L, Bengtsson B, Dong L, Yang Z, EMGT Group. Predictors of long-term progression in the early manifest glaucoma trial. *Ophthalmology*. 2007;114:1965–1972.
2. The AGIS Investigators. The Advanced Glaucoma Intervention Study (AGIS): 7. The relationship between control of intraocular pressure and visual field deterioration. *Am J Ophthalmol*. 2000;130:429–440.
3. DiMatteo MR. Variations in patients' adherence to medical recommendations: a quantitative review of 50 years of research. *Med Care*. 2004;42:200–209.
4. Kass MA, Meltzer DW, Gordon M, et al. Compliance with topical pilocarpine treatment. *Am J Ophthalmol*. 1986;101:515–523.
5. Kass MA, Gordon M, Morley RE, et al. Compliance with topical timolol treatment. *Am J Ophthalmol*. 1987;103:188–193.
6. Tsai T, Robin AL, Smith JP III. An evaluation of how glaucoma patient use topical medications: a pilot study. *Transactions of the AOS*. 2007;105:29–33.
7. Stone JL, Robin AL, Sleath B, Covert DW, Cagle G, Novack GN. Compliance: An Objective Evaluation in Glaucoma Patients of Eye-Drop Instillation Using Video Instillations and Patient Surveys. *Invest Opthalmol Vis Sci*. 2008;49:E-Abstract 1580.
8. Brown MM, Brown GC, Spaeth GL. Improper topical self-administration of ocular medication among patients with glaucoma. *Can J Ophthalmol*. 1984;19:2–5.
9. Kass MA, Hodapp E, Gordon M, et al. Part I. Patient administration of eyedrops: interview. *Ann Ophthalmol*. 1982;14:775–779.
10. Norell SE, Granstrom PA, Wassen R. A medication monitor and fluorescein technique designed to study medication behaviour. *Acta Ophthalmol (Copenh)*. 1980;58:459–467.
11. Kass MA, Hodapp E, Gordon M, et al. Patient administration of eyedrops: observation. Part II. *Ann Ophthalmol*. 1982;14:889–893.
12. Kass MA, Heuer DK, Higginbotham EJ, et al. The Ocular Hypertension Treatment Study: A randomized trial determines that topical ocular hypotensive medicine delays or prevents the onset of POAG. *Arch Ophthalmol*. 2002;120(6):701–713.
13. The AGIS Investigators. The Advanced Glaucoma Study (AGIS):7. The relationship between control of intraocular pressure and visual field deterioration. *Am J Ophthalmol*. 2000;130(4):429–440.
14. Lichter PR, Musch DC, Gillespie BW, et al. Interim clinical outcomes in the Collaborative Initial Glaucoma Treatment Study comparing initial treatment randomized to medications or surgery. *Ophthalmology*. 2001;108:1943–1953.
15. Robin AL, Novack GD, Covert DW, et al. Adherence in glaucoma: Objective measurements of once-daily and adjunctive medication use. *Am J Ophthalmol*. 2007;144:533–540.
16. Sleath B, Robin AL, Covert D, et al. Patient-reported behavior and problems in using glaucoma medications. *Ophthamology*. 2006;113(3):431–436.

17. Taylor SA, Galbraith SM, Mills RP. Causes of non-compliance with drug regimens in glaucoma patients: a qualitative study. *J Ocul Pharmacol Ther.* 2002;18:401–409.
18. Lee MD, Fechtner FR, Fiscella RG, et al. Emerging perspectives on glaucoma: highlights of a roundtable discussion. *Am J Ophthalmol.* 2000;130(4 suppl):S1–S11.
19. Covert D, Robin AL, Novack GD. Systemic medications and glaucoma patients. *Ophthalmology.* 2005;112:1500–1504.
20. Nordstrom BL, Friedman DS, Mozaffari E, et al. Persistence and adherence with topical glaucoma therapy. *Am J Ophthalmol.* 2005;140(4):598–606.
21. Schwartz GF, Platt R, Reardon G, et al. Accounting for restart rates in evaluating persistence with ocular hypotensives. *Ophthalmology.* 2007;114:648–652.
22. Tsai JC, McClure CA, Ramos SE, et al. Compliance barriers in glaucoma: a systematic classification. *J Glaucoma.* 2003;12(5): 393–398.
23. Miller LG, Liu H, Hays RD, et al. How well do clinicians estimate patients' adherence to combination antiretroviral therapy? *J Gen Intern Med.* 2002;17:1–11.
24. Cramer JA. A systematic review of adherence with medications for diabetes. *Diabetes Care.* 2004;27:1218–1224.
25. Crane J. Patient comprehension of doctor-patient communication on discharge from the emergency department. *J Emerg Med.* 1997;15:1–7.
26. Roter DL. The outpatient medical encounter and elderly patients. *Clin Geriatr Med.* 2000;16:95–107.
27. Beisecker AE, Beisecker TD. Patient information-seeking behaviors when communicating with doctors. *Med Care.* 1990;28:19–28.
28. Deber RB, Kraetschmer N, Irvine J. What role do patients wish to play in treatment decision making? *Arch Intern Med.* 1996;156:1414–1420.
29. Strull WM, Lo B, Charles G. Do patients want to participate in medical decision making? *JAMA.* 1984;252:2990–2994.
30. Herndon LW, Brunner TM, Rollins JN. The Glaucoma Research Foundation Patient Survey: patient understanding of glaucoma and its treatment. *Am J Ophthalmol.* 2006;141:22–28.
31. Sleath B, Byrd J, Robin AL, et al. Glaucoma patient receipt of information and instruction on how to use their eye drops. *Int J Pharm Pract.* 2008;16(1):35–40.
32. AAO. *Comprehensive Adult Medical Eye Evaluation, Preferred Practice Pattern.* San Francisco: American Academy of Ophthalmology. <http://www.aao.org/ppp>; 2005.
33. Schwartzberg JG, Cowett A, VanGeest J, et al. Communication techniques for patients with low health literacy: a survey of physicians, nurses, and pharmacists. *Am J Health Behav.* 2007;31(suppl 1):S96–S104.
34. Schillinger D, Piette J, Grumbach K, et al. Closing the loop: physician communication with diabetic patients who have low health literacy. *Arch Intern Med.* 2003;163:83–90.
35. Golin CE, DiMatteo MR, Gelberg L. The role of patient participation in the doctor visit: implications for adherence to diabetes care. *Diabetes Care.* 1996;19:1153–1164.
36. Street RL, Piziak VK, Carpenter WS, et al. Provider-patient communication and metabolic control. *Diabetes Care.* 1993;16:714–721.
37. Roter DL, Hall JL. *Doctors Talking with Patients/Patients Talking with Doctors: Improving Communication in Medical Visits.* Westport, CT: Auburn House; 1992:203.
38. Mead N, Bower P. Patient-centredness: a conceptual framework and review of the empirical literature. *Soc Sci Med.* 2000;51(7): 1087–1110.
39. Sleath B, Roter D, Chewning B, et al. Question-asking about medications: physician experiences and perceptions. *Med Care.* 1999;37(11):1169–1173.
40. Sleath B, Krishnadas R, Cho M, et al. Patient-reported barriers to glaucoma medication access, use, and adherence in Southern India. *Indian J Ophthalmol.* 2009;57(1):63–68.
41. Konstas AGP, Maskaleris G, Gratsonidis S, et al. Compliance and viewpoint of glaucoma patients in Greece. *Eye.* 2000;14:752–756.
42. Spaeth GL. Visual loss in a glaucoma clinic. I. Sociological considerations. *Invest Ophthalmol.* 1970;9:73–82.
43. Olthoff CMG, Schouten JSAG, Van de Borne BW, et al. Noncompliance with ocular hypotensive treatment in patients with glaucoma or ocular hypertension. *Ophthalmology.* 2005;112:953–961.
44. Heijl A, Leske MC, Bengtsson B, Hyman L, Bengtsson B, Hussein M. Reduction of intraocular pressure and glaucoma progression: results from the Early Manifest Glaucoma Trial. *Arch Ophthalmol.* 2002;120(10):1268–1279.
45. Collaborative Normal-Tension Glaucoma Study Group. The effectiveness of intraocular pressure reduction in the treatment of normal-tension glaucoma. *Am J Ophthalmol.* 1998;126(4):498–505.
46. Urquhart J. Patient non-compliance with drug regimens: measurement, clinical correlates, economic impact. *Eur Heart J.* 1996;17(suppl A):S8–S15.
47. DuBiner HB, Sircy MD, Landry T, et al. Comparison of the diurnal ocular hypotensive efficacy of travoprost and latanoprost over a 44-hour period on patients with elevated intraocular pressure. *Clin Ther.* 2004;26:84–91.
48. Garcia-Feijoo J, Martinez-de-la-Casa JM, Castillo A, et al. Circadian IOP-lowering efficacy of travoprost 0.004% ophthalmic solution compared to latanoprost 0.005%. *Curr Med Res Opin.* 2006;22: 1689–1697.
49. Sit AJ, Weinreb RN, Crowston JG, et al. Sustained effect of travoprost on diurnal and nocturnal intraocular pressure. *Am J Ophthalmol.* 2006;141:1131–1133.
50. Neelakantan A, Vaishnav HD, Iyer SA, et al. Is the addition of a third or fourth antiglaucoma medication effective? *J Glaucoma.* 2004;13:130–136.
51. Young TL, Higginbotham EJ, Zou XL, et al. Effects of topical glaucoma drugs on the fistulized rabbit conjunctiva. *Ophthalmology.* 1990;97:1423–1427.
52. Hughes D, Cowell W, Koncz T, et al. Methods for integrating medication compliance and persistence in pharmacoeconomic evaluations. *Value Health.* 2007;10:498–509.
53. Lee PL, Walt JG, Doyle JJ, et al. A multi-center, retrospective pilot study of resource utilization and costs associated with severity of disease in glaucoma. *Arch Ophthalmol.* 2006;124:12–19.
54. Distelhorst JS, Hughes GM. Open-angle glaucoma. *Am Fam Physician.* 2003;67:1937–1944.
55. McKean-Cowdin R, Varma R, Wu J, et al. Severity of visual field loss and health-related quality of life. *Am J Ophthalmol.* 2007;143: 1013–1023.
56. Altangerel U, Spaeth GL, Rhee DJ. Visual function, disability, and psychological impact of glaucoma. *Curr Opin Ophthalmol.* 2003;14:100–105.

# Chapter 56
# Alternative and Non-traditional Treatments of Glaucoma

Joseph R. Zelefsky and Robert Ritch

Glaucoma often exists and progresses at normal or even low intraocular pressure (IOP) levels, on the basis of IOP-independent risk factors. Pressure-independent risk factors have only begun to be explored. Decreased perfusion of the optic nerve head may result from orthostatic hypotension, nocturnal hypotension, atrial fibrillation, migraine, Raynaud's phenomenon, abnormally low intracranial pressure, autoimmune phenomena, and sleep apnea. Hemorheologic abnormalities, such as increased erythrocyte agglutinability, decreased erythrocyte deformability, increased serum viscosity, or increased platelet aggregability, may also play a role. Recent evidence has implicated oxidative stress as playing a significant role in retinal ganglion cell (RGC) damage in glaucoma.[1] Gamma-aminobutyric acid ($GABA_A$) receptors are expressed on RGCs and may play a role in apoptosis induced by oxidative stress.[2]

The aim of neuroprotection in glaucoma is to retard progression by blocking the mechanisms that lead to apoptosis. Many categories of both natural and synthetic compounds that have been reported to have neuroprotective activity include not only antioxidants, N-methyl-D-aspartic acid (NMDA) receptor antagonists, inhibitors of glutamate release, calcium channel blockers, polyamine antagonists, and nitric oxide synthase inhibitors, but also cannabinoids, aspirin, melatonin, and vitamin B-12. The paucity of clinical trials examining the benefits of neuroprotective compounds for glaucoma limit the current use of these agents.

There are, however, many available natural compounds that have actions that may confer neuroprotection. There has been a tendency throughout the twentieth century to denigrate non-pharmaceutical extracts and preparations. However, this was the nature of medicine for millennia, and many valuable compounds still used were originally isolated from plants, including vitamin C from citrus, digitalis from foxglove, quinine from cinchona bark, salicylic acid from willow bark, Taxol from yew bark, and pilocarpine from jaborandi (*Pilocarpus microphyllus*). In the absence of clinical trials, it devolves upon us to make the best possible guess as to what might or might not be effective in glaucoma. This chapter summarizes the potential benefits of natural compounds in the treatment of eye disease.

## 56.1 Alpha-Lipoic Acid

Alpha-lipoic acid is a cofactor in mitochondrial dehydrogenase complexes. When administered exogenously, it has powerful antioxidant properties, which include free radical scavenging, metal chelation, and regeneration of other antioxidants. Alpha-lipoic acid decreases iron uptake from transferrin and reduces the size of the highly reactive iron pool in the cytoplasm of cells of the lens, changes associated with increased cell resistance to oxidative damage.[3] Alpha-lipoic acid may also help to prevent or slow cataract progression.[4-6] It also inhibits the formation of atherosclerotic lesions in mouse models of human atherosclerosis.[7]

Increases in leukostasis/monocyte adhesion to the capillary endothelium and decreased retinal blood flow are implicated in the pathogenesis of diabetic retinopathy. Treatment with alpha-lipoic acid normalizes the amount of leukostasis in diabetic rats.[8] Alpha-lipoic acid corrects decreased retinal ion demand associated with chronic hyperglycemia[9] and may also rectify abnormal retinal oxygenation found in experimental diabetic retinopathy.[10] Alpha-lipoic acid also protects retinal pigment epithelial (RPE) cells from oxidative damage and mitochondrial dysfunction associated with toxins such as cigarette smoke.[11]

## 56.2 Fish Oil and Omega-3 Fatty Acids

Omega-3 fatty acids, such as docosahexaenoic acid (DHA) and eicosapentaenoic acid (EPA), have major health benefits. DHA is thought to play an important role in providing an adequate environment for conformational rhodopsin changes and in modifying the activity of retinal enzymes in photoreceptor cells. Decreased retinal DHA content affects visual function in the monkey.

Oxidative damage induces apoptosis in retinal neurons during their early development in culture and suggests that the loss of mitochondrial membrane integrity is crucial in the apoptotic death of these cells. DHA activates intracellular mechanisms that prevent this loss and by modulating the levels of pro- and antiapoptotic proteins of the Bcl-2 family, selectively protects photoreceptors from oxidative stress.[12] DHA is enriched in RPE cells and is the precursor of neuroprotectin D1 (NPD1), which inhibits oxidative-stress-mediated pro-inflammatory gene induction and apoptosis, and consequently promotes RPE cell survival.[13] NPD1 bioactivity demonstrates that DHA is the precursor to a neuroprotective signaling response to ischemia–reperfusion, thus opening newer avenues of therapeutic exploration in stroke, neurotrauma, spinal cord injury, and neurodegenerative diseases, such as glaucoma, aiming to upregulate this novel cell-survival signaling.[14]

DHA is effective intraperitoneally in protecting the retina against transient retinal ischemia induced by elevated intraocular pressure.[15] Oral DHA can partially counteract retinal neurotoxicity induced by kainic acid.[16] In ischemia–reperfusion injury, DHA protects against cell death, probably by inhibiting the formation of hydroxyl radicals.[17] DHA, in conjunction with lutein and zeaxanthin, promotes survival of rat photoreceptors after oxidative damage.[18]

In the eye, fish oil has been investigated most extensively with regard to age-related macular degeneration (ARMD). In large studies, including the Nurses' Health Study and the Health Professionals' Follow-up Study, increased dietary fish consumption was associated with a 35% lower risk of ARMD.[19,20] Another prospective, multicenter study found that higher intake of specific types of fat – including vegetable, monounsaturated, and polyunsaturated fats, and linoleic acid – rather than total fat intake may be associated with a greater risk for advanced macular degeneration; while diets high in omega-3 fatty acids and fish were inversely associated with risk for macular degeneration when intake of linoleic acid was low.[21]

A combination of DHA, vitamin E, and vitamin B were reported to improve both visual field indices and retinal contrast sensitivity in patients with glaucoma.[22] Intramuscular injections of fish oil containing EPA and DHA significantly lowered intraocular pressure in rabbits.[23] Recent studies in mice demonstrated that an increased diet of omega-3 fatty acids lowers IOP by increasing aqueous outflow facility.[24] Intraperitoneal injection of DHA protected against transient retinal ischemia caused by elevation of intraocular pressure,[15] while dietary supplementation of DHA protected against retinal degeneration caused by N-methyl-N-nitrosourea.[25] DHA also exerts a protective effect against acute light-induced retinal toxicity.[17,26]

## 56.3 Alpha-Tocopherol (Vitamin E) and Tocotrienol

In nature, eight substances have been found to have vitamin E activity: alpha-, beta-, gamma-, and delta-tocopherol; and alpha-, beta-, gamma-, and delta-tocotrienol. In diabetic rats, treatment with the antioxidant alpha-lipoic acid normalized the amount of leukostasis but not retinal blood flow, while treatment with D-alpha-tocopherol prevented the increases in leukostasis and decreases in retinal blood flow in diabetic rats.[8]

Alpha-tocopherol has been reported to protect against retinal phototoxicity,[27] age-related changes in the retina,[28] and ischemic injury of the central nervous system.[29-31] It inhibits human Tenon's capsule fibroblast proliferation[32] and improves the results of filtering surgery in rabbits.[33] Vitamin E appears to protect against cataract formation and progression in animal models and in humans.[34-37]

Tocotrienols possess powerful neuroprotective, anticancer, and cholesterol-lowering properties that are often not exhibited by tocopherols. At nanomolar concentrations, alpha-tocotrienol, not alpha-tocopherol, prevents neurodegeneration.[38] Alpha-tocotrienol increases neuronal resistance to glutamate and homocysteine induced toxicity.[39] Among the vitamin E analogs, alpha-tocotrienol exhibited the most potent neuroprotective actions in rat striatal cultures.[40] Tocotrienols have a cardioprotective effect in ischemia–reperfusion injury[41] and demonstrate antineoplastic effects in gastric and breast cancer cells.[42,43]

## 56.4 Carnitine

Carnitine, an amino acid derivative found in high energy demanding tissues (skeletal muscles, myocardium, liver), is essential for the intermediary metabolism of fatty acids. It plays an important role in those tissues of the eye, such as the ciliary body, where muscle cells are present and may represent an important energy reserve.[44]

Carnitine prevents glutamate neurotoxicity in primary cultures of cerebellar neurons.[45] It has been reported to prevent retinal injury following ischemia–reperfusion injury.[46] In streptozotocin-diabetic rats, carnitine loss in the lens is an initial and important event and may be related to cataract development.[44]

Considerable evidence suggests that mitochondrial dysfunction and oxidative damage may play a role in the pathogenesis of Parkinson's disease and that acetyl-L-carnitine is beneficial in animal models of the disease.[47] Carnitine also protects against selenite-induced cataract[48] and protects RPE cells against hydrogen peroxide-induced oxidative damage.[49]

## 56.5 Citicoline

Citicoline (exogenous CDP-choline) is a nontoxic and well-tolerated drug used in pharmacotherapy of brain insufficiency and other neurological disorders such as stroke, brain trauma, and Parkinson's disease.[50] When administered, citicoline undergoes rapid transformation to cytidine and choline, which are believed to enter brain cells separately and provide neuroprotection by enhancing phosphatidylcholine synthesis. Citicoline activates biosynthesis of structural phospholipids of neuronal membranes, increases brain metabolism, and acts upon different neurotransmitters.[51] It also inhibits apoptosis associated with cerebral ischemia, and, in certain neurodegeneration models, it potentiates neuroplasticity mechanisms.[51]

A similar effect may be expected to occur in glaucomatous retinal ganglion cells (RGCs), but the precise effect of citicoline on damaged RGCs remains to be explained. In RGC tissue culture, citicoline reduces apoptosis and increases the number of regenerating neurites.[52] Citicoline may induce an improvement of the retinal and visual pathway functions in patients with glaucoma, in whom treatment with citicoline induced a significant ($P<0.01$) improvement of visual evoked potential and pattern electroretinography (ERG) parameters.[53-55] Both citicoline and lithium protect RGCs and their axons in vivo against delayed degeneration triggered by optic nerve crush injury and also on retinal cell damage induced by kainic acid.[56,57] The retinoprotective action of both drugs may involve an increase in Bcl-2 expression.[58] Citicoline is as effective as methylprednisolone, previously the only agent having clinically proven beneficial effects on spinal cord injury, in preventing neurodegeneration.[59]

## 56.6 Coenzyme Q10

Tissues that are highly dependent on oxygen such as muscle, the central and peripheral nervous system, kidney, and insulin-producing pancreatic beta-cells are especially susceptible to defective oxidative phosphorylation, which plays an important role in atherogenesis and in the pathogenesis of Alzheimer's disease, Parkinson's disease, diabetes, and aging.[60] Pretreatment of cultured neuronal cells and astrocytes with coenzyme Q10, an essential cofactor in the electron transport chain, inhibits cell death due to glutamate neurotoxicity.[61] It also exhibits anti-apoptotic effects, apparently by stabilizing mitochondrial depolarization.[62] These properties may be beneficial in the treatment of glaucoma, as coenzyme Q10 has been shown to prevent apoptosis in RGCs subjected to ischemia by limiting the release of glutamate.[63] Oral coenzyme Q10 supplementation is effective in treating cardiomyopathies and in restoring plasma levels reduced by the statin type of cholesterol-lowering drugs.[60] Coenzyme Q10 also possesses significant antihypertensive properties.[64] Supplementation with coenzyme Q10 has been reported to slow the development of Parkinson's disease.[65] Patients with open-angle glaucoma may have an increased prevalence of Parkinson's disease.[66] Coenzyme Q10 is beneficial in animal models of neurodegenerative diseases and has shown promising effects both in clinical trials of Parkinson's disease, Huntington's disease, and Friedreich's ataxia.[47]

## 56.7 Curcumin

Curcumin is an antioxidant extracted from the plant *Curcuma longa* and is an important ingredient in Indian cuisine, being present in the commonly used spice turmeric. It is also used in herbal remedies and is reported to possess therapeutic properties against a variety of diseases ranging from cancer to cystic fibrosis.

Turmeric extracts have shown beneficial effects in experimental studies of acute and chronic diseases characterized by an exaggerated inflammatory reaction; they also have strong antioxidant activity and inhibit lipid peroxidation.[67] Curcumin has anticancer, anti-inflammatory, and anti-angiogenesis activities.[68] It also interacts with several molecular targets affecting numerous biochemical cascades. Among these targets are DNA transcription factors, inflammatory cytokines, protein kinases, growth factors, adhesion molecules, anti-apoptotic proteins, and numerous enzymes.[69] Antiulcer activity of curcumin is primarily attributed to MMP-9 inhibition, one of the major pathways of ulcer healing.[70] MMP-9 is the gelatinase B gene, which is activated during angiogenesis by fibroblast growth factor-2 (FGF-2). Curcumin targets the FGF-2 angiogenic signaling pathway and inhibits expression of gelatinase B in the angiogenic process.[71] It also binds metals such as iron and copper and can thus function as an effective chelator.[72]

Al-Omar et al[73] evaluated the neuroprotective effect of curcumin on neuronal death of hippocampal neurons following transient forebrain ischemia in the rat. Treatment with curcumin reduced neuronal damage and increased glutathione, catalase, and superoxide dismutase to normal levels. Numerous other publications have evidenced the neuroprotective activity of curcumin.[74,75] Of particular interest is a recent study that demonstrated that curcumin clears amyloid plaques and reverses neurotoxicity in Alzheimer's disease.[76] Curcumin inhibits chloroquine-resistant *Plasmodium falciparum* growth in culture and reduces blood levels of *Plasmodium berghei* in mice, suggesting its possible use as an antimalarial compound.[77] It accelerates cutaneous wound healing and increases wound tensile strength.[78] Curcumin also prevents heart failure in rats by inhibiting the pathways associated with cardiac myocyte hypertrophy.[79] Several randomized clinical trials investigating curcumin's antineoplastic and anti-inflammatory qualities are currently underway.

In the rat eye, curcumin is effective against the development of diabetic cataract,[80] galactose-induced cataract,[81] and naphthalene-induced cataract.[82] In diabetes, there is a decline in the chaperone-like activity of eye lens alpha-crystallin.

Curcumin, at levels close to dietary consumption, prevents the loss of chaperone-like activity of alpha-crystallin vis-à-vis cataractogenesis due to diabetes in the rat lens.[83] In rat retinal cultures, curcumin reduces N-methyl-D-aspartate-mediated excitotoxic cell damage and decreases apoptosis.[84] Curcumin also inhibits the expression of vascular endothelial growth factor (VEGF) in diabetic rat retinas.[85] Two small studies demonstrated beneficial effects of curcumin on chronic anterior uveitis and inflammatory orbital pseudotumor.[86,87]

## 56.8 Dan Shen (*Salvia miltiorrhiza*)

*Salvia miltiorrhiza* (also known as Asian red sage or Dan shen) contains salviolonic acid B, a potent water-soluble, polyphenolic antioxidant with anti-inflammatory and anti-atherosclerotic properties.[88,89] It has been reported to reduce brain damage in cerebral infarction[90,91] and mitochondrial damage in ischemia–reperfusion injury.[92]

Retinal ganglion cell damage in glaucoma was markedly reduced by intravenous treatment with *Salvia miltiorrhiza*.[93] It has been claimed in one report to stabilize the visual field in patients with glaucoma.[94] A recent study showed that oral administration of Dan shen in diabetic rats restored ocular levels of malondialdehyde, a marker of oxidative stress, to normal levels.[95] Data also demonstrate that it inhibits TNF-alpha-induced activation of NFkB, and in the rabbit model of glaucoma, protects against RGC loss. NMDA receptor antagonist activity may underlie its neuroprotective effects.[96]

## 56.9 Folic Acid

Mild hyperhomocysteinemia is an independent risk factor for premature vascular disease,[97] myocardial infarction,[98] and stroke.[99] Significantly elevated homocysteine levels were also found in patients with Alzheimer's disease as well as in patients with vascular dementia.[100] Homocysteine can induce alterations in extracellular matrix and neuronal cell death that are characteristic findings in glaucoma. Folate supplementation reduces hyperhomocysteinemia.

Culturing embryonic cortical neurons and differentiated SH-SY-5Y human neuroblastoma cells in folate-free medium induced neurodegenerative changes characteristic of those observed in Alzheimer's disease.[101] A significant increase in homocysteine was detected following folate deprivation, which decreased the reduced form of glutathione, indicating a depletion of oxidative buffering capacity.[101] Folic acid (400 µg) associated with vitamin B6 and B12 can reduce homocysteine levels by 30%.[102]

Exfoliation syndrome (XFS) is the most common recognizable cause of open-angle glaucoma overall worldwide.[103] It has been associated in the literature with a history of hypertension, angina, myocardial infarction, stroke,[104] and Alzheimer's disease.[105] Plasma homocysteine levels are elevated in patients with XFS both with and without glaucoma when compared to controls with no ocular disease and to patients with normal-tension glaucoma.[106,107] Plasma levels of vitamin B6, B12, and folate in patients with exfoliative glaucoma are significantly lower than controls.[108] Both XFS and hyperhomocysteinemia share common associations with various disorders. Hyperhomocysteinemia might be a modifiable risk factor for XFS. Homocysteine levels and the frequency of heterozygous methylenetetrahydrofolate reductase (MTHFR) C677T mutation are also increased in primary open-angle glaucoma.[109] In addition to its homocysteine-related effects, the use of folate or vitamin B12 supplements was found to have a strong protective influence on cortical cataract in the Blue Mountains Eye Study.[34]

## 56.10 *Ginkgo biloba* Extract (GBE)

*Ginkgo biloba* extract contains more than 60 known bioactive compounds, about 30 of which are found nowhere else in nature. The standardized extract used most widely in clinical research, EGb 761 (Dr. Willmar Schwabe GmbH & Co, Karlsruhe, Germany), contains 24% ginkgo flavone glycosides (flavonoids), 6% terpene lactones (ginkgolides and bilobalide), approximately 7% proanthocyanidins, and other uncharacterized compounds.[110] GBE has been claimed effective in a variety of disorders associated with aging, including cerebrovascular disease, peripheral vascular disease, dementia, tinnitus, bronchoconstriction, and sexual dysfunction. It appears to have many properties applicable to the treatment of pressure-independent risk factors for glaucomatous damage.[111]

GBE exerts significant protective effects against free radical damage and lipid peroxidation in various tissues and experimental systems. Its antioxidant potential is comparable to water soluble antioxidants, such as ascorbic acid and glutathione, and lipid soluble ones, such as alpha-tocopherol and retinol acetate.[112] It preserves mitochondrial metabolism and adenosine triphosphate (ATP) production in various tissues and partially prevents morphologic changes and indices of oxidative damage associated with mitochondrial aging.[113-115] It can scavenge nitric oxide[116] and possibly inhibit its production.[117]

Substantial experimental evidence exists to support the view that GBE has neuroprotective properties in conditions such as hypoxia/ischemia, seizure activity, cerebral edema, and peripheral nerve damage.[118,119] GBE can reduce glutamate-induced elevation of calcium concentrations[120] and can reduce oxidative metabolism in both resting and calcium-loaded neurons.[121] Neurons in tissue culture are protected from a variety of toxic insults by GBE, which inhibits apoptosis.[122-125] GBE improves both peripheral and cerebral blood flow. It has been reported to protect myocardium against hypoxia and ischemia–reperfusion injury,[126,127] perhaps by uncoupling oxidative phosphorylation in cardiac mitochondria.[128] There is convincing evidence for GBE inducing functional improvement in patients with Alzheimer's-type and multi-infarct dementias.[129,130] Preliminary data suggest that GBE may increase the probability of survival in the elderly population.[131]

In the eye, GBE may have a protective effect against the progression of diabetic retinopathy[132] and reduces ischemia–reperfusion injury in rat retina.[133] GBE protects retinal photoreceptors against light-induced damage by preventing oxidative stress in the retina.[134,135] Chloroquine-induced ERG changes were prevented by simultaneous treatment with GBE.[136] In a rat model of central retinal artery occlusion, GBE reduced edema and necrosis, and blocked the reduction in b-wave amplitude on ERG.[137]

GBE has been reported to improve automated visual field indices.[138,139] In one clinical cross-over study of low-dose, short-term treatment in normal volunteers, GBE increased ophthalmic artery blood flow by a mean of 24%.[140] A more recent study, however, failed to confirm these results.[141]

## 56.11 Ginseng RB1/RG3

Next to GBE, ginseng, a highly valued herb in the Far East, is the most studied plant compound. *Panax ginseng* is one of the most widely used herbs in traditional Chinese medicine. The major active components of ginseng are ginsenosides, a diverse group of steroidal saponins, which demonstrate the ability to target a myriad of tissues, producing an array of pharmacological responses.[142] Of greatest interest are the ginsenoside saponins Rb1 and Rg3, which attenuate or inhibit responses that lead to the apoptotic cascade, including glutamate-induced neurotoxicity, calcium influx into cells in the presence of excess glutamate, and lipid peroxidation.

Ginsenosides Rb1 and Rg3 exert significant neuroprotective effects on cultured cortical cells,[143] and apparently act by inhibiting N-methyl-D-aspartate (NMDA) receptor activity.[144] Central infusion of ginsenoside Rb1 in a gerbil model after forebrain ischemia protects hippocampal CA1 neurons against lethal ischemic damage.[145] Ginsenoside Rb1 has been reported to enhance peripheral nerve regeneration in vitro.[146] Ginsenosides suppress tumor necrosis factor-alpha production in vitro and may have potential therapeutic efficacy against TNF-alpha mediated disease.[147] *Pfaffia paniculata*, a Brazilian ginseng, was effective at inhibiting angiogenesis in mouse corneas.[148]

## 56.12 L-Glutathione

Glutathione is one of the most important antioxidants in the body. Oxidative DNA damage is significantly increased in the trabecular meshwork of glaucoma patients. Glutathione S-transferase M1 polymorphism (GSTM1) gene deletion, which has been associated with an increased risk of cancer at various sites and molecular lesions in atherosclerosis, predisposes to more severe glaucomatous damage.[149]

In a study to identify retinal proteins that are the targets of serum autoantibodies in patients with glaucoma, serum antibodies against glutathione S-transferase antigen were recognized in 34(52%) of 65 patients with glaucoma and 5(20%) of 25 age-matched controls ($P<0.05$). These findings indicate that glutathione S-transferase is targeted by the serum antibodies detected in some patients with glaucoma.[150]

A significant association of the GSTM1 polymorphism with primary open-angle glaucoma has been reported. The risk among the GSTM1-positive individuals of developing glaucoma was even higher among smokers.[151,152] The level of sulfhydryl groups was reported to be significantly lowered in the anterior chamber humor of patients with open-angle glaucoma.[153] Levels of glutathione S-transferases are down-regulated in exfoliation syndrome, suggesting that oxidative damage plays a role in the pathogenesis of exfoliation syndrome and exfoliative glaucoma.[154]

## 56.13 Grape Seed Extract

Grape seed proanthocyanidins have a broad spectrum of pharmacological and medicinal properties against oxidative stress. Grape seed proanthocyanidin extract (GSE) provides excellent protection against free radicals in both in vitro and in vivo models.[155] GSE significantly prevents and postpones development of cataract formation in rats with hereditary cataracts.[156] GSE-induced improvement in myocardial ischemia–reperfusion injury in vitro has also been reported.[157-159] Activin, a new generation antioxidant derived from grape seed proanthocyanidins, reduces plasma levels of oxidative stress and adhesion molecules (ICAM-1, VCAM-1 and E-selectin) in patients with systemic sclerosis.[160] Supplementation of a meal with GSE minimizes postprandial oxidative stress by increasing the antioxidant levels in plasma, and, as a consequence, enhancing the resistance to oxidative modification of low density lipoproteins.[161] Grape seed proanthocyanidins have also been reported to have activity against HIV-1 entry into cells.[162] Grape seed extract has recently been shown to inhibit the growth of prostate cancer tumor cells in mice.[163] In the eye, GSE inhibits key components of cataractogenesis by reducing oxidative stress within lens epithelial cells.[164]

## 56.14 Green Tea Catechins

Tea contains a number of bioactive chemicals and is particularly rich in catechins, of which epigallocatechin gallate (EGCG) is the most abundant[165] and is an extremely potent antioxidant.[166] Catechins and epicatechins are important constituents in human nutrition. There is a concentration-dependent correlation between these compounds and modulation of cell survival/cell death-related gene pathways in vitro.[167] Catechins reduce mitochondrial damage during ischemia reperfusion injury.[168] Green tea extract scavenges free radicals and nitric oxide,[169] and has been reported to both counteract the oxidative insult from cigarette smoke and retard the progression of cataract.[170,171] Oxidative alterations of low-density lipoproteins, scavenging of oxygen free radicals, and inhibition of glutamate toxicity are properties of catechins.[172] EGCG blunts the development of oxidative damage and ischemia/reperfusion damage to retinal photoreceptors, suggesting a potential role for it in the treatment of macular degeneration and glaucoma.[173,174]

## 56.15 Lutein and Zeaxanthine

Lutein is one of the most widely distributed carotenoids in fruits and vegetables. Distribution of lutein among tissues is similar to other carotenoids but, along with zeaxanthin, is found selectively at the center of the retina, being usually referred to as macular pigments. Lutein and zeaxanthin may protect the macula and photoreceptor outer segments throughout the retina from oxidative stress and play a role in an antioxidant cascade that safely disarms the energy of reactive oxygen species.

Age-related macular degeneration is the leading cause of blind registration in the developed world. One etiological hypothesis involves oxidation, and the intrinsic vulnerability of the retina to damage via this process. This has prompted interest in the role of antioxidants, particularly the carotenoids lutein and zeaxanthin, in its prevention and treatment. There is ample epidemiological evidence that the amount of macular pigment is inversely associated with the incidence of ARMD. Dietary supplementation with lutein and zeaxanthin increases macular pigment density.[175]

Several large, randomized, controlled trials, including the highly publicized Age-Related Eye Disease Study, have examined the role of supplements containing lutein, vitamins C and E, zinc, and copper on measures of visual function in people with and without age-related macular disease and have observed a beneficial effect.[176,177] Amplitudes of focal electroretinograms were improved in patients with ARMD receiving supplementation with lutein, vitamin E, and nicotinamide.[178] Zeaxanthin has been reported to protect retinal photoreceptors from acute light-induced toxicity.[179] Lutein and zeaxanthin may[180,181] or may not[176] also retard cataract progression.

## 56.16 Methylcobalamin

In patients with glaucoma, studies have shown possible improvement or stabilization in visual field performance with oral B12 supplementation.[182,183] Methylcobalamin also protects cultured RGCs against glutamate-induced neurotoxicity.[184]

## 56.17 N-Acetyl-L-cysteine

Apoptosis in retinal microvessels in diabetic retinopathy is associated with an increase in cellular ceramide and diacylglycerol levels.[185] The production of diacylglycerol and ceramide is inhibited by N-acetyl-L-cysteine.[185] Protein carbonylation, a nonenzymatic modification that occurs in conditions of cellular oxidative stress, is inhibited by the N-acetyl-L-cysteine.[186] N-Acetyl-L-cysteine increases the neuronal cell survival rate in cultured neurons from embryonic mouse cortex and striatum.[187] N-Acetyl-cysteine decreases the expression of proinflammatory cytokines and adhesion molecules, leading to reduced inflammation in mouse-model of uveitis.[188]

## 56.18 Pycnogenol

Pycnogenol, an extract of French maritime pine bark (*Pinus pinaster*), is primarily composed of procyanidins and phenolic acids, and is a potent antioxidant with strong free-radical-scavenging activity against reactive oxygen and nitrogen species. Procyanidins are biopolymers of catechin and epicatechin subunits, which are recognized as important constituents in human nutrition.[189] Pretreatment with Pycnogenol reduces smoke-induced platelet aggregation.[190] Pycnogenol significantly reduces LDL-cholesterol levels.[191,192] In patients with chronic venous insufficiency, circumference of the lower legs and symptoms of pain, cramps, nighttime swelling, feeling of "heaviness," and reddening of the skin were reduced with Pycnogenol intake.[191] A recent randomized controlled trial revealed that Pycnogenol is an effective treatment for erectile dysfunction.[193]

Pycnogenol is effective in patients with venous microangiopathy[194,195] and accelerates healing in patients' ulcerations of the leg secondary to chronic venous insufficiency[196] and diabetes.[197]

After oral administration, plasma samples significantly inhibited matrix metalloproteinase 9 (MMP-9) release from human monocytes and NFkB activation, indicating that Pycnogenol exerts anti-inflammatory effects by inhibition of proinflammatory gene expression.[198]

Glutamate-induced cytotoxicity in HT-4 neuronal cells has been demonstrated to be due to oxidative stress caused by depletion of cellular glutathione (GSH). More recently, it has been shown to inhibit cyclooxygenases 1 and 2.[199] This cytotoxicity was inhibited by both GBE and Pycnogenol.[200] Pycnogenol can protect vascular endothelial cells from injury induced by amyloid β-peptide (Aβ), suggesting that it may be useful for the prevention and/or treatment of vascular or neurodegenerative diseases associated with Aβ toxicity.[201] Pycnogenol not only suppresses the generation of reactive oxygen species, but also attenuates caspase-3 activation and DNA fragmentation, suggesting protection against Aβ-induced apoptosis.[202] Pycnogenol also demonstrates protective properties against ovarian carcinogenesis.[203]

Pycnogenol has also been reported to have angiotensin-converting enzyme (ACE) inhibiting activity and the ability to enhance the microcirculation by increasing capillary permeability.[204] Pycnogenol inhibits the progression of diabetic retinopathy,[205] and may reduce the risk of formation of both diabetic retinopathy and cataract.[206]

## 56.19 Quercetin

This flavonoid antioxidant, found in GBE and in red wine, inhibits the release of nitric oxide[207] and TNF-alpha,[208] which may be an important factor in the initiation of glaucomatous damage. Quercetin is neuroprotective against oxidative injury in cortical cell cultures, inhibiting lipid peroxidation and scavenging free radicals,[209] and hepatoprotective against ischemia–reperfusion injury when given orally.[210] Apoptosis-promoting substances, including TNF-alpha secreted by activated glial cells after exposure to stress, contribute directly to neuronal cytotoxicity.[211] Quercetin inhibits lipid peroxidation in the mammalian eye,[212] and has been reported to slow the progression of selenite-induced cataract in rats.[213] At low concentrations, quercetin protects human lens epithelial cells in vivo from dimethyl sulfoxide-induced oxidative damage.[214] Treatment of galactose-induced cataracts in rodents with quercetin restored the proper osmotic and ionic equilibrium of the lens, thereby maintaining its transparency, compared to controls.[215]

## 56.20 Resveratrol

Resveratrol is found largely in the skins of red grapes and came to scientific attention as a possible explanation for the low incidence of heart disease among the French, who eat a relatively high-fat diet. Many studies suggest that consuming alcohol (especially red wine) may reduce the incidence of coronary heart disease (CHD). Grape juice, which is not a fermented beverage, is not a significant source of resveratrol.

Resveratrol increases the lifespan of the yeast *Saccharomyces cerevisiae*, the nematode *Caenorhabditis elegans*, and the fruit fly *Drosophila melanogaster*. It was later shown to extend the lifespan of the short-lived killifish *Nothobranchius furzeri*[216]; and has now been shown to significantly increase the health and survival of mice on a high-calorie diet, pointing to a new approach to treating diseases of aging.[217] Among its multiple functions, resveratrol activates sirtuins, a family of proteins that plays an important role in DNA repair, gene silencing, chromosomal stability, and longevity.[218]

Resveratrol is an effective antioxidant.[219-221] It inhibits lipid peroxidation of low-density lipoprotein (LDL), prevents the cytotoxicity of oxidized LDL, and protects cells against lipid peroxidation.[221] Resveratrol protects against the degeneration of neurons after axotomy.[222] A single infusion of resveratrol can elicit neuroprotective effects on cerebral ischemia-induced neuron damage through free radical scavenging and cerebral blood elevation due to nitric oxide release.[223] Its antiapoptotic activity has led to the suggestion that resveratrol may make a useful dietary supplement for minimizing oxidative injury in immune-perturbed states and human chronic degenerative diseases.[224]

Levels of intracellular heme (iron-protoporphyrin IX), a pro-oxidant, increase after stroke. In neuronal cell cultures, resveratrol induces heme oxygenase 1, suggesting that increased heme oxygenase activity is a unique pathway by which resveratrol can exert its neuroprotective actions.[225]

In the eye, resveratrol suppresses selenite-induced oxidative stress and cataract formation in rats.[226] The authors suggested that the presence of oxidative stress in selenite cataract development and its prevention by resveratrol support the possibility that high natural consumption of resveratrol in food can help prevent human senile cataract. Resveratrol also induces dilation of retinal arterioles, suggesting a potential benefit for this compound in the treatment of retinal vascular disease.[227] Sirtuin-1 activators (such as resveratrol) demonstrate neuroprotective properties in mouse models of optic neuritis and multiple sclerosis.[228]

## 56.21 Taurine

Taurine is a free amino acid particularly abundant in the retina. Visual dysfunction in both humans and animals results from taurine deficiency, which can be reversed with nutritional supplementation. The distribution of taurine is tightly regulated in the different retinal cell types throughout the development of the retina. The exact function or functions of taurine in the retina are still unresolved. Nevertheless, taurine depletion results in significant retinal lesions, and taurine release and uptake have been found to employ distinct regulatory mechanisms in the retina.[229]

Taurine supplementation in diabetic rats significantly decreases lipid peroxidation and preserves ATPase activity.[230] Taurine protects against low level radiation-associated protein leakage.[231] In studies of neuritic outgrowth from postcrush goldfish retinal explants, taurine increased length and density of neurites.[232] Treatment with taurine, diltiazem, and vitamin E, has a beneficial effect of decreasing the rate of visual field loss in patients with retinitis pigmentosa, likely through a protective action from free radical reactions in affected photoreceptors.[233] Evidence also suggests that taurine may prevent the development of diabetic cataracts.[234]

## 56.22 Clinical Pearls

1. In patients with normal tension glaucoma or in patients who progress at consistently low pressures, consider IOP-independent factors in the pathogenesis and treatment of the disease.
2. Raynaud's phenomenon is associated with glaucoma and may be a marker for diminished blood flow to the optic nerve head. Treatment with Gingko biloba extract (GBE) may be beneficial in these cases.
3. Because of its blood thinning properties, GBE should be used with caution in patients taking blood thinners such as aspirin, clopidogrel, and warfarin.
4. Explain to your patients that the purpose of supplements for glaucoma is not to reduce IOP but rather to protect the optic nerve via alternate mechanisms.

**Acknowledgments** The authors have no financial interest in products mentioned. From the Einhorn Clinical Research Center, New York Eye and Ear Infirmary, New York, NY, USA and The New York Medical College, Valhalla, NY, USA. Supported in part by the Derald H. Ruttenberg Foundation and the New York Glaucoma Research Institute, New York City

## References

1. Liu Q, Ju WK, Crowston JG, et al. Oxidative stress is an early event in hydrostatic pressure induced retinal ganglion cell damage. *Invest Ophthalmol Vis Sci.* 2007;48:4580–4589.
2. Okumichi H, Mizukami M, Kiuchi Y, et al. GABA(A) receptors are associated with retinal ganglion cell death induced by oxidative stress. *Exp Eye Res.* 2008;86:727–733. Epub ahead of print.
3. Goralska M, Dackor R, Holley B, et al. Alpha lipoic acid changes iron uptake and storage in lens epithelial cells. *Exp Eye Res.* 2003;76:241–248.
4. Kojima M, Sun L, Hata I, et al. Efficacy of alpha-lipoic acid against diabetic cataract in rat. *Jpn J Ophthalmol.* 2007;51:10–13.
5. Maitra I, Serbinova E, Tritschler HJ, et al. Stereospecific effects of R-lipoic acid on buthionine sulfoximine-induced cataract formation in newborn rats. *Biochem Biophys Res Commun.* 1996;221:422–429.
6. Borenshtein D, Ofri R, Werman M, et al. Cataract development in diabetic sand rats treated with alpha-lipoic acid and its gamma-linolenic acid conjugate. *Diabetes Metab Res Rev.* 2001;17:44–50.
7. Zhang WJ, Bird KE, McMillen TS, et al. Dietary alpha-lipoic acid supplementation inhibits atherosclerotic lesion development in apolipoprotein E-deficient and apolipoprotein E/low-density lipoprotein receptor-deficient mice. *Circulation.* 2008;117:421–428.
8. Abiko T, Abiko A, Clermont AC, et al. Characterization of retinal leukostasis and hemodynamics in insulin resistance and diabetes: role of oxidants and protein kinase-C activation. *Diabetes.* 2003;52:829–837.
9. Berkowitz BA, Roberts R, Stemmler A, et al. Impaired apparent ion demand in experimental diabetic retinopathy: correction by lipoic acid. *Invest Ophthalmol Vis Sci.* 2007;48:4753–4758.
10. Roberts R, Luan H, Berkowitz BA. Alpha-lipoic acid corrects late-phase supernormal retinal oxygenation response in experimental diabetic retinopathy. *Invest Ophthalmol Vis Sci.* 2006;47:4077–4082.
11. Jia L, Liu Z, Sun L, et al. Acrolein, a toxicant in cigarette smoke, causes oxidative damage and mitochondrial dysfunction in RPE cells: protection by (R)-alpha-lipoic acid. *Invest Ophthalmol Vis Sci.* 2007;48:339–348.
12. Rotstein NP, Politi LE, German OL, et al. Protective effect of docosahexaenoic acid on oxidative stress-induced apoptosis of retina photoreceptors. *Invest Ophthalmol Vis Sci.* 2003;44:2252–2259.
13. Bazan NG. Cell survival matters: docosahexaenoic acid signaling, neuroprotection and photoreceptors. *Trends Neurosci.* 2006;29:263–271.
14. Bazan NG. Neuroprotectin D1 (NPD1): a DHA-derived mediator that protects brain and retina against cell injury-induced oxidative stress. *Brain Pathol.* 2005;15:159–166.
15. Miyauchi O, Mizota A, Adachi-Usami E, et al. Protective effect of docosahexaenoic acid against retinal ischemic injury: an electroretinographic study. *Ophthalmic Res.* 2001;33:191–195.
16. Mizota A, Sato E, Taniai M, et al. Protective effects of dietary docosahexaenoic acid against kainate-induced retinal degeneration in rats. *Invest Ophthalmol Vis Sci.* 2001;42:216–221.
17. Murayama K, Yoneya S, Miyauchi O, et al. Fish oil (polyunsaturated fatty acid) prevents ischemic-induced injury in the mammalian retina. *Exp Eye Res.* 2002;74:671–676.
18. Chucair AJ, Rotstein MP, Sangiovanni JP, et al. Lutein and zeaxanthin protect photoreceptors from apoptosis induced by oxidative stress: relation with docosahexaenoic acid. *Invest Ophthalmol Vis Sci.* 2007;48:5168–5177.
19. Smith W, Mitchell P, Leeder SR. Dietary fat and fish intake and age-related maculopathy. *Arch Ophthalmol.* 2000;118:401–404.
20. Cho E, Hung S, Willett WC, et al. Prospective study of dietary fat and the risk of age-related macular degeneration. *Am J Clin Nutr.* 2001;73:209–218.
21. Seddon JM, Rosner B, Sperduto RD, et al. Dietary fat and risk for advanced age-related macular degeneration. *Arch Ophthalmol.* 2001;119:1191–1199.
22. Cellini M, Caramazza N, Mangiafico P, et al. Fatty acid use in glaucomatous optic neuropathy treatment. *Acta Ophthalmol Scand.* 1998;227(suppl):41–42.
23. Mancino M, Ohia E, Kulkarni P. A comparative study between cod liver oil and liquid lard intake on IOP in rabbits. *Prostaglandins Leukot Essent Fatty Acids.* 1992;45:239–243.
24. Nguyen CTO, Bui BV, Sinclair AJ, et al. Dietary omega 3 fatty acids decrease intraocular pressure with age by increasing aqueous outflow facility. *Invest Opthalmol Vis Sci.* 2007;48:756–762.
25. Moriguchi K, Yuri T, Yoshizawa K, et al. Dietary docosahexaenoic acid protects against N-methyl-N-nitrosourea-induced retinal degeneration in rats. *Exp Eye Res.* 2003;77:167–173.

26. Reme CE, Malnoe A, Jung HH, et al. Effect of dietary fish oil on acute light-induced photoreceptor damage in the rat retina. *Invest Ophthalmol Vis Sci.* 1994;35:78–90.
27. Aonuma H, Koide K, Masuda K, et al. Retinal light damage: protective effect of alpha-tocopherol. *Jpn J Ophthalmol.* 1997;41:160–167.
28. Tanito M, Yoshida Y, Kaidzu S, et al. Acceleration of age-related changes in the retina in alpha-tocopherol transfer protein null mice fed a vitamin E-deficient diet. *Invest Ophthalmol Vis Sci.* 2007;4:396–404.
29. Van der Worp HB, Bar PR, Kappelle LJ, et al. Dietary vitamin E levels affect outcome of permanent focal cerebral ischemia in rats. *Stroke.* 1998;29:1002–1005.
30. Takahashi H, Kosaka N, Nakagawa S. Alpha-Tocopherol protects PC12 cells from hyperoxia-induced apoptosis. *J Neurosci Res.* 1998;52:184–191.
31. Tagami M, Yamagata K, Ikeda K, et al. Vitamin E prevents apoptosis in cortical neurons during hypoxia and oxygen reperfusion. *Lab Invest.* 1998;78:1415–1429.
32. Haas AL, Boscoboinik D, Mojon DS, et al. Vitamin E inhibits proliferation of human Tenon's capsule fibroblasts in vitro. *Ophthalmic Res.* 1996;28:171–175.
33. Pinilla I, Larrosa JM, Polo V, et al. Alpha-tocopherol derivatives in an experimental model of filtering surgery. *Ophthalmic Res.* 1999;31:440–445.
34. Kuzniarz M, Mitchell P, Cumming RG, et al. Use of vitamin supplements and cataract: the Blue Mountains Eye Study. *Am J Ophthalmol.* 2001;132:19–26.
35. Kojima M, Shui YB, Murano H, et al. Inhibition of steroid-induced cataract in rat eyes by administration of vitamin-E ophthalmic solution. *Ophthalmic Res.* 1996;28(suppl 2):64–67.
36. Rouhiainen P, Rouhiainen H, Salonen JT. Association between low plasma vitamin E concentration and progression of early cortical lens opacities. *Am J Epidemiol.* 1996;144:496–500.
37. Nagata M, Kojima M, Sasaki K. Effect of vitamin E eye drops on naphthalene-induced cataract in rats. *J Ocul Pharmacol Ther.* 1999;15:345–350.
38. Sen CK, Khanna S, Roy S. Tocotrienols: vitamin E beyond tocopherols. *Life Sci.* 2006;78:2088–2098.
39. Khanna S, Roy S, Slivka A, et al. Neuroprotective properties of the natural vitamin E alpha-tocotrienol. *Stroke.* 2005;36:2258–2264.
40. Osakada F, Hashino A, Kume T, et al. Alpha-tocotrienol provides the most potent neuroprotection among vitamin E analogs on cultured striatal neurons. *Neuropharmacology.* 2004;47:904–915.
41. Das S, Powell SR, Wang P, et al. Cardioprotection with palm tocotrienol: antioxidant activity of tocotrienol is linked with its ability to stabilize proteasomes. *Am J Physiol Heart Circ Physiol.* 2005;289:H361–H367.
42. Sun W, Wang Q, Chen B, et al. Gamma-tocotrienol-induced apoptosis in human gastric cancer SGC-7901 cells is associated with a suppression in mitogen-activated protein kinase signalling. *Br J Nutr.* 2008;99:1247–1254. Epub ahead of print.
43. Samant GV, Sylvester PW. Gamma-tocotrienol inhibits ErbB3-dependent PI3K/Akt mitogenic signalling in neoplastic mammary epithelial cells. *Cell Prolif.* 2006;39:563–574.
44. Pessotto P, Valeri P, Arrigoni-Martelli E. The presence of L-carnitine in ocular tissues of the rabbit. *J Ocul Pharmacol.* 1994;10:643–651.
45. Llansola M, Erceg S, Hernandez-Viadel M, et al. Prevention of ammonia and glutamate neurotoxicity by carnitine: molecular mechanisms. *Metab Brain Dis.* 2002;17:389–397.
46. Kocer I, Kulacoglu D, Altuntas I, et al. Protection of the retina from ischemia–reperfusion injury by L-carnitine in guinea pigs. *Eur J Ophthalmol.* 2003;13:80–85.
47. Beal MF. Bioenergetic approaches for neuroprotection in Parkinson's disease. *Ann Neurol.* 2003;53(suppl 3):S39–S47.
48. Geraldine P, Sneha B, Elanchezhian R, et al. Prevention of selenite-induced cataracttogenesis by acetyl-L-carnitine: an experimental study. *Exp Eye Res.* 2006;83:1340–1349.
49. Shamsi FA, Chaudhry IA, Bouton ME, et al. L-carnitine protects human retinal pigment epithelial cells from oxidative damage. *Curr Eye Res.* 2007;32:575–584.
50. Grieb P, Rejdak R. Pharmacodynamics of citicoline relevant to the treatment of glaucoma. *J Neurosci Res.* 2002;67:143–148.
51. Secades JJ, Frontera G. CDP-choline: pharmacological and clinical review. *Methods Find Exp Clin Pharmacol.* 1995;17(suppl B):1–54.
52. Oshitari T, Fujimoto N, Adachi-Usami E. Citicoline has a protective effect on damaged retinal ganglion cells in mouse culture retina. *Neuroreport.* 2002;13:2109–2111.
53. Rejdak R, Toczolowski J, Kurkowski J, et al. Oral citicoline treatment improves visual pathway function in glaucoma. *Med Sci Monit.* 2003;9:PI24–PI28.
54. Parisi V. Electrophysiological assessment of glaucomatous visual dysfunction during treatment with cytidine-5′-diphosphocholine (citicoline): a study of 8 years of follow-up. *Doc Ophthalmol.* 2005;110:91–102.
55. Parisi V, Manni G, Colacino G, et al. Cytidine-5′-diphosphocholine (citicoline) improves retinal and cortical responses in patients with glaucoma. *Ophthalmology.* 1999;106:1126–1134.
56. Park CH, Kim YS, Lee HK, et al. Citicoline reduces upregulated clusterin following kainic acid injection in the rat retina. *Curr Eye Res.* 2007;32:1055–1063.
57. Han YS, Chung IY, Park JM, et al. Neuroprotective effect of citicoline on retinal cell damage induced by kainic acid in rats. *Korean J Ophthalmol.* 2005;19:219–226.
58. Schuettauf F, Rejdak R, Thaler S, et al. Citicoline and lithium rescue retinal ganglion cells following partial optic nerve crush in the rat. *Exp Eye Res.* 2006;83:1128–1134.
59. Yucel N, Cayli SR, Ates O, et al. Evaluation of the neuroprotective effects of citicoline after experimental spinal cord injury: improved behavioral and neuroanatomical recovery. *Neurochem Res.* 2006;31:767–775.
60. Fosslien E. Mitochondrial medicine – molecular pathology of defective oxidative phosphorylation. *Ann Clin Lab Sci.* 2001;31:25–67.
61. Sandhu JK, Pandey S, Ribecco-Lutkiewicz M, et al. Molecular mechanisms of glutamate neurotoxicity in mixed cultures of NT2-derived neurons and astrocytes: protective effects of coenzyme Q10. *J Neurosci Res.* 2003;72:691–703.
62. Papucci L, Schiavone N, Witort E, et al. Coenzyme Q10 prevents apoptosis by inhibiting mitochondrial depolarization independently of its free radical-scavenging property. *J Biol Chem.* 2003;278:28220–28228.
63. Nucci C, Tartaglione R, Cerulli A. Retinal damage caused by high intraocular pressure-induced transient ischemia is prevented by coenzyme Q10 in rat. *Int Rev Neurobiol.* 2007;82:397–406.
64. Rosenfeldt FL, Haas SJ, Krum H, et al. Coenzyme Q10 in the treatment of hypertension: a meta-analysis of the clinical trials. *J Hum Hypertens.* 2007;21:297–306.
65. Shults CW, Oakes D, Kieburtz K, et al. Effects of coenzyme Q(10) in early Parkinson disease – evidence of slowing of the functional decline. *Arch Neurol.* 2002;59:1541–1552.
66. Bayer AU, Keller ON, Ferrari F, et al. Association of glaucoma with neurodegenerative diseases with apoptotic cell death: Alzheimer's disease and Parkinson's disease. *Am J Ophthalmol.* 2002;133:135–137.
67. Tilak JC, Banerjee M, Mohan H, et al. Antioxidant availability of turmeric in relation to its medicinal and culinary uses. *Phytother Res.* 2004;18:798–804.
68. Weber WM, Hunsaker LA, Abcouwer SF, et al. Anti-oxidant activities of curcumin and related enones. *Bioorg Med Chem.* 2005;13:3811–3820.

69. Goel A, Kunnumakkara AB, Aggarwal BB. Curcumin as "Curecumin": from kitchen to clinic. *Biochem Pharmacol.* 2008;75:787–809.
70. Swarnakar S, Ganguly K, Kundu P, et al. Curcumin regulates expression and activity of matrix metalloproteinases 9 and 2 during prevention and healing of indomethacin-induced gastric ulcer. *J Biol Chem.* 2005;280:9409–9415.
71. Mohan R, Sivak J, Ashton P, et al. Curcuminoids inhibit the angiogenic response stimulated by fibroblast growth factor-2, including expression of matrix metalloproteinase gelatinase B. *J Biol Chem.* 2000;275:10405–10412.
72. Hatcher H, Planalp R, Cho J, et al. Curcumin: from ancient medicine to current clinical trials. *Cell Mol Life Sci.* 2008;65:1631–1652.
73. Al-Omar FA, Nagi MN, Abdulgadir MM, et al. Immediate and delayed treatments with curcumin prevents forebrain ischemia-induced neuronal damage and oxidative insult in the rat hippocampus. *Neurochem Res.* 2006;31:611–618.
74. Wang Q, Sun AY, Simonyi A, et al. Neuroprotective mechanisms of curcumin against cerebral ischemia-induced neuronal apoptosis and behavioral deficits. *J Neurosci Res.* 2005;82:138–148.
75. Zbarsky V, Datla KP, Parkar S, et al. Neuroprotective properties of the natural phenolic antioxidants curcumin and naringenin but not quercetin and fisetin in a 6-OHDA model of Parkinson's disease. *Free Radic Res.* 2005;39:1119–1125.
76. Garcia-Alloza M, Borrelli LA, Rozkalne A, et al. Curcumin labels amyloid pathology in vivo, disrupts existing plaques, and partially restores distorted neurites in an Alzheimer mouse model. *J Neurochem.* 2007;102:1095–1104.
77. Reddy RC, Vatsala PG, Keshamouni VG, et al. Curcumin for malaria therapy. *Biochem Biophys Res Commun.* 2005;326:472–474.
78. Panchatcharam M, Miriyala S, Gayathri VS, et al. Curcumin improves wound healing by modulating collagen and decreasing reactive oxygen species. *Mol Cell Biochem.* 2006;290:87–96.
79. Morimoto T, Sunagawa Y, Kawamura T, et al. The dietary compound curcumin inhibits p300 histone acetyltransferase activity and prevents heart failure in rats. *J Clin Invest.* 2008;118:868–878.
80. Suryanarayana P, Saraswat M, Mrudula T, et al. Curcumin and turmeric delay streptozotocin-induced diabetic cataract in rats. *Invest Ophthalmol Vis Sci.* 2005;46:2092–2099.
81. Raju TN, Kumar CS, Kanth VR, et al. Cumulative antioxidant defense against oxidative challenge in galactose-induced cataractogenesis in Wistar rats. *Indian J Exp Biol.* 2006;44:733–739.
82. Pandya U, Saini MK, Jin GF, et al. Dietary curcumin prevents ocular toxicity of naphthalene in rats. *Toxicol Lett.* 2000;115:195–204.
83. Kumar PA, Suryanarayana P, Reddy PY, et al. Modulation of alpha-crystallin chaperone activity in diabetic rat lens by curcumin. *Mol Vis.* 2005;11:561–568.
84. Matteucci A, Frank C, Domenici MR, et al. Curcumin treatment protects rat retinal neurons against excitotoxicity: effect on N-methyl-D: -aspartate-induced intracellular Ca(2+) increase. *Exp Brain Res.* 2005;167:641–648.
85. Mrudula T, Suryanaryana P, Srinivas PN, et al. Effect of curcumin on hyperglycemia-induced vascular endothelial growth factor expression in streptozotocin-induced diabetic rat retina. *Biochem Biophys Res Commun.* 2007;361:528–532.
86. Lal B, Kapoor AK, Agrawal PK, et al. Role of curcumin in idiopathic inflammatory orbital pseudotumours. *Phytother Res.* 2000;14:443–447.
87. Lal B, Kapoor AK, Asthana OP, et al. Efficacy of curcumin in the management of chronic anterior uveitis. *Phytother Res.* 1999;13:318–322.
88. Wu YJ, Hong CY, Lin SJ, et al. Increase of vitamin E content in LDL and reduction of atherosclerosis in cholesterol-fed rabbits by a water-soluble antioxidant-rich fraction of *Salvia miltiorrhiza*. *Arterioscler Thromb Vasc Biol.* 1998;18:481–486.
89. Chen YH, Lin SJ, Ku HH, et al. Salvianolic acid B attenuates VCAM-1 and ICAM-1 expression in TNF-alpha-treated human aortic endothelial cells. *J Cell Biochem.* 2001;82:512–521.
90. Lam BY, Lo AC, Sun X, et al. Neuroprotective effects of tanshinones in transient focal cerebral ischemia in mice. *Phytomedicine.* 2003;10:286–291.
91. Min LQ, Dang LY, Ma WY. Clinical study on effect and therapeutical mechanism of composite Salvia injection on acute cerebral infarction. *Zhongguo Zhong Xi Yi Jie He Za Zhi.* 2002;22:353–355.
92. Zhang WH, Wang JS, Zhou Y, et al. Gadolinium chloride and salvia miltiorrhiza compound ameliorate reperfusion injury in hepatocellular mitochondria. *World J Gastroenterol.* 2003;9:2040–2044.
93. Zhu MD, Cai FY. Evidence of compromised circulation in the pathogenesis of optic nerve damage in chronic glaucomatous rabbit. *Chin Med J.* 1993;106:922–927.
94. Wu ZZ, Jiang YQ, Yi SM, et al. Radix salviae miltiorrhizae in middle and late-stage glaucoma. *Chin Med J.* 1983;96:445–447.
95. Yue KK, Lee KW, Shan KK, et al. Danshen prevents the occurrence of oxidative stress in the eye and aorta of diabetic rats without affecting the hyperglycemic state. *J Ethnopharmacol.* 2006;106:136–141.
96. Sun X, Chan LN, Gong X, et al. N-methyl-D-aspartate receptor antagonist activity in traditional Chinese stroke medicines. *Neurosignals.* 2003;12:31–38.
97. Clarke R, Daily L, Robinson K, et al. Hypermocysteinemia: an independent risk factor for vascular disease. *N Engl J Med.* 1991;324:1149–1155.
98. Stampfer MJ, Malinow MR, Willet WC, et al. A prospective study of plasma homocysteine and risk of myocardial infarction in US physicians. *JAMA.* 1992;268:877–881.
99. Perry IJ, Refsum H, Morris RW, et al. Prospective study of serum total homocysteine concentration and risk of stroke in middle-aged British me. *Lancet.* 1995;346:1395–1398.
100. Leblhuber F, Walli J, Artner-Dworzak E, et al. Hyperhomocysteinemia in dementia. *J Neural Transm.* 2000;107:1469–1474.
101. Ho PI, Ashline D, Dhitavat S, et al. Folate deprivation induces neurodegeneration: roles of oxidative stress and increased homocysteine. *Neurobiol Dis.* 2003;14:32–42.
102. Lobo A, Naso A, Arheart K, et al. Reduction of homocysteine levels in coronary artery disease by low-dose folic acid combined with vitamins B6 and B12. *Am J Cardiol.* 1999;83:821–825.
103. Ritch R. Exfoliation syndrome: the most common identifiable cause of open-angle glaucoma. *J Glaucoma.* 1994;3:176–178.
104. Mitchell P, Wang JJ, Smith W. Association of pseudoexfoliation with increased vascular risk. *Am J Ophthalmol.* 1997;124:685–687.
105. Linnér E, Popovic V, Gottfries CG, et al. The exfoliation syndrome in cognitive impairment of cerebrovascular or Alzheimer's type. *Acta Ophthalmol Scand.* 2001;79:283–285.
106. Leibovitch I, Kurtz S, Shemesh G, et al. Hyperhomocystinemia in pseudoexfoliation glaucoma. *J Glaucoma.* 2003;12:36–39.
107. Vessani RM, Liebmann JM, Jofe M, et al. Plasma homocysteine is elevated in patients with exfoliation syndrome. *Am J Ophthalmol.* 2003;136:41–46.
108. Roedl JB, Bleich S, Reulbach U, et al. Vitamin deficiency and hyperhomocysteinemia in pseudoexfoliation glaucoma. *J Neural Transm.* 2007;114:571–575.
109. Jünemann AG, von Ahsen B, Kornhuber H, et al. MTHFR C677T Polymorphism Is a genetic risk factor for primary open-angle glaucoma. *Invest Ophthalmol Vis Sci.* 2003;35(suppl):748–752.
110. De Feudis FV. *Ginkgo biloba extract (EGb 761): pharmacological activities and clinical applications.* Paris: Elsevier; 1991.
111. Ritch R. A potential role for *Ginkgo biloba* extract in the treatment of glaucoma. *Med Hypotheses.* 2000;54:221–235.

112. Köse K, Dogan P. Lipoperoxidation induced by hydrogen peroxide in human erythrocyte membranes. 1. Protective effect of *Ginkgo biloba* extract (EGb 761). *J Int Med Res*. 1995;23:1–8.
113. Sastre J, Lloret A, Borras C, et al. GBE EGb 761 protects against mitochondrial aging in the brain and in the liver. *Cell Mol Biol*. 2002;48:685–692.
114. Pierre S, Jamme I, Droy-Lefaix MT, et al. *Ginkgo biloba* extract (EGb 761) protects NaK-ATPase activity during cerebral ischemia in mice. *Neuroreport*. 1999;10:47–51.
115. Janssens D, Delaive E, Remacle J, et al. Protection by bilobalide of the ischaemia-induced alterations of the mitochondrial respiratory activity. *Fundam Clin Pharmacol*. 2000;14:193–201.
116. Marcocci L, Maguire JJ, Droy-Lefaix MT, et al. The nitric oxide-scavenging properties of *Ginkgo biloba* extract (EGb 761). *Biochem Biophys Res Commun*. 1994;201:748–755.
117. Kobuchi H, Droy-Lefaix MT, Christen Y, et al. *Ginkgo biloba* extract (EGb 761): inhibitory effect on nitric oxide production in the macrophage cell line RAW 264.7. *Biochem Pharmacol*. 1997;53:897–904.
118. Ahlemeyer B, Krieglstein J. Pharmacological studies supporting the therapeutic use of *Ginkgo biloba* extract for Alzheimer's disease. *Pharmacopsychiatry*. 2003;36(suppl 1):S8–S14.
119. Smith PF, Maclennan K, Darlington CL. The neuroprotective properties of the *Ginkgo biloba* leaf: a review of the possible relationship to platelet-activating factor (PAF). *J Ethnopharmacol*. 1996;50:131–139.
120. Zhu L, Wu J, Liao H, et al. Antagonistic effects of extract from leaves of *Ginkgo biloba* on glutamate neurotoxicity. *Acta Pharmacol Sin*. 1997;18:344–347.
121. Oyama Y, Chikahisa L, Ueha T, et al. *Ginkgo biloba* extract protects brain neurons against oxidative stress induced by hydrogen peroxide. *Brain Res*. 1996;712:349–352.
122. Ahlemeyer B, Mowes A, Krieglstein J. Inhibition of serum deprivation- and staurosporine-induced neuronal apoptosis by *Ginkgo biloba* extract and some of its constituents. *Eur J Pharmacol*. 1999;367:423–430.
123. Zhou LJ, Zhu XZ. Reactive oxygen species-induced apoptosis in PC12 cells and protective effect of bilobalide. *J Pharmacol Exp Ther*. 2000;293:982–988.
124. Guidetti C, Paracchini S, Lucchini S, et al. Prevention of neuronal cell damage induced by oxidative stress in vitro: effect of different *Ginkgo biloba* extracts. *J Pharmacy Pharmacol*. 2001;53:387–392.
125. Lu G, Wu Y, Mak YT, et al. Molecular evidence of the neuroprotective effect of *Ginkgo biloba* (EGb761) using bax/bcl-2 ratio after brain ischemia in senescence-accelerated mice, strain-prone 8. *Brain Res*. 2006;1090:23–28.
126. Punkt K, Welt K, Schaffranietz L. Changes of enzyme activities in the rat myocardium caused by experimental hypoxia with and without ginkgo biloba extract EGb 761 pretreatment, A cytophotometrical study. *Acta Histochem*. 1995;97:67–79.
127. Haramaki N, Aggarwal S, Kawabata T, et al. Effects of natural antioxidant *Ginkgo biloba* extract (EGb 761). on myocardial ischemia–reperfusion injury. *Free Radic Biol Med*. 1994;16:789–794.
128. Trumbeckaite S, Barenatoniene J, Majiene D, et al. Effect of *Ginkgo biloba* extract on the rat heart mitochondrial function. *J Ethnopharmacol*. 2007;111:512–516.
129. Le Bars PL, Katz MM, Berman N, et al. A Placebo-controlled, double-blind, randomized trial of an extract of *Ginkgo biloba* for dementia. *JAMA*. 1997;278:1327–1332.
130. Hofferberth B. The efficacy of EGb 761 in patients with senile dementia of the Alzheimer type. A double-blind, placebo-controlled study on different levels of investigation. *Hum Psychopharmacol*. 1994;9:215–222.
131. Dartigues JF, Carcaillon L, Helmer C, et al. Vasodilators and nootropics as predictors of dementia and mortality in the PAQUID cohort. *J Am Geriatr Soc*. 2007;55:395–399.
132. Droy-Lefaix MT, Szabo-Tosaki ME, Doly MN. Free radical scavenger properties of EGb 761 on functional disorders induced by experimental diabetic retinopathy. In: Cutler RG, Packe L, Bertram J, Mori A, eds. *Oxidative stress and aging*. Basel: Birkhäuser Verlag; 1996.
133. Szabo ME, Droy-Lefaix MT, Doly M, et al. Modification of ischemia/reperfusion-induced ion shifts (Na+, K+, Ca2+ and Mg2+) by free radical scavengers in the rat retina. *Ophthalmic Res*. 1993;25:1.
134. Ranchon I, Gorrand JM, Cluzel J, et al. Functional protection of photoreceptors from light-induced damage by dimethylthiourea and *Ginkgo biloba* extract. *Invest Ophthalmol Vis Sci*. 1999;40:1191–1199.
135. Xie Z, Wu X, Gong Y, et al. Intraperitoneal injection of *Ginkgo biloba* extract enhances antioxidation ability of retina and protects photoreceptors after light-induced retinal damage in rats. *Curr Eye Res*. 2007;32:471–479.
136. Meyniel G, Doly M, Millerin M, et al. Involvement of PAF (Platelet-Activating Factor) in chloroquine-induced retinopathy. *C R Acad Sci III*. 1992;314:61–65.
137. Droy-Lefaix MT, Szabo ME, Doly MN. Ischaemia and reperfusion-induced injury in the retina obtained form normotensive and spontaneously hypertensive rats: effects of free radical scavengers. *Int J Tissue React*. 1993;15:85–91.
138. Quaranta L, Bettelli S, Uva MG, et al. Effect of *Ginkgo biloba* extract on pre-existing visual field damage in normal tension glaucoma. *Ophthalmology*. 2003;110:359–364.
139. Raabe A, Raabe M, Ihm P. Therapeutic follow-up using automatic perimetry in chronic cerebroretinal ischemia in elderly patients, prospective double-blind study with graduated dose *Ginkgo biloba* treatment. *Klin Monatsbl Augenheilkd*. 1991;199:432–438.
140. Chung HS, Harris A, Kristinsson JK, et al. *Ginkgo biloba* extract increases ocular blood flow velocity. *J Ocul Pharmacol Ther*. 1999;15:233–240.
141. Wimpissinger B, Berisha F, Garhoefer G, et al. Influence of *Gingko biloba* on ocular blood flow. *Acta Ophthalmol Scand*. 2007;85:445–449.
142. Attele AS, Wu JA, Yuan CS. Ginseng pharmacology: multiple constituents and multiple actions. *Biochem Pharmacol*. 1999;58:1685–1693.
143. Kim YC, Kim SR, Markelonis GJ, et al. Ginsenosides Rb1 and Rg3 protect cultured rat cortical cells from glutamate-induced neurodegeneration. *J Neurosci Res*. 1998;53:426–432.
144. Kim S, Ahn K, Oh TH, et al. Inhibitory effect of ginsenosides on NMDA receptor-mediated signals in rat hippocampal neurons. *Biochem Biophys Res Commun*. 2002;296:247–254.
145. Lim JH, Wen TC, Matsuda S, et al. Protection of ischemic hippocampal neurons by ginsenoside Rb1, a main ingredient of ginseng root. *Neurosci Res*. 1997;28:191–200.
146. Chen YS, Wu CH, Yao CH, et al. Ginsenoside Rb1 enhances peripheral nerve regeneration across wide gaps in silicone rubber chambers. *Int J Artif Organs*. 2002;25:1103–1108.
147. Cho JY, Yoo ES, Baik KU, et al. In vitro inhibitory effect of protopanaxadiol ginsenosides on tumor necrosis factor (TNF)-alpha production and its modulation by known TNF-alpha antagonists. *Planta Med*. 2001;67:213–218.
148. Carneiro CS, Costa-Pinto FA, da Silva AP, et al. Pfaffia paniculata (Brazilian ginseng) methanolic extract reduces angiogenesis in mice. *Exp Toxicol Pathol*. 2007;58:427–431.
149. Izzotti A, Sacca SC, Cartiglia C, et al. Oxidative deoxyribonucleic acid damage in the eyes of glaucoma patients. *Am J Med*. 2003;114:638–646.
150. Yang J, Tezel G, Patil RV, et al. Serum autoantibody against glutathione S-transferase in patients with glaucoma. *Invest Ophthalmol Vis Sci*. 2001;42:1273–1276.

151. Juronen E, Tasa G, Veromann S, et al. Polymorphic glutathione S-transferase M1 is a risk factor of primary open-angle glaucoma among Estonians. *Exp Eye Res.* 2000;71:447–452.
152. Unal M, Guven M, Devranoglu K, et al. Glutathione S transferase M1 and T1 genetic polymorphisms are related to the risk of primary open-angle glaucoma: a study in a Turkish population. *Br J Ophthalmol.* 2007;91:527–530.
153. Bunin AI, Filina AA, Erichev VP. A glutathione deficiency in open-angle glaucoma and the approaches to its correction. *Vestn Oftalmol.* 1992;108:13–15.
154. Zenkel M, Kruse F, Naumann GO, Schlötzer-Schrehardt U. Impaired cytoprotective mechanisms in eyes with pseudoexfoliation syndrome/glaucoma. *Invest Ophthalmol Vis Sci.* 2007;48:5558–5566.
155. Bagchi D, Bagchi M, Stohs S, et al. Cellular protection with proanthocyanidins derived from grape seeds. *Ann N Y Acad Sci.* 2002;957:260–270.
156. Yamakoshi J, Saito M, Kataoka S, et al. Procyanidin-rich extract from grape seeds prevents cataract formation in hereditary cataractous (ICR/f) rats. *J Agric Food Chem.* 2002;50:4983–4988.
157. Bagchi D, Sen CK, Ray SD, et al. Molecular mechanisms of cardioprotection by a novel grape seed proanthocyanidin extract. *Mutat Res.* 2003;523–524:87–97.
158. Shao ZH, Becker LB, Vanden Hoek TL, et al. Grape seed proanthocyanidin extract attenuates oxidant injury in cardiomyocytes. *Pharmacol Res.* 2003;47:463–469.
159. Pataki T, Bak I, Kovacs P, et al. Grape seed proanthocyanidins improved cardiac recovery during reperfusion after ischemia in isolated rat hearts. *Am J Clin Nutrition.* 2002;75:894–899.
160. Kalin R, Righi A, Del Rosso A, et al. Activin, a grape seed-derived proanthocyanidin extract, reduces plasma levels of oxidative stress and adhesion molecules (ICAM-1, VCAM-1 and E-selectin) in systemic sclerosis. *Free Radical Res.* 2002;36:819–825.
161. Natella F, Belelli F, Gentili V, et al. Grape seed proanthocyanidins prevent plasma postprandial oxidative stress in humans. *J Agric Food Chem.* 2002;50:7720–7725.
162. Nair MP, Kandaswami C, Mahajan S, et al. Grape seed extract proanthocyanidins downregulate HIV-1 entry coreceptors, CCR2b, CCR3 and CCR5 gene expression by normal peripheral blood mononuclear cells. *Biol Res.* 2002;35:421–431.
163. Raina K, Singh RP, Agarwal R, et al. Oral grape seed extract inhibits prostate tumor growth and progression in TRAMP mice. *Cancer Res.* 2007;67:5976–5982.
164. Barden CA, Chandler HL, Lu P, et al. Effect of grape polyphenols on oxidative stress in canine lens epithelial cells. *Am J Vet Res.* 2008;69:94–100.
165. Higdon JV, Frei B. Tea catechins and polyphenols: health effects, metabolism, and antioxidant functions. *Crit Rev Food Sci Nutr.* 2003;43:89–143.
166. Lee SR, Im KJ, Suh SI, et al. Protective effect of green tea polyphenol (-)-epigallocatechin gallate and other antioxidants on lipid peroxidation in gerbil brain homogenates. *Phytother Res.* 2003;17:206–209.
167. Weinreb O, Mandel S, Youdim MB. cDNA gene expression profile homology of antioxidants and their antiapoptotic and proapoptotic activities in human neuroblastoma cells. *FASEB J.* 2003;17:935–937.
168. van Jaarsveld H, Kuyl JM, Schulenburg DH, et al. Effect of flavonoids on the outcome of myocardial mitochondrial ischemia/reperfusion injury. *Res Commun Mol Pathol Pharmacol.* 1996;91:65–75.
169. Nakagawa T, Yokozawa T. Direct scavenging of nitric oxide and superoxide by green tea. *Food Chem Toxicol.* 2002;40:1745–1750.
170. Gupta SK, Halde N, Sivastava S, et al. Green tea (*Camellia sinensis*) protects against selenite-induced oxidative stress in experimental cataractogenesis. *Ophthalmic Res.* 2002;34:258–263.
171. Thiagarajan G, Chandani S, Sundari CS, et al. Antioxidant properties of green and black tea, and their potential ability to retard the progression of eye lens cataract. *Exp Eye Res.* 2001;73:393–401.
172. Kakuda T. Neuroprotective effects of the green tea components theanine and catechins. *Biol Pharm Bull.* 2002;25:1513–1518.
173. Zhang B, Osborne NN. Oxidative-induced retinal degeneration is attenuated by epigallocatechin gallate. *Brain Res.* 2006;1124:176–187.
174. Zhang B, Safa R, Rusciano D, et al. Epigallocatechin gallate, an active ingredient from green tea, attenuates damaging influences to the retina caused by ischemia/reperfusion. *Brain Res.* 2007;1159:40–53.
175. Bone RA, Landrum JT, Guerra LH, et al. Lutein and zeaxanthin dietary supplements raise macular pigment density and serum concentrations of these carotenoids in humans. *J Nutr.* 2003;133:992–998.
176. Age-Related Eye Disease Study Research Group T. A randomized, placebo-controlled, clinical trial of high-dose supplementation with vitamins C and E and beta carotene, and zinc for age-related cataract and vision loss. AREDS report No. 9. *Arch Ophthalmol.* 2001;119:1439–1452.
177. Age-Related Eye Disease Study Research Group. A randomized, placebo-controlled, clinical trial of high-dose supplementation with vitamins C and E, beta carotene, and zinc for age-related macular degeneration and vision loss. AREDS report No. 8. *Arch Ophthalmol.* 2001;119:1417–1436.
178. Falsini B, Piccardi M, Iarossi G, et al. Influence of short-term antioxidant supplementation on macular function in age-related maculopathy: a pilot study including electrophysiologic assessment. *Ophthalmology.* 2003;110:51–60.
179. Thomson LR, Toyoda Y, Delori FC, et al. Long term dietary supplementation with zeaxanthin reduces photoreceptor death in light-damaged Japanese quail. *Exp Eye Res.* 2002;75:529–542.
180. Jacques PF, Chylack LT Jr, Hankinson SE, et al. Long-term nutrient intake and early age-related nuclear lens opacities. *Arch Ophthalmol.* 2001;119:1009–1019.
181. Berendschot TT, Broekmans WM, Klopping-Ketelaars IA, et al. Lens aging in relation to nutritional determinants and possible risk factors for age-related cataract. *Arch Ophthalmol.* 2002;120:1732–1737.
182. Yamazaki Y, Hayamizu F, Tanaka C. Effects of long-term methylcobalamin treatment on the progression of visual field defects in normal-tension glaucoma. *Curr Ther Res.* 2000;61:443–451.
183. Azumi I, Kosaki H, Nakatani H. Effects of metcobalamin (Methylcobal) on the visual field of chronic glaucoma – a multicenter open study. *Folia Ophthalmol Jpn.* 1983;34:873–878.
184. Kikuchi M, Kashii S, Honda Y, et al. Protective effects of methylcobalamin, a vitamin B12 analog, against glutamate-induced neurotoxicity in retinal cell culture. *Invest Ophthalmol Vis Sci.* 1997;38:848–854.
185. Denis U, Lecomte M, Paget C, et al. Advanced glycation end-products induce apoptosis of bovine retinal pericytes in culture: involvement of diacylglycerol/ceramide production and oxidative stress induction. *Free Radic Biol Med.* 2002;33:236–247.
186. England K, O'Driscoll C, Cotter TG. Carbonylation of glycolytic proteins is a key response to drug-induced oxidative stress and apoptosis. *Cell Death Differ.* 2004;11:252–260.
187. Hori K, Katayama M, Sato N, et al. Neuroprotection by glial cells through adult T cell leukemia-derived factor/human thioredoxin (ADF/TRX). *Brain Res.* 1994;652:304–310.
188. Zhang XY, Hayasaka S, Hayasaka Y, et al. Effect of N-acetylcysteine on lipopolysaccharide-induced uveitis in rats. *Jpn J Ophthalmol.* 2007;51:14–20.
189. Rohdewald P. A review of the French maritime pine bark extract (Pycnogenol), a herbal medication with a diverse clinical pharmacology. *Int J Clin Pharmacol Ther.* 2002;40:158–168.
190. Araghi-Niknam M, Hosseini S, Larson D, et al. Pine bark extract reduces platelet aggregation. *Integrative Med.* 2000;2:73–77.
191. Koch R. Comparative study of Venostasin and Pycnogenol in chronic venous insufficiency. *Phytother Res.* 2002;16(suppl 1):S1–S5.
192. Devaraj S, Vega-Lopez S, Kaul NS, et al. Supplementation with a pine bark extract rich in polyphenols increases plasma antioxidant

capacity and alters the plasma lipoprotein profile. *Lipids*. 2002;37:931–934.
193. Stanislavov R, Nikolova V, Rohdewald P. Improvement of erectile function with Prelox: a randomized, double-blind, placebo-controlled, crossover trial. *Int J Impot Res*. 2008;20:173–180.
194. Cesarone MR, Belcaro G, Rohdewald P, et al. Rapid relief of signs/symptoms in chronic venous microangiopathy with pycnogenol: a prospective, controlled study. *Angiology*. 2006;57:569–576.
195. Cesarone MR, Belcaro G, Rohdewald P, et al. Improvement of diabetic microangiopathy with pycnogenol: a prospective, controlled study. *Angiology*. 2006;57:431–436.
196. Belcaro G, Cesarone MR, Errichi BM, et al. Venous ulcers: microcirculatory improvement and faster healing with local use of Pycnogenol. *Angiology*. 2005;56:56.
197. Belcaro G, Cesarone MR, Errichi BM, et al. Diabetic ulcers: microcirculatory improvement and faster healing with pycnogenol. *Clin Appl Thromb Hemost*. 2006;12:318–323.
198. Grimm T, Chovanova Z, Muchova J, et al. Inhibition of NF-kappaB activation and MMP-9 secretion by plasma of human volunteers after ingestion of maritime pine bark extract (Pycnogenol). *J Inflamm (Lond)*. 2006;27:1.
199. Schafer A, Chovanova Z, Muchova J, et al. Inhibition of COX-1 and COX-2 activity by plasma of human volunteers after ingestion of French maritime pine bark extract (Pycnogenol). *Biomed Pharmacother*. 2006;60:5–9.
200. Kobayashi MS, Han D, Packer L. Antioxidants and herbal extracts protect HT-4 neuronal cells against glutamate-induced cytotoxicity. *Free Radic Res*. 2000;32:115–124.
201. Liu F, Lau BH, Peng Q, et al. Pycnogenol protects vascular endothelial cells from beta-amyloid-induced injury. *Biol Pharm Bull*. 2000;23:735–737.
202. Peng QL, Buz'Zard AR, Lau BH. Pycnogenol((R)) protects neurons from amyloid-beta peptide-induced apoptosis. *Brain Res Mol Brain Res*. 2002;104:55–65.
203. Buz'Zard AR, Lau BH. Pycnogenol reduces talc-induced neoplastic transformation in human ovarian cell cultures. *Phytother Res*. 2007;21:579–586.
204. Packer L, Rimbach G, Virgili F. Antioxidant activity and biologic properties of a procyanidin-rich extract from pine (Pinus maritima) bark, pycnogenol. *Free Radic Biol Med*. 1999;27:704–724.
205. Schonlau F, Rohdewald P. Pycnogenol for diabetic retinopathy, a review. *Int Ophthalmol*. 2001;24:161–171.
206. Kamuren ZT, McPeek CG, Sanders RA, et al. Effects of low-carbohydrate diet and Pycnogenol treatment on retinal antioxidant enzymes in normal and diabetic rats. *J Ocul Pharmacol Ther*. 2006;22:10–18.
207. Wadsworth TL, Koop D. Effects of *Ginkgo biloba* extract (EGb 761) and quercetin on lipopolysaccharide-induced release of nitric oxide. *Chem Biol Interact*. 2001;137:43–58.
208. Wadsworth TL, McDonald TL, Koop DR. Effects of *Ginkgo biloba* extract (EGb 761) and quercetin on lipopolysaccharide-induced signaling pathways involved in the release of tumor necrosis factor-alpha. *Biochem Pharmacol*. 2001;62:963–974.
209. Dok-Go H, Lee KH, Kim HJ, et al. Neuroprotective effects of antioxidative flavonoids, quercetin, (+)-dihydroquercetin and quercetin 3-methyl ether, isolated from Opuntia ficus-indica var. saboten. *Brain Res*. 2003;965:130–136.
210. Su JF, Guo CJ, Wei JY, et al. Protection against hepatic ischemia–reperfusion injury in rats by oral pretreatment with quercetin. *Biomed Environ Sci*. 2003;16:1–8.
211. Tezel G, Wax M. Increased production of tumor necrosis factor-alpha by glial cells exposed to simulated ischemia or elevated hydrostatic pressure induces apoptosis in cocultured retinal ganglion cells. *J Neurosci*. 2000;20:8693–8700.
212. Ueda T, Ueda T, Armstrong D. Preventive effect of natural and synthetic antioxidants on lipid peroxidation in the mammalian eye. *Ophthalmic Res*. 1996;28:184–192.
213. Orhan H, Marol S, Hepsen IF, et al. Effects of some probable antioxidants on selenite-induced cataract formation and oxidative stress-related parameters in rats. *Toxicology*. 1999;139:219–232.
214. Cao XG, Li XX, Bao YZ, et al. Responses of human lens epithelial cells to quercetin and DMSO. *Invest Ophthalmol Vis Sci*. 2007;48:3714–3718.
215. Ramana BV, Raju TN, Kumar VV, et al. Defensive role of quercetin against imbalances of calcium, sodium, and potassium in galactosemic cataract. *Biol Trace Elem Res*. 2007;119:35–41.
216. Valenzano DR, Cellerino A. Resveratrol and the pharmacology of aging: a new vertebrate model to validate an old molecule. *Cell Cycle*. 2006;5:1027–1032.
217. Baur JA, Pearson KJ, Price NL, et al. Resveratrol improves health and survival of mice on a high-calorie diet. *Nature*. 2006;444: 337–342.
218. Michan S, Sinclair D. Sirtuins in mammals: insights into their biological function. *Biochem J*. 2007;404:1–13.
219. Shigematsu S, Ishida S, Hara M, et al. Resveratrol, a red wine constituent polyphenol, prevents superoxide-dependent inflammatory responses induced by ischemia/reperfusion, platelet-activating factor, or oxidants. *Free Radic Biol Med*. 2003;34: 810–817.
220. Frankel EN, Waterhouse AL, Kinsella JE. Inhibition of human LDL oxidation by resveratrol. *Lancet*. 1993;341:1103–1104.
221. Chanvitayapongs S, Draczynska-Lusiak B, Sun AY. Amelioration of oxidative stress by antioxidants and resveratrol in PC12 cells. *Neuroreport*. 1997;8:1499–1502.
222. Araki T, Sasaki Y, Milbrandt J. Increased nuclear NAD biosynthesis and SIRT1 activation prevent axonal degeneration. *Science*. 2004;305:954–955.
223. Lu KT, Chiou RY, Chen LG, et al. Neuroprotective effects of resveratrol on cerebral ischemia-induced neuron loss mediated by free radical scavenging and cerebral blood flow elevation. *J Agric Food Chem*. 2006;54:3126–3131.
224. Losa GA. Resveratrol modulates apoptosis and oxidation in human blood mononuclear cells. *Eur J Clin Invest*. 2003;33:818–823.
225. Zhuang H, Kim YS, Koehler RC, et al. Potential mechanism by which resveratrol, a red wine constituent, protects neurons. *Ann NY Acad Sci*. 2003;993:276–286.
226. Doganay S, Borazan M, Iraz M, et al. The effect of resveratrol in experimental cataract model formed by sodium selenite. *Curr Eye Res*. 2006;31:147–153.
227. Nagaoka T, Hein TW, Yoshida A, et al. Resveratrol, a component of red wine, elicits dilation of isolated porcine retinal arterioles: role of nitric oxide and potassium channels. *Invest Ophthalmol Vis Sci*. 2007;48:4232–4239.
228. Shindler KS, Verntura E, Rex TS, et al. SIRT1 activation confers neuroprotection in experimental optic neuritis. *Invest Ophthalmol Vis Sci*. 2007;48:3602–3609.
229. Militante JD, Lombardini JB. Taurine: evidence of physiological function in the retina. *Nutr Neurosci*. 2002;5:75–90.
230. Di Leo MA, Santini SA, Cercone S, et al. Chronic taurine supplementation ameliorates oxidative stress and Na+ K+ ATPase impairment in the retina of diabetic rats. *Amino Acids*. 2002;23:401–406.
231. Bantseev V, Bhardwaj R, Rathbun W, et al. Antioxidants and cataract: (cataract induction in space environment and application to terrestrial aging cataract). *Biochem Mol Biol Int*. 1997;42:1189–1197.
232. Cubillos S, Fazzino F, Lima L. Medium requirements for neuritic outgrowth from goldfish retinal explants and the trophic effect of taurine. *Int J Dev Neurosci*. 2002;20:607–617.
233. Pasantes-Morales H, Quiroz H, Quesada O. Treatment with taurine, diltiazem, and vitamin E retards the progressive visual field reduction in retinitis pigmentosa: a 3-year follow-up study. *Metab Brain Dis*. 2002;17:183–197.
234. Son HY, Kim H, Kwon Y. Taurine prevents oxidative damage of high glucose-induced cataractogenesis in isolated rat lenses. *J Nutr Sci Vitaminol (Tokyo)*. 2007;53:324–330.

# Chapter 57
# Intravitreal Steroids and Glaucoma

Yousuf Khalifa and Sandra M. Johnson

## 57.1 Current Indications for IVTA

Intravitreal injection of pharmaceuticals has gained widespread acceptance. As the roles of inflammation and neovascularization in eye pathologies are being elucidated, the indications for intravitreal triamcinolone (IVTA) are expanding. First introduced in 1974 as a treatment for proliferative vitreoretinopathy,[1] IVTA is currently employed in the treatment of diabetic macular edema,[2] macular edema associated with branch[3] and central[4,5] retinal vein occlusion, exudative age-related macular degeneration,[6,7] pseudophakic cystoid macular edema,[8] and uveitic cystoid macular edema.[9]

## 57.2 Pharmacokinetics of IVTA

The concentration of IVTA needed to achieve therapeutic results is not clear, and the dosage of triamcinolone acetonide administered in a single intravitreal injection ranges from 4 mg in the United States to 20 mg in Europe. The mechanism of IVTA clearance is ill-defined, but studies measuring aqueous and vitreous samples in nonvitrectomized eyes revealed the half-life of a single 4 mg IVTA injection to be 18.6 days. This extrapolates to up to 3 months of intraocular presence.[10,11] Using a single injection dosage of 20–25 mg, detectable levels of IVTA are found up to 1.5 years after injection.[12]

In vitrectomized eyes, animal studies have shown clearance of IVTA is 50% faster than in control eyes.[13] In eyes filled with silicone oil, detectable levels of IVTA after a 20–25 mg injection have been found for up to 8 months.[14]

## 57.3 Intraocular Pressure and IVTA

The intraocular pressure (IOP) elevating effects of IVTA may best be discussed by considering time of onset. This time dependent perspective effects etiologies, prognosis and treatment.

### 57.3.1 Immediate

Typically, the delivery of IVTA involves a volume of 0.1 ml injected directly through the pars plana into the vitreous cavity causing a sudden increase in IOP.[15] IOP has been shown to increase immediately to an average of 40.6 ± 12.1 mmHg (Kotliar et al[15]) and to equilibrate within 15 min.[16] Eyes with longer axial lengths have greater volumes to buffer the IOP elevating effects. Shorter eyes show a more profound IOP spike.[15] In addition, patients with uveitic macular edema have a 2.5 odds ratio of adverse IOP events with IVTA administration compared with nonuveitic patients.[17]

Some have recommended lowering IOP preoperatively[18] while others have suggested postinjection paracentesis. It has been shown that the IOP equilibrates regardless of whether a paracentesis is performed or not.[16] The consequences of IVTA-associated transient elevations in IOP are not clearly defined, but optic nerve insult is suspected and no consensus has been reached on the proper management. The authors are aware of one case of glaucomatous vision loss associated with intermittent IOP elevations associated with IVTA treatment. In eyes with significant glaucomatous optic atrophy, consideration should be given to prophylactic IOP lowering agents preinjection and postinjection IOP evaluation and possible paracentesis to avoid further disc damage. Patients undergoing serial injections should have monitoring of the optic disc. Filtration surgery should be considered for progression of glaucoma and need for continued IVTA injection.

### 57.3.2 Early

Significant IOP rise within 1 week of IVTA has been reported to result from blockage of the trabecular meshwork with triamcinolone particulate matter.[19] The cases in the report were all pseudophakic, which allowed for migration of the material into the anterior segment. It has also been suggested that vitrectomized eyes are at increased risk of this early IOP rise.

Methods to prevent kenalog particles from blocking the trabecular meshwork include filtering the triamcinolone and asking patients to sleep on their backs for a few days after the IVTA injection.[20] None of the reported cases of early IOP elevation associated with particulate blockage of the trabecular meshwork were amenable to medical management, and all patients in the report received a tube shunt.

### 57.3.3 Delayed

As with topical and systemic administration of corticosteroids, IVTA causes a reduction in matrix metalloproteinases, increases deposition of substances in the TM, and depresses TM endothelial cell phagocytosis; therefore, an increase in trabecular meshwork resistance to outflow ensues.[21] IVTA injection delivers a potent dose of intraocular corticosteroid leading to IOP elevation in 28–52% of patients.[21-25]

In one study, patients receiving a 4 mg dosage of IVTA had a mean time to IOP elevation of approximately 100.6 days, and the mean IOP increase was 8 mmHg with 40.4% having an IOP increase of 24 mmHg or more. Glaucoma patients with a baseline IOP of 15 mmHg and who underwent IVTA had a 60% chance of developing a pressure greater than or equal to 24 mmHg while nonglaucomatous eyes with the same baseline IOP had a 22.7% chance. In this series, the underlying diagnosis and the number of injections did not correlate with IOP elevation.[26] Filtration surgery should be considered if the IOP is not controlled medically. As always, the decision about whether or not to intervene needs to be based upon the status of the optic nerve. If there is a reservoir of IVTA that has achieved its therapeutic endpoint pars plana vitrectomy may be of benefit.

## References

1. Graham OR, Peyman GA. Intravitreal injection of dexamethasone: treatment of experimentally induced endophthalmitis. *Arch Ophthalmol.* 1974;92:149–154.
2. Patelli F, Fasolino G, Raice P, et al. Time course of changes in retinal thickness and visual acuity after intravitreal triamcinolone acetonide for diffuse diabetic macular edema with and without previous macular laser treatment. *Retina.* 2005;25:840–844.
3. Ozkiris A, Everklioglu C, Erkilic K, Dogan H. Intravitreal triamcinolone acetonide for treatment of persistent macular oedema in branch retinal vein occlusion. *Eye.* 2006;20:13–17.
4. Bashshur ZF, Ma'luf RN, Allam S, et al. Intravitreal triamcinolone for the management of macular edema due to nonischemic central retinal vein occlusion. *Arch Ophthalmol.* 2004;122:1137–1140.
5. Gregori NZ, Rosenfeld PJ, Puliafito CA, et al. One-year safety and efficacy of intravitreal triamcinolone acetonide for the management of macular edema secondary to central retinal vein occlusion. *Retina.* 2006;26(8):889–895.
6. Schadlu R, Kymes SM, Apte RS. Combined photodynamic therapy and intravitreal triamcinolone for neovascular age-related macular degeneration: effect of initial visual acuity on treatment response. *Graefes Arch Clin Exp Ophthalmol.* 2007;245:1667–1672.
7. Spaide RF, Sorenson J, Maranan L. Photodynamic therapy with verteporfin combined with intravitreal injection of triamcinolone acetonide for choroidal neovascularization. *Ophthalmology.* 2005;112:301–304.
8. Benhamou N, Massin P, Haouchine B, et al. Intravitreal triamcinolone for refractory pseudophakic macular edema. *Am J Ophthalmol.* 2003;135:246–249.
9. Kok H, Lau C, Maycock N, et al. Outcome of intravitreal triamcinolone in uveitis. *Ophthalmology.* 2005;112:1916–1921.
10. Beer PM, Bakri SJ, Singh RJ, et al. Intraocular concentration and pharmacokinetics of triamcinolone acetonide after a single intravitreal injection. *Ophthalmology.* 2003;110:681–686.
11. Mason JO, Somaiya MD, Singh RJ. Intravitreal concentration and clearance of triamcinolone acetonide in nonvitrectomized human eyes. *Retina.* 2004;24:900–904.
12. Jonas JB. Intraocular availability of triamcinolone acetonide after intravitreal injection. *Am J Ophthalmol.* 2004;137:560–562.
13. Chin H, Park T, Moon Y, Oh J. Difference in clearance of intravitreal triamcinolone between vitrectomized and nonvitrectomized eyes. *Retina.* 2005;25:556–560.
14. Jonas JB. Concentration of intravitreally injected triamcinolone acetonide in intraocular silicone oil. *Br J Ophthalmol.* 2002;86:1450–1451.
15. Kotliar K, Maier M, Bauer S, et al. Effect of intravitreal injections and volume changes on intraocular pressure: clinical results and biomechanical model. *Acta Ophthalmol Scand.* 2007;85(7):777–781.
16. Chang W, Chung M. Efficacy of anterior chamber paracentesis after intravitreal triamcinolone injection. *Eur J Ophthalmol.* 2007;17(5):776–779.
17. Galor A, Margolis R, Brasil OM, et al. Adverse events after intravitreal triamcinolone in patients with and without uveitis. *Ophthalmology.* 2007;114(10):1912–1918.
18. Hernaez-Ortega MC, Soto-Pedre E. Use of the Honan balloon as a compression device for intravitreal triamcinolone acetonide injection. *Ophthalmic Surg Lasers Imaging.* 2007;38(1):87–88.
19. Singh IP, Ahmad SI, Yeh D, et al. Early rapid rise in intraocular pressure after intravitreal triamcinolone acetonide injection. *Am J Ophthalmol.* 2004;138:286–287.
20. Vendantham V. Intraocular pressure rise after intravitreal triamcinolone. *Am J Ophthalmol.* 2005;139(3):575.
21. Wang YS, Friedrichs U, Eichler W, et al. Inhibitory effects of triamcinolone acetonide on bFGF-induced migration and tube formation in choroidal microvascular endothelial cells. *Graefes Arch Clin Exp Ophthalmol.* 2002;240:42–48.
22. Gillies MC, Kuzniarz M, Craig J, et al. Intravitreal triamcinolone-induced elevated intraocular pressure is associated with the development of posterior subcapsular cataract. *Ophthalmology.* 2005;112:139–143.
23. Jonas JB, Degenring RF, Kreissig I, et al. Intraocular pressure elevation after intravitreal triamcinolone acetonide injection. *Ophthalmology.* 2005;112:593–598.
24. Gillies MC, Simpson JM, Billson FA, et al. Safety of an intravitreal injection of triamcinolone. *Arch Ophthalmol.* 2004;122:336–340.
25. Jonas JB, Kreissig I, Degenring R. Intraocular pressure after intravitreal injection of triamcinolone acetonide. *Br J Ophthalmol.* 2003;87:24–27.
26. Smithen LM, Ober MD, Maranan L, Spaide RF. Intravitreal triamcinolone acetonide and intraocular pressure. *Am J Ophthalmol.* 2004;138:740–743.

# Chapter 58
# Pregnancy and Glaucoma

Jeff Martow

Glaucoma, in most cases, is a disease of the elderly. As ophthalmologists, however, we treat women of childbearing age who have glaucoma. The treatment of glaucoma in women who are attempting to conceive, are pregnant, or are lactating raises many challenging questions with respect to management options for the care and safety of the mother and child. This chapter will discuss issues related to glaucoma management during pregnancy and lactation.

## 58.1 Intraocular Pressure During Pregnancy

Pregnancy is known to have a wide variety of effects on the pregnant woman's eye which have been reviewed in an article by Sunness.[1] Changes can be physiological, pathological, or the modification of a preexisting disease. Intraocular pressure (IOP), with rare exception,[2,3] has been reported to decrease during pregnancy. This decrease has been reported to occur throughout pregnancy[4-6] or during the second half of pregnancy,[7,8] and these changes tend to persist for several months postpartum.[7] The ocular hypotensive effect of late pregnancy was found to be equivalent in systemically hypertensive and nonhypertensive women.[8] Proposed mechanisms to explain the IOP reduction include increased facility of outflow[4,9] with hormonally mediated enhancement of uveoscleral outflow. Reduced episcleral venous pressure,[10] secondary to a general decrease of venous pressure in the upper extremities,[11] has also been suggested. Another proposed reason for the decreased IOP is the acidosis of pregnancy.[5]

Preexisting glaucoma has been reported to improve during pregnancy with rare exception. It is unusual for glaucoma to be first noted during pregnancy.[5] In contrast to this observation, there are reports of pregnant women who had glaucoma with unstable IOPs despite various forms of therapeutic intervention. Vaideanu recently surveyed all consultant ophthalmologists in the UK and found 26% had previously treated pregnant women with glaucoma.[12] Interestingly, 31% of the ophthalmologists were unsure how to treat a patient whose IOP was felt likely to cause disease progression during pregnancy.

Brauner et al published a retrospective case series on 15 pregnant women with glaucoma. As one might anticipate, most of the diagnoses were forms of glaucoma typical of a young age group, including: congenital forms of glaucoma, juvenile open angle glaucoma, aniridic glaucoma, juvenile rheumatoid arthritis with uveitic glaucoma and pigmentary glaucoma.[13] In 16 (57.1%) of 28 eyes with glaucoma, there was no increase in IOP and no change of visual fields during pregnancy. Many of these women were maintained on fewer IOP-lowering medications during pregnancy compared to before pregnancy, and no progression of the disease was observed. However, in 10 (35.7%) of 28 eyes in the study, there was an increase in IOP or progression of visual field loss. Many of these women required additional medication to control their IOP. It is therefore apparent that, although most women with glaucoma remain stable or improve during pregnancy, a significant proportion will worsen and require therapy.

## 58.2 Glaucoma Therapy in the Peripregnancy Period

As with the initiation of any form of therapy, a discussion of the risks and benefits of treatment must be undertaken. This discussion may need to be lengthier than usual. Because lipid-soluble, nonionized, low-molecular-weight drugs (this includes most antiglaucoma medications) readily cross the placenta (or into the breast milk) and enter the fetal circulation,[14] this issue is complicated by the risks of treatment to the fetus (or newborn in the case of breastfeeding mothers). It is very difficult to predict the level of risk a patient is willing to accept; as such, this discussion with the patient is critical. Furthermore, contemplation of therapeutic options should include a discussion with the patient's obstetrician, as she/he will view issues from a different perspective and may offer important considerations not otherwise anticipated. While discussion with the patient is essential in order to achieve informed consent, we are limited in our knowledge of these medications' effects during pregnancy as a result of the paucity of studies investigating their effects on the pregnant woman, fetus, and newborn because designing ethical studies to investigate this area is all but impossible. Counseling of patients should include all women who are capable of becoming pregnant because 50% of pregnancies in the United States are unplanned, which creates a significant potential for exposure to medication prior to the diagnosis of pregnancy.[15]

The US Food and Drug Administration (FDA) has classified medication safety during pregnancy into the following groups (see Table 58.1): Category A: safety established using human studies; Category B: presumed safety based on animal studies; Category C: uncertain safety; no human studies; animal studies show adverse effects; Category D: unsafe, evidence of risk that in certain clinical circumstances may be justifiable; and Category X: highly unsafe. At present, there are no antiglaucoma medications that fall into Category A. Brimonidine is the only antiglaucoma medication classified as Category B. While this may make it a relatively safe choice during pregnancy, it is important to consider discontinuing brimonidine treatment in breastfeeding women because it may be secreted in breast milk and has been known to cause CNS effects on infants, including severe hypotension and apnea.

Other antiglaucoma medications, including β-blockers, prostaglandin analogs, α-agonists, carbonic anhydrase inhibitors, epinephrine derivatives, and miotics, have been classified as Category C. β-Blockers have been shown to produce fetal bradycardia, arrhythmia,[16] and apnea.[17] Despite their potential side effects, β-blockers are probably the first choice of topical antihypertensive therapy in pregnant women. In fact, Vaideanu's survey of UK ophthalmologists found that 45% named topical β-blockers as their first choice in pregnant women with glaucoma,[12] despite the fact that ophthalmologists are increasingly using topical prostaglandin agonists as their first-line drug to lower IOP in the nonpregnant population.[18] The reason for choosing β-blockers first line is likely because of the long-standing experience that ophthalmologists have with these medications (although the important risks associated with prostaglandin analog use may have played a role and will be discussed shortly). Furthermore, obstetricians frequently use β-blockers to treat systemic hypertension during pregnancy. A recent paper by Parvaz et al showed that timolol in breast milk was noted to be at levels unlikely to cause systemic side effects to the healthy breastfed baby.[19] Case reports of harmful cardiorespiratory events from timolol maleate suggest that predisposed neonates may experience dramatic adverse effects after exposure to timolol eye drops[17,20]; these infants must be carefully monitored.

Brauner et al select topical carbonic anhydrase inhibitors as their third choice (after β-blockers and α2-adrenergic agents).[13] Despite the associations of sacrococcygeal teratoma and transient renal tubular acidosis in neonates with oral carbonic anhydrase inhibitors,[21,22] there are no reported adverse effects during pregnancy due to treatment with topical carbonic anhydrase inhibitors.

Prostaglandin analogs have generally been avoided during pregnancy because this class of medications is used to induce labor and/or therapeutic abortion. In fact, Phase 3 clinical trials for the prostaglandin medications specifically excluded pregnant women or women who could become pregnant and did not have a reliable form of birth control. While no documented cases of abortion related to topical prostaglandin analog use in glaucoma have been reported, many experts feel that extreme caution is advised in pregnant women. However, one should note that even if one was to fully absorb one drop of prostaglandin analog in each eye, the maximum systemic dose would be 1,500–7,500 times less than the dose associated with clinically induced abortions. Furthermore, DeSantis found no evidence of adverse effects on pregnancy or neonatal outcomes in 11 women exposed to latanoprost.[23] Interestingly, Vaideanu's UK survey found that 25% of respondents would be willing to use topical prostaglandins in pregnant women.[12]

Miotics are not generally well tolerated by young phakic patients because of induced miosis and ciliary spasm. Pseudophakic and aphakic patients seen with the congenital and juvenile glaucomas, however, may be good candidates for their use. Miotics should be avoided close to delivery because of reports of neonatal hyperthermia, seizures, and diaphoresis.[24]

When any topical medications are used, efforts should be made to minimize systemic absorption. In the case of pregnant or breastfeeding women, it is especially important to minimize toxicity to the mother, fetus, and breastfed child. Using the lowest effective concentration and frequency are recommended. Punctal occlusion, maintaining eyelid closure for 5 min, and possibly including the use of punctal plugs may all be beneficial. Blowing the nose immediately after

**Table 58.1** Categories of risk and glaucoma medication

| FDA category | | Antiglaucoma medications |
| --- | --- | --- |
| A | No risk | None |
| B | Animal studies: no risk<br>Human studies: not adequate | Brimonidine |
| C | Animal studies: toxicity<br>Human studies: not adequate | β-blockers<br>Carbonic anhydrase inhibitors<br>Miotics<br>Prostaglandin analogs |
| D | Human studies: risk<br>(benefits may outweigh risk if no suitable alternative) | Fixed-combination timolol 0.05%/dorzolamide 2% |
| X | Highly unsafe: risks of use outweigh possible benefits | None |

eye drop installation in order to clear the nasopharynx can be suggested. If drops are being used bilaterally, then waiting 15 min between applications will help to reduce the peak plasma concentration.

## 58.3 Another Option to Consider Is Laser Therapy

### 58.3.1 Laser Trabeculoplasty

ALT or SLT offers the potential benefits of IOP lowering and/or reducing the need for antiglaucoma medications. It has very limited risk to the patient and the fetus. However, if a patient has a susceptible optic nerve, perioperative medications may be required to control a perioperative IOP spike. Additionally, the delayed onset of IOP lowering experienced with laser treatment may not make it ideal when more immediate reduction is required. Laser is probably optimally used in anticipation of pregnancy should one desire to discontinue medications during the upcoming pregnancy. Laser therapy is more likely to be effective in a patient with pigment dispersion glaucoma than some of the more recalcitrant forms of glaucoma (congenital, juvenile, and uveitic) typical of this population.

When medical and laser options are unacceptable and/or inadequate, incisional surgery provides another alternative. Glaucoma surgery in pregnant patients carries additional risks though, including topical/local anesthetics, lying in a supine position, and postoperative medications. Reports of anesthetic use in pregnant patients are limited. Retrobulbar bupivicaine[25] and general anesthesia[26] cases were reported without complications arising from the anesthesia. A large multicenter retrospective study demonstrated no significant increase in malformations despite exposure to local anesthetics during early pregnancy.[27] Moore reported, in the dental literature, that while bupivacaine induced fetal bradycardia, lidocaine was not associated with any fetal effects.[28] This would suggest that local (topical and/or subconjunctival) administration of lidocaine for incisional glaucoma surgery would present little risk to the mother and fetus. Furthermore, Shamus demonstrated that anesthesia with local lidocaine was equal in efficacy to retrobulbar lidocaine during phacoemulsification and had fewer complications.[29] Jonathan Myers recommends that surgery be deferred until after the first trimester, when possible, to reduce the risk of exposing the fetus to potentially teratogenic agents.[30] Surgery offered to a nursing mother would be best timed immediately after nursing in order to avoid significant accumulation of the administered lidocaine in the breast milk.

Although antimetabolite usage might be tempting in this young population at increased risk for surgical failure, they must be used with extreme caution (if at all) because of the possible impact on a growing fetus/newborn. Intraoperative patient positioning can present problems for patients who are more advanced in their pregnancy because the uterus can compress the aorta and vena cava.[31]

## 58.4 Conclusion

Glaucoma and pregnancy may be complicated enough to treat in isolation; together they can pose an especially complex challenge. Thankfully, most pregnant glaucoma patients will experience an improvement in their condition, while those who require treatment to prevent visual loss will have to make some difficult decisions. There is little evidence-based medicine to support the clinical situations encountered in these circumstances. Consensus guidelines from experts in the area would be of great benefit to physicians and patients dealing with glaucoma during pregnancy.

## References

1. Sunness JS. The pregnant woman's eye. *Surv Ophthalmol.* 1988;32:219–238.
2. Avashi P, Sethi MB, Mithal S. Effects of pregnancy and labor on intraocular pressure. *Int Surg.* 1976;61:82–84.
3. Stefanini, Ricci. Bassini 9:68, 1964, cited in Duke-Elder S. *System of Ophthalmology.* Vol. IV. St Louis: CV Mosby; 1968:279–280.
4. Becker B, Friedenwald JS. Clinical aqueous outflow. *Arch Ophthalmol.* 1953;50:557–571.
5. Imre J. Pregnancy and the eye, their endocrinological relations. *XV Concilium Ophthalmol Egypt.* 1937;III:213–226.
6. Kass MA, Sears ML. Hormonal regulation of intraocular pressure. *Surv Ophthalmol.* 1977;22:153–176.
7. Horven I, Gjonnaess H. Corneal indentation pulse and intraocular pressure in pregnancy. *Arch Ophthalmol.* 1974;91:92–98.
8. Phillips CI, Gore SM. Ocular hypotensive effect of late pregnancy with and without high blood pressure. *Br J Ophthalmol.* 1985;69: 117–119.
9. Paterson GL, Miller SJH. Hormonal influences in simple glaucoma. *Br J Ophthalmol.* 1963;47:129–137.
10. Wilke L. Episclereal venous pressure and pregnancy. *Acta Ophthalmol Suppl.* 1975;125:40–41.
11. Horven I, Gjonnaess H, Kroese A. Blood circulation changes in the eyes and limbs with relation to pregnancy and female sex hormones. *Acta Ophthalmol.* 1976;54:203–214.
12. Vaideanu D, Fraser S. Glaucoma management in pregnancy: a questionnaire survey. *Eye.* 2007;21:341–343.
13. Brauner SC, Chen TC. The course of glaucoma during pregnancy. *Arch Ophthalmol.* 2006;124:1089–1094.
14. Kooner KS, Zimmerman TJ. Antiglaucoma therapy during pregnancy-part 1. *Ann Ophthalmol.* 1988;20:166–169.
15. Meadows M. Pregnancy and the drug dilemma. *FDA Consumer Magazine.* 2001; May–June.
16. Wagenvoort AM, van Vugt JM, Sobotka M, et al. Topical timolol therapy in pregnancy: is it safe for the fetus? *Teratology.* 1998;58: 258–262.

17. Olson RJ, Bromberg BB, Zimmerman TJ. Apneic spells associated with timolol therapy in a neonate. *Am J Ophthalmol.* 1979;88:120–122.
18. Kaiserman I, Kaiserman N, Nakar S, et al. The effect of combination pharmacotherapy on the prescription trends of glaucoma medications. *J Glaucoma.* 2005;14(2):157–160.
19. Madadi PB, Koren G. Timolol concentrations in breast milk of a women treated for glaucoma: calculation of neonatal exposure (case report). *J Glaucoma.* 2008;17(4):329–331.
20. Williams T, Ginther WH. Hazard of ophthalmic timolol. *N Engl J Med.* 1982;306:1485–1486.
21. Ozawa H, Azuma E, Shindo K, et al. Transient renal tubular acidosis in a neonate following transplacental acetazolamide. *Eur J Prediatr.* 2001;160:321–322.
22. Worsham F Jr, Beckham EN, Mitchell EH. Sacrococcygeal teratoma in a neonate. *JAMA.* 1978;240:251–252.
23. De Santis M, Lucchese A, Carducci B, et al. Latanoprost exposure in pregnancy. *Am J Ophthalmol.* 2004;138:305–306.
24. Davis EA, Dana MR. Pregnancy and the eye. In: Albert DM, Jakobiec FA, Azar DT, et al., eds. *Principles and Practice of Ophthalmology.* 2nd ed. Philadelphia: WB Saunders; 2000: 4767–4783.
25. Smith RB, Linn JG Jr. Retrobulbar injection of bupivacaine (marcaine) for anesthesia and akinesia. *Invest Ophthalmol.* 1974; 13:157–158.
26. Birks DA, Prior VJ. Echothiophate iodide treatment of glaucoma in pregnancy. *Arch Ophthalmol.* 1968;79:283-285.
27. Heinonen OP, Sloane D, Shapiro S. *Birth Defects and Drugs in Pregnancy.* Littleton, MA: Publishing Science Group; 1977: 357–365.
28. Moore PA. Selecting drugs for the pregnant dental patient. *J Am Dent Assoc.* 1998;129:1281–1286.
29. Shammas HJ, Milkie M. Topical and subconjunctival anesthesia for phacoemulsification: prospective study. *J Cataract Refract Surg.* 1997;23:1577–1580.
30. Johnson SM, Martinez M. Management of glaucoma in pregnancy and lactation. *Surv Ophthalmol.* 2001;45(5):449-454.
31. Rosen MA. Management of anesthesia for the pregnant surgical patient [see comments]. *Anesthesiology.* 1999;91:1159–1163.

# Chapter 59
# Systemic Side Effects of Glaucoma Medications

Paul Lama

Direct ophthalmic administration is the usual method by which ophthalmologists medically manage most ocular diseases. Topical instillation of pharmacologic agents in the management of ocular disease offers the advantages of rapidly achieving high intraocular drug levels, particularly in the aqueous humor, using significantly smaller doses than that used to treat systemic disease. The management of chronic disease states such as glaucoma, in particular, involves long-term or lifelong administration of often multiple topical agents. Thus, chronic exposure to agents that are systemically active are of great importance from the perspective of safety. This is especially true in glaucoma since the prevalence of disease increases with age as does the prevalence of significant comorbidities that not only can influence the disease process, but can also pose limitations on various treatments due to potential systemic interactions leading to undesired side effects and toxicity. Although the total dosage relative to a comparable systemic agent is far lower, a topical agent is directly absorbed into the systemic circulation via the nasopharyngeal mucosa following passage through the nasolacrimal duct. Thus, in contrast to an orally administered agent, no first-pass hepatic metabolism occurs with a topically administered ophthalmic drug. The small doses notwithstanding, there may be significant systemic accumulation causing untoward systemic side effects, rarely with lethal potential. It is good to know and understand the full spectrum of systemic effects of ophthalmic agents as well as their interactions with other concomitantly administered systemic agents to minimize the risk of an adverse event.

## 59.1 Beta-Adrenergic Blockers

Since the introduction of timolol ophthalmic solution 30 years ago in 1978, ophthalmic beta-adrenergic blockers have been an important class of agents in the management of glaucoma and ocular hypertension. While the efficacy of ophthalmic beta-adrenergic blockers in the management of glaucoma is indisputable, there has been mounting concern and debate amongst practitioners regarding their chronic use due to potentially serious systemic side effects. This class of agents in the management of glaucoma has thus been viewed upon in many ways as a paradox. Though second in efficacy to prostaglandin analogs,[1] the concern regarding systemic safety has often relegated this class to a much lower order of preference with the treating physician selecting an agent from another class despite lesser published efficacy as single agents by comparison to nonselective beta-adrenergic blockers.[1] Clearly, thorough review of the peer-reviewed literature is necessary to properly guide the practitioner with respect to systemic safety and tolerability. The following sections will discuss the pharmacology of beta-blockers, present an update regarding the evolving and changing role of beta-blockade in cardiovascular medicine, followed by systemic effects following beta-blocker administration based on data from the peer-reviewed literature and recommendations with respect to safety of beta-adrenergic blocker administration in the management of glaucoma or ocular hypertension.

### 59.1.1 Pharmacology and Physiology

There are three beta-adrenergic receptor subtypes $\beta 1$, $\beta 2$, and $\beta 3$. Beta-3 adrenoreceptor subtypes are located mostly in adipose tissue and are involved in thermogenesis.[2,3] Mutations in the $\beta 3$ receptor gene may be implicated in the development of insulin resistance and obesity.[4] Since the beta receptors of interest, from the safety vantage point, are found in cardiovascular and pulmonary tissue, and since most beta-adrenergic receptor blocking agents are agonists or antagonists of $\beta 1$ and $\beta 2$ receptors, we will be focusing exclusively on interactions at these receptor subtypes.

Commercially available beta-adrenergic antagonists are either selective ($\beta 1$ only), nonselective, or nonselective with intrinsic sympathomimetic activity (ISA). Selective beta-adrenergic blockers are incompletely selective with varying ratios of beta-1/beta-2 selectivity. Most ophthalmic beta-adrenergic antagonists are nonselective with the exception of betaxolol, which is selective, and carteolol, which is nonselective with ISA. As with all ophthalmically administered agents, there is no first-pass hepatic metabolism. Because the kinetics of nasopharyngeal absorption may be similar to an intravenous bolus, blood levels are achieved very quickly with topical administration. The highest plasma concentration will occur soon after entry into the circulation before significant dilution occurs, and the drug is spread over its known volume of distribution. Peak plasma levels of ophthalmically administered timolol have been shown to occur 10 min after instillation as compared to 1–2 h following oral ingestion.[5,6] With timolol gel, the drug is released more slowly than timolol solution, and the kinetics the kinetics may more closely resemble oral dosing.[6] The slope of the rise and peak plasma levels achieved with a drug administered orally or topically reflects the difference between the absorption constant and the elimination constant and may show considerable interindividual variation. In one study, the mean peak plasma concentration following chronic use (7 days) in seven normal volunteers was $64 \pm 4$ ng/ml.[7] However, when 20 mg was administered as a single dose in seven normal volunteers (mean body weight = 67.5 kg), the range of peak values was between 50 and 103 ng/ml and trough levels were between 0.8 and 7.2 ng/ml.[5] In another study in which the oral dose administered was 0.4 mg/kg, the mean peak plasma concentration was $123 \pm 14$ ng/ml.[8] In stark contrast, when timolol solution was administered topically OU BID, the peak plasma levels were 0.5 ng/ml and after 4 h decreased to 0.3 ng/ml.[9] Review of the pharmacokinetic data demonstrates that the peak plasma levels following ingestion of oral timolol range from 100 to 246 times that achieved with topical administration.[7–9]

### 59.1.2 Beta-Adrenergic Blockers in Cardiovascular Medicine

Systemic beta-adrenergic blockers are one of the most important agents used in cardiovascular medicine. There has often been great confusion amongst noninternists regarding the role of beta-blockers with respect to indications and contraindications in cardiovascular disease. While there have been numerous clinical trials, from the early 1980s onward that have consistently demonstrated mortality reduction in patients prescribed beta-adrenergic blockers with a history of myocardial infarction, the benefits in heart failure have been identified and recognized only in the past decade.[10–17]

Confounding the issue is the dramatic about-face regarding the use of beta-blockers in the management of congestive heart failure (CHF) in the past decade, which although once a contraindication is now recognized as an important life-saving indication.

The mortality reduction in heart failure appears to be largely because of a reduction in sudden arrhythmic death.[18,19] However, reduced pathological ventricular remodeling and improved ejection fraction are also felt to be important.[12,20] Reduction in antioxidant activity and plasma renin as well as angiotensin-converting enzyme (ACE) inhibition even in patients on ACE inhibitors are also potentially important contributory beneficial effects in heart failure patients. While several beta-adrenergic blocker subtypes have been shown to reduce the incidence of sudden death in susceptible individuals such as those with a history of myocardial infarction and heart failure, there has been variability demonstrated between subtypes.[10,11,20,21] Lipophilic beta-blockers such as timolol, metoprolol, bisoprolol, carvedilol, and propranolol appear to reduce sudden death better than the hydrophilic beta-adrenergic antagonists. This is felt to be due to CNS beta-1 receptor blockade, which modulates cardiac vagal tone and perhaps myocardial electrical stability.[19] Similarly, though controversial, the Carvedilol or Metoprolol European Trial (COMET) study has shown that carvedilol, a nonselective beta antagonist with alpha blocking properties, may be particularly advantageous in heart failure over the beta-1 selective metoprolol.[21] This may be explained by carvedilol's antioxidant effects and alpha blocking vasodilating properties. Though further studies are necessary to further delineate class differences amongst beta-adrenergic blocker subtypes in heart failure, beta-adrenergic blockers, as a class, are now considered standard of care in the management of CHF as has been for two-and-a-half decades in postmyocardial infarction patients.[20,22] Beta-blockers are disease-modifying agents in patients with CHF. It is important to note that decompensated CHF manifest by pulmonary edema and/or systemic hypotension is a contraindication to beta-blocker administration topical or systemic.

In addition to patients with myocardial infarction and CHF, recent studies have demonstrated that beta-antagonists administered in the perioperative period in those with cardiovascular disease reduce postoperative cardiac morbidity because of ischemia and arrhythmia, and possibly mortality in patients undergoing noncardiac surgical intervention under general anesthesia.[22–24] The reduction in mortality, however, was not substantiated in a recently published meta-analysis.[25]

## 59.2 Systemic Reactions and Clinical Recommendations

Hypotension, bronchospasm, bradycardia, dizziness, and fatigue are potentially serious treatment-limiting adverse effects associated with beta-adrenergic blockade. However, prospective studies have shown that systemic beta-adrenergic blockers can be safely used even in patients with traditional contraindications such as asthma and chronic obstructive pulmonary disease (COPD).[26,27] Furthermore, elderly patients (>70 years of age) also appear to be able to tolerate systemic beta-adrenergic blockers and should not be withheld from use of these agents if clinically indicated.[27-31] These trials have demonstrated the cardiac survival benefit in elderly patients who have had a myocardial infarction and CHF. The data regarding beta-blockers in elderly patients with CHF, however, are not as robust as those in younger patients. Two third-generation beta-blockers carvedilol and nebivolol, the latter a novel beta-blocker with nitric oxide-mediated vasodilatory properties, have been demonstrated in well-designed clinical trials to be of benefit in the elderly group with CHF.[30,31] However, unlike a patient with a history of myocardial infarction and CHF, there is no optic nerve survival advantage associated with the use of an ophthalmic beta-adrenergic blocker over other ocular hypotensive agents beyond their individual efficacy with respect to IOP lowering. The efficacy of an ocular hypotensive agent is thus far attributed only to its IOP lowering efficacy. Additional non-IOP related neuroprotective benefits have not been substantiated with any glaucoma agent in human studies.

### 59.2.1 Bradycardia and Dysrhythmia

The goal of glaucoma therapy is to safely reduce IOP and restrict the amount of undesired systemic absorption. Noninternist practitioners often regard a diagnosis of "cardiac arrhythmia" as a contraindication to beta-blocker use. This broad statement is, in fact, grossly incorrect. Beta-blockers have been an important class of agents in the pharmacological treatment for many tachyarrhythmias of supraventricular origin and first-line therapy in some ventricular arrhythmias or diseases associated with potentially lethal ventricular arrhythmias such as the prolonged QT syndromes.[32-34] Beta-blockers are effective antiarrhythmic agents because they suppress catecholamine-mediated hyperactivity, suppress automaticity, and slow myocardial conduction in those with predominant slow response activity.[35] Beta-adrenergic blocker use in *bradyarrhythmias*, in contrast, would be problematic and contraindicated. Patients with symptomatic bradycardia or heart block of any etiology; newly discovered asymptomatic bradycardia not associated with aerobic conditioning; and a history of unexplained syncope, dizziness or presyncope, should not be prescribed a beta-blocker, topical or systemic. The latter patient should be referred without delay to the patient's internist if such symptoms are new, or were never discussed or presented by the patient to their primary care physician. Those with a bradyarrhythmia but have a functioning pacemaker implanted can be safely prescribed a topical or systemic beta-adrenergic blocker.

### 59.2.2 Asthma and Obstructive Lung Disease

Blockade of bronchodilating beta-2 receptors in the lung can exacerbate or trigger bronchospasm in susceptible patients who have asthma or obstructive lung disease with a significant reactive component. Patients with asthma should not be prescribed a beta-adrenergic blocker unless other therapeutic options have been exhausted, and the patient has stable mild–moderate disease. In such a situation, betaxolol, the beta-1 selective beta-adrenergic blocker, is the preferred agent. Close communication with the patient's internist or pulmonologist is recommended. Those with protracted or unstable disease manifested by frequent exacerbations, emergency room visits, or steroid dependency should not be prescribed a beta-blocker, selective or nonselective. Since COPD patients do not have the same degree of reactive airways disease as an asthmatic, ophthalmic beta-adrenergic blocker administration may be considered in these patients with concomitant glaucoma. There are data from a published meta-analysis demonstrating that systemic beta-1 selective blocker administration is safe in patients with mild–moderate stable COPD.[36,37] In this meta-analysis, administration of systemic beta-1 selective beta-adrenergic blockers in patients with COPD did not provoke an exacerbation, worsen symptoms, increase the need for inhalers, or reduce 1-second forced expiratory volume (FEV1). The reversibility of the FEV1 change from acute to chronic use in asthma patients and the tolerability in COPD patients was felt in part to be due to rapid upregulation of beta-2 receptors, thus suggesting that there are differential pharmacological effects depending upon the degree and persistency of receptor–ligand activity.[37] These data notwithstanding, coordination of care with the patient's internist or pulmonologist is encouraged and highly recommended, especially if a nonselective beta-blocker is being considered. Patients should be instructed in following once daily administration and nasolacrimal punctal occlusion to reduce systemic exposure. Otherwise, beta-1 selective betaxolol would be the preferred agent in this class in the COPD patient.

### 59.2.3 Depression

For many years, beta-blockers as a class were associated with depression, cognitive dysfunction, insomnia, and memory loss, as well as other neuropsychiatric disturbances. The widely held opinion of causality with respect to beta-blockers and depression is essentially based on case reporting beginning with the first in 1967 by Waal in the *British Medical Journal*.[38] Since then there have been numerous case reports and small case series disseminated throughout the literature.[39–45] Most of them related to propranolol, a highly lipophilic early generation beta-blocker. The dogma that beta-blockers cause depression has been widely disseminated in the medical community and essentially became accepted as fact from the evidence largely presented in these case reports. With time, however, the relationship became muddied as evidence from clinical trials and systematic analyses became available.[46] In fact, pindolol, a beta-blocker with 5HT-1A serotonin receptor antagonist activity has been shown to accelerate and augment the response of selective serotonin reuptake inhibitors (SSRIs) in the treatment of depression[47]; hence, underscoring the complexity of the pharmacology of beta-blockers as a class with some beta-blockers possessing unique receptor activity over others. Population-based studies that explored antidepressant use concomitant or following beta-blocker therapy has been split between association and nonassociation, perhaps slightly favoring nonassociation.[46,48] However, results of randomized clinical trials, and meta-analyses now strongly argue against the notion of causality between beta-blockers and depression.[49–52] Ko et al. published a quantitative review of all the randomized trials that tested beta-blockers in myocardial infarction, heart failure, and hypertension.[50] There were 15 trials that reported on depression. They found no association between beta-blocker use and incidence of depressive symptoms. In separate prospective randomized placebo-controlled clinical trials, Perez Stable and Sorgi reported no association between systemic beta-blockers and depression.[51,52] Both trials were done specifically to evaluate whether propranolol or nadolol respectively are associated with depression. The disparity between clinical case reports or short case series and clinical trials is likely attributable to multiple reasons, including lack of control for confounders such as age and other demographics, comorbidities, previous history of affective disorders, and nonuniformity in the description and definition of what constitutes a diagnosis of depression or depressive symptoms. Standardized depression-rating instruments such as Beck, Hamilton, and Zung scales, and Diagnostic and Statistical Manual of Mental Disorders 4th edition (DSM IV) criteria were not used in the case reports to make a diagnosis of depression or quantify depressive symptoms. Furthermore, case reports are often inherently biased because of preexisting associations between depression and beta-blockers that influence whether an association between beta-blocker use and depression actually exists.

To date the information regarding topical beta-blocker use and depression is sparse and until a recent study by Kaiserman et al., there have been no well-designed studies that specifically addressed whether ophthalmic beta-blocker administration is associated with an increased risk of depression.[53] The study by Kaiserman and coworkers was a population-based cohort study that defined at least four antidepressant prescriptions filled over the observation period as a surrogate marker for a diagnosis of depression. They found no difference in incidence of depression between beta-blocker users and nonusers even after adjusting for age. Their results add to the accumulating data from clinical trials and population-based studies that beta-blockers do not cause depression.

### 59.2.4 Other Systemic Interactions

Other traditional systemic adverse effects related to beta-adrenergic blocker use have not been substantiated by controlled prospective studies or have only been demonstrated with systemically administered doses and not following ophthalmic use. Many such traditionally accepted associations have been propagated for decades by single case reports or short case series. Thus far, placebo-controlled prospective studies have failed to show that beta-adrenergic blockers exacerbate symptoms of intermittent claudication in those with mild-moderate peripheral vascular disease or cause prolonged hypoglycemia or hypoglycemic unawareness in patients with noninsulin-dependent diabetes (NIDDM).[54,55] Both systemic and ophthalmic beta-blockers have been shown to reduce serum high density lipoprotein (HDL) and increase total triglycerides by about 8–10%.[56–60] These changes are largely mediated by inhibition of lipoprotein lipase. Nonselective beta-adrenergic blockers have the greatest propensity for these metabolic changes followed by selective beta-blockers, and least in those with ISA. Studies with ophthalmic beta-blockers, however, lacked a placebo control, were short duration (6 weeks), and only one pretreatment measurement was made at baseline and one posttreatment measurement for comparison.

Systemic beta-adrenergic blockers may reduce sexual function in male patients.[61] Exercise capacity is also affected by beta-adrenergic blockers when used systemically.[62,63] However, there are no prospective data to show that either occurs following ophthalmic administration. Although ophthalmic administration of beta-adrenergic blockers has been shown to reduce heart rate and systolic blood pressure, workload performed was not affected.[64] This seemingly enigmatic finding is because exercise capacity modulated by beta-blockade has been theorized to be due to its effect on electrolyte metabolism, potassium in particular, and the reduced availability of energy substrate to the exercising muscles rather than simply its effect on hemodynamic parameters such as heart rate and blood pressure. In one study, despite a reduction in heart rate and blood pressure with a systemically administered beta-blocker, cardiac output actually remained unchanged but work capacity was reduced by 29% as compared to controls.[63] The reduction in heart rate with a beta-adrenergic blocker actually improves stroke volume with increased ventricular filling time and improves blood flow because of a reduction in peripheral vascular resistance or afterload, thereby preventing a decrease in cardiac output.

## 59.3 Carbonic Anhydrase Inhibitors

In 1949, Friedenwald postulated that aqueous humor secretion occurred via a redox process in the ciliary body and that the fluid secreted was alkaline in composition.[65] Several years later, Becker serendipitously discovered that the oral carbonic anhydrase inhibitor (CAI) acetazolamide can also lower intraocular pressure following oral administration to lower systemic blood pressure.[66] Since the 1950s, CAI have continued to play an important role in the management of glaucoma and ocular hypertension. However, the relatively narrow therapeutic index of oral/systemic CAI prompted the development of a topical version. In the mid 1990s, dorzolamide was the first topical CAI to come to market, followed by brinzolamide. Currently, topical CAI agents are used primarily second- or third-line in combination with beta-adrenergic blockers and prostaglandin analogs. Though often highly effective, because of significant systemic side effects, systemic CAI agents are predominantly reserved in the management of acute uncontrolled glaucoma, in chronic open angle glaucoma as a last resort before surgical intervention, or as a temporizing measure prior to surgical intervention.

### 59.3.1 Physiology and Pharmacology

There are at least seven carbonic anhydrase (CA) isoenzymes in the human body, and though CA-II is the predominant isoenzyme in the ciliary epithelium, CA-IV is also present in the nonpigmented ciliary epithelium. Carbonic anhydrase catalyzes the reversible conversion of $CO_2$ and $H_2O$ to carbonic acid. Hydrogen ion and bicarbonate ion produced by this reaction is transported by facilitated diffusion via antiport and symport systems on the ciliary epithelium. Energy for transport is driven by the sodium electrochemical gradient, which is maintained by sodium/potassium ATPase on the plasma membrane. Effective CAI-mediated suppression of aqueous humor production requires more than 99% inhibition of carbonic anhydrase.[67] Acetazolamide, the prototype systemic CAI, has been shown to be ineffective in those with autosomal recessive CA-II deficiency.[68] Acetazolamide administered orally is rapidly absorbed from the gastrointestinal (GI) tract and has a relatively rapid onset of action with a duration of action of about 6–8 h. Acetazolamide is also extensively protein bound (>90%) and excreted virtually unchanged in the urine. Though plasma levels of acetazolamide are dose dependent, there is considerable variability noted experimentally following single dose administration.[69,70] Since elimination of acetazolamide occurs via the kidney, plasma concentration is strongly dependent upon glomerular filtration rate (GFR) – with declining renal function, plasma levels will increase. Despite dose-dependency, plasma levels exceeding 10 μg/ml were not consistently found to provide additional IOP-lowering benefit.[69] However, in another study, 250-mg tablets administered four times daily or 500 mg extended-release capsules BID produced maximal IOP lowering efficacy at plasma concentrations between 15 and 20 μg/ml. Thus, based on the dose response studies collectively, maximal therapeutic plasma concentrations should remain less than 20 μg/ml with a target range of 10–15 μg/ml.[70]

Methazolamide has different pharmacological and chemical properties as compared to acetazolamide and is extensively metabolized before excretion, leaving only about 25% excreted unchanged in the urine. It is also more lipophilic with less plasma protein binding (55% with methazolamide versus >90% with acetazolamide) and thus penetrates ocular tissues at smaller doses.[71] Since, the renal/metabolic effects of CAI primarily depend upon carbonic anhydrase inhibition at the level of the proximal convoluted tubule in the nephron and since most of the methazolamide is metabolized to inactive form prior to glomerular filtration, the corresponding renal/metabolic effects of methazolamide will be necessarily attenuated as compared to acetazolamide.

### 59.3.2 Systemic Reactions

The systemic effects of carbonic anhydrase inhibition on electrolyte, acid–base, and fluid metabolism are dependent upon the amount of active drug filtered by the glomerulus as inhibition of renal CA occurs at the level of the proximal convoluted tubule. Inhibition of renal CA causes rapid excretion of bicarbonate leading to urinary alkalinization and a concomitant obligate reduction in sodium absorption.[72] Increased delivery of bicarbonate and sodium to the distal tubule will also reduce potassium absorption and hence cause potassium wasting. Thus, CAI agents cause a metabolic acidosis and will reduce total body sodium and potassium.[72] The effects on water, sodium, and potassium metabolism are transient, however, for several reasons. First, despite persistent CA inhibition, the loss of plasma bicarbonate plateaus. This is because as plasma bicarbonate concentration decreases the filtered load at the glomerulus (plasma concentration of bicarbonate mg/ml × GFR ml/min = mg/min filtered bicarbonate through the glomerulus) likewise decreases. Eventually, the filtered load of bicarbonate "matches" the level of carbonic anhydrase activity in the proximal tubule leading to cessation of further bicarbonate wasting and a steady state plasma concentration of bicarbonate is achieved. This is analogous to reaching the "transport maximum" of a filtered substance that is normally reabsorbed at the proximal convoluted tubule. Second, as bicarbonate wastage ceases so do sodium and water loss, as they are linked to bicarbonate loss. Third, the initial inhibition of sodium and water absorption in the proximal tubule leads to a compensatory increase in sodium and water absorption at the ascending thick limb of Henle and the distal convoluted tubule, which also limits the degree of sodium and water loss. Finally, the increase in solute delivery from proximal to distal tubule during the early phase of renal CA inhibition activates a process called tubuloglomerular feedback, which lowers GFR by vasoconstriction of the afferent arterioles and hence the filtered load of bicarbonate.[72]

CAI agents also reduce urinary citrate in addition to raising urinary pH, both of which are important in maintaining calcium solubility, hence leading to an increased propensity to the development of urolithiasis.[72,73] Concomitant administration of loop or thiazide diuretics in the management of systemic hypertension or edema with a CAI agent can magnify and perpetuate each agent's systemic metabolic effect on fluid and electrolyte metabolism as well as stone formation. Other reported renal effects include acute renal failure, which appears to be mediated by tubular obstruction.[74] Even though patients with end-stage renal disease are functionally anephric, preexisting renal failure associated acidosis may be worsened by acetazolamide as a result of inhibition of extrarenal buffers in bone.[75,76]

The systemic effects of CAI agents are protean, but the most common effects involve the gastrointestinal tract. Gastrointestinal complaints related to systemic CAI agents include nausea, vomiting, diarrhea, constipation, and anorexia.[77] Inhibition of gastric CA will also disrupt the composition of the protective barrier on the gastric mucosal surface, thus increasing the risk of gastrointestinal bleeding. In one case report, massive GI bleeding in a patient with end-stage renal disease and plasma levels of acetazolamide exceeding 70 μg/ml resulted in development of disseminated intravascular coagulation and death, despite dialysis to lower plasma levels.[78] Patients with end-stage renal disease are at risk for bleeding due to dysfunctional uremic platelets.[79] The loss of the protective alkaline mucosal barrier promoted the GI bleed, which was compounded by the patient's renal failure associated hemorrhagic diathesis.

Paresthesias of the fingers and toes are also extremely common. Central nervous system (CNS) penetration leads to lethargy, somnolence, fatigue, and, in the elderly, confusion is very common. CAI agents also reduce libido. Bone marrow toxicity, the most serious adverse event is an idiosyncratic effect and not dose or time dependent. Aplastic anemia involves suppression of all cellular blood elements. However, leukopenia, thrombocytopenia, and agranulocytosis may occur in the absence of anemia.[80] Since the therapeutic index with systemically administered CAI agents is narrow, the minimal dose necessary to reach the maximal effect on IOP lowering is recommended, especially if acetazolamide is used. Based on previous pharmacologic experiments correlating plasma levels with IOP response, plasma levels of acetazolamide exceeding 10 μg/ml should yield a maximal to near maximal benefit.[69,70] Despite individual variability in plasma levels, healthy patients without renal disease may be dosed up to 1,000 mg daily in divided doses to achieve maximal IOP lowering, if well-tolerated, as this dose will result in plasma levels that may exceed 15 μg/ml.[70] However, since lower doses may still be equally effective, routine plasma level determination in the patient without renal disease is unnecessary. Thus, starting at lower doses and escalating as tolerated is appropriate. On the other hand, if the patient is symptomatic, dose reduction is appropriate with close monitoring of IOP.

However, in the patient with renal insufficiency, as previously illustrated, plasma accumulation can be quite dramatic and in some cases leading to potentially serious toxicity and profound CNS depression – in some cases necessitating urgent dialysis to lower plasma levels. Thus, patients at known risk for renal insufficiency, such as diabetics and hypertensives, should have baseline measurement of blood urea nitrogen (BUN) and creatinine levels at the time of initiation of acetazolamide. If levels are in normal range, the clinician should proceed as previously described. However, in the presence of renal insufficiency, dose adjustment guided by determination of plasma levels is mandated to prevent unwanted toxicity. Although, dose-related side effects are reversible with cessation and if necessary accelerated with hemodialysis, severe CNS depression with altered sensorium may cause serious secondary problems such as aspiration pneumonia, especially in elderly patients. Because renal failure prolongs the half-life, reducing frequency of administration is most important to prevent the accumulation of acetazolamide to undesired high levels. With greater loss of renal function dosage should be reduced as well. There are specific recommendations published guiding the use of acetazolamide in the patient with end-stage renal disease on hemodialysis.[81,82] In a pharmacokinetic study, the authors recommended an initial dose of 250 mg the first day then 125-mg QD for 4 days.[82] If therapy for more than 1 week is necessary, then plasma levels should be obtained and the dose adjusted accordingly. Because the efficiency of dialysis in removing acetazolamide is only 30% of the efficiency of eliminating urea nitrogen, the dose frequency may need to be spaced at intervals greater than 24 h.[83] Though, not validated without measuring plasma levels, one possible maintenance dose regimen of acetazolamide is 125–250 mg after each dialysis session. Assistance in dosing with a nephrologist in patients with renal insufficiency is strongly advocated if acetazolamide is necessary for a prolonged period of time in the management of glaucoma in the patient with end-stage renal disease.[1]

Elderly patients without overt renal disease should likely be prescribed doses less than 1,000 mg/day. First, lower plasma levels than that achieved with this dose can result in maximal IOP lowering response. Second, even elderly patients with normal levels of creatinine have a GFR that is reduced compared with younger adults, and thus a given dose will achieve higher steady state plasma levels than a younger patient. And, third, the CNS depressant effects may potentially be worse in these patients who may have other comorbid conditions. A rule of thumb relating age with renal function is that GFR is reduced by 50% between the third and ninth decades, or by about 1 ml/min for every year over the age of 30.[84] Though this rule of thumb is subject to debate, nevertheless, elderly patients still have lower numbers of functioning nephrons such that lower doses such as 250 mg twice daily or 500-mg sequels once daily are likely to be sufficient in providing maximal ciliary body CA inhibition.

Aside from renal failure, patients with limited pulmonary reserve as a result of COPD may develop respiratory failure during the physiologic hyperventilatory respiratory compensatory response to metabolic acidosis induced by acetazolamide. Thus, caution needs to be exercised in such patients, especially those who are chronic retainers of $CO_2$. The combination of respiratory acidosis from chronic $CO_2$ retention and metabolic acidosis may lead to a severe reduction in plasma pH, with dangerous consequences.

Topically administered CAI agents achieve plasma levels that are 1/200 those achieved with the systemic agents, thus do not cause the metabolic changes seen with the oral agents. There are no reports in the literature that suggest that topical administration leads to any of the side effects reported with the systemic CAI agents.[85]

## 59.4 Selective Alpha Agonists

Apraclonidine and brimonidine are ocular hypotensive alpha 2 agonists. Although both agents are alpha 2 selective, brimonidine has much greater selectivity at the alpha 2 receptor. At high concentrations, apraclonidine can bind alpha 1 receptors and cause vasoconstriction. Brimonidine, which in contrast to apraclonidine is lipophilic, can penetrate the CNS.[86]

### 59.4.1 Pharmacology and Physiology

Both apraclonidine and brimonidine lower intraocular pressure through alpha 2 agonist mediated aqueous suppression and a secondary mechanism that improves aqueous outflow. Following topical administration of apraclonidine, plasma levels are low but can be detectable for up to 8 h.[87] While the effect of apraclonidine on IOP is independent of plasma levels, it can bind to peripheral alpha 2 receptors, potentially affecting cardiovascular activity. The high lipophilicity of brimonidine results in increased CNS penetration relative to apraclonidine. The physiologic changes mediated by alpha 2 agonist activity accounts for the systemic effects following topical administration of these agents. The dilute plasma concentration and high receptor selectivity for the alpha 2 receptor, especially with brimonidine, greatly lessens the probability of developing manifestations related to alpha 1 binding.

### 59.4.2 Systemic Reactions

Both agents have been shown to be safe in clinical trials.[86] However, their ability to bind to alpha receptors may result in unwanted cardiovascular side effects. Alpha 2 receptor agonist activity inhibits neuronal release of norepinephrine. Thus, systemic toxicity from these agents would be expected to resemble the antihypertensive agent clonidine. Bradycardia and hypotension are potential reactions following topical apraclonidine administration. Robin, however, showed that topical administration of apraclonidine did not affect heart rate or mean arterial blood pressure and minimally blunted exercise-induced tachycardia in healthy volunteers.[87] The changes in these parameters were statistically significantly less than the effect of ophthalmic timolol on heart rate and blood pressure. Similarly, brimonidine has been shown to have minimal effects on heart rate and did not reduce blood pressure.[86] These actions, as expected, are due to alpha 2 binding. As stated previously, the alpha 1 affects are not seen systemically because of the low plasma concentration and their relative selectivity for the alpha 2 receptor. Vasoconstriction, however, is noted locally on the conjunctiva following topical administration with either agent, because the local ocular concentration is high enough to cause significant activity at the alpha 1 receptor and mediate conjunctival vasoconstriction. Dryness of the oral and nasopharyngeal mucosa is also because of local passage of the drop via the nasolacrimal duct and direct binding to mucosal alpha receptors. Like conjunctival blanching, dryness is mediated by alpha 1 mediated vasoconstriction because local concentrations are high following direct contact with the mucosal surface. Thus, despite the selectivity of both of these agents for the alpha 2 receptor, selectivity is incomplete; and if local concentrations are high enough, the vasoconstrictive effects of these agents become manifest.

Unlike apraclonidine, brimonidine is lipophilic allowing brimonidine to penetrate the CNS. Central alpha 2 agonist activity can cause CNS depression and somnolence. This is particularly evident and has been reported to occur more frequently and more severely in the pediatric age group as compared to adults, especially with toddlers and infants because of their small size. In fact, it is contraindicated in young children specifically because of its potentially severe CNS depressant effect.[88] In a retrospective study, 4/22 children under age 14 (mean age of 8 years) had to discontinue brimonidine because of fatigue and fainting spells.[89]

## 59.5 Sympathomimetics

### 59.5.1 Nonselective Agonists

This class of agents was an important and commonly used class of glaucoma agents and had dual mechanism of action to lower IOP via aqueous suppression as well as an enhancing conventional and uveoscleral outflow. However, with the development of newer safe and effective topical glaucoma agents in the past decade, use of nonselective adrenergic agonists has steadily declined. Epinephrine 1% and 2% formulations were the most commonly used until the prodrug dipivalyl epinephrine was developed to reduce both local and systemic toxicity without compromising its ocular hypotensive effect.

### 59.5.2 Pharmacology and Physiology

These agents are nonselective alpha- and beta-adrenergic agonists. The dipivalyl prodrug has 100–600 times greater lipophilicity than epinephrine and thus has higher intraocular penetration by 17 times over epinephrine.[90] The drug is converted to epinephrine by corneal stromal esterases resulting in free epinephrine in the anterior chamber. Thus, the concentration of epinephrine in the prodrug is 0.1% as compared to the 1% and 2% formulations.

Systemic absorption of these agents, as with all topically administered ophthalmic agents, involves passage through the nasolacrimal duct and direct absorption through the nasopharyngeal mucosa, avoiding first-pass hepatic metabolism. The systemic effect of adrenergic agents on the cardiovascular system would be expected to be variable and not only dependent upon the bioavailability of these agents but also dependent, in part, upon basal catecholamine activity. Thus, it is no surprise that the reported effects of this class of agents as described later, particularly the nonprodrug agents, have been quite variable. In addition, the relatively wide but normal fluctuations in the hemodynamic parameters potentially affected by these agents, such as heart rate and blood pressure, necessitates adequate assessment of the diurnal mean variation in these parameters with a placebo control as well as controlling for variation in physical activity before conclusive statements can be made about changes in these cardiovascular parameters.

### 59.5.3 Systemic Reactions

While Kerr et al. reported an increase in systolic blood pressure and mean arterial blood pressure in 5/20 patients receiving epinephrine, and one patient had "significant ventricular ectopy," Kohn et al., however, did not report any such changes.[91,92] In a single dose study Blondeau and Cote reported a slight increase in diastolic blood pressure with epinephrine 2% as compared to dipivalyl epinephrine or placebo in patients already on timolol topically.[93] The lack of systemic esterases that can cleave the prodrug to active epinephrine and the significantly lower systemic plasma levels have rendered the drug essentially devoid of unwanted cardiovascular changes. Thus, if this class of agents is necessary in the individual glaucoma patient, the prodrug is the drug of choice.

## 59.6 Miotics

### 59.6.1 Pharmacology and Physiology

Miotic agents as a class increase cholinergic activity at the synapse via direct agonist activity at the postsynaptic receptor, enhanced release of acetylcholine at the neural junction, or indirectly via cholinesterase inhibition (anti-ChE), which prolongs the half-life of endogenous acetylcholine activity. Thus, there are three classes of cholinomimetics for ocular use: direct agonists such as pilocarpine or acetylcholine, indirect agonists such as ecthiophate (phospholine iodide), and mixed direct agonist/acetylcholine releasing agents such as carbachol. Ocular use of this class of agents is primarily in the management of glaucoma.

The cholinergic neural pathway has both muscarinic and nicotinic cholinergic receptors. The effects of cholinomimetics thus depend upon whether they bind primarily to muscarinic or nicotinic receptors, or both, and whether such binding is preganglionic or postganglionic. Muscarinic receptors are postganglionic and are present on smooth muscle cells that are involved in involuntary activity-autonomic effector cells. This is the autonomic parasympathetic pathway.[94] In contrast, nicotinic receptors are found primarily on striated muscle and also in cholinergic sympathetic ganglia. Typical muscarinic effects include miosis, flushing, bradycardia, bronchospasm, increased bronchial secretions, involuntary urination and defecation, nausea, vomiting, sweating, lacrimation, salivation, hypotension, hypothermia, and seizures. Nicotinic toxic effects on striated muscle include muscle cramps, fasciculations, weakness, and paralysis due to persistent depolarization. Nicotinic agents at low doses stimulate the postsynaptic receptor and at higher doses cause blockade such as the anti-ChE nerve-blocking agents. Nicotinic sympathetic ganglionic effects lead to tachycardia and hypertension.[94,95]

### 59.6.2 Systemic Reactions

Systemic toxicity from topical applied cholinergic agonists have been rarely reported. However, systemic pilocarpine used in the treatment of Sjogrens syndrome to promote salivary activity and lacrimal activity has been reported to cause systemic adverse reactions.[96] Signs and symptoms of cholinergic toxicity from pilocarpine involve muscarinic receptor binding and include hypersalivation, diaphoresis, diarrhea, bradycardia, hypotension, and seizures.[94,95] Pilocarpine, however, in the lung binds selectively to inhibitory M2 muscarinic receptors (inhibitory autoreceptors), which experimentally prevent vagally mediated bronchoconstriction by blocking release of acetylcholine.[97-99] Thus, unlike the other cholinergic agents, prolonging acetylcholine activity in preganglionic and postganglionic receptors by pilocarpine have a wider range of effects as a result of modulation of both muscarinic and nicotinic receptor activity. In the medical literature, cholinergic toxicity following ophthalmic application of pilocarpine is rarely seen. Kushnick et al. reported a case of cholinergic toxicity leading to a seizure following sudden release of pilocarpine from an ocusert.[100]

There is clinical and experimental evidence that echothiophate iodide ophthalmic solution can reduce plasma cholinesterase significantly, especially in the pediatric age group.[101,102] Systemic toxicity due to this agent has been reported and included cardiac arrest.[103] In one report, echothiophate iodide (phospholine iodide) eye drops administered in an adult patient apparently led to severe muscle weakness prompting a preliminary diagnosis of myasthenia gravis.[104] However, red blood cell and serum cholinesterase levels were severely depressed consistent with anti-ChE activity. Discontinuation of echothiophate iodide eyedrops resulted in resolution of symptoms. Caution must be exercised in patients on anti-ChE agents when undergoing anesthesia with depolarizing agents such as succinylcholine. The paralytic effects of these nerve blocking agents may be prolonged and profound.[105-108] Atropine is the drug of choice in treatment of cholinergic toxicity, especially the cardiovascular depression that occurs with muscarinic agonist activity. However, toxicity due to anti-ChE agents cannot be treated with atropine because it will only serve to exacerbate the paralytic effects of these depolarizing agents. Cholinesterase reactivators such as pralidoxime are the drugs of choice in this scenario.[71]

In a life-threatening situation (respiratory depression), cholinesterase reactivators would have been appropriate. Although toxicity from echothiophate iodide is due to its anti-ChE activity, in one report the iodide portion of the agent was associated with the development of thyroid disease as a result of iodide accumulation in the thyroid gland.[109]

## 59.7 Prostaglandin Analogs

Prostaglandin analogs include latanoprost, travoprost, bimatoprost, and unoprostone. All of these agents have variable activity at the prostaglandin F2 alpha receptor. The most potent agonist is travoprost and the weakest, with little to no activity at the F2 alpha receptor, is unoprostone. The prostaglandin analogs, with the exception of unoprostone, are potent IOP-lowering agents and have surpassed beta-adrenergic blockers in terms of efficacy. Toxicity associated with these agents has been primarily due to their local ocular effects causing iris and periocular pigmentation as well as conjunctival hyperemia and ocular discomfort.[110]

### 59.7.1 Pharmacology and Physiology

Latanoprost and travoprost are potent F2 alpha agonists and lower IOP via increased uveoscleral outflow. This increase in uveoscleral outflow appears to be mediated by increased matrix metalloproteinase activity.[111] Bimatoprost, a prostamide, is hydrolyzed to free acid by corneal, scleral, and uveal amidases. Presumably, though controversial, its mechanism of action, once hydrolyzed to free acid, is also via agonist activity at the F2 alpha receptor like latanoprost and travoprost. Unoprostone, a docasonoid, has very poor binding to F2 alpha receptors. Its mechanism of action has not been fully elucidated.

The half-life following systemic absorption of latanoprost is rapid and was calculated to be 17 min whether administered topically or intravenously. Following systemic absorption, these agents are metabolized in the liver via beta oxidation and the inactive metabolites are then excreted by the kidney.[77]

### 59.7.2 Systemic Reactions and Clinical Recommendations

Because these agents are prostaglandin analogs, systemic toxicity, if it occurs, would theoretically be related to their stimulatory contractile effects on smooth muscle. In the lungs, this may manifest as tracheobronchial spasm. Uterine contractions may also theoretically occur and thus in pregnancy there is a theoretical risk of triggering a spontaneous abortion. The most common adverse event reported during clinical trials with latanoprost was upper respiratory/influenza-like symptoms. To date, there have been no systemic adverse events reported that would be consistent with the pharmacological activity of these agents. Latanoprost administered to asthmatics in a double-masked placebo controlled crossover study failed to show clinical symptomatic exacerbations of their asthma, did not result in increased use of inhalers, had no effect on the responsiveness to inhalers, and did not reduce FEV1.[112,113] In fact, intravenous infusion of up to 3 µg/kg in healthy human volunteers produced plasma concentrations up to 200 times greater than that achieved via ophthalmic administration without reported systemic adverse events.[77] Administration of prostaglandin analogs are not only safe in asthmatics, but largely devoid of systemic adverse events. As addressed elsewhere in this text, it would be prudent to withhold these agents during pregnancy, if possible, due to the theoretical but unproven effect on uterine contractile activity with topical administration and the unknown teratogenic effects in human embryos.

## References

1. van der Valk R, Webers CA, Schouten JS, et al. Intraocular pressure-lowering effects of all commonly used glaucoma drugs: a meta-analysis of randomized clinical trials. *Ophthalmology*. 2005;112(7):1177–1185.
2. Lipworth BJ. Clinical pharmacology of beta 3-adrenoceptors. *Br J Clin Pharmacol*. 1996;42(3):291–300.
3. Weyer C, Gautier JF, Danforth E Jr. Development of beta 3-adrenoceptor agonists for the treatment of obesity and diabetes–an update. *Diabetes Metab*. 1999;25(1):11–21.
4. Kobayashi I, Ishigami T, Umemura S. Insulin resistance and beta 3-adrenergic receptor function. *Nippon Rinsho*. 2000;58(2):333–337.
5. Vuori ML, Kaila T. Plasma kinetics and anatgonist activity of topical ocular timolol in elderly patients. *Arch Clin Exp Ophthalmol*. 1995;233:131–134.
6. *Physicians' Desk Reference*. 53rd ed. Montvale, NJ: Medical Economics Co.; 1999:1741.
7. Bobik A, Jennings GL, Asley P, et al. Timolol pharmacokinetics and effects on heart rate and blood pressure after acute and chronic administration. *Eur J Clin Pharmacol*. 1979;16:243–249.
8. Wilson TW, Fior WB, Johnson GE, et al. Timolol and propranolol: bioavailability, plasma concentration, and beta blockade. *Clin Pharmacol Ther*. 1982;32:676–685.
9. Shedden A, Laurence J, Tipping R, et al. Efficacy and tolerability of timolol maleate gel-forming solution versus timolol ophthalmic solution in adults with open angle glaucoma and ocular hypertension: a 6-month, double-masked, multicenter study. *Clin Ther*. 2001;23:440–450.
10. The MIAMI Trial Research Group. Metoprolol in acute myocardial infarction (MIAMI). A randomised placebo-controlled international trial. The MIAMI Trial Research Group. *Eur Heart J*. 1985;6:199–226.
11. First International Study on Infarct Survival Collaborative Group. Randomised trial of intravenous atenolol among 16, 027 cases of suspected acute myocardial infarction: ISIS-1. First international study of infarct survival collaborative group. *Lancet*. 1986;2: 823–827.
12. Teerlink JR, Massie BM. Beta-adrenergic blocker mortality trials in congestive heart failure. *Am J Cardiol*. 1999;84:94R–102R.
13. CIBIS II Investigators and Commitees. The cardiac insufficiency bisoprolol study II (CIBIS II). *Lancet*. 1999;353:9–13.
14. MERIT-HF Study Group. Effect of metoprolol CR/XL in chronic heart failure: Metoprolol CR/XL randomised intervention trial in congestive heart failure (MERIT-HF). *Lancet*. 1999;353: 2001–2007.
15. Packer M, Bristow MR, Cohn JN, et al. The effect of carvedilol on morbidity and mortality in patients with chronic heart failure. U.S. Carvedilol Heart Failure Study Group. *N Engl J Med*. 1996;334: 1349–1355.
16. Packer M, Coats AJ, Fowler MB, et al. Effect of carvedilol on survival in severe chronic heart failure. *N Engl J Med*. 2001; 344:1651–1658.
17. Beta-Blocker Evaluation of Survival Trial Investigators. A trial of the beta-blocker bucindolol in patients with advanced chronic heart failure. *N Engl J Med*. 2001;344:1659–1667.
18. Klein L, O'Connor CM, Gattis WA, et al. Pharmacologic therapy for patients with chronic heart failure and reduced systolic function: review of trials and practical considerations. *Am J Cardiol*. 2003;91(9A):18F–40F.
19. Hjalmarson A. Prevention of sudden cardiac death with beta blockers. *Clin Cardiol*. 1999;22(suppl 5):V11–V15.
20. Domanski MJ, Krause-Steinrauf H, Massie BM, et al. A comparative analysis of the results from 4 trials of beta-blocker therapy for heart failure: BEST, CIBIS-II, MERIT-HF, and COPERNICUS. *J Card Fail*. 2003;9(5):354–363.
21. McBride BF, White CM. Critical differences among beta-adrenoreceptor antagonists in myocardial failure: debating the MERIT of COMET. *J Clin Pharmacol*. 2005;45(1):6–24.
22. Finley AC, Elliott BM, Robison JJ, Brothers TE. Prophylactic beta-blocker use to prevent perioperative morbidity and mortality. *J S C Med Assoc*. 2004;100(8):223–226.
23. Kertai MD, Boersma E, Westerhout CM, et al. A combination of statins and beta-blockers is independently associated with a reduction in the incidence of perioperative mortality and nonfatal myocardial infarction in patients undergoing abdominal aortic aneurysm surgery. *Eur J Vasc Endovasc Surg*. 2004;28(4): 343–352.
24. Lindenauer PK, Fitzgerald J, Hoople N, Benjamin EM. The potential preventability of postoperative myocardial infarction: underuse of perioperative beta-adrenergic blockade. *Arch Intern Med*. 2004;164(7):762–766.
25. Wiesbauer F, Schlager O, Domanovits H, et al. Perioperative beta-blockers for preventing surgery-related mortality and morbidity: a systematic review and meta-analysis. *Anesth Analg*. 2007;104(1): 27–41.
26. Glaab T, Weiss T. Use of beta blockers in cardiovascular diseases and bronchial asthma/COPD. *Internist (Berl)*. 2004;45(2): 221–227.
27. Chen J, Radford MJ, Wang Y, Marciniak TA, Krumholz HM. Effectiveness of beta-blocker therapy after acute myocardial infarction in elderly patients with chronic obstructive pulmonary disease or asthma. *J Am Coll Cardiol*. 2001;37(7):1950–1956.
28. Gutierrez ME, Labovitz AJ. Underutilization of beta-adrenoceptor antagonists post-myocardial infarction. *Am J Cardiovasc Drugs*. 2005;5(1):23–29.
29. Fu M. Beta-blocker therapy in heart failure in the elderly. *Int J Cardiol*. 2008;125(2):149–153.

30. Coats AJ. Beta-adrenoceptor antagonists in elderly patients with chronic heart failure: therapeutic potential of third-generation agents. *Drugs Aging*. 2006;23(2):93–99.
31. Dobre D, van Veldhuisen DJ, Mordenti G, et al. SENIORS Investigators. Tolerability and dose-related effects of nebivolol in elderly patients with heart failure: data from the Study of the Effects of Nebivolol Intervention on Outcomes and Rehospitalisation in Seniors with Heart Failure (SENIORS) trial. *Am Heart J*. 2007;154(1):109–115.
32. Lévy S, Ricard P. Using the right drug: a treatment algorithm for regular supraventricular tachycardias. *Eur Heart J*. 1997;18(suppl C):C27–C32.
33. Akhtar M, Jazayeri MR, Sra J, et al. Atrioventricular nodal reentry. Clinical, electrophysiological, and therapeutic considerations. *Circulation*. 1993;88(1):282–295. Review.
34. Chiang CE. Congenital and acquired long QT syndrome. Current concepts and management. *Cardiol Rev*. 2004;12(4):222–234.
35. Dorian P. Antiarrhythmic action of beta-blockers: potential mechanisms. *J Cardiovasc Pharmacol Ther*. 2005;10(suppl 1): S15–S22.
36. Salpeter SR, Ormiston TM, Salpeter EE, Poole PJ, Cates CJ. Cardioselective beta-blockers for chronic obstructive pulmonary disease: a meta-analysis. *Respir Med*. 2003;97(10):1094–1101.
37. Salpeter SR, Ormiston TM, Salpeter EE. Cardioselective beta-blockers in patients with reactive airway disease: a meta-analysis. *Ann Intern Med*. 2002;137(9):715–725.
38. Waal HJ. Propranolol-induced depression. *Br Med J*. 1967; 2(5543):50.
39. Fitzgerald JD. Propranolol-induced depression. *Br Med J*. 1967; 2(5548):372–373.
40. Nolan BT. Acute suicidal depression associated with use of timolol. *JAMA*. 1982;247(11):1567.
41. Avorn J, Everitt DE, Weiss S. Increased antidepressant use in patients prescribed beta-blockers. *JAMA*. 1986;255(3):357–360.
42. Parker WA. Propranolol-induced depression and psychosis. *Clin Pharm*. 1985;4(2):214–218.
43. Griffin SJ, Friedman MJ. Depressive symptoms in propranolol users. *J Clin Psychiatry*. 1986;47(9):453–457.
44. Acosta Artiles F, Suárez Cabrera M, Acosta Artiles M, Acosta Artiles P. Beta blocker induced depression. A case report [Spanish]. *Actas Esp Psiquiatr*. 2006;34(5):352–354.
45. Steffensmeier JJ, Ernst ME, Kelly M, Hartz AJ. Do randomized controlled trials always trump case reports? A second look at propranolol and depression. *Pharmacotherapy*. 2006;26(2):162–167.
46. Ried LD, McFarland BH, Johnson RE, Brody KK. Beta-blockers and depression: the more the murkier? *Ann Pharmacother*. 1998;32(6):699–708.
47. Artigas F, Adell A, Celada P. Pindolol augmentation of antidepressant response. *Curr Drug Targets*. 2006;7(2):139–147.
48. Gerstman BB, Jolson HM, Bauer M, et al. The incidence of depression in new users of beta-blockers and selected antihypertensives. *J Clin Epidemiol*. 1996;49(7):809–815.
49. van Melle JP, Verbeek DE, van den Berg MP, et al. Beta-blockers and depression after myocardial infarction: a multicenter prospective study. *J Am Coll Cardiol*. 2006;48(11):2209–2214.
50. Ko DT, Hebert PR, Coffey CS, et al. Beta-blocker therapy and symptoms of depression, fatigue, and sexual dysfunction. *JAMA*. 2002;288(3):351–357.
51. Sorgi P, Ratey J, Knoedler D, et al. Depression during treatment with beta-blockers: results from a double-blind placebo-controlled study. *J Neuropsychiatry Clin Neurosci*. 1992;4(2):187–189.
52. Pérez-Stable EJ, Halliday R, Gardiner PS, et al. The effects of propranolol on cognitive function and quality of life: a randomized trial among patients with diastolic hypertension. *Am J Med*. 2000;108(5):359–365.
53. Kaiserman I, Kaiserman N, Elhayany A, Vinker S. Topical beta-blockers are not associated with an increased risk of treatment for depression. *Ophthalmology*. 2006;113(7):1077–1080.
54. Radack K, Deck C. Beta-adrenergic blocker therapy does not worsen intermittent claudication in subjects with peripheral arterial disease. A meta-analysis of randomized controlled trials. *Arch Intern Med*. 1991;151(9):1769–1776.
55. Umited Kingdom Prospective Diabetes Study Group. Efficacy of atenolol and captopril in reducing risk of macrovascular and microvascular complications in type 2 diabetes. *Br Med J*. 1998;317:713–720.
56. Madu EC, Reddy RC, Madu AN, et al. Review: the effects of antihypertensive agents on serum lipids. *Am J Med Sci*. 1996;312: 76–84.
57. Lakshman R, Reda DJ, Materson BJ, et al. Diuretics and beta-blockers do not have adverse effects at 1 year on plasma lipid and lipoprotein profiles in men with hypertension. *Arch Intern Med*. 1999;159:551–558.
58. Coleman AL, Diehl DLC, Jampel HD, et al. Topical timolol decreases plama high-density lipoprotein cholesterol level. *Arch Ophthalmol*. 1990;108:1260–1263.
59. Stewart WC, Dubiner HB, Mundorf TK, et al. Effects of carteolol and timolol on plasma lipid profiles in older women with ocular hypertension or primary open-angle glaucoma. *Am J Ophthalmol*. 1999;127:142–147.
60. Freedman SF, Freedman NF, Shields MB, et al. Effects of ocular carteolol and timolol on plasma high-density lipoprotein cholesterol level. *Am J Ophthalmol*. 1993;116:600–611.
61. Ko DT, Hebert PR, Coffey CS, Sedrakyan A, Curtis JP, Krumholz HM. Beta-blocker therapy and symptoms of depression, fatigue, and sexual dysfunction. *JAMA*. 2002;288(3):351–357.
62. Gordon NF, Duncan JJ. Effect of beta-blockers on exercise physiology: implications for exercise training. *Med Sci Sports Exerc*. 1991;23:668–676.
63. Vanhees L, Defoor JG, Schepers D, et al. Effect of bisoprolol and atenolol on endurance exercise capacity in healthy men. *J Hypertens*. 2000;18:35–43.
64. Dickstein K, Aarsland T. Comparison of the effects of aqueous and gellan ophthalmic timolol on peak exercise performance in middle-aged men. *Am J Ophthalmol*. 1996;121(4):367–371.
65. Friedenwald JS. The formation of intraocular fluid. *Am J Ophthalmol*. 1949;32:9.
66. Becker B. Chemical composition of human aqueous humor; effects of acetazoleamide. *AMA Arch Ophthalmol*. 1957;57(6):793–800.
67. Maren TH. The relation between enzyme inhibition and physiologic response in the carbonic anhydrase system. *J Pharmacol Exp Ther*. 1963;139:140.
68. Krupin T, Sly WS, Whyte MP, Dodgson SJ. Failure of acetazolamide to decrease intraocular pressure in patients with carbonic anhydrase II deficiency. *Am J Ophthalmol*. 1985;99(4):396–399.
69. Friedland BR, Mallonee J, Anderson DR. Short-term dose response characteristics of acetazolamide in man. *Arch Ophthalmol*. 1977;95(10):1809–1812.
70. Berson FG, Epstein DL, Grant WM, Hutchinson BT, Dobbs PC. Acetazolamide dosage forms in the treatment of glaucoma. *Arch Ophthalmol*. 1980;98(6):1051–1054.
71. Stone RA, Zimmerman TJ, Shin DH, Becker B, Kass MA. Low-dose methazolamide and intraocular pressure. *Am J Ophthalmol*. 1977;83(5):674–679.
72. Ellison DH, Okusa MD, Schrier RW. Mechanisms of diuretic action. In: Schrier RW, ed. *Diseases of the Kidney and Urinary Tract*. 7th ed. Philadelphia, PA: Lippincott, Williams, & Wilkins; 2001:2426–2429.
73. Kass MA, Kolker AE, Gordon M, et al. Acetazolamide and urolithiasis. *Ophthalmology*. 1981;88(3):261–265.

74. Rossert J, Rondeau E, Jondeau G, et al. Tamm-Horsfall protein accumulation in glomeruli during acetazolamide-induced acute renal failure. *Am J Nephrol.* 1989;9(1):56–57.
75. Elinav E, Ackerman Z, Gottehrer NP, Heyman SN. Recurrent life-threatening acidosis induced by acetazolamide in a patient with diabetic type IV renal tubular acidosis. *Ann Emerg Med.* 2002;40(2):259–260.
76. De Marchi S, Cecchin E. Severe metabolic acidosis and disturbances of calcium metabolism induced by acetazolamide in patients on haemodialysis. *Clin Sci (Lond).* 1990;78(3):295–302.
77. *Physician's Desk Reference for Ophthalmology.* 28th ed. Montvale, NJ: Medical Economics Co.; 1999.
78. Takeda K, Nakamoto M, Yasunaga C, et al. Acute hemorrhagic gastritis associated with acetazolamide intoxication in a patient with chronic renal failure. *Clin Nephrol.* 1997;48(4):266–268.
79. Boccardo P, Remuzzi G, Galbusera M. Platelet dysfunction in renal failure. *Semin Thromb Hemost.* 2004;30(5):579-589.
80. Fraunfelder FT, Meyer SM, Bagby GC Jr, Dreis MW. Hematologic reactions to carbonic anhydrase inhibitors. *Am J Ophthalmol.* 1985;100(1):79–81.
81. Schwenk MH, St Peter WL, Meese MG, Singhal PC. Acetazolamide toxicity and pharmacokinetics in patients receiving hemodialysis. *Pharmacotherapy.* 1995;15(4):522–527.
82. Roy LF, Dufresne LR, Legault L, Long H, Morin C. Acetazolamide in hemodialysis patients: a rational use after ocular surgery. *Am J Kidney Dis.* 1992;20(6):650–652.
83. Vaziri ND, Saiki J, Barton CH, Rajudin M, Ness RL. Hemodialyzability of acetazolamide. *South Med J.* 1980;73(4):422–423.
84. Aronheim JC. Special problems in the Geriatric patient. In: Bennet JC, Plum F, eds. *Cecil Textbook of Medicine.* Philadelphia: WB Saunders Co.; 1996:21–22.
85. Maren TH, Conroy CW, Wynns GC, Levy NS. Ocular absorption, blood levels, and excretion of dorzolamide, a topically active carbonic anhydrase inhibitor. *J Ocul Pharmacol Ther.* 1997;13(1):23–30.
86. Robin AL. The role of alpha-agonists in glaucoma therapy. *Curr Opin Ophthalmol.* 1997;8(2):42–49.
87. Robin AL, Coleman AL. Apraclonidine hydrochloride: an evaluation of plasma concentrations, and a comparison of its intraocular pressure lowering and cardiovascular effects to timolol maleate. *Trans Am Ophthalmol Soc.* 1990;88:149–159.
88. Walters G, Taylor RH. Severe systemic toxicity caused by brimonidine drops in an infant with presumed juvenile xanthogranuloma. *Eye.* 1999;13(Pt 6):797–798.
89. Bowman RJ, Cope J, Nischal KK. Ocular and systemic side effects of brimonidine 0.2% eye drops (Alphagan) in children. *Eye.* 2004;18(1):24–26.
90. Wei CP, Anderson JA, Leopold I. Ocular absorption and metabolism of topically applied epinephrine and adipivalyl ester of epinephrine. *Invest Ophthalmol Vis Sci.* 1978;17(4):315–321.
91. Kerr CR, Hass I, Drance SM, Walters MB, Schulzer M. Cardiovascular effects of epinephrine and dipivalyl epinephrine applied topically to the eye in patients with glaucoma. *Br J Ophthalmol.* 1982;66(2):109–114.
92. Kohn AN, Moss AP, Hargett NA, Ritch R, Smith H Jr, Podos SM. Clinical comparison of dipivalyl epinephrine and epinephrine in the treatment of glaucoma. *Am J Ophthalmol.* 1979;87(2):196–201.
93. Blondeau P, Cote M. Cardiovascular effects of epinephrine and dipivefrin in patients using timolol: a single-dose study. *Can J Ophthalmol.* 1984;19(1):29–32.
94. Taylor P. Cholinergic agonists. In: Gilman AG, Goodman LS, Gilman A, eds; Mayer SE, Melmon KL, Assoc. eds. *Goodman and Gilman's Pharmacological Basis of Therapeutics.* New York: Macmillan Publishing Co., Inc.; 1980:90–119.
95. Mayer SE. Neurohumoral transmission and the autonomic nervous system. In: Gilman AG, Goodman LS, Gilman A, eds; Mayer SE, Melmon KL, Assoc. eds. *Goodman and Gilman's Pharmacological Basis of Therapeutics.* 6th ed. New York: Macmillan Publishing Co., Inc.; 1980:56–91.
96. Hendrickson RG, Morocco AP, Greenberg MI. Pilocarpine toxicity and the treatment of xerostomia. *J Emerg Med.* 2004;26(4):429–432.
97. Fryer AD, Okanlami OA. Neuronal M2 muscarinic receptor function in guinea-pig lungs is inhibited by indomethacin. *Am Rev Respir Dis.* 1993;147(3):559–564.
98. Fryer AD, Wills-Karp M. Dysfunction of M2-muscarinic receptors in pulmonary parasympathetic nerves after antigen challenge. *J Appl Physiol.* 1991;71(6):2255–2261.
99. Golkar L, Yarkony KA, Fryer AD. Inhibition of neuronal M(2) muscarinic receptor function in the lungs by extracellular nitric oxide. *Br J Pharmacol.* 2000;131(2):312–318.
100. Kushnick H, Liebmann JM, Ritch R. Systemic pilocarpine toxicity from Ocusert leakage. *Arch Ophthalmol.* 1996;114(11):1432.
101. Wahl JW, Tyner GS. Echothiophate iodide. The effect of 0.0625 per cent solution on blood cholinesterase. *Am J Ophthalmol.* 1965;60(3):419–425.
102. De Roetth A, Jr WA, Dettbarn W, Rosenberg P, Wilensky JG. Blood cholinesterase activity of glaucoma patients treated with phospholine iodide. *Am J Ophthalmol.* 1966;62(5):834–838.
103. Hiscox PE, McCulloch C. Cardiac arrest occurring in a patient on echothiophate iodide therapy. *Am J Ophthalmol.* 1965;60(3):425–427.
104. Manoguerra A, Whitney C, Clark RF, Anderson B, Turchen S. Cholinergic toxicity resulting from ocular instillation of echothiophate iodide eye drops. *J Toxicol Clin Toxicol.* 1995;33(5):463–465.
105. Donati F, Bevan DR. Controlled succinylcholine infusion in a patient receiving echothiophate eyedrops. *Can Anaesth Soc J.* 1981;28(5):488–490.
106. Packman PM, Meyer DA, Verdun RM. Hazards of succinylcholine administration during electrotherapy. *Arch Gen Psychiatry.* 1978;35(9):1137–1141.
107. Cavallaro RJ, Krumperman LW, Kugler F. Effect of echothiophate therapy on the metabolism of succinylcholine in man. *Anesth Analg.* 1968;47(5):570–574.
108. Gesztes T. Prolonged apnoea after suxamethonium injection associated with eye drops containing an anticholinesterase agent. *Br J Anaesth.* 1966;38(5):408–409.
109. Mezer E, Krivoy N, Scharf J, Miller B. Echothiophate iodide induced transient hyper- and hypothyroidism. *J Glaucoma.* 1996;5(3):191–192.
110. Parrish RK, Palmberg P, Sheu WP, XLT Study Group. A comparison of latanoprost, bimatoprost, and travoprost in patients with elevated intraocular pressure: a 12-week, randomized, masked-evaluator multicenter study. *Am J Ophthalmol.* 2003;135(5):688–703.
111. Weinreb RN, Lindsey JD, Marchenko G, Marchenko N, Angert M, Strongin A. Prostaglandin FP agonists alter metalloproteinase gene expression in sclera. *Invest Ophthalmol Vis Sci.* 2004;45(12):4368–4377.
112. Hedner J, Everts B, Moller CS. Latanoprost and respiratory function in asthmatic patients: randomized, double-masked, placebo-controlled crossover evaluation. *Arch Ophthalmol.* 1999;117(10):1305–1309.
113. Hedner J, Svedmyr N, Lunde H, Mandahl A. The lack of respiratory effects of the ocular hypotensive drug latanoprost in patients with moderate-steroid treated asthma. *Surv Ophthalmol.* 1997;41(suppl 2):S111–S115.

# Chapter 60
# Systemic Diseases and Glaucoma

Paul Lama

Although, the level of intraocular pressure (IOP) is presently the most important and only modifiable risk factor in the development and progression of open-angle glaucoma, disease progression in many patients may occur with average IOP while others with ocular hypertension never develop glaucoma. Clearly then, non-pressure-related factors are playing an important role in modifying risk of disease progression. While the Ocular Hypertension Treatment Study (OHTS) served to identify age and central corneal thickness in addition to IOP as important factors in determination of risk to glaucomatous progression, the association between nonocular systemic factors and glaucoma has been controversial. Perplexingly, data from the OHTS in fact, found that having diabetes was "protective" of progression to glaucoma.[1] Confounding the relationship between glaucoma and systemic disease is the fact that prevalence of glaucoma and systemic diseases such as cardiovascular disease and hypertension, diabetes, and thyroid dysfunction also increase with age. What then is the relationship between various systemic disease conditions and open-angle glaucoma risk and are there shared pathogenetic mechanisms involved? The relationship between various systemic disorders and glaucomatous nerve damage is intriguing and has been studied for the last three decades.

## 60.1 Cardiovascular Disease and Tissue Injury

The spectrum of cardiovascular disease is broad and encompasses varied etiologies and pathogenetic mechanisms. The most common causes of cardiovascular disease are hypertension and ischemic heart disease due to atherosclerosis. Cardiac dysfunction may be manifest with left-sided or right-sided pump failure, cardiac diastolic dysfunction, or arrhythmia. Atherosclerosis may affect the coronary arteries, the aorta, and its branches leading to coronary artery, cerebrovascular, renal, and peripheral vascular disease; the final common pathway being tissue ischemia with injury or death.

In a simple anatomic model, the factors that determine blood flow and delivery of nutrients and oxygen to a tissue include the anatomic pattern of the blood vessels, blood pressure, resistance to flow within the blood vessels, and the vessels' dynamic autoregulatory capacity. With respect to the ocular circulation, there is no one standard pattern of the blood supply in all human eyes and significant interindividual variation exists in the pattern of the posterior ciliary artery (PCA) circulation – the main source of blood supply to the optic nerve head. The variations in the pattern of PCA circulation include the variations in the number of PCAs supplying an eye, area of supply to the optic nerve head by each PCA, the location of the watershed zones between the various PCAs in relation to the optic nerve head, and the blood pressure in various PCAs as well as short PCAs.[2] These variations in the anatomic pattern may likewise result in variable risk of ischemia. In addition to blood pressure and vascular resistance, vascular autoregulatory capacity is critical in maintaining adequate delivery of oxygen and nutrients as metabolic demand increases or when pathologic disease states threaten to reduce blood flow, such as loss of the pressure head (heart failure), development of arterial stenosis, or alteration of the rheologic properties of blood. Autoregulation involves a change in downstream resistance at the level of the arterioles and is under neurogenic control by the autonomic nervous system as well as local and systemic hormonal and metabolic factors. For example, for a given blood pressure differential, if there is stenosis in a coronary artery that leads to 60% narrowing of that artery, resistance to flow will expectedly increase, resulting in lower blood flow and ischemia unless the arterioles distal to the stenosis dilate to maintain the overall resistance to flow to the myocardium constant. This can be thought about schematically as a pair of resistors in series. Once the degree of stenosis surpasses a critical level, however, the capacity for autoregulation distal to the stenosis will be surpassed with no further compensation resulting in a drop in blood flow and corresponding ischemia, unless collateral blood vessels develop circumventing the stenotic artery. In the eye, intraocular pressure is an important component of the blood flow equation as it raises venous pressure and correspondingly lowers perfusion pressure to the optic nerve and retinal circulation – a factor unique to the ocular circulation as compared to perfusion of other tissues.

The relationship between "cardiovascular disease" as a risk factor in the development of the glaucomatous optic neuropathy has not been firmly established. Studies that have investigated cardiovascular disease and glaucoma have largely been epidemiologic prevalence-based studies that sought to determine the relationship between a history of cardiac disease or hypertension and glaucoma.[3-9] Potential low blood flow states as potential risk factors were also investigated.[5,6,8,9] Unfortunately, a causal link is extremely difficult to establish on prevalence data alone when there are multiple confounders and covariates that may be difficult to control for. If cardiovascular disease is indeed important in the development of glaucomatous optic nerve damage, then by what mechanism does injury occur to the optic nerve? Is it inadequate blood flow due to low perfusion pressure, small vessel pathology, atherosclerosis, vasospasm, and autonomic dysregulation or are there shared pathogenetic mechanisms linking glaucoma and cardiovascular disease?

### 60.1.1 Hypertension and Cardiovascular Risk

Hypertension is the most prevalent cardiovascular condition in the United States. It is estimated that more than 50 million Americans and 60% of persons older than age 65 have arterial hypertension.[10] The definition of hypertension, which has been traditionally classified as blood pressure ≥140/90 mmHg, has evolved over the last decade. The Sixth Report of the Joint National Committee on Detection, Prevention, Evaluation, and Treatment of High Blood Pressure (JNC-VI) has modified the "normal" category by stratifying this group into "optimal," "normal," and "high normal"[11] (Table 60.1). The JNC-VII report has further defined high-normal as prehypertension and recommended lifestyle adjustments and blood pressure-lowering intensity adjusted to the level of absolute cardiovascular risk.[12]

The JNC-VII report also determined that the risk of cardiovascular complications secondary to arterial hypertension escalates in a graded, continuous, and predictable manner with no threshold value. The cardiovascular event risk doubles with each increment of 20/10 mmHg, beginning at a pressure of 115/75 mmHg. It also deemphasized diastolic blood pressure and found that systolic blood pressure and pulse pressure is more important, particularly in those over 50 years of age. The reclassification of "normal" blood pressure values by the JNC-VI and VII reports, and the emphasis for tighter blood pressure control with the virtual elimination of a threshold blood pressure value distinguishing hypertensive from normotensive, represents a distillation of emerging data pooled from various clinical as well as epidemiologic studies. Vasan et al showed that high-normal blood pressure was associated with a risk-factor-adjusted hazard ratio of 2.5 as compared to optimal blood pressure.[13] In the Framingham Offspring Study, patients with high-normal blood pressure had a two- to threefold increased risk of developing a coronary event as compared to those with optimal blood pressure.[14]

At diagnosis, identifying the stage of hypertension with assessment for target organ damage is now the standard. As stated previously, emphasis for more intensive treatment of hypertension is in those patients who are at higher risk since they are the group with greater expected benefit, specifically those with manifest target organ damage.[11] Data from multiple studies including the Hypertension Optimal Treatment Study (HOTS) and the United Kingdom Prospective Diabetes Study (UKPDS) recommend lower target pressures in diabetics since diabetes is considered a coronary risk equivalent.[15-17] Even tighter control is recommended (target blood pressure <125/75) for diabetics with elevated creatinine, microalbuminuria, or overt proteinuria, especially those with a greater than 1 g/day of proteinuria.[18-20]

Analogous to some extent with intraocular pressure, blood pressure also follows a circadian rhythm and can be described and categorized by four distinct patterns (Table 60.2). The normal pattern is defined by a nocturnal dip in mean systolic and diastolic blood pressure by great than 10% but less than 20%. Multiple studies have shown that nondippers and reverse dippers (i.e., those with sustained blood pressure elevations) are at significantly increased risk of ischemic and hemorrhagic stroke.[20-29] In Japan, the Ohasama epidemiologic study reported the prognostic significance of blood

**Table 60.1** Classification of blood pressure based on the Sixth Report of the Joint National Committee on prevention, detection, evaluation, and treatment of high blood pressure.[11]

| Category | Systolic BP (mmHg) | Diastolic BP (mmHg) |
|---|---|---|
| Hypertension | | |
| Stage 1 | 140–159 | or 90–99 |
| Stage II | 160–179 | or 100–109 |
| Stage III | ≥180 | or ≥110 |
| Prehypertension | 130–139 | or 85–89 |
| Normal | <130 | and <85 |
| Optimal | <120 | and <80 |

**Table 60.2** Nocturnal blood pressure variability patterns

| Category | Mean decrease in systolic and diastolic BP[a] |
|---|---|
| Normal | >10% but <20% |
| Nondipper | <10% |
| Reverse dipper | Nocturnal BP > diurnal BP |
| Over dipper | >20% |

[a]Reflects change from mean diurnal blood pressure.

pressure variability in a population cohort followed for 20 years.[27] Using ambulatory and home blood pressure monitoring data, the investigators found that flattening of the blood pressure profile (i.e., loss of the normal nocturnal dip) as well as wide blood pressure variability characterized by morning blood pressure surges and nocturnal hypotension are both associated with cerebral hemorrhagic strokes. Patients with the lowest risk for stroke are those with a normal nocturnal dip. Hence stroke risk, with respect to the circadian blood pressure pattern, follows a J-shaped curve.[23,27] These and other similar studies have contributed to the emerging paradigm in the pharmacologic treatment of arterial hypertension in which the goal is not only achievement of lower target pressures according to level of cardiovascular risk, but also the attainment of the normal circadian blood pressure profile whereby the normal nocturnal dip is restored. Indeed, some physicians have utilized data obtained from results of ambulatory blood pressure monitoring to plan tailored dosing and administration of antihypertensive agents.[30,31] This newer concept of targeted blood pressure control derived from modeling of the patient's circadian blood pressure profile and then using specific antihypertensive agents based on differences in kinetics and the benefits and side effects of each agent to achieve 24-h blood pressure control is called chronotherapy (see Sidebar 60.1). At the moment, this mode of treatment is predominantly conducted in a research setting and not yet the standard of care. Further clinical studies will help determine the feasibility of adopting this method in general practice and its impact on stroke and heart attack prevention. There is an ongoing clinical trial, currently in its fourth year, designed to investigate chronotherapy and its potential impact on cardiovascular, cerebrovascular, and renal risk.[32] Data from this trial are not yet available.

### Sidebar 60.1 Antihypertensive medications and glaucoma

Kevin C. Leonard and Cindy M. L. Hutnik

There are a variety of well-established risk factors for primary open-angle glaucoma (POAG) including age, race, positive family history, myopia, and, most importantly, ocular hypertension. However, a significant subgroup of patients with glaucoma lack any of these known risk factors. Other potential risk factors have been proposed and investigated. Most of these are vascular risk factors, and include both systemic hypertension and hypotension, low diastolic perfusion pressure, as well as altered ocular blood flow[1]. A risk factor that has garnered notable attention is the effect that treatment of systemic hypertension may have on the incidence or progression of open-angle glaucoma. The potential impact of a demonstrated effect of antihypertensive treatment in glaucoma would be great, given the number of patients with glaucoma who are also being treated for systemic hypertension.

### Rationale

Several concepts relevant to understanding the potential effect of systemic antihypertensives on glaucoma are important. Diastolic ocular perfusion pressure (DOPP) is the diastolic blood pressure (DBP) minus the intraocular pressure (IOP). It can be regarded as the "driving force" to move blood into the eye. The Baltimore eye survey[2] revealed an increased prevalence of POAG in the presence of systemic hypotension and low DOPP. Several major longitudinal studies have confirmed DOPP as a risk factor[2-4]. Decreasing IOP will improve DOPP while decreasing DBP will worsen DOPP. Medications that manipulate either BP or IOP can have an effect on the perfusion pressure. This provides a rationale for the possibility that systemic antihypertensive treatments may be linked to the progression of glaucoma due to the effect on DOPP.

There is considerable evidence that nocturnal hypotension may be important in the pathogenesis of glaucoma. Many studies have shown that it is associated with increased incidence of glaucoma, increased severity of disease at diagnosis, and increased progression of the disease[1,5]. Increased progression of visual field loss has been reported in patients with nocturnal hypotension linked to the use of systemic antihypertensives[6]. Angiotensin-converting enzyme (ACE) inhibitors and calcium channel blockers (CBB) exaggerate the normal nocturnal hypotensive episodes, while the same has not been found for β-blockers and angiotensin receptor blockers. The effect of diuretics on the exaggerated nocturnal hypotensive dip is variable.

The concept of vascular dysregulation has also been associated with the pathogenesis of glaucoma. This concept can be defined as an imbalance between the blood supply to a tissue and its metabolic demands, resulting in either overperfusion or underperfusion. An imbalance between vasodilator and vasoconstrictor substances may result in vascular dysregulation. This phenomenon has been identified in subgroups of glaucoma patients, resulting in unstable ocular blood flow. The end result is a perfusion/reperfusion injury and oxidative stress[7,8].

## Evidence

Several studies have examined systemic antihypertensive use as a risk factor for the development or progression of glaucoma. The Thessaloniki Eye Study, which was a population-based cross-sectional study, measured the effect of BP status on optic disk structure in 232 patients without glaucoma using Heidelberg Retina Tomograph (HRT). This study revealed that diastolic BP <90 mmHg, specifically resulting from antihypertensive treatment in nonglaucomatous patients, was associated with increased cupping and decreased rim area of the optic disk[10]. Similarly, a positive association between low DOPP (<50 mmHg) and high-tension glaucoma (OR 4.68) was identified only for patients receiving systemic antihypertensive treatment in the Rotterdam Study[11]. Interestingly, an inverse association was noted for normal tension glaucoma (OR 0.25). Another study used confocal scanning laser ophthalmoscopy to evaluate the effect of systemic antihypertensive treatment on progression of optic nerve parameters in glaucoma suspects. In comparison to age-matched normotensive controls, statistically significant increases were identified in cup area and cup-to-disk area ratio, while rim area, rim-to-disk area ratio, and global Retinal Nerve Fiber Layer (RNFL) thickness were all decreased[12].

Population data have provided some conflicting results. Data from the Barbados Eye Study Group suggested that hypertensive patients on treatment had a decreased risk of developing glaucoma over a 4-year span as compared to normotensive controls (RR 0.49). Hypertensive patients using antihypertensive medications were shown to have a decreased risk in comparison to nonusers (RR 0.74), although this was not a statistically significant effect[13]. Several authors have suggested that these contradictory results are likely attributable to different study designs and study populations.

Langman et al.[9] have presented data suggesting that systemic hypertension was significantly more common in patients with glaucoma based on a case–control study with a very large sample size. Oral β-blockers were shown to have a statistically significant protective effect (OR 0.77), while oral calcium channel blockers and angiotensin-converting enzyme (ACE) inhibitors were associated with a significant increase in the risk of developing glaucoma (OR 1.34 and 1.16). Diuretics were not identified to have any significant effect either way in this study. The Rotterdam Study was a prospective population-based cohort study that revealed the effect of antihypertensive medications on the incidence of open-angle glaucoma over a 6.5-year period. Patients using calcium channel antagonists were found to have a statistically significant 1.8-fold higher risk. β-Blocker treatment was associated with a nonsignificant risk reduction (OR 0.60), while other types of antihypertensive agents were not significantly associated with the incidence of open-angle glaucoma[14]. This apparent risk associated with the use of calcium channel blockers contradicts the results of several other studies, including the initial reports of the Rotterdam study. The initial Rotterdam study demonstrated a lower IOP and protective effect on OAG in patients using systemic β-blockers, while ACE inhibitors and calcium channel blockers showed no effect on IOP.[15] Results from the European Glaucoma Prevention Study (EGPS) provided some additional insight into the effects of the various antihypertensive agents. The EGPS was a randomized, double-masked controlled clinical trial designed to assess treatment with dorzolamide versus placebo. Intercurrent factors that were associated with the development of open-angle glaucoma were examined. This study was the first to suggest systemic diuretics as a risk factor (HR 2.41) for the development of glaucoma[4].

## Clinical Recommendations

Based on the studies done to date it appears that systemic antihypertensive therapy may have an effect on the progression of optic nerve damage in glaucoma. A possible mechanism may be the reduction in DBP associated with antihypertensive therapy with exaggerations in the nocturnal dipping of DOPP. Vascular dysregulation may be an essential element linking systemic antihypertensive use and hypotension to the pathophysiology of glaucoma.

The available evidence suggests that β-blockers are the most well-tolerated systemic antihypertensive agents from a glaucoma standpoint and may even have a protective effect. Other agents, including diuretics, ACE inhibitors, and calcium channel antagonists have been associated with an increased risk of glaucoma.

Collectively, this evidence brings the importance of systemic blood pressure into the realm of the ophthalmologist. Patients demonstrating glaucomatous progression at low intraocular pressures may benefit from 24-h ambulatory blood pressure monitoring. Collaboration may be required between the ophthalmologist and internist to select the ideal antihypertensive medication and dosing regimen. Long-lasting medications may be preferred. If short-acting medications are required, evening doses may need to be eliminated. However, it should be cautioned that although the evidence is growing, it may still be insufficient to make solid recommendations regarding appropriate blood pressure management for patients with glaucoma. At present, the recommendation may be to obtain a relatively stable blood pressure over 24 h with increased attention to hypotensive episodes, especially at night. The ophthalmologist must work closely with other care providers to balance the potential progression of glaucoma with other risk factors for systemic disease requiring control of hypertension.

## Bibliography

1. Deokule S, Weinreb RN. Relationships among systemic blood pressure, intraocular pressure, and open-angle glaucoma. *Can J Ophthalmol*. 2008;43(3):302–307.
2. Tielsch JM, Katz J, Sommer A, Quigley HA, Javitt JC. Hypertension, perfusion pressure, and primary open-angle glaucoma. A population-based assessment. *Arch Ophthalmol*. 1995;113(2):216–221.
3. Leske MC, Heijl A, Hyman L, Bengtsson B, Dong L, Yang Z. Predictors of long-term progression in the early manifest glaucoma trial. *Ophthalmology*. 2007;114(11):1965–1972.
4. Miglior S, Torri V, Zeyen T, Pfeiffer N, Vaz JC, Adamsons I. Intercurrent factors associated with the development of open-angle glaucoma in the European glaucoma prevention study. *Am J Ophthalmol*. 2007;144(2):266–275.
5. Pache M, Flammer J. A sick eye in a sick body? Systemic findings in patients with primary open-angle glaucoma. *Surv Ophthalmol*. 2006;51(3):179–212.
6. Hayreh SS, Zimmerman MB, Podhajsky P, Alward WL. Nocturnal arterial hypotension and its role in optic nerve head and ocular ischemic disorders. *Am J Ophthalmol*. 1994;117(5):603–624.
7. Nicolela MT. Clinical clues of vascular dysregulation and its association with glaucoma. *Can J Ophthalmol*. 2008;43(3):337–341.
8. Flammer J, Mozaffarieh M. Autoregulation, a balancing act between supply and demand. *Can J Ophthalmol*. 2008;43(3):317–321.
9. Langman MJ, Lancashire RJ, Cheng KK, Stewart PM. Systemic hypertension and glaucoma: mechanisms in common and co-occurrence. *Br J Ophthalmol*. 2005;89(8):960–963.
10. Topouzis F, Coleman AL, Harris A, et al. Association of blood pressure status with the optic disk structure in non-glaucoma subjects: the Thessaloniki eye study. *Am J Ophthalmol*. 2006;142(1):60–67.
11. Hulsman CA, Vingerling JR, Hofman A, Witteman JC, de Jong PT. Blood pressure, arterial stiffness, and open-angle glaucoma: the Rotterdam study. *Arch Ophthalmol*. 2007;125(6):805–812.
12. Punjabi OS, Stamper RL, Bostrom AG, Lin SC. Does treated systemic hypertension affect progression of optic nerve damage in glaucoma suspects? *Curr Eye Res*. 2007;32(2):153–160.
13. Leske MC, Wu SY, Nemesure B, Hennis A. Incident open-angle glaucoma and blood pressure. *Arch Ophthalmol*. 2002;120(7):954–959.
14. Muskens RP, de Voogd S, Wolfs RC, et al. Systemic antihypertensive medication and incident open-angle glaucoma. *Ophthalmology*. 2007;114(12):2221–2226.
15. Dielemans I, Vingerling JR, Algra D, Hofman A, Grobbee DE, de Jong PT. Primary open-angle glaucoma, intraocular pressure, and systemic blood pressure in the general elderly population. The Rotterdam Study. *Ophthalmology*. 1995;102(1):54–60.

## 60.2 Vascular Factors and Glaucoma

### 60.2.1 Hypertension, Blood Flow, and Glaucoma Risk

The current evidence in the medical literature has firmly established that hypertension is an important risk factor in the development of stroke, heart disease, and renal failure, with increasing risk of developing target organ injury or death and disability with higher blood pressures. In contrast, cross-sectional data from population-based studies linking hypertension and glaucoma have been mixed.[3–9] To complicate matters, recently published data from the Early Manifest Glaucoma Treatment Study (EMGTS) and the Barbados Eye Study have shown an inverse relationship with respect to blood pressure and risk of glaucoma progression, results that are paradoxical as compared to data from the medical literature.[33,34] Analyzing the data from the EMGTS, Leske et al identified lower ocular systolic perfusion pressure (defined as systolic blood pressure minus IOP ≤125 mmHg) in all patients (HR 1.42) and lower systolic blood pressure (SBP ≤ 160 mmHg) in patients with lower baseline IOP as new baseline predictors of glaucoma progression in their study cohort.[33] Conversely, the risk of progression was halved (HR 0.46) in patients with SBP>160 mmHg. In stark contrast, the Systolic Hypertension in the Elderly Program (SHEP), the Systolic Hypertension in Europe (Syst-Eur) Trial, and the Systolic Hypertension in China (Syst-China) study have all shown that those with isolated SBP of greater than 160 mmHg have a significantly increased cardiovascular event rate and benefit from antihypertensive therapy.[35–37] Pooled estimates from the three trials demonstrated that active treatment, compared with placebo, reduced all-cause mortality by 17%, cardiovascular mortality by 25%, all cardiovascular end-points by 32%, total stroke by 37%, and myocardial infarction including sudden death by 25%.[38] Furthermore, patients with optimal blood pressure (<120/80 mmHg) have a two- to threefold lower cardiovascular event risk rate as compared to those with high-normal blood pressure.[13,14] In other words, in terms of blood pressure as a vascular risk factor, it appears that high blood pressure may be "neuroprotective" from the glaucoma perspective but detrimental to the heart, brain, and kidney, and vice versa thus creating an untenable therapeutic dilemma. In fact, Leske et al suggested maintaining elevated blood pressures in hypertensive patients (Barbados Eye Study)[34] while clinicians who treat arterial hypertension and follow the prevailing guidelines will ideally aim for lower target blood pressures based on cardiovascular risk with restoration of a normal 10–20% nocturnal dip in mean blood pressure. This contradictory or paradoxical relationship between glaucoma and hypertension needs further clarification. There are two distinctly separate but interrelated pathophysiologic mechanisms at hand that when treated separately may help resolve this apparent paradox: the relationship between hypertension and glaucoma and low perfusion and glaucoma. At the moment, it appears from the available evidence, mostly from prevalence-based epidemiological studies, that high blood pressure, at the very least, does not appear to increase the risk of future development of glaucoma. The logic in this observation is that high blood pressure is necessary to maintain perfusion to the optic nerve particularly in those with elevated IOP, which counteracts the driving force for perfusion. One must be careful, however, not to reflexively assume that a higher systolic pressure translates to greater perfusion to the optic nerve or any other tissue, especially in patients with known cardiovascular disease. Blood flow depends not only upon perfusion pressure but also vascular resistance. Patients with hypertension, particularly those who have higher blood pressures, often have correspondingly elevated catecholamine levels contributing to increased peripheral vascular resistance. Furthermore, intimal damage from chronic hypertension further compromises vascular integrity as well as resistance, thereby increasing the risk of hemorrhage or ischemic injury. What then might cause failure of finding an association between hypertension and glaucoma? In some of the glaucoma epidemiologic studies a diagnosis of hypertension was considered to be present based on verbal history or on isolated blood pressure measurements in the clinical trial.[3-9] The white coat syndrome is a well-described cause of misclassification of normotensive individuals as hypertensives. Pickering reported that as many as 20% of normotensives may be misclassified as hypertensives.[39] Such misclassification can certainly confound the data and underestimate the relationship. Also, since the incidence of glaucoma is low, it is possible that if only a subset of patients with more severe or labile hypertension are at higher risk of developing glaucoma the association will be missed. Long-term incidence studies may identify an association that prevalence studies have failed to do. In contrast to high blood pressure, low blood pressure or low ocular perfusion pressure has been identified as a potential vascular risk factor in glaucoma.[5,6,8,9,33,34,40–44] In the Barbados Eye Study, low systolic, diastolic, and mean ocular perfusion pressures have been associated with an increased relative risk of developing glaucoma.[34] These data complement other evidence in the ophthalmic literature to show that nocturnal hypotension is associated with progressive injury in both normal tension and open-angle glaucoma. Moreover, low perfusion is consistent with increased brain ischemia and stroke as well as myocardial injury in hypertensive patients with an overdipping circadian rhythm. As shown in the Ohasama study, wide variability in blood pressure with nocturnal overdipping is also associated with an increased risk of cerebral hemorrhage.[27] Thus, it is likewise reasonable to presume that independent of IOP, similar episodes of extreme nocturnal blood pressure dipping due to unstable hypertension or autonomic dysfunction can lead to ocular hypoperfusion and visual field progression in glaucoma patients. Graham, Follman, Collignon, Kaiser, and Meyer all reported increased nocturnal dips or overdipping in both primary open-angle glaucoma (POAG) and normal tension glaucoma (NTG) patients with disease progression.[40–42,45,46] Bechetoille found lower blood pressures but the number of nocturnal low readings was no different in patients with focal ischemic NTG than in POAG patients.[47] Complementary to data from the medical literature, Collignon, Kashiwagi, and Detry found that disease progression may also be associated with absent or insufficient nocturnal dip.[45,48,49]

Thus, labile hypertension with episodes of hypotension or overaggressive treatment of hypertension may create a low flow state especially in those with elevated IOP, thereby contributing to glaucomatous optic nerve damage. Also, dysregulation of the normal circadian blood pressure rhythm with absent or reverse nocturnal dip may also contribute to optic nerve injury. Further prospective studies investigating circadian blood pressure variability and risk to the optic nerve in glaucoma patients is warranted. At this time, it appears from both the ophthalmic and medical literature, that episodes of exaggerated nonphysiologic nocturnal hypotension are likely detrimental and should be avoided as they appear to increase the risk of progressive optic nerve damage as well as stroke and cardiac ischemia. Thus, until further data are available, low perfusion states but not physiologic nocturnal dipping are bad and the connection between hypertensive patients and glaucoma progression risk, at the moment, may be related to an overdipper circadian pattern in some patients caused by intrinsic autonomic instability or overaggressive antihypertensive treatment. Aggressive control of intraocular pressure, as well as coordination of targeted blood pressure therapy with the patient's primary care physician or internist, to avoid nonphysiologic nocturnal hypotension would be appropriate management in these patients. Overly simplistic measures such as advising a high-salt diet or high-salt beverages and foods before bedtime in the absence of blood pressure data from ambulatory blood pressure monitoring, knowledge of the patient's antihypertensive regimen, and appropriate supervision and input from the patient's internist may in fact be detrimental.

## 60.3 Hypothyroidism and Glaucoma

Hypothyroidism is a common condition that increases in prevalence with age but is overwhelmingly more common in females than males. The prevalence of hypothyroidism depends upon the geographic area as it relates to iodine availability. In areas of adequate iodine supply the prevalence is 0.8–1.0%. The diagnosis is often elusive due to the nonspecific nature of the symptoms such as fatigue, weight gain, constipation, depressed mood, and cold intolerance. Biochemically, cellular metabolism is considerably slowed and there is increased tissue deposition of mucopolysaccharides. In advanced cases, myxedema develops, which imparts swelling and a change in skin texture to a doughy consistency that is nonpitting.[50] The relationship between hypothyroidism and glaucoma was first suggested by Hertel nearly 90 years ago.[51] Mucopolysaccharide deposition in the trabecular meshwork is thought to belie the mechanism of outflow obstruction. Indeed there have been multiple studies that have shown reduced tonographic outflow facility or elevated IOP in patients with hypothyroidism.[52–55] Smith et al demonstrated in a series of 25 consecutive patients with hypothyroidism that treatment with thyroid hormone improved tonographic outflow facility, reduced IOP, and hence reduced the pressure/outflow facility ratio.[54] They also describe an anecdotal case report of a patient with hypothyroidism and glaucoma with refractory IOP elevation that improved only following treatment of hypothyroidism and which also resulted in reduction of the medical regimen to treat IOP.[56] As opposed to trabecular meshwork dysfunction, vasculopathy causing altered ocular blood flow and weakening of the lamina cribrosa are also theoretical mechanisms by which hypothyroidism can contribute to the development of glaucomatous optic neuropathy in patients in the absence of elevated IOP.

Although, mucopolysaccharide deposition causing trabecular dysfunction and elevated IOP is certainly biologically plausible, review of the literature reveals mixed data regarding the clinical relationship of glaucoma and hypothyroidism.[55–65] Most of the published data essentially arises from case–control epidemiologic studies, consecutive case series, or a case report, which often demonstrate flaws in design and introduce bias. Unfortunately, as expected, the low annual incidence of glaucoma in the general population precludes the availability of prospective incidence data and thus, scientific assessment of the relationship can only be practically made through case–control studies. Most of these studies, whether case–control or consecutive case series, however, identified fewer than 100 cases of hypothyroidism or glaucoma.[55,57–62] There are only three published trials with greater than 100 patients and only two available in print.[63–65] The Blue Mountain Eye Study showed that of 147 patients on thyroxine replacement therapy, 6.8% had glaucoma as compared to 2.8% of age-matched controls.[63] The largest of the case–control epidemiologic studies in print was a nested case–control study conducted in men at a US Veterans Administration (VA) medical center by Girkin et al[64] In this study 590 newly diagnosed patients with glaucoma matched with 5,897 nonglaucoma controls were found to be more likely to have a prior diagnosis of hypothyroidism as compared to the control group: 6.4% versus 4.0%. The diagnosis of glaucoma was made between 1997 and 2001 and was based on identifying glaucoma cases from recorded ICD-9 diagnoses. Similarly hypothyroidism was based on ICD-9 diagnosis and or concurrent thyroxine use as determined by prescriptions filled. Although the study findings were intriguing and support the potential relationship between hypothyroidism and glaucoma, there are significant weaknesses in the study design. The study was done only in men and cannot be extrapolated to women who are significantly more likely to be diagnosed with hypothyroidism. The diagnosis was made by identifying an ICD-9 diagnosis recorded between a specified time interval; and perhaps with a longer follow-up interval, the incidence of glaucoma between the hypothyroid group and nonhypothyroid group may even out. There are many patients with significantly high TSH (biochemical hypothyroidism) but are clinically asymptomatic and not under treatment with thyroxine replacement, thus potentially underestimating the pool of patients that are hypothyroid and who may not have been coded as hypothyroid. Moreover, only a diagnosis of glaucoma made after the start of the observation period was considered. Since glaucoma does not start abruptly it is possible that a "delayed" diagnosis of glaucoma resulted in a left bias as the authors conceded, thus questioning the veracity of the timing of the development of hypothyroidism preceding the diagnosis of glaucoma. The most recent and by far the largest epidemiologic study (EPUB publication), in contrast, failed to show an association between a prior diagnosis of hypothyroidism and development of glaucoma.[65] In that study Motsko and Jones, using a similar case–control study design as Girkin et al, identified 4,728 newly diagnosed patients and matched them with 14,184 controls. Prior hypothyroidism in open-angle glaucoma patients was found in 17.2% versus 17.6% in controls, which is significantly higher in both cases and controls as compared to the VA study by Girkin. This finding is as might be expected due to the inclusion of women in the study by Motsko and Jones. Although both studies shared similar weaknesses, the strengths of the Motsko and Jones study as compared to the Girkin et al study was the larger number of cases of glaucoma and the demographically more diverse study group in the former; hence a better representation of the population.

At this juncture, a causal or permissive relationship between hypothyroidism and glaucoma is intriguing but the available data have failed to prove this relationship. Even though elevated IOP has been demonstrated in patients with hypothyroidism, Bahcesi et al have recently shown that there is a reversible decrease in central corneal thickness that may completely account for the observed improvement in IOP before and after hormone replacement therapy.[54,55] Additional investigation, preferably prospective in nature, is therefore warranted to determine whether hypothyroidism potentially increases the risk of development of open-angle glaucoma.

## 60.4 Diabetes and Glaucoma

Diabetes affects 6–8% of the population and 95% of all diabetics have type 2 diabetes.[66] Beginning with the Framingham Heart Study, the relationship between diabetes and the development of cardiovascular, cerebrovascular, and peripheral vascular disease has been firmly corroborated by numerous studies that followed.[67,68] Most diabetics will die a cardiac death and the risk of an acute coronary event in a diabetic is high enough that the National Cholesterol Education Program – Adult Treatment Panel III (NCEP-ATPIII) guidelines on the treatment of hyperlipidemia recommend aggressive lowering of LDL cholesterol to the same target levels as in patients with manifest coronary artery disease.[15,69,70] The American Diabetes Association and the American Heart Association likewise categorize diabetes as a coronary artery disease risk equivalent.[69,70] Furthermore, the metabolic syndrome, which includes insulin resistance as a feature, confers a significantly increased risk of developing a coronary event.[69,70] Target organ damage due to diabetes is related to development of micro and macrovascular disease with accelerated atherosclerosis.

While diabetes is an established risk factor for vascular disease and end-stage renal failure, and low blood flow has been implicated as a potential risk factor in the pathophysiology of glaucoma, the relationship between diabetes and glaucoma has been subject to much debate and controversy. In the streptozotocin-induced diabetic mouse and rat model there are experimental data that show retinal ganglion cell loss as well as abnormal morphology and increased numbers of dendritic terminals in the surviving retinal ganglion cells after 3 months.[71,72] In addition, retrograde axoplasmic flow has also been shown to be reduced in large and medium-type retinal ganglion cells.[73] Clinically, Soares et al, in a prospective cohort study of 137 patients with primary open-angle glaucoma, found that diabetes is significantly associated with development of optic disk hemorrhages, with a hazard ratio of 4.4 as compared to nondiabetics.[74] Elisaf et al studied metabolic abnormalities amongst patients with known primary open-angle glaucoma and showed that elevated glucose as well as uric acid levels were significantly higher as compared to a matched control group.[75] Similarly, Oh et al found that insulin resistance in patients with the metabolic syndrome was associated with elevated IOP, and that mean IOP increased linearly with the presence of increasing numbers of components for the metabolic syndrome.[76] These and other experimental and clinical studies have provided evidence for diabetes as a causative or permissive factor in the development of glaucoma. Unfortunately, much of the controversy regarding the relationship between diabetes and glaucoma stems from the inconsistent results obtained from larger clinical and population-based epidemiologic studies.[1,77–89] The OHTS initially showed that having diabetes, in fact, was surprisingly protective of the development of glaucoma.[1] In this study, however, the diagnosis of diabetes was identified by self-reporting without validation by record review, blood tests, or treatment history. The protocol also specifically excluded those with diabetic retinopathy since diabetic retinopathy could influence results of visual field testing and confound the specificity of visual field changes. Unfortunately, such exclusion creates an obvious selection bias in favor of diabetics with less severe disease, and hence a prognostically different subgroup. Gordon et al, recognizing the methodological shortcomings of the study, reran the data using more detailed information regarding the diagnosis of diabetes as well as the details of their treatment.[77] During this follow-up study, 409 patients responded positively to the same question originally posed as compared to 191 in the original publication, but were now divided into three sensitivity/specificity subgroups based on what type of treatment was recommended. Using the same Cox proportional hazards prediction model, this follow-up study determined that a history of diabetes mellitus was not statistically significantly predictive for the development of POAG and failed to support the original conclusion that diabetes was protective of glaucoma in patients with ocular hypertension. A smaller cohort of ocular hypertensives from the Diagnostic Innovations in Glaucoma Study yielded similar hazard ratios as in the OHTS analysis for all reported risk factors for progression, except that diabetics who progressed to glaucoma had an increased hazard ratio as compared to those that did not progress.[90] In the European Glaucoma Prevention Study (EGPS) only 4.7% of 1,077 randomized participants with ocular hypertension reported diabetes, a number too small to determine prospectively the effect of diabetes on progression to glaucoma.[91,92]

The majority of the published data regarding the relationship between diabetes and glaucoma are derived from population-based cross-sectional studies, case–control studies, and cohort studies with fewer prospective population-based incidence studies such as the Barbados Eye Study.[78,80–89] In aggregate, there was considerable heterogeneity with respect to race and ethnicities, though the individual studies came from predominantly homogeneous population groups. Vijaya et al did not find diabetes to be associated with glaucoma in a South Indian population in Chennai.[80] Neither de Voogd in a prospective cohort study in Rotterdam nor Ellis in the DARTS/MEMO (Diabetes Audit and Research in Tayside Study/Medicines Monitoring Unit) in Scotland found an association between diabetes and glaucoma.[81,82] The latter study population was comprised of 6,631 diabetics and 166,144 nondiabetic participants.[82] The Baltimore Eye Survey, a predominantly African-American population, failed to show that diabetes was associated in the development of glaucoma.[78,79] In an 11 county area of southern Wisconsin, a predominantly Caucasian population with diabetes was compared to a smaller group of nondiabetics and were found to have a tendency toward a greater mean intraocular pressure than nondiabetics and higher rates of a positive history of glaucoma than in diabetic participants.[83] In a 10-year follow-up prospective study of the same cohort of diabetic participants, multivariate analysis of risk factors associated with increased self-reporting of glaucoma identified age in younger patients, age, baseline intraocular pressure, and insulin use in older diabetics as statistically significant risk factors.[84] The Los Angeles Latino Eye Study (LALES), a population-based cross-sectional study, recently showed that in Latinos over 40 years of age who were never on any glaucoma hypotensive therapy, diabetes was one of several systemic factors independently and positively correlated with elevated IOP on clinical examination. Furthermore, those with type 2 diabetes mellitus, defined as having diabetes after the age of 30, the prevalence of glaucoma was 40% higher than those without type 2 diabetes.[85,86] The patient was determined to be diabetic in the LALES if the participant had a history of being treated for diabetes, the glycosylated hemoglobin was measured at 7.0% or higher, or a random blood glucose was 200 mg or higher. The Barbados Eye Study, a prospective population-based incidence study, described the temporal changes in intraocular pressure over a 9-year time period in a population of participants of African descent and identified a history of diabetes in a multivariate analysis as one of several systemic risk factors correlated with increasing intraocular pressure.[87] These data were consistent with a previously published report in the same study population that also identified diabetes as a significant risk factor in longitudinal increases in intraocular pressure after a 4-year follow-up.[88] In another recent prospective analysis of a cohort of women over 40 years of age from the Nurses' Health Study observed between 1980 and 2000, Pasquale et al found that type 2 diabetes mellitus was positively associated with development of primary open-angle glaucoma as confirmed by record review with a relative rate ratio of 1.82.[89] In this study, a diagnosis of diabetes was validated on a supplemental questionnaire. Confounders such as age, race, hypertension, body mass index, family history, alcohol intake, smoking, and physical activity were controlled for including the potential for detection bias based on the number of eye exams (see Sidebar 60.2). The latter is a factor commonly held by many as the reason for finding a positive association between diabetes and glaucoma or ocular hypertension.

The data are conflicting and the only meta-analysis published to date regarding the association between diabetes and glaucoma, prior to the availability of the results of the LALES and the Nurses' Health Study, failed to identify diabetes as a potential risk factor.[93] Furthermore, interestingly, one study showed that changes in the biomechanical properties of the cornea due to increased glycosylated hemoglobin may artificially influence intraocular pressure measurements leading to a false-positive association between diabetes and elevated intraocular pressure.[94] Krueger and Ramos-Esteban proposed that corneal stiffening due to glucose-mediated collagen cross-linking may account for higher intraocular pressure readings in diabetics. Notwithstanding, more recent prospective well-designed studies such as the Barbados Eye Study and the Nurses' Health Study are showing a positive association. The LALES, which also showed a positive association in a cross-sectional study of a predominantly Mexican Hispanic population and thus subject to inherent biases of similar prevalence-based studies, appeared to reduce patient recall bias as well as misclassification by validating a diabetes diagnosis through both medical history and blood testing. Selection bias, however, remains a potential confounder in a restricted population study set. Other reasons for the conflicting data regarding diabetes and glaucoma is the low prevalence of both diabetes and glaucoma as compared to cardiovascular diseases, and the often equivocal nature of a glaucoma diagnosis leading to potential misclassification and underreporting, thus biasing against an association. This is unlike coronary artery or cerebrovascular disease where an ischemic event when it occurs is clearly evident. At the moment, the available evidence regarding the effect of diabetes on the development of glaucoma is equivocal. More prospective studies will be necessary to determine whether a causal or permissive relationship exists between diabetes and glaucoma.

### Sidebar 60.2 Glaucoma, diet, exercise, and life style

Janet Betchkal and Rick Bendel

Anyone treating glaucoma patients is used to facing questions about how a patient's lifestyle, habits, and/or emotional state may affect his or her intraocular pressure (IOP) or, more accurately, their risk of glaucomatous progression.

As with most chronic diseases, glaucoma risk factors can be divided into "nonmodifiable" and "modifiable" categories. The former would include family history, age, gender, underlying pathology, and genetics. The modifiable category includes the life style issues over which we might be able to exert some level of "control."

Through the years, there have been numerous studies that have demonstrated the relationship between IOP and the development of and/or progression of open-angle glaucoma[1-3]. Therefore, most research and review articles have focused on the affects of various lifestyle factors on IOP. Some of the factors examined include diet, exercise, systemic hypertension, cigarette smoking, alcohol consumption, caffeine ingestion, marijuana usage, and various types of stress.[4]

There are a plethora of non-Food and Drug Administration (FDA)-approved "supplements" on the market that tout their effectiveness for various disease states of the body[5-6], including the eye. However, these herbal or nutritional supplements are not regulated by the FDA as are prescription drugs, and, as such, the makers of these products can make statements that are not based on evidence-based scientific data.[7]

There are several well-designed studies indicating that the use of zinc and oral antioxidant food supplements may help prevent progression in patients with age-related macular degeneration. However, there is no similar evidence to indicate that nutritional supplemental therapy will help prevent the progression of damage to the optic nerve, visual field, or vision in patients with primary open-angle glaucoma[8,9]. Nonetheless, there are several supplements that are specifically marketed to the glaucoma patient to help stabilize or improve their disease[10-12]. These include bilberry, lutein, and ginkgo[13]. In our opinion, there is no clear evidence that these help in the treatment of glaucoma; at this time, there is also no data to suggest that they are harmful to the glaucomatous eye. We recognize that there are different opinions about the validity of the literature.

Some studies have shown that obesity is a risk factor for elevated IOP,[14-15] while other studies have determined that caloric restriction may be neuroprotective in rats and other animal models.[16-18]

While there is no denying the overall health benefits of a well-balanced diet and a regular exercise routine[19], the advantages, if any, to glaucoma patients are less clear. Aerobic exercise has been shown to reduce IOP more in glaucoma patients than in healthy individuals.[20-22] This effect is greatest in sedentary individuals starting an exercise program for the first time. The acute IOP reduction may be as great as 7–13 mmHg in primary open-angle glaucoma patients. However, the effect is short-lived and IOP has been shown to return to baseline in as little as 40 min.[20-21]

Interestingly, physically fit glaucoma patients and individuals participating in as little as 3 months of conditioning have been shown to have lower resting IOP levels,[23-24] however, these same individuals show much less of an acute decrease in IOP after bouts of aerobic exercise than do their sedentary counterparts.[25-26] The mechanism responsible for the decrease in IOP in these two subsets of glaucoma patients is not fully understood.[27-29]

In contrast, any activities involving the Valsalva maneuver and/or anaerobic or isotonic exercise are associated with an acute increase in IOP.[30] One activity that should clearly be avoided in glaucoma patients would be any regimen that involves total-body inversion or head stands, as the immediate increase in IOP can be as high as 16 mmHg.[31-32]

There are many good reasons to stop smoking cigarettes that have nothing to do with glaucoma. And, while cigarette smoking has been shown to cause a mild and transient increase in IOP in some primary open-angle glaucoma patients,[33-34] several large studies have failed to demonstrate a link between cigarette smoking and increased incidence or prevalence of ocular hypertension or glaucoma.[35-36]

In 1965, Pecson and Grant[37] first reported that alcohol consumption caused a much greater decrease in the IOP of primary open-angle glaucoma patients than in the normal population. The effect is transient and tends to dissipate in 2–5 h.[37-38] The clinician would be advised to exercise caution in relating this information to the patient, as he or she would not want to encourage binge drinking, or worse, create a situation whereby the patient is in a constant state of inebriation. In known alcoholics and/or in any patient who has alcohol on the breath, it is probably worth noting the time since ingestion of alcohol in relationship to the time of IOP measurement. A word of caution here: we have noted several incidences where the physician and staff have noted the typical aroma of alcohol (presumably on the patient's breath), only to later realize that the odor is secondary to the use of hand sanitizers (an increasingly popular product on the market).

A majority of the population consumes caffeine in some form on a regular basis. In fact, it is estimated that in the United States, 80% of people over the age of 50 consume caffeine on a daily basis.[38] More than two billion pounds of caffeine-containing beverages are consumed annually in the United States alone.[39] It is contained in numerous beverages such as coffee, tea, and soft drinks, and in foods and various medications.[40] Caffeine's effects on the human body are well known and include increased blood pressure, decreased heart rate, increased wakefulness, and reduced cerebral blood flow.[41–42]

Overall, most studies have shown that caffeine causes a transient increase in the IOP of normal, ocular hypertensive, and open-angle glaucoma subjects.[43–48] However, there are a few studies that did not reach this same conclusion.[49–51] Despite the fact that most studies demonstrated a statistically relevant elevation in IOP in response to caffeine ingestion, some investigators like Higginbotham et al.[44] did not feel that this was "clinically relevant" and went so far as to recommend that glaucoma patients not be dissuaded from consuming caffeinated beverages, while others recommended that patients with glaucoma or ocular hypertension limit their daily caffeine consumption to a specified amount.[47] It may be that patients vary in response to caffeine and that it has more of an effect on select individuals than others based on a host of unstudied factors.

Just about everyone knows (or think they know) that marijuana (cannabis) is useful in the treatment of glaucoma. Ever since Hepler and Frank first reported the effects of marijuana smoking on IOP in 1971,[52] this has a been a hot topic that resurfaces every few years – usually when some celebrity is diagnosed with glaucoma or a law favoring legalization of marijuana is up for consideration.

Since 1971, numerous studies have shown that marijuana smoking will reduce IOP for up to three to 4 h.[53–56] Besides marijuana, various derivatives of tetrahydrocannabinol (THC) in oral and intravenous[58] forms have also been shown to affect similar reductions in IOP. However, this has to be weighed against evidence that marijuana can reduce blood flow and, thus, optic disk perfusion.[59]

The problem with the use of marijuana for the treatment of glaucoma is that glaucoma is a 24-h disease and as such, marijuana, with a duration of action of 3–4 h, would have to be smoked eight to ten times per day in order to maintain a lowered pressure throughout the 24-h period. On top of that, there is a suggestion that frequent marijuana smokers build up a tolerance to the drug, requiring more and more to achieve the same results.[60] That would mean susceptible patients would need to smoke a minimum of 2,920–3,650 marijuana cigarettes annually.[54,61] Besides the acute effects of marijuana including increased heart rate, conjunctival hyperemia, hypotension, euphoria, and cognitive disorders,[62–64] long-term side effects can involve many organ systems throughout the body – not the least of which involves the brain.[63–70] Even the staunchest supporter of marijuana legalization would have to concede that such massive and regular doses of marijuana would render the individual mentally and physically debilitated. Who would want one of these frequent smokers driving a bus, piloting an airplane, operating machinery, or performing surgery in our society?

When specifically asked about the advisability of marijuana use in the treatment of glaucoma, we do not recommend it and "warn" the individual that if he or she is caught with possession of an "illegal" substance he or she should expect to pay the legal consequences. Having a diagnosis of glaucoma would not suffice as a legal defense.

All of the questions about the issues addressed previously, do not begin to equal the number of inquires we receive about the effect of "stress" (in any or all forms) on IOP. We live in a stressful world – or, at least we believe we do. Patients – young and old – are quick to explain away most adverse events in their lives as being related to some sort of stressful event under which they are living.

In fact, there have been numerous studies that support the notion that physical, psychological, and psychosocial stress can increase IOP.[71–77] In these studies, stress was induced in various ways including hard physical activity, the solving of difficult mental arithmetic problems, and exposure to loud continuous noises. More recently, Yamamoto et al, developed and validated an inventory to measure psychosocial stress (IMPS).[76] They showed that the IMPS-measured stress score was correlated with increased IOP in women; however, the same association was not seen in men.[77] They postulated that stress may raise IOP by increasing blood cortisol levels that have been found to be temporally related to IOP diurnal variation.[78] Stress also increases circulating catechols, and has been mentioned elsewhere in this text, catechols drive aqueous production in the ciliary body.

So having discussed how events in each of our daily lives affect IOP and, by extension, primary open-angle glaucoma, what do we advise our patients with or at risk for developing primary open-angle glaucoma? We advise them to take "good care" of themselves by seeing their doctor regularly, taking their prescribed medications according to instructions, eating a diet rich in fruits and green-leafy vegetables, watching their weight and caloric intake, getting enough sleep, following an aerobic exercise program, limiting participation in isotonic exercises (that cause the Valsalva maneuver), quitting or severely reducing cigarette (and other tobacco product) smoking, avoiding the use of illicit drugs (of any kind), using alcohol and caffeine in moderation (and NOT within 3 h of their glaucoma follow-up office visits), and NEVER doing total-body inversion therapy (including Yoga head stands).

## Bibliography

1. Gordon MO, Beiser JA, Brandt, JD, et al. The ocular hypertension treatment study: baseline factors that predict the onset of primary open angle glaucoma. *Arch Ophthalmol.* 2002;120:714–720.
2. The AGIS Investigators. The Advanced Glaucoma Intervention Study (AGIS):7. The relationship between control of intraocular pressure and visual field deterioration. *Am J Ophthalmol.* 2000;130:429–440.
3. Leske MC, Connell AM, Wu SY, et al. Risk factors for open angle glaucoma. The Barbados Eye Study. *Arch Ophthalmol.* 1995;113:918–924.
4. Stewart WC. The effect of lifestyle on the relative risk to develop open-angle glaucoma. *Curr Opin Ophthalmol.* 1995;6:3–9.
5. Eisenberg DM, Davis RB, Ettner SL, et al. Trends in alternative medicine use in the United States, 1990-1997: results of a follow up national survey. *JAMA.* 1998;280:1569–1575.
6. Morris CA, Avorn J. Internet marketing of herbal products. *JAMA.* 2003;290:1505–1509.
7. Hampton T. More scrutiny for dietary supplements? *JAMA.* 2005;293:27–28.
8. West AL, Oren GA, Moroi SE. Evidence for the use of nutritional supplements and herbal medicines in common eye diseases. *Am J Ophthalmol.* 2006;141:157–166.
9. Kang JH, Pasquale LR, Willett W, et al. Antioxidant intake and primary open-angle glaucoma: a prospective study. *Am J Epidemiol.* 2003;158:337–346.
10. Rhee DJ, Spaeth GL, Myer JS, et al. Prevalence of the use of complementary and alternative medicine for glaucoma. *Ophthalmology.* 2002;109:438–443.
11. Rhee DJ, Katz LJ, Spaeth GL, et al. Complementary and alternative medicine for glaucoma. *Surv Ophthalmol.* 2001;46:43–55.
12. West AL, Fetters MD, Hemmila MR, et al. Herb and vitamin supplementation use among a general ophthalmology practice population. *Am J Ophthalmol.* 2005;139:522–529.
13. Chung HS, Harris A, Kristinsson JK, et al. Ginkgo biloba extract increases ocular blood flow velocity. *J Ocul Pharmacol Ther.* 1999;15:233–240.
14. Shiose Y. The aging effect on intraocular pressure in an apparently normal population. *Arch Ophthalmol.* 1984;102:883–887.
15. Shiose Y, Kawase Y. A new approach to stratified normal intraocular pressure in a general population. *Am J Ophthalmol.* 1986;101:714–721.
16. Kawai SI, Vora S, Das S, et al. Modeling of risk factors for the degeneration of retinal ganglion cells following ischemia/reperfusion in rats: effects of age, caloric restriction, diabetes, pigmentation, and glaucoma. *FASEB J.* Express article 10.1096/fj.-0666fje (online March 2001).
17. Masoro EJ. Caloric restriction and aging: an update. *Exp Gerontol.* 2000;35:299–305.
18. Nicolas AS, Lanzmann-Petithory D, Villas B. Caloric restriction and aging. *J Nutr Health Aging.* 1999;3:77–83.
19. Guyton AC. Sports physiology. In: Guyton AC, ed. *Guyton Textbook of Medical Physiology.* 8th edn. Philadelphia: W.B. Saunders Company: Philadelphia; 1991.
20. Lempert P, Cooper KH, Culver JF, et al. The effect of exercise on intraocular pressure. *Am J Ophthalmol.* 1967;63:1673–1676.
21. Stewart RH, LeBlanc R, Becker B. Effects of exercise on aqueous dynamics. *Am J Ophthalmol.* 1970;69:245–248.
22. Leighton DA, Phillips CI. Effect of moderate exercise on ocular tension. *Br J Ophthalmol.* 1970;54:599–605.
23. Passo MS, Goldberg L, Elliot DL, et al. Exercise conditioning and intraocular pressure. *Am J Ophthalmol.* 1987;103:754–757.
24. Passo MS, Elliot DL, Goldberg L. Long-term effects of exercise conditioning on intraocular pressure in glaucoma suspects. *J Glaucoma.* 1992;1:39–41.
25. Passo MS, Goldberg L, Elliot DL, et al. Exercise training reduces intraocular pressure among subjects suspected of having glaucoma. *Arch Ophthalmol.* 1991;109:1096–1110.
26. Qureshi IA. Effects of exercise on intraocular pressure in physically fit subjects. *Clin Exp Pharm Phys.* 1996;23:648–652.
27. Sargent TG, Blair SN, Magun JC, et al. Physical fitness and intraocular pressure. *Am J Optom Physiol Opt.* 1981;58:460–466.
28. Kielar RA, Teraslinna P, Rowe DG, et al. Standardized aerobic and anaerobic exercise: differential effects on intraocular tension, blood pH, and lactate. *Invest Ophthalmol.* 1975;14:132–145.
29. Ashkenazi I, Melamed S, Blumenthal M. The effect of continuous strenuous exercise on intraocular pressure. *Invest Ophthalmol Vis Sci.* 1992;33:2872–2877.
30. Oggel K, Sommer G, Neuhann T, et al. Veränderungen des augeninnendruckes bei intratherakaler druckerhöhung in abhägigkeit von der körperposition und der achsenlänge des augapfels. *Graefes Arch Clin Exp Ophthalmol.* 1982;218:51–54.
31. Weinreb RN, Cook J, Friberg TR. The effect of inverted body position on intraocular pressure. *Am J Ophthalmol.* 1984;98:784–787.
32. Carlson KH, McLaren JW, Topper JE, et al. Effect of body body position on intraocular pressure and aqueous flow. *Invest Ophthalmol Vis Sci.* 1987;28:1346–1352.
33. Mehra KS, Roy PN, Khare BB. Tobacco smoking and glaucoma. *Ann Ophthalmol.* 1976;8:462–464.
34. Shepard RJ, Ponsford E, Basu PF, et al. Effects of cigarette smoking on intraocular pressure and vision. *Br J Ophthalmol.* 1978;62:682–687.
35. Steward WC, Crinkley CMC, Murrell HP. Cigarette smoking in normal subjects, ocular hypertensive, and chronic open angle glaucoma patients. *Am J Ophthalmol.* 1994;117:267–268.
36. Klein BE, Klein R, Ritter LL. Relationship of drinking alcohol and smoking to prevalence of open-angle glaucoma: The Beaver Dam Eye Study. *Ophthalmology.* 1993;100:1609–1613.
37. Pecson JD, Grant WM. Glaucoma, alcohol, and intraocular pressure. *Arch Ophthalmol.* 1965;73:495–501.
38. Massey LK. Caffeine and the elderly. *Drugs Aging.* 1998;13:43–50.
39. Ritchie JM, Central nervous system stimulants [continued]: the xanthines. In: Goodman L, Gilman A, eds. *The Pharmacological Basis of Therapeutics.* 5th ed. New York: MacMillan Publishing Company, Inc.; 1975:367–378.
40. Bunker ML, McWiliams M. Caffeine content of common beverages. *J Am Diet Assoc.* 1979;74:28–32.
41. Whitsett TL, Manien CV, Christensen HD. Cardiovascular effects of coffee and caffeine. *Am J Cardiol.* 1984;53:918–922.
42. Casiglia E, Bongiovi S, Paleari CD, et al. Haemodynamic effects of coffee and caffeine in normal volunteers: a placebo-controlled clinical study. *J Intern Med.* 1191;229:501–504.

43. Peczon JD, Grant WM. Sedatives, stimulants, and intraocular pressure in glaucoma. *Arch Ophthalmol.* 1964;72:178–188.
44. Higginbotham EJ, Kilimanjaro HA, Wilenski JT, et al. The effect of caffeine on intraocular pressure in glaucoma patients. *Ophthalmol.* 1989;96:624–626.
45. Okimi PH, Sportsman S, Pickard MR, et al. Effects of caffeinated coffee on intraocular pressure. *Appl Nurs Res.* 1991;4:72–76.
46. Ajayi OB, Ukwade MT. Caffeine and intraocular pressure in a Nigerian population. *J Glaucoma.* 2001;10:25–31.
47. Avisar R, Avisar E, Weinberger D. Effect of coffee consumption on intraocular pressure. *Ann Pharmacother.* 2002;36:992–995.
48. Chandrasekaran S, Rochtchina E, Mitchell P. Effects of caffeine on intraocular pressure. *J Glaucoma.* 2005;14:504–507.
49. Ricklefs G. [Studies on the ways of life of glaucoma patients]. *Doc Ophthalmol.* 1968;25:43–99 [in German].
50. Ricklefs G, Pohls EU. [Effect of caffeine containing tablets and Coca Cola on intraocular pressure of patients without glaucoma and patients with regulated glaucoma]. *Klin Monatsbl Augenheklkd.* 1969;154:545–551 [in German].
51. Adams BA, Brubaker RF. Caffeine has no clinically significant effect on aqueous humor flow in the normal human eye. *Ophthalmology.* 1990;97:1031–1041.
52. Hepler RS, Frank IR. Marijuana smoking and intraocular pressure. *JAMA.* 1971;271:1392.
53. Merritt JC, Crawford WJ, Alexander PC, et al. Effect of marihuana on intraocular and blood pressure in glaucoma. *Ophthalmology.* 1980;87:222–228.
54. Green K. Marihuana and the eye: a review. *J Toxicol Cutan Ocul Toxicol.* 1982;1:3–32.
55. Green K. Marijuana effects on intraocular pressure. In: Drance SM, Neufeld AH, eds. *Glaucoma: Applied Pharmacology in Medical Treatment.* Orlando, FL: Grune and Stratton, Inc.; 1984:507–526.
56. Jarvinen T, Pate DW, Laine K. Cannabinoids in the treatment of glaucoma. *Pharmacol Ther.* 2002;95:203–220.
57. Tiedeman JS, Shields MD, Weber PA, et al. Effect of synthetic cannabinoids on elevated intraocular pressure. *Ophthalmology.* 1981;88:270–277.
58. Green K, Pederson JE. Effect of Δ′ 1-tetrahydrocannabinol aqueous dynamics and ciliary body permeability in the rabbit. *Exp Eye Res.* 1973;15:499–507.
59. Shields MB. *Textbook of Glaucoma.* 3rd ed. Baltimore, MD: Williams and Wilkins; 1992:515–516.
60. Flom MC, Adams AJ, Jones RT. Marijuana smoking and reduced pressure in human eyes: drug action or epiphenomenon? *Invest Ophthalmol.* 1975;14:52–55.
61. Green K, McDonald TF. Ocular toxicity of marijuana: an update. *J Toxicol Cutan Ocul Toxicol.* 1987;6:309–334.
62. Agurell S, Dewey WL, Willette RE, eds. *The Cannibinoids: Chemical, Pharmacological and Therapeutic Aspects.* Orlando, FL: Academic Press Inc.; 1984.
63. Graham IDP. *Cannibis and Health.* Orlando, FL: Academic Press, Inc. 1976.
64. Dewey WL. Cannibinoid pharmacology. *Pharmacol Rev.* 1986;38:151–178.
65. Rosenkrantz H, Fleishman RW. Effects of cannibis on lungs. In: Nahas GG, Palon WDM, eds. *Marihuana: Biological Effects.* Elmsford, NY: Dergamon Press, Inc.; 1979:279–299.
66. Murray JB. Marijuana effects on human cognitive functions, psychomotor functions, and personality. *J Gen Psychol.* 1986;113:23–55.
67. Leon-Carrion J. Mental performance in long-term heavy cannabis: a preliminary report. *Psychol Rep.* 1990;67:947–952.
68. Solowij N. Cognitive impairments recover following cessation of cannibis use? *Life Sci.* 1995;5:2119–2126.
69. Fletcher JM, Page JB, Francis DJ, et al. Cognitive correlates of long-term cannibis use in Costa Rican men. *Arch Gen Psychiatry.* 1996;53:1051–1057.
70. Pope HG, Yurgelun-Todd D. The residual cognitive effects of heavy marijuana use in college students. *JAMA.* 1996;275:521–527.
71. Buckingham T, Young R. The rise and fall of intraocular pressure: the influence of physiological factors. *Ophthal Physiol.* 1986;6:95–99.
72. Shily BG. Psychophysiological stress, elevated intraocular pressure, and acute closed angle glaucoma. *Am J Optom Physiol Opt.* 1987;64:866–870.
73. Sauerborn G, Schmitz M, Franzen U, et al. Stress and intraocular pressure in myopes. *Psychol Health.* 1992;6:61–68.
74. Kaluza G, Strempel I, Mauer I. Stress reactivity of intraocular pressure after relaxation training in open-angle glaucoma patients. *J Behav Med.* 1996;19:587–598.
75. Leung JP, Yap MKH. The relationship between stress and intraocular pressure of the eye. *Psychologia.* 1999;42:51–58.
76. Yamamoto K, Irie M, Sakamoto Y, et al. The relationship between IMPS-measured stress score and biomedical parameters regarding health status among public school workers. *J Physiol Anthropol.* 2007;26:149–158.
77. Yamamoto K, Sakamoto Y, Masahiro I, et al. The relationship between IMPS-measured stress score and intraocular pressure among public school workers. *J Physiol Anthropol.* 2008;27:43–50.
78. Weitzman ED, Henkind P, Leitman M, et al. Correlative 24-hour relationships between intraocular pressure and plasma cortisol in normal subjects and patients with glaucoma. *Br J Ophthalmol.* 1975;59:566–572.

## 60.5 Sleep Apnea and Glaucoma

Obstructive sleep apnea (OSA) represents the largest group of sleep apneas.[95] Sleep apnea can also occur as a result of central and peripheral neurologic or neuromuscular disorders. The prevalence of sleep apnea in cross-sectional studies has been reported to be in the vicinity of 3–7% in adult men and 2–5% in adult women but as high as 15% overall, in some reviews.[96–98] The prevalence is higher in different population subsets such as obese people, minorities, and elderly individuals.[96] The true prevalence of OSA has been difficult to estimate because many affected persons remain undiagnosed. Differences in methodologies regarding case identification, disparities in techniques used to monitor sleep and breathing, and patient selection bias have contributed to the large variability in reported disease prevalence.[96] Typically, OSA occurs predominantly in males between ages of 40–70 years of age and is associated with obesity or increased body mass index (BMI). It is characterized clinically by nocturnal episodes of apnea lasting at least 10 s followed by arterial desaturation and sleep disturbances due to hypoxia.[95,96,99] The diagnosis of OSA or sleep-disordered breathing is based on results of polysomnography – the gold standard; and its severity is measured with the apnea–hypopnea index (AHI), which is the number of apneas and hypopneas per hour of sleep. The severity can also be characterized by the degree of nocturnal hypoxemia (oxyhemoglobin desaturation) or sleep fragmentation (arousal frequency).[96] The risk of worsening sleep apnea is correlated with increasing age and body mass index, with weight change being one of the most important determinants of disease progression or regression.[100,101] Obstructive sleep apnea has been associated with development of arterial hypertension, pulmonary hypertension, stroke, and other cardiovascular abnormalities such as arterial stiffness, endothelial dysfunction, and echocardiographic evidence of increased left ventricular mass and left ventricular systolic dysfunction.[99,102–106] In a prospective study of 709 participants of the Wisconsin Sleep Cohort Study, there was a dose–response association between OSA and development of hypertension at both 4 and 8 years of follow-up.[104,105] Increasing AHI was associated with an increased risk of developing hypertension independent of known confounders. Derangements in glucose metabolism have also been attributed to OSA.[107] OSA is thus associated with significant cardiovascular and cerebrovascular morbidity, and there is accumulating data from population-based prospective cohort studies that OSA is independently associated with increased mortality.[108,109] Continuous positive airway pressure (CPAP) therapy is the primary treatment modality in patients with OSA. There are strong data from clinical and research trials showing its benefit in reducing daytime sleepiness and blood pressure as well as other risks associated with OSA.[110]

Since reduced ocular perfusion pressure due to nocturnal hypotension can potentially influence glaucomatous disease progression, likewise, hypoxemia due to arterial desaturation can potentially result in reduced oxygen delivery to the optic nerve head and retinal ganglion cells resulting in injury and axonal loss. Furthermore, disordered autoregulation and blood pressure fluctuation have been implicated as potential mechanisms for sleep apnea-related glaucomatous optic nerve damage.[111] Elevation of intraocular pressure in patients on CPAP therapy may also be a factor. As expected, most of the information evaluating the association between sleep apnea and glaucoma is derived from a small cross-sectional case series of patients with either a sleep apnea syndrome diagnosis who underwent ophthalmologic evaluation, perimetry, and disk evaluation to determine the prevalence of glaucoma, or, vice versa, patients with a glaucoma diagnosis who then underwent polysomnography to determine the prevalence of sleep apnea.[111–120] The percentage of patients with sleep apnea who were found to have glaucoma in these studies was as high as 27%.[114] Mojon et al performed the first systematic cross-sectional observational study of 114 patients suspected of having sleep apnea referred for polysomnography.[111] Sixty nine (60.5%) patients met the criteria for sleep apnea and five were also identified as having glaucoma, three of whom were previously undiagnosed. It is interesting to note that three of the five patients with glaucoma had very high respiratory disturbance index (apnea–hypopnea index) indicating more severe disease. In a more recent small case–control study by Karakucuk et al of 31 patients with OSA, all 4 patients identified as having glaucoma also were classified as having severe OSA.[112] The prevalence of glaucoma in these small observational studies were 7.2 and 12.9% and thus higher than expected in the general population. The strength of both of these small studies was the masked status of the examiners performing the ophthalmologic evaluation to minimize bias. Mojon et al later published two additional papers of 16 patients with established normal tension glaucoma undergoing polysomnography and 30 consecutive patients with primary open-angle glaucoma who underwent transcutaneous oximetry as a surrogate marker for a diagnosis of sleep apnea.[113,119] In the former, 8/16 (50%) were found to have a respiratory disturbance index of greater than 10. In the latter, 20% were found to have sleep apnea by oximetry data. Other small case–control observational series and small consecutive case series provided additional evidence linking sleep apnea and glaucoma. In contrast, however, two of the three largest of the published studies failed to show an association.[117,118] Girkin et al, in a nested case–control study of an exclusively male population at a VA hospital, found that a previous diagnosis of OSA was not statistically significantly increased in glaucoma patients as compared to controls.[117] The authors concluded that their study does not support sleep apnea as having a significant impact on the eventual development of glaucoma. Geyer et al performed a cross-sectional study of 228 patients with confirmed sleep apnea – the largest group of sleep apnea patients to date.[118] The prevalence of glaucoma in their sleep apnea cohort was 2%, similar to the general population. Furthermore, they found no correlation between respiratory disturbance index and the presence of glaucoma. The large study sample, having two highly experienced glaucoma experts perform the eye examinations, standardization of the criteria used to identify glaucoma, and the requirement that visual field data had to match disk findings, were important study strengths, especially since the latter three would expectedly improve the sensitivity and specificity of a glaucoma diagnosis. One other case–control study with 212 open-angle glaucoma patients and 218 controls used a questionnaire to indirectly determine symptoms of sleep-disordered breathing by evaluating the prevalence of snoring, excessive daytime sleepiness, and insomnia.[121] When all three symptoms were included, the prevalence decreased to 14.6% in glaucoma patients, but was still statistically significantly greater than nonglaucoma controls.

However, the lack of definitive diagnostic criteria to establish a sleep apnea syndrome (i.e., lack of gold standard polysomnographic data) significantly reduces the specificity of this association.

The relationship between sleep apnea and glaucoma is intriguing and while the potential association is physiologically plausible, the data are conflicting and insufficient. Small study size, selection bias, lack of control groups, unmasked evaluations, lack of confirmatory data to strengthen a glaucoma diagnosis, variability in sleep-monitoring techniques, potential inaccurate case identification due to lack of standardized diagnostic criteria for sleep apnea, and use of surrogate information to determine whether sleep apnea is present are factors that significantly limit the interpretation of the data. Furthermore, due to the observational nature of the studies that identified a positive association between sleep apnea and glaucoma, causality still cannot be inferred. It is possible, however, that those with more severe sleep apnea with a high AHI and associated blood pressure fluctuations are at greatest risk while those with mild-moderate disease are at average risk. A mixed-risk study population may hence reduce the strength of an association between sleep apnea and glaucoma. In summary, further studies are necessary to establish the true relationship between glaucoma and sleep apnea (see Chap. 12).

## 60.6 Other Factors Possibly Affecting Glaucoma Risk

### 60.6.1 Statins and Glaucoma

Following the publication of the report of the NCEP-ATPIII emphasizing aggressive lipid lowering for both primary and secondary prevention of coronary artery disease, statins have emerged as the most important class of lipid-lowering agents in the treatment of hyperlipidemia.[69,70] Statins belong to a class of agents known as HMG-CoA (3-hydroxy 3-methylglutaryl-Coenzyme A) inhibitors, the prototype being lovastatin. More potent statins with respect to LDL (low-density lipoprotein) lowering potential have emerged including pravastatin, atorvastatin, simvastatin, and rosuvastatin. It was presumed that the reduction in mortality associated with statin use was related solely to its lipid-lowering ability. However, clinical studies evaluating the salutary benefits of statins in patients with coronary artery disease have shown that some of the cardiovascular benefits associated with statins appear to be unaccounted for by the reduction in LDL activity alone, and in some cases, appear to be independent of the patient's baseline lipid profile.[122,123] The MIRACL (Myocardial Ischemia Reduction with Aggressive Cholesterol Lowering) study, PROVE-IT (PRavastatin Or atorVastatin Evaluation and Infection Therapy), and IDEAL-ACS (Incremental Decrease in End-Points Through Aggressive Lipid-Lowering Acute Coronary Syndromes) studies outline the benefits of high-dosage atorvastatin therapy initiated within 24–96 h, 10 days, or 2 months, respectively, of an acute coronary syndrome.[124-127] Moreover, the ARMYDA (Atorvastatin for Reduction in MYocardial DAmage during angioplasty) and ARMYDA-3 trials demonstrated that 7 days of administration of atorvastatin 40 mg/day before coronary intervention significantly reduced the risks of peri-procedural myocardial damage, postprocedural myocardial infarction (MI), and atrial fibrillation as compared to placebo.[128,129] From the clinical data previously cited, it appears that statins must have pleiotropic effects that extend beyond their capacity to reduce LDL levels in order to explain the cardiovascular benefits achieved soon after an acute ischemic event or during invasive cardiac intervention. It has been proposed that heightened inflammation following an acute coronary syndrome increases the risk of a subsequent ischemic event.[130,131] Increased levels of C-reactive protein (CRP) have been associated with arterial wall inflammation, which promotes lipid deposition, plaque growth, and plaque instability. Use of statins has been shown to modulate expression of anti-inflammatory mediators, reduce proinflammatory function, and abrogate the levels of several inflammatory markers including CRP, serum amyloid A (SAA) and interleukin-6 (IL-6).[123,130–133] Hence, statin-mediated anti-inflammatory activity has been suggested as a potential mechanism in secondary prevention of an acute ischemic event independent of its lipid-lowering capabilities.

Like coronary artery disease, the pathophysiology of glaucoma is multifactorial and aberrant immune activity may be one of multiple non-pressure-related mechanisms linked to retinal ganglion cell apoptosis. Tezel and Wax proposed that instability in immune regulation may tip the balance between the neuroprotective and neurodegenerative mechanisms, favoring the latter, thus leading to ganglion cell death and optic nerve atrophy.[134-137] While experimental data have shown that upregulation of the heat shock proteins hsp 27, hsp 60, and hsp 70 are cytoprotective and promote ganglion cell survival under a variety of cellular stresses, Tezel et al postulated that dysregulation in the production and activity of this family of proteins may, in fact, lead to optic nerve injury.[134,135,138,139] Since heat shock proteins are highly antigenic, overexpression can lead to antibody-mediated neutralization of the natural antiapoptotic activity of these proteins as well as induction of autoimmune injury. If autoimmune inflammatory injury could be pathogenetically linked to glaucomatous optic nerve damage, then suppression of inflammatory activity may help preserve ganglion cell survival and axonal loss.

Furthermore, if dysregulation of heat shock protein expression can lead to optic nerve injury then pharmacologic intervention to reregulate expression may protect ganglion cells from death. Statin delivery in a rat transient ischemia model has been shown to modulate expression of alpha B-crystalline and heat shock proteins with prolongation of retinal ganglion cell survival.[140] In an in vivo axotomized rat optic nerve model, intravitreal injection of simvastatin was shown to increase ganglion cell survival with increased expression of hsp 27; hence, implying that the neuroprotective effect of statins may be related to modulation of heat shock protein production during various mechanisms of neuronal injury.[141] At the moment, there is a paucity of clinical data regarding the effects of statins and lipid-lowering agents on optic nerve health and glaucoma progression. De Castro et al in a retrospective review of glaucoma suspects who had been on statins plus aspirin for greater than 23 months showed reduced progression of several CSLO (confocal scanning laser ophthalmoscopy) parameters in the glaucoma suspect group on statins as compared to glaucoma suspects not on statins.[142] In a case–control study conducted in a male VA population, long duration (greater than 24 months) statin use, was associated with a reduced risk of having open-angle glaucoma.[143] Curiously, reduced glaucoma risk was also associated with use of nonstatin lipid-lowering agents. Further clinical investigation would help determine whether there is indeed a neuroprotective benefit in statin users with glaucoma (Sidebar 60.3).

### Sidebar 60.3 Statin medications and glaucoma

Kevin C. Leonard and Cindy M. L. Hutnik

Statin medications were first introduced more than 20 years ago, and are currently indicated for reduction of serum cholesterol levels in the prevention of coronary artery disease and stroke. These drugs are the most effective medications for treating dyslipidemia and have an excellent tolerability profile, resulting in their widespread use. More recently, statins have been investigated for other indications based on their pleiotropic effects including anti-inflammatory, antiapoptotic and antiproliferative properties. Several studies have provided evidence for statins having a neuroprotective function in the central nervous system, specifically for cerebral ischemia and stroke, Alzheimer's dementia, and multiple sclerosis.[1] Evidence from both clinical and basic research studies have suggested that statins may be protective against age-related macular degeneration[2], diabetic retinopathy[3], nuclear cataract[4], and open-angle glaucoma[5,6].

### Rationale

Targeting either the aqueous outflow system or the optic nerve could potentially affect glaucomatous progression. There is a rationale suggesting that statins may mediate a protective effect by acting at both of these sites where disease may manifest. Statins are competitive inhibitors of the 3-hydroxy-3-methylglutaryl-Coenzyme A (HMG-CoA) reductase enzyme, which catalyzes an early and rate-limiting step in cholesterol biosynthesis. This mediates a reduction in both total cholesterol and low-density lipoprotein (LDL), while the protective high-density lipoprotein (HDL) is increased. This primary mechanism suggests that statins are protective against any component of disease, cardiovascular or otherwise, that is mediated or exacerbated by excess total cholesterol or LDL. Their known inhibitory effect on atherosclerotic processes and subsequent vascular diseases has caused some to postulate that statins could protect optic nerve head (ONH) vasculature, resulting in improved ocular blood flow.

In addition to the primary effect of statin drugs, inhibition of the HMG-CoA reductase enzyme also limits the synthesis of other intermediate metabolites involved in cellular functions, which is thought to mediate many of the pleiotropic effects. In particular, statins have been shown to inhibit the production of various nonsteroidal isoprenoids. The isoprenoid molecules play an important role in basic cell biology by regulating the activity of various cellular proteins, including the Rho subfamily of molecules. These molecules are involved in regulating cellular contraction, actin cytoskeletal organization, and cell–cell and cell–ECM interactions[7]. Evidence exists that inhibition of Rho kinase leads to enhanced aqueous outflow and decreased IOP. Additional rationale for statins having an ocular hypotensive effect comes from knowing that statins enhance vascular endothelial cell function, and thus they may similarly enhance trabecular endothelial cell function and mediate enhanced aqueous outflow.

Recent evidence also suggests that statin drugs may have neuroprotective effects, for which several potential mechanisms have been put forth. These include decreasing glutamate mediated excitotoxicity, and exerting anti-inflammatory effects by inhibiting leukocyte–endothelium interaction following ischemic injury. Another recent study has suggested a role for heat shock proteins as a target of statin-mediated neuroprotective effects in ocular diseases[8]. Of course it is also likely that there are other undiscovered or indirect effects of statin drugs that may mediate some neuroprotective effect.

## Evidence

The first study to demonstrate a beneficial effect in glaucoma was a case–control matched study, using a clinical database to identify previous statin use in patients newly diagnosed with primary open-angle glaucoma. A lower risk of open-angle glaucoma was associated with statin use, especially in those who used the medication for more than 2 years (OR 0.60), or in those with cardiovascular and lipid diseases (OR 0.63 for both conditions). Interestingly though, a protective effect was also identified among those who used nonstatin cholesterol-lowering agents (OR 0.59). While these results raise some question as to whether it was the improved lipid profile or the statin causing the effect, use of the medications did seem to have a beneficial effect[5].

There is also evidence that systemic administration of a statin may directly improve retinal circulation. Laboratory-based studies have shown that simvastatin may exert a neuroprotective effect that is mediated by inhibition of leukocyte–endothelium interaction through nitric oxide release from the endothelium[9, 10]. A small Japanese study carried out on healthy volunteers revealed that daily administration of simvastatin for 7 days significantly increased blood velocity and flow in retinal arteries and veins, without a significant effect on vessel diameter. These changes were also associated with a significant reduction in intraocular pressure ($14.3 \pm 0.4$ mmHg at baseline, $12.6 \pm 0.5$ mmHg at 90 min, and $12.4 \pm 0.6$ mmHg at 7 days), as well as an increase in plasma nitrite/nitrate levels reflecting an increase in nitric oxide, both at 90 min and 7 days after starting systemic statin therapy[11]. These results provide additional evidence for a beneficial effect of statins, and suggest that the mechanism may be a nitric oxide mediated increase in retinal blood flow as well as a reduction in intraocular pressure.

Song et al[7] have provided evidence that statins can function as ocular hypotensive agents, and revealed some potential mechanisms for this action. The statin drugs lovastatin and compactin were shown to induce changes in cell shape and actin cytoskeletal organization and decrease myosin light chain phosphorylation in cultured porcine trabecular meshwork and ciliary body cells. It was postulated that these events could lead to cellular and tissue relaxation, and thereby increase aqueous outflow. Their studies also demonstrated that lovastatin increased aqueous outflow in an organ-cultured anterior eye segment perfusion model. Evidence was provided that the effects were mediated by inhibition of isoprenylation of the small guanosine triphosphate (GTP)-binding proteins such as Rho-GTPase. A strong relationship was also identified between decreased myosin light chain phosphorylation induced by statins and increased aqueous outflow facility, suggesting another potential mechanism. A previous cell culture study provided additional evidence, demonstrating that statins increased retinal ganglion cell axonal growth through inhibition of Rho-GTPase and Rho kinase[12].

The most recent work in this area employed confocal scanning laser ophthalmoscopy to assess the effect of statins on the progression of open-angle glaucoma suspects[6]. Outcome measures included rim volume, retinal nerve fiber layer cross-sectional area and mean global retinal nerve fiber layer thickness as assessed by confocal scanning laser ophthalmoscopy (CSLO). All of these parameters were significantly preserved in patients using statins for greater than 23 months. Despite this slower rate of progression in optic disk parameters, no significant difference in progression to glaucoma was identified based on glaucoma hemi-field measurements.

## Clinical Recommendations

While there is insufficient evidence at this point in time to make any major changes to the management of glaucoma patients, several important comments can be made regarding the concept of statin use as a treatment for glaucoma. Research done to date does suggest that statins may have a protective effect in glaucoma, however, there have been only a handful of studies published and those available have all had limitations. Since all studies done to date have been retrospective, an inherent limitation is that patients will also have other risk factors requiring them to use a statin, specifically dyslipidemia, and often systemic hypertension and coronary artery disease. Statin medications are widely used already and are very well-tolerated. However, the side effects of these medications are not benign and include systemic adverse effects such as abnormal liver function tests, myopathy, and, rarely, rhabdomyolysis. Other factors that must be considered include the cost of these medications and lack of efficacy data for topical administration. Based on the currently available evidence, systemic statin therapy does not appear to increase the risk of glaucoma progression, and there may be some potential benefit for patients on these drugs. A larger, randomized clinical trial will be necessary before stronger recommendations can be made.

## Bibliography

1. Schmeer C, Kretz A, Isenmann S. Statin-mediated protective effects in the central nervous system: general mechanisms and putative role of stress proteins. *Restor Neurol Neurosci.* 2006;24(2):79-95.
2. Guymer RH, Chiu AW, Lim L, Baird PN. HMG CoA reductase inhibitors (statins): do they have a role in age-related macular degeneration? *Surv Ophthalmol.* 2005;50(2):194-206.
3. Gordon B, Chang S, Kavanagh M, et al. The effects of lipid lowering on diabetic retinopathy. *Am J Ophthalmol.* 1991;112(4):385-391.
4. Klein BE, Klein R, Lee KE, Grady LM. Statin use and incident nuclear cataract. *JAMA.* 2006;295(23):2752-2758.
5. McGwin G Jr, McNeal S, Owsley C, Girkin C, Epstein D, Lee PP. Statins and other cholesterol-lowering medications and the presence of glaucoma. *Arch Ophthalmol.* 2004;122(6):822-826.
6. De Castro DK, Punjabi OS, Bostrom AG, et al Effect of statin drugs and aspirin on progression in open-angle glaucoma suspects using confocal scanning laser ophthalmoscopy. *Clin Experiment Ophthalmol.* 2007;35(6):506-513.
7. Song J, Deng PF, Stinnett SS, Epstein DL, Rao PV. Effects of cholesterol-lowering statins on the aqueous humor outflow pathway. *Invest Ophthalmol Vis Sci.* 2005;46(7):2424-2432.
8. Schmeer C, Kretz A, Isenmann S. Therapeutic potential of 3-hydroxy-3-methylglutaryl coenzyme a reductase inhibitors for the treatment of retinal and eye diseases. *CNS Neurol Disord Drug Targets.* 2007;6(4):282-287.
9. Miyahara S, Kiryu J, Yamashiro K, et al. Simvastatin inhibits leukocyte accumulation and vascular permeability in the retinas of rats with streptozotocin-induced diabetes. *Am J Pathol.* 2004;164(5):1697-1706.
10. Honjo M, Tanihara H, Nishijima K, et al. Statin inhibits leukocyte-endothelial interaction and prevents neuronal death induced by ischemia-reperfusion injury in the rat retina. *Arch Ophthalmol.* 2002;120(12):1707-1713.
11. Nagaoka T, Takahashi A, Sato E, et al. Effect of systemic administration of simvastatin on retinal circulation. *Arch Ophthalmol.* 2006;124(5):665-670.
12. Swiercz JM, Kuner R, Behrens J, Offermanns S. Plexin-B1 directly interacts with PDZ-RhoGEF/LARG to regulate RhoA and growth cone morphology. *Neuron.* 2002;35(1):51-63.

## 60.7 Conclusion

Currently, the most important and only modifiable risk factor in the development and progression of glaucoma is intraocular pressure. However, given the varying susceptibilities among individuals with respect to the development of glaucoma, it is clear that non-pressure-related factors must be involved. The studies cited show that certain concurrent systemic conditions may potentially significantly impact retinal ganglion cell survival. Although unfortunately, limitations in study design in the past have often failed to identify a permissive or causative effect of a certain systemic condition and glaucoma, future studies may provide such evidence. At the moment, lack of definitive evidence notwithstanding, the health of the eye must continue to be viewed in the context of an individual's overall health status. The clinician must remain mindful of systemic factors that are remediable, but if untreated, may influence the development or progression of glaucoma. Failure to appreciate the patient's clinical status and its potential impact on optic nerve survival may be detrimental to the preservation of vision.

## References

1. Gordon MO, Beiser JA, Brandt JD, et al. The Ocular Hypertension Treatment Study: baseline factors that predict the onset of primary open-angle glaucoma. *Arch Ophthalmol.* 2002;120(6):714–720; discussion 829-830.
2. Hayreh SS. Inter-individual variation in blood supply of the optic nerve head. Its importance in various ischemic disorders of the optic nerve head, and glaucoma, low-tension glaucoma and allied disorders. *Doc Ophthalmol.* 1985;30;59(3):217–246.
3. Mitchell P, Lee AJ, Rochtchina E, Wang JJ. Open-angle glaucoma and systemic hypertension: the Blue Mountains Eye Study. *J Glaucoma.* 2004;13(4):319–326.
4. Hennis A, Wu SY, Nemesure B, Leske MC, Barbados Eye Studies Group. Hypertension, diabetes, and longitudinal changes in intraocular pressure. *Ophthalmology.* 2003;110(5):908–914.
5. Leske MC, Wu SY, Nemesure B, Hennis A. Incident open-angle glaucoma and blood pressure. *Arch Ophthalmol.* 2002;120(7):954–959.
6. Hulsman CA, Vingerling JR, Hofman A, et al. Blood pressure, arterial stiffness, and open-angle glaucoma: the Rotterdam study. *Arch Ophthalmol.* 2007;125(6):805–812.
7. Suzuki Y, Iwase A, Araie M, et al, Tajimi Study Group. Risk factors for open-angle glaucoma in a Japanese population: the Tajimi Study. *Ophthalmology.* 2006;113(9):1613–1617.
8. Bonomi L, Marchini G, Marraffa M, et al. Vascular risk factors for primary open angle glaucoma: the Egna-Neumarkt Study. *Ophthalmology.* 2000;107(7):1287–1293.
9. Tielsch JM, Katz J, Sommer A, et al. Hypertension, perfusion pressure, and primary open-angle glaucoma. A population-based assessment. *Arch Ophthalmol.* 1995;113(2):216–221.
10. Oparil S. Arterial hypertension. In: Wyngaarden JB, Smith LH Jr, Bennet JC, eds. *Cecil Textbook of Medicine.* 20th ed. Philadelphia: W.B. Saunders; 1996:256–270.
11. The sixth report of the Joint National Committee on prevention, detection, evaluation, and treatment of high blood pressure. *Arch Intern Med.* 1997;157:2413–2446.
12. Chobanian AV, Bakris GL, Black HR, et al. The seventh report of the Joint National Committee on prevention, detection, evaluation, and treatment of high blood pressure: the JNC 7 report. *JAMA.* 2003;289(19):2560–2572.
13. Atilla K, Vasan RS. Prehypertension and risk of cardiovascular disease. *Expert Rev Cardiovasc Ther.* 2006;4(1):111–117.
14. Vasan RS, Larson MG, Leip EP, et al. Impact of high normal blood pressure on the risk of cardiovascular disease. *N Engl J Med.* 2001;345(18):1291–1297.
15. Haffner SM, Lehto S, Ronnemaa T, et al. Mortality from coronary heart disease in subjects with type 2 diabetes and in non-diabetic

subjects with and without prior myocardial infarction. *N Eng J Med.* 1998;339(4):229–234.
16. Hansson L, Zanchetti A, Carruthers SG, et al. Effects of intensive blood-pressure lowering and low-dose aspirin in patients with hypertension: principal results of the Hypertension Optimal Treatment (HOT) randomised trial. HOT Study Group. *Lancet.* 1998;351(9118):1755–1762.
17. Tight blood pressure control and risk of macrovascular and microvascular complications in type 2 diabetes: UKPDS 38. UK Prospective Diabetes Study Group. *BMJ.* 1998;317(7160):703–713.
18. Mann JF, Gerstein HC, Pogue J, et al. Renal insufficiency as a predictor of cardiovascular outcomes and the impact of ramipril: the HOPE randomized trial. *Ann Intern Med.* 2001;134(8):629–636.
19. Mann JF, Yi QL, Gerstein HC. Albuminuria as a predictor of cardiovascular and renal outcomes in people with known atherosclerotic cardiovascular disease. *Kidney Int Suppl.* 2004;(92):S59–S62.
20. Duka I, Bakris G. Influence of microalbuminuria in achieving blood pressure goals. *Curr Opin Nephrol Hypertens.* 2008;17(5):457–463.
21. Kario K, Pickering TG, Matsuo T, et al. Stroke prognosis and abnormal nocturnal blood pressure falls in older hypertensives. *Hypertension.* 2001;38(4):852–857.
22. Kario K, Shimada K. Risers and extreme-dippers of nocturnal blood pressure in hypertension: antihypertensive strategy for nocturnal blood pressure. *Clin Exp Hypertens.* 2004;26(2):177–189.
23. Kario K. [Blood pressure variation and cardiovascular risk in hypertension]. *Nippon Rinsho.* 2004;62(11):2145-2156 [in Japanese].
24. Tsivgoulis G, Vemmos KN, Zakopoulos N, et al. Association of blunted nocturnal blood pressure dip with intracerebral hemorrhage. *Blood Press Monit.* 2005;10(4):189–195.
25. Giles TD. Circadian rhythm of blood pressure and the relation to cardiovascular events. *J Hypertens Suppl.* 2006;24(2):S11–S16.
26. Izzedine H, Launay-Vacher V, Deray G. Abnormal blood pressure circadian rhythm: a target organ damage? *Int J Cardiol.* 2006;107(3):343–349.
27. Metoki H, Ohkubo T, Kikuya M, et al. Prognostic significance for stroke of a morning pressor surge and a nocturnal blood pressure decline: the Ohasama study. *Hypertension.* 2006;47(2):149–154.
28. Cicconetti P, Donadio C, Pazzaglia MC, et al. [Circadian rhythm of blood pressure: non-dipping pattern and cardiovascular risk]. *Recenti Prog Med.* 2007;98(7-8):401–406 [in Italian].
29. Schwartz GL, Bailey KR, Mosley T, et al. Association of ambulatory blood pressure with ischemic brain injury. *Hypertension.* 2007;49(6):1228–1234.
30. Hermida RC, Ayala DE, Portaluppi F. Circadian variation of blood pressure: the basis for the chronotherapy of hypertension. *Adv Drug Deliv Rev.* 2007;59(9-10):904–922.
31. Hermida RC, Calvo C, Ayala DE, et al. Dose- and administration time-dependent effects of nifedipine gits on ambulatory blood pressure in hypertensive subjects. *Chronobiol Int.* 2007;24(3):471–493.
32. Hermida RC. Ambulatory blood pressure monitoring in the prediction of cardiovascular events and effects of chronotherapy: rationale and design of the MAPEC study. *Chronobiol Int.* 2007;24(4):749–775.
33. Leske MC, Heijl A, Hyman L, et al. EMGT Group. Predictors of long-term progression in the early manifest glaucoma trial. *Ophthalmology.* 2007;114(11):1965–1972.
34. Leske MC, Wu SY, Hennis A, et al, BESs Study Group. Risk factors for incident open-angle glaucoma: the Barbados Eye Studies. *Ophthalmology.* 2008;115(1):85–93.
35. Prevention of stroke by antihypertensive drug treatment in older persons with isolated systolic hypertension. Final results of the Systolic Hypertension in the Elderly Program (SHEP). SHEP Cooperative Research Group. *JAMA.* 1991;265(24):3255–3264.
36. Black HR. Isolated systolic hypertension in the elderly: lessons from clinical trials and future directions. *J Hypertens Suppl.* 1999;17(5):S49–S54.
37. Wang JG, Staessen JA. The benefit of treating isolated systolic hypertension. *Curr Hypertens Rep.* 2001;3(4):333–339.
38. Staessen JA, Wang JG, Thijs L, Fagard R. Overview of the outcome trials in older patients with isolated systolic hypertension. *J Hum Hypertens.* 1999;13(12):859–863.
39. Pickering TG. Clinical applications of ambulatory blood pressure monitoring: the white coat syndrome. *Clin Invest Med.* 1991; 14(3):212–217.
40. Follman P, Palotas C, Suveges I, Petrovits A. Nocturnal blood pressure and intraocular pressure measurement in glaucoma patients and healthy controls. *Int Ophthalmol.* 1996-1997;20(1-3):83-87.
41. Graham SL, Drance SM, Wijsman K, et al. Ambulatory blood pressure monitoring in glaucoma patients: the nocturnal dip. *Ophthalmology.* 1995;102(1):61–69.
42. Kaiser HJ, Flammer J. Systemic hypotension: risk factor for glaucomatous damage? *Ophthalmologica.* 1991;203(3):105–108.
43. Hayreh SS, Zimmerman MB, Podhajsky P, Alward WL. Nocturnal arterial hypotension and its role in optic nerve head and ocular ischemic disorders. *Am J Ophthalmol.* 1994;117(5):603–624.
44. Orgül S, Kaiser HJ, Flammer J, Gasser P. Systemic blood pressure and capillary blood-cell velocity in glaucoma patients: a preliminary study. *Eur J Ophthalmol.* 1995;5:88-91.
45. Collignon N, Dewe W, Guillaume S, Collignon-Brach J. Ambulatory blood pressure monitoring in glaucoma patients. The nocturnal systolic dip and its relationship with disease progression. *Int Ophthalmol.* 1998;22(1):19–25.
46. Meyer JH, Brandi-Dohrn J, Funk J. Twenty-four hour blood pressure monitoring in normal tension glaucoma. *Br J Ophthalmol.* 1996; 80(10):864–867.
47. Bechetoille A, Bresson-Dumont H. Diurnal and nocturnal blood pressure drops in patients with focal ischemic glaucoma. *Graefes Arch Clin Exp Ophthalmol.* 1994;232(11):675–679.
48. Kashiwagi K, Hosaka O, Tsukahara S. Comparison of nocturnal dip of blood pressure and other blood circulatory parameters in normal tension glaucoma and normal subjects (abstract). *Invest Ophthalmol Vis Sci.* 1997;38(suppl):S274.
49. Detry M, Boschi A, Ellinghaus G, De Plaen JF. Simultaneous 24-hour monitoring of intraocular pressure and arterial blood pressure in patients with progressive and non-progressive primary open-angle glaucoma. *Eur J Ophthalmol.* 1996;6(3):273–278.
50. Dillman WH. The thyroid. In: Wyngaarden JB, Smith LH Jr, Bennet JC, eds. *Cecil Textbook of Medicine,* vol. 2. 20th ed. Philadelphia: W.B. Saunders; 1996:1237–1240.
51. Hertel G. Einiges uber den Augendruck und Glaukom. *Klin Monatsbl Augenheilkd.* 1920;64:390–392.
52. Becker B, Kolker AE, Ballin N. Thyroid function and glaucoma. *Am J Ophthalmol.* 1966;61:997–999.
53. Pohjanpelto P. The thyroid gland and intraocular pressure. Tonographic study of 187 patients with thyroid disease. *Acta Ophthalmol (Copenh).* 1968:suppl 97:1–70.
54. Smith KD, Tevaarwerk GJ, Allen LH. An ocular dynamic study supporting the hypothesis that hypothyroidism is a treatable cause of secondary open-angle glaucoma. *Can J Ophthalmol.* 1992;27(7): 341–344.
55. Bahçeci UA, Ozdek S, Pehlivanli Z, et al. Changes in intraocular pressure and corneal and retinal nerve fiber layer thicknesses in hypothyroidism. *Eur J Ophthalmol.* 2005;15(5):556–561.
56. Smith KD, Tevaarwerk GJ, Allen LH. Reversal of poorly controlled glaucoma on diagnosis and treatment of hypothyroidism. *Can J Ophthalmol.* 1992;27(7):345–347.
57. Smith KD, Arthurs BP, Saheb N. An association between hypothyroidism and primary open-angle glaucoma. *Ophthalmology.* 1993;100(10):1580–1584.
58. Gillow JT, Shah P, O'Neill EC. Primary open angle glaucoma and hypothyroidism: chance or true association? *Eye.* 1997;11(Pt 1):113–114.
59. Muñoz-Negrete FJ, Rebolleda G, Almodóvar F, et al. Hypothyroidism and primary open-angle glaucoma. *Ophthalmologica.* 2000;214(5): 347–349.

60. Tahat AA, al-Khawaldeh AM. Hypothyroidism and open-angle glaucoma: an accidental or an essential coexistence? *East Mediterr Health J*. 2000;6(2-3):299–303.
61. Karadimas P, Bouzas EA, Topouzis F, et al. Hypothyroidism and glaucoma. A study of 100 hypothyroid patients. *Am J Ophthalmol*. 2001;131(1):126–128.
62. Gawaii H, Friedrich Y, Dickstein G, Friedman Z. [Does hypothyroidism contribute to the etiology of primary open angle glaucoma or is it just a coincidence?] *Harefuah*. 2003;142(4):246–248, 320 [in Hebrew].
63. Lee AJ, Rochtchina E, Wang JJ, et al. Open-angle glaucoma and systemic thyroid disease in an older population: The Blue Mountains Eye Study. *Eye*. 2004;18(6):600–608.
64. Girkin CA, McGwin G Jr, McNeal SF, et al. Hypothyroidism and the development of open-angle glaucoma in a male population. *Ophthalmology*. 2004;111(9):1649–1652.
65. Motsko SP, Jones JK. Is there an association between hypothyroidism and open-angle glaucoma in an elderly population? An epidemiologic study. *Ophthalmology*. 2008;115(9):1581–1584.
66. Sherwin RS. Diabetes mellitus. In: Wyngaarden JB, Smith LH Jr, Bennet JC, eds. *Cecil Textbook of Medicine*, vol. 2. 20th ed. Philadelphia: W.B. Saunders; 1996:1258–1277.
67. Kannel WB, McGee DL. Diabetes and cardiovascular risk factors: the Framingham study. *Circulation*. 1979;59(1):8-13.
68. Kannel WB, McGee DL. Diabetes and glucose tolerance as risk factors for cardiovascular disease: the Framingham study. *Diabetes Care*. 1979;2(2):120–126.
69. Brewer HB Jr. New features of the National Cholesterol Education Program Adult Treatment Panel III lipid-lowering guidelines. *Clin Cardiol*. 2003;26(4 suppl 3):III19–III24.
70. Grundy SM, Cleeman JI, Merz CN, et al. Coordinating Committee of the National Cholesterol Education Program Implications of recent clinical trials for the National Cholesterol Education Program Adult Treatment Panel III Guidelines. *J Am Coll Cardiol*. 2004;44(3):720–732.
71. Kohzaki K, Vingrys AJ, Bui BV. Early inner retinal dysfunction in streptozotocin-induced diabetic rats. *Invest Ophthalmol Vis Sci*. 2008;49(8):3595–3604.
72. Qin Y, Xu G, Wang W. Dendritic abnormalities in retinal ganglion cells of three-month diabetic rats. *Curr Eye Res*. 2006;31(11):967–974.
73. Zhang L, Ino-ue M, Dong K, Yamamoto M. Retrograde axonal transport impairment of large- and medium-sized retinal ganglion cells in diabetic rat. *Curr Eye Res*. 2000;20(2):131–136.
74. Soares AS, Artes PH, Andreou P, et al. Factors associated with optic disc hemorrhages in glaucoma. *Ophthalmology*. 2004;111(9):1653–1657.
75. Elisaf M, Kitsos G, Bairaktari E, et al. Metabolic abnormalities in patients with primary open-angle glaucoma. *Acta Ophthalmol Scand*. 2001;79(2):129–132.
76. Oh SW, Lee S, Park C, Kim DJ. Elevated intraocular pressure is associated with insulin resistance and metabolic syndrome. *Diabetes Metab Res Rev*. 2005;21(5):434–440.
77. Gordon MO, Beiser JA, Kass MA, Ocular Hypertension Treatment Study Group. Is a history of diabetes mellitus protective against developing primary open-angle glaucoma? *Arch Ophthalmol*. 2008;126(2):280–281.
78. Tielsch JM, Katz J, Quigley HA, et al. Diabetes, intraocular pressure, and primary open-angle glaucoma in the Baltimore Eye Survey. *Ophthalmology*. 1995;102(1):48–53.
79. Sommer A. Glaucoma risk factors observed in the Baltimore Eye Survey. *Curr Opin Ophthalmol*. 1996;7(2):93–98.
80. Vijaya L, George R, Baskaran M, et al. Prevalence of primary open-angle glaucoma in an urban south Indian population and comparison with a rural population. The Chennai Glaucoma Study. *Ophthalmology*. 2008;115(4):648–654.
81. de Voogd S, Ikram MK, Wolfs RC, et al. Is diabetes mellitus a risk factor for open-angle glaucoma? The Rotterdam Study. *Ophthalmology*. 2006;113(10):1827–1831.
82. Ellis JD, Evans JM, Ruta DA, et al. Glaucoma incidence in an unselected cohort of diabetic patients: is diabetes mellitus a risk factor for glaucoma? DARTS/MEMO collaboration. Diabetes Audit and Research in Tayside Study. Medicines Monitoring Unit. *Br J Ophthalmol*. 2000;84(11):1218–1224.
83. Klein BE, Klein R, Moss SE. Intraocular pressure in diabetic persons. *Ophthalmology*. 1984;91(11):1356–1360.
84. Klein BE, Klein R, Moss SE. Incidence of self-reported glaucoma in people with diabetes mellitus. *Br J Ophthalmol*. 1997;81(9):743–747.
85. Memarzadeh F, Ying-Lai M, Azen SP, Varma R, Los Angeles Latino Eye Study Group. Associations with intraocular pressure in Latinos: the Los Angeles Latino Eye Study. *Am J Ophthalmol*. 2008;146(1):69–76.
86. Chopra V, Varma R, Francis BA, et al, Los Angeles Latino Eye Study Group. Type 2 diabetes mellitus and the risk of open-angle glaucoma the Los Angeles Latino Eye Study. *Ophthalmology*. 2008;115(2):227–232.e1.
87. Hennis A, Wu SY, Nemesure B, Leske MC, Barbados Eye Studies Group. Hypertension, diabetes, and longitudinal changes in intraocular pressure. *Ophthalmology*. 2003;110(5):908–914.
88. Leske MC, Wu SY, Hennis A, et al, Barbados Eye Studies Group. Nine-year incidence of age-related macular degeneration in the Barbados Eye Studies. *Ophthalmology*. 2006;113(1):29–35.
89. Pasquale LR, Kang JH, Manson JE, et al. Prospective study of type 2 diabetes mellitus and risk of primary open-angle glaucoma in women. *Ophthalmology*. 2006;113(7):1081–1086.
90. Medeiros FA, Weinreb RN, Sample PA, et al. Validation of a predictive model to estimate the risk of conversion from ocular hypertension to glaucoma. *Arch Ophthalmol*. 2005;123(10):1351–1360.
91. Miglior S, Zeyen T, Pfeiffer N, et al, European Glaucoma Prevention Study Group. The European glaucoma prevention study design and baseline description of the participants. *Ophthalmology*. 2002;109(9):1612–1621.
92. Miglior S, Zeyen T, Pfeiffer N, et al, European Glaucoma Prevention Study (EGPS) Group. Results of the European Glaucoma Prevention Study. *Ophthalmology*. 2005;112(3):366–375.
93. Bonovas S, Peponis V, Filioussi K. Diabetes mellitus as a risk factor for primary open-angle glaucoma: a meta-analysis. *Diabet Med*. 2004;21(6):609–614.
94. Krueger RR, Ramos-Esteban JC. How might corneal elasticity help us understand diabetes and intraocular pressure? *J Refract Surg*. 2007;23(1):85–88.
95. Plum F. Disorders of sleep and arousal. In: Wyngaarden JB, Smith LH Jr, Bennet JC, eds. *Cecil Textbook of Medicine*. 20th ed. Philadelphia: W.B. Saunders; 1996:1982–1985.
96. Punjabi NM. The epidemiology of adult obstructive sleep apnea. *Proc Am Thorac Soc*. 2008;5(2):136–143.
97. Ferini-Strambi L, Fantini ML, Castronovo C. Epidemiology of obstructive sleep apnea syndrome. *Minerva Med*. 2004;95(3):187–202.
98. Stradling JR, Davies RJ. Obstructive sleep apnoea/hypopnoea syndrome: definitions, epidemiology, and natural history. *Thorax*. 2004;59(1):73–78.
99. Dorasamy P. Obstructive sleep apnea and cardiovascular risk. *Ther Clin Risk Manag*. 2007;3(6):1105–1111.
100. Peppard PE, Young T, Palta M, et al. Longitudinal study of moderate weight change and sleep-disordered breathing. *JAMA*. 2000;284(23):3015–3021.
101. Newman AB, Foster G, Givelber R, et al. Progression and regression of sleep-disordered breathing with changes in weight: the Sleep Heart Health Study. *Arch Intern Med*. 2005;165(20):2408–2413.
102. Yilmaz F, Ozyildirim S, Talay F, et al. Obstructive sleep apnea as a risk factor for cardiovascular diseases. *Cardiol J*. 2007;14(6):534–537.

103. Chami HA, Devereux RB, Gottdiener JS, et al. Left ventricular morphology and systolic function in sleep-disordered breathing: the Sleep Heart Health Study. *Circulation*. 2008;117(20):2599–2607.
104. Peppard PE, Young T, Palta M, Skatrud J. Prospective study of the association between sleep-disordered breathing and hypertension. *N Engl J Med*. 2000;342(19):1378–1384.
105. Young T, Peppard P, Palta M, et al. Population-based study of sleep-disordered breathing as a risk factor for hypertension. *Arch Intern Med*. 1997;157(15):1746–1752.
106. Valham F, Mooe T, Rabben T, et al. Increased risk of stroke in patients with coronary artery disease and sleep apnea: a 10-year follow-up. *Circulation*. 2008;118(9):955–960.
107. Punjabi NM, Polotsky VY. Disorders of glucose metabolism in sleep apnea. *J Appl Physiol*. 2005;99:1998–2007.
108. Young T, Finn L, Peppard PE, et al. Sleep disordered breathing and mortality: eighteen-year follow-up of the Wisconsin sleep cohort. *Sleep*. 2008;31(8):1071–1078.
109. Marshall NS, Wong KK, Liu PY, et al. Sleep apnea as an independent risk factor for all-cause mortality: the Busselton Health Study. *Sleep*. 2008;31(8):1079–1085.
110. Sanders MH, Montserrat JM, Farré R, Givelber RJ. Positive pressure therapy: a perspective on evidence-based outcomes and methods of application. *Proc Am Thorac Soc*. 2008;5(2):161–172.
111. Mojon DS, Hess CW, Goldblum D, et al. High prevalence of glaucoma in patients with sleep apnea syndrome. *Ophthalmology*. 1999;106(5):1009–1012.
112. Karakucuk S, Goktas S, Aksu M. Ocular blood flow in patients with obstructive sleep apnea syndrome (OSAS). *Graef Arch Clin Exp Ophthalmol*. 2008;246(1):129-134.
113. Mojon DS, Hess CW, Goldblum D, et al. Primary open-angle glaucoma is associated with sleep apnea syndrome. *Ophthalmologica*. 2000;214(2):115–118.
114. Bendel RE, Kaplan J, Heckman M, Fredrickson PA, Lin SC. Prevalence of glaucoma in patients with obstructive sleep apnoea across-sectional case-series. *Eye*. 2007;22(9):1105–1109.
115. Sergi M, Salerno DE, Rizzi M, et al. Prevalence of normal tension glaucoma in obstructive sleep apnea syndrome patients. *J Glaucoma*. 2007;16(1):42–46.
116. Batisse JL, Vix J, Swalduz B, et al. Sleep-related breathing disorders and normal or high-tension glaucoma: 35 patients with polysomnographic records. *J Fr Ophtalmol*. 2004;27(6 Pt 1):605–612.
117. Girkin CA, McGwin G Jr, McNeal SF, Owsley C. Is there an association between pre-existing sleep apnoea and the development of glaucoma? *Br J Ophthalmol*. 2006;90(6):679–681.
118. Geyer O, Cohen N, Segev E, et al. The prevalence of glaucoma in patients with sleep apnea syndrome: same as in the general population. *Am J Ophthalmol*. 2003;136(6):1093–1096.
119. Mojon DS, Hess CW, Goldblum D, et al. Normal-tension glaucoma is associated with sleep apnea syndrome. *Ophthalmologica*. 2002;216(3):180–184.
120. Marcus DM, Costarides AP, Gokhale P, et al. Sleep disorders: a risk factor for normal-tension glaucoma? *J Glaucoma*. 2001;10(3):177–183.
121. Onen SH, Mouriaux F, Berramdane L, et al. High prevalence of sleep-disordered breathing in patients with primary open-angle glaucoma. *Acta Ophthalmol Scand*. 2000;78(6):638–641.
122. Shaw SM, Fildes JE, Yonan N, Williams SG. Pleiotropic effects and cholesterol-lowering therapy. *Cardiology*. 2008;112(1):4–12.
123. Schönbeck U, Libby P. Inflammation, immunity, and HMG-CoA reductase inhibitors: statins as antiinflammatory agents? *Circulation*. 2004;109(21 suppl 1):II18–II26.
124. Correia LC. Is there a true beneficial effect of statin therapy in the acute phase of unstable angina or myocardial infarction? *Curr Vasc Pharmacol*. 2007;5(3):221–225.
125. Arca M, Gaspardone A. Atorvastatin efficacy in the primary and secondary prevention of cardiovascular events. *Drugs*. 2007;67(Suppl 1):29–42.
126. Schwartz GG, Olsson AG, Ezekowitz MD, et al, Myocardial Ischemia Reduction with Aggressive Cholesterol Lowering (MIRACL) Study Investigators. Effects of atorvastatin on early recurrent ischemic events in acute coronary syndromes: the MIRACL study: a randomized controlled trial. *JAMA*. 2001;285(13):1711–1718.
127. Pedersen TR, Faergeman O, Kastelein JJ, et al, Incremental Decrease in End Points Through Aggressive Lipid Lowering (IDEAL) Study Group. High-dose atorvastatin vs usual-dose simvastatin for secondary prevention after myocardial infarction: the IDEAL study: a randomized controlled trial. *JAMA*. 2005;294(19):2437–2445.
128. Patti G, Pasceri V, Colonna G, et al. Atorvastatin pretreatment improves outcomes in patients with acute coronary syndromes undergoing early percutaneous coronary intervention: results of the ARMYDA-ACS randomized trial. *J Am Coll Cardiol*. 2007;49(12):1272–1278.
129. Patti G, Chello M, Candura D, et al. Randomized trial of atorvastatin for reduction of postoperative atrial fibrillation in patients undergoing cardiac surgery: results of the ARMYDA-3 (Atorvastatin for Reduction of MYocardial Dysrhythmia After cardiac surgery) study. *Circulation*. 2006;114(14):1455–1461.
130. Tokaç M, Ozeren A, Aktan M, et al. The role of inflammation markers in triggering acute coronary events. *Heart Vessels*. 2003;18(4):171–176.
131. Blake GJ, Ridker PM. C-reactive protein and other inflammatory risk markers in acute coronary syndromes. *J Am Coll Cardiol*. 2003;41(4 suppl S):37S–42S.
132. Kinlay S, Schwartz GG, Olsson AG, et al, Myocardial Ischemia Reduction with Aggressive Cholesterol Lowering Study Investigators. High-dose atorvastatin enhances the decline in inflammatory markers in patients with acute coronary syndromes in the MIRACL study. *Circulation*. 2003;108(13):1560–1566.
133. Chan KY, Boucher ES, Gandhi PJ, Silva MA. HMG-CoA reductase inhibitors for lowering elevated levels of C-reactive protein. *Am J Health Syst Pharm*. 2004;61(16):1676–1681.
134. Tezel G, Yang J, Wax MB. Heat shock proteins, immunity and glaucoma. *Brain Res Bull*. 2004;62(6):473–480.
135. Wax MB, Tezel G. Neurobiology of glaucomatous optic neuropathy: diverse cellular events in neurodegeneration and neuroprotection. *Mol Neurobiol*. 2002;26(1):45–55.
136. Wax M, Yang J, Tezel G. Autoantibodies in glaucoma. *Curr Eye Res*. 2002;25(2):113–116.
137. Wax MB, Tezel G, Kawase K, Kitazawa Y. Serum autoantibodies to heat shock proteins in glaucoma patients from Japan and the United States. *Ophthalmology*. 2001;108(2):296–302.
138. Franklin TB, Krueger-Naug AM, et al. The role of heat shock proteins Hsp70 and Hsp27 in cellular protection of the central nervous system. *Int J Hyperthermia*. 2005;21(5):379–392.
139. Whitlock NA, Lindsey K, Agarwal N, et al. Heat shock protein 27 delays Ca2+-induced cell death in a caspase-dependent and -independent manner in rat retinal ganglion cells. *Invest Ophthalmol Vis Sci*. 2005;46(3):1085–1091.
140. Schmeer CW, Gamez A, Tausch S, et al. Statins modulate heat shock protein expression and enhance retinal ganglion cell survival after transient retinal ischemia/reperfusion in vivo. *Invest Ophthalmol Vis Sci*. 2008;49(11):4971–4981.
141. Kretz A, Schmeer C, Tausch S, Isenmann S. Simvastatin promotes heat shock protein 27 expression and Akt activation in the rat retina and protects axotomized retinal ganglion cells in vivo. *Neurobiol Dis*. 2006;21(2):421–430.
142. De Castro DK, Punjabi OS, Bostrom AG, et al. Effect of statin drugs and aspirin on progression in open-angle glaucoma suspects using confocal scanning laser ophthalmoscopy. *Clin Experiment Ophthalmol*. 2007;35(6):506–513.
143. McGwin G Jr, McNeal S, Owsley C, et al. Statins and other cholesterol-lowering medications and the presence of glaucoma. *Arch Ophthalmol*. 2004;122(6):822–826.

# Part V
# The Surgical Treatment

# Chapter 61
# Laser Therapies: Iridotomy, Iridoplasty, and Trabeculoplasty

Douglas Gaasterland

The name "laser" is an acronym for Light Amplification by Stimulated Emission of Radiation. In 1960, Theodore Maiman built the first working laser; the medium was a ruby crystal.[1] Due to unique properties of the laser beam, the intensity of the focused output from lasers was an early, recognized attraction for treating the eye. Photons from the laser source had the same direction of travel, with minimal divergence, and were all of the same wavelength (monochromatic), coherence, and polarization. This reduced aberrations when directed to a focus. These properties minimized the focus spot diameter. Useful summaries of laser light properties for eye applications are available.[2] Within a short interval after laser introduction, systems to treat the eye were under study. The initial applications were reported by Zaret et al for iris and retina in rabbits in 1961[3]; and for human retina by Campbell et al and Kapany et al in 1963.[4,5]

Depending on the instrument design, the output beam from a laser is either *continuous*, resembling light from a light bulb, or *pulsed*. With electronic switches, continuous laser output can be turned on and off rapidly and precisely. By contrast, pulsed output is repetitive, with numerous repeated pulses generated by the system, each pulse with a short on-time and a longer off-time. Alternatively, the output of the system can be manipulated within the laser cavity to be in the form of single, brief, high energy pulses. These pulses are identified as *Q-switched* when the laser cavity geometry results in a single "giant" pulse output, with duration measured in nanoseconds ($10^{-9}$ s). The pulses are identified as *mode-locked* when the laser cavity geometry results in a short train of brief pulses with picosecond ($10^{-12}$ s) duration all enclosed within a nanosecond envelope. The wavelength of the output photons depends on the type of atoms or molecules forming the active media within the laser cavity. For medical applications, wavelengths are available from the deep ultraviolet, as from excimer systems, to the far infrared, as from carbon dioxide lasers. Excimer laser systems represent the special case of deep ultraviolet light emitted as long trains of brief (nanosecond) pulses from a cavity containing rare gas halides; the wavelength varies with the type of halide (for example, 193 nm from argon fluoride to 308 nm from xenon chloride).

The output of continuous wave and repetitively pulsed lasers is measured in watts, the quotient of the total energy out per duration of on-time. Single-pulsed laser output is measured in joules per pulse.

Photons from lasers either traverse or are absorbed by target tissue, depending on the photon wavelength and the pigmented chromatophores in the tissue. Absorption is wavelength dependent and can cause local heating. If exposure is long enough, the result is *coagulation* of proteins within the target and spread of heat to nearby tissue. This is the usual interaction with continuous wave laser light and with repetitive, low-energy pulsed laser light, provided the interval between pulses is sufficiently short that the target tissue does not cool before the next pulse arrives. By contrast, Q-switched and excimer pulses deliver massive numbers of photons at the focus during the short on-time interval. If enough photons are present during this interval, electrons are stripped away from molecules within the focal volume, with the resultant ionization causing a local microexplosion with Q-switched laser light and photochemical ablation with excimer laser light.[6,7] If the Q-switched interaction is strong enough, the target tissue undergoes *disruption*. Two tissue interactions due to photon absorption – *coagulation* and *disruption* – are the underlying bases for glaucoma laser treatments. Studies of excimer systems for glaucoma interventions have not yet yielded clinical systems or methods.

## 61.1 Trabecular Meshwork

Trabeculoplasty – trabecular meshwork laser treatment – is a beneficial, effective laser treatment for several, yet not for all, types of open-angle glaucoma. Delivery of laser energy for this treatment requires a clear gonioscopic view, with unequivocal identification of the trabecular meshwork within the anterior chamber angle recess.

### 61.1.1 Indications and Contraindications

The patient with glaucoma has, by definition, optic nerve damage. The management goal is to inhibit progression of the damage. Reduction of intraocular pressure (IOP) to a target range substantially lower than the baseline in eyes with high-risk ocular hypertension and those with established glaucoma preserves visual function (as measured by the optic nerve morphology or the visual field), no matter what the sustained baseline elevation of IOP or how early, or advanced, the stage of the nerve damage.[8–12]

The goal of laser trabeculoplasty in glaucoma is to lower IOP from the pretreatment level. There are several eligibility and exclusion criteria for an eye to be treatable and to have an expected beneficial response.

*First, the eye should have glaucoma and be at a stage where something should be done to further lower IOP.* Either there has been a demonstration of advancing visual system damage at the current sustained level of IOP, or there is high risk for worsening to occur – usually there is a threatening elevation of the IOP (this is a criterion difficult to define; it usually encompasses a sustained IOP elevation to a level at which visual system damage is likely to occur) – despite treatment already prescribed. Sometimes trabeculoplasty is considered as an alternative to escalation of topical or systemic medical treatment or for eyes already prescribed maximum-tolerated, effective, and acceptable (to the patient) medical treatment.

*Second, the eye considered for trabeculectomy must be treatable.* This, of course, seems obvious; yet it is important that the eye have an open angle with identifiable trabecular meshwork in most, if not all, of the anterior segment circumference. If the doctor cannot see the target tissue, then it will not be amenable to laser treatment. The treating physician's gonioscopic skill is important. The anterior chamber angle structures, particularly trabecular meshwork, must be identifiable. Trabecular meshwork, which overlies Schlemm's canal, should be distinguished from the deposition in some eyes of pigment in the inferior angle recess forming Sampaolesi's line anterior to Schwalbe's line. Treating Sampaolesi's line is not beneficial.

*Third, the patient must be treatable, including having given informed consent.* Patient cooperation is needed during treatment. If the patient cannot cooperate then there is reduced ability to apply the laser energy accurately to the target tissue. Squirming, squeezing, nystagmus, and easy fatigue all make treatment difficult or impossible. This alone excludes most children, who typically get minimal benefit from trabeculoplasty anyway.

*Fourth, some types of open-angle glaucoma are unlikely to get a meaningful or durable response to trabeculoplasty in any of its forms.* Eyes with these types of glaucoma should not be treated. For example, eyes with congenital glaucoma, the juvenile onset glaucoma associated with unusual angle structure, uveitic glaucoma, glaucoma associated with angle recession, and neovascular glaucoma seldom respond sufficiently or favorably.[13] Eyes with primary open-angle glaucoma, serious optic nerve damage, a target pressure in the midteens or lower, and extreme IOP elevation despite medical treatment (above 35 mmHg is a useful guideline) are not good candidates. Early reports indicated aphakic eyes were not likely to derive a beneficial response from argon laser trabeculoplasty (ALT).[14] By contrast, clinical experience has indicated that pseudophakic eyes respond like phakic eyes to the various forms of laser trabeculoplasty. Eyes with previous continuous wave laser trabeculoplasty seldom respond meaningfully to repeat continuous wave laser trabeculoplasty, with the response being time-limited in the minority of eyes that respond at all. By contrast, primary open-angle glaucoma without extreme IOP elevation, normal pressure glaucoma, residual open-angle glaucoma after iridotomy, and secondary open-angle glaucoma due to pigment dispersion or pseudoexfoliation are, in general, responsive to one or another form of laser trabeculoplasty.[13]

### 61.1.2 History

The early investigators of trabeculoplasty in glaucomatous eyes – including Hans Hager using continuous wave lasers[15] and Michail Krasnov using high-power, Q-switched pulsed lasers – believed they would be able to drill holes in the trabecular meshwork, enhancing aqueous humor outflow.[16] These early treatment reports, and those of others, demonstrated a useful IOP lowering that tended to persist in some eyes. Although early animal and human eye histologic studies indicated healing of treatment sites in the trabecular tissue, with local scarring, the early investigators continued to believe that their treatment methods opened the trabecular mesh; they showed that for a meaningful proportion of eyes, the laser treatment method was beneficial for the long-term.[17] Widespread and enthusiastic acceptance of continuous wave argon laser treatment followed introduction by Wise and Witter in 1979 of a trabeculoplasty method employing circumferential trabecular treatment with 100 evenly spaced, short (0.1 s duration), small spot size (50 µm in air) laser applications of 1.0–1.5 W to the pigmented trabecular band.[14] They used an antireflective-coated three-mirror Goldmann contact lens for anterior chamber examination and treatment. The laser power was selected based on amount of trabecular pigmentation – higher power for lightly pigmented tissue – and on target tissue response, blanching at the threshold of bubble formation being ideal. There followed a long-term drop of IOP in most treated eyes. With a few modifications and enhancements, this method has continued in use for continuous wave laser trabeculoplasty.[18] Subsequent reports indicated that slightly lower power was usually sufficient and that eyes often responded favorably with treatment limited to half the trabecular circumference.[19] This allowed divided treatment, the second step being applied to a new location in the trabecular tissue circumference, when a second step became needed. It reduced the potential for treatment-related problems and avoided the scarring related to retreatment of the same site.[20] It was known that scarring from heavy, aggressive retreatment could actually cause glaucomatous IOP elevations in normal monkey eyes.[21] Later clinical studies showed that second trabeculoplasties, with retreatment of the same part of the trabecular circumference, were seldom beneficial in the long-term.

This early work was with argon laser systems with blue–green output (mixed 488 nm and 514.5 nm wavelengths) or green output (514.5 nm). Subsequent clinical studies have shown that other continuous wave lasers – including frequency-doubled neodymium/yttrium–aluminum–garnet (YAG) (532 nm), krypton yellow (568.2 nm) and red (647.1 nm), and near-infrared diode (810 nm) – are effective for trabeculoplasty; these wavelengths are all relatively high on the absorption spectrum of melanin, though the shorter wavelengths are slightly better absorbed.

Trabeculoplasty increases outflow of aqueous humor. What is the mechanism? The initial impression, proposed by Wise,[22] soon after his initial paper, was that laser-induced "…microscars reduced the diameter of the trabecular ring, tightening the meshwork, and restoring function…" This led to the name of the procedure as "trabeculoplasty."

Histologic studies have clarified that treatment with continuous wave lasers does not create persistent new holes through the trabecular meshwork to Schlemm's canal. Treatment sites heal with smooth scars covered by cells resembling corneal endothelium.[23] As time has passed, an alternative hypothesis has gained credence. Laser applications cause altered biochemical function with trabecular cellular division and spreading not only at the target site but also within trabecular tissue distant from the target. The resultant tissue changes, both biochemical and cellular, restore trabecular function and improve aqueous drainage.[24,25] This explanation is now more widely accepted, particularly so since demonstration that trabeculoplasty methods with low-energy, pulsed lasers improve aqueous outflow without coagulating target tissue or causing trabecular scarring.

Capitalizing on the observation of Anderson and Parish that low-energy, brief laser pulses caused selective photothermolysis of targeted cells,[26] Latina and Park studied laser effects on cultured pigmented and nonpigmented trabecular cells.[27] They sought a form of laser delivery that would selectively damage trabecular cells containing melanin pigment granules, sparing adjacent nonpigmented cells. They learned that frequency-doubled neodymium (Nd)-YAG, large diameter (400 μm), Q-switched, low-energy pulses caused this effect on pigmented trabecular cells with no collateral thermal damage. They applied these observations to development of a clinical system for trabecular treatment that they named *selective laser trabeculoplasty* (SLT); clinical studies demonstrated efficacy similar to that of continuous wave, coagulative laser trabeculoplasty, yet lacking thermal effects and avoiding scarring of target trabecular tissue.[28–30]

Recent, preliminary clinical studies indicate a similar beneficial trabeculoplasty effect after micropulsed diode laser delivery. In this modality, the laser energy is delivered as large diameter (300 μm) applications of about 100 brief pulses each with a duration of 0.3 ms, or 300 μs, with a comparatively long off-time (1.7 ms) between pulses, with all the pulses delivered in a 0.2 s (200 ms) envelope (Fig. 61.1)

In summary, the continuous wave laser system trabeculoplasty techniques use small focal spot sizes with large energy coagulation that spreads from the treatment sites. The short-pulsed systems use large spot sizes with relatively

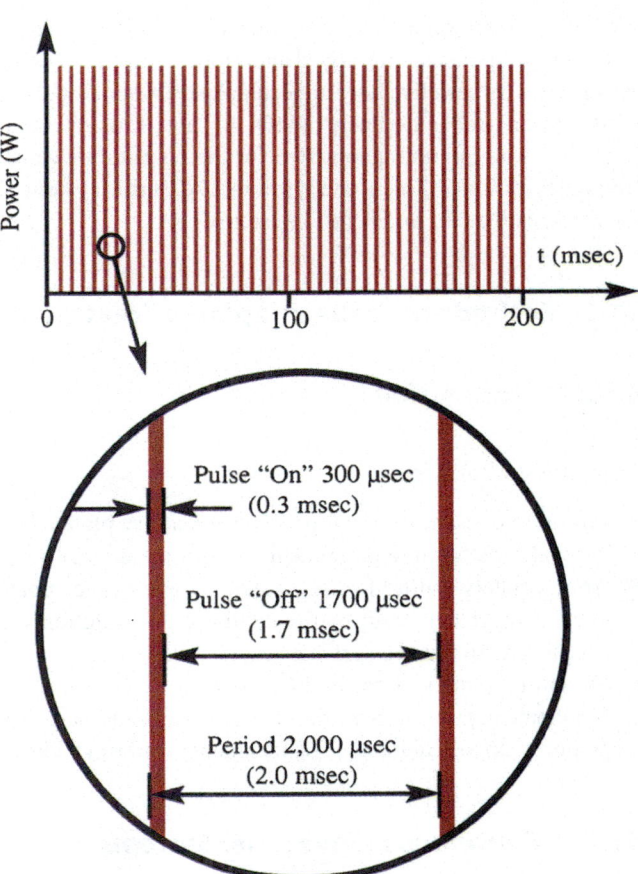

**Fig. 61.1** Diagram illustrating micropulsed diode laser energy delivery in a 15% duty cycle. Laser turned on for 300 μs and off for 1,700 μs, thus on for 15% of 2,000 μs envelope of cycle. Power of each application, 2.0 W, consists of 100 pulses, each of 4.0 mJ, delivered in 200 ms (0.2 s). Thus, 400 mJ (0.4 J) in 0.2 s, which is equal to 2.0 W. (Illustration courtesy of IRIDEX Corp., Mountain View, CA)

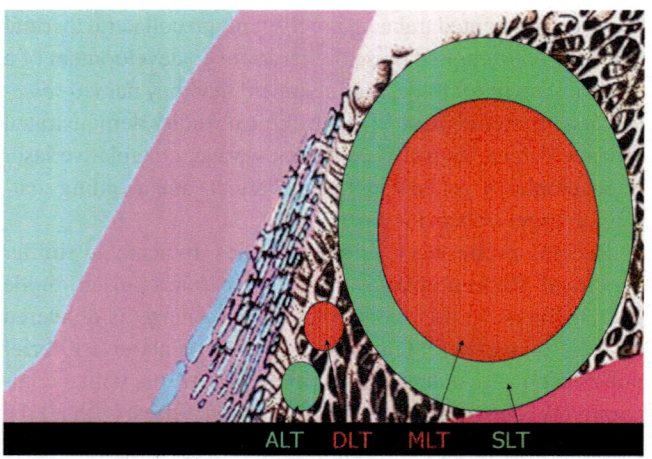

**Fig. 61.2** Laser spot sizes on trabecular meshwork during trabeculoplasty. Spot size for Selective Laser Trabeculoplasty (SLT) (400 μm) is larger than for Micropulsed Diode Laser Trabeculoplasty (MDLT) (300 μm). Both are much larger than coagulative trabeculoplasty spot sizes (50–75 μm). (Illustration courtesy of IRIDEX Corp., Mountain View, CA)

low-energy interaction that is confined to the treatment sites. The relative spot sizes for argon and diode continuous wave systems and for selective laser trabeculoplasty and micropulsed diode laser trabeculoplasty (MDLT) are illustrated in Fig. 61.2. The treatment spot size for the continuous wave, frequency-doubled green neodymium:YAG laser system is the same as that for argon laser systems.

## 61.2 Methods of Trabeculoplasty Treatment

### 61.2.1 Preparation

There are several steps:

- Informed consent for the type of laser surgery planned.
- Topical anesthesia (e.g., tetracaine or proparacaine).
- Appropriately antireflective-coated, gonioscopic treatment contact lens with methylcellulose 1% solution for coupling with the eye surface.
- Slit lamp biomicroscope delivery system.
- Anticipating posttreatment pressure spikes, some surgeons pretreat with topical Iopidine (apraclonidine) or brimonidine.

### 61.2.2 Continuous Wave Laser Systems

#### 61.2.2.1 Treatment and Suggested Settings

- Set laser system at spot size 50–75 μm, 0.4–1.0 W power, 0.1 s duration.
- Decide the extent of the circumference to be treated – 50 or 100%.
- Apply approximately 50 (for one-half the circumference treatment) or 100 (for circumferential treatment) evenly spaced laser applications, each aimed at the anterior border of the pigmented trabecular meshwork.
- Adjust power during treatment for local blanching at the threshold for small bubble formation during laser applications.[18]
- Record the approximate percent of applications with blanching, bubble formation, or both in the procedure note.

#### 61.2.2.2 Postoperative Care

For the first postoperative days, add topical steroid medication to the continued use of preoperative glaucoma medications

### 61.2.3 Selective Laser Trabeculoplasty

#### 61.2.3.1 Treatment and Suggested Settings

- The Selective Laser Trabeculoplasty (SLT) laser system (Lumenis, Inc., Santa Clara, CA) has a spot size of both the low-power helium–neon aiming beam and the treatment beam of 400 μm; the aiming beam is directed to cover the entire meridional height of the pigmented trabecular meshwork.
- The initial energy setting for each treatment pulse is 0.8 mJ, with pulse energy adjustable from 0.2 to 1.7 mJ; pulse energy is adjusted during treatment to the threshold for small "champagne" bubbles within target tissue, which should occur in about half of the applications.[30]
- Decide the extent of the circumference to be treated: 50 or 100%.
- Using an appropriate treatment contact lens, apply approximately 50 (for one-half the circumference treatment) or 100 (for circumferential treatment) adjacent, nonoverlapping, evenly spaced laser applications, each aimed at the center of the pigmented trabecular meshwork.
- In the procedure note include the treatment parameters, including pulse energy, amount, and location of trabecular circumference treated, and number of applications.

#### 61.2.3.2 Postoperative Care

For the first postoperative days, add topical nonsteroidal anti-inflammatory medication or steroid to the continued use of preoperative glaucoma medications; because the treatment effect depends upon a macrophage response, aggressive suppression of the inflammatory response is relatively contraindicated.

## 61.2.4 Micropulsed Diode Laser Trabeculoplasty

### 61.2.4.1 Treatment and Suggested Settings

- The IQ 810 diode laser system with slit lamp adaptor (IRIDEX Inc., Mountain View, CA) has an adjustable spot size of both the low-power helium–neon aiming beam and the treatment beam from 50 to 300 μm; use the 300 μm diameter and direct the aiming beam to center on the meridional height of the pigmented trabecular meshwork. This size usually covers the entire pigmented trabecular meshwork.
- The laser system is set during system initiation to deliver individual applications consisting of a series of 100 micropulses, each with a duration of 0.3 ms (300 μs) and each followed by a 1.7 ms off time (this is a 15% "duty cycle"), all within a 200 ms (0.2 s) envelope. Each pulse delivers about 4 mJ. The power indicated in the system console represents the sum of the energy of all the pulses divided by the duration of the envelope; it is typically about 2,000 mW (2.0 W) (see Fig. 61.1). The short duration of each pulse of light within the envelope, followed by the comparatively long off-time, ensures localization of light energy to pigment granules within cells in the irradiated zone, without spread of coagulative heat to adjacent structures (Fig. 61.3). Thus this treatment interaction resembles the tissue effect of SLT. These applications cause no observable change in the target tissue, so

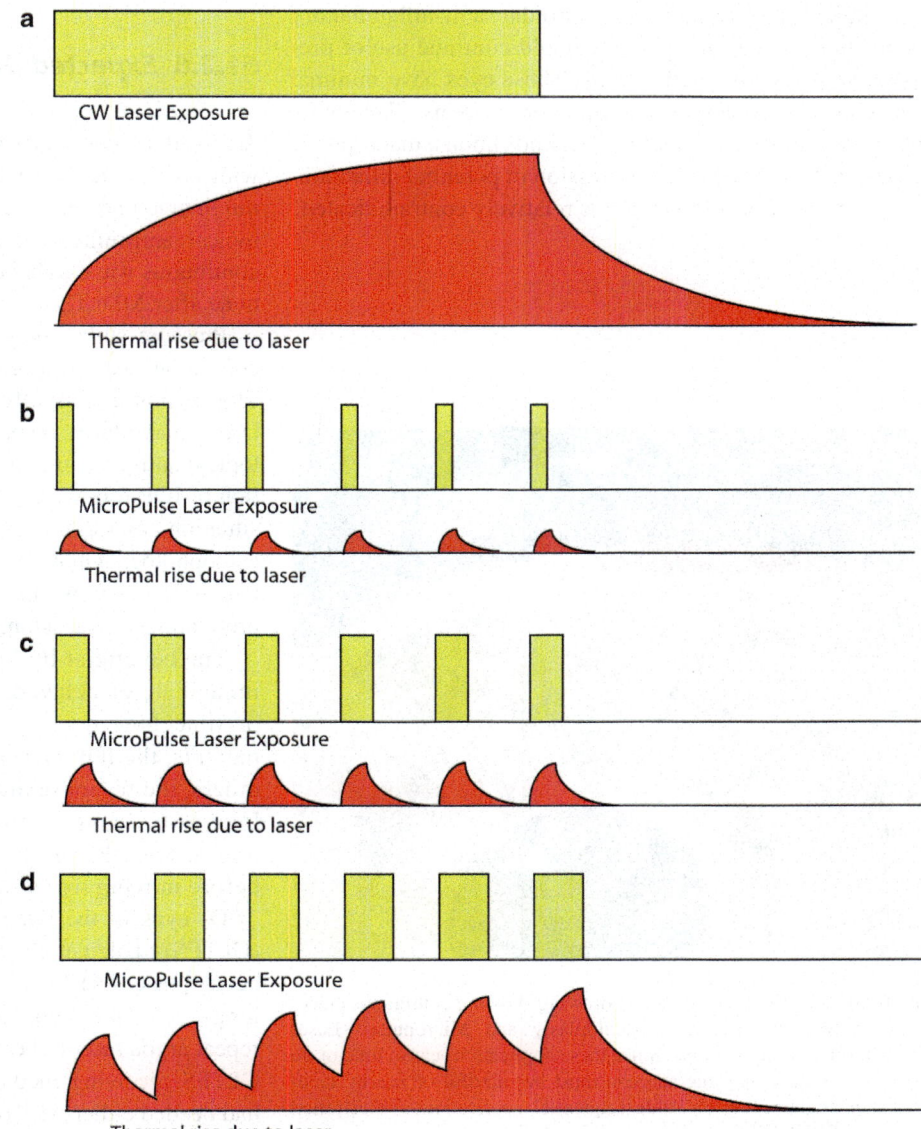

**Fig. 61.3** Schematic interpretation of target tissue temperature elevation during and after trabecular laser treatment. Continuous wave (CW) laser treatment (**a**) causes rise to a plateau that decays when laser is turned off. Micropulsed responses (**b**–**d**) vary according to duty cycle. Short pulses with a long interval between pulses (low duty cycle) (**b**, **c**) cause brief thermal rise followed by decay before the next pulse arrives. Longer pulses (**d**) eventually cause buildup of tissue target thermal response. (Illustration courtesy of IRIDEX Corp., Mountain View, CA)

the doctor must pay diligent attention to the location of each application in order to achieve confluent coverage.

- Decide the extent of the circumference to be treated: 50 or 100%.
- Similar to SLT, apply approximately 50 (for one-half the circumference treatment) or 100 (for circumferential treatment) adjacent, nonoverlapping yet confluent, evenly spaced laser applications, each aimed at the center of the pigmented trabecular meshwork (Fig. 61.4).
- In the procedure note, describe the treatment parameters including system power setting, duration, duty cycle, amount, and location of trabecular circumference treated, and number of applications

#### 61.2.4.2 Postoperative Care

There is usually no need during the postoperative days to add topical nonsteroidal or steroidal anti-inflammatory medication, though the patient should continue use of preoperative glaucoma medications. These eyes have minimal to no clinically detectable inflammatory response. Treatment effect, similar to that after SLT, depends upon a macrophage response, thus aggressive suppression of potential inflammation after the laser intervention is relatively contraindicated.

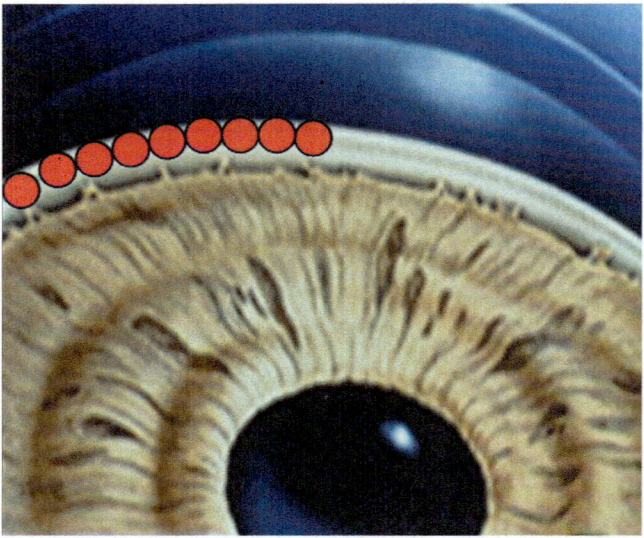

**Fig. 61.4** Anterior chamber angle drawing showing contiguous placement of Selective Laser Trabeculoplasty and Micropulsed Laser Trabeculoplasty applications. Since these applications cause little or no marks on angle tissue, the surgeon must be mindful of nearby landmarks in angle recess to guide sequential applications. (Illustration courtesy of IRIDEX Corp., Mountain View, CA)

### 61.2.5 Complications and Problems

There may be one, or more, complications as follows:

- Transient, or, rarely, permanent blurred vision.
- Transient inflammation (treat with anti-inflammatory medications, as discussed later).
- Spike of IOP, may be due to trabecular blockage from debris or inflammatory precipitates (treat with increased antiglaucoma medications, as discussed later).
- Formation of PAS after continuous wave laser trabeculoplasty; may be numerous, though usually localized and with a pillar shape, extending from the iris base to the middle of the pigmented trabecular meshwork.
- Insufficient reduction of treated IOP from the preoperative baseline, may require alternative management; if persistent there may follow worsening of the visual field loss.

### 61.2.6 Expected Outcomes

Trabeculoplasty causes inflammation – more after treatment with continuous wave laser systems, some after SLT, and minimal to undetectable after MDLT. Most doctors prescribe topical anti-inflammatory medications for 4–7 days after continuous wave trabeculoplasty, a few days after SLT, and none after MDLT.

Pressure spikes may occur within an hour or two after continuous wave trabeculoplasty and occasionally after SLT. This response is usually of small magnitude, and, even if of larger magnitude, responds quickly to additional doses of topical antiglaucoma medications. Rarely, a sustained elevation of IOP follows continuous wave trabeculoplasty. In this situation, expedited filtering surgery or transscleral laser cyclophotocoagulation may be required. It is good if the patient has been warned about pressure elevation during the pretreatment discussion.

The beneficial IOP response to trabeculoplasty can be immediate or delayed. There is no way to predict ahead of time how quickly the response will start. In some patients, the IOP is lower within hours after treatment. In others, the response may develop slowly, over a period as long as 6 weeks. If possible, it is sensible to wait for as long as 6 weeks when there is no early beneficial response before moving to another treatment modality.

Of eyes in the Glaucoma Laser Trial Follow-up Study (GLTFS) treated at glaucoma diagnosis with argon laser trabeculoplasty (ALT), 11% had progressed by the end of the long-term follow-up, either needing filtering surgery or repeat argon laser trabeculoplasty. By contrast, of eyes in the GLTFS receiving medication as initial management, 34% had needed either ALT or filtering surgery.[31] This result indicates an acceptable long-term effectiveness of initial ALT compared with initial medical treatment. In the Advanced Glaucoma Intervention Study (AGIS), which enrolled patients with medically uncontrolled, elevated IOP open-angle glaucoma, analysis of results was divided by self-reported race. Of eyes receiving ALT as the first surgical intervention, by Kaplan–Meier survival analysis at 5 years there was a 30% rate of failure among black patients and a 40% rate of failure among white patients. In both subgroups the rate increased to about 50% by 10 years.[32] Thus about half of eyes treated with ALT at the time of failure of medical management in the AGIS still had a successful status, with continued medical management, 10 years later. A similar assessment of long-term success is not yet available for eyes treated with SLT or MDLT (see Sidebars 61.1 and 61.2).

### Sidebar 61.1. Comparing laser instruments

Yara Catoira-Boyle

The current traditional therapy algorithm for open-angle glaucomas includes laser trabeculoplasty (LTP), usually as the next step after medical therapy is insufficient to reach desired intraocular pressure (IOP). The laser energy is directed at the trabecular meshwork; it lowers IOP by improving the facility of outflow. LTP is a brief, minimally uncomfortable procedure with little risk of visual loss. It may be performed in the office setting or in an ambulatory surgery center. The most common postoperative complications are inflammation and a usually brief spike in IOP. These spikes are most often dealt with in a "routine" manner and should be discussed with the patient when obtaining informed consent to do the procedure. Because it is easy to perform and relatively risk free for a surgical procedure, it is an important tool in the armamentarium of the glaucoma specialist and also for the general ophthalmologist who is comfortable with doing gonioscopy.

The indications for laser trabeculoplasty continue to evolve as newer laser modalities are developed. Despite the fact that the 1988 GLT (Glaucoma Laser Trial) and its follow-up study have shown Argon Laser Trabeculoplasty (ALT) to be safe and as effective as medical therapy, ALT has not achieved the status of a primary therapy in the USA during the past 20 years. The newer Selective Laser Trabeculoplasty (SLT) has been imputed to have some advantages over ALT and is currently been evaluated as primary therapy by many ophthalmologists.

Gonioscopy is performed on all patients who are being considered for laser treatment of their anterior chamber angles, to ensure that all structures are easily visible before performing LTP. The typical patient who may benefit from laser trabeculoplasty has mild-to-moderate glaucoma. They are aware that treatment options include medical therapy, laser treatment, and possibly incisional surgery. Patients in the United States will usually have failed to reach "target IOP" on medical therapy alone. Patients are told that laser therapy for their open-angle glaucoma should be thought of as an additional treatment, which if successful, may or may not allow them to use less topical glaucoma medication postoperatively. They are also informed that even when successful, the IOP-lowering benefits of laser trabeculoplasty may only last for a period of months to years, but are not likely to be permanent.

In addition to glaucoma poorly controlled with the medical therapy, other important indications for LTP include poor compliance with drop regimens; difficulty using eye drops due to intolerance, allergic reaction, lifestyle considerations, or financial issues. Some patients may just prefer laser therapy over the need for chronic use of eye drops. SLT has been shown to successfully replace some medical therapy (average decrease from 2.79 to 1.5 drops) in patients with a target IOP of $16 \pm 2$ mmHg, with stable IOP 12 months later. Recently, SLT has also been shown to reduce IOP in patients with steroid-induced glaucoma after intravitreal Kenalog injections. It is reasonable to perform LTP even on patients with advanced disease, who have baseline IOP in the teens, and a desired target pressure in the single digits. Some of those instances include patients who are poor surgical candidates, or patients with glaucoma progression who are very reluctant to undergo incisional surgery and need a stepped approach or "last chance" for a conservative treatment. Patients with advanced glaucoma with IOP in the low teens (11–13 mmHg) on medical therapy can often achieve consistent IOPs of 9–10 mmHg after undergoing SLT.

Some patients are poor candidates for incisional surgery. They may be blind in one eye, they may have difficulty complying with postoperative instructions and necessary postoperative examinations, and they may simply refuse incisional surgery. Some elderly patients, while they have moderately advanced glaucoma, are not likely to suffer much additional functional loss or go blind for the remainder of their expected lifetimes. They really do not require the very low pressures that might be achieved with incisional surgery. For these patients, laser trabeculoplasty, while not the ideal procedure to lower intraocular pressure, may nonetheless be the best alternative.

Laser trabeculoplasty is not recommended for patients with IOPs higher than 35 mmHg, for those people who need their eye pressure lowered very quickly, or for those patients who have shown rapid progression of visual field defects or optic nerve damage.

## Choices of Laser

Argon laser trabeculoplasty (ALT) was introduced in 1979. Diode laser trabeculoplasty (DLT) was shown to effectively lower IOP in 1990, and selective laser trabeculoplasty (SLT) was initially reported in 1995, becoming commercially available in 2002. Micropulse diode laser trabeculoplasty (MDLT) was first reported in 2005 using the same DLT diode laser set in the micropulse emission mode – instead of the conventional continuous wave (CW) emission mode – to minimize tissue damage, collateral effects, and avoid scarring with the application of repetitive short diode laser pulses. MDLT was recently shown to control IOP for up to 12 months in 75% of medically insufficiently controlled open-angle glaucoma (OAG) eyes that responded to treatment with an IOP reduction of ≥3 mmHg and maintaining IOP≤21 mmHg.

Currently there are three main options for laser trabeculoplasty: (a) the 514-nm CW argon laser or the newer 532-nm CW frequency-doubled Nd:YAG laser both used to perform ALT; (b) the 532-nm Q-Switched and frequency-doubled Nd:YAG laser used to perform SLT; and (c) the 810-nm CW and micropulsed diode laser that can be used to perform both DLT and MDLT.

Studies comparing the three laser modalities have shown IOP lowering to be comparable. Naturally, there is much more long-term experience with ALT. Due to the thermal coagulative damage that ALT and DLT cause to the trabecular meshwork (TM), the treatments should not be overlapped and should not be repeated in the same area of the TM because it may lead to elevation of IOP. For some physicians it is routine to treat only 180° of angle, while some treat all 360° at one session. Thirty-four percent of patients in the GLT developed peripheral anterior synechiae (PAS), but the clinical implications of this are not clear. A similar amount of patients developed an IOP spike greater than 5 mmHg in the immediate postoperative period as opposed to 25% reported for SLT, without pretreatment of IOP. With the addition of prophylactic topical apraclonidine or brimonidine, IOP spikes are cut to less than half.

The SLT stands out due to histopathologic studies that show absence of thermal or collateral damage to the non-pigmented cells or structure of the TM. The tissue effects of ALT, SLT, and MDLT in cadaver eyes have been compared in a study at the Wills Eye Institute in Philadelphia, Pennsylvania, with ALT showing coagulative and structural damage and both SLT and MDLT showing no morphologic change detectable at scanning electron microscopy. There is no formation of PAS with both SLT and MDLT. This absence of structural thermal damage makes the SLT and MDLT procedures theoretically repeatable without the pressure spikes that are common with repeat ALT. The immediate postoperative IOP spikes of greater than 5 mmHg are usually reported at about 10% or less.

It has been reported that SLT reduces IOP in patients with a history of ALT. A study done at the Indianapolis Veterans Administration Hospital Eye Clinic, with patients on maximum-tolerated medical therapy who were poor surgical candidates, showed an additional average IOP reduction of 13% after SLT. All patients had a history of at least 180° ALT.

ALT has been reported to work better in more pigmented angles, as in pigmentary glaucoma or pseudoexfoliation glaucoma. That is not the case with SLT, so those cases might do better with ALT, at least as initial laser therapy. SLT has been reported to have similar effect in pseudophakic and phakic patients. Finally, SLT requires less precise aiming of the laser beam, which makes it technically easier for training physicians and ophthalmologists with less experience in gonioscopy and angle surgery.

## What Results to Expect

The long-term magnitude of IOP lowering with ALT and SLT has been found to be basically comparable in patients who have failed medical therapy or prior laser, with responses from 19 to 29%. When used as primary therapy, SLT's average IOP reduction was 31% at 12 months. It seems primary therapy and higher baseline IOP (upper 20s) are factors that lead to lower IOP results.

Regarding survival of response in patients on maximal medical therapy, success rates for IOP decreases of >3 mmHg and ≥20% reduction without additional drops at 1, 3, and 5 years were 58, 38, and 31% for SLT and 46,

23, and 13% for ALT, but not statistically different. Another study showed success of SLT at 1, 2, 3, and 4 years at 60, 53, 44, and 44% with failure defined as need for any additional therapy, including another drop. Long-term evaluation of SLT as primary therapy is currently under way.

The rate of responders who achieved at least 20% IOP reduction at 12 months was 59.7% for SLT and 60.3% for ALT. Those patients were on maximal medical therapy. When receiving SLT as primary therapy, responder rates with IOP lowering of ≥20 and ≥30% at 12 months were 83 and 55%. In the same study, patients who had been washed out of medications prior to SLT did not obtain as good results as primary SLT patients.

In conclusion, SLT and ALT are the most common modalities of laser trabeculoplasty currently used. Most of the time, the choice of laser will be dictated by what machine is available to the treating physician. The studies show that both lasers are probably good primary therapy modalities with the potential to reduce cost, side effects, and noncompliance with medications. Nevertheless, due to lack of scarring of the trabecular meshwork, SLT has a theoretical potential to be repeated several times on patients who had prior ALT or SLT and it is also technically easier to perform treatment with this device. LTP should be considered in patients who are not good candidates for surgical therapy. The effects of both laser treatments have been shown to last with decreasing effect after 1 year.

## Bibliography

Chung PY, Schuman JS, Netland PA, et al. Five-year results of a randomized, prospective, clinical trial of diode vs Argon laser trabeculoplasty for open-angle glaucoma. *Am J Ophthalmol*. 1998;126(2):185–190.

Damji KF, Bovell AM, Hodge WG, et al. Selective laser trabeculoplasty versus argon laser trabeculoplasty: results from a 1-year randomized clinical trial. *Br J Ophthalmol*. 2006;90:1490–1494.

Damji KF, Shah KC, Rock WJ, et al. Selective laser trabeculoplasty vs argon laser trabeculoplasty: a prospective randomized clinical trial. *Br J Ophthalmol*. 1999;83:718–722.

Fea AM, Bosone A, Rolle T, Brogliatti B, Grignolo FM. Micropulse diode laser trabeculoplasty (MDLT): A phase II clinical study with 12 months follow-up. *Clin Ophthalmol* 2008;2(2):247–252.

Francis BA, Ianchulev T, Schofield JK, et al. Selective Laser trabeculoplasty as a replacement for medical therapy in open-angle glaucoma. *Am J Ophthalmol*. 2004;140(3):524–525.

Fudemberg SJ, Myers JS, Katz LJ. Trabecular meshwork tissue examination with scanning electron microscopy: a comparison of Micropulse diode Laser (MLT), Selective Laser (SLT), and Argon Laser (ALT) Trabeculoplasty in human cadaver tissue. *Invest Ophthal Vis Sci*. 2008;49:ARVO E-Abstract 1236.

Glaucoma Laser Trial Research Group. The Glaucoma Laser Trial (GLT). 2. Results of argon laser trabeculoplasty versus topical medicines. *Ophthalmology*. 1990;97(11):1403–1413.

Glaucoma Laser Trial Research Group. The Glaucoma Laser Trial (GLT) and Glaucoma Laser Trial Follow-up Study: 7. Results. *Am J Ophthalmol*. 1995;120(6):718–731.

Hodge WG, Damji KF, Rock W, et al. Baseline IOP predicts selective laser trabeculoplasty success at 1 year post-treatment: results of a randomized clinical trial. *Br J Ophthalmol*. 2005;89:1157–1160.

Ingvoldstad DD, Krishna R, Willoughby L. Micropulse diode laser trabeculoplasty. *Invest Ophthal Vis Sci*. 2005;46:ARVO E-Abstract 123.

Juzych MS, Chopra V, Banitt MR, et al. Comparison of long-term outcomes of selective laser trabeculoplasty versus argon laser trabeculoplasty in open-angle glaucoma. *Ophthalmology*. 2004;111(10):1853–1859.

Latina MA, Sibayan SA, Shin DH, et al. Q-switched 532-nm Nd:YAG laser trabeculoplasty (selective laser trabeculoplasty): a multicenter, pilot, clinical study. *Ophthalmology*. 1998;105(11):2082–2088.

Lunde M. Argon laser trabeculoplasty in pigmentary dispersion syndrome with glaucoma. *Am J Ophthalmol*. 1983;96:721–725.

McHugh D, Marshall J, Jffytche T, et al. Diode laser trabeculoplasty (DLT) for primary open-angle glaucoma and ocular hypertension. *Br J Ophthalmol*. 1990;74:743–747.

McIlraith I, Strasfeld M, Colev G, et al. Selective laser trabeculoplasty as initial and adjunctive treatment for open-angle glaucoma. *J Glaucoma*. 2006;15(2):124–130.

Melamed S, Simon GJB, Levkovitch-Verbin H. Selective laser trabeculoplasty as primary treatment for open-angle glaucoma. *Arch Ophthal*. 2003;121:957–960.

Ritch R, Liebermann J, Robin A, et al. Argon laser trabeculoplasty in pigmentary glaucoma. *Ophthalmology*. 1993;100:909.

Robin AL, Pollack IP. Argon laser trabeculoplasty in secondary forms of open angle glaucoma. *Arch Ophthalmol*. 1983;101:382–384.

Rubin B, Taglienti A, Rothman RF, et al. The effect of selective laser trabeculoplasty on intraocular pressure in patients with intravitreal steroid-induced elevated intraocular pressure. *J Glaucoma*. 2008;17(4):287–292.

Vishnu S, Catoira-Boyle Y, WuDunn D, et al. Efficacy of selective laser trabeculoplasty after argon laser trabeculoplasty in open angle glaucoma. Indianapolis, IN: Indiana University; 2007:ARVO poster 3971/B951.

Weinand FS, Althen F. Long-term clinical results of selective laser trabeculoplasty in the treatment of primary open angle glaucoma. *Eur J Ophthalmol*. 2006;16(1):100–104.

### Sidebar 61.2. New forms of trabeculoplasty

Giorgio Dorin and John Samples

In addition to the present modalities of laser trabeculoplasty (ALT, SLT, and MDLT), laser iridoplasty, laser iridotomy, laser iridectomy, and transscleral or endoscopic laser cyclophotocoagulation, there are a number of new potential laser applications for the treatment of glaucoma. These include transscleral application of infrared laser energy (a) to the pars plana to create a lowering of pressure, which we speculate may be due to increased uveoscleral outflow, and (b) to the Schlemm's canal and nearby regions, a sort of trabeculoplasty *ab-externo*, which would work in angle closure or narrow angle situations. Finally, a deeper form of laser trabeculoplasty capable to interact with the deepest juxtacanalicular trabecular meshwork layers is considered.

### Pars Plana Application of 810-nm Diode Laser in the Micropulse Emission Mode

Application of laser to the pars plana to lower the intraocular pressure is not a new idea and, in fact, may be unknowingly performed by default with many transscleral laser cyclophotocoagulation procedures. In an animal study performed on monkey eyes, Liu and coworkers demonstrated that contact transscleral cyclophotocoagulation with the 1,064-nm Nd:YAG laser directed at the pars plana decreased IOP and resulted in tracer particles detectable in the suprachoroidal space. The same treatment over the pars plicata also resulted in IOP reduction, but without tracer particles detectable in the suprachoroidal space, suggesting two mechanisms of IOP reduction: lowering the production of aqueous humor with the treatment over the pars plicata and increasing the uveoscleral outflow with the treatment over the pars plana.

Studies done with transscleral applications of infrared laser energy at the pars plana showed that coagulative necrosis can occur with these treatments. A study presented at the World Glaucoma Congress 2007 in Singapore suggested that micropulse diode laser applications over the pars plana can produce significant and long-lasting reduction of IOP without causing the destruction of any ocular structure. As a result, clinical trials are presently underway to study the lowering of pressure through the nondestructive micropulse laser application over the pars plana, whose mechanism of action remains to be elucidated.

### External Laser Trabeculoplasty

Laser trabeculoplasty delivered *ab-externo* through the sclera has the potential of overcoming some anatomic and physical disadvantages common to all present laser trabeculoplasty techniques with *ab-interno* gonioscopic laser delivery.

A first obvious disadvantage is the prerequisite of an open angle to be applied. Another disadvantage, from an anatomic viewpoint, is that trabecular beams and less dense filtrating meshwork obstruct the delivery and the interaction of the laser energy with the deeper layers of the trabecular meshwork involved in the obstruction of the outflow.

It has been suggested, though perhaps it is counterintuitive, that the application of infrared laser energy through the sclera could actually more effectively reach and interact with the walls of the Schlemm's canal and perhaps with the juxtacanalicular meshwork, which are hypothesized as the site of origin of outflow resistance.

### A Deeper Laser Trabeculoplasty

From a gonioscopic approach, it seems intuitive that the deeper one is able to treat tissue the more likely the trabeculoplasty can produce a more pronounced hypotensive effect. At present the lasers most likely to have a deep interaction are those with infrared emission such as the 790-nm Titanium-Sapphire used for TLT and the 810-nm diode laser used in continuous wave emission for diode laser trabeculoplasty (DLT) and in micropulse emission for micropulse diode laser trabeculoplasty (MDLT). It could well be that these infrared lasers will be effective when conventional more superficial trabeculoplasty with visible emitting lasers (488/514 nm Argon laser, 532-nm CW frequency-doubled Nd:YAG laser and with 532-nm Q-switched frequency-doubled Nd:YAG laser) fails.

### Staging of Treatment

Laser treatments offer unique advantages in glaucoma management including flattening of the diurnal curve, elimination of compliance-related issues, decrease cost on a long-term basis, and difference in whether or not insurances will reimburse a treatment, usually favoring the laser. It is possible to visualize a time when the first treatment for glaucoma might be SLT followed by MDLT or TLT, followed by either nondestructive micropulse transscleral applications of trabeculoplasty *ab-externo* or pars plana cyclophotocoagulation or even both. This would occur in a stepwise fashion, and would have considerable advantage in terms of compliance and overall cost.

However, much more clinical information is needed before this type of protocol is implemented. It is undeniably cost-effective.

## Conclusion

Newer laser applications may reposition laser treatments with respect to invasive surgical treatments and medications in the management of glaucoma. The evolution of a laser-only protocol for treatment in select instances is anticipated.

## Bibliography

Aquino MCD, Tan A, Chew PTK. The initial experience with micropulse diode laser transscleral cyclophotocoagulation for severe glaucoma. World Glaucoma Congress 2007: Abstract P428.

Ho Ching Lin, Wong EYM, Chew PTK. Effect of diode laser contact transscleral pars plana photocoagulation on intraocular pressure in glaucoma. *Clin Experiment Ophthalmol.* 2002;30:343–347.

Liu GJ, Mizukawa A, Okisaka S. Mechanism of intraocular pressure decrease after contact transscleral continuous wave Nd:YAG laser cyclophotocoagulation. *Ophthalmic Res.* 1994;26:65–79.

## 61.3 The Iris

Early in the 1960s some of the first-tested applications of laser for the eye were iris treatment to create an iridotomy.[3] Iridotomy and iridoplasty are now among the more frequent laser treatments for glaucoma. These interventions are usually done for eyes with elevated IOP and angle closure, or for eyes with high-risk anatomic narrow angle. As with laser treatment for open-angle glaucoma, here again gonioscopic skill is important. The surgeon has to recognize that the angle is closed, partly or completely, and whether the closure is appositional or due to formation of peripheral anterior synechiae (PAS), or a mix of the two. If PAS are present it is important to determine the extent of the angle circumference involved.

In addition to iridotomy and iridoplasty as iris treatments, the occasional patient with miosis benefits from laser photomydriasis or laser sphincterotomy. These two laser treatments are usually justified by a need to improve vision or fundus visualization rather than a need to improve glaucoma status.

### 61.3.1 Iridotomy Indications and Contraindications

Angle closure may be acute, subacute, or chronic. Patients with angle closure often present with a chronic, indolent condition, suspected based on the van Herrick sign during slit lamp examination.[33] Often, yet not always, these patients are hyperopic. They can be of any age, although the condition is more frequent among older individuals. The IOP is usually elevated, though it may be normal. Gonioscopy clarifies the extent of the anterior chamber angle blockage.

Occasionally the presentation is acute and dramatic. In the event of acute, marked IOP elevation, the cornea may have stromal or epithelial edema, and be hazy. The patient may have disabling pain and nausea. This interferes with gonioscopy and laser iridotomy (see Sidebar 61.3). Breaking the acute attack medically becomes important, as this relieves the pressure elevation and allows the cornea to clear. The patient may need systemic hyperosmotic agents in addition to topical agents to break the acute attack. In subacute presentations, the patient may have undergone repeated episodes of angle closure, and have sector iris atrophy and numerous, small subcapsular lens opacities (glaucomflecken).

---

**SIDEBAR 61.3. Corneal edema following angle closure: how to perform laser iridotomy**

Peter T. Chang

Corneal edema is a common sign in an acute angle-closure attack. The sudden and severe elevation of intraocular pressure (IOP) forces fluid into the cornea, overwhelming the capability of the endothelial pumps. While the edema may provide helpful information regarding the acute nature of IOP elevation, further ophthalmic examination may be impeded by the corneal opacity. Visualization of the anterior segment structures is often critical to an accurate, prompt diagnosis because other entities, such as neovascular glaucoma and other secondary angle-closure glaucomas, may also present with elevated IOP and corneal edema yet require different management modalities than pupillary-block glaucomas. Inappropriate peripheral iridotomy could potentially exacerbate these other conditions. And of course significant corneal edema in the case of angle closure secondary to pupillary block, may preclude the ability to perform a laser peripheral iridotomy and necessitate incisional surgical intervention.

Any attempt to improve corneal edema should include antiglaucoma medications to lower the IOP. Aqueous suppressants and parasympathomimetics are preferred due to their quicker onset and mechanisms of action. Additionally, corneal edema can be reduced with the use of topical hypertonic agents, such as glycerin, as they draw water from the cornea by osmosis. Instillation of topical glycerin causes significant burning or stinging, and it should, therefore, be preceded by use of a topical anesthetic agent. If glycerin is not readily available or if the use of glycerin does not yield significant reduction of corneal edema, anterior chamber paracentesis may be performed to lower IOP and to reduce corneal edema. Both the use of topical hyperosmotic agents and anterior chamber paracentesis may only temporarily clear the cornea, but they may do so for a sufficient amount of time to allow laser iridotomy to be performed

My preferred technique for anterior chamber paracentesis was taught to me by my mentor, Dr. Paul Palmberg, at the Bascom Palmer Eye Institute. A half-inch, 30-gage needle is attached to a tuberculin syringe with the plunger removed. Following instillation of a topical anesthetic agent and a prep of the conjunctival sac and lashes with a povidone–iodine solution, the patient is positioned at the slit lamp with the lids held open either manually or with a wire speculum. A long entry path through the corneal stroma with this size needle almost eliminates the risk of wound leak. Entry into the anterior chamber through the limbus near 6-o'clock reduces the possibility of inadvertent injury to the crystalline lens in a phakic eye. The needle is withdrawn from the anterior chamber after approximately 20 s with the resultant IOP around 10 mmHg, as the small lumen of the 30-gage needle apparently prohibits flow against the atmospheric pressure at a lower IOP.

Paracentesis should be performed with caution as these patients often have severe pain and nausea. Overtly short entry through the cornea may result in a leaky wound and, consequently, hypotony and increased risk for intraocular infection. Inadvertent trauma to the crystalline lens is also possible. Moreover, paracentesis in an eye with rubeosis irides may result in a significant hyphema and further elevation of IOP and worsening of visualization of anterior and posterior segment structures.

Alternatively to peripheral iridotomy, which requires reasonably clear cornea, laser gonioplasty or iridoplasty can be performed even through a relative hazy cornea. Laser iridoplasty may resolve the acute angle-closure attack in addition to facilitating a subsequent laser iridotomy by reducing corneal edema, and should therefore be a part of an armamentarium of any glaucomatologist.

## Bibliography

Arnavielle S, Creuzot-Garcher C, Bron AM. Anterior chamber paracentesis in patients with acute elevation of intraocular pressure. *Graefes Arch Clin Exp Ophthalmol*. 2007;245:345–350.
Lai JS, Tham CC, Lam DS. Limited argon laser peripheral iridoplasty as immediate treatment for an acute attack of primary angle-closure glaucoma: a preliminary study. *Eye*. 1999;13:26–30.
Lam DS, Lai JS, Tham CC. Immediate argon laser peripheral iridoplasty as treatment for acute attack of primary angle-closure glaucoma: a preliminary study. *Ophthalmology*. 1998;105:2231–2236.
Luxenberg MN, Green K. Reduction of corneal edema with topical hypertonic agents. *Am J Ophthalmol*. 1971;71:847–853.

## 61.4 Mechanism of Angle Closure

Angle closure is usually the result of block of flow of aqueous humor from the posterior chamber through the pupil to the anterior chamber-pupillary block. This is more likely when the pupil is in a middilated state, as occurs when the patient is in a location with dim illumination (the theater or driving an automobile at night come to mind). The midperipheral iris balloons due to the slightly higher pressure in the posterior chamber; then the ballooned iris may come into contact with the trabecular meshwork. The IOP becomes elevated when there is sufficient trabecular blockage by this "flap valve" effect. Creation of a small hole through the iris relieves the pressure inequality, and allows the ballooned iris to return to a more normal location.

Other patients have a normal IOP associated with a narrow, yet slit open, crowded anterior chamber recess. Iridotomy will often relieve the high risk status for these patients.

Despite a successful iridotomy, some patients have a persistent appositional angle closure due to plateau iris with forward rotation of the ciliary body. These patients are often hyperopic. The condition is discovered during gonioscopy after iridotomy and can be definitively diagnosed with ultrasonic biomicroscopy. In this situation, *iridoplasty* is often helpful (see Chap. 62). Iridoplasty seldom relieves synechial angle closure.

## 61.4.1 Iridectomy and Iridotomy

### 61.4.1.1 History

Iridectomy as an effective treatment for glaucoma dates to 1857, when Albrecht von Graefe made the initial report.[34] Not all glaucomatous eyes responded. Understanding the mechanism of pupillary block as the principal cause of angle closure was delayed until the publication of an explanation by Curran in 1920.[35] Meyer-Schwickerath developed the xenon arc photocoagulator in the early 1950s, and reported creating iridotomies with this noninvasive instrument in 1956.[36] The instrument was cumbersome and the focused spot size large; it burned through the iris tissue in some patients, yet often caused burns of the nearby cornea and lens. With the availability of ophthalmic laser systems starting in the late 1960s there followed a plethora of publications reporting iridotomy methods, success rates, long-term success, and complications with both continuous wave and high-power pulsed laser systems. These early studies are summarized.[37]

Focusing treatment contact lenses, developed with high dioptric power and antireflective coating, facilitated the procedure.[38-40] After the original designs, eye surgeons developed lenses with features to enhance the iridotomy procedure, and many surgeons have readily adopted use of these special lenses. The Abraham lens has a 63-diopter treatment button. The Wise–Munnerlyn–Erickson lens has a 103-diopter treatment button. Lenses are available from commercial sources (Fig. 61.5). By the 1990s, techniques for iridotomy, iridoplasty, and pupilloplasty using these lenses were in wide use.

Goins et al furthered the laser iridotomy procedure in 1990 with description of a method for iridotomy using argon laser pretreatment followed by high-power pulsed laser applications. This reduced the occurrence of bleeding that accompanied iridotomies done with pulsed laser systems alone, and the complication of frequent late closure that followed argon laser iridotomy as it was done at that time.[41]

The surgeon should be familiar with the guidance provided by the American Academy of Ophthalmology in the Preferred Practice Pattern for Primary Angle Closure, available online at http://one.aao.org/CE/PracticeGuidelines/default.aspx under Glaucoma in the Subspecialty Browser.[42]

### 61.4.1.2 Methods of Iridotomy

#### 61.4.1.2.1 Preparation

- A hazy cornea, as in an acute angle closure attack, precludes laser iridotomy. Topical or systemic medical glaucoma treatment, including hyperosmotic agents, to break the acute attack and lower the elevated IOP often clears the cornea allowing treatment to proceed.

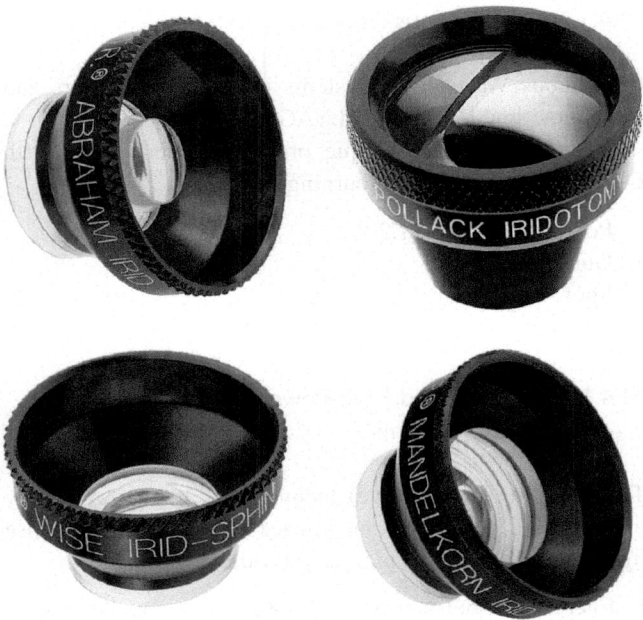

**Fig. 61.5** Lenses for iridotomy. Abraham lens (*upper left*) has eccentric 66-diopter treatment button providing 1.5× image magnification and 0.67× treatment spot diameter reduction. Wise lens (*lower left*) has an eccentric 103-diopter treatment button providing 2.6× image magnification and 0.38× treatment spot diameter reduction. Pollack lens (*upper right*) combines a treatment button similar to the Abraham lens with a gonioscopic mirror to allow intraoperative anterior chamber angle viewing. Mandelkorn lens (*lower right*) has a large diameter viewing surface providing 1.2× image magnification and 0.83× laser treatment spot diameter reduction for iris periphery or lens capsule. (Photographs courtesy of Ocular Instruments, Inc., Bellevue, WA)

- Informed consent for the type laser surgery planned.
- Obtain a presurgery measurement of IOP.
- Pretreatment with a miotic – typically pilocarpine 1 or 2% – drops to the eye to be treated about one-quarter to one-half hour before laser treatment.
- Topical anesthesia (e.g., tetracaine or proparacaine).
- Appropriate antireflective-coated, iridotomy treatment contact lens of choice with methylcellulose 1% solution for coupling with the eye surface.
- Slit lamp biomicroscope delivery system adjusted with aiming beam centered in the on-axis slit beam and with laser confocal with microscope focus.
- Anticipating posttreatment pressure spikes, some surgeons pretreat with Iopidine (apraclonidine) or brimonidine.

#### 61.4.1.2.2 Treatment and Suggested Laser System Settings

The surgeon may find it advantageous to vary laser settings based on observation of tissue response during treatment.

### 61.4.1.2.3 Continuous Wave Laser Systems

Continuous Wave (CW) systems include argon lasers and frequency-doubled green Nd:YAG systems

The "chipping" technique provides better results with CW systems than slower, burning techniques.

- Power 1,200 mW (1.2 W)
- Duration 0.05 s
- Spot size 50 μm

### 61.4.1.2.4 Q-switched, High-Power, Nd:YAG Laser Systems

The "blasting" (disruptive) technique is better for lightly pigmented irides with noncompact stroma than for dense light-colored or deeply pigmented irides.

- Energy per pulse usually 4.0–6.0 mJ (may be higher, though this approaches levels potentially causing crystalline lens damage).
- Single pulses or bursts of three pulses.
- Duration and spot size are an automatic characteristic of the system.
- With the Q-switched pulsed system (prepared as indicated previously) ready to treat and the treatment site selected, make an initial tissue-disrupting application and observe the effect.
- Make additional applications to exactly the same site, drilling deeper into the tissue.
- Oozing of blood from disrupted small vessels will stop spontaneously or faster when pressure is applied to the eye with the treatment contact lens. Wait until the treatment site is again clearly visible. Subsequent applications may start the ooze again.
- If brisk bleeding develops, stop it with pressure on the treatment contact lens and either choose another site or discontinue and postpone treatment to another day. The patient who has been forewarned about this rare possibility is not surprised if this situation develops during treatment.

### 61.4.1.2.5 The Combined CW and Pulsed Laser Technique

This is reliable and nearly always successful in one treatment session.

- Start with the CW system (prepared as indicated previously) ready to treat.
- Make two or three "chipping" applications close together on the tissue in a row parallel to the limbus to start a linear incision. Subsequent applications aimed at pigmented tissue in exactly the same site carry the opening into the iris stroma, deepening the cut.
- About 30–50 applications will usually create small perforations to the posterior chamber, and puffs of pigmented debris enter the laser-created crypt. This often leaves devitalized, depigmented, or lightly pigmented strands across the base of the opening.
- Next, move the patient to the Q-switched laser system, or move the system to the patient, with the system prepared as indicated previously and ready to treat. Reapply the treatment contact lens if it has come off the eye. Warn the patient that the laser makes a "snapping" sound when it comes to focus.
- Provided the initial chipping burns have opened the tissue nearly to the posterior chamber, one laser Q-switched laser pulse, aimed carefully upon devitalized strands bridging the base of the treatment site, often suffices to open the iridotomy widely; if so, treatment is complete. Sometimes more than one application is required. Successful applications often cause a large cloud of pigment particles and pigmented cellular debris to migrate from the posterior chamber to the anterior chamber, which usually deepens.

### 61.4.1.2.6 Treatment Site

- The far peripheral, upper nasal iris, under the lid is first choice – approximately the 12:30–1:30 meridian for the right eye and the 10:30–11:30 meridian for the left eye. Avoid the 12 o'clock meridian as bubbles formed during treatment will not move out of the way.
- The far peripheral upper temporal iris is an attractive alternative.
- Treatment should not be so far peripheral that arcus senilis or the peripheral corneal vascular arcade interfere with the view of the treatment site.
- Treat in an iris crypt if one is available; alternatively treat in another, thin location. When treating with a continuous wave laser, seek a site that contains some pigment (to absorb the laser energy) – nevi are nice in this regard.

### 61.4.1.2.7 Postoperative Care

- Rinse methylcellulose remnant from the tear film.
- Apply an anti-inflammatory agent (e.g., prednisolone 1%). Do not dilate the pupil.
- Consider doing repeat gonioscopy with a four-mirror lens (Zeiss or Sussman) to assess effect of treatment on the anterior chamber angle recess.
- Record the lens type used, laser settings, treatment site(s), and number of laser applications in note in medical record.

- Check IOP 1–2 h after treatment to assess for a pressure spike.[43] A rise of IOP 5–10 mmHg above pretreatment level may justify supplemental topical glaucoma eyedrops immediately and for several postoperative days. Continue to monitor the patient until worrisome spikes are resolving with the additional medical treatment.
- Discharge the stable patient on continued, unchanged use of preoperative medications supplemented with 4 days of topical anti-inflammatory drops t.i.d. or q.i.d. Plan to check status within a week to 10 days.
- During the follow-up visit check IOP and do postoperative gonioscopy. When there is a need for the second eye to have iridotomy, this can be accomplished on the same day as the follow-up visit for the first eye iridotomy.
- Adjust medical treatment as justified by findings.
- The second follow-up visit can be 1–4 weeks later. Dilate the pupil during this visit to reduce the chance of formation of posterior synechiae and to allow thorough fundus examination.

### 61.4.1.2.8 Complications and Problems

These are infrequent, yet important, and those amenable to altered treatment should be managed promptly.

- Blurred vision – this is almost always transient and arises from the after image due to retinal pigment epithelial bleaching from the bright, visible laser beam, from pigment dispersion in the aqueous, or inflammation. There is a single report of loss of central vision from "snuffing."
- Pupil distortion – from peaking toward the treatment site – usually transient, occasionally persistent, yet is usually minor.
- Monocular diplopia or glare from light entering the eye through the small iridotomy opening – this symptom usually decreases with time.
- Inflammation – this usually responds to the anti-inflammatory agent, though persistent inflammation may cause posterior synechiae formation; pupil dilation within several weeks of laser surgery usually averts this.
- Corneal epithelial or endothelial burns – these are the result of absorption of light energy at the corneal interface and may worsen if treatment is continued after they appear. Select a different site and restart the procedure.
- Bleeding has already been mentioned and is more likely after pulsed laser iridotomy.
- IOP spiking has also been mentioned – early postoperative monitoring reveals its occurrence. It usually responds to more aggressive antiglaucoma medication.
- "Malignant" glaucoma due to unrelieved angle closure occurs rarely after laser iridotomy – it is the result of cilio-lenticular block. Management, including cycloplegia and additional laser and invasive surgical procedures, is presented elsewhere in this book.
- Closure of the treatment site happens occasionally – if it occurs early postoperative it is usually from debris occluding the opening. Or, if it is delayed or late, it is usually from newly formed cellular structures that bridge the depth of the opening. These closures respond to application of one or two Q-switched laser pulses.
- Local lens opacities – may follow energy deposition and tissue heating next to the lens surface. These persist yet do not progress.
- Retinal burns – can arise from a focused laser beam encountering the retinal pigment epithelium. During treatment the path of the laser light should not point through the treatment lens directly toward the macula and the focus should be held tightly on the target iris tissue, ensuring divergence of the laser beam should it get past the target.

## 61.4.2 Iridoplasty Indications and Contraindications

After patent iridotomy is achieved, the postoperative indentation, four-mirror, gonioscopy may show persistent appositional angle closure without PAS. This justifies a probable diagnosis of plateau iris. The diagnosis can be confirmed with ultrasound biomicroscopy, if available, which shows forward rotation of the ciliary body. Untreated persistent appositional angle closure has the potential to cause sustained elevation of IOP, trabecular meshwork damage, PAS formation, and secondary glaucomatous optic neuropathy. While medical treatment of IOP often helps, it does not solve this problem.

### 61.4.2.1 History

The approach advocated years ago by Robert Ritch has proven effective and is widely accepted.[44] It has proven effective to open the appositionally closed angle in plateau iris, and helpful to open the angle sufficiently to relieve an acute attack of angle closure.

### 61.4.2.2 Surgery and Postoperative Care

#### 61.4.2.2.1 Preparation

- While a treatment contact lens will stabilize the eye during the procedure, it is not required.
- Otherwise, preparation including pretreatment with a miotic is as outlined for iridotomy.

#### 61.4.2.2.2 Suggested Laser System Settings

Treatment is done with a continuous wave laser system (argon laser system or frequency-doubled green neodymium:YAG system). A low-power, slow application technique provides better results.

- Power 150–500 mW (0.15–0.5 W)
- Duration 0.2–0.5
- Spot size 200–500 μm

The surgeon may find it advantageous to vary settings based on observation of tissue response during treatment – for example, a higher power and smaller diameter for lightly pigmented irides. The goal is to produce contraction of the iris stroma at and surrounding each application site.

#### 61.4.2.2.3 Treatment

- Make 30 or more evenly spaced applications to the far peripheral iris, leaving 1–2 application diameters between burns.
- Postoperative monitoring and care.
- Gonioscopy assures that there has occurred successful opening of the anterior chamber angle recess.
- Topical anti-inflammatory agent immediately, and then t.i.d. to q.i.d. for 4 days.

#### 61.4.2.2.4 Complications and Problems

- Transient or, rarely, permanent blurred vision.
- Transient iritis (treat with anti-inflammatory medications).
- Spike of IOP (treat with increased antiglaucoma medications).
- Transient or permanent change of pupil shape or diameter (rare and usually self-healing).
- Need for retreatment in the event of persistent or recurrent crowding of the anterior chamber angle recess.

### 61.4.3 Other Iris Laser Procedures: Pupilloplasty and Pupillary Sphincterotomy

#### 61.4.3.1 Indications and Contraindications

The usual cause of mydriatic-resistant miosis is previous long-term use of cholinergic medications as medical treatment for glaucoma. Surgical after effects causing pupillary sphincter fibrosis explain other cases. In this regard there are relatively young aphakic glaucoma patients after surgery for congenital cataract who have small, poorly dilating pupils. Other patients have formed hammock pupil after lens surgery, with the iris covering the visual axis. The small or misplaced pupil in these eyes inhibits vision, especially in reduced light, and inhibits examination of the ocular fundus, handicapping glaucoma, or diabetes mellitus monitoring. Pupilloplasty and sphincterotomy are procedures that address this problem, and provide relief.

#### 61.4.3.2 History

Soon after xenon and argon systems were available, surgeons who applied photocoagulation to the retina noted side effects on the pupil in some cases. Eye movements during treatment resulted in light energy applications on the iris near the pupil border, with focal areas of stromal atrophy and subsequent irregular or enlarged pupil.[45,46] The name *photomydriasis* and a description of a method first appeared in a publication by James et al in 1976.[47] These investigators developed a method involving a double row of contiguous coagulative laser burns around the pupil margin, applied over the iris sphincter muscle. Clinically, the treatment doubled the diameter of the miotic pupil from 1.5 to 3.1 mm on average. This treatment also proved helpful for pseudophakic pupillary block.[47] The method developed by L'Esperance and associates[47] is still used occasionally.

Wise in 1985 reported a method to make linear cuts in iris with multiple short-duration, relatively high-power argon laser burns delivered through an iridotomy lens.[48] He illustrated cuts across the pupillary sphincter for treatment of miosis. Clinicians have subsequently used a combined continuous wave laser pretreatment followed by high-power, Q-switched pulsed laser to open a cut across the pupillary sphincter in several meridians, yielding a permanently enlarged, dilatable pupil and relief from miosis.

#### 61.4.3.3 Methods of Pupilloplasty and Pupillary Sphincterotomy

##### 61.4.3.3.1 Preparation

- Warn the patient that several treatment sessions may be needed to achieve the desired endpoint.
- Apply dilating medications (for example, a combination of Neo-Synephrine and tropicamide).
- An iridotomy treatment contact lens stabilizes the eye for pupilloplasty. The laser energy is applied through the 63.0-diopter (Abraham lens) or 103.0-diopter (Wise–Munnerlyn–Erickson lens) focusing button of the lens.

### 61.4.3.4 Pupilloplasty

#### 61.4.3.4.1 Treatment and Suggested Settings

- Continuous wave argon or frequency-double neodymium: YAG laser system with 200–500 μm spot size and 0.2 s duration. The required power is 200–600 mW, selected according to iris pigmentation and observed tissue reaction.
- Apply multiple, contiguous, solitary laser burns to encircle the pupil margin in two concentric circles. The first circle, at the pupil margin is with the 200-μm spot size, and the outer circle is with the 500-μm spot size. The outer circle applications require the higher power setting to achieve the desired tissue reaction.
- After healing, a second step of applications may be needed to combat recurrent miosis.

### 61.4.3.5 Sphincterotomy

#### 61.4.3.5.1 Treatment and Suggested Settings

- Initial steps of treatment are with continuous wave argon or green frequency-doubled Nd:YAG laser system with 50-μm spot size and 0.05 s duration. The required power is 1.2–1.4 W, selected according to iris pigmentation and observed tissue reaction.
- Completion of treatment is with a Q-switched high-power pulsed neodymium:YAG laser system with one, two, or three pulses per burst at energy of 3.0–7.0 mJ per pulse. Lower energy settings in the range are for phakic eyes with miosis.
- Select the meridian for a cut across the sphincter.
- Apply multiple chipping continuous wave laser burns to the iris tissue in a line starting about 1 mm distal to the margin and extending toward the edge of the pupil, creating a cut line deep into the pupil margin tissue.
- Make similar preparatory cuts in one, two, or three more evenly spaced meridians around the pupil.
- Switch to the Q-switched laser system and apply disruptive pulses to the strands bridging the base of the meridional cuts. Avoid applications that hit the lens surface.

### 61.4.3.6 Postoperative Monitoring and Care for Both Procedures

- Apply anti-inflammatory steroids and a strong cycloplegic (e.g., atropine 1%).
- Monitor for 1–2 h to identify and treat any posttreatment IOP spikes.
- Discontinue miotics; continue other antiglaucoma medications; supplement as needed for spikes of IOP.
- Topical cycloplegic once daily for 1 week and anti-inflammatory steroids t.i.d. to q.i.d. for 1 week, then taper to b.i.d. for another week; can then restart miotic, if needed.

### 61.4.3.7 Complications and Problems

The occasional lightly pigmented, yet thick, iris is difficult to penetrate with either chipping CW laser burns or high-power pulsed laser applications. The surgeon may find it useful to move to an alternative treatment site, preferably one with some iris stromal pigment.

Bleeding may follow disruptive laser applications to the iris. This is usually minor and transient, and stops spontaneously. It stops faster if the surgeon applies light pressure to the treatment contact lens on the eye.

If the iris is close to the corneal inner surface during CW or pulsed laser iridotomy the laser applications may cause corneal endothelial damage. The damaged corneal site can interfere with the view of the iris treatment site. This can be sufficient to make it needed to move to a new site to do the treatment.

Postoperative treatment-induced iritis may occur. Prophylactic topical steroids for 3–5 postoperative days are usually sufficient to suppress this problem. It may be sufficient to induce formation of posterior synechiae. This is also averted by postoperative pupil dilation about 1–3 weeks after iridotomy and pupilloplasty treatment. Dilation with a long-lasting mydriatic is indicated after pupillary sphincterotomy; this averts posterior synechiae formation.

Closure of an iridotomy by liberated tissue debris or proliferated iris pigment epithelium occurs rarely. An iridotomy may be discovered to be imperforate during an early postoperative follow-up examination. Both these respond to one or two disruptive high-power laser pulses applied through a treatment contact lens.

### 61.4.3.8 Expected Outcomes

Once established, laser iridotomies persist. The iris will settle back from the anterior chamber angle recess after successful iridotomy in cases of pupillary block, except in sites where there are peripheral anterior synechiae. Peripheral anterior synechiae are detected during postoperative indentation gonioscopy. If there is plateau iris, the angle may not open spontaneously after iridotomy. It will open with indentation gonioscopy, which is an indication to consider iridoplasty.

## 61.5 Ciliary Body

Effective laser treatment of the ciliary processes and ciliary body reduces aqueous humor inflow, and secondarily reduces intraocular pressure – similar to the effect of beta blockers, carbonic anhydrase inhibitors, or alpha adrenergic agents. The laser treatment can be accomplished transsclerally with CW red and near-infrared lasers, or by invasive, direct application of infrared CW laser energy.

### 61.5.1 Indications and Contraindications

These procedures are indicated to reduce aqueous inflow in glaucomatous eyes. The laser energy can be applied to an intact eye through the anterior sclera or can be applied directly to the ciliary processes during an invasive procedure. The goal is to reduce the formation of aqueous humor, bringing inflow into better balance with outflow resistance in eyes with a severe outflow handicap.

Transscleral laser treatment of the ciliary body – transscleral cyclophotocoagulation (TSCPC) – is usually reserved for eyes with some vision potential and refractory glaucoma after failure of previous trabeculectomies or tube-shunt procedures; for eyes with limited vision and highly elevated IOP despite maximum acceptable medical treatment; for painful glaucomatous eyes with highly elevated IOP and little or no vision potential; for eyes with severe surface scarring precluding additional filtration procedures; and for eyes with recent onset of neovascular glaucoma, preferably prior to formation of circumferential occlusive peripheral anterior synechiae. Attractive success rates have been reported in small series of eyes with refractory glaucoma after penetrating keratoplasty,[49] uveitic glaucoma,[50] glaucoma after intravitreal silicone oil,[51] refractory pediatric glaucoma,[52,53] after failure of a previous tube-shunt procedure,[54] and as a primary treatment in challenging situations.[55] Transscleral cyclophotocoagulation may also be helpful for patients with a debilitated general medical condition that precludes invasive surgery, or those who refuse invasive surgery.

Eyes with good vision are not excluded, though patients with these seriously affected eyes at any level of vision should be warned that in about 25% of cases – depending upon the preoperative vision and the diagnosis – postoperative vision will be somewhat worse than the pretreatment level and only rarely improved after surgery.[56,57] Often, these eyes are at risk of imminent loss of vision from glaucoma.

Treatment is less likely to be helpful for eyes with total occlusion of outflow, because these eyes would need near total stoppage of inflow in order for IOP to come to acceptable levels. While this treatment is often done in an office setting, it requires profound local, usually retrobulbar, anesthesia, or general anesthesia in an operating room setting; the patient must be cooperative and medically fit for this.

Endoscopic photocoagulation (ECP) is for eyes with refractory glaucoma and some eyes with neovascular glaucoma. It has also been used widely for eyes with medically controlled glaucoma undergoing phacoemulsification. In the last group, the goal is to reduce dependence on medical glaucoma treatment. ECP is an invasive procedure. As with TSCPC it requires profound local, usually peribulbar, anesthesia, or general anesthesia in an operating room setting, with the usual associated requirements for patient cooperation and medial clearance.

### 61.5.2 History

Ciliary ablation for glaucoma dates to the early twentieth century. Ciliary ablation has been done with nearly every imaginable method of energy delivery to the eye, including coagulation with chemicals, diathermy, freezing, xenon light, laser light delivered directly to the ciliary processes or across the sclera, and ultrasound.[58] In the 1970s, cyclocryotherapy had largely replaced the earlier methods of ciliary ablation for recalcitrant glaucoma. The many postoperative problems associated with cyclocryotherapy[59] led to interest in laser methods of ciliary ablation. In 1972, Beckman and coworkers were first to report using a laser method for transscleral cyclophotocoagulation.[60] By the mid-1980s, commercial free-running neodymium:YAG laser systems had become available and were employed successfully for transscleral procedures.[61–63] Success with ruby and neodymium:YAG systems was based on the high transmission through sclera of longer wavelength ruby (red) and neodymium:YAG (infrared) light coupled with relatively high absorbance of these wavelengths by pigment in ciliary tissue.[64,65] Diode laser systems for eye treatment were commercially available starting in the late 1980s. These small, portable systems provided continuous output in the near-infrared part of the spectrum, thus meeting the requirement for good scleral transmission and melanin absorption. The energy could be delivered through fiber optics to a treatment handpiece. The fiber-optic tip compressed both surface vasculature over the sclera and the sclera itself, enhancing transmission of the treatment beam. Gaasterland, working with Buzawa of Iridex Corporation (Mountain View, CA) developed the G-Probe fiber-optic delivery device and methods for this diode laser treatment in the late 1980s; Gaasterland and Pollack reported on the method and initial results of treatments in 1992.[58] The method has come into use for both early and late glaucoma of all varieties throughout the world. While there are some intraoperative and postoperative problems related to this approach to ciliary ablation, they are less than after cyclocryotherapy and somewhat less than after the neodymium:YAG method, both of which are now less frequently done.[58]

Endophotocoagulation of the ciliary processes, though an invasive procedure, offers direct visualization of location and effect on target tissue, adjustment of treatment parameters to optimize tissue response, and relative sparing of underlying pigmented tissue.[66–68] Uram, in the early 1990s, developed a clinical method and commercial system for this treatment.[69] This procedure has been adopted for eyes with glaucoma undergoing phacoemulsification as an alternative to combined cataract and glaucoma-filtering surgery.

### 61.5.3 Surgery and Postoperative Care

As with all surgical procedures, the patient should understand the plan, requirements, benefits, risks, and alternatives, and give informed consent for the proposed procedure. For TSCPC, warn the patient about the potential for postoperative pain and some reduction of vision. The patient should also understand that more than one step of TSCPC treatment may be needed to achieve the desired control of glaucoma.

### 61.5.4 Preparation

For TSCPC, local peribulbar and retrobulbar anesthesia is needed. In the treatment room, using an Atkinson needle and 10-mL syringe, administer 2 mL of a 50% mix of Marcaine 0.5% and plain lidocaine 2% (without epinephrine) in the peribulbar space in the lateral half of the lower lid, followed by 3–4 mL in the retrobulbar space. Lesser amounts of anesthesia are seldom sufficient.

- For ECP, standard operating room preparation is used with peribulbar or retrobulbar anesthesia.
- Allow sufficient time before starting treatment for the local anesthetic agent to spread. Test gently for adequate numbing with forceps before starting TSCPC.

### 61.5.5 TSCPC

#### 61.5.5.1 Treatment and Suggested Settings

Set up the IRIS Medical Instruments OcuLight® SLx system or the IRIDEX IQ 810 system with G-Probe™ delivery; there are two treatment approaches for energy delivery:

- "Slow Coagulation Technique" for eyes with dark and light brown iris color – 1.25 W and 4.0–4.5 s duration (5.0–5.6 J per application); and for eyes with all other degrees of iris pigmentation – 1.5 W and 3.5–4.0-s duration (5.25–6.0 J per application).
- "Standard Technique" uses a starting power of 1.75 W and 2.0-s duration (3.5 J per application); power is adjusted upward or downward in 0.25-W increments according to whether there are excessive tissue "pops" during applications; eyes with darker pigmentation require slightly lower energies to obtain equivalent results.
- Clean the delivery probe and fiber optic scrupulously with alcohol wipes before and after treatment.
- With slit lamp biomicroscope or another form of magnified observation, treat three quadrants, with about seven applications per quadrant. For the first step of treatment, omit the temporal quadrant; and for a second step of treatment on a later date, if needed, omit either the upper temporal or lower temporal quadrant.
- The location of each laser application is guided by the footplate of the G-Probe, which is positioned with the curved anterior edge of the footplate on the anterior border of the limbus and with each subsequent application spaced one-half the width of the footplate. The fiber-optic protrudes 0.7 mm from the footplate, causing a slight indentation at the treatment site in the paralimbal tissue, which serves as a mark for the sequential applications (during the next application the trailing edge of the footplate bisects the indentation of the fiber optic at the site of the previous application).
- Observe for "pops" or surface burns and adjust power and technique accordingly. The probe tip must be clean throughout treatment, as charred debris on the tip can heat and burn into or through the sclera.

### 61.5.6 Endoscopic Photocoagulation

#### 61.5.6.1 Treatment and Suggested Settings

Set up the Medtronic Ophthalmics Endo Optiks system with the 20-gage endoscopic probe containing the fiber-optic light source, helium–neon aiming beam, and the 810-nm diode laser treatment source; power is from 0.5 to 0.9 W and duration is surgeon controlled:

- Laser applications to the ciliary processes are typically from 0.5 to 2.0-s duration, depending upon observed tissue reaction of whitening and shrinkage.
- This is an invasive procedure and is carried out in operative suite. Patients should be informed of risk and benefits, and indicate understanding of the alternatives of filtration surgery or transscleral cyclophotocoagulation.
- Uram has described the method.[69] The pupil is dilated widely.
- The 20-gage fiber-optic probe – inserted through a limbal 2.5 mm paracentesis, after extra deepening of the anterior

chamber and elevation of the iris to expand the ciliary sulcus of the posterior chamber of the phakic, aphakic, or pseudophakic eye with viscoelastic – rovides an endoscopic view to a monitor. In addition to the viewing function, the probe contains a light source, a helium–neon aiming beam, and the 810-nm diode laser treatment laser beam.
- Alternatively, in aphakic or pseudophakic eyes the probe may be introduced through the pars plana after a limited anterior vitrectomy.
- Long duration, about 0.5–2.0 s, laser applications are directed onto individual ciliary processes to produce whitening and shrinkage of the entire anterioposterior extent of the ciliary process, omitting scar or disrupted tissue.
- Power, duration, or both are adjusted downward if, due to boiling of tissue water, bubble formation is seen or "popping" occurs.
- From 180° to 360° of the ciliary body circumference is treated, usually requiring two or three paracentesis sites.
- The viscoelastic is removed from the anterior segment of the eye and, if needed, the paracentesis wounds closed with a single suture.

### 61.5.7 Postoperative Care

- For both procedures, apply a strong, long-lasting cycloplegic (e.g., atropine) and a topical steroid at the conclusion of the procedure. Give a topical antibiotic for eyes after ECP; a soft eye patch protects the eye until the local anesthesia wears off.
- The cycloplegic b.i.d. and steroid drops q.i.d. are continued for at least 2 weeks, and may be required for a longer time. Severe postoperative inflammation may require more aggressive use of steroids. The antibiotic given t.i.d. to q.i.d. may be discontinued after a week.
- Acetaminophen (Tylenol) may be taken for pain; stronger analgesics are seldom needed. Some patients may benefit from short-term use of an ice pack.
- As with all surgical procedures, patients are monitored at a decreasing frequency to assure safe healing during several months after the procedure.

### 61.5.8 Problems and Complications

#### 61.5.8.1 Intraoperative

- Surface burns during TSCPC. These may occur if the fiber-optic tip is contaminated with charred debris[58]; clean the tip.

- "Pops" during TSCPC or ECP. Occasional popping sounds will occur normally. Repeated pops, with every application, indicate power is too high, which brings cellular water to a boil during the application; reduce the power. Consider lengthening duration of applications at the lower power.
- Laser energy transmission to the posterior retina during diode TSCPC treatment appears to be well within safety guidelines.[70]

#### 61.5.8.2 Postoperative

- Pain – found in one-third to one-half of eyes undergoing TSCPC, this is usually mild, yet may be severe. Treatment is with topical cycloplegics, topical nonsteroidal anti-inflammatory medications, icepacks, and systemic analgesics, as needed.
- Inflammation – this is to be expected and should be treated appropriately. Severe inflammation with formation of a protein clot occurs occasionally after TSCPC, particularly in eyes with neovascular glaucoma, and requires more aggressive anti-inflammatory management.
- Bleeding – this is rare, more often in eyes with neovascular glaucoma. It usually is sufficiently mild to resolve spontaneously with passage of time.
- Change of visual acuity[56,57] – decrease of two Snellen lines or more has been reported in various studies in anywhere from 12 to 40% (mean about 25%) of eyes treated with TSCPC. It appears more likely in eyes with preexisting poor vision. Improved vision has also occurred (though it is seldom discussed). The falloff, which sometimes improves with healing, has to be considered in comparison with the expected deterioration that would occur in the absence of intervention.
- Sympathetic ophthalmia – has occurred in a small number of eyes after ciliary destructive procedures, including penetrating cyclodiathermy,[71-s75] though none are reported yet after diode laser TSCPC.
- Malignant glaucoma – was found in an eye after diode laser cyclophotocoagulation.[76] By way of contrast, there are reports of successful treatment for malignant glaucoma with laser cyclotherapy,[77] including treatment for malignant glaucoma with TSCPC.[78]

### 61.5.9 Expected Outcomes

The goal of TSCPC is to reduce IOP by reducing aqueous humor inflow. When treatment ablates a large portion of the ciliary processes, less aqueous humor is formed thereafter.

More extensive damage is followed by more reduction in aqueous production. Provided there is no increase of resistance to aqueous outflow through the trabecular meshwork and the uveoscleral route, the IOP will fall. The reported rates of lack of failure of the TSCPC intervention vary from about 50 to >90% after 1–2 years.[79,80] Failure is more likely in eyes with zero or minimal outflow before treatment. The rates are dependent upon diagnosis and ethnic background of the patients. For example, patients with neovascular glaucoma often require a second step of treatment during the first 3 months after the initial step; with this they have about a 50–60% rate of long-term success. Often after TSCPC, patients are able to reduce topical and systemic medical glaucoma treatment slightly, yet most still need some continued medical treatment for satisfactory IOP control. A second step of TSCPC treatment for eyes with insufficient response to a first step is often helpful, though the rates of success are not established and appear to be lower than after the initial step of intervention (see Chap. 63).

## 61.6 Other Laser Procedures for Glaucoma

### 61.6.1 Laser Suture Lysis

This laser intervention allows the surgeon to divide one or more scleral flap sutures, with the goal to enhance insufficient aqueous bleb formation and filtration after trabeculectomy. This procedure and trabeculectomy with releasable scleral flap sutures have a similar efficacy.[81] Eligible eyes have had recent trabeculectomy yet have elevated IOP and a low or flat filtration bleb with a deep anterior chamber and a patent inner ostium seen during gonioscopy. If no adjunctive antifibrotic was used during trabeculectomy, this procedure should be done during the first few postoperative days; after that the fibrosis during healing reduces the likelihood of improvement with suture lysis. For trabeculectomy performed with 5-fluorouracil, the time to expect benefit from suture lysis is extended to several postoperative weeks; when it was done with adjunctive mitomycin-C postoperative suture lysis may be beneficial for up to 2 months. After these intervals there is a decreasing likelihood of enhancement of bleb function.

Suture lysis is done with topical anesthesia, usually with a treatment lens to enhance visualization of the sutures to be cut.[82] Several lenses have been designed for this purpose. The lens compresses the bleb tissue over the suture. The lens for this can be the flat between mirrors of a four-mirror gonioscopy lens or one of several lenses specially designed to enhance suture visibility and a tight focus of the laser beam (Fig. 61.6). Occasionally the sutures cannot be located through thick overlying conjunctiva and Tenon's tissues, in which case an invasive procedure may be justified.

Most surgeons use an argon or frequency-doubled continuous wave neodymium-YAG laser for this procedure. Krypton red laser systems are an alternative. Diode systems at 810 nm are less likely to be successful because the dye of black nylon sutures is poorly absorbent at this wavelength.

#### 61.6.1.1 Laser System Settings and Laser Applications

The power setting for blue–green (argon) or green (frequency-doubled neodymium:YAG) systems is 200–1,000 mW with duration of 0.05–0.2 s (usually 0.1 s) and a spot size of 50 or 100 μm.

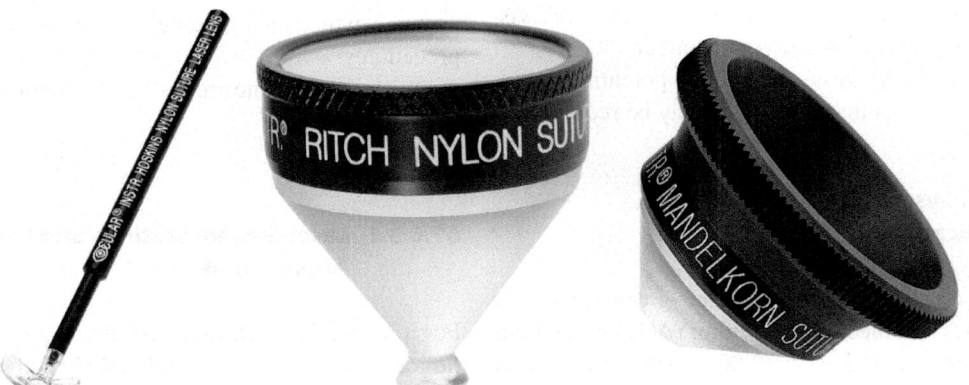

**Fig. 61.6** Lenses for lysis of nylon sutures. All provide compression of conjunctiva and blanching of blood vessels overlying buried sutures. Hoskins lens (*left*) has 3.0 mm diameter glass button centered in a flange designed to retract lids; button yields 1.2× image magnification and 0.83× laser treatment spot diameter reduction. Ritch lens (*center*) is cone shaped with a 5.94 mm diameter convex contact surface and a frosted, nonreflective external surface; flange and lens cone enhance lid retraction; lens does not alter image magnification or laser treatment spot size. Mandelkorn lens (*right*) has 5.6 mm diameter base; lens yields 1.32× image magnification and 0.76× laser treatment spot diameter reduction; wide handpiece provides lid separation. (Photographs courtesy of Ocular Instruments, Inc., Bellevue, WA)

Slightly lower power is sufficient during treatment with red (krypton) continuous wave laser systems. One or two precisely placed applications to a clearly visible suture usually suffices to divide the suture; the surgeon can see the successfully cut ends of the suture separate.

Formation or elevation of the bleb usually follows. Sometimes local pressure on the flap or massage of the eye is needed to initiate flow into the bleb through the site of the cut suture. If this is not successful, cutting another suture may help.

Problems that may arise after suture lysis include lack of success to enhance filtration, overfiltration with hypotony or even a shallow or flat anterior chamber, burns or perforation of the bleb wall with potential for a local leak, bleeding, iris incarceration, malignant glaucoma, and dellen formation adjacent to a high bleb.

## 61.6.2 Sealing Hypotonous Cyclodialysis Clefts

This condition usually follows ocular trauma. A small cleft can cause excessive hypotony, choroidal effusion, shallowing of the anterior chamber, cataract, retinal and choroidal folds, optic disk edema, and secondary decline of vision.[83] Such clefts, when located with gonioscopy, are amenable to laser photocoagulation of the inner surface of the cleft at its entrance in the anterior chamber recess. Large clefts are not eligible because laser treatment of this type is almost never successful; other management is indicated. For small clefts, noninvasive laser treatment with the continuous wave argon or frequency-doubled neodymium:YAG laser energy can be done using a gonioscopic lens, or invasive laser treatment can be done using an endoscopic diode laser system. Both approaches require that the entrance to the cleft be surgically visible, which may require adjunctive intracameral viscoelastic to deepen a shallow anterior chamber.

Treatment must be aggressive, which is potentially painful. Peribulbar or retrobulbar anesthesia may be required.

### 61.6.2.1 Laser System Settings and Laser Applications

Recommended treatment starts with blue–green (argon) or green (frequency-doubled neodymium:YAG) continuous wave laser system set at 2–3 W (2,000–3,000 mW) power using a spot size of 50–100 μm with 0.1-s duration. Laser applications are in contiguous rows parallel to the limbus onto the visible outer scleral surface of the cleft starting at the scleral spur. The entire visible inner scleral surface of the cleft is treated. Next the spot size is increased to 100–200 μm and power reduced to 1 W, while duration is unchanged at 0.1 s.

Overlapping rows of laser applications are made to the choroid and ciliary body inner surface of the cleft; these rows are made parallel to the limbus starting at the visible depth of the cleft and moving anteriorly toward the base of the iris.

Postoperative treatment is with topical atropine BID to enhance apposition of the walls of the cleft; topical corticosteroids are avoided in order to enhance healing with fibrosis.

Because the trabecular drainage pathways may have collapsed during hypotony, there is a possibility that several days following cleft closure the IOP will become elevated due to cleft healing with resumption of aqueous production. The elevation is usually transient, resolving as the outflow pathways resume function; the transient rise of IOP is managed with standard glaucoma medications.

Failure of a first session of treatment to provoke closure can be approached with a second session of laser treatment. Thereafter alternative surgical management becomes justified.

## 61.6.3 Treatment to Reopen an Occluded Inner Ostium of a Filtering Site

Occasionally, early in the postoperative period, a filtering operation fails to function adequately due to occlusion of the inner ostium of the filtering tract by iris incarceration, PAS formation, or a membrane across the inner opening.

An early iris occlusion may be opened with coagulative, followed by high-power pulsed disruptive laser applications onto the juncture of the occluding iris tissue and the endothelial surface of the cornea at the border of the inner ostium.[84]

Thin membranes occluding the inner ostium can be opened with disruptive laser applications.[85] Early laser treatments preceded availability of high-power pulsed laser systems, which have enhanced the ease and success of these procedures.

Apply topical anesthesia for the gonioscopic laser treatment contact lens.

### 61.6.3.1 Laser System Settings and Laser Applications

For iris occluding the inner ostium, begin with a blue–green (argon) or green (frequency-doubled neodymium:YAG) continuous wave laser system with power of 400–1,000 mW, spot diameter of 50–100 μm, and duration of 0.1–0.2 s. The laser applications cause local shrinkage when applied to the iris tissue at the edge of the adhesion to the cornea. During treatment, adjust spot size, power, or duration to achieve a blanching tissue reaction. Apply a double row of treatment spots to the adhesion site. This will ensure against bleeding during the next step.

Next, with the gonioscopic lens in place, switch to a Q-switched neodymium:YAG system set to deliver single pulses at 3.0–6.0 mJ. Direct sufficient applications to disrupt the coagulated tissue at the edge of the inner ostium and separate the adhesion.

For thin membranes occluding the inner ostium, use settings as in the second step of iris occlusions and make laser applications directly to the center of the membrane with the Q-switched neodymium:YAG laser system.

In successful cases, with local massage, the filtering bleb inflates and the IOP falls. For several days treat with increased frequency of topical steroid medication. If the bleb does not inflate after successful clearing of the inner ostium and massage, another, nonlaser, management option is justified.

### 61.6.4 Coagulation of Bleeders Located in the Internal Aspect of Surgical Wounds

Small, pesky bleeders occasionally follow trabeculectomy or other surgeries that are completed with full thickness limbal wounds.[86] Sometimes the bleeder is located in the iris at the site of the iridectomy or behind the iris from a damaged ciliary process. Wherever located, these bleeders often leak intermittently and cause a postoperative hyphema. The bleeding site in the anterior chamber angle is found with gonioscopy and with the slit lamp when in the iris. When found, provided the optical pathway to the site is clear, the bleeder can be coagulated with a continuous wave argon or frequency-doubled neodymium:YAG laser system. It is helpful for localization when there is a small clot of blood at the site of origin of the bleeding, which occurs when there has been recent leakage.

#### 61.6.4.1 Laser System Settings and Laser Applications

Make single applications of blue–green (argon) or green (frequency-doubled neodymium:YAG) continuous wave laser energy onto and adjacent to the bleeding site using power of 600–1,000 mW, a spot size of 50 or 100 μm, and 0.1–0.2-s duration. Make sufficient applications to blanch the bleeding site thoroughly. Occasionally, on another day, a second session of treatment may be required – warn the patient about this during the preoperative discussion before the first treatment session.

Usually no escalation of the postoperative medication regimen is needed. If successful, the recurrent bleeding stops.

### 61.6.5 Direct Treatment of New Vessels on Trabecular Meshwork in Neovascular Glaucoma

The early pathophysiology in neovascular glaucoma is formation of fine, new vessels on the inner surface of the open trabecular meshwork. The retraction of the fibrosis that follows pulls the base of the iris onto the trabecular tissue, forming PAS. Although contemporary management of this condition rests upon panretinal photocoagulation and, more recently, intravitreal administration of an anti-VEGF agent, the ophthalmologist encounters an occasional case of early rubeosis after ischemic retinal vein occlusion or diabetic retinopathy that would benefit from immediate inhibition of fibrovascular tissue proliferating in the anterior chamber angle recess. The goal is to coagulate the small new vessels traversing the angle recess and thus interrupt formation of PAS. More than one session of treatment is often required as new vessels form after the first session.[87]

Apply topical anesthesia for the gonioscopic laser treatment contact lens.

#### 61.6.5.1 Laser System Settings and Applications

Make applications of blue–green (argon) or green (frequency-doubled neodymium:YAG) continuous wave laser energy directly onto the small vessels in the anterior chamber angle recess using power of 600–1,000 mW, a spot size of 50 or 100 μm, and 0.1–0.2 s duration. Adjust power and duration to cause observable blanching of the vessels. Use sufficient applications to blanch vessels in at least one-third to one-half the circumference of the angle, treat even more if the neovascularization is circumferential.

Most treated eyes do not require a modified medication regimen. Long-term, persistent avoidance of angle closure with normalization of IOP are reported for about three-quarters of treated eyes, in reports from the days before panretinal photocoagulation and anti-VEGF agents.[87] Nowadays, this procedure should be considered adjunctive to these newer modalities of management and applied in early cases of rubeosis when the clinical course justifies it.

### 61.7 Conclusion

Table 61.1 compares the five types of laser trabeculoplasty that are presently approved. Two of these are continuous wave (CW) using argon laser (ALT) or diode laser (DLT). Three of the present trabeculoplasties are pulsed treatments. These include selective laser trabeculoplasty (SLT) using a

**Table 61.1** Comparison of laser trabeculoplasty techniques and treatment parameters

Comparison of various laser trabeculoplasty techniques and treatment parameters within the range considered typical for average patients

| Characteristics and parameter | Units | CW-laser trabeculoplasty | | Pulsed-laser trabeculoplasty | | |
|---|---|---|---|---|---|---|
| | | ALT[88–90] | DLT[88–90] | SLT[89,90] | MLT[91–ww93] | TLT[94] |
| Indication(s) for use (IFU) | –/– | Laser trabeculoplasty | Laser trabeculoplasty | Laser trabeculoplasty | Laser trabeculoplasty | Laser trabeculoplasty |
| Contact gonio lens (laser magnification) | –/– | Goldmann 3-mirror lens (1.08×) | Ritch trabeculoplasty (0.71×) | Latina laser gonio lens (1.0×) | Latina laser gonio lens (1.0×) | Goldmann 3-mirror lens (1.08×) |
| Laser wavelength | nm | 488/514 (or 532) | 810 | 532 | 810 | 790 |
| (Spot diameter in air) spot diameter at tissue | μm | (50) 54 | (75) 53 | (400) 400 | (200–300) 200–300 | (200) 216 |
| Laser power | W | 0.4–0.7 | 0.6–1.0 | 200–400×0³ | 2 | 4.3–17.1×10³ |
| Laser irradiance | W/cm² | 20–36×10³ | 30–50×10³ | 160–320×10⁶ | 2.83–6.37×10³ | 13.7–54.5×10⁶ |
| Laser pulse length | s | 0.1 | 0.1–0.2 | 3×10⁻⁹ | 300×10⁻⁶ | 7×10⁻⁶ |
| Pulses/application site (time – % duty factor) | # (s) | 1 (0.1s – 100%) | 1 (0.1–0.2s – 100%) | 1 (3×10⁻⁹s – 100%) | 100 (0.2s at 15%) | 1 (7×10⁻⁶s – 100%) |
| Laser energy per pulse (per application site) | J | 40–70×10⁻³ | 60–200×10⁻³ | 0.6–1.2×10⁻³ | 0.6×10⁻³(60×10⁻³) | 40–80×10⁻³ |
| Laser fluence per pulse (per application site) | J/cm² | 2.0–3.6×10³ | 3.0–10×10³ | 0.5–1.0 | 0.85–1.91 (85–191) | 4.1–16.3×10³ |
| Number of applications and placement over the TM | # | 50 (or 100) spaced over 180° (or 360°) | 50 (100) spaced over 180° (360°) | 50 (or 100) confluent over 180° (or 360°) | 66–100 (132–200) confluent over 180° (360°) | 50 spaced over the inferior 180° |
| Treated fraction (%) of the TM circumference | –/– | 6.5–13% | 6.5–13% | 50% (or 100%) | 50% (or 100%) | 25% |
| Total energy per eye | J | 2.0–7.0 | 3.0–20.0 | 30–120×10⁻³ | 3.96–12.0 | 2.0–4.0 |
| Expected endpoint | –/– | Blanching (mild) to bubbles (intense) | Blanching to no visible reaction (in lightly pigmented TM) | No visible tissue reaction to small bubbles | No visible tissue reaction | Visible TM tissue reaction with microbubbles |

frequency-doubled laser and based upon the notion that the laser selectively affects pigmented cells in the meshwork; microdiode laser trabeculoplasty (MLT); and Titanium laser trabeculoplasty (TLT), which was approved in the Fall of 2008. Both MLT and TLT use frequencies that would be expected to reach into the deeper aspects of the trabecular meshwork, and could, theoretically have more effect upon the juxtacanalicular meshwork.

In terms of treatment applications, the table describes what has appeared in the literature to date. Generally all of the treatments have involved 50–66 treatments in 180°. Some clinicians favor treating 360° at once while others favor treating only 180° at a time. One of the most valuable aspects of this table is that it compares what one sees as an endpoint. Traditionally ALT treatment has resulted in blanching or bubbles. Virtually no tissue reaction is seen with MLT. With the other treatments, some type of tissue reaction is usually seen.

## References

1. Maiman TH (1960) Stimulated optical radiation in ruby. Nature 187:493–497
2. Steinert RF, Puliafito CA. The Nd-YAG Laser in Ophthalmology. Principles and Clinical Applications of Photodisruption. 1985. W.B. Saunders Company, Philadelphia, chapters 1, 2.
3. Zaret MM, Breinin GM, Schmidt H et al (1961) Ocular lesions produced by an optical maser (laser). Science 134:1525–1528
4. Campbell CJ, Rittler MC, Koestler CJ (1963) The optical maser as retinal photocoagulator: an evaluation. Trans Am Acad Ophthalmol Otolaryngol 67:58–67
5. Kapany NS, Peppers NA, Zweng HC et al (1963) Retinal photocoagulation by lasers. Nature 199:146–149
6. Mainster MA, Sliney DH, Belcher CD et al (1983) Laser photodisruptors. Damage mechanisms, instrument design and safety. Ophthalmology 90:973–991
7. Trokel SL, Srinivasan R, Braren B (1983) Eximer laser surgery of the cornea. Am J Ophthalmology 96:710–715
8. Kass MA, Heuer DK, Higginbotham EJ, et al, Ocular Hypertension Treatment Study Group. The Ocular Hypertension Treatment Study: a randomized trial determines that topical ocular hypotensive medication delays or prevents the onset of primary open-angle glaucoma. *Arch Ophthalmol.* 2002;120:701–713
9. Collaborative Normal-Tension Glaucoma Study Group (1998) Comparison of glaucomatous progression between untreated patients with normal-tension glaucoma and patients with therapeutically reduced intraocular pressures. Am J Ophthalmol 126:487–497
10. Leske MC, Heijl A, Husssein M, et al, Early Manifest Glaucoma Trial Group. Factors for glaucoma progression and the effect of treatment. The Early Manifest Glaucoma Trial. *Arch Ophthalmol.* 2003;121:48–56.
11. Lichter PR, Musch DC, Gillespie BW, et al, CIGTS Study Group. Interim clinical outcomes in the Collaborative Initial Glaucoma Treatment Study comparing initial treatment randomized to medications or surgery. *Ophthalmology.* 2001;108:1943–1953
12. The AGIS Investigators (2000) The Advanced Glaucoma Intervention Study (AGIS): The relationship between control of intraocular pressure and visual field deterioration. Am J Ophthalmol 130:429–440
13. Robin AL, Pollack IR (1983) Argon laser trabeculoplasty in secondary forms of open-angle glaucoma. Arch Ophthalmol 101:382–384
14. Wise JB, Witter SL (1979) Argon laser therapy for open-angle glaucoma. A pilot study. Arch Ophthalmol 97:319–322
15. Hager H. [Special microsurgical interventions. 2. First experiences with the argon laser apparatus 800] *Klin Monatsbl Augenheilkd.* 1973;162:437–450 [in German].
16. Krasnov MM (1973) Laseropuncture of anterior chamber angle in glaucoma. Am J Ophthalmol 75:674–678
17. Wickham MG, Worthen DM (1979) Argon laser trabeculotomy: long-term follow-up. Ophthalmology 86:495–503
18. Schwartz AL, Del Priore LV (1991) The evolving role of argon laser trabeculoplasty in glaucoma. Ophthalmol Clin North Am 4:827–838
19. Weinreb RN, Ruderman J, Juster R et al (1983) Influence of the num ber of laser burns administered on the early results of argon laser trabeculoplasty. Am J Ophthalmol 95:287–292
20. Weinreb RN, Ruderman J, Juster R et al (1983) Immediate intraocular pressure response to argon laser trabeculoplasty. Am J Ophthalmol 95:279–286
21. Gaasterland DE, Kupfer C (1974) Experimental glaucoma in the rhesus monkey. Invest Ophthalmol 13:455–457
22. Wise JB (1981) Long-term control of adult open angle glaucoma by Argon laser treatment. Ophthalmology 88:197–202
23. Rodriques MM, Spaeth GL, Donohoo P (1982) Electron microscopy of argon laser therapy in phakic open-angle glaucoma. Ophthalmology 89:198–210
24. Acott TS, Kingley PD, Samples JR et al (1988) Human trabecular meshwork organ culture: morphology and glycoaminoglycan synthesis. Invest Ophthalmol Vis Sci 29:90–100
25. Bylsma SS, Samples JR, Acott TS et al (1988) Trabecular cell division after argon laser trabeculoplasty. Arch Ophthalmol 106:545–547
26. Anderson RR, Parish JA (1983) Selective photothermolysis: precise microsurgery by selective absorption of pulsed radiation. Science 29(220):524–527
27. Latina MA, Park C (1995) Selective targeting of trabecular meshwork cells: in vitro studies of pulsed and CW laser interactions. Exp Eye Res 60:359–371
28. Latina MA, Sibayan SA, Shin DH et al (1998) Q-switched 532-nm Nd:YAG laser trabeculoplasty (Selective Laser Trabeculoplasty): a multicenter, pilot, clinical study. Ophthalmology 105:2082–2090
29. Latina MA, de Leon JM (2005) Selective laser trabeculoplasty. Ophthalmol Clin North Am 18:409–419
30. Barkana Y, Belkin M (2007) Selective laser trabeculoplasty. Diagnostic and surgical techniques. Surv Ophthalmol 52:634–654
31. Glaucoma Laser Trial Research Group (1995) The Glaucoma Laser Trial (GLT) and Glaucoma Laser Trial Follow-up Study: 7. Results. Am J Ophthalmol 120:718–731
32. The AGIS Investigators (2004) The Advanced Glaucoma Intervention Study (AGIS) 13. Comparison of treatment outcomes within race: 10-year results. Ophthalmology 111:651–664
33. Van Herrick W, Shaffer RN, Schwartz A. Estimation of width of angle of anterior chamber. Incidence and significance of the narrow angle. Am J Ophthalmol. 1969 Oct;68(4):626–9
34. Von Graefe A (1857) Ueber die Iridectomie die Glaucom; und uber den glaucomatosen process. Graefes Arch Clin Exp Ophthalmol 3(pt 2):456–555
35. Curran EJ (1920) A new operation for glaucoma involving a new principle in the etiology and treatment of chronic primary glaucoma. Arch Ophthalmol 49:695–716
36. Meyer-Schwickerath G (1956) Erfahrungen mit der Lichtkoagulation der Netzhuat und der Iris. Doc Ophthalmol 10:91–131
37. American Academy of Ophthalmology (1994) Laser peripheral iridotomy for pupillary-block glaucoma. Arch Ophthalmol 101:1749–1758
38. Abraham RK (1981) Protocol for single-session argon laser iridectomy for angle closure glaucoma. Int Ophthalmol Clin 21:145–166

39. Schirmer KE (1983) Argon laser surgery of the iris, optimized by contact lenses. Arch Ophthalmol 101:1130–1132
40. Wise JB, Munnerlyn CR, Erickson PJ (1986) A high effeciency laser iridotomy-sphincterotomy lens. Am J Ophthalmol 101:546–553
41. Goins K, Schmeisser E, Smith T (1990) Argon laser pretreatment in Nd:YAG iridotomy. Ophthalmic Surg 21:497–500
42. American Academy of Ophthalmology (2005) Preferred Practice Pattern. Primary Angle Closure. American Academy of Ophthalmology, San Francisco, CA
43. Krupin T, Stone RA, Cohen BH et al (1985) Acute intraocular pressure response to argon laser iridotomy. Ophthalmology 92:922–926
44. Ritch R (1982) Argon laser treatment fo medically unresponsive attacks of angle-closure glaucoma. Am J Ophthalmol 94:197–204
45. Zweng HC, Little HL, Hammond AH (1974) Complications of argon laser photocoagulation. Trans Am Acad Ophthalmol Otolaryngol 78:195–204
46. Thomas NE, Morse PH (1976) Anterior segment complications of argon laser therapy. Ann Ophthalmol 8:299–301
47. James WA Jr, deRoeth A Jr, Forbes M, et al. Argon laser photomydriasis. Am J Ophthalmol. 1976;81:62–70
48. Wise JB (1985) Iris sphincterotomy, iridotomy, and synechiotomy by linear incision with the argon laser. Ophthalmology 92:641–645
49. Shah P, Lee GA, Kirwan JK et al (2001) Cyclodiode photocoagulation for refractory glaucoma after penetrating keratoplasty. Ophthalmology 108:1986–1991
50. Schlote T, Derse M, Zierhut M (2000) Transscleral diode laser cyclophotocoagulation for the treatment of refractory glaucoma secondary to inflammatory eye diseases. Br J Ophthalmol 84:999–1003
51. Kan SK, Park KH, Kim DM et al (1999) Effect of diode laser transscleral cyclophotocoagulation in the management of glaucoma after intravitreal silicone oil injection for complicated retinal detachments. Br J Ophthalmol 83:713–717
52. Izgi B, Demirci H, Ysim F et al (2001) Diode laser cyclophotocoagulation in refractory glaucoma. Comparison between pediatric and adult glaucomas. Ophthalmic Surg Lasers 32:100–107
53. Kirwan JF, Shah P, Khaw PT (2002) Diode laser cyclophothocoagulation. Role in the management of refractory pediatric glaucomas. Ophthalmology 109:316–323
54. Semchyshyn TM, Tsai JC, Joos KM (2002) Supplemental transscleral diode laser cyclophtotcoagulation after aqueous shunt placement in refractory glaucoma. Ophthalmology 109:1078–1084
55. Egbert PR, Fiadoyor S, Budenz DL et al (2001) Diode laser transscleral cyclophotocoagulation as a primary surgical treatment for primary open-angle glaucoma. Arch Ophthalmol 119:345–350
56. Wilensky JT, Kammer J (2004) Long-term visual outcome of transscleral laser cyclotherapy in eyes with ambulatory vision. Ophthalmology 111:1389–1392
57. Pokroy R, Greenwald Y, Pollack A et al (2008) Visual loss after transscleral diode laser cyclophotocoagulation for primary open-angle and neovascular glaucoma. Ophthalmic Surg Lasers Imaging 39:22–29
58. Gaasterland D, Pollack I (1992) Initial experience with a new method of laser transscleral cyclophotocoagulation for ciliary ablation in severe glaucoma. Trans Am Ophthalmol Soc 90:225–246
59. Caprioli J, Strang SL, Spaeth GL (1985) Cyclocryotherapy in the treatment of advanced glaucoma. Ophthalmology 92:947–954
60. Beckman H, Kinsshita A, Rota AN et al (1972) Transscleral ruby laser irradiation of the ciliary body in the treatment of intractable glaucoma. Trans Am Acad Ophthalmol Otolaryngol 76:423–435
61. Wilensky JT, Welch D, Mirolovich M (1985) Transscleral cyclocoagulation using a neodymium:YAG laser. Ophthalmic Surg 16:95–98
62. Fankhauser F, van der Zypen E, Kwasniewska S et al (1986) Transscleral cyclophtocoagulation using a neodymium:YAG laser. Ophthalmic Surg 17:94–100
63. Federman JL, Ando F, Schubert HD et al (1987) Contact laser for transscleral photocoagulation. Ophthalmic Surg 18:182–184
64. Smith RS, Stein MN (1968) Ocular hazards of transscleral laser radiation: I. Spectral reflection and transmission of the sclera, choroid and retina. Am J Ophthalmol 66:21–31
65. Rol P, Niederer P, Dürr U et al (1990) Experimental investigations on the light scattering properties of the; human sclera. Lasers Light Ophthalmol 3:201–202
66. Charles S (1981) Endophotocoagulation. Retina 1:117–120
67. Patel A, Thompson JT, Michels RG et al (1986) Endolaser treatment of the ciliary body for uncontrolled glaucoma. Ophthalmology 93:825–830
68. Zarbin MA, Michels RG, de Bustros S et al (1988) Endolaser treatment of the ciliary body for severe glaucoma. Ophthalmology 95:1639–1647
69. Uram M (1995) Endoscopic cyclophotocoagulation in glaucoma management. Curr Opin Ophthalmol 6:19–29
70. Myers JS, Trevisani MG, Imami N et al (1998) Laser energy reaching the posterior pole during transscleral cyclophotocoagulation. Arch Ophthalmol 116:488–491
71. Bodian M (1953) Sympathetic ophthalmia following cyclodiathermy. Am J Ophthalmol 36:217–225
72. Harrison TJ (1993) Sympathetic ophthalmia after cyclocryotherapy of neovascular glaucoma without ocular penetration. Ophthalmic Surg 24:44–46
73. Edward DP, Brown SVL, Higginbotham E et al (1969) Sympathetic ophthalmic following Neodymium:YAG cyclotherapy. Ophthalmic Surg 20:644–646
74. Lam S, Tessler HH, Lam BL et al (1992) High incidence of sympathetic ophthalmia after contact and noncontact Neodymium:YAG cyclotherapy. Ophthalmology 99:1818–1822
75. Bechrakis NE, Müller-Stolzenburg NW, Helbig H et al (1994) Sympathetic ophthalmia following laser cyclocoagulation. Arch Ophthalmol 112:80–84
76. Azuara-Blanco A, Dua HS (1999) Malignant glaucoma after diode laser cyclophotocoagulation. Am J Ophthalmol 127:467–469
77. Herschler J (1980) Laser shrinkage of the ciliary processes: a treatment for malignant (ciliary block) glaucoma. Ophthalmology 87:1155–1159
78. Carassa RG, Bettin P, Fiori M et al (1999) Treatment of malignant glaucoma with contact transscleral cyclophotocoagulation. Arch Ophthalmol 117:688–690
79. Pastor SA, Singh K, Lee DA et al (2001) Cyclophotocoagulation. A report by the American Academy of Ophthalmology. Ophthalmology 108:2130–2138
80. Kaushik S, Pandav SS, Jain R et al (2008) Lower energy levels adequate for effecdtive transscleral diode laser cyclophotocoagulation in Asian eyes with refractory glaucoma. Eye 22:398–405
81. Aykan U, Bilge AH, Akin T et al (2007) Laser suture lysis or releasable sutures after trabeculectomy. J Glaucoma 16:240–245
82. Hoskins HD Jr, Migliazzo C (1984) Management of failing filtering blebs with the argon laser. Ophthalmic Surg 15:731–733
83. Ormerod LD, Baerveldt G, Sunalp MA et al (1991) Management of the hypotonous cyclodialysis cleft. Ophthalmology 98:1384–1393
84. Ticho U, Ivry M (1977) Reopening of occluded filtering blebs by argon laser photocoagulation. Am J Ophthalmol 84:413–418
85. Van Buskirk EM (1982) Reopening filtration fistulas with the argon laser. Am J Ophthalmol 94:1–3
86. Sharpe ED, Simmons RJ (1986) Argon laser therapy of occult recurrent hyphema from anterior segment wound neovascularization. Ophthalmic Surg 17:283–285
87. Simmons RJ, Dueker DK, Kimbrough RL et al (1977) Goniophotocoagulation for neovascular glaucoma. Trans Am Acad Ophthalmol Otolaryngol 83:80–89

88. American Academy of Ophthalmology. Committee on Ophthalmic Procedures Assessment. Laser trabeculoplasty for primary open-angle glaucoma. *Ophthalmology.* 1996;103(10):1706–1712.
89. Park CH, Latina MA, Schuman JS (2000) Developments in laser trabeculoplasty. Ophthalmic Surgery and Lasers 30(4):315–322
90. Olivier MMG (2004) Glaucoma laser treatment: where are we now? Techniques in Ophthalmology 2(3):118–123
91. Fea AM, Bosone A, Rolle T, Brogliatti B, Grignolo FM (2008) Micropulse diode laser trabeculoplasty (MDLT): a phase II clinical study with 12 months follow-up. Clin Ophthalmol 2(2):247–252
92. Ingvoldstad DD, Krishna R, Willoughby L. Micropulse diode laser trabeculoplasty versus argon laser trabeculoplasty in the treatment of open angle glaucoma [abstract]. *Invest Ophthal Vis Sci.* 2005;46:ARVO E-Abstract 123.
93. Fea AM, Dorin G (2008) Laser treatment of glaucoma: evolution of laser trabeculoplasty techniques. Tech Ophthalmol 6(2):45–52
94. Garcia-Sanchez j, Garcia-Fiejoo J, Saenz-Frances F et al. Titanium sapphire laser trabeculoplasty: hypotensive efficacy and anterior chamber inflammation. *Invest Ophthal Vis Sci.* 2007;48:E-Abstract 3975.

# Chapter 62
# Laser Iridoplasty Techniques for Narrow Angles and Plateau Iris Syndrome

Baseer U. Khan

The apparent mechanism of intraocular pressure (IOP) elevation in primary angle closure (PAC) is straightforward: the obstruction of aqueous to the trabecular meshwork (TM) by the peripheral iris, usually interacting with the lens, which is therefore termed *papillary block*. With age, the crystalline lens increases in diameter, moving the peripheral iris forward and/or increasing pupil block, thus narrowing the angle.[1–4] The conundrum that arises is determining when the threshold of occludability has been reached. Most epidemiological studies have chosen to define this point as when 270° or more of the posterior (pigmented) trabecular meshwork is not visible on gonioscopy; however, this threshold is arbitrary and has not been validated.[5] The issue of angle compression has not been addressed. Nevertheless, at this time, the literature does not purport any other definition to be of greater accuracy and thus this is the operational definition used in this chapter.

Laser peripheral iridotomy (LPI) is almost universally accepted as the first-line management of PAC (Fig. 62.1). However, performing an LPI does not guarantee resolution of occludability. In a study of PAC suspects (eyes deemed occludable without signs of increased IOP), 20% of eyes demonstrated persistent occludability following LPI.[6] There are two significant implications of these findings: It is imperative to reexamine the angle following LPI, and that PAC can be multifactorial in a significant number of patients.

Persistent occludability may be managed with medication, surgery, or further laser therapy. Chronic miotic therapy may adequately open the angle; however, this is not generally tolerated well by the prepresbyopic patient. Brow ache, cataract formation, posterior synechiae formation, and retinal detachment are all possible undesirable side effects. Crystalline lens removal with or without adjunctive procedures will be very effective in increasing angle width. Concomitant presence of a cataract makes this approach highly desirable, but the removal of a lens without cataractous changes remains controversial. Argon laser peripheral iridoplasty (ALPI) is the final option and is discussed in further detail in this chapter.

## 62.1 Pathophysiology and Mechanism of Action

In 1995, Ritch et al described four anatomic levels of force causing the iris to obstruct the trabecular meshwork: (1) the iris (pupil block), (2) the ciliary body (plateau iris), (3) the lens (phacomorphic glaucoma), and (4) posterior to the lens (malignant glaucoma).[7]

Pupil block results when the pupil margin abuts another structure 360°, thereby limiting the flow of aqueous from the posterior to anterior chamber.[8] In the phakic eye, the interacting structure is the anterior lens capsule, but pupil block can also be seen in aphakic and pseudophakic eyes (the discussion of which is beyond the scope of this chapter). In the absence of an alternative communication between the two chambers, the pressure in the posterior chamber rises relative to the anterior chamber causing the midperipheral iris to bow anteriorly (iris bombe). The arching of the iris can significantly narrow the angle, obstructing the TM and resulting in an increase in IOP. LPI creates an alternative pathway for aqueous to flow from the posterior to anterior chamber, thereby equalizing pressure and allowing the iris to move posteriorly to its natural position, resulting in widening of the angle.[6,9,10]

LPI effectively manages pupil block but does not alter the lens position or anterior chamber depth[6]; therefore, persistent occludability indicates a secondary or alternate mechanism. Plateau iris is secondary to large or anteriorly positioned pars plicata[11,12] that push the peripheral iris anteriorly against the TM. Phacomorphic glaucoma is secondary to a large or subluxed crystalline lens that moves the entire iris diaphragm forward.[13,14] Malignant glaucoma, resulting from posteriorly directed aqueous flow, is rare in previously unoperated eyes.

Originally described by Kimbrough et al in 1979[15] to treat angle closure in nanophthalmos, ALPI has been primarily described in the management of persistent appositional closure following LPI,[16–18] be it secondary to plateau iris[19] or phacomorphic glaucoma.[20,21] More recently, ALPI has been used in the setting of acute angle closure.[16,22–28]

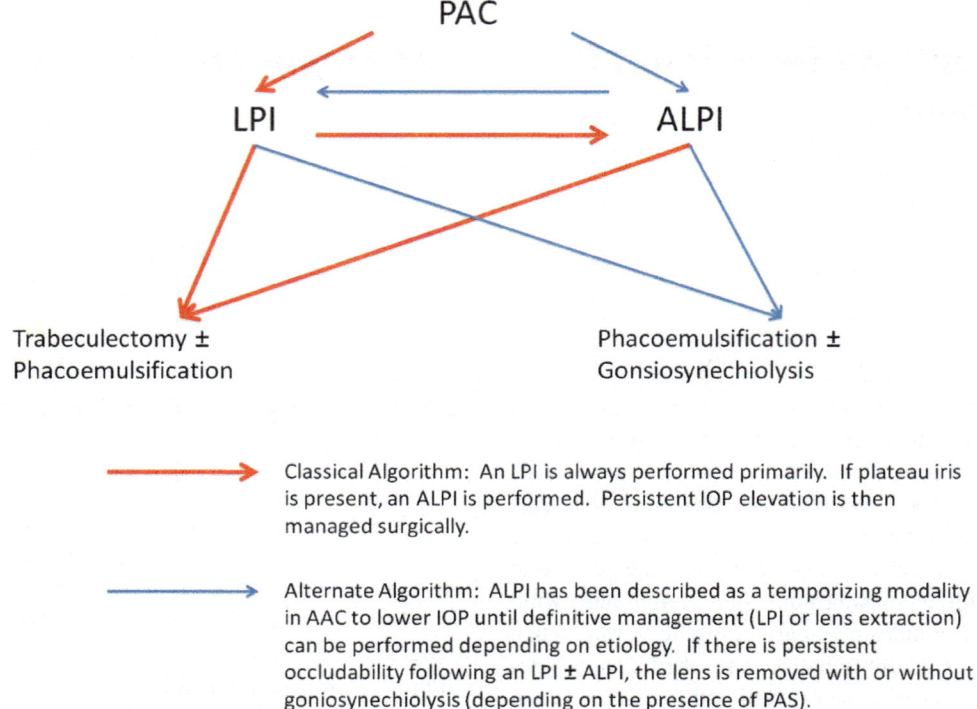

**Fig. 62.1** Management algorithm for primary angle closure (PAC) glaucoma. *LPI* laser peripheral iridotomy; *ALPI* argon laser peripheral iridoplasty

ALPI contracts the peripheral iris stroma, which physically opens the angle.[16–18] Histopathology suggests that the initial effect is due to heat-induced collagen shrinkage and that the long-term effect is secondary to contraction of a fibroblastic membrane in the region of laser application.[29]

## 62.2 Indications

### 62.2.1 Plateau Iris Syndrome

Plateau iris configuration is a result of large or anteriorly positioned pars plicata.[11,12] Clinically, this is manifest by a relatively normal central anterior chamber depth, but a narrow angle peripherally. Plateau iris syndrome is defined as PAC in the presence of a patient LPI.[30] In a long-term study of 23 eyes with appositional PAC following LPI (mean follow-up of 79 months), 20 eyes remained open over the course of follow-up. Three patients required retreatment due to gradual reclosure, 5–9 years after initial treatment.[19] None of these eyes required filtration surgery. Antiglaucoma medications were reduced from 1.2 to 0.6 after treatment.

Lens extraction will remove any pupil block and phacomorphic contribution to angle closure but will not relieve the plateau iris configuration[31,32]; ALPI is thus also indicated in plateau iris configuration in the pseudophakic eye. ALPI has also successfully been used in eyes with iridociliary cysts that resulted in a pseudoplateau iris configuration.[33]

### 62.2.2 Acute Angle Closure

ALPI has been used to break attacks of acute angle closure primarily[22–28] or in cases that were recalcitrant to medical therapy and/or LPI.[16] In a randomized trial, 77 eyes in acute angle closure with IOPs over 40 mmHg in which an LPI could not be performed due to corneal edema, received topical pilocarpine and timolol.[28] They were then randomized to receive either ALPI or systemic acetazolamide (and intravenous mannitol if the IOP was greater than 60 mmHg). There were no significant differences in IOP between the two groups at the initiation of therapy and at 2 and 24 h posttherapy. However, there was a significantly lower IOP in the ALPI group at 15 min, 30 min, and 1 h after initiation of therapy. As the underlying pupil block had not been corrected, all patients underwent an LPI within 48 h of initial therapy. Long-term follow-up (mean 15.7 months) failed to show any significant differences between groups with respect to IOP, PAS formation, or antiglaucoma medication requirement.[25] ALPI appears to be a safe alternative in the management of acute angle closure and should be given particular consideration when systemic therapy may adversely affect a patient.

### 62.2.3 Phacomorphic Glaucoma

A large or anteriorly subluxed crystalline lens, particularly in a smaller eye, can cause significant narrowing of the angle, leading to occlusion. Definitive management is lens removal; however, these eyes can present in acute angle closure and are often not amenable to LPI. ALPI has been suggested as a fast and safe alternative to medical management to lower IOP and functions as a temporizing modality until cataract surgery can be performed under more favorable circumstances.[20,21] A prospective series of 10 patients presenting with acute phacomorphic induced angle closure, with IOPs greater than 40 mmHg, underwent ALPI.[21] The IOP was reduced to a mean of 25.5 mmHg by 2 h and 13.6 mmHg by 24 h. Uneventful cataract surgery was then performed within 4 days of presentation.

### 62.2.4 Other Indications

Lens extraction has been described as an effective modality in managing PAC. When concomitant PAS are present, especially when greater than 270°, goniosynechiolysis has been proven to augment the IOP lowering effect[34–36] (Fig. 62.2a, b). Due to the phenomenon of "iris memory," the unabated iris has a propensity to reform PAS. To reduce the incidence of PAS reformation, postoperative miotics are prescribed to patients to draw the peripheral iris away from the TM. Performing ALPI following cataract surgery combined with goniosynechiolysis further increases angle width.[36]

Malignant or ciliary block glaucoma occurs due to posterior misdirection of aqueous flow. In a previously unoperated eye, this is usually associated with a choroidal effusion that may occur secondary to nanophthalmos,[15] panretinal photocoagulation, sulfa-based agents, etc. ALPI can also be useful in managing angle-closure in these cases.[37]

Though described in one study,[38] ALPI is generally thought to not lyse PAS and is therefore not helpful or indicated in chronic angle closure glaucoma (CACG).[37]

## 62.3 Clinical Assessment

### 62.3.1 History

Symptoms consistent with PAC after undergoing an LPI should alert the examiner to assessing the eye for persistent occludability.

### 62.3.2 Clinical Examination

The examiner should be careful to note any anomalies that may suggest secondary angle closure issues such as neovascularization of the iris, prior panretinal photocoagulation, iris abnormalities, etc. Acutely, the cornea will often be edematous upon an acutely high rise in IOP, requiring topical glycerin to adequately examine and possibly initiate laser therapy. The presence (and patency) or absence of an LPI should be determined. Gonioscopy is then performed to assess for occludability. Dynamic gonioscopy, using a handheld Posner or similar lens, with indentation is critical to determine the presence of PAS, which has implications on the utilization of ALPI and the necessity of goniosynechiolysis if cataract surgery is to be performed. Dynamic gonioscopy will also assess for the presence of the "double hump" sign created by the anterior ciliary body processes in plateau iris configuration.[39] A light touch is useful in performing routine gonioscopy; putting pressure on the lens to create indentation is very useful, but the examiner needs to be cognizant of how the lens is being held.

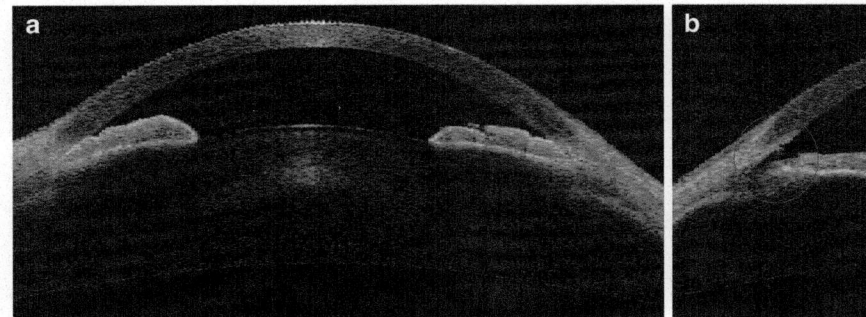
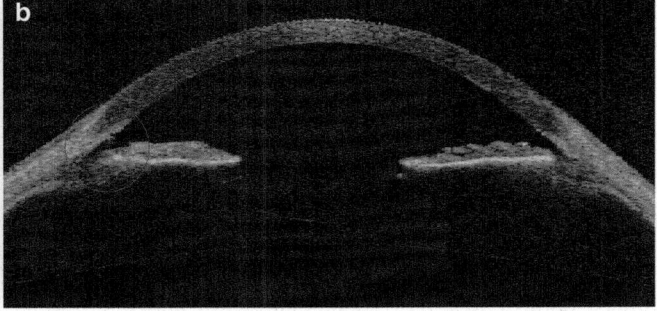

**Fig. 62.2** (a) Visante image of chronic angle closure with PAS formation before goniosynechiolysis. (b) Postoperative imagine demonstrates a deeper chamber and open angles. The *red circle* identifies a trace amount of residual iris tissue following goniosynechiolysis

Central anterior chamber depth will be relatively normal in plateau iris configuration. Conversely, a shallow central anterior chamber depth, increased lens thickness, and advanced maturity of the lens indicate a lenticular contribution to occludability. The relative health of the optic nerve and the IOP will determine the urgency and aggressiveness of any intervention that is required.

## 62.3.3 Ancillary Testing

As indicated earlier, the definition of occludability is arbitrary and has been suggested by some to be not sensitive enough. Furthermore, clinical exam is hindered by variable amounts of ambient light that can constrict the pupil, making an occludable angle appear open. Ancillary testing may be useful in cases that are deemed suspect or borderline on clinical examination.

### 62.3.3.1 Provocative Testing

Physiologic or pharmacologic dilation of the pupil will cause crowding of the angle and result in an increase in IOP if occludability is present. Dark room prone provocative testing involves having a patient sitting in a chair in a dark room with their head down for a duration of 1 h. An IOP elevation at the end of this time greater than 8 mmHg indicates a positive result.[39,40] The sensitivity and specificity of dark room testing, however, has not been validated in the literature; one consideration being the lability of IOP can be a function of POAG and unrelated to angle closure.[41] Pharmacologic testing utilizes a weak mydriatic such as cyclopentolate or phenylepinephrine. This dilation, however, is nonphysiologic and results in low sensitivity. Furthermore, patients can suffer an acute attack hours after instillation after being discharged home. Overall, provocative testing has not been validated and poses a potential safety concern for patients.[41]

### 62.3.3.2 Imaging

The advantage of imaging is the ability to view and objectively quantify anatomical structures under virtually no ambient light – minimizing angle opening by pupil constriction. Ultrasound biomicroscopy (UBM) is the gold standard in anterior segment imaging and was instrumental in understanding and describing pupil block and plateau iris configuration.[40] While providing excellent resolution of the iris and ciliary body, UBM is a contact modality and requires an experienced technician (usually a physician) to perform. Anterior segment optical coherence tomography (AS-OCT) is an optical diagnostic device operating at 1,310 nm, which provides good penetration into the anterior segment – angle imaging is excellent while ciliary body visualization is variable. This is a result of absorption of the imaging light by pigmented uveal tissue, thereby attenuating the image signal beyond these structures. The AS-OCT has the advantage of being a noncontact modality and requires little training to perform. Two studies have demonstrated UBM and AS-OCT to yield comparable results in quantifying angle anatomy and width[42,43] (Figs. 62.3a, b and 62.4a, b), though there has been no standardization of what quantitatively constitutes an occludable angle or an angle at risk. No doubt this will be an area of research in the years to come. Schleimpflug photography has also been described, but its relatively low resolution inadequately visualizes angle anatomy.[2,44]

## 62.4 Technique

Like most techniques, the parameters vary from clinician to clinician. Those that are presented here are those of the author's but are within the reported variance of the stated parameters.

### 62.4.1 Pretreatment

The eye is pretreated with pilocarpine 1% and then 15 min later again with pilocarpine 1% and brimonidine 0.2%. Others have described the use of pilocarpine 4%[37]; however, in the author's experience, the degree of pupil constriction is equivalent with the lower concentration, which yields a lower incidence and severity of brow ache and nausea. Higher doses of pilocarpine may shift the lens–iris diaphragm forward so the author advises that they be avoided. If any corneal edema exists, the eye is also instilled with other IOP lowering medication and topical glycerin.

### 62.4.2 Treatment

Treatment is conducted at least 15 min after the second instillation of pretreatment drops. Patients should be advised that they may feel discomfort, but they should avoid movement during laser application. Either an Abraham[37] iridotomy lens or an SLT gonio laser lens can be used to place the laser burns. A gonioscopy lens results in a tangential application of energy, resulting in a more diffuse delivery, leading to less peripheral stromal contraction and thinning,[37] which then requires more injury. There is also a risk of inadvertent

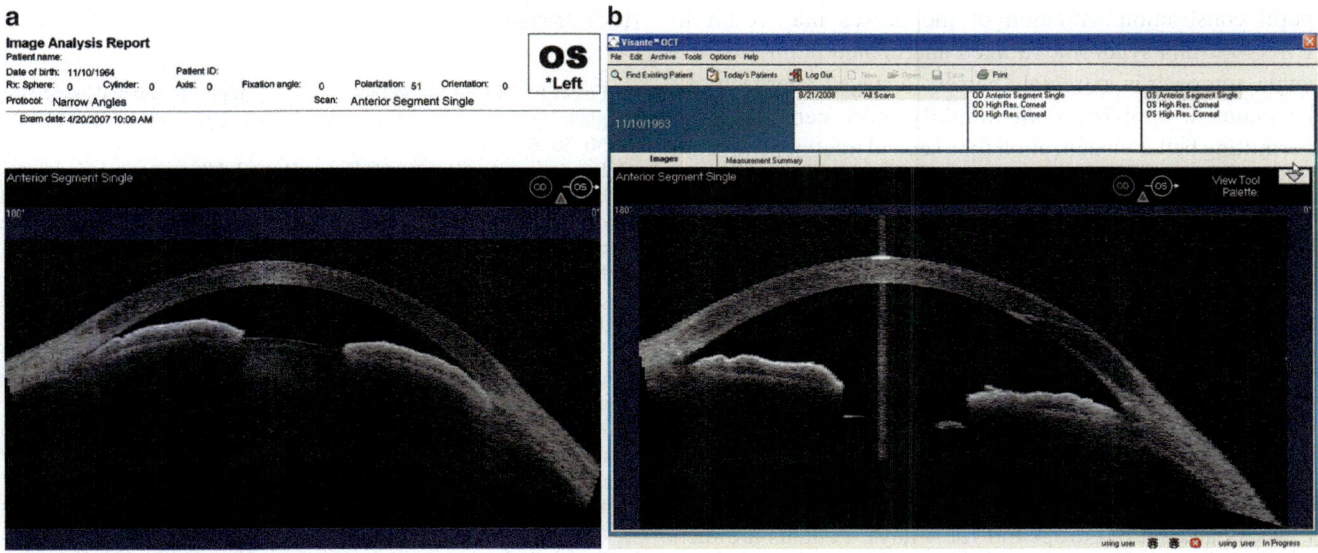

**Fig. 62.3** Visante optical coherence tomography image of the anterior segment (**a**) precataract surgery and (**b**) postcataract surgery. Figures courtesy of Robert J. Noecker, MD, University of Pittsburgh School of Medicine

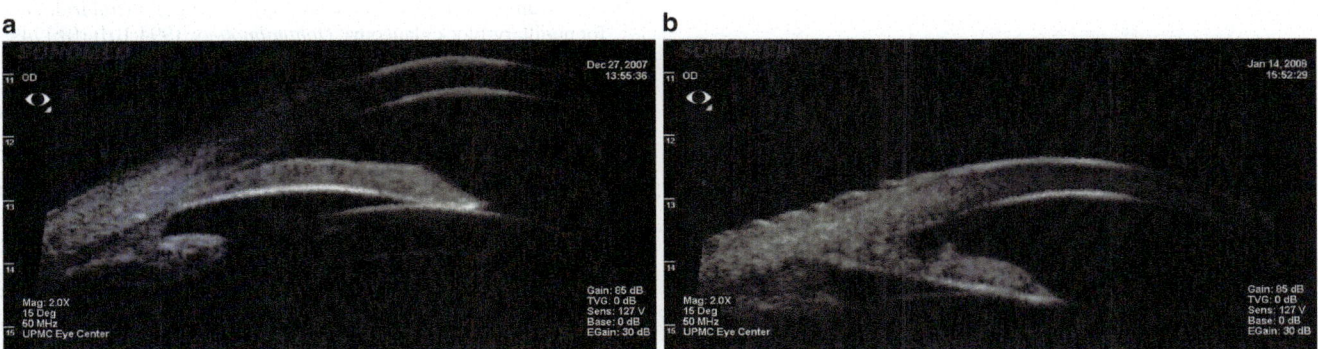

**Fig. 62.4** Laser peripheral iridotomy (LPI). (**a**) Scan of angle before LPI and (**b**) post LPI. Figures courtesy of Robert J. Noecker, MD, University of Pittsburgh School of Medicine

damage to the TM. However, a gonioscopy lens provides better access to the peripheral angle and allows the clinician to see the efficacy of the contraction burns as they are applied – unlike the Abraham lens, which requires the clinician to examine the patient immediately after with a goniolens to assess the effect of the treatment. Furthermore, a goniolens provides access to areas of the angle that might be obstructed by peripheral corneal pathology when viewed through an Abraham lens such as marked arcus senilis or a pterygium. The author's preference is to use a goniolens.

The laser is set for a spot size of 500 μm and a duration of 0.5 s. The power is set at 200 mJ to start with and titrated up until the iris stroma begins to contract approximately halfway through duration of the burn. Bubble formation or pigment release indicates a suprathreshold power that should be reduced. Lighter irides may fail to demonstrate an effect up to 500 mJ, at which point the spot size is reduced – increasing the power delivery per unit area.[37] It is important to depress the laser pedal or trigger for the full duration of the burn; there is a propensity to simply depress and release, which will result in a subtherapeutic and variable application of energy.

The contraction burns should be placed as peripheral as possible, being careful not to apply energy to the TM if using the SLT lens. The space between burns should be approximately 2 spot diameters – closer burns may result in iris tissue necrosis.[37] This results in approximately 12–14 burns per 180°. Care should be taken to avoid placing burns over large vessels, which may bleed, as well as on the horizontal axis where the long ciliary nerves enter the iris and contribute to pupil constriction. Ablation of the nerves may result in Urrets-Zavalia syndrome (a fixed and dilated pupil).[45] If the angle approach is extremely narrow, a staged approach can be planned; applying burns slightly more centrally first, permitting better visualization for a second treatment directed more peripherally at another time.[37] The author treats 180° at a time beginning with the inferior half, which is usually narrower. At the follow-up appointment, the angle is reassessed and the second half is treated if necessary.

### 62.4.3 Posttreatment

One hour posttreatment, the IOP is checked to ensure no IOP spike has occurred. Patients are given pilocarpine 1% qid for 2 weeks and steroid drops qid for 4 days. Patients are then examined in 4–6 weeks to reassess the angle.

### 62.4.4 Complications

Complications from ALPI are almost always mild and self-limited. Patients almost always develop a mild iritis that subsides within a few days. Rarely, patients may demonstrate a protracted anterior chamber inflammation that is amenable to steroid therapy. Endothelial burns can occur, especially when using the Abraham iridotomy lens, and resolve within several days with no sequelae.[28] Pigmented scars often develop at the site of burn placement but are of no consequence. Finally, an enlarged or atonic pupil can sometimes result[4,37] – the theory being that ciliary nerves are damaged during laser application; however, this likely is also self-limited but may take months to resolve.

## 62.5 Conclusion

Although the mechanism is well understood, the quantitative definition of occludability continues to challenge the clinician in the management of angle closure. Quantitative imaging techniques show promise in being able to properly define these parameters, but thorough and evidence-based research is required before adopting these as the gold standards for evaluation and diagnosis. These measures will also be cost prohibitive in many parts of the world. Until that time, the clinician needs to continue to rely heavily on clinical examination and acumen to determine which eyes require treatment for what is generally a curable condition when identified early. ALPI is a safe and effective procedure that can be used primarily or adjunctively to manage angle closure.

## References

1. Foster PJ. The epidemiology of primary angle closure and associated glaucomatous optic neuropathy. *Semin Ophthalmol.* 2002;17(2):50–58. Review.
2. Friedman DS, Gazzard G, Foster P, et al. Ultrasonographic biomicroscopy, Scheimpflug photography, and novel provocative tests in contralateral eyes of Chinese patients initially seen with acute angle closure. *Arch Ophthalmol.* 2003;121(5):633–642.
3. Markowitz SN, Morin JD. The clinical course in primary angle-closure glaucoma: a reassessment. *Can J Ophthalmol.* 1986;21(4):130–133.
4. Wojciechowski R, Congdon N, Anninger W, Teo Broman A. Age, gender, biometry, refractive error, and the anterior chamber angle among Alaskan Eskimos. *Ophthalmology.* 2003;110(2):365–375.
5. Foster PJ, Buhrmann R, Quigley HA, Johnson GJ. The definition and classification of glaucoma in prevalence surveys. *Br J Ophthalmol.* 2002;86(2):238–242, Review.
6. He M, Friedman DS, Ge J, et al. Laser peripheral iridotomy in primary angle-closure suspects: biometric and gonioscopic outcomes: the Liwan Eye Study. *Ophthalmology.* 2007;114(3):494–500.
7. Ritch R, Liebmann JM, Tellow C. A construct for understanding angle closure glaucoma: the role of ultrasound biomicroscopy. *Ophthalmol Clin North Am.* 1995;8:281–293.
8. Pavlin CJ, Harasiewicz K, Foster FS. An ultrasound biomicroscopic dark-room provocative test. *Ophthalmic Surg.* 1995;26(3):253–255.
9. American Academy of Ophthalmology. Laser peripheral iridotomy for pupillary-block glaucoma. *Ophthalmology.* 1994;101(10):1749–1758, Review, No abstract available.
10. Fleck BW, Dhillon B, Khanna V, Fairley E, McGlynn C. A randomised, prospective comparison of Nd:YAG laser iridotomy and operative peripheral iridectomy in fellow eyes. *Eye.* 1991;5(Pt 3):315–321.
11. Pavlin CJ, Ritch R, Foster FS. Ultrasound biomicroscopy in plateau iris syndrome. *Am J Ophthalmol.* 1992;113(4):390–395.
12. Ritch R. Plateau Iris is caused by abnormally positioned ciliary processes. *J Glaucoma.* 1992;1:23–26.
13. Jain IS, Gupta A, Dogra MR, Gangwar DN, Dhir SP. Phacomorphic glaucoma – management and visual prognosis. *Indian J Ophthalmol.* 1983;31(5):648–653.
14. Epstein DL. Diagnosis and management of lens-induced glaucoma. *Ophthalmology.* 1982;89(3):227–230.
15. Kimbrough RL, Trempe CS, Brockhurst RJ, Simmons RJ. Angle-closure glaucoma in nanophthalmos. *Am J Ophthalmol.* 1979;88(3 Pt 2):572–579.
16. Ritch R. Argon laser treatment for medically unresponsive attacks of angle-closure glaucoma. *Am J Ophthalmol.* 1982;94(2):197–204.
17. Ritch R. Argon laser peripherl iridoplasty: an overview. *J Glaucoma.* 1992;1:206–213.
18. York K, Ritch R, Szmyd LJ. Argon laser peripheral iridotoplasty: indications, techniques and results. *Invest Ophthalmol Vis Sci.* 1984;25(suppl):94.
19. Ritch R, Tham CC, Lam DS. Long-term success of argon laser peripheral iridoplasty in the management of plateau iris syndrome. *Ophthalmology.* 2004;111(1):104–108.
20. Yip PP, Leung WY, Hon CY, Ho CK. Argon laser peripheral iridoplasty in the management of phacomorphic glaucoma. *Ophthalmic Surg Lasers Imaging.* 2005;36(4):286–291
21. Tham CC, Lai JS, Poon AS, et al. Immediate argon laser peripheral iridoplasty (ALPI) as initial treatment for acute phacomorphic angle-closure (phacomorphic glaucoma) before cataract extraction: a preliminary study. *Eye.* 2005;19(7):778–783.
22. Chew P, Chee C, Lim A, et al. Laser treatment of severe acute angle-closure glaucoma in dark Asian irides: the role of iridoplasty. *Lasers Light Ophthalmol.* 1991;4:41–42.

23. Lim AS, Tan A, Chew P, et al. Laser iridoplasty in the treatment of severe acute angle closure glaucoma. *Int Ophthalmol.* 1993;17:33–36.
24. Matai A, Consul S. Argon laser iridoplasty. *Indian J Ophthalmol.* 1987;35(5–6):290–292.
25. Lai JS, Tham CC, Chua JK, et al. To compare argon laser peripheral iridoplasty (ALPI) against systemic medications in treatment of acute primary angle-closure: mid-term results. *Eye.* 2006;20(3):309–314.
26. Lai JS, Tham CC, Chua JK, Lam DS. Immediate diode laser peripheral iridoplasty as treatment of acute attack of primary angle closure glaucoma: a preliminary study. *J Glaucoma.* 2001;10(2):89–94.
27. Lai JS, Tham CC, Chua JK, Poon AS, Lam DS. Laser peripheral iridoplasty as initial treatment of acute attack of primary angle-closure: a long-term follow-up study. *J Glaucoma.* 2002;11(6):484–487.
28. Lam DS, Lai JS, Tham CC, Chua JK, Poon AS. Argon laser peripheral iridoplasty versus conventional systemic medical therapy in treatment of acute primary angle-closure glaucoma: a prospective, randomized, controlled trial. *Ophthalmology.* 2002;109(9):1591–1596.
29. Sassani JW, Ritch R, McCormick S, et al. Histopathology of argon laser peripheral iridoplasty. *Ophthalmic Surg.* 1993;24(11):740–745.
30. Wand M, Grant WM, Simmons RJ, Hutchinson BT. Plateau iris syndrome. *Trans Sect Ophthalmol Am Acad Ophthalmol Otolaryngol.* 1977;83(1):122–130.
31. Tran HV, Liebmann JM, Ritch R. Iridociliary apposition in plateau iris syndrome persists after cataract extraction. *Am J Ophthalmol.* 2003;135(1):40–43.
32. Azuara-Blanco A. Iridociliary apposition in plateau iris syndrome persists after cataract extraction. *Am J Ophthalmol.* 2003;136(2):395.
33. Crowston JG, Medeiros FA, Mosaed S, Weinreb RN. Argon laser iridoplasty in the treatment of plateau-like iris configuration as result of numerous ciliary body cysts. *Am J Ophthalmol.* 2005;139(2):381–383.
34. Teekhasaenee C, Ritch R. Combined phacoemulsification and goniosynechialysis for uncontrolled chronic angle-closure glaucoma after acute angle-closure glaucoma. *Ophthalmology.* 1999;106(4):669–674.
35. Harasymowycz PJ, Papamatheakis DG, Ahmed I, et al. Phacoemulsification and goniosynechialysis in the management of unresponsive primary angle closure. *J Glaucoma.* 2005;14(3):186–189.
36. Lai JS, Tham CC, Lam DS. The efficacy and safety of combined phacoemulsification, intraocular lens implantation, and limited goniosynechialysis, followed by diode laser peripheral iridoplasty, in the treatment of cataract and chronic angle-closure glaucoma. *J Glaucoma.* 2001;10(4):309–315.
37. Ritch R, Tham CC, Lam DS. Argon laser peripheral iridoplasty (ALPI): an update. *Surv Ophthalmol.* 2007;52(3):279–288, Review.
38. Wand M. Argon laser gonioplasty for synechial angle closure. *Arch Ophthalmol.* 1992;110(3):363–367.
39. Kiuchi Y, Kanamoto T, Nakamura T. Double hump sign in indentation gonioscopy is correlated with presence of plateau iris configuration regardless of patent iridotomy. *J Glaucoma.* 2009;18(2):161–164.
40. Friedman Z, Neumann E. Comparison of prone-position, darkroom, and mydriatic tests for angle-closure glaucoma before and after peripheral iridectomy. *Am J Ophthalmol.* 1972;74(1):24–27.
41. Epstein DL, Allingham RR, Schuman JS, eds. In: *Chandler and Grant's Glaucoma.* 4th ed. Baltimore: Lippincott Williams & Wilkins, 1997;279–280.
42. Dada T, Sihota R, Gadia R, Aggarwal A, Mandal S, Gupta V. Comparison of anterior segment optical coherence tomography and ultrasound biomicroscopy for assessment of the anterior segment. *J Cataract Refract Surg.* 2007;33(5):837–840.
43. Radhakrishnan S, Goldsmith J, Huang D, et al. Comparison of optical coherence tomography and ultrasound biomicroscopy for detection of narrow anterior chamber angles. *Arch Ophthalmol.* 2005;123(8):1053–1059.
44. Böker T, Sheqem J, Rauwolf M, Wegener A. Anterior chamber angle biometry: a comparison of Scheimpflug photography and ultrasound biomicroscopy. *Ophthalmic Res.* 1995;27(Suppl 1):104–109.
45. Espana EM, Ioannidis A, Tello C, Liebmann JM, Foster P, Ritch R. Urrets-Zavalia syndrome as a complication of argon laser peripheral iridoplasty. *Br J Ophthalmol.* 2007;91(4):427–429.

# Chapter 63
# Laser Therapies: Cyclodestructive Procedures

Christopher J. Russo and Malik Y. Kahook

## 63.1 Introduction

Early attempts to reduce intraocular pressure (IOP) through treating the ciliary body utilized the process of diathermy to destroy aqueous-producing cells.[1] This method quickly fell out of favor due to a high rate of hypotony as well as lack of efficacy. Cryotherapy was another early method of ciliary body ablation, and, while the results were more successful and repeatable than diathermy, freezing of the ciliary body never achieved widespread acceptance.[2-4] The use of cyclophotocoagulation (CPC) was first reported in the early 1960s using a xenon arc photocoagulator for ciliary body destruction. A decade later, the arc photocoagulator was replaced by a laser and development of the present form of cycloablation began its evolution.[5]

There were several shortcomings with early CPC methodologies, particularly the transpupillary method. Due to minimal visualization of the ciliary processes through a dilated pupil, treatment was limited to a fraction of the total ciliary body with subsequent suboptimal IOP reduction.[6] A solution to this problem was found when the ciliary body was targeted via a transscleral route. While the ciliary body was not directly visualized, treatment of a much larger area was achieved while remaining a noninvasive procedure. In the 1970s, the Nd:YAG laser with a sapphire-tipped contact probe was used via a transscleral approach and found a place in the armamentarium for treatment of refractory glaucoma.[7,8] The procedure continued to evolve when the solid-state diode laser replaced the Nd:YAG laser and a disposable probe was introduced. Today a new form of cycloablation utilizing the solid-state diode laser in combination with an endoscope has greatly enhanced the precision of the procedure while minimizing the destructive forces applied to adjacent structures. This procedure, known as endoscopic cyclophotocoagulation (ECP), provides the ophthalmologist better control of laser application to the targeted tissue and may represent a more viable option for earlier treatment of glaucoma refractory to standard medical or laser trabeculoplasty therapy.

## 63.2 Indications

The goal of all cycloablative procedures is to lower IOP by reducing aqueous production via destruction of the nonpigmented ciliary epithelium. In the past, CPC was often considered only in cases of refractory glaucoma. Patients on maximum medical therapy showing continued progression of disease were often considered as appropriate candidates. Other indications were in patients who had failed filtration surgery or were considered at high risk for failure or complications post-traditional filtration procedures. Commonly treated glaucomas included neovascular glaucoma, glaucoma associated with penetrating keratoplasty, and aphakic glaucoma. Reasons that CPC remained one of the last lines of treatment in these cases often centered on the complications of the procedure. These included the expected collateral damages associated with transscleral ablation: chronic inflammation, pain, and hemorrhage, as well as a relative or perceived higher incidence of hypotony. Additionally, the lack of ability to titrate or target treatment through the transscleral route often resulted in incomplete ablation and suboptimal reduction in IOP.

Several of these concerns have been addressed with the development of ECP, and, as such, the indications for ECP have evolved compared to CPC. Visualization of the area undergoing treatment has been a breakthrough in the emergence of cycloablative procedures. The endoscopic approach allows both a precise titration of treatment and a decrease in collateral damage. While great advances have been made since the beginning days of CPC, both CPC and ECP are certainly not risk-free. Complications for both include pain, chronic inflammation, vitreous hemorrhage, hypotony, macular edema, serous choroidal detachments, development of phthisis bulbi, and ineffectiveness. ECP is an invasive procedure carrying the risk of postoperative leak from surgical wounds as well as the possibility of endophthalmitis. Thus, it is imperative that the patient population is selected with great care and undergoes thorough preoperative counseling.

## 63.3 Cyclophotocoagulation

### 63.3.1 *Techniques/Features*

Transscleral laser CPC comprises treatment with both the Nd:YAG laser and the diode laser. The mechanism of action is ciliary body destruction by absorption of the wavelengths of the corresponding lasers. While the ciliary epithelium is ablated, it is important to realize that the underlying ciliary body muscle and blood vessels are also destroyed. At this point, the diode laser offers several advantages over the Nd:YAG laser including smaller size (portability) and balance of emitted energy to absorbed energy; thus the diode laser has found wider use.

Noncontact Nd:YAG laser cyclophotocoagulation (NCYC) is no longer in use in most centers. Historically, it was performed at the slit lamp with a LASAG Microruptor laser. Contact Nd:YAG laser cyclophotocoagulation (CYC) employs a 2.2-mm sapphire tip coupled with a fiber-optic probe. Both methods carry the risks and complications previously discussed including chronic inflammation, pain, and hypotony. Despite its drawbacks, several studies have confirmed some success with NCYC and CYC. Several investigators independently found success rates from 45 to 86% in the intermediate term (6–22 months) among recipients of NCYC.[9–12] Schuman found similar results with CYC with success rates of 56–72% in the intermediate term (12–36 months).[13] Long-term results of CYC were reported by Lin.[14] Mean pretreatment IOP was 36.3 mmHg and mean posttreatment IOP was 18.9 mmHg at 10 years. However, 62.5% of eyes with initial visual acuity better than 20/200 on the Snellen chart lost at least two lines at the end of follow-up. Additional findings included need for retreatment in approximately 44% and a failure rate above 50%.

Transscleral diode laser CPC utilizing the contact method has been shown to have similar results to CYC. At a wavelength of 810 nm, the light emitted from the diode laser enables a better coupling of emitted energy and absorbed energy due to the intrinsic physical properties of the ciliary epithelium and surrounding pigmentation. This allows for less application time and a decreased energy per application spot. Long-term data from Kosoko et al showed an average 44% decrease in IOP after 270° treatment with average follow-up of 19 months.[15] Success rates dropped from an average of 80% at 1 year to approximately 57% at 2 years. Carassa on the other hand, increased treatment to 360° and achieved an average 50% lowering of IOP in all 12 eyes reported.[16] Such encouraging results led to greater acceptance of cycloablation as a modality of treatment for glaucoma, especially in refractory cases.

### 63.3.2 *Endoscopic Cyclophotocoagulation*

With visualization of the tissue being treated and a less destructive method of applying the laser, ECP has achieved successful outcomes while minimizing some of the complications associated with a transscleral approach. ECP employs the same 810-nm diode laser as CPC, but allows the surgeon to precisely aim and deploy the laser to cause effective cycloablation while avoiding damage to adjacent structures.

Pantcheva examined histopathological changes in human autopsy eyes after ECP and CPC.[17] Light and electron microscopy were used to examine autopsy eyes that underwent either procedure and untreated control eyes. Changes were found at the histological level in both treatment groups, with the CPC group exhibiting disruption of the ciliary body muscle and stroma as well as changes in the ciliary processes (both the pigmented and nonpigmented ciliary epithelium). In the ECP group, extensive contraction of the ciliary processes was observed as well as changes to the ciliary body epithelium. There was much less destruction (if any) to the ciliary body muscle and deformation of structures in the ECP group. It was concluded that the higher degree of selectivity implicit in ECP results in less photocoagulative damage to structures adjacent to the targeted tissues.

The technique utilized in ECP is critical to successful outcomes. Good exposure facilitates better treatment, and this can be achieved with injection of a cohesive viscoelastic between the iris and anterior lens capsule. A curved probe is employed allowing for better access to the ciliary body. Most of the early reports on use of ECP were performed through a single clear corneal wound; however, a study by Kahook and Noecker has shown that two-site treatment allows for better exposure and treatment under the initial subincisional site allowing for 360° ablation.[18] A distance of 2 mm between the probe and ciliary processes is ideal as shown by Yu and colleagues who examined the effectiveness of the diode laser used in ECP at different distances and with different viscoelastics.[19] While results with the various viscoelastics were not statistically significant, it was shown that 2 mm was the optimal treatment distance between the target tissue and laser probe. This corresponds to six ciliary processes in view on the endoscope monitor. Initial power is 0.25 W titratable to 1.2 W. Pulse mode is possible but continuous laser is preferable, utilizing a painting technique. Evidence of appropriate treatment delivery is tissue whitening and contraction.

ECP has been performed with both pars plana and clear cornea approaches. The pars plana approach works adequately in pseudophakic or aphakic eyes that have been vitrectomized. However, the pars plana approach becomes technically difficult in phakic eyes or eyes that have not previously undergone vitrectomy. Viscoelastic has often been used with ECP to help elevate the iris for increased exposure of ciliary epithelium.

There have been reported cases of postoperative IOP spikes secondary to retained viscoelastics. Iris hooks may be an effective alternative, especially in cases of aphakia or compromised posterior capsule where viscoelastic removal is more complicated.[20] The current standard approach is through a clear cornea incision. It is, thus, easy to understand why ECP is increasingly being paired with cataract surgery in glaucoma patients. Indications for ECP currently include cases of glaucoma where filtering surgery is contraindicated, patients maintained on multiple topical therapies who are scheduled for cataract extraction, and pediatric glaucoma refractory to other modalities of treatment.

Long-term data for ECP performed concurrently with phacoemulsification has been reported by Berke.[21] This study included both a large amount of patients and an extended follow-up period. The phaco/ECP group was compared to a group of glaucoma patients that had phaco alone. Over a mean follow-up period of 3.2 years, the ECP group was found to have an average decrease in IOP of 3.4 mmHg – from 19.1 to 15.7 mmHg. The phaco group actually had an IOP rise from 18.2 to 18.9 mmHg. The ECP group was also found to have a decrease in the number of glaucoma medications needed while the phaco group was unchanged. The postoperative rate of CME was unchanged. This data is particularly valuable because it examines the usefulness of ECP in the setting of medically controlled glaucoma.

Lima et al examined the results of ECP versus Ahmed valve glaucoma drainage devices in cases of advanced glaucoma. Sixty-eight eyes of patients with refractory glaucoma were randomized to either arm of treatment.[22] The procedures were all performed by a single surgeon. None of the eyes had previously undergone cycloablation or glaucoma drainage device implantation. Preoperative IOP was approximately 41 mmHg in both groups. Results showed significant IOP reductions in both groups to around 14 mmHg with the ECP group being slightly lower. Overall, complications were higher in the Ahmed valve arm of the study.

Chen et al evaluated the IOP lowering effects of ECP. Successful treatment was defined as posttreatment IOP of less than 21 mmHg. Treatment was successful for 94% of patients at 1 year and 82% at 2 years.[23] Average IOP reduction of all study participants was 34% from pretreatment levels. Only 6% of patients lost two or more lines on the Snellen chart during the average 12.9 months of follow-up.

Neely and Plager have reported on the use of ECP in children. One study details the results of ECP on 34 aphakic or pseudophakic eyes with pediatric glaucoma.[24] Success was defined as postoperative IOP of less than 24 mmHg with associated decrease in IOP of at least 15% from pretreatment levels. The pretreatment mean IOP was 32.6 mmHg. Success was achieved in a total of 18 out of 34 eyes, or 53%. Patients were followed an average of 44 months. Of note, retinal detachment occurred in two eyes within 1 month of treatment. They used 360° treatment in 23.5% of eyes and no cases of hypotony were noted.

Another study by Neely and Plager included 36 eyes of 29 pediatric glaucoma patients who received ECP. Treatment success was defined as IOP less than 21 mmHg with or without glaucoma medications. Pretreatment IOP was 35.06 mmHg with a posttreatment IOP of 23.63. An average 30% decrease in IOP was appreciated. Several eyes required multiple treatments for an average of 1.42 treatments per eye. Overall success was 43% of eyes. Retinal detachment was reported in two eyes with complications of hypotony and vision loss from hand motion to no light perception in one patient each.[25] All complications were seen in aphakic eyes.

Gayton et al examined the increasingly popular combination of ECP with cataract extraction. It was compared against combined trabeculectomy and cataract extraction. Success was defined as posttreatment IOP less than 19 mmHg and was achieved in 30% of ECP eyes and 40% of trabeculectomy eyes. When patients were also treated with topical glaucoma medications in addition to their respective surgeries, the ECP arm showed a success rate of 65% compared to 52% in the trabeculectomy arm.[26] ECP in combination with cataract extraction was found to be a viable option for lowering IOP to a similar degree as filtering surgery while avoiding some of the complications associated with trabeculectomy. The advantages of ECP over previous methods of cycloablation seem obvious, but head-to-head, well-controlled trials comparing the endoscopic versus the transscleral route have not been performed. Such studies are needed to better delineate the advantages and disadvantages of both modalities.

## 63.4 Conclusion

Cycloablative procedures have evolved from their first introduction and will continue to improve with the introduction of new technologies and laser capabilities. CPC and the transscleral approach involved targeting the ciliary epithelium without direct visualization, an increased amount of energy delivered to the intraocular structures, and inability to titrate treatment. While ECP does have several benefits over CPC, including less damage to adjacent structures, direct visualization of targeted tissue, and lower frequency of complications, it is still an intraocular procedure with all of the associated risks (Table 63.1).

Cycloablative therapies have not been utilized as first-line or even second-line treatments in glaucoma. However, with the advancements in ECP and the recent published results revealing substantial efficacy and safety, it is possible that ECP will become an increasingly appealing option earlier and in more instances than previously accepted. One limitation is the lack of stand-alone data for ECP since most reports

**Table 63.1** Advantages and disadvantages of CPC and ECP

|     | Advantages | Disadvantages |
| --- | --- | --- |
| CPC | Avoid intraocular surgery | Destruction of adjacent tissues |
|     | Can be performed in clinic | Higher amount of energy delivered |
|     | Easy to perform | Higher complication rate |
| ECP | Less collateral damage | Risk factors associated with intraocular surgery |
|     | Titratable | Spikes in IOP postoperatively |
|     | Direct visualization | Requires expensive equipment |

detailing efficacy of ECP often combine cataract extraction at the time of surgery. Long-term studies of ECP are ongoing and will help in better understanding where it fits in our treatment algorithm of glaucoma.

# References

1. Weve H. Die Zyklodiatermie das Corpus ciliare bei Glaukorm. *Zentralbl Ophthalmol*. 1933;29:562–569.
2. deRoetth A. Cryosurgery for the treatment of glaucoma. *Trans Am Ophthalmol Soc*. 1964;63:189–204.
3. deRoetth A. Cryosurgery for the treatment of advanced simple glaucoma. *Am J Ophthalmol*. 1968;66:1034–1041.
4. Bellows AR, Grant WM. Cyclocryotherapy in advanced inadequately controlled glaucoma. *Am J Ophthalmol*. 1973;75:679–684.
5. Weekers R, Lavergne G, Watillion M, et al. Effects of photocoagulation of ciliary body upon ocular tension. *Am J Ophthalmol*. 1961;52:156–163.
6. Lee P-F, Pomerantzeff O. Transpupillary cyclophotocoagulation of rabbit eyes; an experimental approach to glaucoma surgery. *Am J Ophthalmol*. 1971;71:911–920.
7. Beckman H, Kinoshita A, Rona AN, et al. Transscleral ruby laser irradiation of the ciliary body in the treatment of intactable glaucoma. *Trans Am Acad Ophthalmol Otolatnygol*. 1972;76:423–436.
8. Schuman JS. Nd:YAG laser transscleral cyclophotocaogulation. In: Thomas JV, Belcher CD, Simmons RJ, eds. *Glaucoma Surgery*. St Louis: Mosby-Yearbook; 1992.
9. Hampton C, Shields MB, Miller KN, Blasin M. Evaluation of a protocol fro transscleral neodymium: YAG cyclophotocoagulation in one hundered consecutive patients. *Ophthalmology*. 1990;97:910–917.
10. Devenyi RG, Trope GE, Hunter WH, et al. Neodymium-YAG transscleral cyclophotocaulation in human eyes. *Ophthalmology*. 1987;94:1519–1522.
11. Trope GE, Ma S. Mid term effects of neodymium:YAG thermal cyclophotocoagulation in glaucoma. *Ophthalmology*. 1990;97:73–75.
12. Klapper RM, Wandel T, Donnenfeld E, et al. Transscleral neodymium:YAG thermal cyclophotocoagulation in refractory glaucoma, a preliminary report. *Ophthalmology*. 1988;95:719–722.
13. Schuman JS, Belows AR, Shingleton BJ, et al. Contact transscleral Nd:YAG laser cyclophotocaogulation: midterm results. *Ophthalmology*. 1992;99;1089–1094, discussion 1095.
14. Gaasterland D, Abrams D, Belcher C, et al. A multicenter study of contact diode laser transscleral cyclophotocoagulation in glaucoma patients. *Invest Ophthalmol Vis Sci*. 1992;33(Suppl):1019
15. Kosoko O, Gaasterland DE, Pollack IP, et al. Long term outcome of initial ciliary ablation with contact diode laser transscleral cyclophotocoagulation for severe glaucoma. *Ophthalmology*. 1996;103:1924–1302.
16. Carassa RG Trabucchi G, Bettin P, et al. Contact transscleral cyclophotocagulation (CTCP) with diode laser: a pilot clinical study. *Invest Ophthalmol Vis Sci*. 1992;33(Suppl):1019.
17. Pantcheva MB, Kahook MY, Schuman JS, et al. Comparison of acute structural and histopathological changes in human autopsy eyes after endoscopic cyclophotocoagulation and trans-scleral cyclophotocoagulation. *Br J Ophthalmol*. 2007;91:248–252.
18. Kahook MY, Lathrop KL, Noecker RJ. One-site versus two-site endoscopic cyclophotocoagulation. *J Glaucoma*. 2007;16:527–530.
19. Yu JY, Kahook MY, Lathrop KL Noecker RJ. The effect of probe placement and type of viscoelastic material on endoscopic cyclophotocoagulation laser energy transmission. *Ophthalmic Surg Lasers Imaging*. 2008;39:133–136.
20. Kahook MY, Schuman JS, Noecker RJ. Endoscopic cyclophotocaogulation using iris hooks versus viscoelastic devices. *Ophthalmic Surg Lasers Imaging*. 2007;38:170–172.
21. Berke SJ, Sturm RT, Caronia RM, et al. Phacoemulsification combined with endoscopic cyclophotocoagulation (ECP) in the management of cataract and medically controlled glaucoma: a large, long term study. Presented at the AGS Annual Meeting; March 2006; Charleston, SC.
22. Lima FE, Magacho L, Carvalho DM, et al. A prospective, comparative study between endoscopic cyclophotocoagulation and the Ahmed drainage implant in refractory glaucoma. *J Glaucoma*. 2004;13:233–237.
23. Chen J, Cohn RA, Lin SC, et al. Endoscopic photocoagulation of the ciliary body for treatment of refractory glaucoma. *Am J Ophthalmol*. 1997;124:787–796.
24. Carter BC, Plager DA, Neely DE, et al. Endoscopic diode laser cyclophotocoagulation in the management of aphakic and pseudophakic glaucoma in children. *J AAPOS*. 2007;11:34–40.
25. Neely DE, Plager DA. Endocyclophotocoagulation for management of difficult pediatric glaucomas. *J AAPOS*. 2001;5:221–229.
26. Gayton JL, Van Der Karr M, Sanders V. Combined cataract and glaucoma surgery; trabeculectomy versus endoscopic laser cycloablation. *J Cataract Refract Surg*. 1999;25:1214–1219.

# Chapter 64
# Laser Therapies: Newer Technologies

Michael S. Berlin and Kevin Taliaferro

The treatment of glaucoma with lasers has been one of the earliest applications of laser technology in medicine. Progress in laser technology has led to the development of several new glaucoma therapies. This chapter reviews basic laser light properties, current laser applications, and the latest developments in the use of lasers to treat glaucoma: Excimer Laser Trabeculostomy (ELT), an alternative to trabeculectomy; Titanium:Sapphire Laser Trabeculoplasty (TLT) and Micropulse Diode Laser Trabeculoplasty (MDLT), alternatives to Selective Laser Trabeculoplasty (SLT); Diode Laser Cyclophotocoagulation (DCPC) and Endoscopic Cyclophotocoagulation (ECP), alternatives to cyclocryotherapy.

## 64.1 Laser Light Properties and Parameters

Lasers are devices that concentrate electromagnetic energy and radiate light as a monochromatic beam. Laser light is comprised of photons that propagate as coherent, minimally divergent electromagnetic waves through space. Its interaction with tissue varies depending on the parameters of the light – such as wavelength, pulse duration and fluence (Fig. 64.1) – and the properties of the tissue. The characteristics of the laser and the various components of the target tissue determine the relative amounts of absorbance, scattering, transmission, and reflection of incident laser radiation (Fig. 64.2).

The *absorption path length*, or the distance into the target tissue in which photon absorption occurs, is also essential in determining the laser–tissue interaction. Photons with higher energy levels are generally absorbed at a much deeper plane than those with lower energy levels. Also affecting the absorption path length is the molecular composition of the target tissue. When photons possess a similar wavelength to the absorption profile of the tissue's components they are absorbed at a higher rate. This causes the photons to have a shorter penetration depth.

Another important component of laser–tissue interaction is *irradiance*, or the number of photons delivered to the target area per unit time (Fig. 64.3). When irradiance is increased, more energy is delivered. Under certain conditions, when laser energy is applied to tissue, heat may be generated at the local target site from increased molecular vibrations. This heat is then conducted away from the local site to cooler regions of the tissue. If the diffusion rate of heat in the target tissue is slower than the rate at which heat is being generated by laser radiation, thermal events will occur in local sites of the target tissue.[1] When parameters are carefully chosen, laser–tissue interactions can also occur without thermal change to the target tissue. These situations enable surgical procedures that are unique to specific lasers, such as the non-thermal, nonscar-producing tissue ablation with excimer lasers for refractive corneal surgery and ELT.

Understanding these laser–tissue interaction parameters determines if the tissue phase change will occur through (1) *photovaporization*: thermal molecular fragmentation; (2) *photodisruption*: plasma expansion leading to mechanical molecular fragmentation; or (3) *photodissociation*: direct, nonthermal, molecular decomposition.

Photovaporization occurs when high energy laser light is delivered to the target tissue resulting in carbonization of tissue. Carbonization occurs when the target tissue has been converted to carbon from the heat of laser energy absorption. Photodisruption describes the optical breakdown of molecules. Molecules are fragmented into ionic components creating rapidly expanding ionic "plasma." The fragmentation, expanding plasma, along with subsequent shock-wave effects, cause the mechanical disruption of the adjacent tissue.[2] Photodissociation is the process in which chemical bonds are broken nonthermally through the absorption of photons. The energy absorbed by the tissue is sufficient to dissociate carbon–carbon and carbon–nitrogen bonds directly. The resultant fragments expand and are rapidly expelled, dissipating heat.[3]

## 64.2 Lasers for Outflow

One of the primary factors causing elevated intraocular pressure (IOP) in open-angle glaucoma is the obstruction of outflow at the juxtacanalicular trabecular meshwork and inner

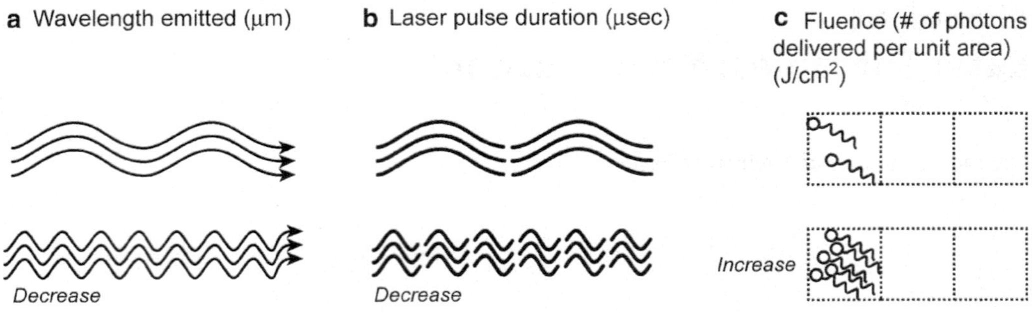

**Fig. 64.1** Wavelength, pulse duration, and fluence

**a** Wavelength emitted (μm)

**b** Laser pulse duration (μsec)

**c** Fluence (# of photons delivered per unit area) (J/cm²)

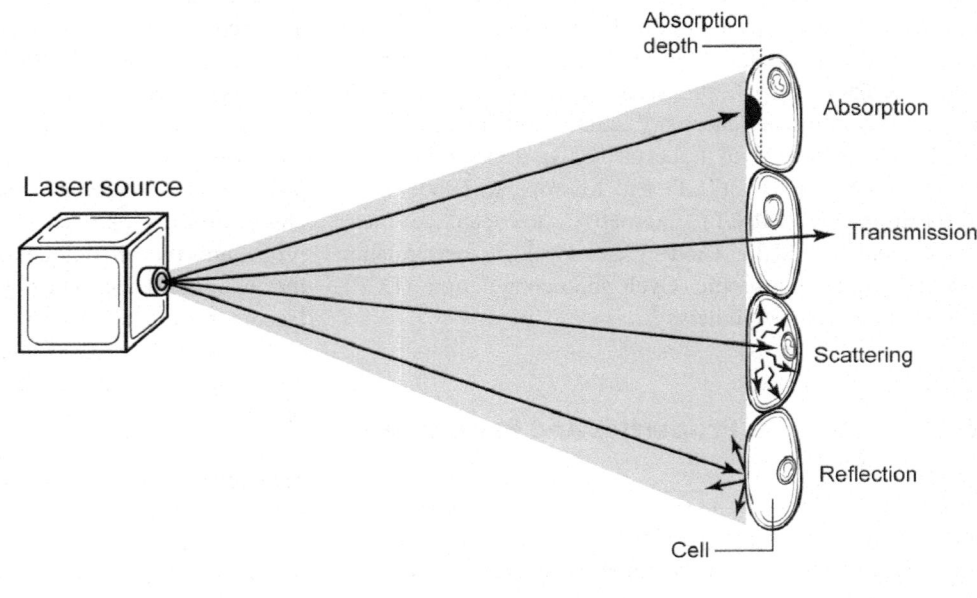

**Fig. 64.2** Light absorption, transmission, scattering, and reflection

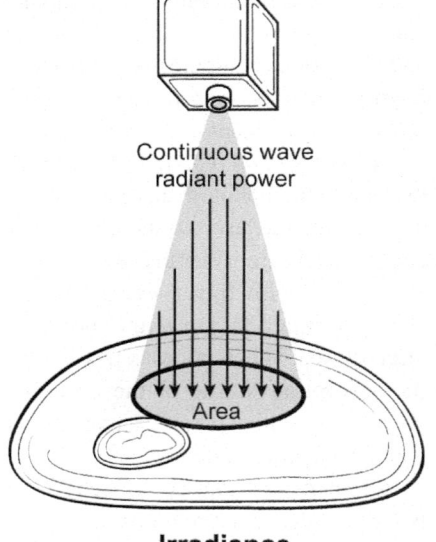

**Fig. 64.3** Irradiance

wall of Schlemm's canal. Many attempts have been made to bypass this outflow obstruction through the utilization of lasers. Early work by Krasnov et al showed only moderate success using a ruby laser (943 nm) to perform trabeculopuncture.[4] Other laser trabeculopuncture attempts, including Hager's study using an argon laser (488+514 nm) and Fankhauser's study using an Nd:YAG laser (1,064 nm), have also been unsuccessful.[5] Following these initial attempts, Wise et al determined that a continuous wave, essentially long pulsed argon laser (488+514 nm) could successfully modify the trabecular meshwork to increase outflow without perforation.[6] However, this argon laser trabeculoplasty (ALT) causes thermal damage to the trabecular meshwork and repetition of the procedure is not effective in lowering pressure. The next generation of laser trabeculoplasty was the development of the short pulse length SLT (see chap. 27). The SLT procedure has shown to be as effective as ALT with less thermal damage. This allows SLT to be clinically appropriate as initial therapy. However, like ALT, SLT is limited in both the extent of IOP lowering and the duration of efficacy. Generally, when SLT is repeated, clinical effectiveness is noticeably decreased. Alternatives to SLT include TLT and MDLT.

The subsequent generation of laser therapy targets the site of the identified anatomic pathology, the juxtacanalicular trabecular meshwork, and inner wall of Schlemm's canal, rather than the trabecular meshwork to increase outflow. The goals are to normalize IOP and to increase the duration of effectiveness while minimizing invasiveness and eliminating the patient compliance issues of medication therapies.

### 64.2.1 Excimer Laser Trabeculostomy

During the development of nonthermal, short-pulsed excimer 193 nm ArF lasers for corneal refractive surgery, it was discovered that these lasers could also remove angle tissue, trabecular meshwork, and sclera with almost no thermal damage – unlike all prior lasers used to treat angle tissue – thereby minimizing inflammation and scar tissue formation. To treat the angle tissue and to be clinically useful, the lasers needed a delivery system into the eye since the ultraviolet (UV) wavelengths are readily absorbed by the cornea. Since 193 nm ArF cannot be transmitted through fiber optics, 308 nm XeCl UV excimer lasers were used in preclinical trials, which began in the 1980s, initially designed for nonthermal, full-thickness, *ab interno* sclerectomy. Histology confirmed that this laser caused minimal thermal damage when compared to visible or infrared lasers. Unlike ALT, SLT, and other lasers in which the laser–tissue interaction is thermal and "treats" the tissue, ELT, like LASIK, precisely excises tissue without thermal injury or scarring of the surrounding tissue, enabling the creation of an anatomic opening connecting the anterior chamber directly to Schlemm's canal (Fig. 64.4a–f). With this advantage in mind and the exquisite accuracy of depth of tissue removal, early developers saw that it was possible to use this 308 nm XeCl laser to precisely excise the juxtacanalicular trabecular meshwork and inner wall of Schlemm's canal to increase internal outflow by creating ostia into Schlemm's canal instead of creating a full thickness sclerectomy. The first human clinical trial for ELT was performed by Vogel et al in Germany in 1997.[7] In 22 eyes with open-angle glaucoma, the median IOP reduction was 7 mmHg. Furthermore, the minimal trauma to the eye from this procedure left all other options of surgery open.

Another advantage of ELT is that this procedure enables pneumatic canaloplasty. As ELT is performed, both coaxial endoscopic views and gonioscopic views reveal gas bubble expansion at the previous ostium created as Schlemm's canal is entered at each subsequent ELT site, confirming patency and continuity of flow into Schlemm's canal (Fig. 64.5a–c).

As a result of ELT converting trabecular meshwork tissue into gas by photoablation, the pressure of this gas is proposed to dilate Schlemm's canal and collector channels to improve aqueous outflow.

Numerous clinical studies have demonstrated ELT's ability to achieve the long-term reduction of IOP and the elimination of glaucoma medications in patients with open-angle glaucoma or ocular hypertension. In a study by Giers et al, ELT was performed on 33 patients with phakic eyes.[8] After 3 years, there was a mean IOP reduction of 36% among the subjects in addition to a mean medications reduction of 91%. In the same study, 15 patients with pseudophakic eyes underwent ELT. After 3 years, the mean IOP reduction among this group was 47%, and the mean medications reduction was 77%. In another study, Babighian et al followed 21 patients who underwent ELT for a 2-year period.[9] Patients had a mean preoperative IOP of 24.8±2.0 mmHg. Two years later, they had a mean IOP of 16.9±2.1 mmHg, a reduction of 32%.

When ELT is combined with cataract surgery, the same corneal incision is used. After phacoemulsification is performed, ELT sites (current protocol=10 sites) are created in the inferior quadrants. In a study by Pache et al, in which this combined procedure was performed on 60 patients by Georgaras, at the postoperative 1-year visit, 91% of patients continued to have a ≥20% reduction in IOP from baseline levels.[10] Giers et al also conducted a study in which 33 patients underwent combined ELT and phacoemulsification/IOL implantation procedures.[11] At the 3-year follow-up visit, there was a 39% IOP reduction and a 70% medications reduction.

ELT has been approved for use in the European Union since 1998. Thousands of ELT procedures have been successful in lowering and maintaining lower IOP for years in Europe. Currently, clinical studies are pending in both Canada and the United States, and the next generation of ELT devices is under development.[1]

---

[1]EyeLight, Inc.

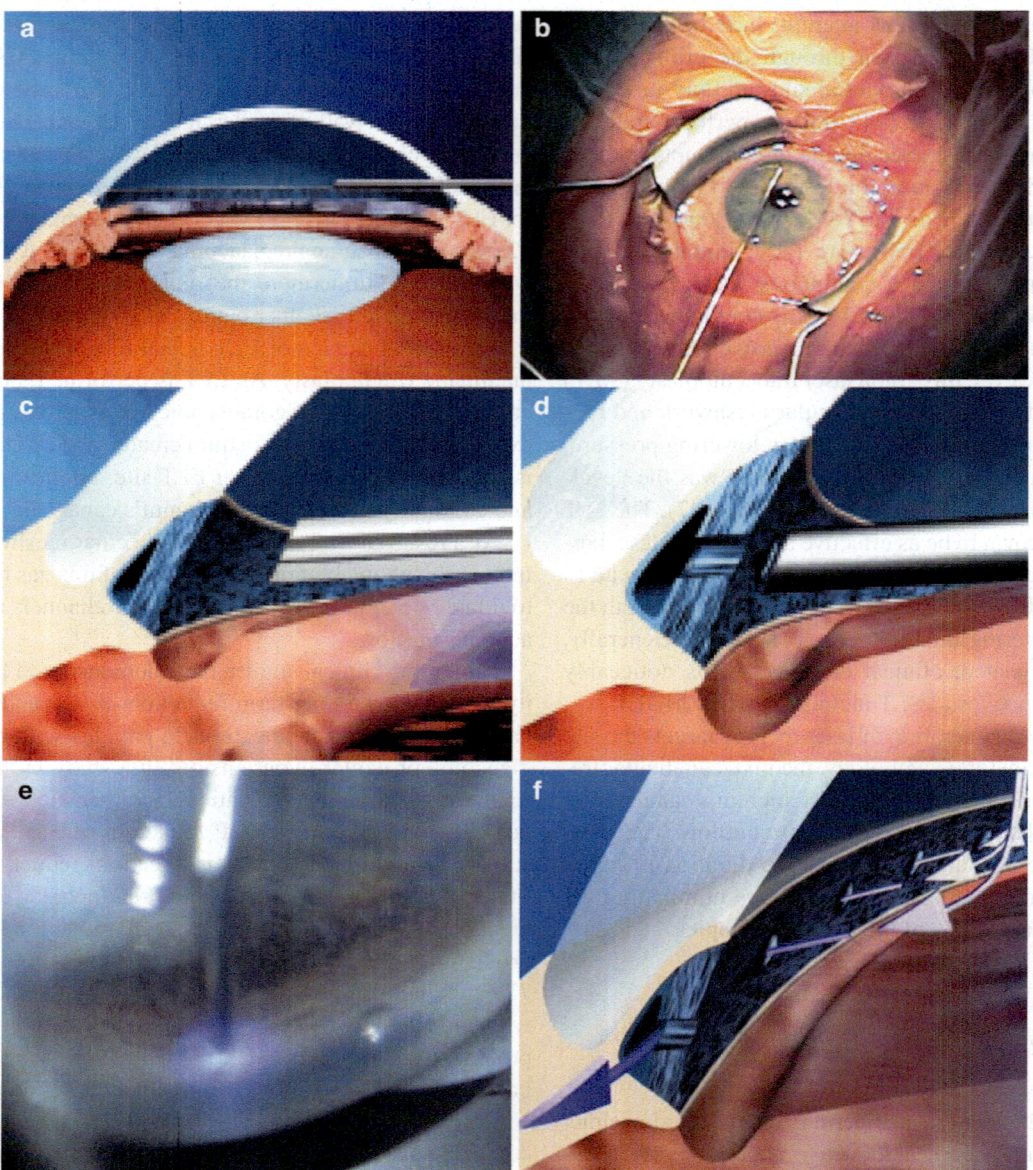

**Fig. 64.4** Schematic and photos of Excimer Laser Trabeculostomy (ELT) procedure. (**a**) Paracentesis, viscoelastic, and probe across chamber. (**b**) Probe across chamber. (**c**) Probe contacts trabecular meshwork, laser pulses ablate tissue into gas. (**d**) Second opening created into Schlemm's canal. (**e**) Laser pulses excising the trabecular meshwork. (**f**) Patent trabeculostomies enable outflow into Schlemm's canal. (Animation stills courtesy of Rudolf G. Peschke)

## 64.3 Alternatives to Argon Laser Trabeculoplasty

Several newer alternatives to ALT have a common goal of achieving equivalent IOP lowering with less damage to the trabecular meshwork. With the development of SLT (q-switched, 532 nm), thermal damage is minimized by decreasing the pulse duration to 3 ns vs. 100,000,000 ns (0.1 s) for ALT while maintaining almost the same wavelength and therefore the same tissue absorption and penetration depth.[122] With SLT, the target chromophore, the region responsible for light absorption, is intracellular pigment that

---

[2] Note: the terminology "Argon" Laser Trabeculoplasty is commonly used, although most lasers used for this procedure are no longer Argon ($\lambda = 488 + 514$ nm), but solid state, frequency doubled Nd:YAG (532 nm). The laser-tissue effects are similar in spite of the difference in wavelength.

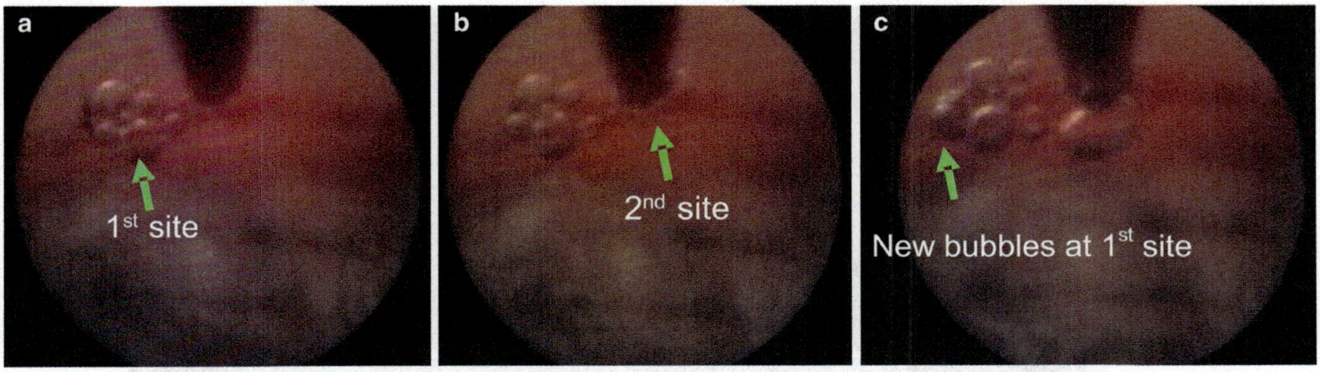

**Fig. 64.5** Photos of ELT procedure. (**a**) Coaxial endoscopic view of the trabecular meshwork. (**b**) As second ostium is created into Schlemm's canal, (**c**) bubble expansion is observed at the adjacent ELT site confirming flow and patency into Schlemm's canal. (Photos courtesy of Professor J. Funk)

limits the spread of laser-induced thermal damage resulting in much less structural damage to the trabecular meshwork. This short pulse duration ensures that the heat diffusion is limited. SLT has proven as successful as ALT in decreasing IOP for several years, but, like ALT, both the extent of IOP lowering and the duration of efficacy are limited.

### 64.3.1 Titanium:Sapphire Laser Trabeculoplasty

Another alternative to ALT is the 790 nm Titanium:Sapphire laser (SOLX, Inc., Waltham, Massachusetts) with a pulse duration of 7,000 ns. This laser was originally developed in the 1990s for *ab interno* laser sclerostomy; however, it was noted that IOP decreased when the laser energy was focused on the trabecular meshwork.[13] Similar to 532 nm SLT, histologic analysis has shown that the laser is selective for targeting pigmented trabecular meshwork cells causing less thermal damage and scarring to surrounding tissue than ALT, but slightly more than SLT due to the deeper absorption depth of this 790 nm wavelength (Fig. 64.6 a–c).

In the pilot clinical trial, 206 eyes underwent TLT and were followed for 12 months.[14][3] All of the eyes were treated with approximately 50 pulses at 30–80 mJ using a 200 μm diameter spot over 180° of the meshwork. Results showed a reduction from a mean preoperative IOP of $22.5 \pm 5.1$ to $17.0 \pm 3.3$ mmHg at 12 months. This represents a 24% reduction in IOP. Harasymowycz et al randomized 181 patients with primary open-angle glaucoma to receive either TLT or ALT. They found an insignificant difference between the two groups. Both had a mean IOP reduction of approximately 25% after 12 months.[15]

TLT was approved for use in the European Union in November 2003, and approved in Canada in January 2006. It is currently considered an investigational device in the United States and is undergoing a multicenter clinical trial to evaluate its safety and efficacy.

### 64.3.2 Micropulse Diode Laser Trabeculoplasty

Yet another alternative to ALT is MDLT. Unlike other trabeculoplasty procedures that utilize continuous wave lasers, MDLT uses an 810 nm diode laser to deliver a repetitive series of short, subthreshold pulses (Fig. 64.7a, b; see also, Chap. 61: Figs. 61.1 and 61.4). In a typical MDLT procedure, a series of 100 pulses are delivered to the eye with 300 ns of "on" time and 1,700 ns of "off" time. Due to the short "on" time pulse, and the low irradiance, less heat disperses to adjacent tissue, and the thermal event is restricted to the chromophore.[16]

MDLT has shown to be effective in reducing IOP with less of the side effects associated with ALT. Several studies have shown insignificant differences in IOP reduction between MDLT and ALT, but intraoperative and postoperative discomfort was significantly reduced with MDLT.[17] A limited study by Ingvoldstad et al randomized 21 patients with primary open-angle glaucoma to receive either MDLT or ALT and found that MDLT was equally as effective in reducing IOP as ALT after three months, with a reduction of 4.5 mmHg in the MDLT group and 4.6 mmHg in the ALT group.[18] In another study, conducted by Fea et al,

---

[3] Gabriel Simon Ophthalmic Institute, Madrid, Spain.

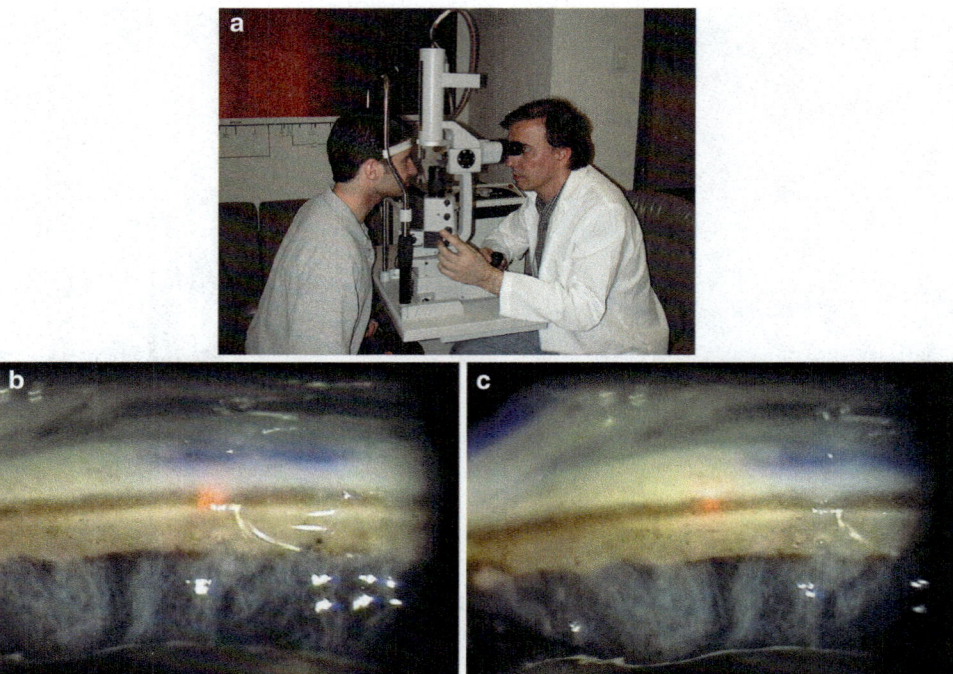

**Fig. 64.6** (a) Titanium:Sapphire Laser Trabeculoplasty (TLT) being performed for primary open angle glaucoma. (b) Slit lamp view of trabecular meshwork during TLT. (c) Slit lamp view of trabecular meshwork immediately post-TLT. (Photos courtesy of Solx, Inc., Waltham, Massachusetts)

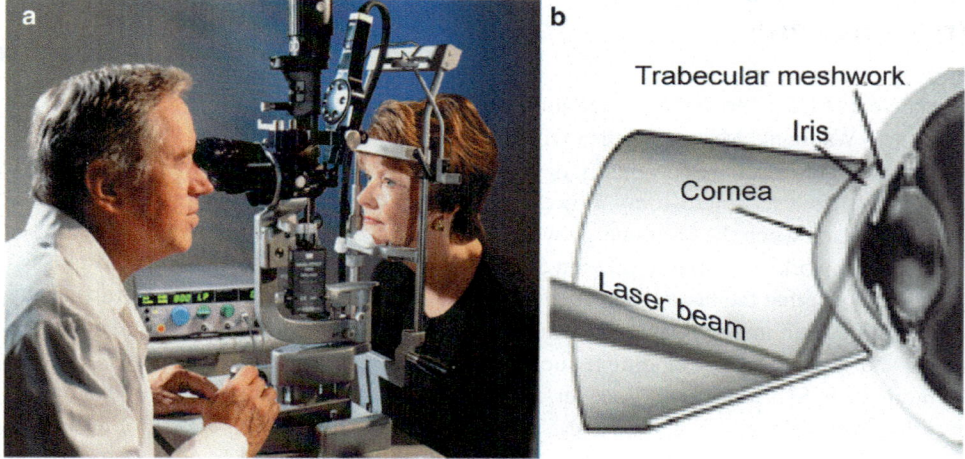

**Fig. 64.7** (a) Micropulse Diode Laser (OcuLight SLX 810 nm Laser) attached to a Haag Streit slit lamp prior to insertion of goniolens (Photo courtesy of IRIDEX Corp., Mountain View, California). (b) Diagram of goniolens optics

MDLT was found to be effective in reducing IOP in 75% of eyes with open-angle glaucoma after 12 months of follow-up.[17]

MDLT has been proven to reduce IOP with limited complications and side effects. In addition, this same laser can be used for retinal photocoagulation and transscleral cyclophotocoagulation by altering the pulse duration and thereby modifying the thermal laser–tissue interactions. Additional clinical studies are currently being conducted to determine the long-term efficacy of MDLT.

### 64.3.3 IOPtima $CO_2$ Laser Assisted Nonpenetrating Deep Sclerectomy

Trabeculectomy, the standard surgical procedure for filtration surgery, is known to be associated with numerous postoperative complications. Nonpenetrating deep sclerectomy (NPDS) procedures have gained much attention in efforts to achieve filtration without penetration into the anterior chamber to reduce the risk profile.

In NPDS procedures, a scleral flap is created and most of the underlying sclera is removed until only the trabecular meshwork remains, without actually entering the anterior chamber (Fig. 64.8). This technique entails a steep learning curve for the surgeon to become accustomed to both the anatomy and the precision needed. If an insufficient amount of sclera is removed, filtration will not occur. Conversely, if the surgeon removes too much, the thin trabecular membrane may be punctured, requiring conversion of the procedure to a standard trabeculectomy. This intraoperative complication occurs in as many as 30–50% of cases. Because of this high rate of complications, researchers have explored several methods to achieve repeatable and satisfactory results while shortening the procedure's learning curve.

A variety of lasers, including 193 nm excimer, 2,100 nm holmium, and 2,940 nm erbium:YAG lasers have been used in NPDS trials; however, none of these lasers was clinically practical for this application. In 2006, Assia et al evaluated the use of a $CO_2$ laser (10,600 nm) for performing a deep sclerectomy in a manner identical to that described by Seiler et al in 1989.[19] In his partial external trabeculectomy (PET) procedure, Seiler used the 193 nm excimer laser under flap *ab externo* to excise scleral tissue until aqueous percolating through the base of the treatment site absorbed the energy and prevented perforation.[20] Assia chose the $CO_2$ laser because of its controlled penetration depth and because its radiation is also absorbed and dissipated rapidly in water. These characteristics are useful in NPDS because the laser energy would be absorbed by percolating fluid flowing through the trabecular membrane and prevent the perforation of the trabecular membrane (Fig. 64.9). Additional clinical studies are currently being conducted to determine the long-term efficacy of this $CO_2$ laser in performing NPDS.

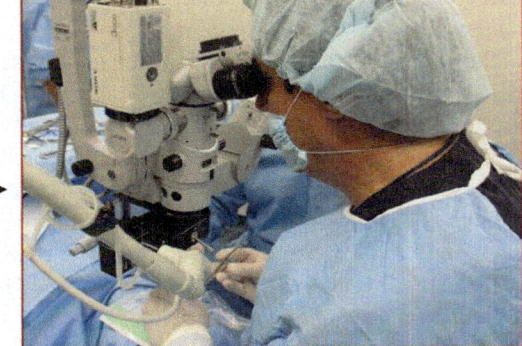

**Fig. 64.8** Nonpenetrating deep sclerectomy procedure performed under direct observation with $CO_2$ laser and scanner attached to a micromanipulator mounted on the surgical microscope. (Photo courtesy of Dr. Ehud Assia) — Delivery tube from $CO_2$ laser to surgical microscope

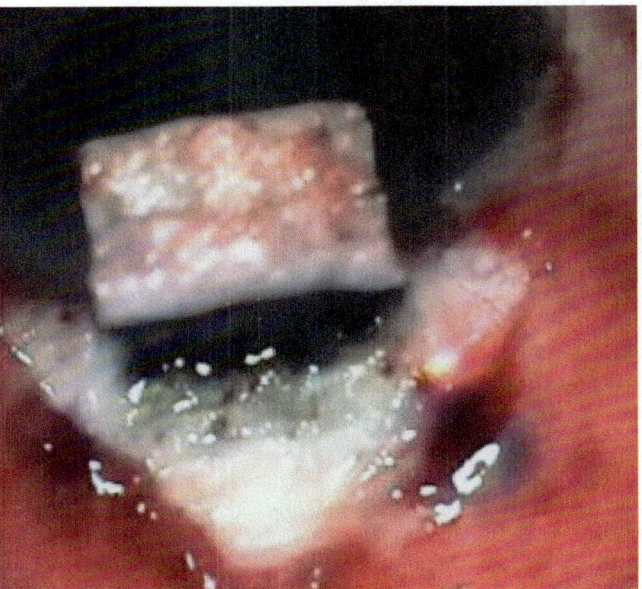

**Fig. 64.9** IOPtima $CO_2$ laser assisted nonpenetrating deep sclerectomy. Percolation of aqueous in the area treated by the $CO_2$ laser. (Photo courtesy of Dr. Ehud Assia)

## 64.4 Lasers for Inflow

### 64.4.1 Cyclophotocoagulation

The goal of cyclophotocoagulation is to reduce the inflow of aqueous humor through the destruction of the ciliary body. However, titration is critical and very difficult to estimate to achieve control without hypotony. In addition, short-term postoperative pressure spikes may occur and the blood aqueous barrier is often compromised with resultant chronic uveitis. Insufficient destruction of ciliary processes results in inadequate reduction in IOP. Therefore, the therapeutic window is a narrow one.

Using laser light for ciliary body destruction was found to be as effective as cyclocryotherapy, more easily titrated, and less painful. The continuous wave, long pulse duration (20 μm) photocoagulative Nd:YAG laser (1,064 nm), is used in the majority of cyclophotocoagulation procedures in contrast to the short pulse duration, q-switched photodisruptive Nd:YAG laser used for posterior capsulotomy. This wavelength is able to deeply penetrate the sclera due to its minimal absorption and backscatter. In addition, the Nd:YAG laser can be used via both a contact, fiber optic probe or noncontact slit-lamp delivery system.

Subsequently, the use of the infrared diode laser (810 nm) to perform transscleral cyclophotocoagulation has gained popularity. This diode laser has practically replaced cyclocryotherapy and Nd:YAG lasers for cyclodestruction. One of the most common diode laser systems is the continuous-wave 810 nm semiconductor diode laser with a fiber-optic G-Probe (OcuLight SLx, IRIS Medical Instruments, Mountain View, California). The G-Probe is a 400-μm diameter fiber optic delivery device specifically designed to facilitate transscleral cyclophotocoagulation (Fig. 64.10a–d).

DCPC, like other cyclodestructive procedures is reserved for glaucomas resistant to other treatments and is indicated for late stage glaucoma patients who experience pain and discomfort because of their elevated IOP.

Studies have shown that DCPC is successful in controlling IOP in eyes with refractory glaucoma. Iliev et al found a 55% reduction in IOP and a 65% reduction in glaucoma medications over a 3-year follow-up period.[21] However, similar to Nd:YAG laser therapy, clinical studies have shown that the effectiveness of diode cyclophotocoagulation may decrease over time, requiring additional treatments. In seven recent clinical studies, additional treatments were necessary in 25–45% of patients who underwent cyclophotocoagulation.[21]

Complications of diode laser transscleral cyclophotocoagulation commonly observed are chronic uveitis, ocular discomfort, headache, hyphema, vitreous hemorrhage, hypotony, and phthisis. According to the study conducted by Iliev et al, hypotony occurred in 17.6% of cases and was not correlated to increased laser energy, repeat treatments, or type of glaucoma. Staging photocoagulation with fewer initial treatment sites and lower laser power may reduce this risk of hypotony.[21]

### 64.4.2 Endoscopic Cyclophotocoagulation

ECP follows the same concepts for the reduction of inflow as transscleral cyclophotocoagulation, but the laser energy delivery to the ciliary process is *ab interno* under direct observation via an endoscope, rather than transscleral (Fig. 64.11a–c). The advantage is the direct observation of the cyclodestruction process. The disadvantage is the requirement of incisional surgery. Therefore, ECP is usually performed concurrent with cataract surgery.

Similar to transscleral cyclophotocoagulation, ECP uses an 810-nm semiconductor diode laser. In addition to this laser, the ECP unit includes a video camera, a xenon light source, and a helium–neon laser aiming beam (Endo Optiks,

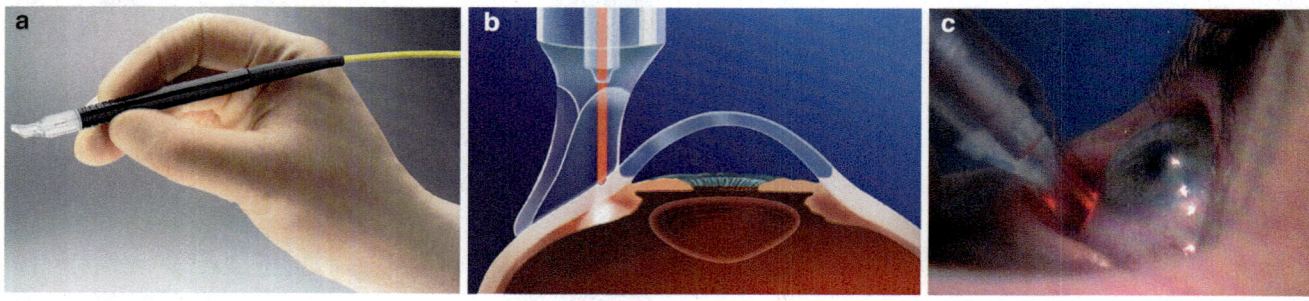

**Fig. 64.10** (a) Cyclophotocoagulation via noncontact slit lamp delivery. (b) G-Probe fiberoptic delivery device (Photo courtesy of IRIDEX Corp., Mountain View, California). Diagram (c) and (d) photograph of G-Probe delivery device applied to an eye (Illustration and photograph courtesy of IRIDEX Corp., Mountain View, California)

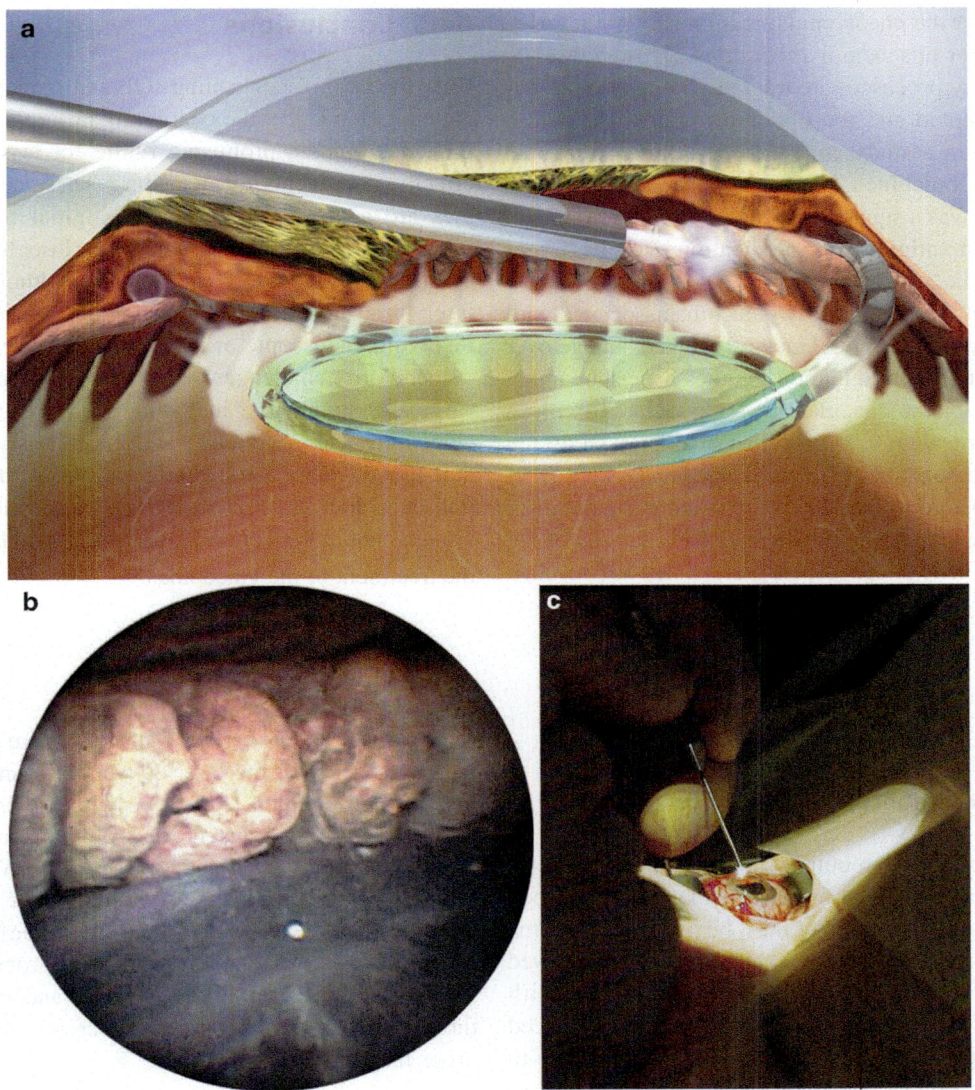

**Fig. 64.11** (a) Endoscopic cyclophotocoagulation of the ciliary body. Coaxial probe crosses anterior chamber into posterior chamber to view and treat ciliary processes. (b) Endoscopic view of ciliary body during ECP. (c) Endoscopic cyclophotocoagulation procedure being performed on patient. (Diagram and photos courtesy of Endo Optiks, Little Silver, New Jersey)

Little Silver, New Jersey). These elements are combined in a 20-gauge fiber optic cable and endoscope probe. The endoscope allows for a 70° field of vision for the surgeon. The laser is focused 0.75 mm beyond the tip of the probe. Titration of the directly observed photocoagulative thermal cyclodestruction is controlled by modulating the duration of the laser pulse, switched by a foot pedal.

There are two approaches for performing ECP: a limbal approach and a pars plana entry. More common is the limbal approach since an anterior vitrectomy is required for a pars plana entry. Also, risks of choroidal and retinal detachment are associated with a pars plana entry.

Multiple studies have shown ECP to have comparable results to DCPC in reducing IOP and glaucoma medications. In one study, 68 eyes with refractory glaucoma underwent ECP. Over a 1-year period, IOP was reduced 34% and glaucoma medications were decreased by 33%.[22] However, even with this significant pressure reduction, there were a considerable number of complications associated with this procedure. These complications included fibrin exudates (24%), hyphema (12%), cystoid macular edema (10%), vision loss (6%), and choroidal detachment (4%).

Most ECP procedures are performed concurrent with phacoemulsification cataract surgery. The same limbal incisions used for the phacoemulsification surgery are used for the ECP. After phacoemulsification is performed, 180–270° of the ciliary processes are treated. Then, an intraocular lens is implanted and the operation is concluded in a typical fashion. In a study conducted by Berke et al, 626 eyes underwent combined ECP and phacoemulsification surgery.[23] There was a significant 18% reduction in IOP and 53% reduction in antiglaucoma medication over the 3-year study period.

In patients who have refractory glaucoma associated with a penetrating keratoplasty, ECP may offer an advantage over transscleral cyclophotocoagulation. Studies have shown that transscleral cyclophotocoagulation is associated with a higher rate of corneal graft failures. In a small pilot study, ten patients who had penetrating keratoplasties underwent ECP. At 30 months postprocedure, 80% of the patients maintained an IOP less than 22 mmHg with an average reduction of 1.4 medications and none of the corneal grafts failed as a result.[22]

## 64.5 Conclusions

With the goal of controlling IOP and reducing the need for patient compliance, the continuing progress in clinical laser therapies holds a promising future for less invasive, more effective treatments for glaucoma. These newer laser therapies are appropriate as first-line, initial treatment having resolved concerns that arose in earlier laser therapies without compromising IOP lowering efficacy. Although many of the laser procedures under development, particularly those involving endoscopic or *ab interno* laser delivery, are difficult and offer challenges to even experienced surgeons, their surgical counterparts, including such procedures as trabeculectomy and goniotomy, are difficult as well. We anticipate that the demonstrated effectiveness of these procedures will accelerate their inclusion into the ophthalmic surgery armamentaria and continue to make a significant impact on the treatment of the glaucomas.

### Sidebars

### Excimer laser trabeculostomy procedure

ELT is performed as an outpatient procedure under topical anesthesia. Since 308 nm laser radiation is absorbed by the cornea, an optical fiber must be used to deliver the energy intracamerally. A paracentesis is created, followed by the stabilization of the anterior chamber with viscoelastic. The fiber optic probe is then advanced through the paracentesis across the anterior chamber to contact the trabecular meshwork. This placement is visualized through gonioscopy or via an endoscope. Pulsed photoablative energy is then applied. In most protocols, 10 sites are created in an inferior quadrant. A small amount of blood reflux from Schlemm's canal is commonly observed and confirms each opening's patency. The probe is then removed from the eye, and the viscoelastic is exchanged for balanced salt solution. Postoperatively, topical antibiotics and steroid drops are generally continued for 1–2 weeks. Following ELT, IOP decreases immediately. Additionally, pressure lowering medications are rarely needed.[24]

### Micropulse diode laser trabeculoplasty

The IRIDEX OcuLight SLx 810 diode is the most commonly used device for MDLT procedures. Preoperatively, topical anesthesia is applied to the operative eye, and the patient is seated at the laser delivery slit lamp. A gonio lens is then coupled to the eye with Goniosol and an aiming beam is focused on the anterior trabecular meshwork. The laser is set at a power of 2 W with 2 ms duration and 60–65 spots are applied over the inferior 180° or 120–130 applications are made over 360°. Postoperatively, 0.1% indomethacin eye drops are administered immediately after the treatment and are continued throughout the first day. In some cases topical steroid drops may be indicated.[16]

### Titanium:sapphire laser trabeculoplasty procedure

Preoperatively, topical anesthesia is applied to the operative eye and the patient is seated at a slit-lamp. A gonio lens is then coupled to the eye with Goniosol. Following visualization of the trabecular meshwork, an He–Ne aiming laser is focused on the pigmented region. Initial laser settings should start at a power of 25 mJ and duration of 8 µm. If this is insufficient in producing slight movements of the trabecular meshwork and depigmentation, or "micro-bubbles" in the meshwork, the power may be increased in 25 mJ steps. In most protocols, initial treatment should include 180° of the trabecular meshwork. Postoperatively, topical steroid eye drops are continued for 1–2 weeks.[15]

### Diode laser cyclophotocoagulation procedure

This procedure is performed under retrobulbar or, occasionally, topical anesthesia. The anterior ciliary body is approximated to be 1.5–3.0 mm posterior to the corneoscleral limbus. However, in cases where the ciliary body's location is assumed to be abnormal, transillumination may be used to localize the ciliary body. Once its location is determined or approximated, the surgeon applies a slight amount of pressure to the sclera via the G-probe over the ciliary body. The number of treatment sites should range from 15 to 30 spots. The laser's pulse power ranges from 1,500 to 2,000 mW. These power levels should be adjusted to prevent excessive damage. Pulse duration is fixed at 2 s. No more than 270° of the ciliary body's circumference is treated, leaving the superior sector (the common site of most filtration surgeries) intact.

The immediate postoperative care for DCPC is the instillation of antibiotic/steroid ointment with an overnight eye patch. For patients with severe glaucomatous optic neuropathy, use of an oral carbonic anhydrase inhibitor overnight may decrease the risk of postoperative pressure spikes. Oral analgesics are also prescribed. On postoperative day 1, the patient is started on topical antibiotics and steroid drops. In addition, all glaucoma medications are restarted except for miotics and prostaglandin analogues, which may worsen inflammation. In cases of moderate inflammation, cycloplegics, such as 1% atropine sulfate, are used. Glaucoma medications may be discontinued when deemed appropriate.[21]

### IOPtima $CO_2$ laser-assisted nonpenetrating deep sclerectomy procedure

Preoperatively the patient is prepared in a similar fashion to trabeculectomy surgery. The procedure is performed under retrobulbar anesthesia. A local peritomy is followed by the creation of a 4×5-mm partial thickness scleral flap. The sclera under the flap is then ablated with the carbon dioxide laser. Initially, the laser power is set to 10 W. After every 5–10 laser shots, a noticeable amount of charred tissue may accumulate. This charred tissue is removed with a damp surgical sponge. At the initial sign of fluid percolation, the laser power should be decreased to 5 W. Once fluid is seen, there should be delays between each laser pulse to ensure that only dry tissue continues to be ablated. If the tissue appears to be ablated unevenly, the fluid should be allowed to percolate until it fills the deeper troughs, revealing only the elevated tissue regions.

Once clinically adequate filtration is observed, the surgeon closes the scleral flap with 10–0 nylon sutures.[19]

### Endoscopic cyclophotocoagulation procedure: limbal approach

In the limbal approach, the pupil is dilated with topical 2% cyclopentolate. Under retrobulbar anesthesia with bupivacaine, a limbal paracentesis is made at the 3 o'clock position for a right eye and at 9 o'clock for a left eye. Viscoelastic is used to stabilize the anterior chamber. The surgeon also injects enough viscoelastic into the posterior chamber to sufficiently inflate the ciliary sulcus and break any posterior synechiae that would preclude access from an anterior approach. The probe is then advanced through the paracentesis, across the anterior chamber and into the posterior chamber. Once the ciliary processes are visualized the treatment is initiated. The laser power is set according to the surgeon's preference, usually in the 60–90 mW range. The beam is focused on the raised processes rather than the valleys between them. The photocoagulative laser energy is applied to each ciliary process. The thermal effect causes the tissue to shrink and turn white. This transformation signals the endpoint of the treatment. If excessive energy is used, the ciliary process will visibly rupture with an audible "pop." This rupture can cause the blood aqueous barrier to be further compromised leading to an increased risk of inflammation and hyphema. Depending on the level of IOP reduction required, 180–270° of the ciliary process are treated. The probe is then removed and the viscoelastic is exchanged for balanced salt solution.[19] Following ECP, antibiotic/steroid ointment is applied and the eye is patched. For patients with severe glaucomatous optic neuropathy, use of an oral carbonic anhydrase inhibitor overnight may decrease the risk of postoperative pressure spikes. Oral analgesics are also prescribed. On postoperative day 1, the patient is started on topical antibiotics and steroid drops. In addition, all glaucoma medications are restarted except for miotics and prostaglandin analogues, which may worsen inflammation. In cases of moderate inflammation, cycloplegics, such as 1% atropine sulfate, are used. Glaucoma medications may be discontinued when deemed appropriate.[22]

### Endoscopic cyclophotocoagulation procedure: pars plana approach

In the pars plana approach, three ports are created: one for infusion in the inferior pars plana and two superior ports for illumination and vitrectomy. An anterior vitrectomy is initially performed to allow access to the ciliary processes. Then, the endoscope is inserted and the same end point of treatment is observed as with the limbal approach. Following ECP, antibiotic/steroid ointment is applied and the eye is patched. For patients with severe glaucomatous optic neuropathy, use of an oral carbonic anhydrase inhibitor overnight may decrease the risk of postoperative pressure spikes. Oral analgesics are also prescribed. On postoperative day 1, the patient is started on topical antibiotics and steroid drops. In addition, all glaucoma medications are restarted except for miotics and prostaglandin analogues, which may worsen inflammation. In cases of moderate inflammation, cycloplegics, such as 1% atropine sulfate, are used. Glaucoma medications may be discontinued when deemed appropriate.[22]

## References

1. Sliney DH, Mainster MA. Opthalmic laser safety: tissue interactions, hazards, and protection. In: Stamper RL, Berlin MS, eds. *Lasers in Ophthamology*. Philadelphia, PA: W.B. Saunders Company; 1998:157-164.
2. Berlin MS. General aspects of laser therapy. In: Stamper RL, Lieberman MF MF, Drake MV, eds. *Becker-Shaffers's Diagnosis and Therapy of the Glaucomas*. St. Louis, MO: Mosby, Inc.; 1999:522-524.
3. Berlin MS. Current options in laser sclerotomy. In: Ritch R, Shields MB, Krupin T, eds.*The Glaucomas: Glaucoma Therapy*. St. Louis, Missouri: Mosby, Inc. 1996; 1591-1604.
4. Krasnov MM. Laseropuncture of anterior chamber angle in glaucoma. *Am J Ophthalmol*. 1973;75:674.
5. Berlin MS. Re-thinking glaucoma surgery: ELT present and future. Lecture for ALCON vs. Irvine. Irvine, California. May, 2008.
6. Wise JB. Long-term control of adult open angle glaucoma by argon laser treatment. *Ophthalmology*. 1981;88:197.
7. Vogel M, Lauritzen K. Selective excimer laser ablation of the trabecular meshwork. Clinical results. *Der Ophthalmologe*. 1997; 94(9):665-667.
8. Giers et al. Personal communication.
9. Babighian S, Rapizzi E, Galan A. Efficacy and safety of ab interno excimer laser trabeculotomy in primary open-angle glaucoma: two years of follow-up. *Ophthalmologica*. 2006;220(5):285-290.
10. Pache M, Wilmsmeyer S, Funk J. Laser surgery for glaucoma: excimer-laser trabeculotomy. *Klin Monatsbl Augenheilkd*. 2006; 223(4):303-307.
11. Giers et al. Personal communication.
12. Kramer TR, Noecker RJ. Comparison of the morphologic changes after selective laser trabeculoplasty and argon laser trabeculoplasty in human eye bank eyes. *Ophthalmology*. 2001;108:773-779.
13. Lewandowski JT. Exploring uveoscleral outflow: a new treatment system seeks to take the bleb out of glaucoma surgery. *Glaucoma Today*. http://glaucomatoday.com/pages/current/innovators.html Accessed April 5, 2007.
14. Groves N. Investigational device in United States: titanium-sapphire laser procedure reduces IOP by 25%. *Ophthalmology Times*. http://www.solx.com/pdf/254200.pdf Accessed April 7, 2007
15. Harasymowycz P, Ahmed I, Perez B. Initial results from a multicenter, randomized clinical trial comparing argon laser and Titanium:Sapphire laser trabeculoplasty in primary open-angle glaucoma. Paper presented at: The 2008 ASCRS Symposium on Cataract, IOL and Refractive Surgery; April 7, 2008; Chicago, IL.
16. Fea AM, Dorin G. Laser treatment of glaucoma: evolution of laser trabeculoplasty techniques. *Tech Ophthalmol*. 2008; 6(2):45-52.
17. Fea AM, Bosone A, Rolle T, Brogliatti B, Grignolo FM. Micropulse diode laser trabeculoplasty (MDLT): A phase II clinical study with 12 months follow-up. *Clin Ophthalmol*. 2008; 2(2):247-252
18. Ingvoldstad DD, Krishna R, Willoughby L. MicroPulse diode laser trabeculoplasty versus argon laser trabeculoplasty in the treatment of open angle glaucoma. *Invest Ophthalmol Vis Sci*. 2005;46. E-Abstract 123.
19. Assia EI, Rotenstreich Y, Barequet IS, Apple DJ, Rosner M, Belkin M. Experimental studies on nonpenetrating filtration surgery using the $CO_2$ laser. *Graefes Arch Clin Exp Ophthalmol*. 2007;245(6):847-854.
20. Seiler T, Kriegerowski M, Bende T, Wollensak J. Partial external trabeculectomy. *Klin Monatsbl Augenheilkd*. 1989;195(4):216-220.
21. Iliev ME, Gerber S. Long-term outcome of trans-scleral diode laser cyclophotocoagulation in refractory glaucoma. *Br J Ophthalmol*. 2007;91:1631-1635.
22. Lin S. Endoscopic cyclophotocoagulation. *Br J Ophthalmol*. 2002; 86:1434-1438.
23. Boyle, E.L. Combined phaco-ECP procedure lowers IOP, number of medications. *Ocular Surgery News*. http://www.endooptiks.com/articles/berke_ecp_phaco_4.pdf Accessed April 22, 2007.
24. Berlin MS, Giers U, Kleineberg L, Taliaferro K. ELT: excimer laser trabeculostomy: clinical update, 2008. American Glaucoma Society Annual Meeting; March 2008.

# Chapter 65
# Incisional Therapies: Trabeculectomy Surgery

Shlomo Melamed and Daniel Cotlear

Trabeculectomy with an antimetabolite is considered the "gold standard" for the surgical management of glaucoma.

Surgical management for glaucoma was first described in 1857 by Von Graefe, who reported that by removing a large piece of the iris he could help many patients with glaucoma. In 1909, Elliot described a full-thickness filtering procedure by using a trephine to make an anterior sclerectomy under a conjunctival flap, coupled with a peripheral iridectomy. Uncontrolled transclerostomy flow with resulting hypotony was the trigger for most surgeons to switch from full-thickness sclerostomy to a partial-thickness fistula. The guarded fistula was first suggested in 1961 by Sugar but was only published in 1968 by Cairns. The obstruction of the aqueous humor was assumed to be at the juxtacanalicular portion of the trabecular meshwork, and the outflow system distal to the juxtacanalicular meshwork (primarily Schlemm's canal and the distal collector channels) was thought to be normal in patients with glaucoma. Therefore, the primary goal of the trabeculectomy was to eliminate the obstruction to aqueous humor outflow at the inner aspect of Shlemm's canal[1] (Figs. 65.1 and 65.2).

Although Cairns intention was to avoid "unnecessary and a non physiologic bypass" of the collector channels by excising a portion of the trabecular meshwork and adjusted Schlemm's canal, we know today that the mechanism responsible for lowering intraocular pressure (IOP) after guarded filtration procedure is a through-and-through fistula, through the scleral flap borders, connecting the anterior chamber with the subconjunctival space.

Possible alternative routes of filtration after trabeculectomy surgery (Fig. 65.3) are through:

1. The cut ends of Schlemm's canal
2. Suprachoroidal space
3. Scleral vessels
4. Thin scleral flap
5. The scleral flap borders

Since then, many surgical and wound-healing modifications were added to the procedure. In order to keep the fistula open and functional, these modifications mainly address the wound-healing process in order to minimize the fibroblast proliferation and secondary scar tissue formation.

At this point, it is necessary to define that all the trabeculectomy modifications still use a common concept to lower the IOP by creation of a fistula between the anterior chamber of the eye and the sub-Tenon and subconjunctival space. The aqueous humor is diverted by this fistula from the anterior chamber outside of the eye into the sub-Tenon and subconjunctival space, and finally collected into the episcleral and conjunctival veins.

In order to guide the reader systematically through the trabeculectomy procedure and all controversial aspects of this procedure (see Sidebar 65.1), we will explain the procedure step by step, in chronological order.

## 65.1 Anesthesia

General anesthesia is reserved for noncooperative patients.

Topical anesthesia with eye drops – Localin (oxybuprocaine hydrochloride 0.4%), tetracaine/amethocaine (2-(dimethylamino) ethyl p-(butylamino) benzoate monohydrochloride 0.5%), lidocaine 2% (lignocaine hydrochloride 2%) – and jelly (Xylocaine – lidocaine 2%) should be preferred in most cases. When compared to peribulbar or retrobulbar anesthesia, there was no difference regarding pain control or surgical complication.[2,3] Another option is to inject nonpreserved lidocaine 1% into the anterior chamber.

In addition to the anesthetic effect, intracameral lidocaine dilates the pupil. Although there is an advantage in combined surgery (cataract extraction combined with trabeculectomy), this effect is unwanted in trabeculectomy alone.

The main disadvantage of the topical anesthesia is the lack of akinesia, which can be achieved with retrobulbar injections, or partial akinesia with peribulbar or sub-Tenon injections. Subconjunctival injection at the bleb site is to be avoided because it delivers poorer surgical outcomes.[4]

For retrobulbar or peribulbar injections, a mixture of 50% lidocaine and 50% bupivacaine 0.75% is used in order to

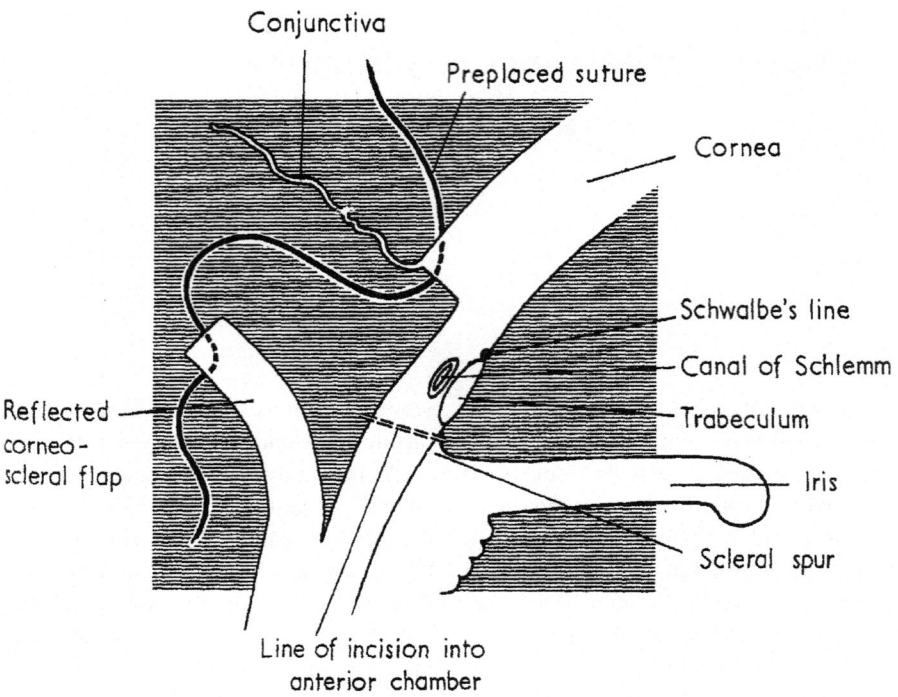

**Fig. 65.1** Line of incision into anterior chamber. Reprinted with permission from Cairns JE[1]; Elsevier

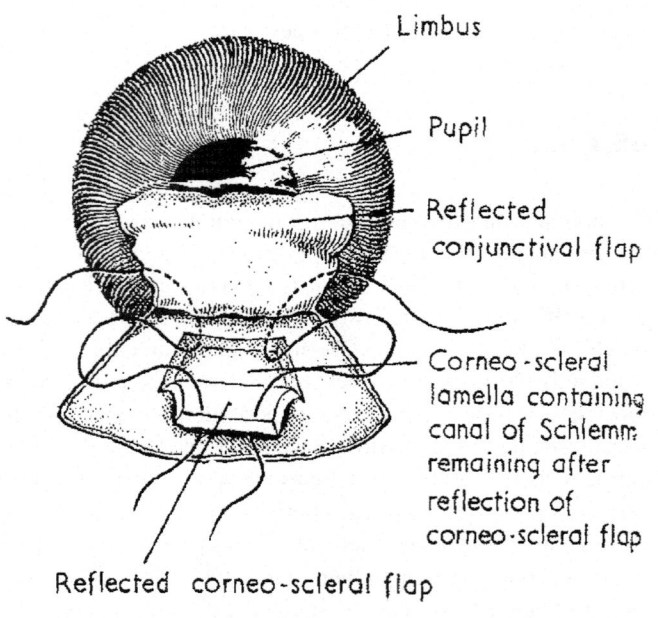

**Fig. 65.2** Elevation of the corneoscleral flap. Reprinted with permission from Cairns JE[1]; Elsevier

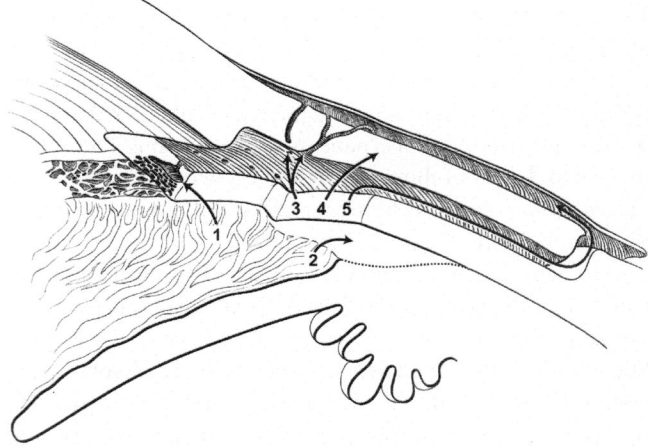

**Fig. 65.3** Possible alternative routes of filtration after trabeculectomy surgery

prolong the anesthetic effect up to 6 h from 15 to 30 min with lidocaine only. It is recommended not to inject more than 5 ml of anesthetic volume around or behind the globe in order to avoid a "positive" pressure on the globe, which may add to the ischemic damage of the already compromised optic nerve. Complications of injections are globe perforation, optic nerve damage, and peri/retrobulbar hemorrhage.

## 65.2 Eye Exposure

A good exposure of the surgical field is mandatory, and is achieved with a lid speculum, which opens the eye, preferably without creating pressure on the globe.

**SIDEBAR 65.1 Incisional glaucoma surgery: making the decision to operate**

Claudia U. Richter

Glaucoma is a group of diseases with patients who present with varying degrees of optic nerve damage and visual field loss as well as individually varied general medical, ophthalmic, and social issues. All of these factors combine to make the risk/benefit ratio and the decision to do glaucoma surgery different for each patient. Incisional glaucoma surgery, whether by filtering surgery, aqueous tube shunt, or nonpenetrating procedures, lowers intraocular pressure (IOP) by providing an alternative path for aqueous humor outflow, and often stops or limits progression of the disease. The decision to perform incisional glaucoma surgery is based upon our knowledge of the natural history of glaucoma progression correlated with a particular patient's history and status, the patient's response to medical and laser therapy, the benefits of surgery, and contraindications to and risks of surgery.

Glaucoma is frequently a slowly progressive illness with a long disease period before optic nerve damage and visual loss are detectable. However, once glaucoma damage is present, progression of damage may occur at lower IOPs and more rapidly than earlier in the disease course. Glaucoma progression may occur more rapidly with greater IOP elevation above the targeted pressure. Additionally, the greater the degree of glaucoma damage, the lower is the pressure required to minimize future vision loss. Patients with advanced glaucoma may require IOPs approximating 12 mmHg to minimize the risk of further glaucomatous damage, a level difficult to reach and maintain with only medical and laser therapy. Conversely, patients with little glaucomatous damage and few risk factors may tolerate higher pressures.

Patients with advanced glaucoma who have not reached a targeted low IOP are appropriately managed surgically in order to reach the clinically indicated low target IOP. Incisional glaucoma surgery is typically recommended only when medical and laser therapies have failed to prevent optic nerve damage or visual field loss, or lower IOP to a level that will prevent such loss. Initial glaucoma surgery without prior medical or laser therapy is rarely appropriate or performed in the USA, but may be for a patient presenting with advanced glaucoma damage and high IOP for whom urgent IOP control is the best hope to salvage vision. Most patients are tried on multiple topical antiglaucomatous medications, often in combination, including a prostaglandin analog, a beta-adrenergic blocker, an alpha-agonist, and a topical carbonic anhydrase inhibitor. Pilocarpine, phospholine iodide and oral carbonic anhydrase inhibitors may be tried, but their side effects frequently preclude long-term use. All the topical antiglaucomatous medications may cause side effects that limit their use: allergic reactions, precipitation of asthma, keratitis, and decreased vision, for example. Some patients may experience annoying side effects such as increased skin pigmentation, hyperemia, and ocular irritation. Should these patients have glaucoma surgery to relieve their symptoms? That question can be answered only after an extensive discussion of the possible benefits and complications of surgery. The complex medication schedule and the cost of chronic medical therapy may prevent a patient's persistence with an otherwise successful medication plan. If these barriers to chronic successful management of glaucoma cannot be overcome, glaucoma surgery may be necessary to provide long-term control of the disease.

Laser trabeculoplasty (LTP) often lowers IOP for a number of years, reportedly as often as 75% after initial laser treatment, and is indicated prior to incisional glaucoma surgery in those patients with a type of glaucoma that may respond. LTP may be performed prior to initiating topical glaucoma medications or after a trial of one to several medications. There is currently no consensus as to the best time in the disease course for laser intervention, with some ophthalmologists using it as first-line therapy. The efficacy of LTP in controlling glaucoma fades with time, and 30–50% of eyes require additional surgical therapy within 5 years of treatment. Additional sessions of LTP are less successful than initial therapy. However, even considering the limitations of this procedure, LTP does lower IOP for an extended time in many patients with fewer complications than incisional surgery and should be considered prior to incisional surgery. However, LTP is not indicated prior to incisional glaucoma surgery in those patients with advanced glaucoma and high IOP because it is not always successful, takes time to be effective, and may cause IOP elevations – these patients require urgent glaucoma control to prevent progression.

Incisional glaucoma surgery is successful in 70–80% of patients in reducing IOP and preserving vision. It also frequently eliminates or reduces the need for antiglaucomatous medications, reducing ocular side effects, compliance problems, and the ongoing cost of disease management for the patient. However, glaucoma surgery may fail 20–30% of the time and carries risks of significant complications. Therefore, the recommendation for surgery should include an extensive discussion with the patient of the proposed procedure, the postoperative management necessary to maximize success, and the potential complications. For most patients with uncontrolled IOP or progressive optic nerve damage and visual field loss, surgery will be the correct decision. Some patients with compliance difficulties or medication side effects will choose to improve their compliance or endure side effects and therefore delay or avoid surgery. The physician and patient must carefully weigh the risks of vision loss in the patient's lifetime without surgery, which is often difficult and always imprecise. If a patient appears to have a life-threatening disease or a limited life expectancy, consultation with the patient's other physicians may be helpful in the decision-making process.

In summary, incisional glaucoma surgery is usually required when the IOP in uncontrolled or optic nerve cupping is progressing or visual field loss is progressing despite a comprehensive medication trial and LTP. The greater degree of glaucoma damage and the more elevated the IOP, the more urgent the surgery. While frequently successful, glaucoma surgery may also have vision threatening complications, both in the early postoperative period and later, and requires careful counseling of the prospective surgical patient of the potential risks as well as benefits and the postoperative care necessary.

## Bibliography

Migdal C, Gregory W, Hitchings R. Long-term functional outcome after early surgery compare with laser and medicine in open-angle glaucoma. *Ophthalmology*. 1994;101:1651–1656.

Richter CU, Shingleton BJ, Bellows AR, et al. Retreatment with argon laser trabeculoplasty. *Ophthalmology*. 1987;94: 1085–1089.

Shingleton BJ, Richter CU, Dharma SK, et al. Long-term efficacy of argon laser trabeculoplasty. A 10-year follow-up study. *Ophthalmology*. 1993;100:1324–1329.

Spaeth GL, Baez KA. Argon laser trabeculoplasty controls one third of cases of progressive, uncontrolled, open angle glaucoma for 5 years. *Arch Ophthalmol*. 1992;110:491–494.

The Advanced Glaucoma Intervention Study (AGIS): 13. Comparison of treatment outcomes within race: 10-year results. *Ophthalmology*. 2004;111:651–664.

The AGIS Investigators. The Advanced Glaucoma Intervention Study (AGIS): 7. The relationship between control of intraocular pressure and visual field deterioration. *Am J Ophthalmol*. 2000;130:429–440.

The Glaucoma Laser Trial (GLT) and Glaucoma Laser Trial follow-up study: 7. Results. Glaucoma Laser Trial Research Group. *Am J Ophthalmol*. 1995;120:718–731.

Weber PA, Burton GD, Epitropoulos AT. Laser trabeculoplasty retreatment. *Ophthalmic Surg*. 1989;20:702–706.

It is important not to drag the conjunctiva with the speculum arms because this may tighten the conjunctiva and create an unnecessary surgical difficulty.

## 65.3 Traction Suture

This step is useful since it helps to keep the eye in the desired inferior position throughout the surgery. The suture can be placed in clear cornea or underneath the superior rectus muscle. For the clear corneal traction suture, a 7/0 spatulated Vicryl or silk corneal traction suture is placed half thickness and 2 mm anterior to the limbus. The eye is rotated inferiorly, and the suture is affixed to the drape inferior to the eye (Fig. 65.4a–c).

In the superior rectus muscle traction suture technique, a 4/0 silk suture is passed approximately 12 mm behind the superior limbus, underneath the superior rectus muscle, and attached to the drape over the patient's forehead.

The clear corneal traction suture is preferred because it provides better exposure (more firmly attached), no risk for subconjunctival hemorrhage or conjunctival damage, no risk of postoperative proptosis due to the superior rectus damage, and has been found to provide a better surgical outcome by the UK National Survey of Trabeculectomy.[5]

## 65.4 Conjunctival Incision

The bleb surgical site is in the upper globe, preferably under the upper eyelid in order to reduce infections or bleb leakage.[6] It is advised to use a topical vasoconstrictive agent, like adrenaline 0.01%. Efrin 10% can also be used but provides less vasoconstriction. The vasoconstrictive agent is used before conjunctival dissection in order to minimize conjunctival bleeding. The conjunctival incision can be performed in a limbal base or fornix base fashion.[7,8] In general, the limbal base technique first described by Cairns was abandoned due to higher rate of postoperative complications (Table 65.1). The higher rates of complications are probably related to the differences in bleb morphology, with limbus-based flap cases more likely to develop cystic blebs.[7]

Limbal base bleb creation is more time-consuming, has more risk of buttonhole formation, and allows poorer surgical exposure, which prevents diffuse antibiotic application. A large and diffuse antibiotic treated area results in a

**Table 65.1** Postoperative complications of limbal-base versus fornix-base techniques

| Complication | Limbal base | Fornix base |
|---|---|---|
| Cystic bleb | 90% | 20% |
| Blebitis | 20% | None |
| Leakage | 24% | 65% |

### Sidebar 65.2 Anticoagulants and glaucoma surgery

Siva S. Radhakrishnan Iyer, Sarwat Salim, and Peter A. Netland

Many patients requiring glaucoma surgery are concomitantly receiving anticoagulation therapy for other comorbidities, including arrhythmia, cardiac prosthetic valve, or thromboembolic disease resulting from various etiologies. The alternative of complete discontinuation of anticoagulation therapy before surgical intervention has raised concerns about the risk of serious thromboembolic events in the perioperative period in these patients. Glaucoma surgeons are usually concerned about hemorrhagic complications of anticoagulation that can ultimately affect surgical success.

Anticoagulation therapy is commonly categorized in two groups: those undergoing therapy with warfarin, and those undergoing therapy with an antiplatelet agent (clopidogrel and aspirin [acetylsalicylic acid]). The antiplatelet agents, which inhibit activation of the lipid peroxidation system in the platelet wall, are usually regarded as less severe drugs for blood thinning. Warfarin and aspirin should usually not be mixed. The common intraoperative and postoperative surgical complications associated with blood thinning medications include retrobulbar hemorrhage, hyphema, vitreous hemorrhage, and suprachoroidal hemorrhage.

A few retrospective studies have analyzed hemorrhagic complications of glaucoma surgery in patients using anticoagulation therapy. Law and colleagues reported a higher incidence of complications following glaucoma surgery in patients who were on either warfarin or antiplatelet therapy compared to controls, with the highest rate of complication noted in patients who continued warfarin therapy through surgery. In this study, there were less hemorrhagic complications in patients who discontinued Coumadin compared with those who continued anticoagulation; however, the difference failed to reach statistical significance. Similarly, in a retrospective examination of 367 trabeculectomies, Cobb et al observed that continuation of either warfarin or aspirin therapy in those undergoing surgery had approximately twice the risk of hyphema. However, the use of aspirin did not adversely affect the eventual surgical outcomes, whereas warfarin's use ultimately resulted in poor surgical outcomes and intraocular pressure (IOP) control.

Alwitry and colleagues reported that most glaucoma surgeons in the United Kingdom do not routinely stop anticoagulation therapy prior to glaucoma surgery. A smaller percentage of these surgeons chose to discontinue long-term anticoagulation therapy and initiate heparin therapy.

Bleeding complications secondary to anticoagulation therapy are not limited to the glaucoma surgical patient, as there have been concerns among surgeons in other subspecialties including vitreoretinal surgery and oculoplastic surgery. However, a unique aspect of glaucoma surgery is the risk of hypotony and hypotony-related complications, including suprachoroidal hemorrhage, during the early postoperative period. In high-risk eyes, glaucoma surgeons may choose to discontinue anticoagulation during the perioperative period or use other techniques to reduce the risks of hemorrhagic complications during and after surgery.

When surgeons choose to discontinue anticoagulant therapy, the approaches vary and can be individualized to each patient. In patients treated with warfarin, the drug can be discontinued for a minimum of 3 days prior to surgery to improve coagulation intraoperatively and postoperatively. The patient's primary care practitioner may allow withholding warfarin for an additional several days after surgery, which may avoid postoperative complications in high-risk eyes. It is worth noting that warfarin cessation may lead to a rise in clotting factors that put the patient in a hypercoagulable state, shown to peak at 1 week afterwards. Because aspirin has a prolonged antiplatelet aggregation effect, some surgeons recommend cessation of aspirin therapy 1 or 2 weeks prior to surgery, with approval by the patient's primary care provider. Discontinuation of aspirin on the day of surgery probably has little or no influence on the antiplatelet effect of the drug during the perioperative and immediate postoperative period.

There are risks associated with discontinuation of long-term anticoagulation therapy in patients undergoing surgery. The risk of thromboembolic events is probably low (less than 1%). However, some of these problems such as pulmonary embolus or stroke can be life-threatening. In each patient, the ocular risk of continuation of anticoagulant therapy should be weighed against the systemic risk of life-threatening hemorrhagic complications. Communication and coordination with the physician who is managing the long-term anticoagulant therapy is strongly recommended, along with a frank discussion with the patient of the risks and benefits of altering anticoagulation therapy in the perioperative period.

Alternatives to discontinuation of anticoagulation therapy may be tried in order to reduce the risk of bleeding complications. Modifying anesthetic methods may be helpful, including use of topical and local anesthesia in order to minimize the risk of retrobulbar hemorrhage associated with retrobulbar injection of anesthetic. Surgical techniques, also, may be modified to avoid hemorrhagic complications. Meticulous use of hemostasis during flap dissection, anterior placement of sclerotomy to avoid the ciliary body, and omitting surgical iridectomy have been shown to avoid bleeding. Tightly securing the scleral flap to prevent bleeding and postoperative hypotony has been advocated. Postoperative hypotony increases the risk of bleeding complications, specifically suprachoroidal hemorrhage. In glaucoma drainage implant surgery, use of suture ligatures around the tube or two-stage surgery can reduce the rate of postoperative hypotony. Intraoperative and postoperative use of viscoelastics may avoid or mitigate problems associated with hypotony. Gradual reduction of the IOP during surgery may avoid dramatic fluctuations in IOP, which increase the risk of bleeding complications.

In summary, the current literature suggests that patients receiving anticoagulation therapy with warfarin and/or antiplatelet agents who are candidates for glaucoma surgery are at increased risk for serious hemorrhagic complications. Many glaucoma subspecialists continue anticoagulation through surgery, although surgeons may modify their anesthetic and surgical techniques to minimize complications. In patients at high risk for ocular hemorrhagic complications, the surgeon may recommend withholding anticoagulant therapy during the perioperative period. In all instances, ophthalmologists should collaborate with the patient's physician and other medical specialists in assessing the patient's risk of hemorrhagic ocular complications, the systemic risk of discontinuing anticoagulant therapy, and the perioperative plan for use of anticoagulant drugs.

## Bibliography

Alwitry A, King AJ, Vernon SA. Anticoagulation in glaucoma surgery. *Graefes Arch Clin Exp Ophthalmol*. 2008;246(6):891–896.

Baudo F, de Cataldo F, Mostarda G, et al. Management of patients on long-term oral anticoagulant therapy undergoing elective surgery: survey of the clinical practice in the Italian anticoagulation clinics. *Intern Emerg Med*. 2007;2:280–284.

Cobb CJ, Chakrabarti S, Chadha V, Sanders R. The effect of aspirin and warfarin therapy in trabeculectomy. *Eye*.2007;21(5):598–603.

Grip L, Blomback M, Schulman S. Hypercoaguable state and thromboembolism following warfarin withdrawal in post-myocardial-infarction patients. *Eur Heart J*. 1991;12(11):1225–1233.

Jampel H. Glaucoma surgery in the patient undergoing anticoagulation. *J Glaucoma*. 1998;7(4):278–281.

Jeganathan VS, Ghosh S, Ruddle JB, Gupta V, Coote MA, Crowston JG. Risk factors for delayed suprachoroidal hemorrhage following glaucoma surgery. *Br J Ophthalmol*. 2008;92(10):1393–1396.

Konstas AGP, Jay JL. Modification of trabeculectomy to avoid postoperative hyphema. The 'guarded anterior fistula' operation. *Br J Ophthalmol*. 1992;76:353–357.

Law SK, Song BJ, Yu F, Kurbanyan K, Yang TA, Caprioli J. Hemorrhagic complications from glaucoma surgery in patients on anticoagulation therapy or antiplatelet therapy. *Am J Opthalmol*. 2008;145(4):736–746.

McCormack P, Simcock PR, Tullo AB. Management of the anticoagulated patient for ophthalmic surgery. *Eye*. 1993;7:749–750.

Narendran N, Williamson TH. The effects of aspirin and warfarin therapy on haemorrhage in vitreoretinal surgery. *Acta Ophthalmol Scand*. 2003;81:38–40.

Parkin B, Manners R. Aspirin and warfarin therapy in oculoplastic surgery. *Br J Ophthalmol*. 2000;84:1426–1427.

The Flurouracil Filtering Surgery Study Group. Risk factors for suprachoroidal hemorrhage after filtering surgery. *Am J Ophthalmol*. 1992;113:501–507.

Tuli SS, WuDunn D, Ciulla TA, Cantor LB. Delayed suprachoroidal hemorrhage after glaucoma filtration procedures. *Ophthalmology*. 2001;108(10):1808–1811.

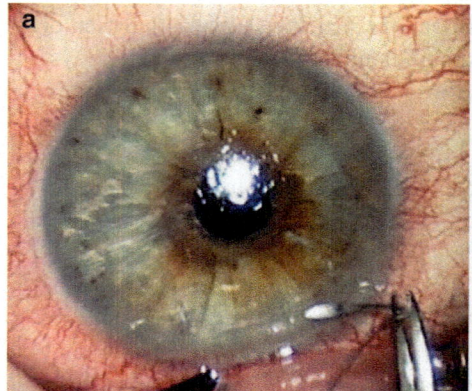 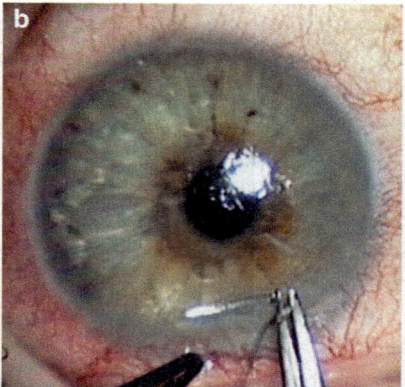 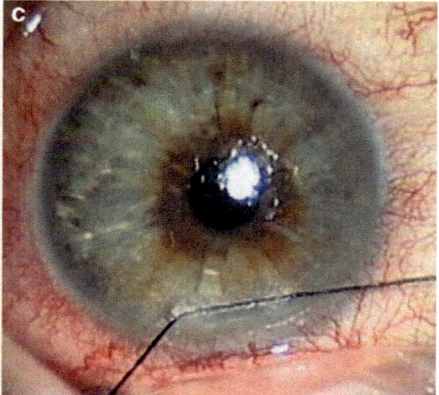

**Fig. 65.4** Clear corneal traction suture. (**a, b**) a corneal traction suture is placed half thickness and 2 mm anterior to the limbus. (**c**) The eye is rotated inferiorly, and the suture is affixed to the drape inferior to the eye

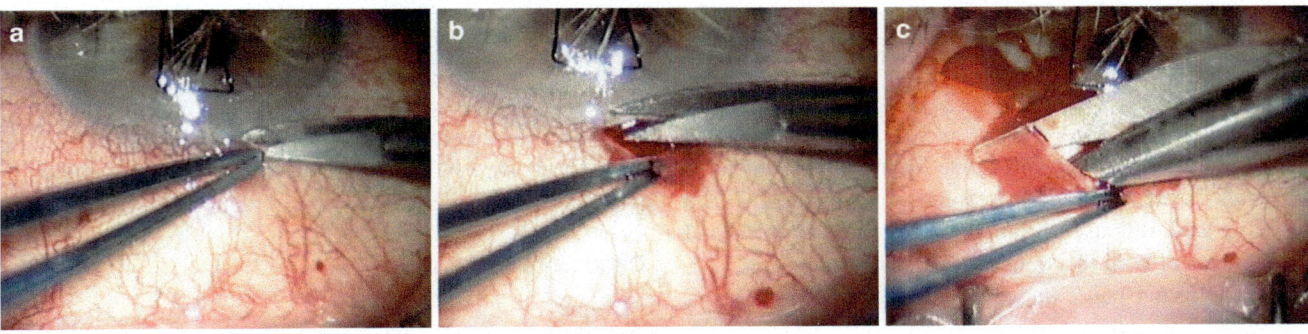

**Fig. 65.5** Tight suture techniques. (**a**) The conjunctiva is grasped close to the limbus. (**b**) The conjunctiva is then lifted and an initial small incision parallel to the limbus is made with Vannas or Westcott scissors. (**c**) The incision is extended parallel to the limbus

postoperative diffuse posterior filtering bleb and an increase in bleb survival.[7,9]

One of the risks with fornix base opposed to limbal base may be a higher rate of early leakage, but this was not found to be a risk factor of bleb failure.[10] This leakage can be minimized with new surgical methods of tight suture techniques[11-13] (Fig. 65.5a–c).

The conjunctiva is grasped close to the limbus at the selected superior nasal or temporal quadrant, with a nontraumatic fine forceps. Toothed forceps that can cut the conjunctiva should not be used. The conjunctiva is then lifted and an initial small incision parallel to the limbus is made with Vannas or Westcott scissors (preferable blunt tip instruments). The incision is extended parallel to the limbus up to two clock hours.

The 12 o'clock or superior nasal quadrant is preferred unless the conjunctiva is scarred from previous surgery. The first reason for selecting these positions is to reserve the nearby areas, mainly the temporal or superotemporal quadrant for subsequent cataract surgery. Another reason is that these sites provide lower IOPs at long-term follow-up compared to the superior or superotemporal positions.[14]

The Tenon's capsule can be separated together with the conjunctiva or in two steps. Performing a separate incision and separation of the Tenon's capsule improves the ability to enter the sub-Tenon space. A blunt and, as much as possible, nontraumatic undermining of the Tenon is carried out with Westcott scissors, in order to minimize inflammatory mediator release and to reduce the post scar formation.[15] The sub-Tenon's space should be dissected at least 8 mm posterior from the limbus. Meticulous care must be made to prevent conjunctiva buttonhole formation, and it is advised to grasp just the Tenon layer as this may result in a button-hole. An area of approximately 5.5 mm exposed sclera is desired.

Bleeding episcleral blood vessels should be gently diathermized, in order to minimize clot and fibrin formation and to reduce the postop inflammation. Wet field cautery with or without the use of a Weck-cell sponge is the preferred technique (Fig. 65.6). Care must be taken not to cauterize the conjunctiva. Smaller tipped cautery units are preferable. This can be achieved by pushing the conjunctiva away from the cautery tip with the Weck-cell sponge.

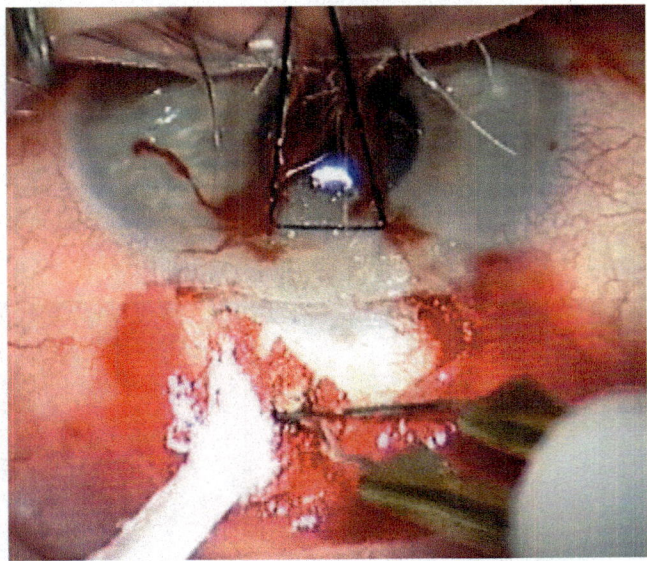

**Fig. 65.6** Wet field cautery

Cautery of deep scleral blood vessels is not necessary and may also just increase inflammatory mediators in the field. Excessive and loose episcleral tissue should be removed with a sharp blade to minimize postop scar tissue formation.

Small incision trabeculectomy (SIT)[16] avoids Tenon dissection. A limbal parallel conjunctival incision of 2.5 mm is performed and then a scleral pocket extending posteriorly is carried out and the subconjunctival space is entered (see Sidebar 65.3). There are still not enough published reports of success rates or prevalence of cystic bleb or scar tissue development around these small blebs.

### Sidebar 65.3. Fornix versus limbal based flaps

Kenneth B. Mitchell

Surgeons become comfortable with either limbal or fornix-based flaps and it becomes their "fastball." That being said, it is useful to note the advantages and disadvantages of both incisions for trabeculectomy.

The fornix-based flap

### Advantages

The fornix-based incision can be quickly made (Fig. 65.3-1a–d). Conjunctiva and Tenon's are fused at the limbus and Tenon's is thinnest anteriorly. There is much less manipulation of the conjunctiva and Tenon's after the initial incision and dissection. Vessel transection is anterior where the vessel diameter is smallest. This relates to less bleeding, which may be controlled by application of brimonidine with or without light wet-field cautery. There is usually no need for dissecting Tenon's from the limbal zone and visualization is excellent. Closure may be quicker. The surgeon may be less in need of an experienced assistant.

A fornix-based flap is easily combined with a single site phaco-trabeculectomy.

### Disadvantages

Any posterior hemorrhage from tissue plane dissection with scissors is more difficult to visualize and treat with fornix-based flaps.

Closure of the flap is less routine than with a limbal-based flap. If no relaxing incisions were made, there is some judgment call as to where to approximate the flap to the corneal periphery. Is one suture enough? Is a running suture necessary? Any tightness on reapproximating the flap to the cornea may result in a button-hole or tear from the suture needle. These holes are anterior and must be closed with interrupted sutures. Their anterior location may interfere with filtration in that region.

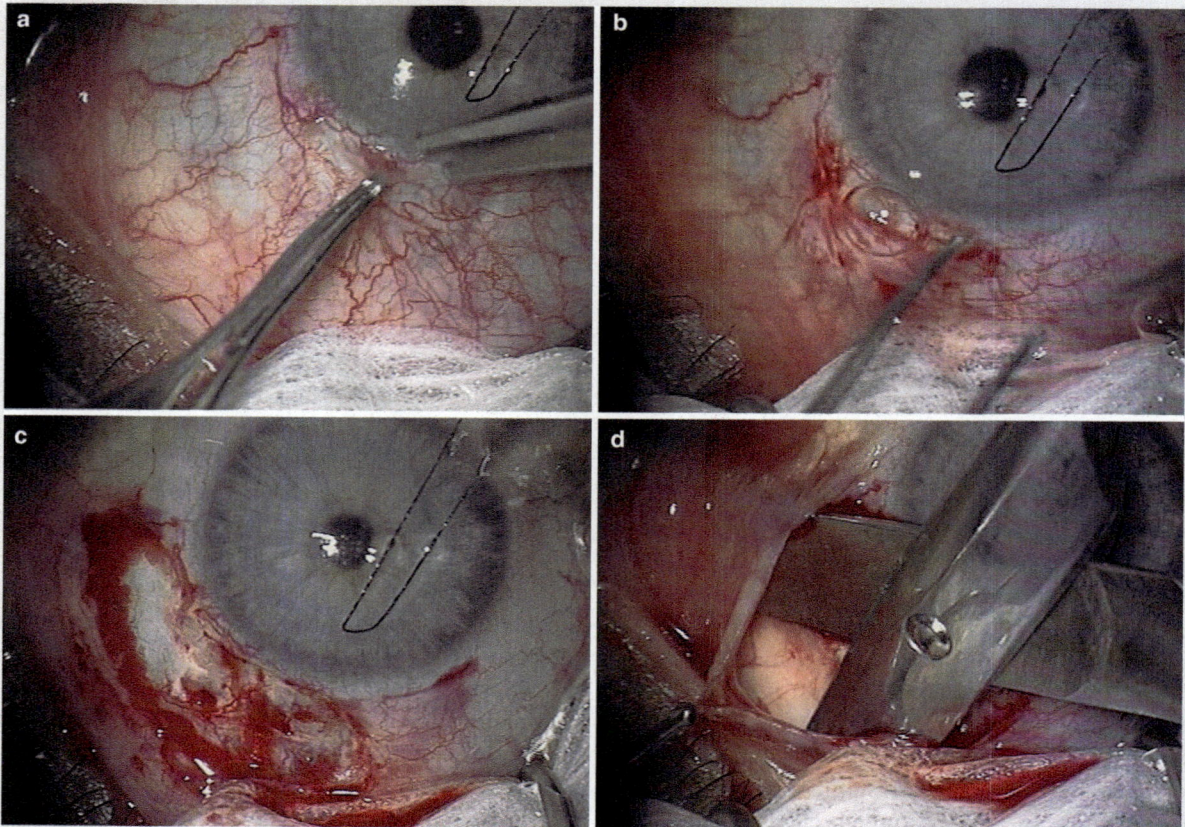

**Fig. 65.3-1** Steps in creating a fornix-based flap. (**a**) Beginning the fornix-based flap with nontoothed forceps and scissors tenting the fused conjunctiva and Tenon's up at the limbus. (**b**) Ending the curvilinear limbal incision. (**c**) Exposing the scleral bed. (**d**) Blunt dissection posteriorly for antimetabolite or tube shunt plate insertion

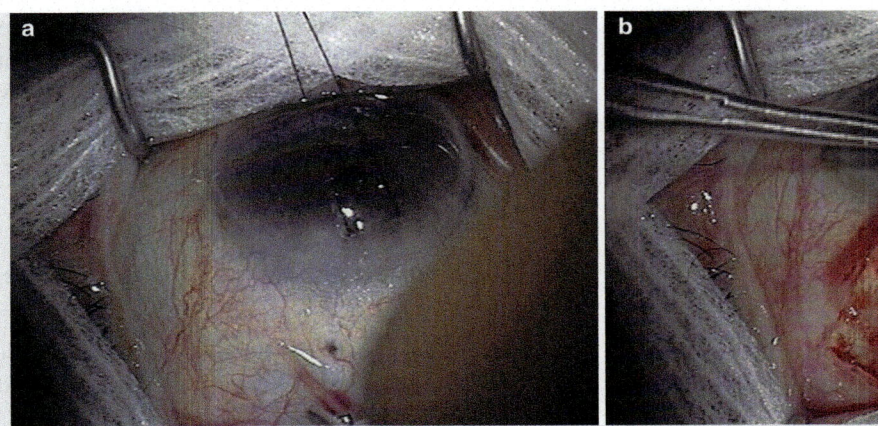

**Fig. 65.3-2** Creating a limbal-based flap. (**a**) Starting the limbal based flap in a patient with thin conjunctiva and scant Tenon's. (**b**) Reflecting the limbal-based flap onto the cornea

At the end of the case, when these flaps are challenged with a balanced salt solution infusion into the anterior chamber, slight leakage is often seen. Is that significant? Does it always translate into a positive Seidel the next day? No, but early bleb leaks are more common with fornix-based flaps. Fortunately, they tend to be small and resolve, or can be treated with bandage soft lenses, fibrin sealant, or suture reinforcement, and IOP control is usually not compromised.

If suture knots are not buried or if buried knots come to the surface, they may cause irritation, which tempts their removal perhaps a bit earlier than the surgeon would like.

Limbal-based flaps

### Advantages

Closure of a limbal-based flap is usually straightforward (Fig. 65.3-2a, b). Whether Tenon's and conjunctiva are closed separately or together, a snug running suture with locking bites usually balloons up nicely after infusion challenge and are water-tight. Any gape can usually be closed with additional interrupted bites. These gapes are located posteriorly and may not interfere with filtration elsewhere.

The suture closure located posteriorly is not associated with irritative symptoms as much as an anterior suture closure.

### Disadvantages

The creation of the flap or its extension may bring the surgeon into the neighborhood of the superior rectus. Bleeding, an inadvertent tenotomy, or disinsertion may result. Even without tendon injury, bleeding is encountered as the vascular diameter of the conjunctival vessels is greatest posteriorly. Tenon's capsule is thickest posteriorly and a decision to excise Tenon's may be made. This can result in thinner flaps posteriorly; particularly with antimetabolite use.

The dissection anteriorly to clear the limbal region requires sharp dissection or scraping Tenon's off the corneal-scleral surface, both in the region of the flap's insertion. The more the manipulation, the greater is the risk of pressure compression from forceps, inadvertent cautery burn, and button-holes.

A surgeon usually needs an experienced assistant to elevate the conjunctiva and Tenon's flap for the scleral dissection and the intracameral steps.

A limbal-based flap requires more manipulation during one-site phaco-trabeculectomy surgery.

A "ring of steel" appearance with the use of antimetabolites occurs occasionally in limbal-based flaps and is rare after fornix-based flaps.

Thin-walled blebs are more often seen after limbal based flaps with antimetabolite use. In association, blebitis has been described more often with limbal-based flaps.

## Conclusion

Both flaps have their champions, advantages, and disadvantages. With care, either can result in acceptable, diffuse, posterior blebs and acceptable IOP control.

## Bibliography

Kohl D, Walton D. Limbus-based versus fornix-based conjunctival flaps in trabeculectomy: 2005 Update. *Int Ophthalmol Clin*. 2005;45(4):107–113.

## 65.5 Anterior Chamber Paracentesis

A paracentesis is performed – prior to the fistula creation in order to manage intraoperative complications – mainly to prevent anterior chamber collapse. The secondary goal is to check if the fistula is functional and the bleb is without leakage at the end of the surgery by injecting a small amount of fluid into the anterior chamber. This is performed by injecting balanced salt solution (BSS) through a 30-gauge blunt-tipped needle into the anterior chamber, which should cause an elevation of the bleb without conjunctival leak along the limbal border or from a conjunctival buttonhole (Fig. 65.7). The most preferred paracentesis sites are at 11 or 1 o'clock vertically down or horizontally at 3 or 9 o'clock and parallel over the iris to minimize possible lens damage. The paracentesis is made either with a disposable 25- or 27-gauge needle, or a 15° or a stiletto knife. If an anterior chamber maintainer is used, then the desired position is at 6 o'clock and the paracentesis is performed with a 25-gauge stiletto knife. The anterior chamber system provides many advantages during the operation, mainly keeping a deep anterior chamber and lowering the chance for IOP fluctuations.

The advantage of the 3, 6, and 9 o'clock positions is that hypotony with a flat anterior chamber postoperatively can be managed at the slit lamp by injecting a viscoelastic material.

## 65.6 Scleral Flap Size and Shape

There are two popular scleral flap shapes: triangle or rectangular. Some prefer trapezoids, and even other shapes are not unknown, although some investigators suggest that from clinical observation more posterior large flaps are associated with thicker (noncystic) and more diffuse blebs then anterior small flaps.[17] No scleral flap size or shape has been proven to be superior. The pitfalls with more posterior large flaps are ciliary body damage – mainly ciliary body hemorrhage.

### 65.6.1 Rectangular Scleral Flap Technique

A straight, partial thickness, scleral cut is made 4 mm behind and tangential to the limbus to create the posterior border of the scleral flap (Fig. 65.8a–g).

The initial cut is dissected anterior toward the limbus with an angled crescent blade. The knife should be advanced as parallel to the sclera while carefully monitoring the flap thickness, and then converted by cutting down the sides to a 4 mm to 4 mm half-thickness scleral flap with a diamond blade or straight Vannas scissors. In order to minimize leakage and to maximize posterior flow, it is recommended to leave a 1 mm border between the scleral flap edges and the limbus.

### 65.6.2 Triangular Scleral Flap Technique

An isosceles triangle partial thickness scleral cut is made (Fig. 65.9a–g). The triangle base is positioned 1 mm posterior to the limbus with the triangle apex pointed toward the fornix. The triangle dimensions are: 3 mm base length and each side length of 3–4 mm. The flap edge is lifted at the apex with a nontoothed forceps, and slight traction is applied in order to cut the collagen scleral fibers and to create a smooth flap bed. The flap is dissected best by a beaver, diamond, or crescent blade. Throughout the dissection, the flap can be adjusted to the proper thickness. The desired scleral flap thickness is one-half to two-thirds to prevent flap dehiscence or suture cheese wiring. Throughout the flap creation, it is best to keep the surgical area dry, because it allows better visualization of the flap details. Only if bleeding, which obscures the surgical site, occurs at this stage must irrigation with BSS be carried out. The flap is extended 1–2 mm and anterior to the anatomical limbus.

The next steps apply for both scleral flap shapes.

A circumferential cut is made at the scleral bed – underneath the partial thickness scleral flap at the most anterior border – with a sharp instrument like a diamond, 15°, or stiletto knife, and the anterior chamber is entered. Another cutting technique is to make a parallel incision into the anterior chamber with a keratome to create a corneal tunnel; this should reduce injury to the structures underneath, which could be damaged using a perpendicular cut. The incision is made anterior or at the corneolimbal junction and extended

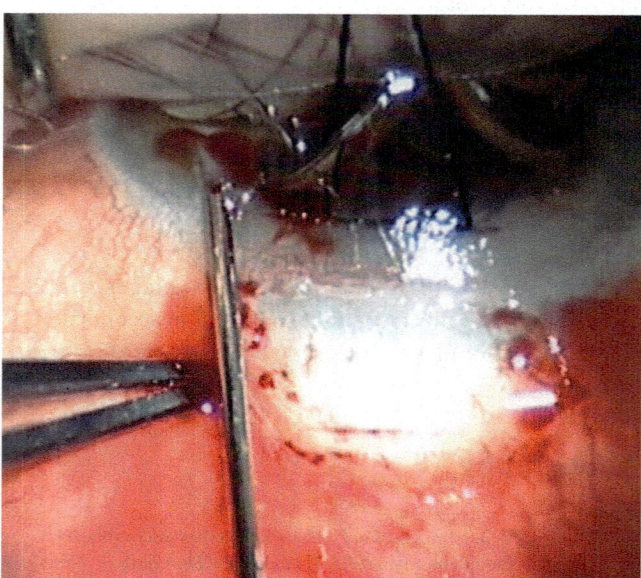

**Fig. 65.7** Anterior chamber paracentesis

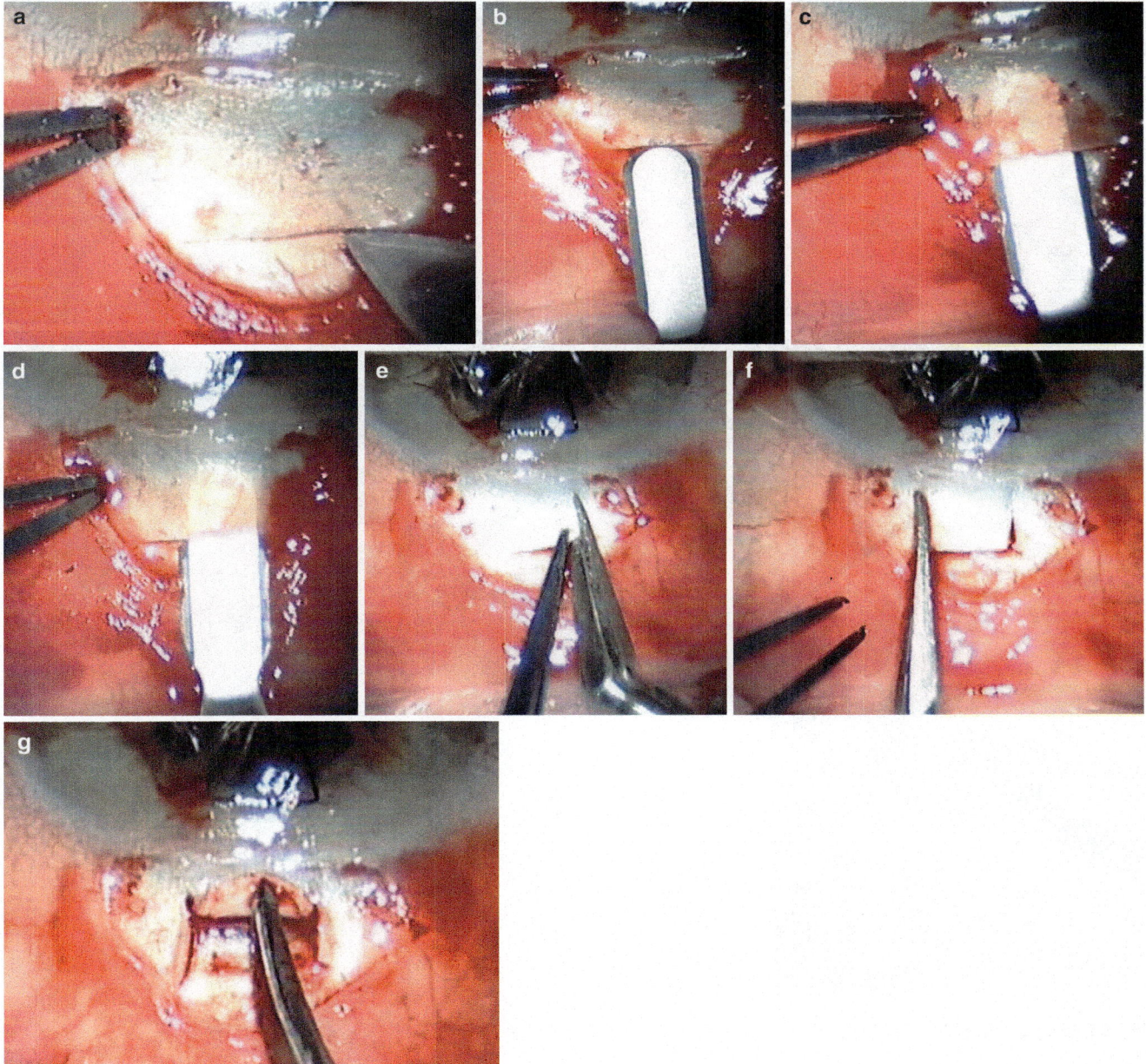

**Fig. 65.8** (a–g) Rectangular scleral flap technique

posterior toward the sclerolimbal junction (Fig. 65.10). This junction is also known as the surgical limbus and is visible as the transfer zone from the translucent bluish-gray cornea and the white sclera (Fig. 65.11). This junction is an important anatomical landmark because failure to perform a well-localized trabeculectomy by excessive posterior extension may result in ciliary body damage with subsequent hemorrhage or ostium blockage by uveal tissue.

The fistula is created by removing a portion of the scleral bed underneath the flap. It can be performed by hand cut or with the use of a punch like the Kelly-Descemet's punch.

The desired size of the ostium should be more then 40–50 μm in diameter, because below that size, significant resistance to the physiological aqueous outflow[18] can still remain. Since each punch bite removes tissue sections of approximately 0.25×0.30 mm, one punch bite is enough. Proper technique is vital to create a functional ostium. The punch must be rotated vertically so that it is perpendicular to the bed of the flap, in order to avoid a tunnel-like ostium that might close. Another important consideration is to make sharp cuts and to remove the excised tissue to prevent secondary blockage of the ostium. The scleral flap is sutured

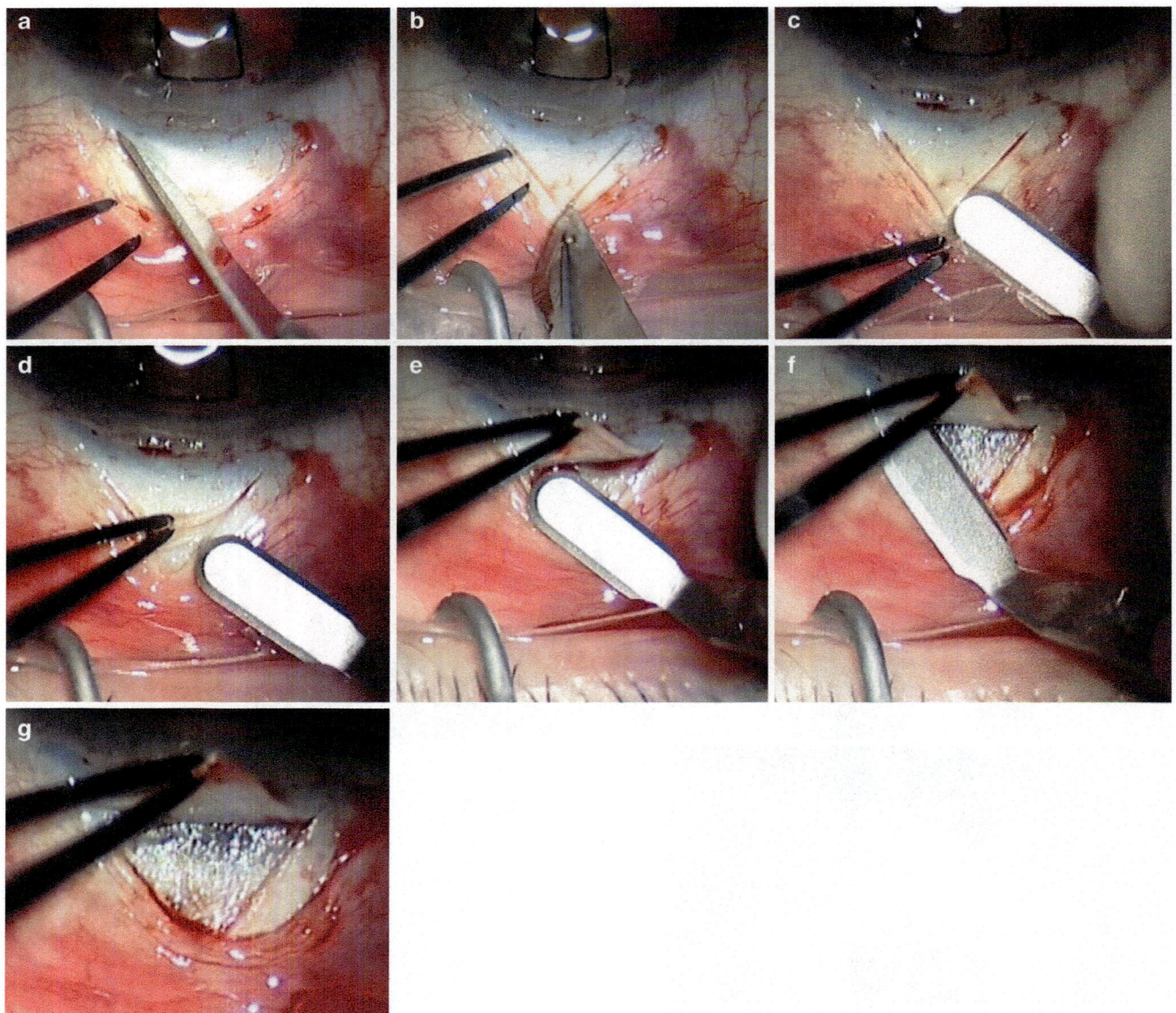

**Fig. 65.9** (a–g) Triangular scleral flap technique

tight to allow a minimal desired fluid flow rate through the flap borders. The control of the resistance to outflow is determined by flap construction, suture position, and tension.[19]

## 65.7 Flap Suturing Techniques

There are many flap closure suturing variations. A large survey in the United Kingdom reported that scleral flap shape is most often rectangular and most commonly secured with two interrupted 10–0 nylon sutures at the upper two corners[5] (Fig. 65.12).

Nylon suture is preferred because of its low tendency to create an inflammatory response. It is better to create a tight wound closure that can be reopened with similar results, by suture lysis[20] or removal of a releasable suture in the postoperative period, rather than a loose overfiltrating bleb with hypotony.[21]

The releasable suture is released simply by pulling the exteriorized corneal loop with a suture-holding forceps under topical anesthesia with the patient seated at the slit lamp. The use of releasable sutures in filtration surgery originated by Schaffer et al[22], and since then, many technique modifications have been reported.[23,24]

There are several releasable suture techniques. All have in common an exterior suture end (exterior loop or buried

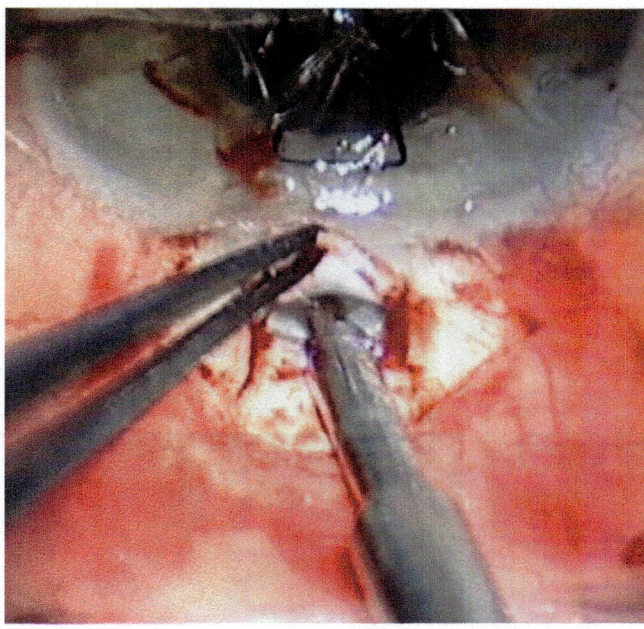

**Fig. 65.10** Creating a corneal tunnel

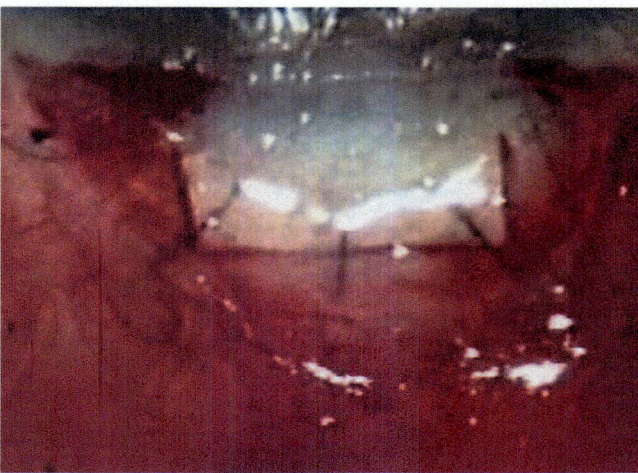

**Fig. 65.12** Flap suturing technique. In this picture, two interrupted 10–0 nylon sutures were placed at the each corner and one halfway between them

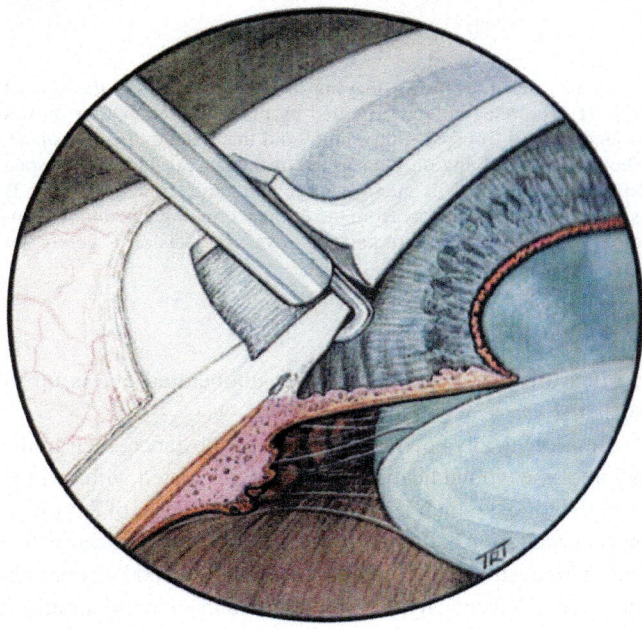

**Fig. 65.11** The surgical limbus. Reprinted with permission from Salmon JF, Kanski J. *Textbook of Glaucoma*. 3rd ed. Elsevier Butterworth-Heinemann; 2004

in the corneal stroma) that can be pulled at the slit lamp (Fig. 65.13a–f). When the wound and the anterior chamber are believed to be stabilized, the sutures can be removed serially to increase filtration.

Peng Khaw's adjustable suture technique allows a titrated outflow compared to the releasable or suture lysis technique but requires specially designed forceps (Khaw Transconjunctival Adjustable Suture Forceps No 2-502, manufactured by Duckworth and Kent) to allow transconjunctival suture tension release.[19] This maneuver, although reported as safe, may have the potential complications of conjunctival buttonhole formation, especially through thin conjunctiva encountered after antimetabolite use.

In patients with thick or scarred conjunctivae, suture lysis or adjustable suture maneuvers may not be possible, and releasable sutures are preferred.

A formed anterior chamber must be established and results of collapsed anterior chamber and hypotony must be avoided. Additional sutures are placed until a well-formed anterior chamber is achieved.

## 65.8 Antimetabolites

The most commonly used antimetabolites are mitomycin C (MMC) and 5-fluorouracil (5-FU). Both were introduced as adjuncts to trabeculectomy in the early 1980s.[25,26] Their main action is inhibition of the fibroblast proliferation and activity. MMC is an alkaloid synthesized by *Streptomyces caespitosus* that affects fibroblast proliferation by cross-linking their DNA. 5-FU is a phase-specific pyrimidine analog that blocks DNA synthesis by inhibiting thymidylate synthesis.

The drug produces a direct cell-cycle nonspecific cytotoxic effect by reducing fibroblast collagen synthesis. The use of antimetabolites provides lower postop IOP and better long-term success rates of filtrating surgery. In the hand of experts, the success rate of filtering surgery – alone or with adjunctive

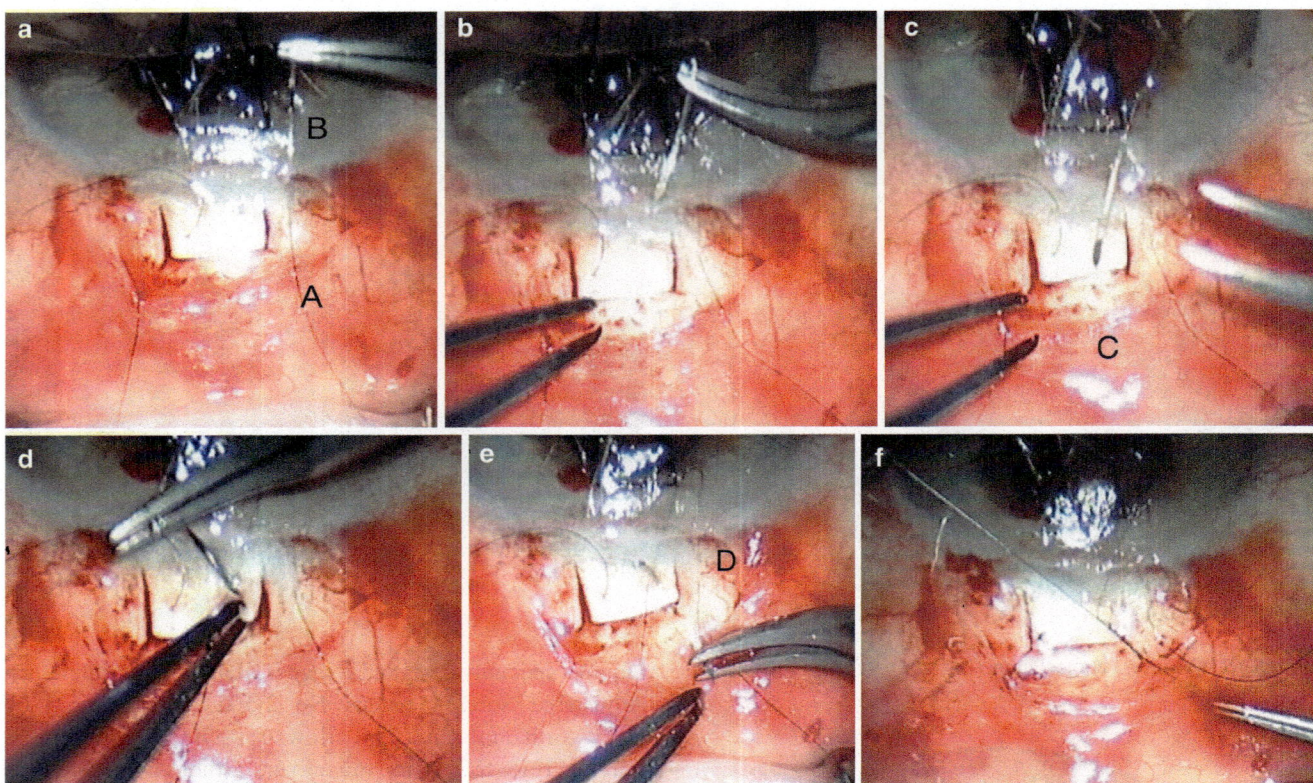

**Fig. 65.13** (a) A spatulate needle enters the sclera at *point A* and is advanced trough the episclaral/scleral tissue into clear cornea, and exit at *point B*. (b) The tip of the needle is then rotated towards the limbus and advanced through the corneal stoma into the scleral flap. (c) The needle exits near the scleral flap border at *point C*. The suture is pulled so that the loop is tightened against the cornea. (d) The needle is passed through the scleral flap edge and across the cut scleral flap into the adjustant sclera at 45° to the flap edges and (e) comes out at *point D*, leaving a small loop above the scleral flap. (f) The releasable knot is tied by placing three or four throws around a tying forceps of the suture end that extends from *point D*. The suture loop lying on the surface of the scleral flap was grasped with a forcep. End *D* is then pulled towards the cornea, and loop B is pulled posteriorly away from the cornea, creating a hemibow slipknot. The end of the suture knot tied over the incision is gently cut with the Vannas scissors

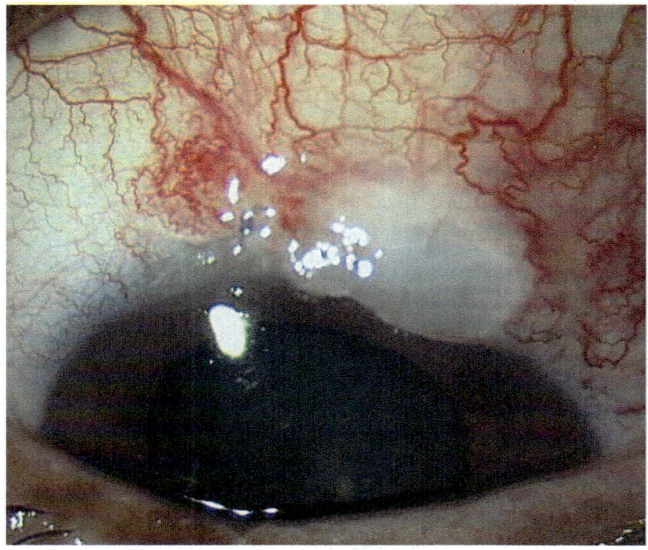

**Fig. 65.14** Avascular cystic bleb

medical therapy – in a previously unoperated eye is up to 90% at 2 years.[27]

But as with any potential antifibrotic substance, their mutilation of the wound healing process is associated with serious complications, which are related to the duration of exposure and concentration of the antimetabolite. Those agents cause thin avascular cystic blebs (Fig. 65.14) with early and late complications like leakage, hypotony, blebitis, and endophthalmitis.[28] Additional antimetabolite complications include corneal toxicity, uveitis, and suprachoroidal hemorrhage.

An isolated bleb leak must be carefully observed. Fortunately, the majority of them resolve with antibiotic prophylaxis alone, and do not develop into blebitis or endophthalmitis.[29]

Blebitis and endophthalmitis are hazardous complications of glaucoma filtering surgery frequently associated with bleb failure and loss of functional vision. In a retrospective study using MMC, a 1.3% annual risk of endophthalmitis was

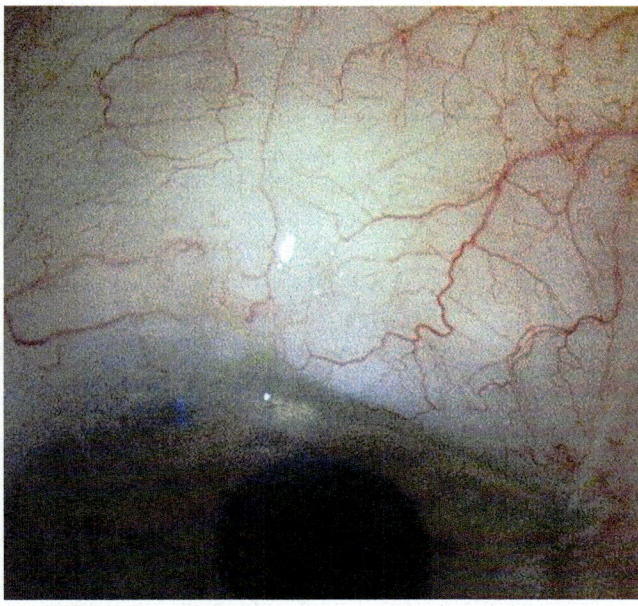

**Fig. 65.15** Tenon's cyst or encapsulated bleb

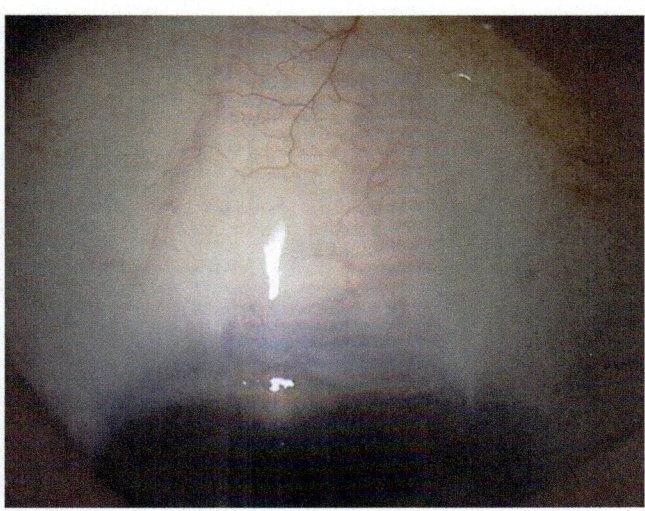

**Fig. 65.16** Antimetabolite should be applied over a large scleral area

found along with a 4.4% risk of at least one of the following complications: bleb leakage, blebitis, or endophthalmitis.[30]

Although intraoperative MMC is more effective than 5-FU in reducing IOP, and prevention of Tenon's cyst or encapsulated bleb[31] (Fig. 65.15), both agents are effective and equally safe adjuvants intraoperatively if used by an expert glaucoma specialist.

The success or complication rates after 1 year were not found to be statistically significant in a recent study.[32] Long-term result studies have shown a decline of IOP control over time. One study found success rates of 61% at 5 years, 44% at 10 years, and 41% at 14 years in eyes treated with 5-FU.[33]

Concentration and exposure time varies among surgeons, depending on the desired postoperative IOP and the patient's risk profile of bleb failure.[34] MMC concentration of 0.2–0.5 mg/ml and exposure time of up to 5 min have been advocated. Regarding 5-FU, the recommended concentration is 50 mg/ml for 5 min. The antimetabolite is soaked in pieces made from a Weck-cell sponge preferably made from polyvinyl alcohol and not from methylcellulose, which tends to fragment.[35] Those soaked pieces are placed underneath the Tenon and some surgeons also apply the antimetabolites under the scleral flap, since this appears to be advantageous.[36] To do so, the scleral flap needs to be created before applying the antimetabolite. The main disadvantage is that if the anterior chamber is entered prematurely, the antimetabolite should not be used.

In order to achieve diffuse posterior blebs, it is advocated to apply the antimetabolite over a large scleral area (Fig. 65.16). The conjunctival edges should be lifted and kept away from the antimetabolite to minimize postop leakage and late cystic limbal bleb formation. Special conjunctival forceps (No2-686, Duckworth and Kent) have been produced for this step.

After their usage, the soaked antimetabolite pieces are removed and disposed of as any other antimetabolite substance. The eye is irrigated thoroughly with 20–60 ml of BSS and the irrigation fluid is absorbed by preplaced surgical pads. After the irrigation, those pads are discarded in the toxic waste container, and some surgeons also change their gloves too for the next steps of the operation.

Other antiscarring agents were tested: mushroom lectins,[37] methylxanthines,[38] matrix metalloproteinases,[39,40] and an antibody that neutralizes transforming growth factor-beta 2 (TGF-ß2).

Regarding Trabio (lerdelimumab CAT-152 – human monoclonal antibody to TGF-ß2, which is believed to be responsible for the formulation of excessive scar tissue), Cambridge Antibody Technology UK announced that it has terminated further development since Trabio failed to meet the primary endpoint of improving the outcome of surgery for glaucoma in its second pivotal ("International" Phase III) clinical trial.

See Sidebar 65.4 for further discussion of antimetabolites.

### Sidebar 65.4 Antimetabolites and glaucoma surgery

Claudia U. Richter

Glaucoma filtration surgery is performed when the surgeon judges that vision preservation is more likely with better glaucoma control than the risks of vision loss with surgery. The outcome of filtration surgery is improved by the use of the antimetabolites 5-fluorouracil and mitomycin-C with higher success rates, lower IOP, and fewer glaucoma medications. Unfortunately, these adjunctive agents increase the risk of vision threatening complications including hypotony maculopathy, bleb leaks, and bleb infections and endophthalmitis. How does the surgeon weigh the risks of complications – some of which may not occur for years – with the chance for improved success? There are two observations that make the case for the use of antimetabolites in primary filters: the better outcomes of primary filters compared to those performed after previous conjunctival-scarring surgery and the lower IOPs obtained by filtering surgery performed with antimetabolites.

Numerous studies show that primary glaucoma filtering surgery has higher success rates than surgery that follows conjunctival scarring surgery, and great effort is made to maximize successful results with filtration surgery. Meticulous surgical procedure to minimize tissue handling and obtain adequate subconjunctival aqueous humor flow is essential but not sufficient for surgical success. Postoperative steroid therapy results in better outcomes and is nearly universally used. Despite these efforts, some glaucoma filtering operations are not successful, usually because fibrosis and vascularization develop between the conjunctiva and sclera, preventing subconjunctival flow of aqueous humor and reduction of IOP. 5-Fluorouracil inhibits fibroblast growth because it antagonizes pyrimidine metabolism, inhibits DNA synthesis, and results in cell death. Mitomycin-C inhibits the proliferative phase of wound healing by its inhibition of DNA replication, mitosis, and protein synthesis. Both agents reduce subconjunctival fibrosis and vascularization, improving the development of filtering blebs and the successful outcome of filtering surgery, both for primary and secondary filters.

The importance of setting and achieving a low-target IOP, rather than just reaching an IOP at or below 21 mmHg to minimize the risk of further glaucoma damage, is one of the important advances in glaucoma management. The Advanced Glaucoma Intervention Study demonstrated that those patients whose IOPs were always below 18 mmHg, and averaged 12 mmHg, had minimal visual field progression compared with patients who had higher IOPs. Antimetabolite therapy in glaucoma filtering surgery results in lower IOPs. Lower long-term IOP is expected to result in better long-term preservation of vision and is a powerful argument for the use of antimetabolites in primary filtering surgery.

Unfortunately, antimetabolite therapy in filtering surgery has both short-term and long-term risks. 5-FU frequently causes corneal toxicity including punctate keratopathy, filamentary keratopathy, frank epithelial defects, and whorl-like or striate melanokeratosis. These toxic corneal effects frequently resolve without reducing vision but may lead to bacterial corneal ulceration and corneal melting. Both 5-FU and mitomycin-C can cause thin-walled, avascular blebs. These types of blebs may develop focal bleb leaks, often years after glaucoma surgery, and are more common with the use of mitomycin-C. The thin-walled avascular blebs are also associated with an increased risk of developing endophthalmitis. The lower IOPs achieved with antimetabolite therapy can result in hypotony, which may lead to choroidal effusions, suprachoroidal hemorrhage, shallowing of the anterior chamber, and hypotony maculopathy. Hypotony maculopathy is characterized by folds in Bruch's membrane and retina secondary to choroidal thickening and may persist after normalization of IOP. It has been reported sporadically following 5-FU use and more commonly, but at variable rates, following mitomycin-C. Young myopic individuals are more prone to the development of maculopathy, and the incidence appears to be affected by trabeculectomy flap design.

Dealing with the difficult complications of hypotony maculopathy, bleb leaks, and bleb infections and endophthalmitis is arduous and difficult for both the glaucoma surgical patient and surgeon. Undoubtedly, these complications can be catastrophic and life-changing for the patient. However, these complications are significantly less common than the overall success rate of filtering surgery enhanced by antimetabolite therapy. The greater risk for patients facing primary filtering surgery is failure of the surgery or partial success with still inadequate IOP control, continuing glaucoma damage, and vision loss throughout their lifetime. Antimetabolite therapy with 5-fluoruracil or mitomycin-C significantly enhances the chance for successful glaucoma control and is appropriately used in primary filtering surgery.

### Bibliography

Andreanos D, Georgopoulos GT, Vergados J, et al. Clinical evaluation of the effect of mitomycin-C in re-operation for primary open angle glaucoma. *Eur J Ophthalmol.* 1997;7:49–54.

Costa VP, Comegno PE, Vasconcelos JP, et al. Low-dose mitomycin C trabeculectomy in patients with advanced glaucoma. *J Glaucoma*. 1996;5:193–199.
Greenfield DS, Liebmann JM, Jee J, Ritch R. Late-onset bleb leaks after glaucoma filtering surgery. *Arch Ophthalmol*. 1998;116: 443–447.
Gross RL, Feldman RM, Spaeth GL, et al. Surgical therapy of chronic glaucoma in aphakia and pseudophakia. *Ophthalmology*. 1988;95:1195–1201.
Heuer DK, Gressel MG, Parrish RK II, et al. Trabeculectomy in aphakic eyes. *Ophthalmology*. 1984;91:1045–1051.
Jacobi PC, Dietlein TS, Krieglstein GK. Adjunctive mitomycin C in primary trabeculectomy in young adults: a long-term study of case-matched young patients. *Graefes Arch Clin Exp Ophthalmol*. 1998;236:652–657.
Martini E, Laffi GL, Sprovieri C, Scorolli L. Low-dosage mitomycin C as an adjunct to trabeculectomy. A prospective controlled study. *Eur J Ophthalmol*. 1997;7:40–48.
Rasheed el-S. Initial trabeculectomy with intraoperative mitomycin-C application in primary glaucomas. *Ophthalmic Surg Lasers*. 1999;30:360–366.
Robin AL, Ramakrishnan R, Krishnadas R, et al. A long-term dose-response study of mitomycin in glaucoma filtration surgery. *Arch Ophthalmol*. 1997;115:969–974.
Roth SM, Spaeth GL, Starita RJ, et al. The effects of postoperative corticosteroids on trabeculectomy and the clinical course of glaucoma: five-year follow-up study. *Ophthalmic Surg*. 1991;22:724–729.
Shirato S, Kitazawa Y, Mishima S. A critical analysis of the trabeculectomy results by a prospective follow-up design. *Jpn J Ophthalmol*. 1982;26:468–480.
Singh K, Mehta K, Shaikh N, et al. Trabeculectomy with intraoperative mitomycin C versus 5-fluorouracil. Prospective randomized clinical trial. *Ophthalmology*. 2000;107:2305–2309.
Soltau JB, Rothman, RF, Budenz DL, et al. Risk factors for glaucoma filtering bleb infections. *Arch Ophthalmol*. 2000;118:338–342.
Stamper RL, McMenemy MG, Lieberman MF: Hypotonous maculopathy after trabeculectomy with subconjunctival 5-fluorouracil. *Am J Ophthalmol*. 1992;114:544–553.
Starita RJ, Fellman RL, Spaeth GL, et al. Short- and long-term effects of postoperative corticosteroids on trabeculectomy. *Ophthalmology*. 1985;92:938–946.
Suner IJ, Greenfield DS, Miller MP, et al. Hypotony maculopathy after filtering surgery with mitomycin C. Incidence and treatment. *Ophthalmology*. 1997;104:207-14;discussion 214–215.
The Advanced Glaucoma Intervention Study (AGIS): 7. The relationship between control of intraocular pressure and visual field deterioration. The AGIS Investigators. *Am J Ophthalmol*. 2000;130:429–440.
The advanced glaucoma intervention study (AGIS);13. Comparison of treatment outcomes within race: 10-year results. *Ophthalmology*. 2004;111:651–64.
Wilkins M, Indar A, Wormald R. Intra-operative mitomycin C for glaucoma surgery. *Cochrane Database Syst Rev*. 2001;(1): CD002897.
WuDunn D, Cantor LB Palanca-Capistrano AM, et al. A prospective randomized trial comparing intraoperative 5-fluorouracil vs mitomycin C in primary trabeculectomy. *Am J Ophthalmol*. 2002;134:521–528.
Zacharia PT, Deppermann SR, Schuman JS. Ocular hypotony after trabeculectomy with mitomycin C. *Am J Ophthalmol*. 1993;116:314–326.

## 65.9 Peripheral Iridectomy

A peripheral iridectomy (PI) (Fig. 65.17) is performed with Vannas scissors to prevent iris incarceration and ostium blockage, which may lead to bleb failure. In pseudophakic patients, the PI may not be mandatory.[41] Intracameral Miochol (acetylcholine chloride) can be used to constrict the pupil before the iridectomy, in order to achieve a well-sized peripheral iridectomy. Encroaching the pupillary borders must be prevented to eliminate visual complaints like monocular diplopia, halos, and photophobia, which are associated with a large iridectomy.

Peripheral iridectomy complications include iris bleeding with secondary hyphema, increased postoperative intracameral inflammation, damage to the underlying zonules, and possible vitreous loss through the peripheral iridectomy from excessive intrusion of a surgical instrument.

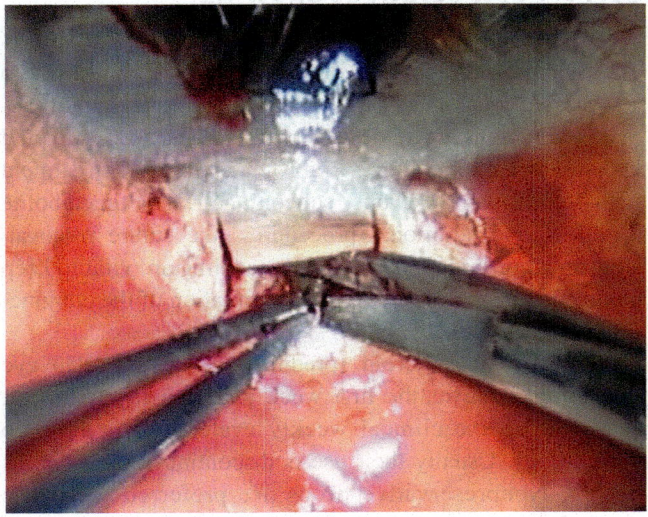

**Fig. 65.17** A peripheral iridectomy is performed with Vannas scissors, to prevent iris incarceration and ostium blockage, which may lead to bleb failure

## 65.10 Conjunctival Closure

Meticulous closure of the conjunctival flap is mandatory to reduce the risk of leakage. Nylon or absorbable 10 to 9/0 sutures like Vicryl may be used for this task (Fig. 65.18a–f).

Various techniques including horizontal mattress sutures or tight wing sutures are practiced to achieve this goal by creation of a water-tight border at the limbus. Another tip is to precauterize or scrape the epithelium adjacent to the

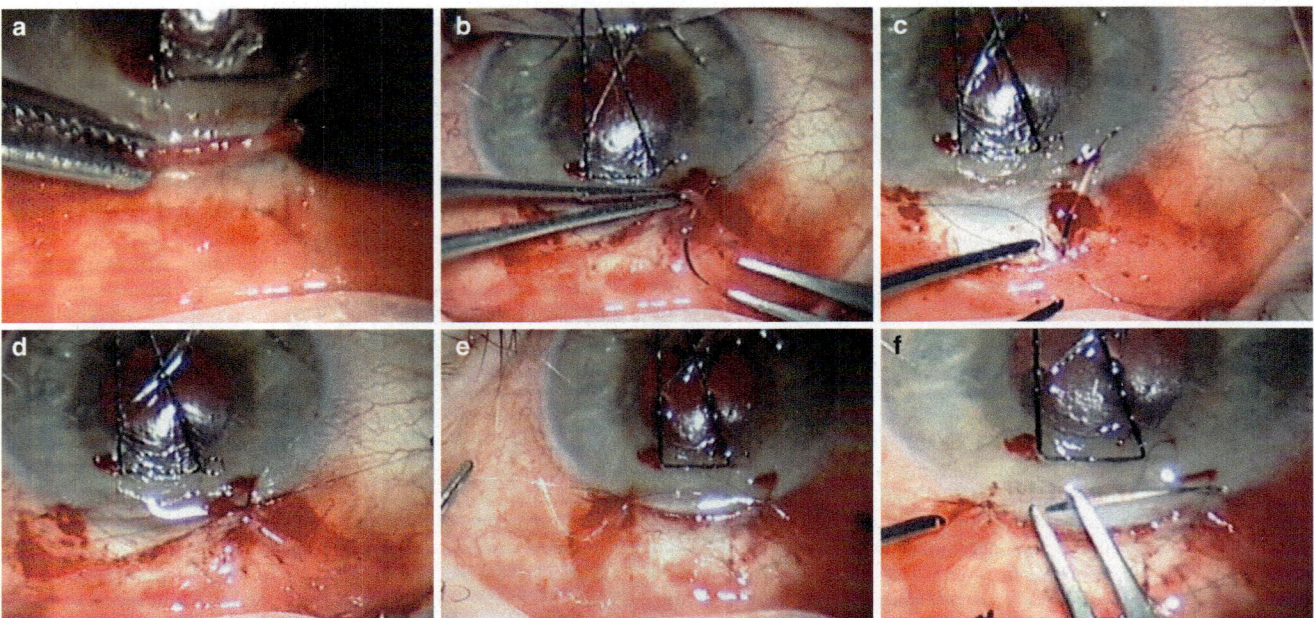

**Fig. 65.18** (a–f) Conjunctival closure

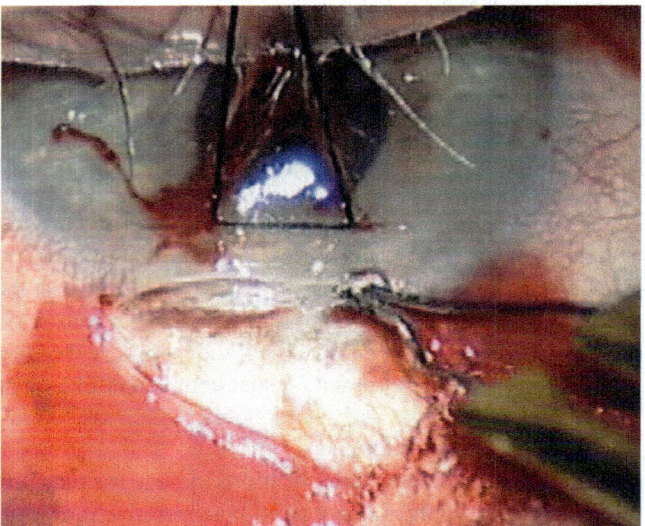

**Fig. 65.19** Precauterizing the epithelium adjacent to the limbus to promote wound healing at the conjunctival corneal border

limbus in order to promote wound healing at the conjunctival corneal border (Fig. 65.19).

For conjunctival closure, only tapered noncutting needles are preferred, but if corneoscleral anchoring sutures are performed, a spatulated needle is preferred. Leakage can be best tested with the Seidel Technique. The conjunctiva is painted with fluorescein drops and examined under a blue light to determine whether there is any leakage. The bleb potency is checked by injecting BCC through the paracentesis (Fig. 65.20a). An ideal result is a well-formed and posterior filtering diffuse bleb without signs of leakage (Fig. 65.20b).

At the end of the surgery, a subconjunctival injection containing steroid and antibiotics is injected into the inferior fornix (Fig. 65.21).

The eye is patched and an eye shield applied until first dressing. The eye shield is recommended for the first 24 h and then at bedtime for another 2–4 weeks.

## 65.11 Postoperative Follow-up

Thorough postop treatment and follow-up are mandatory to a successful outcome. Weekly visits, and clinical and treatment evaluations are not less important than a successful and uncomplicated operation. Rigorous antifibrotic treatment with topical steroid drops, subconjunctival antimetabolite injection, and additional procedures like suture removal/adjustment or laser lysis, and bleb needling are vital to keep the fistula open and to prevent the formation of the conjunctival "ring of steel."[11,34]

Hourly topical steroid (prednisolone acetate 1%) eye drops are given for the first week and then tapered down according to the clinical weekly evaluation of the bleb morphology. Usually their use is discontinued 1–3 months postop. Nonpreservative drops are preferred to reduce the inflammatory response.[42] Systemic steroid treatment carries systemic side effects and should not be adopted routinely.[43]

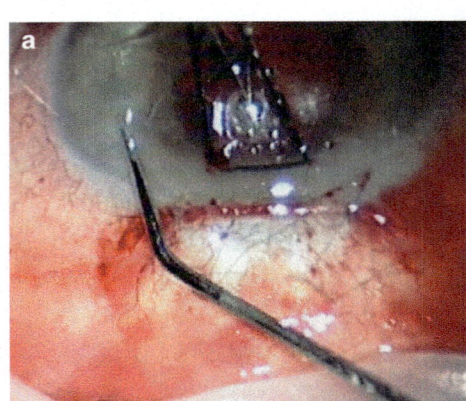
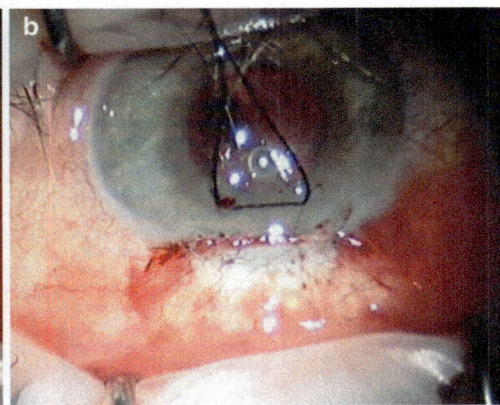

**Fig. 65.20** (a) Bleb potency is checked by injecting BCC through the paracentasis. (b) A well-formed and posterior filtering diffuse bleb without signs of leakage

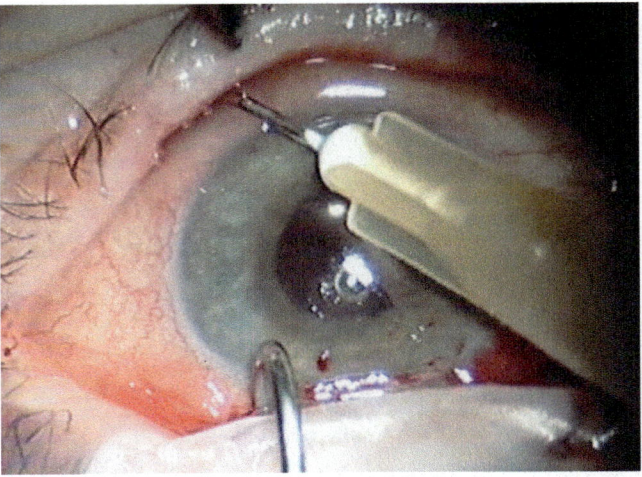

**Fig. 65.21** A subconjunctival injection containing steroid and antibiotics is injected into the inferior fornix

Broad-spectrum antibiotic eye drops are usually prescribed for the first postoperative week. Topical cycloplegic (1% cyclopentolate hydrochloride) drops may be given for 2–4 weeks.[44]

### 65.11.1 Complications

Complications and bleb failure are described in detail in Chap. 70. This section is intended to guide the reader to a few important points in postoperative management.

Complications are secondary to improper surgical technique or usage of the antimetabolites. Overfiltration may produce a flat anterior chamber, choroidal detachment, persistent hypotony, hypotony maculopathy, aqueous misdirection, cataract, and suprachoroidal hemorrhage.

Antimetabolite complications (described in detail in the antimetabolite paragraph) are mainly hypotony, bleb leak, blebitis, and endophthalmitis.

A large population survey from the UK of first-time trabeculectomies performed on chronic open angle glaucoma patients revealed the following complications (listed in Fig. 65.22a, b)[5] at 1 year from the trabeculectomy.

The complications were divided into early (less than 2 weeks from the operation) and late. In this survey, flat anterior chamber refers only to corneolenticular touch, and hypotony was defined as an intraocular pressure (IOP) equal to or less than 6 mmHg.

Hyphema was the most frequent complication in the early period, and the majority resolved within a week (Fig. 65.23). Cataract was the most frequent complication in the late period and the most common cause of visual loss cases.

Other complications encountered in various reports include: conjunctival buttonholes and tears [3%], scleral flap disinsertion, vitreous loss, and acute visual loss known as "wipe out syndrome," with a prevalence of 5% in advanced glaucoma optic neuropathy patients.

### 65.11.2 Postoperative Bleb Evaluation

The desired bleb appearance has been described previously. Important signs to look for are: extension, elevation, conjunctival vessel appearance, microcysts, and leakage. Diffuse elevation is associated with a functional filtering bleb, whereas corkscrew conjunctival vessels and flat blebs are signs of early bleb failure. The anatomical sites of bleb failure are:

1. Extraocular, due to fibrosis and subsequent scarring of the subconjunctival and Tenon's tissue. This is the most common cause of filter failure, with the typical "ring of steel" appearance. In order to reduce this complication rate and

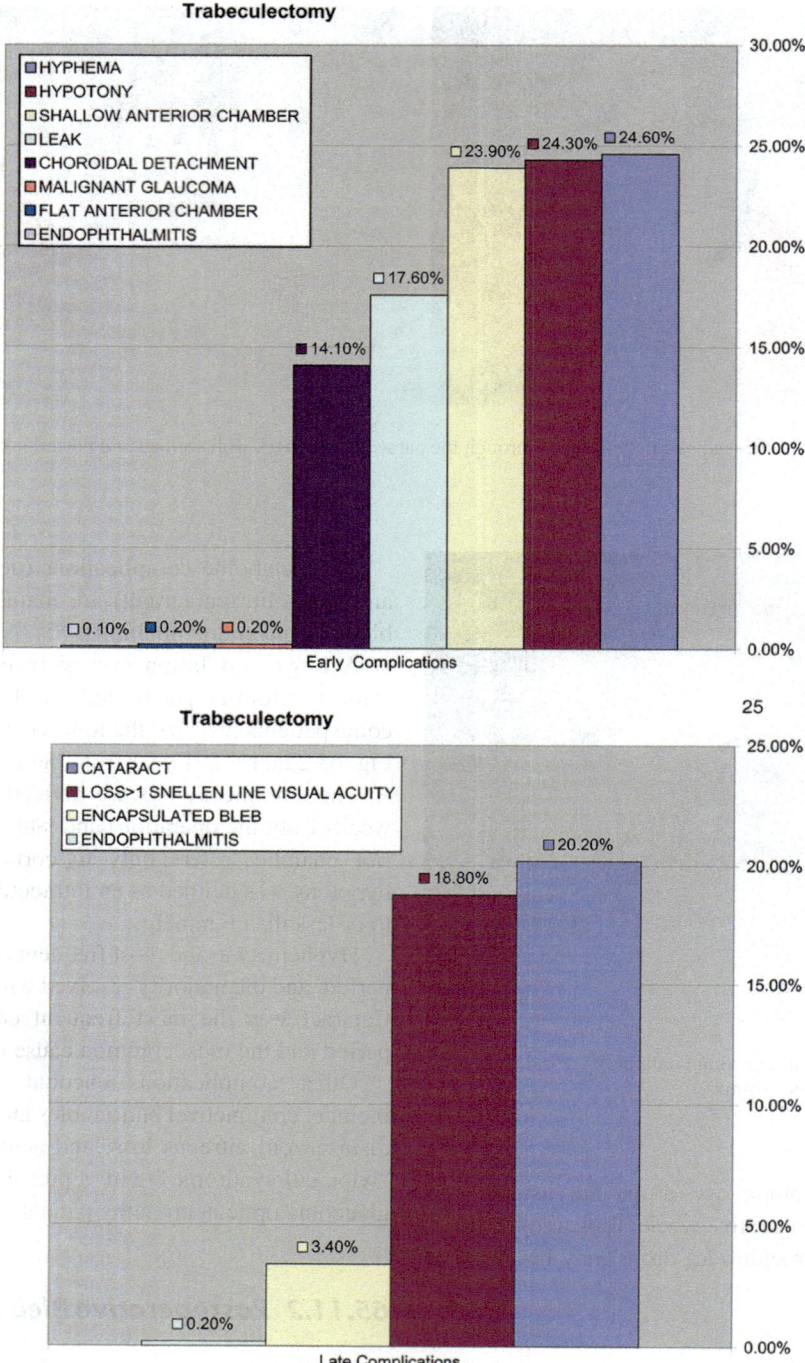

**Fig. 65.22** (a) Early and (b) late complications following first-time trabeculectomies for chronic open angle glaucoma as reported in a large population survey from the UK[5]

to improve the surgical outcome, the following tips are suggested[17] (Fig. 65.24):

- Good exposure and antimetabolite application over a large area.
- Tight adjustable sutures.
- Large scleral flaps, not cut to the limbus.
- Single scleral punch sclerostomy.

2. Scleral, due to tight flap sutures, or pronounced fibrosis along the flap edges.
3. Sclerostomy. The ostium is blocked by one of the following: uveal tissue, blood clot, vitreous, fibrosis, or remnant corneoscleral membrane left from an incomplete tissue removal.

Following are a few points concerning early bleb failure examples and possible treatment regimens.

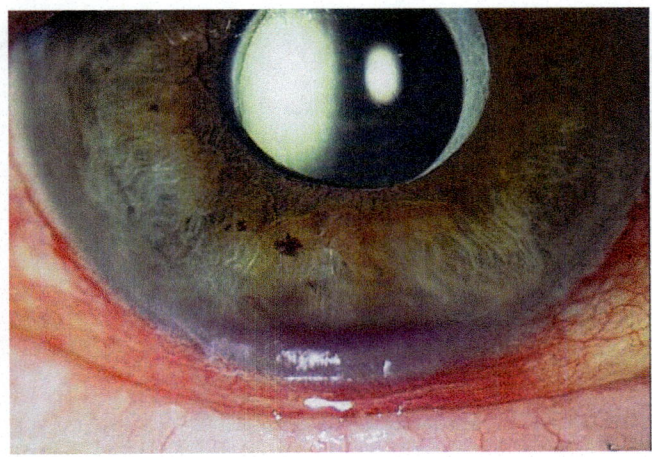

**Fig. 65.23** Hyphema was the most frequent complication in the early period following trabeculectomy

### 65.11.2.1 Flat Blebs

In the immediate postoperative period, suture lysis – removal of a releasable suture or local digital or cotton tip pressure adjacent to the scleral flap borders (Carlo Traverso maneuver)[45] – is performed to encourage refiltration. These maneuvers may be coupled with subconjunctival 5 mg 5-FU antimetabolite injection near the bleb border (Fig. 65.25a, b).

High IOP may result in worsening of the glaucomatous optic neuropathy. Massage of the flap borders results in a gush of aqueous and increase of bleb area and depth. This may be a transient lowering of the IOP unless there is loosening of the sutures at the same time. Excessive pressure could lead to occlusion of the internal ostium, for example, by iris tissue or vitreous, which would lead to secondary raised IOP.[19] This can be solved surgically by release of the incarcerated iris tissue (Fig. 65.26).

Suture release or lysis is an effective method of decreasing scleral resistance to flow and lowering IOP.[46] This suture maneuver can be performed successfully before the healing of the tissues – within a week from the operation if no antimetabolite was used and months if MMC was used.[47]

### 65.11.2.2 Bleb Leakage

Prophylactic antibiotic treatment is sufficient if there is a well-established anterior chamber without further complications. But if there is hypotony with a shallow anterior chamber or hypotony maculopathy, supplementary measures (tissue adhesive, cryotherapy, therapeutic bandage contact lens, or autologous blood injection) with or without ophthalmic viscoelastic device (OVD) injection into the anterior chamber are advised to close the conjunctival leak.

Injection of a dense viscoelastic – such as Healon 5 (sodium hyaluronate 2.3%) – into a hypotonous flat anterior chamber can be used as a temporary step in keeping a deep anterior chamber with elevation of the IOP.[48]

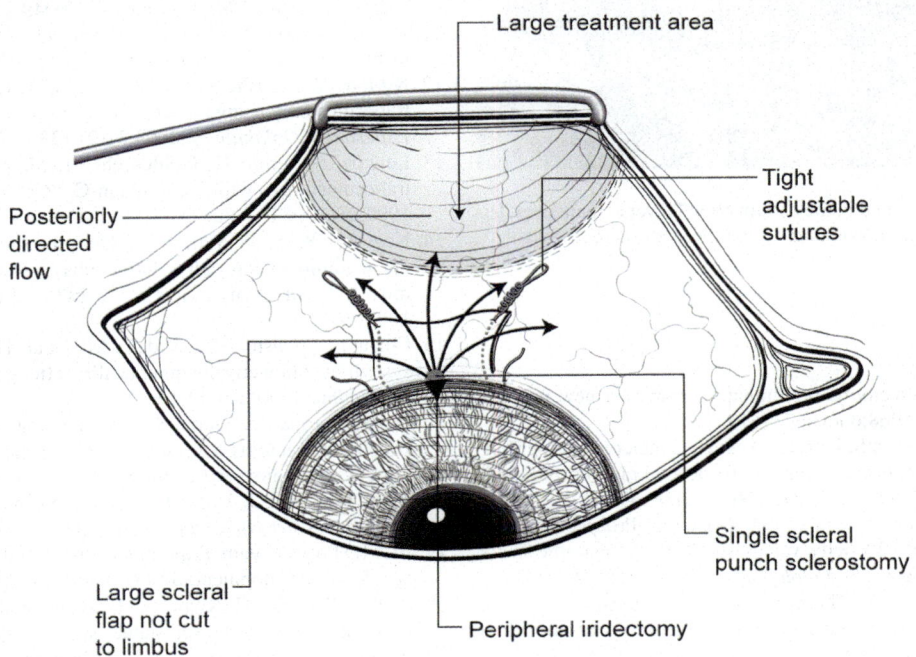

**Fig. 65.24** Techniques that reduce complications

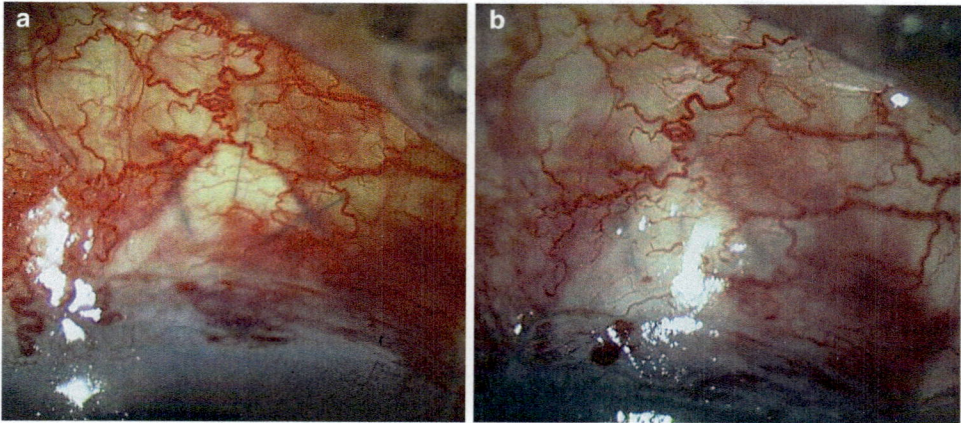

**Fig. 65.25** (a) Flat bleb. (b) Bleb elevation after a successful traverse maneuver

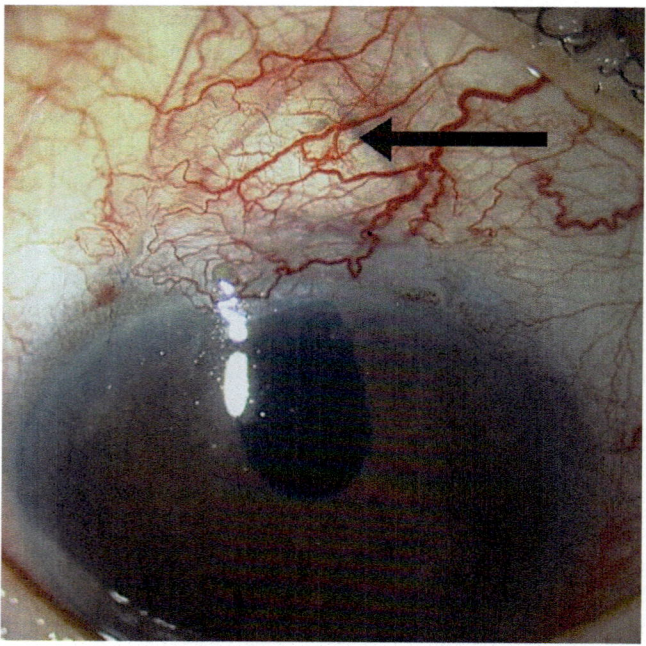

**Fig. 65.26** Iris incarcerated in the ostium after Traverso maneuver. Iris tissue is visible through the conjunctiva flap border (*black arrow*)

## References

1. Cairns JE. Trabeculectomy. preliminary report of a new method. *Am J Ophthalmol*. 1968;66(4):673–679.
2. Pablo LE, Perez-Olivan S, Ferreras A, et al. Contact versus peribulbar anaesthesia in trabeculectomy: a prospective randomized clinical study. *Acta Ophthalmol Scand*. 2003;81:486–490.
3. Carrillo MM, Buys YM, Faingold D, Trope GE. Prospective study comparing lidocaine 2% jelly versus sub-Tenon's anaesthesia for trabeculectomy surgery. *Br J Ophthalmol*. 2004;88:1004–1007.
4. Edmunds B, Bunce CV, Thompson JR, et al. Factors associated with success in first-time trabeculectomy for patients at low risk of failure with chronic open angle glaucoma. *Ophthalmology*. 2004;111:97–103.
5. Edmunds B, Thompson JR, Salmon JF, Wormald RP. The National Survey of Trabeculectomy. III. Early and late complications. *Eye*. 2002;16:297–303.
6. Hu CY, Matsuo H, Tomita G, et al. Clinical characteristics and leakage of functioning blebs after trabeculectomy with mitomycin-C in primary glaucoma patients. *Ophthalmology*. 2003;110:345–352.
7. Wells AP, Cordeiro MF, Bunce C, Khaw PT. Cystic bleb formation and related complications in limbus- versus fornix-based conjunctival flaps in pediatric and young adult trabeculectomy with mitomycin C. *Ophthalmology*. 2003;110:2192–2197.
8. Kohl DA, Walton DS. Limbus-based versus fornix-based conjunctival flaps in trabeculectomy: 2005 update. *Int Ophthalmol Clin*. 2005;45(4):107–113.
9. Agbeja AM, Dutton GN. Conjunctival incisions for trabeculectomy and their relationship to the type of bleb formation: a preliminary study. *Eye*. 1987;1:738–743.
10. Henderson HW, Ezra E, Murdoch IE. Early postoperative trabeculectomy leakage: incidence, time course, severity, and impact on surgical outcome. *Br J Ophthalmol*. 2004;88:626–629.
11. Jones E, Clarke J, Khaw PT. Recent advances in trabeculectomy technique. *Curr Opin Ophthalmol*. 2005;16(2):107–113.
12. Ng PW, Yeung BY, Yick DW, Tsang CW, Lam DS. Fornix-based trabeculectomy using the 'anchoring' corneal suture technique. *Clin Experiment Ophthalmol*. 2003;31(2):133–137.
13. Levkovitch-verbin H, Goldenfeld M, Melamed S. Fornix-based trabeculectomy with mitomycin-C. *Ophthalmic Surg Lasers*. 1997;28(10):818–822.
14. Negi AK, Kiel AW, Vernon SA. Does the site of filtration influence the medium to long term intraocular pressure control following microtrabeculectomy in low risk eyes? *Br J Ophthalmol*. 2004;88:1008–1011.
15. Chang L, Crowston JG, Cordeiro MF, et al. The role of the immune system in conjunctival wound healing after glaucoma surgery. *Surv Ophthalmol*. 2000;45:49–68.
16. Das J, Sharma P, Chaudhuri Z. A comparative study of small incision trabeculectomy avoiding Tenon's capsule vis-a-vis trabeculectomy with mitomycin-C. *Indian J Ophthalmol*. 2004;52:23–27.
17. Jones E, Clarke J, Khaw PT. Recent advances in trabeculectomy technique. *Curr Opin Ophthalmol*. 2005;16:107–113.
18. AGFID Project Team. Experimental flow studies in glaucoma drainage device development. *Br J Ophthalmol*. 2001;85:1231–1236.
19. Wells AP, Bunce C, Khaw PT. Flap and suture manipulation after trabeculectomy with adjustable sutures: titration of flow and intraocular pressure in guarded filtration surgery. *J Glaucoma*. 2004;13:400–406.

20. Melamed S, Ashkenagi I, Glorinski J, Blumenthal M. Tight scleral flap trabeculectomy with post operative laser suture lysis. *Am J Ophthalmol*. 1990;109:303–309.
21. Aykan U, Bilge AH, Akin T, Certel I, Bayer A. Laser suture lysis or releasable sutures after trabeculectomy. *J Glaucoma*. 2007;16(2): 240–245.
22. Schaffer RN, Hetherington J, Hoskins HD. Guarded thermal sclerostomy. *Am J Ophthalmol*. 1971;72:769–772.
23. Kolker AE, Kass MA, Rait JL. Trabeculectomy with releasable sutures. *Arch Ophthalmol*. 1994;112:62–66.
24. Raina UK, Tuli D. Trabeculectomy With releasable sutures a prospective, randomized pilot study. *Arch Ophthalmol*. 1998;116: 1288–1293.
25. Heuer DK, Parrish RK II, Gressel MG, Hodapp E, et al. 5-Fluorouracil and glaucoma filtering surgery, II: a pilot study. *Ophthalmology*. 1984;91:384–394.
26. Chen CW. Enhanced intraocular pressure controlling effectiveness of trabeculectomy by local application of mitomycin C. *Trans Asia Pac Acad Ophthalmol*. 1983;9:172.
27. European Glaucoma Society. *Terminology and Guidelines for Glaucoma*. 2nd ed. Savona, Italy: DOGMA; 2003.
28. Rothman RF, Liebmann JM, Ritch R. Low-dose 5-fluorouracil trabeculectomy as initial surgery in uncomplicated glaucoma: long-term followup. *Ophthalmology*. 2000;107:1184–1190.
29. DeBry PW, Perkins TW, Heatley G, Kaufman P, Brumback LC. Incidence of late-onset bleb-related complications following trabeculectomy with mitomycin. *Arch Ophthalmol*. 2002;120(3):297–300.
30. Debry PW, Perkins TW, Heatley G, et al. Incidence of late-onset bleb-related complications following trabeculectomy with mitomycin. *Arch Ophthalmol*. 2002;120:297–300.
31. Membrey WL, Poinoosawmy DP, Bunce C, Hitchings RA. Glaucoma surgery with or without adjunctive antiproliferatives in normal tension glaucoma: 1 intraocular pressure control and complications. *Br J Ophthalmol*. 2000;84:586–590.
32. Singh K. Trabeculectomy with intraoperative mitomycin C versus 5-fluorouracil prospective randomized clinical trial *Ophthalmology*. 2000;107(12):2305–2309.
33. Suzuki R, Dickens CJ, Iwach AG, et al. Long-term follow-up of initially successful trabeculectomy with 5-fluorouracil injections. *Ophthalmology*. 2002;109:1921–1924.
34. Khaw PT, Jones E, Mireskandari K, et al. Modulating wound healing after glaucoma surgery. *Glaucoma Today*. July/August: 12–19, 2004.
35. Khaw PT. Advances in glaucoma surgery: evolution of antimetabolite adjunctive therapy. *J Glaucoma*. 2001;10(5 Suppl 1):S81–S84.
36. El Sayyad F, Belmekki M, Helal M, et al. Simultaneous subconjunctival and subscleral mitomycin C application in trabeculectomy. *Ophthalmology*. 2000;107:298–301.
37. Batterbury M, Tebbs CA, Rhodes JM, Grierson I. Agaricus bisporus (edible mushroom lectin) inhibits ocular fibroblast proliferation and collagen lattice contraction. *Exp Eye Res*. 2002;74:361–370.
38. Saika S, Yamanaka O, Okada Y, et al. Pentoxifylline and pentifylline inhibit proliferation of human Tenon's capsule fibroblasts and production of type-I collagen and laminin in vitro. *Ophthalmic Res*. 1996;28:165–170.
39. Mead AL, Wong TT, Cordeiro MF, et al. Evaluation of anti-TGF-beta2 antibody as a new postoperative anti-scarring agent in glaucoma surgery. *Invest Ophthalmol Vis Sci*. 2003;44:3394–3401.
40. Wong TT, Mead AL, Khaw PT. Matrix metalloproteinase inhibition modulates postoperative scarring after experimental glaucoma filtration surgery. *Invest Ophthalmol Vis Sci*. 2003;44: 1097–1103.
41. Shingleton BJ, Chaudhry IM, O'Donoghue MW. Phacotrabeculectomy: peripheral iridectomy or no peripheral iridectomy? *J Cataract Refract Surg*. 2002;28(6):998–1002.
42. Baudouin C, Pisella PJ, Fillacier K, et al. Ocular surface inflammatory changes induced by topical antiglaucoma drugs: human and animal studies. *Ophthalmology*. 1999;106:556–563.
43. Vote B, Fuller JR, Bevin TH, Molteno AC. Systemic anti-inflammatory fibrosis suppression in threatened trabeculectomy failure. *Clin Exp Ophthalmol*. 2004;32:81–86.
44. Raina UK, Tuli D. Trabeculectomy with releasable sutures a prospective, randomized pilot study. *Arch Ophthalmol*. 1998;116:1288–1293.
45. Traverso CE, Greenidge KC, Spaeth GL, et al. Focal pressure: A new method to encourage filtration after trabeculectomy. *Ophthalmic Surg*. 1984;15:62.
46. Khaw PT, Sherwood MB, Doyle JW, et al. Intraoperative and post operative treatment with 5-fluorouracil and mitomycin-c: long term effects in vivo on subconjunctival and scleral fibroblasts. *Int Ophthalmol*. 1992;16:381–385.
47. Hoffman RS, Fine IH, Packer M. Stabilization of flat anterior chamber after trabeculectomy with Healon5. *J Cataract Refract Surg*. 2002;28(4):712–714.
48. Savage JA, Condon GP, Lytle RA, et al. Laser suture lysis after trabeculectomy. *Ophthalmology*. 1988;95:1631–1638.

# Chapter 66
# Incisional Therapies: Trabeculotomy Surgery in Adults

Ronald L. Fellman

Glaucoma patients who require incisional glaucoma surgery and who neither are optimal candidates for filtering surgery nor need an intraocular pressure (IOP) as low as 10 mmHg may be candidates for trabeculotomy. Trabeculotomy *ab externo* is an anterior chamber angle procedure designed to increase conventional trabecular outflow. IOP is lowered without creating a filtering bleb. Patients with only mild to moderate disc damage and with uncontrolled IOPs greater than 21 mmHg may do well with postoperative IOPs in the mid- to late teens and perhaps just one antiglaucoma medication – the typical scenario post-trabeculotomy surgery (Fig. 66.1a, b).

It is well known that trabeculotomy is effective for congenital glaucoma, but it is also useful for select cases of juvenile and adult glaucomas,[1] as well as steroid-induced glaucoma. It also works well when combined with phacoemulsification.[2,3] In Europe and Asia, where angle and canal surgery are popular, trabeculotomy remains an option to filtration surgery for adult and juvenile glaucomas.[4] In many parts of the world, angle and/or canal surgery is carried out earlier in the disease process than in the USA. Surgeons in these locales believe that surgery that addresses the collector system has a better chance of long-term function than does more conventional glaucoma surgery. Decades of topical medications, as seen typically with the US treatment paradigm, along with continued collapse of the collector system with progressive disease, probably create a more unfavorable environment for procedures that theoretically reestablish normal outflow, such as trabeculotomy, and other nonpenetrating novel canal procedures, such as canaloplasty. Intervening earlier may increase the success with these alternative surgeries.

Trabeculotomy is a more difficult and complicated operation than trabeculectomy and does not lower IOP as much. Most US eye surgeons prefer an easier surgical procedure that also achieves lower IOPs. Trabeculotomy is technically more demanding because the surgeon must find, cannulate, and manipulate the canal compared to just removing a block of corneoscleral tissue as done with a glaucoma filtering surgery. Because there is no bleb formation, the trabeculotomy site may be selected anywhere at the limbus but is typically placed slightly off the 12 o'clock position.

Because no bleb is formed, future superiorly placed conjunctival surgery is usually not a problem. However, postoperative day 1 hyphema is common, and treatment to blunt postoperative IOP spike is often necessary.

Adult patients with primary open angle glaucoma (POAG) who are not optimal candidates for filtration surgery, and who require incisional glaucoma surgery, may be reasonable candidates for trabeculotomy, especially if they require combined cataract and glaucoma surgery (Table 66.1).

## 66.1 Surgical Technique for Trabeculotomy Ab Externo

The following describes trabeculotomy from an external approach (*ab externo*) as this is the most common approach worldwide. The ultimate success of trabeculotomy is highly dependent on the following:

1. Intraoperative localization of Schlemm's canal
2. Accurate identification of Schlemm's canal
3. The successful cannulation of Schlemm's canal
4. Opening of the canal either by a metal trabeculotome or suture technique
5. Adequate closure of the scleral flap and wound to prevent bleb formation
6. A permanent cleft into Schlemm's canal with minimal peripheral anterior synechiae (PAS) formation

### 66.1.1 Exposing Schlemm's Canal

There are currently two popular techniques to expose the canal. The classic T-shaped cut-down in the scleral bed remains a steadfast method of exposing the canal (Fig. 66.2a, b). Another technique gaining in popularity is the exposure of the canal similar to that used with other nonpenetrating surgical techniques such as viscocanalostomy, deep sclerectomy, and canaloplasty.

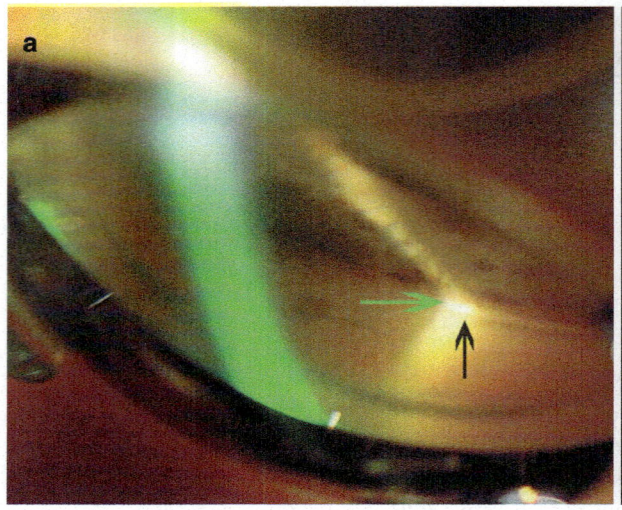 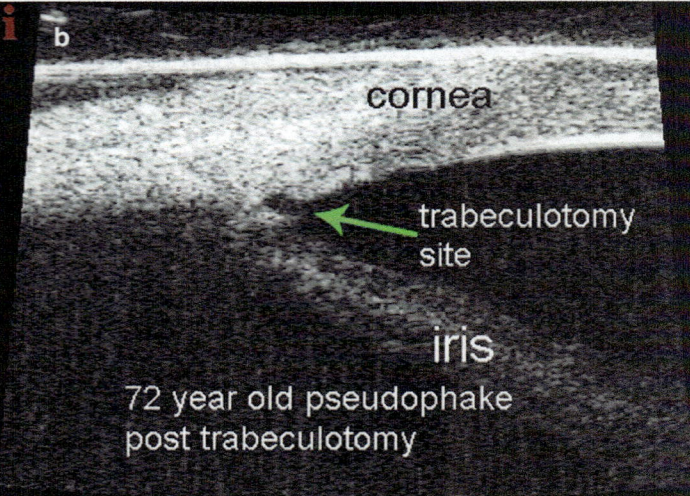

**Fig. 66.1** Goniophotograph and high-resolution ultrasound of Schlemm's canal post-trabeculotomy in a 72-year-old patient with pseudophakic glaucoma. (**a**) Goniophotograph of chamber angle post trabeculotomy. The *green arrow* designates the opening into Schlemm's canal. The inner wall of the canal is cleaved open during trabeculotomy exposing its posterior wall. The *black arrow* designates anterior trabecular pigment. Preoperative IOP on two medications was 26 mmHg and postoperative IOP control at 2 years was excellent at 14 mmHg on one medication. This 72-year-old pseudophake had moderate disc damage and mild field loss. (**b**) High frequency ultrasound of trabeculotomy site in (**a**). The opening into Schlemm's canal can easily be seen with this 100 MHz high frequency ultrasound system from iScience Interventional (Menlo Park, California). The site of greatest resistance in glaucoma, the trabecular meshwork and juxtacanalicular tissue, is cleaved open allowing flow to the downstream collector system. This trabeculotomy was successful because the cleaved anterior leaflets remained open and did not fuse back together, a likely cause of failure

**Table 66.1** Potential candidates for trabeculotomy

1. Severe ocular surface disease (blepharitis, ocular rosacea, cicatrizing diseases)
2. Juvenile glaucoma with classis trabeculodysgenesis
3. Steroid-induced glaucoma
4. Failed filter under optimal circumstances in fellow eye
5. Symptomatic filtering bleb in fellow eye
6. Poor candidate for a filter; e.g., uveitic disease
7. History of suprachoroidal hemorrhage in the fellow eye
8. History of blebitis in the fellow eye
9. History of chronic hypotony with visual loss in the fellow eye
10. Patients with post scleral buckle with severe conjunctival scarring
11. Need for combined cataract glaucoma surgery with mild to moderate glaucoma damage
12. Congenital glaucoma with trabeculodysgenesis (classic example)

The T-shaped cut-down is the classic technique used to expose the canal and is the same for pediatric, juvenile, and adult cases. The absolute essential landmark for all *ab externo* glaucoma surgery is the accurate identification of the scleral spur. The scleral spur is the location where the ciliary body attaches to the sclera. Limbal anatomy is highly variable from patient to patient and the location of the canal varies considerably. Due to this variability, a nylon suture, as seen in Fig. 66.2a, may be used to help verify the exact location. The limbal zone is a 1.5 mm transition area between sclera and cornea (Fig. 66.3a, b). The scleral spur lies underneath this zone and is a circumferential ring of white scleral fibers identified in stark contrast to the juxtaposed longitudinal fibers of the scleral bed. The difference in the direction of the fibers is easy to appreciate under the microscope.

### 66.1.2 Single Scleral Flap with T Cut Technique

1. Create a fornix-based conjunctival flap in the desired location and follow with very light wet-field cautery.
2. Create a 2/3 thickness scleral flap, dimensions approximately 4–5 mm at its base and 5 mm posterior extent (Fig. 66.4). Make sure the flap extends anteriorly into clear cornea in order to adequately uncover an anterior displaced canal and posteriorly to uncover a posteriorly displaced canal. The most common error is to make the scleral flap too superficial, leaving a great deal of tissue to dissect through to reach the canal, or failure to make the flap large enough to gain access to the canal. In other words, do not make a wimpy scleral flap!
3. In a very meticulous and deliberate manner, make a radial cut 1 mm anterior to the proposed site of the spur and extend one millimeter posteriorly (Fig. 66.5a).

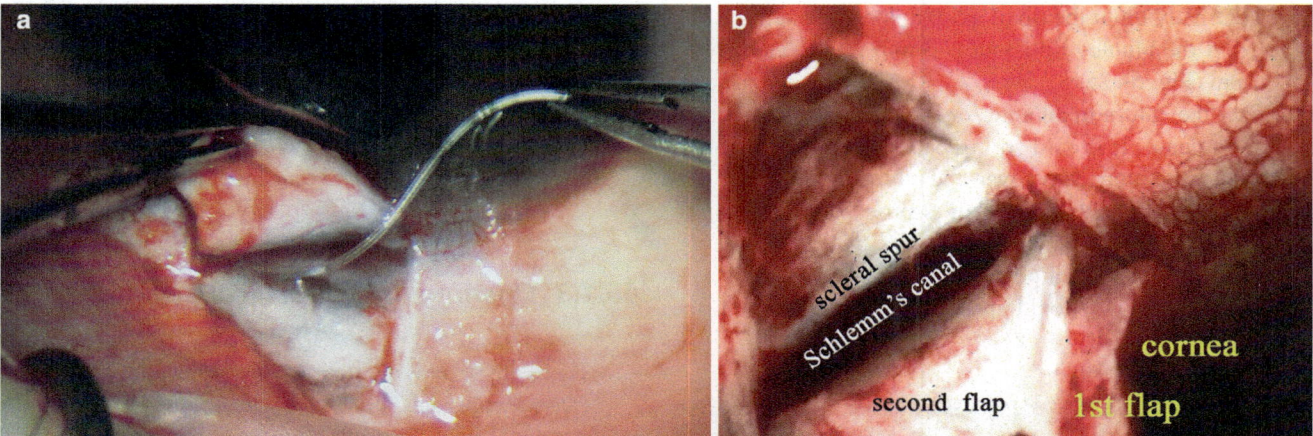

**Fig. 66.2** Alternate approaches to expose Schlemm's canal for trabeculotomy. (**a**) Classic T cut approach with single flap. A single scleral flap is fashioned to expose the canal. Several meticulous radial cuts are made through the layers of sclera over the proposed site of the canal. Once the canal is exposed, a lateral cut is made on each side to gain better access to the canal. A 5-0 nylon suture is used to probe the canal and verify its identity and location. (**b**) Nonpenetrating surgery dual flap approach. Nonpenetrating surgery typically calls for a two flap technique to unroof the canal. The first flap is 300 μm thick and the second deep flap is generally 600 μm thick. Careful forward dissection of the deep flap usually unroofs the canal. Note the smooth transition of endothelium as seen on the back side of the deep flap. Note (**a**). Thermally blunt the tip of a 5-0 clear nylon suture to use as a canal probe. This will prevent a sharp edge from perforating the floor of the canal. Insert the tip of the blunted suture into the proposed canal site for 2–3 mm. Flex the suture anteriorly over the cornea and release it, it should spring back to its original position if in the canal. If not, it will stay over the cornea indicating the suture is likely in the suprachoroidal space. Now flex it posteriorly, over the sclera. Again, it should spring back to its original position if in the canal. If not, the suture is likely in the anterior chamber

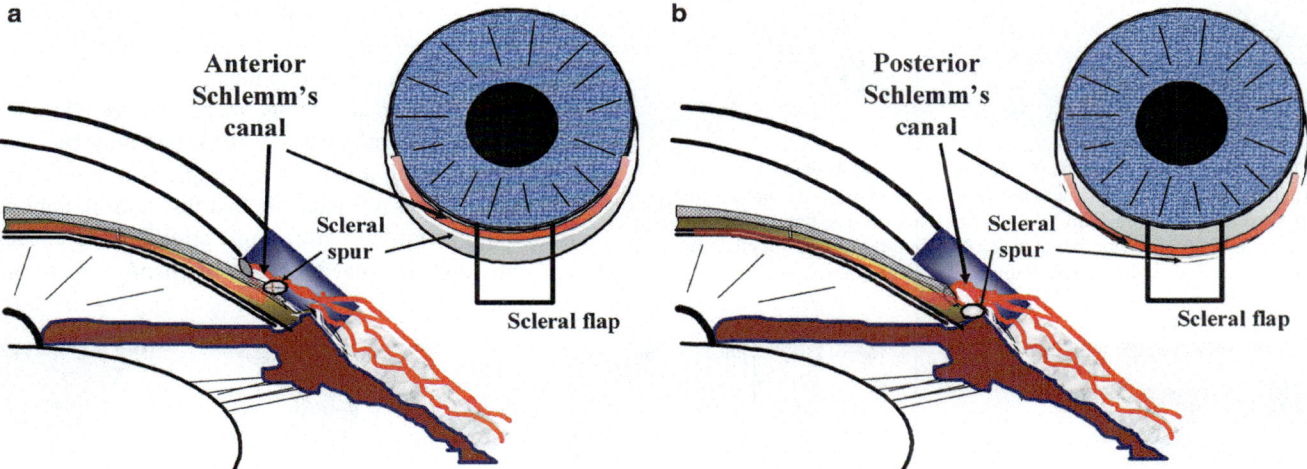

**Fig. 66.3** Variable location of Schlemm's canal. (**a**) Anteriorly located Schlemm's canal. The location of Schlemm's canal is highly variable as limbal anatomy is quite different based on genetics, refractive error, developmental abnormalities, and other factors. The key is to always make the scleral flap large enough so that the posterior border will still cover a posteriorly located canal. (**b**) Posteriorly located Schlemm's canal. Prior to dissection, the location of the canal is a guess. The proper construction of the flap is critical in order to successfully find the canal

4. Deepen the cut, fiber by fiber, as you approach the roof of the canal (Figs. 66.5b, c).
5. Once in the canal, the texture of the floor of the canal is very different than the prior dissection. Pigment may be seen in the floor of the canal; the tissue is slightly darker as well. If in the wrong location, which may happen, these landmarks will not present themselves, and the case becomes exponentially more difficult. The chamber may be perforated and collapse.
6. No matter how convinced one is that one has found the canal, it behooves you to verify the exact location with a suture technique. Initially, avoid using a metal trabeculotome at this stage to probe the canal until you are convinced you have located the canal.

7. Thermally blunt the tip of a 5-0 nylon clear suture.
8. Insert the blunted tip about 2–3 mm into the suspected canal (Fig. 66.2a).
9. Flex the suture in an anterior direction over the cornea and release. It should spring back into position. If not, the suture may stay over the cornea, indicating the suture is not in the canal but is probably in the suprachoroidal space.
10. Flex the suture in a posterior direction over the sclera and let it go. It should spring back; if it does not, the suture is probably somewhere in the anterior chamber and not in the canal. These very simple maneuvers may help identify the canal.
11. Another simple method is to place a blue 6-0 Prolene blunted suture in the canal, and if the cornea is clear, the blue suture may be seen gonioscopically.

### 66.1.3 Opening the Canal (Trabeculotomy)

1. There are several methods to open the canal from an *ab externo* approach: filamentary technique with a suture, standard metal trabeculotome, microcatheter rupture of canal wall, and viscodilation and canal rupture.
2. The filamentary suture technique is widely used in the pediatric glaucomas and is popular because the entire angle or 360° can be opened at one sitting. Occasionally, less of the angle is opened due to altered anatomy. This same technique, either a 180 or 360° filamentary trabeculotomy, can be used in the pediatric, juvenile, or adult open angle glaucomas (Fig. 66.6a–e).
3. The classic method of using a metal trabeculotome is still very popular throughout the world, especially in Japan and Germany. The metal probe is inserted into the canal (Fig. 66.7a–c) and the canal walls are ruptured with a single rotating movement into the anterior chamber, and the process may be repeated in the opposite direction.
4. The iTrack 250A canaloplasty microcatheter (iScience Interventional, Menlo Park, California) may be used as a "suture," with a similar technique (Fig. 66.8a, b). The microcatheter advantage is that viscoelastic may be inserted throughout the entire angle prior to rupture. This may cut down on bleeding and hyphema formation.

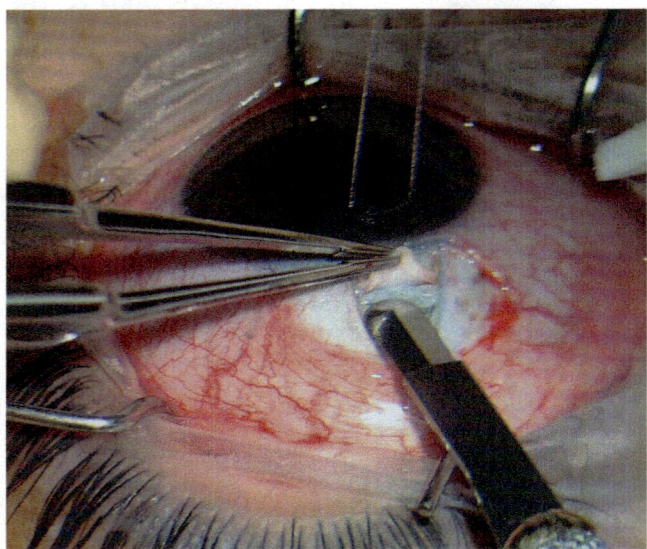

**Fig. 66.4** Fashion scleral flap. After making a fornix-based conjunctival flap, dissect a 2/3 thickness uniform scleral flap – this is not the time to be skimpy on your flap. The anterior extent of the flap is into clear cornea and the posterior extent of the flap should be posterior enough to allow an adequate dissection of the flap prior to discovering the canal

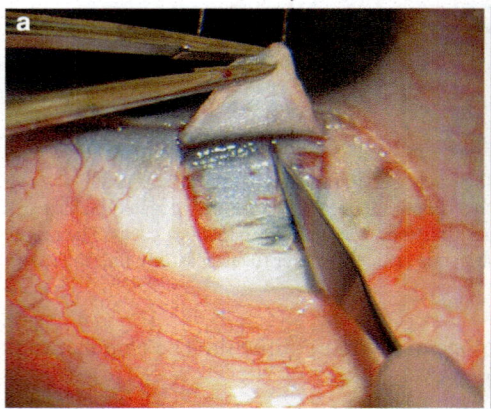 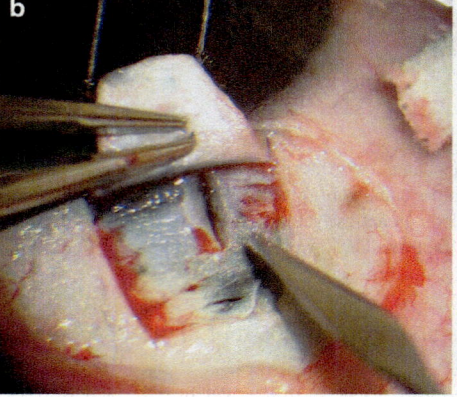 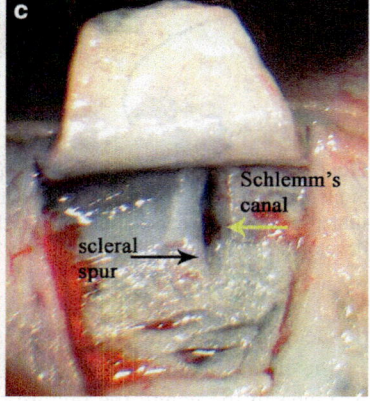

**Fig. 66.5** Scleral bed radial cut down technique. (**a**) Initiate radial cut down. Estimate the position of the scleral spur, and the length of the cut should be approximately 1 mm anterior and 1 mm posterior to the proposed site of the scleral spur and canal. (**b**) Radial cut down progress. A careful fiber by fiber cut down seeking the canal will eventually expose it. This part of the procedure is very meticulous and methodical. (**c**) Full radial cut down to canal. The scleral spur is finally exposed and is noted by its circumferential nature and compactness. There is blood noted in the canal, which is directly anterior to the spur

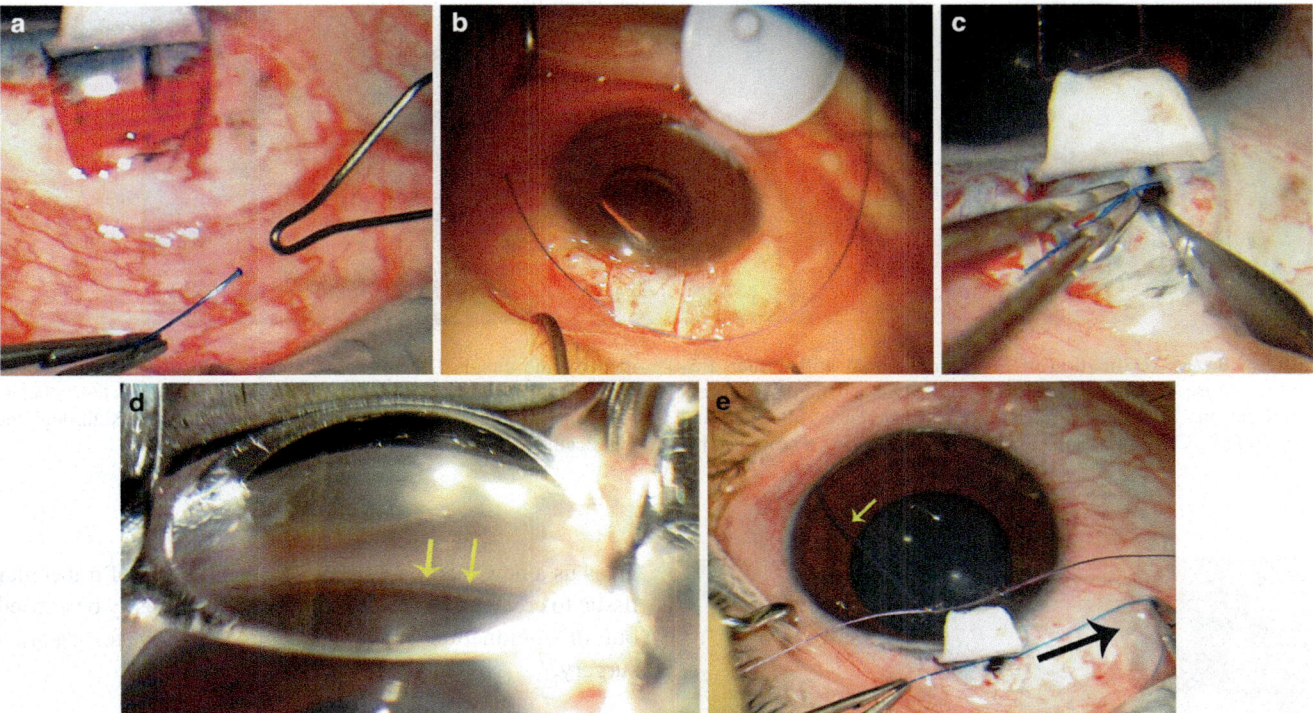

**Fig. 66.6** Filamentary trabeculotomy with Prolene suture. (**a**) Thermally blunt a 6-0 Prolene suture in order to produce a small bulb on the end of the suture so it will not be sharp. (**b**) Note the blunt end of the suture. The arc of the suture is utilized to the surgeon's advantage by placing the suture on the globe prior to inserting into the canal. This allows a less traumatic insertion of the suture into the canal. (**c**) Cannulate the canal for 360° and pull the opposite end of the suture out of the canal. (**d**) If possible, follow the position of the suture by gonioscopy to note its progress. Note the blue Prolene suture in Schlemm's canal verified by gonioscopy. (**e**) The trabeculotomy is performed by grasping both ends of the Prolene suture. Pull in opposite directions to bow-string the suture into the anterior chamber creating the trabeculotomy (*yellow arrow*). This method allows opening the entire angle at one sitting. If the suture does not go all the way around, a 180° may also be accomplished

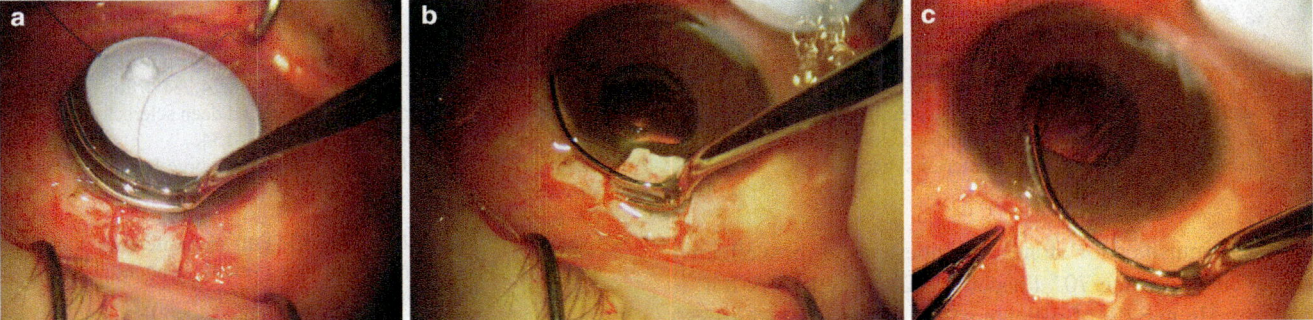

**Fig. 66.7** Trabeculotomy performed with traditional metal trabeculotome. (**a**) Trabeculotomy probe positioned over limbus to visualize the surgical maneuver necessary to open the canal. (**b**) Trabeculotomy probe gently inserted into the canal and carefully threaded several millimeters until the majority of the probe is in the canal. (**c**) Rotation of probe into the anterior chamber by breaking through the inner wall of the canal creating the trabeculotomy

The opening is larger with the microcatheter with the potential advantage that the anterior leaflets of the trabecular meshwork are less likely to close back up, months later.

5. Close the scleral flap in a water-tight fashion. If the iris prolapses at any stage, perform a small basal iridotomy (Fig. 66.9).
6. Close the conjunctiva in standard fashion.
7. Patch and shield the eye.

Obviously, the technique varies depending on surgeon training and preference.[5–7] The results combined with phacoemulsification work well with either a one- or two-site technique.[8] Postoperative IOP control with phacotrabeculotomy is superior

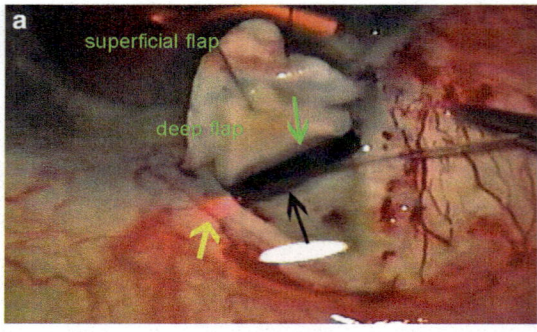
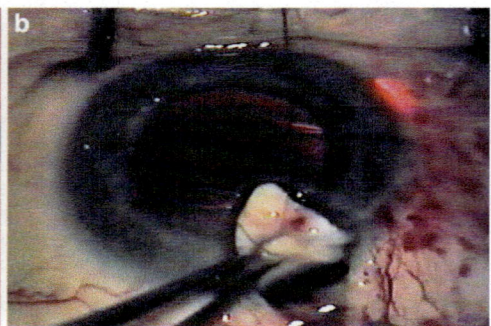

**Fig. 66.8** (a) Verification of Schlemm's canal with either a 5-0 nylon suture or microcatheter. (b) An advanced method of canal verification. A special microcatheter (iScience Interventional, Menlo Park, California) with an illuminated tip acts as a beacon to help identify the canal. The microcatheter is able to travel the entire circumference of the canal and the illuminated tip verifies the catheters position at all times. Viscoelastic may also be administered through the microcatheter

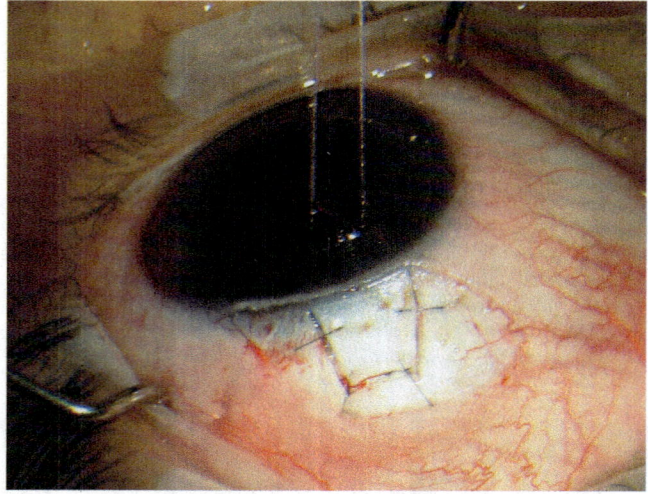

**Fig. 66.9** Closure of scleral flap. The scleral flap is always closed tightly following a trabeculotomy because excess filtration may shallow the chamber and lead to peripheral anterior synechiae

to phacoemulsification alone[9] and appears to be most effective in patients over age 70.[9] Phacotrabeculotomy lowers IOP to ≤21°mmHg in 84% of patients with medications and in 36% of patients without at 3 years.[10] Postoperative IOP spikes up to 40 mmHg may occur due to postoperative hyphema.[10]

The postoperative care for trabeculotomy is simple. The main theme is to blunt the IOP rise usually associated with postoperative day 1 hyphema. Miotics may be useful for the first two postoperative months, but not mandatory, to help keep open the drainage area and probably keep the anterior leaflets from reapproximating. Inflammation is usually minimal. Try to use as little postoperative steroids as possible for a steroid IOP response may occur.

A novel way of performing a trabeculotomy using a goniotomy transchamber-like approach with a Trabectome gives us a new method to remove a small piece of trabecular tissue to create the trabeculotomy. This may easily be carried out in conjunction with phacoemulsification for cataract surgery.[11]

# References

1. Chihara E, Nishida A, Kodo M, et al. Trabeculotomy ab externo: an alternative treatment in adult patients with primary open-angle glaucoma. *Ophthalmic Surg*. 1993;24:746–749.
2. Tanito M, Ohira A, Chihara E. Factors leading to reduced intraocular pressure after combined trabeculotomy and cataract surgery. *J Glaucoma*. 2002;11:3–9.
3. Honjo M, Tanihara T, Inatani M, et al. Phacoemulsification, intraocular lens implantation, and trabeculotomy to treat pseudoexfoliation syndrome. *J Cataract Refract Surg*. 1998;24:781–786.
4. Abdelrahman AM. Trabeculotome-guided deep sclerectomy. A pilot study. *Am J Ophthalmol*. 2005;140:152–154.
5. Fellman RL. Trabeculotomy. In: Spaeth George L, ed. *Ophthalmic Surgery: Principles and Practice*. 3rd ed. Philadelphia: Saunders; 2003.
6. Lynn JR, Fellman RL, Starita RJ. Full circumference trabeculotomy: an improved procedure for primary congenital glaucoma (Abstr). *Ophthalmology*. 1988;95(Suppl):168.
7. Beck AD, Lynch MG. 360 degress trabeculotomy for primary congenital glaucoma. *Arch Ophthalmol*. 1995;113:1200–1202.
8. Tanihara H, Honjo M, Inatani M, et al. Trabeculotomy combined with phacoemulsification and implantation of an intraocular lens for the treatment of primary open angle glaucoma and coexisting cataract. *Ophthalmic Surg Lasers*. 1997;28:810–817.
9. Tanito M, Ohira A, Chihara E. Surgical outcome of combined trabeculotomy and cataract surgery. *J Glaucoma*. 2001;10:302–308.
10. Park M, Hayashi K, Takahashi H, Tanito M, Chichara E. Phacoviscanalostomy versus phacotrabeculotomy: a middle term study. *J Glaucoma*. 2006;15:456–461.
11. Minckler DS, Baerveldt G, Alfaro MR, Francis BA. Clinical results with the Trabectome for treatment of open-angle glaucoma. *Ophthalmology*. 2005;112:962–967.

# Chapter 67
# Incisional Therapies: Canaloplasty and New Implant Devices

Diamond Y. Tam and Iqbal "Ike" K. Ahmed

Incisional surgery for the treatment of glaucoma was first described in 1896 with surgical iridectomy,[1] followed by corneo–scleral trephination in the 1920s[2] and full thickness procedures in the 1950s.[3] In 1968, Cairns described the technique of trabeculectomy,[4] still considered by many today to be the gold standard of glaucoma surgery. Techniques have been modified and the addition of adjunctive antimetabolites has perhaps improved the original procedure to enhance long-term success and survival, as measured by intraocular pressure reduction and control, but the common final goal remains to create and maintain a nonphysiologic fistula from the anterior chamber to the subconjunctival space. Although lowering of intraocular pressure (IOP) is undisputable and well established, the generous complication profile of these procedures is well known. Both short-term and long-term risks of blebitis, endophthalmitis, hypotony, overfiltration, bleb leaks, dysesthesia, overhang, encapsulation, corneal dellen, endothelial cell loss, episcleral fibrosis, aqueous misdirection, and accelerated cataract formation are some of the many potential complications, most of which are lifetime risks for patients undergoing trabeculectomy.[5]

Prior to the advent of trabeculectomy, the first glaucoma drainage device emerged in 1906 with the implantation of a horse hair through a corneal paracentesis in a patient with a blind painful hypertensive eye.[6] While this had fairly obvious limitations and risks, the first tube and plate device was introduced in the late 1960s by Molteno.[7,8] This was followed by several variations including the Krupin eye disc,[9] Baerveldt tube and plate shunt,[10] and the Ahmed valve.[11] These long tube shunt devices are designed to allow a conduit for aqueous humor to flow from the anterior chamber to a reservoir in the posterior subconjunctival space, usually 10–12 mm posterior to the limbus. Like trabeculectomy, these procedures, while effective, have a significant risk of hypotony and suprachoroidal hemorrhage. Tube shunts, although filtering aqueous posteriorly, share some similar postoperative challenges with trabeculectomy, such as bleb encapsulation and fibrosis. While posterior filtration may be less likely to encounter these issues, as the bleb is further from the metabolically active limbal zone, tube shunts have their own unique set of postoperative risks, such as tube or plate exposure, tube lumen occlusion, corneal endothelial loss even with proper tube positioning, tube migration, ptosis, and diplopia.

Because of the unpredictability of wound healing modulation, flow control, the nonphysiologic nature of subconjunctival filtration, the significant risk of hypotony and other visually devastating complications, new glaucoma surgical approaches have emerged toward the enhancement of physiologic mechanisms of aqueous outflow.

In 1893, De Vicentiis first described surgery of the iridocorneal angle in patients with congenital glaucoma. Goniotomy followed in the 1940s, described by Barkan.[12,13] Since then procedures involving the iridocorneal angle have continued to emerge, from laser trabeculopuncture, to goniocurretage, to the Trabectome microelectrocautery device (NeoMedix Corp. San Juan Capistrano, California) and the trabecular microbypass stent (Glaukos Corp., Laguna Hills, California). *Ab externo* approaches to Schlemm's canal have also been developed such as the nonpenetrating canaloplasty using the iScience microcatheter device (iScience Interventional Inc., Menlo Park, California).

Aqueous humor alternatively exits the anterior chamber via the uveoscleral outflow pathway, consisting of the interstitium of the ciliary body, the suprachoroidal space, and choroidal and scleral vasculature. While this pathway, reportedly comprising anywhere from 20 to 54% of total aqueous outflow,[14,15] is commonly augmented medically by prostaglandin analogs, surgical approaches to enhance suprachoroidal draining have also been attempted first with cyclodialysis, followed by suprachoroidal seton devices and implants. Recently, a gold micro-shunt has been developed to act as a conduit between the anterior chamber and the suprachoroidal space (SOLX Inc., Waltham, Massachusetts).

This chapter reviews the various new surgical devices except for the trabecular micro-bypass stent (Glaukos Corp., Laguna Hills, California), which is discussed in another chapter.

## 67.1 Basic Review of Anatomy and Physiology of Aqueous Outflow

Aqueous humor production begins with the epithelium of the ciliary body behind the iris, travels forward through the pupillary aperture into the anterior chamber, and exits the eye through the anterior chamber angle. The delicate regulation of this pathway is responsible for the control of IOP. Overproduction or decrease in egress or filtration results in elevated IOP, commonly leading to optic neuropathy. While surgical approaches directed at decreasing aqueous production involve cyclodestruction via transscleral diode laser, transscleral cryoablation, or more recently endoscopic diode laser cycloablation, many novel techniques and devices have emerged to enhance outflow.

The two physiologic outflow pathways in the normal human eye are the conventional pathway and the uveoscleral outflow pathway. The conventional pathway consists of the trabecular meshwork, Schlemm's canal, and distal intrascleral and episcleral venous plexi. The uveoscleral outflow pathway consists of the interstitium of the ciliary body, the suprachoroidal space, and ultimately scleral or choroidal vasculature. Alternatively, while subconjunctival filtration is nonphysiologic, it still remains the most widely utilized means of surgical IOP reduction via trabeculectomy and tube shunt procedures.

### 67.1.1 Subconjunctival Filtration

#### 67.1.1.1 Anterior Subconjunctival Filtration

Filtration of aqueous humor into the anterior subconjunctival space is achieved by the procedure of trabeculectomy, where a fistula is created from the anterior chamber under a scleral flap, to the subconjunctival space to form what is commonly known as a bleb. Once entering this space, aqueous humor is absorbed by episcleral and scleral vasculature to eventually enter the orbital circulation. This procedure thus bypasses both the conventional and uveoscleral outflow pathways and results in a nonphysiologic means of IOP lowering.

The success of anterior subconjunctival filtration depends upon both intra- and postoperative factors. During surgery, ostium size and scleral flap suture tension determine the amount of aqueous egress, while postoperatively, episcleral fibrosis and wound healing ultimately determine bleb survival. Although surgical techniques have improved and postoperative care has evolved with the use of adjustable sutures, postoperative laser suture lysis, the advent of antimetabolites such as mitomycin-C and 5-fluorouracil, achieving a therapeutically low IOP whilst avoiding hypotony, remains a major challenge. In a recent 5-year follow-up report of trabeculectomy with adjunctive mitomycin-C, a surprising 42% rate of hypotony, defined as an IOP lower than 6 mmHg at 6 months postoperatively, was reported.[16] Additionally, antimetabolite-related complications must also be considered, including endothelial cell toxicity; delayed conjunctival wound healing; avascular encapsulated limbal blebs, which are at risk of leaking, especially with small intraoperative application zones; and perhaps most significantly, persistent long-term hypotony.[17-20]

Despite these potentially visually devastating early and late complications of trabeculectomy, its technical ease of performance, familiarity to all glaucoma surgeons, and well-documented efficacy in IOP lowering cause it to remain arguably the most commonly performed glaucoma surgical procedure today.

#### 67.1.1.2 Posterior Subconjunctival Filtration

The Molteno, Krupin, Ahmed, Baerveldt, and OptiMed glaucoma drainage devices share the tube and plate design whereby a tube is placed into the anterior chamber connecting to a plate reservoir fixated to the postequatorial sclera. This design allows aqueous humor to egress from the anterior chamber to the posterior subconjunctival space away from the active limbal zone with the potential advantages of less extensive subconjunctival fibrosis, a potentially larger reservoir for aqueous fluid, and lower incidence of bleb dysesthesia.

Although traditionally reserved for patients who have failed primary trabeculectomy or who have conjunctival pathology, which makes such a procedure less likely to succeed, recent reports have shown that the long nonvalved tube shunt devices have a lower incidence of postoperative complications, avoid persistent hypotony, and maintain good IOP control over a 1-year period when compared to a repeat trabeculectomy with adjunctive mitomycin-C.[21,22] Current studies are ongoing comparing primary trabeculectomy versus primary tube shunt procedures as well as comparing valved versus nonvalved long tube shunt devices.

### 67.1.2 Schlemm's Canal Outflow

#### 67.1.2.1 Proximal Outflow System

The conventional outflow system can be thought of as consisting of a proximal and a distal component. The proximal outflow system includes the uveoscleral, corneoscleral and juxtacanalicular trabecular meshwork, Schlemm's canal and its collector channels. The distal outflow system includes aqueous veins and the episcleral and scleral venous plexi. Early work by Grant in the 1950s yielded strong evidence that the juxtacanalicular trabecular meshwork (JTM) and the extracellular matrix accounted for 75% of aqueous outflow resistance with elevation of IOP in glaucoma due to resistance at the JTM and/or collapse of Schlemm's canal.[23-25]

Because of the nonphysiologic nature of subconjunctival filtration surgery and the significant risk profile in both the short- and long-term, the quest for a safer alternative has been ongoing since the 1950s. *Ab externo* Schlemm's canal surgery and nonpenetrating glaucoma surgery first emerged in the 1960s as "sinusotomy,"[26-29] followed by guarded deep scleral flaps in the 1980s,[30-32] viscodilation of Schlemm's canal in the 1990s,[33] and then various implants and drainage devices under a scleral flap in the late 1990s and early 2000s.[34-38] While early nonpenetrating procedures have been able to avoid some of the risks of fistulizing surgery, success of these early procedures still relied on the formation of a bleb. More recently, viscocanalostomy attempted to re-expand a segment of Schlemm's canal, but expansion of the entire circumference was not possible until recently with the development of a microcatheter to cannulate the entire 360° (iScience Interventional Inc., Menlo Park, California). The 200 μm microcatheter allows for 360° viscodilation of Schlemm's canal as well as suture passage to maintain mechanical expansion of the canal. Recent studies have revealed effectiveness in IOP reduction as well as proportional decrease in IOP in relation to the degree of distension of Schlemm's canal.[39] In addition, data released by iScience has shown an increase in trans-trabecular aqueous flow with increased centripetal tension of the canal suture (Fig. 67.1).

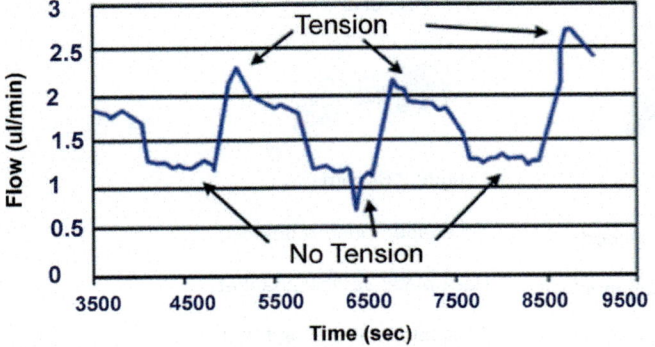

**Fig. 67.1** A graph comparing the aqueous flow across the trabecular meshwork and the inner wall of Schlemm's canal with and without tension on a Prolene suture in the canal. Reprinted from Tam DY, Ahmed IK. New glaucoma surgical devices. In: Franz Grehn F, Stamper R, eds. Glaucoma [Essentials in Ophthalmology series]. Berlin: Springer; 2009 with permission from Springer

*Ab interno* Schlemm's canal surgery has also emerged with the premise that if the major resistance point in aqueous outflow is the JTM, devices which result in bypass of this point of resistance should result in lowering of IOP. Although goniotomy in adults and laser trabeculopuncture have been largely unsuccessful as a result of scarring in the surgical area,[40-44] new devices such as the trabecular microbypass stent (Glaukos Corp., Laguna Hills, California) and the Trabectome microelectrocautery device (NeoMedix Corp., San Juan Capistrano, California) have been designed to allow aqueous humor to bypass the resistance of the JTM and enter Schlemm's canal directly. The trabecular microbypass stent is a titanium L-shaped half pipe designed to rest in Schlemm's canal with a snorkel into the anterior chamber.[45] The Trabectome microelectrocautery device is designed with the purpose of removing trabecular meshwork to allow aqueous to directly contact Schlemm's canal. Initial studies and clinical data have shown these devices to be effective in IOP reduction and in decreasing the number of glaucoma medications required for IOP control.[46-49]

### 67.1.2.2 Distal Outflow System

After entrance into Schlemm's canal and its collector channels, aqueous humor enters the surrounding circulation through aqueous veins and ultimately episcleral and intrascleral venous plexi. The relationship between episcleral venous pressure (EVP) and IOP has been established since the 1950s.[50] As further evidence that elevated IOP was indeed correlated to raised EVP, patients in an inverted posture were found to have an elevated IOP.[51] While the normal EVP varies between individuals, it may range from 8 to 13 mmHg, theoretically being the lowest possible attainable IOP from Schlemm's canal surgery. Patients with conditions predisposing to elevated EVP such as Sturge–Weber syndrome, venous obstructive disease, arteriovenous malformations in the orbit, head, neck, or mediastinum are prone to elevated IOP resulting in glaucomatous optic atrophy.[52,53] Surgical approaches and attempts at reducing EVP have yet to be described or reported.

### 67.1.3 *Suprachoroidal Outflow*

Aqueous humor exits the anterior chamber also via the uveoscleral pathway, consisting of the interstitium of the ciliary body, the suprachoroidal space, and ultimately choroidal and scleral vasculature. Augmentation of outflow via this pathway is achieved using prostaglandin analogues medically, and, historically, by creation of a cyclodialysis cleft separation of the ciliary body from the sclera via both *ab externo* and *ab interno* approaches.[54-58] Although this often resulted in early successful lowering of IOP, these procedures had several limitations and risks including possible prolonged irreversible hypotony, intraoperative and postoperative hemorrhage due to the vascular nature of uveal tissue, and late closure with scarring of the cleft leading to rapid onset of IOP spikes. One study reported that 75% of patients undergoing *ab interno* cyclodialysis cleft creation required further surgical intervention at just 60 days postoperatively.[55] Yet others have attempted to prevent closure and fibrosis of a created cyclodialysis cleft with use of implants such as high molecular weight hyaluronic acid, Teflon tube implants, hydroxyethyl methacrylate capillary strip, and a scleral strip.[59-62] However, these implants have yet to demonstrate successful long-term control of IOP in human eyes with glaucoma. Suprachoroidal seton device implantation has also been reported but likewise without successful long-term control of IOP. Furthermore, implantation of sizeable devices in the suprachoroidal space carries risks of suprachoroidal hemorrhage, choroidal detachment and atrophy, and exudative retinal detachment.[63,64] The gold suprachoroidal shunt (SOLX Inc., Waltham, Massachusetts) is a new *ab externo* device designed to provide a pathway for aqueous to travel through and around the shunt from the anterior chamber into the suprachoroidal space to augment uveoscleral outflow.

## 67.2 The EX-PRESS Shunt: A Subconjunctival Filtration Device

While trabeculectomy has been well established as a potent IOP lowering procedure, late hypotony, defined as an IOP of less than 6 mmHg at 6 months, has been reported in 42% of patients.[16] Although a well established procedure and technically familiar to all glaucoma surgeons, inconsistency even between cases of the same surgeon may yield differing ostium sizes and thus, differing amounts of flow. Because of these challenges, as well as the unacceptably high rate of hypotony, the Ex-PRESS Mini Glaucoma Shunt (Optonol Ltd., Neve Ilan, Israel) has been developed to attempt to improve performance and consistency in trabeculectomy.

Four designs of this stainless steel device exist (R-50, X-50, T-50, X-200) with the same functional design, but differing in dimensions and lumen size with the X-200 shunt having a 200 µm wide lumen while the others with 50 µm lumens (Fig. 67.2). The tip of the shunt consists of one or multiple orifices, which sit in the anterior chamber and allow aqueous to drain through the 27-gauge shaft, designed to approximate the thickness of human sclera. On the underside of the shaft, a spur is present to prevent extrusion of the device out of the anterior chamber, while the scleral side of the shunt consists of an external plate, which prevents the shunt from migrating into the anterior chamber. While the original intent of the shunt was for placement directly under the conjunctiva into the anterior chamber, the high incidence of resultant hypotony, conjunctival erosion and shunt migration required placement of the shunt under a trabeculectomy style scleral flap.[66,67] The device appears to be safe in patients undergoing magnetic resonance imaging (MRI) as well as biocompatible to human ocular tissue.[70]

The surgical placement of the shunt begins as if one were to perform a trabeculectomy, with a conjunctival peritomy, gentle cautery, and creation of a scleral flap. Because of the size of the external footplate of the shunt, the scleral flap may have to be slightly larger in dimension than that performed during standard trabeculectomy in order to attain full coverage of the footplate. After the scleral flap has been constructed, the anterior chamber is inflated with viscoelastic or air, particularly in the

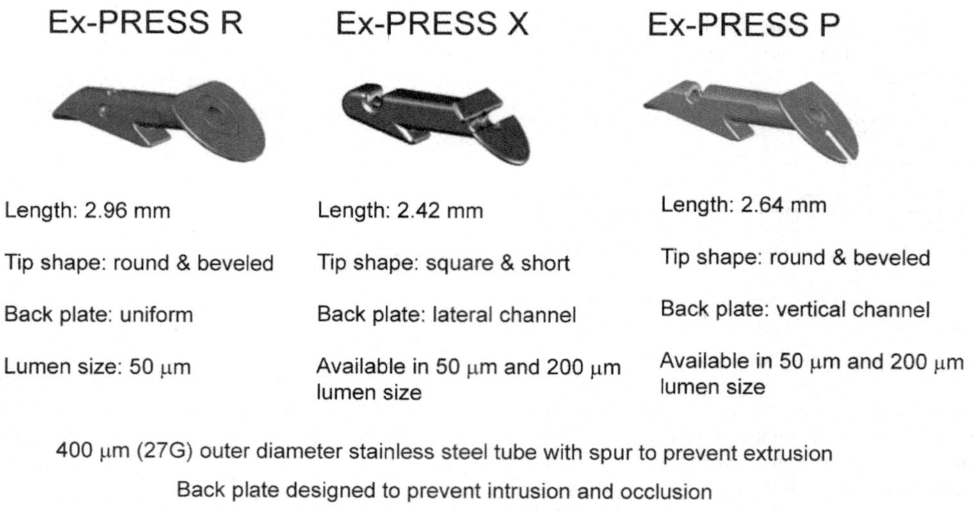

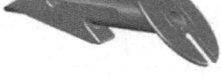

| Ex-PRESS R | Ex-PRESS X | Ex-PRESS P |
|---|---|---|
| Length: 2.96 mm | Length: 2.42 mm | Length: 2.64 mm |
| Tip shape: round & beveled | Tip shape: square & short | Tip shape: round & beveled |
| Back plate: uniform | Back plate: lateral channel | Back plate: vertical channel |
| Lumen size: 50 µm | Available in 50 µm and 200 µm lumen size | Available in 50 µm and 200 µm lumen size |

400 µm (27G) outer diameter stainless steel tube with spur to prevent extrusion

Back plate designed to prevent intrusion and occlusion

**Fig. 67.2** A schematic diagram of the different models of the Ex-PRESS shunt with specifications listed below each

area where the shunt will be placed. Identification of the scleral spur is critical to the correct placement of the shunt. At the base of the scleral flap, this anatomical landmark should be readily identifiable, and intraoperative gonioscopy can be used to confirm this. At this point, an entry is made into the anterior chamber exactly at the level of the scleral spur with a 27-gauge needle or sapphire blade (manufactured by Optonol) (Fig. 67.3). The angle of entry must be parallel to the iris in order to ensure proper shunt positioning. An entry that is angled toward the iris results in the shunt embedded in the iris, risking incarceration; and likewise an entry toward the cornea may result in shunt-to-cornea touch and endothelial trauma. The shunt is preloaded on an injector system and is released by the surgeon using the index finger once it has been successfully placed in the previously created needle track entry (Figs. 67.4 and 67.5). Flow through the shunt is then assessed by dry removal of viscoelastic from the anterior chamber using a blunt cannula and irrigation of balanced saline solution (BSS) through the anterior chamber. A peripheral surgical iridectomy is not required. Scleral flap and conjunctival flap closure is then performed in the same manner as standard trabeculectomy. Although the shunt itself is designed to restrict flow, diligent assessment of scleral flap tension must still be performed as excess flow may still occur in the presence of the shunt (Figs. 67.6 and 67.7). Once satisfactory flow has been achieved, watertight conjunctival closure must also be achieved.

As the Ex-PRESS shunt relies on a subconjunctival bleb for IOP control, it too may require similar postoperative adjunctive procedures as trabeculectomy such as laser suture lysis and bleb needling with or without anti-metabolites. While similar to standard trabeculectomy in the mode of filtration and reliance on a bleb, the Ex-PRESS shunt has the advantages of providing a constant orifice size for filtration, requiring a smaller entry into the anterior chamber, obviating the need for

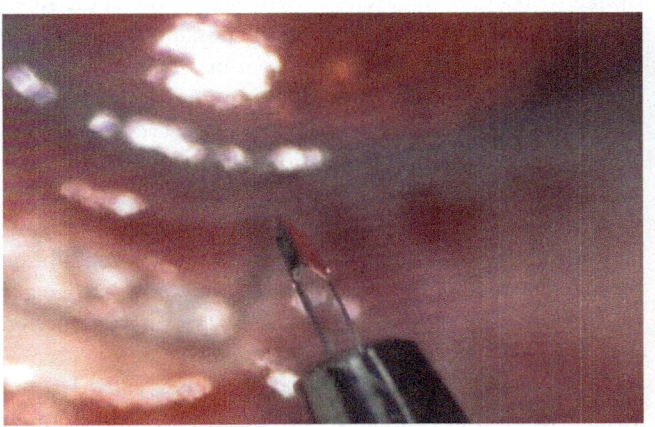

**Fig. 67.3** The sapphire blade specifically manufactured for creating the entrance into the anterior chamber for the Ex-PRESS shunt

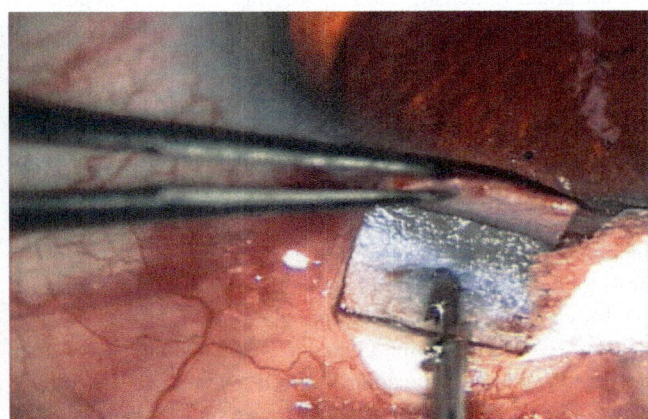

**Fig. 67.5** The Ex-PRESS shunt is inserted into the opening at the level of the scleral spur. Turning the shunt 90° may facilitate its entry

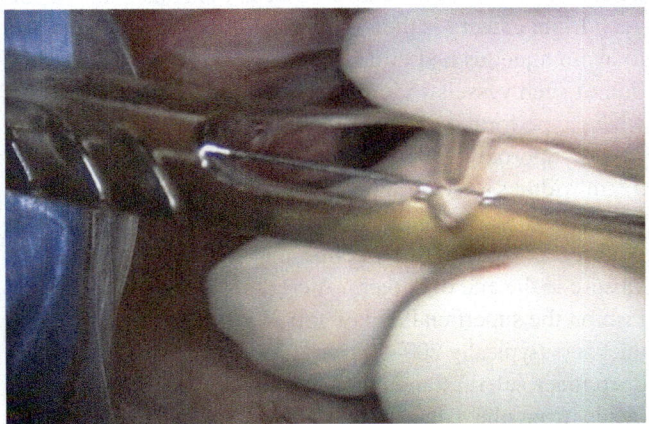

**Fig. 67.4** The handle of the Ex-PRESS shunt injector showing the metal wire under the plastic apparatus that is to be depressed by the surgeon's index finger when the shunt is to be released from the tip

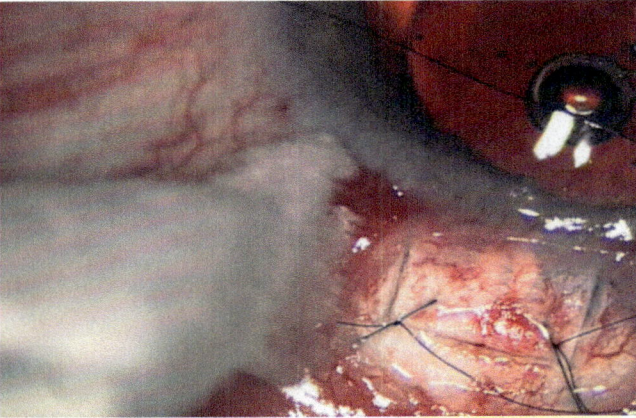

**Fig. 67.6** Two interrupted 10–0 nylon sutures are placed into the scleral flap. Tension is adjusted via a slipknot technique. The Ex-PRESS shunt footplate can be seen through the scleral flap with the tip of the shunt visible in the anterior chamber

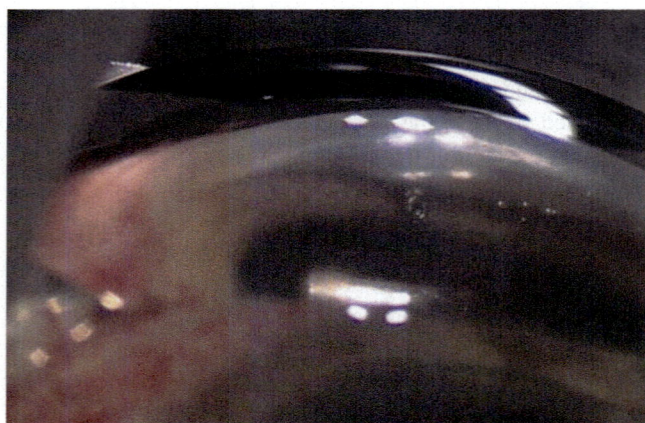

Fig. 67.7 A gonioscopic view of the Ex-PRESS shunt in the anterior chamber

a surgical iridectomy, and providing two-tiered control of IOP via the shunt lumen size and scleral flap tension. It is possible to inject the device in a highly controlled manner.[65] However, despite the design of the shunt to regulate flow, hypotony and overfiltration remain postoperative risks; although when compared to trabeculectomy, some studies have shown that the complication profile, hypotony, and related complications are less frequent in the early postoperative period.[66] Although exclusion criteria advised for the use of the Ex-PRESS shunt includes narrow and closed angle glaucoma, it has been our anecdotal experience that it is as well suited for this angle morphology as it is for the open angle glaucomas.

The Ex-PRESS Mini Glaucoma Shunt is a new device designed to improve the control of IOP and reduce the complication profile of subconjunctival filtration surgery. However, the shunt still relies on a nonphysiologic bleb as the mechanism of IOP lowering, much like trabeculectomy, and therefore the same short-term and long-term complications associated with blebs apply also to the Ex-PRESS shunt. Advantages of the shunt over trabeculectomy include a possibly lowered early postoperative incidence of hypotony, the elimination of the need for a surgical iridectomy, and ease of learning the procedure due to its similarity to performing a standard trabeculectomy. Although it was initially implanted without a scleral flap, the use of a "trabeculectomy-like" flap has made the insertion of this device more appealing.[68] Furthermore, the efficacy of the device has been demonstrated when combined with phacoemulsification.[69]

## 67.3 Schlemm's Canal Devices

### 67.3.1 Nonpenetrating Ab Externo Schlemm's Canaloplasty

Canaloplasty is the procedure by which catheterization of Schlemm's canal is achieved via an *ab externo* approach in order to restore and enhance physiologic aqueous outflow through the conventional pathway thus avoiding a subconjunctival bleb. Expansion of Schlemm's canal was first described by Stegmann as viscocanalostomy, a nonpenetrating procedure, wherein two cut ends of the canal were inflated with viscoelastic spanning a few clock hours.[33] Various implants were used in an attempt to enhance the success of nonpenetrating surgery in the early 2000s, but these procedures continued to rely on a bleb for IOP control.[34-36] Recently, a device has been developed to allow 360° cannulation of Schlemm's canal to expand the entire circumference with viscoelastic and also to allow a suture to be delivered within the canal to exert centripetal force maintaining expansion of the canal. This procedure, termed canaloplasty, aims to restore physiologic outflow via the conventional pathway with suture-assisted canal distension, foregoing the need for a bleb or fistula.

Although in theory Schlemm's canal can be accessed from any location, the usual chosen surgery site is the superior sclera, for eyelid coverage, in the possible event of bleb formation, as well as for patient comfort. This requires the patient to maintain a downgaze position for the majority of the procedure. While, in the authors' experience, topical anesthesia and patient cooperation usually is sufficient for successful performance of the surgery, a traction suture may be utilized to assist in globe positioning, and retrobulbar or peribulbar block as well. In some cases, general anesthesia may be required. If a corneal traction suture is utilized, careful site selection is required to ensure the suture is placed several clock hours away from the intended surgical site.

A fornix-based conjunctival peritomy is created leaving an anterior skirt of conjunctiva attached to the limbus. Blunt dissection is carried out posteriorly to ensure that the posterior edge is relaxed sufficiently to allow for creation of a 5 mm × 5 mm parabolic scleral flap. The posterior conjunctiva should also be easily brought forward to appose to the anterior lip to allow for easy closure at the conclusion of surgery. Light cautery is then applied to the sclera, being careful to avoid aqueous and ciliary veins. Observation of the location of such vessels should also affect the initial selection of where to perform the dissection. A superficial parabolic scleral flap of approximately 5 mm anterior–posterior length by 5 mm width is then outlined on the scleral surface (Fig. 67.8). Although this scleral flap may be any shape, it is the authors' preference to create a parabolic flap to facilitate watertight closure at the end of surgery. A crescent knife is then used to fashion the superficial flap of approximately one-third scleral thickness (typically 200–300 µm) forward into clear cornea. A deep inner scleral flap is then outlined approximately 1 mm inside from the edge of the superficial scleral flap. Once again, the crescent knife is used to fashion the deep flap and carry it forward directly into Schlemm's canal. An approximately 100 µm thick layer of sclera should be left covering the choroid at the base of the deep dissection (Fig. 67.9).

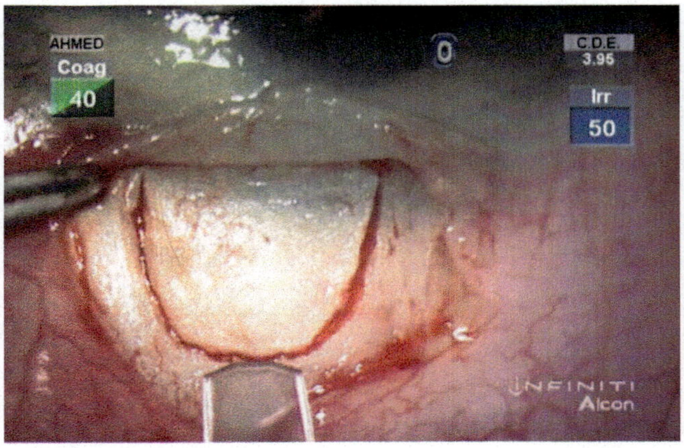

# 67 Incisional Therapies: Canaloplasty and New Implant Devices

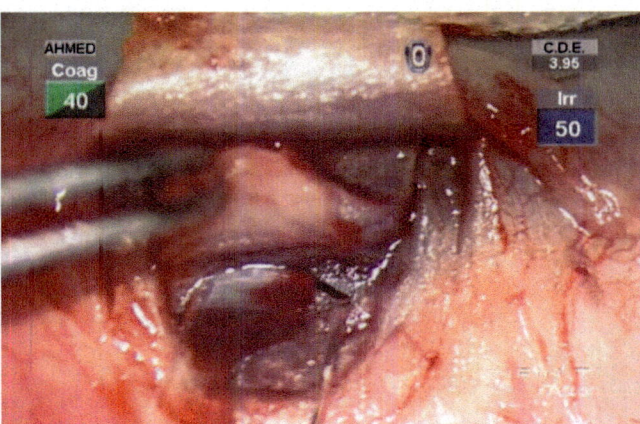

**Fig. 67.8** The scleral flap for canaloplasty is outlined in a parabolic shape

**Fig. 67.10** Schlemm's canal is exposed with a crescent blade

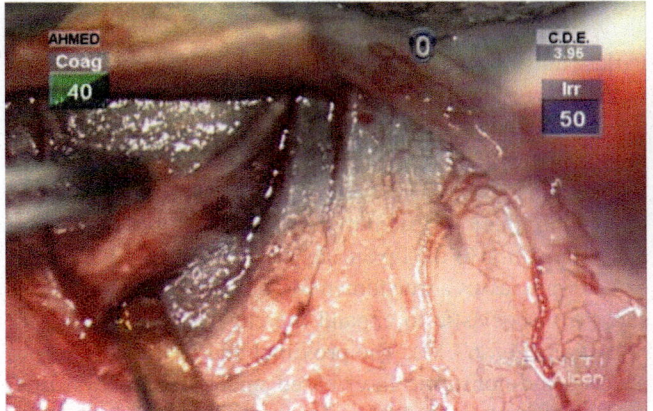

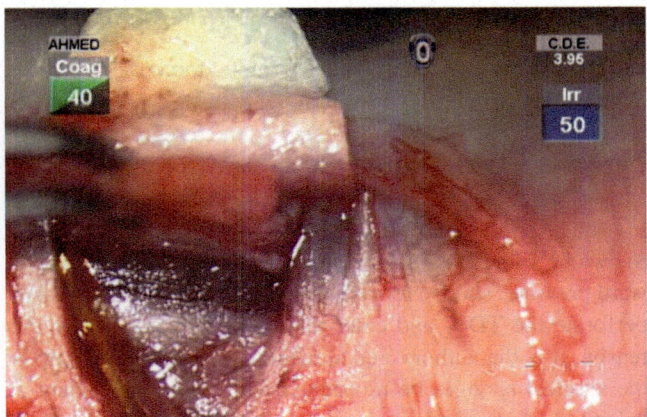

**Fig. 67.9** After a superficial flap has been fashioned, a deeper scleral flap is created with slightly smaller dimensions than that of the superficial flap

**Fig. 67.11** The radial edges of the deep scleral flap are then released being careful not to penetrate into the globe

It is not uncommon to be left with a full thickness dissection at some points of the dissection of the deep flap. Care must then be taken to reestablish a tissue plane leaving a thin layer of sclera in the bed of the dissection. It is of utmost importance that the surgeon maintains an adequate depth during the deep flap dissection in order to unroof Schlemm's canal (Figs. 67.10 and 67.11). If the dissection is too deep, then penetration into the globe occurs, while if the dissection is too superficial, which is more common, it is possible to dissect and pass right over Schlemm's canal into clear cornea without exposing the canal itself. This results in a difficult situation where a deeper plane of dissection needs to be established with only a thin layer of residual sclera in the bed. Identification of the proper anatomical landmarks is often challenging in these situations and there is a resultant higher likelihood of penetration into the anterior chamber unintentionally.

Once the white limbus-parallel fibers of the scleral spur are visible at the deep dissection, fibers of the outer wall of Schlemm's canal should be visible by lifting of the deep flap with a toothed forceps. Aqueous humor may be observed to percolate through the Schlemm's canal and blood regurgitation may be encountered from the cut ends of the canal (Fig. 67.12). A paracentesis incision should be made in the clear cornea away from the surgical site to lower the IOP to single digits levels to prevent outward bulging of Descemet's membrane and the inner wall of Schlemm's canal, lowering the likelihood of penetration into the anterior chamber during the ensuing delicate dissection. The deep flap is now advanced forward approximately another 1 mm to expose Descemet's membrane. Aqueous humor may again be observed to percolate through Descemet's membrane in the anterior bed of the deep dissection commonly known as the trabeculodescemet window (TDW). In some instances, to increase aqueous

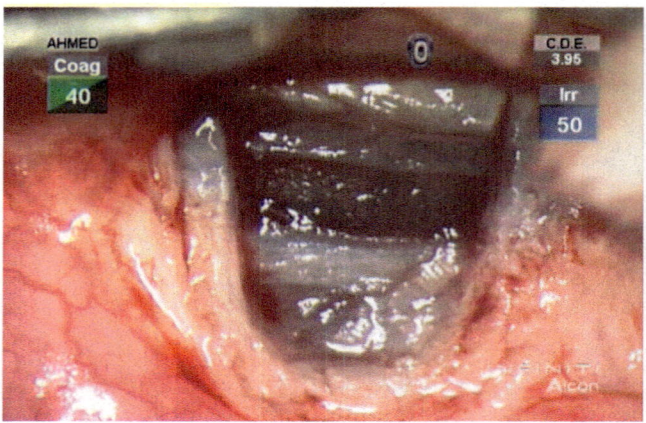

**Fig. 67.12** Once the deep flap has been excised, the trabeculodescemet window (TDW) can be seen. Note than heme is emerging from the two cut ends of Schlemm's canal

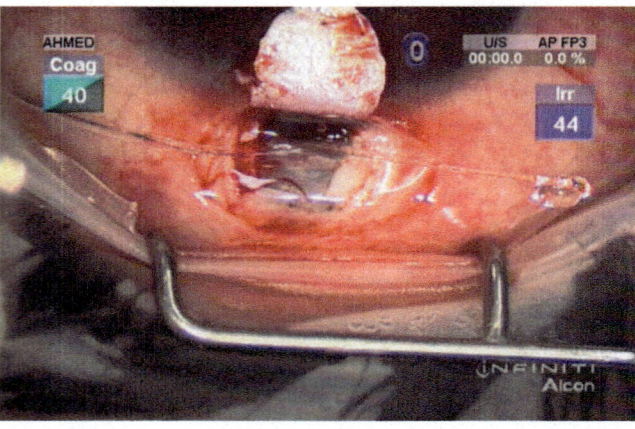

**Fig. 67.13** Once the entire circumference of the canal has been cannulated with the iScience microcatheter, the device is primed with ophthalmic viscosurgical device, which can be seen emerging from the tip of the device on the right

percolation through the TDW, a Mermoud forceps can be used to delicately strip the inner wall of Schlemm's canal away. The corneal stroma should be separated from Descemet's window with surgical sponges such as Merocel (Merocel Corp., North Mystic, Connecticut) and Weck-cel (Medtronic, Jacksonville, Florida) sponges carefully and gently pushing down on Schwalbe's line and Descemet's membrane. Excessive downward pressure, sudden movements, or a dry sponge may easily perforate the TDW and enter the anterior chamber. For this reason, it is the authors' recommendation that the very tip of the surgical sponges be moistened with a minute amount of balanced saline solution prior to use on the surgical field. Once the TDW has been satisfactorily fashioned, the underside of the deep flap is scored with a sharp tip blade at the very anterior aspect and cut off with Vannas scissors. Each cut end of Schlemm's canal is then intubated with a 150-μm outer bore viscocanalostomy cannula, and a very small amount of high viscosity sodium hyaluronate, such as Healon GV (Advanced Medical Optics Inc., Santa Ana, California), is injected into each end to dilate the ostia and facilitate entrance of the iScience device into the canal.

In the normal human eye, Schlemm's canal is known to be of 300 μm in diameter. Studies have shown evidence to suggest that the canal, however, collapses in glaucoma as a result of increased trabecular meshwork and inner wall resistance.[71] A vicious cycle may then be set up, wherein the elevated IOP further compresses Schlemm's canal because of the reduced circumferential flow of aqueous from the canal into its collector channels. The iScience device aims to restore the patency and re-expand the canal using a 45-mm working length flexible polymer microcatheter of 200-μm shaft diameter with a rounded 250-μm tip diameter designed to be atraumatic to, and to guide the 360° passage and catheterization of, Schlemm's canal (iScience Interventional Inc., Menlo Park, California). The catheter consists of a central support wire designed to provide a backbone for guidance during advancement and to add resistance to potential kinking of the microcatheter. The optical fibers in the microcatheter allow for transmission of a red blinking light from a laser-based micro-illumination system to the tip to assist in visualization and localization of the tip during passage. Thirdly, the microcatheter possesses a true lumen for the delivery of substances such as viscoelastic to expand the canal during passage or retraction (Fig. 67.13). The proximal end of the device connects to the nonsterile laser-based micro-illumination light source on a mayo stand from one arm, with another arm connected to a sterile screw-mechanism syringe designed to assist in controlled injection of viscoelastic into Schlemm's canal. The microcatheter is then secured to the surgical drape with surgical tape such as Steri-strips (3M, St. Paul, Minnesota). Two nontoothed forceps are then used to introduce the microcatheter into one of the cut ends of Schlemm's canal and advanced 360° until the tip emerges from the other cut end of the canal. Although in the vast majority of patients, this passage is possible, a minority of patients will not allow successful catheter passage through the entirety of the canal. In addition, the authors have observed the microcatheter pass into the suprachoroidal space posterior to Schlemm's canal. In these cases, early recognition of unusual location of the blinking red light is of utmost importance and the catheter retracted to attempt passage again with scleral depression or removal of the entire microcatheter and passage attempted in the opposite direction.

Once the microcatheter has been passed 360° and the tip has emerged, a 10–0 Prolene suture with the needles cut off is tied around the shaft of the device near the tip with the two loose ends tied to the loop (Fig. 67.14). The device is then withdrawn carefully in the reverse direction to which it was

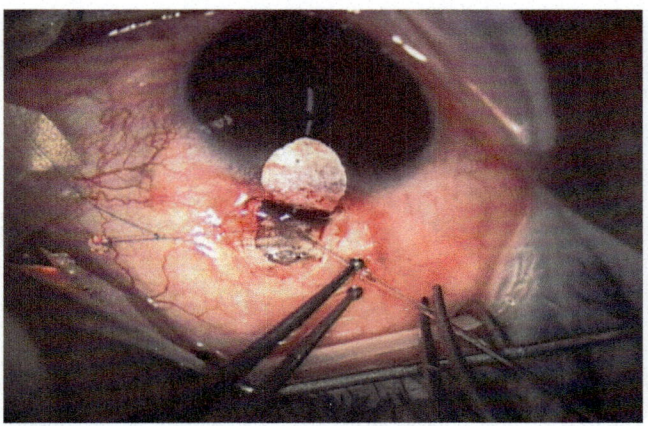

**Fig. 67.14** A 10–0 Prolene suture is tied around the end of the device prior to its retraction

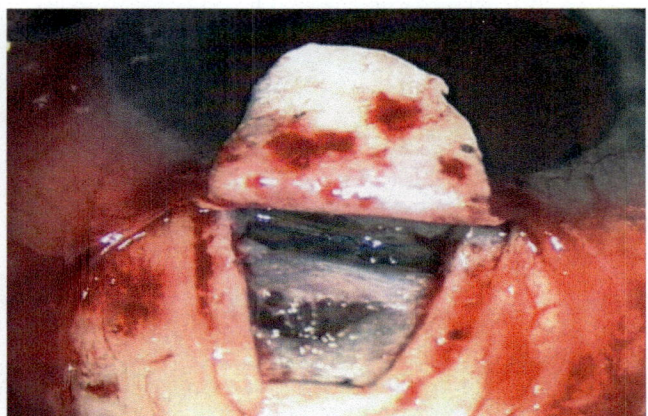

**Fig. 67.16** The two suture knots can be seen resting on the TDW

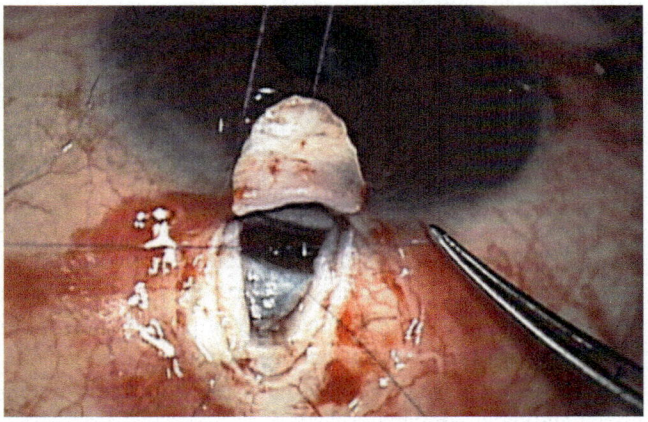

**Fig. 67.15** Once the suture has been delivered and cut away from the microcatheter, the two cut ends must be matched and tied together

passed, with controlled injection of viscoelastic into the canal by a surgical assistant. Care must be taken not to inject an excessive amount of viscoelastic into Schlemm's canal as a Descemet's detachment can occur. Regurgitation of heme into the anterior chamber is also commonly seen during passage or withdrawal of the microcatheter. Once the catheter has been removed, the 10–0 Prolene is cut from the tip, essentially leaving two single 10–0 Prolene sutures in the canal with two loose ends emerging from each cut end of Schlemm's canal. The surgeon must then identify the corresponding ends and each suture is tied to itself in a slipknot fashion with some back and forth movement in the canal, known as "flossing," to ensure that the suture sits anteriorly in Schlemm's canal. Suture tension is then assessed by observing the amount of indentation of the TDW, as well as by pulling the suture knot posteriorly, until it is only barely able to reach the scleral spur (Figs. 67.15 and 67.16). The suture is postulated to produce a surgical pilocarpine-like effect by putting the trabecular meshwork on tension and thus enhancing flow through Schlemm's canal and its collector channels. Suture tension is felt to play an important role in canaloplasty, where a greater suture tension results in more distension of Schlemm's canal with resultant greater IOP reduction and increased flow.[39]

The superficial scleral flap is then placed back into position and sutured in a watertight fashion with five interrupted 10–0 nylon sutures. High viscosity sodium hyaluronate is then injected under the superficial scleral flap using the viscocanalostomy cannula in order to maintain the scleral lake – the space where aqueous humor that has percolated through the TDW accumulates and is then absorbed into episcleral, scleral, and choroidal circulation. The conjunctiva is then closed over the surgical site in a watertight fashion with a 10–0 Vicryl suture in a running horizontal mattress fashion.

Canaloplasty seeks to restore aqueous outflow through the conventional outflow pathway into Schlemm's canal and its collector channels to control IOP. However, the potential space under the superficial scleral flap, or the scleral lake, also allows for aqueous humor to drain into multiple pathways such as the cut ends of Schlemm's canal, the surrounding scleral and episcleral vasculature, the suprachoroidal space, and even subconjunctivally in some patients, resulting in a bleb despite a watertight closure. It has been the authors' experience that fibrosis of the TDW can occur postoperatively with a resultant elevated IOP that requires YAG (yttrium–aluminum–garnet) laser to puncture the TDW, restoring aqueous flow to the scleral lake and resulting in IOP control (Figs. 67.17 and 67.18). A recent study demonstrated that 94 patients who underwent canaloplasty had an IOP reduction from 24.6 to 14.9 mmHg with a decrease in medication usage from 1.9 to 0.6 medications.[39] A similar efficacy was observed in patients undergoing combined phacoemulsification and intraocular lens implantation surgery with canaloplasty.[72] Complications reported were elevated IOP and hyphema, most commonly, with

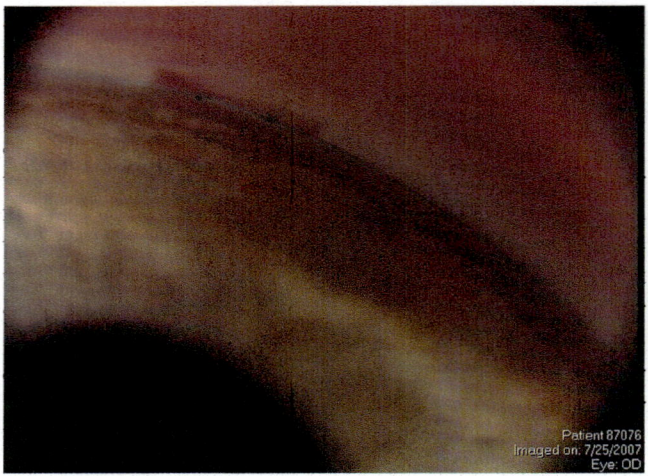

**Fig. 67.17** Postoperative gonioscopic photograph of the TDW with the two suture knots

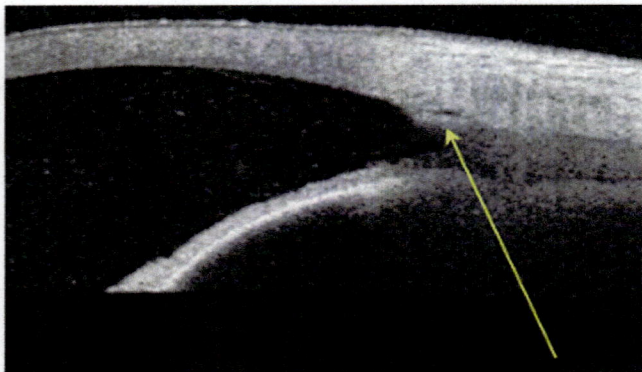

**Fig. 67.19** An anterior segment OCT image showing the anterior distension and expansion of Schlemm's canal induced by the intracanalicular suture. Reprinted from Tam DY, Ahmed IK. New glaucoma surgical devices. In: Franz Grehn F, Stamper R (eds). Glaucoma [Essentials in Ophthalmology series]. Berlin: Springer; 2009 with permission from Springer

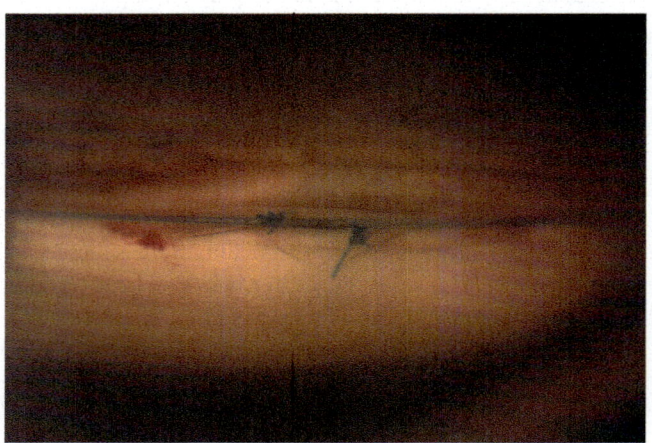

**Fig. 67.18** Postoperatively, Nd:YAG laser goniopuncture may be required to break the TDW membrane to augment aqueous egress from the anterior chamber. Note the scrolled edges of the Descemet's membrane around the suture knots revealing the puncture sites. Reprinted from Tam DY, Ahmed IK. New glaucoma surgical devices. In: Franz Grehn F, Stamper R, eds. Glaucoma [Essentials in Ophthalmology series]. Berlin: Springer; 2009 with permission from Springer

reported were elevated IOP and hyphema, most commonly, with Descemet's detachment, hypotony, and choroidal effusion also being reported.

Careful patient selection must occur for successful canaloplasty. As the suture in Schlemm's canal places centripetal tension on the inner wall, it draws the trabecular meshwork in toward the pupil (Fig. 67.19). Although this is a minute distance, in narrow angle patients or those with crowded anterior segments, this may result in constant or intermittent iridotrabecular touch, peripheral anterior synechiae, and angle closure. As a result, it is advisable to exclude patients with narrow angles or crowded anterior segments from being potential candidates for canaloplasty. Preoperative gonioscopy and in some cases adjunctive anterior segment imaging is of great importance in assessing the angle and iris profile when a patient is being considered for this procedure. It has been the authors' experience that postoperatively even the patient who had an unequivocally open angle may develop peripheral anterior synechiae and iris incarceration into microperforations in the TDW. An intact Schlemm's canal is also a prerequisite to successful canaloplasty; thus, patients with prior surgery such as a trabeculectomy or patients with obvious scarring in Schlemm's canal due to prior medication use, laser, surgery, corneoscleral trauma at the limbus may not be good candidates for canaloplasty.

In summary, canaloplasty is the procedure of catheterizing and distending Schlemm's canal with an *ab externo* non-penetrating dissection and using a microcatheter to deliver viscoelastic and sutures to restore aqueous outflow through the conventional pathway and into a scleral lake created at the surgical site. The aim is to lower IOP in glaucomatous eyes without the reliance on a subconjunctival bleb, thus avoiding both short- and long-term complications of subconjunctival filtration surgery. Studies have shown efficacy at 1 year in terms of IOP reduction and dependence on glaucoma medications with a low complication profile and minimal postoperative management. However, canaloplasty remains technically challenging and other issues remain to be studied such as the optimal tension of the suture in Schlemm's canal, the yet-undetermined long-term implications of a suture in the canal, fibrosis of the TDW resulting in the need for postoperative YAG laser, closure and contraction of the intrascleral lake, and its implications are yet poorly understood. Finally, because of episcleral venous pressure, it would seem that in theory, a ceiling to the maximal amount of physiologic outflow should exist, and thus a limit in the lowest IOP attainable by this procedure. This too, is yet to be well understood and requires further investigation.

## 67.4 Ab Interno Devices: The Trabecular Micro-bypass Stent and the Trabectome

While canaloplasty seeks to access Schlemm's canal from an *ab externo* approach, devices have also emerged for access to Schlemm's canal via an *ab interno* approach. Because studies have shown the juxtacanalicular tissue and inner wall of Schlemm's canal to be the site of greatest resistance to aqueous outflow,[71,73] it follows that bypassing this point of resistance allowing aqueous humor to access Schlemm's canal directly should produce IOP lowering with the resultant resistance point being episcleral venous pressure (EVP). One device that seeks to provide a direct passage from the anterior chamber to the lumen of Schlemm's canal is the trabecular micro-bypass iStent (Glaukos Corp., Laguna Hilla, California). This 1-mm long titanium stent is an L-shaped stent designed to partially sit inside Schlemm's canal and has a "snorkel," which sits in the anterior chamber.[74,75] This Glaukos device is reviewed in detail in another chapter of this textbook.

Traditionally, goniotomy has been a procedure that has been attempted to remove the resistance point of the trabecular meshwork and inner wall of Schlemm's canal. A blade is used to create an incision in the angle along several clock hours to, in theory, allow aqueous humor direct access to collector channels. Success has been attainable, however, only in the pediatric population[77] and similar results seemingly unattainable in the adult population.[40,76,79] Although procedures such as goniotomy and trabeculotomy, used when the view to the angle is poor,[78] have not found success in IOP control in adults, these procedures have led to innovative advances such as laser trabecular ablation, laser goniopuncture, and goniocurretage.[44,80,81] The Trabectome (NeoMedix Corp., San Juan Capistrano, California) is a new device that is a microelectrocautery handpiece designed to ablate trabecular meshwork and Schlemm's canal inner wall tissue over an area of several clock hours.

The device is a disposable handpiece that is activated by foot pedal control connected to a console that allows the surgeon to adjust infusion, aspiration, and dissipated electrosurgical energy. A 19-gauge infusion sleeve, 25-gauge aspiration port, and bipolar electrocautery unit located 150 μm away from an insulated footplate make up the components of the handpiece. The length of the footplate is 800 μm from heel to tip with a maximum width of 230 μm and maximum thickness of 110 μm (Fig. 67.20). The tapered design of the footplate leads to a pointed tip to aid penetration through trabecular meshwork tissue. Cross-sectional view of the footplate reveals an elliptical shape with an anterior–posterior dimension of 5 μm at the tip, widening to 50 μm at the heel with a meridional diameter from 350 μm at the tip to 500 μm at the bend, designed to fit into Schlemm's canal. Once the tip of the footplate is inserted into the canal, trabecular tissue is guided into the electrocautery unit by the footplate, while the insulated smooth design, along with continuous irrigation, protect the outer wall of Schlemm's canal and the collector channel ostia from trauma and injury.

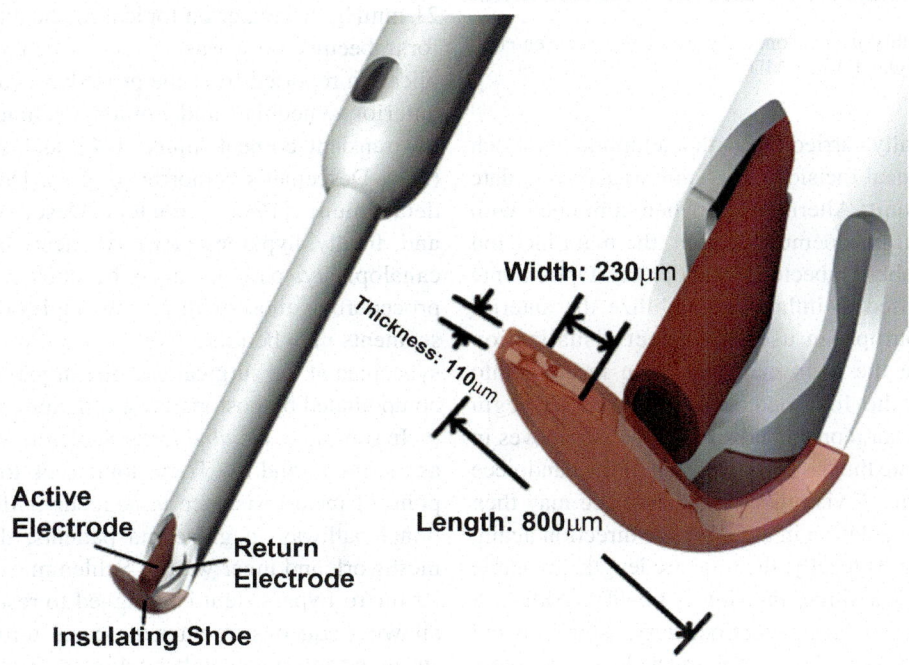

**Fig. 67.20** The Trabectome handpiece and footplate

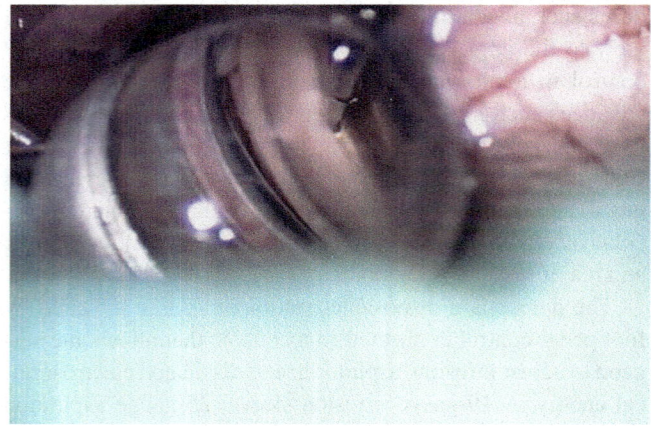

**Fig. 67.21** Under direct gonioscopic view, the meshwork is incised by the tip of the Trabectome handpiece. Photo courtesy of Douglas J. Rhee, MD

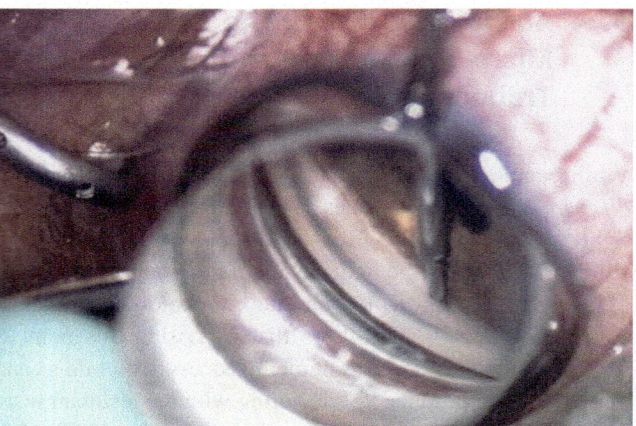

**Fig. 67.23** The Trabectome actively ablating angle tissue. Photo courtesy of Douglas J. Rhee, MD

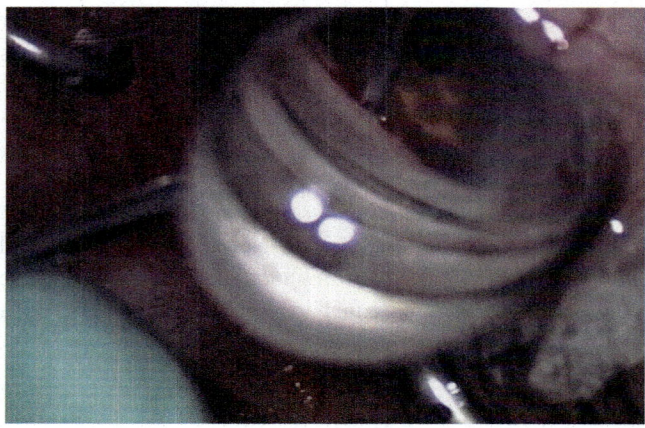

**Fig. 67.22** Heme reflux is seen once the canal has been entered. Photo courtesy of Douglas J. Rhee, MD

Surgery is typically carried out with a temporal approach through a clear corneal incision of 1.6 mm to accommodate the electrocautery unit. Alternatively, when combined with clear cornea coaxial phacoemulsification, the main incision may be used for the Trabectome handpiece. Ophthalmic visco-devices are used to inflate and stabilize the anterior chamber and a gonioprism used for direct visualization of the angle. Once the instrument has been inserted into Schlemm's canal, the foot pedal is depressed to begin electrocautery. The surgeon's hand simultaneously moves in one direction to ablate the tissue until the tip of the handpiece has reached the limit of visibility. The handpiece may then be turned to achieve ablation in the opposite direction again, to the limits of view. Typically, the total arc length amenable to treatment through a single incision is 60–90°. Although tissue debris is released during electrocautery, aspiration and continuous irrigation assist in maintaining a clear view to the angle (Figs. 67.21–67.23). With irrigation maintaining pressure in the eye, reflux of heme is not typically seen during ablation, but commonly seen when the handpiece is withdrawn from the anterior chamber and the IOP drops. It is advisable to place a clear corneal suture and intracameral air at the conclusion of Trabectome ablation as these maneuvers seemed to correlate with less postoperative hyphema.[49]

A recent study reported 101 patients undergoing the procedure with an IOP reduction from 27.6 mmHg preoperatively to a maximum follow-up of 30 months in ten patients with a mean postoperative IOP of 16.3 mmHg.[47] The same group also reported a decrease in medication usage from 1.2 to 0.4 at 6 months follow-up.[49] Despite the excellent outcome in some patients, a 16% failure rate, defined as an IOP of 21 mmHg or greater on topical medical therapy or the need for trabeculectomy, was reported. The most significant complication reported from the procedure was partial peripheral anterior synechiae and goniosynechiae (14%), followed by transient corneal injury (6%) such as epithelial defect (3%), Descemet's hemorrhage (1%), Descemet's scrolling/detachment (1%), persistent Descemet's injury (1%), and, finally, hypotony (1%). As mentioned previously with canaloplasty, patients must be chosen carefully for this procedure as those with narrow angles or crowded anterior segments may be more likely to develop peripheral anterior synechiae at the surgical site due in part to tissue proximity compounded by postoperative inflammation.

In summary, the *ab interno* Schlemm's canal devices such as the iStent and the Trabectome seek to bypass the known point of most resistance in aqueous outflow in the conventional pathway in glaucoma patients, the juxtacanalicular meshwork and inner wall of Schlemm's canal. The trabecular micro-bypass stent is designed to rest in the canal itself, allowing aqueous to enter the canal through a snorkel that sits in the anterior chamber, while the Trabectome ablates the trabecular tissue and inner wall of Schlemm's canal to allow aqueous to access collector channels directly in a treated arc length of the iridocorneal angle. These procedures are advantageous in their use of a small incision, the avoidance of a subconjunctival bleb, minimal postoperative management, and preservation of conjunctival tissues in the event that a filter is indeed required for IOP control in the long term. Although these devices resemble other prior innovations in goniosurgery in their aim to provide direct access of aqueous humor to Schlemm's canal and its collector channels, they differ in that there is preservation of the outer wall and the collector channel ostia, which are critical to aqueous egress and filtration. Previous procedures have been more likely to damage and cause fibrosis of these structures, ultimately resulting in failure to control IOP and creating a distal resistance point to aqueous egress. Histopathologic studies appear to support the notion that the insulated footplate on the Trabectome protects the outer wall and collector channels.[48] While the studies to date seem to show promising IOP control and decreased medication usage in some patients, longer follow-up for a larger number of patients is required, the formation of peripheral anterior goniosynechiae postoperatively is of concern, and histochemical work to assess the role and implications of inflammatory mediators in Schlemm's canal and the collector channels following electrocautery remains to be done. As with canaloplasty and *ab externo* Schlemm's canal approaches, a similar question remains about the lowest attainable IOP with these procedures because of downstream factors such as EVP.

## 67.5 The Gold Microshunt: A Suprachoroidal Device

The gold microshunt (SOLX Inc., Occulogix, Waltham, Massachusetts) is a 24-karat gold device designed to be surgically placed in an *ab externo* fashion with the anterior aspect of the device situated in the anterior chamber, the body to sit intrascleral, and the posterior aspect to rest in the suprachoroidal space (Fig. 67.24a, b). The device is composed of two leaflets fused together vertically concealing nine channels within the body that connect the anterior openings to the posterior ones (Fig. 67.25). Two different models of the device exist, the GMS (XGS-5) and the GMS Plus (XGS-10), both measuring 5.2 mm long, 2.4 mm wide anteriorly and 3.2 mm wide posteriorly, but differing in weight and channel size. The XGS-5 model weighs 6.2 mg and is 60 μm in thickness with the channels measuring 25 μm in width and 44 μm in height while the XGS-10 model weighs 9.2 mg and the channels measure 25 μm in width by 68 μm in height. Aqueous humor from the anterior chamber exiting through the uveoscleral pathway to the suprachoroidal space is enhanced by this device by allowing fluid to travel both through the channels in the shunt and also around the body of the shunt (Fig. 67.26). Gold has been chosen because it is an inert, noncorrosive metal, and because of its known biocompatibility, especially as a intraocular foreign body, even after many years.[82,83]

Implantation of the gold shunt, in theory, can be in any location around the circumference of the globe. However, due to ease of access and technical performance of the surgery, superotemporal and inferotemporal are the most commonly chosen locations. Angle anatomy should be relatively preserved in the location of choice and thus, preoperative gonioscopy is imperative. One must also use caution in highly myopic eyes and with large anterior segments as the scleral spur may be further posterior on the sclera than usual, mandating a more posteriorly placed shunt. Intraoperative gonioscopy is also an important tool in implantation of the gold microshunt.

A fornix-based conjunctival peritomy is fashioned to approximately 4 mm in length leaving a short 1 mm skirt of conjunctiva attached to the limbus. Then, typically 2 mm posterior to the limbus, a perpendicular 3.5 mm scleral incision is created to near full thickness leaving only a thin layer of sclera visible covering the blue hue of the choroid

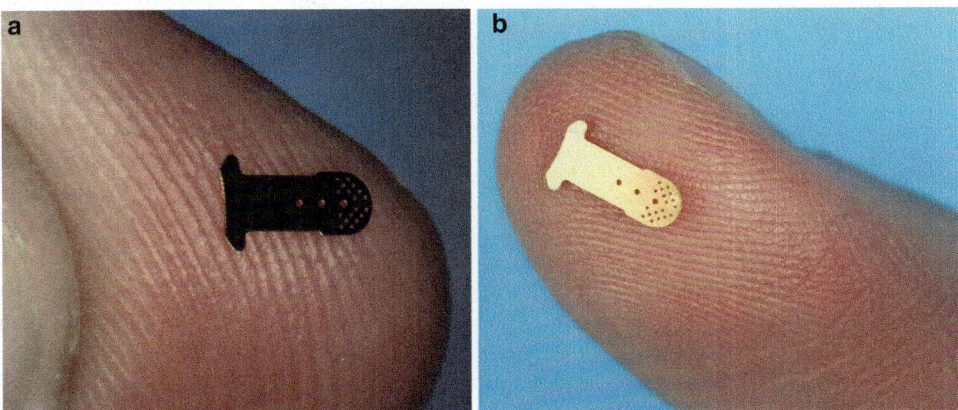

**Fig. 67.24** (a, b) The SOLX suprachoroidal gold microshunt on fingertip. The shown is a different model from the one discussed in this chapter. Illustrations courtesy of SOLX Inc., Waltham, Massachusetts

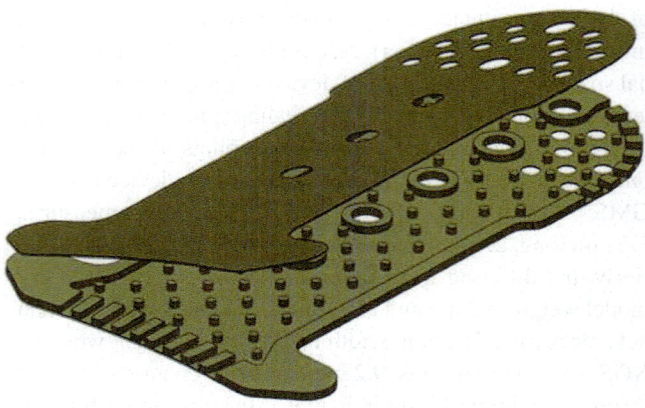

**Fig. 67.25** An interior view of the gold shunt revealing the channels connecting the anterior openings with the posterior ones. The shunt shown is a different model from the one discussed in this chapter. Illustration courtesy of SOLX Inc., Waltham, Massachusetts

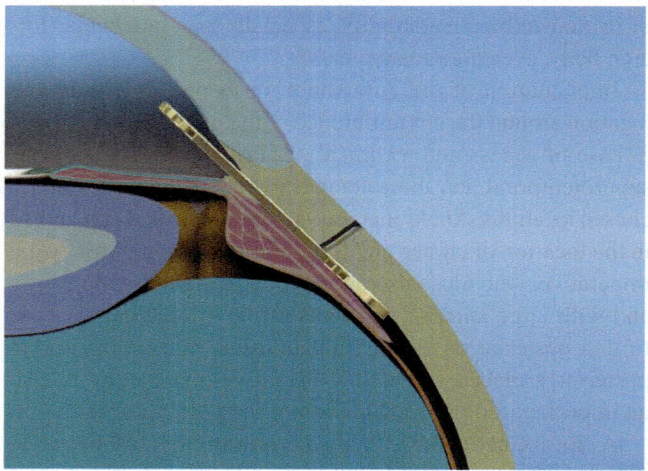

**Fig. 67.26** A schematic diagram of the intended position of the gold shunt. Reprinted from Tam DY, Ahmed IK. New glaucoma surgical devices. In: Franz Grehn F, Stamper R, eds. Glaucoma [Essentials in Ophthalmology Series]. Berlin: Springer; 2009 with permission from Springer

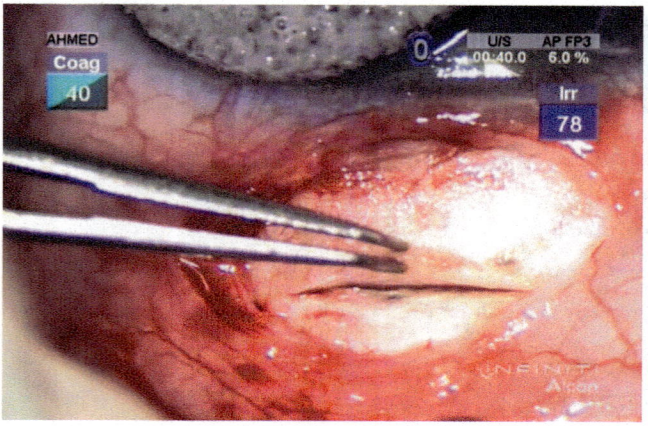

**Fig. 67.27** A scleral cutdown is initiated to near full thickness with the *blue* choroidal hue seen at the base of the dissection

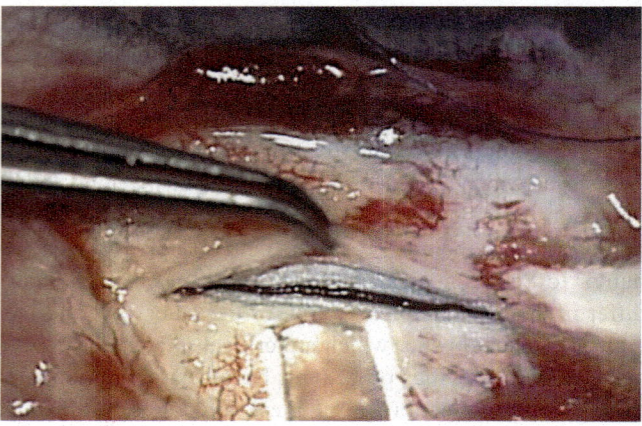

**Fig. 67.28** The toothed forceps reveals the layers of scleral dissection including a full thickness cutdown with a near full thickness scleral tunnel

(Fig. 67.27). A scleral tunnel incision is then fashioned toward the clear cornea at this 95% plane created by the perpendicular incision. Once the tip of the crescent blade is visible at the limbus and has clearly passed the scleral spur, the tunnel is adequately anterior. The original perpendicular incision is then completed to full thickness revealing choroidal tissue (Fig. 67.28). A paracentesis incision may be required at this point to lower the IOP and lessen bulging of the choroidal tissue through the full thickness incision. A blunt cannula is then used to administer nonpreserved xylocaine very gently into the suprachoroidal space posterior to the incision. The cannula need not be advanced very far into the highly vascular suprachoroidal space. A small amount of viscoelastic should also be injected gently into the suprachoroidal space to provide space for the posterior edge of the shunt. The anterior chamber at this point should be filled with viscoelastic in the area of anticipated shunt placement. An entry wound should then be created into the anterior chamber at the level of the scleral spur to allow for the anterior edge of the shunt to be placed. Note that this may be slightly posterior to the anterior aspect of the scleral tunnel. Intraoperative gonioscopy is at this step, very useful in determining the position of the entry into the anterior chamber.

The shunt is then brought onto the field and very gently removed from its housing. A nontoothed forceps is recommended as well as avoidance of grasping the shunt body as the delicate channels in the body are easily crushed (Fig. 67.29). A 27-gauge needle on the body of the shunt can then be used to guide the posterior aspect of the shunt into the suprachoroidal space. Alternatively, two positioning holes on the posterior edge of the shunt are available for use by a Sinskey hook (Figs. 67.30 and 67.31). The posterior openings of the shunt should not be visible and should be wholly in the suprachoroidal space. The anterior aspect of the shunt is then placed into the anterior chamber through the previously created entry at the level of the scleral spur. A positioning hole

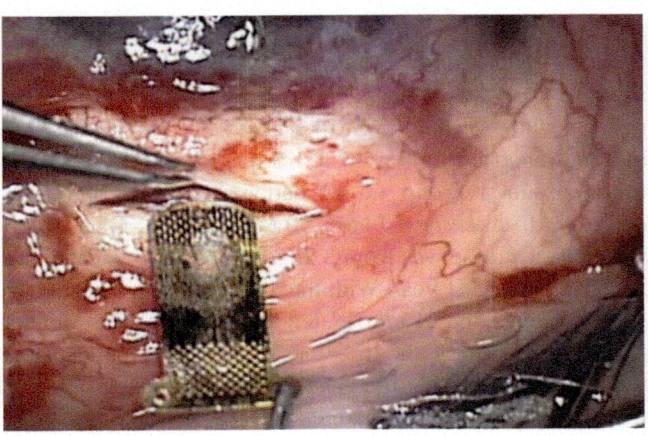

**Fig. 67.29** The gold shunt is gently inserted into the scleral tunnel with a non-toothed forceps

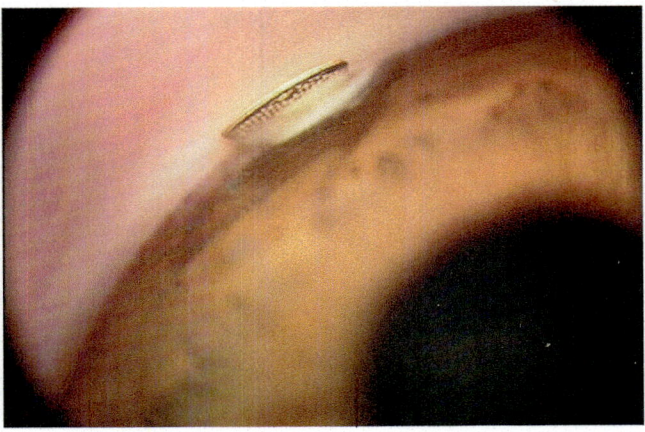

**Fig. 67.32** Postoperative goniophotograph of the gold shunt

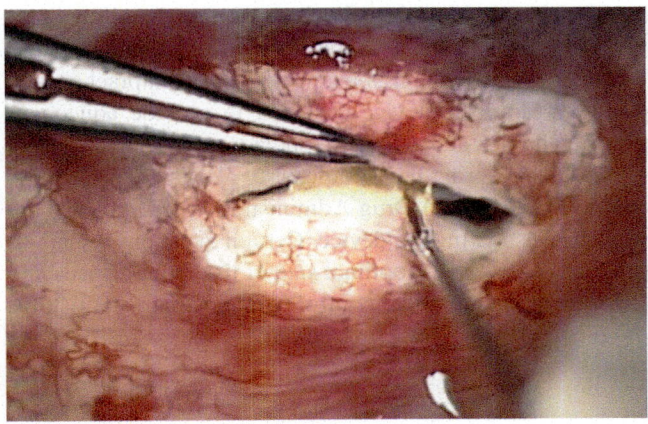

**Fig. 67.30** A 27-gauge needle is gently used on the body of the shunt to encourage it into the proper position

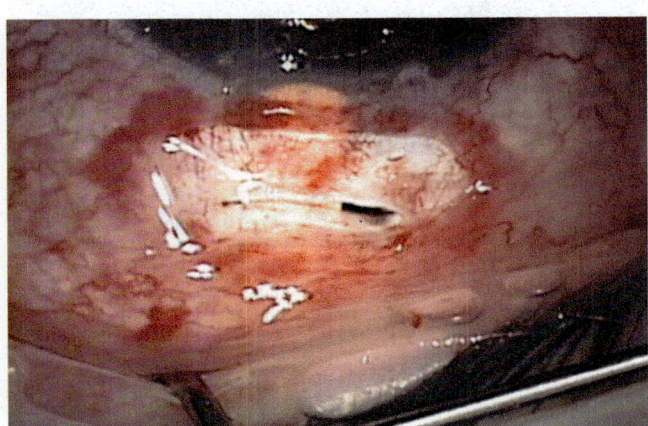

**Fig. 67.33** The posterior openings of the shunt are fully located in the suprachoroidal space and not visible

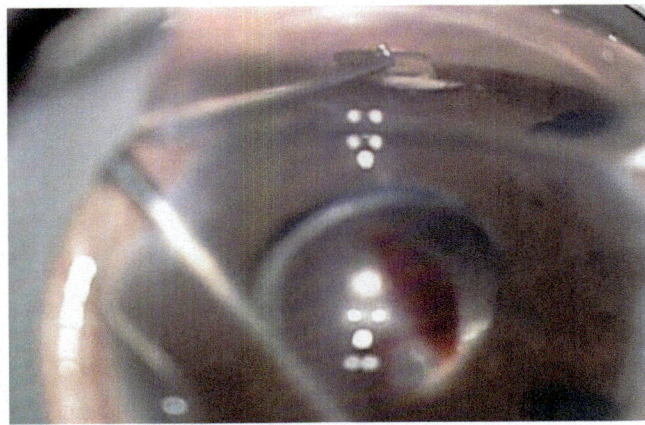

**Fig. 67.31** A gonioscopic view intraoperatively with a Sinskey hook assisting the gold shunt into position

is present at the head of the shunt to allow for positioning assistance again by a Sinskey hook through the anterior chamber. The shunt is in satisfactory position when all of the anterior drainage openings can be seen on intraoperative gonioscopy just anterior to or at the scleral spur while all of the posterior openings are fully in the suprachoroidal space (Figs. 67.32 and 67.33). The scleral incision is then closed in a watertight fashion using four to five interrupted 10–0 nylon sutures (Fig. 67.34). A 10–0 Vicryl suture is then used to close the overlying conjunctiva in a running horizontal mattress fashion to ensure watertight closure as well. Postoperative imaging of the shunt by anterior segment optical coherence tomography has indeed shown a suprachoroidal reservoir of fluid surrounding the body of the shunt (Fig. 67.35).

Nonrandomized clinical data released by SOLX, in patients with at least one prior failed incisional glaucoma procedure,

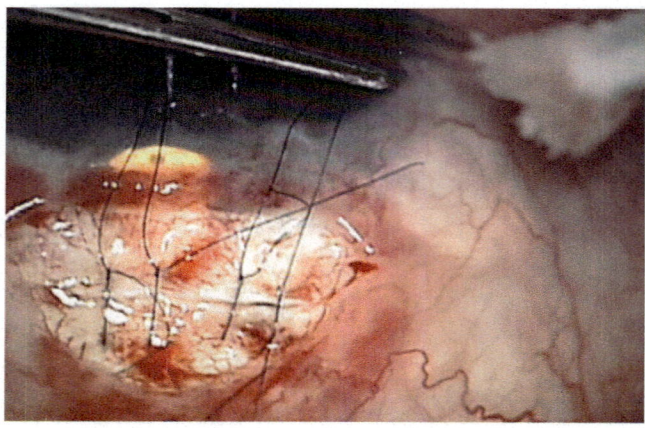

**Fig. 67.34** Interrupted nylon sutures are used to close the scleral incision in a watertight fashion

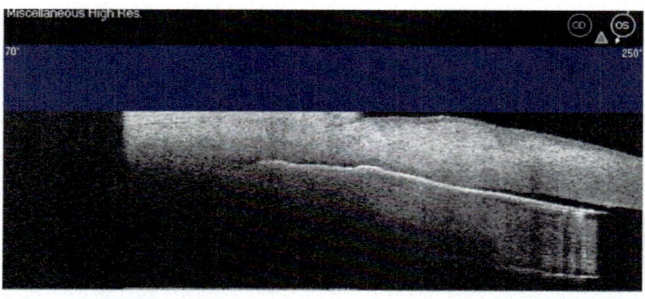

**Fig. 67.35** Anterior segment OCT image showing the gold shunt in position with a small amount of fluid around the shunt body

for the XGS-5 model of the shunt showed an IOP reduction from 27.4 ± 4.7 preoperatively to 18.1 ± 4.7 postoperatively at a 1-year follow-up, accounting for a 33% reduction in 39 patients who received the GMS. The XGS-10 model showed a reduction from 25.5 ± 6.0 to 18.0 ± 2.5 also at a 1-year follow-up in a group of 40 patients. Medication usage decreased from 1.97 ± 0.74 to 1.50 ± 0.94 in the XGS-5 group while the decrease was from 2.25 ± 0.84 to 0.85 ± 0.90 in the XGS-10 group at 1 year. With the definition of success as an IOP between 5 and 21 mmHg, ten out of the final 36 patients in the XGS-5 group and three out of the final 13 patients in the XGS-10 were classified as failures. Reported complications of shunt placement include cataract formation, choroidal detachment, shunt-cornea touch, shunt-iris touch, shunt exposure, shunt migration, peripheral anterior synechiae formation around the shunt, anterior chamber inflammation, hyphema, hypotony, vitreous hemorrhage, infection, pain, and blurred vision. Fibrosis and membrane growth over the anterior shunt orifices has also been observed and may prevent aqueous from entering the channels of the shunt.

The gold microshunt is a new *ab externo* suprachoroidal glaucoma drainage device designed to provide aqueous a pathway through and around the shunt into the suprachoroidal space, thus lowering IOP. While early results are promising, current US Food and Drug Administration (FDA) trials are further investigating the device. Certain questions remain to be studied such as the optimal size of the shunt orifices and channels to maintain IOP control without significant risk for

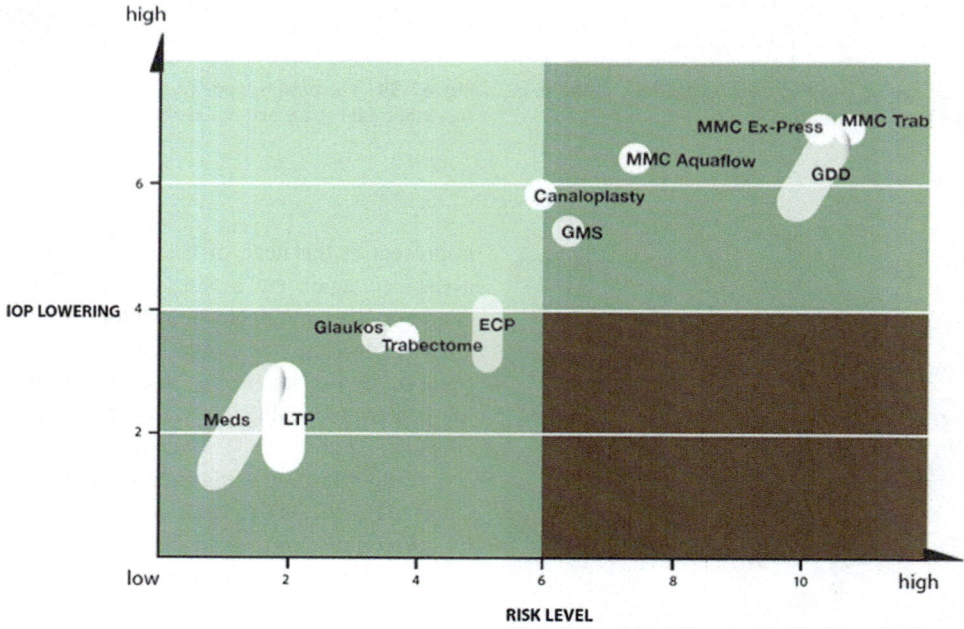

**Fig. 67.36** Current treatment landscape comparing glaucoma treatment modalities in terms of efficacy in IOP lowering versus risk. Reprinted from Tam DY, Ahmed IK. New glaucoma surgical devices. In: Franz Grehn F, Stamper R, eds. Glaucoma [Essentials in Ophthalmology series]. Berlin: Springer; 2009 with permission from Springer

hypotony. It is also unknown whether flow around the shunt into the suprachoroidal space plays a significant role in IOP reduction and if, as such, fibrosis and scarring in this effect cyclodialysis cleft plays a role in long-term success of this procedure.

## 67.6 Conclusion

Trabeculectomy was first described 40 years ago, and to this day, this nonphysiologic bleb-forming procedure is still considered widely to be the gold standard of glaucoma surgery. Although potent in IOP lowering, and relatively simple to learn and perform, this procedure is fraught with short-term and potential lifetime risks with visually devastating consequences. Combined with the task of attempting to modulate wound healing both intraoperatively and postoperatively, glaucoma surgeons have begun to search for alternative procedures to achieve IOP control. Several new devices have emerged, attempting to make trabeculectomy safer (the Ex-PRESS shunt), to augment physiologic conventional outflow (canaloplasty, trabecular micro-bypass stent, Trabectome), and suprachoroidal outflow (gold microshunt). Although studies are ongoing and long-term successes still have yet to be demonstrated from these procedures, early results are promising in the quest for a safe, reliable, and predictable glaucoma surgical procedure Fig. 67.36.

## References

1. Richey SO. Management of glaucoma. *Trans Am Ophthalmol Soc.* 1896;7:723–730.
2. Davenport RC. The after results of corneo-scleral trephining for glaucoma. *Br J Ophthalmol.* 1926;10(9):478–484.
3. Scheie HG. Retraction of scleral wound edges; as a fistulizing procedure for glaucoma. *Am J Ophthalmol.* 1958;45(4, Part 2):220–229.
4. Cairns JE. Trabeculectomy. Preliminary report of a new method. *Am J Ophthalmol.* 1968;66(4):673–679.
5. Borisuth NS, Phillips B, Krupin T. The risk profile of glaucoma filtration surgery. *Curr Opin Ophthalmol.* 1999;10(2):112–116.
6. Rollett M, Moreau M. Le drainage au crin de la chambre anterieure contre l'hypertonie et la douleur. *Rev Gen Ophtalmol.* 1907;26:289–292.
7. Molteno ACB. New implant for drainage in glaucoma: animal trial. *Br J Ophthalmol.* 1969;53:161–168.
8. Molteno ACB. New implant for drainage in glaucoma: clinical trial. *Br J Ophthalmol.* 1969;53:606–615.
9. Krupin T, Podos SM, Becker B, Newkirk JB. Valve implants in filtering surgery. *Am J Ophthalmol.* 1976;81(2):232–235.
10. Lloyd MA, Baerveldt G, Heuer DK, Minckler DS, Martone JF. Initial clinical experience with the Baerveldt implant in complicated glaucomas. *Ophthalmology.* 1994;101(4):640–650.
11. Coleman AL, Hill R, Wilson MR, et al. Initial clinical experience with the Ahmed Glaucoma Valve implant. *Am J Ophthalmol.* 1995;120(1):23–31.
12. Barkan O. Goniotomy for the relief of congenital glaucoma. *Br J Ophthalmol.* 1948;32(9):701–728.
13. Scheie HG. Goniotomy in the treatment of congenital glaucoma. *Trans Am Ophthalmol Soc.* 1949;47:115–137.
14. Bill A, Phillips CI. Uveoscleral drainage of aqueous humor in human eyes. *Exp Eye Res.* 1971;12:275–281.
15. Toris CB, Yablonski ME, Wang YL, et al. Aqueous humor dynamics in the aging human eye. *Am J Ophthalmol.* 1999;127:407–412.
16. Bindlish R, Condon GP, Schlosser JD, D'Antonio J, Lauer KB, Lehrer R. Efficacy and safety of mitomycin-C in primary trabeculectomy: five-year follow-up. *Ophthalmology.* 2002;109(7):1336–1341.
17. Palmer SS. Mitomycin as adjunct chemotherapy with trabeculectomy. *Ophthalmology.* 1991;98(3):317–321.
18. Fluorouracil Filtering Surgery Study one-year follow-up. The Fluorouracil Filtering Surgery Study Group. *Am J Ophthalmol.* 1989;108(6):625–635.
19. Kupin TH, Juzych MS, Shin DH, Khatana AK, Olivier MM. Adjunctive mitomycin C in primary trabeculectomy in phakic eyes. *Am J Ophthalmol.* 1995;119(1):30–39.
20. Ticho U, Ophir A. Late complications after glaucoma filtering surgery with adjunctive 5-fluorouracil. *Am J Ophthalmol.* 1993;115(4):506–510.
21. Gedde SJ, Schiffman JC, Feuer WJ, Herndon LW, Brandt JD, Budenz DL. Treatment outcomes in the tube versus trabeculectomy study after one year of follow-up. *Am J Ophthalmol.* 2007;143(1):9–22.
22. Gedde SJ, Herndon LW, Brandt JD, Budenz DL, Feuer WJ, Schiffman JC. Surgical complications in the Tube Versus Trabeculectomy Study during the first year of follow-up. *Am J Ophthalmol.* 2007;143(1):23–31.
23. Grant WM. Further studies on facility of flow through the trabecular meshwork. *AMA Arch Ophthalmol.* 1958;60(4 part 1):523–533.
24. Rosenquist R, Epstein D, Melamed S, Johnson M, Grant WM. Outflow resistance of enucleated human eyes at two different perfusion pressures and different extents of trabeculotomy. *Curr Eye Res.* 1989;8(12):1233–1240.
25. Ethier CR, Kamm RD, Palaszewski BA, Johnson MC, Richardson TM. Calculations of flow resistance in the juxtacanalicular meshwork. *Invest Ophthalmol Vis Sci.* 1986;27(12):1741–1750.
26. Epstein E. Fibrosing response to aqueous; its relation to glaucoma. *Br J Ophthalmol.* 1959;43:641–647.
27. Krasnov MM. Externalization of Schlemm's canal (sinusotomy) in glaucoma. *Br J Ophthalmol.* 1968;52:157–161.
28. Ellingsen BA, Grant WM. Trabeculotomy and sinusotomy in enucleated human eyes. *Invest Ophthalmol.* 1972;11:21–28.
29. Johnstone MA, Grant WM. Microsurgery of Schlemm's canal and the human aqueous outflow system. *Am J Ophthalmol.* 1973;76:906–917.
30. Koslov VI, Bagrov SN, Anisimova SY, et al. [Nonpenetrating deep sclerectomy with collagen] [Russian]. *Oftalmokhirurgiia.* 1990;3:44–46.
31. Fyodorov SN, Ioffe DI, Ronkina TI. Deep sclerectomy: technique and mechanism of a new antiglaucomatous procedure. *Glaucoma.* 1984;6:281–283.
32. Zimmerman TJ, Kooner KS, Ford VJ, et al. Trabeculectomy vs. nonpenetrating trabeculectomy: a retrospective study of two procedures in phakic patients with glaucoma. *Ophthalmic Surg.* 1984;15:734–740.
33. Stegmann R, Pienaar A, Miller D. Viscocanalostomy for open angle glaucoma in black African patients. *J Cataract Refract Surg.* 1999;25:316–322.
34. Sourdille P, Santiago P-Y, Villain F, et al. Reticulated hyaluronic acid implant in nonperforating trabecular surgery. *J Cataract Refract Surg.* 1999;25:332–339.
35. Ambresin A, Shaarawy T, Mermoud A. Deep sclerectomy with collagen implant in one eye compared with trabeculectomy in the other eye of the same patient. *J Glaucoma.* 2002;11:214–220.

36. Sanchez E, Schnyder CC, Sickenberg M, Chiou AG, Hédiguer SE, Mermoud A. Deep sclerectomy: results with and without collagen implant. *Int Ophthalmol.* 1996/97;20:157–162.
37. Spiegel D, Kobuch K. Trabecular meshwork bypass tube shunt: initial case series. *Br J Ophthalmol.* 2002;86:1228–1231.
38. Yablonski ME. Trabeculectomy with internal tube shunt: a novel glaucoma surgery. *J Glaucoma.* 2005;14:91–97.
39. Lewis RA, von Wolff K, Tetz M, et al. Canaloplasty: circumferential viscodilation and tensioning of Schlemm's canal using a flexible microcatheter for the treatment of open-angle glaucoma in adults: interim clinical study analysis. *J Cataract Refract Surg.* 2007;33(7): 1217–1226.
40. Luntz MH, Livingston DG. Trabeculotomy ab externo and trabeculectomy in congenital and adult-onset glaucoma. *Am J Ophthalmol.* 1977;83:174–179.
41. Tanihara H, Negi A, Akimoto M, et al. Surgical effects of trabeculectomy ab externo on adult eyes with primary open angle glaucoma and pseudoexfoliation syndrome. *Arch Ophthalmol.* 1993;111: 1653–1661.
42. Krasnov MM. Q-switched laser goniopuncture. *Arch Ophthalmol.* 1974;92:37–41.
43. Wickham MG, Worthen DM. Argon laser trabeculotomy: long-term follow-up. *Ophthalmology.* 1970;86:495–503.
44. Epstein DL, Melamed S, Puliatio CA, Steinert RF. Neodymium: YAG laser trabeculopuncture in open-angle glaucoma. *Ophthalmology.* 1985;92:931–937.
45. Bahler CK, Smedley GT, Zhou J, Johnson DH. Trabecular bypass stents decrease intraocular pressure in cultured human anterior segments. *Am J Ophthalmol.* 2004;138(6):988–994.
46. Spiegel D, Wetzel W, Haffner DS, Hill RA. Initial clinical experience with the trabecular micro-bypass stent in patients with glaucoma. *Adv Ther.* 2007;24(1):161–170.
47. Minckler D, Baerveldt G, Ramirez MA, et al. Clinical results with the Trabectome, a novel surgical device for treatment of open-angle glaucoma. *Trans Am Ophthalmol Soc.* 2006;104:40–50.
48. Francis BA, See RF, Rao NA, Minckler DS, Baerveldt G. Ab interno trabeculectomy: development of a novel device (TrabectomeTM) and surgery for open-angle glaucoma. *J Glaucoma.* 2006;15:68–73.
49. Minckler DS, Baerveldt G, Alfaro MR, Francis BA. Clinical results with the Trabectome for treatment of open-angle glaucoma. *Ophthalmology.* 2005;112:962–967.
50. Bain WE. Variations in the episcleral venous pressure in relation to glaucoma. *Br J Ophthalmol.* 1954;38(3):129–135.
51. Friberg TR, Sanborn G, Weinreb RN. Intraocular and episcleral venous pressure increase during inverted posture. *Am J Ophthalmol.* 1987;103(4):523–526.
52. Phelps CD. The pathogenesis of glaucoma in Sturge-Weber syndrome. *Ophthalmology.* 1978;85(3):276–286.
53. Bigger JF. Glaucoma with elevated episcleral venous pressure. *South Med J.* 1975;68(11):1444–1448.
54. Suguro K, Toris CB, Pederson JE. Uveoscleral outflow following cyclodialysis in the monkey eye using a fluorescent tracer. *Invest Ophthalmol Vis Sci.* 1985;26:810–813.
55. Jordan JF, Dietlein TS, Dinslage S, et al. Cyclodialysis ab interno as a surgical approach to intractable glaucoma. *Graefes Arch Clin Exp Ophthalmol.* 2007;245:1071–1076.
56. Shields MB, Simmons RJ. Combined cyclodialysis and cataract extraction. *Ophthalmic Surg.* 1976;7(2):62–73.
57. Galin MA, Baras I. Combined cyclodialysis cataract extraction: a review. *Ann Ophthalmol.* 1975;7(2):271–275.
58. Gills JP Jr, Paterson CA, Paterson ME. Action of cyclodialysis utilizing an implant studied by manometry in a human eye. *Exp Eye Res.* 1967;6:75–78.
59. Klemm M, Balazs A, Draeger J, Wiezorrek R. Experimental use of space-retaining substances with extended duration: functional and morphological results. *Graefes Arch Clin Exp Ophthalmol.* 1995;233(9):592–597.
60. Nesterov AP, Batmanov YE, Cherkasova IN, Egorov EA. Surgical stimulation of the uveoscleral outflow: experimental studies on enucleated human eyes. *Acta Ophthalmol (Copenh).* 1979;57(3):409–417.
61. Pinnas G, Boniuk M. Cyclodialysis with teflon tube implants. *Am J Ophthalmol.* 1969;68(5):879–883.
62. Krejci L. Cyclodialysis with hydroxyethyl methacrylate capillary strip. *Ophthalmologica.* 1972;164:113–121.
63. Ozdamar A, Aras C, Karacorlu M. Suprachoroidal seton implantation in refractory glaucoma: a novel surgical technique. *J Glaucoma.* 2003;12:354–359.
64. Jordan JF, Engels BF, Dinslage S, et al. A novel approach to suprachoroidal drainage for the surgical treatment of intractable glaucoma. *J Glaucoma.* 2006;15:200–205.
65. Sarkisian SR. Use of an Injector for the Ex-PRESS™ Mini Glaucoma Shunt. *Ophthalmic Surg Lasers Imaging.* 2007;38(5):434–436.
66. Coupin A, Li Q, Riss I. Ex-PRESS miniature glaucoma implant inserted under a scleral flap in open-angle glaucoma surgery: a retrospective study. *Fr J Glaucoma.* 2007;30(1):18–23.
67. Maris PJG, Ishida K, Netland PA. Comparison of trabeculectomy with Ex-PRESS miniature glaucoma device implanted under scleral flap. *J Glaucoma.* 2007;16:14–19.
68. Dahan E, Carmichael TR. Implantation of a miniature glaucoma device under a scleral flap. *J Glaucoma.* 2005;14(2):98–102.
69. Traverso CE, De Feo F, Messas-Kaplan A, et al. Long term effect on IOP of a stainless steel glaucoma drainage implant (Ex-PRESS) in combined surgery with phacoemulsification. *Br J Ophthalmol.* 2005;89(4):425–429.
70. Nyska A, Glovinsky Y, Belkin M, Epstein Y. Biocompatibility of the Ex-PRESS miniature glaucoma drainage implant. *J Glaucoma.* 2003;12(3):275–280.
71. Moses RA, Grodzki WJ Jr, Etheridge EL, Wilson CD. Schlemm's canal: the effect of intraocular pressure. *Invest Ophthalmol Vis Sci.* 1981;20(1):61–68.
72. Shingleton B, Tetz M, Korber N. Circumferential viscodilation and tensioning of Schlemm's canal (canaloplasty) combined with temporal clear corneal phacoemulsification cataract surgery for the treatment of open angle glaucoma and visually significant cataract – one year results. *J Cataract Refract Surg.* 2008;34(3):433–440.
73. Grant WM. Experimental aqueous perfusion in enucleated human eyes. *Arch Ophthalmol.* 1963;69:783–801.
74. Zhou J, Smedley GT. A trabecular bypass flow hypothesis. *J Glaucoma.* 2005;14(1):74–83.
75. Zhou J, Smedley GT. Trabecular bypass: effect of Schlemm canal and collector channel dilation. *J Glaucoma.* 2006;15(5):446–455.
76. Herschler J, Davis EB. Modified goniotomy for inflammatory glaucoma. Histologic evidence for the mechanism of pressure reduction. *Arch Ophthalmol.* 1980;98:684–687.
77. Gramer E, Tausch M, Kraemer C. Time of diagnosis, reoperations and long-term results of goniotomy in the treatment of primary congenital glaucoma: a clinical study. *Int Ophthalmol.* 1996;20: 117–123.
78. Mendicino ME, Lynch MG, Drack A, et al. Long-term surgical and visual outcomes in primary congenital glaucoma: 360 degrees trabeculotomy versus goniotomy. *J AAPOS.* 2000;4:205–210.
79. Dickens CS, Hoskins HD Jr. Epidemiology and pathophysiology of congenital glaucoma. In: Ritch R, Shields MB, Krupin T, eds. *The Glaucomas*, vol. 2. 2nd ed. St. Louis: Mosby; 1996:729–738.
80. Hill RA, Baerveldt G, Ozler SA, et al. Laser trabecular ablation (LTA). *Lasers Surg Med.* 1991;11:341–346.
81. Jacobi PC, Dietlein TS, Krieglstein GK. Technique of goniocurettage: a potential treatment for advanced chronic open angle glaucoma. *Br J Ophthalmol.* 1997;81:302–307.
82. Eisler R. Mammalian sensitivity to elemental gold (Au). *Biol Trace Elem Res.* 2004;100:1–17.
83. Sen SC, Ghosh A. Gold as an intraocular foreign body. *Br J Ophthalmol.* 1983;67:398–399.

# Chapter 68
# Incisional Therapies: Shunts and Valved Implants

John W. Boyle IV and Peter A. Netland

The earliest attempts to drain fluid out of the anterior chamber into the subconjunctival space consisted of implanting a variety of foreign objects into the eye extending from the anterior chamber to the subconjunctival space. These early operations failed because of excessive fibrosis over the subconjunctival portion of the implant at the limbus, seton migration, or conjunctival erosion. Dr. Anthony Molteno introduced the concept of draining fluid away from the anterior chamber to a plate posterior to the limbus.[1] The Molteno implant had an episcleral plate positioned in the equatorial region, which was connected to the anterior chamber by means of an elongated silicone tube.

Additional modifications of glaucoma drainage implants have improved the safety and efficacy of the devices. Dr. Theodore Krupin developed a pressure-sensitive, slit valve that provided resistance to the flow of aqueous, reducing the occurrence of early postoperative hypotony.[2] Dr. Mateen Ahmed introduced the Ahmed Glaucoma Valve, which is a pressure-sensitive glaucoma drainage device with a valve designed to open when the intraocular pressure is approximately 8 mmHg.[3] Implants with increased surface area have been intended to increase the surface area of the end-plate and possibly lower the intraocular pressure. Thus, double-plate versions of the Molteno implant[4] and the Ahmed Glaucoma Valve[5] have been introduced. Also, Dr. George Baerveldt introduced a nonvalved silicone tube attached to a large barium-impregnated silicone plate.[6]

Essential steps of glaucoma drainage implant surgery include suturing an episcleral plate with an attached tube posterior to the limbus and placing the other end of a tube in the anterior chamber. The tube is covered with allograft or autograft material to prevent erosion of the tube through the conjunctiva. Drainage implants have been useful in treating patients who have failed or are at high risk for failure of other glaucoma surgical procedures, including trabeculectomy. There is increasing interest in use of these devices for primary glaucoma surgery (Sidebar 68.1).

## 68.1 Current Glaucoma Drainage Devices

Current glaucoma drainage devices can be classified into two broad categories, valved or nonvalved (Table 68.1). Valved implants or flow-restrictive drainage devices provide resistance to aqueous flow and prevent hypotony during the early postoperative period. Nonvalved implants or open tube drainage devices provide little resistance to aqueous flow during the early postoperative period until a fibrous capsule forms around the plate. Various techniques have been devised for use during the early postoperative period to prevent hypotony associated with open tube implants.

The Ahmed Glaucoma Valve and the Eagle Vision implant with a modified Krupin slit valve are examples of flow-restrictive drainage devices. The nonvalved implants or open tube drainage devices include the Baerveldt glaucoma implant and the Molteno implant.

### 68.1.1 Ahmed Glaucoma Valve

The Ahmed Glaucoma Valve (New World Medical, Inc., Rancho Cucamonga, California) consists of a silicone tube attached to a valve mechanism on an end plate, comprised of either polypropylene or silicone. The valve consists of two thin silicone elastomer membranes (8 mm long × 7 mm wide) positioned in a venturi-shaped chamber. The elastic membranes of the valve restrict flow up to a pressure of approximately 8–12 mmHg, which is intended to reduce the incidence of early postoperative hypotony. Early results suggested that the Ahmed Glaucoma Valve restricts aqueous flow,[7] while subsequent studies have demonstrated true valve function of the device.[8,9]

### Sidebar 68.1 Trabeculectomy or tube shunt surgery – which to perform?

Daniel A. Jewelewicz

Until fairly recently, tube shunt surgery was considered a "surgical last resort" in patients who had failed prior trabeculectomy. This has changed recently, with tube shunt surgery gaining in popularity and even becoming the primary glaucoma surgery of choice for some surgeons. The Tube Versus Trabeculectomy Study (TVT) is the first study to prospectively compare the results of trabeculectomy to tube shunt surgery. The investigators followed up 212 patients aged 18–85 with intraocular pressure (IOP) ranging from 18 to 40 mmHg who were on maximally tolerated medical therapy. One half received a trabeculectomy with 4 min of 0.4-mg/cc mitomycin C (MMC). The other half received a Baerveldt 350 implant (BGI). IOP, visual acuity, complications, and need for reoperation were compared for both groups over the course of 1 year. The three most salient points to be gleaned from the treatment outcomes in the *Tube Versus Trabeculectomy Study After 1 Year of Follow-Up* are:

1. Tube shunt surgery was more likely to maintain IOP control at 1 year. The cumulative probability of failure was 3.9% in the tube group and 13.5% in the trabeculectomy group, indicating that a trabeculectomy was more than four times as likely to fail at 1 year. Failure was defined as:

   (a) IOP>21 mmHg or not reduced by 20% below baseline on two consecutive visits after 3 months
   (b) IOP < or equal to 5 mmHg on two consecutive visits after 3 months
   (c) Reoperation for glaucoma
   (d) Loss of light perception

2. Tube shunt surgery is more likely to require supplemental medication at 1 year. The number of medications in the tube group was 1.3, and 0.5 in the trabeculectomy group.
3. Tube shunt surgery is more likely to avoid hypotony. Three trabeculectomy patients failed because of hypotony; none did in the tube group.

The authors then examined more closely the nature of the complications in a second paper, the *Surgical Complications in the Tube Versus Trabeculectomy Study During the First Year of Follow Up*. They noted:

1. Postoperative complications were higher in the trabeculectomy group – 57% in the trabeculectomy group and 34% in the tube group.
2. The rates of intraoperative surgical complications and re-operation were similar between the two groups.

It is tempting to conclude that tube shunt surgery is a superior form of surgical reduction of IOP – it is reported as more likely to work and it has fewer complications, albeit with the possible need for continued medication. It is also worth noting that the single case of endophthalmitis in the entire study occurred in the trabeculectomy group. As with all studies, though, data must be interpreted cautiously. Other studies offer differing results. In October 2007, Stein et al published the *Longitudinal Rates of Postoperative Adverse Outcomes After Glaucoma Surgery Among Medicare Beneficiaries 1994 to 2005*. This was an excellent retrospective study that examined a nationally representative longitudinal sample by examining Medicare claims. They compared Medicare beneficiaries older than or equal to 68 years who underwent primary trabeculectomy, trabeculectomy with excision of scar tissue, or tube shunt surgery. In contradistinction to the TVT study they noted that:

1. Rates of severe adverse outcomes, less severe adverse outcomes, corneal edema and low vision/blindness were higher in the tube shunt group – 2% in the tube shunt group experienced severe adverse outcomes, versus 0.6% in the trabeculectomy group, and 1.3% in the trabeculectomy with scarring group.
2. Rates of re-operation were highest in the trabeculectomy scarring group.

It is somewhat alarming to note that within 6 years of undergoing tube shunt surgery, more than 40% experienced an adverse outcome, and nearly 30% received a code indicating low vision or blindness. However, these data must be taken in context. This was a retrospective study, and as such there were no screening criteria. Patients in the tube shunt group may very well have had prior trabeculectomy surgery, possibly even more than once. Furthermore, this study examined charts from 1990 onward, when tube shunt surgery was not nearly as commonplace as now (and was therefore often reserved for complicated cases that had failed prior surgical intervention). Lastly, this study examined Medicare claims; the codes used may have been appropriate for billing but not necessarily for accurate diagnosis. Nonetheless, this study does suggest that tube shunt surgery may not be as safe as the TVT study leads us to believe.

We must also exercise similar caution when interpreting the results from the TVT Study. The TVT study looked only at BGI 350 implants compared with trabeculectomy using 0.4 mg/cc MMC for 4 min. Glaucoma surgery is an art, and an experienced glaucoma surgeon will choose not only which procedure to perform, but also modify the procedure in order to achieve the best result for an individual patient. One might use only 30 s for MMC if the conjunctiva is thin, or as long as 5 min if there is scarring from prior failed surgeries. One may choose to use a valved implant if there is concern about hypotony, or if one does not need an especially low target IOP. Some surgeons use MMC with tube shunts to prevent encapsulation. Some might place the implant inferonasally rather than superotemporally.

These are excellent studies that offer clinically relevant information – but how should they be applied to your practice? Should you favor one procedure over the other?

As with any study, careful consideration should be given to individual cases, using the study results as one potential piece of information in the decision-making process. The following issues should be considered when deciding on the most appropriate surgical approach.

Factors that may favor trabeculectomy

Does the patient have a history of intolerance to many glaucoma medications? Does the patient have difficulty administering eyedrops? Is he or she arthritic? If so, a trabeculectomy may be a better option, as there is less likelihood of requiring supplemental medication.

Does the surgeon have access to a surgical assistant? Most glaucoma surgeons place a BGI beneath the superior and lateral rectus muscles, requiring extensive dissection that is greatly facilitated by an assistant. If no assistant is available, trabeculectomy may be a better option. (Note that Ahmed and Molteno implants require less dissection, as they are placed between the muscles and may be an alternative.)

Does the patient have endothelial disease that may be potentially worsened by placing a tube near the corneal endothelium? Has the patient had a Descemet's Stripping Automated Endothelial Keratoplasty (DSAEK), or will he or she need one in the future? Having a tube in the anterior chamber makes this significantly more difficult. If so, a trabeculectomy would be a better choice.

Does the patient have a scleral buckle or other hardware in the eye? This may make placement of the plate difficult with tube shunt surgery.

Is the eye unusually short with a crowded anterior chamber? In a short, crowded, phakic eye it may be difficult to place a tube without jeopardizing the cornea or lens.

Factors that may favor tube shunt surgery

Does the patient have extensive scarring from prior superior surgery such as extracapsular cataract extraction (ECCE)? If so, the necessary conjunctival dissection for a trabeculectomy could be difficult.

Does the patient have an inflammatory or uveitic glaucoma that would induce scarring and render a trabeculectomy more likely to fail?

Does the patient intend to wear contact lenses? An avascular bleb is a contraindication to contact lens wear due to the increased risk of infection, and a tube shunt may be a better option.

Is the patient at risk for hypotony (high myope, scleral disorder, etc.)? If so, a ligated, nonfenestrated tub shunt may be a better option.

Does the patient have difficulty returning to the office for regular postop visits? Is he or she elderly, frail, or live far away? Trabeculectomy generally requires more postop visits in the first 3 months, and so tube shunt surgery may be a better option.

Is the patient exposed to dirty conditions due to occupation or recreation that might increase the risk of infection through a thin bleb?

Above and beyond all these considerations is each individual surgeon's expertise and level of comfort performing these procedures. We do what we feel would be best for our patients in our hands. But the TVT study has certainly demonstrated that tubes should no longer be relegated to last resort status in eyes that have had multiple prior surgeries. They deserve a place in our surgical armamentarium as a viable alternative to trabeculectomy in the correct patient.

## Bibliography

Gedde SJ, Herndon LW, Brandt JD, Budenz DL, Feuer WJ, Schiffman JC. Surgical complications in the tube versus trabeculectomy study during the first year of follow-up. *Am J Ophthalmol.* 2007;143(1):23–31.

Gedde SJ, Schiffman JC, Feuer WJ, Herndon LW, Brandt JD, Budenz DL and the Tube Versus Trabeculectomy Study Group. Treatment outcomes in the tube vs trabeculectomy study. *Am J Ophthalmol.* 2007;143(1):9–22.

Jamil A, Mills R. Glaucoma tube or trabeculectomy? That is the question. *Am J Ophthalmol.* 2007;143(1):141–142

Stein JD, Ruiz D Jr, Belsky D, Lee PP, Sloan FA. Longitudinal rates of postoperative adverse outcomes after glaucoma surgery among medicare beneficiaries 1994 to 2005. *Ophthalmology.* 2008;115(7):1109–1116.e7.

**Table 68.1** Design features of current glaucoma drainage implants

| Implant type | Size | Material | Valved/nonvalved |
|---|---|---|---|
| Ahmed Glaucoma Valve | 184 mm$^2$ | Polypropylene | Valved |
| | 364 mm$^{2a}$ | Polypropylene | Valved |
| | 96 mm$^2$ | Polypropylene | Valved |
| | 184 mm$^2$ | Silicone | Valved |
| | 364 mm$^{2a}$ | Silicone | Valved |
| | 96 mm$^2$ | Silicone | Valved |
| Eagle Vision implant | 209 mm$^2$ | Silicone | Valved |
| Baerveldt implant | 250 mm$^2$ | Silicone | Nonvalved |
| | 350 mm$^2$ | Silicone | Nonvalved |
| Molteno implant | 134 mm$^2$ | Polypropylene | Nonvalved |
| | 268 mm$^{2a}$ | Polypropylene | Nonvalved |

[a]Indicates double-plate model.

The plate of the Ahmed Glaucoma Valve varies in size and composition, depending on the model. A hard, polypropylene plate is used in the single-plate (S2 model) and the double-plate (B1 model). Both models have a surface area of 184 mm$^2$ (16 × 13 mm) and are 1.9 mm thick. A soft, silicone plate is used in the flexible single-plate (FP7 model) and the flexible double-plate (FX1 model). Advantages of the flexible silicone model include ease of implantation and likely improved biocompatibility compared with polypropylene.[10,11] The double-plate (Bi-Plate) Ahmed Glaucoma Valve allows for greater surface area (364 mm$^2$) for aqueous drainage, and may be implanted on either the right or left side of the eye.[5] Both single-plated models (S2 and FP7) exist in smaller sizes (S3 and FP8) intended for pediatric patients, although many clinicians use the larger-sized plates for children.

### 68.1.2 Eagle Vision Glaucoma Valve

The Eagle Vision glaucoma valve (Eagle Vision, Inc., Memphis, Tennessee) consists of a silicone tube attached to a valve mechanism on a silicone disc with a surface area of 209 mm$^2$. The valve is a pressure-sensitive slit valve that is calibrated to close at approximately 8–10 mmHg.

### 68.1.3 Baerveldt Glaucoma Implant

The Baerveldt Glaucoma Implant (Advanced Medical Optics, Inc., Santa Ana, California) consists of a nonrestrictive silicone tube attached to a soft barium-impregnated silicone plate with a surface area of 250 mm$^2$ (20 × 13 mm), 350 mm$^2$ (32 × 14 mm), or 500 mm$^2$ (36 × 17.5 mm). The plate has fenestrations that allow growth of fibrous tissue through the plate to reduce the height of the bleb, which may reduce the incidence of postoperative diplopia. The 350 mm$^2$ implant is the preferred size because it appears safer and slightly more effective than the 500 mm$^2$ implant.[12,13] Unlike the Ahmed and Krupin valves, which fit between the rectus muscles, the Baerveldt implant must be positioned under two adjacent rectus muscles.

### 68.1.4 Molteno Implant

The single plate Molteno Implant (IOP, Inc., Costa Mesa, California, and Molteno Ophthalmic Limited, Dunedin, New Zealand) consists of a nonrestrictive silicone tube attached to a 13-mm polypropylene end-plate with a surface area of 134 mm$^2$. The double-plate Molteno Implant consists of two plates connected by a 10-mm silicone tube, providing an increased surface area of 270 mm$^2$. The double plate Molteno Implant can be implanted on the right or left side of the eye. A pediatric-size plate (8 mm diameter) is available. The Molteno dual ridge device incorporates a modification that attempts to minimize overfiltration and early hypotony without tube occlusion. The upper surface of the plate is divided into two separate spaces by a V-shaped ridge that encases an area of 10.5 mm$^2$ around the opening of the silicone tube. Theoretically, aqueous must overcome the conjunctival resistance to flow across the ridge into the bleb. While one earlier study supported the benefit of this modification, a more recent study found unpredictable results.[14,15]

## 68.2 Indications

The indications for glaucoma drainage device implantation include the following: previous failure of primary surgery (usually trabeculectomy), extensive conjunctival scarring, and likely failure of trabeculectomy (Table 68.2). Glaucoma drainage implants can be considered for use in primary glaucoma surgery.

**Table 68.2** Indications for glaucoma drainage implants

| |
|---|
| Failed trabeculectomy |
| Extensive conjunctival scarring |
| Likely failure of trabeculectomy, including |
|   Neovascular glaucoma |
|   Uveitic glaucoma |
|   Glaucoma associated with penetrating keratoplasty |
|   ICE syndrome |
|   Epithelial downgrowth |
|   Refractory pediatric glaucoma |
|   Glaucoma following retinal detachment surgery |
| Primary surgery[a] |

[a]Currently under investigation.

### 68.2.1 Failed Trabeculectomy

Glaucoma drainage implants may be considered in eyes that have failed to achieve control of intraocular pressure after trabeculectomy, with or without mitomycin C. Some patients may be candidates for a second trabeculectomy, but conjunctival scarring or rapid failure of trabeculectomy may hasten the decision to proceed to a drainage implant.

### 68.2.2 Extensive Conjunctival Scarring

Drainage implant surgery may be warranted in cases with inadequate conjunctiva because of scarring from previous surgical procedures. Conjunctival scarring near the limbus may preclude the trabeculectomy procedure. In contrast, glaucoma drainage implants may be performed despite extensive conjunctival scarring posterior to the limbus. In some patients, such as those with severe ocular surface disease, it is not possible to perform trabeculectomy, whereas glaucoma drainage implants may be effective.[16] Patients who have undergone multiple previous ocular surgeries may have extensive conjunctival scarring that may preclude trabeculectomy.

### 68.2.3 Poor Prognosis for Trabeculectomy

In some instances, primary surgical treatment with trabeculectomy has a poor prognosis for success. In patients with neovascular glaucoma and uveitic glaucoma, filtration surgery has a high failure rate. In these settings, surgeons may choose to implant a drainage device rather than to perform a trabeculectomy, in order to improve the likelihood of long-term success. Other glaucomas that may be associated with poor long-term success for trabeculectomy include iridocorneal endothelial (ICE) syndrome, epithelial downgrowth, and refractory pediatric glaucomas.

### 68.2.4 Primary Surgery

Glaucoma drainage implants are indicated for primary surgery when trabeculectomy is judged likely to fail by the surgeon. In addition, drainage devices can be considered for broader use for primary surgery, rather than trabeculectomy. One-year results from a randomized, prospective trial comparing trabeculectomy versus Baerveldt implant in patients who have undergone previous trabeculectomy and/or cataract extraction with intraocular lens implantation showed similar success rates.[17] The trabeculectomy group required fewer glaucoma medications but had a higher rate of postoperative complications.[18] A randomized, prospective trial comparing trabeculectomy to the Ahmed Glaucoma Valve for primary surgery has also been reported.[19,20] In this trial, despite lower intraocular pressures for the trabeculectomy group during the first year, longer follow-up showed similar intraocular pressure control and success rates in comparisons between the two groups. Contact lens wearers who require glaucoma surgery should also be considered for primary drainage implant surgery. Although clinicians are concerned about the long-term complications associated with filtration blebs – such as bleb leaks, hypotony, and endophthalmitis – it is not known whether long-term complication rates would be improved after drainage implant surgery compared with trabeculectomy.

### 68.2.5 Contraindications

There are no known absolute contraindications for glaucoma drainage implants. Glaucoma drainage implant surgery and other glaucoma surgical procedures are relatively contraindicated in patients who are noncompliant with self-care in the postoperative period. Borderline corneal endothelial function may worsen after glaucoma drainage implant surgery or other types of glaucoma surgery.[21]

## 68.3 Surgical Techniques

### 68.3.1 Basic Techniques

Retrobulbar anesthesia is administered in most cases. In order to achieve adequate exposure, a 6-0 silk or polyglactin traction suture on a spatula (side-cutting) needle is placed through the cornea near the limbus. Maximal exposure for suturing the plate is achieved by placing the bridle suture adjacent to the quadrant chosen for implantation.

The basic techniques for drainage implant surgery are similar for different types of devices (Fig. 68.1a–c). In most instances, the device is placed in a superior quadrant, usually the superotemporal quadrant. In the quadrant chosen for implantation of the device, a fornix-based incision is made through the conjunctiva and Tenon's capsule. Radial relaxing incisions on one or both sides of the conjunctival flap are frequently required to improve surgical exposure. For implantation of the double-plate devices, a 180° superior conjunctival flap is created. Blunt Westcott scissors are used to dissect between the episclera and Tenon's capsule. The closed blades

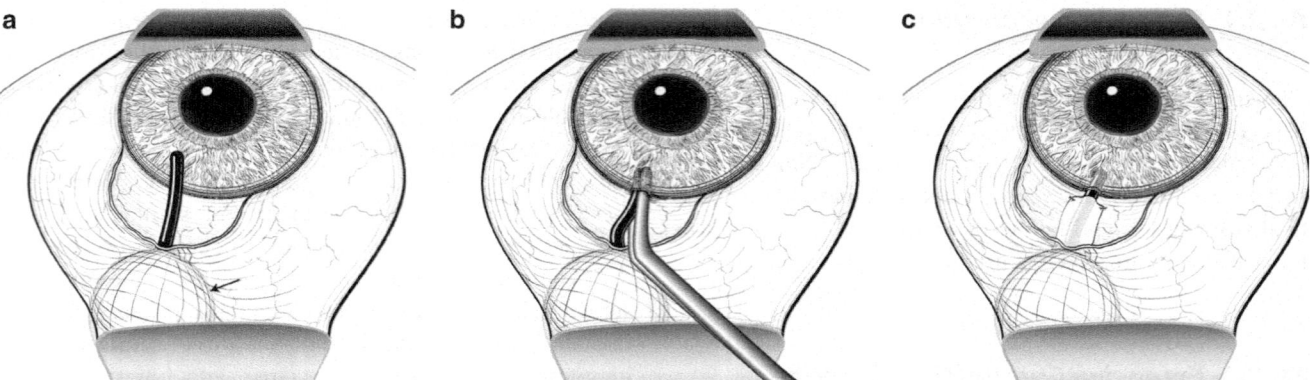

**Fig. 68.1** Glaucoma drainage implant surgical procedure. (**a**) The plate (*arrow*) is sutured to the sclera in the equatorial region. (**b**) The tube is inserted into the anterior chamber through a needle tract. (**c**) The tube is covered with patch material

of Stevens tenotomy scissors (curved or straight) are inserted posteriorly and spread, creating a pocket between the rectus muscles. Wet-field cautery is used sparingly, usually around the site of the tube insertion at the limbus. In the unusual instance when bleeding seems to persist, a Weck-cell sponge soaked in epinephrine-containing solution can provide hemostasis and facilitate posterior dissection.

Prior to implantation, valved implants should be examined and primed. During the sterilization process, the membranes in the valve may adhere to each other. Intraoperative priming of the valve is performed by using a 27- or 30-gauge cannula to irrigate balanced salt solution (BSS) through the tube, ensuring that the valve is functioning properly. In the open tube implants, it is advisable to flush the tubes to confirm that the tube is open.

The Ahmed Glaucoma Valve, Eagle Vision implant, and single-plate Molteno Implant are placed into the pocket between the muscles. For the Baerveldt Glaucoma Implant, the superior and lateral or medial rectus muscles are identified with muscle hooks, and the plate is placed between and beneath the muscles. The valve mechanisms of the Ahmed and Eagle Vision valves should not be grasped with toothed forceps when inserting the plates into the sub-Tenon pocket, because this may damage the devices.[22] The valve is positioned 8–9 mm posterior to the limbus, and the plate is anchored to the sclera with 8-0 or 9-0 nylon suture on a spatula needle though the openings on the anterior edge of the plate. Other permanent suture material with similar or greater tensile strength may be substituted for 8-0 or 9-0 nylon. Care should be taken to avoid scleral perforation, especially in buphthalmic eyes with thin sclera. Implants placed in the superonasal quadrant should not be positioned further than 8 mm posterior to the limbus. Evaluation of postmortem eyes implanted with the Ahmed valve in the superonasal quadrant have shown that the posterior edge of the plate may be close to the optic nerve with further posterior placement of the plate.[23]

The drainage tube is then cut bevel up to permit the tube tip to extend approximately 3 mm into the anterior chamber. The anterior chamber is entered with a 23-gauge needle approximately 0.5 mm posterior to the limbus, parallel or angling slightly forward to the iris plane. The 23-gauge needle provides an adequate size track for tube insertion while minimizing leakage of aqueous around the tube postoperatively. Entry into the anterior chamber posterior to Schwalbe's line and anterior to the iris plane will minimize the risk of contact with the cornea or iris, respectively. The drainage tube is inserted into the anterior chamber through the needle track using nontoothed forceps. An instrument designed for tube insertion (Tube Inserter, New World Medical, Inc., Rancho Cucamonga, California) facilitates this step. The tube is then loosely secured to the sclera using a single 9-0 or 10-0 nylon suture, avoiding constriction of the tube.

To prevent erosion of the tube through the conjunctiva near the limbus, a rectangular flap of processed pericardium (Tutoplast, New World Medical, Inc., Rancho Cucamonga, California; or IOP, Inc., Costa Mesa, California) or preserved donor sclera is sutured over the tube. Other suitable patch graft materials may be used, such as fascia lata, dura, or cornea. Both autograft and allograft patch materials have been used successfully for this application. Although some surgeons use up to four sutures to anchor the patch graft, only two interrupted 9-0 or 10-0 nylon sutures placed on either side of the graft are required to secure the patch graft to the sclera. Fibrin glue may also be used to secure the patch graft, which reduces the need for suturing.[24]

As an alternative to the use of patch materials, a partial-thickness limbal-based scleral flap can be made. A needle tract can be made under the flap through which the tube is placed. The flap is sutured over the flap using 10-0 nylon sutures. Alternatively, a long needle tract may be created with the 23-gauge needle, which minimizes the risk of postoperative erosion of the conjunctiva over the tube.

The conjunctiva is closed using 9-0 or 8-0 polyglactin suture on a tapered needle. The monofilament 9-0 polyglactin suture is preferred because it has a smaller diameter but a higher tensile strength compared with 8-0 braided polyglactin suture. Relaxing incisions are also closed using interrupted or continuous 9-0 polyglactin sutures. Fibrin glue is an alternative to sutures for conjunctival closure, especially when the conjunctiva can be re-approximated with minimal tension. Subconjunctival steroids and antibiotics are injected, preferably 180° away from the plate. Topical steroid and antibiotics are started on postoperative day 1 and tapered over the next 6–8 weeks.

### 68.3.2 Modifications

Following implantation of a glaucoma drainage device, aqueous humor flows from the anterior chamber through a tube connected to a posterior episcleral plate reservoir in the subconjunctival space. Unless a flow-restrictive or valved device is used, no resistance to aqueous humor outflow exists during the early postoperative period, until the formation of a capsule around the plate that resists aqueous flow. To avoid overfiltration and hypotony in the early postoperative period, a two-stage implantation[25-27] or temporary ligation of the tube[15,28-30] may be utilized. In the first stage of a two-stage implantation, the plate is secured to the episclera without inserting the tube into the anterior chamber. The tube is folded back and placed under the patch graft or beneath an adjacent rectus muscle and can be attached to the episclera with a nylon or silk suture to facilitate identification during the second stage. In the second stage, the tube is inserted 4–6 weeks later after a fibrous capsule (pseudocyst) has formed around the plate. This technique minimizes the risk of postoperative hypotony, but disadvantages include transient postoperative intraocular pressure elevation requiring antiglaucoma medication and a second surgical procedure and its attendant inconvenience and risk.

In routine cases, most clinicians implant open tube devices with transient flow restriction techniques (Fig. 68.2a–c). Aqueous flow can be limited in the early postoperative period by internal and external occlusion techniques. In the "rip-cord" technique, a 5-0 nylon or Prolene suture can be placed into the tube lumen at the plate end, providing additional restriction of flow with an absorbable 6-0 or 7-0 Vicryl suture around the tube. The end of the rip-cord suture is placed subconjunctivally near the inferior limbus for subsequent removal. Alternatively, a 6-0 or 7-0 Vicryl suture can be tied tightly approximately 2 mm from the junction of the plate and the tube. This technique prevents any aqueous flow until 4–6 weeks later, when the suture loses tensile strength and the fibrous capsule has formed. Some surgeons also choose to create a slit anterior to the Vicryl suture so that some fluid can escape – maintaining a low IOP during the early postoperative period.[31] A 10-0 Prolene suture can be placed around the tube tip prior to tube insertion into the anterior chamber to restrict flow during the postoperative period. This suture can be opened with a laser, providing additional control of the intraocular pressure during the postoperative period.

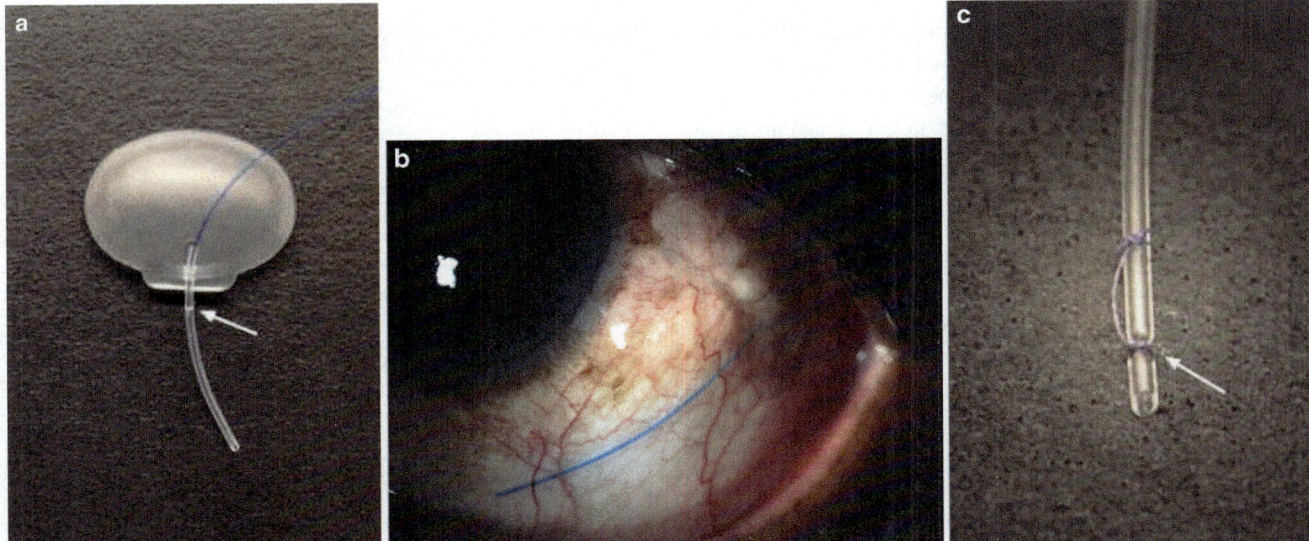

**Fig. 68.2** Flow-restriction techniques for open-tube implants. (**a**) Rip-cord suture. A Prolene suture in the lumen of the tube, and a polyglactin suture around the outside of the tube (*arrow*) reduces or eliminates aqueous flow. (**b**) Rip-cord suture in a patient with a Baerveldt implant. The suture can be visualized under the inferior bulbar conjunctiva at the slit lamp. The 4-0 Prolene suture can be removed at the slit lamp after making a small conjunctival incision with topical anesthesia. (**c**) Prolene suture ligature at tip of tube. The 8-0 to 10-0 Prolene suture is tied tightly near the tip of the tube (*arrow*) and loosely at another proximal position on the tube. The suture at the tip of the tube can be cut with a laser during the postoperative period, thereby allowing aqueous flow through the tube

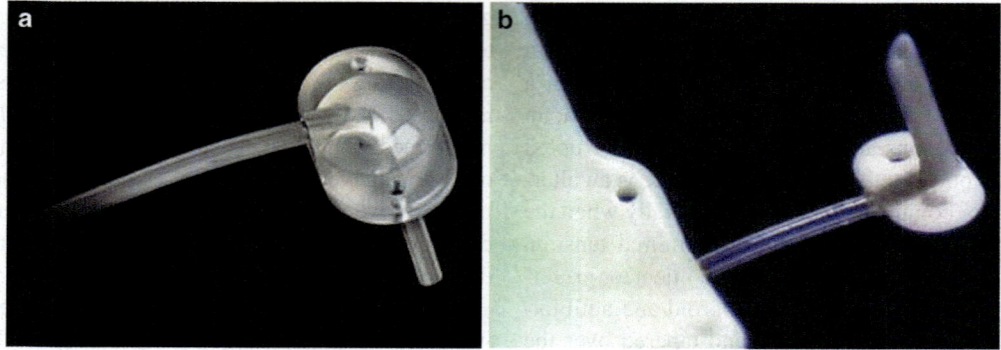

**Fig. 68.3** Pars plana tube insertion devices. (**a**) Pars Plana Clip (New World Medical, Inc., Rancho Cucamonga, California). (**b**) Hoffman elbow (Advanced Medical Optics, Inc., Santa Ana, California)

Viscoelastic is not required for routine cases. However, in certain patients, surgeons may make a self-sealing stab incision (paracentesis) into the anterior chamber near the limbus, usually temporally, and inject viscoelastic into the anterior chamber. Prior to tube insertion, the viscoelastic may help avoid shallowing of the anterior chamber, which can occur when the anterior chamber is later entered with a 23-gauge needle. After tube placement, viscoelastic may help minimize the risk of hypotony in eyes the surgeon considers to be at risk for this problem.

In eyes that contain silicone oil, viscoelastic may avoid intraoperative loss of oil through the tube.[32] Also, placement of the plate in an inferior quadrant (usually inferotemporal) may minimize the loss of silicone oil through the tube during the postoperative period.

In certain patients who are pseudophakic or aphakic and who have had a vitrectomy performed previously, it may be preferable to place the tube into the vitreous cavity rather than the anterior chamber (Fig. 68.3a, b). The Pars Plana Clip (Model PC, New World Medical, Inc., Rancho Cucamonga, California) provides for tube insertion through the pars plana, and can be used with any glaucoma drainage implant. The Pars Plana Clip is easily sutured to the sclera and eliminates kinking of the tube.[33] Pars plana insertion also eliminates the possibility of tube-cornea touch, which may be a consideration in patients with preexisting corneal grafts. The Hoffman Elbow (Advanced Medical Optics, Inc., Santa Ana, California) has been designed for pars plana insertion of the Baerveldt Implant through the pars plana.[34] Repositioning of the Baerveldt implant tube from the anterior chamber into the vitreous cavity may avoid tube-related anterior segment complications.[35]

Some surgeons apply mitomycin C to the area around the plate during surgery, in an attempt to improve the success of the procedure. However, a randomized, prospective, multicenter trial showed no benefit of intraoperative mitomycin C during Ahmed Glaucoma Valve implantation compared with controls in various clinical outcome measures, including postoperative intraocular pressure, number of postoperative medications, and postoperative success rates (Fig. 68.4).[36] Similarly, the use of mitomycin C during Baerveldt implant surgery failed to show an improvement in postoperative intraocular pressure compared to controls.[37]

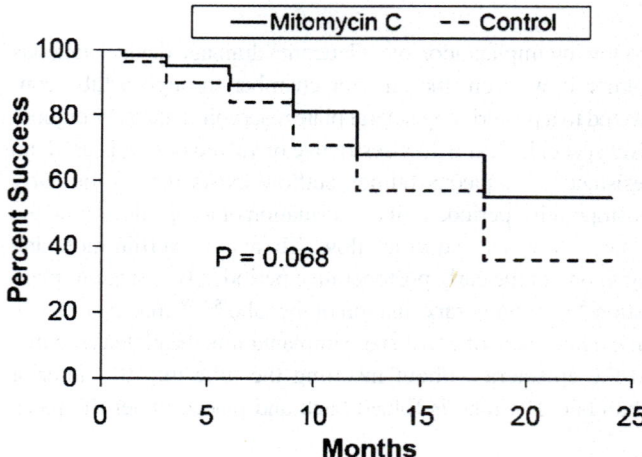

**Fig. 68.4** Mitomycin C and Ahmed Glaucoma Valve implantation. Cumulative probability of success (Kaplan–Meier analysis) from a randomized, controlled, multicenter clinical trial (Reprinted from Costa et al.,[36] with permission from Elsevier)

## 68.4 Clinical Outcomes

Multiple studies have reported the short- and long-term results of the more commonly implanted drainage implants, such as the Ahmed Glaucoma Valve (Fig. 68.5a, b), the Baerveldt Implant (Fig. 68.6a, b), and the Molteno Implant. In these studies, success was typically characterized as an intraocular pressure less than 21 or 22 mmHg and greater than 4 or

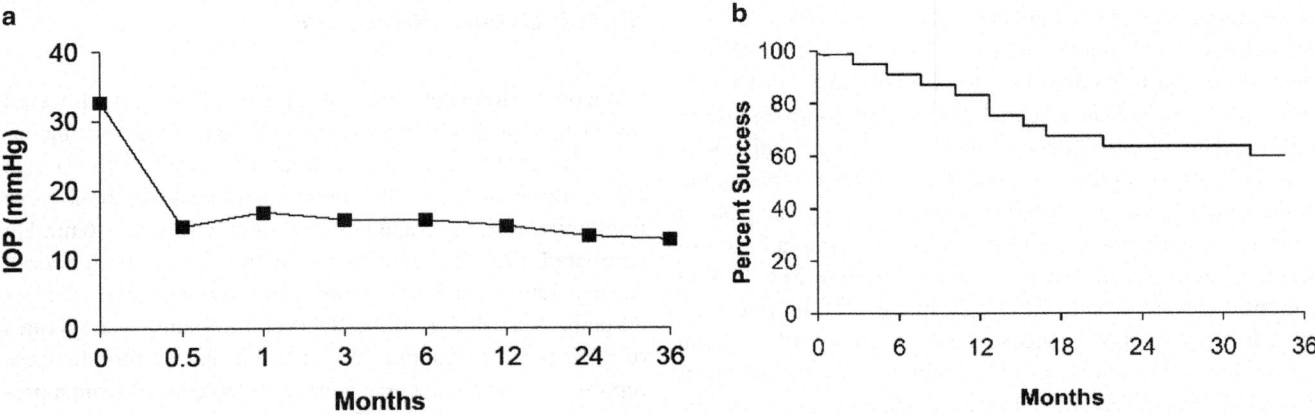

**Fig. 68.5** Clinical outcomes after the Ahmed Glaucoma Valve. (**a**) Mean intraocular pressure after the Ahmed Glaucoma Valve. (**b**) Cumulative probability of success after the Ahmed Glaucoma Valve (Figures reprinted from Huang et al.,[40] with permission from Elsevier)

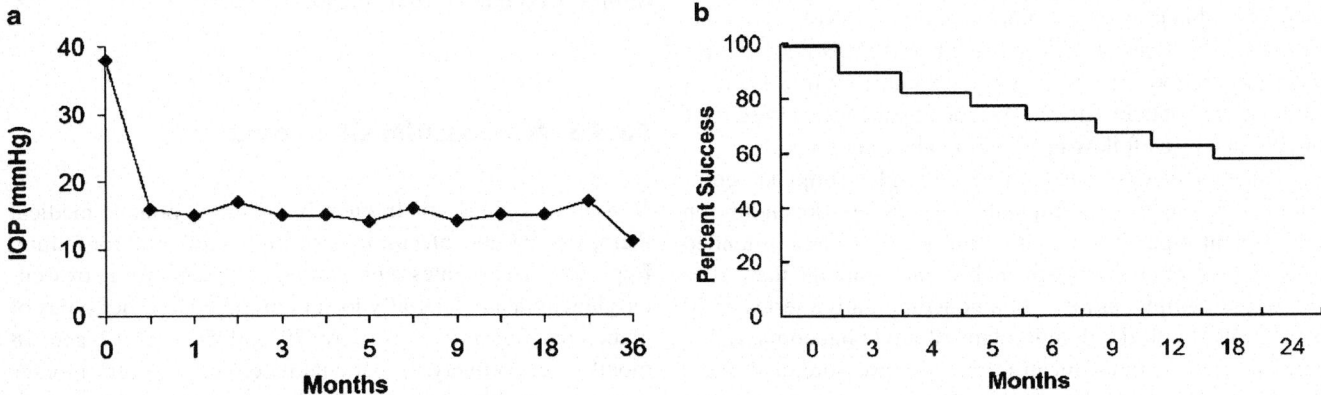

**Fig. 68.6** Clinical outcomes after the Baerveldt implant. (**a**) Mean intraocular pressure. (**b**) Cumulative probability of success after the Baerveldt implant (Figures reprinted from Siegner et al.,[42] with permission from Elsevier)

5 mmHg, with or without medicines, and without further glaucoma surgery or loss of light perception. These studies usually reported outcomes based on the cumulative probability of success. Most of these studies are retrospective, noncomparative case series; and direct comparison of surgical outcomes between different drainage implants is difficult because of the lack of uniformity in the studies.

In long-term follow-up of patients after drainage implant surgery for refractory glaucoma, the intraocular pressure usually ranges in the mid-teens, occasionally reaching the low-teens.[38-46] The intraocular pressure may vary before stabilizing in this range. Initially, the intraocular pressure is low, often less than 10 mmHg, before the formation of a capsule around the implant plate. This hypotensive phase may be followed by a rise of the intraocular pressure, typically at 3–6 weeks after surgery. When the increased intraocular pressure is transient, improving after nonsurgical therapy, it has been described as a "hypertensive phase." When the increased intraocular pressure persists, it can be described as "failure" of the drainage implant surgery.

The hypertensive phase is presumably due to the formation of a thickened capsule around the plate of the implant. The increased intraocular pressure may be severe in rare instances, requiring surgical treatment. The incidence of the hypertensive phase has varied in different reports, occurring in 30–82% of patients following polypropylene (Model S2) Ahmed Glaucoma Valve implantation.[40,41,47-49] The incidence of the hypertensive phase may be lower after silicone plate (Model FP7) compared with polypropylene plate (Model S2) implantation.[48] A hypertensive phase has not been commonly observed after treatment with the Baerveldt or double-plate Molteno implants.[42,50]

Patients often require adjunctive medical therapy for IOP control after surgery, and most studies allow additional medical therapy in their success criteria. The average number of postoperative glaucoma medications required is usually around one.[40,42] In studies with the Ahmed Glaucoma Valve, success rates of IOP control ranged from 76 to 87% at 1 year and from 68 to 77% at 2 years.[38-41] One study with long-term follow-up found success rates at 4 years of 76%.[41] Similar success and complication rates were observed after implantation of the silicone plate compared with the polypropylene plate of Ahmed valve. For the Baerveldt implant, the cumulative probability of success reported in studies ranges from 73 to 92% at 6 months and from 60 to 79% at 24 months.[42,51] In trials with the Molteno implant, success rates of 74% with a mean follow-up of 33 months and 57% with a mean follow-up of 44 months were found.[43,44] Reported success rates with the Krupin valve have ranged from 66 to 80% at 1–2 years.[45,46]

Multiple studies have shown that African-American race is a risk factor for surgical failure of trabeculectomy with adjunctive mitomycin C. In a retrospective, comparative study, African-American race was also shown to be a risk factor for failure of glaucoma drainage device implantation.[47] Success for white patients and African-American patients was 100% and 91% at 1 year and 96 and 79% at 3 years, respectively. In a study of Molteno implants in African-American patients, success rates of 72% at a mean follow-up of 30 months were found.[52]

Reported success rates after double-plate implants compared with single-plate implants have varied, depending on the implant type. Postoperative intraocular pressure tended to be lower after double-plate Molteno implant than after single-plate implantation.[53] In a noncomparative series of 50 eyes treated with the double-plate Ahmed Glaucoma Valve, surgical success rates, mean intraocular pressure, and mean number of medicines were comparable to previous studies reported after implantation of the single-plate Ahmed Glaucoma Valve.[5] The 350 mm$^2$ and 500-mm$^2$ Baerveldt implants also have had similar surgical success rates in studies that compared the different models.[13]

### 68.4.1 Pediatric Glaucoma

In patients with congenital or aphakic glaucoma, cumulative probabilities of success have ranged from 70 to 94% at year 1 and from 56 to 86% at year 2.[54-60] Children may be treated with trabeculectomy with mitomycin C or glaucoma drainage implant, depending on surgeon preference. In some patients judged to be at high risk for complications, such as those with advanced buphthalmos or Sturge–Weber syndrome associated with glaucoma, two-stage implantation over a 4- to 6-week period is probably safer than one-stage implantation, even when valved devices are implanted.[59,60] This approach allows capsule formation around the plate, thereby providing additional protection against postoperative hypotony, and its associated complications.

### 68.4.2 Uveitic Glaucoma

Glaucoma drainage implants have effectively lowered intraocular pressure in patients with controlled and uncontrolled uveitic glaucoma. In a study of 21 eyes with average follow-up of 24.5 months following Ahmed Glaucoma Valve implantation, the average postoperative IOP was 11.6 mmHg compared with 35.1 mmHg preoperatively, with an overall success rate of 94% at 4 years.[61] In a retrospective study of 24 patients treated with the Baerveldt implant, success rates of 96% at 3 months and 92% at 6, 12, and 24 months were reported.[62] The intraocular pressure was reduced from a preoperative mean of 30 mmHg on three antiglaucoma medications to a postoperative mean at 1 year of 13 mmHg on one medication. In patients with uveitis and uncontrolled glaucoma, the success rates are usually improved in patients treated with intensive antiuveitis therapy, including the use of immunomodulatory medications.[61,63,64]

### 68.4.3 Neovascular Glaucoma

Neovascular glaucoma frequently fails to respond to medical therapy, and trabeculectomy has a high likelihood for failure. Reported success rates with drainage implants for neovascular glaucoma are generally lower compared to other types of glaucoma. Success rates were 79 and 56% at 12 and 18 months, respectively, in patients receiving different models of the Baerveldt Glaucoma Implant, with loss of light perception in nearly one-third of patients.[65] In a study of the Ahmed Glaucoma Valve, the success rate was 68% at an average follow-up of 13 months.[40] Studies are pending showing the potential benefit of antivascular endothelial growth factor (VEGF) medicines prior to glaucoma drainage implantation.

### 68.4.4 Glaucoma Associated with Penetrating Keratoplasty

Eyes that undergo corneal transplantation frequently develop elevated intraocular pressure, and conventional filtration surgery may have an increased likelihood for failure.[66-68] In 31 eyes treated with the Ahmed Glaucoma Valve, the success rate at 12 and 20 months was 75 and 52%, respectively.[69] Eyes with a history of infectious keratitis or keratouveitis had 5.8 times the risk of graft failure after placement of the Ahmed Glaucoma Valve. In some instances, the risk of graft failure may be increased after glaucoma drainage device implantation because of mechanical endothelial trauma or inflammation associated with multiple surgeries. Other glaucoma surgical treatments besides glaucoma drainage implants have been associated with increased risk of graft failure. In patients with corneal grafts, there was no significant difference in graft failure rate after glaucoma drainage implant surgery, trabeculectomy, or cyclophotocoagulation.[21]

### 68.4.5 Glaucoma Associated with Severe Ocular Surface Disease

A keratoprosthesis is an alternative for visual rehabilitation in patients with severe ocular surface disease, including ocular cicatricial pemphigoid, Stevens–Johnson syndrome, severe dry eye disease, severe chemical burns, and repeated failure of penetrating keratoplasty. These patients have a high incidence of both open-angle and closed-angle glaucoma before surgery, and many without glaucoma preoperatively develop elevated intraocular pressure after keratoprosthesis surgery. In a study of 55 eyes with severe ocular surface disease treated with keratoprostheses, there was an incidence of glaucoma of 64%.[16] These patients then underwent Ahmed Glaucoma Valve implantation at the same time as the keratoprosthesis if they were previously diagnosed with glaucoma (20 of 35 eyes) or underwent Ahmed Glaucoma Valve implantation at a later time if a diagnosis of postkeratoprosthesis glaucoma was made (15 of 35 eyes). Intraocular pressure was controlled in 81% of patients with 25% requiring additional medications. Vision was improved in 63%, worse in 20%, and unchanged in 17% of eyes.

### 68.4.6 Glaucoma Following Retinal Detachment

Elevated intraocular pressure can occur after pars plana vitrectomy and silicone oil injection for complicated retinal detachments. Most of these cases can be managed with antiglaucoma medicines. Trabeculectomy has a poor prognosis in this clinical situation due to significant conjunctival scarring, possible blockage of sclerostomy by silicone oil, and other adverse effects. In a study including eyes that failed medical therapy, elevated intraocular pressure was managed with the Ahmed Glaucoma Valve.[32] Viscoelastic was injected into the anterior chamber, and the implants were placed in an inferior quadrant to prevent loss of silicone oil. Of 450 eyes treated with pars plana vitrectomy and silicone oil, 51 (11%) developed elevated intraocular pressure. Of these eyes, the majority were treated medically, while the remaining eyes that failed medical therapy were treated surgically with the Ahmed Glaucoma Valve. The intraocular pressure was reduced from a mean of 44 mmHg preoperatively to 14 mmHg postoperatively, with a reduction of antiglaucoma medicines from 3.5 to 1.2. A need for prolonged steroid therapy in eyes containing silicone oil was observed. Silicone oil, observed at the tip of the tube in the anterior chamber in approximately 20% of cases, did not cause obstruction or loss of function of the tube.

## 68.5 Complications

Complications may occur after glaucoma drainage implant surgery (Table 68.3), although most problems occurring with drainage implants can be treated effectively.

### 68.5.1 Hypotony

Hypotony and complications associated with hypotony may occur during the immediate postoperative period after glaucoma drainage implant surgery. Options to restrict aqueous flow include two-stage implantation technique, suture ligature around the tube, and temporary occlusion of the tube lumen with a stent. In a study of 103 eyes treated with the Baerveldt implant, hypotony and choroidal effusions occurred in 32% and 20% of eyes, respectively.[42] Similarly, hypotony-induced choroidal detachments and shallow anterior chamber occurred in 20% of eyes after placement of the Molteno implant.[70] In eyes treated with the Ahmed Glaucoma Valve, hypotony occurred less frequently compared with nonvalved implants, presumably because of the flow-restrictive device on the Ahmed Glaucoma Valve.[38,40]

Hypotony and choroidal effusions may resolve without surgical treatment. When hypotony occurs with a flat chamber and lens-corneal touch, the anterior chamber may be reformed with viscoelastic injected into the anterior chamber in the clinic or may be treated in the operating room. Choroidal effusions may be treated with topical corticosteroid and cycloplegic medications, while large or persistent choroidal

**Table 68.3** Complications of drainage implants

| |
|---|
| Hypotony |
| Choroidal effusion |
| Obstruction of tube by fibrin, blood, iris, vitreous |
| Tube retraction and erosion |
| Tube kink |
| Motility disturbance |
| Corneal decompensation and graft failure |
| Endophthalmitis |
| Retinal detachment |
| Valve malfunction (rare)[a] |

[a]Associated with Ahmed Glaucoma Valve.

effusions may be drained surgically. Removal of the tube can be considered in severe cases.

## 68.5.2 Elevated Intraocular Pressure Due to Other Causes

Elevated intraocular pressure in the postoperative period may occur due to thickening of the capsule or "encapsulation" of the bleb around the drainage implant plate (see Sidebar 68.2).

In one study, encapsulated blebs were observed in 23% of patients, occurring at a median of 32 days after surgery, with a mean intraocular pressure of 34.4 mmHg.[47] Initial treatment of elevated intraocular pressure due to encapsulated bleb consists of adjunctive medical therapy. Other methods to lower persistent elevated intraocular pressure include digital ocular compression, needling with or without 5-fluorouracil (5-FU) injection, or surgical excision of the capsule around the implant plate. Laser cyclophotocoagulation or a second glaucoma drainage device can also be considered.

---

**SIDEBAR 68.2. Encapsulated filtering blebs after glaucoma shunt surgery**

Sandra M. Johnson

The hypertensive phase (HP) is a well-known clinical entity that has been associated with glaucoma filtration surgery such as trabeculectomy, the Ahmed Valve (New World Medical, Rancho Cucamonga, California) as well as other glaucoma tube implants. Like many clinical entities, this one lacks a well-accepted, specific definition and criteria for diagnosis. Hypertensive phase, encapsulated bleb, or Tenon's cyst (Fig. 68.2-1) following trabeculectomy has been described as a thick-walled bleb with prominent vascularity that is localized with associated elevated intraocular pressure (IOP). The thick wall causes the bleb to become more of an extension of the anterior chamber rather than a filtration site. It generally occurs 1–6 weeks following surgery and lasts up to 3 months. The intraocular pressure becomes elevated and some have defined the elevation in general terms such as an IOP over 21 mmHg, but we would benefit from better definitions. Patient risk factors have been sought for Tenon's cysts following trabeculectomy and have included male gender, prior laser trabeculoplasty, prior conjunctival surgery, type of conjunctival incision, and prior beta-blocker usage. There is a suggestion that long-term IOP control is not as good in eyes that have experienced the HP.

In a series of 62 patients who underwent a polypropylene Ahmed glaucoma tube shunt surgery, 23% developed Tenon's cysts over a median time of 32 days postoperative and the IOP rose to the preop level for a duration up to 108 days. In a series of 85 patients, reported by Ayyala, 82% of patients developed an HP. Caprioli sought to characterize the HP following the insertion of polypropylene Ahmed valves. In his series of 156 surgical cases, 56.4% developed HP. He reported that 40.9% of eyes had IOP reach 30 mmHg or higher, which is the preoperative level for his series.

Etiology

The etiology of the hypertensive phase may be related to the flow and/or characteristics of the aqueous itself, because it develops in both eyes having had trabeculectomies or those with implanted glaucoma drainage devices. There also are likely patient factors, as suggested previously, that have yet to be exactly determined. It is known that there is greater bleb failure in eyes with disrupted blood aqueous barrier such as uveitic and neovascular glaucoma. Molteno proposes that opposing "fibro proliferative" and "fibro degenerative" factors in aqueous determine the ultimate bleb histology. For example, Tripathi has described the finding of proinflammatory transforming

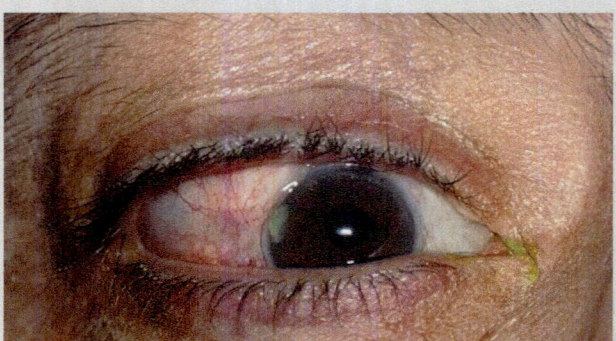

**Fig. 68.2-1** Case of Tenon's cyst. This patient had IOP of 23 mmHg pre-op on four topical medications. He had an Ahmed placed, and 12 days postoperative his IOP was 37 mmHg with a congested thick-walled bleb that deviated his eye nasally. An area of corneal dellen developed adjacent to this elevated thick-walled bleb. Aqueous suppression was instituted and IOP gradually stabilized in the teens over the next 6 weeks

growth factor-alpha 2 (TGF-α2) in the aqueous of glaucoma eyes, and Jampel has suggested that uric acid levels in aqueous influence the outcome of trabeculectomy. The successful blebs around a glaucoma tube implant are the ones that develop a collagen stroma that becomes less compact, as supported by rabbit studies.

There is a mechanical theory that relates to compression of the Tenon's layer from the flow of aqueous into a bleb. Of note, early flow restriction is commonly used with nonvalved implants like the Molteno (IOP, Inc., Costa Mesa, California) and Baerveldt (Advanced Medical Optics, Inc., Santa Ana, California) compared to a valved design like the Ahmed. This also supports a mechanical compression of the inner wall of the filtration bleb as a contributing factor to HP development. Support for restriction of flow is derived from reports on the Baerveldt implant by Siegner and one from Tsai. The case series of Siegner describes no HP following the use of the nonvalved Baerveldt implant and Tsai reported 27% for his Baerveldt group compared to 60% for his Ahmed group. Ayyala also reported 84% HP with Ahmed versus 44% with the implantation of double-plate Molteno devices. As previously mentioned, the exposure of the developing capsule to aqueous and pressure of its flow is limited early on in the healing cascade following surgery when a nonvalved implant is used. Also, the healing of an eye following a tube implant has been thoroughly studied by Molteno on eyes with the Molteno device. The fibro degenerative layer is dependent of aqueous flow as is the fibro vascular layer. The early flow restriction used in the nonvalved implants may have a role in the interaction of the aqueous and the forming capsule layers.

Additionally, the degress of surface area of an implant may play a role in the HP associated with the tube implants. Evidence related to surface area is also presented in the study by Ayyala who compared the HP in patients following implantation of a double-plate Molteno implant to those who received an Ahmed implant. Fewer patients in the Molteno group experienced an HP compared to those in the Ahmed cohort. Both of these implants are constructed of similar material: polypropylene. The surface area of a double-plate Molteno is 270 mm$^2$ and that of the Ahmed is 185 mm$^2$. The smaller surface area of the Ahmed implant may have a role in the HP noted. Support for surface area as a factor for HP development is also derived from the reports on the Baerveldt implant by Siegner and Tsai, where the Ahmed groups with smaller surface area for filtration had more HP reported than the Baerveldt groups. The Baerveldt has a surface area of 350 mm$^2$.

The Baerveldt implant is constructed of silicone. Thus, we need to consider the material of the implant as another variable that may be a factor in the development of HP, as compared to the Ahmed implant. In fact, Baerveldt implants were less reactive in the subconjunctival space compared to polypropylene implant plates. Direct comparison of HP associated with the silicone Baerveldt and the polypropylene Molteno are not available. However, comparison of the silicone and the polypropylene Ahmed has shown no difference in the HP in a report by Ayyala. A report by Mackenzie defined HP as IOP over 21 mmHg and 48% of HP developed with the silicone Ahmed versus 51% in the polypropylene in the cohorts reported.

## Treatment

Some authors suggest intraoperative techniques to influence the development of HP. A report by Susanna, in his prospective study of 92 eyes with neovascular glaucoma, also suggests some modulation of the HP with posterior tenonectomy intraoperative when mitomycin C (MMC) was used as an adjunct in Ahmed placement. The HP was 40% versus 46.8%. Ellingham suggests that the use of MMC over the second Molteno plate at the time of surgery reduces the incidence of HP.

Costa completed a prospective randomized study on management of Tenon's cysts following trabeculectomy. He compared needling to medical management and found no difference in the outcomes of filtration surgery. This suggests that medical management should be first-line treatment, because it is simpler and noninvasive. Of course, in a nonvalved implant, the first-line treatment of the development of elevated IOP would be removal of stints or ligature sutures that are restricting flow, just as laser suture lysis is done with trabeculectomy patients who have rising intraocular pressure. In persistent HP in these eyes and in postoperative Ahmed cases, the medical management is utilized as described for Tenon's cysts following trabeculectomy. Aqueous suppressants are the medical treatment of choice with additional digital massage a further option. As with other conditions, how aggressive one is with treatment depends upon the status of the optic nerve. Moroi and her coworkers described a cohort with a high incidence of failures with medical management, and they utilized needling in most of their cases with some success and excision of the capsule for failures of needling also with some success.

Chen and Palmberg described a technique of needling the encapsulated glaucoma implant with the use of 5-fluorouracil. However, one patient in their series developed endophthalmitis, supporting the use of this as a second-line treatment. Freedman described serial tapping of the bleb to remove the reactive aqueous. Excision of the encapsulation can be undertaken, although this is likely not to be successful if the fibrosis is so extensive as to have a complete failure of filtration prior to excision.

## Conclusions

HP can occur after any filtration surgery and occurs frequently following the Ahmed glaucoma implant. This surgery is notable for a smaller surface area for the filtration reservoir versus other glaucoma tube implants. Although, polypropylene is more reactive than silicone, using a silicone Ahmed has not eliminated HP. The other factor in Ahmed surgery is unrestricted flow in patients who may have reactive aqueous and/or early high flow of aqueous. Mitomycin C has not had a great impact on the development of HP nor has surgical intervention once it occurs. Initial aggressive treatment of inflammation in the anterior chamber should theoretically create a less proinflammatory aqueous. Early use of aqueous suppressants in the postoperative period for a valved design, once the brief hypotensive period passes, is recommended. This can create a medical ligature or stent to decrease aqueous in the early bleb and contribute to the milieu created by the nonvalved implants and theoretically reduce HP in this procedure. Needling and surgical revision remain alternatives for failure to control the HP with medical therapy with some success reported.

## Bibliography

Ayyala RS, Harman LE, Michelini-Norris B, et al. Comparison of different biomaterials for glaucoma drainage devices. Arch Ophthalmol. 1999;117:233–236.

Ayyala RS, Michelini-Norris B, Flores A, et al. Comparison of different biomaterials for glaucoma drainage devices: part 2. Arch Ophthalmol. 2000;118:1081–1084.

Ayyala RS, Zurakowski D, Monshizadeh R, et al. Comparison of double plate Molteno and Ahmed glaucoma valve in patients with advanced uncontrolled glaucoma. Ophthalmic Surg Lasers. 2002;33:94–101.

Ayyala RS, Zurakowski D, Smith JR, et al. A clinical study of the Ahmed Glaucoma valve implant in advanced glaucoma. Ophthalmology. 1998;105:1968–1976.

Campagna JA, Munden PM, Alward WL. Tenon's cyst formation after trabeculectomy with mitomycin C. Ophthalmic Surg. 1995;26:57–60.

Chen PP, Palmberg PF. Needling revision of glaucoma drainage device filtering blebs. Ophthalmology. 1997;104:1004–1010.

Costa VP, Correa MM, Kara-Jose N. Needling versus medical treatment in encapsulated blebs. A randomized prospective study. Ophthalmology. 1997;104:1215–1220.

Eibschitz-Tsimhoni M, Schertzer RM, Musch DC, Moroi SE. Incidence and management of encapsulated cysts following Ahmed glaucoma valve insertion. J Glaucoma. 2005;14:276–279.

Ellingham RB, Morgan WH, Westlake W, House PH. Mitomycin C eliminates the short-term intraocular pressure rise found following Molteno tube implantation. Clin Experiment Ophthalmol. 2003;31:191–198.

Freedman J, Rubin B. Molteno implants as a treatment for refractory glaucoma in black patients. Arch Ophthalmol. 1991;109:1417–1420.

Hinkle DM, Zurakowski D, Ayyala RS. A comparison of the polypropylene plate Ahmed glaucoma valve to the silicone plate Ahmed glaucoma flexible valve. Eur J Ophthalmol. 2007;17:696–701.

Jampel HD, Moon J, Quigley HA, Barron Y, Lam K. Aqueous humor uric acid and ascorbic acid concentrations and the outcome of trabeculectomy. Arch Ophthalmol. 1998;116:281–285.

Kouros N, Caprioli J. Evaluation of the hypertensive phase after insertion of the Ahmed Glaucoma Valve. Am J Ophthalmol. 2003;136:1001–1008.

Lloyd MA, Baerveldt G, Nguyen QH, Minckler DS. Long-term histologic studies of the Baerveldt implant in a rabbit model. J Glaucoma. 1996;5:334–339.

Mackenzie PJ, Schertzer RM, Isbister CM. Comparison of silicone and polypropylene Ahmed glaucoma valves: 2 year follow-up. Can J Ophthalmol. 2007;42:227–232.

Molteno ACB, Fucik M, Dempster AG, Bevin TH. Otago Glaucoma Surgery Outcome Study. Facotrs controlling capsule fibrosis around Molteno implants with histopathologic correlation. Ophthalmology. 2003;110:2198–2206.

Molteno ACB, Suter AJ, Fenwick M, Bevin TH, Dempster AG. Otago Glaucoma Surgery Outcome Study: cytology and immunohistochemical staining of bleb capsules around Molteno implants. Invest Ophthalmol Vis Sci. 2006;47(5):1975–1981.

Richter CU, Shingleton BJ, Bellows AR, Hutchinson BT, O'Connor T, Brill I. The development of encapsulated filtering blebs. Ophthalmology. 1988;95:1163–1168.

Schwartz AL, Van Veldhuisen PC, Gaasterland DE, et al. The Advanced Glaucoma Intervention Study (AGIA): 5. Encapsulated bleb after initial trabeculectomy. Am J Ophthalmol. 199;127:8–19.

Scott DR, Quigley HA. Medical management of a high bleb phase after trabeculectomy. Ophthalmology. 1988;95:1169–1173.

Seigner SW, Netland PA, Urban RC, et al. Clinical experience with the Baerveldt glaucoma drainage implant. Ophthalmology. 1995;102:1298–1307.

Shah AA, WuDunn D, Cantor LB. Shunt Revision versus additional tube shunt implantation after failed tube shunt surgery in refractory glaucoma. Am J Ophthalmol. 2000;129:455–460.

Sherwood MB, Spaeth GL, Simmones ST, et al. Cysts of Tenon's capsule following filtration surgery. Arch Ophthalmol. 1987;105:1517–1521.

Susanna R, Latin America Glaucoma Society Investigators. Partial Tenon's capsule resection with adjunctive mitomycin C in Ahmed glaucoma valve implant surgery. Br J Ophthalmol. 2003;87:994–998.

Tripathi RC, Li J, Ghan WF, Tripathi BJ. Aqueous in glaucomatous eyes contains and increased level of TGF-beta 2. Exp Eye Res. 1994;59:723–729.

Tsai JC, Johnson CC, Dietrich MS. The Ahmed shunt versus the Baerveldt shunt for refractory glaucoma. Ophthalmology. 2003;110:1814–1821.

Yarangumeli A, Koz OG, Kural G. Encapsulated blebs following primary standard trabeculectomy: course and treatment. J Glaucoma. 2004;13:251–255.

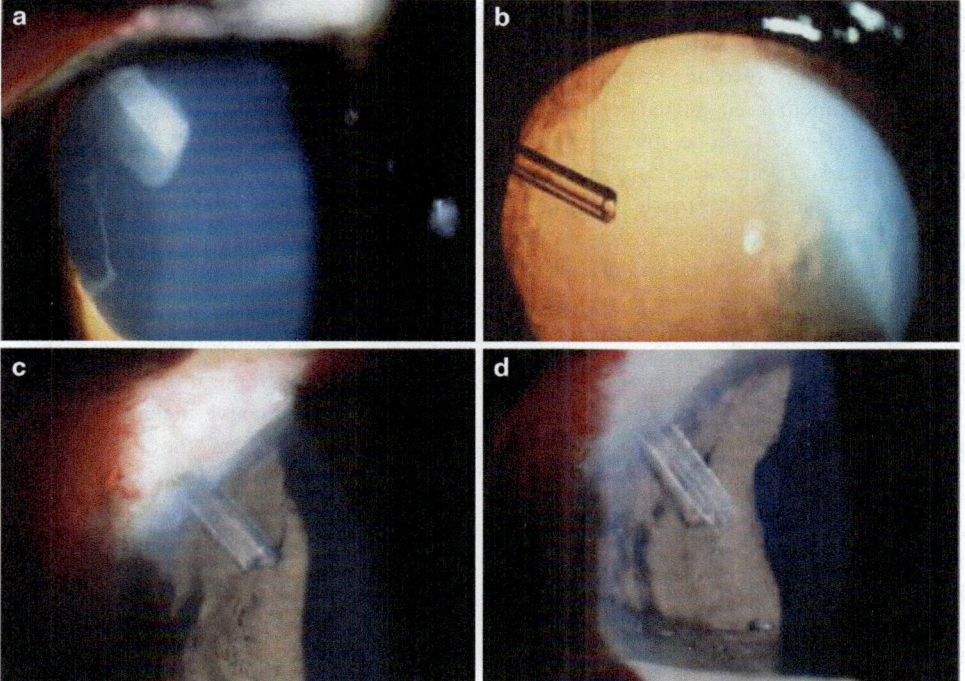

**Fig. 68.7** Obstruction of drainage implant tube. (**a**) Patient with elevated intraocular pressure and blockage of drainage implant tube with fibrin during the immediate postoperative period. (**b**) Same eye as shown in (**a**), a short time after treatment with 10 μg tissue plasminogen activator (TPA) in 0.1 cc. The intraocular pressure remained in the normal range after injection of TPA. (**c**) Patient with shallow anterior chamber during the immediate postoperative period developed blockage of drainage implant tube with iris tissue. (**d**) Same eye as shown in (**c**), immediately after injection of viscoelastic in the anterior chamber

## 68.6 Elevated Pressure Following Implantation

Failure to prime the Ahmed Glaucoma Valve with balanced salt solution intraoperatively can lead to increased intraocular pressure postoperatively. Fibrosis of the valve and postoperative valve failure is rare, but has been reported.[71] Fibrovascular ingrowth into the Ahmed Glaucoma Valve is uncommon, but has been documented as a cause of late failure in adults and pediatric patients.[72]

Elevated intraocular pressure may be caused by obstruction of the tube by fibrin, blood, iris, vitreous, or other substances (Fig. 68.7a–d). This was found to occur in 11% of eyes, most frequently by blood in patients with neovascular glaucoma.[40] Occlusion of the tube by the posterior capsule has also been reported after Ahmed Glaucoma Valve implantation.[73] Intracameral injection of tissue plasminogen activator (0.1–0.2 cc of 5–20 μg) may dissolve a fibrin or blood clot. Neodymium:yttrium aluminum garnet (Nd:YAG) laser can be used to ablate iris tissue or the posterior capsule occluding the tube. A vitrectomy may be required for vitreous in the tube.

Tube obstruction may be due to kinking of the tube after pars plana insertion. This complication can be managed by reinserting the tube in a different scleral entry site or by using a Pars Plana Clip.[32] The Pars Plana Clip has a smooth curvature that avoids kinking. Utilizing the clip during the initial insertion of the tube through the pars plana will avoid this potential complication.

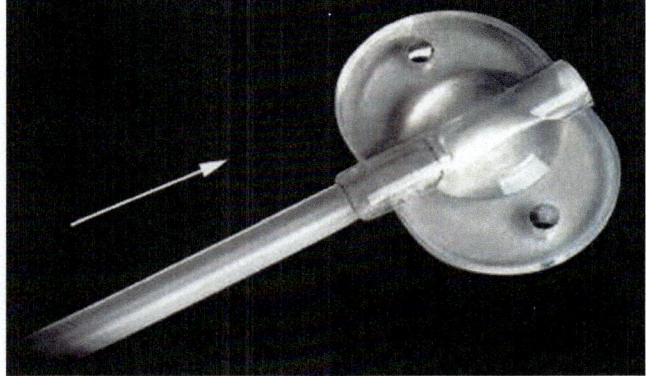

**Fig. 68.8** Tube extender (New World Medical, Inc., Rancho Cucamonga, California). The tube extender can be used for any type of glaucoma drainage device, and has been used for treatment of tube retraction. *Arrow* shows the direction of aqueous flow

### 68.6.1 Tube Migration, Retraction, and Erosion

Tube migration and retraction can occur after any type of glaucoma drainage implant surgery. Inadequate anchoring of the tube or plate may lead to tube-cornea touch, lens injury, obstruction of the tube, or tube retraction. If tube retraction occurs and the tube is too short to reposition, a new valve can be reinserted, the tube can be reinserted in the pars plana, or a tube extender can be utilized to lengthen the tube. The Tube Extender (New World Medical, Inc., Ranch Cucamonga, California) has been shown to be an effective device to lengthen the tube from either an Ahmed Glaucoma Valve, Baerveldt implant, or Molteno implant (Fig. 68.8).[74] Erosion of the tube through the overlying conjunctiva is another recognized complication. As previously described, the tube should be covered with preserved pericardium or preserved donor sclera to prevent this complication. Melting or thinning of the patch graft can occur, potentially leading to an exposed tube. Erosion of the tube should be repaired immediately by surgical debridement, and by covering the area with patch graft and conjunctiva. Erosion of the implant plate may necessitate explantation of the device.

### 68.6.2 Motility Disturbances and Diplopia

In the early postoperative period, transient motility disturbances, including diplopia and restriction of gaze, are attributed to periocular swelling and typically resolve in weeks. Permanent motility disorders may result from mechanical displacement (mass effect) by the implant and bleb, fat adherence syndrome, or posterior fixation suture (Faden) effect associated with scarring under the rectus muscles. This complication has been reported more frequently following implantation of larger drainage devices, such as the Baerveldt and double-plate Molteno implants, but may occur after any type of drainage implant.[6,75-78] Common presentations include exotropia, hypertropia, limitation of rotations, muscle palsies, and acquired Brown's syndrome.

### 68.6.3 Vision-Threatening Complications

Complications that threaten vision are not common after glaucoma drainage implant surgery. Suprachoroidal hemorrhage, choroidal effusions, and retinal detachments are potential complications following surgery. They have been reported to occur in up to 2–5% of patients.[40,41] Endophthalmitis is a rare complication of glaucoma drainage implant surgery that can be associated with any type of glaucoma drainage device. The incidence in one study, which examined 542 eyes with Ahmed Glaucoma Valves, was 1.7%, with *Haemophilus influenzae* and *Streptococcus* species as the most common isolated organisms.[79] The majority of cases of endophthalmitis occurred at least 6 weeks after implantation. Conjunctival erosion overlying the Ahmed Glaucoma Valve tube was found to be the most important risk factor. Surgical revision with a patch graft is recommended in all cases with an exposed tube.

## 68.4 Conclusion

Glaucoma drainage implants are effective for the treatment of patients who have a variety of refractory or intractable glaucomas, including failure to respond to trabeculectomy, extensive conjunctival scarring, or poor prognosis of trabeculectomy for primary surgery. Broader use drainage implants, including use for primary surgery, can be considered. Glaucoma drainage implants can be classified as valved or nonvalved implants. The Ahmed Glaucoma Valve is a popular valved implant, while the Baerveldt and Molteno implants are representative open-tube devices. The valve mechanism of the Ahmed Glaucoma Valve may minimize the incidence of hypotony and its associated complications, while open-tube devices use adjunctive flow-restrictive techniques to minimize the risk of hypotony during the immediate postoperative period. Vision-threatening complications are uncommon after drainage implant surgery.

## References

1. Molteno AC, Straughan JL, Ancker E, et al. Long tube implants in the management of glaucoma. *S Afr Med J*. 1976;50:1062–1066.
2. Krupin T, Podos SM, Becker B, et al. Valve implants in filtering surgery. *Am J Ophthalmol*. 1976;81:232–235.
3. Tam MM, Choplin N, Coleman A, et al. Preliminary results of glaucoma valve implant clinical trial. *Invest Ophthalmol Vis Sci*. 1994;35:1914.
4. Molteno AC. The optimal design of drainage implants for glaucoma. *Trans Ophthalmol Soc N Z*. 1981;33:29–41.
5. Al-Aswad LA, Netland PA, Bellows AR, et al. Clinical experience with the double-plate Ahmed glaucoma valve. *Am J Ophthalmol*. 2006;141:390–391.
6. Smith MF, Starita RJ, Fellman RL, et al. Early clinical experience with the Baerveldt 350-mm² glaucoma implant and associated extraocular muscle imbalance. *Ophthalmology*. 1993;100:914–918.
7. Prata JA Jr, Mermoud A, LaBree L, et al. In vitro and in vivo flow characteristics of glaucoma drainage implants. *Ophthalmology*. 1995;102:894–904.
8. Francis BA, Cortes A, Chen J, et al. Characteristics of glaucoma drainage implants during dynamic and steady-state flow conditions. *Ophthalmology*. 1998;105:1708–1714.
9. Eisenberg DL, Koo EY, Hafner G, et al. In vitro flow properties of glaucoma implant devices. *Ophthalmic Surg Lasers*. 1999;30:662–667.
10. Ayyala RS, Harman LE, Michelini-Norris B, et al. Comparison of different biomaterials for glaucoma drainage devices. *Arch Ophthalmol*. 1999;117:233–236.
11. Ayyala RS, Michelini-Norris B, Flores A, et al. Comparison of different biomaterials for glaucoma drainage devices: part 2. *Arch Ophthalmol*. 2000;118:1081–1084.
12. Lloyd MA, Baerveldt G, Fellenbaum PS, et al. Intermediate-term results of a randomized clinical trial of the 350- versus the 500-mm² Baerveldt implant. *Ophthalmology*. 1994;101:1456–1463.

13. Britt MT, LaBree LD, Lloyd MA, et al. Randomized clinical trial of the 350-mm² versus the 500-mm² Baerveldt implant: longer term results: is bigger better? *Ophthalmology*. 1999;106:2312–2318.
14. Freedman J. Clinical experience with the Molteno dual-chamber single-plate implant. *Ophthalmic Surg*. 1992;23:238–241.
15. Gerber SL, Cantor LB, Sponsel WE. A comparison of postoperative complications from pressure-ridge Molteno implants versus Molteno implants with suture ligation. *Ophthalmic Surg Lasers*. 1997;28:905–910.
16. Netland PA, Terada H, Dohlman CH. Glaucoma associated with keratoprosthesis. *Ophthalmology*. 1998;105:751–757.
17. Gedde SJ, Schiffman JC, Feuer WJ, et al. Treatment outcomes in the tube versus trabeculectomy study after one year of follow-up. *Am J Ophthalmol*. 2007;143:9–22.
18. Gedde SJ, Herndon LW, Brandt JD. Surgical outcomes in the tube versus trabeculectomy study durgin the first year of follow-up. *Am J Ophthalmol*. 2007;143:23–31.
19. Wilson MR, Mendis U, Smith SD, et al. Ahmed glaucoma valve implant vs trabeculectomy in the surgical treatment of glaucoma: a randomized clinical trial. *Am J Ophthalmol*. 2000;130:267–273.
20. Wilson MR, Mendis U, Paliwal A, et al. Long term follow-up of primary glaucoma surgery with Ahmed glaucoma valve implant versus trabeculectomy. *Am J Ophthalmol*. 2003;136:464–470.
21. Ayyala RS, Pieroth L, Vinals AF, et al. Comparison of mitomycin C trabeculectomy, glaucoma drainage device implantation, and laser neodymium:YAG cyclophotocoagulation in the management of intractable glaucoma after penetrating keratoplasty. *Ophthalmology*. 1998;105:1550–1556.
22. Hill RA, Pirouzian A, Liaw L. Pathophysiology of and prophylaxis against late Ahmed glaucoma valve occlusion. *Am J Ophthalmol*. 2000;129:608–612.
23. Leen MM, Witkop GS, George DP. Anatomic considerations in the implantation of the Ahmed glaucoma valve. *Arch Ophthalmol*. 1996;114:223–224.
24. Kahook MY, Noecker RJ. Fibrin glue-assisted glaucoma drainage device surgery. *Br J Ophthalmol*. 2006;90:1486–1490.
25. Molteno AC, Van Biljon G, Ancker E. Two stage insertion of glaucoma drainage implants. *Trans Ophtalmol Soc N Z*. 1979;31:17–26.
26. Bilson F, Thomas R, Aylward W. The use of two-stage Molteno implants in developmental glaucoma. *J Pediatr Ophthalmol Strabismus*. 1989;26:3–8.
27. Budenz DL, Sakamoto D, Eliezer R, et al. Two-staged Baerveldt glaucoma implant for childhood glaucoma associated with Sturge-Weber syndrome. *Ophthalmology*. 2000;107:2105–2110.
28. Latina MA. Single stage Molteno implant with combination internal occlusion and external ligature. *Ophthalmic Surg*. 1991;22:444–446.
29. Sherwood MB, Smith MF. Prevention of early hypotony associated with Molteno implants by a new occluding stent technique. *Ophthalmology*. 1993;100:85–90.
30. Price FW, Whitson WE. Polypropylene ligatures as a means of controlling intraocular pressure with Molteno implants. *Ophthalmic Surg Lasers*. 1989;20:781–783.
31. Trible JR, Brown DB. Occlusive ligature and standardized fenestrations of a Baerveldt tube with and without antimetabolites for early postoperative intraocular pressure control. *Ophthalmology*. 1998;105:2243–2250.
32. Al-Jazzaf AM, Netland PA, Charles S. Incidence and management of elevated intraocular pressure after silicone oil injection. *J Glaucoma*. 2005;14:40–46.
33. Netland PA, Schuman S. Management of glaucoma drainage implant tube kink and obstruction with pars plana clip. *Ophthalmic Surg Lasers Imaging*. 2005;36:167–168.
34. Joos KM, Lavina AM, Tawansky KA, et al. Posterior repositioning of glaucoma implants for anterior segment complications. *Ophthalmology*. 2001;108:279–284.
35. Luttrull JK, Avery RL, Baerveldt G, et al. Initial experience with pneumatically stented Baerveldt implant modified for pars plana insertion for complicated glaucoma. *Ophthalmology*. 2000;107:143–149.
36. Costa VP, Azuara-Blanco A, Netland PA, et al. Efficacy and safety of adjunctive mitomycin C during Ahmed glaucoma valve implantation: a prospective randomized clinical trial. *Ophthalmology*. 2004;111:1071–1076.
37. Irak I, Moster MR, Fontanarosa J. Intermediate-term results of Baerveldt tube shunt surgery with mitomycin C use. *Ophthalmic Surg Lasers Imaging*. 2004;35:189–196.
38. Coleman AL, Hill R, Wilson MR, et al. Initial clinical experience with the Ahmed glaucoma valve implant. *Am J Ophthalmol*. 1995;120:23–31.
39. Topouzis F, Coleman AL, Choplin N, et al. Follow-up of the original cohort with the Ahmed glaucoma valve implant. *Am J Ophthalmol*. 1999;128:198–204.
40. Huang MC, Netland PA, Coleman AL, et al. Intermediate-term clinical experience with the Ahmed glaucoma valve implant. *Am J Ophthalmol*. 1999;127:27–33.
41. Ayyala RS, Zurakowski D, Smith JA, et al. A clinical study of the Ahmed glaucoma valve implant in advanced glaucoma. *Ophthalmology*. 1998;105:1968–1976.
42. Siegner SW, Netland PA, Urban RC, et al. Clinical experience with the Baerveldt glaucoma drainage implant. *Ophthalmology*. 1995;102:1298–1307.
43. Price FW, Wellemeyer M. Long-term results of Molteno implants. *Ophthalmic Surg*. 1995;26:130–135.
44. Mills RP, Reynolds A, Emond MJ, et al. Long-term survival of Molteno glaucoma drainage deices. *Ophthalmology*. 1996;103:299–305.
45. Krupin eye valve with disk for filtration surgery: The Krupin Eye Valve Filtering Study Surgery Group. *Ophthalmology*. 1994;101:651–658.
46. Fellenbaum PS, Almedia AR, Minckler DS, et al. Krupin disk implantation for complicated glaucomas. *Ophthalmology*. 1994;101:1178–1182.
47. Ishida K, Netland PA. Ahmed glaucoma valve implantation in African-American and white patients. *Arch Ophthalmol*. 2006;124:800–806.
48. Ishida K, Netland PA, Costa VP, et al. Comparison of polypropylene and silicone Ahmed glaucoma valves. *Ophthalmology*. 2006;113:1320–1326.
49. Nouri-Mahdavi K, Caprioli J. Evaluation of the hypertensive phase after insertion of the Ahmed glaucoma valve. *Am J Ophthalmol*. 2003;136:1001–1008.
50. Ayyala RS, Zurakowski D, Monshizadeh R, et al. Comparison of double plate Molteno and Ahmed glaucoma valve in patients with advanced glaucoma. *Opthalmic Surg Lasers*. 2002;33:94–101.
51. WuDunn D, Phan AD, Cantor LB, et al. Clinical experience with the Baerveldt 250-mm² Glaucoma implant. *Ophthalmology*. 2006;113:766–772.
52. Freedman J, Rubin B. Molteno implants as a treatment for refractory glaucoma in black patients. *Arch Ophthalmol*. 1991;109:1417–1420.
53. Heuer DK, Lloyd MA, Abrams DA, et al. Which is better? One or two? A randomized clinical trial of single-plate versus double-plate Molteno implantation for glaucomas in aphakia and pseudophakia. *Ophthalmology*. 1992;99:1512–1519.
54. Chen TC, Bhatia LS, Walton DS. Ahmed valve surgery for refractory pediatric glaucoma: a report of 52 eyes. *J Pediatr Ophthalmol Strabismus*. 2005;42:274–283.
55. Djodeyre MR, Calvo JP, Gomez JA. Clinical evaluation and risk factors of time to failure of Ahmed glaucoma valve implant in pediatric patients. *Ophthalmology*. 2001;108:614–620.
56. Englert JA, Freedman SF, Cox TA. The Ahmed valve in refractory pediatric glaucoma. *Am J Ophthalmol*. 1999;127:34–42.
57. Coleman AL, Smyth RJ, Wilson MR, et al. Initial clinical experience with the Ahmed glaucoma valve implant in pediatric patients. *Arch Ophthalmol*. 1997;115:186–191.

58. Netland PA, Walton DS. Glaucoma drainage implants in pediatric patients. *Ophthalmic Surg.* 1993;24:723–729.
59. Ishida K, Mandal AK, Netland PA. Glaucoma drainage implants in pediatric patients. *Ophthalmol Clin North Am.* 2005;18:431–442.
60. Mandal AK, Netland PA. *The Pediatric Glaucomas.* Edinburgh: Elsevier; 2006.
61. Da Mata A, Burk SE, Netland PA, et al. Management of uveitic glaucoma with Ahmed glaucoma valve implantation. *Ophthalmology.* 1999;106:2168–2172.
62. Ceballos EM, Parrish RK, Schiffman JC. Outcome of Baerveldt glaucoma drainage implants for the treatment of uveitic glaucoma. *Ophthalmology.* 2002;109:2256–2260.
63. Netland PA, Denton NC. Uveitic glaucoma. *Contemp Ophthalmol.* 2006;5:1–8.
64. Papadaki TG, Zacharopoulos IP, Pasquale LR, et al. Long-term results of Ahmed glaucoma valve implantation for uveitic glaucoma. *Am J Ophthalmol.* 2007;144:62–69.
65. Sidoti PA, Duphy TR, Baerveldt G, et al. Experience with the Baerveldt glaucoma implant in treating neovascular glaucoma. *Ophthalmology.* 1995;102:1107–1118.
66. Foulks GN. Glaucoma associated with penetrating keratoplasty. *Ophthalmology.* 1987;94:871–874.
67. Franca ET, Arcieri ES, Arcieri RS, et al. A study of glaucoma after penetrating keratoplasty. *Cornea.* 2002;21:284–288.
68. Insler MS, Cooper HD, Kastl PR, et al. Penetrating keratoplasty with trabeculectomy. *Am J Ophthalmol.* 1985;100:593–595.
69. Coleman AL, Mondino BJ, Wilson MR, et al. Clinical experience with the Ahmed glaucoma valve implant in eyes with prior or concurrent penetrating keratoplasties. *Am J Ophthalmol.* 1997;123:54–61.
70. Wilson RP, Cantor L, Katz LJ, et al. Aqueous shunts. Molteno versus Schocket. *Ophthalmology.* 1992;99:672–678.
71. Feldman RM, el-Harazi SM, Villanueva G. Valve membrane adhesion as a cause of Ahmed glaucoma valve failure. *J Glaucoma.* 1997;6:10–12.
72. Trigler L, Proia AD, Freedman SF. Fibrovascular ingrowth as a cause of Ahmed glaucoma valve failure in children. *Am J Ophthalmol.* 2006;141:388–389.
73. Tessler Z, Jluchoded S, Rosenthal G. Nd: YAG laser for Ahmed tube shunt occlusion by the posterior capsule. *Ophthalmic Surg Lasers.* 1997;28:69–70.
74. Sarkisian SR, Netland PA. Tube extender for revision of glaucoma drainage implants. *J Glaucoma.* 2007;16:637–639.
75. Munoz M, Parrish RK. Strabismus following implantation of Baerveldt drainage devices. *Arch Ophthalmol.* 1993;111:1096–1099.
76. Dobler-Dixon AA, Cantor LB, Sondhi N, et al. Prospective evaluation of extraocular motility following double-plate Molteno implantation. *Arch Ophthalmol.* 1999;117:1155–1160.
77. Christmann LM, Wilson ME. Motility disturbances after Molteno implants. *J Pediatr Ophthalmol Strabismus.* 1992;29:44–48.
78. Frank JW, Perkins TW, Kushner BJ. Ocular motility defects in patients with Krupin valve implant. *Ophthalmic Surg.* 1995;26:228–232.
79. Al-Torbak AA, Al-Shahwan S, Al-Jadaan I, et al. Endophthalmitis associated with the Ahmed glaucoma valve implant. *Br J Ophthalmol.* 2005;89:454–458.

# Chapter 69
# Incisional Therapies: What's on the Horizon?

Richard A. Hill and Don S. Minckler

For decades, the primary resistance to aqueous outflow has been thought to reside in the outer one-third of the trabecular meshwork including the juxtacanalicular connective tissue in continuity with the inner wall of Schlemm's canal. Dysfunction of this portion of the trabecular outflow system has been considered to be the main cause of open-angle glaucoma (COAG).[1,2] Surgical therapies have either targeted this tissue directly or bypassed it via scleral fistulas such as trabeculectomy. Goniotomy and ab externo trabeculotomy, still considered the mainstay of surgeries for congenital glaucoma worldwide, have not been considered useful by North American surgeons in adult open-angle glaucoma, but have remained popular in Europe and especially Japan. Other types of microincisional surgery utilizing lasers, such as Q-switched neodymium:YAG, have also been attempted but not been found successful because of a posttreatment healing process described as tissue filling-in whether utilizing micropuncture or strip-ablations. The amount of tissue removed during laser ablation has been increased and thermal damage minimized through the application of erbium:YAG lasers still being clinically utilized in Europe.

The ultimate goal of all nonaesthetic surgery is the restoration of physiologic function. Trabeculectomy and tube shunt surgery have not addressed the primary dysfunction involved in open-angle glaucoma. As an alternative to restoration of function, aqueous is shunted away from physiologic outflow structures into new reservoirs, which allows for passive diffusion. These reservoirs are associated with complications unique to their function and location. Limbal filtering blebs cause bleb-related dysesthesia, and wound leaks or overfiltration may be associated with hypotony maculopathy and bleb-related endophthalmitis. Aqueous drainage shunts produce equatorial filtering blebs, which pose little risk of infection unless the device extrudes, but they can create muscle interference with secondary diplopia. The capsule that forms around the equatorial explant may become over-collagenized with clinically inadequate diffusional capacity.

In terms of the restoration of function of the filtering organ, respect must be shown to the tissues while treating the defect which is present. Healing responses must be integrated into the surgical plan so that filling-in will not cause operative failure. Native tissue functions, such as pumping effects secondary to the ocular pulse (choroidal piston), should be preserved.

Recently, there have been two additional novel surgical approaches to the trabecular portion of the outflow system. One involves trabecular stenting, (Glaukos, iStent, Fig. 69.1). Another technique removes an arc of trabecular meshwork and inner wall of Schlemm's via electro-ablation with simultaneous infusion of fluid and aspiration of tissue debris (NeoMedics, Trabectome, Fig. 69.2).

## 69.1 Developing a Microstent

The concept for the iStent was developed from the observation that trabecular tissues would fill in to apposition after injury or focal removal. The iStent is actually a family of devices to enhance the physiologic outflow of the eye. This device makes a bypass opening in the trabecular meshwork and allows trabecular meshwork to fill into the edge of the device inlet but prevents closure of the opening (Fig. 69.3).

The development of the trabecular stent was not possible until recent engineering improvements in micro machining. The size of the device is based on the scale imposed by the trabecular meshwork and Schlemm's canal. The iStent, which resides in the lumen of Schlemm's canal, is 1,000 μm long and 250 μm in width. It has an open, arched body (Fig. 69.1). The iStent design is intended to perform two functions: providing direct access of aqueous into Schlemm's from the anterior chamber (the snorkel effect) (Fig. 69.4), and pushing the anterior trabecular meshwork away from the posterior wall of Schlemm's canal, where aqueous collector channel openings are located. The arch precludes occlusion of a collector channel opening should it lie behind the iStent (Fig. 69.5).

The device is self-trephining with the aid of an angled tip and open in its tail portion to allow for bidirectional flow. The arch portion of the device also has elevated retention features to limit movement or backing out (self-retaining) from its placement in Schlemm's canal. The device is made out of medical grade titanium (6AL4V) and is heparin-coated (Duraflow). The weight is approximately 60 µg, and mirror image left and right eye devices are required because of anatomical considerations.

## 69.2 Surgical Techniques

Both procedures (Glaukos iStent or Trabectome) can be performed either as a stand-alone surgery or in combination with cataract surgery. Trabecular surgery at the same time as cataract surgery may be performed before or after cataract

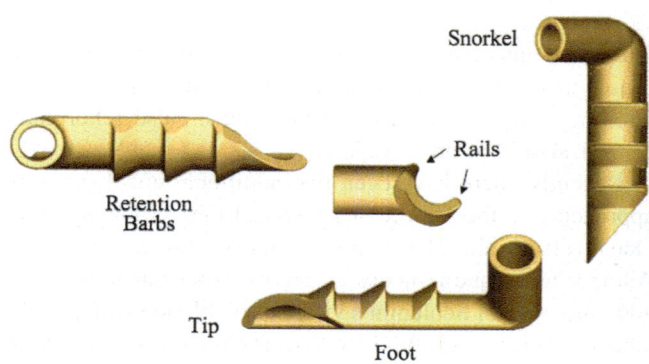

**Fig. 69.1** Glaukos trabecular iStent. Courtesy of Glaukos Corp., Laguna Hills, California

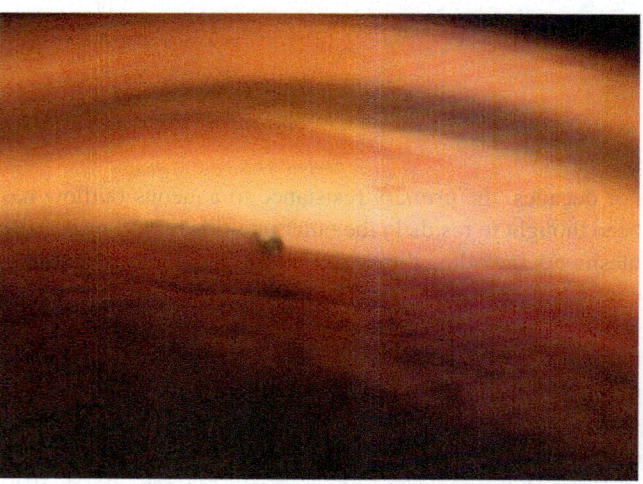

**Fig. 69.3** In vivo goniophotograph of the first iStent implantation, 6 months postoperatively. Courtesy of Glaukos Corp., Laguna Hills, California

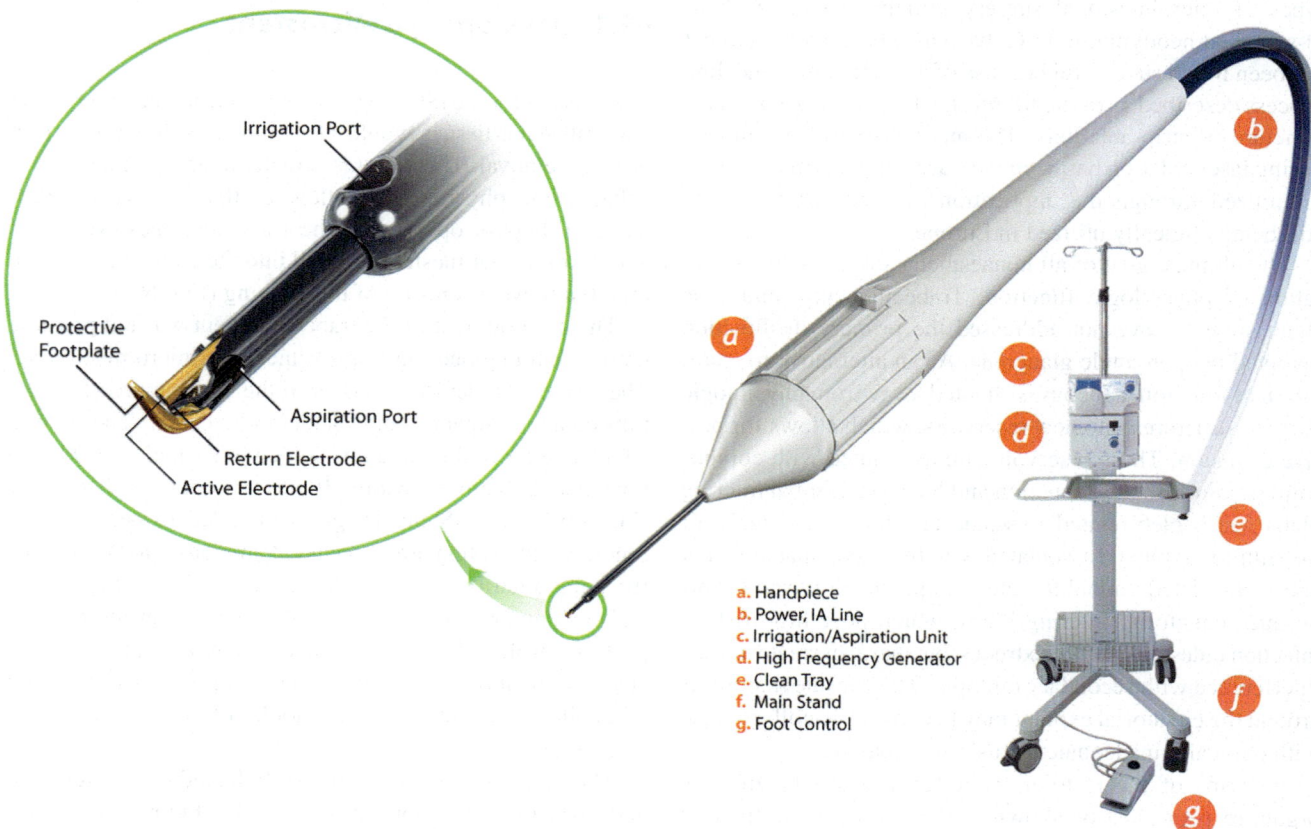

**Fig. 69.2** Trabectome surgical unit and handpiece. Illustration courtesy of NeoMedix, Tustin, California

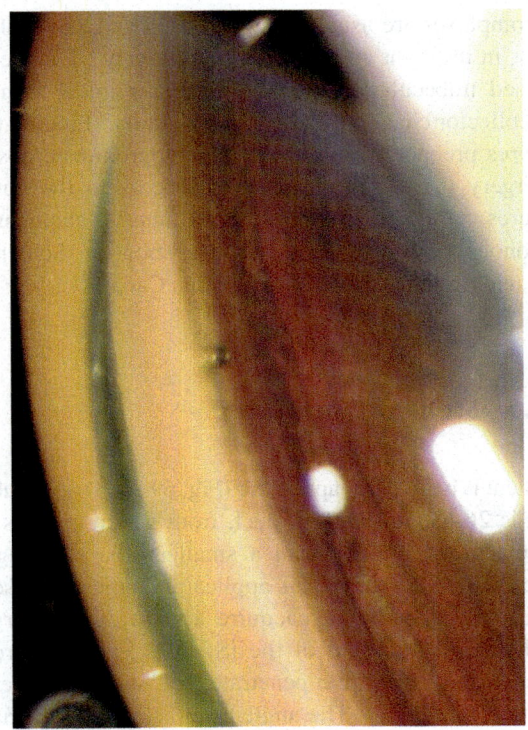

**Fig. 69.4** In vivo goniophotograph 6 months postimplantation. Note trabecular meshwork has filled in to edge of snorkel and stopped. Courtesy of Dr. Jonathan Meyers, Wills Eye Hospital

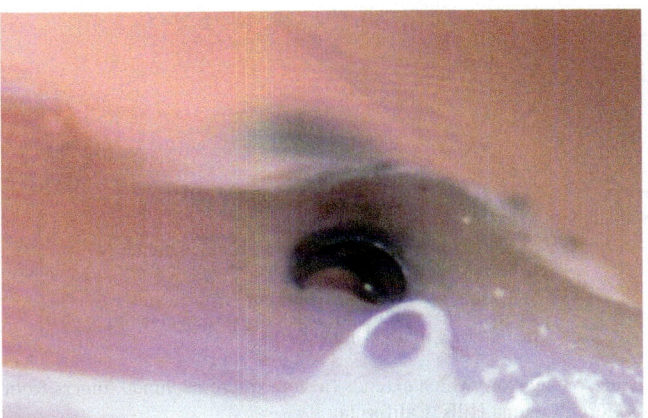

**Fig. 69.5** An iStent implanted in eye bank tissue, showing stenting of Schlemm's canal. Courtesy of Glaukos Corp., Laguna Hills, California

and loss of view when the iStent applicator or Trabectome instrument is placed through the cornea.

Gonioscopes were designed (RAH) in conjunction with Ocular Instruments (Bellevue, Washington) for both procedures (Fig. 69.6), and provide excellent wide-angle views. Both lenses are modified Swan–Jacobs direct gonioscopes for comfortable right- or left-handed manipulation with an elongated handle moved to the side of the lens. On the side facing away from the surgeon, a metal flange facilitates stabilization of the eye and negates the need for traction sutures.

After the creation of the corneal wound, viscoelastic is usually instilled into the anterior chamber to overdeepen it. This allows excellent access to the filtering angle and maximizes the safety in phakic adult and pediatric patients. Alternatively, the Trabectome hand piece includes an infusion sleeve for continual irrigation with balanced salt solution, which is usually adequate in pseudophakic eyes to maintain a deep anterior chamber. The Trabectome surgical pack includes a Simcoe irrigation cannula for use if necessary to ensure removal of all viscoelastic after angle surgery. For iStent, the applicator/hand piece tip is advanced through the wound up to the pupillary margin and the gonioscope placed on the eye. For both procedures, the patient's head should be tilted away at approximately a 45° angle and the microscope body and oculars adjusted toward the operator as necessary to optimize the view. Taping the patient's head is avoided to allow head adjustments intraoperatively. With the gonioscope on the eye, a light touch is used to view the filtering angle. Care should be taken not to indent the cornea as this distorts the view. The site for surgery is selected based

surgery and lens implantation. Potential advantages of angle surgery first before cataract surgery include greater clarity of the peripheral cornea for improved visualization of the filtering angle. In addition, reflux hemorrhage, highly likely, with either can be easily removed during the cataract removal. Both surgeries are started by making a small, temporal, clear corneal incision, with a 15° degree knife or appropriately sized keratome. This incision is made as close to the limbus as possible to prevent lifting of the gonioscope

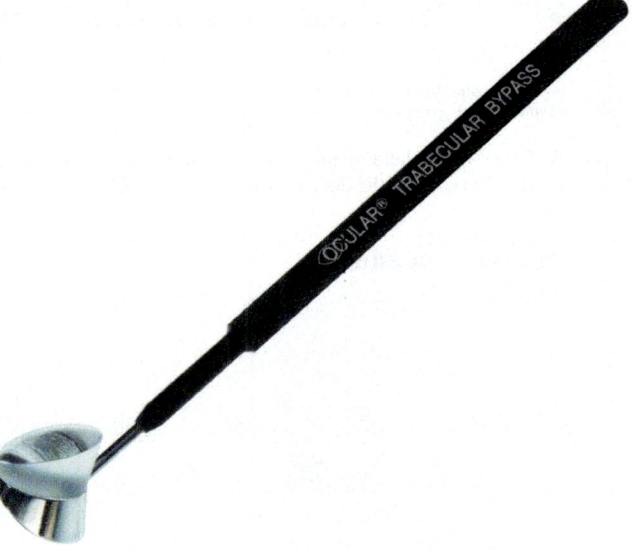

**Fig. 69.6** The trabecular bypass surgical gonioscope. Courtesy of Ocular Instruments, Bellevue, Washington

on observed positions of external aqueous vein complexes (Fig. 69.7) and areas of increased trabecular pigmentation. Aqueous veins may originate with a "C" or "S" shape at the limbus, and their episcleral portion tends to be more linear in which tri-laminar flow often can be seen. The large aqueous vein complexes are usually found at 3:30 and 8:30, inferior nasally, in the right and left eyes respectively.[3] The areas of increased trabecular pigmentation are a clinical sign that large collector channel ostia are in proximity.[4] Finding these structures preoperatively will give an approximate position for surgery that will give maximal access to the outflow structures. Viscoelastic support of the anterior chamber at a hypotonous pressure leads to congestion of Schlemm's Canal, aiding in identifying Schlemm's Canal.

### 69.2.1 iStent Implantation

The iStent is held by the applicator (Fig. 69.8a, b) outer tubing, which is 26-gauge stainless steel, from which extends four micromachined fingers from a smaller tube securing the device by the inlet tube. This applicator can also be used to reposition a stent or to reacquire a stent during surgery. The distal, pointed end of the iStent is inserted through trabecular meshwork in a penetrate, lift, and slide insertion technique (Fig. 69.9). The angle of attack is approximately 30° and the stent is passed through trabecular meshwork at a

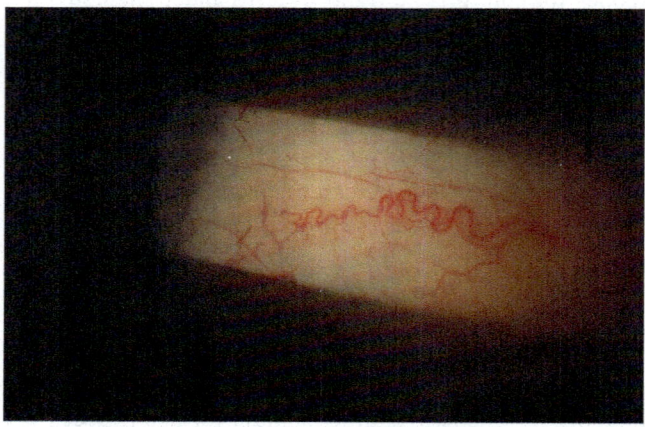

**Fig. 69.7** A large aqueous vein at approximately 3:30 in a right eye. The origin is "C" or "S" shaped – they tend to be more linear and tri-laminar flow can be seen. Courtesy of Glaukos Corp., Laguna Hills, California

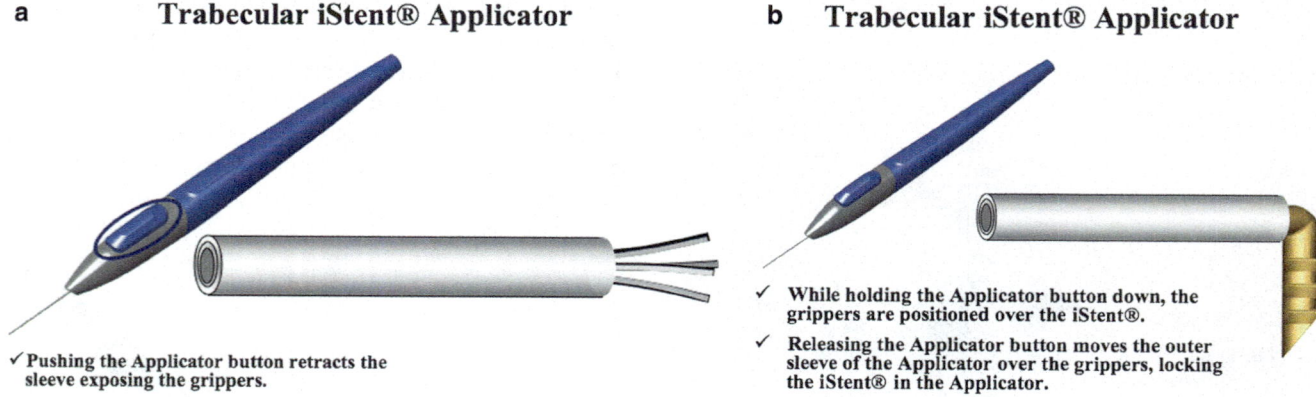

**Fig. 69.8** The iStent is held by the applicator tubing, which is 26-gauge stainless steel from which extends (**a**) four micromachined fingers from a smaller tube (**b**) securing the device by the inlet tube. Courtesy of Glaukos Corp., Laguna Hills, California

### surgical procedure

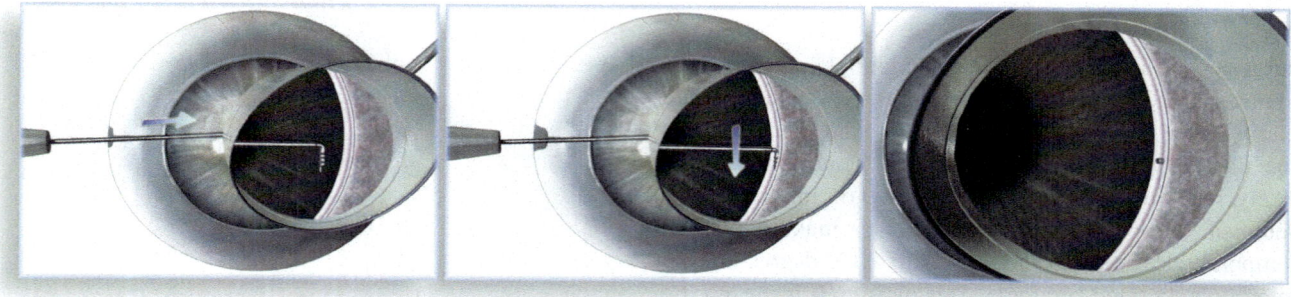

**Fig. 69.9** The pointed end of the iStent is inserted through trabecular meshwork in a penetrate, lift, and slide insertion technique

position of about one-half of the way down the pigmented portion of the trabecular meshwork band (uveal-scleral meshwork). The initial penetration usually goes through trabecular meshwork and the inner wall of Schlemm's canal lodging in the outer wall of Schlemm's canal. At this point, there is a definite sticking sensation and the eye itself can be moved without the implant advancing. A small lifting or a small backing motion is utilized to disengage the posterior wall of Schlemm's canal and a sliding motion is then used to advance the device into Schlemm's canal. Once this has occurred, the release button on the applicator is pushed and the applicator fingers holding the snorkel of the device are released. At this part of the implantation sequence, the heel of the device compresses trabecular meshwork focally and the implant is not locked into Schlemm's canal. Using the applicator, the device must be advanced slightly further to allow the heel to pass beyond trabecular meshwork and the body of the device to sit entirely within Schlemm's canal (Fig. 69.10a–e).

### a  Trabecular Bypass Surgery

- ✓ The Largest Aqueous Collector Channels are Just Under the Horizontal Midline.
- ✓ Clear Cornea Incision is Made and Viscoelastic Added.
- ✓ The iStent® is Pointed at Meshwork with a 20-30 degree Angle of Attack.

### b  Trabecular Bypass Surgery

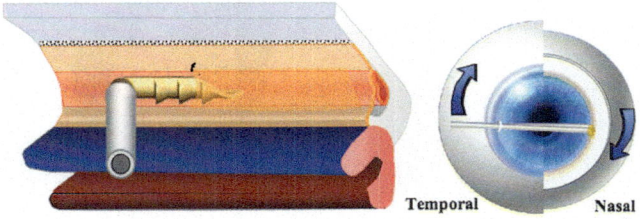

- ✓ The Tip of the iStent® Passes Through the Trabecular Meshwork and Lodges in the Posterior Wall of Schlemm's Canal. A Slight Backing or lifting Motion Will Disengage the Posterior Wall of the Canal.

### c  Trabecular Bypass Surgery

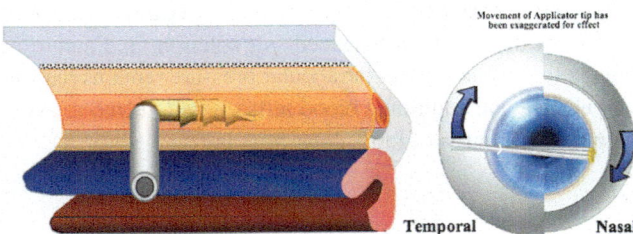

- ✓ Using the Penetrate, Lift/Back-up and Slide Technique Will Allow the iStent® to Intubate Schlemm's canal.
- ✓ Significant Resistance Indicates a False Passage is Being Created.

### d  Trabecular Bypass Surgery

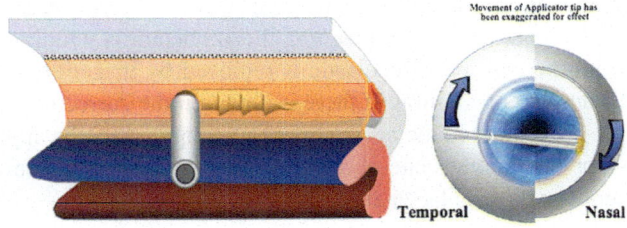

- ✓ Once Intubated, the iStent® Should Slide without Significant Resistance.
- ✓ Advance Only Until the Snorkel Shaft Meets the Meshwork.
- ✓ Push the Button on the Applicator to Release the iStent®.

### e  Trabecular Bypass Surgery

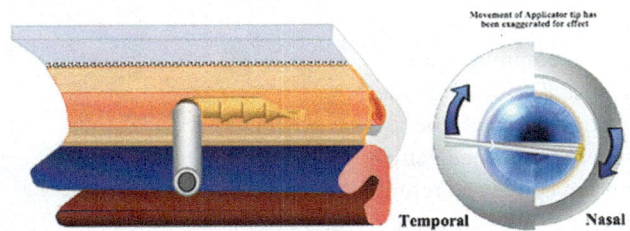

- ✓ Once Intubated, the iStent® Should Slide without Significant Resistance.
- ✓ Advance Only Until the Snorkel Shaft Meets the Meshwork.
- ✓ Push the Button on the Applicator to Release the iStent®.

**Fig. 69.10** (a–e) Implantation sequence of the Glaukos iStent. Illustrations courtesy of Glaukos Corp., Laguna Hills, California

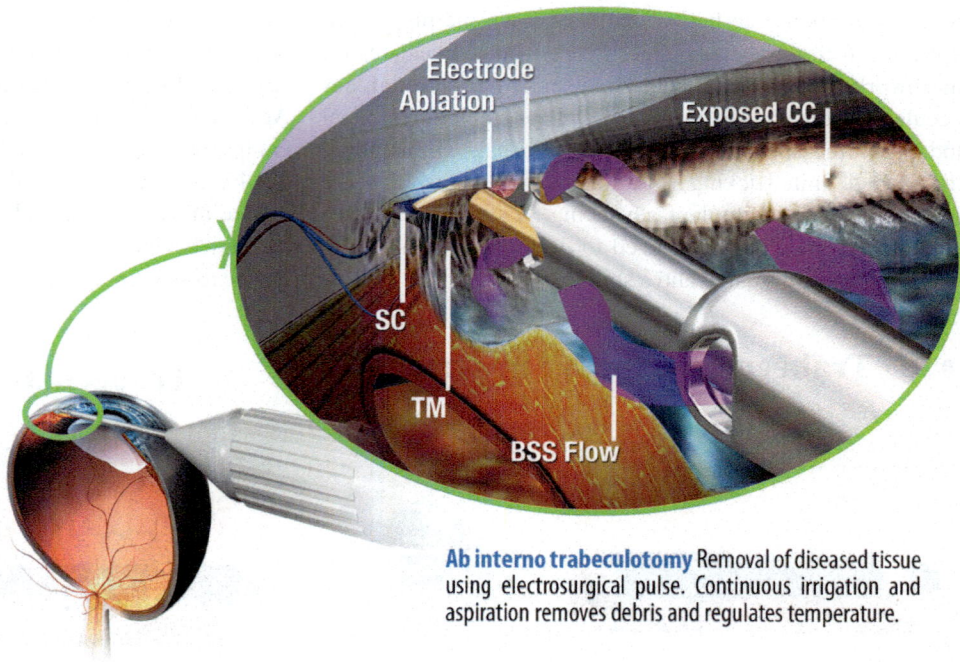

**Fig. 69.11** Trabectome in use. The footplate acts as a guide within Schlemm's canal as the hand piece is rotated. Simultaneous aspiration removes tissue debris and infusion both maintains the anterior chamber and provides cooling as additional protection from thermal injury to adjacent tissues. Illustration courtesy of NeoMedix, Tustin, California

This is accomplished by pushing on the snorkel of the device with the tip of the empty applicator. Reflux of blood may not occur at this point in time as it is tamponaded by viscoelastic in the anterior chamber. When the operator is sure that the device is in the correct position, the applicator is withdrawn from the eye and viscoelastic is removed by irrigation with balanced salt solution. If there is doubt on the correctness of the implantation, the device may be reacquired by the applicator and another site chosen for implantation. The gonioscope is then replaced and the device viewed.

### 69.2.2 Trabectome Trabecular Excision

The Trabectome hand piece – currently cleared for single-use only by the US Food and Drug Administration (FDA) – includes a foot-pedal controlled infusion sleeve and an aspiration function (Fig. 69.2). The tip of the hand piece is passed through trabecular meshwork in a compression and rotation maneuver, using primarily visual clues. Gentle compression of the mesh creates a fold into which the tip can be rotated. The Trabectome tip incorporates an electro-ablation function utilizing a spark between active and return electrodes, shielded from the posterior wall of Schlemm's by the ceramic coated footplate. The footplate acts as a guide within Schlemm's canal as the hand piece is rotated. Simultaneous aspiration removes tissue debris and infusion maintains both the anterior chamber and provides cooling as additional protection from thermal injury to adjacent tissues (Fig. 69.11). Most Trabectome surgeons are attempting to treat at least 3 clock hours (Fig. 69.12).

After both surgeries, it is important to irrigate any viscoelastic used from the eye with balanced salt solution, and suture or hydrate the wound so that intraocular pressure remains reasonably normal and additional blood reflux is minimized to avoid temporary elevation of intraocular pressure.

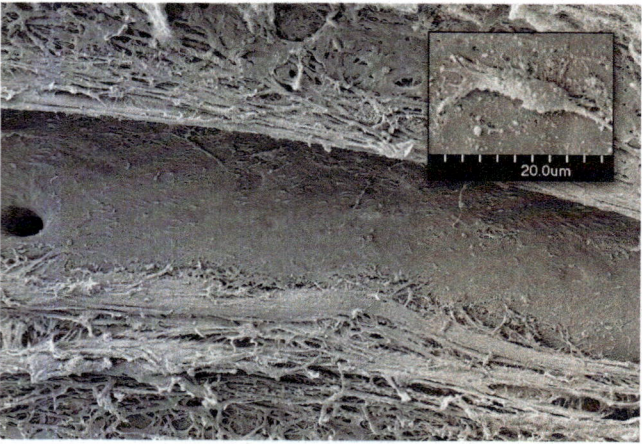

**Fig. 69.12** Scanning electron micrograph; the Trabectome hand piece then utilizes an electric spark to ablate the meshwork and inner wall of Schlemm's canal and aspirate tissue debris for approximately 3 clock hours. Courtesy of Doug Johnson

## 69.3 Results

### 69.3.1 iStent Implantation

The first Glaukos iStent currently has completed a multicenter randomized trial in the US comparing IOP outcomes after iStent and phacoemulsification to phacoemulsification alone; these results have been submitted to the FDA for approval for use in the United States. The Glaukos iStent is CE marked for use in Europe. Peer-reviewed published studies include basic science studies and initial clinical case series.[5-10] The initial proof of concept study ($N=6$) utilized a silicone transtrabecular tube.[8] In cultured autopsy eye perfusion experiments, adding successive bypass shunts produced dramatic step-wise increases in outflow, an encouraging demonstration of the potential for titrating therapy and achieving lower pressures with multiple iStents.[6] A follow-up series, which actually used an early model titanium iStent ($N=6$), established that both pressures and medications could be reduced with stent stability at a follow-up of 1 year.[9]

After the initial proof of principle studies, the device has been studied further as a stand-alone device, in combination with cataract surgery and with two or three iStent implants per eye.

Studies of iStent implantation alone include De Feo et al,[11] who studied 45 patients who had iStent implantation without cataract surgery. The authors found that IOP dropped from a mean preoperative level of $28.4 \pm 6.39$ to $17.9 \pm 3.62$ mmHg at 18 months, and medications decreased from $2.1 \pm 0.94$ to $1.2 \pm 1.18$. The most common adverse events were transient iStent lumen occlusion (seven eyes) and malpositioning (nine eyes). Transient occlusion or malpositioning did not always preclude function. The iStent was also studied in a multicenter open label refractory population by Simmons et al[12] with a total of 45 patients whom had failed filtering surgery. Thirty of the 45 subjects had reached 18 months of a 24-month study. Preoperative mean IOP of $28.4 \pm 6.39$ was reduced to $17.9 \pm 3.62$ mmHg at month 18 ($P<0.0001$). Ninety percent of the 30 eyes remaining in the study at 18 months had IOPs $\leq 21$ mmHg. Ten eyes (33%) achieved IOPs $\leq 21$ without medications. The most common adverse event was safety exit to trabeculectomy in 13 eyes.

IStent implantation has also been studied in combination with cataract surgery. Craven et al[13] updated the GC 002 study, which reported on 59 patients with 24 months follow-up. Intraocular pressure was reduced from a baseline of $21.5 \pm 4.07$ to $15.8 \pm 2.08$ mmHg. Medication usage dropped from $1.7 \pm 0.9$ to $0.5 \pm 0.7$. The most commonly reported adverse event was transient stent lumen obstruction in seven eyes. IStent malpositioning was noted in nine eyes but did not lead to failure in the majority of cases.

Buznego and Tratter also reported 12-month interim results of a 2-year study of iStent and cataract extraction.[14] In 42 patients IOP dropped from $21.7 \pm 3.98$ to $17.4 \pm 2.99$ mmHg at 12 months, and medications used dropped from $1.6 \pm 0.8$ to $0.4 \pm 0.62$ mm Hg. Twenty-one subjects achieved an IOP $\leq 18$ mmHg and had discontinued all topical medications. The most commonly reported adverse event was stent lumen obstruction in seven eyes. IStent malpositioning without IOP failure was noted in six eyes.

Multiple iStent implantations have also been shown to offer additional benefits. This was studied initially in an anterior segment perfusion model and later in human implantations. Doug Johnson showed that adding successive bypass stents produced step-wise increases in outflow.[1] This in vitro experiment provided an enticing demonstration of the potential for achieving very low IOP with such devices, not yet demonstrated in vivo.[1] Although the first stent has the largest effect, dropping IOP from $21.4 \pm 3.8$ to $12.4 \pm 4.2$ mmHg, successive addition of up to four stents placed into Schlemm's canal produced step-wise reduction in system pressure ($13.6 \pm 4.1$ to $10.0 \pm 4.3$ mmHg). After complete excision of the trabecular meshwork, IOP was reduced to $6.3 \pm 3.2$ mmHg.[1] After these initially encouraging results, Ahmed[15] reported on a prospective study of 25 patients undergoing two or three iStent implantation and cataract extraction. Intraocular pressure was reduced from a baseline of 20.5 to 13.2 mmHg. Medication usage dropped from 2.9 to 1.1. IOP drops were similar in the two groups, with the three stent group requiring less medication.

Reflux bleeding from Schlemm's canal after successful iStent implantation and viscoelastic removal intraoperatively is expected.

### 69.3.2 Trabectome Surgery

Trabectome surgery has been cleared by the FDA in the US and has been extensively studied with more than 1,100 surgeries reported.[16-20] Kaplan–Meier survival curves defining "failure" as IOP greater than 21 mmHg and not reduced by 20% below baseline on two consecutive visits beyond 2 weeks postoperatively or additional surgery indicate a "success" rate of 70% out to 52 months ($N=1,127$; $n$ at 60 months $=2$).[20]

In combination with cataract surgery, a sustained drop of 5 mmHg over 2 years has also been demonstrated. Mean preoperative IOP among combined Trabectome-phaco cases, with or without medications, decreased 21% at 6 months ($n=143$), 18% at 12 months ($n=45$), and an overall mean of 20% from $20.0 \pm 6.2$ to $15.5 \pm 4.0$ mmHg at 30 months. Medication use decreased from a preoperative mean of $2.6 \pm 1.1$ to $1.7 \pm 1.5$ at 30 months.

The decrease in IOP among Trabectome-only cases with or without medications was 40% at 24 months ($n=46$), 41% at 36 months ($n=35$) and 35% at 60 months ($n=2$) to $16.4 \pm 4.5$ mmHg down from a mean preoperative IOP of $25.7 \pm 7.7$ mmHg (Fig. 69.13). The mean decrease in adjunctive medications for Trabectome-only cases was 39% from a preoperative mean of $2.9 \pm 1.30$ to a mean postoperative utilization of $1.8 \pm 1.4$ antiglaucoma medications (Fig. 69.14).

Failure defined as additional glaucoma surgery has been reported in 100/738 (14%) of Trabectome-only cases.

In studies to date, only a weak association between treatment arc length and IOP outcomes has been demonstrated.[21] Complications and adverse events among all cases to date have included transient IOP elevation, defined as IOP exceeding 10 mmHg above baseline at day 1, reported in 65/1,127 cases (5.8%).

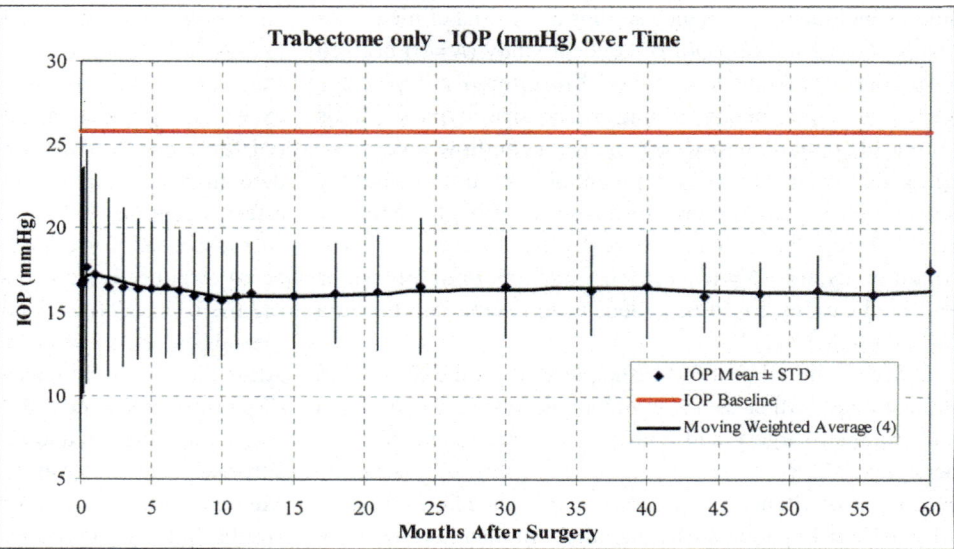

**Fig. 69.13** The decrease in IOP among Trabectome-only cases with or without medications was 40% at 24 months ($n=46$), 41% at 36 months ($n=35$) and 35% at 60 months ($n=2$). Reprinted from Minckler D, Mosaed S, Dustin L, Francis B, and the Trabectome study group. Trans Am Ophthalmol Soc 2008;106:149-160 with permission from the American Ophthalmological Society

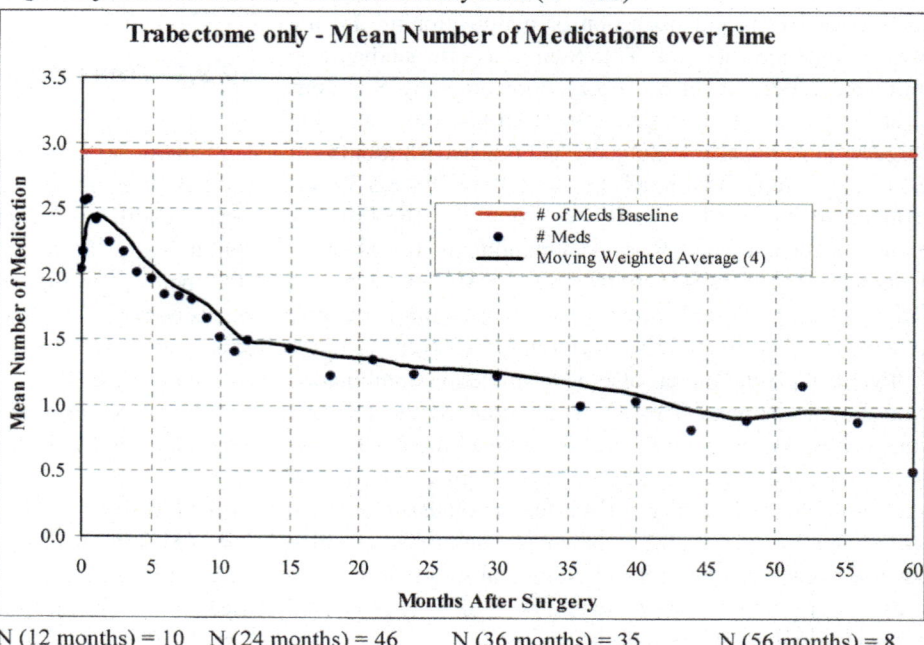

**Fig. 69.14** The mean decrease in adjunctive medications for Trabectome-only cases was 39% from a preoperative mean of $2.9 \pm 1.30$ to a mean postoperative utilization of $1.8 \pm 1.4$ antiglaucoma medications. Reprinted from Minckler D, Mosaed S, Dustin L, Francis B, and the Trabectome study group. Trans Am Ophthalmol Soc 2008;106:149-160 with permission from the American Ophthalmological Society

## 69.4 Discussion

Both techniques in preliminary reports have low complication rates and significant and sustained IOP decreases, usually in the mid-teens. These pressures are probably satisfactory for most early and some moderate glaucomas. The low morbidity associated with these techniques will encourage their early application in both pseudophakic and phakic eyes and will lead to a marked reduction in patients' medical burden. These procedures may also be especially desirable in high myopia, or in cases of hypotony maculopathy or choroidal hemorrhage following prior surgery in the same or opposite eye. Traditionally, the high morbidity associated with filtering surgery has dictated that surgery be deferred in patients with moderate to advanced uncontrolled disease and low intraocular pressure targets. Trabectome and iStent may not be appropriate choices for patients with more moderate to advanced disease. To date, no evidence suggests that either iStent or Trabectome appear to accelerate cataract formation. These techniques do not create conjunctival incisions or scarring, which would compromise subsequent filtering surgery with or without implants. These early techniques to bypass resistance to outflow are passive in nature. Numerous variations in the devices are possible. Experience and computer modeling of the intrascleral collector channels and the outflow organ as a whole should help us better understand why postoperative pressures are in the mid to upper teens with these procedures. In order to achieve lower pressures without trabeculectomy or tube-shunt surgeries, different surgical approaches will have to be utilized. These approaches may include shunting to the uveal-scleral outflow system or the creation of nonpassive devices.

The ultimate goal in the evolution of glaucoma surgery is the early and safe restoration of physiologic function. These two approaches enhance the passive filtration of aqueous through the trabecular outflow organ. They are clinically important, low morbidity options for surgical intervention in the treatment of open angle glaucoma.

### 69.4.1 Clinical Pearls

1. Gonioscopy: Intraoperatively, no single landmark will always accurately locate Schlemm's canal across adult or pediatric eyes. Viscoelastic support of the anterior chamber at a pressure below episcleral venous leads to reflux of blood into Schlemm's canal. This can aid in identifying Schlemm's canal as a red line when overlying trabecular meshwork is nonpigmented or angle structures are poorly defined. As more viscoelastic is added to the anterior chamber, the refluxed blood disappears; and scleral spur or pigmented meshwork may be best for surgical orientation. In the presurgical evaluation of the patient, scleral spur may not be well defined, or trabecular meshwork may be nonpigmented. If this is found, then another technique may be useful for orientation. Under gonioscopic observation, a very bright and thin slit beam creates a parallelpiped of light. This can be seen tracking downward through cornea, terminating at Schwalbe's line.
2. Compression gonioscopy can differentiate between appositional and synechial angle closure.
3. The gonioscope is held lightly against the cornea with only capillary attraction holding it in place. A blink by the patient should easily dislocate the gonioscope. Folds in the cornea may be from excessive force or low intraocular pressure.
4. Hyper pigmented areas of trabecular meshwork logically mark the areas of most active flow through the meshwork and imply the proximity of aqueous collector channels.
5. If the corneal section is made too far from the limbus or too long, the hand piece or applicator will lift the gonioprism off the eye, making the view of the angle difficult and lead to excessive leak of aqueous around the instrument.

## References

1. Grant WM. Experimental aqueous perfusion in enucleated human eyes. *Arch Ophthalmol.* 1963;69:783–801.
2. Johnson DH, Johnson M. How does non-penetrating glaucoma surgery work? Aqueous outflow resistance and glaucoma surgery. *J Glaucoma.* 2001;10:55–67.
3. Ascher KW. *The Aqueous Veins.* Springfield: Charles C. Thomas; 1961.
4. Tanchel NA et al. IOVS 1984;25: ARVO Abstract 7
5. Spiegel D, Kobuch K. Trabecular meshwork bypass tube shunt: initial case series. *Br J Ophthalmology.* 2002;86:1228–1231.
6. Bahler C, Smedley G, Zhou J, Johnson D. Trabecular bypass stents decrease intraocular pressure in cultured human anterior segments. *Am J Ophthalmol.* 2004;138:988–994.
7. Zhou J, Smedley GT. A trabecular bypass flow hypothesis. *J Glaucoma.* 2005;14:74–83.
8. Zhou J, Smedley GT. Trabecular bypass effect of schlemm's canal and collector channel dilation. *J Glaucoma.* 2006;15:446–455.
9. Spiegel D, Haffner WW, DS HRA. Initial clinical experience with the trabecular micro-bypass iStent in patients with glaucoma. *Adv Ther.* 2007;24:161–170.
10. Spiegel D, Garcia-Feijoo J, Garcia-Sanchez J, Lamielle H. Coexistent primary open-angle glaucoma and cataract: preliminary analysis of treatment by cataract surgery and the iStent trabecular micro-bypass stent. *Adv Ther.* 2008;25:453–464.
11. De Feo F et al. ARVO 2008; poster A235.
12. Simmons et al. American Glaucoma Society 2008; poster #72.
13. Craven R et al. Updated the GC 002 study. American Glaucoma Society 2009; Poster 4.
14. Buznego, Tratter. ISRS 2007; poster 101052.
15. Ahmed. American Glaucoma Society 2009; paper 20.
16. Minckler DS, Baerveldt G, Alfaro MR, Francis BA. Clinical results with the trabectome for treatment of open-angle glaucoma. *Ophthalmology.* 2005;112:962–967.

17. Francis BA, See RF, Rao NA, Minckler DS, Baerveldt G. Ab interno trabeculectomy: development of a novel device (trabectome) and surgery for open-angle glaucoma. *J Glaucoma*. 2006;15:68–73.
18. Minckler DS, Baerveldt G, Ramirez MA, et al. Clinical results with the trabectome, a novel surgical device for treatment of adult open-angle glaucoma. *Trans Am Ophthalmol Soc*. 2006;104: 40–50.
19. Francis BA, Minckler D, Mosaed S, Dustin L. Combined trabectome and cataract surgery. *J Cataract Refract Surg*. 2008;34(7):1096-1103.
20. Minckler DS, Mosaed S, Dustin L, Francis BA, The Trabectome Study Group. Trabectome (trabeculectomy-internal approach) additional experience and extended follow-up. *Trans Am Ophthalmol Soc*. 2008. in-press.
21. Khaja HA, Hodge DO, Sit A. ARVO 2008; poster #4191.

# Chapter 70
# Incisional Therapies: Complications of Glaucoma Surgery

Marlene R. Moster and Augusto Azuara-Blanco

A guarded filtration procedure, frequently called trabeculectomy, has been the gold standard for initial surgery for glaucoma almost since its inception in the late 1960s (Fig. 70.1). The current form of this procedure has been attributed to Cairns. Overall, severe visual loss is uncommon, but the incidence of transient complications is high. For example, in the Collaborative Initial Glaucoma Treatment Study (CIGTS), early complications occurred in 50% of 465 trabeculectomies. The most frequent complications were shallow or flat anterior chamber (13%), encapsulated bleb (12%), ptosis (12%), serous choroidal detachment (11%), and hyphema (10%). Suprachoroidal hemorrhage occurred in 0.7% of cases, and there were no cases of endophthalmitis.[2] In the United Kingdom, a national survey of trabeculectomy was conducted, and of 1,240 reported cases, early complications were reported in 46% and late complications in 42% of cases.[3] The most common early complications were hyphema (24%), shallow anterior chamber (23%), hypotony (24%), wound leak (17%), and choroidal detachment (14%). The most frequent late complications were cataract (20%), visual loss (18%), and encapsulated bleb (3%). Recently, the tube versus trabeculectomy (TVT) study in 212 patients found intraoperative complications in 10 and 7% of cases during trabeculectomy and tube surgery, respectively, and postoperative complications in 57 and 34% of patients after trabeculectomy and tube surgery, respectively. Most complications were self-limited.[4]

In this chapter, we review the practical aspects for preventing and managing the complications after glaucoma surgery in general and, specifically, of filtration surgery.

## 70.1 Hypotony and Overfiltration

Hypotony can be caused by excessive aqueous outflow (related to excessive filtration, wound leak, or cyclodialysis cleft) and/or to reduced aqueous production (due to ciliochoroidal detachment, inflammation, inadvertent use of aqueous suppressants, or extensive cyclodestruction). Transient hypotony is very common after glaucoma surgery, but it may lead to other possible complications including flat anterior chamber (Fig. 70.2), corneal edema, Descemet's membrane folds (Fig. 70.3), choroidal effusions (Fig. 70.4), suprachoroidal hemorrhage, visual loss, cataract, macular and optic disc edema, and chorio-retinal folds (predominantly in young myopic patients).[2,3,5]

The initial management of early postoperative hypotony with a formed anterior chamber is conservative, with the use of topical steroids and cycloplegics. Restrictions in activity (bending, weight lifting) and avoidance of Valsalva-positive conditions are recommended. For example, patients might be advised to use bulk stool softeners such as Metamucil. Intervention is indicated in cases when hypotony is associated with other complications such as persistent low intraocular pressure (IOP) with loss of visual acuity and hypotony maculopathy. Treatment should be aimed at correcting the specific cause of hypotony. When there is a flat anterior chamber with lens–corneal touch, immediate surgical intervention is necessary to prevent corneal endothelial damage and cataract formation (see Sidebar 70.1). Reformation of the anterior chamber with viscoelastic can be done in the clinic at the slit lamp or under the operating microscope through the paracentesis that was made intraoperatively.

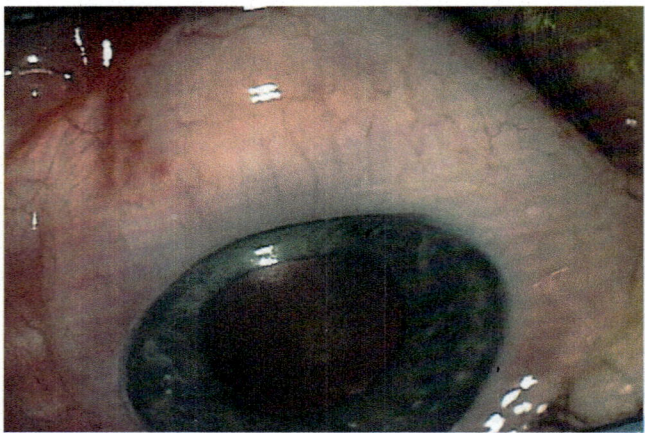

**Fig. 70.1** Low diffuse bleb with large surface area is the goal of glaucoma surgery

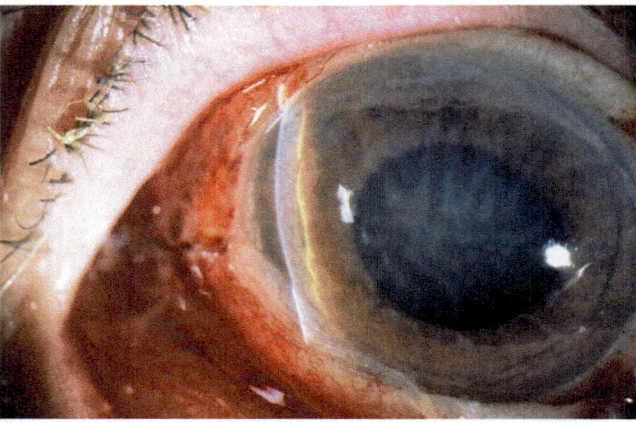

**Fig. 70.3** Corneal edema and Descemet's folds are seen in this hypotonous eye

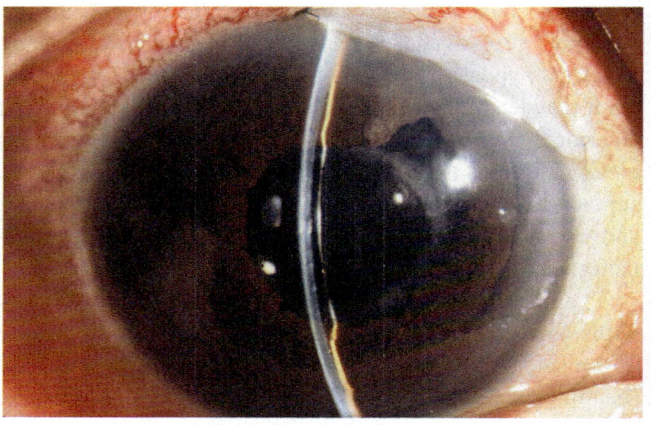

**Fig. 70.2** Shallow chamber after trabeculectomy. Note that there is contact between the cornea and the iris but no lens–cornea touch within the pupillary area

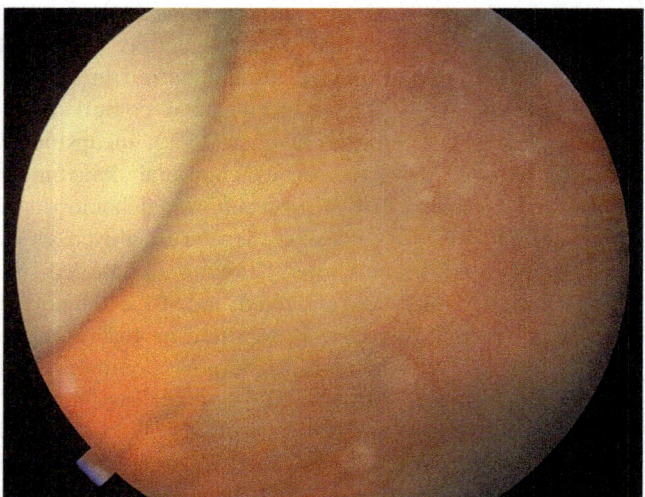

**Fig. 70.4** Serous choroidal detachment noted after a trabeculectomy when the IOP was initially 43 mmHg and fell to 12 mmHg. The chamber shallowed and the choroidal detachment was observed in the periphery

---

**SIDEBAR 70.1 Postoperative flat anterior chamber**

Janet Betchkal and Rick Bendel

You have done the surgery, applied the patch, and have a really good feeling about it. Then you take off the patch the next morning and the anterior chamber is shallow, or, even worse, FLAT. Now you have got a problem that needs more of your attention and the real work begins. How quickly you recognize, diagnose, treat, and *fix* the problem can have a direct bearing not only on the patient's long-term filtering success, but also on the patient's postoperative visual acuity. With respect to glaucoma filtering surgery, the surgery is often the "easy" part and the postoperative care is really the "difficult" part.

This dreaded, often preventable, complication has been reported in as few as 2% to more than 40% of all posttrabeculectomy surgical cases. A large host of variables likely influence its occurrence. Flat anterior chamber most commonly occurs in the early postoperative period; however, it can occur in the later postoperative period (and even years after successful filtering surgery). Early recognition of the problem is the key to the management of flat or shallow anterior chambers.

Some of the more common causes include overfiltration, bleb leak, ciliary body shutdown, pupillary block, aqueous misdirection, and suprachoroidal hemorrhagic effusion, while less common causes include retinal detachment, anterior choroidal detachment, and various patient activities resulting in trauma and/or Valsalva maneuver, often resulting in a choroidal effusion.

For the purposes of defining shallow or flat anterior chambers, we shall use the Spaeth classification where grade I is defined as peripheral anterior iris–corneal endothelial touch, grade II denotes iris–corneal endothelial touch extending all the way from the angle to the pupillary margin, and grade III involves a totally flat anterior chamber with lenticular (or vitreous)–corneal endothelial touch.

The key to determining the etiology of the flat/shallow anterior chamber is most often related to bleb appearance and intraocular pressure (IOP) level. Flat anterior chamber (AC) with a high bleb and low IOP is most commonly associated with overfiltration or ciliary body shutdown. Presence of a bleb leak will also have a low IOP, but it will have a low or flat bleb.

Flat anterior chambers in the presence of ("relatively") elevated IOP are most commonly seen in cases of papillary block or aqueous misdirection – the former associated with a variable bleb appearance and the latter with a low bleb.

Overfiltration (or "too much of a good thing" as we like to think of it) is relatively straightforward to diagnose. The key is a low IOP and flat AC with or without slowly developing choroidal effusions. The only thing it can be confused about is ciliary body shutdown, which is characterized by progressively increasing anterior choroidal effusions (seen at slit lamp and/or on ultrasound).

All blebs should be checked carefully for leaks – with a strip of fluorescein applied directly to the bleb surface, the suture line, and along the limbus. With strict adherence to this policy, a bleb leak should rarely, if ever, be missed.

In eyes with a flat AC, relatively high IOP, and low bleb, the differential diagnosis has to include both pupillary block and aqueous misdirection. Pupillary block should be considered in eyes without a patent full thickness peripheral iridotomy (PI) as in cases utilizing the Express Mini Shunt and/or other anterior chamber tube shunt.

Aqueous misdirection (often referred to as "malignant glaucoma" in the older literature, because of its seemingly "malignant" response to most forms of therapy) is probably the most serious cause of flat AC. In cases of aqueous misdirection, one finds a shallow AC, a patent peripheral iridotomy (without pupillary block), and the absence of choroidal effusions. It is referred to as aqueous misdirection because the aqueous is misdirected posteriorly and ends up in or posterior to the vitreous.

Classically, in cases of aqueous misdirection, the IOP is described as "elevated," but this is a "relative" IOP elevation (i.e., too high for the clinical presentation). Failure to realize that may result in delay in diagnosis, or worse, failure to diagnose. Remember that a filtered eye has a hole in it! Therefore, a "normal" pressure as low as 8–12 mmHg might be significant.

Recognizing the underlying cause of the flat AC is key to implementing the appropriate treatment. In most cases the "best" therapy is prevention (however, once the complication has occurred this will only be helpful in your next case). For example, overfiltration is probably best prevented by limiting the size of the sclerostomy, careful scleral flap closure, the filling of the AC with a viscous agent at the conclusion of the case, the use of topical cycloplegic agents, and possibly by lowering the preoperative IOP (as some have suggested that eyes with lower pre-op IOPs are less likely to experience overfiltration).

In cases of overfiltration, without progressive AC shallowing (grade I AC) one can often get by with simple observation and/or medical treatment with cycloplegic agents (delivered in "pulses"). However, if the AC is progressively shallowing (still grade I), more aggressive treatment may be called for, such as a large diameter soft contact lens (16–22 mm), pressure patch, or Simmons shell. In general, grade I anterior chambers are observed and/or treated noninvasively with pharmacologic agents only.

There is somewhat less agreement about the treatment of a grade II anterior chamber. Recently, the first randomized, prospective study of three methods of treating grade II flat anterior chambers secondary to early overfiltration was reported. This study compared (1) AC reformation with a viscoelastic agent; (2) AC reformation with balanced salt solution (BSS) accompanied by drainage of choroidal effusions using posterior sclerostomies; and (3) medical therapy consisting of atropine or phenylephrine (and, in some cases, an oral carbonic anhydrase inhibitor was required) was reported. The results demonstrated that the grade II anterior chambers treated medically were less likely to lose vision after surgery than those treated surgically with AC reformation with or without drainage of choroidal effusions. While not statistically significant, there seemed to be a trend toward lower postoperative IOP levels in cases undergoing AC reformation with a viscoelastic substance.

Once the AC is totally flat (grade III), there is general agreement that surgical intervention (sooner rather than later) is indicated in order to prevent cataract formation, corneal decompensation, and/or synechiae formation. This most often takes the form of AC reformation with a viscoelastic substance with or without a concurrent posterior sclerostomy.

Ciliary body shutdown occurs in the presence of an excessively inflamed ciliary body resulting in a decrease in aqueous humor production. Therefore, treatment is aimed at reducing that inflammation with increased steroid administration – most commonly topically, but in rare cases, the use of sub-Tenon's and/or oral steroids may be used. Reformation of the anterior chamber is often required while you wait out this process.

Most bleb leaks could be prevented with careful conjunctival dissection, meticulous wound closure, and the use of an appropriate flap type (limbal-based versus fornix-based). Once the leak is identified, if possible, reduce the frequency and dosage of topical steroids. Some of the same therapies employed in the treatment of overfiltration might be useful here, including a pressure patch or large diameter bandage contact lens. Depending on the location of the leak, you can try to use cyanoacrylate glue – always with the use of an underlying bandage contact lens. Other potential treatments aimed at increasing local "inflammation" in the area of the bleb leak include subconjunctival autologous blood injection, topical pilocarpine, cryotherapy, sclerosing agents, or thermocoagulation. Surgical revision is usually the treatment of last resort since suturing of conjunctiva treated with intraoperative antimetabolite therapy can lead to buttonhole formation and increased bleb leakage. Other surgical options include anterior advancement of the conjunctiva or even a "free" conjunctival patch.

Aqueous misdirection is the most frustrating cause of flat AC to treat. Once the diagnosis has been made, adequate cycloplegic therapy must be instituted along with aqueous suppressants (either topically or orally) and increased dosing of topical steroids. In cases with markedly elevated IOP, it is often necessary to use oral hyperosmotic agents (if you can get them). In aphakic eyes or in pseudophakic eyes with an intact posterior capsule, one can do a laser iridotomy accompanied by laser rupture of the anterior hyaloid face or posterior capsulotomy. If all of these measures fail to reverse the trend, then it is necessary to refer the patient to a vitreo–retina specialist for a vitrectomy (with or without a lensectomy).

Suprachoroidal hemorrhagic effusions are a relatively uncommon cause of flat AC. In these cases, one needs to treat the patient's symptoms and continue topical steroids. As long as the IOP is adequately controlled, there is no corneal–lenticular touch, and the patient is comfortable, these eyes can be observed. Otherwise, it becomes necessary to drain the hemorrhage.

Very often as you wait out the protracted course of a flat or shallow anterior chamber, the bleb will begin to fail. In order to "protect" the bleb, one can consider additional use of postoperative antimetabolites and/or elevation of the bleb with a viscous agent (usually at time of AC reformation).

The frequent use of adjunctive antimetabolites in filtering surgery and the rush to achieve lower and lower target IOP levels will ensure that this problem is not going to go away. Therefore, careful attention to detail during the actual filtering procedure as well as vigilance in recognizing the symptoms, identifying the cause(s), and instituting treatment as soon as possible is essential. In all cases, the goal is good IOP, halting the progression of glaucomatous damage, and preserving vision and quality of life.

## Bibliography

Beck AD. Review of recent publications of the advanced glaucoma intervention study. *Curr Opin Ophthalmol.* 2003;14:83–85.

Bellows J, Lieberman H, Abrahamson I. Flattened anterior chamber. *AMA Arch Ophthalmol.* 1955;54:170–178.

Borisuth NS, Phillips B, Krupin T. The risk profile of glaucoma filtration surgery. *Curr Opin Ophthalmol.* 1999;10:112–116.

Brown RH, Lynch MG, Tearse JE, et al. Neodymium-YAG vitreous surgery for phakic and pseudophakic malignant glaucoma. *Arch Ophthalmol.* 1986;104:1464–1466.

Burnstein A, WuDunn D, Ishii Y, et al. Autologous blood injection for the late-onset filtering bleb leak. *Am J Ophthalmol.* 2001;132:36–40.

Byrnes GA, Leen MM, Wong TP, et al. Vitrectomy for ciliary block (malignant) glaucoma. *Ophthalmology.* 1995;102:1308–1311.

Chandler PA, Grant WM. Mydriatic-cycloplegic treatment in malignant glaucoma. *Arch Ophthalmol.* 1962;62:353–359.

Chandler PA, Simmons RJ, Grant WM. Malignant glaucoma medical and surgical treatment. *Am J Ophthalmol.* 1968;66:495–502.

Chandler PA. Malignant glaucoma. *Am J Ophthalmol.* 1951;34:993–1000.

Costa VP, Smith M, Spaeth, GL, et al. Loss of visual acuity after trabeculectomy. *Ophthalmology.* 1993;100:599–612.

Edmunds B, Thompson, JR, Salmon JF, et al. The national survey of trabeculectomy III. Early and late complications. *Eye.* 2002;16:297–303

Epstein DL. Pseudophakic malignant glaucoma – is it really pseudomalignant? *Am J Ophthalmol.* 1987;103:231–233.

Epstein DL, Steinert RF, Puliafito, CA. Neodymium-YAG laser therapy to the anterior hyaloids in aphakic malignant glaucoma. *Am J Ophthalmol.* 1984;98:137–143.

Fontana H, Nouri-Mahdavi K, Lumba J, et al. Trabeculectomy with mitomycin C: outcomes and risk factors for failures in phakic open-angle glaucoma. *Ophthalmology.* 2006;113:930–936.

Gerber SL, Cantor LB. Slit lamp reformation of the anterior chamber following trabeculectomy. *Ophthalmic Surg.* 1990;21:404–406.

Harbour JW, Rubsamon PE, Palmberg P. Pars plana vitrectomy in the management of phakic and pseudophakic malignant glaucoma. *Arch Ophthalmol.* 1996;114:1073–1079.

Jampel HD, Musch DC, Gillespie BW, et al. Perioperative complications of trabeculectomy in the Collaborative Initial Glaucoma Treatment Study (CIGTS). *Am J Ophthalmol.* 2005;140:16–22.

Kim YY, Yung HR. The effect of flat anterior chamber on the success of trabeculectomy. *Acta Ophthalmol Scand.* 1995;73:268–272.

Monteiro de Barros DS, Navano JBV, Mantravadi AV, et al. The early flat anterior chamber after trabeculectomy. A randomized, prospective study of 3 methods of management. 2009;18:13–20.

Osher RH, Cionni LB, Cohen JS. Reforming the flat anterior chamber with Healon. *J Cataract Refract Surg.* 1996;22:411–415.

Parc, CE, Johnson DH, Oliver JE, et al. The long-term outcome of glaucoma filtration surgery. *Am J Ophthalmol.* 2001;132:27–35.

Shaffer RN. The role of vitreous detachment in aphakic and malignant glaucoma. *Trans Am Acad Ophthalmol Otolaryngol.* 1954;58:217–238.

Simmons RJ, Kimbrough RL. Shell tamponade in filtering surgery for glaucoma. *Ophthalmic Surg.* 1979;10(9):17–34.

Smith MF, Magauran III RG, Betchkal JA, et al. Treatment of postfiltration bleb leaks with autologous blood. *Am J Ophthalmol.* 1995;102:868–871.

Spaeth GL. Glaucoma surgery. In: Spaeth GL, ed. *Ophthalmic Surgery: Principles and Practice.* 2nd ed. Philadelphia: WB Saunders; 1990.

Stewart WC, Shields MB. Management of anterior chamber depth after trabeculectomy. *Am J Ophthalmol.* 1988;106:41–44.

The AGIS Investigators. The advanced glaucoma intervention study (AGIS) 7. The relationship between control of intraocular pressure and visual field deterioration. *Am J Ophthalmol.* 2000;130:429–440.

Weiss H, Shin DH, Kollarits CR. Vitrectomy for ciliary block (malignant) glaucoma. *Ophthalmology.* 1981;21:113–119.

WuDunn D, Ryser D, Cantor LB. Surgical drainage of choroidal effusions following glaucoma surgery. *J Glaucoma.* 2005;14: 103–108.

Zalta AH, Wieder RH. Closure of leaking filtering blebs with cyanoacrylate tissue adhesive. *Br J Ophthalmol.* 1991;175(3): 170–173.

## 70.2 Hypotony and Choroidal Effusions

When there are large appositional ("kissing") choroidal effusions and the bleb is threatened, drainage of the fluid is recommended (Fig. 70.5).[5] Large, nonkissing, choroidal effusions may be managed by watchful waiting, but frequent (e.g., every week) monitoring is necessary to make sure that apposition does not occur. Patients should be advised that if central vision decreases, they should notify their surgeon immediately.

Most commonly, hypotony is due to overfiltration of a filtering bleb. Several treatment options are available. Localized compression of the filtration site with a large bandage contact lens or a Simmons shell may be helpful.[6,7] Several treatments have been used to induce an inflammatory or healing reaction in the filtering bleb, which modifies the morphology of the filtering blebs and increases the IOP. These procedures include topical application of chemicals to the bleb surface, cryotherapy, or thermal lasers, but are not very popular.[8,9] Injection of autologous blood into the bleb may reduce overfiltration and resolve bleb leaks, but in our experience, the results are disappointing.[10–12] Finally, surgical revision is the most efficacious option. Resuturing the scleral flap (occasionally associated with use of a scleral patch graft when resuturing is not possible) is our favored option.[13–15]

### 70.2.1 Hypotony Maculopathy

Some patients with intraocular hypotony develop loss of central vision secondary to marked irregular folding of the

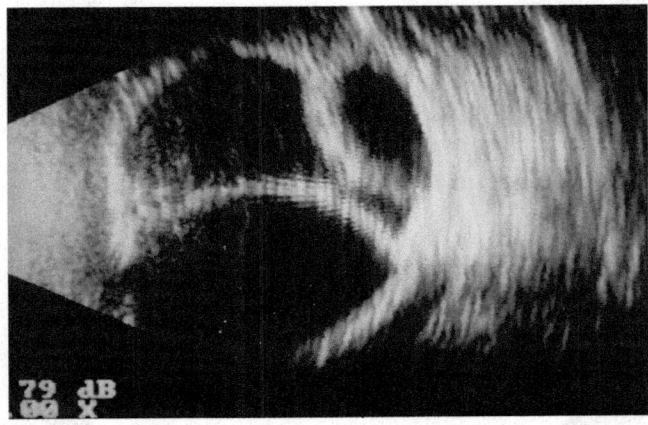

**Fig. 70.5** B-scan of large kissing choroidals (serous choroidal effusions)

choroid and retina. The incidence of hypotony maculopathy after glaucoma surgery has increased with the use of antifibrotic agents, specifically mitomycin-C. The maculopathy is most likely to occur in young myopic patients, who may have a sclera more susceptible to swelling and contraction.[16–18]

The retina often shows a series of stellate folds around the center of the fovea (Figs. 70.6 and 70.7). The retinal vessels are tortuous and sometimes engorged. There may be swelling of the peripapillary choroid simulating papilledema. Visual loss is due to the marked folding of the central retina. Early detection of this condition is a key to preventing permanent visual loss, because long-standing retinal folds will not revert to normal anatomy and normal vision will not be restored.

To prevent postoperative hypotony, intraoperative and postoperative control of outflow drainage is essential. During a

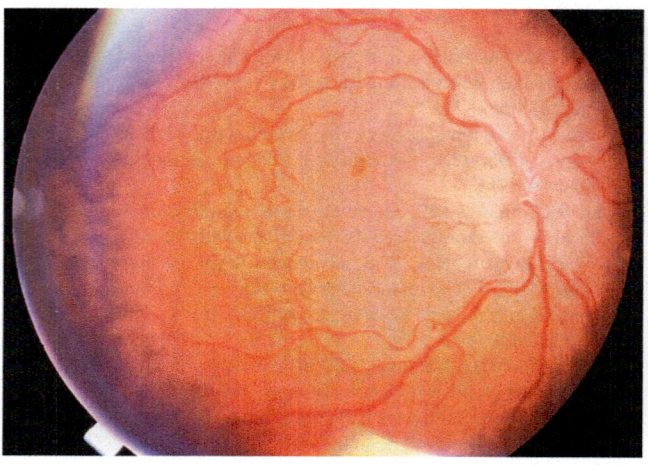

**Fig. 70.6** Disc edema with hypotony maculopathy. The border of the optic disc is swollen due to the low intraocular pressure and disruption of axoplasmic flow. The vessels are tortuous and there are chorio-retinal folds, with edema

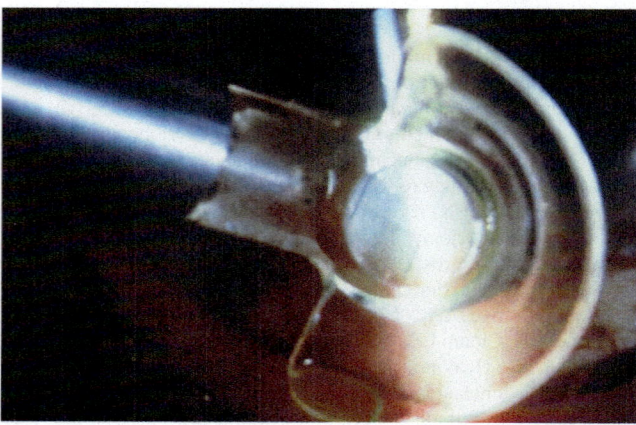

**Fig. 70.8** Laser suture lysis with the Hoskins lens

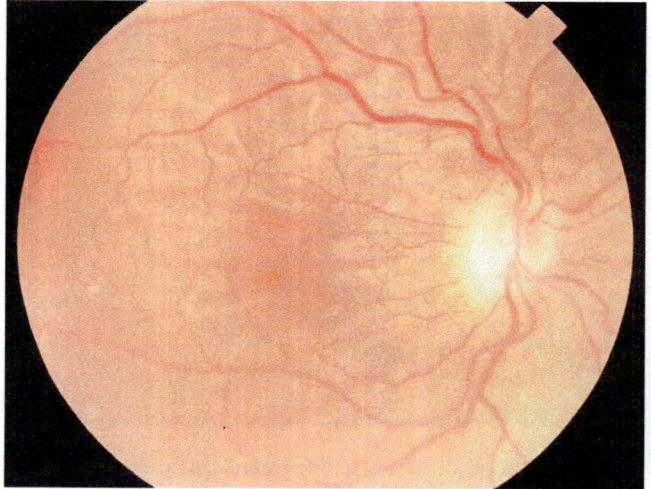

**Fig. 70.7** Chorioretinal folds are often noted in hypotonous eyes of long duration. After the IOP is normalized, the folds often regress and vision can return to normal

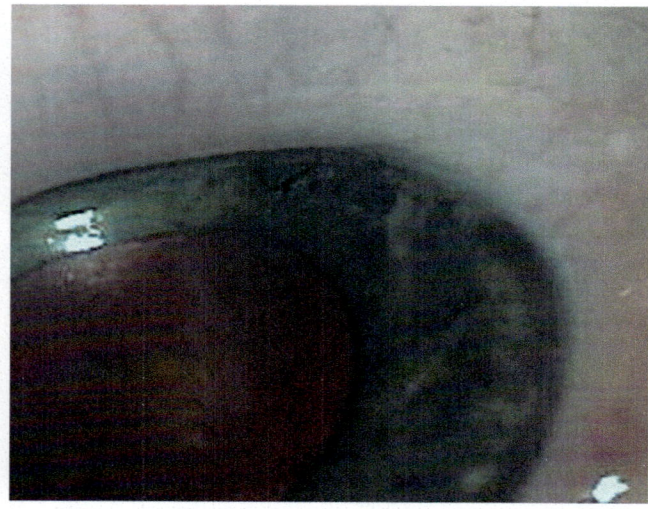

**Fig. 70.9** Releasable suture of 10-0 nylon near the limbus helps control flow in the postoperative period. These can be easily removed at the slit lamp

glaucoma filtration procedure, the surgeon will try to provide sufficient outflow of aqueous, to lower intraocular pressure to the desired target level but also try to avoid complications: specifically hypotony, flat anterior chamber, choroidal detachment, and pressure spikes. Repeated injections of balanced salt solution (BSS) through the paracentesis or use of an anterior chamber maintainer is recommended to test the outflow after initial suturing of the scleral flap. The flow can then be adjusted by loosening or tightening the sutures as needed.

The possibility of removing or cutting a scleral flap suture postoperatively, allows the surgeon to tightly close the scleral flap intraoperatively to decrease the probability of developing profound hypotony and a flat anterior chamber, especially if mitomycin-C has been used. Permanent and/or releasable scleral–flap sutures can be cut or adjusted in the clinic during the postoperative period to enhance the outflow (Figs. 70.8 and 70.9)[19–23] (see Sidebar 70.2)

### SIDEBAR 70.2 Hypotony maculopathy after glaucoma surgery

Raghu C. Mudumbai and Sarwat Salim

Hypotony maculopathy (HM) was first described in 1954 by Dellaporta. This syndrome occurs in patients who develop anatomic distortions of the sclera, choroid, retina, and optic nerve from low intraocular pressure (less than 6–8 mmHg) that is poorly tolerated and which eventually leads to retinal dysfunction. While multiple clinical settings may result in HM, the most common scenario is post filtering surgery. Antifibrotic agents employed at the time of surgery have increased the relative risk of HM. Prompt recognition and treatment is important in preventing visual sequelae.

Clinically, patients may be asymptomatic or experience a loss of central visual acuity with intraocular pressure less than 6–8 mmHg. Conversely, hypotony is not always associated with maculopathy. Fundus exam may reveal vessel tortuosity, chorioretinal folds, cystoid macular edema (CME), and optic nerve swelling. It is important to recognize that accompanying disc swelling is not secondary to raised intracranial pressure but is due to axonal stasis from forward bowing of the lamina cribrosa. Chorioretinal folds center around the fovea, leading to characteristic alternating bands of black and white stripes thought secondary to folding of the retinal pigment epithelium (RPE) into peaks and valleys. An older, less accepted alternative theory ascribes the folds from pulling on the retina by the elevated, swollen optic nerve. Induced hyperopic shift may also be observed from a decrease in axial length.

In subtle cases, ancillary testing may be of benefit. Fluorescein angiography can accentuate detection of chorioretinal folds along with selective leakage from capillaries supplying the optic nerve head but not retinal capillaries. Contrast between background choroidal fluorescence and darker zones is secondary to wrinkling of the choroid and RPE.

Optical Coherence Tomography (OCT) may increasingly be of benefit both in the diagnosis of HM and to evaluate the success of treatment in patients with HM. OCT typically reveals retinal macular thickening along with less often encountered intraretinal cysts and serous retinal detachment. Reduction of thickness of the retinal nerve fiber layer (rNFL) may indicate that the HM is resolving.

Other ophthalmic disease may mimic the fundus findings found in HM but should be straightforward to exclude, especially when associated with normal or high intraocular pressure. These entities include retrobulbar mass, posterior scleritis, thyroid eye disease, choroidal neovascularization, and placement of a scleral buckle. Patients with idiopathic chorioretinal folds typically have normal visual acuity.

HM most typically is encountered postglaucoma filtration surgery. Careful preoperative assessment of associated risk factors and meticulous attention to surgical technique may be invaluable in preventing this complication. Factors that increase the risk include male gender, young age, myopia, and patients undergoing primary surgical procedures. Caucasians have a higher risk than African-Americans

Intraoperative antimetabolite use is also a factor with higher risk associated with increased concentration and application time. HM may develop by either excessive filtration or possibly direct toxicity to the ciliary body. Mitomycin C extends a higher risk compared with 5-flurouracil.

In the postoperative setting, care should be taken to rule out factors that may exacerbate hypotony including choroidal effusions and other treatable complications, such as a wound leak or the presence of a cyclodialysis cleft. Trauma, chronic uveitis, and cyclitic membranes leading to ciliary body detachment may also play a role.

In high risk patients, tighter scleral flap suturing intraoperatively to prevent excessive filtration and anticipated postoperative suture lysis/suture release may prevent hypotony and associated maculopathy.

Once identified, prompt correction of the factors leading to hypotony is key to reversal of the maculopathy. A bleb leak may initially be treated with aqueous suppressants, bandage contact lens, and irritating topical antibiotics like gentamicin in an effort to close the leak. More aggressive interventions include topical glue, autologous blood injections, and low energy argon laser cauterization.

If conservative management fails, surgical intervention may be indicated. Surgical treatment includes conjunctival compression sutures and bleb revision with excision to treat bleb leaks. Scleral patch grafting with conjunctival advancement or autologous free graft placement can be used for overfiltration through the scleral flap.

Visual recovery is variable and delayed improvement may occur. Permanent changes in the RPE pigmentation may persist despite recovery of visual acuity. Reports of long standing HM (years) that respond with improved vision to correction of hypotony should at least lead to consideration of intervention.

## Bibliography

Dellaporta A. Fundus changes in post-operative hypotony. *Am J Ophthalmol.* 1955;40:781–785.

Gass JD. Hypotony maculopathy. In: Bellows JG, ed. *Contemporary Ophthalmology. Honoring Sir Stewart Duke-Elder.* Baltimore: Williams and Wilkins; 1972:343–366.

Fannin LA, Schiffman JC, Budenz DL. Risk factors for hypotony maculopathy. *Ophthalmology.* 2003;110:1185–1191.

Nuyts RM, Felten PC, Pels E, et al. Histopathologic effects of mitomycin C after trabeculectomy in human glaucomatous eyes with persistent hypotony. *Am J Ophthalmol.* 1994;118:225–237.

Oyakhire JO, Moroi SE. Clinical and anatomical reversal of long-term hypotony maculopathy. *Am J Ophthalmol.* 137:953–955.

Shields MB, Scroggs MW, Sloop CM, Simmons RB. Clinical and histopathologic observations concerning hypotony after trabeculectomy with adjunctive mitomycin C. *Am J Ophthalmol.* 1993;116:673–683.

## 70.3 Releaseable suture to avoid complications

Releasable sutures to close the scleral flap have some practical advantages as the externalized sutures are easily removed, they are effective in cases of hemorrhagic or thickened bleb (that would make difficult suture lysis), and they do not require laser equipment to be cut.[24–26] There are some potential disadvantages of releasable sutures, including additional operating time, potential discomfort if they are not buried, and, rarely, ocular infection. If antimetabolites are used, there may be a risk of an aqueous leak around the suture site, especially if there is a limbal closure (fornix-based flap). The timing for cutting/releasing sutures is important. If antimetabolites are *not* used, sutures may still be effectively cut within the first 2 weeks.[27] Later on, fibrosis of the scleral flap may negate any potential increase in outflow due to cutting. The window of opportunity is expanded when antimetabolites have been associated with the surgery, although the response decreases with a longer interval until suture release.[1]

Suture release/lysis should be performed in a conservative step-wise manner. Usually only one suture is released at a time to avoid overfiltration.

## 70.4 Postoperative Suprachoroidal Hemorrhage

Suprachoroidal hemorrhage after surgery is rare, but can be devastating. Risk factors for suprachoroidal hemorrhage include glaucoma, aphakia, previous vitrectomy, myopia, and postoperative hypotony. Systemic risk factors are arteriosclerosis, high blood pressure, tachycardia, bleeding disorders, and anticoagulant therapy.[28–31]

Postoperative suprachoroidal hemorrhage usually occurs within the first week after glaucoma surgery and is usually associated with hypotony. The development of a suprachoroidal hemorrhage is typically acute and associated with the sudden onset of severe pain. Often this follows exertion with a Valsalva maneuver. Examination of the anterior segment frequently reveals a shallow anterior chamber (Fig. 70.10)

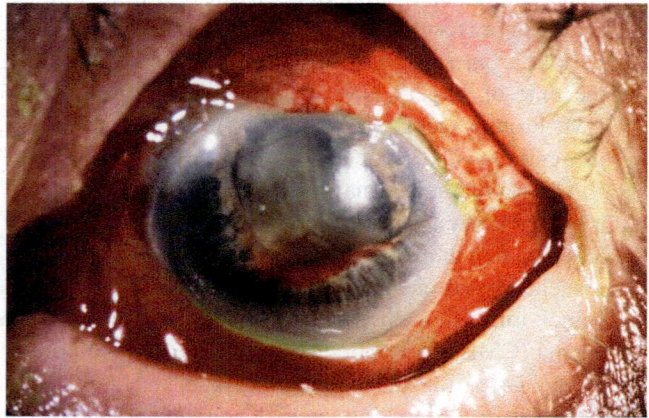

**Fig. 70.10** Delayed suprachoroidal hemorrhage in a patient on chronic anti-platelet therapy

and either a low, normal, or high intraocular pressure depending on the extent of the hemorrhage. On fundus exam a detached and dark choroid is noted. Some cases present with bleeding into the vitreous cavity. Bleeding into the vitreous cavity at the time of the hemorrhage and retinal detachment greatly worsen the visual prognosis.[32]

Treatment of postoperative suprachoroidal hemorrhage is directed toward control of the IOP and relief of pain. The majority of these eyes will do well with this conservative management, and surgical drainage is not usually necessary. The indications for drainage through a sclerotomy include intolerable pain, a persistent flat anterior chamber, failure of bleb filtration, and massive choroidal detachments. A waiting period of at least 7–10 days following a suprachoroidal hemorrhage is advised for the fibrinolytic response to liquefy the clot and allow for more effective evacuation of the suprachoroidal space.[33]

## 70.5 Hyphema

In general, hyphema presents at surgery or within the first 2 or 3 days following surgery (Fig. 70.11). Hyphema commonly arises from the ciliary body or cut ends of the

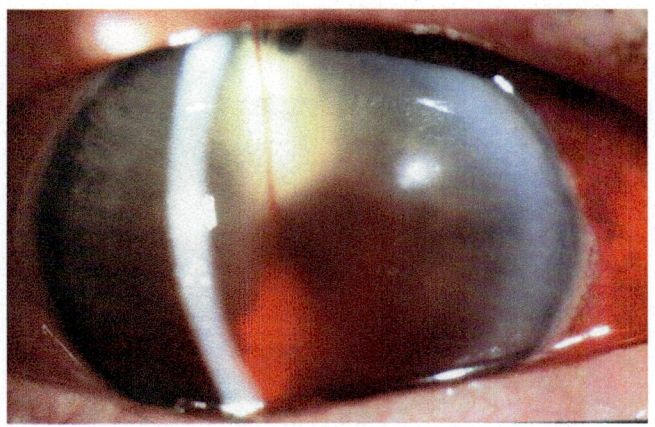

**Fig. 70.11** Hyphema photographed in the development stage following filtration surgery. The source of the hyphema was the edge of the trabectomy flap

Schlemm's canal, though it might also arise from the corneoscleral incision or iris. The probability of having postoperative hyphema is decreased during filtration surgery bleeding by performing the internal fistula as far anterior as possible (i.e., at the cornea). Some surgeons recommend stopping oral anticoagulants or antiaggregants before glaucoma surgery. We prefer to confirm that the anticoagulation (INR) is within the therapeutic range before the surgery. In addition, in patients with open angles, we choose not to do peripheral iridotomy.

In the vast majority of cases, no treatment is necessary and the blood will be absorbed within a brief period of time. Cycloplegics, corticosteroids, restriction of activity, and elevation of head of the bed 30–45° (to prevent blood from obstructing a superior sclerostomy) are recommended. Increased IOP can occur, particularly if the filtering site is obstructed by a blood clot, and it should be treated if necessary with oral and/or topical aqueous suppressants.

Surgical evacuation is considered depending on the level of IOP, size of hyphema, severity of optic nerve damage, likelihood of corneal blood staining, and the presence of sickle trait or sickle cell anemia (infarction of the optic nerve can occur at relatively low IOP, and carbonic anhydrase inhibitors are contraindicated). Liquid blood can easily be removed with irrigation. If a clot has formed, it can be removed by expression with viscoelastic or with a vitrectomy instrument set at low vacuum.

## 70.6 Malignant Glaucoma

Malignant glaucoma (also called aqueous misdirection or ciliary block glaucoma) is characterized by a shallowing or flattening of the anterior chamber without pupillary block (i.e., in presence of a patent iridectomy) or choroidal pathology (such as suprachoroidal hemorrhage), commonly with an accompanying rise in intraocular pressure (IOP). It is more common after surgery for angle closure glaucoma, in phakic, hyperopic (small) eyes[34,35] (see Chap. 37).

In this condition, an increased pressure at the vitreous cavity displaces the lens forward, shallowing the anterior chamber (Figs. 70.12a, b). In malignant glaucoma, a relative resistance to the anterior movement of fluid from the vitreous cavity to the anterior chamber probably occurs.[34]

Aqueous misdirection usually occurs in the early postoperative period. The anterior chamber is shallow and the intraocular pressure is high. However, with a functioning filtration bleb, the intraocular pressure may not be high.

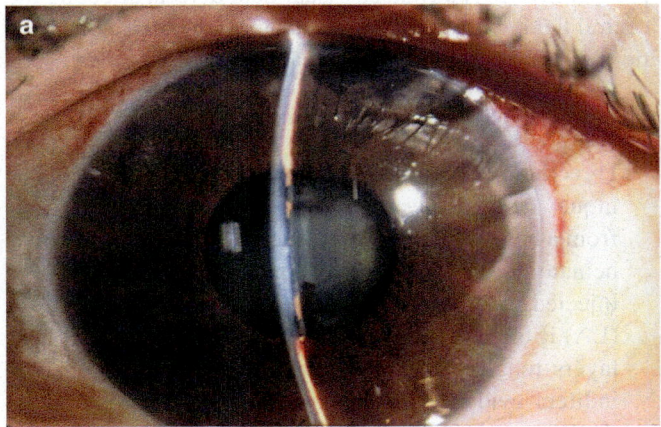
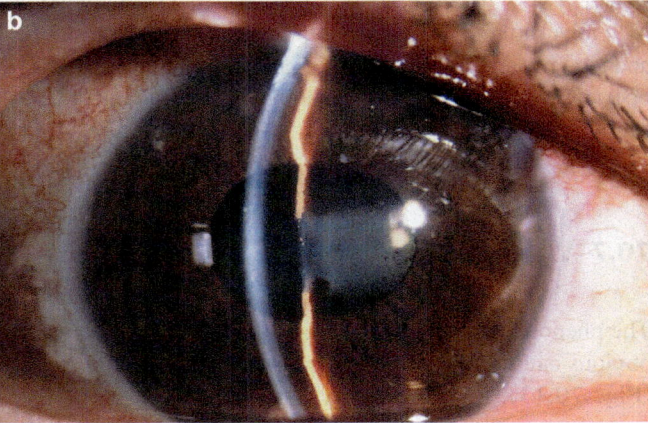

**Fig. 70.12** Aqueous misdirection, historically called malignant glaucoma, is characterized by a flat chamber and increased IOP after pupillary block has been ruled out. (**a**) Appearance before treatment and (**b**) after atropine 1% drops. Note the deepening of the anterior chamber with posterior movement of the lens–iris diaphragm after dilation

The peripheral iridectomy is patent, and there are no chorioretinal abnormalities.

Malignant glaucoma is initially managed with mydriatic–cycloplegic drops, aqueous suppressants, and hyperosmotic agents. If the condition is relieved (e.g., the anterior chamber has deepened), the hyperosmotic agents are discontinued first, then the aqueous suppressants are reduced or even stopped over several days. Cycloplegic drops should be continued for weeks to months.[35]

In pseudophakic eyes, a peripheral hyaloidotomy with the Nd:YAG laser may be efficient and can often be accomplished through an existing peripheral iridectomy.[36] Often times, breaking the hyaloid face with the Nd:YAG laser can be done at the edge of the optic through the posterior capsule. If not successful, zonulo–hyaloido–vitrectomy via the anterior segment has been successfully used in a series of pseudophakic patients.[37]

Pars plana vitrectomy should be considered when other therapies fail.[38,39] A standard 3-port pars plana vitrectomy, removing the anterior vitreous and part of the anterior hyaloid, is done. In phakic patients, the lens can sometimes be spared, but the probability of recurrence is higher. Pars plana tube-shunt insertion with vitrectomy has been recommended to treat patients with aqueous misdirection, especially in cases with angle closure glaucoma. The implantation of the tube shunt through pars plana can help prevent recurrence of this condition and can help in long-term control of IOP.[39]

### 70.6.1 Prevention

In high-risk eyes undergoing cataract or filtration surgery, rapid decompression and shallowing of the anterior chamber should be minimized if at all possible. Postoperative overfiltration should be avoided with a thick scleral flap, sutured tighter and with more sutures than usual. Postoperatively, judicious suture lysis or cutting/pulling of releasable sutures and slow tapering of cycloplegics are recommended. A postoperative shallow anterior chamber due to overfiltration should be vigorously treated.

## 70.7 Wipe-Out

The phenomenon of severe visual loss after surgery, with no obvious cause, is known as "wipe-out" or "snuff syndrome" (Fig. 70.13). Wipe-out may affect patients who have very severe glaucomatous damage, and overall is a very uncommon complication but remains an important concern among glaucoma surgeons.[42] Wipe-out was probably more common after full-thickness filtration surgery.[40] However, it is not known whether patients who had been diagnosed with wipe-out could have had another undetected cause such as macular edema, hypotonous maculopathy, or inflammation. With modern surgical techniques, it is becoming increasingly rare.[41,43]

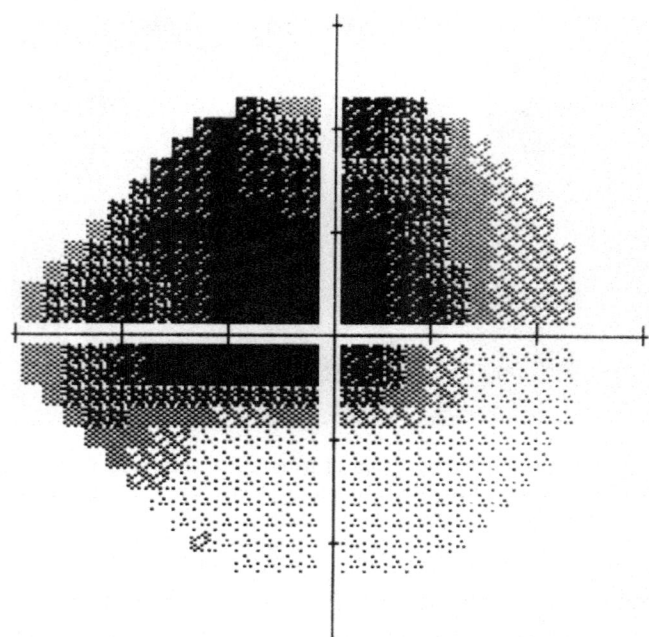

**Fig. 70.13** Visual field test. Loss of the central visual field is a rare occurrence following glaucoma filtering surgery and is characterized by decreased central vision (wipe out) that cannot otherwise be explained

There are a few studies that have evaluated the incidence of wipe-out after trabeculectomy. The reported incidence ranged from 0 to 0.95% of surgeries. A retrospective study of 508 trabeculectomies identified four cases of wipe-out, all of which had retrobulbar anesthesia.[41] Older patients with high preoperative IOP, advanced visual field defects affecting the central field, with split fixation, and postoperative complications would appear to be at increased risk.

Possible mechanisms and prevention strategies of wipe-out:

- Direct damage to the optic nerve from anesthetic technique – Local pressure to the optic nerve may result from a hematoma in the optic nerve sheath, a retrobulbar hematoma, or simply from the volume of anesthetic injected,[44] even with a low volume of local anesthetic (LA) if the LA were to become trapped between fascial layers to give a "compartment syndrome." Additional indirect evidence of the possible effect of local anesthetic was noted in a small series of three cases of hyaluronidase-associated orbitopathy, in which the most severe and long-lasting visual loss occurred in the one patient who had glaucoma.[45] Doppler imaging studies have shown that retrobulbar injections can cause a marked reduction in blood flow in the arteries supplying the anterior optic nerve, particularly if epinephrine is included in the LA mixture.[46] This effect is not seen with anterior placement of local anesthetic, for example by sub-conjunctival anesthesia.[47]

- Pressure spike – Early undiagnosed postoperative IOP spikes could potentially inflict further insult to a very severely damaged optic nerve with end-stage glaucoma. Thus, it seems logical to associate an early and severe pressure spike with the occurrence of wipe-out. Pressure spikes may occur if the scleral flap has been sutured very tightly or the fistula is blocked by iris tissue or a blood clot. In patients with advanced glaucomatous damage undergoing trabeculectomy, IOP should be monitored a few hours after surgery, and also the following day. Thus, if there is an early IOP spike, it can be treated accordingly.
- Postoperative hypotony – Postoperative profound hypotony has been associated with "wipe-out," and it seems that this complication was more common when full-thickness filtration procedures were the standard surgeries for glaucoma. In the recent tube versus trabeculectomy study (TVT), choroidal effusion was an independent risk factor for unexplained visual acuity loss after surgery.[4] Choroidal effusion is generally considered a relatively mild problem, but the TVT study results suggested that this complication may not be always benign in nature.[4]

## 70.8 Early Bleb Leak

An inadvertent buttonhole in the conjunctiva during a filtering procedure or a wound leak, through the conjunctival incision, can be responsible for an early leaking bleb. Early leaking can flatten the bleb and lead to subconjunctival-to-episcleral fibrosis, which would jeopardize a satisfactory long-term filtration. Bleb leaks are detected with the Seidel test (Fig. 70.14).

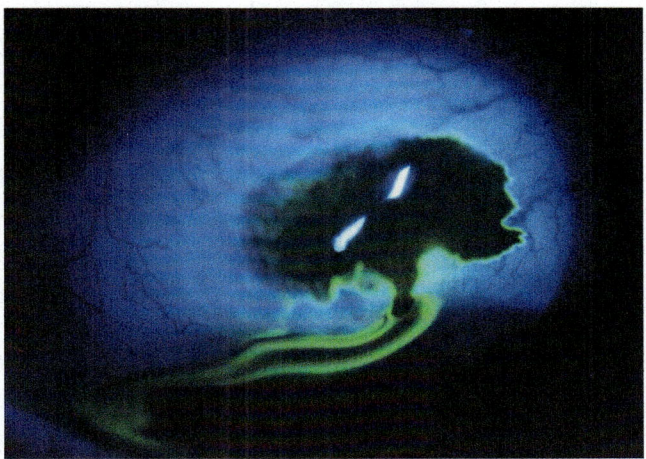

**Fig. 70.14** A bleb leak at the limbus can occur early in the postoperative course either from poor wound healing or inadvertent trauma

The usual cause for conjunctival buttonholes is penetration of the tissue by the tip of a sharp instrument (needle, scissors, blade) or the teeth of a forceps. Buttonholes and tears are more likely to occur in cases with extensive conjunctival scarring. To diagnose a buttonhole intraoperatively the conjunctiva should be carefully examined at the end of the procedure by filling the anterior chamber and raising the filtering bleb. If recognized, the buttonhole should be closed at the time of surgery. If it is located in the center of the conjunctival flap, a "purse string" closure is attempted either internally on the undersurface of the conjunctiva or externally if the flap has already been reapproximated. A 10-0 or 11-0 nylon on a tapered ("vascular") needle should be used. When the conjunctival buttonhole or tear occurs at the limbus, it can be sutured directly to the corneal–limbal junction.[4]

Early bleb leaks usually heal spontaneously, but discontinuation of topical steroids may accelerate the spontaneous closure. Prophylactic wide spectrum antibiotics are indicated. If there are associated complications, such as shallow or flat anterior chamber, active intervention is recommended. Our preferred therapeutic modalities to treat leaking blebs include bandage contact lens, fibrin tissue glue (see Sidebar 70.3), and surgical revision.[5,48]

---

**SIDEBAR 70.3. Fibrin glue and glaucoma surgery**

Andrew M. Hendrick and Malik Y. Kahook

The use of fibrin glue has been reported in ophthalmic literature for nearly 20 years beginning with its utilization in sealing perforated corneal ulcers. Reports also described the use of fibrin glue for strabismus surgery and to secure conjunctival grafts during pterygium surgery. There have been reports of fibrin glue use both intraoperatively and for postoperative bleb leaks or overfiltration post trabeculectomy. More recently, glaucoma drainage device implantation using fibrin glue has been described with short-term follow-up.

Fibrin glue is a two-part admixture containing a protein base and thrombin–calcium chloride activating solution. The protein base contains fibrinogen, plasminogen, fibronectin, and factor XIII in bovine aprotonin solution. Collagen crosslinking lends strength to tissue adherence through fibrin–fibronectin bonds. It activates rapidly, within 20–30 s, lending to its intraoperative appeal for conjunctival wound closure.

There are several techniques to combine the protein base and calcium solution to allow collagen crosslinking. One method involves application of each component independently and mixing them at the site of action passively or with a blunt instrument. Another technique involves the manufacturer's syringe that accompanies the package. In one step, the mixture is combined and applied to the surgical site through the Duploject device that holds two syringes with a single terminal lumen. However, partial occlusion of the lumen can lead to an unequal component ratio negatively affecting proper congealing of the mixture. The terminal cannula may be changed out in case of occlusion. It is necessary to visually confirm proper mixing has occurred by noting a gelatinous consistency. Lastly, a new preparation of fibrin glue is currently available that does not require heating and can be ready in 2 min, which can reduce operating room time and cost.

Concern regarding the proinflammatory potential of fibrin glue was expressed by several groups and subsequently addressed. Bahar et al examined posttrabeculectomy rabbit eyes for histologic changes after either fibrin adhesive or nylon suture were used for conjunctival closure. The glue was histologically identified as an amorphic eosinophilic material present for 3 days but had completely disappeared by day 7 postoperatively, indicating the glue was not inciting a vigorous chronic immune response. However, it was hypothesized that the temporary nature of the glue may lead to an increase in late onset leakage and hypotony.

Specifically in glaucoma literature, Asrani and Wilensky described the use of autologous fibrin tissue glue to treat bleb leaks. They noted successful healing of bleb leak in nine of their 12 patients that was comparable to their other treatment modalities, which included bandage contact lenses, patching the eye, suturing the leak, cyanoacrylate glue, and injecting autologous blood into the bleb. Based on their experience, they recommended fibrin glue as a consideration for safe and effective treatment of postoperative bleb leaks.

Grewing and Mester reported on the use of fibrin glue for post-trabeculectomy hypotony. They described two patients with lens–cornea touch with large choroidal detachments that resolved with single application of subconjunctival fibrin glue to the scleral flap. Subsequent formation of filtering bleb was noted in both patients with resolution of both choroidal detachment and improvement of intraocular pressure.

Fibrin glue was used in trabeculectomies both alone and combined with suture by O'Sullivan et al in a small set of patients. Watertight closure was achieved in all cases. This was one of the first suggestions of using fibrin glue as suture replacement in glaucoma surgery.

Thereafter, fibrin glue was used as suture substitute for Baerveldt tube implantation by Kahook and Noecker. In a retrospective, nonrandomized comparative consecutive case series they described 28 patients in whom fibrin glue was used to replace suture in fastening the tube to the sclera, securing the pericardial patch graft, and, lastly, in closure of the conjunctiva. They found no difference between complication rates, intraocular pressure control, or the need for glaucoma drops for the suture group and fibrin glue group. However, they did appreciate less conjunctival inflammation along with significantly less surgical time in the fibrin glue group. It was noted that the added cost of the fibrin glue was offset by the reduced intraoperative time.

Valimaki described 11 eyes in a noncomparative consecutive case series of adjunctive fibrin glue use during Molteno implantation when peritubular aqueous humor leakage was noted. No postoperative hypotony, flattening of the anterior chamber, or choroidal detachments were noted in the patients who received intraoperative fibrin glue.

Because of its track record of safety and efficacy, fibrin glue is becoming more accepted both as adjunctive to and replacement of sutures in various ophthalmic surgeries. However, its utility is not without risk – both proven and speculative. Caution must be employed in certain situations when a suture is truly necessary for proper tissue securing as is the case with scarred poorly mobile conjunctiva. Additionally, since fibrin glue is derived from blood products, there is a theoretical possibility of transmission of human immunodeficiency virus (HIV), hepatitis C virus (HCV), and prion-related diseases; although to date, this has not been reported. New formulations of fibrin glue with slower setting characteristics as well as synthetic glues are currently being studied for future use in ophthalmic surgery. Research in this field may allow for safer more physiologic closure of wounds while allowing for improved patient comfort and less morbidity postoperatively.

## Bibliography

Asrani SG, Wilensky JT. Management of bleb leaks after glaucoma filtering surgery. Use of autologous fibrin tissue glue as an alternative. *Ophthalmology.* 1996;103:294–298.

Bahar I, Weinberger D, Lusky M, et al. Fibrin glue as a suture substitute: histological evaluation of trabeculectomy in rabbit eyes. *Curr Eye Res.* 2006;31:31–36.

Biedner B, Rosenthal G. Conjunctival closure in strabismus surgery: vicryl versus fibrin glue. *Ophthalmic Surg Lasers.* 1996;27:967.

Cohen RA, McDonald MB. Fixation of conjunctival autografts with an organic tissue adhesive. *Arch Ophthalmol.* 1993;111:1167–1168.

Grewing R, Mester U. Fibrin sealant in the management of complicated hypotony after trabeculectomy. *Ophthalmic Surg Lasers.* 1997;28:124–127.

http://www.glaucomatoday.com/articles/0508/GT0508_02.pdf. Accessed April 5, 2009.

Kahook MY, Noecker RJ. Fibrin glue-assisted glaucoma drainage device surgery. *Br J Ophthalmol.* 2006;90:1486–1489.

Lagoutte FM, Gauthier L, Comte PR. A fibrin sealant for perforated and preperforated corneal ulcers. *Br J Ophthalmol.* 1989;73:757–761.

O'Sullivan F, Dalton R, Rostron CK. Fibrin glue: an alternative method of wound closure in glaucoma surgery. *J Glaucoma.* 1996;5:367–370.

Seligsohn A, Moster MR, Steinmann W, Fontanarosa J. Use of Tisseel fibrin sealant to manage bleb leaks and hypotony: case series. *J Glaucoma.* 2004;13(3):227.

Valimaki J. Fibrin glue for preventing immediate postoperative hypotony following glaucoma drainage implant surgery. *Acta Ophthalmol Scand.* 2006;84:372–374.

## 70.9 Late Bleb Leak

Spontaneous late bleb leaks are more frequent in avascular, thin blebs, which occur more frequently when antimetabolites are used in the filtering procedure (Fig. 70.15). Leakage of the filtering bleb can be associated with hypotony, shallow-flat anterior chamber, and choroidal detachment, and may increase the chances for bleb infection and subsequent endophthalmitis.[5]

Bleb leaks can heal spontaneously, and conservative management with prophylactic antibiotics is recommended if there are no associated problems. Patient education regarding symptoms of bleb-related ocular infection is crucial for prompt diagnosis and management. The need and timing for surgical repair of bleb leaks depend on the presence of other complications such as severe hypotony, flat anterior chamber, vision loss, or previous episodes of bleb-related infections.[48–55]

Multiple techniques have been proposed such as the use of a Simmons shell, injection of autologous blood, cryopexy, or thermal Nd:YAG laser. Our preferred intervention is surgical revision, attempting to save the established initial filtration site (Fig. 70.16).[54,55] Due to the friable nature of the conjunctiva in long-established filtering blebs, it is often impossible to close the defect directly with sutures and, therefore, healthy conjunctival tissue is needed. First, the ischemic and thin-walled bleb tissue is denuded of conjunctival epithelium by blade debridement or cautery to allow long-term adherence of the grafted conjunctiva. Fresh conjunctiva adjacent to the bleb is then mobilized to cover the de-epithelialized bleb by rotational, sliding, or free conjunctival grafts, depending on the dimension of the avascular area of the bleb and the quality of the surrounding conjunctiva. For conjunctival advancement, separate dissection of conjunctiva and Tenon's capsule sometimes aids in closure, because although conjunctiva can often be stretched further than Tenon's capsule, the closure of the latter provides more

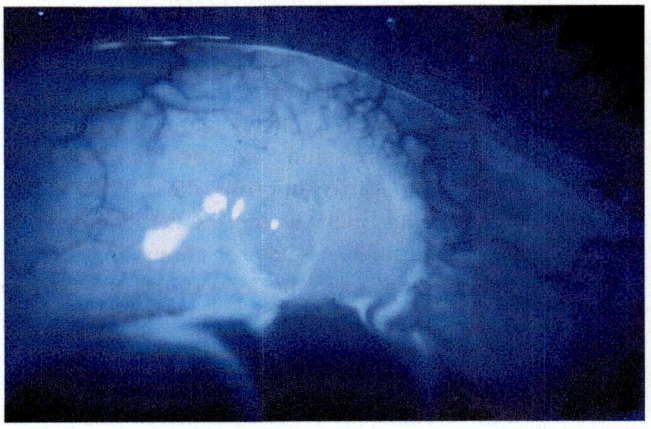

**Fig. 70.15** Bleb leak, Seidel (+). Often times, a wound leak may go undetected, especially late in the postoperative period. A Seidel test should be done in avascular, cystic blebs

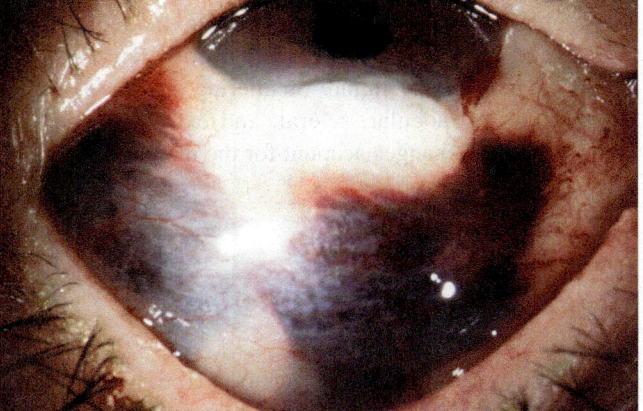

**Fig. 70.16** Injection of autologous blood in the bleb can be helpful to reverse a hypotonous situation, and on occasion heal a bleb leak

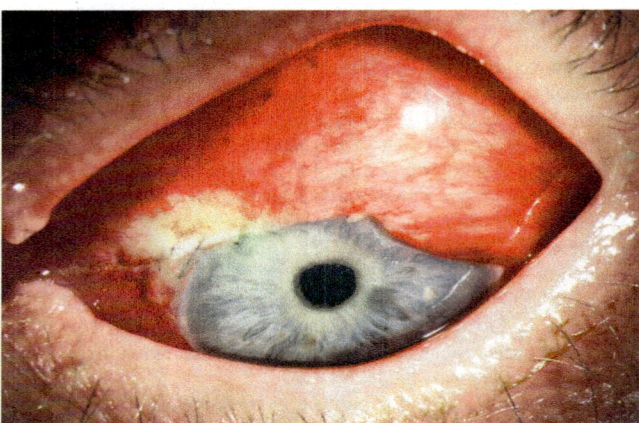

**Fig. 70.17** Repair of a nasal leaking bleb with additional 10-0 nylon sutures. The formation of a Seidel negative bleb is critical to the success of the procedure

support. The conjunctiva is sutured over the previously abraded peripheral cornea, providing a watertight seal. With these methods, bleb function frequently can be preserved. Some surgeons prefer to remove completely the avascular area, but this approach may compromise the function of the filtering bleb. Alternatively, a free conjunctival graft from the inferior bulbar conjunctiva or amniotic membrane can be used as an alternative substrate. Hypotony associated with bleb leak presents difficult challenges. To plan a surgical intervention, it must be determined whether the hypotony is caused directly by the leak or not. In the latter situation, additional sutures (Fig. 70.17) to the scleral flap or scleral reinforcement with a patch graft would be necessary. The use of a donor patch graft (e.g., sclera, pericardium, or cornea) is likely to compromise the function of the filtering bleb.

## 70.10 Failure of the Filtering Bleb

Failed blebs are those associated with inadequate IOP control and impending or established obstruction of aqueous outflow. The cause of failure of filtering operations can be divided into intraocular, scleral, and extraocular factors. The extraocular changes account for the majority of failures of external filtering operations.[5,56]

### 70.10.1 Early Failure of Filtering Bleb

Early failure of filtering blebs is characterized by a high IOP, deep anterior chamber, and low and hyperemic bleb. Failing blebs should be recognized promptly because if obstruction is not relieved permanent adhesions between conjunctiva and episcleral can lead to closure of the fistula. A tight scleral flap and episcleral fibrosis are the most common causes of early bleb failure. Internal obstruction of the fistula by blood clot, vitreous, iris, or incompletely excised Descemet's membrane is also possible.

To reduce postoperative subconjunctival fibrosis and preserve bleb function, postoperative topical steroids are routinely used.[57] In phakic eyes without high risk for failure we use 0.1% dexamethasone drops four times a day for 1 month, tapering them over the following 4–6 weeks, depending on the appearance of the bleb. In pseudophakic eyes or for patients with high risk of failure, the initial dose is six to eight times a day. The use of antifibrotic agents in filtering procedures is associated with a higher success but also with a higher complication rate (hypotony due to overfiltration, bleb leak, and ocular infection). For this reason, an individualized consideration of the risk/benefit ratio is recommended. A survey of glaucoma specialists in the American Glaucoma Society indicated that antifibrotic agents are used in the majority of operations,[58] but in the UK they are used less frequently.[59] The agent 5-fluorouracil (5-FU) is usually administered intraoperatively as a subconjunctival sponge soaked with 50 mg/ml 5 FU for 5 min. 5-FU is also used in 5-mg aliquots injected subconjunctivally during the first 2 weeks after surgery.[60,61] The dosage is adjusted according to the tolerance of the corneal epithelium of each eye.

Complications associated with the use of postoperative 5-FU include corneal and conjunctival epithelial toxicity, corneal ulcers, conjunctival wound leaks, subconjunctival hemorrhage, or inadvertent intraocular spread of 5-FU. The frequency of complications is reduced with lower dosages of 15–50 mg administered in three to ten injections, according to individual response. Mitomycin-C is approximately 100 times more potent than 5-FU. Postoperative complications associated with overfiltration, hypotony maculopathy, bleb leak, and bleb-related ocular infections are more likely to occur when mitomycin-C is used.[62,63] Current technique of mitomycin-C application involves the treatment of a large subconjunctival area with multiple sponges, and avoiding the treatment of the conjunctival edge. Thus, the bleb morphology is typically more diffuse.

Digital ocular compression and focal compression can be used to temporarily improve the function of a nonfunctioning filtering bleb. Digital ocular compression can be applied to the inferior sclera or cornea through the inferior eyelid, or to the sclera posterior to the scleral flap through the superior eyelid. Focal compression is applied with a moistened cotton tip at the edge of the scleral flap.[21] In the early postoperative period, laser suture lysis or removal of an externalized releasable suture can enhance the filtration. Gonioscopy performed prior to the laser can confirm an open sclerostomy with no tissue or clot occluding its entrance.

Specially designed lenses (such as Hoskins, Ritch, or Mandelkorn lenses), the central button edge of the Zeiss and Sussman lenses, the Goldmann lens, glass rods, or glass pipettes can be used to visualize sutures that need to be cut. After the suture is cut, if the bleb and IOP are unchanged, ocular massage or focal pressure can be applied. Usually only one suture is cut at a time to avoid the possible complications of overfiltration, hypotony, and flat anterior chamber. The timing of suture release is critical. As stated earlier in this chapter, suture lysis is effective within the first 2 weeks after surgery without antimetabolites; later, fibrosis of the scleral flap may negate any beneficial effect of this procedure. If antimetabolites have been used at the time of surgery, suture lysis can be effective up to several months after surgery.

Releasable sutures are as effective as laser suture lysis (Figs. 70.8 and 70.9). The use of releasable sutures allows the surgeon to tightly close the scleral flap knowing that the flow can be increased postoperatively. The externalized sutures are easily removed and are effective in cases of hemorrhagic conjunctiva or thickened Tenon's tissue (that would make difficult suture lysis due to poor visualization). The disadvantages of releasable sutures include the need for additional intraoperative manipulation and postoperative discomfort from the externalized suture, corneal epithelial defects, and possibly increased risk of ocular infection.

### 70.10.2 Late Failure of Filtering Bleb

A filtering bleb can fail, after months–years of adequate function, with subconjunctival-episcleral fibrosis the most common cause.[56]

There are several factors that accelerate fibrosis such as black race, childhood, postoperative subconjunctival hemorrhage, the presence of reactive sutures, and inflammation.[64] Less commonly, internal closure of the sclerostomy can occur. A classic example would be late closure of the internal sclerostomy by a membrane in patients with iridocorneal endothelial (ICE) syndrome. "Warning signs" of failing filtration are increased bleb vascularization, bleb inflammation, and/or bleb thickening. The IOP is typically high.

In cases of subconjunctival-episcleral fibrosis, an external revision or bleb needling can be tried.[65–68] A 27- or 25-gauge needle is used to cut the edge of the scleral flap and restore aqueous outflow. Entry of the needle tip into the anterior chamber beneath the flap is important, but should be undertaken with extreme caution in phakic eyes. The technique can be repeated as needed. The outcome may be more favorable if there was a previously well-established filtration bleb before the fistula became occluded. Repeated subconjunctival injections in the superior fornix of 5–10 mg of 5-FU in 0.1 ml may increase the probability of success. Mitomycin-C before or after needling has been used also in conjunction with needling of blebs. The most common complications are associated with postoperative hypotony (see previous entry on hypotony).[65–68] We are currently using 0.1 cc of nonpreserved 1% lidocaine mixed with 0.1 ml of 0.4 mg/ml-mitomycin C at the time of the needling.

### 70.10.3 Encapsulated Blebs

Encapsulated blebs are localized, elevated, and tense filtering blebs, with vascular engorgement of the overlying conjunctiva and a thick connective tissue (Fig. 70.18). This type of bleb commonly appears within 2–6 weeks following surgery. Encapsulation of the filtering bleb is associated with a rise of IOP after an initial period of pressure control following glaucoma surgery. They can interfere with upper lid movement and tear film distribution leading to corneal complications such us dellen and astigmatism. Often it is seen through the eyelid simulating a lid mass. The frequency of bleb encapsulation after trabeculectomies without antimetabolites ranges from 8.3 to 28%. The frequency of encapsulated blebs after guarded filtering procedures with mitomycin-C is lower. Predisposing factors may include male gender, glove powder, and prior treatment with sympathomimetics, argon laser trabeculoplasty, and surgery involving the conjunctiva.[69–71] The causes of encapsulation are not clearly identified, but inflammatory mediators are probably involved in their development. The long-term prognosis for IOP control in eyes that develop encapsulated blebs is relatively good.[72]

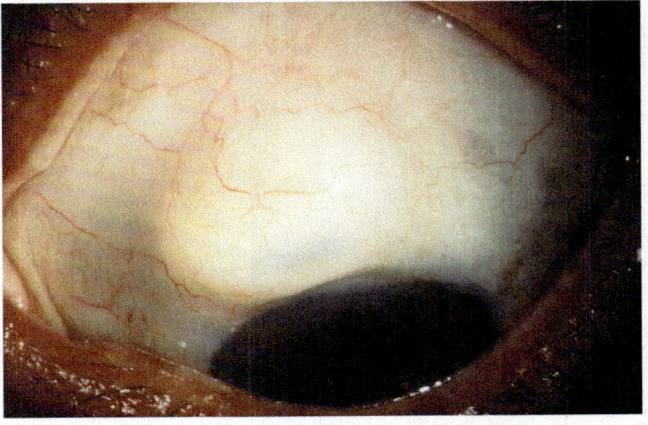

**Fig. 70.18** An encapsulated bleb with a tight Tenon's capsule can prevent posterior aqueous flow. The IOP is 35 mmHg yet the internal osteum is wide open

Initial management of encapsulated blebs includes antiglaucoma medications in cases of elevated IOP and topical steroids. Deciding between conservative management (medical) or a surgical revision is usually dependent upon the severity of glaucomatous damage, the level of IOP, and the response to medical management. When surgical revision is needed, the simplest technique is to cut the fibrotic wall with a 27-gauge needle, a Ziegler knife, or an MVR blade.

### 70.10.4 Symptomatic Blebs

Filtering blebs are usually free of unpleasant symptoms. Some patients do have discomfort, which is most common with nasally located, large blebs that extend onto the cornea. Tear film abnormalities with dellen formation and superficial punctate keratopathy may occur.

Artificial tears and ocular lubricants can be helpful, especially in cases with abnormal tear films. As noted previously, several chemical and thermal methods have been used to shrink blebs. Large blebs that extend onto the cornea can be freed by blunt dissection. The corneal extension can be excised with a cut, parallel to the limbus, usually with excellent results. Partial surgical excision and conjunctival flap reinforcement are usually helpful, although there is the possibility of bleb failure. Placement of large X compression sutures with either 9-0 or 10-0 nylon on the conjunctiva directly over the flap can often flatten the bleb so it no longer cause the patient discomfort. The tear film can then more easily cover the cornea, decreasing the localized dry eye symptoms. The sutures can be removed after a number of weeks (Fig. 70.19)

### 70.10.5 Bleb-Related Ocular Infection

Ocular infections related to filtration procedures can occur months to years after the initial surgery.[73–83] The incidence of bleb-related ocular infections after filtration procedures not supplemented with antifibrotic agents ranges from 0.2 to 1.5% after mid- and long-term follow-up. Thin bleb walls and, most importantly, bleb leaks are associated with a higher risk of infection. Another surprising risk factor that has been detected is the long-term use of topical antibiotics. Bleb-related ocular infections can affect three compartments: the subconjunctival space, the anterior segment, and the vitreous cavity. Usually, the spread of infection proceeds in that order. Because the fluid within the bleb is continuous with the anterior chamber, the bleb may be considered an exteriorized portion of the anterior chamber. Therefore, an infection of the bleb affecting the subconjunctival space ("blebitis") has a very real potential to rapidly spread posteriorly.

Patients with bleb-related ocular infection usually present with ocular pain, sensitivity to light, blurred vision, tearing, redness, and discharge. Examination often reveals conjunctival and ciliary injection, most intense around the bleb edge, purulent discharge, and variable intensity of periorbital chemosis, corneal edema, and anterior chamber reaction including keratic precipitates and, in some cases, hypopyon (Fig. 70.20). The most common causative organisms are streptococcus and staphylococcus. The bleb typically has a milky-white appearance with loss of clarity; a pseudohypopyon within the bleb can be observed. A positive Seidel's test is common, and some patients may have a substantial leak, hypotony, and even flat anterior chamber. Alternatively, an increased IOP is possible due to internal closure of sclerostomy site with purulence and debris. Vitreous reaction is not evident in early cases of blebitis, but if left untreated, the infection spreads to the posterior segment.

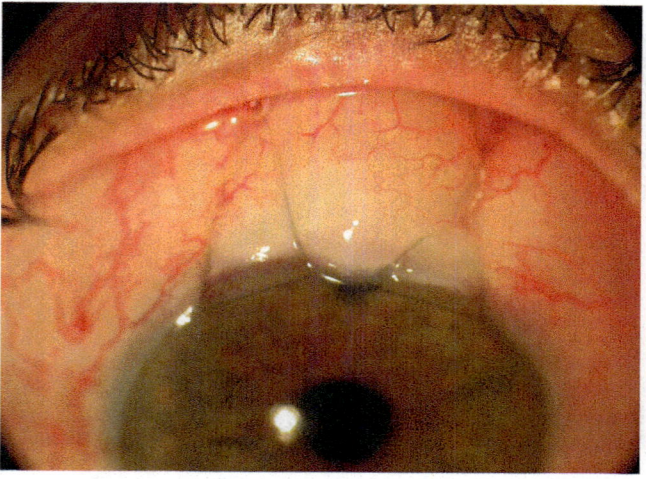

**Fig. 70.19** Compression sutures for large dysesthetic bleb ("Palmberg sutures")

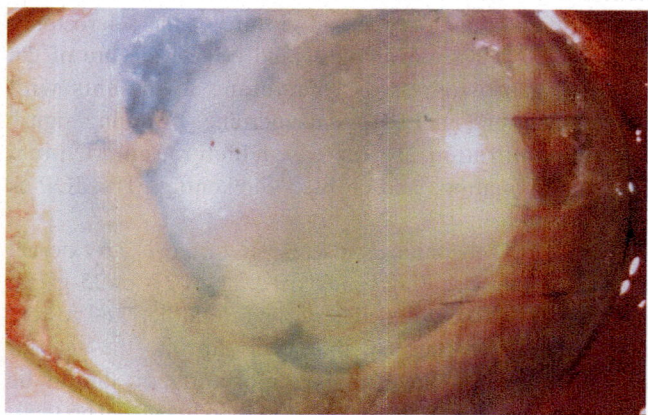

**Fig. 70.20** Infectious blebitis can lead to endophthalmitis if not diagnosed and treated early. Gram-positive organisms are the most frequent cause

The general principles that guide the management of ocular infections apply to this condition as well. It is important to try to identify the organism responsible for the infection as soon as possible to allow for specific antimicrobial therapy. A conjunctival sample is routinely collected, stained, and cultured. However, conjunctival culture in the etiologic diagnosis of bleb-related endophthalmitis may not always be helpful.

In blebitis without anterior chamber reaction, frequent topical application of a commercially available broad-spectrum antibiotic can be used under very close supervision. If the anterior segment but not the posterior segment is involved, treatment as an outpatient, with fortified topical antibiotics around the clock, is advisable. Topical fortified cefazoline or vancomycin (25 mg/ml) associated with fortified tobramycin (14 mg/ml), or amikacin (50 mg/ml) are likely to be effective against most gram-positive and gram-negative microorganisms. Another alternative is one of the fourth-generation topical fluoroquinolones, which have a broad gram-positive and gram-negative coverage. Additional systemic antibiotics such as oral ofloxacin or moxifloxacin can be used. In bleb-related endophthalmitis with vitreous activity, a vitreous sample should be obtained associated with injection of intravitreal antibiotics. We are currently using 1 mg of vancomycin (10 mg/ml) and 400 μg. of amikacin (5 mg/ml). Oral ofloxacin (400 mg p.o. twice daily) and fortified topical eyedrops of the same antibiotics that were injected into the vitreous cavity should be used. The visual outcome is usually good in cases with anterior segment involvement; and poor when the vitreous is involved, especially with virulent bacteria such as streptococci, coagulase-positive staphylococci, and gram-negative organisms.

Prevention of bleb-related ocular infection is important. It seems reasonable to use antibiotics in some cases of leaking blebs, or recurrent bleb-related infections, but routine long-term use of topical antibiotics is not recommended. Conjunctivitis and blepharitis should be treated promptly, and soft contact lens wear should be avoided. Patient education about early symptoms of infection is currently the most important approach to minimize the chances of severe visual loss.[75,76] It may also be useful giving patients with thin, avascular, localized blebs an undated prescription for a wide-spectrum topical antibiotic to be filled emergently by the patient at the first possible sign of infection, while an appointment to see the glaucoma surgeon is arranged.

## 70.11 Conclusion

Glaucoma surgery can be associated with a variety of complications. This chapter reflects a comprehensive review of the literature and the authors' experiences, which summarize the best current practice for the prevention, recognition, and management of such complications.

## References

1. Cairns JE. Trabeculectomy. Preliminary report of a new method. *Am J Ophthalmol.* 1968;66:673–679.
2. Jampel HD, Musch DC, Gillespie BW, et al. Perioperative complications of trabeculectomy in the Collaborative Initial Glaucoma Treatment Study (CIGTS). *Am J Ophthalmol.* 2005;140:16–22.
3. Edmunds B, Thompson JR, Salmon JF, et al. The national survey of trabeculectomy. III. Early and late complications. *Eye.* 2002;16:297–303.
4. Gedde SJ, Herndon LW, Brandt JD, et al. Surgical complications in the tube versus trabeculectomy study during the first year of follow up. *Am J Opthalmol.* 2007;143:23–31.
5. Azuara-Blanco A, Katz LJ. Dysfunctional filtering blebs. *Surv Ophthalmol.* 1998;43:93–126.
6. Blok MDW, Kok JHC, van Mil C, et al. Use of the megasoft bandage lens for treatment of complications after trabeculectomy. *Am J Ophthalmol.* 1990;110:264–268.
7. Simmons RJ, Kimbrough RL. Shell tamponade in filtering surgery for glaucoma. *Ophthalmic Surg.* 1984;10:17–34.
8. Fink AJ, Boys-Smith JW, Brear R. Management of large filtering blebs with the argon laser. *Am J Ophthalmol.* 1986;101:695–699.
9. Lynch MG, Roesch M, Brown RH. Remodeling filtering blebs with the Neodynium:YAG laser. *Ophthalmology.* 1986;103:1700–1705.
10. Leen MM, Moster MR, Katz LJ, et al. Management of overfiltering and leaking blebs with autologous blood injection. *Arch Ophthalmol.* 1995;113:1050–1055.
11. Wise JB. Treatment of chronic postfiltration hypotony by intrableb injection of autologous blood. *Arch Ophthalmol.* 1993;111:827–830.
12. Lu DW, Azuara-Blanco A, Katz LJ. Severe visual loss after autologous blood injection for mitomycin-associated hypotony maculopathy. *Ophthalmic Surg Lasers.* 1997;28:244–245.
13. Schwartz GF, Robin AL, Wilson RP, et al. Resuturing the scleral flap leads to resolution of hypotony maculopathy. *J Glaucoma.* 1996;5:246–251.
14. Haynes WL, Alward WLM. Rapid visual recovery and long-term intraocular pressure control after donor scleral-patch grafting for trabeculectomy-induced hypotony maculopathy. *J Glaucoma.* 1994;4:200–201.
15. Suner IJ, Greenfield DS, Miller MP, et al. Hypotony maculopathy after filtering surgery with mitomycin-C: incidence and treatment. *Ophthalmology.* 1997;104:207–215.
16. Zacharia PT, Deppermann SR, Schuman JS. Ocular hypotony after trabeculectomy with mitomycin C. *Am J Ophthalmol.* 1993;116:314–326.
17. Shields MB, Scroggs MW, Sloop CM, et al. Clinical and histopathologic observations concerning hypotony after trabeculectomy with adjunctive mitomycin C. *Am J Ophthalmol.* 1993;116:673–683.
18. Costa VP, Wilson RP, Moster MR, et al. Hypotony maculopathy following the use of topical mitomycin C in glaucoma filtration surgery. *Ophthalmic Surg.* 1993;24:389–394.
19. Melamed S, Ashkenazi I, Glovinski J, et al. Tight scleral flap trabeculectomy with postoperative laser suture lysis. *Am J Ophthalmol.* 1990;109:303–309.
20. Chopra H, Goldenfeld M, Krupin T, et al. Early postoperative titration of bleb function: argon laser suture lysis and removable sutures in trabeculectomy. *J Glaucoma.* 1992;1:54–57.
21. Traverso CE, Greenidge KC, Spaeth GL, et al. Focal pressure: a new method to encourage filtration after trabeculectomy. *Ophthalmic Surg.* 1984;15:62–65.

22. Morinelli EN, Sidoti PA, Heuer DK, et al. Laser suture lysis after mitomycin C trabeculectomy. *Ophthalmology*. 1996;103:306–314.
23. Pappa KS, Derick RJ, Weber PA, et al. Late argon laser suture lysis after mitomycin C trabeculectomy. *Ophthalmology*. 1993;100:1268–1271.
24. Wilson RP. Technical advances in filtration surgery. In: McAllister JA, Wilson RP, eds. *Glaucoma*. Boston: Butterworths; 1986:243–350.
25. Cohen JS, Osher RH. Releasable scleral flap suture. *Ophthalmol Clin North Am*. 1988;1:187–197.
26. Johnstone MA, Wellington DP, Ziel CJ. A releasable scleral-flap tamponade suture for guarded filtration surgery. *Arch Ophthalmol*. 1993;111:398–403.
27. Tezel G, Kolker AE, Kass MA, Wax MB. Late removal of releasable sutures after trabeculectomy or combined trabeculectomy with cataract extraction supplemented with antifibrotics. *J Glaucoma*. 1998;7:75–81.
28. Cantor LB, Katz LJ, Spaeth GL. Complications of surgery in glaucoma: suprachoroidal expulsive hemorrhage in glaucoma patients undergoing intraocular surgery. *Ophthalmology*. 1985;92:1266–1270.
29. Ruderman JM, Harbin TS, Campbell DG. Postoperative suprachoroidal hemorrhage following filtering procedures. *Arch Ophthalmol*. 1986;104:201–205.
30. Givens K, Shields MB. Suprachoroidal hemorrhage after glaucoma filtering surgery. *Am J Ophthalmol*. 1987;103:689–694.
31. Frenkel REP, Shin DH. Prevention and management of delayed suprachoroidal hemorrhage after filtration surgery. *Arch Ophthalmol*. 1986;104:1459–1463.
32. Spaeth GL, Baez KA. Long-term prognosis of eyes having had operative suprachoroidal expulsive hemorrhage. *Ger J Ophthalmol*. 1994;3:159–163.
33. WuDunn D, Ryser D, Cantor LB. Surgical drainage of choroidal effusions following glaucoma surgery. *J Glaucoma*. 2005;14:103–108.
34. Quigley HA, Frieadman DS, Congdon NG. Possible mechanisms of primary angle-closure and malignant glaucoma. *J Glaucoma*. 2003;12:167–180.
35. Ruben S, Tsai J, Hitchings RA. Malignant glaucoma and its management. *Br J Ophthalmol*. 1997;81:163–167.
36. Epstein DL, Steinert RF, Puliafito CA. Neodynium:YAG laser therapy to the anterior hyaloid in aphakic malignant (ciliary block) glaucoma. *Ophthalmology*. 1980;87:1155–1159.
37. Lois N, Wong D, Groenwald C. New surgical approach in the management of pseudophakic malignant glaucoma. *Ophthalmology*. 2001;108:780–783.
38. Byrnes GA, Leen MM, Wong TP, et al. Vitrectomy for ciliary block (malignant) glaucoma. *Ophthalmology*. 1995;102:1308–1311.
39. Azuara-Blanco A, Katz LJ, Gandham S, et al. Pars plana tube insertion of aqueous shunt with vitrectomy in malignant glaucoma. *Arch Ophthalmol*. 1988;116:808–810.
40. Lichter PR, Ravin JG. Risk of sudden visual loss after glaucoma surgery. *Am J Ophthalmol*. 1974;78:1009–1013.
41. Costa VP, Smith M, Spaeth GL, et al. Loss of visual acuity after trabeculectomy. *Ophthalmology*. 1993;100:599–612.
42. Law SK, Nguyen AM, Coleman AL, et al. Severe loss of central vision in patients with advanced glaucoma undergoing trabeculectomy. *Arch Ophthalmol*. 2007;125:1044–1050.
43. Moster MR, Moster ML. Wipe-out: a complication of glaucoma surgery or a just a blast from the past. *Am J Ophthalmol*. 2005;140:705–706.
44. Eke T. Anesthesia for glaucoma surgery. *Ophthalmol Clin North Am*. 2006;19:245–255.
45. Kumar CM, Dowd TC, Dodds C, et al. Orbital swelling following peribulbar and sub Tenon's anaesthesia. *Eye*. 2004;18:418–420.
46. Hulbert MF, Yang YC, Pennefather PM, et al. Pulsatile ocular blood flow and intraocular pressure during retrobulbar injection of lignocaine: influence of additives. *J Glaucoma*. 1998;7:413–416.
47. Huber KK, Remky A. Effect of retrobulbar versus subconjunctival anaesthesia on retrobulbar haemodynamics. *Br J Ophthalmol*. 2005;89:719–723.
48. Zalta AH, Wieder RH. Closure of leaking filtering blebs with cyanoacrylate tissue adhesive. *Br J Ophthalmol*. 1991;75:170–173.
49. Asrani SG, Wilenski JT. Management of bleb leaks after glaucoma filtering surgery. Use of autologous fibrin tissue glue as an alternative. *Ophthalmology*. 1996;103:294–298.
50. Kajiwara K. Repair of a leaking bleb with fibrin glue. *Am J Ophthalmol*. 1990;109:599–601.
51. Wilensky JT. Management of late bleb leaks following glaucoma filtering surgery. *Trans Am Ophthalmol Soc*. 1992;93:161–168.
52. Wadhwani RA, Resham A, Bellows AR, et al. Surgical repair of leaking filtering blebs. *Ophthalmology*. 2000;107:1681–1687.
53. Burnstein AL, WuDunn D, Knotts L, et al. Conjunctival advancement versus nonincisional treatment for late-onset glaucoma filtering bleb leaks. *Ophthalmology*. 2002;109:71–75.
54. Catoria Y, Wudunn D, Cantor LB. Revision of dysfunctional filtering blebs by conjunctival advancement with bleb preservation. *Am J Ophthalmol*. 2000;130:574–579.
55. Harris L, Yang G, Feldman RN, et al. Autologous conjunctival resurfacing of leaking filtering blebs. *Ophthalmology*. 2000;107:1675–1680.
56. Maumenee AE. External filtering operations for glaucoma: the mechanism of function and failure. *Trans Am Acad Ophthalmol Soc*. 1960;58:319–328.
57. Starita RJ, Fellman RL, Spaeth GL, et al. Short- and long-term effects of postoperative corticosteroids on trabeculectomy. *Ophthalmology*. 1985;92:938–946.
58. Joshi AB, Parrish RK 2nd, Feuer WF. 2002 survey of the American Glaucoma Society: practice preferences for glaucoma surgery and antifibrotic use. *J Glaucoma*. 2005;14:172–174.
59. Siriwardena D, Edmunds B, Wormald RP, et al. National survey of antimetabolite use in glaucoma surgery in the United Kingdom. *Br J Ophthalmol*. 2004;88:873–876.
60. Goldenfeld M, Krupin T, Ruderman JM, et al. 5-fluorouracil in initial trabeculectomy. A prospective, randomized, multicenter study. *Ophthalmology*. 1994;101:1024–1029.
61. The Fluorouracil Filtering Surgery Study Group. Five-year follow-up of the Fluorouracil Filtering Surgery Study. *Am J Ophthalmol*. 1996;121:349–366.
62. Kitazawa Y, Suemori-Matsushita H, Yamamoto T, et al. Low-dose and high-dose mitomycin trabeculectomy as an initial surgery in primary open-angle glaucoma. *Ophthalmology*. 1993;100:1624–1628.
63. Wu-Dunn D, Cantor LB, Palanca-Capistrano AM, et al. A prospective randomized trial comparing intraoperative 5-fluorouracil versus mitomycin C in primary trabeculectomy. *Am J Ophthalmol*. 2002;134:521–528.
64. Borisuth NS, Phillips B, Krupin T. The risk profile of glaucoma filtration surgery. *Curr Opin Ophthalmol*. 1999;10:112–116.
65. Ewing RH, Stamper RL. Needle revision with and without 5-fluorouracil for the treatment of failed filtering blebs. *Am J Ophthalol*. 1990;110:254–259.
66. Greenfield DS, Miller MP, Suner IJ, et al. Needle revision of failed filtering blebs using mitomycin-C. *Ophthalmology*. 1996;122:195–204.
67. Mardelli PG, Lederer CM, Murrary PL, et al. Slit-lamp needle revision of filtering blebs using mitomycin C. *Ophthalmology*. 1996;103:1946–1955.
68. Shetty RK, Wartluft L, Moster MR. Slit-lamp needle revision of failed filtering blebs using high-dose mitomycin C. *J Glaucoma*. 2005;14:52–56.
69. Feldman RM, Gross RL, Spaeth GL, et al. Risk factors for the development of Tenon's capsule cysts after trabeculectomy. *Ophthalmology*. 1989;96:336–341.
70. Scott DR, Quigley HA. Medical management of a high bleb phase after trabaculectomies. *Ophthalmology*. 1988;95:1169–1173.

71. Azuara-Blanco A, Bond BJ, Wilson RP, et al. Encapsulated filtering blebs after trabeculectomy with mitomycin-C. *Ophthalmic Surg Lasers*. 1997;28:805–809.
72. Yarangümeli A, Köz OG, Kural G. Encapsulated blebs following primary standard trabeculectomy: course and treatment. *J Glaucoma*. 2004;13:251–255.
73. Katz LJ, Cantor LB, Spaeth GL. Complications of surgery in glaucoma. Early and late bacterial endophthalmitis following glaucoma filtering surgery. *Ophthalmology*. 1985;92:959–963.
74. Caronia RM, Liebmann JM, Friedman R, et al. Trabeculectomy at the inferior limbus. *Arch Ophthalmol*. 1996;114:387–391.
75. Greenfield DS, Suner IJ, Miller MP, et al. Endophthalmitis after filtering surgery with mitomycin. *Arch Ophthalmol*. 1996;114:943–949.
76. Mandelbaum S, Forster RK, Gelender H, et al. Late onset endophthalmitis associated with filtering blebs. *Ophthalmology*. 1985;92:964–972.
77. DeBry PW, Perkins TW, Heatley G, et al. Incidence of late-onset bleb-related complications following trabeculectomy with mitomycin. *Arch Ophthalmol*. 2002;120:297–300.
78. Soltau JB, Rothman RF, Budenz DL, et al. Risk factors for glaucoma filtering bleb infections. *Arch Ophthalmol*. 2000;118:338–342.
79. Jampel HD, Quigley HA, Kerrigan-Baumrid LA, et al. The Glaucoma Surgical Outcomes Study Group. Risk factors for late-onset infection following glaucoma filtration surgery. *Arch Ophthalmol*. 2001;119:1001–1008.
80. Song A, Scott IU, Flynn HW Jr, et al. Delayed-onset bleb-associated endophthalmitis: clinical features and visual acuity outcomes. *Ophthalmology*. 2002;109:985–991.
81. Kangas TA, Greenfield DS, Flynn HW Jr, et al. Delayed-onset endophthalmitis associated with conjunctival filtering blebs. *Ophthalmology*. 1997;104:746–752.
82. Reynolds AC, Skuta GL, Monlux R, et al. Management of blebitis by members of the American Glaucoma Society: a survey. *J Glaucoma*. 2001;10:340–347.
83. Wand M, Quintiliani R, Robinson A. Antibiotic prophylaxis in eyes with filtration blebs: survey of glaucoma specialists, microbiological study, and recommendations. *J Glaucoma*. 1995;4:103–109.

# Chapter 71
# Amniotic Membrane Grafts for Glaucoma Surgery

Hosam Sheha, Lingyi Liang, and Scheffer C.G. Tseng

Human amniotic membrane (AM) is the innermost layer of the placental membrane. While the tough, semitransparent nature of AM is valuable as a graft for ocular surface reconstruction, it is the unique inherent biological action of AM during embryogenesis that has spawned increasing interests over the past decade in ophthalmology. The biological actions known to AM include antiinflammatory, antiscarring, anti-angiogenic, and growth-promoting effects.[1-3] Several investigators have explored the clinical efficacy of deploying AMT as an adjunctive therapy to improve the surgical outcome of various glaucoma procedures including high-risk trabeculectomy, repair of conjunctival buttonholes during trabeculectomy, repair of early- and late-onset bleb leak, and covering of the shunt tube in glaucoma drainage devices (GDDs) during primary insertion or exposure.

## 71.1 High-Risk Trabeculectomy

The success rate of trabeculectomy has been limited by postoperative fibrosis that leads to bleb failure months or years after surgery.[4] To inhibit this fibrosis and hence improve the surgical outcome of trabeculectomy, antifibrotic agents such as 5-fluorouracil (5-FU) and mitomycin C (MMC) are commonly used.[5-8] Adjunctive uses of these two antifibrotics have improved the outcome in previously unoperated eyes, but still achieve a limited success in eyes with previously failed filtering surgery. This is particularly true in eyes carrying such high-risk factors as aphakia, pseudophakia, anterior segment neovascularization, uveitis, young age, and black race.[4,9,10] For glaucoma with these high-risk factors, GDDs or cyclodestructive procedures are frequently advocated, but may be associated with complications.

To circumvent these complications, one new approach is to use AM to reduce the fibrosis while halting rapid drainage of aqueous humor and its associated hypotony during the immediate postoperative period. Indeed, many investigators have used amniotic membrane transplantation (AMT) during trabeculectomy with or without MMC in both experimental and clinical studies with promising results[11-22] (summarized in Tables 71.1 and 71.2). The aforementioned favorable outcomes could be attributed to a synergistic beneficial effect of MMC and AMT on controlling fibrosis at the trabeculectomy site. MMC is known to enhance the success of trabeculectomy by inhibiting fibroblast proliferation at the filtering site.[23] AM has also been shown to down-regulate transforming growth factor-β signaling in cultured normal conjunctival and pterygium fibroblasts.[24,25] Furthermore, AM can facilitate macrophage apoptosis.[26] Therefore, AM inserted under and around the scleral flap might further enhance the success of MMC-treated trabeculectomy. This notion was suggested by the experimental rabbit data showing that AM reduces the number of subconjunctival fibroblasts at trabeculectomy sites even without MMC.[12,27] Moreover, numbers of both fibroblasts and macrophages around trabeculectomy sites in rabbits are significantly reduced by either MMC or AM,[13] and such suppression of fibroblasts is comparable between AMT and MMC in rabbit eyes.[17] Promising results of adding AMT in trabeculectomy surgery have also been noted in several clinical studies (Table 71.2). They have shown that transplantation of a single[11,15,16,19,22] or folded[20,21] AM under the scleral flap[11,16,19,20,22] and/or under the conjunctiva[16,19-22] with[11,19,20,22] or without[15,16,20,21] additional MMC reduces IOPs in eyes with refractory glaucoma that are associated with variable high-risk factors. Particularly, in a randomized control clinical trial of 48 eyes, Zheng et al[18] reported that the success rate in trabeculectomy with either AM or MMC is similar. Recently, in a randomized controlled clinical trial including 37 eyes, Sheha et al[22] added AM to trabeculectomy with MMC and achieved a significantly higher complete success (IOP≤21 mmHg without medications) and qualified success (IOP≤21 mmHg with or without additional medications) at postoperative 6 and 12 months, respectively. Furthermore, over a period of 1-year follow-up, a better control of IOP and bleb morphology (i.e., diffuse and translucent bleb with normal vascularity) is also more often observed in eyes with AM, while there is no such complications as hypotony, shallow anterior chamber, and choroidal effusion that are more frequently observed in eyes using

**Table 71.1** Animal studies of AMT in trabeculectomy

| | No. of rabbit eyes | Trab | Trab+AMT | Trab+MMC | Location of AM | Findings |
|---|---|---|---|---|---|---|
| Zhong et al[12] | 24 | X | X | | NA | Less fibroblast and more inflammatory cells in AMT[a] |
| Demir et al[13] | 30 | X | X | X | NA | Less fibroblast and macrophage in MMC and AMT Same macrophage but less fibroblast in MMC compared to AMT[a] |
| Demir et al[14] | 20 | X | X | | Under flap | Less macrophage and fibroblast in AMT |
| Wang et al[17] | 48 | | X | X | Under flap | Same fibroblast but more inflammatory cell in AMT[a] |

[a]Note: It is known that human AM transplanted in rabbits can produce inflammation due to xenograft reaction.[27]

**Table 71.2** Human studies of AMT in trabeculectomy

| | No. of eyes | Glaucoma | Control | MMC | Location of AMT | Mean FU (m) | Outcome |
|---|---|---|---|---|---|---|---|
| Fujishima et al[11] | 14 | NA | − | + | Under flap | NA | Controlled IOP in 13 cases |
| Lu et al[15] | 17 | NA | − | − | NA | 11.2 | Controlled IOP in 16 and 14 eyes after 3 and 6 months |
| Yue et al[16] | 67 | High risk | − | − | Under flap and under conjunctiva | 19.5 | Functional bleb in 80.6% |
| Zheng et al[18] | 48 | NA | + (MMC+) | − | NA | 6 | Similar success rate but less complications in AMT |
| Bruno et al[20] | 17 | High risk | − | +/− | Under flap (16) or under conjunctiva (1) | 6 | Controlled IOP in nine cases |
| Eliezer et al[21] | 63 | Primary | + (MMC−) | − | Under conjunctiva | 12 | AMT: more thin avascular blebs, less flat vascularized blebs |
| Drolsum et al[19] | 9 | High risk | − | + | Under flap and under conjunctiva | 9.8 | Significant reduction in IOP and glaucoma medications |
| Sheha et al[22] | 37 | High risk | + (MMC+) | + | Under and around flap | 12 | Higher success rates and less complications in AMT |

MMC alone at the early postoperative period. These beneficial effects may be attributed to the fact that AM inserted under the scleral flap effectively halts rapid drainage of aqueous humor from the trabeculectomy site.[22] Although human AM dissolves at 1 month postoperatively in experimental rabbits,[17] such a finding was not noted in humans. Collectively, these encouraging results warrant further investigation of AM's utility in glaucoma filtrating procedures, especially in high-risk refractory glaucoma.

## 71.2 Intraoperative Conjunctival Buttonholes

Conjunctival buttonholes are not uncommon complications during trabeculectomy,[28] but might ensue when the eye has prior surgeries and/or receives MMC, where scarred tissue limits conjunctival advancement to the limbal region. Buttonholes are usually detected during inspection of the conjunctiva before wound closure. Once identified, closure of buttonholes is traditionally achieved by direct suturing. However, additional suture passes through fragile conjunctiva may result in multiple buttonholes, rendering this technique ineffective. Alternatively, the buttonhole area may be excised if adjoining the conjunctival incision. Sutureless AM using fibrin glue (Baxter Bioscience, Deerfield, Illinois) has been successfully used to achieve closure of intraoperative buttonholes in fragile conjunctiva not amenable to primary closure.[29] AMT over leaking filtration blebs may not only promote epithelial healing of conjunctival leaks, but also reduces scarring and may enhance bleb survival. It is also possible to apply the AM in the subconjunctival space before closure with or without fibrin glue. However, using fibrin glue in the subconjunctival space may alter the bleb function. The role of the orientation of the AM in enhancing successful filtration while promoting wound closure is not clear. In ophthalmic surgery, the epithelial or basement membrane side is generally applied facing up whereas the stromal side faces the ocular surface. With this orientation, the AM serves as a scaffold and provides a suitable basement membrane upon which epithelial cells can grow.[2] Therefore, we believe that applying the stromal side toward the conjunctiva is ideal for either over or under the conjunctiva in repairing buttonholes.

## 71.3 Bleb Leak

Bleb leak is one of the increasing complications after trabeculectomy with adjunctive use of antimetabolites, and may lead to sight-threatening complications. Several authors have reported success rates of surgical revision being 83–96%, either with conjunctival advancement or with a free autologous conjunctival graft for repairing late-onset bleb leak, although each author used different definitions of success.[30-32] Although these types of surgical intervention can resolve bleb leak, they share the risk of loss of bleb function.[31-33]

An ideal procedure to repair leaking bleb, therefore, is one that can both support the fragile conjunctival tissue and suppress the exaggerated bleb scarring. In this regard, investigators have used AMT to repair bleb leak with promising results. They used single[34-38] or double[39] layers with the epithelial side up[36,38] or down[35,38] over[35,36] or under[38] the conjunctiva with[34,37-39] or without[35,36,38] bleb excision (summarized in Table 71.3).

After excision of the preexisting bleb, AM can be applied in single or double layers. To ensure success, the membrane is fashioned to cover the conjunctival defect with the epithelial side up when a single layer is used. The limbal side of AM is sutured to the sclera, while the fornix side is inserted underneath healthy conjunctiva posterior to the conjunctival incision line and sutured with the underlying Tenon's capsule.[38] Fantes and Palmberg[39] folded the AM with the epithelial/basement membrane surfaces facing outward and the mesenchymal surfaces in apposition on the inside. Successful closure was achieved immediately after surgery and reepithelialization is usually completed on AM in 3 weeks in eyes with ischemic and scarred conjunctiva.

As late bleb leaks often occur in avascular, thin-walled blebs after antimetabolite use, failure of AMT to heal bleb leaks after bleb excision is likely related to the devitalized and ischemic nature of the conjunctiva.[34,37,40] Such a complication has not been noted when AM is used to reconstruct large conjunctival defects after removal of pterygia and symblepharon.[2,41,42] If the bordering conjunctiva is not ischemic and has a normal epithelium and subconjunctival stroma, successful closure can be achieved by AM.[43] Recently, it has been reported that scleral melt because of ischemia can be corrected by AMT if a vascularized thin Tenon pedicle graft is used as tenonplasty.[44] It remains unclear whether such a thin Tenon pedicle graft can also be used to correct bleb ischemia.

Other authors have reported successful repair of late bleb leaks using AM without bleb excision. They cover the bleb with a single layer of AM with the epithelial side up using sutures or fibrin glue[1], or apply a single layer of AM, epithelial side down, underneath the conjunctiva through a limbal-based flap while the preexisting scleral flap is revised.[38] The AMT-assisted bleb revision not only halts bleb leak but also maintains functioning blebs extending posteriorly beyond the conjunctival incision without bleb leak.

Because there is a high chance of maintaining a functioning bleb, AMT can be considered the first option before conjunctival advancement.

**Table 71.3** Human studies of AMT in bleb leak

| | No. of eyes | Control | Bleb leak | AMT | | | Mean FU (m) | Outcome |
| | | | | Layers | Orientation | Location | | |
| --- | --- | --- | --- | --- | --- | --- | --- | --- |
| Budenz et al[34] | 15 | +15 (Conj. advancement) | Late-onset | Single | NA | Over bare sclera | 19 | Releakage/failure in 7/15 |
| Rauscher et al[37] | 15 | +15 (Conj. advancement) | NA | – | NA | Over bare sclera/stitch | 80 | Earlier failure, higher releakage with AMT |
| Fantes and Palmberg[39] | 2 | – | Late-onset | Double | Stroma to stroma | Over bare sclera | NA | Bleb leaks were closed, and bleb function was maintained |
| Kee and Hwang[35] | 2 | – | Late-onset | Single | Epithelium down | Over bleb/stitch | 24 | In both patients, bleb leaks were closed, and bleb function was maintained |
| Kiuchi et al[36] | 1 | – | Late-onset | Single | Epithelium up | Over bleb/stitch | 6 | Well-functioning bleb was maintained/no recurrence |
| Nagai et al[38] | 6 | – | Late-onset | Single 5/ Double1 | Epithelium down 5/up 1 | Under conjunctiva 5/over bare sclera1 | 49 | Bleb leaks were closed, and bleb function was maintained/no recurrence |

---

[1]Dr. Brian Francis, personal communication October 2008

**Table 71.4** Human studies of AMT in covering shunt tube

| | No. of eyes | Exposed shunt tube | Patch graft | AMT | Mean FU (m) | Outcome |
|---|---|---|---|---|---|---|
| Rai et al[58] | 9 | Yes | Sclera | Single layer | 42 | Tube remained covered with intact conjunctival epithelium in all cases in seven cases |
| Ainsworth et al[57] | 3 | Yes | Sclera | Double layer | 30 | Tube remained covered with intact conjunctival epithelium in all cases |
| Papadaki et al[59] | 1 | Yes | – | Single layer | 6 | Tube remained covered with intact conjunctival epithelium |

## 71.4 Glaucoma Drainage Devices

### 71.4.1 To Repair Conjunctival Erosion and Tube Exposure

Glaucoma drainage devices are being used more frequently in the treatment of refractory and other high-risk glaucomas to channel the aqueous humor from the anterior chamber to an equatorial plate.[10,45,46] If left uncovered, the extraocular portion of the tube is relatively long and may erode through the conjunctiva, presenting the eye with a risk of intraocular infection.[47] Several patch grafts have been used to cover the tube including human sclera,[48] pericardium,[49] dura,[50] autologous fascia lata,[51] and cornea.[52] The advent of these patches has decreased the tube exposure rate from 30% to 5%.[46] However, the incidence of thinning and/or melting of graft materials, leading to tube exposure, is about 25% in 2 years.[53-55] Repair of these eroded tubes usually requires replacement of the scleral or pericardial patch and covering of this patch with conjunctiva. If inadequately covered with conjunctiva, the donor patch will melt again, leading to reexposure of the tube. In eyes with prior multiple ocular surface surgeries, however, closure of the conjunctival covering can be very difficult, if not impossible, because of the fragile nature of the tissue similar to aforementioned conjunctival buttonholes.[56] Several studies have demonstrated the efficacy of using cryopreserved AM as a conjunctival substitute to cover the exposed tube. It was used as double[57] or single layer[58] in conjunction with or without[59] scleral patch (Table 71.4). All these cases retained good short- and long-term results during the follow-up of 6 months to 2.5 years without epithelial defects.

### 71.4.2 To Cover Shunt Tube in Primary Surgery

To circumvent the limitation of scleral or pericardial patch, a thicker cryopreserved AM with an average thickness of 300–600 μm has been developed (Bio-Tissue, Inc., Miami, Florida) to cover the shunt tube in primary GDD surgery or secondarily exposed tube. Preliminary results are promising in reducing tube exposure and supporting the hypothesis that AM patch can promote host cell infiltration into it to form a Tenon-like layer over the shunt tube. Additional advantages include a better esthetic appearance (without a whitish patchy appearance) and allowing laser suture lysis. A prospective study is underway to evaluate its clinical efficacy in preventing conjunctival erosion and tube exposure compared with the existing patch grafts.

## References

1. Tseng SCG, Espana EM, Kawakita T, et al. How does amniotic membrane work? *Ocul Surf.* 2004;2:177–187.
2. Dua HS, Gomes JA, King AJ, Maharajan VS. The amniotic membrane in ophthalmology. *Surv Ophthalmol.* 2004;49:51–77.
3. Bouchard CS, John T. Amniotic membrane transplantation in the management of severe ocular surface disease: indications and outcomes. *Ocul Surf.* 2004;2:201–211.
4. Skuta GL, Parrish RK. Wound healing in glaucoma filtering surgery. *Surv Ophthalmol.* 1987;32:149–170.
5. Chen C. Enhanced intraocular pressure controlling effectiveness of trabeculectomy by local application of mitomycin C. *Trans Asia Pac Acad Ophthalmol.* 1983;9:172–177.
6. Heuer DK, Parrish RK, Gressel MG, Hodapp E, Palmberg PF, Anderson DR. 5-fluorouracil and glaucoma filtering surgery. II. A pilot study. *Ophthalmology.* 1984;91:384–394.
7. Lama PJ, Fechtner RD. Antifibrotics and wound healing in glaucoma surgery. *Surv Ophthalmol.* 2003;48:314–346.
8. Yoon PS, Singh K. Update on antifibrotic use in glaucoma surgery, including use in trabeculectomy and glaucoma drainage implants and combined cataract and glaucoma surgery. *Curr Opin Ophthalmol.* 2004;15:141–146.
9. Sturmer J, Broadway DC, Hitchings RA. Young patient trabeculectomy. Assessment of risk factors for failure. *Ophthalmology.* 1993;100:928–939.
10. Broadway DC, Chang LP. Trabeculectomy, risk factors for failure and the preoperative state of the conjunctiva. *J Glaucoma.* 2001;10:237–249.
11. Fujishima H, Shimazaki J, Shinozaki N, Tsubota K. Trabeculectomy with the use of amniotic membrane for uncontrolled glaucoma. *Ophthalmic Surg Lasers.* 1998;29:428–431.
12. Zhong Y, Zhou Y, Wang K. [Effect of amniotic membrane on filtering bleb after trabeculectomy in rabbit eyes]. *Yan Ke Xue Bao.* 2000;16:73–76. 83.

13. Demir T, Turgut B, Akyol N, Ozercan I, Ulas F, Celiker U. Effects of amniotic membrane transplantation and mitomycin C on wound healing in experimental glaucoma surgery. *Ophthalmologica.* 2002;216:438–442.
14. Demir T, Turgut B, Celiker U, Ozercan I, Ulas F, Akyol N. Effects of octreotide acetate and amniotic membrane on wound healing in experimental glaucoma surgery. *Doc Ophthalmol.* 2003;107:87–92.
15. Lu H, Mai D. [Trabeculectomy combined amniotic membrane transplantation for refractory glaucoma]. *Yan Ke Xue Bao.* 2003; 19:89–91.
16. Yue J, Hu CQ, Lei XM, Qin GH, Zhang Y. [Trabeculectomy with amniotic membrane transplantation and combining suture lysis of scleral flap in complicated glaucoma]. *Zhonghua Yan Ke Za Zhi.* 2003;39:476–480.
17. Wang L, Liu X, Zhang P, Lin J. [An experimental trial of glaucoma filtering surgery with amniotic membrane]. *Yan Ke Xue Bao.* 2005;21:126–131.
18. Zheng K, Huang Z, Zou H, Li H, Huang Y, Xie M. [The comparison study of glaucoma trabeculectomy applying amniotic membrane or mitomycin C]. *Yan Ke Xue Bao.* 2005;21:84–87. 91.
19. Drolsum L, Willoch C, Nicolaissen B. Use of amniotic membrane as an adjuvant in refractory glaucoma. *Acta Ophthalmol Scand.* 2006;84:786–789.
20. Bruno CA, Eisengart JA, Radenbaugh PA, Moroi SE. Subconjunctival placement of human amniotic membrane during high risk glaucoma filtration surgery. *Ophthalmic Surg Lasers Imaging.* 2006;37:190–197.
21. Eliezer RN, Kasahara N, Caixeta-Umbelino C, Pinheiro RK, Mandia C Jr, Malta RF. Use of amniotic membrane in trabeculectomy for the treatment of glaucoma: a pilot study. *Arq Bras Oftalmol.* 2006;69:309–312.
22. Sheha H, Kheirkhah A, Taha H. Amniotic membrane transplantation in trabeculectomy with mitomycin C for refractory glaucoma. *J Glaucoma.* 2008;17:303–307.
23. Jampel HD. Effect of brief exposure to mitomycin C on viability and proliferation of cultured human Tenon's capsule fibroblasts. *Ophthalmology.* 1992;99:1471–1476.
24. Tseng SCG, Li D-Q, Ma X. Suppression of transforming growth factor isoforms, TGF-b receptor II, and myofibroblast differentiation in cultured human corneal and limbal fibroblasts by amniotic membrane matrix. *J Cell Physiol.* 1999;179:325–335.
25. Lee S-B, Li D-Q, Tan DTH, Meller D, Tseng SCG. Suppression of TGF-b signaling in both normal conjunctival fibroblasts and pterygial body fibroblasts by amniotic membrane. *Curr Eye Res.* 2000;20:325–334.
26. Li W, He H, Kawakita T, Espana EM, Tseng SCG. Amniotic membrane induces apoptosis of interferon-gamma activited macrophages in vitro. *Exp Eye Res.* 2006;82:282–292.
27. Barton K, Budenz D, Khaw PT, Tseng SCG. Glaucoma filtration surgery using amniotic membrane transplantation. *Invest Ophthalmol Vis Sci.* 2001;42:1762–1768.
28. Levkovitch-verbin H, Goldenfeld M, Melamed S. Fornix-based trabeculectomy with mitomycin-C. *Ophthalmic Surg Lasers.* 1997; 28:818–822.
29. Li G, O'Hearn T, Yiu S, Francis B. Amniotic membrane transplantation for intraoperative conjunctival repair during trabeculectomy with mitomycin C. *J Glaucoma.* 2007;16:521–526.
30. Wadhwani RA, Bellows AR, Hutchinson BT. Surgical repair of leaking filtering blebs. *Ophthalmology.* 2000;107:1681–1687.
31. Schnyder CC, Shaarawy T, Ravinet E, Achache F, Uffer S, Mermoud A. Free conjunctival autologous graft for bleb repair and bleb reduction after trabeculectomy and nonpenetrating filtering surgery. *J Glaucoma.* 2002;11:10–16.
32. Tannenbaum DP, Hoffman D, Greaney MJ, Caprioli J. Outcomes of bleb excision and conjunctival advancement for leaking or hypotonous eyes after glaucoma filtering surgery. *Br J Ophthalmol.* 2004;88:99–103.
33. Burnstein AL, WuDunn D, Knotts SL, Catoira Y, Cantor LB. Conjunctival advancement versus nonincisional treatment for late-onset glaucoma filtering bleb leaks. *Ophthalmology.* 2002;109: 71–75.
34. Budenz DL, Barton K, Tseng SCG. Amniotic membrane transplantation for repair of leaking glaucoma filtering blebs. *Am J Ophthalmol.* 2000;130:580–588.
35. Kee C, Hwang JM. Amniotic membrane graft for late-onset glaucoma filtering leaks. *Am J Ophthalmol.* 2002;133:834–835.
36. Kiuchi T, Okamoto H, Ishii K, Oshika T. Amniotic membrane transplantation for late-onset bleb leakage with scleritis. *Jpn J Ophthalmol.* 2005;49:56–58.
37. Rauscher FM, Barton K, Budenz DL, Feuer WJ, Tseng SC. Long-term outcomes of amniotic membrane transplantation for repair of leaking glaucoma filtering blebs. *Am J Ophthalmol.* 2007;143: 1052–1054.
38. Nagai-Kusuhara A, Nakamura M, Fujioka M, Negi A. Long-term results of amniotic membrane transplantation-assisted bleb revision for leaking blebs. *Graefes Arch Clin Exp Ophthalmol.* 2008;246: 567–571.
39. Fantes F, Palmberg PF. Late complications of glaucoma surgery. In: Rhee DJ, Rapuano CJ, eds. *Glaucoma: Color Atlas and Synopsis of Clinical Ophthalmology.* Chicago: McGraw-Hill Professional; 2003:338–363.
40. Skuta GL, Beeson CC, Higginbotham EJ, et al. Intraoperative mitomycin versus postoperative 5-fluorouracil in high-risk glaucoma filtering surgery. *Ophthalmology.* 1992;99:438–444.
41. Ma DH-K, See L-C, Liau S-B, Tsai RJF. Amniotic membrane graft for primary pterygium: comparison with conjunctival autograft and topical mitomycin C treatment. *Br J Ophthalmol.* 2000;84:973–978.
42. Solomon A, Pires RTF, Tseng SCG. Amniotic membrane transplantation after extensive removal of primary and recurrent pterygia. *Ophthalmology.* 2001;108:449–460.
43. Francis BA, Du LT, Najafi K, et al. Histopathologic features of conjunctival filtering blebs. *Arch Ophthalmol.* 2005;123:166–170.
44. Casas V, Kheirkhah A, Blanco G, Tseng SCG. Scleral approach for scleral ischemia and melt. *Cornea.* 2008;27:196–201.
45. Ayyala RS, Zurakowski D, Smith JA, et al. A clinical study of the Ahmed glaucoma valve implant in advanced glaucoma. *Ophthalmology.* 1998;105:1968–1976.
46. Heuer DK, Lloyd MA, Abrams DA, et al. Which is better? One or two? A randomized clinical trial of single-plate versus double-plate Molteno implantation for glaucomas in aphakia and pseudophakia. *Ophthalmology.* 1992;99:1512–1519.
47. Gedde SJ, Scott IU, Tabandeh H, et al. Late endophthalmitis associated with glaucoma drainage implants. *Ophthalmology.* 2001;108: 1323–1327.
48. Freedman J. Scleral patch grafts with Molteno setons. *Ophthalmic Surg.* 1987;18:532–534.
49. Raviv T, Greenfield DS, Liebmann JM, Sidoti PA, Ishikawa H, Ritch R. Pericardial patch grafts in glaucoma implant surgery. *J Glaucoma.* 1998;7:27–32.
50. Brandt JD. Patch grafts of dehydrated cadaveric dura mater for tube-shunt glaucoma surgery. *Arch Ophthalmol.* 1993;111:1436–1439.
51. Tanji TM, Lundy DC, Minckler DS, Heuer DK, Varma R. Fascia lata patch graft in glaucoma tube surgery. *Ophthalmology.* 1996;103:1309–1312.
52. Rojanapongpun P, Ritch R. Clear corneal graft overlying the seton tube to facilitate laser suture lysis. *Am J Ophthalmol.* 1996;122: 424–425.
53. Smith MF, Doyle JW, Tierney JW Jr. A comparison of glaucoma drainage implant tube coverage. *J Glaucoma.* 2002;11:143–147.
54. Jacob T, LaCour OJ, Burgoyne CF, LaFleur PK, Duzman E. Expanded polytetrafluoroethylene reinforcement material in glaucoma drain surgery. *J Glaucoma.* 2001;10:115–120.

55. Lama PJ, Fechtner RD. Tube erosion following insertion of a glaucoma drainage device with a pericardial patch graft. *Arch Ophthalmol*. 1999;117:1243–1244.
56. Heuer DK, Budenz D, Coleman A. Aqueous shunt tube erosion. *J Glaucoma*. 2001;10:493–496.
57. Ainsworth G, Rotchford A, Dua HS, King AJ. A novel use of amniotic membrane in the management of tube exposure following glaucoma tube shunt surgery. *Br J Ophthalmol*. 2006;90:417–419.
58. Rai P, Lauande-Pimentel R, Barton K. Amniotic membrane as an adjunct to donor sclera in the repair of exposed glaucoma drainage devices. *Am J Ophthalmol*. 2005;140:1148–1152.
59. Papadaki TG, Siganos CS, Zacharopoulos IP, Panteleontidis V, Charissis SK. Human amniotic membrane transplantation for tube exposure after glaucoma drainage device implantation. *J Glaucoma*. 2007;16:171–172.

# Chapter 72
# Treating Choroidal Effusions After Glaucoma Surgery

Jody Piltz-Seymour

Serous choroidal detachments that develop after glaucoma surgery can be an annoyance to both patient and doctor, but most cases resolve spontaneously without permanent sequelae. The use of antimetabolites, however, has increased the incidence of persistent choroidals, complicating the postoperative course with prolonged visual compromise, shallow anterior chambers, cataract formation, and bleb failure. The best "treatment" for choroidal detachments is prevention. Prevention avoids the potential roller coaster of choroidalrelated complications, and every effort should be made throughout the postoperative period to avoid slipping down the road to choroidals. Once choroidals develop, careful consideration should be given to deciding when conservative treatment is indicated versus when the situation warrants surgical drainage of the serous choroidals.

Understanding the underlying mechanism of serous choroidal formation is vital to prevention. Hypotony is the main factor causing the development of serous choroidals after glaucoma surgery. Hypotony leads to transudation of fluid into the suprachoroidal space causing quadratic bullous elevations of the retina and choroid tethered by the four vortex veins. Unfortunately, choroidals themselves cause aqueous shutdown and worsening of the hypotony. This leads to a vicious cycle of hypotony causing choroidals, and persistent choroidals causing hypotony, and so on.[1,2]

Hypotony after glaucoma surgery is most often caused by overfiltration, but inflammation also plays a key role in the process. Inflammation causes aqueous shutdown, which contributes to hypotony. Other conditions that can predispose patients to postoperative choroidals include cyclodialysis cleft, posterior scleritis, nanophthalmos, and any condition with elevated episcleral venous pressure such as Sturge Weber disease or thyroid ophthalmopathy.[2]

Initiating topical or systemic carbonic anhydrase inhibitors, beta-blockers, or prostaglandin analogues have been associated with the onset or exacerbation of serous choroidals after trabeculectomy. This phenomenon can occur even when the offending medication is initiated months or years after surgery and even when topically administered to the contralateral eye.[3-9]

Occasionally, choroidals can be very peripheral and low-lying, requiring ultrasound examination to accurately make the diagnosis.[10] These develop most commonly after topiramate or other sulfabased medication is prescribed.[11,12] These shallow uveal effusions cause swelling of the ciliary body, forward rotation of the lens iris diaphragm, myopic shift in refraction, and ultimately angle closure. Patients may present as if in aqueous misdirection with shallow anterior chamber, angle closure, elevated intraocular pressure (IOP), and no evidence of serous choroidals on clinical examination. Ultrasound examination is needed to diagnose these shallow choroidals. While bullous choroidals are more common postoperatively, low-lying choroidals still should be considered in the differential of shallow anterior chamber following glaucoma filtration surgery.

The symptomatology of serous choroidals after trabeculectomy varies greatly. Small bullous peripheral choroidals may be asymptomatic causing minimal shallowing of the anterior chamber. Larger choroidals can cause markedly decreased vision secondary to uncorrected refractive shifts associated with forward displacement of the lens and shallowing of the anterior chamber. Choroidals cause absolute scotoma where they are located, and patients may notice dark absolute blind regions in their peripheral vision. Vision can fall dramatically as choroidals enlarge and encroach on the macula.

Serous choroidals develop painlessly, which distinguishes them from hemorrhagic choroidals. Hemorrhagic choroidals typically present with sudden onset of severe pain, severe visual compromise, and dusky appearance to the choroidals. Hemorrhagic choroidals are usually devastating with poor long-term visual prognosis.

Every effort should be made perioperatively to avoid the development of serous choroidal developments. Physicians should proceed cautiously in high-risk cases, such as nanophthalmos or Sturge Weber cases. Some advocate prophylactically performing scleral windows or sclerotomies at the time of trabeculectomy in these high-risk cases. Meticulous surgical technique to avoid postoperative hypotony will minimize the risk of choroidals in all patients. Good flap architecture involves employing modest cautery and adequate flap thickness.

The sclerostomy should be placed anteriorly to avoid cleft formation and bleeding, which can incite inflammation. The sclerostomy should be centered under the scleral flap so that there is overlap between the flap and bed on both sides of the sclerostomy. The lowest dose of antimetabolites should be used and applied diffusely with a wide pledget. A Merocel sponge works better than cut surgical spears, which can fray, leaving behind a subconjunctival foreign body. The flap should be closed with multiple adjustable sutures and filtration should be evaluated intraoperatively, readjusting the sutures until there is gentle flow with a deep anterior chamber and IOP roughly in the mid to early teens. The author prefers to aim for a goal IOP to minimize the need for early suture lysis. Meticulous closure of the conjunctival wound minimizes the risk of wound leak. The bleb should be inflated through a limbal paracentesis to identify and close any wound leaks prior to leaving the operating room.

Postoperatively, avoid early suture lysis if possible, particularly if antimetabolites were used. Minimizing postoperative inflammation with liberal use of topical steroids is also key to preventing choroidals. Discontinue glaucoma meds in the operative eye, and discontinue systemic carbonic anhydrase inhibitors if used. If the IOP is low postoperatively, consider discontinuing contralateral topical betablockers if possible, or minimize systemic absorption with strict punctal occlusion and 5 min of eyelid closure.

Even the most meticulous surgeon will encounter choroidal detachments occasionally. Most physicians favor conservative management since the majority of choroidals are selflimited and will resolve within 2–3 weeks.[2,13] Conservative management is aimed primarily at minimizing hypotony and inflammation, and secondarily at the treatment of shallow anterior chambers. As mentioned in the prevention section, be sure topical glaucoma drops were discontinued in the operative eye, discontinue oral carbonic anhydrase inhibitors, discontinue or minimize systemic absorption of contralateral betablockers, and consider discontinuing systemic betablockers if medically permissible. Treat vigorously with topical steroids if inflammation is prominent, or decrease steroid dosing if overfiltration is the underlying cause of the choroidals. Cycloplegics can also help deepen the anterior chamber. Some advocate a short course of systemic steroids.

If the shallow anterior chamber is moderate with iridocorneal touch but formed chamber between the lens and cornea, a large diameter contact lens (18–24 mm) can be placed with or without pressure patching to diminish outflow through the bleb. Compression shells are rarely used any longer. If the situation does not improve or if there is risk of iridolenticular touch, the anterior chamber can be reformed with viscoelastic[14]; however, if overfiltration remains the instigating cause of the choroidals, the viscoelastic may rapidly exit the eye, and the chamber may reshallow. A high-density viscoelastic such as Healon 5 (Advanced Medical Optics, Inc., Santa Ana, California) may remain in the anterior chamber better, but it also has the risk of resulting in a dramatic IOP spike if the filter has become compromised.

The optimal time to drain postoperative choroidal effusions is a highly controversial topic. Few would dispute the need for emergency choroidal drainage if lenticular–corneal touch or corneal decompensation develops. Drainage can be performed earlier if there is need for more rapid visual recovery. Hypotony increases the risk of cataract formation with or without shallow chamber.[15,16] Permanent peripheral anterior synechiae may develop from shallow chambers causing diminished outflow after the choroidals resolve. Since long-term bleb development requires aqueous percolation, choroidals can lead to bleb scarring by causing aqueous shutdown. Earlier intervention should be considered if there is evidence of bleb failure, development of peripheral anterior synechiae, or cataract. Some also advocate earlier drainage with kissing choroidals particularly if there is any blood in the vitreous.

Consideration must be given to the status of the filtering bleb at the time of choroidal drainage. If the bleb is still at risk for overfiltering, it is vital to revise the bleb at the time of choroidal drainage to prevent the choroidals from reforming. In cases with overfiltration, the conjunctiva should be incised and the scleral flap reassessed. Additional sutures can be placed in the scleral flap to decrease outflow. It is important to place multiple sutures if possible so that the flow can be slowly titrated with suture removal postoperatively if the pressure should become elevated. If sutures cannot be visualized sufficiently to perform laser suture lysis postoperatively, releasable sutures should be used. In some cases, the scleral flap is too friable to resuture, and a graft of scleral or pericardium can be placed over the filtration site and secured with a mattress suture to apply direct pressure to the scleral flap. Not all trabeculectomy sites need to be revised; sometimes, even blebs that started out with excessive flow can heal or scar enough during the observation period to maintain adequate IOP.

Choroidal drainage is a much less delicate procedure than most ophthalmic surgeons are used to. A selfsealing anterior chamber maintainer helps keep the eye pressurized throughout the procedure. A horizontal conjunctival incision is made 3–6 mm from the limbus in the quadrant with the greatest choroidal elevation, usually one of the inferior quadrants. Cautery is applied to the sclera. Radially, a blade is used to scratch down gradually through the sclera centered 3–4 mm from the limbus until the suprachoroidal space is reached. A copious amount of strawcolored fluid drains when the choroidal space is entered. The indelicate portion of the procedure includes grasping the sides of the scleral incision to pull the wound open while rolling cotton applicators over the sclera toward the wound to "milk" the residual fluid out of the choroidal space. An indirect ophthalmoscope can be used to check if the choroidals have been adequately drained. Additional expression with the applicators can be performed until adequate flattening of the choroidals is achieved. Occasionally, a second sclerotomy needs to be performed in another quadrant to achieve adequate drainage. The edges of the sclerotomy can be cauterized to help gape the incision, or some advocate using a scleral punch on one side of the wound. The scleral incision is left unsutured, and the conjunctiva is closed with absorbable suture.

Choroidals can reform after drainage, particularly if there is continued overfiltration or inflammation.[1,17] If overfiltration persists, limit topical steroids and consider inserting a large diameter contact lens. If inflammation is active, treat aggressively postoperatively with steroids and continue cycloplegics. While some studies have shown little long-term effects of serous choroidals on vision or IOP,[18,19] the hypotony and aqueous shutdown from the choroidals may compromise bleb development causing IOP to rise after the choroidals resolve. Some have also observed an increased risk of encapsulated blebs after choroidal detachments causing elevated IOP to overshadow the prior problem of hypotony.

In their series of 94 choroidal drainage procedures, WuDunn and associates noted complete resolution of choroidals in 59% of eyes by month 1, and 90% of eyes by 4 months postoperatively. Surgical drainage resulted in resolution of hypotony and improved vision, but cataracts developed in 77% of phakic eyes.[17]

The treatment of serous choroidal detachments needs to proceed in a logical fashion. However, there can be great variability in the approach and timing of the progressive interventions, allowing ophthalmologists to express the art as well as the science of their medical practice.

## References

1. Bellows AR, Chaylack LT, Hutchinson BT. Choroidal detachment. Clinical manifestation, therapy and mechanism of formation. *Ophthalmology.* 1981;88:1107–1115.
2. Brubaker RF, Pederson JE. Ciliochoroidal detachment. *Surv Ophthalmol.* 1983;27:281–289.
3. Callahan C, Ayyala RS. Hypotony and choroidal effusion induced by topical timolol and dorzolamide in patients with previous glaucoma drainage device implantation. *Ophthalmic Surg Lasers Imaging.* 2003;34:467–469.
4. Davani S, Delbosc B, Royer B, et al. Choroidal detachment induced by dorzolamide 20 years after cataract surgery. *Br J Ophthalmol.* 2002;86:1457–1458.
5. Fineman MS, Katz LJ, Wilson RP. Topical dorzolamide-induced hypotony and ciliochoroidal detachment in patients with previous filtration surgery. *Arch Ophthalmol.* 1996;114:1031–1032.
6. Geyer O, Neudorfer M, Lazar M. Recurrent choroidal detachment following timolol therapy in previously filtered eye. *Acta Ophthalmol.* 1992;70:702–703.
7. Pereira Marques ML, Katz LJ. Choroidal detachment after the use of topical latanoprost. *Am J Ophthalmol.* 2001;132:928–929.
8. Sharma T, Salmon JF. Hypotony and choroidal detachment as a complication of topical combined timolol and dorzolamide. *J Ocul Pharmacol Ther.* 2007;23:202–205.
9. Vela MA, Campbell DG. Hypotony and ciliochoroidal detachment following pharmacologic aqueous suppressant therapy in previously filtered patients. *Ophthalmology.* 1985;92:50–57.
10. Sugimoto K, Ito K, Edaki K, et al. Supraciliochoroidal fluid at an early stage after trabeculectomy. *Nippon Ganka Gakkai Zasshi.* 2001;105:766–770.
11. Panday VA, Rhee DJ. Review of sulfonamide-induced acute myopia and acute bilateral angle-closure glaucoma. *Compr Ophthalmol Update.* 2007;8:271–276.
12. Banta JT, Hoffman K, Budenz DL, et al. Presumed topiramate-induced bilateral acute angle-closure glaucoma. *Am J Ophthalmol.* 2001;132:112–114.
13. Burney EN, Quigley HA, Robin AL. Hypotony and choroidal detachment as late complications of trabeculectomy. *Am J Ophthalmol.* 1987;103:685–688.
14. Fisher YL, Turtz AI, Gold M, et al. Use of sodium hyaluronate in reformation and reconstruction of the persistent flat anterior chamber in the presence of severe hypotony. *Ophthalmic Surg.* 1982;13:819–821.
15. Mills K. Trabeculectomy: a retrospective long-term follow-up of 444 cases. *Br J Ophthalmol.* 1981;65:790–795.
16. Shin DH. Management of flat anterior chamber with hypotony after glaucoma surgery. *Glaucoma.* 1982;4:193–197.
17. WuDunn D, Ryser D, Cantor LB. Surgical drainage of choroidal effusions following glaucoma surgery. *J Glaucoma.* 2005;14:103–108.
18. Altan C, Azturker C, Bayraktar S, et al. Post-trabeculectomy choroidal detachment: not an adverse prognostic sign for either visual acuity or surgical success. *Eur J Ophthamol.* 2008;18:771–777.
19. Stewart WC, Crinkley CM. Influence of serous suprachoroidal detachments on the results of trabeculectomy surgery. *Acta Ophthalmol.* 1994;72:309–314.

# Chapter 73
# Cyclodialysis Clefts: Surgical and Traumatic

George R. Reiss

## 73.1 Anatomy

Cyclodialysis (CDC) describes the separation between the uveal tissue and the sclera that can occur via blunt injury or be inadvertently caused during ocular surgery. This condition was first described by Fuchs in 1900,[1] and based on his observation was even proposed as surgical treatment for glaucoma by Heine in 1905.[2] A firm attachment which exists between the ciliary body and the sclera can be broken when the meridional ciliary muscle insertion into the sclera is ruptured. If this occurs, even at a pinpoint location, aqueous humor can leave the anterior chamber and enter the suprachoroidal space. Ciliochoroidal detachments can occur, which are potentially large enough to hold large volumes of aqueous, thus causing ocular hypotony. The low intraocular pressure (IOP) that results can cause visual changes that are extremely disturbing to the patient.

## 73.2 Pathogenesis

Most cases of CDC occur as a result of some type of trauma, both surgical and accidental.[3-6] Most recently, reports of air bag-induced cases have been described and will likely become more prevalent.[7] The energy from blunt trauma is conducted into the eye through tissues and fluids. The elastic stretching of the iris root as the globe expands and then contracts, if significant, can result in detachment of the ciliary body from sclera. In cases of cataract surgery, the suction of iris root into the aspiration port followed by dragging this tissue in toward the center of the eye can result in either tearing of the iris (iridodialysis) or separation of the iris base and ciliary body from the overlying sclera (cyclodialysis) (Figs. 73.1 and 73.2). CDC has also been reported in other surgeries. Most recently, CDC has been reported to occur in small port vitrectomies, where fluid intended for the vitreous chamber is instead injected into the suprachoroidal space. This again separates the ciliary body from the overlying sclera but from a more posterior location. CDC can vary in location, size, and in number (Figs. 73.3a–d).

## 73.3 Signs and Symptoms

If the CDC is significant enough to cause the IOP to drop to hypotonous levels, visual blurring can occur on the basis of several mechanisms. Low IOP can cause macular edema or thickening as retinal capillaries leak unopposed by normal IOP. These retinal changes may become permanent if long-standing, with fixed submacular folds or even pigmentary abnormalities, although visual recovery is possible even after several years of hypotony.[8] Another cause for visual blurring is the instability of the hypotonous globe during blinking, which can cause corneal contortions and irregular astigmatism.

CDC-related hypotony could occasionally occur months or years after surgical insults for reasons that are uncertain. For that reason, it is important to obtain a complete history, including previous surgical and traumatic events, in any patient who presents with unexplained hypotony.

### 73.3.1 Diagnostic Considerations

Many cases of CDC can be diagnosed by findings seen on the gonioscopic examination of the angle where a space or cleft is found at the interface of the ciliary body and the sclera. Unfortunately, the diagnosis of CDC can be problematic in some patients when the clefts are small, the anterior chamber shallow, or if the cornea is so edematous that clear gonioscopy is impossible (Fig. 73.3e). Occasionally, a CDC can be hidden alongside a broad-based peripheral anterior synechia (PAS). Such synechiae are often the only clue as to the cleft location and act as a "sentinel cleft" (Fig. 73.3f).

One reported method of diagnosis is intraoperative use of a powerful transillumination probe, which can reveal a patch of red reflex associated with the location of the cleft.[9] Ultrasound biomicroscopy (UBM) has proven to be a valuable modality to identify the presence of a cleft as well as its location.[10-15] Unfortunately, the present generation of UBM

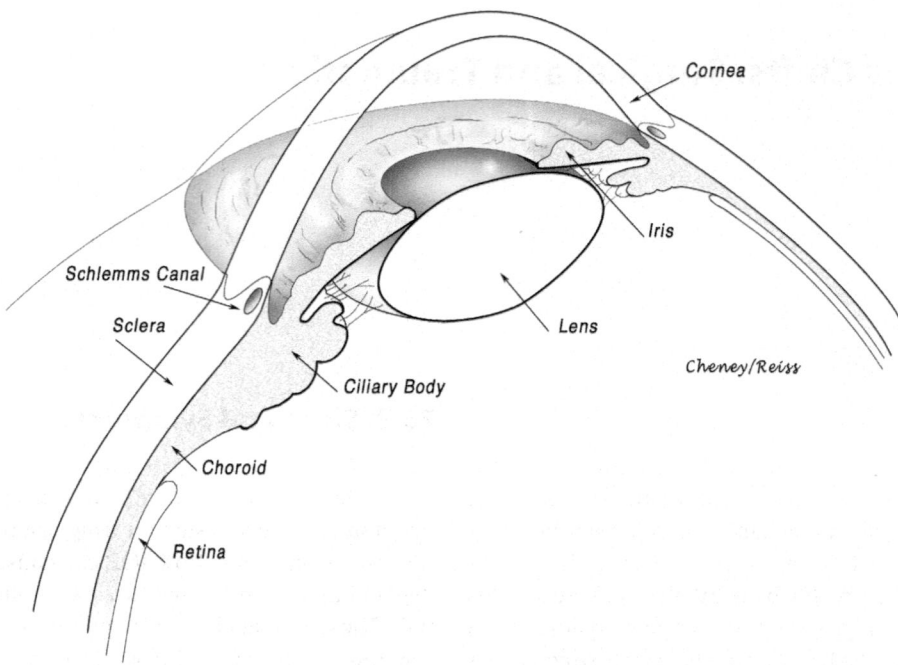

**Fig. 73.1** Normal anatomy of the eye

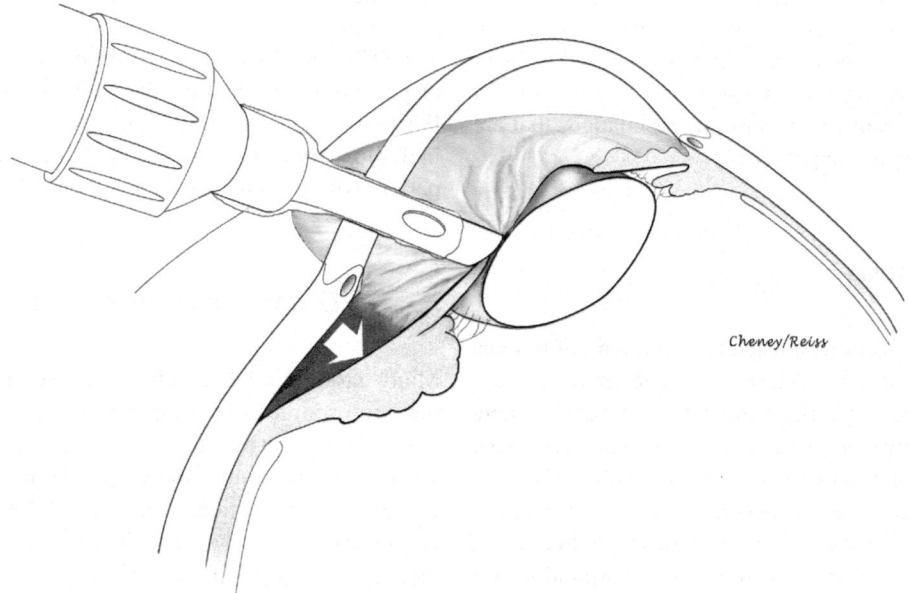

**Fig. 73.2** Cyclodialysis cleft created by inadvertent suction of iris into phaco tip

devices is expensive and many communities do not have one. Other options include the endoscope, a device that has become more available owing to its increasing popularity for cyclophotocoagulation during cataract extraction. Both UBM and endoscopic evaluation have the advantage of not being affected by a cloudy cornea.

## 73.4 Treatment

Closure of the cleft will prevent the escape of aqueous humor from the anterior chamber into the suprachoroidal space, thus restoring normal IOP. Once a cleft is identified and localized, a wide array of treatments have been successfully

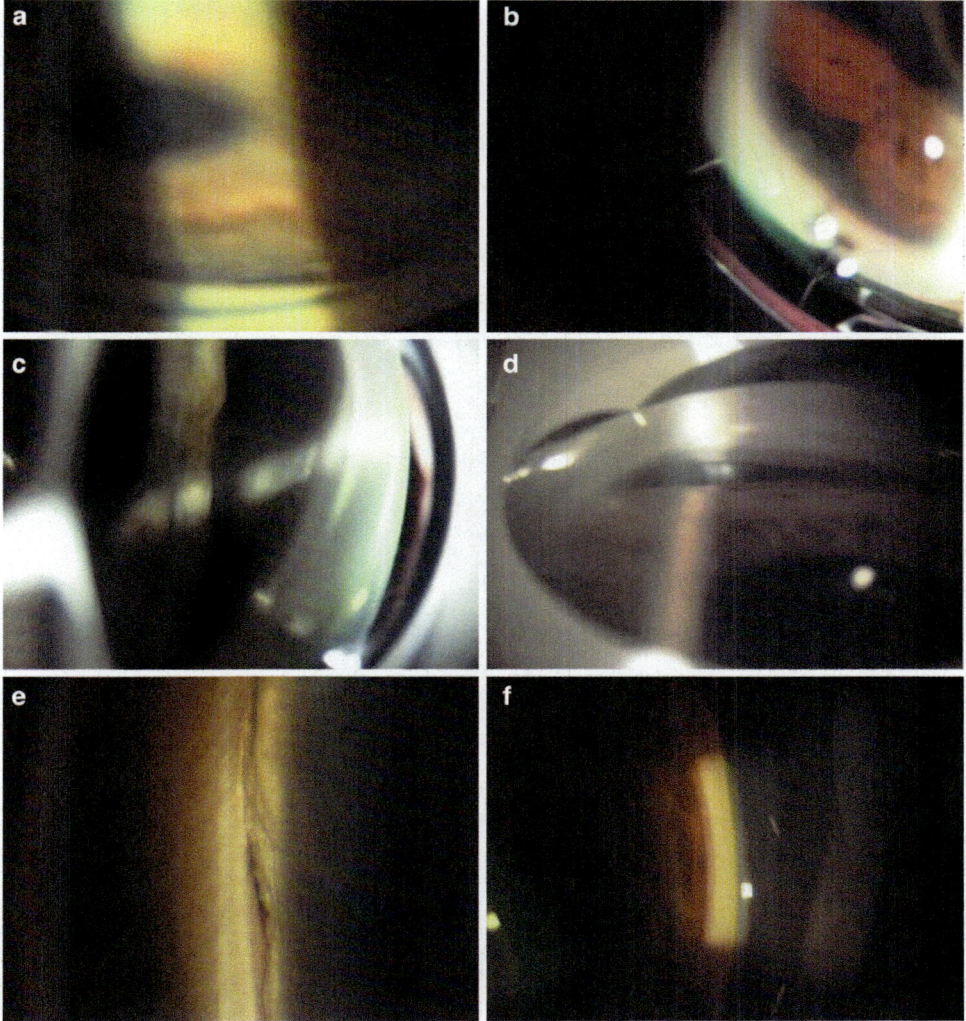

**Fig. 73.3** (**a–d**) Cyclodialysis clefts can vary in location, size, and number. (**e, f**) Note the small "sentinel cleft" apparent just alongside a PAS, which at times can camouflage a CDC

used to resolve the disorder. Medical treatment alone using cycloplegia is usually the first method tried.[16] The dilation of the pupil and backing off any topical steroids has been reported to close off the cleft, after which time the cycloplegic agent can be tapered.

Argon laser treatment to the cleft has also been successful in closing smaller clefts.[17-20] This most likely works by inducing an inflammation and "stickiness" of the choroidal tissue that promotes an adhesion between choroid and sclera, thus sealing the cleft. Cycloplegia should be continued in these patients to encourage sustained contact between the ciliary body and sclera during the healing phase. Transcleral applications of cyclocryotherapy,[21] diathermy,[22] external application of the YAG laser,[23] and diode laser[24] have been reported as methods of inducing cleft closure. These have the advantage of not requiring incisional surgery. Intraocular endoscopy has also been used to close clefts by applying direct laser application intraocularly.[25,26] This has the advantage of more precisely directing high energy into the cleft, and unlike gonioscopic technique, is not affected by corneal edema.

Surgical treatments are almost always successful in those clefts that remain recalcitrant to medical and laser treatments, and in those where the clefts are several clock hours large.[27-29]

Direct cycloplexy (Fig. 73.4) involves raising a partial thickness limboscleral flap over the site of the cleft. The deep scleral bed is then incised to provide a view of the underlying ciliary body, which can then be imbricated to the overlying sclera by passing a 10-0 or 9-0 nylon of Prolene suture from posterior sclera through ciliary body and out through anterior sclera all under the flap. After a sufficient number of sutures are passed, the scleral flap can be closed.

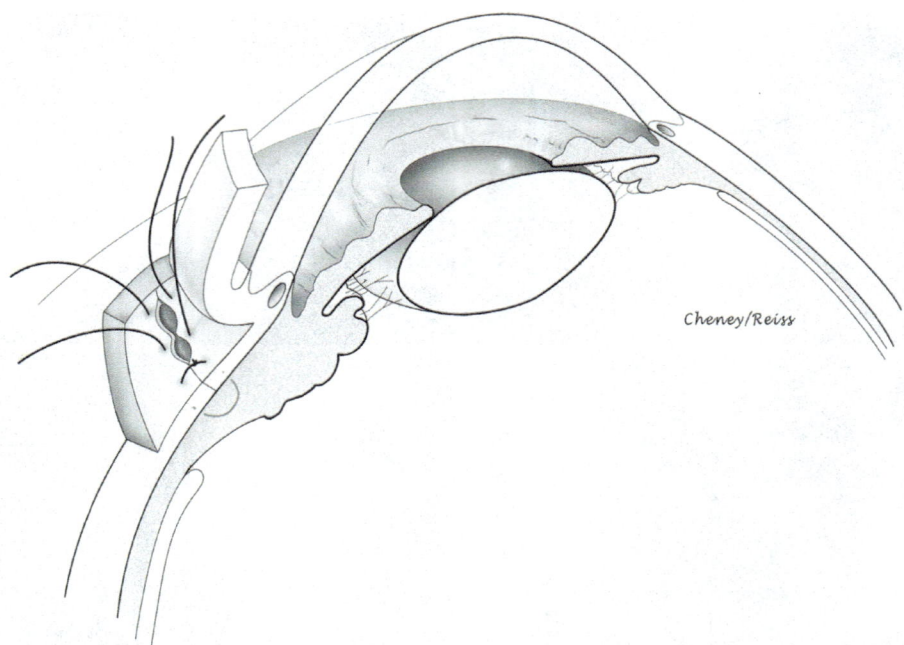

**Fig. 73.4** Direct cycloplexy involves raising a partial thickness limboscleral flap over the site of the cleft. The deep scleral bed is incised to provide a view of the underlying ciliary body, which is imbricated to the overlying sclera by passing a 10-0 or 9-0 nylon or Prolene suture from posterior sclera through ciliary body and out through anterior sclera all under the flap

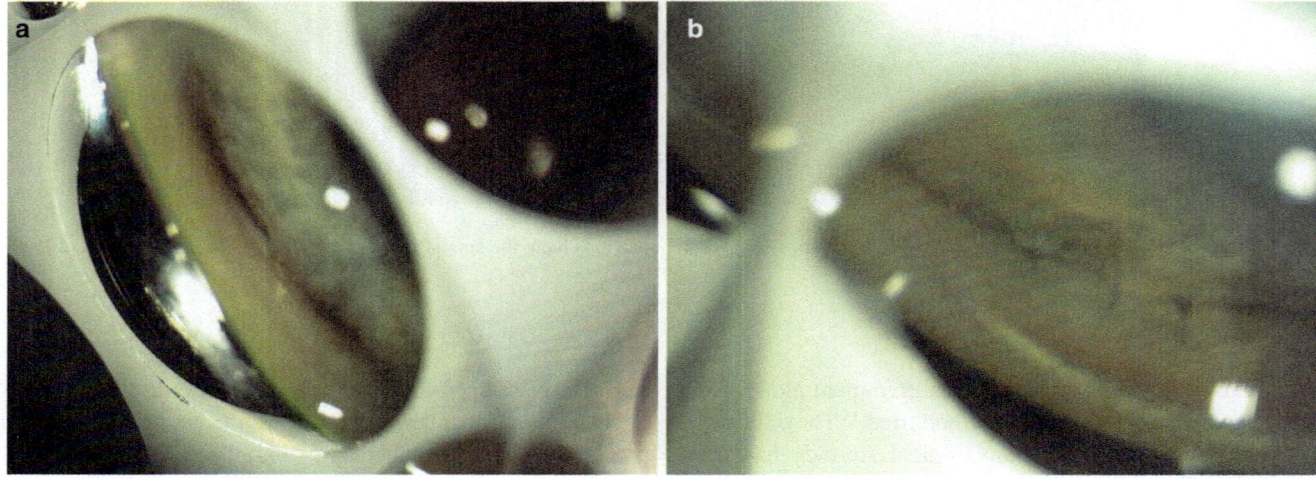

**Fig. 73.5** (**a**) Cleft prior to McCannel suture technique, which passes larger needles from cornea through the anterior chamber, imbricating iris root before passing out through sclera approximately 2 mm behind the limbus. (**b**) Sutured cleft

McCannel-type techniques have also been described passing larger needles from cornea through the anterior chamber, imbricating iris root before passing out through sclera approximately 2 mm behind the limbus (Figs. 73.5a, b). Clear corneal incisions are then made just in front of the limbus and a small intraocular lens (IOL) hook is used to grab the transcameral suture, which can then be brought out of the eye. The two ends of the suture can then be tied to create a loop that compresses the ciliary body and iris root to the overlying sclera thus closing off the cleft.[30]

In cases of CDC where the clefts are too large to repair using any of the previously mentioned techniques or if success is not achieved, several other techniques have been reported. Anterior scleral buckling has been used to compress the sclera overlying the detached choroid, which had been treated with cryopexy thus closing the cleft.[31] A sclerally fixated capsular tension ring has been reported to internally push the choroid against the overlying sclera successfully closing off the cleft.[32] Finally, vitrectomy, cryotherapy, and gas tamponade has been used to treat a CDC.[33,34] This technique has been successful in the author's experience with an aphake who demonstrated a 180° CDC and choroidal detachment that was judged to be too large to suture.

Combinations of techniques are also possible and sometimes necessary. This author uses endoscopy to precisely identify the cleft location that is then marked at the limbus before the overlying scleral flap is created. In some cases, residual cleft or additional clefts can be treated with argon laser post surgery once the cornea has cleared.

## 73.5 Conclusion

CDC is an oft-missed anatomical defect that can cause severe and prolonged hypotony, which in turn can cause permanent loss of vision. It should be ruled out in all cases of unexplained hypotony and treated appropriately. Treatment should be advanced from medical to laser or surgical as needed. In some cases, a combination of treatment modalities may be required to successfully repair CDC.

## References

1. Fuchs E. Ablosung der Aderhaut nach Staaroperation. *Graefes Arch Clin Exp Ophthalmol*. 1900;51:199–224.
2. Heine L. Die Cyklodialyse, eine neue Glaucomoperation. *Deutsche Med Wehnschr*. 1905;31:824–826.
3. Maffett M, O'Day D. Cyclodialysis cleft following a scleral tunnel incision. *Ophthalmic Surg*. 1994;25(6):387–388.
4. Small E, Solomon J, Prince A. Hypotonus cyclodialysis cleft following suture fixation of a posterior chamber intraocular lens. *Ophthalmic Surg*. 1994;25(2):107–109.
5. Parnes R, Aminlari A, Dailey J. Hypotonus cyclodialysis cleft following anterior chamber intraocular lens removal. *Ophthalmic Surg*. 1994;25(6):386–387.
6. Espana E, Tello C, Liebmann J, Ritch R. Cyclodialysis cleft secondary to removal of an anterior chamber phakic intraocular lens. *J Cataract Refract Surg*. 2007;33:542–544.
7. Greenfield D, Parrish R II, Scott I. Airbag-associated injury producing cyclodialysis cleft and ocular hypotony. *Ophthalmic Surg Lasers*. 1996;27(11):955–957.
8. Delgado M, Daniels S, Pascal S, Dickens C. Hypotony maculopathy: improvement of visual acuity after 7 years. *Am J Ophthalmol*. 2001;132(6):931–933.
9. Jewelewicz D, Liebman J, Ritch R. The use of scleral transillumination to localize the extent of a cyclodialysis cleft. *Ophthalmic Surg Lasers*. 1999;30:571–574.
10. Karawatowski W, Weinreb R. Imaging of cyclodialysis cleft by ultrasound biomicroscope. *Am J Ophthalmol*. 1994;117(4):541–543.
11. Kaushik S, Arya S, Dhir S, Kochhar S. Cyclodialysis cleft diagnosed by conventional ultrasonography. *Ophthalmic Surg Lasers*. 2000;31(4):346–349.
12. Gentile R, Pavlin C, Liebmann J, Easterbrook M, Foster S, Ritch R. Diagnosis of traumatic cyclodialysis by ultrasound biomicroscopy. *Ophthalmic Surg Lasers*. 1996;27:97–105.
13. Park M, Kondo T. Ultrasound biomicroscopic findings in a case of cyclodialysis. *Ophthalmologica*. 1998;212:194–197.
14. Chialant D, Kamji K. Ultrasound biomicroscopy in diagnosis of a cyclodialysis cleft in a patient with corneal edema and hypotony after an air bag injury. *Can J Ophthalmol*. 2000;35:148–150.
15. Shah V, Majji A. Ultrasound biomicroscopic documentation of traumatic cyclodialysis cleft closure with hypotony by medical therapy. *Eye*. 2004;18:857–858.
16. Aminlari A, Callahan C. Medical, laser and surgical management of inadvertent cyclodialysis cleft with hypotony. *Arch Ophthalmol*. 2004;122:399–404.
17. Bauer B. Argon laser photocoagulation of cyclodialysis clefts after cataract surgery. *Acta Ophthalmol Scand*. 1995;73:283–284.
18. Harbin T. Treatment of cyclodialysis clefts with argon laser photocoagulation. *Ophthalmology*. 1982;88:1082–1083.
19. Alward W, Anderson D, Hodapp E, Parel J. Argon laser endophotocoagulator closure of cyclodialysis clefts. *Am J Ophthalmol*. 1998;106(6):748–749.
20. Partamian L. Treatment of a cyclodialysis cleft with argon laser photocoagulation in a patient with a shallow anterior chamber. *Am J Ophthamol*. 1985;99:5–7.
21. Krohn J. Cryotherapy in the treatment of cyclodialysis cleft induced hypotony. *Acta Ophthalmol Scand*. 1997;75:96–98.
22. Ormerod D, Baerveldt G, Sunalp M, Riekhof T. Management of the hypotonous cyclodialysis cleft. *Ophthalmology*. 1991;98:1384–1393.
23. Brooks A, Troski M, Gillies W. Noninvasive closure of a persistent cyclodialysis cleft. *Ophthalmology*. 1996;103:1943–1945.
24. Amini H, Razeghinejad M. Transscleral diode laser therapy for cyclodialysis cleft induced hypotony. *Clin Experiment Ophthalmol*. 2005;33:348–350.
25. Caronia R, Sturm R, Marmor M, Berke S. Treatment of a cyclodialysis cleft by means of ophthalmic laser microendoscope endophotocoagulation. *Am J Ophthalmol*. 1999;128(6):760–761.
26. Gnanaraj L, Lam W, Rootman D, Levin A. Endoscopic closure of a cyclodialysis cleft. *J AAPOS*. 2005;9(6):592–594.
27. Kuchle M, Naumann G. Direct cyclopexy for traumatic cyclodialysis with persisting hypotony. *Ophthalmology*. 1995;102:322–333.
28. Kato T, Hayasaka S, Nagaki Y, Matsumoto M. Management of traumatic cyclodialysis cleft associated with ocular hypotony. *Ophthalmic Surg Lasers*. 1999;30:469–472.
29. Hwang J, Ahn K, Kim C, Kee C. Ultrasonic biomicroscopic evaluation of cyclodialysis before and after direct cyclopexy. *Arch Ophthalmol*. 2008;126(9):1222–1225.
30. Jaffe NS, Jaffe MS, Jaffe GF. In: Hypotension. Cataract Surgery and its Complications. 5th ed. St. Louis: Mosby; 1990:374–375.
31. Mandava N, Kahook M, Olson J. Anterior scleral buckling procedure for cyclodialysis cleft with chronic hypotony. *Ophthalmic Surg Lasers Imaging*. 2006;37:151–153.
32. Yuen N, Hui S, Woo D. New method of surgical repair for 360-degree cyclodialysis. *J Cataract Refract Surg*. 2006;32:13–17.
33. Hoerauf H, Roider J, Laqua H. Treatment of traumatic cyclodialysis with vitrectomy, cryotherapy, and gas endotamponade. *J Cataract Refract Surg*. 1999;25:1299–1301.
34. Takaya K, Suzuki Y, Nakazawa M. Four cases of hypotony maculopathy caused by traumatic cyclodialysis and treated by vitrectomy, cryotherapy, and gas tamponade. *Graefes Arch Clin Exp Ophthalmol*. 2006;244(7):855–858.

# Chapter 74
# Epithelial Downgrowth

Matthew C. Willett, Sami Al-Shahwan, and Deepak P. Edward

Epithelial downgrowth is a disastrous complication of ocular surgery or trauma in which corneal or conjunctival epithelium invades the anterior chamber and other intraocular structures. The epithelial growth patterns are categorized as diffuse or cystic growth, with diffuse growth being up to four times more common and occurring more frequently after trauma.[1] The current incidence of epithelial downgrowth is difficult to determine. Previous literature has cited cataract surgery as the most common cause[1-4] with an incidence of 0%[5] to 0.076%[2] and up to 1.1%.[5] Most authors agree the incidence of epithelial downgrowth has decreased secondary to improvements in surgical technique, instrumentation, and suture material.[2] Other surgical procedures cited as predisposing to epithelial downgrowth are listed in Table 74.1. The time to onset is highly variable and dependent on etiology. For example, epithelial downgrowth following cataract surgery has been reported 4 days[11] to 56 years[12] into the postoperative period, with a mean onset of presentation ranging from 5 months[2] to 10 months.[3] In one study, epithelial downgrowth occurred 4–7 months following penetrating keratoplasty.[11] Glaucoma is variably present in patients with epithelial downgrowth. In Küchle and Green's review of 207 histopathologically proven cases, they reported a rate of glaucoma of 43.1%.[1]

## 74.1 Etiology and Pathogenesis

The factors suggested to predispose an eye to this condition include gaping wound edges, iris or vitreous incarceration, delayed wound healing, full thickness sutures, and aspiration of aqueous.[12] It is therefore not surprising that epithelial downgrowth is more often reported following surgeries with intraoperative and postoperative complications.[2,5] The true mechanism and predisposing factors necessary for epithelial cells to proliferate inside the eye remains elusive. In a review by Smith and Doyle,[5] their evaluation of experimental models showed epithelial inhibition by healthy endothelium and fibrin. Multiple other studies based on enucleated specimens and animal models have suggested an inability of epithelium to grow over healthy endothelium, possibly due to contact inhibition.[8,13] In other models, this appears to be a complex interaction, and although damaged or absent endothelium promotes downgrowth, it is not essential.[1] A possible mechanism of the interaction was reported by Zavala and Binder.[8] In reviewing electron micrographs, they noted pseudopodial extensions of the basal epithelial cells "pulling" the cells forward. The underlying endothelial cells degenerate and the basal cells produce a collagenous basement membrane. The epithelial cells then attach to this basement membrane with hemidesmosomes. This results in degeneration of the endothelial cells underlying the epithelial downgrowth. A recent report of epithelial downgrowth following Descemet's-stripping automated endothelial keratoplasty (DSAEK) raises an important point, namely that removal of diseased host endothelium and Descemet's membrane provides an excellent opportunity for rapid epithelial downgrowth.[7] Given the increasing use of DSAEK, careful attention will be needed to determine the incidence of epithelial downgrowth with this procedure.

Another point of debate has been the importance of a fistula as an essential factor in epithelial downgrowth. Multiple cases of epithelial downgrowth have been described that have a fistula or incarcerated material in the wound. Originally it was believed that these were a key factor in the etiology.[4] The rate of fistulas involved with epithelial downgrowth ranges from around 3%[1] to 26%[2] to 50%,[8,14] and are reported more commonly after trauma. The fact that many cases lack a fistula, along with reports of epithelial downgrowth with McCannel suture,[8] argue against their being an absolute predisposing factor.

It has also been suggested that anticoagulation may facilitate epithelial downgrowth through inhibition of fibroblast formation in the wound,[2] which if true has serious implications as large numbers of ageing patients are now on chronic anticoagulation therapy. However, it is likely that the reasons for proliferation of epithelium within the eye are multifactorial.

**Table 74.1** Surgical causes of epithelial downgrowth

| |
|---|
| Intracapsular cataract extraction |
| Extracapsular cataract extraction |
| Phacoemulsification with clear corneal incision[6] |
| Penetrating keratoplasty |
| DSAEK[7] |
| Pterygium excision[2] |
| McCannel suture[8] |
| Glaucoma drainage implant[9] |
| Aspiration of aqueous[2] |
| Congenital glaucoma surgery[10] |

## 74.2 Signs and Symptoms

A correct and prompt diagnosis is rooted in high clinical suspicion. A review of the literature shows that the correct referral diagnosis is present in only 50–67.5%[3] of patients, with the decrease to 50% based on review of cases in the 1990s.[1] Patient complaints are often non-specific, including pain, photophobia, blurred vision, and epiphora among others.

The classic finding on clinical examination is the presence of retrocorneal membrane (Fig. 74.1). This is described as gray-white with an advancing scalloped border[5] (Fig. 74.2). In cases following penetrating keratoplasty, this can be differentiated from graft failure by the trace to absent edema between the line and graft wound, which is common after rejection.[11] Stromal vascularization is frequently noted in the overlying cornea, and believed to be important as a source of nutrition.[2] The epithelium grows on the posterior cornea as well as the nutrient-rich iris, angle structures, and vitreous. Rarely, the proliferation of epithelium may be extensive resulting in its extension into the posterior segment. Smoothing of the normal iris architecture and decreased motility as a result of the membrane may be noted.[5,11,15] As a result of epithelial downgrowth on the iris, ectropion uvea may also be present

Ocular inflammation is a cardinal sign. Iritis is common, showing minimal ciliary flush, minimal to absent keratic precipitates, and poor response to corticosteroid treatment.[11] Clumps of anterior chamber cellular debris typify this iritis. This can also aid in differentiation of epithelial downgrowth versus transplant rejection after penetrating keratoplasty (Table 74.2), in which keratic precipitates and subepithelial infiltrates are more common.[11]

Intraocular pressure may be low, normal, or high depending on the presence of a fistula. As a result, some reports list 50% of patients as never having shown increased pressure.[15] Seidel testing with 2% fluorescein may reveal a leaking wound. If Seidel is negative initially, a dynamic test should be performed with appropriate pressure to elicit subclinical leaks. As stated previously, the incidence of glaucoma following epithelial downgrowth is variable. Glaucoma is more frequent in eyes with diffuse growth.[12] Vision loss and eventual enucleation of eyes with epithelial downgrowth is usually secondary to intractable glaucoma. Glaucoma in epithelial downgrowth may occur through multiple mechanisms, as listed in Table 74.3. Early in the disease it may

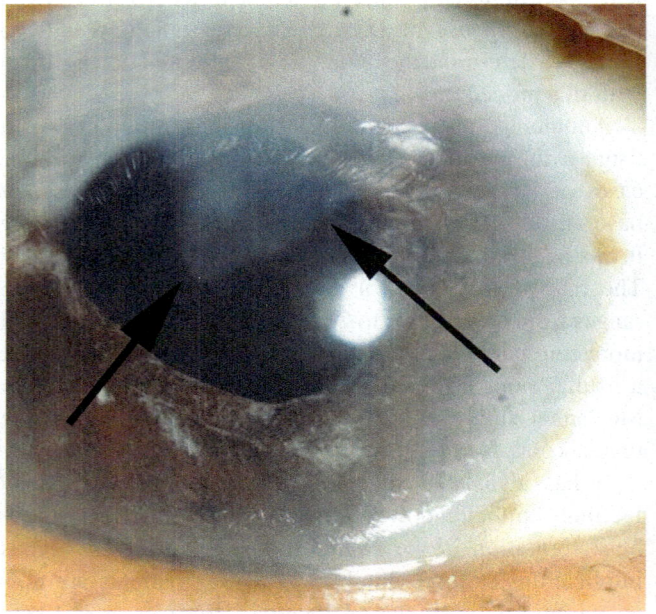

**Fig. 74.1** Slit lamp photo in a pseudophakic patient after complicated surgery showing whitish membrane with sharp edge behind the corneal surface (*arrows*) consistent with epithelial downgrowth

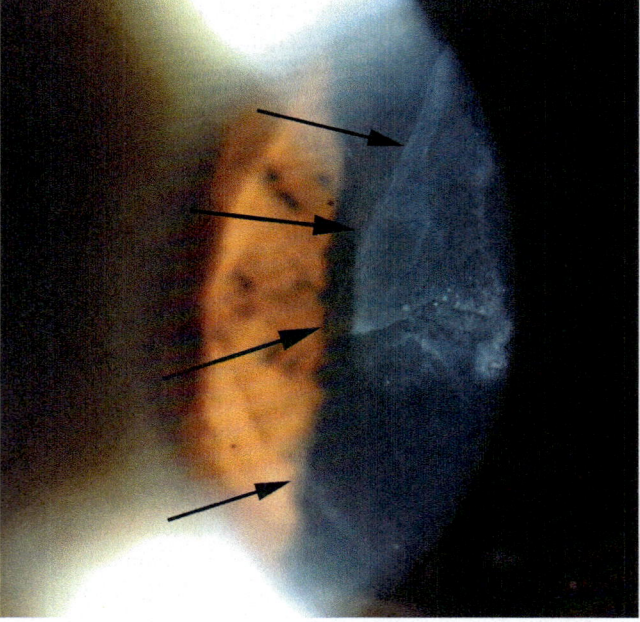

**Fig. 74.2** Scalloped edge of epithelial downgrowth (*arrows*) at higher magnification

**Table 74.2** Differentiating between epithelial downgrowth and graft rejection after penetrating keratoplasty

| Epithelial downgrowth | Graft rejection |
|---|---|
| Few or absent keratic precipitates | Prominent keratic precipitates |
| Trace or absent corneal edema between retrocorneal line and graft wound | Clear ahead of the rejection line and cloudy and edematous behind it |
| Poor response to topical steroids | Often good response |

**Table 74.3** Mechanisms of glaucoma in epithelial downgrowth

| |
|---|
| Peripheral anterior synechiae (PAS) |
| Angle closure |
| Trabeculitis |
| Neovascular glaucoma |
| Hemorrhagic glaucoma |
| Steroid induced secondary glaucoma |
| Pupillary-block |
| Secondary mucogenic open-angle glaucoma |

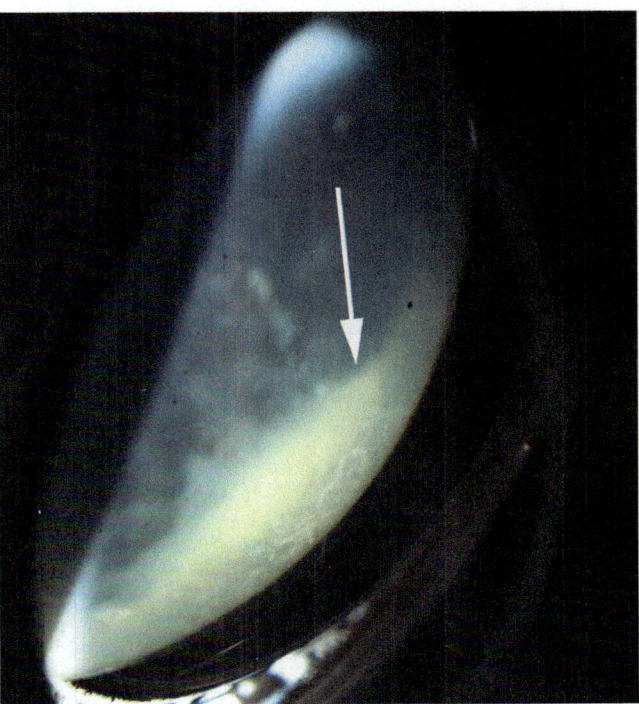

**Fig. 74.3** Gonioscopy showing angle occluded by whitish heaped up epithelium (*arrow*)

cause trabeculitis and in cases of extensive epithelial downgrowth, peripheral anterior synechiae may form due to growth of the epithelial membrane over the anterior chamber angle with resultant partial or total angle closure.[13,16] Often patients have been on topical corticosteroid treatment, which may result in steroid-related elevation of intraocular pressure, further complicating the issue. Other causes include direct extension of the fibrous sheet of cells over the trabecular meshwork (Fig. 74.3), or through mechanical plugging by circulating epithelial cells or macrophages.[1,13] Less frequent causes include secondary mucogenic open-angle glaucoma from circulating mucinous products,[17] as well as pupillary-block.[16]

## 74.3 Diagnosis

The diagnosis is often based on clinical examination. In addition, if the epithelial downgrowth has extended onto the iris surface, creating argon laser burns on the surface of the iris may aid in the diagnosis (500 μm, 0.1 s, 200 mW). In the normal iris, argon laser burns result in discoloration of the iris surface with contraction of the stroma. However, in an iris with overlying epithelium, the iris surface turns white following laser application. Other diagnostic options include specular microscopy, fluorophotometry, and aqueous humor aspiration. The pattern noted on specular microscopy involves sharply defined borders between endothelium and the epithelial downgrowth. When the instrument is focused to a deeper plane, it then shows interlacing borders of the epithelial cells.[14] The appearance of epithelial cells on specular microscopy is reversed (when compared to normal corneal endothelium) with dark centers and a lighter periphery.[18] Fluorophotometry shows increased disappearance time from the overlying stroma secondary to decreased permeability caused by the epithelial membrane, but is an indirect test.[18] Aqueous fluid cytopathology is performed using one or more of the following methods: the celloidin bag technique,[19] modified Papaniculaou-staining technique, as well as air-dried and wet-fixed smears.[20] Clusters of typical epithelial cells with or without goblet cells are observed. These may be superficial rectangular type, rounded basal type, or vacuolated. Vacuolated cells represent goblet cells or degenerated epithelial cells.[11] Of note, in one case, diagnostic vitrectomy ruled out a suspected recurrence, showing instead new fibrous tissue proliferation.[20]

In the rare cases where the above means of diagnosis are insufficient, a biopsy may be taken. This can then be analyzed using light microscopy, electron microscopy as well as immunohistochemical staining with a pancytokeratin marker (Fig. 74.4).

### 74.3.1 Differential Diagnosis

Maumenee described the likely entities to be confused with epithelial downgrowth, which are listed in Table 74.4.[4] One of the most likely pathologies to be confused with epithelial

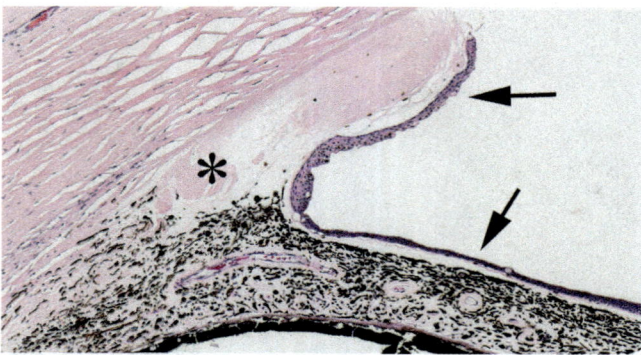

**Fig. 74.4** Microphotograph showing epithelial downgrowth covering posterior surface of the cornea and iris surface (*arrows*) and occluding anterior chamber angle (*)

**Table 74.4** Differential diagnosis of epithelial downgrowth

Very shelved corneal cataract wound
Vitreous–corneal touch
Invasion of the anterior chamber by connective tissue and blood vessels
Peeling of Descemet's
Reduplication of Descemet's

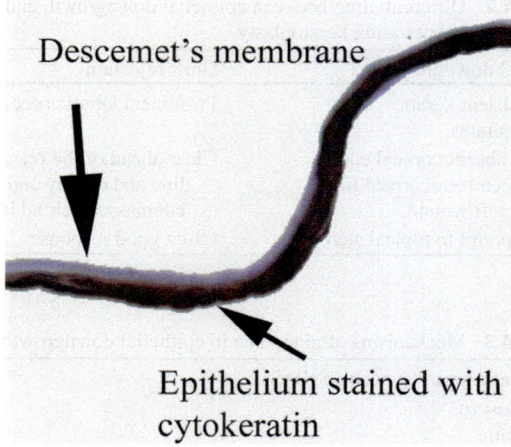

**Fig. 74.5** Biopsy of Descemet's membrane stained with cytokeratin showing epithelial replacing endothelial cells

downgrowth is fibrous proliferation or ingrowth. It is also more common with complicated surgeries, and it also presents with a retrocorneal membrane. Features that differentiate fibrous ingrowths from epithelial downgrowth include its (normally) slow growth, vascularity, and infrequent association of inflammation and refractory glaucoma. Duplication of Descemet's membrane can also be confusing. In cases where doubt exists, an argon laser can be utilized, where absence of whitening on the iris surface will be noted.

### 74.3.2 Pathology

Light microscopy reveals single or multiple layers of nonkeratinized stratified squamous epithelium that line the posterior cornea, iris, and angle structures (Fig. 74.5). The cells are often elongated in the direction of migration.[8] The leading edge is sloping, and superficial cells contain more numerous and prominent intercellular junctions.[8] Multiple epithelial layers are usually found on more nutrient rich areas such as the iris. Goblet cells are less frequently observed. In Küchle and Green's review, goblet cells were observed in only around 9% of specimens.[1] It is important to note that some experimental models have shown an inability to distinguish whether corneal or conjunctival epithelium was implanted to cause epithelial downgrowth based on histological review.[21] Therefore, the presence or absence of goblet cells should not be used to ultimately determine the source of epithelial downgrowth.

Scanning electron microscopy (SEM) shows the same characteristics as light microscopy and may demonstrate the presence of surface microvilli.[8] Transmission electron microscopy (TEM) may show differentiation into three distinct layers. The basal layer shows desmosomes, dilated rough endoplasmic reticulum, and Golgi vacules.[8] The middle layer is more loosely arranged with infrequent desmosomes, and the superficial layer contains numerous apical microvilli and a glycoprotein matrix.[1,8] Tonofilaments are present in all layers but more prominent at the leading edge. There is also loss of the normal architecture of the underlying endothelium.[8]

### 74.4 Treatment

If diffuse epithelial downgrowth is present, prompt surgical treatment is suggested.[22] Following the degree of corneal involvement by the epithelial membrane is inadequate, as it may progress slower than iris involvement.[22] Furthermore, an earlier diagnosis and smaller amount of downgrowth may allow less extensive surgery to be performed and improve the final outcome.[22] Many treatment modalities have been advocated over the years – most involving radiation or surgery. Radiation therapy has now been abandoned. Despite surgical intervention, the prognosis remains poor in many cases and may be related to late detection of the disease. In Maumenee et al's series of 40 cases, 27.5% of patients achieved visual acuity of 20/50 or better and normal intraocular pressure or glaucoma controlled with topical medication alone.[3] A simplified outline of Maumenee's treatment involves identification of involved iris either at the slit lamp, if possible, or through photocoagulation. The lower margin of the corneal involvement is marked by scratching the anterior corneal epithelium with a knife. Dynamic Seidel is then performed, and if a fistula is present it is excised. This would be followed by excision of the involved iris, removal of vitreous in the anterior chamber, and cryoprobe to the involved cornea.[3] Stark et al[22] modified this technique. Argon photocoagulation was used to mark the interface of the membrane with normal iris; each spot half white and half burn to delineate the involved iris. Vitrectomy equipment was utilized to remove involved iris and then perform an anterior vitrectomy, followed by instillation of an air bubble. The air bubble enhanced the cryotherapy, both via a thermal insulating effect and by acting as a goniolens to allow visualization of the angle for cryotherapy. A freeze–refreeze technique was then used. Using this technique in a series of ten cases, 40% of patients achieved visual acuity of 20/40 or better.

In a paper by Naumann and Rummelt, they suggested block excision of both the involved tissue and adjacent pars plicata, sclera, and cornea.[12] In their series of 32 patients, a postoperative visual acuity of 20/60 or better was found in 37.5%. Of note, 28 of the 32 patients in their study had cystic rather than diffuse growth. En bloc excision was also used in a series of three patients described by Friedman, with the postoperative visual acuity being 20/60 or better in two of the three patients.[23]

If only small epithelial cysts are noted, many advocate observation, as cases of diffuse downgrowth have resulted from attempts to remove them.[1,24,25] Indications to remove the cysts include enlargement, visual obstruction, inflammation, glaucoma, corneal decompensation, or cyst rupture. Treatment modalities reported range from argon laser photocoagulation to conservative surgery to en bloc resection.[4,12,22,24-29] If possible, cysts should be removed without rupture. In the event this seems unlikely, such as those with adherence to both iris and cornea, they may be decompressed with a needle, and then the cyst and any associated iris, cornea, vitreous, and other affected structures removed.[25] Haller et al[24] reported a small series of four eyes with satisfactory results after aspiration or excision of cyst contents and subsequent photocoagulation of remaining cyst structure to devitalize remaining cells. Jadav et al[26] reported a case treated by endoscopic photocoagulation, penetrating keratoplasty, and cryoablation of the remaining cornea. There was no recurrence after 1 year, and they suggested this method as a minimally invasive alternative. In the end, treatment is based on the individual case and the comfort of the surgeon with these different techniques

### 74.4.1 Treatment of Glaucoma

Treatment is first directed at topical medications, which is inadequate in most patients.[5] Surgical treatment of the epithelial downgrowth as described previously is initiated if appropriate. Despite these measures, cases of postoperative refractory glaucoma are frequent.[13,16,30,31] Several methods have been attempted to address this. Shaikh et al[29] reported one case treated by viscodissection of the membrane from the posterior of the cornea using 5-fluorouracil mixed with sulfate-sodium hyaluronate after a previous anterior chamber injection. In this patient, there was no recurrence 14 months later. Despite this case, most studies have failed to show a prolonged benefit of antimetabolite agents, and one showed rapid progression of the membrane after discontinuation of 5-flourouracil injections.[31] As a result, trabeculectomies often fail as epithelial sheets close the sclerostomy.[5] Other treatment options include ciliodestructive procedures and implanted tube shunts. Studies have shown successful control of intraocular pressure using drainage-seton implants. One study showed 78% of patients achieved an IOP less than 22 mmHg, with the remaining patients controlled with the addition of topical beta-blockers.[13] In this study, visual acuity of 1/200 was maintained in 56% of patients. Rubin et al[16] evaluated an eye enucleated 2 years after implantation of a Molteno implant for epithelial downgrowth. They showed no growth of epithelium in the lumen of the tube and continued patency, suggesting the epithelial cells are unable to grow on tube material.[16] It has also been suggested that drainage devices be used as a palliative measure in eyes that are poor candidates for attempted full removal of all epithelial downgrowth.[13] With successful control of IOP possible, combined or secondary penetrating keratoplasty can be performed to improve visual acuity where appropriate.

## 74.5 Conclusion

Epithelial downgrowth is a rare complication of ocular surgery or trauma. Glaucoma secondary to epithelial downgrowth occurs through multiple mechanisms and is often refractory to topical medications. If appropriate, treatment should first be aimed at complete removal of all epithelial downgrowth. Specific treatment for glaucoma can then be tailored to the situation and may include a seton procedure or cyclodestruction. Early treatment as a result of high clinical suspicion for this disorder is likely to lead to the best outcome.

## References

1. Küchle M, Green WR. Epithelial ingrowth: a study of 207 histopathologically proven cases. *Ger J Ophthalmol.* 1996;5(4):211–223.
2. Weiner MJ, Trentacoste J, Pon DM, Albert DM. Epithelial downgrowth: a 30-year clinicopathological review. *Br J Ophthalmol.* 1989;73:6–11.
3. Maumenee AE, Paton D, Morse PH, Butner R. Review of 40 histologically proven cases of epithelial downgrowth following cataract

extraction and suggested surgical management. *Am J Ophthalmol.* 1970;69(4):598–603.
4. Peyman GA, Peralta E, Ganiban GJ, Kraut R. Endoresection of the iris and ciliary body in epithelial downgrowth. *J Cataract Refract Surg.* 1998;24(1):130–133.
5. Smith MF, Doyle JW. Glaucoma secondary to epithelial and fibrous downgrowth. *Semin Ophthalmol.* 1994;9(4):248–253.
6. Lee BL, Gaton DD, Weinreb RN. Epithelial downgrowth following phacoemulsification through a clear cornea. *Arch Ophthalmol.* 1999;117:283.
7. Walker BM, Hindman HB, Ebrahimi KB, et al. Epithelial downgrowth following Descemet's-stripping automated endothelial keratoplasty. *Arch Ophthalmol.* 2008;126(2):278–280.
8. Zavala EY, Binder PS. The pathologic findings of epithelial ingrowth. *Arch Ophthalmol.* 1980;98(11):2007–2014.
9. Jewelewicz DA. Epithelial downgrowth following insertion of an Ahmed glaucoma implant. *Arch Ophthalmol.* 2003;121(2):285–286.
10. Giaconi JA, Coleman AL, Aldave AJ. Epithelial downgrowth following surgery for congenital glaucoma. *Am J Ophthalmol.* 2004;138(6):1075–1077.
11. Feder RS, Krachmer JH. The diagnosis of epithelial downgrowth after keratoplasty. *Am J Ophthalmol.* 1985;99:697–703.
12. Naumann GOH, Rummelt V. Block excision of cystic and diffuse epithelial ingrowth of the anterior chamber. Report on 32 consecutive patients. *Arch Ophthalmol.* 1992;110:223–227.
13. Fish LA, Heuer DK, Baerveldt G, et al. Molteno implantation for secondary glaucoma associated with advanced epithelial ingrowth. *Ophthalmology.* 1990;97:557–561.
14. Smith RE, Parrett C. Specular microscopy of epithelial downgrowth. *Arch Ophthalmol.* 1978;96(7):1222–1224.
15. Chee PH. Epithelial downgrowth. *Arch Ophthalmol.* 1967;78(4):492–495.
16. Rubin B, Chan CC, Burnier M, et al. Histopathologic study of the Molteno glaucoma implant in three patients. *Am J Ophthalmol.* 1990;110:371–379.
17. Kuchle M, Naumann GOH. Mucogenic secondary open-angle glaucoma in diffuse epithelial ingrowth treated by block-excision. *Am J Ophthalmol.* 1991;111:230–234.
18. Holliday JN, Buller CR, Bourne WM. Specular microscopy and fluorophotometry in the diagnosis of epithelial downgrowth after sutureless cataract operation. *Am J Ophthalmol.* 1993;116:238–240.
19. Green WR. Diagnostic cytopathology of ocular fluid specimens. *Ophthalmology.* 1984;91:726–749.
20. Engel HM, Green WR, Michaels RG, et al. Diagnostic vitrectomy. *Retina.* 1981;1:121–129.
21. Burris TE, Nordquist RE, Rowsey JJ. Long-term evaluation of epithelial downgrowth models. *Cornea.* 1986;5:211–221.
22. Stark WJ, Michaels RG, Maumenee AE, et al. Surgical Management of epithelial ingrowth. *Am J Ophthalmol.* 1978;85:772–780.
23. Friedman AH. Radical anterior segment surgery for epithelial invasion of the anterior chamber: report of three cases. *Trans Sect Ophthalmol Am Acad Ophthalmol Otolaryngol.* 1977;83(2):216–223.
24. Haller JA, Stark WJ, Azab A, Thomsen RW, Gottsch JD. Surgical approaches to the management of epithelial cysts. *Trans Am Ophthalmol Soc.* 2002;100:79–84.
25. Taylor HR, Michaels RG, Stark WJ. Vitrectomy methods in anterior segment surgery. *Ophthalmic Surg.* 1979;10:25–58.
26. Jadav DS, Rylander NR, Vold SD, Fulcher SF, Rosa RH Jr. Endoscopic photocoagulation in the management of epithelial downgrowth. *Cornea.* 2008;27(5):601–604.
27. Maumenee AE. Treatment of epithelial downgrowth and intraocular fistula following cataract extractions. *Trans Am Opthalmol Soc.* 1964;62:153.
28. Bangert A, Bialasiewicz AA, Engelmann K, Schäfer HJ, Domarus DV. Intraocular epithelial downgrowth – report on 14 cases from 1986 to 2000. *Klin Monatsbl Augenheilkd.* 2004;221(3):197–203.
29. Shaikh AA, Damji KF, Mintsioulis G, Gupta SK, Kertes PJ. Bilateral epithelial downgrowth managed in one eye with intraocular 5-fluorouracil. *Arch Ophthalmol.* 2002;120(10):1396–1398.
30. McAllister IL, Meyers SM, Meisler DM, et al. Epithelial downgrowth. *Ophthalmic Surg.* 1988;19(10):713–714.
31. Costa VP, Katz LJ, Cohen EJ, Raber IM. Glaucoma associated with epithelial downgrowth controlled with Molteno tube shunts. *Ophthalmic Surg.* 1992;23:797–800.

# Chapter 75
# Penetrating Keratoplasty and Glaucoma

Michele L. Scott and Peter A. Netland

Multiple mechanisms can lead to the development of glaucoma following penetrating keratoplasty (PK), including open and closed angle mechanisms. Previously controlled glaucoma can become uncontrolled or elevated intraocular pressure (IOP) can develop following penetrating keratoplasty.[1] Treatment in these patients can be complex, and the glaucoma is often refractory to medical therapy.[2]

The incidence of glaucoma following penetrating keratoplasty varies in the literature, with the prevalence ranging from 10% up to 53%.[3] In a prospective series of 137 consecutive eyes with follow-up ranging from 7 to 30 months, 27% developed chronically elevated IOP after PK.[4] Kirkness and Ficker[5] reported a 14% incidence of glaucoma in 1,122 post-keratoplasty eyes. Risk factors for developing post-keratoplasty glaucoma were preexisting glaucoma, aphakia, inflammation, intraocular lens removal, vitrectomy, and certain corneal diagnoses, including iridocorneal endothelial (ICE) syndrome, bullous keratopathy, anterior segment trauma, and anterior segment dysgenesis syndromes.[3,5]

Mechanisms involved in post-keratoplasty glaucoma can include pupillary block, retained viscoelastic agents, inflammatory mechanisms, lens induced mechanisms, and progressive angle closure due to peripheral anterior synechiae.[6] Another possible mechanism is trabecular collapse leading to decreased outflow, which can be minimized by oversizing the corneal donor button.[7]

A common cause for chronic elevated IOP after keratoplasty is synechial angle closure. Kirkness and Ficker[5] reported open-angle glaucoma in 13% of eyes with PK, with synechial angle closure in the remaining eyes. The incidence of glaucoma was related to the amount of synechial angle closure, and a higher degree of closure was correlated with a higher incidence of surgery for the control of the glaucoma.

Medical therapy is usually initiated with aqueous suppressants, especially beta-adrenergic antagonists and alpha$_2$-adrenergic agonists. Miotics are avoided in the early postoperative period, due to further breakdown of the blood aqueous barrier and shallowing of the anterior chamber, which further increases the risk of synechial closure.[6] Although topical carbonic anhydrase inhibitors (CAI) may be used safely in post-PK eyes, the enzyme carbonic anhydrase is present in the corneal endothelium, and may play a role in the endothelium pump function.[8] In post-keratoplasty patients with signs of corneal decompensation, topical CAI should be used with caution.[8] Prostaglandin analogs should be avoided in patients with a history of herpetic eye disease who have received a corneal transplant, due to the risk of recurrence of herpetic eye disease.[9]

The surgical management of post-PK glaucoma can be challenging and is complicated by risks to corneal graft survival. In cases of suspected pupillary block, a laser iridotomy should be performed to break the block and help control the intraocular pressure. There is little or no role for laser trabeculoplasty in glaucoma associated with penetrating keratoplasty. Effective surgical procedures include trabeculectomy with antimetabolites, glaucoma drainage implants, and cyclodestructive procedures[10-17] (Fig. 75.1).

The use of antimetabolites with trabeculectomy has been reported to increase the success of trabeculectomy after PK. In a retrospective study of 34 eyes, eyes that were treated with trabeculectomy with mitomycin C had better control of intraocular pressure than eyes that did not receive the antimetabolite (73% vs. 25%, respectively), with graft survival of 69.2% in the mitomycin C group and 37.5% in the group that did not receive mitomycin C. Combined filtration surgery and PK has been associated with a higher graft survival rate compared with staged surgery.[18]

Glaucoma drainage implants are an alternative surgical treatment in post-keratoplasty glaucoma, with reported success rates for control of IOP ranging from 65 to 96%.[11-14] Cornea-tube touch is one possible mechanism for corneal graft failure with glaucoma drainage implants placed in the anterior chamber. Arroyave et al.[13] compared the corneal graft survival rates in eyes after PK with the glaucoma drainage implant tube placed in the anterior chamber versus the implant tube placed in the vitreous cavity, finding a higher corneal graft survival after 1 year in the eyes with the glaucoma drainage implant in the vitreous cavity. Pars plana tube insertion may be associated with an increased rate of posterior segment complications, including suprachoroidal hemorrhage,

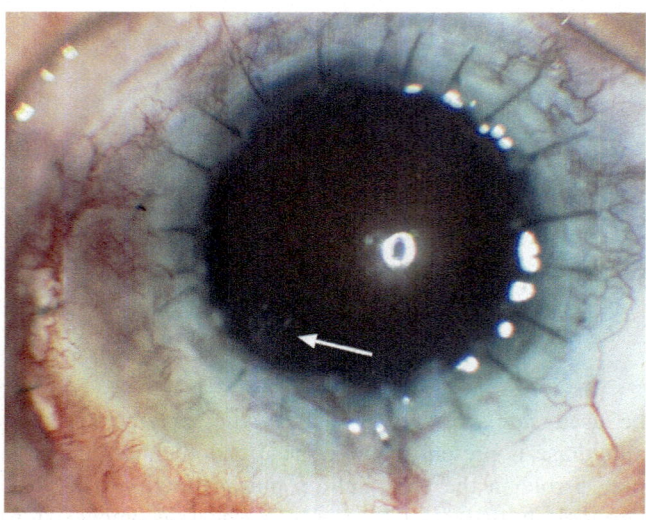

**Fig. 75.1** Clear graft in a patient with Aniridia and glaucoma who has been treated with penetrating keratoplasty, limbal stem cell transplant, and glaucoma drainage implant. The drainage implant tube (*arrow*) is visible in the inferotemporal anterior chamber angle

retinal detachment, epiretinal membrane, and cystoid macular edema.[14] Patients with a corneal graft who develop tube-graft touch should be treated with tube repositioning.

Cyclodestructive procedures may be used in eyes with glaucoma associated with penetrating keratoplasty, especially in eyes with poor visual potential or as adjunctive treatment after other glaucoma surgical procedures. Cohen et al.[15] reported results from 28 eyes that underwent Nd:YAG cyclophotocoagulation (CPC) for uncontrolled glaucoma after PK. Control of IOP was achieved in 64% at 3 months, and 73% at 2 years, but 46% of the eyes required multiple treatments. Of the grafts that were clear prior to therapy, 46% failed after the initial treatment. In a study of 28 eyes with glaucoma after PK treated with diode cyclophotocoagulation, 79% achieved IOP control with a follow up of 30 months.[16] Another approach is endoscopic cyclophotocoagulation to selectively treat the ciliary body.

Ayyala et al.[17] compared trabeculectomy with mitomycin C, glaucoma drainage implant surgery, and Nd:YAG cyclophotocoagulation in a retrospective study of 38 patients. In this study, no significant differences in IOP control or graft survival were found when comparing these surgical options for glaucoma after penetrating keratoplasty, but CPC was associated with a higher complication rate.

## 75.1 Conclusion

Glaucoma after penetrating keratoplasty may be due to multiple mechanisms and is often refractory to medical therapy. Corneal graft failure can occur in many of these patients as a result of treatment or as a result of the glaucoma if left untreated. Surgical management may include use of trabeculectomy with mitomycin C, glaucoma drainage implants, or cyclophotocoagulation, and should be individualized to the patient.

## References

1. Ficker LA, Kirkness CM, Steele ADM, et al. Intraocular surgery following penetrating keratoplasty: the risks and advantages. *Eye*. 1990;4:693–697.
2. Beebe WE. Management of glaucoma in penetrating keratoplasty patients. *Refract Corneal Surg*. 1991;7:67–69.
3. Al-Mohamimeed M, Al-Shahwan S, Al-Torbak A, Wagoner MD. Escalation of glaucoma therapy after penetrating keratoplasty. *Ophthalmology*. 2007;114:2281–2286.
4. Goldberg DB, Schanzlin DJ, Brown SI. Incidence of increased of intraocular pressure after keratoplasty. *Am J Ophthalmol*. 1981;92:372–377.
5. Kirkness CM, Ficker LA. Risk Factors for the development of postkeratatplasty glaucoma. *Cornea*. 1992;11:427–432.
6. Brandt JD, Lim MC, O'Day DG. Glaucoma after penetrating keratoplasty. In: Krachmer JH, Mannis MJ, Holland EJ, eds. *Cornea*. 2nd ed. CV Mosby: St. Louis; 2004:1575–1589.
7. Foulks GN, Perry HD, Dohlman CH. Oversize corneal donor grafts in penetrating keratoplasty. *Ophthalmology*. 1979;86:490–494.
8. Konowal A, Morrison JC, Brown SV, et al. Irreversible corneal decompensation in patients treated with topical dorzolamide. *Am J Ophthalmol*. 1999;129:403–406.
9. Wand M, Gilbert CM, Liesegang TJ. Latanoprost and herpes simplex keratitis. *Am J Ophthalmol*. 2002;133:393–397.
10. Ishioka M, Shimazaki J, Yamagami J, Fujishima H, Shimmura S, Tsubota K. Trabeculectomy with mitomycin C for post-keratoplasty glaucoma. *Br J Ophthalmol*. 2000;84:714–717.
11. Kwon YH, Taylor JM, Hong S, et al. Long-term results of eyes with penetrating keratoplasty and glaucoma drainage tube implant. *Ophthalmology*. 2001;108:272–278.
12. Alvarenga LS, Mannis MJ, Brandt JD, Lee WB, Schwab IR, Lim MC. The long-term results of keratoplasty in eyes with a glaucoma drainage device. *Am J Ophthalmol*. 2004;13:200–205.
13. Arroyave CP, Scott IU, Fantes FE, Feuer WJ, Murray TG. Corneal graft survival and intraocular pressure control after penetrating keratoplasty and glaucoma drainage device implantation. *Ophthalmology*. 2001;108:1978–1985.
14. Sidoti PA, Mosny AY, Ritterband DC, Seedor JA. Pars plana tube insertion of glaucoma drainage implants and penetrating keratoplasty in patients with coexisting glaucoma and corneal disease. *Ophthalmology*. 2001;108:1050–1058.
15. Cohen EJ, Schwartz LW, Luskind RD, et al. Neodymium:YAG Laser transscleral cyclophotocoagulation for glaucoma after penetrating keratoplasty. *Ophthalmic Surg*. 1989;20:713–716.
16. Shah P, Lee GA, Kirwan JK, et al. Cyclodiode photocoagulation for refractory glaucoma after penetrating keratoplasty. *Ophthalmology*. 2001;108:1986–1991.
17. Ayyala RS, Pieroth L, Vinals AF, et al. Comparison of mitomycin C trabeculectomy, glaucoma drainage device implantation, and laser neodymium:YAG cyclophotocoagulation in the management of intractable glaucoma after penetrating keratoplasty. *Ophthalmology*. 1998;105:1550–1556.
18. Kirkness CM, Steele AD, Ficker LA, Rice NS. Coexistent corneal disease and glaucoma managed by either drainage surgery and subsequent keratoplasty or combined drainage surgery and penetrating keratoplasty. *Br J Ophthalmol*. 1992;76:146–152.

# Chapter 76
# Descemet's Stripping Endothelial Keratoplasty (DSEK) and Glaucoma

Theodoros Filippopoulos, Kathryn A. Colby, and Cynthia L. Grosskreutz

Posterior lamellar corneal procedures are gaining widespread acceptance as the surgical procedure of choice in cases of endothelial dysfunction. These offer more rapid visual recovery and more predictable refractive outcomes compared to penetrating keratoplasty.[1] Originally developed by Melles[2,3] and modified by Terry,[4,5] deep lamellar endothelial keratoplasty (DLEK) evolved into Descemet stripping endothelial keratoplasty with (DSAEK)[6,7] or without (DSEK) the use of an automated microkeratome.[8,9] As the procedure and the pertinent instrumentation are undergoing refinements, little is known about the management of glaucoma that may coexist or arise as a result of posterior lamellar corneal procedures. We will review the available information on the incidence of glaucoma after DSEK/DLEK, the error of measurement in intraocular pressure (IOP) with the Goldmann applanation tonometer (GAT) and summarize considerations about the surgical management of glaucoma in patients after DSEK/DLEK.

## 76.1 Glaucoma after Keratoplasty

The incidence of glaucoma after penetrating keratoplasty (PKP) has been reported as between 9% and 35% depending on patient selection and length of follow-up.[10] The pathogenesis of glaucoma after penetrating keratoplasty is likely multifactorial and related to the distortion of the angle architecture secondary to surgical manipulations, to inflammation giving rise to peripheral anterior synechiae, and to the long-term steroid use to prevent rejection. Incidence data of glaucoma in patients after DSEK/DLEK from prospective studies with sufficient follow-up are not available yet. However, we can infer that the incidence may be in fact smaller than after PKP since there is significantly less distortion of the angle architecture and potentially less postoperative inflammation. On the other hand, due to fewer concerns about postoperative wound integrity, many DLEK/DSEK patients may receive steroids postoperatively for a longer period of time.[1,11] While current indications for DSEK/DLEK include endothelial dysfunction such as Fuchs endothelial dystrophy or pseudophakic bullous keratopathy, it is also being performed in patients at risk of developing glaucoma such as in iridocorneal endothelial syndrome.[12] As experience with these procedures increases, the procedure may also be offered to patients with coexisting glaucoma.[13,14] In a retrospective study of 44 patients after DLEK, 10 of whom (22.7%) had elevated intraocular pressure (IOP) preoperatively, elevated IOP was encountered in 13 patients (29.5%) in the early postoperative period including the 10 patients with preexisting glaucoma.[13] The IOP rise necessitated discontinuation of steroids in one patient with subsequent graft rejection, trabeculectomy in one patient, and insertion of a glaucoma drainage device in another.[13] These prevalence data derived from IOP measurements alone should be interpreted with caution as measurement errors introduced by the lamellar corneal surgery in the readings obtained with the commonly employed GAT are unknown. More recently, Vajaranant et al. retrospectively reviewed 400 consecutive patients after DSEK, 85 of whom had preexisting glaucoma defined as previous glaucoma surgery, preoperative IOP≥24 mmHg, cup-to-disc ratio≥0.6, or history of glaucoma and/or glaucoma medications.[15] She determined that peak IOP occurred at 3 months postoperatively, which may be consistent with a steroid response, and that the glaucoma group had a higher prevalence of increased intraocular pressures compared with the control group. About 20% of patients in the control group required glaucoma medications postoperatively, and 0.3% required a glaucoma procedure to adequately control IOP. The percentage of patients in the glaucoma group that required medication adjustments or a subsequent glaucoma procedure was higher.

In the immediate postoperative period, pupillary block glaucoma may be encountered as a result of a large residual intraoperative air bubble that is used to unfold and float the posterior corneal donor lenticule and to facilitate attachment to the host corneal stroma.[7,16] While some authors advocate a peripheral iridectomy in certain cases,[16] keeping the intraoperative air bubble of reasonable size along with cycloplegia appears to be effective in preventing pupillary block.[17] Aqueous misdirection has been also described after DSEK.[7] Recently, 5 late cases (3–18 weeks after the procedure) of peripheral anterior iridocorneal synechiae to the edge of the donor lenticule were reported in phakic patients undergoing DSEK resulting in increased IOP and requiring operative intervention; since this complication occurred during the first 104 cases of a single surgeon, a steep learning curve may be responsible for such an occurrence.[18]

## 76.2 Dsek and Intraocular Pressure

So far, the precise effect of DSEK or similar procedures on the intraocular pressure (IOP) measurement error with the currently available tonometers has not been precisely determined. Central Corneal Thickness (CCT) increases to an average value of 690–700 μm after DSEK.[16,19,20] A direct comparison between pre- and post-operative values would not be valid as the preexisting corneal edema leads to underestimation of the IOP at least with the more commonly used GAT.[21] It is also known that Dynamic Contour tonometry (DCT) compared with Goldmann Applanation tonometry (GAT) may be less affected by changes in corneal thickness induced by surgical procedures such as LASIK,[22] which may be suggestive of a similar benefit after DSEK. In a recent comprehensive comparison of DCT and GAT in a cohort of eyes after DSEK, the average discrepancy in the IOP readings (DCT-GAT) was estimated as $3.9 \pm 2.4$ mmHg[20] which is higher than what is reported in population-based studies of normal eyes.[23,24] In the same study, the average GAT reading was $15.9 \pm 4.9$ mmHg for the cohort after DSEK.[20] It has also been established that the difference in IOP readings between the DCT and GAT (DCT-GAT) tends to be more pronounced in thin corneas.[24,25] We may therefore conclude that corneas after DSEK tend to behave from a biomechanical standpoint like thin corneas as if only the relatively thin recipient bed of $502 \pm 46$ μm on average[20] would contribute to their elastic properties, and the value of central corneal thickness would be irrelevant (Fig. 76.1).

## 76.3 Surgical Management

The preferred surgical management option for patients with glaucoma that is not adequately controlled with medications after a posterior corneal lamellar procedure has not been established. Both trabeculectomies[13,26] and glaucoma drainage devices[13] have been reported, apparently with successful outcomes but after only limited follow-up. Considerations about the most effective and safe management option are pertinent to the preoperative state of the conjunctiva, especially in the setting of multiple previous surgeries and to endothelial cell survival.

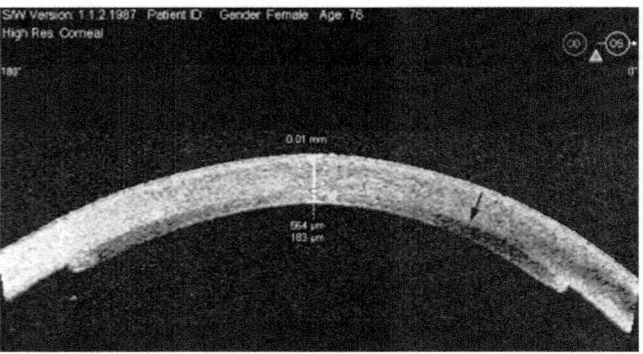

**Fig. 76.1** High resolution anterior segment optical coherence tomography image of a patient after DSEK. The *black arrow* indicates the interface between the recipient bed and the donor lenticule. (Reprinted with permission from Vajaranant TS, Price MO, Price FW, et al. Intraocular pressure measurements following Descemet stripping endothelial keratoplasty. *Am J Ophthalmol* 2008; 145(5):780-6. Copyright© 2008, Elsevier. All rights reserved.)

Posterior corneal lamellar surgery is most frequently performed through a temporal 5 mm sclerocorneal incision that can be self-sealing[7] and therefore advantageous during the surgical procedure. Viscoelastic is also used with prudence in order to facilitate graft adherence.[16] The procedure can also be performed through a clear corneal incision, which may be beneficial with respect to endothelial cell survival and may be utilized to perform phacoemulsification concurrently.[17] Either approach usually leaves conjunctiva available to perform a superior trabeculectomy. Known risk factors for failure after trabeculectomy include previous ocular surgery, young age, secondary glaucomas such as neovascular or uveitic glaucoma, black race, and chronic therapy with topical glaucoma medications – all of which are associated with a higher number of fibroblasts, macrophages, and lymphocytes in the conjunctival stroma accounting for an intensified wound healing response.[27] As a result, trabeculectomy in the presence of a previous posterior lamellar corneal procedure should be viewed as a procedure with a relative higher risk for failure similar to pseudophakia or aphakia.

### 76.3.1 Glaucoma Drainage Devices

There is evidence supporting a substantial (25–34%) endothelial cell loss during the first 6 months after DSEK/DSAEK[17,28] and DLEK[29] and a slower rate of endothelial cell loss thereafter. This raises the concern of the added effect of glaucoma drainage devices on long-term endothelial cell survival. Glaucoma drainage devices are an independent risk factor for graft failure in patients after penetrating keratoplasty[30] but are, in general, associated with fair outcomes with respect to corneal clarity after a follow-up of 2 or 3 years.[30,31] Recent studies evaluating corneal clarity after penetrating keratoplasty in the presence of pars plana tubes are suggestive of superior results at 1 and 2 years, respectively, compared with historical controls.[32,33] This is probably a result of the increased distance between the tube and the posterior corneal surface, which virtually eliminates the risk of tube-corneal touch or other mechanically induced endothelial trauma. It has to be noted that the anterior chamber can be potentially crowded after DSEK, especially in the rare phakic patient, as a result of the volume of the donor lenticule. A possible effect therefore of anterior chamber tubes on long-term corneal clarity in DSEK patients cannot be excluded, although there is not sufficient evidence yet to support exclusive pars plana placement or trabeculectomy as the glaucoma procedure of choice in these patients.

Another issue that has arisen is the feasibility of DSEK to restore corneal clarity in the presence of an anterior chamber tube. These are usually patients with an extensive previous surgical history. Published reports[14] and the consensus among glaucoma specialists as it is reflected in an online discussion through the American Glaucoma Society (Ramesh Ayyala and Robert Feldman) indicate that DSEK in the presence of anterior chamber tubes with a mature bleb is feasible, although technically more difficult, and no special precautions need to be taken to prevent the anterior chamber air bubble from escaping prematurely. In that context, DSEK has been employed to treat corneal decompensation as a result of lenticular–corneal touch after a glaucoma drainage device.[14]

## 76.4 Conclusion

Glaucoma in patients with previous DSEK/DLEK will become a growing concern as the procedure becomes more popular among cornea specialists. Further study is needed to formulate specific recommendations regarding the glaucoma procedure of choice following DSEK/DLEK.

## References

1. Price MO, Price FW. Descemet's stripping endothelial keratoplasty. *Curr Opin Ophthalmol.* 2007;18(4):290–294.
2. Melles GR, Eggink FA, Lander F, et al. A surgical technique for posterior lamellar keratoplasty. *Cornea.* 1998;17(6):618–626.
3. Melles GR, Lander F, van Dooren BT, et al. Preliminary clinical results of posterior lamellar keratoplasty through a sclerocorneal pocket incision. *Ophthalmology.* 2000;107(10):1850–6. discussion 7.
4. Terry MA, Ousley PJ. Deep lamellar endothelial keratoplasty in the first United States patients: early clinical results. *Cornea.* 2001;20(3):239–243.
5. Terry MA, Ousley PJ. Small-incision deep lamellar endothelial keratoplasty (DLEK): six-month results in the first prospective clinical study. *Cornea.* 2005;24(1):59–65.
6. Gorovoy MS. Descemet-stripping automated endothelial keratoplasty. *Cornea.* 2006;25(8):886–889.
7. Price FW Jr, Price MO. Descemet's stripping with endothelial keratoplasty in 200 eyes: early challenges and techniques to enhance donor adherence. *J Cataract Refract Surg.* 2006;32(3):411–418.
8. Melles GR, Wijdh RH, Nieuwendaal CP. A technique to excise the descemet membrane from a recipient cornea (descemetorhexis). *Cornea.* 2004;23(3):286–288.
9. Price FW Jr, Price MO. Descemet's stripping with endothelial keratoplasty in 50 eyes: a refractive neutral corneal transplant. *J Refract Surg.* 2005;21(4):339–345.
10. Ayyala RS. Penetrating keratoplasty and glaucoma. *Surv Ophthalmol.* 2000;45(2):91–105.
11. Allan BD, Terry MA, Price FW Jr, et al. Corneal transplant rejection rate and severity after endothelial keratoplasty. *Cornea.* 2007;26(9):1039–1042.
12. Price MO, Price FW Jr. Descemet stripping with endothelial keratoplasty for treatment of iridocorneal endothelial syndrome. *Cornea.* 2007;26(4):493–497.
13. Hyams M, Segev F, Yepes N, et al. Early postoperative complications of deep lamellar endothelial keratoplasty. *Cornea.* 2007;26(6):650–653.
14. Duarte MC, Herndon LW, Gupta PK, Afshari NA. DSEK in eyes with double glaucoma tubes. *Ophthalmology.* 2008;115(8):1435.e1.
15. Vajaranant TS. Vision and IOP after Descemet-stripping endothelial keratoplasty in patients with preexisting glaucoma. *Paper Presented at American Academy of Ophthalmology*; November 10, 2008 PA040.
16. Koenig SB, Covert DJ. Early results of small-incision Descemet's stripping and automated endothelial keratoplasty. *Ophthalmology.* 2007;114(2):221–226.
17. Price MO, Price FW Jr. Endothelial cell loss after descemet stripping with endothelial keratoplasty influencing factors and 2-year trend. *Ophthalmology.* 2008;115(5):857–865.
18. Basak SK, et al. Late secondary angle-closure glaucoma following Descemet stripping endothelial keratoplasty. *Paper Presented at American Academy of Ophthalmology*; November 10, 2008 PA040 PA039.
19. Price MO, Price FW Jr. Descemet's stripping with endothelial keratoplasty: comparative outcomes with microkeratome-dissected and manually dissected donor tissue. *Ophthalmology.* 2006;113(11):1936–1942.
20. Vajaranant TS, Price MO, Price FW, et al. Intraocular pressure measurements following Descemet stripping endothelial keratoplasty. *Am J Ophthalmol.* 2008;145(5):780–786.
21. Whitacre MM, Stein R. Sources of error with use of Goldmann-type tonometers. *Surv Ophthalmol.* 1993;38(1):1–30.
22. Pepose JS, Feigenbaum SK, Qazi MA, et al. Changes in corneal biomechanics and intraocular pressure following LASIK using static, dynamic, and noncontact tonometry. *Am J Ophthalmol.* 2007;143(1):39–47.
23. Pache M, Wilmsmeyer S, Lautebach S, Funk J. Dynamic contour tonometry versus Goldmann applanation tonometry: a comparative study. *Graefes Arch Clin Exp Ophthalmol.* 2005;243(8):763–767.
24. Francis BA, Hsieh A, Lai MY, et al. Effects of corneal thickness, corneal curvature, and intraocular pressure level on Goldmann applanation tonometry and dynamic contour tonometry. *Ophthalmology.* 2007;114(1):20–26.
25. Doyle A, Lachkar Y. Comparison of dynamic contour tonometry with goldman applanation tonometry over a wide range of central corneal thickness. *J Glaucoma.* 2005;14(4):288–292.
26. Terry MA, Ousley PJ. Deep lamellar endothelial keratoplasty: early complications and their management. *Cornea.* 2006;25(1):37–43.
27. Broadway DC, Chang LP. Trabeculectomy, risk factors for failure and the preoperative state of the conjunctiva. *J Glaucoma.* 2001;10(3):237–249.

28. Price MO, Baig KM, Brubaker JW, Price FW Jr. Randomized, prospective comparison of precut vs surgeon-dissected grafts for descemet stripping automated endothelial keratoplasty. *Am J Ophthalmol*. 2008;146(1):36–41.
29. Terry MA, Ousley PJ. Deep lamellar endothelial keratoplasty visual acuity, astigmatism, and endothelial survival in a large prospective series. *Ophthalmology*. 2005;112(9):1541–1548.
30. Alvarenga LS, Mannis MJ, Brandt JD, et al. The long-term results of keratoplasty in eyes with a glaucoma drainage device. *Am J Ophthalmol*. 2004;138(2):200–205.
31. Kwon YH, Taylor JM, Hong S, et al. Long-term results of eyes with penetrating keratoplasty and glaucoma drainage tube implant. *Ophthalmology*. 2001;108(2):272–278.
32. Ritterband DC, Shapiro D, Trubnik V, et al. Penetrating keratoplasty with pars plana glaucoma drainage devices. *Cornea*. 2007;26(9):1060–1066.
33. Sidoti PA, Mosny AY, Ritterband DC, Seedor JA. Pars plana tube insertion of glaucoma drainage implants and penetrating keratoplasty in patients with coexisting glaucoma and corneal disease. *Ophthalmology*. 2001;108(6):1050–1058.

# Chapter 77
# Cataract and Glaucoma Surgery

Joseph R. Zelefsky and Stephen A. Obstbaum

Cataract and glaucoma are leading causes of worldwide blindness and are among the most common ocular conditions associated with the aging process. Because the worldwide population is aging, the prevalence of cataract and glaucoma are increasing, and these conditions will require greater allocations of resources to achieve favorable outcomes and positive influences on quality-of-life measures. Cataract surgery and intraocular lens (IOL) implantation has become the most successful rehabilitative microsurgical procedure in modern medicine. Our success with the management of glaucoma, either medically or surgically, has not achieved similar success. Nonetheless, we are increasingly forced to deal with situations in which patients have both cataract and glaucoma; and we frequently contend with our patients' expectations of a functional result similar to that achieved by modern cataract surgery. The perplexing question is how to manage these coexisting conditions to promote the best possible outcome.

For the purposes of this chapter, we will define the patient population under discussion as individuals with a characteristic optic neuropathy, accompanied by visual field loss and elevated intraocular pressure (IOP) or an IOP level deemed sufficient to produce damage to a particular optic nerve. These patients are glaucoma patients and glaucoma suspect patients, respectively. We will also assume that we are dealing with a visually disabling cataract that is capable of impairing functional activity in the absence of visual field loss. We recognize that it is often difficult to distinguish between the functional disability induced by the glaucomatous state and the effects of glaucoma treatment from the influence of the cataract. Because of this question, it is important for the patient to have as much information about realistic expectations of a functional outcome so that he or she can make a reasoned decision about any proposed intervention. Patients need to be made to understand that they and their physician are dealing with two distinct clinical entities. Surgical correction of a visually disabling cataract will not rehabilitate glaucomatous loss of visual field and visual acuity.

## 77.1 Evidence-Based Information

Evidence-based medicine is the disciplined approach of applying the best available evidence to the clinical decision-making process. In the field of glaucoma, we have benefited from several randomized controlled studies that have either confirmed our earlier practice patterns or have provided new information that we have applied to patient care. Some of the recommendations from randomized controlled trials such as AGIS, EMGT, CIGTS, and OHTS (see Chap. 3) have already become part of our current treatment practices. We now know with some certainty that lowering of intraocular pressure, either via medicine, laser treatments, or incisional surgery, halts or at least retards the progression of optic nerve damage due to glaucoma. Unfortunately, the evidence-based information regarding the management of coexisting cataract and glaucoma is less certain.[1] It has been shown that there is an increased risk of nuclear sclerotic cataract related to elevated IOP and also the use of glaucoma medications may increase this risk.[2]

There is a vast body of literature on the topic of coexisting cataract and glaucoma that dates to the use of both intracapsular and extracapsular cataract surgery. Where the information is pertinent to our discussion, we will cite these earlier reports. A systematic assessment of the literature undertaken a few years ago indicated that most of the published information had either weak or moderate strength with regard to the questions posed about patterns of care.[1]

## 77.2 Preoperative Considerations

Patients with coexisting cataract and glaucoma should be evaluated to determine if the cataract is responsible for a significant component of the vision loss. Careful slit-lamp examination to determine the clinical appearance of the lens in conjunction with subjective testing such as visual acuity, potential acuity meter (PAM), or glare testing may help clarify the role that the cataract plays in the patient's visual impairment. Coexisting glaucomatous optic neuropathy or retinal pathology such as macular degeneration must be considered as to the degree these pathologies contribute to reduced visual acuity and contrast.

Necessary modifications in surgical maneuvers to ensure optimum outcome should be considered in advance of the operation and notes made in the patient's chart that will be brought into the operating room. A detailed slit-lamp examination is performed on all potential cataract surgery patients (whether with or without trabeculectomy). Make particular note of patients with pseudoexfoliation syndrome, chronic angle-closure glaucoma, or those who have been on chronic miotic therapy (Sidebar 77.1), as they often have small pupils that may poorly dilate. Such advance knowledge allows the surgeon to plan a suitable medical and surgical strategy prior to the operating room.

Careful consideration must be given to the severity of the patient's glaucoma. Patients with mild to moderate glaucoma are likely to be able to withstand both intra- and postoperative transient elevations of intraocular pressure. Patients with more advanced glaucomatous disease may be at risk for further damage with high intraoperative pressures or early or late postoperative pressure spikes. Elevations in IOP after extracapsular cataract extraction (ECCE) have been well-documented.[3] While IOP tends to decrease after phacoemulsification in the long term, transient spikes in IOP can arise after phacoemulsification within the first few hours or days after surgery.[4,5] The patient should, therefore, be carefully evaluated to determine if the glaucoma is controlled to the point that he or she can withstand a transient spike in IOP after cataract extraction.

### Sidebar 77.1 Flomax: implications for glaucoma and cataract surgery

#### Maria Basile and John Danias

Intraoperative Floppy-Iris Syndrome (IFIS) is a condition characterized by a triad of intraoperative findings: (1) iris fluttering occurring under normal fluidic conditions, (2) iris billowing and prolapse to the phaco and side port incisions despite proper wound construction, and (3) progressive miosis. Poor preoperative dilation and failure of dilation despite mechanical stretching of the pupil are additional characteristics. IFIS was first described in 2005 by Chang et al in patients undergoing phacoemulsification while being treated with tamsulosin. The intraoperative findings make cataract surgery in eyes with IFIS difficult and lead to increased risk of complications. More recently, IFIS has been reported to complicate routine trabeculectomy surgery in patients taking alpha-antagonists.

Tamsulosin hydrochloride (Flomax) is the most commonly prescribed medication for treatment of benign prostatic hyperplasia (BPH) and associated symptoms of lower urinary tract obstruction (LUTS). It is reported that 50 and 80% of men over the age of 50 and 85, respectively, require treatment for LUTS. Over the last decade, pharmacotherapy as opposed to surgery has become a first-line treatment for BPH/LUTS and tamsulosin is considered a first-line therapeutic agent. Therefore, it is not surprising that more patients undergoing cataract surgery are using tamsulosin, thus accounting for the progressive increase in the incidence of IFIS. In fact, IFIS associated with the use of tamsulosin occurs in approximately 2% of cataract cases.

Tamsulosin is a selective $\alpha_1$-adrenergic-receptor (AR) blocker with a tenfold greater affinity for $\alpha_{1a}$ and $\alpha_{1d}$ receptors than for $\alpha_{1b}$-adrenergic receptors. This distinguishes tamsulosin from other alpha-blockers available in the United States – terazosin, doxazosin, alfuzosin – that all have similar affinity for all three $\alpha_1$-receptor subtypes. Studies have shown that (alpha)$\alpha_{1a}$ AR-selective antagonists relieve obstructive symptoms of LUTS via relaxation of the prostate smooth muscle, whereas (alpha) $\alpha_{1d}$ AR-selective antagonists relieve bladder-based irritability symptoms. In contrast, blockade of the $\alpha_{1b}$-adrenergic receptors leads to orthostatic hypotension; a side effect associated with nonselective alpha blockers.

Two $\alpha_1$-ARs have been identified in the iris: $\alpha_{1a}$ and $\alpha_{1b}$. Several studies have confirmed the presence of the $\alpha_{1a}$-AR in the rabbit iris dilator muscle, as well as its role in the sympathetic mediation of mydriasis. In contrast, $\alpha_{1b}$AR has been localized to the iris arterioles. Although $\alpha_1$-AR localization has not been reported for the human eye, it is on the basis of these animal studies that IFIS has been proposed to develop. Specifically, it has been proposed that the blockade of the postsynaptic $\alpha_{1a}$AR in the iris dilator smooth muscle by tamsulosin causes IFIS. This theory is further supported by a report of intraoperative reversal of miosis and possible increase in iris tone after intracameral administration of phenylephrine (an $\alpha_1$-AR agonist that competes with tamsulosin for $\alpha_{1a}$-ARs).

However, this proposed mechanism cannot explain all the features of IFIS. While it is likely that tamsulosin blockade of $\alpha_{1a}$-AR causes miosis, it does not explain well the iris floppiness or the elasticity of the pupillary margin. In describing the syndrome, Chang et al proposed that the iris propensity to billow and prolapse was caused by disuse iris dilator atrophy. They suggested that tamsulosin's long half-life and a relatively constant receptor blockade leads to disuse atrophy of the iris, which in turn contributes to low iris tone and the presence of a small pupil long after tamsulosin cessation. Although this concept has been disputed by Schwinn et al based on previous work demonstrating denervation supersensitivity of the $\alpha_1$-AR in rabbits, it is still quite popular.

In addition to the $\alpha_{1a}$-AR blockade, an interaction between the $\alpha_1$-AR blockers and melanin has been postulated to contribute to IFIS. $\alpha_1$-ARs appear to be significant in melaninogenesis, as their blockade in the neonatal period causes a decrease in iris pigmentation. More recently, Goseki et al reported structural changes in the irides of patients with IFIS. These changes included vacuolation of the dilator muscle cells, as well as irregularity of melanocyte pigment granules and presence of lipofuscin-like granules in the iridal clump cells – giant pigment cells in the iris stroma that are believed to be resident macrophages. The authors hypothesized that high local concentration of the $\alpha_1$-AR blocker in the melanocytes of pigment epithelium contributes to the atrophy of the intimately proximal dilator smooth muscle cells and causes IFIS. However, studies in rabbit irides did not find increased binding of $\alpha_{1a}$-AR drugs to melanin, as evidenced by similar binding of $\alpha_{1a}$-AR agonist in pigmented and albino irides.

The theory of iris dilator muscle atrophy as the cause of IFIS was also investigated by Kim et al In this study, the authors demonstrated lack of identifiable myofibrils in iris dilator muscle on electron microscopy of peripheral iridectomy samples from patients on tamsulosin. This finding was in contrast to lack of observed difference on light microscopy in iris dilator muscle thickness between tamsulosin-treated and control iridectomy samples. Also of importance was the lack of direct relationship between duration of tamsulosin use and dilator muscle thickness.

Finally, contrary to the previous reports and based on histopathological evidence, we have proposed that the main site of IFIS pathology is the muscularis of the iris arterioles (in review).

According to a recently published survey, 95% of the American Society of Cataract and Refractive Surgery (ASCRS) members found that tamsulosin makes cataract surgery more difficult, and 77% reported that it increases the risk of complications. In the original report by Chang et al, vitreous loss occurred in 12% of IFIS cases. Posterior capsular rupture was reported in 22% of resident cataract surgery in patients taking tamsulosin. Significant intraoperative iris trauma was also reported by 52% of surveyed cataract surgeons in eyes with IFIS.

IFIS-associated posterior capsular rupture and vitreous loss were reported to be much lower (0.6% only) in a follow-up report by Chang et al suggesting that as surgeons become more aware of the syndrome and anticipate it, the risk of surgical complications decreases.

There appears to be a spectrum of severity of tamsulosin-associated IFIS. In one study, mild, moderate, and severe IFIS was reported in 17, 30, and 43% of patients on tamsulosin, respectively, with no IFIS in 10%. Other studies confirmed the spectrum of IFIS severity in patients on tamsulosin but reported a much lower incidence of IFIS (with only 43–57% of patients on tamsulosin showing any signs of IFIS).

Various management strategies have been proposed in an effort to ensure safe surgery in patients with IFIS. Preoperative discontinuation of tamsulosin was originally recommended, but has been found to be ineffective. It is currently routinely employed by only 20% of surveyed cataract surgeons. This lack of effect of short-term discontinuation of tamsulosin on IFIS severity can be explained by the presence of significant levels of tamsulosin in the aqueous humor of 60% of patients who discontinue the drug for up to 4 weeks. Another preoperative strategy is the topical administration of atropine 1% three times daily for 1–2 days prior to surgery. It should be noted that when administering atropine, discontinuation of systemic alpha blockers is not recommended because of the risk of acute urinary retention. The most important of the preoperative strategies by far, however, is obtaining a careful present and past drug use history and recognition of the potential problem.

Various intraoperative maneuvers have been suggested for use in IFIS cases. Strategies include careful wound construction, use of gentle hydrodissection, directing irrigating currents away from the pupillary margin and lowering the irrigation, aspiration rates, and vacuum levels. All of these maneuvers help decrease turbulence in the anterior chamber and decrease washout of the ocular viscosurgical device (OVD). In addition, 38% of surveyed cataract surgeons routinely administer dilute intracameral unpreserved $\alpha_1$ agonists such as phenylephrine and epinephrine (0.25 ml of 2.5% unpreserved phenylephrine diluted with 2 ml of BSS, or unpreserved epinephrine 1:2,500–1:4,000).

Use of the viscoadaptive agent, sodium hyaluronate 2.3% (Healon 5, AMO, Santa Ana, CA), is another widely used strategy. Fifteen percent of cataract surgeons reported its use in IFIS cases. As a super-cohesive OVD, Healon 5 aids in mydriasis and blocks iris prolapse through the wound. Unlike other cohesive agents, however, its pseudodispersive quality allows Healon 5 to remain in the eye and maintain anterior chamber depth at higher flow rates. It is reported that 95% of IFIS cases that utilized Healon 5 did not require the use of adjunctive mechanical devices.

Mechanical devices include iris hooks and pupil expansion rings and are employed to dilate the pupil and prevent iris prolapse. Iris hooks are generally preferred to the expansion rings (23% versus 4%). Positioning the hooks in a diamond configuration with one of the retractors placed through a separate paracentesis just below the main corneal incision, further minimizes iris prolapse and trauma. However, once capsulorhexis has been performed, it becomes difficult to place iris hooks safely without capturing the capsular edge. Therefore, the ability to anticipate IFIS and the placement of mechanical devices early in surgery becomes very important. Two other common techniques for small pupil management – mechanical stretching of the pupil and partial thickness sphincterotomies – are ineffective in IFIS and may exacerbate it.

Following the original description of IFIS and its association with tamsulosin, other case reports of IFIS occurring in patients on nonselective $\alpha_1$-AR blockers, as well as saw palmetto (*Serona repens* – an over-the-counter alternative therapy for BPH, believed to act via 5-alpha reductase pathway and also found to have $\alpha_1$-AR-inhibitory properties), have been described. One retrospective study reported a 15.4% risk of IFIS in patients on alfuzosin compared to an 86.4% risk in patients on tamsulosin. However, two prospective studies failed to show any significant associations between nonselective $\alpha_1$-AR blockers and IFIS. Alfuzosin's ability to antagonize phenylephrine-induced contraction of the iris dilator muscle in pigmented rabbits is much lower than that of tamsulosin and in addition its serum concentrations may be too low to antagonize the effect of perioperative alpha-agonist administration on the dilator muscle.

In 2007, Au et al reported the first case of IFIS during trabeculectomy in a patient on doxazosin. The authors described excessive iris prolapse through the sclerostomy and the paracentesis site. They also reported difficulty to reposition the iris into the anterior chamber after peripheral iridectomy during routine trabeculectomy with the use of an anterior chamber (AC) maintainer. Intraoperative management of IFIS included switching off the AC maintainer in order to decompress the eye and suturing of the sclerostomy with releasable sutures prior to resumption of the AC infusion. Postoperatively, the location of peripheral iridectomy was noted to be less basal than desired without ostium obstruction. The authors recommended thorough preoperative assessment on prior alpha-antagonist use if planning to use the AC maintainer during trabeculectomy. They also suggested lowering the infusion rate or omitting the use of the maintainer altogether if the risk of IFIS exists, as well as preoperative use of pilocarpine or intraoperative use of Miochol.

Since the initial report of IFIS during trabeculectomy, other cases have been reported in patients on tamsulosin and alfusozin. The authors described similar iris prolapse through the ostium after sclerostomy during trabeculectomy without the use of an AC maintainer in a patient with history of tamsulosin use and preoperative use of pilocarpine 4%. Certain intraoperative strategies such as cutting a large peripheral iridectomy, stroking the cornea, sweeping the iris with a Rycroft cannula through the paracentesis incision, and using intracameral injections of viscoelastic and Miochol exacerbated the iris prolapse. Final iris repositioning was achieved by using bimanual irrigation/aspiration probes to sweep the iris into the anterior chamber after creation of a second sideport incision. In the second case report, the authors recommended use of two iris hooks in what is described to be a "fish mouth" configuration in order to prevent iris prolapse. They created two paracentesis incisions at the 3 and 9 o'clock positions through which they placed iris hooks and used them to create a "fish mouth" pupil configuration prior to sclerostomy. This step stretched tight the superior iris and allowed the surgeon to perform an uncomplicated peripheral iridectomy. The iris was then described to return to its preoperative position.

In our own practice, we encountered a case of IFIS during trabeculectomy in a patient taking tamsulosin. Excessive iris prolapse through the ostium was observed immediately after sclerostomy despite prior administration of an OVD. The iris continued to prolapse even after a broad basal peripheral iridectomy was created. Final repositioning of the iris into the anterior chamber was achieved by sweeping the iris with an iris spatula through the paracentesis incision aided by a cohesive OVD and subsequent closure of the sclerostomy with interrupted nylon sutures (in review).

It is important to point out that there are multiple other disease states and drugs that can potentially cause similar iris findings. In diabetics, surgically induced miosis has been reported to occur with greater frequency compared to normal controls during routine cataract surgery. Resting pupil size in diabetic patients has also been noted to be smaller than that in healthy subjects – a finding attributed to sympathetic neuropathy. More recently, changes in the distribution and concentration of the potent vasoconstrictor endothelin-1 (ET-1) that mediates iris dilator contraction via endothelin-A (ETA) receptors have been proposed to occur in patients with diabetes and hypertension. In addition, ETA-selective inhibitors have been shown to relax smooth muscle contraction, as demonstrated by a blockade of norepinephrine- and angiotensin II-mediated vasoconstriction in human subjects. It, thus, appears that control of iris dilation and contraction is a multifactorial process. Therefore, rather than focusing on one drug as the cause of IFIS of variable severity, perhaps multiple factors should be considered in order to determine the risk of IFIS and its severity.

In summary, IFIS is an important risk factor for cataract surgery complications. Although the exact mechanism of IFIS has yet to be elucidated, several preoperative and intraoperative strategies can be employed to reduce the rate of complications. Of these, by far the most important risk-reducing strategy is preoperative recognition of the patient at risk. Therefore, careful history taking remains crucial to surgical success.

**Acknowledgments** Supported by NEI EY 01867 and an unrestricted grant from RPB

## Bibliography

Akhtar RA, Abdel-Latif AA. Surgical sympathetic denervation increases alpha 1-adrenoceptor-mediated accumulation of myoinositol trisphosphate and muscle contraction in rabbit iris dilator smooth muscle. *J Neurochem*. 1986;46:96–104.

Au L, Wechsler D, Fenerty C. Alpha antagonists and intraoperative floppy iris syndrome (IFIS) during trabeculectomy. *Eye*. 2007;21:671–6722.

Blouin M, Blouin J, Perreault S, et al. Intraoperative floppy iris syndrome associated with Alpha-1 adrenoreceptors. Comparison of tamsulosin and alfuzosin. *J Cataract Refract Surg*. 2007;33:1227–1234.

Chadha V, Borooah S, Tey A, et al. Floppy iris behaviour during cataract surgery: associations and variations. *Br J Ophthalmol*. 2007;91:40–42.

Chang DF, Braga-Mele R, Mamalis N, et al. Clinical experience with intraoperative floppy-iris syndrome. Results of the 2008 ASCRS member survey. *J Cataract Refract Surg*. 2008;34:1201–1209.

Chang DF, Campbell JR. Intraoperative floppy iris syndrome associated with tamsulosin. *J Cataract Refract Surg*. 2005;31:664–673.

Chang DF, Osher RH, Wang L, Koch DD. A prospective multicenter evaluation of cataract surgery in patients taking tamsulosin (Flomax). *Ophthalmology*. 2007;114:957–964.

Dhingra N, Rajkumar KN, Kumar V. Intraoperative floppy iris syndrome with doxazosin. *Eye*. 2007;21:678–679.

Goepel M, Hecker U, Krege S. Saw palmetto extracts potently and noncompetitively inhibit human alpha1-adrenoceptors in vitro. *Prostate*.1999;38:208–215.

Goseki T, Shimizu K, Ishikawa H, et al. Possible mechanism of intraoperative floppy iris syndrome: a clinicopathological study. *Br J Ophthalmol*. 2008;92:1156–1158.

Gurbaxani A, Packard R. Intracameral phenylephrine to prevent floppy iris syndrome during cataract surgery in patients on tamsulosin. *Eye*. 2007;21:331–332.

http://stream.expoplanner.com/ascrs2006/handouts/076414_powerpointtamsulosin.ppt. Accessed March 10, 2009.

Koike T, Kitazumi H, Mukai H. Tissue distribution of NS-49, a phenethylamine class alpha1A-adrenoceptor agonist, in pigmented rates. *Arzneimittelforschung*. 2001;51:402–407.

Manvikar S, Allen D. Cataract surgery management in patients taking tamsulosin staged approach. *J Cataract Refract Surg*. 2006; 32:1611–1614.

Masket S, Belani S. Combined preoperative topical atropine sulfate 1% and intracameral nonpreserved epinephrine hydrochloride 1:2500 for management of intraoperative floppy-iris syndrome. *J Cataract Refract Surg*. 2007;33:580–582.

Mirza SA, Alexandridou A, Marshall T, et al. Surgically induced miosis during phacoemulsification in patients with diabetes mellitus. *Eye*. 2003;17:194–199.

Norris JH, Mall S, Burnett CAM. Floppy iris syndrome hull hooks (FISH Hooks): a new technique for managing IFIS in trabeculectomy surgery. *Eye*. 2009;23(3):743–744.

Odin L, O'Donnell. Adrenergic influence on iris stromal pigmentation: evidence for alpha-adrenergic receptors. *Invest Ophthalmol Vis Sci*. 1982;23:528–530.

Oshika T, Ohashi Y, Inamura M, et al. Incidence of intraoperative floppy iris syndrome in patients on either systemic or topical alpha (1)-adrenoceptor antagonist. *Am J Ophthalmol*. 2007;143:150–151.

Palea S, Chang DF, Rekik M, et al. Comparative effect of alfuzosin and tamsulosin on the contractile response of isolated rabbit prostatic and iris dilator smooth muscles. Possible model for intraoperative floppy iris syndrome. *J Cataract Refract Surg*. 2008;34:489–496.

Parssinen O, Leppanen E, Keski-Rahkonen P, Mauriala T, Dugué B, Lehtonen M. Influence of tamsulosin on the iris and its implication for cataract surgery. *Invest Ophthalmol Vis Sci*. 2006;47: 3766–3771.

Schwinn DA, Afshari NA. Alpha-1-Adrenergic receptor antagonists and the iris: new mechanistic insights into floppy iris syndrome. *Surv Ophthal*. 2006;51:501–512.

Schwinn DA, Roehrborn CG. Alpha-1-Adrenoceptor subtypes and lower urinary tract symptoms. *Int J Urol*. 2008;15:193–199.

Settas G, Fitt AW. Intraoperative floppy iris syndrome in a patient taking alfuzosin for benign prostatic hypertrophy. *Eye*. 2006;20:1431–1432.

Smith SA, Smith SE. Evidence for a neuropathic etiology in the small pupil of diabetes mellitus. *Br J Ophthalmol*. 1983;67: 89–93.

Suzuki F, Taniguchi T, Nakamura S, et al. Distribution of alpha-1 adrenoceptor subtypes in RNA and protein in rabbit eyes. *Br J Pharmacol*. 2002;135:600–608.

Takmaz T, Can I. Clinical features, complications, and incidence of intraoperative floppy iris syndrome in patients taking tamsulosin. *Eur J Ophthalmol*. 2007;6:909–913.

Venkatesh R, Veena K, Gupta S, Ravindran RD. Intraoperative floppy iris syndrome associated with terazosin. *Indian J ophthalmol*. 2007;55:395–396.

Wenzel RR, Ruthemann J, Bruck H, et al. Endothelin-A receptor antagonist inhibits angiotensin II and noradrenaline in man. *Br J Clin Pharmacol*. 2001;52:151–157.

Wollensak G, Schaefer HE, Ihling C. An immunohistochemical study of endothelin-1 in the human eye. *Curr Eye Res*. 1998;17: 541–545.

Yamada T, Okuyama Y, Mukai H. In vitro melanin binding of NS-49, a phenethylamine class alpha 1A-adrenoceptor agonist. *Arzneimittelforschung*. 2001;51:299–303.

Yeu E, Grostern R. Saw palmetto and intraoperative floppy-iris syndrome. *J Cataract Refract Surg*. 2007;33:927–928.

Yu Y, Koss MC. Studies of alpha-adrenoceptor antagonists on sympathetic mydriasis in rabbits. *J Ocul Pharmacol Ther*. 2003;19: 255–263.

Zaczek A, Zetterstrom C. Cataract surgery and pupil size in patients with diabetes mellitus. *Acta Ophthalmol Scand*. 1997;75:429–432.

Ziada A, Rosenblum M, Crawford ED. Benign prostatic hyperplasia: an overview. *Urology*. 1999;53:1–6.

## 77.3 Surgical Options for the Management of Cataract and Glaucoma

Three standard surgical options for the management of patients with cataract and glaucoma are generally acknowledged:

1. Cataract extraction with IOL implantation alone
2. Sequential surgery – trabeculectomy followed by cataract extraction with IOL implantation
3. Combined surgery – cataract extraction with IOL implantation combined with trabeculectomy

### 77.3.1 Cataract Extraction with IOL Implantation Alone

The option of cataract extraction with IOL implantation alone is appropriate for patients with a visually disabling cataract whose glaucoma is considered mild based on the appearance of the optic disk and minimal visual field loss. Generally speaking these patients have their IOP readily controlled on one or two topical medications and they are compliant with the medical regimen. They are stable with respect to their glaucoma and surgical intervention is needed only for coexisting cataract. It should be noted, that laser trabeculoplasty does appear to be a bit more effective in patients before they undergo cataract surgery, although the reason for this is not well understood.[6] Therefore, for patients with marginal intraocular pressure control, but who are not considered candidates for incisional glaucoma surgery, it may be advisable to perform laser trabeculoplasty first, wait several months, and then consider cataract surgery. Current techniques for phacoemulsification and IOL insertion are associated with excellent functional outcomes and are easier to perform than combined procedures. Phacoemulsification alone in glaucomatous eyes has been associated with a long-term reduction of IOP as well as less need for postoperative medications. This reduction in IOP is long-lasting; several studies have reported reduction in pressure persisting up to 5 years postoperatively.[7-10] With clear-corneal phacoemulsification, especially when performed temporally, the superior conjunctival tissue is preserved should trabeculectomy be required in the future.

The major concern with this option is the possibility of a significant IOP elevation in the immediate postoperative period. Transient elevations in IOP after cataract surgery are associated either with acutely altered aqueous outflow (secondary to inflammation or retained viscoelastic material) or develop as a consequence of the glaucoma process itself. Significant elevations in IOP are common within the first 24 h after ECCE. With phacoemulsification, the level of elevation and the magnitude of IOP spikes are considerably less than with ECCE. Glaucoma patients who have cataract surgery alone should be adequately controlled preoperatively, with the expectation that if elevation of IOP occurs postoperatively it can be easily treated and that the period of elevated IOP should not have an adverse affect on the optic nerve (Sidebar 77.2).

---

**Sidebar 77.2 Anterior chamber intraocular lenses, pupillary block and peripheral iridectomy**

Christopher C. Shen, Sarwat Salim, and Peter A. Netland

Despite advances in instrumentation and surgical techniques for cataract surgery, glaucoma following cataract surgery remains a common problem. Elevation of intraocular pressure may occur early or late in the postoperative course due to a variety of mechanisms, resulting in either open- or closed-angle glaucoma. Angle-closure glaucoma after ACIOL implantation is usually preventable and, when it does occur, can be effectively treated.

In pseudophakic pupillary block glaucoma, the implanted intraocular lens (IOL) is involved in the obstruction of the aqueous flow through the pupil, resulting in iris bombe with subsequent closure of the drainage angle. This condition is more frequently encountered in the presence of an anterior chamber intraocular lens (ACIOL) than with a posteriorly implanted IOL (PCIOL). Potential mechanisms include obstruction by the smooth round optical portion of the IOL or development of adhesions between vitreous and the posterior iris.

While the role of routine surgical iridectomy is controversial in posterior chamber implants, it is widely accepted as standard of care in anterior chamber implants. Surgical iridectomy performed at the time of an ACIOL implant provides an alternate route for aqueous to pass from the posterior into the anterior chamber if the pupil becomes blocked by an intact vitreous face or the IOL itself. This critical step is often neglected intraoperatively due to elevated anxiety and distraction from the impetus for ACIOL implantation (prolapsed vitreous, ruptured capsule, zonule instability) or in haste to complete the case (Figs. 77.2-1–77.2-3).

Although prior studies have demonstrated effective elimination of pupillary block following ACIOL

# 77 Cataract and Glaucoma Surgery

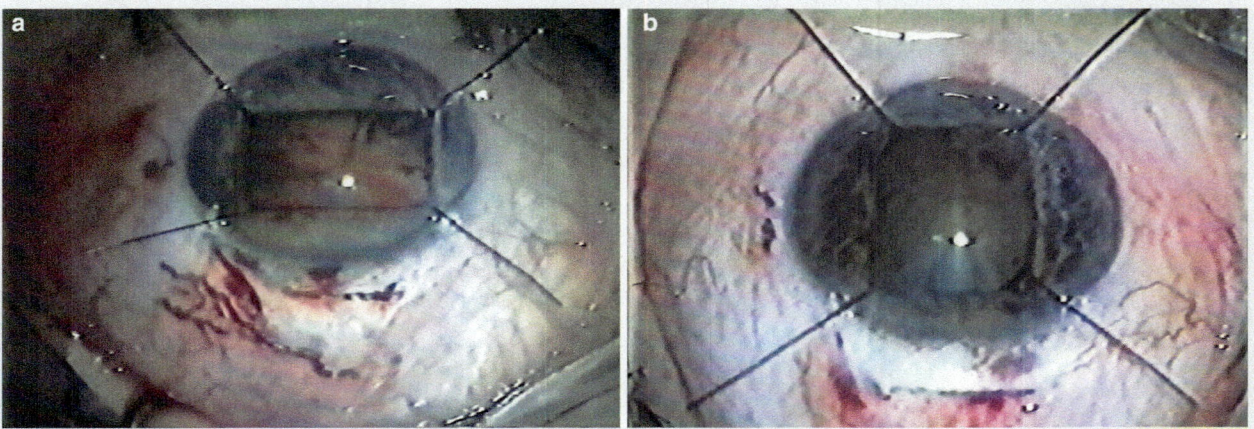

**Fig. 77.2-1** A patient referred for evaluation and treatment 1 day after unplanned anterior chamber intraocular lens (ACIOL) implantation, without surgical iridectomy. The cornea is edematous and the intraocular pressure is markedly elevated

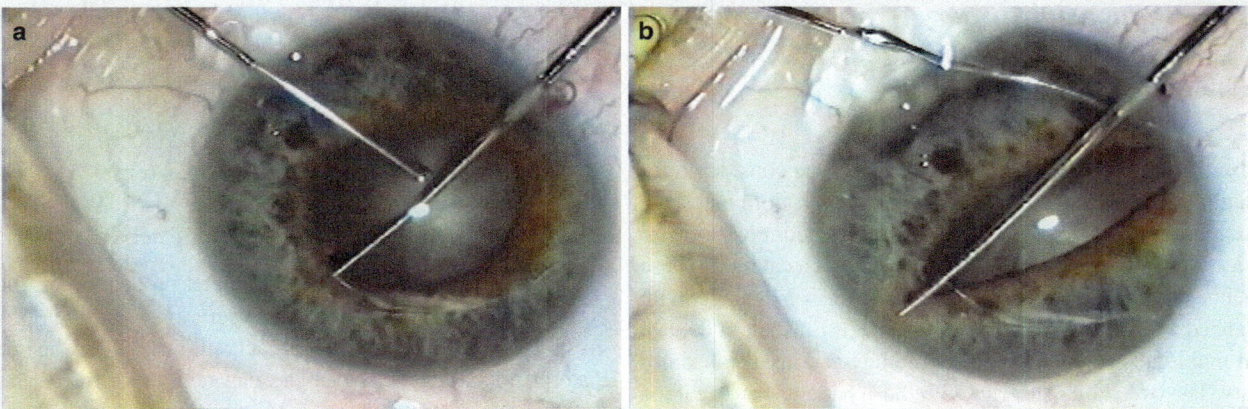

**Fig. 77.2-2** Slit lamp view shows a shallow anterior chamber, with both the iris and the edge of the anterior chamber intraocular lens (ACIOL) optic in contact with the corneal endothelium

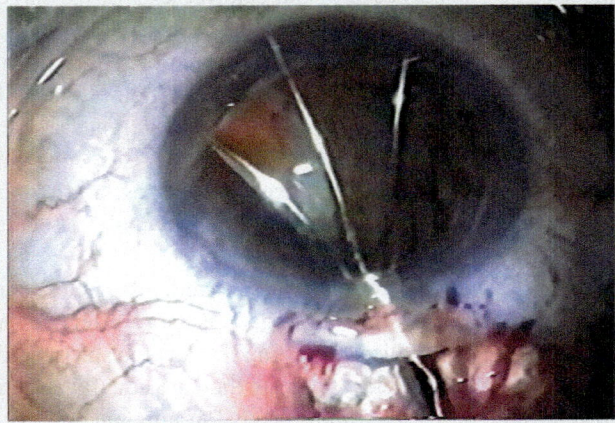

**Fig. 77.2-3** A short time after Nd:YAG iridotomy (*arrows*), the corneal edema has improved, the anterior chamber has deepened, and the intraocular pressure has returned to normal

implantation with postoperative laser iridotomy, the availability of laser iridotomy should not tempt the surgeon to neglect iridectomy during cataract surgery. Postoperative laser iridotomies may be at increased risk for occlusion due to intraocular inflammation present after complicated cataract extraction. Medical therapy is the same compared with treatment of phakic angle-closure glaucoma due to pupillary block. Those patients with ACIOLs who present with acutely elevated IOP and irs bombe should have emergent laser iridotomies placed, preferably in more than one area of the iris. Multiple PIs are helpful because the ACIOL optic may shift in the future and occlude a single irditomy site.

Pseudophakic pupillary block glaucoma in the setting of ACIOL implantation is unpredictable in its onset, ranging from an acute form in the immediate postoperative period to an occult form presenting months to years following surgery. This entity should be treated prophylactically by surgical iridectomy to prevent angle-closure glaucoma.

## Bibliography

Chandler PA. Glaucoma from pupillary block in aphakia. *Trans Am Ophthalmol Soc*. 1961;59:96–105.

Gaton DD, Mimouni K, Lusky M, et al. Pupillary block following posterior chamber intraocular lens implantation in adults. *Br J Opthalmol*. 2003;87:1109–1111.

Kalina PH, Shingleton BJ. Glaucoma after cataract surgery. In. Steinert, R, ed. *Cataract Surgery: Technique, Complications, and Management*. 2nd ed. Philadelphia, PA: Elsevier; 2004:515.

Melamed S. Recurrent closure of neodymium: YAG laser iridotomies requiring multiple treatments in pseudophakic pupillary block. *Ann Ophthalmol*. 1988;20:105–108.

Van Buskirk EM. Pupillary block after intraocular lens implantation, *Am J Ophthalmol*. 1983;95:55–59

## 77.4 Sequential Surgery versus Combined Surgery

### 77.4.1 Sequential Surgery: Trabeculectomy Followed by Cataract Extraction and IOL Implantation

Trabeculectomy followed by cataract surgery is considered for situations in which the state of the glaucoma dominates the clinical picture. These eyes usually need glaucoma surgery to reduce the IOP independent of the presence of a cataract. These patients typically have significant optic nerve damage with advanced visual field loss and an IOP that is difficult to control with maximally tolerated medical therapy and laser trabeculoplasty. The overriding strategy with these patients is to treat the vision-threatening condition first, and achieve IOP levels low enough to protect an already compromised optic nerve. There are situations in which reduction of IOP after trabeculectomy improves the visual acuity, even in the face of a cataract.

Concerns related to sequential surgery include the need for two separate surgical procedures, the possibility that filtration surgery might hasten cataract development, and that cataract surgery might have an adverse effect on the filtering bleb. The earlier literature using ECCE as the method of cataract surgery did indeed demonstrate a reduction of bleb function even when clear-corneal incisions were performed anterior to the bleb.[11] As we will discuss later, phacoemulsification through a temporal clear-corneal incision has fared better in preserving bleb function.[12]

### 77.4.2 Combined Surgery

Support for the strategy that combines cataract extraction/IOL implantation with trabeculectomy has waxed and waned over the past 30 years, being largely dependent upon the surgical techniques that prevailed at the time. Clear-corneal phacoemulsification has had a major influence on the trend to popularize combined cataract and filtration surgery for patients with a visually significant cataract and either:

- Glaucoma that fails to respond to a maximally tolerated medical regimen
- Glaucoma with a history of noncompliance with medications
- Glaucoma with appreciable visual field loss and disk change independent of medical control, or
- Conditions in which transient elevations of IOP postoperatively might cause significant optic nerve damage

The major advantages of a combined procedure are that it eliminates the need for separate operations and it improves visual acuity associated with cataract removal. IOP in the immediate postoperative period is less elevated and there are fewer IOP spikes greater than 30 mmHg in combined cases.[13] There is insufficient evidence to support the concept that sequential surgery is better than combined surgery or vice versa.[1] The decision with respect to which option is adopted should be based on the specific clinical scenario and comfort level of the surgeon after discussion of the options with the patient.

In the early days of phacoemulsification, a scleral tunnel incision at the 12 o'clock position was employed. This incision site could then be easily used to create a scleral flap for trabeculectomy. Now that many surgeons have switched to temporal clear-corneal incisions, a "two-site" approach for combined cataract extraction with trabeculectomy has become quite popular.

To date, there has been no randomized, prospective study demonstrating that one-site surgery is more effective than two-site surgery or vice versa. In fact, a recent prospective, randomized 3-year study suggests they are equally effective in IOP reduction with similar needs for antiglaucoma medications.[14] There are several advantages and disadvantages of each technique worth mentioning. Performing the procedure through separate sites may be advantageous in that less tissue manipulation occurs near the site of the trabeculectomy incision, which may affect filtration. In addition, should laser suture lysis or removal of a releasable suture be required, this would not involve manipulation near the cataract incision.[15]

One disadvantage of a two-site approach is longer operating time, as the surgeon must move from a temporal to superior position and adjust the operating microscope accordingly. The increased surgical time leads to a longer duration of the need for anesthesia and an increased risk of phototoxicity. These issues are practical considerations for the surgeon who performs combined cataract and glaucoma surgery infrequently.

## 77.5 Recent Trends in the Management of Patients with Cataract and Glaucoma

- Influence of clear-corneal phacoemulsification on surgical strategies
- Influence of the effectiveness of topical glaucoma medications
- Influence of the emergence of selective laser trabeculoplasty (SLT)

### 77.5.1 Clear-Corneal Phacoemulsification

An essential element in managing coexisting cataract and glaucoma is preserving the potential glaucoma surgery without any difficulties caused by first having cataract extraction. With ECCE and a scleral tunnel approach for phacoemulsification, the conjunctiva is incised. This frequently leads to scarring of the conjunctiva to the underlying episcleral tissues, making it difficult to perform an adequate dissection for a trabeculectomy and often compromising its outcome.

Clear-corneal phacoemulsification obviates the need for conjunctival dissection and preserves the conjunctiva should glaucoma surgery be subsequently required. A temporal incision avoids the necessity of operating over the brow, especially in deeply set eyes, and reduces induced astigmatism. In addition, patients who are taking anticoagulants can, if medically indicated, proceed with surgery without stopping their medications. Performing the corneal incision correctly is important in maintaining the stability of the wound and preventing endophthalmitis. An ocular coherence tomography (OCT) study of clear-corneal incisions demonstrated that appropriately performed incisions were self-sealing and that stromal hydration lasted up to 24 h after surgery.[16] Because of the technical advantages of temporal, clear-corneal phacoemulsification – in addition to its effect on IOP reduction – many surgeons have adopted this method for cataract surgery in eyes with mild-to-moderate glaucoma.

### 77.5.2 Topical Medications

The introduction of the prostaglandin analogs to the US market in 1996 has led to a significant effect on the practice pattern recommendations for the medical treatment of glaucoma. The prostaglandin analogs latanoprost, bimatoprost, and travoprost effectively reduce IOP with virtually no systemic side effects. Once-daily dosing simplifies the usage regimen and promotes better compliance and adherence. These drugs reduce IOP primarily through an increase in uveoscleral outflow, which distinguishes their mechanism of action from other outflow enhancing drugs. Following their introduction, the effectiveness with which prostaglandin analogs controlled IOP (either alone or with other glaucoma medications) resulted in a reduction in the incidence of glaucoma surgeries.[17,18]

Drug formulations that combine beta-blockers with prostaglandin analogs (not available in the USA), carbonic anhydrase inhibitors, or alpha-agonists have also gained in popularity and are welcomed agents for medically controlling IOP. The availability of the variety of these drugs for reducing IOP has influenced the trend toward performing cataract surgery alone as an initial step for patients with coexisting disease. If the IOP cannot be controlled after clear-corneal phacoemulsification, glaucoma surgery can be performed as a staged procedure.

### 77.5.3 Selective Laser Trabeculoplasty

Selective laser trabeculoplasty (SLT) utilizes a frequency-doubled, Q-switched Nd:YAG laser applied to the trabecular meshwork to treat eyes with ocular hypertension. Studies comparing SLT with argon laser trabeculoplasty (ALT) demonstrate equal IOP reduction, but patients report greater comfort with the SLT procedure.[19,20] The laser energy in SLT is absorbed by intracytoplasmic pigment granules resulting in trabecular cell destruction. This mechanism of action does not produce coagulative damage as seen with ALT, and may be the rationale behind the observation that SLT can be performed multiple times even in eyes that have had previous ALT. SLT can be used preoperatively to reduce the IOP prior to cataract surgery. Cataract surgery alone can frequently be performed in eyes treated with SLT alone or in addition to topical medications.

The goal of any surgical intervention is to perform a procedure that is technically akin to a standard operation. In the case of cataract surgery, this technique is clear-corneal phacoemulsification. If we can create an environment in which most of the surgery in eyes with coexisting conditions permits us to do this operation, the outcomes should be optimal. Using a clear-corneal incision, newer glaucoma medications, and SLT when necessary can help achieve this goal.

## 77.6 Surgical Techniques

### 77.6.1 Pupil Management

Many patients with glaucoma have pupils that do not dilate adequately to perform cataract surgery without difficulty. In some instances, dilation is poor because the patient has chronically been on miotic agents. Other eyes may have posterior synechiae as a consequence of inflammation, chronic angle closure, or prior laser procedures. The pupils of older patients may not dilate well. Many patients with pseudoexfoliation syndrome have inadequate pupil dilation because of infiltration of the iris with the pseudoexfoliation material. Preoperative assessment to determine the cause of an inadequately dilated pupil is important in planning the surgical procedure. In each of these situations, the goal is to achieve a pupil of adequate dimension to make an appropriately sized capsulorhexis for an uncomplicated phacoemulsification to be performed.

#### 77.6.1.1 Preoperative Steps for Pupil Management

Prior to cataract surgery, any miotic drug the patient may have been using should be discontinued. The ability of the pupil to dilate well should be determined in the office during the preoperative visit. Both topical cycloplegic-mydriatics and sympathomimetic agents should be administered to assess dilation of the pupil. Pharmacologic dilation might break posterior synechiae preoperatively and make intraoperative maneuvers easier. Even if adequate pupil dilation is not achieved by this preoperative office regimen, it allows the surgeon to plan an intraoperative pupil management strategy. Preoperative use of nonsteroidal anti-inflammatory drugs, starting 3–5 days before the scheduled surgery, as well as on the day of surgery, is also beneficial in promoting pupil maintenance during the procedure. Also, there is the potential benefit of topical nonsteroidal anti-inflammatory drugs helping to prevent postoperative cystoid macular edema that may occur after cataract extraction.[21]

#### 77.6.1.2 Operative Measures

Miotic pupils are frequently a consequence of inflammatory membranes that form between the iris and the anterior lens capsule. The presence of a membrane may not be recognized until all posterior synechiae are lysed. A cyclodialysis spatula is introduced through the paracentesis incision. It passes over the iris, parallel to the iris plane, until the tip of the spatula engages the synechiae at the pupil margin. Gently placing the tip of the spatula under the iris will separate the synechiae. Moving the instrument around the circumference of the pupil – at times via an additional incision – will free the pupil. In the presence of a pupillary membrane, it may be difficult to engage the synechiae and separate them. In this instance, first fill the anterior chamber with an ophthalmic viscoelastic device (OVD), then try to mobilize an edge with fine forceps and strip the membrane. If the cyclodialysis spatula cannot accomplish this maneuver, the hooked end of a 25-gage needle can be used to make a tiny nick in the membrane, which can then be grasped with fine forceps in order to peel the membrane. Care must be taken to ensure that the anterior capsule is not damaged.

Another method of obtaining additional mydriasis intraoperatively is by instilling nonpreserved 1:10,000 epinephrine beneath the iris sphincter. OVDs are extremely helpful in widening the pupil and in maintenance of pupil dilation throughout the procedure. We have had our best success with viscoadaptive and viscodispersive agents. Once the OVD is instilled around the circumference of the pupil margin, the surgeon can determine whether the pupil is adequately sized or if other surgical options should be undertaken.

#### 77.6.1.3 Mechanical Pupil Widening

- Radial sphincterotomy
- Multiple sphincterotomies
- Partial radial sphincterotomy with preplaced suture
- Multiple incomplete mini-sphincterotomies
- Pupil-stretching techniques
- Pupil maintainers

There are several techniques for widening the pupil that were popular when the extracapsular technique was the predominant method for cataract extraction. A *radial sphincterotomy* is made by extending an incision from a peripheral iridectomy through the sphincter. The iridectomy would either be left open, if adequately covered by the upper lid, or would be sutured to reconstruct the iris. This method is satisfactory for producing a large pupil intraoperatively, but often causes unwanted images and glare. If this option is chosen it is best done through a superior approach. Performing *multiple sphincterotomies* is another way to widen the pupil and yet retain its circular shape. While this technique produces a good surgical field, it often leaves the eye with a large pupil that lacks the normal pupillary response to light. Although these methods offer intraoperative benefits, they each have postoperative side effects, including prolonged inflammation and glare.

There are currently newer techniques to enlarge the pupil and retain pupillary function. One method is a *partial radial sphincterotomy with a preplaced suture*. This technique was originally described by Sam Masket. A suture is placed through the distal iris in the following fashion: The suture passes into the anterior chamber through the cornea and into iris substance. The needle then passes out of the iris and then out through clear cornea. A central loop of suture is retrieved through a peripheral corneal incision. A partial sphincterotomy is then made to widen the pupil. After phacoemulsification and IOL implantation, the suture is tied and the iris reconstructed.

Another method is the creation of *multiple incomplete mini-sphincterotomies*. This technique, introduced by Howard Fine, involves widening the pupil by making small incomplete sphincterotomies with a Rapazzo scissors. The incisions are made superficially so that they do not involve the full extent of the sphincter. Once the incisions have been made, the pupil is stretched to the iris root using either a Kuglen or a Graether hook. After IOL implantation, a Sinskey hook is used to engage the iris to reform the pupil.

Perhaps the most popular method of dealing with the miotic pupil is via *pupil stretching*. There are several methods for stretching the pupil. The simplest technique involves using iris hooks – such as Kuglen, Barrett, or Graether hooks – to perform bimanual, bidirectional pupil dilation (Fig. 77.1a, b). Two paracentesis incisions are placed about 90° from the phacoemulsification incision. The anterior chamber is filled with an OVD. Two hooks are introduced through the incisions so that the right hand hook engages the sphincter on the left side and vice versa (Fig. 77.2a). Steady, smooth movement of the hooks in opposite directions mechanically dilates the pupil bidirectionally (Fig. 77.2b). One hook is then removed and placed through the main incision. Each hook engages the sphincter and stretches the pupil in a direction at right angles to the initial stretch. The hooks are then removed and OVD is injected at the edge of the pupillary margin to ensure adequate pupil size for the remainder of the procedure.

There are also mechanical devices – such as the Beehler two- or three-point pupil dilators or the Keuch two-point dilator – that effectively widen the pupil. These devices are introduced through the phacoemulsification incision into an OVD-filled chamber. Each device contains a small hook that engages the proximal iris and upon activation of a sliding device, two or three arms (depending on the specific device) extend to engage the pupil margin and then stretch it to the iris root (Fig. 77.3). These devices effectively dilate the pupil. As with dilation with iris hooks some bleeding may occur, particularly with very small pupils. Regardless of the specific set of hooks or device employed, slow deliberate stretching minimizes the development of significant sphincter tears.

If the pupil cannot be adequately dilated by the methods previously mentioned, another option is to use a *pupil maintainer*. The most frequently used pupil maintainers are *flexible iris retractors*. These are placed in a diamond-shaped pattern at the 3, 6, 9, and 12 o'clock positions. Assuming that the cataract procedure is being performed from a temporal approach, the phaco incision is made anterior to the clear-corneal incision for the temporal retractor. Once the flexible retractors

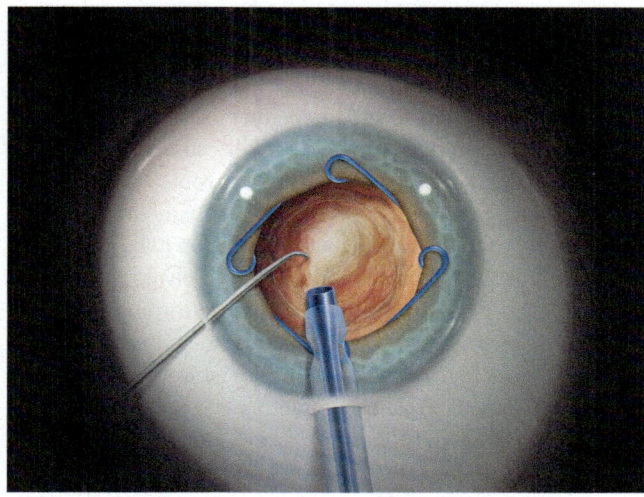

**Fig. 77.1** (**a**, **b**) Iris hooks used to expand the pupil

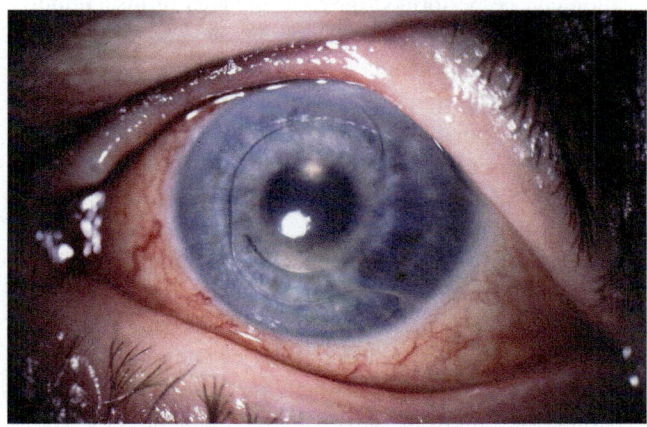

**Fig. 77.2** Pupil-stretching technique. (**a**) The right hand hook engages the sphincter on the left side and vice versa. (**b**) Movement of the hooks in opposite directions dilates the pupil bidirectionally

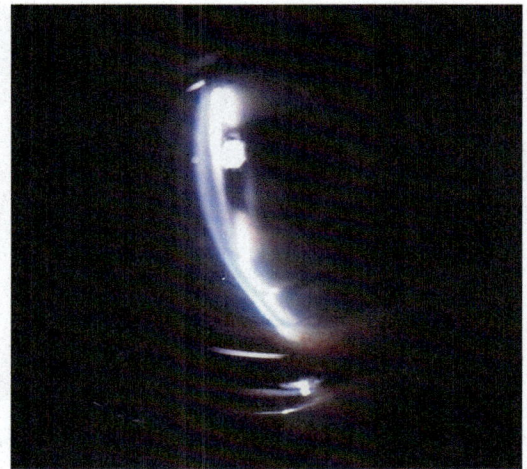

**Fig. 77.3** The Beehler three-point pupil dilator

have been introduced with their hooked ends engaging the sphincter, they are retracted to stretch the pupil by sliding the plastic disk along the shaft of the retractor into the proper position. The incisions should neither be too beveled nor positioned too anteriorly, since this will cause the iris to tent upward rather than be moved to the iris root. The diamond-shaped pupil opening (as opposed to a square-shaped pupillary aperture) allows for phacoemulsification to be performed over a relatively flat area of the iris, which minimizes the potential for iris chafing and iris prolapse through the main wound.[22] Richard Mackool has also designed self-retaining metal iris retractors that are used in a fashion similar to that described for the flexible iris retractors.

The *Morcher pupil dilating ring* is a device loaded into a syringe-like introducer that is placed in an OVD-filled anterior chamber. The dilating ring resumes its circular shape while engaging the pupillary margin when the plunger is depressed. The ring does not form a complete circle so that phacoemulsification can be performed through this area of discontinuity. Upon completion of IOL implantation, one end of the device is elevated and the cannula is reintroduced to engage a positioning hole on the ring that is then withdrawn into the cannula and removed from the anterior chamber.

The *Malyugin ring* is a new device that utilizes the principle of the diamond-shaped pupil (Fig. 77.4). The ring collapses into a flattened introducer. When the ring is inserted, four separate two-planed loop-like protrusions at the 12, 3, 6, and 9 o'clock positions engage the iris to form a diamond-shaped pupil. The ring is removed by mobilizing the temporal loop, reengaging the insertion device and retracting it.

The different methods available to dilate a pupil for phacoemulsification are all satisfactory.[23] Each surgeon should try these various methods to decide which one works best for him or her.

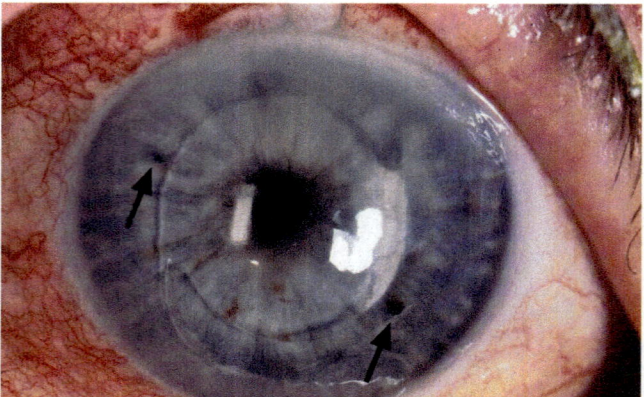

**Fig. 77.4** A pupil maintainer, such as the Malyugin ring, can be used to dilate the pupil. (Illustration courtesy of Microsurgical Technology, Redmond, WA)

## 77.6.2 Combined Surgery

### 77.6.2.1 Single-Site Surgery

Single-site surgery incorporates both the phacoemulsification and trabeculectomy procedures within a superiorly situated incision. Anesthesia can be achieved via either retrobulbar injection, peribulbar injection, or with the application of topical 4% Xylocaine and intracameral nonpreserved Xylocaine introduced through the paracentesis incision. A fornix-based flap is bluntly dissected superiorly to accommodate the placement of multiple pledgets of antimetabolite when indicated. The anterior portion of the dissection leaves a portion of the conjunctiva attached to the cornea. Light cautery is applied to produce hemostasis in the area intended for creating the superficial scleral flap. An incision about 2.5 mm posterior to the limbus and 4 mm in length is made with a diamond blade to about 50% scleral depth. An angulated crescent blade is used to dissect the entire width of the scleral pocket forward into clear cornea. If antimetabolites are being employed, two small portions of a corneal shield soaked in mitomycin-C (0.4 mg/ml) or 5-FU (50 mg/ml) are then placed beneath the conjunctiva, superior to the scleral incision. They are usually left in place for 2 min, although there are many different approaches to dose, exposure time, and technique for the application of mitomycin-C. It is important not to expose the conjunctival edge to the mitomycin-C. After removing the pledgets, the area is copiously irrigated with balanced salt solution.

A clear-corneal paracentesis incision is made for the second instrument. One percent nonpreserved Xylocaine is instilled intracamerally through this incision and an OVD is injected. A keratome enters the anterior chamber at the anterior aspect of the scleral tunnel. If the pupil is adequately dilated, a capsulorhexis is performed using a cystotome and capsulorhexis forceps. (Should the pupil not be adequately dilated the options outlined in the section on *Pupil Management* can be undertaken.) Hydrodissection and hydrodelineation using balanced saline and a 26-gage cannula are performed. The authors make an effort to perform sufficient hydrodelineation so that the nucleus is easily rotated. This is particularly important in eyes with pseudoexfoliation syndrome.

Phacoemulsification is then performed by the surgeon's favored technique. This subject has currently engendered significant debate, with one group favoring a bimanual technique while others prefer coaxial phacoemulsification. It is beyond the scope of this chapter to enter into this debate. Regardless of the specific technique used, best efforts should be made to remove the cataract as efficiently as possible. Following phacoemulsification of the nucleus, the cortex is removed by the irrigation/aspiration handpiece. The posterior capsule should be polished or vacuumed of any remaining cortical or posterior subcapsular remnants. The anterior chamber and capsular bag are filled with an OVD and the desired IOL is implanted within the capsular bag either with lens forceps or an inserting device. The authors currently implant an acrylic IOL with aspheric properties, a lens which enhances contrast sensitivity. There are several intraocular lenses available that have the potential for multifocal vision but there is little published data reporting how these lenses behave in eyes with visual field defects. Until these data become available, we have opted to provide our glaucoma patients with the best quality vision that can be provided with a monofocal IOL.

After IOL implantation, the authors make two radial incisions at the extremities of the scleral pocket, toward but not reaching the limbus, with Vannas scissors. A Kelly punch is used to create a sclerostomy by removing one or more pieces of tissue. The OVD is then removed by irrigation and aspiration. Miochol is instilled into the anterior chamber to constrict the pupil. A peripheral iridectomy is performed using a nontoothed jeweler's forceps and Vannas scissors, and the area is then irrigated to remove as much pigment as possible to assess the patency of the iridectomy. The superior corners of the scleral flap are sutured in place with interrupted 10-0 nylon sutures. The conjunctiva is apposed to the limbus using two peripheral wing 10-0 nylon sutures and a central horizontal mattress suture. Balanced saline solution is then injected through the paracentesis site to deepen the anterior chamber and to assess filtration by observing fluid accumulation under the conjunctiva in the area of the sclerostomy. Using sterile fluorescein, a Seidel test is performed to confirm water-tight closure of the conjunctiva. The paracentesis incision is then hydrated to ensure a good seal.

### 77.6.2.2 Two-Site Surgery

The two-site procedure separates the cataract operation from the trabeculectomy. Phacoemulsification is performed through a temporal clear-corneal incision following the surgeon's standard fashion. The steps for pupil management as have previously been described are followed. After IOL implantation, the OVD is removed and Miochol is instilled into the anterior chamber. The authors prefer to suture the corneal incision with a single 10-0 nylon suture.

The surgeon then moves superiorly to perform the trabeculectomy at the 12 o'clock position. The trabeculectomy is done as described for the single-site operation. Care should be taken that the incision into the anterior chamber is constructed in a fashion that allows easy placement of the Kelly punch so that an adequate piece of tissue is removed. Frequently, the entry incision is too beveled, making it difficult to use the punch. A modification of this technique described by Gary Condon involves placing the incision in a slightly more posterior location so that the Kelly punch can be reversed and the punch made anteriorly. This maneuver removes an adequate piece of tissue and minimizes the risk of damaging the ciliary body. Closure of the scleral flap and conjunctiva is performed as previously described.

### 77.6.3 Cataract Surgery in the Presence of a Filtering Bleb

Cataract surgery in patients with a filtering bleb should be approached with special care and an abundance of caution. Inadvertent trauma to the bleb may lead to bleb leaks, and postoperative inflammation can induce bleb failure. When performing phacoemulsification in the presence of a filtering bleb, we recommend a temporal clear-corneal incision to minimize the risk of trauma to the bleb. For the same reason, it is important to place the paracenteses at appropriate locations to minimize bleb contact. During phacoemulsification, the bottle height and fluidics should be managed appropriately to avoid intraoperative hypotony and collapse of the bleb. At the conclusion of the case, we recommend suturing the main wound to avoid any risk of postoperative leaks.

Postoperative subconjunctival injections of 5-fluorouracil or mitomycin-C are helpful in preventing bleb failure after cataract surgery. These agents are of particular importance in cases where bleb filtration was already limited prior to cataract extraction. These eyes often require intense topical steroids (often hourly or every 2 h) to avoid excessive inflammation leading to bleb failure.

In cases where the filtration is minimal, a few options exist. One is to perform a bleb revision combined with cataract extraction. This can be done by inserting a 27- or 30-gage needle through the conjunctiva posterior to the bleb and advancing it toward the bleb in order to break up any episcleral scar tissue. Care should be taken to avoid creating a conjunctival buttonhole. The needle can then be advanced underneath the scleral flap and into the anterior chamber to break up any fibrotic tissue within the scleral flap. Another surgical option is to perform an *ab interno* bleb revision. After completing cataract extraction, the anterior chamber is filled with viscoelastic. A cyclodialysis spatula is inserted through a paracentesis incision, into the sclerostomy, and under the scleral flap. Gentle side-to-side motion is used to elevate the scleral flap and separate the conjunctival tissue adjacent to the bleb. Alternatively, if bleb fibrosis is very advanced, cataract extraction combined with a new trabeculectomy can be preformed as previously described. As described elsewhere in the text, bleb needling has been used as well.

### 77.6.4 Other Types of Combined Surgery

Trabeculectomy is the glaucoma procedure most commonly combined with a cataract operation today. Other procedures that provide favorable outcomes with respect to visual acuity and IOP control have recently been described. In recent years, trabeculotomy, deep sclerectomy, viscocanalostomy, canaloplasty, and the use of tube-shunt devices have all been combined with phacoemulsification. For the most part, the evidence-based data on these procedures is limited to case reports and consequently reflect the experience of a few skilled surgeons. Whether ophthalmologists will adopt one or more of these procedures will depend on the relative ease of performing the procedure (since several of them have greater complexity than trabeculectomy) and demonstration that the results obtained are equal to or better than those currently published.

## 77.7 Prostaglandin Analogs and Pseudophakic Cystoid Macular Edema

Cystoid macular edema (CME) is a known complication of cataract extraction. It has been suggested that aphakic and pseudophakic CME occurs due to the synthesis of endogenous prostaglandins. Prostaglandins are metabolic products that are derived from the breakdown of arachidonic acid. They function as inflammatory mediators and promote the breakdown of the blood–ocular barrier. Surgical trauma to the iris, ciliary body, or lens epithelial cells induces the synthesis of prostaglandins in the aqueous humor. This can be particularly significant in individuals with preexisting breakdown of the blood–aqueous barrier as is the case in patients with diabetes, uveitis, and multiple ocular surgeries.

The synthesis of prostaglandins can be suppressed by treatment with nonsteroidal anti-inflammatory drugs (NSAIDs). Reduction of circulating prostaglandins is associated with fewer disruptions in the blood–aqueous and blood–retinal barriers, thereby decreasing the incidence of CME. For this reason, NSAIDS have become a first-line treatment for CME and are frequently being used preoperatively for the prevention of CME.

Does prostaglandin analog use for the treatment of glaucoma and ocular hypertension contribute to the development of pseudophakic CME? Evidence-based data in the literature is conflicting on this issue. Several isolated case reports have noted a correlation between prostaglandin analog use and pseudophakic CME. This has led to speculation that prostaglandin analogs may promote CME the same way that endogenous prostaglandins do. Based on this, some ophthalmologists advocate discontinuing prostaglandin analog therapy after cataract surgery, particularly in diabetics, patients who underwent complicated cataract surgery, and others who may be prone to developing CME.

However, the association between prostaglandin analog use and CME is not so clear-cut. Although Miyake and colleagues conducted a randomized study that implicated prostaglandin analogs in postcataract extraction CME,[24] a similar study that they conducted 2 years later found the same results with preserved timolol.[25] They concluded that the preservative benzalkonium chloride was responsible for the development of pseudophakic CME, as opposed to timolol or a prostaglandin analog. On the other hand, another recent randomized study reported breakdown of the blood–aqueous barrier after initiation of prostaglandin analog therapy in 80 aphakic and pseudophakic eyes. In this study, six eyes developed cystoid macular edema; and in each instance there was an open or absent posterior capsule confirming previous observations. All cases of CME resolved after discontinuation of the prostaglandin analog and treatment with NSAIDs.[26]

Because CME is reversible upon discontinuation of a prostaglandin analog, we do not advocate routinely discontinuing them after cataract surgery, particularly in situations where they are required to control IOP. Patients should be closely monitored for inflammation and visual acuity; frequent examinations of the posterior pole should be performed. Appropriate use of nonsteroidal and steroidal anti-inflammatory agents is essential in the postoperative period.

## References

1. Jampel H, Friedman DS, Lubomski LH, et al. Effect of technique on intraocular pressure after combined cataract and glaucoma surgery. *Ophthalmology*. 2002;109:2215–2224.
2. Panchapakesan J, Mitchell P, Tumuluri K, Rochtchina E, Foran S, Cumming RG. Five year incidence of cataract surgery: the Blue Mountains Eye Study. *Br J Ophthalmol*. 2003;87(2):168–172.
3. Krupin T, Feitl ME, Bishop KI. Postoperative intraocular pressure rise in open-angle glaucoma patients after cataract or combined cataract-filtration surgery. *Ophthalmology*. 1989;96:579–584.
4. Levkovitch-Verbin H, Habot-Wilner Z, Burla N, et al. Intraocular pressure elevation within the first 24 hours after cataract surgery in patients with glaucoma or exfoliation syndrome. *Ophthalmology*. 2008;115:104–108.
5. Pohjalainen T, Vesti E, Uusitalo RJ, et al. Phacoemulsification and intraocular lens implantation in eyes with open-angle glaucoma. *Acta Ophthalmol Scand*. 2001;79:313–316.
6. Brown SV, Thomas JV, Budenz DL, Bellows AR, Simmons RJ. Effect of cataract surgery on intraocular pressure reduction obtained with laser trabeculoplasty. *Am J Ophthalmol*. 1985;100(3): 373–376.
7. Tennen DG, Masket S. Short and long-term effect of clear corneal incision on intraocular pressure. *J Cataract Refract Surg*. 1996;22: 568–570.
8. Tong JT, Miller KM. Intraocular pressure change after sutureless phacoemulsification and foldable posterior chamber lens implantation. *J Cataract Refract Surg*. 1998;24:256–262.

9. Shingleton BJ, Gamell LS, O'Donoghue MW. Long-term changes in intraocular pressure after clear corneal phacoemulsification: normal patients versus glaucoma suspect and glaucoma patients. *J Cataract Refract Surg.* 1999;25:885–890.
10. Shingleton BJ, Pasternak JJ, Hung JW, et al. Three and five year changes in intraocular pressures after clear corneal phacoemulsification in open angle glaucoma patients, glaucoma suspects, and normal patients. *J Glaucoma.* 2006;15:494–498.
11. Kass MA. Cataract extraction in an eye with filtering bleb. *Ophthalmology.* 1982;89:871–874.
12. Rebolleda G, Muñoz-Negrete FJ. Phacoemulsification in eyes with functioning filtering blebs: a prospective study. *Ophthalmology.* 2002;109(12):2248–2255.
13. Hopkins JJ, Apel A, Trope GE, et al. Early intraocular pressure after phacoemulsification combined with trabeculectomy. *Ophthalmic Surg Lasers.* 1998;29:273–279.
14. Cotran PR, Roh S, McGwin G. Randomized comparison of 1-site and 2-site phacotrabeculectomy with 3-year follow-up. *Ophthalmology.* 2008;115:447–454.
15. Weitzman M, Caprioli J. Temporal corneal phacoemulsification with separate-incision superior trabeculectomy. *Ophthalmic Surg.* 1995;26:271–273.
16. Fine IH, Hoffman RS, Packer M. Profile of clear corneal cataract incisions demonstrated by ocular coherence tomography. *J Cataract Refract Surg.* 2007;33:94–97.
17. Bateman DN, Clark R, Azuara-Blanco A, et al. The effects of new topical treatments on management of glaucoma in Scotland: an examination of ophthalmological health care. *Br J Ophthalmol.* 2002;86:551–554.
18. Strutton DR, Walt JG. Trends in glaucoma surgery before and after the introduction of new topical glaucoma pharmacotherapies. *J Glaucoma.* 2004;13(3):221–226.
19. Damji KF, Shah KC, Rock WJ, et al. Selective laser trabeculoplasty v argon laser trabeculoplasty: a prospective randomised clinical trial. *Br J Ophthalmol.* 1999;83(6):718–722.
20. Martinez-de-la-Casa JM, Garcia-Feijoo J, Castillo A, et al. Selective vs argon laser trabeculoplasty: hypotensive efficacy, anterior chamber inflammation, and postoperative pain. *Eye.* 2004;18(5): 498–502.
21. O'Brien TP. Emerging guidelines for use of NSAID therapy to optimize cataract surgery patient care. *Curr Med Res Opin.* 2005;21(7): 1131–1137.
22. Oetting TA, Omphroy LC. Modified technique using flexible iris retractors in clear corneal cataract surgery. *J Cataract Refract Surg.* 2002;28:596–598.
23. Akman A, Yilmaz G, Oto S, et al. Comparison of various pupil dilatation methods for phacoemulsification in eyes with a small pupil secondary to pseudoexfoliation. *Ophthalmology.* 2004;111: 1693–1698.
24. Miyake K, Ota I, Maekuba K, et al. Latanoprost accelerates disruption of the blood-aqueous barrier and the incidence of angiographic cystoid macular edema in early postoperative pseudophakias. *Arch Ophthalmol.* 1999;117:34–40.
25. Miyake K, Ota I, Ibaraki N, et al. Enhanced disruption of the blood-aqueous barrier and the incidence of angiographic cystoid macular edema by topical timolol and its preservative in early postoperative pseudophakia. *Arch Ophthalmol.* 2001;119:387–394.
26. Arcieri ES, Santana A, Rocha FN, et al. Blood-aqueous barrier changes after the use of prostaglandin analogues in patients pseudophakia or aphakia. *Arch Ophthalmol.* 2005;123:186–192.

# Chapter 78
# Cataract Extraction as Treatment for Acute and Chronic Angle Closure Glaucomas

Baseer U. Khan

Many cases of primary angle closure glaucoma remain undetected or misdiagnosed obviating appropriate and optimal treatment. The value of routine gonioscopy in all patients to screen for occludable angles should not be understated. Early recognition and subsequent management of primary angle closure is almost always effectively curative.

The challenge in the management of primary angle closure begins with its definition. The criteria of glaucomatous optic neuropathy are fairly well defined; however, the classification of primary angle closure is not universally agreed upon. Foster et al[1] proposed a classification scheme that recognized pre-glaucomatous eyes: primary angle closure suspects and primary angle closure. In a meta-analysis of primary angle closure management, this classification was expanded by Saw et al[2] to create additional categories for acute presentations of primary angle closure. The resultant classification scheme is presented in Table 78.1. and used in this chapter.

The management of PAC (see Chap. 62, Fig. 62.1) is initiated with a laser peripheral iridotomy. Subsequent therapy may include argon laser peripheral iridoplasty for recalcitrant occludability and/or IOP lowering medication to treat elevated IOP secondary to synechial angle closure or a mixed mechanism etiology. Classically, patients requiring further surgical intervention have undergone trabeculectomy with or without a combined crystalline lens extraction. However, trabeculectomy in PAC has been reported to exhibit an increased risk of flat anterior chamber and malignant glaucoma, as well as higher rates of inflammation, particularly in the context of a past angle closure attack, all factors lending to a reduced success rate.[3]

## 78.1 The Lens in Angle Closure

In the absence of an anterior pulling mechanism or posterior segment pathology, the lens is central to the development of angle closure. With age, the anterior–posterior dimension of the lens increases along with an anterior shift in lens position potentiating angle closure in predisposed eyes.[1,4-9] The resultant mechanism of angle closure is pupil block, plateau iris, phacomorphic angle closure, or a combination of these entities.[10] If angle closure is primarily appositional, the first two entities are usually adequately treated by peripheral iridotomy and possible peripheral iridoplasty. However, persistent IOP elevation often exists if synechial closure is greater than 180° and surgical intervention is often required when greater than 270°.[11] Lens extraction, with or without the presence of a cataract, has emerged as an alternative or adjunctive modality in the management of PAC.

## 78.2 Mechanism of Action

The most recent evidenced-based review of angle closure management[2] rated the evidence for all surgical interventions (including both cataract extraction and trabeculectomy) to be C, III – the weakest rating (C: the recommendation may be relevant but cannot be definitely related to clinical outcome; III: a weak body of evidence insufficient to provide support for or against the efficacy of a test or therapy and that would generally apply to panel consensus or individual opinions, small non-comparative case series, and individual case reports). However, there is a growing body of evidence supporting crystalline lens extraction in the management of angle closure. The principal mechanism of action is readily apparent; replacement of the crystalline lens with a significantly thinner IOL effectively debulks the anterior segment, increasing angle depth, thereby exposing trabecular meshwork leading to increased outflow of aqueous.[12-14]

There is often a lowering of IOP following phacoemulsification in non-angle closure patients. These mechanisms would also likely contribute to IOP-lowering effect of phacoemulsification in PAC in addition to the primary mechanism. Irrigation of the anterior chamber during phacoemulsification is thought to flush out debris from the trabecular meshwork, thus reducing resistance to outflow.[15] Pressure from the haptics on the

**Table 78.1** Classification of angle closure[1,2]

| Diagnosis | Definition |
|---|---|
| Primary angle closure suspect | An eye in which appositional contact between the peripheral iris and posterior trabecular meshwork is considered possible[a] |
| Acute angle closure (AAC) | At least two of the following symptoms: ocular or periocular pain, nausea and/or vomiting, a history of intermittent blurring of vision with haloes, IOP 21 mmHg; and at least three of the following signs: conjunctival injection, corneal epithelial edema, mid-dilated unreactive pupil, shallow AC, presence of an occludable angle |
| Acute angle-closure glaucoma (AACG) | AAC with evidence of glaucoma (GON) as defined by Foster et al[1b] |
| Primary angle closure (PAC) | An eye with an occludable drainage angle and features indicating that trabecular obstruction by the peripheral iris has occurred, such as PAS, increased IOP, iris whorling, "glaucomfleken," lens opacities, or excessive pigment deposition on the trabecular surface, and the optic disc does not have glaucomatous damage |
| Primary angle closure glaucoma (PACG) | PAC with evidence of glaucoma (GON) as defined by Foster et al[1] |

[a]In epidemiological research, this has most often been defined as an angle in which >270° of the posterior trabecular meshwork (the part which is often pigmented) cannot be seen. This definition is arbitrary and its evaluation in longitudinal study is an important priority. Producing a more evidence based definition of this parameter is a major research priority.[1]

[b]Foster et al[1] defined glaucoma by both structural and functional evidence. Eyes with a CDR or CDR asymmetry >97.5th percentile for the normal population, or a neuroretinal rim width reduced to <0.1 CDR (between 11 and 1 o'clock or 5–7 o'clock) that also showed a definite visual field defect consistent with glaucoma. They also provided guidelines if structural and/or functional evaluation was not possible.

ciliary body is suggested to have a number of IOP-lowering effects; decrease in aqueous production, stretching of trabecular meshwork, traction on the zonules preventing collapse of Schlemm's canal as well as biochemical changes leading to alterations in the blood-aqueous barrier.[16-20]

## 78.3 Indications

### 78.3.1 Acute Angle Closure/Glaucoma

There is a paucity of literature evaluating the utility of phacoemulsification in the management of AAC. The only randomized control trial addressing this topic compared phacoemulsification to peripheral iridotomy in 62 eyes.[21] However, either intervention was only undertaken after the IOP had been reduced to less than 22 mmHg and anterior chamber inflammation had been settled with medical intervention; a mean of 5 days. Eyes undergoing phacoemulsification were significantly more likely to have an untreated IOP of less than 21 mmHg. Secondary outcomes demonstrated significant differences in Shaffer Gonioscopy grading and PAS formation in favor of phacoemulsification. There were no significant differences with respect to vertical cup-to-disc ratio, mean deviation, or pattern standard deviation at the 18-month conclusion of the study.

The rest of the literature evaluating the lens extraction to treat AAC consists of case reports and small series. It is thus not possible to stipulate the indications for lens extraction in the AAC, and more research is needed in this area to evaluate the efficacy and safety of this treatment algorithm.

### 78.3.2 Chronic Angle Closure/Glaucoma

Several studies have described phacoemulsification performed as a solo procedure to manage PAC/PACG.[22-26] All studies reported a significant reduction in IOP and in the number of medications required to lower IOP. Only one study[25] required that the lens have visually significant cataractous changes. The same study also reported a reduction PAS post-operatively, suggesting a passive lysis of PAS from irrigation and other mechanical forces generated during surgery. In all studies, patients included those that had controlled and elevated IOPs and did not stratify results as such – one study, however, reported that a higher pre-operative IOP and relatively deep AC pre-operatively correlated with a higher post-operative IOP.[23] It is worth noting that the mean (treated) preoperative IOP in all these studies was less than 21 mmHg, suggesting that the degree of angle closure and compromise was mild to moderate. The study duration ranged from 3 to 26 months in these studies, during which time none of the studies reported that the patient required further filtration surgery.

### 78.3.3 Adjunctive Procedures

#### 78.3.3.1 Goniosynechialysis

Three studies described performing goniosynechialysis (GSL) adjunctive to lens extraction in uncontrolled ACG secondary to near total or complete angle closure.[27-29] Only Lai et al[29] required that the eye manifest a visually significant cataract. This study also performed post-operatively laser iridoplasty to the inferior half of the iris where GSL was performed.

Teekhasanee et al[27] and Haraysymowycz[28] evaluated patients who had suffered AAC and had not been successfully treated with laser and medical therapy, with a mean time from AAC to surgery of 3 and 2 months respectively. The mean preoperative (and postoperative) IOPs were 29.7 (13.2), 40.7 (15.6), and 33.0(13.3) mmHg respectively. There was a significant reduction in the degree of PAS present and the number of medications required in each study – the majority of patients not requiring any postoperative medications. Across all three studies, only 2 of 75 eyes required subsequent filtration surgery. Complications were rare and were limited to increased postoperative inflammation and limited hyphemas. There is a general agreement that GSL is only effective if performed within 1 year of PAS formation; prolonged PAS formation is felt to be associated with scarring of the meshwork and iris proliferation into the meshwork.[11] However, the author has reported on the effectiveness of goniosynechialysis up to 720 days after first diagnosis.[36] Part of the difficulty with respect to timing is the determination of when PAS formation began.

### 78.3.3.2 Limited Pars Plana Vitrectomy

The AC in PAC eyes is often very shallow and crowded, increasing the complexity and risk of lens extraction. A limited pars plana vitrectomy (LPPV) can be performed to debulk the anterior vitreous enough to allow the anterior chamber to deepen.[30,31] These eyes are also susceptible to intraoperative aqueous misdirection giving rise to extensive posterior pressure. Performing an LPPV in this context can also be very effective. However, a choroidal hemorrhage must be considered with this presentation and must be ruled out before performing an LPPV.

### 78.3.3.3 Endocyclophotocoagulation (ECP)

ECP has been described as an adjunctive procedure to lens extraction to reduce aqueous production in mild to moderate glaucoma. It can potentially be employed in PAC eyes in which there is a plateau component to reduce the size of the anterior ciliary processes contributing to the plateau configuration.

### 78.3.3.4 Filtering Procedures

Combined lens extraction with a filtering procedure should be considered when significant optic neuropathy already exists. Both trabeculectomy[32] and deep sclerectomy[33] have been evaluated in the literature for this purpose. Both studies reported significant reduction in IOP; however, the deep sclerectomy study reported no cases of hypotony whereas the trabeculectomy study reported a rate of 19%. Performing deep sclerectomy in PACG requires that the closure that is appositional be relieved with lens extraction as synechial angle closure is a contraindication to non-penetrating surgery.

See Table 78.2. for a summary of indications for adjunctive procedures.

## 78.4 Technique

Performing phacoemulsification in the context of PAC warrants a number of considerations to minimize the risk of complications and adverse events that occur and a higher frequency as compared to routine cataract extraction.

**Table 78.2** Indications for adjunctive therapies

| Procedure | Indications | Special consideration and cautions |
|---|---|---|
| Lens removal only | • Persistent appositional closure despite LPI or ALPI. Minimal or no ACG or well controlled IOP on topical medications prior to surgery. | • Removal of a non-cataractous lens requires additional discussion with patient to explain rational for surgery. Hyperopic patients in this scenario are generally very happy patients post-operatively. |
| + Goniosynechialysis | • Synechial angle closure > 180° | • Increase post operative steroids<br>• Requires post-operative miotics<br>• Consider post-operative ALPI |
| + Limited Par Plana Vitrectomy | • Very shallow anterior chamber<br>• Excessive positive posterior pressure<br>• History of malignant glaucoma in fellow eye | • Careful not to damage posterior capsule<br>• Avoid over decompression<br>• Must rule out choroidal hemorrhage if performing due to build up of posterior pressure during surgery |
| + Endocyclophotocoagulation | • Prominent plateau iris configuration<br>• Mild to moderate ACG | • Titration of energy crucial<br>• Increase post-operative steroids |
| + Filtering procedures | • Advanced ACG | • Non-penetrating procedures should only be performed if appositional closure only<br>• Err on side of suturing flap tightly to avoid hypotony and aqueous misdirection |

These indications are based on the experience and practice of the author.

## 78.4.1 Principles

### 78.4.1.1 Anterior Chamber Stability

At all times the anterior chamber should remain pressurized. These eyes are particularly susceptible to choroidal hemorrhages and aqueous misdirection. Loss of anterior chamber pressure may result in either of these complications.

### 78.4.1.2 Manage Positive Posterior Pressure

Due to high IOP and crowded anterior segments, these patients invariably demonstrated positive posterior pressure. Attention to proper wound construction and usage of ophthalmic-viscoelastic devices is imperative. Occasionally, adjunctive procedures maybe required to further decompress the eye. Constant attention to the development of iris prolapse is also required as post-AAC irides are often atrophic and floppy.

### 78.4.1.3 Corneal Endothelium

These eyes are at a greater risk of post-operative corneal decompensation. The anterior chambers are typically shallow and therefore endothelial cells are more susceptible to phaco-injury. Furthermore, if the eye has already suffered an AAC attack, the endothelium has already been traumatized.

### 78.4.1.4 Beware of Zonular Compromise

Zonular incompetence is often present either as a cause or result of PAC. Zonular laxity can result in the anterior movement of the lens precipitating angle narrowing or AACG can result in compromise to the zonules. In the author's opinion, a capsular tension ring should be placed prior to IOL insertion in any eye that has suffered a previous AAC.

## 78.4.2 Preoperative Considerations

Preoperative treatment with IV mannitol or acetazolamide will reduce IOP and deturgess the vitreous minimizing the risk of choroidal hemorrhage and aqueous direction and reducing posterior pressure. Placing the patient in a slight reverse-Trendelenburg position on the operating table and using the minimal amount of tension on the lid speculum will also help to reduce posterior positive pressure.

While useful in routine cases, preoperative dilation of the pupil should be avoided, because it could exacerbate angle closure. Instead intra-cameral, non-preserved, 1% lidocaine injected in the anterior chamber would provide adequate dilation; non-preserved 0.5% phenylepinephrine can also be used.

## 78.4.3 Incisions

With the initial incision, care should be taken not to allow the chamber to shallow. Wound length should err on the side of being longer. Increased wound length will reduce OVD or irrigation solution loss when instruments are placed through the wound, also the anteriorization of the internal ostomy of the wound will reduce the incidence of iris prolapse. Consideration should be given to performing the capsulorhexis using intra-ocular microforceps, which can be inserted through a paracentesis prior to creating the main incision. This will further minimize loss of OVD during this step. Alternatively, the capsulorhexis can be performed using a cystotome through a paracentesis.

## 78.4.4 OVDs

The viscoelastic soft-shell technique[34] optimizes the various properties of cohesive and dispersive OVDs and is of particular utility in challenges that may present in phacoemulsification in a PAC eye. Briefly, the soft shell technique calls for the injection of a dispersive agent first and then the injection of a cohesive agent centrally and just anterior to the lens – pushing the dispersive against the cornea and peripherally. The cohesive OVD assists in deepening the anterior chamber and maintaining the space. The dispersive OVD coats the endothelium, protecting it from trauma from irrigating fluids and phacoemulsification energy. Coating iris with a dispersive agent will also reduce the risk of iris prolapse. Finally, dispersive agent will effectively trap the cohesive OVD centrally, reducing the risk of sudden expression of the cohesive agent through the main wound, thereby improving anterior chamber stability. Used instead of the cohesive agent, a super-cohesive OVD, such as Healon-5 (AMO) is particularly useful in these cases.

During phacoemulsification, the dispersive agent should be injected intermittently toward the cornea especially if the anterior chamber is particularly shallow, the lens very dense or there is a history of an AACG episode. Upon completion of phacoemulsification, before withdrawing the hand-piece, the cohesive agent should be injected into the eye to maintain the anterior chamber and prevent collapse while the hand-piece is exchanged for the irrigation and aspiration (IA) equipment. Finally, a cohesive agent should be injected at conclusion of irrigation and aspiration, to prevent collapse as well as to prepare for lens insertion. The use of a cohesive is especially important here as it mitigates the need to go posterior to the lens with the IA hand piece – a maneuver that requires a partial or complete collapse of the AC.

### 78.4.5 Capsulorhexis

Due to the anterior vaulting and positive posterior pressure in PAC eyes, there is greater propensity of the capsulorhexis to run out. To reduce this risk, size of the capsulorhexis should err on the smaller side – the capsulorhexis can be enlarged after lens insertion more safely. The use of a super-cohesive OVD, aside for the advantages listed above, will also help to lower the risk of running out the capsulorhexis. If vision blue is to be used, it should be injected under the OVD and not prior to OVD injection as the later can result in instability of the anterior chamber.

### 78.4.6 Iris

Chronic cholinergic usage may result in a phimotic pupil with posterior synechiae. Standard measures for managing small pupils may be under taken, but care should be made to minimize iris manipulation as much as possible as these eyes are at greater risk for post-operative inflammation, especially if there has been a recent history of AACG.

Conversely, the pupil may be atrophic and enlarged, increasing the risk of iris prolapse. A single iris hook, placed through a paracentesis made just posterior to the main incision will alleviate iris prolapse through the main wound.

### 78.4.7 Phacoemulsification and Irrigation and Aspiration

The author is of the opinion that a surgeon should not change flow and power parameters for challenging cases as this adds increased variability in a case that presents with altered characteristics. Rather attention to meticulous surgical technique should be observed. Keeping the phaco tip within the pupil margin will minimize dispersive OVD removal – maintaining the seal at the main wound and reducing iris floppiness. Minimizing posterior forces induced by the phaco tip and second instrument during nuclear manipulation will minimize iatrogenic trauma to the zonular complex.

Leakage through the main wound is usually minimal, however than can be considerable leakage through the paracentesis through which the second instrument is inserted in the eye. Though this leakage is usually inconsequential in routine cases and can be minimized by appropriate wound sizing, alternatively consideration should be given to bimanual phacoemulsification. This technique offers enhanced anterior chamber stability through minimizing leakage around instrumentation at the corneal wounds, especially at the second instrument site. While bimanual phacoemulsification is optional, bimanual IA is necessary. There is significant leakage around co-axial IA hand pieces. Bimanual IA significantly reduces leakage and improves anterior chamber stability. The creation of a second paracentesis to provide sub-paracentesis access to the primary site is often necessary and is inconsequential.

### 78.4.8 Postoperative Management

Routine postoperative medical management with an antibiotic, NSAID and steroid is often adequate. However, if there has been a past history of AAC or intra-operative iris manipulation was required, the frequency of steroid dosing should be increased. Post-operative corneal edema, if present, may be ameliorated with topical hypertonic solution or ointment. If goniosynechialysis was performed (see below), postoperative pilocarpine should be administered until post-operative inflammation has subsided to prevent reformation of peripheral anterior synechiae.

Postoperative laser peripheral iridoplasty has also been described. See Chap. 61 for indications and techniques.

## 78.5 Adjunctive Procedures

### 78.5.1 Goniosynechialysis

After insertion of IOL, a miosis-inducing agent such as Miochol is injected into the anterior chamber. Mechanical manipulation of the iris may be required if the pupil is atonic after an AAC. The chamber is then deepened using a cohesive viscoelastic – if the PAS are weak, this alone may result in GSL.[35] Inspection and view of the angle require an intraoperative gonio lens. Classically, this was done with direct lenses such as the Swan-Jacob or Barkan lens. While these lenses provide good visualization of the angle, they require intraoperative tilting of the patient's head and microscope to gain view to the entire angle. Alternatively, the author's preference is to use an indirect intraoperative gonio lens such as the Maxfield AC Four Mirror or the Osher Surgical Gonio Posterior Pole Lenses. Once the PAS have been identified intraoperatively, a blunt instrument, such as a Swan knife, under visualization is pressed against the most peripheral iris adjacent to the point of adhesion, and then a posterior sweeping motion is made, lysing the PAS, until the trabecular meshwork is exposed.[27] The technique requires precise placement of the tip of the knife; if the tip is too proximal, tissue may be left, if too distal the trabecular mesh work or ciliary body may be damaged. The author's preference is to use the intraocular Ahmed Micro-graspers (MST, Redmond, Washington). In this technique, peripheral iris is grasped with the forceps, and under visualization, a centripetal and slightly posterior force is applied to the iris, disinserting the iris, until the scleral spur is exposed.[36] This is done up to 360°, as required, inserting the forceps through either the main wound or the side port incision.

The most common complication in GSL is a localized hyphema usually a result of overly aggressive disinsertion of the iris. This is easily managed by tamponading the hemorrhage by pressuring the AC with a cohesive OVD. Overly aggressive manipulation of the iris can result in irido- or cyclo-dialysis; however, this is very uncommon. As mentioned, post-operative management should include increased steroid dosing, topical miotic therapy, and possible peripheral laser iridoplasty – all modalities directed to minimize recurrence of PAS formation.

### 78.5.2 Limited Pars Plana Vitrecomy

The LPPV can be performed at any point of the procedure according to the indications discussed above. The optimal location to perform a LPPV is in the infero-temporal quadrant. Here access is optimized while preserving superior conjunctiva that will be important if a filtering procedure is required subsequently. Sub-conjunctival injection of anesthetic should provide adequate anesthesia, although patient may feel the MVR incision and should be advised as such. The MVR incision should be 4 mm posterior to the limbus and therefore the peritomy should be created accordingly. The MVR blade should be aimed toward the optic nerve and inserted until visualized posterior to the lens if the density of the cataract permits visualization. If there is significant liquification of the vitreous, fluid may be liberated – the surgeon should look for a flow of fluid out of the sclerostomy site. Digital assessment of the anterior chamber pressure and observed deepening of the AC are objective signs that will indicate to the surgeon if the posterior segment has been significantly decompressed.

If minimal to no change has occurred, a LPPV is required. The cut rate should be at the highest frequency setting, the flow rate low (20 cc/min), and vacuum should be minimal (100 mmHg). Bottle height is irrelevant as there is no infusion of fluid into the eye in this procedure. The vitrectomy sequence should be set to ICA (Irrigation-Cut-Aspiration). The vitrector only (any irrigation sleeve should be removed) should be inserted carefully in the same direction as wound was created – toward the optic nerve to avoid inadvertent damage to the lens. This can be minimized, in the author's opinion, if the vitrector is positioned so that the cutter is facing posteriorly. Often the lip of the incision must be grasped by a 0.12 forceps to facilitate insertion of the vitrector. The vitrector should be inserted until the tip can be visualized posterior to the lens. The vitrectomy should then be performed in 5 s increments – every 5 s, the surgeon should reassess AC depth and IOP as described previously. This should be continued until a reasonable outcome has been achieved. Excessive debulking of vitreous will result in an undesirably deep AC, particularly if there is zonular instability, which presents a separate set of technical challenges.

Once an acceptable end point has been reached, OVD should be injected in the AC to ensure adequate AC depth and pressurization. The sclerostomy should be checked to ensure it is free of vitreous. If vitreous is present, the vitrector can be used on the surface of the sclera to remove it. The sclerostomy should be closed with an 8–0 Vicryl in a shoe tie knot – this can be released and a further vitrectomy can be performed later in the case if required. Upon completion of the case, the suture is then permanently tied and the conjunctiva closed in a routine fashion. The newer 25 gauge systems do not require sutured closure.

### 78.5.3 Endocyclophotocoagulation

After insertion of the endocapsular IOL insertion, a cohesive OVD is injected in the sulcus. The ECP probe is then inserted through the main wound and the tip is positioned in the sulcus. Through the endoscopic view, laser energy is applied to the ciliary processes, particularly anteriorly to shrink and rotate the processes away from the posterior iris. The energy applied to the ciliary process needs to be titrated to achieve the desired outcome: too little energy will induce little to no effect; too much energy will cause the ciliary process to burst and bleed. The titration of energy is achieved by establishing the correct distance from the tip of the probe to the ciliary process; the distance is inversely proportional to degree of burn.

Complications from ECP are usually minimal and self-limiting; small hyphema and prolonged inflammation. Patients should receive a higher frequency of steroids in the immediate post-operative phase until inflammation subsides.

### 78.5.4 Filtration Procedures

Any number of filtration procedures can be performed adjunctive to lens removal, the descriptions of which are beyond the scope of this chapter. One procedural consideration worth mentioning is to err on the side of suturing the scleral flap too tight (where applicable). This reduces the risk of post-operative hypotony, flat anterior chamber, and aqueous misdirection; adverse events to which PAC eye are more susceptible.

## 78.6 Conclusion

Primary angle closure glaucoma is a subset of glaucoma that can be cured by the appropriate interventions. The earlier the risk of PAC and PACG are realized by the clinician, the lower the morbidity associated with required intervention, once again emphasizing the vigilance of both establishing better diagnostic criteria as well as performing routine gonioscopy.

The aging changes that the crystalline undergoes are central to the pathophysiology of PAC. The age of the patient at the time of presentation often coincides with the development of visual deterioration and presbyopia. Replacement of the crystalline lens with an IOL offers patients a relatively safe and curative procedure that has the ancillary benefit of improving a patient's vision.

## References

1. Foster PJ. The epidemiology of primary angle closure and associated glaucomatous optic neuropathy. *Semin Ophthalmol.* 2002;17(2): 50–58. Review.
2. Saw SM, Gazzard G, Friedman DS. Interventions for angle-closure glaucoma: an evidence-based update. *Ophthalmology.* 2003;110(10): 1869–1878. quiz 1878–9, 1930. Review.
3. Aung T, Tow SL, Yap EY, Chan SP, Seah SK. Trabeculectomy for acute primary angle closure. *Ophthalmology.* 2000;107(7):1298–1302.
4. Lowe RF. Causes of shallow anterior chamber in primary angle-closure glaucoma. Ultrasonic biometry of normal and angle-closure glaucoma eyes. *Am J Ophthalmol.* 1969;67(1):87–93.
5. Lowe RF. Aetiology of the anatomical basis for primary angle-closure glaucoma. Biometrical comparisons between normal eyes and eyes with primary angle-closure glaucoma. *Br J Ophthalmol.* 1970;54(3): 161–169.
6. Friedman DS, Gazzard G, Foster P, et al. Ultrasonographic biomicroscopy, Scheimpflug photography, and novel provocative tests in contralateral eyes of Chinese patients initially seen with acute angle closure. *Arch Ophthalmol.* 2003;121(5):633–642.
7. Markowitz SN, Morin JD. The ratio of lens thickness to axial length for biometric standardization in angle-closure glaucoma. *Am J Ophthalmol.* 1985;99(4):400–402.
8. Markowitz SN, Morin JD. Angle-closure glaucoma: relation between lens thickness, anterior chamber depth and age. *Can J Ophthalmol.* 1984;19(7):300–302.
9. Wojciechowski R, Congdon N, Anninger W, Teo Broman A. Age, gender, biometry, refractive error, and the anterior chamber angle among Alaskan Eskimos. *Ophthalmology.* 2003;110(2):365–375.
10. Ritch R, Liebmann JM, Tellow C. A construct for understanding angle closure glaucoma: the role of ultrasound biomicroscopy. *Ophthalmol Clin North Am.* 1995;8:281–293.
11. Campbell DG, Vela A. Modern goniosynechialysis for the treatment of synechial angle-closure glaucoma. *Ophthalmology.* 1984;91(9): 1052–1060.
12. Hayashi K, Hayashi H, Nakao F, Hayashi F. Changes in anterior chamber angle width and depth after intraocular lens implantation in eyes with glaucoma. *Ophthalmology.* 2000;107(4):698–703.
13. Kurimoto Y, Park M, Sakaue H, Kondo T. Changes in the anterior chamber configuration after small-incision cataract surgery with posterior chamber intraocular lens implantation. *Am J Ophthalmol.* 1997;124(6):775–780.
14. Meyer MA, Savitt ML, Kopitas E. The effect of phacoemulsification on aqueous outflow facility. *Ophthalmology.* 1997;104(8):1221–1227.
15. Kim DD, Doyle JW, Smith MF. Intraocular pressure reduction following phacoemulsification cataract extraction with posterior chamber lens implantation in glaucoma patients. *Ophthalmic Surg Lasers.* 1999;30(1):37–40.
16. Kooner KS, Cooksey JC, Perry P, Zimmerman TJ. Intraocular pressure following ECCE, phacoemulsification, and PC-IOL implantation. *Ophthalmic Surg.* 1988;19(9):643–646.
17. Steuhl KP, Marahrens P, Frohn C, Frohn A. Intraocular pressure and anterior chamber depth before and after extracapsular cataract extraction with posterior chamber lens implantation. *Ophthalmic Surg.* 1992;23(4):233–237.
18. Hansen TE, Naeser K, Rask KL. A prospective study of intraocular pressure four months after extracapsular cataract extraction with implantation of posterior chamber lenses. *J Cataract Refract Surg.* 1987;13(1):35–38.
19. Hansen TE, Naeser K. Nilsen NE Intraocular pressure 2 1/2 years after extracapsular cataract extraction and sulcus implantation of posterior chamber intraocular lens. *Acta Ophthalmol (Copenh).* 1991;69(2):225–228.
20. Miyake K, Asakura M, Kobayashi H. Effect of intraocular lens fixation on the blood-aqueous barrier. *Am J Ophthalmol.* 1984;98(4):451–455.
21. Lam DS, Leung DY, Tham CC, et al. Randomized trial of early phacoemulsification versus peripheral iridotomy to prevent intraocular pressure rise after acute primary angle closure. *Ophthalmology.* 2008;115(7):1134–1140.
22. Hata H, Yamane S, Hata S, Shiota H. Preliminary outcomes of primary phacoemulsification plus intraocular lens implantation for primary angle-closure glaucoma. *J Med Invest.* 2008;55(3–4):287–291.
23. Liu CJ, Cheng CY, Wu CW, Lau LI, Chou JC, Hsu WM. Factors predicting intraocular pressure control after phacoemulsification in angle-closure glaucoma. *Arch Ophthalmol.* 2006;124(10):1390–1394.
24. Euswas A, Warrasak S. Intraocular pressure control following phacoemulsification in patients with chronic angle closure glaucoma. *J Med Assoc Thai.* 2005;88(suppl 9):S121–S125.
25. Lai JS, Tham CC, Chan JC. The clinical outcomes of cataract extraction by phacoemulsification in eyes with primary angle-closure glaucoma (PACG) and co-existing cataract: a prospective case series. *J Glaucoma.* 2006;15(1):47–52.
26. Kubota T, Toguri I, Onizuka N, Matsuura T. Phacoemulsification and intraocular lens implantation for angle closure glaucoma after the relief of pupillary block. *Ophthalmologica.* 2003;217(5):325–328.
27. Teekhasaenee C, Ritch R. Combined phacoemulsification and goniosynechialysis for uncontrolled chronic angle-closure glaucoma after acute angle-closure glaucoma. *Ophthalmology.* 1999;106(4):669–674.
28. Harasymowycz PJ, Papamatheakis DG, Ahmed I, et al. Phacoemulsification and goniosynechialysis in the management of unresponsive primary angle closure. *J Glaucoma.* 2005;14(3): 186–189.
29. Lai JS, Tham CC, Lam DS. The efficacy and safety of combined phacoemulsification, intraocular lens implantation, and limited goniosynechialysis, followed by diode laser peripheral iridoplasty, in the treatment of cataract and chronic angle-closure glaucoma. *J Glaucoma.* 2001;10(4):309–315.

30. Dada T, Kumar S, Gadia R, Aggarwal A, Gupta V, Sihota R. Sutureless single-port transconjunctival pars plana limited vitrectomy combined with phacoemulsification for management of phacomorphic glaucoma. *J Cataract Refract Surg.* 2007;33(6):951–954.
31. Chalam KV, Gupta SK, Agarwal S, Shah VA. Sutureless limited vitrectomy for positive vitreous pressure in cataract surgery. *Ophthalmic Surg Lasers Imaging.* 2005;36(6):518–522.
32. Tham CC, Kwong YY, Leung DY, et al. Phacoemulsification versus combined phacotrabeculectomy in medically controlled chronic angle closure glaucoma with cataract. *Ophthalmology.* 2008;115(12):2167–2173.
33. Yuen NS, Chan OC, Hui SP, Ching RH. Combined phacoemulsification and nonpenetrating deep sclerectomy in the treatment of chronic angle-closure glaucoma with cataract. *Eur J Ophthalmol.* 2007;17(2):208–215.
34. Arshinoff SA. Dispersive-cohesive viscoelastic soft shell technique. *J Cataract Refract Surg.* 1999;25(2):167–173.
35. Razeghinejad MR. Combined phacoemulsification and viscogoniosynechialysis in patients with refractory acute angle-closure glaucoma. *J Cataract Refract Surg.* 2008;34(5):827–830.
36. Khan B, Ahmed II. *Phaco and Goniosynechiolysis using Microforceps for Synechial Angle Closure GlaucomaAmerican Glaucoma Society Meeting*; 2006.

# Chapter 79
# Refractive Surgery and Glaucoma

Sarwat Salim and Peter A. Netland

The demand for refractive surgery has escalated over the past decade, and surgical options have been developed for various refractive errors. Although secondary glaucoma is uncommon after refractive surgery, there are concerns related to patients who are glaucoma suspects or who have been diagnosed with glaucoma. This review will address preoperative, intraoperative, and postoperative considerations that clinicians need to be aware of in refractive surgery patients.

## 79.1 Preoperative Considerations

Refractive surgery is most commonly performed in young myopes. In some population-based studies, myopia has been identified as a risk factor for the development of glaucoma. In the Blue Mountains Eye Study, glaucoma was almost three times more prevalent in myopes when compared with non-myopes.[1] In addition, myopia is a risk factor for steroid-induced ocular hypertension and glaucoma.[2] Topical steroids are routinely used in patients after refractive surgery. In photorefractive keratectomy (PRK), steroids may be required for an extended period of time to combat stromal haze and regression, further prolonging the risk – especially in glaucoma suspects and patients with glaucoma.

## 79.2 Intraoperative Considerations

During laser in situ keratomileusis (LASIK), intraocular pressure (IOP) is markedly elevated in the range of 60–90 mmHg to provide mechanical support and stability to the eye for the microkeratome to form a corneal flap. Although the duration of this dramatic IOP rise is transient, it can vary between surgeons and patients. Cases of optic neuropathy and visual field loss associated with LASIK have been attributed to the effect of markedly high IOP rise on the optic nerve.[3,4] Although the exact mechanism of optic nerve damage is not clearly understood, some investigators have speculated that the damage may be due to ischemia from compromised blood flow or direct trauma to the optic nerve head.[5] Therefore, in patients with susceptible optic nerves, LASIK may not be the ideal procedure, and PRK may be a better alternative since there is no elevated IOP phase in this surgery. In patients presenting with a functional bleb after trabeculectomy, the microkeratome pass during LASIK may destroy the bleb integrity. In such cases, PRK may also be preferable.

### 79.2.1 Postoperative Considerations

A significant challenge after refractive surgery relates to obtaining accurate IOP measurements for follow-up visits. It has been well established that corneal thickness has a major influence on IOP measurements.[6,7] The Goldmann applanation tonometer (GAT) uses a prism of 3.06 mm in diameter with an estimated average corneal thickness of 520 microns to cancel the opposing forces of surface tension and corneal rigidity to allow indentation. It is now known that a wide variation exists in corneal thickness among individuals. In general, IOP is overestimated in thicker corneas and underestimated in thinner corneas with GAT, depending on the amount of force required to indent the cornea.

Excimer laser ablation reshapes the central cornea and alters corneal thickness, curvature, and structure.[8,9] The power change of central cornea depends on the degree of treatment, and the resultant thinning leads to underestimation of IOP by GAT. Because error results from both changes in corneal thickness and to a lesser degree, curvature, underestimation of IOP cannot be calculated from nomograms based on thickness alone.[10] Although many formulas for IOP correction have been proposed, there is no general consensus on a particular algorithm. One reasonable recommendation is to record the difference between the preoperative IOP and that measured at 3 or 6 months after surgery – allowing adequate time interval for the cornea to heal and stabilize – and use this difference as a correction factor. Another way to overcome imprecise recordings is to use different modalities for IOP measurements, which are less likely to be affected by surface properties of the cornea. The pneumotonometer, Tono-Pen, and dynamic contour tonometer have been shown to be less or not affected when compared with GAT readings in eyes after refractive surgery.[11-13]

Because of the difficulties in measuring IOP after procedures that thin the cornea, physicians should be attentive to other parameters of glaucoma evaluation, such as stereoscopic optic nerve assessment, nerve fiber analysis, and visual field testing. In certain patients, it may be helpful to include strategies designed to detect early visual loss, such as short wavelength automated perimetry and frequency-doubling technology perimetry. When ordering scanning laser polarimetry, physicians need to be mindful that corneal refractive surgery may alter the corneal birefringence, affecting the accuracy of this device, especially with the earlier models that lack the variable corneal compensator.[14] Recent studies, using individualized corneal polarization compensation or alternative techniques such as optical coherence tomography (OCT), have shown that LASIK-induced corneal alterations did not affect mean nerve fiber layer thickness measurements.[15-17]

Other concerns in the postoperative period are steroid-induced ocular hypertension and flap-associated complications. Case reports of end stage glaucoma resulting from masking of steroid response due to inaccurate IOP measurement by standard methods have been reported both after PRK and LASIK.[18,19] Another condition that may lead to underestimation of IOP after LASIK is the interface cyst.[20] The accumulation of fluid under the LASIK flap renders the cornea softer and easily distensible. Lower IOP measurements due to flap interface fluid can mask steroid-induced IOP elevation, resulting in optic nerve damage.

Davidson et al described a distinct entity called pressure-induced interlamellar stromal keratitis (PISK) in a patient after uncomplicated LASIK.[21] Although the clinical presentation of this condition is similar to diffuse lamellar keratitis (DLK), it usually presents beyond the first postoperative week. Unlike DLK, which resolves with corticosteroid therapy, PISK results from steroid response. Elevated IOP in PISK does not respond to IOP lowering medications, while discontinuation of steroids leads to resolution of both keratitis and elevated IOP.

### 79.2.2 Other Considerations

Glaucoma patients who have had refractive surgery may become candidates for combined cataract and glaucoma surgery at a later time. Availability of accurate lens power calculations is improving, which helps predict the correct intraocular lens (IOL) choice for an individual patient. If unexpected refractive errors are found postoperatively after combined surgery, management choices will include intraocular lens exchange, contact lens, refractive corneal surgery, and piggy-back IOLs.

Clear lens extraction may be performed for high myopia, but can be associated with vision loss during the postoperative period. In addition to other potential complications, including retinal detachment, endophthalmitis, and cystoid macular edema, elevated IOP and glaucoma can occur after clear lens extraction for high myopia. In a retrospective study of highly myopic eyes treated with clear lens extraction (without intraocular lens implantation), Rodriguez and coworkers[22] reported treatment of 11 of 33 eyes (33%) with anti-glaucoma medications, with secondary glaucoma developing in 8 of 33 (24%) eyes. Severe vision loss with legal blindness due to glaucoma has been reported following clear lens extraction for high myopia.[23] Patients treated with lens extraction for high myopia require continued monitoring for glaucoma after the refractive procedure.

## 79.3 Conclusion

Refractive surgery is a rapidly growing sector of ophthalmology. In the average patient, there is probably little or no change of the nerve fiber layer or the optic nerve after the procedure. However, patients with preexisting glaucoma may be more sensitive to transient alterations of IOP during the refractive procedure. IOP should be monitored in patients requiring long-term treatment with steroid drops after refractive procedures. Measurement of IOP should take into account the decreased corneal thickness that occurs after certain refractive procedures, especially LASIK and PRK.

Refractive surgery is not contraindicated for glaucoma suspects or glaucoma patients, although opinions vary among corneal and glaucoma specialists about the suitability of individual patients for certain procedures. With multiple choices now available for refractive correction, both patients and physicians have more options. With vigilant screening, detailed informed consent, and meticulous postoperative surveillance, adverse effects can be circumvented and patients are more likely to enjoy the benefits of this advancing technology.

## References

1. Mitchell P, Hourihan F, Sandbach J, et al. The relationship between glaucoma and myopia: The Blue Mountains eye Study. *Ophthalmology*. 1999;106:2010–2015.
2. Podos SM, Becker B, Morton WR. High myopia and primary open-angle glaucoma. *Am J Ophthalmol*. 1966;62:1038–1043.

3. Lee AG, Kohnen T, Ebner R, et al. Optic neuropathy associated with laser in situ keratomileusis. *J Cataract Refract Surg.* 2000;26:1581–1584.
4. Bushley DM, Parmley VC, Paglen P. Visual field defect associated with laser in situ keratomileusis. *Am J Ophthalmol.* 2000;129:668–671.
5. Lim MC. Refractive surgery and the glaucoma patient: caveat emptor. *Int Ophthalmol Clin.* 2004;44(2):137–150.
6. Ehlers N, Bramsen T, Sperling S. Applanation tonometry and central corneal thickness. *Acta Ophthalmol (Copenh).* 1975;53:34–43.
7. Whitacre MM, Stein RA, Hassanein K. The effect of corneal thickness on applanation tonometry. *Am J Ophthalmol.* 1993;115:592–596.
8. Chatterjee A, Shah S, Bessant DA, et al. Reduction in intraocular pressure after excimer laser photorefractive keratectomy. Correlation with pretreatment myopia. *Ophthalmology.* 1997;104:355–359.
9. Fournier AV, Podtetenev M, Lemire J, et al. Intraocular pressure change measured by Goldmann tonometry after lasik in situ keratomileusis. *J Cataract Refract Surg.* 1998;24:905–910.
10. Mark HH. Corneal curvature in applanation tonometry. *Am J Ophthalmol.* 1973;223–224.
11. Zadok D, Tran DB, Twa M, et al. Pneumotonometry versus Goldman tonometry after laser in situ keratomileusis for myopia. *J Cataract Refract Surg.* 1999;25:1344–1348.
12. Garzozi HJ, Chung HS, Lang Y, et al. Intraocular pressure and photorefractive keratectomy: a comparison of three different tonometers. *Cornea.* 2001;20:33–36.
13. Kaufman C, Bachmann LM, Thiel MA. Intraocular pressure measurements using dynamic contour tonometry after laser in situ keratomileusis. *Invest Ophthalmol.* 2003;44:3790–3794.
14. Gurses-Ozden R, Liebmann JM, Schuffner D, et al. Retinal nerve fiber layer thickness remains unchanged following laser-assisted in situ keratomileusis. *Am J Ophthalmol.* 2001;132:512–516.
15. Choplin NT, Schallhorn SC, Sinai M, et al. Retinal nerve fiber layer measurements do not change after LASIK for high myopia as measured by scanning laser polarimetry with custom compensation. *Ophthalmology.* 2005;112:92–97.
16. Zangwill LM, Abunto T, Bowd C, Angeles R, et al. Scanning laser polarimetry retinal nerve fiber layer thickness measurements after LASIK. *Ophthalmology.* 2005;112:200–207.
17. Halkiadakis I, Anglionto L, Ferensowicz M, et al. Assessment of nerve fiber layer thickness before and after laser in situ keratomileusis using scanning laser polarimetry with variable corneal compensation. *J Cataract Refract Surg.* 2005;31:1035–1041.
18. Shaikh NM, Shaikh S, Singh K, et al. Progression to end-stage glaucoma after laser in situ keratomileusis. *J Cataract Refract Surg.* 2002;28:356–359.
19. Kim JH, Sah WJ, Hahn TW, et al. Some problems after photorefractive keratectomy. *J Refract Corneal Surg.* 1994;10(2 suppl):226–230.
20. Hamilton DR, Manche EE, Rich LF, et al. Steroid induced glaucoma after laser in situ keratomileusis associated with interface fluid. *Ophthalmology.* 2002;109:659–665.
21. Davidson RS, Brandt JD, Mannis MJ. Intraocular pressure-induced interlamellar keratitis after LASIK surgery. *J Glaucoma.* 2003;12:23–26.
22. Rodriguez A, Guierrez E, Alvira G. Complications of clear lens extraction in axial myopia. *Arch Ophthalmol.* 1987;105:1522–1523.
23. King JS, Priester B, Netland PA. Pseudophakic glaucoma and vision loss after clear lens extraction for high myopia. *Ann Ophthalmol.* 2004;36:53–54.

# Chapter 80
# Glaucoma after Retinal Surgery

Annisa L. Jamil, Scott D. Lawrence, David A. Saperstein, Elliott M. Kanner, Richard P. Mills, and Peter A. Netland

Following vitreoretinal surgery, patients may develop elevated intraocular pressure (IOP), which may be due to multiple different mechanisms. Preexisting glaucoma may be a potential cause of any postoperative IOP elevation in patients undergoing treatment for retinal disorders. Neovascularization of the anterior segment from underlying ischemic retinopathy may lead to neovascular glaucoma during the perioperative and postoperative periods. Also, prolonged treatment with topical or intravitreal steroids following retinal surgery can cause a steroid-induced glaucoma in susceptible patients.

It is estimated that ocular hypertension occurs after vitreoretinal surgery in 19–28% of cases.[1] The increased intraocular pressure may be acute or chronic depending on the underlying pathophysiologic mechanism. Additionally, multiple ocular surgeries increase the risk of temporary or sustained ocular hypertension.[2] Frequently, this complication can be easily managed by medical therapy alone; however, some cases may go on to develop a secondary glaucoma requiring surgical intervention. Various vitreoretinal surgical techniques and their relation to elevated intraocular pressure will be examined to define their mechanisms and consider possible interventions for the establishment of intraocular pressure control.

## 80.1 Scleral Buckle

The occurrence of primary open angle glaucoma (POAG) in patients with rhegmatogenous retinal detachments is higher than in the general population alone.[3] The prevalence of POAG in patients with retinal detachments is 4.0–5.8% compared to that in the general population which is between 1.1 and 3.0%.[4,5] In addition, the placement of a scleral buckle to repair a retinal detachment often results in an elevation of intraocular pressure or secondary glaucoma due to a closed angle mechanism. Postoperative narrowing of the angle has been found in 14.4% of patients after the use of a scleral buckle. In the same study, permanent abnormal intraocular pressure elevation and narrowing of the angle was seen in 3.75% of cases.[6] The incidence of acute angle-closure glaucoma was 1.4% over a 6-year period following scleral buckle.[7]

Patients with narrow angles or those treated with anteriorly placed buckles or encircling bands may be predisposed to develop angle-closure glaucoma.[6] Ciliary body congestion has been postulated as one mechanism, with impaired venous drainage from direct pressure of the buckle, swelling and anterior rotation of the ciliary body, and choroidal effusions, leading to anterior movement of the lens–iris diaphragm, and narrowing of the anterior chamber angle.[8] Angle closure in the late postoperative period may occur due to peripheral anterior synechiae.

Sato et al. described three cases where there was development of glaucoma despite normal intraocular pressure and normal angle anatomy after scleral buckling surgery.[9] Scanning laser Doppler flowmetry at the optic nerve head was measured in eyes with an encircling element and found to be significantly lower than that of the comparable area in fellow eyes. These patients demonstrated visual field defects and glaucomatous optic neuropathy. After the scleral buckle was removed, blood flow improved with no further progression of the disease.

When the anterior chamber shallows following scleral buckle, most cases resolve spontaneously within a few days. Acute IOP elevations can be managed with topical or systemic anti-glaucoma medications. Cycloplegics are often employed to deepen the anterior chamber and rotate the ciliary body posteriorly. Adjunctive use of topical steroids may also help to decrease inflammation and prevent the formation of peripheral anterior synechiae. Miotics should be avoided due to the risk of increased inflammation and anterior movement of the lens–iris diaphragm. Surgical treatments include argon laser peripheral iridoplasty as well as drainage of large choroidal effusions. Laser peripheral iridotomy is usually not indicated, as pupillary block is uncommon following scleral buckling procedures. Persistent elevations in intraocular pressure may require revision of the buckle or loosening of the encircling band.

## 80.2 Panretinal Photocoagulation

Panretinal photocoagulation is routinely used to treat potential or active neovascularization of the anterior and posterior segments. Profound elevations of intraocular pressure at the time of photocoagulation were common with the xenon arc and ruby lasers. Argon laser is considered a safer modality, but the transfer of thermal energy causes an inflammatory cascade that can lead to ciliochoroidal effusions and detachments with anterior rotation of the ciliary body. Subsequent forward shifting of the lens–iris diaphragm may lead to narrowing of the anterior chamber angle with the potential for angle-closure glaucoma.[10] The majority of cases of secondary glaucoma following panretinal photocoagulation resolve within several days to 2 weeks.[11] However, IOP spikes during the acute postoperative period should be treated with cycloplegics as well as topical and systemic anti-glaucoma medications. Topical steroids may help to decrease the inflammatory stimulus of choroidal effusions.

## 80.3 Pars Plana Vitrectomy

Simple pars plana vitrectomy may be associated with elevated intraocular pressures due to either open angle or closed angle mechanisms. In one study, 43.3% of patients undergoing pars plana vitrectomy had intraocular pressures above 30 mmHg in the acute postoperative period.[12] Subjects who demonstrated early IOP spikes had a tendency to sustain high IOP 6 weeks or more after surgery. In another study examining the effects of simple pars plana vitrectomy on IOP in the early postoperative period, 92% of eyes experienced a rise in IOP 2 h after surgery. However, only 39% of them reached an IOP of at least 30 mmHg.[13] These findings suggest that there are a significant number of patients with acute elevations in IOP in the first 24 h after surgery followed by normalization of the pressure curve in many patients.

The underlying causes of these pressure elevations after vitrectomy may be, in part, related to the interventions performed at the time of surgery. In one series, among the open angle mechanisms, gas expansion without angle closure was the most common cause of acute postvitrectomy IOP elevation followed in descending order by inflammation, silicone oil related (without pupillary block), corticosteroid response, and erythroclastic glaucoma.[12] For those who experienced closed angle glaucoma, ciliary body edema causing pupillary block was the most common mechanism followed in descending order by pupillary block secondary to fibrin, gas, and, lastly, silicone oil. Risk factors for IOP elevation delineated in this study include intraoperative or previous scleral buckling, intraoperative scatter endophotocoagulation, intraoperative lensectomy, and postoperative fibrin formation. Surprisingly, a preexisting history of glaucoma did not increase the overall rate of IOP elevation after a vitrectomy.[12] In contrast, Desai and coworkers had found that 60% of ocular hypertensives required pressure reducing medications postoperatively compared to 35% of normotensive patients.[13]

Medical management can help abate postoperative pressure elevation, and surgical intervention is infrequently required. Although Han et al reported the need for surgical treatment in 11.3% of subjects, no patients required any surgical intervention in the study conducted by Desai et al[12,13] When required, surgical interventions included anterior chamber paracentesis, laser peripheral iridotomy, and laser iridoplasty or membranectomy.[12]

## 80.4 Intravitreal Gas

Intravitreal gas tamponade for repair of retinal detachment can be associated with a significant intraocular pressure spike during the rapid phase of gas expansion. Patients with advanced glaucomatous optic nerve damage or compromised retinal vasculature may be particularly vulnerable to vision-threatening sequelae from increased IOP. Sulfur hexafluoride ($SF_6$) and perfluoropropane ($C_3F_8$) achieve retinal tamponade by expanding within the vitreous cavity. Elevated IOP is directly related to the expansile property and final volume of the intraocular gas bubble. Perfluoropropane ($C_3F_8$) and sulfur hexafluoride ($SF_6$) are commonly used high molecular weight gases in nonexpansile concentrations of 14% and 18%, respectively.[14,15] However, despite these concentrations, pressure spikes are common in the early postoperative period.[16,17]

The incidence of high intraocular pressure after pars plana vitrectomy and long acting gas tamponade has been reported by Chen and Thompson who found a 43% incidence of pressures greater than 25 mmHg.[16] These gases can remain in the eye for 10–14 days for sulfur hexafluoride and up to 55–65 days for perflouropropane.[15] Mittra and coworkers found that 52% of their subjects experienced an elevation greater than 25 mmHg and 29% experienced an elevation over 30 mmHg in the first 4 to 6 h after surgery.[18]

Certain tonometers are preferred when monitoring the IOP after retinal gas tamponade. A gas-filled eye has altered rigidity, which can provide false readings if using the Schiotz tonometer. Also, pneumatic tonometry can underestimate the IOP. Recommended tonometers include the Perkins or Goldmann applanation tonometers. The Tono-Pen (Mentor Inc, Norwell, Massachusetts) is commonly used in practice because of its portability and facility of use in patients with corneal aberrations. It has demonstrated good correlation when compared with a monometer except for cases with pressures exceeding 30 mmHg where it falls short by underestimating the actual intraocular pressure.[19]

Elevated pressure after the use of intravitreal gas develops by both open and closed angle mechanisms. Angle closure with pupillary block occurs when the anterior displacement of the lens–iris diaphragm results in iris bombe and iridocorneal touch. This mechanism can occur despite the patient assuming a prone position. There are also cases of closed angle glaucoma with the enlarging gas bubble causing iridocorneal apposition without pupillary block. In addition, open angle glaucoma occurs when the rate of expansion of the gas exceeds the rate of egress of the aqueous humor through the trabecular meshwork. Anterior chamber fibrinous exudation has been reported in some patients following intravitreal gas injection. The incidence is increased in diabetics and may lead to pupillary block with angle closure.[20]

Risk factors for increased intraocular pressure after intravitreal gas tamponade include the concentration of gas used, older patient, postoperative fibrin in the anterior chamber, concurrent use of a scleral buckle, and intraoperative endophotocoagulation.[12,16] Nitrous oxide inhaled anesthetics will elute from the blood stream into adjacent gas filled spaces and increase the volume of these spaces. Patients with intraocular gas who receive nitrous oxide during surgery can develop intraocular pressures in excess of 70 mmHg, which can result in artery occlusion, retinal ischemia, and/or infarction.

The US Food and Drug Administration (FDA) mandates that all patients treated with intraocular gases wear a medic alert bracelet warning medical practitioners that the patient has gas in their eye and that inhaled nitrous oxide should be avoided during all anesthetic procedures. Patients with intraocular gas should be cautioned against travelling to places where the atmospheric pressure decreases significantly as this can result in dangerous IOP elevations. Generally, it is suggested that these patients do not increase their elevation by 2,500 feet or travel by air where changes in the cabin pressure can instantaneously cause severe elevation of intraocular pressure.[21]

Mittra and coworkers found that the use of topical aqueous suppressants immediately after surgery significantly reduced the intraocular pressure 4–6 h and one day after surgery when compared against a control group.[18] In their study, 9.5% of the control group and none of those who had postoperative instillation of aqueous suppressants required an anterior chamber tap.

All patients undergoing intravitreal gas injection should maintain a face-down position following surgery in order to augment the tamponade effect of the gas bubble as well as to decrease anterior displacement of the lens–iris diaphragm. IOP elevations in the initial postoperative period should be treated with topical and systemic anti-glaucoma agents. The treatment of high elevation of IOP is based on the underlying causative mechanisms. If pupillary block is present, an inferior laser peripheral iridotomy is necessary. Angle closure without pupillary block resulting in iridocorneal touch must be treated promptly to prevent the establishment of peripheral anterior synechiae. This can be accomplished by partial removal of the intravitreal gas and reformation of the anterior chamber with the help of a viscoelastic. In addition, a paracentesis can immediately lower pressures in the setting where topical medications are ineffective. Air travel in patients who have undergone intravitreal gas tamponade should be avoided until the gas bubble has been completely absorbed.[22]

## 80.5 Silicone Oil

Silicone oil endotamponade for complex retinal detachments is a common cause of secondary glaucoma. The reported incidence of postoperative IOP elevation following silicone injection has varied, with one report exceeding 50%.[23] The highly purified silicone oils that are now available have less toxicity with a presumed reduction in secondary glaucoma. A recent study found a lower incidence (11%) of glaucoma after pars plana vitrectomy with injection of highly purified silicone oil (5,000 centistokes).[24] Postoperative IOP elevation was attributed to preexisting glaucoma in 31% of cases and neovascular glaucoma in 29% of patients. Twenty-five percent of patients with postoperative IOP elevation were determined to have silicone oil-related glaucoma due to the presence of silicone oil in the anterior chamber and/or anterior chamber angle. Notably, no eye developed pupillary block with angle closure due to silicone oil, all patients were aphakic or pseudophakic at the time of surgery, and all were exposed to steroids postoperatively.[24] Thus, elevated IOP in patients with silicone oil endotamponade may be due to multiple mechanisms.

In aphakic patients treated with pars plana vitrectomy and silicone oil injection, inferior peripheral iridectomy has become standard, and has greatly reduced pupillary block as a cause of secondary glaucoma.[25] Removal of the entire lens capsule with forceps at the time of vitrectomy may help to eliminate late closure of the iridectomy. A prone position is advocated postoperatively to prevent forward movement of the lens–iris diaphragm. Since it has a lower density than water, the silicone oil tends to accumulate superiorly. Follow-up slit lamp exams should focus on the superior angle, looking for oil droplets.

In eyes developing an increased IOP, the IOP increases during the first 3 months following surgery.[23,24] Topical and systemic anti-glaucoma medications achieve effective control of intraocular pressure in a majority of patients, and topical steroids are often administered after surgery to control inflammation. Guarded filtration surgery (trabeculectomy) is generally not recommended due to the upward migration of silicone oil as well as conjunctival scarring following pars plana vitrectomy. However, a glaucoma drainage implant is useful for the treatment of elevated IOP in eyes that do not respond to medical therapy.[24,26] Transscleral diode cycloablation is recommended for patients with a poor visual prognosis and can achieve a reduction in IOP of approximately 49% from baseline IOP with success rates of 44%.[27]

In patients with elevated IOP after silicone oil endotamponade, removal of the silicone oil may not be enough to resolve the underlying problem.[28,29] In a study by Moisseiev and colleagues, removal of the emulsified oil did not change the intraocular pressure in 91% of subjects.[29] Silicone oil removal and medications offered IOP control in only 25% of patients in another study.[28] Budenz and coworkers found that patients who underwent silicone oil removal with or without glaucoma surgery and those with glaucoma surgery alone experienced satisfactory IOP control.[30] Decisions to surgically manage glaucoma in these patients must be thoroughly discussed with the retinal specialist because removal of silicone oil prematurely is associated with a re-detachment rate in 11–33% of eyes.[28]

In eyes with intractable elevation of IOP after pars plana vitrectomy and silicone oil injection, glaucoma drainage implant surgery can control the IOP in the majority of eyes, when implanted in the inferonasal or inferotemporal quadrant.[26] Viscoelastic is used intraoperatively to prevent the loss of silicone oil. This technique is especially helpful in eyes that cannot have the oil removed due to the risk of recurrent retinal detachment. Silicone oil may accumulate around the tube, which is a benign finding that occurs in approximately 40% of eyes (Fig. 80.1).[26] Eyes containing silicone oil require prolonged treatment with topical corticosteroids during the postoperative period.

## 80.6 Conclusion

Glaucoma after vitreoretinal surgery is a common reality in clinical practice. Understanding the underlying process helps to determine the required therapy. In most cases, intraocular pressure can be controlled medically with surgery as a secondary option. However, as illustrated previously, some chronic pressure elevations may need a surgical intervention. Regardless, these complicated cases necessitate judicious communication with the retina specialist to ensure that all therapeutic goals are achieved on a case-by-case basis.

## References

1. Weinberg RS, Peyman GA, Huamonte FU. Elevation of intraocular pressure after pars plana vitrectomy. *Arch Klin Exp Ophthalmol*. 1976;200:157–161.
2. Tranos P, Asaria R, Aylward W, Sullivan P, Franks W. Long term outcome of secondary glaucoma following vitreoretinal surgery. *Br J Ophthalmol*. 2004;88:341–343.
3. Scott IU, Gedde SJ, Budenz DL, et al. Baerveldt drainage implants in eyes with a preexisting sclera buckle. *Arch Ophthalmol*. 2000;118:1509–1513.
4. Becker B. In discussion of: Smith JL. Retinal detachment and glaucoma. *Trans Am Acad Ophthalmol Otolaryngol*. 1963;67:731–732.
5. Phelps CD, Burton TC. Glaucoma and retinal detachment. *Arch Ophthalmol*. 1977;95:418–422.
6. Sebestyen JG, Schepens CL, Rosenthal ML. Retinal detachment and glaucoma. I Tonometric and gonioscopic study of 160 cases. *Arch Ophthalmol*. 1962;67:736–745.
7. Perez RN, Phelps CD, Burton TC. Angle closure glaucoma following sclera buckling procedures. *Trans Am Acad Ophthalmol Otolaryngol*. 1976;81:247–252.
8. Chandler PA, Grant WM. *Lectures on glaucoma*. Philadelphia: Lea and Febiger; 1965:204–207.
9. Sato EA, Shinoda K, Inoue M, Ohtake Y, Kimura I. Reduced choroidal blood flow can induce visual field defect in open angle glaucoma patients without intraocular pressure elevation following encircling scleral buckling. *Retina*. 2008;28:493–497.
10. Blondeau P, Pavan PR, Phelps CD. Acute pressure elevation following panretinal photocoagulation. *Arch Ophthalmol*. 1981;99:1239–1241.
11. Liang JC, Huamonte FU. Reduction of immediate complications after panretinal photocoagulation. *Retina*. 1984;4:166–170.
12. Han DP, Lewis H, Lambrou FH, Mieler WF. Mechanisms of intraocular pressure elevation after pars plana vitrectomy. *Ophthalmology*. 1989;96:1357–1362.
13. Desai UR, Alhalel AA, Schiffman RM, Campen TJ, Sundar G, Muhich A. Intraocular pressure elevation after simple pars plana vitrectomy. *Ophthalmology*. 1997;104:781–785.
14. Peters MA, Abrams GW, Hamilton LH. The nonexpansile, equilibrated concentration of perfluoropropane gas in the eye. *Am J Ophthalmol*. 1985;100:831–839.
15. Chang S. Intraocular gases. In: Ryan SJ, ed. *Retina*, vol. 3. St. Louis: CV Mosby; 1989:245.
16. Chen PP, Thompson JT. Risk factors for elevated intraocular pressure after the use of intraocular gases in vitreoretinal surgery. *Ophthalmic Surg Lasers*. 1997;28:37–42.
17. Chen CJ. Glaucoma after macular hole surgery. *Ophthalmology*. 1998;105:94–9.
18. Mittra RA, Pollack JS, Dev S, et al. The use of topical aqueous suppressants in the prevention of postoperative intraocular pressure elevation after pars plana vitrectomy with long-acting gas tamponade. *Ophthalmology*. 2000;107:588–592.
19. Lim JI, Blair NP, Higginbotham EJ, Farber MD, Shaw WE, Garretson BR. Assessment of intraocular pressure in vitrectomized gas-containing eyes. A clinical and monometric comparison of the

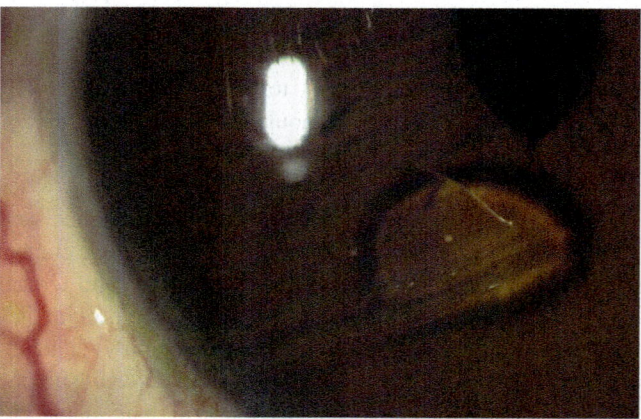

**Fig. 80.1** Patients who are treated with silicone oil endotamponade and glaucoma drainage implant may accumulate silicone oil adjacent to the tube, which usually does not require treatment

Tono-Pen to the pneumotonometer. *Arch Ophthalmol.* 1990;108: 684–688.
20. Abrams GW, Swanson DE, Sabates WI, Goldman AI. The results of sulfur hexafluoride gas in vitreous surgery. *Am J Ophthalmol.* 1982;94:165–171.
21. Mills MD, Devenyi RG, Lam WC, Berger AR, Beijer CD, Lam SR. An assessment of intraocular pressure rise in patients with gas-filled eyes during simulated air flight. *Ophthalmology.* 2001;108:40–44.
22. Diecket JP, O'Connor PS, Schacklett DE, et al. Air travel and intraocular gas. *Ophthalmology.* 1986;93:642–645.
23. deCorral LR, Cohen SB, Peyman GA. Effect of intravitreal silicone oil on intraocular pressure. *Ophthalmic Surg.* 1987;18:446–449.
24. Al-Jazzaf AM, Netland PA, Charles S. Incidence and management of elevated intraocular pressure after silicone oil injection. *J Glaucoma.* 2005;14:40–46.
25. Ando F. Intraocular hypertension resulting from pupillary block by silicone oil. *Am J Ophthalmol.* 1985;99:87–88.
26. Ishida K, Ahmed IK, Netland PA. Ahmed glaucoma valve surgical outcomes in eyes with and without silicone oil endotamponade. *J Glaucoma.* 2009;18:325–330.
27. Sivagnanavel V, Ortiz-Hurtado A, Williamsom TH. Diode laser trans-scleral cyclophotocoagulation in the management of glaucoma in patients with long-term intravitreal silicone oil. *Eye.* 2005;19:253–257.
28. Honavar SG, Goyal M, Majji AB, Sen PK, Naduvilath T, Dandona L. Glaucoma after pars plana vitrectomy and silicone oil injection for complicated retinal detachments. *Ophthalmology.* 1999;106:169–177.
29. Moisseiev J, Barak A, Manaim T, Triester G. Removal of silicone oil in the management of glaucoma in eyes with emulsified silicone. *Retina.* 1993;13:290–295.
30. Budenz DL, Taba KE, Feuer WJ, et al. Surgical management of secondary glaucoma after pars plana vitrectomy and silicone oil injection for complex retinal detachment. *Ophthalmology.* 2001;108: 1628–1632.

# Part VI
# The Future

# Chapter 81
# Immunology and Glaucoma

Michal Schwartz and Anat London

Glaucoma, although once thought of as a single disease, is actually a group of diseases of the optic nerve involving loss of retinal ganglion cells. The process of cell death occurs in a characteristic pattern of optic neuropathy – a broad term for a certain pattern of damage to the optic nerve (the bundle of nerve fibers that carries information from the eye to the brain). Untreated glaucoma leads to permanent damage of the optic nerve and resultant visual field loss that can progress to permanent blindness.

## 81.1 Glaucoma as a Neurodegenerative Disease

Traditionally, elevation in intraocular pressure (IOP) has been considered to be the main cause of glaucoma.[1] IOP is determined by the balance between secretion and drainage of aqueous humor. In glaucoma, this balance is interrupted, as insufficient fluid drains out of the eye, leading to increased IOP. As a result, the retina and the optic nerve heads are subjected to mechanical,[2,3] hypoxic,[4] and oxidative tissue stress.[5]

Over the past decades, scientists have focused on elevated IOP as a primary therapeutic target, trying to diminish this major risk factor,[6–10] while totally disregarding the process of damage that derives from it. Consequently, the currently approved glaucoma medications and surgical therapies are directed at lowering IOP; and, indeed, there is evidence from several clinical trials for a significant attenuation of progressive visual field loss among the treated patients.[6–8,11]

However, some patients continued to suffer from an ongoing visual field loss even after their IOP was effectively controlled.[12–14] Even more confusing is the case of normal tension glaucoma (NTG), in which progressive retinal ganglion cell death and subsequent glaucomatous damage occurs in the absence of any elevated IOP. Moreover, some studies have reported a negligible relationship between mean IOP and vision loss in glaucoma.[15–17] These observations indicate the possible contribution of IOP-independent mechanisms to disease progression.

It seems, therefore, that glaucoma is a complex multivariate disease, initiated by several risk factors (with elevated IOP as only one of them), whose individual contributions to glaucomatous destruction have not yet been fully elucidated. As a result, the efforts of researchers have shifted toward understanding and subsequently preventing the disease progression, regardless of the primary cause. Thus, the major goal of glaucoma treatment is moving to neuroprotection, preventing the spread of damage, and protection from the progressive loss of the nerve fiber layers.[18,19]

There are many molecular and cellular elements that contribute to the pathological progression and neuronal loss in glaucoma, even after the primary risk factor no longer exists. Following the initial insult, there is a progressive self-perpetuating secondary degeneration of neurons that were spared from the primary injury. This secondary damage is an outcome of the hostile environment produced by the degenerating neurons. The noxious extracellular environment includes mediators of oxidative stress and free radicals, excessive amounts of glutamate and excitotoxicity, increased calcium concentration, deprivation of neurotrophins and growth factors, abnormal accumulation of proteins, and apoptotic signals (Scheme 81.1), all of which are universal features of many neurodegenerative diseases.[20] These characteristics place glaucoma among the common neurodegenerative disorders.

### 81.1.1 Oxidative Stress and Free Radicals

Oxidative stress is involved in the pathogenesis of many neurodegenerative disorders.[21–27] The central nervous system (CNS) has a unique sensitivity to oxidative stress. Its function requires electrical excitability, transsynaptic chemical connections, and a high metabolic rate, that involves the augmented use of oxygen and adenosine triphosphate (ATP) synthesis. In addition, the CNS lacks an appropriate defense system against the elevated levels of reactive oxygen species (ROS) produced in these tissues. These ROS, accumulating in cells that undergo oxidative stress, react with nitric oxide

> **SCHEME 81.1 Immune protection in glaucoma**
>
> Degenerating neurons create a noxious milieu, which consists of oxidative stress and free radicals, excessive amounts of glutamate and excitotoxicity, increased calcium concentration, deprivation of neurotrophins and growth factors, abnormal accumulation of proteins, and apoptotic signals. These features are characteristics of a hostile microenvironment to the remaining neurons that leads to secondary degeneration and further loss of neurons.
>
> The immune system plays a key role in the ability of the optic nerve and the retina to withstand these threatening conditions, by recruiting both innate (resident and blood-borne macrophages) and adaptive (self-antigens specific T cells) cells that together create a protective niche and, thereby, halt disease progression. The spontaneous immune response might not be sufficient, and therefore boosting it by immunization (with the appropriate antigen, in specific timing and dosing) may be a suitable therapeutic vaccination to treat glaucoma.

to produce free radicals, leading to a chain of reactions that result in mitochondrial dysfunction, DNA degradation, and eventually cell death. As in Alzheimer's disease,[24,27] Parkinson's,[23] and amyotrophic lateral sclerosis (ALS),[21,22] the association of oxidative stress with neurodegeneration has been increasingly reported in glaucoma. Free radicals cause extensive damage to the retinal ganglion cells and their axons[28–30]; they contribute to the secondary degeneration by either a direct neurotoxic effect, or indirectly through the induction of glial dysfunction,[31] oxidative modification of proteins,[32] and activation of apoptotic pathways.[33] Oxygen-derived free radicals are therefore an important therapeutic target for treating glaucoma. A variety of antioxidants[34,35] and nitric oxide synthase (NOS)-inhibitors[36] are currently being investigated as potential therapeutic agents.

### 81.1.2 Excessive Glutamate, Increased Calcium Levels, and Excitotoxicity

Glutamate is an essential neurotransmitter, participating in a variety of neurological processes in the CNS.[37,38] It is also the main excitatory neurotransmitter in the retina and is involved in photo-transduction.[39]

Excessive levels of glutamate are toxic and detrimental to neurons; an excess of glutamate can hyperactivate the $N$-methyl-D-aspartate (NMDA) receptor, resulting in a poisonous influx of calcium[40] – a phenomenon termed *excitotoxicity*.[41,42] In glaucoma, the initially degenerating neurons expel their glutamate stores into the extracellular environment, thereby damaging their still healthy neighboring neurons. Moreover, Muller glial cells, which normally take up glutamate, fail to do so in glaucoma,[43] and thus glutamate levels continue to escalate, leading to retinal ganglion cell death.[44,45] Excitotoxicity is also common in other neurodegenerative diseases and neurological disorders including ALS,[46] Alzheimer's,[47,48] Parkinson's,[49,50] stroke, and Huntington's disease.[38,51] Blocking NMDA receptors by a glutamate antagonist can prevent the glaucomatous excitatory damage.[52]

However, because glutamate is a fundamental neurotransmitter vital for the normal maintenance of the retina and essential to many CNS functions,[37] the blockage of its receptor is accompanied by many side effects.

Another approach is to focus on the increased influx of calcium, caused by the excess of glutamate and the hyperstimulation of voltage-gated calcium channels.[51,53] Indeed, some calcium channel blockers have been shown to reduce retinal damage.[54,55]

### 81.1.3 Deprivation of Neurotrophins and Growth Factors

Neurotrophins are crucial for the normal maintenance of the CNS. These factors are required by all types of neurons including retinal ganglion cells (RGCs). They are produced in the superior colliculus and lateral geniculate nucleus in the brain and delivered along the optic nerve to the RGCs. Any interference with this neurotrophin supply could lead to neuronal damage. Ganglion cells are supported by brain-derived neurotrophic factor (BDNF), which delays apoptosis and prevents secondary degeneration.[56–60] Moreover, retinal cells respond to ciliary nerve trophic factor (CNTF) and fibroblast growth factor (FGF).[61] In glaucoma, retrograde and anterograde axonal transport are defective, often resulting in an insufficient supply of neurotrophins and growth factors to the retinal ganglion cells, leading to their apoptotic breakdown. Administration of neurotrophins can protect the retinal ganglion cells and prevent their programmed cell death.[56–60]

### 81.1.4 Abnormal Accumulation of Proteins

A shared feature among many of the neurodegenerative diseases is the abnormal increased accumulation of certain self-proteins during disease progression. The accumulation of beta-amyloid protein in the senile plaques in Alzheimer's and of alpha synuclein protein in Parkinson's are among the main characteristics of each of these diseases.[62] The abnormal processing of amyloid precursor protein has also been reported in glaucoma.[63] This is in addition to the oxidatively modified proteins that are produced during glaucomatous neurodegeneration.[32] Drug candidates that inhibit aggregation are now being tested in the clinic for the treatment of Alzheimer's and Parkinson's, and might also serve in the future as a therapy for glaucoma.[62,64]

### 81.1.5 Apoptotic Signals

The final outcome of disease progression is the enhanced activation of programmed cell death pathways among retinal ganglion cells. In a normal cell, a balance is maintained between pro-apoptotic and anti-apoptotic proteins. During disease progression, this balance is interrupted and there is an increase in the proportion of pro-apoptotic signals. This is manifested by the upregulation of the expression of pro-apoptotic genes, such as *bax*,[65] in parallel to the downregulation of the anti-apoptotic genes, such as *bcl-xL*.[66] Following the initial death signal, there is a rapid cascade of caspase activation that eventually results in a noninflammatory cell death.[67–69] The programmed cell death cycle of retinal cells is an interesting potential therapeutic target, though caution should be taken when considering this approach, since any anti-apoptotic agent can also serve as a potential carcinogen.

## 81.2 Pharmacological Neuroprotection for Glaucoma

The features described previously, presenting the toxic environment that is one of the well-known characteristics of neurodegenerative diseases, are also associated with glaucoma. This hostile environment might explain the fact that in glaucoma, as in other neurodegenerative disorders, primary cell death is followed by the secondary degeneration of surrounding neurons that were affected by the toxic microenvironment caused by the initial dying cells. This spread of damage, as a part of disease progression, is one of the hallmarks of neurodegenerative diseases, and can be clearly seen in glaucoma. We, as well as others, have proposed that the factors contributing to this ongoing degeneration are physiological compounds emerging in toxic quantities from the injured fibers or their cell bodies. Studies along these lines have revealed that some of the compounds identified in the pathogenesis of glaucoma are already known to be active in other neurodegenerative diseases. The many common features between the neurodegenerative diseases and glaucoma have led to the recognition of glaucoma as a neurodegenerative disease, rather than simply a disease of elevated ocular pressure.[70–72] This raises the possibility of utilizing similar therapeutic approaches for glaucoma that are currently being used in other neurodegenerative disorders.[20] Indeed, treatments used for Alzheimer's and Parkinson's are becoming more relevant to glaucoma; for example, Memantine, an NMDA channel blocker, used as a therapy for Alzheimer's and Parkinson's diseases, was evaluated for glaucoma treatment but ultimately failed to meet critical endpoints. It is likely that as our recognition of glaucoma as a neurodegenerative disease increases, more of the newly developed therapies will be based on neuroprotection,[73,74] fighting against the spread of damage and degeneration of retinal ganglion cells.

## 81.3 Protection of the Retinal Ganglion Cells Involves the Immune System

The CNS was always viewed as an "immune privileged" site, in which any immune response was considered harmful, and was usually associated with a disease or other malfunction. Our own studies of acute and chronic injuries to the rodent optic nerve led us to the unexpected discovery that the immune system plays a key role in the ability of the optic nerve and the retina to withstand injurious conditions.

Our first observations that the immune system (in the form of T cells directed to certain self-antigens) can protect injured neurons from death came from studies in rodents showing that passive transfer of T cells specific to myelin basic protein (MBP) reduces the loss of retinal ganglion cells (RGCs) after traumatic optic nerve injury.[75] We found that these T cells are also effective when directed to either cryptic or pathogenic epitopes of MBP, as well as toward other myelin-derived antigens or their epitopes.[76,77] These findings raised a number of critical questions. For example, are myelin antigens capable of protecting the visual system from all types of acute or chronic insults? Is the observed neuroprotective activity of immune cells merely an artifact of our experimental system, or does it indicate the critical participation of the immune system in fighting off injurious conditions in the visual system and in the CNS in general? If the latter is true, does that mean that glaucoma is a systemic disease? And if so, can this finding be translated into a systemic therapy that would protect the eye?

In a series of experiments carried out over almost a decade, we have learned much about the role of the immune response in neuroprotection. We first learned that the injury-induced response of T cells reactive to specific self-antigens residing in the site of stress (eye or brain) is a spontaneous physiological response that protects the nerve against the degenerative effects of the hostile environment – a concept that was established in our lab and named "protective autoimmunity."[78] Unfortunately, this protective response might not always be sufficient or properly controlled, which might explain the minimal spontaneous recovery following many severe CNS insults, including the damage that occurs in glaucoma. Secondly, we discovered that the specificity of such protective T cells depends on the site of the insult and type of cells damaged. Thus, for example, the protective effect of vaccination with myelin-associated antigens is restricted to injuries of the white matter; i.e., to myelinated axons.[77,79,80] If the insult is to the retina, which contains no myelin, myelin-related antigens have no effect.

We also sought to identify the phenotype of the beneficial autoimmune T cells, and to understand what determines the balance between a beneficial (neuroprotective) outcome of the T cell-mediated response to a CNS injury and a destructive effect causing autoimmune disease. Finally, we examined ways of translating the beneficial response into a therapy for glaucoma.

Some critical aspects of this approach had to be addressed along the way: (1) We verified that the loss of RGCs in a rat model of high intraocular pressure (IOP), simulating some types of glaucoma, is T cell-dependent[81]; (2) We attempted to determine whether the specific self-antigens that are harnessed by the protective autoimmune T cells in our rat model of chronic glaucoma, and which can be boosted for therapeutic purposes, reside in the retina or the optic nerve[82]; and, finally, (3) We searched for an antigen that would be able to safely boost the physiological response without causing autoimmune disease.

Using a rat model of elevated intraocular pressure, we showed that a protective response could be obtained only with an antigen residing in the retina, suggesting that, at least in this model, the site of self-perpetuating degeneration, and therefore the site in need of protection, is not the optic nerve but the retina.[79,82] We further determined that in immune-deficient animals, the number of surviving retinal ganglion cells following an insult of elevated IOP is significantly lower than in matched controls with an intact immune system. This suggests that the ability to withstand insult to the optic nerve or to the retina depends on the integrity of the immune system, and particularly on the specific cell population within the immune system that recognizes the site-specific self-antigens. Interestingly, treatment with steroids, which have an immunosuppressant effect, caused a significant loss of RGCs.[82] Moreover, in a model of RGC loss induced by non-IOP conditions (for example uveitis), steroids, which alleviate the inflammatory manifestations of the uveitis, not only failed to protect RGCs but even caused further death. These results prompted us to suggest that the well-controlled boosting of the T cell response might protect RGCs, even under conditions of normal tension glaucoma as well as in uveitis.

### 81.3.1 T cells Specific to Antigens Residing in the Site of Damage Help Clean and Heal

To manifest their protective effects, anti-self T cells should home to the site of damage and be locally activated. This is why only those antigens that are present at the site of lesion can be used for the vaccination. Once activated, the T cells provide a source of cytokines and growth factors, which create the proper niche for microglia and infiltrating blood-borne monocytes, so as to make them active protective cells that the eye can tolerate (Scheme 81.1). Namely, such activated microglia/macrophages can take up glutamate, remove debris, and produce growth factors; additionally, they do not produce agents that are part of their cytotoxic mechanism, such as TNFα, which the eye, like the brain tolerates poorly.[83–87] Such T cells are constitutively controlled by regulatory T cells that are part of the physiological immune network and are themselves amenable to control upon need.[88,89]

## 81.4 Searching for an Antigen for Potential Glaucoma Therapy

Among the many immunomodulatory compounds that we tested for therapy of glaucoma was glatiramer acetate (GA), also known as Copaxone, a synthetic 4-amino-acid copolymer, currently used as a treatment (administered according to a daily regimen) for multiple sclerosis. We chose to test this compound because of its low-affinity cross-reaction with a wide range of self-antigens residing in the CNS. In the rat model of chronically high IOP, vaccination with GA significantly reduces RGC loss even if the IOP remains high. Vaccination does not prevent disease onset, but rather slows down the progression of the RGC loss by controlling the milieu of the nerve and retina, making it less hostile to neuronal survival and allowing the RGCs to better withstand the stress.[79,88,90–92] In our initial studies, we used GA emulsified in complete Freund's adjuvant (CFA).[79] We subsequently found that in models of optic nerve insults and in models of spinal cord injury, regardless of the choice of the antigens, the type of adjuvant (amount of mycobacteria), the timing of the vaccination, and the dosing critically affect the outcome.[93–95] In subsequent studies in a model of IOP, we tested adjuvant-free GA, and found that GA is effective even without an adjuvant, but the onset of the treatment, the frequency, and the dosing are critical.[94] Given that a self-perpetuating degeneration is a multiparameter disease in which numerous factors are participating, it seems that a therapy involving the well-controlled activation of the immune system can provide a multidimensional effectual treatment. For chronic

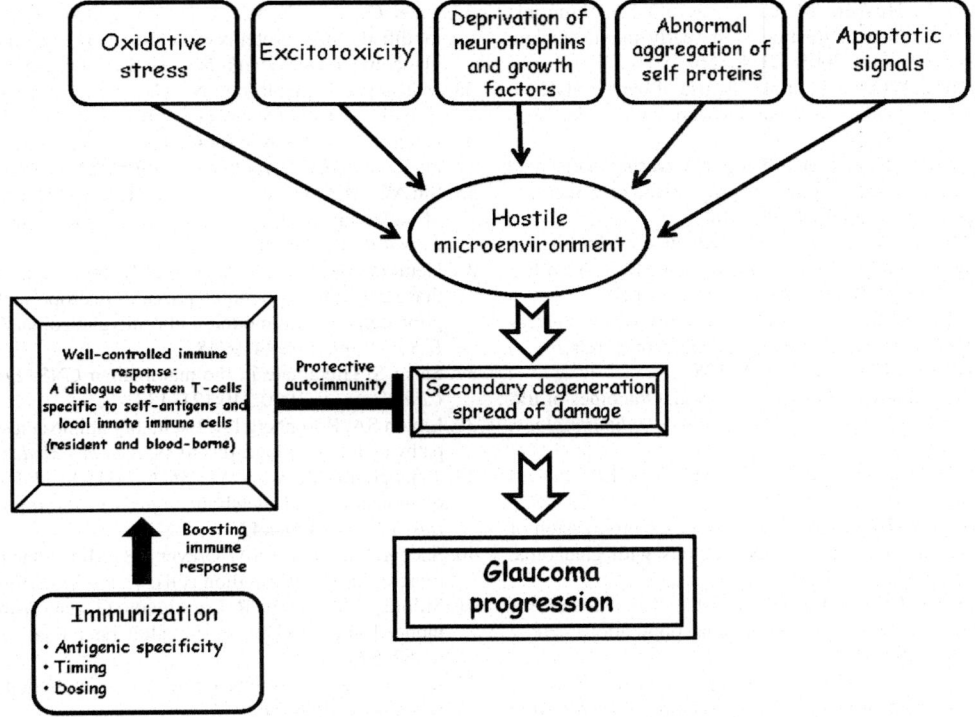

**Fig. 81.1** Factors contributing to glaucoma versus immune responses

treatment, daily, weekly, and monthly regimens were tested; no benefit was found in daily injection, while weekly and monthly treatments were effective.[94]

## 81.5 Conclusion

During the past decade, scientists and clinicians began to accept that glaucoma should not be viewed as a distinct syndrome with its own peculiar features, but as one of the large group of neurodegenerative disorders of the central nervous system (CNS). Regardless of the primary source of tissue injury, degeneration may continue due to the loss of equilibrium that exists between the initial insult and the ability of the eye to withstand it. As described previously, this stage of equilibrium is generally managed by the immune system (Fig. 81.1). According to our view, rather than or in addition to fighting off the risk factor(s), there is a need to protect the tissue from the ongoing spread of damage, an approach collectively termed "Neuroprotection."[18] This view of glaucoma has led to major changes in the nature of glaucoma research, the way in which clinicians perceive the disease, and the approach to therapy. One comprehensive approach is to harness the immune system, which if properly controlled can be used to modulate the local milieu, so as to become protective rather than hostile to the RGCs (Scheme 81.1). Such selective immune activation can address the multiple risk factors contributing to the glaucomatous degeneration process. Currently, more specific antigens are being tested as possible candidates for specific immune therapy of glaucoma.

## References

1. Weinreb RN, Khaw PT. Primary open-angle glaucoma. *Lancet*. 2004;363:1711–1720.
2. Burgoyne CF, Downs JC, Bellezza AJ, et al. The optic nerve head as a biomechanical structure: a new paradigm for understanding the role of IOP-related stress and strain in the pathophysiology of glaucomatous optic nerve head damage. *Prog Retin Eye Res*. 2005;24:39–73.
3. Sigal IA, Flanagan JG, Ethier CR. Factors influencing optic nerve head biomechanics. *Invest Ophthalmol Vis Sci*. 2005;46:4189–4199.
4. Tezel G, Wax MB. Hypoxia-inducible factor 1alpha in the glaucomatous retina and optic nerve head. *Arch Ophthalmol*. 2004;122:1348–1356.
5. Tezel G, Hernandez R, Wax MB. Immunostaining of heat shock proteins in the retina and optic nerve head of normal and glaucomatous eyes. *Arch Ophthalmol*. 2000;118:511–518.
6. Quigley HA, Maumenee AE. Long-term follow-up of treated open-angle glaucoma. *Am J Ophthalmol*. 1979;87:519–525.
7. Kass MA, Heuer DK, Higginbotham EJ, et al. The Ocular Hypertension Treatment Study: a randomized trial determines that topical ocular hypotensive medication delays or prevents the onset of primary open-angle glaucoma. *Arch Ophthalmol*. 2002;120:701–713. discussion 829–730.

8. Leske MC, Heijl A, Hussein M, et al. Factors for glaucoma progression and the effect of treatment: the early manifest glaucoma trial. *Arch Ophthalmol*. 2003;121:48–56.
9. Johnson EC, Cepurna WO, Jia L, et al. The use of cyclodialysis to limit exposure to elevated intraocular pressure in rat glaucoma models. *Exp Eye Res*. 2006;83:51–60.
10. Nickells RW, Schlamp CL, Li Y, et al. Surgical lowering of elevated intraocular pressure in monkeys prevents progression of glaucomatous disease. *Exp Eye Res*. 2007;84:729–736.
11. Heijl A, Leske MC, Bengtsson B, et al. Reduction of intraocular pressure and glaucoma progression: results from the Early Manifest Glaucoma Trial. *Arch Ophthalmol*. 2002;120:1268–1279.
12. Jay JL, Allan D. The benefit of early trabeculectomy versus conventional management in primary open angle glaucoma relative to severity of disease. *Eye*. 1989;3(Pt 5):528–535.
13. Nouri-Mahdavi K, Brigatti L, Weitzman M, et al. Outcomes of trabeculectomy for primary open-angle glaucoma. *Ophthalmology*. 1995;102:1760–1769.
14. Brubaker RF. Delayed functional loss in glaucoma. LII Edward Jackson Memorial Lecture. *Am J Ophthalmol*. 1996;121:473–483.
15. Richler M, Werner EB, Thomas D. Risk factors for progression of visual field defects in medically treated patients with glaucoma. *Can J Ophthalmol*. 1982;17:245–248.
16. Schulzer M, Drance SM, Carter CJ, et al. Biostatistical evidence for two distinct chronic open angle glaucoma populations. *Br J Ophthalmol*. 1990;74:196–200.
17. Chauhan BC, Drance SM. The relationship between intraocular pressure and visual field progression in glaucoma. *Graefes Arch Clin Exp Ophthalmol*. 1992;230:521–526.
18. Schwartz M, Belkin M, Yoles E, et al. Potential treatment modalities for glaucomatous neuropathy: neuroprotection and neuroregeneration. *J Glaucoma*. 1996;5:427–432.
19. Schwartz M. Neurodegeneration and neuroprotection in glaucoma: development of a therapeutic neuroprotective vaccine: the friedenwald lecture. *Invest Ophthalmol Vis Sci*. 2003;44:1407–1411.
20. Schwartz M. Lessons for glaucoma from other neurodegenerative diseases: can one treatment suit them all? *J Glaucoma*. 2005;14:321–323.
21. Beckman JS, Carson M, Smith CD, et al. ALS, SOD and peroxynitrite. *Nature*. 1993;364:584.
22. Abe K, Pan LH, Watanabe M, et al. Induction of nitrotyrosine-like immunoreactivity in the lower motor neuron of amyotrophic lateral sclerosis. *Neurosci Lett*. 1995;199:152–154.
23. Giasson BI, Duda JE, Murray IV, et al. Oxidative damage linked to neurodegeneration by selective alpha-synuclein nitration in synucleinopathy lesions. *Science*. 2000;290:985–989.
24. Castegna A, Thongboonkerd V, Klein JB, et al. Proteomic identification of nitrated proteins in Alzheimer's disease brain. *J Neurochem*. 2003;85:1394–1401.
25. Andersen JK. Oxidative stress in neurodegeneration: cause or consequence? *Nat Med*. 2004;10(Suppl):S18–S25.
26. Potashkin JA, Meredith GE. The role of oxidative stress in the dysregulation of gene expression and protein metabolism in neurodegenerative disease. *Antioxid Redox Signal*. 2006;8:144–151.
27. Sultana R, Poon HF, Cai J, et al. Identification of nitrated proteins in Alzheimer's disease brain using a redox proteomics approach. *Neurobiol Dis*. 2006;22:76–87.
28. Oku H, Yamaguchi H, Sugiyama T, et al. Retinal toxicity of nitric oxide released by administration of a nitric oxide donor in the albino rabbit. *Invest Ophthalmol Vis Sci*. 1997;38:2540–2544.
29. Levkovitch-Verbin H, Harris-Cerruti C, Groner Y, et al. RGC death in mice after optic nerve crush injury: oxidative stress and neuroprotection. *Invest Ophthalmol Vis Sci*. 2000;41:4169–4174.
30. Tezel G. Oxidative stress in glaucomatous neurodegeneration: mechanisms and consequences. *Prog Retin Eye Res*. 2006;25:490–513.
31. Tezel G, Wax MB. Glial modulation of retinal ganglion cell death in glaucoma. *J Glaucoma*. 2003;12:63–68.
32. Tezel G, Yang X, Cai J. Proteomic identification of oxidatively modified retinal proteins in a chronic pressure-induced rat model of glaucoma. *Invest Ophthalmol Vis Sci*. 2005;46:3177–3187.
33. Martindale JL, Holbrook NJ. Cellular response to oxidative stress: signaling for suicide and survival. *J Cell Physiol*. 2002;192:1–15.
34. Ritch R. Potential role for Ginkgo biloba extract in the treatment of glaucoma. *Med Hypotheses*. 2000;54:221–235.
35. Siu AW, Maldonado M, Sanchez-Hidalgo M, et al. Protective effects of melatonin in experimental free radical-related ocular diseases. *J Pineal Res*. 2006;40:101–109.
36. Neufeld AH, Sawada A, Becker B. Inhibition of nitric-oxide synthase 2 by aminoguanidine provides neuroprotection of retinal ganglion cells in a rat model of chronic glaucoma. *Proc Natl Acad Sci U S A*. 1999;96:9944–9948.
37. Sahai S. Glutamate in the mammalian CNS. *Eur Arch Psychiatry Clin Neurosci*. 1990;240:121–133.
38. Lipton SA, Rosenberg PA. Excitatory amino acids as a final common pathway for neurologic disorders. *N Engl J Med*. 1994;330:613–622.
39. Tsacopoulos M, Poitry-Yamate CL, MacLeish PR, et al. Trafficking of molecules and metabolic signals in the retina. *Prog Retin Eye Res*. 1998;17:429–442.
40. Sucher NJ, Lipton SA, Dreyer EB. Molecular basis of glutamate toxicity in retinal ganglion cells. *Vision Res*. 1997;37:3483–3493.
41. Siliprandi R, Canella R, Carmignoto G, et al. N-methyl-D-aspartate-induced neurotoxicity in the adult rat retina. *Vis Neurosci*. 1992;8:567–573.
42. Dreyer EB. A proposed role for excitotoxicity in glaucoma. *J Glaucoma*. 1998;7:62–67.
43. Napper GA, Pianta MJ, Kalloniatis M. Reduced glutamate uptake by retinal glial cells under ischemic/hypoxic conditions. *Vis Neurosci*. 1999;16:149–158.
44. Olney JW. Glutaate-induced retinal degeneration in neonatal mice. Electron microscopy of the acutely evolving lesion. *J Neuropathol Exp Neurol*. 1969;28:455–474.
45. Olney JW, Price MT, Samson L, et al. The role of specific ions in glutamate neurotoxicity. *Neurosci Lett*. 1986;65:65–71.
46. Van Den Bosch L, Van Damme P, Bogaert E, et al. The role of excitotoxicity in the pathogenesis of amyotrophic lateral sclerosis. *Biochim Biophys Acta*. 2006;1762:1068–1082.
47. Riederer P, Hoyer S. From benefit to damage. Glutamate and advanced glycation end products in Alzheimer brain. *J Neural Transm*. 2006;113:1671–1677.
48. Lipton SA. Pathologically-activated therapeutics for neuroprotection: mechanism of NMDA receptor block by memantine and S-nitrosylation. *Curr Drug Targets*. 2007;8:621–632.
49. Beal MF. Excitotoxicity and nitric oxide in Parkinson's disease pathogenesis. *Ann Neurol*. 1998;44:S110–114.
50. Lancelot E, Beal MF. Glutamate toxicity in chronic neurodegenerative disease. *Prog Brain Res*. 1998;116:331–347.
51. Choi DW. Glutamate neurotoxicity and diseases of the nervous system. *Neuron*. 1988;1:623–634.
52. Stuiver BT, Douma BR, Bakker R, et al. In vivo protection against NMDA-induced neurodegeneration by MK-801 and nimodipine: combined therapy and temporal course of protection. *Neurodegeneration*. 1996;5:153–159.
53. Choi DW. Calcium-mediated neurotoxicity: relationship to specific channel types and role in ischemic damage. *Trends Neurosci*. 1988;11:465–469.
54. Takahashi K, Lam TT, Edward DP, et al. Protective effects of flunarizine on ischemic injury in the rat retina. *Arch Ophthalmol*. 1992;110:862–870.
55. Bath CP, Farrell LN, Gilmore J, et al. The effects of ifenprodil and eliprodil on voltage-dependent $Ca^{2+}$ channels and in gerbil global cerebral ischaemia. *Eur J Pharmacol*. 1996;299:103–112.
56. Mansour-Robaey S, Clarke DB, Wang YC, et al. Effects of ocular injury and administration of brain-derived neurotrophic factor on

56. [continued] survival and regrowth of axotomized retinal ganglion cells. *Proc Natl Acad Sci U S A*. 1994;91:1632–1636.
57. Peinado-Ramon P, Salvador M, Villegas-Perez MP, et al. Effects of axotomy and intraocular administration of NT-4, NT-3, and brain-derived neurotrophic factor on the survival of adult rat retinal ganglion cells. A quantitative in vivo study. *Invest Ophthalmol Vis Sci*. 1996;37:489–500.
58. Gao H, Qiao X, Hefti F, et al. Elevated mRNA expression of brain-derived neurotrophic factor in retinal ganglion cell layer after optic nerve injury. *Invest Ophthalmol Vis Sci*. 1997;38:1840–1847.
59. Klocker N, Cellerino A, Bahr M. Free radical scavenging and inhibition of nitric oxide synthase potentiates the neurotrophic effects of brain-derived neurotrophic factor on axotomized retinal ganglion cells in vivo. *J Neurosci*. 1998;18:1038–1046.
60. Rocha M, Martins RA, Linden R. Activation of NMDA receptors protects against glutamate neurotoxicity in the retina: evidence for the involvement of neurotrophins. *Brain Res*. 1999;827:79–92.
61. Unoki K, LaVail MM. Protection of the rat retina from ischemic injury by brain-derived neurotrophic factor, ciliary neurotrophic factor, and basic fibroblast growth factor. *Invest Ophthalmol Vis Sci*. 1994;35:907–915.
62. Lansbury PT, Lashuel HA. A century-old debate on protein aggregation and neurodegeneration enters the clinic. *Nature*. 2006; 443:774–779.
63. McKinnon SJ, Lehman DM, Kerrigan-Baumrind LA, et al. Caspase activation and amyloid precursor protein cleavage in rat ocular hypertension. *Invest Ophthalmol Vis Sci*. 2002;43:1077–1087.
64. Weydt P, La Spada AR. Targeting protein aggregation in neurodegeneration – lessons from polyglutamine disorders. *Expert Opin Ther Targets*. 2006;10:505–513.
65. Oltvai ZN, Korsmeyer SJ. Checkpoints of dueling dimers foil death wishes. *Cell*. 1994;79:189–192.
66. Levin LA, Schlamp CL, Spieldoch RL, et al. Identification of the bcl-2 family of genes in the rat retina. *Invest Ophthalmol Vis Sci*. 1997;38:2545–2553.
67. Thornberry NA. Caspases: key mediators of apoptosis. *Chem Biol*. 1998;5:R97–103.
68. Thornberry NA, Lazebnik Y. Caspases: enemies within. *Science*. 1998;281:1312–1316.
69. Quigley HA. Neuronal death in glaucoma. *Prog Retin Eye Res*. 1999;18:39–57.
70. Gupta N, Yucel YH. Glaucoma as a neurodegenerative disease. *Curr Opin Ophthalmol*. 2007;18:110–114.
71. Mozaffarieh M, Flammer J. Is there more to glaucoma treatment than lowering IOP? *Surv Ophthalmol*. 2007;52(Suppl 2):S174–179.
72. Nickells RW. From ocular hypertension to ganglion cell death: a heoretical sequence of events leading to glaucoma. *Can J Ophthalmol*. 2007;42:278–287.
73. Hartwick AT. Beyond intraocular pressure: neuroprotective strategies for future glaucoma therapy. *Optom Vis Sci*. 2001;78:85–94.
74. Chidlow G, Wood JP, Casson RJ. Pharmacological neuroprotection for glaucoma. *Drugs*. 2007;67:725–759.
75. Moalem G, Leibowitz-Amit R, Yoles E, et al. Autoimmune T cells protect neurons from secondary degeneration after central nervous system axotomy. *Nat Med*. 1999;5:49–55.
76. Fisher J, Levkovitch-Verbin H, Schori H, et al. Vaccination for neuroprotection in the mouse optic nerve: implications for optic neuropathies. *J Neurosci*. 2001;21:136–142.
77. Mizrahi T, Hauben E, Schwartz M. The tissue-specific self-pathogen is the protective self-antigen: the case of uveitis. *J Immunol*. 2002; 169:5971–5977.
78. Yoles E, Hauben E, Palgi O, et al. Protective autoimmunity is a physiological response to CNS trauma. *J Neurosci*. 2001;21:3740–3748.
79. Schori H, Kipnis J, Yoles E, et al. Vaccination for protection of retinal ganglion cells against death from glutamate cytotoxicity and ocular hypertension: implications for glaucoma. *Proc Natl Acad Sci U S A*. 2001;98:3398–3403.
80. Avidan H, Kipnis J, Butovsky O, et al. Vaccination with autoantigen protects against aggregated beta-amyloid and glutamate toxicity by controlling microglia: effect of CD4+CD25+ T cells. *Eur J Immunol*. 2004;34:3434–3445.
81. Bakalash S, Kipnis J, Yoles E, et al. Resistance of retinal ganglion cells to an increase in intraocular pressure is immune-dependent. *Invest Ophthalmol Vis Sci*. 2002;43:2648–2653.
82. Bakalash S, Kessler A, Mizrahi T, et al. Antigenic specificity of immunoprotective therapeutic vaccination for glaucoma. *Invest Ophthalmol Vis Sci*. 2003;44:3374–3381.
83. Moalem G, Gdalyahu A, Shani Y, et al. Production of neurotrophins by activated T cells: implications for neuroprotective autoimmunity. *J Autoimmun*. 2000;15:331–345.
84. Butovsky O, Hauben E, Schwartz M. Morphological aspects of spinal cord autoimmune neuroprotection: colocalization of T cells with B7-2 (CD86) and prevention of cyst formation. *FASEB J*. 2001;15:1065–1067.
85. Barouch R, Schwartz M. Autoreactive T cells induce neurotrophin production by immune and neural cells in injured rat optic nerve: implications for protective autoimmunity. *FASEB J*. 2002;16: 1304–1306.
86. Butovsky O, Talpalar AE, Ben-Yaakov K, et al. Activation of microglia by aggregated beta-amyloid or lipopolysaccharide impairs MHC-II expression and renders them cytotoxic whereas IFN-gamma and IL-4 render them protective. *Mol Cell Neurosci*. 2005;29:381–393.
87. Shaked I, Tchoresh D, Gersner R, et al. Protective autoimmunity: interferon-gamma enables microglia to remove glutamate without evoking inflammatory mediators. *J Neurochem*. 2005;92:997–1009.
88. Kipnis J, Mizrahi T, Hauben E, et al. Neuroprotective autoimmunity: naturally occurring CD4+CD25+ regulatory T cells suppress the ability to withstand injury to the central nervous system. *Proc Natl Acad Sci USA*. 2002;99:15620–15625.
89. Kipnis J, Cardon M, Avidan H, et al. Dopamine, through the extracellular signal-regulated kinase pathway, downregulates CD4+CD25+ regulatory T-cell activity: implications for neurodegeneration. *J Neurosci*. 2004;24:6133–6143.
90. Kipnis J, Yoles E, Porat Z, et al. T cell immunity to copolymer 1 confers neuroprotection on the damaged optic nerve: possible therapy for optic neuropathies. *Proc Natl Acad Sci U S A*. 2000;97:7446–7451.
91. Benner EJ, Mosley RL, Destache CJ, et al. Therapeutic immunization protects dopaminergic neurons in a mouse model of Parkinson's disease. *Proc Natl Acad Sci U S A*. 2004;101:9435–9440.
92. Schwartz M. Modulating the immune system: a vaccine for glaucoma? *Can J Ophthalmol*. 2007;42:439–441.
93. Hauben E, Agranov E, Gothilf A, et al. Posttraumatic therapeutic vaccination with modified myelin self-antigen prevents complete paralysis while avoiding autoimmune disease. *J Clin Invest*. 2001; 108:591–599.
94. Bakalash S, Shlomo GB, Aloni E, et al. T-cell-based vaccination for morphological and functional neuroprotection in a rat model of chronically elevated intraocular pressure. *J Mol Med*. 2005;83:904–916.
95. Blair M, Pease ME, Hammond J, et al. Effect of glatiramer acetate on primary and secondary degeneration of retinal ganglion cells in the rat. *Invest Ophthalmol Vis Sci*. 2005;46:884-890.

# Chapter 82
# How the Revolution in Cell Biology Will Affect Glaucoma: Biomarkers

Paul A. Knepper, Michael J. Nolan, and Beatrice Y. J. T. Yue

Multiple biomarker panels of common, multifactorial diseases – such as cardiovascular[1-3] and Alzheimer's disease[4,5] – have recently been described, facilitating the diagnosis and risk management of these diseases. In principle, a biomarker is an indicator of a biochemical feature or facet that can be used to diagnose or monitor the progress of a disease.[6] Detection technology has been identified for possible types of biomarkers in primary open-angle glaucoma (POAG).[7] We will summarize known biomarkers with the intent of cataloging the biomarkers in the aqueous humor, trabecular meshwork (TM), optic nerve, and blood in patients with POAG. To facilitate comparisons and to offer mechanistic clues, biochemical changes such as up- or downregulation of proteins that have been reported in POAG are organized into three categories: namely, extracellular matrix (ECM) changes, cytokine/signaling molecules, and aging/stress (listed respectively in Tables 82.1,[8-23] 82.2,[24-33] and 82.3[34-46]).

POAG is the most common type of glaucoma, particularly in populations with European and African ancestry. This disease is the leading cause of blindness in African-Americans. The major ocular risk factors for POAG include intraocular pressure (IOP) elevation and aging. The prevalence of POAG increases from 0.02% at ages 40 to 49 to 2% to 3% for persons over the age of 70[47]; and incidence of ocular hypertension increases from 2 to 9% over the same time span.[48] Although the relationship between Alzheimer's disease and POAG remains obscure, more than 20% of Alzheimer's patients also have POAG.[49] The plasma concentration of a variety of signaling proteins differs between patients with Alzheimer's and normal control subjects,[4] indicating that systemic plasma changes take place along with central nervous dysfunction. It is likely that cellular insults or molecular defects intersect, leading to neurodegeneration. Similar scenarios may also occur in POAG.

## 82.1 ECM Changes in POAG

ECM components in the TM are essential for maintenance of the normal aqueous humor outflow.[50-53] In the TM of POAG eyes, excessive, abnormal accumulations as well as decreases of other ECM materials (Table 82.1) have been documented.[8,50-53] The ECM produced by the cells is composed of multidomain macromolecules such as collagens, cell-binding glycoproteins, and proteoglycans that link together to form a structurally stable composite. Recent studies have revealed that ECM is a dynamic entity determining and controlling the behavior and biologic characteristics of the cells.

One key component of the ECM in TM is proteoglycans, which are macromolecules consisting of a core protein to which glycosaminoglycan side chains are covalently attached. This class of molecules has been implicated in the maintenance of resistance to aqueous humor outflow ever since Barany,[54] in the 1950s, demonstrated that perfusion of the anterior chamber with testicular hyaluronidase greatly reduced the outflow resistance in enucleated bovine eyes. In the TM tissue, proteoglycans form gel-like networks that may function as a gel filtration system. The major types identified include chondroitin, dermatan, and heparan sulfate proteoglycans that may represent decorin, biglycan, versican, perlecan, and syndecan.[50-52]

The relative amounts of each type of glycosaminoglycan in the TM tissue have been determined.[10,50-52] Hyaluronic acid and chondroitin–dermatan sulfates are the major constituents, with heparan sulfate and keratan sulfate present in smaller amounts. A depletion in hyaluronic acid and an accumulation of chondroitin sulfates and undigestible glycosaminoglycan material have been associated with POAG conditions.[10] Both chondroitin sulfate and hyaluronic acid have been shown to contribute to flow resistance and influence flow rate in vitro.[55] The flow rate was decreased when hyaluronic acid and chondroitin sulfate were used at POAG concentrations.[56] Disrupting glycosaminoglycan chain biosynthesis by sodium chlorate or β-xyloside increases outflow facility in perfusion culture.[57] Of note, the level of an ectodomain fragment of hyaluronic acid receptor CD44 (sCD44) was found to be elevated (Table 82.2) in the aqueous humor of POAG patients,[29] and the concentration was correlated with visual field loss.[29] sCD44 is cytotoxic to TM cells, but the toxicity can be blocked by hyaluronic acid.[58] The decreased hyaluronic acid may thus result in diminished protective capacity and further deterioration in POAG conditions.

**Table 82.1** Extracellular matrix changes in POAG

| | Aqueous humor | Trabecular meshwork | Optic nerve | Systemic (blood) |
|---|---|---|---|---|
| ECM Elements | | | | |
| CD44 | | ↓[8] | | |
| Cochlin | | ↑[9] | | |
| Chondroitin sulfate | | ↑[10] | | |
| Collagen type IV | | nc[11] | | |
| Elastin | | ↑[12] | ↑[13] | |
| Fibronectin | nc[14] | nc[11] | | |
| Hyaluronic acid | ↓↓[15] | ↓↓↓↓[10] | ↓[16] | |
| GAGase-resistant material | | ↑↑↑↑[10] | | |
| Tenascin | | | ↑[17] | |
| Thrombospondin-1 | | ↑[18] | | |
| ECM Remodeling Enzymes and Inhibitors | | | | |
| MMP-1 | | ↑[19] | ↑[20] | |
| MMP-3 | nc[21] | ↑[19] | ↑[20] | |
| MT1-MMP | | | | ↑[22] |
| TIMP-1 | nc[21] | ↑[19] | | |
| TIMP-2 | ↑[23] | | | |

The increase or decrease in the reported biochemical changes in POAG are expressed as statistically significant ↑ or ↓. Whenever possible, a twofold change is denoted by two *arrows*, a threefold change by three *arrows*, and a fourfold change by four *arrows*, and nc indicates no change. GAGase – glycosaminoglycan-degrading enzyme; MMP – matrix metalloproteinase; MT1-MMP – membrane type 1-MMP; TIMP – tissue inhibitor for MMP

Fibronectin, laminin, vitronectin, and matricellular proteins that include tenascin and thrombospondin-1 have been localized in the TM.[18,50,51] These glycoproteins are crucial in biologic processes such as cell attachment, spreading, and cell differentiation. Overexpression of fibronectin and laminin, as well as collagen type IV, results in a decrease in the TM cell monolayer permeability.[50,59] The expression of thrombospondin-1 has in addition been shown to be increased[18] in the TM of POAG eyes (Table 82.1).

Elastin is localized to the central core of sheath-derived plaques or elastic-like fibers in the TM.[50] Fibrillin-1, a component of microfibrils, is found in both the core and the surrounding sheath of the elastic-like fibers. Fibrillin-1 and type VI collagen are also constituents of long-spacing collagens in the TM.[50,53] It is believed that the collagen fibers and elastic-like fibers are organized in the TM to accommodate resilience and tensile strength, providing a mechanism for reversible deformation in response to cyclic hydrodynamic loading. In trabecular lamellae and in juxtacanalicular (JCT) regions, accumulation of long spacing collagens and sheath-derived plaques has been documented in POAG and aged eyes.[50,53]

The ECM is constantly modified by the surrounding cells through enzymes such as matrix metalloproteinase (MMP) family members and inhibitors such as tissue inhibitors for matrix metalloproteinase (TIMPs) found in the TM.[52] Ongoing ECM turnover, initiated by MMPs, appears to be essential for maintenance of the aqueous outflow homeostasis. MMP-3, and possibly also MMP-9, may be responsible for the efficacy of laser trabeculoplasty, an alternative treatment to reduce IOP in patients with glaucoma.[50,52] Addition or induction of MMP-3 in perfused human anterior segment organ cultures increases the aqueous humor outflow facility, whereas blocking the endogenous activity of the MMPs in the TM reduces it.[52]

The ECM in the TM may also be remodeled in response to exogenous stimuli such as glucocorticoids and oxidative stress.[50,51] Mechanical stretch caused an increase in MMP-1 and MMP-3 activities and alteration of ECM molecules including proteoglycans and matricellular proteins.[60] The ECM is modulated by cytokines. The most studied cytokine in the TM is transforming growth factor-beta (TGF-β). A higher than normal level[30] of TGF-β2 was found in the aqueous humor of patients with POAG (Table 82.2). TGF-β2 upregulated ECM-related genes in TM cell cultures. In TGF-β2-perfused organ cultures, focal accumulation of fine fibrillar extracellular material was observed in TM tissues. Furthermore, TGF-β2 perfusion reduced outflow facility and elevated IOP.[61] These results suggest that the increased TGF-β2 level in the aqueous humor may be related to the pathogenesis of glaucoma. Other cytokines such as tumor necrosis factor-α (TNF-α) that is increased in the optic nerve head of POAG (Table 82.2) also modulate the ECM, probably via regulation of MMP and TIMP expressions.[50,51,62] The cochlin deposits in the glaucomatous TM (Table 82.1) appear to increase with age and are associated with proteoglycans. Such deposits have been proposed to contribute to the increase of ECM resistance to outflow and the POAG pathology.[9]

## 82.2 Cytokine/Signaling Molecules in POAG

The TM and optic nerve utilize local and probably systemic cell signaling pathways to maintain cell viability. Locally in the TM, the Rho family of small guanosine triphosphatase (GTPase) has been shown to be of vital importance in the outflow system.[54,63,64] In the active GTP-bound state, Rho GTPases interact with and activate downstream effectors such as Rho kinase to modulate the assembly of actin structures. In TM cells, a decrease in actin stress fibers and focal adhesions has been shown to occur with treatment of Rho kinase inhibitors and gene transfer of dominant negative RhoA and dominant negative Rho-binding domain of Rho kinase.[64] These cellular changes are associated with reduced myosin light chain (MLC) phosphorylation and/or enhanced outflow facility.[53] Conversely, molecules including sphingosine-1-phosphate and endothelin-1 that activate Rho/Rho kinase signaling pathway through G-protein coupled receptors promote MLC phosphorylation, and in turn decrease the aqueous humor outflow facility.[54,63,64] Endothelial-1 has been reported to be increased in the aqueous humor[24] and blood[25] of POAG patients (Table 82.2).

The aqueous humor that also modulates TM cell signaling contains albumin as a major constituent. Other components encompass hydrogen peroxide ($H_2O_2$), ascorbic acid, cytokines such as TGF-β, heptocyte growth factor, and vascular endothelial growth factor (VEGF), and molecules including MMPs, proteinase inhibitors, sCD44, and hyaluronic acid.[50] A recent study has demonstrated that addition of normal aqueous humor rather than the standard fetal bovine serum to monolayers of TM cultures decreases cell proliferation and produces changes in cellular and molecular characteristics to mimic more closely the TM physiologic profiles in situ.[65]

Increased levels of TGF-β2, sCD44, interleukin-2, phospholipase 2, thymulin (Table 82.2), glutathione, ascorbic acid (Table 82.3), and a decreased level of hyaluronic acid

**Table 82.2** Changes in cell signaling molecules in primary open angle glaucoma

|  | Aqueous humor | Trabecular meshwork | Optic nerve | Systemic (blood) |
|---|---|---|---|---|
| Endothelin-1 | ↑[24] | | | ↑[24,25] |
| Hepatocyte growth factor | ↑[26] | | | |
| Interleukin 2 | | | | ↑[27] |
| Phospholipase A2 | ↑[28] | | | |
| Soluble CD44 | ↑↑[29] | | | |
| Transforming growth factor-β2 | ↑[30] | | | |
| Thymulin | | | | ↑↑↑[31] |
| Tumor necrosis factor-α | | | ↑[20] | |
| Vascular endothelial growth factor | ↑[32] | | | ↑[33] |

The increase or decrease in the reported changes in POAG are expressed as statistically significant ↑ or ↓. Whenever possible, a twofold change is denoted by two *arrows*, a threefold change by three *arrows*, and a fourfold change by four arrows.

**Table 82.3** Changes related to stress and aging in POAG

|  | Aqueous humor | Trabecular meshwork | Optic nerve | Systemic (blood) |
|---|---|---|---|---|
| Acetylcholinesterase | | | | ↑[34] |
| αB-Crystallin | | ↑[35] | | |
| 3-α-Hydroxysteroid dehydrogenase | | | | ↓[36] |
| Ascorbic acid | ↑↑↑[37] | | | |
| Cortisol | | | | ↑[38] |
| Fatty acid | | | | |
| Eicosapentaenoic | | | | ↓[39] |
| Docosahexaenoic | | | | ↓[39] |
| Omega 3 | | | | ↓[39] |
| Glutathione | ↑↑↑[40] | | | ↓[41] |
| Hypoxia inducible factor-1α (HIF-1α) | | | ↑[42] | |
| Nuclear factor-kB (NF-kB) | | ↑[43] | | |
| Nitric oxide | ↑[44] | | | |
| Senescence associated β-galactosidase | ↑[45] | | | |
| Serum amyloid A | | ↑↑[46] | | |

The increase or decrease in the reported changes in POAG is expressed as statistically significant ↑ or ↓. Whenever possible, a twofold change is denoted by two *arrows*, a threefold change by three *arrows*, and a fourfold change by four *arrows*.

(Table 82.1) have been reported in the aqueous humor of POAG eyes. Since TM cells are in constant contact with the aqueous humor, it is expected that altered levels and/or activities of aqueous humor components would have an impact on the behavior and activities of these cells. The sCD44 found in the POAG aqueous humor is hypophosphorylated.[66] The hypophosphorylated form has high cytotoxicity and low hyaluronic acid-binding affinity and is suggested to represent a pathophysiologic feature of the disease process.[66]

## 82.3 Stress and Aging in POAG

TM cellularity is reduced with aging.[67,68] Morphologic studies have also revealed thickened basement membranes and accumulation of sheath-derived plaques and long spacing collagens in the TM of aged eyes.[52] The number of senescent cells that stain positive for senescence-associated β-galactosidase is increased (Table 82.3) in the TM of POAG eyes,[45] supporting further that POAG is an age-related disease.[51,69] Oxidative damage has been implicated to contribute to the morphologic and physiologic alterations in the aqueous outflow pathway in aging and glaucoma.[70] The TM is known to be exposed to 20–30 μM $H_2O_2$ present in the aqueous humor and is subjected to chronic oxidative stress.[50] Superoxide dismutase, an enzyme involved in the protection against oxidative damage, has been shown to decline with age in human TM tissues.[69] TM cells also synthesized a specific set of proteins, such as αB-crystalline, that may act as molecular chaperones to prevent oxidative or heat shock damage.[35] Markers of oxidative damage,[70,71] abnormalities in mitochondrial DNA,[72] and diminished blood levels of oxidant scavengers glutathione[41] are found in POAG patients. It appears that oxidative stress that exceeds the capacity of TM cells for detoxification is involved in damaging the cells and alteration of the aqueous humor outflow. Upregulation of acute stress response protein amyloid in blood of POAG patients[46] underscores the notion that POAG has ocular and systemic altered protein expression.

## 82.4 Conclusions and Perspectives

This chapter summarizes the current knowledge of possible biomarkers in POAG. The exact role of each biomarker is sketchy at present, and a direct link to POAG remains to be established. While individual biomarkers are only indicative of POAG, combining multiple biomakers for the risk assessment in POAG is a goal for the future. The regulation of TGF-β, CD44, and Wnt[73] signaling cascades is areas of active research. A theme applicable perhaps to both POAG and other neurodegenerative diseases is emerging that selective cell vulnerability occurs as a result of dysfunctional pathways, stress, aging, or other insults, eventually leading to the disease process. Biochemical changes (listed in Tables 82.1, 82.2, and 82.3) indicate that diverse pathways/mechanisms/molecules including pro-inflammatory cytokines may trigger dysregulation of normal defense mechanisms, faulty signaling, and/or progressive fibrosis, leading to the disease process. A deeper understanding of the various mechanisms is a prerequisite for designing novel gene therapies or treatment modalities for POAG.

## References

1. de Lemos JA, Lloyd-Jones DM. Multiple biomarker panels for cardiovascular risk assessment. *N Eng J Med.* 2008;358:2172–4.
2. Parikh SV, de Lemos JA. Biomarkers in cardiovascular disease: integrating pathophysiology into clinical practice. *Amer J Med Sci.* 2006;332:186–97.
3. Wang TJ, Gona P, Larson MG, et al. Multiple biomarkers for the prediction of first major cardiovascular events and death. *N Eng J Med.* 2006;355:2631–9.
4. Ray S, Britschgi M, Herbert C, et al. Classification and prediction of clinical Alzheimer's diagnosis based on plasma signaling proteins. *Nature Med.* 2007;13:1359–62.
5. Simonsen AH, McGuire J, Hansson O, et al. Novel panel of cerebrospinal fluid biomarkers for the prediction of progression to Alzheimer dementia in patients with mild cognitive impairment. *Arch Neurol.* 2007;64:366–70.
6. Ross JS, Symmans WF, Pusztai L, Hortobagyi GN. Pharmacogenomics and clinical biomarkers in drug discovery and development. *Amer J Clin Path.* 2005;124(Suppl):S29–41.
7. Golubnitschaja O, Flammer J. What are the biomarkers for glaucoma? *Surv Ophthalmol.* 2007;52(Suppl 2):S155–61.
8. Knepper PA, Goossens W, Mayanil CS. CD44H localization in primary open-angle glaucoma. *Invest Ophthalmol Vis Sci.* 1998;39: 673–680.
9. Picciani R, Desai K, Guduric-Fuchs J, et al. Cochlin in the eye. *Prog Retin Eye Res.* 2007;26:453–469.
10. Knepper PA, Goossens W, Hvizd M, et al. Glycosaminoglycans of the human trabecular meshwork in primary open-angle glaucoma. *Invest Ophthalmol Vis Sci.* 1996;37:1360–1367.
11. Hann CR, Springett MJ, Wang X, et al. Ultrastructural localization of collagen IV, fibronectin, and laminin in the trabecular meshwork of normal and glaucomatous eyes. *Ophthalmic Res.* 2001;33:314–324.
12. Umihira J, Nagata S, Nohara M, et al. Localization of elastin in the normal and glaucomatous human trabecular meshwork. *Invest Ophthalmol Vis Sci.* 1994;35:486–494.
13. Pena JD, Netland PA, Vidal I, et al. Elastosis of the lamina cribrosa in glaucomatous optic neuropathy. *Exp Eye Res.* 1998;67:517–524.
14. Vesaluoma M, Mertaniemi P, Mannonen S, et al. Cellular and plasma fibronectin in the aqueous humour of primary open-angle glaucoma, exfoliative glaucoma and cataract patients. *Eye.* 1998;12:886–890.
15. Navajas EV, Martins JR, Melo LA Jr, et al. Concentration of hyaluronic acid in primary open-angle glaucoma aqueous humor. *Exp Eye Res.* 2005;80:853–857.
16. Gong H, Ye W, Freddo TF, et al. Hyaluronic acid in the normal and glaucomatous optic nerve. *Exp Eye Res.* 1997;4:587–595.
17. Pena JD, Varela HJ, Ricard CS, et al. Enhanced tenascin expression associated with reactive astrocytes in human optic nerve heads with primary open angle glaucoma. *Exp Eye Res.* 1999;68:29–40.
18. Flugel-Koch C, Ohlmann A, Fuchshofer R, et al. Thrombospondin-1 in the trabecular meshwork: localization in normal and glaucomatous

eyes, and induction by TGF-β1 and dexamethasone in vitro. *Exp Eye Res.* 2004;79:649–663.
19. Ronkko S, Rekonen P, Kaarniranta K, et al. Matrix metalloproteinases and their inhibitors in the chamber angle of normal eyes and patients with primary open-angle glaucoma and exfoliation glaucoma. *Graefes Arch Clin Exp Ophthalmol.* 2007;245:697–704.
20. Yan X, Tezel G, Wax MB, et al. Matrix metalloproteinases and tumor necrosis factor-α in glaucomatous optic nerve head. *Arch Ophthalmol.* 2000;118:666–673.
21. Schlotzer-Schrehardt U, Lommatzsch J, Kuchle M, et al. Matrix metalloproteinases and their inhibitors in aqueous humor of patients with pseudoexfoliation syndrome/glaucoma and primary open-angle glaucoma. *Invest Ophthalmol Vis Sci.* 2003;44:1117–1125.
22. Golubnitschaja O, Yeghiazaryan K, Liu R, et al. Increased expression of matrix metalloproteinases in mononuclear blood cells of normal-tension glaucoma patients. *J Glaucoma.* 2004;13:66–72.
23. Maatta M, Tervahartiala T, Harju M, et al. Matrix metalloproteinases and their tissue inhibitors in aqueous humor of patients with primary open-angle glaucoma, exfoliation syndrome, and exfoliation glaucoma. *J Glaucoma.* 2005;14:64–69.
24. Tezel G, Kass MA, Kolker AE, et al. Plasma and aqueous humor endothelin levels in primary open-angle glaucoma. *J Glaucoma.* 1997;6:83–89.
25. Emre M, Orgul S, Haufschild T, et al. Increased plasma endothelin-1 levels in patients with progressive open angle glaucoma. *Br J Ophthalmol.* 2005;89:60–63.
26. Hu DN, Ritch R. Hepatocyte growth factor is increased in the aqueous humor of glaucomatous eyes. *J Glaucoma.* 2001;10:152–157.
27. Yang J, Patil RV, Yu H, et al. T cell subsets and sIL-2R/IL-2 levels in patients with glaucoma. *Am J Ophthalmol.* 2001;31:421–426.
28. Ronkko S, Rekonen P, Kaarniranta K, et al. Phospholipase A2 in chamber angle of normal eyes and patients with primary open angle glaucoma and exfoliation glaucoma. *Mol Vis.* 2007;13:408–417.
29. Nolan MJ, Giovingo MC, Miller AM, et al. Aqueous humor sCD44 concentration and visual field loss in primary open-angle glaucoma. *J Glaucoma.* 2007;16:419–429.
30. Picht G, Welge-Luessen U, Grehn F, et al. Transforming growth factor β2 levels in the aqueous humor in different types of glaucoma and the relation to filtering bleb development. *Graefes Arch Clin Exp Ophthalmol.* 2001;239:199–207.
31. Noureddin BN, Al-Haddad CE, Bashshur Z, et al. Plasma thymulin and nerve growth factor levels in patients with primary open angle glaucoma and elevated intraocular pressure. *Graefes Arch Clin Exp Ophthalmol.* 2006;244:750–752.
32. Hu DN, Ritch R, Liebmann J, et al. Vascular endothelial growth factor is increased in aqueous humor of glaucomatous eyes. *J Glaucoma.* 2002;1:406–410.
33. Lip PL, Felmeden DC, Blann AD, et al. Plasma vascular endothelial growth factor, soluble VEGF receptor FLT-1, and von Willebrand factor in glaucoma. *Br J Ophthalmol.* 2002;86:1299–1302.
34. Zabala L, Saldanha C, Martins e Silva J, et al. Red blood cell membrane integrity in primary open angle glaucoma: ex vivo and in vitro studies. *Eye.* 1999;13:101–103.
35. Lutjen-Drecoll E, May CA, Polansky JR, et al. Localization of the stress proteins αB-crystallin and trabecular meshwork inducible glucocorticoid response protein in normal and glaucomatous trabecular meshwork. *Invest Ophthalmol Vis Sci.* 1998;39:517–525.
36. Weinstein BI, Iyer RB, Binstock JM, et al. Decreased 3α-hydroxysteroid dehydrogenase activity in peripheral blood lymphocytes from patients with primary open angle glaucoma. *Exp Eye Res.* 1996;62:39–45.
37. Lee P, Lam KW, Lai M. Aqueous humor ascorbate concentration and open-angle glaucoma. *Arch Ophthalmol.* 1977;95:308–310.
38. McCarty GR, Schwartz B. Reduced plasma cortisol binding to albumin in ocular hypertension and primary open-angle glaucoma. *Curr Eye Res.* 1999;18:467–476.
39. Ren H, Magulike N, Ghebremeskel K, et al. Primary open-angle glaucoma patients have reduced levels of blood docosahexaenoic and eicosapentaenoic acids. *Prostaglandins Leukot Essent Fatty Acids.* 2006;74:157–163.
40. Ferreira SM, Lerner SF, Brunzini R, et al. Oxidative stress markers in aqueous humor of glaucoma patients. *Am J Ophthalmol.* 2004;137:62–69.
41. Gherghel D, Griffiths HR, Hilton EJ, et al. Systemic reduction in glutathione levels occurs in patients with primary open-angle glaucoma. *Invest Ophthalmol Vis Sci.* 2005;46:877–883.
42. Tezel G, Wax MB. Hypoxia-inducible factor-1α in the glaucomatous retina and optic nerve head. *Arch Ophthalmol.* 2004;122:1348–1356.
43. Tsai DC, Hsu WM, Chou CK, et al. Significant variation of the elevated nitric oxide levels in aqueous humor from patients with different types of glaucoma. *Ophthalmologica.* 2002;216:346–350.
44. Wang N, Chintala SK, Fini ME, et al. Activation of a tissue-specific stress response in the aqueous outflow pathway of the eye defines the glaucoma disease phenotype. *Nature Med.* 2001;7:304–309.
45. Liton PB, Challa P, Stinnett S, et al. Cellular senescence in the glaucomatous outflow pathway. *Exp Geront.* 2005;40:745–748.
46. Wang WH, McNatt LG, Pang IH, et al. Increased expression of serum amyloid A in glaucoma and its effect on intraocular pressure. *Invest Ophthalmol Vis Sci.* 2008;49:1916–23.
47. Mukesh BN, McCarty CA, Rait JL, Taylor HR. Five-year incidence of open-angle glaucoma: the visual impairment project. *Ophthalmology.* 2002;109:1047–1051.
48. Quigley HA. Open-angle glaucoma. *N Eng J Med.* 1993;328:097–1106.
49. Tamura H, Kawakami H, Kanamoto T, et al. High frequency of open-angle glaucoma in Japanese patients with Alzheimer's disease. *J Neuro Sci.* 2006;246:79–83.
50. Yue BYJT. Cellular mechanisms in the trabecular meshwork affecting the aqueous humor outflow pathway. In: Albert DM, Miller JW, eds. *Albert and Jacobiec's principles and practice of ophthalmology.* Chap. 192. 3rd ed. Oxford, UK: Elsevier; 2007:2457–2474.
51. Knepper PA, Yue BYJT: Cellular mechanisms in the trabecular meshwork affecting the aqueous humor outflow pathway. In: Levine LA, Albert DM (eds) Ocular disease: mechanisms and management. Elsevier, Oxford, UK (In Press).
52. Acott TS, Kelley MJ. Extracellular matrix in the trabecular meshwork. *Exp Eye Res.* 2008;86:543–61.
53. Lutjen-Drecoll RJW. Morphology of aqueous outflow pathways in normal and glaucomatous eyes. In: Ritch R, Shields MB, Krupin T, eds. *The Glaucomas,* vol. 1. 2nd ed. CV Mosby: St. Louis; 1996:89–123.
54. Tan JCH, Peters DM, Kaufman PL. Recent developments in understanding the pathophysiology of elevated intraocular pressure. *Curr Opin Ophthalmol.* 2006;17:168–174.
55. Barany EH. The effect of different kinds of hyaluronidase on the resistance to flow through the angle of the anterior chamber. *Acta Ophthalmol.* 1956;33:397–403.
56. Knepper PA, Fadel JR, Miller AM, et al. Reconstitution of trabecular meshwork GAGs: influence of hyaluronic acid and chondroitin sulfate on flow rates. *J Glaucoma.* 2005;14:230–238.
57. Keller KE, Bradley JM, Kelley MJ, Acott TS. Effects of modifiers of glycosaminoglycan biosynthesis on outflow facility in perfusion culture. *Invest Ophthalmol Vis Sci.* 2008;49:2495–505.
58. Choi J, Miller AM, Nolan MJ, et al. Soluble CD44 is cytotoxic to trabecular meshwork and retinal ganglion cells in vitro. *Invest Ophthalmol Vis Sci.* 2006;46:214–222.
59. Tane N, Dhar S, Roy S, et al. Effect of excess synthesis of extracellular matrix components by trabecular meshwork cells: Possible consequence on aqueous outflow. *Exp Eye Res.* 2007;84:832–842.
60. Vittal V, Rose A, Gregory KE, et al. Changes in gene expression by trabecular meshwork cells in response to mechanical stretching. *Invest Ophthalmol Vis Sci.* 2005;46:2857–2868.
61. Gottanka J, Chan D, Eichhorn M, Lutjen-Drecoll E, Ethier CR. Effects of TGF-β2 in perfused human eyes. *Invest Ophthalmol Vis Sci.* 2004;45:153–8.

62. Kelley MJ, Rose AY, Songg K, et al. Synergism of TNF and IL-1 in the induction of matrix metalloproteinases-3 in the trabecular meshwork. *Invest Ophthalmol Vis Sci*. 2007;48:2634–2643.
63. Tian B, Geiger B, Epstein DL, Kaufman PL. Cytoskeletal involvement in the regulation of aqueous humor outflow. *Invest Ophthalmol Vis Sci*. 2000;41:619–623.
64. Rao PV, Epstein DL. Rho GTPase/Rho kinase inhibition as a novel target for the treatment of glaucoma. *BioDrugs*. 2007;21:167–177.
65. Fautsch MP, Howell KG, Vrabel AM, et al. Primary trabecular meshwork cells incubated in human aqueous humor differ from cells incubated in serum supplements. *Invest Ophthalmol Vis Sci*. 2005;46:2848–2856.
66. Knepper PA, Miller AM, Wertz CJ, et al. Hypophosphorylation of aqueous humor sCD44 and primary open angle glaucoma. *Invest Ophthalmol Vis Sci*. 2005;46:2829–2837.
67. Alvarado JA, Murphy CG, Polansky JR, Juster R. Age-related changes in trabecular meshwork cellularity. *Invest Ophthalmol Vis Sci*. 1981;21:714–727.
68. Alvarado J, Murphy C, Juster R. Trabecular meshwork cellularity in primary open-angle glaucoma and non-glaucomatous normals. *Ophthalmology*. 1984;91:564–579.
69. Gabelt BT, Kaufman PL. Changes in aqueous humor dynamics with age and glaucoma. *Prog Retina Eye Res*. 2005;24:612–637.
70. Sacca SC, Izzotti A, Rossi P, Traverso C. Glaucomatous outflow pathway and oxidative stress. *Exp Eye Res*. 2007;84:389–399.
71. De La Paz MA, Epstein DL. Effect of age on superoxide dismutase activity of human trabecular meshwork. *Invest Ophthalmol Vis Sci*. 1996;37:1849–1853.
72. Abu-Amero KK, Morales J, Bosley TM. Mitochondrial abnormalities in patients with primary open-angle glaucoma. *Invest Ophthalmol Vis Sci*. 2006;47:2533-2541.
73. Wang WH, McNatt LG, Pang IH, et al. Increased expression of the WNT antagonist sFRP-1 in glaucoma elevates intraocular pressure. *J Clin Invest*. 2008;118:1056-64.

# Chapter 83
# CD44 and Primary Open Angle Glaucoma

Paul A. Knepper, Michael J. Nolan, and Beatrice Y.J.T. Yue

In our view, primary open-angle glaucoma (POAG) is a common neurodegenerative disease caused by a variety of molecular defects and/or cellular insults that result in cell stress and death of the trabecular meshwork (TM) and retinal ganglion cells (RGC). One potential biological marker of POAG is CD44, which is one of the adhesion/homing molecules. Direct evidence for CD44's very central role in POAG includes: (1) aqueous humor of patients with POAG contains an increased amount of the soluble extracellular 32-kDa fragment of CD44 (sCD44) in comparison with the aqueous humor of age-matched normal individuals[1]; (2) increased levels of sCD44 in the aqueous correlates with the extent of visual field loss in POAG patients[2]; (3) sCD44, particularly hypo-phosphorylated sCD44, is a potent and specific toxic protein to TM and RGC in vitro[3]; and (4) overexpression of both full-length CD44 and truncated sCD44 in transgenic mouse eyes is sufficient to cause ocular hypertension. The increase in intraocular pressure (IOP) lasted more than 90 days accompanied by optic nerve damage. The overexpression of CD44 may thus be the first documented animal model that closely mimics the human disease POAG.[4] Other models have been cytodestructive and nonphysiologic. These data suggest that the elevated sCD44 levels documented in POAG compared with secondary glaucoma or normal aqueous is not just an epiphenomenon but plays a causal role in the POAG disease process. In this chapter, we will focus on CD44's role in cell signaling pathways, immune status, response to cell stress, and their impact on cell viability. The question that is asked is: "Are CD44 and its ectodomain sCD44 life or death factors in POAG?"

## 83.1 CD44 Functions as a Receptor

CD44 is a type 1 transmembrane glycoprotein expressed in many cell types of neuroectodermal and mesenchymal origin. CD44 is a receptor for hyaluronic acid (HA). Our biochemical studies of POAG TM have revealed a significant decrease in HA and an increase in chondroitin sulfate.[5] In addition, computer-aided microscopy studies of the juxtacanicular tissue of POAG post-mortem eyes have also confirmed the loss of HA and the increase in the amount of chondroitin sulfate.[6] The cell mechanisms causing the decrease of HA in aging[5–10] or the further loss of HA in POAG are unknown. It is now recognized that HA, even at low concentrations, has important regulatory functions in cellular differentiation.[8,11] Emerging evidence suggests that HA is a key factor in promoting cell motility, adhesion, and proliferation. These cell events are orchestrated by three HA cell receptors – CD44, RHAMM (receptor for HA-mediated motility), and intercellular adhesion molecule (ICAM-1) – all of which have been identified in the human TM.[12]

### 83.1.1 CD44 Interactions

CD44, the principal receptor for HA, is well characterized and increases in aging.[13–15] CD44 plays major roles in multiple physiological processes including autoimmunity,[16–18] phagocytosis,[19,20] and cell survival.[21–23] CD44 vaccination has recently been reported to be useful in treating insulin-dependent diabetes mellitus[24] and inflammatory central nervous system (CNS) diseases like multiple sclerosis.[25] While there is no clinically available vaccination for POAG, the possibility is intriguing. CD44 is an 80–250 kDa transmembrane protein; its ectodomain is released as sCD44[26–28] (see Fig. 83.1). The nucleotide sequence of CD44 cDNA predicts a 37-kDa protein with homology to cartilage link protein.[29] CD44 is multifunctional due to sequence differences arising from alternate splicing of mRNA, as well as posttranslational modifications. CD44 (standard) is the most common form. CD44 proteins are differentially phosphorylated and glycosylated.[30] The structure of CD44 is remarkable for its versatility[32] and is a molecule with a thousand faces due to its surprising number of numerous functions, interactions, and isoforms.[32]

In addition to HA, CD44 has multiple ligands – chondroitin sulfate,[33] collagen types I and IV, fibronectin,[34] osteopontin,[35]

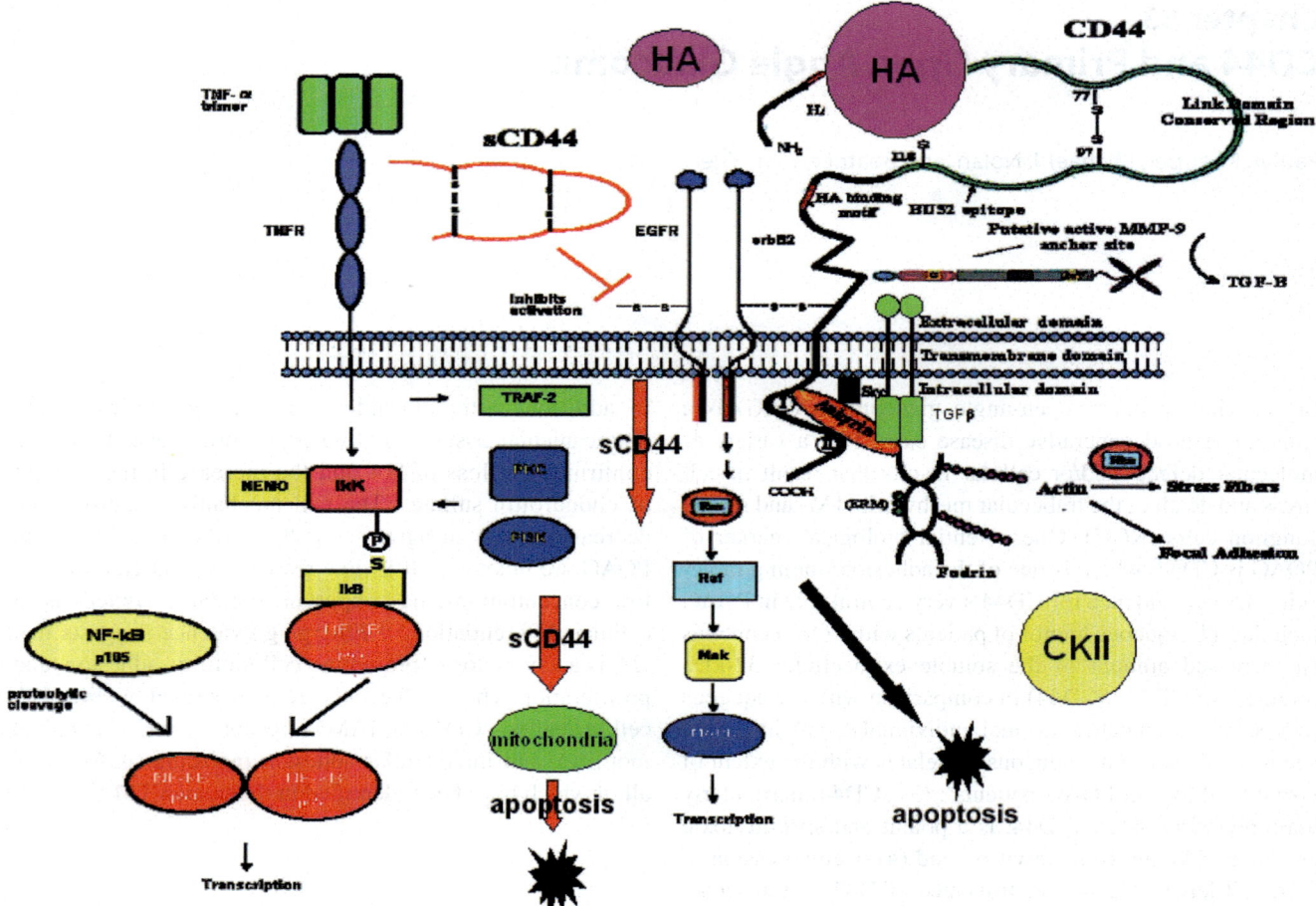

Fig. 83.1 Interactions and signal transduction pathways involving CD44. CD44 associates with HA, matrix metalloproteinase-9 (MMP-9), erbB2, erbB3, EGFR, and TGFβ in the extracellular domain. CD44 is shed as soluble CD44 (sCD44), which does not have variable spliced inserts and is highly conserved. sCD44 may be internalized into mitochondria leading to apoptosis or disrupt membrane interactions, especially the CD44-mediated heterodimer that forms between erbB2 and erbB3 and also TGFβ. sCD44 release causes decreased signal transduction through erbB2–erbB3 leading also to apoptosis. Signal transduction through the EGFR receptor family involves tyrosine kinase activation, Ras, Raf, Mek, and Map kinase (MAPK) activation, leading to transcription. In addition to the MAPK cascade, the EGFR family is involved with the NF-κB signal transduction pathway. TNF-α receptor associated factor-2 (TRAF-2) is the link between the TNF-α pathway and EGFR. Both CD44 and EGFR function through Ras, phosphoinositide-3-kinase (PI3K), protein kinase C (PKC), which leads through the inhibitor of NF-κB kinase (IKK) complex, which consists of IKK-1, IKK-2, and NEMO. TNF-α binds to the TNF-α receptor, which results in signal transduction through IKK, IκB, and NF-κB. Casein kinase II (CKII) activity is negatively regulated in part by TGFβ1. Smaller molecular weight HA (smaller pinkish HA) is pro-inflammatory and has low affinity binding to sCD44

TGF-β receptor,[36] and matrix metalloproteinases.[37,38] CD44 undergoes a variety of activation-dependent, cell-type specific, posttranslational modifications that can affect its ligand specificity and affinity. CD44 plays a critical role in the cell survival of many cell types through its interaction with multiple signaling pathways, including Ras, PKC NF-κB, MAPK, and the PI3K–PKB/Akt pathways.[3] In several cell types, CD44, HA, and androgen receptor stimulation enhance cell survival.[3] Heparan sulfate side chains on CD44 bind and sequester growth factors and chemokines. Each ligand interaction is influenced by CD44 exons and by glycosylation patterns.[39] sCD44 is the ectodomain fragment of CD44 and does not have variable spliced inserts typical of CD44, and the N-terminus of sCD44 ectodomain is highly conserved. ERM (ezrin, radixin, moesin) family members are located just beneath the plasma membrane and act as molecular linkers between a cytoplasmic domain of CD44 and the actin-based cytoskeleton.[40] CD44 participates in the uptake and degradation of HA.[41]

CD44 is expressed on a variety of ocular cells and tissues including RGC and axons.[42] Aging leads to altered T cells, increases in CD44 expression, and the accumulation of cells with signal transduction defects.[43] Functional analysis of CD44 as a receptor for the ECM and its role in signal transduction in cells depends on many factors including: matrix interaction,[14] cell type,[44] extracellular ligands,[45] and cytoplasmic interaction of CD44. Emerging evidence indicates that the ectodomain fragment, sCD44, is functionally distinct from the membrane CD44.[27] The expression and proteolytic release of sCD44 by cells allows the nascent membrane CD44 to bind and internalize HA as well as other HA binding proteins.[46]

CD44 and HA are also involved in the activity of adenosine triphosphate (ATP)-binding cassette (ABC) transporters that remove potentially toxic proteins from cells. A number of the genes implicated in glaucoma have a relationship to the ABC transporters. TM cells express functionally active ABC transporters.[47] ATP-binding cassette transporter superfamily members respond to stressors such as hypoxia, cytokine signaling, increased pressure, mechanical stretch, and aging, which are collectively vital to the function of the TM. The ABCB1 transporter (multidrug resistance protein, p-glycoprotein) expression and function are controlled by HA and CD44, both of which are altered in POAG. Notably, ABC transporter genes ABCB1, ABCA6, ABCA8, ABCA2, ABCF2, and ABCA5 are all flagged as present in TM tissue by Affymetrix microarray analysis.[47] ABCF2 maps to 7q36, a published glaucoma loci GLC1F (7q35-36). In a calcein–AM functional assay of MDR, TM cells incorporate calcein–AM, and MDR activity is inhibited by metabolic stress. These results support the hypothesis that MDR is expressed in cells relevant to the POAG disease process, and abnormal stress may lead to decreased MDR activity and TM cell dysfunction in POAG.

### 83.1.2 CD44 Localization in POAG

We have determined the CD44H profile in normal and in POAG anterior segments by Western blot analysis and computer-assisted densitometry.[48] Western blot analysis of POAG eyes demonstrated a marked increase of CD44H ($P>0.001$) in the ciliary body in all cases of POAG (Fig. 83.2). Immunocytochemical studies also showed a marked change in CD44 in POAG eyes. In normal eyes, the CD44 profile indicated that the highest concentration of CD44 was in the ciliary body stroma. When sections were pretreated with Triton X-100, all of the normal anterior segment regions exhibited a substantial increase in CD44 staining. In contrast, significant decreases in the amount of CD44 were present in POAG eyes compared with normal eyes. As evidenced by scattergram plots (Fig. 83.3), individual cases of normal and POAG eyes are clustered into distinctive patterns in ciliary body stroma and TM. Results of these studies indicate that the concentration of CD44H is increased in the anterior segment of POAG eyes.[48] Triton X-100 is useful in solubilizing a number of integral membrane proteins,[49] such as CD44,[50] which are associated with lipid rafts.[51] Triton X-100 binds

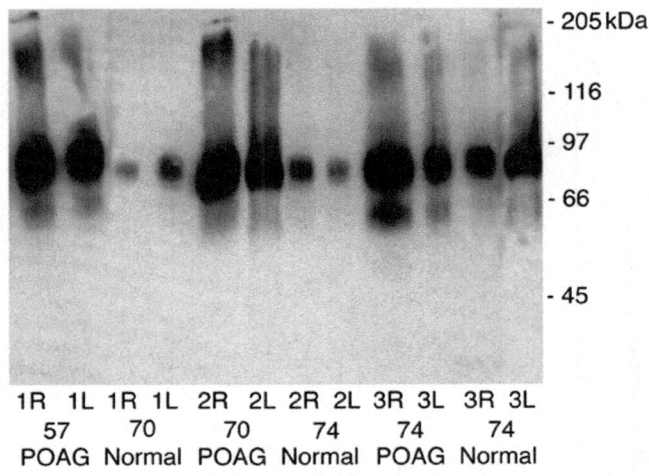

**Fig. 83.2** Western blot of micro-dissected normal and POAG ciliary body solubilized in 1% Triton X-100 and using CD44H antibody which recognizes all forms of CD44. Right: molecular weight (in kilodaltons). Bottom: individual specimen number, age, and clinical status. Note the marked increase in CD44H (~85 kDa) in POAG as compared to normal

to the hydrophobic domains of proteins without disrupting protein–protein interactions. POAG CD44H is increased on Western blots because it is extracted and quantitated, whereas POAG CD44 is decreased on histological sections because it is extracted and removed from the section. Thus, the immunocytochemical studies and Western blot analysis of CD44H[1,48] support the notion that the expression and regulation of CD44 is changed in POAG.

## 83.2 sCD44 and POAG

### 83.2.1 Ectodomain Shedding of sCD44

The 32-kDa ectodomain fragment of CD44 is released from the membrane CD44 by proteolytic cleavage as sCD44.[27] sCD44 is shed from the cell surface in response to ligand binding. The ectodomain has been shown to be released from the cell surface by MT1-MMP, a membrane bound metalloprotease[28] in junction with ADAMS 10 and 17.[52-54]

### 83.2.2 Parallel in Processing of sCD44 and Alzheimer's β-Amyloid

An emerging concept in cell biology, applicable to neurodegenerative diseases such as POAG and Alzheimer's disease is that a specific population of cells becomes vulnerable to a toxic protein. Often the protein is misfolded or aggregated

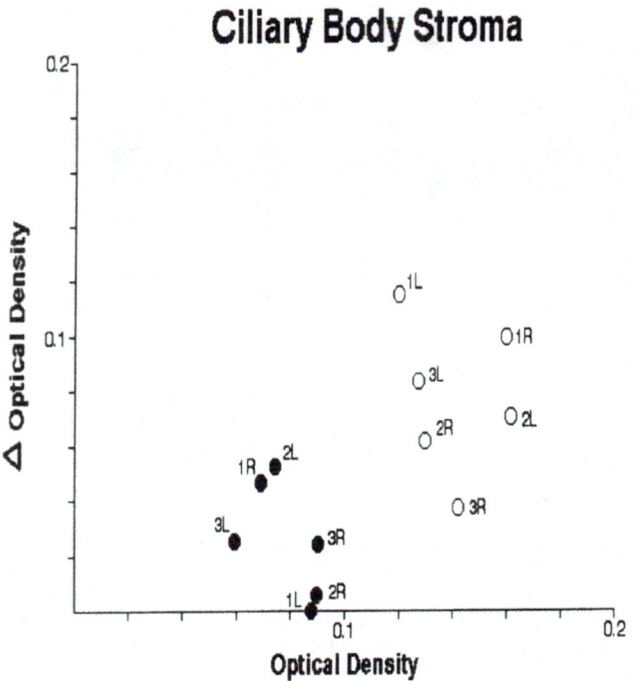

**Fig. 83.3** Scattergram plots of ciliary body and TM of the optical density of CD44H immunostaining without Triton X-100 pretreatment (x axis) versus the change in optical density of CD44 between pretreatment with Triton X-100 and without Triton X-100 (y-axis). Individual cases of POAG eyes are indicated by solid, numbered circles ●, and individual cases of normal eyes are indicated by open, numbered circles ○. Note clear separation of normal from POAG

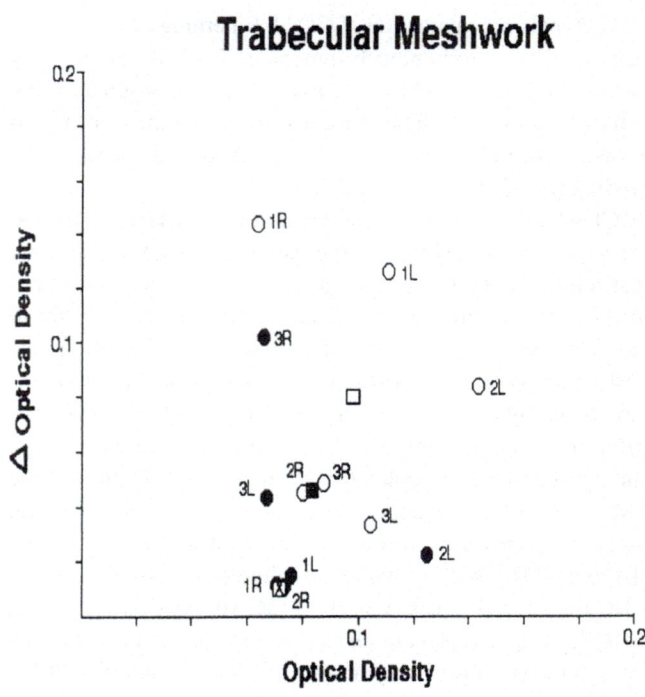

**Fig. 83.4** Ectodomain shedding of CD44 and amyloid precursor protein by initial cleavage of the ectodomain and a second cleavage in the transmembrane domain. Potential ectodomain cleavage of CD44 is shown by MT1-MMP and of amyloid precursor protein by b- and a-secretase. Putative phosphorylation sites are noted by CK II, PKC, APPK, and MAPK. The beta-amyloid like protein fragments are shown in red

with a change in its tertiary, three-dimensional structure. As a consequence, the target cells die. There is a marked parallel in the processing of CD44 and β-amyloid (Fig. 83.4). In both diseases, the intramembrane portion is cleaved by a presenilin γ-secretase which occurs close to the cytoplasmic border to release an intracellular fragment that translocates to the nucleus and promotes transcription; A second cleavage occurs extracellularly to generate an amyloid-like peptide.[55] β-amyloid in Alzheimer's disease is phosphorylated on its ectodomain, analogous to sCD44, and aberrant phosphorylation of the β-amyloid precursor protein enhances the secretion of the β-peptide by γ-secretase.[56]

Clinically, the prevalence of POAG is high in patients with Alzheimer's disease.[57,58] β-secretase is a second enzyme used in the processing of amyloid precursor protein. It is a transmembrane aspartyl protease,[59] the rate-limiting step in the production of toxic β-amyloid, and is active within endosomal/lysosomal compartments. Significantly, β-secretase is up-regulated by cell stress.[60] Whether CD44 is cleaved by β-secretase is not known, but it is an attractive unifying hypothesis that cell stress is a basic element in the pathogenesis of POAG. There are common mechanisms in ectodomain processing. First, the majority of shedding events of the ectodomain are inhibited by metalloproteinase inhibitors[61,62] that interfere with the maturation and the transport of the transmembrane proteins. Second, the ectodomains are shed in response to protein kinase C activators, a stress responder. Third, domain swap constructs of the extracellular domain adjacent to the transmembrane region result in shedding of transmembrane proteins that are normally not shed.

Although the phosphorylation sites are yet to be identified in sCD44, phosphorylation is a key to stress response in several neurodegenerative diseases.[63] We anticipate critical phosphorylation sites within the α-helix portion of sCD44. Regulation of phosphorylation may prove to be a key posttranslational modification. If phosphorylation is downregulated, the charge on sCD44 is changed to create a mitochondrial signaling domain. For example, the net charge on the α-helix portion of sCD44 is zero, but with reduced or absent phosphorylation, the charge becomes basic and the sCD44 would be directed to the mitochondria and cause cell death (Table 83.1).

### 83.2.3 sCD44 Concentration in POAG Aqueous Humor

We determined amounts of sCD44 in the aqueous humor of normal and glaucoma patients using microscale methods developed in our laboratory.[1,2,64] In this ongoing study, we have excluded any patient with recent (6 months) intraocular surgery. As shown in Table 83.2, POAG aqueous without filtration surgery contained a highly significant increase in

**Table 83.1** Putative phosphorylation and influence on theoretical isoelectric point of the HA binding sites in the ectodomain of sCD44

| HA binding site | Example | Amino acid sequence and charge | Phosphorylation sites | Theoretical isoelectric point |
|---|---|---|---|---|
| 1st helix sCD44 | Normal | + . . + . - . - + - | 3 | 4.02 |
| | Normal | + . . + . - . - + - | 2 | 5.03 |
| | | K N G R Y S I S R T | | |
| | POAG | + . . + . . . - + . | 1 | 8.55 |
| | POAG | + . . + . . . . + . | 0 | 11.0 |
| 2nd helix sCD44 | Normal | . + - . - + . . . + | 1 | 8.71 |
| | | N R D G T R Y V Q K | | |
| | POAG | . + - . . + . . . + | 0 | 9.99 |

The amino acid sequence of the first helix of sCD44 is shown with positive charge (+) representing basic amino acids, the negative charge (-) representing acidic amino acids, and neutral (.) representing neutral amino acids. Phosphorylation of serine or threonine residues results in a negative charge (-) whereas lack of phosphorylation of serine or threonine results in a neutral charge. The theoretical isoelectric point was determined by www.nihilnovus.com.

**Table 83.2** Aqueous sCD44* concentration in normal and glaucoma patients

| Clinical status | Subset | n† | sCD44 concentration | Comparison | P value |
|---|---|---|---|---|---|
| Normal | None | 124 | 5.88(0.27) | | |
| Ocular hypertension | None | 5 | 9.82(2.82) | vs. Normal | 0.15‡ |
| POAG | POAG, No filtration surgery | 90 | 12.76(0.66) | vs. Normal | <0.000001§ |
| | POAG, With filtration surgery and medications ‖ | 10 | 5.86(1.26) | vs. POAG, no filtration surgery | 0.001‡ |
| | POAG, With filtration surgery and no medications | 3 | 12.62(3.81) | vs. Normal | 0.05 |
| | Normal pressure | 12 | 9.19(1.75) | vs. Normal | 0.02‡ |
| | | | | vs. POAG, no filtration surgery | 0.04‡ |
| | Myocilin mutation | 2 | 4.77 (0.11) | vs. POAG, no filtration surgery | 0.05‡ |
| JOAG | None | 7 | 6.79(1.67) | vs. POAG, no filtration surgery | 0.01‡ |
| Secondary glaucoma | Secondary glaucoma, no filtration surgery | 36 | 8.98(0.65) | vs. Normal | 0.001‡ |
| | | | | vs. POAG, no filtration surgery | 0.002‡ |
| | Secondary glaucoma, with filtration surgery‖ | 11 | 6.84(0.56) | vs. all secondary glaucoma, no filtration surgery | 0.11‡ |
| | Steroid induced | 2 | 10.92(0.67) | | |
| | Pigmentary | 3 | 9.00(2.54) | | |
| | PXG, no filtration surgery | 19 | 7.97(0.86) | vs. POAG, no filtration surgery | 0.001‡ |
| | PXG, with filtration surgery | 8 | 6.73 (0.75) | vs. PXG, no filtration surgery | 0.3 |
| | Uveitic | 7 | 12.39(1.21) | | |
| | Angle recession(Trauma) | 3 | 8.87(2.56) | | |
| | Chronic angle closure | 2 | 4.98(1.04) | | |

sCD44 concentration of aqueous was determined by ELISA and is expressed as ng/ml (±SEM). †n=number, ‡ Significance using nonparametric Mann Whitney test, § Significance using Student's *t* test. Prior successful surgery defined as IOP of less than 20 mmHg with or without glaucoma medications. *POAG* primary open-angle glaucoma, *JOAG* juvenile open-angle, *PXG* pseudoexfoliation glaucoma.

sCD44 compared with normal aqueous ($P>0.000001$). Successful POAG filtration surgery decreased sCD44 concentration. The increased concentration of sCD44 was observed in POAG patients with or without a positive family history and was not influenced by glaucoma medications. Significantly, normal pressure glaucoma and ocular hypertension also contained increased sCD44, whereas juvenile open angle glaucoma patients did not have an increased concentration of sCD44. Interestingly, patients with diabetes and POAG with mild to moderate visual field loss have a significantly lower sCD44 aqueous concentration.[65]

We sought to determine if there was a relationship between known risk factors for POAG and aqueous sCD44 concentration. A review of the literature disclosed age, gender, hypertension, increased IOP, and race as risk factors for developing POAG. In the current analysis of the cohort, race was the only identifiable glaucoma risk factor that correlated with the extent of visual field loss and sCD44 concentration (see Fig. 83.5). sCD44 concentration was greater in African-Americans than in white patients with mild and moderate visual field loss. In both subsets, sCD44 concentration correlated to the stage of visual field loss. In POAG aqueous of white patients, the sCD44 concentration increased as the visual field loss progressed from mild to moderate to severe. Of note, the sCD44 concentration significantly decreased in African-American patients with severe visual field loss in comparison with white patients. African-Americans with severe visual field loss also had a significantly shorter known duration of the disease and higher IOP. The decrease in sCD44 in the aqueous of African-American POAG patients could be the result of end-stage glaucomatous damage to the ciliary epithelium caused by an accelerated disease process.

### 83.2.4 sCD44 in POAG Disease Process

We considered several factors that would influence sCD44 concentration and the POAG disease process and extensively explored phosphorylation as a key posttranslation control. In normal aqueous humor samples, the apparent isoelectric point (pI) of the 32-kDa sCD44 was $6.38 \pm 0.08$ with an isoelectric variance of 5.4–7.0 (see Fig. 83.6). In contrast, in POAG aqueous humor samples, the apparent pI of sCD44 was $6.96 \pm 0.07$ ($P<0.0004$) with an isoelectric variance of 5.4–8.6, and in normal pressure glaucoma aqueous humor samples, the apparent pI is 6.83 with an isoelectric variance of 5.2–8.6. In juvenile open-angle glaucoma and exfoliation glaucoma aqueous humor samples, the apparent pI of sCD44 are 6.28 and 6.40, respectively. The apparent pI and presence of isoelectric variants of the 32-kDa sCD44 protein clearly distinguishes POAG aqueous humor from that of patients without glaucoma or other clinical forms of glaucoma. Thus, POAG is distinguished from normal or secondary glaucoma aqueous by an increased concentration of sCD44 and the change in the pI of sCD44.[65]

We considered four reasons why phosphorylation could change sCD44 function. Phosphorylation is (1) a critical factor in toxic proteins of Alzheimer's and Parkinson's diseases, (2) a factor in protein aggregation, (3) a factor in sCD44 binding to HA, and (4) a posttranslational modification that would change the pI of sCD44. In order to determine the possible mechanisms for a more basic pI in POAG aqueous humor sCD44, pooled normal and pooled POAG aqueous humor samples were isolated and immunoblotted with phospho-specific antiserine/threonine antibodies.

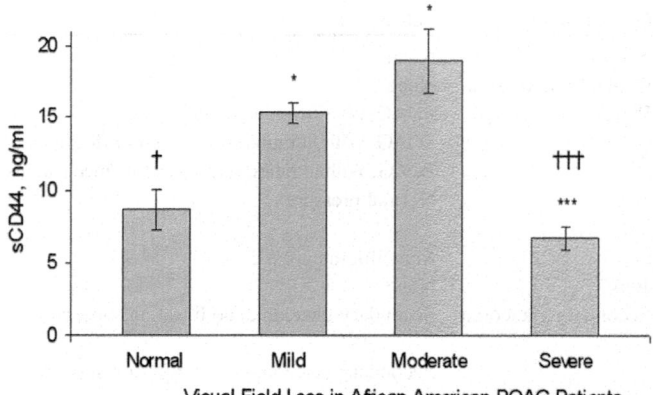

**Fig. 83.5** Aqueous sCD44 and visual field loss in white and African-American POAG patients. The sCD44 in aqueous humor samples was measured in duplicate by soluble CD44 ELISA and compared in white patients and African-American patients. Three stages of visual field loss for POAG patients were mild, arcuate defect; moderate, abnormal in one hemifield and not within 5° of fixation; and, severe, abnormal in both hemifields or within 5° of fixation. The sCD44 concentration in white and African-American POAG patients was analyzed by comparing each stage to normal subjects and to the respective visual field stage. Asterisk indicates significance based on visual field progression; i.e., normal versus mild; mild versus moderate; and moderate versus severe, One asterisk – $P<0.05$; two asterisks – $P<0.01$; three asterisks – $P<0.001$. Dagger indicates significance of African-American POAG patients who were compared to white POAG patients at each stage of visual field loss: one dagger – $P<0.05$, three daggers – $P<0.001$

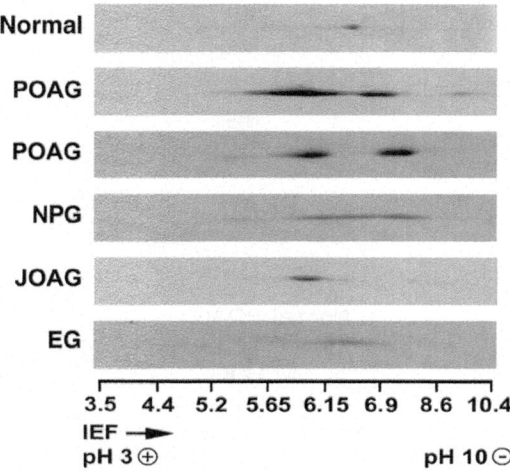

**Fig. 83.6** Aqueous aliquots equivalent to 5 μg protein were separated by electrophoresis and immunoblotted with anti-CD44 antibody to identify isoelectric variants of 32-kDa sCD44. A representative Western blot is shown for a 72-year-old normal white patient with a normal cup/disc ratio and visual fields. Two representative Western blots are shown for POAG: an 86-year-old black patient with a 0.8 cup/disc ratio and moderate visual field loss and a 77-year-old white patient with a 0.7 cup/disc ratio and moderate visual field loss. Representative Western blots are shown for normal pressure glaucoma (NPG): a 59-year-old white patient with a 0.8 cup/disc ratio and moderate visual field loss; Juvenile open-angle glaucoma (JOAG): a 30-year-old Hispanic patient with a 0.9 cup/disc ratio and severe visual field loss; Exfoliation glaucoma (EG): a 74-year-old white patient with a 0.9 cup/disc ratio and severe visual field loss

These results demonstrated that aqueous sCD44 in POAG is hypophosphorylated (Fig. 83.7).

To explore further the role of hypophosphorylation of sCD44 in POAG, pooled aqueous humor of normal and POAG samples was phosphorylated with casein kinase II (CKII) in vitro. To verify the specificity of CK II phosphorylation, aliquots were also treated with CK II in the presence of specific CK II inhibitors. The CK II treated aqueous humor samples were immunoblotted with phospho-specific antiserine/threonine antibodies (Fig. 83.7). After CK II phosphorylation of sCD44, the immunoblots of POAG were identical to normal, indicating that the hypophosphorylation of POAG sCD44 is the result of decreased CK II activity.[66] CK II activity is downregulated in part by transforming growth factor-β (TGF-β).[67] As TGF-β is reported to be upregulated in POAG,[68] the CK II activity is likely to be decreased and result in decreased phosphorylation of CD44.

The ectodomain of CD44 contains seven possible CK II consensus phosphorylation sites. Although the phosphorylation sites are yet to be identified in sCD44, phosphorylation is known to be a regulatory element in several neuro-degenerative diseases. For example, in spino-cerebellar degeneration, hypophosphorylation of the mutant, polyglutamine-containing ataxin-1 decreases toxicity because of increased degradation of the mutant protein.[69] Interestingly, phosphorylation of many proteins by phosphatidyl 3-kinase/protein kinase B neuroprotective pathway is stimulated by insulin-like growth factor-1[70] and prevents neuronal death caused by β-amyloid.[71] Alterations in the phosphorylation of sCD44 may involve metabolic stress, free radicals, or age-related modification of kinase/phosphatase regulation mechanism that may result in the release of the more toxic hypophosphorylated sCD44.

## 83.3 Multiple Roles of CD44 and sCD44

### 83.3.1 Cell Signaling

CD44 interacts with several proteins involved in cell survival and ECM remodeling. CD44 mediates heterodimer formation involving erbB2 and erbB3.[72] In the absence of CD44 function, erbB2 does not properly interact with erbB3, signal transduction is interrupted, and cells undergo apoptosis. Ligands to epidermal growth factor receptor (EGFR) include EGF, TGF-β, amphiregulin, betacellulin, epiregulin, and heparan binding-EGF (HB-EGF).[73] In addition to interactions with erbB receptors, CD44 acts as a docking molecule for matrix metalloproteinases MMP-9 and MMP-7.[56] Overexpression of sCD44 such as in POAG or in adenoviral manipulation in the mouse eye[4] presumably leads to sCD44 binding to multiple proteins, which interfere with cell signaling. Exactly which proteins are involved in the animal model of CD44 overexpression is currently an active area of research in our laboratory.

### 83.3.2 Cell Growth and Survival

The CD44 transmembrane receptor is also implicated in cell growth and survival. We therefore tested: (a) the effects of exogenous sCD44 on cell viability and cell expression of erbB2 in bovine TM cells and (b) the rescue of TM cells from the cytotoxicity of sCD44 by the androgen 17-α-methyl testosterone (17-α-MT). Western analysis was performed using antibodies specific for erbB2, phosphorylated erbB2, erbB3, CD44H and MMP-9. By immunofluorescence microscopy, immunoprecipitation, and Western blotting, CD44H has been shown to associate with erbB2 and erbB3. sCD44 significantly reduced cell viability, erbB2 phosphorylation, and 17-α-MT blocked sCD44 toxicity.[3] From a neuroprotective perspective, preventing sCD44 from binding cell signaling partners or reducing its production in response to cell stress may prove to be useful in preventing cell death of TM and RGC.

Through studies involving TM and organ cultured ciliary epithelium, the cytokines TNF-α and IL-1α were observed

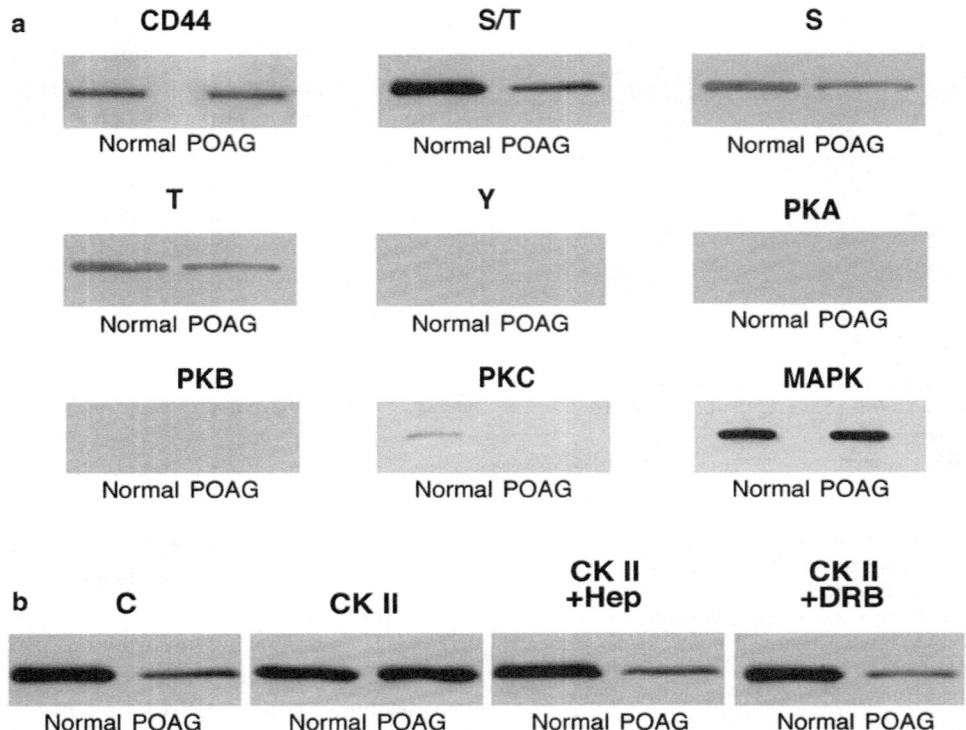

**Fig. 83.7** Phospho-specific Western blot analysis of immunoprecipitated sCD44 from pooled normal and POAG aqueous humor. A 20 pg equivalent of sCD44 was subjected to PAGE and immunoblotted with (**a**) CD44 antibody to ensure equal sCD44 loads and sCD44 transfer (CD44) and with phospho-specific antibodies against the following motifs: serine/threonine (S/T); Serine (S); Threonine (T); Tyrosine (Y); Protein kinase A (PKA); protein kinase B (PKB); protein kinase C (PKC); and Mitogen activated protein kinase (MAPK). (**b**) 20 pg equivalents of sCD44 from normal and POAG samples were treated with 50 ng of casein kinase II alone or in the presence of casein kinase II inhibitors, subjected to PAGE and immunoblotted with antiphospho-serine/threonine antibody. C, control, sCD44 with no enzyme treatment; CK II, sCD44 treated with casein kinase II; CK II + Hep, sCD44 treated with casein kinase II and casein kinase inhibitor, heparin; CK II + DRB, sCD44 treated with casein kinase II and casein kinase inhibitor, DRB

to influence CD44 expression. TNF-α increases MMP-9 expression in cultured TM cells,[74,75] which would modulate ECM turnover, at least in part through a CD44-mediated mechanism. MMP-9 expression is increased by prostaglandin agonists, which are used for the treatment of increased IOP, and by activation of c-Fos, a nuclear regulatory protein.[76,77] Notably, the highest tissue concentration of CD44 is in the ciliary body.[48]

Emerging evidence suggests that sCD44 inhibits cell growth by binding to CD44 and interrupting critical survival pathways.[3] To examine the biological significance of sCD44 hypophosphorylation in POAG, we isolated the sCD44 from human sera and modified its phosphorylation state in vitro. sCD44 was hypophosphorylated with alkaline phosphatase and also hyperphosphorylated with CK II. Alkaline phosphatase treatment caused a more basic pI shift, as observed in sCD44 in POAG and normal pressure glaucoma aqueous humor. Human TM and RGC were treated with the standard, hypo-phosphorylated and hyperphosphorylated forms of sCD44 (Fig. 83.8). After 24 h, the cell viability of human TM cells treated with standard sCD44 was 66% and hypophosphorylated sCD44 was 58% ($P<0.0002$). In contrast, hyperphosphorylated sCD44 was less toxic than standard sCD44. The viability of cells treated with hyperphosphorylated sCD44 was 88% ($P<0.001$) in comparison with cells treated with standard sCD44. Of particular note is the dose of 10 ng/ml, which is within the range of normal human aqueous sCD44 concentration (~6 ng/ml) and POAG (~13 ng/ml).

We also tested the effects of sCD44 on RGC-5 survival (Fig. 83.8). Hypophosphorylated sCD44 was significantly more toxic than the standard sCD44. At a low dose, 0.1 ng/ml, hypophosphorylated sCD44 decreased cell viability to 71% after only 24 h ($P<0.05$). At this dose, it took 48 h for the standard and hyperphosphorylated sCD44 to cause a significant decrease. The viability of cells treated with 10 ng/ml hypophosphorylated sCD44 was 31% after 48 h. In comparison, the viability of cells treated with 10-ng/ml standard sCD44 was 76% after 24 h ($P<0.02$) and 59% after 48 h ($P<0.000002$). The cell viability of RGC treated with hyperphosphorylated sCD44 was similar to that of standard sCD44.

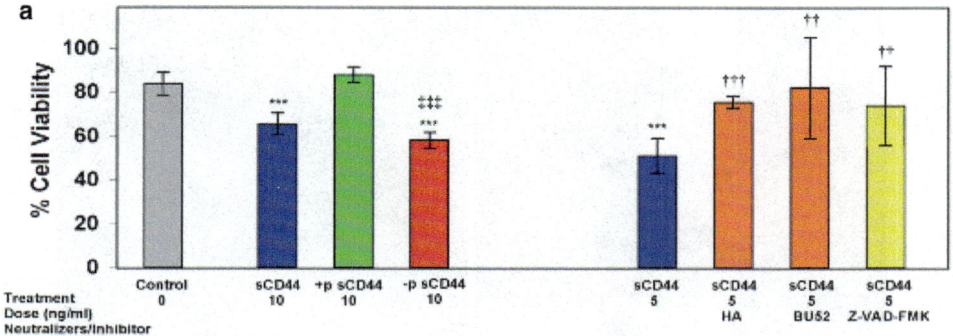

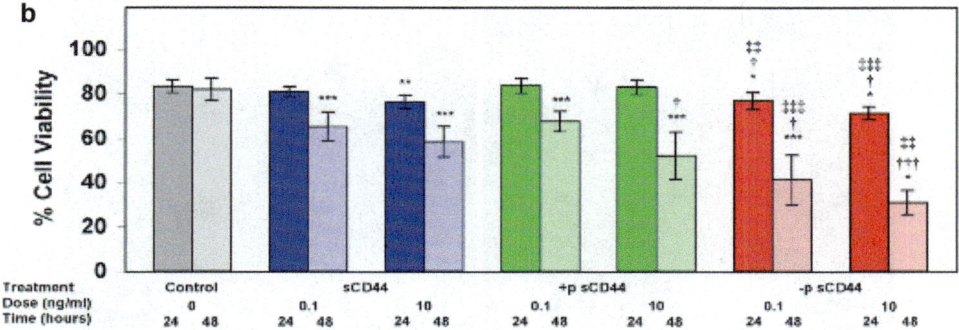

**Fig. 83.8** sCD44 effects on TM, and RGC cell viability. (**a**) Human TM cells were plated at 20,000–40,000 cells/well. The cells were incubated in medium containing 0.1% fetal calf sera (FCS) with 10-ng/ml standard (sCD44), 10-ng/ml hyperphosphorylated (+p sCD44), and 10-ng/ml hypophosphorylated (-p sCD44) for 24 h. Human TM cells were also treated with inhibitors to block the cytotoxicity of 5-ng/ml sCD44; 5-ng/ml sCD44 plus 1 μg HA; 5-ng/ml sCD44 plus 10-μg of anti-CD44 antibody (BU52); 5-ng/ml sCD44 plus 40 μM pan-caspase inhibitor (Z-VAD-FMK). (**b**) RGC-5 cells were plated at 20,000–40,000 cells/well. The cells were then incubated in medium containing 0.1% FCS with 0.1-ng/ml or 10-ng/ml standard (sCD44), hyperphosphorylated (+p sCD44), or hypophosphorylated (-p sCD44) for 24 h and 48 h. Data represent the means ± SD of at least three experiments; $*P<0.05$, $**P<0.01$, $***P<0.001$ compared with control; $†P<0.05$, $††P<0.01$, $†††P<0.001$ compared with standard sCD44; $‡P<0.05$, $‡‡P<0.01$, $‡‡‡P<0.001$ compared with hyperphosphorylated sCD44

### 83.3.3 Antagonists of sCD44: HA Blocks sCD44

In order to verify the cytotoxicity of sCD44, four controls were utilized to determine that sCD44 was cytotoxic to human TM cells: (1) boiling the sCD44 preparation for 5 min to inactivate the preparation (data not shown); (2) premixing CD44 preparation with HA for 2 h; (3) premixing sCD44 preparation with anti-CD44 antibody (BU52); and (4) pretreatment with 40-μM pan-caspase inhibitor (Z-VAD-FMK). All four manipulations inactivated or blocked the cytotoxic effects of sCD44 ($P<0.01$) (see Fig. 83.8).

### 83.3.4 Internalization of sCD44

The HA binding motif of sCD44 is on the ectodomain. Xu et al have convincingly shown that a 42-amino acid HA binding protein is cytotoxic.[78] In addition, recombinant version of sCD44,[79] viral overexpression of sCD44,[26] RHAMM,[80] TSG-6,[81] C1q,[82] a synthetic version of trypsin fragments of aggrecan and link protein named metastatin,[83] and a synthetic polypeptide P4[36] have all been documented to exhibit antitumor activity. Notably, the cytotoxic activity of sCD44[3] and metastatin[83] is inhibited by HA, and cells that have higher pericellular concentrations of HA are resistant to metastatin.

The most compelling evidence for the possible functional role of sCD44 in cell death is from Bryan Toole's laboratory.[10,26,84,85] Stable transfection of murine mammary carcinoma cells with cDNA expressing the sCD44 caused 80% of cells to undergo apoptosis; the surviving cells displayed a marked reduction in their ability to internalize HA. Toole suggests that cell surface CD44 functions to promote cell survival[26] and increased sCD44 leads to apoptosis. When sCD44 is increased, it binds to cell surface CD44 and blocks signal transduction. Toole's results of overexpression of sCD44 parallel our results in POAG; namely, sCD44 is increased in POAG aqueous, sCD44 is cytotoxic to cells and induces apoptosis.[2,3]

Recently, it has been reported that a synthetic peptide containing the HA binding motif inhibited tumor growth by targeting mitochondria and triggering the intrinsic pathway

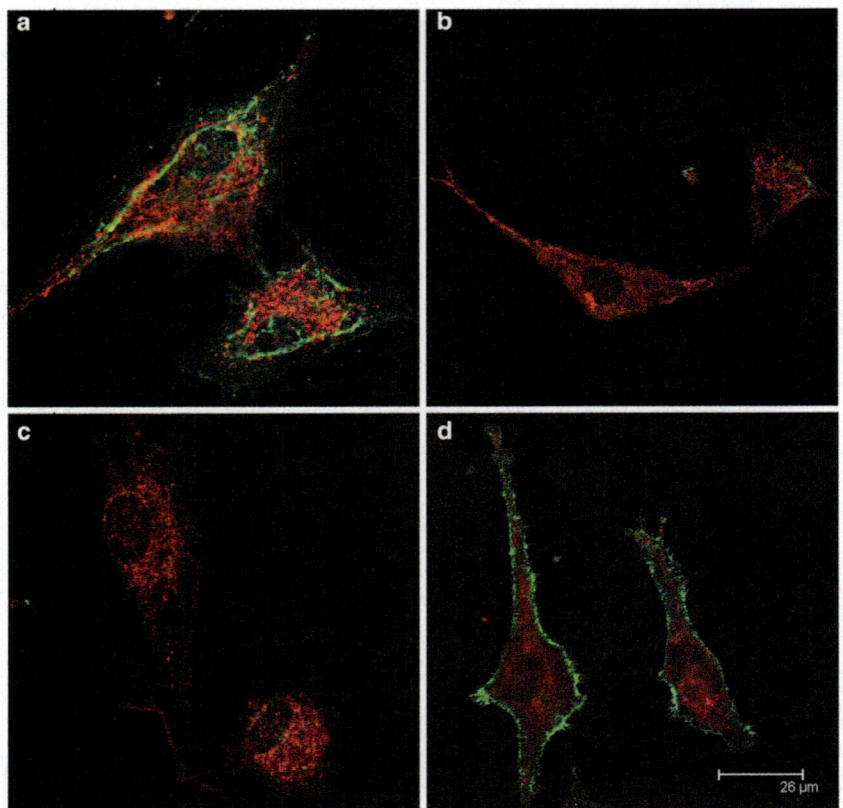

**Fig. 83.9** Internalization of biotinylated-sCD44 (b-sCD44) in TM cells. TM cells were treated with b-sCD44 for 2 h, treated with 125 nM MitoTracker Red, fixed in methanol, permeabilized with 0.1% saponin and treated with mouse anti-biotin and goat FITC labeled anti-mouse IgG antibodies. Cells were photographed with a confocal microscope at the mid-level by optical sectioning. (**a**) 0.1 ng b-sCD44. (**b**) 0.1 ng b- sCD44 coadministered with 1-ug hyaluronic acid. (**c**) Initial administration of 1 ng of selected 10-mer HA binding peptide (KNGRKYSISRT) and then 5 min later followed with 0.1-ng b-sCD44. (**d**) Initial administration of 0.1 ng of unlabelled sCD44 and then 5 min later followed with 0.1 ng b-sCD44 saturated cell surface receptors and prevented intracellular accumulation of biotinylated sCD44

of apoptosis.[46] We therefore tested whether sCD44 is internalized (see Fig. 83.9). sCD44 was biotinylated and the biotin-sCD44 was internalized. The biotin-sCD44 appeared to partially colocalize with mitochondria. The internalization was blocked by preadministrating HA or a 10-mer HA binding peptide. These results suggest that extracellular sCD44 may be partially directed to mitochondria and interact with mitochondrial regulation of cell survival pathways and apoptosis.

### 83.3.5 NF-κB and Lactate Stress

Schuman's group has found increased activation of NF-κB, a transcription factor involved in stress response, in all types of glaucoma.[86] Significantly, CD44 is up-regulated by NF-κB activation[87] and sheds in response to lactate stress.[88] NF-κB is involved in signaling pathways downstream of cytokine receptors, such as TNF-α. Cytokine binding to its receptor results in activation of intracellular kinase cascades including inhibitor of NF-κB kinase (IKK). The IKK complex consists of IKK-1, IKK-2, and NF-κB essential modulator (NEMO).[89] This complex is responsible for phosphorylating the inhibitor of NF-κB, which allows for translocation of NF-κB to the nucleus to initiate transcription. Metabolic stress such as lactate accumulation causes release of sCD44[88,90] and damaged cells are known to express increased amounts of CD44. Altered CD44 transcripts such as CD44v6/v7 have been implicated in autoimmune disorders.[13] Thus, an underlying molecular defect, compounded with metabolic stress and/or a compromised immune response, may lead to cell death and all the sequelae of POAG.

## 83.4 Conclusion

An emerging concept in cell biology, applicable to neurodegenerative diseases such as POAG, is that a specific population of cells becomes vulnerable to a toxic protein as the result of targeted cell stress, free radicals, aging, or other insults. The susceptible cells may lack the putative protective element that normally keeps a toxic protein in check. As a result of the imbalance, the susceptible cells die. Is CD44 the life or death factor in POAG? Certainly this chapter presents ample evidence for a pathophysiological role for sCD44 in POAG, although clinical evidence also indicates the involvement of the cardiovascular, autonomic nervous, and immune system.[91] Consequently, POAG is an ocular disease with systemic features. Upregulation of acute stress response protein amyloid in blood of POAG patients[92] underscores the notion that POAG has ocular and systemic altered protein expression. This is an area that merits substantial future research.

How sCD44 ectodomain shedding occurs, what are the posttranslational modifications (i.e., phosphorylation in sCD44), and exactly why sCD44 is cytotoxic to TM and RGC remain open unanswered questions. It is likely that in normal aqueous, the bioavailability of sCD44 depends on the presence of HA, either in the aqueous or at the cell surface and the degree of its aggregation. Our observation of a hypophosphorylated form of sCD44 in the aqueous humor of POAG and normal pressure glaucoma patients, which was not observed in any of the secondary glaucomas, indicates a change in the synthesis and release of sCD44. The hypophosphorylated sCD44 is highly cytotoxic to TM and RGC in vitro. Therefore, a hypophosphorylated sCD44 in POAG aqueous humor is a possible cell stress related protein candidate that causes cell death in POAG. The presence of hypophosphorylated sCD44 clearly distinguishes POAG from other types of glaucoma, suggesting a specific pathophysiology and a biochemical hallmark of the POAG disease process. The potential clinical significance of these findings is great. CD44 may have diagnostic utility in the future offering several potential methods of treating glaucoma.

## References

1. Knepper PA, Mayanil CSK, Goossens W, et al. Aqueous humor in primary open-angle glaucoma contains an increased level of CD44S. *Invest Ophthalmol Vis Sci.* 2002;343:133–139.
2. Nolan MJ, Giovingo MC, Miller AM, et al. Influence of race on visual field loss and aqueous humor soluble CD44 concentration in primary open-angle glaucoma. *J Glaucoma.* 2007;16:419–429.
3. Choi J, Miller AM, Nolan MJ, et al. Soluble CD44 is cytotoxic to trabecular meshwork and retinal ganglion cells in vitro. *Invest Ophthalmol Vis Sci.* 2005;46:214–222.
4. Shepard AR, Nolan MJ, Millar JC, et al. CD44 Overexpression Causes Ocular Hypertension in the Mouse. ARVO annual meeting; 2008
5. Knepper PA, Goossens W, Palmberg PF. Glycosaminoglycan profile of the human trabecular meshwork in primary open-angle glaucoma. *Invest Ophthalmol Vis Sci.* 1996;37:1360–1367.
6. Knepper PA, Goossens W, Palmberg PF. Glycosaminoglycan stratification in normal and primary open-angle glaucoma juxtacanalicular tissue. *Invest Ophthalmol Vis Sci.* 1996;37:2414–2425.
7. Tammi MI, Day AJ, Turley EA. Hyaluronan and homeostasis: a balancing act. *J Biol Chem.* 2002;277:4581–4584.
8. Lee JY, Spicer AP. Hyaluronan: a multifunctional, megaDalton, stealth molecule. *Curr Opin Cell Biol.* 2000;12:581–586.
9. Gong H, Ye W, Freddo TF, Hernandez MR. Hyaluronic acid in the normal and glaucomatous optic nerve. *Exp Eye Res.* 1997;64:587–595.
10. Toole BP. Hyaluronan is not just a goo! *J Clin Invest.* 2000;106:335–338.
11. Day AJ, Prestwich GD. Hyaluronan-binding proteins: tying up the giant. *J Biol Chem.* 2002;277:4585–4588.
12. Knepper PA, Lukas R, Wills J, Goossens W, Mayanil CSK. Hyaluronic acid receptors of the human trabecular meshwork. *Invest Ophthalmol Vis Sci.* 1997;38:S451.
13. Gunthert U, Johansson B. CD44-a protein family involved in autoimmune diseases and apoptosis. *Immunologist.* 2001;8:4–5.
14. Lokeshwar VB, Iida N, Bourguignon LY. The cell adhesion molecule, GP116, is a new CD44 variant (ex4/v10) involved in hyaluronic acid binding and endothelial cell proliferation. *J Biol Chem.* 1996;271:23853–23864.
15. Gunthert U. CD44 in malignant disorders. *Curr Top Microbiol Immunol.* 1996;213:271–285.
16. Gee K, Kryworuchko M, Kumar A. Recent advances in the regulation of CD44 expression and its role in inflammation and autoimmune diseases. *Arch Immunol Ther Exp (Warsz).* 2004;52:13–26.
17. Naor D, Nedvetzki S, Walmsley M, et al. CD44 involvement in autoimmune inflammations: the lesson to be learned from CD44-targeting by antibody or from knockout mice. *Ann N Y Acad Sci.* 2007;1110:233–247.
18. Eshkar Sebban L, Ronen D, Levartovsky D, et al. The involvement of CD44 and its novel ligand galectin-8 in apoptotic regulation of autoimmune inflammation. *J Immunol.* 2007;179:1225–1235.
19. Vachon E, Martin R, Plumb J, et al. CD44 is a phagocytic receptor. *Blood.* 2006;107:4149–4158.
20. Vachon E, Martin R, Kwok V, et al. CD44-mediated phagocytosis induces inside-out activation of complement receptor-3 in murine macrophages. *Blood.* 2007;110:4492–4502.
21. Ghatak S, Misra S, Toole BP. Hyaluronan oligosaccharides inhibit anchorage-independent growth of tumor cells by suppressing the phosphoinositide 3-kinase/Akt cell survival pathway. *J Biol Chem.* 2002;277:38013–38020.
22. Singleton PA, Salgia R, Moreno-Vinasco L, et al. CD44 regulates hepatocyte growth factor-mediated vascular integrity. Role of c-Met, Tiam1/Rac1, dynamin 2, and cortactin. *J Biol Chem.* 2007;282:30643–30657.
23. Zhang M, Wang MH, Singh RK, Wells A, Siegal GP. Epidermal growth factor induces CD44 gene expression through a novel regulatory element in mouse fibroblasts. *J Biol Chem.* 1997;272:14139–14146.
24. Weiss L, Botero-Anug AM, Hand C, Slavin S, Naor D. CD44 gene vaccination for insulin-dependent diabetes mellitus in non-obese diabetic mice. *Isr Med Assoc J.* 2008;10:20–25.
25. Garin T, Rubinstein A, Grigoriadis N, et al. CD44 variant DNA vaccination with virtual lymph node ameliorates experimental autoimmune encephalomyelitis through the induction of apoptosis. *J Neuro Sci.* 2007;258:17–26.
26. Yu Q, Toole BP, Stamenkovic I. Induction of apoptosis of metastatic mammary carcinoma cells in vivo by disruption of tumor cell surface CD44 function. *J Exp Med.* 1997;186:1985–1996.
27. Cichy J, Pure E. The liberation of CD44. *J Cell Biol.* 2003;161:839–843.
28. Kajita M, Itoh Y, Chiba T, et al. Membrane-type 1 matrix metalloproteinase cleaves CD44 and promotes cell migration. *J Cell Biol.* 2001;153:893–904.
29. Lesley J, Hyman R. CD44 structure and function. *Front Biosci.* 1998;1:616–630.

30. Kincade PW, Zheng Z, Katoh S, Hanson L. The importance of cellular environment to function of the CD44 matrix receptor. *Curr Opin Cell Biol.* 1997;9:635–642.
31. Isacke CM, Yarwood H. The hyaluronan receptor, CD44. *Int J Biochem Cell Biol.* 2002;34:718–721.
32. Naor D, Wallach-Dayan SB, Zahalka MA, Sionov RV. Involvement of CD44, a molecule with a thousand faces, in cancer dissemination. *Semin Cancer Biol.* 2008 [Epub ahead of print]
33. Toyama-Sorimachi N, Miyasaka M. A sulfated proteoglycan as a novel ligand for CD44. *J Dermatol.* 1994;21:795–801.
34. Jalkanen S, Jalkanen M. Lymphocyte CD44 binds the COOH-terminal heparin-binding domain of fibronectin. *J Cell Biol.* 1992; 116:817–825.
35. Weber GF, Ashkar S, Glimcher MJ, Cantor H. Receptor-ligand interaction between CD44 and osteopontin (Eta-1). *Science.* 1996; 271:509–512.
36. Lukashev ME, Werb Z. ECM signalling: orchestrating cell behaviour and misbehaviour. *J Cell Biol.* 1998;8:438–442.
37. Clark AF. New discoveries on the roles of matrix metalloproteinases in ocular cell biology and pathology. *Invest Ophthalmol Vis Sci.* 1998;39:2514–2516.
38. Bradley JMB, Vranka J, Colvis CM, et al. Effect of matrix metalloproteinases activity on outflow in perfused human organ culture. *Invest Ophthalmol Vis Sci.* 1998;39:2649–2658.
39. Sherman L, Sleeman J, Dall P, et al. The CD44 proteins in embryonic development and in cancer. *Curr Top Microbiol Immunol.* 1996;213:249–269.
40. Tsukita A, Oishi K, Sato N, et al. ERM family members are molecular linkers between the cell surface glycoprotein CD44 and actin-based cytoskeleton. *J Cell Biol.* 1994;126:391–401.
41. Jiang H, Peterson RS, Wang W, et al. A requirement for the CD44 cytoplasmic domain for hyaluronan binding, pericellular matrix assembly, and receptor-mediated endocytosis in COS-7 cells. *J Biol Chem.* 2002;277:10531–10533.
42. Sretavan DW, Feng L, Pure E, Reichardt LF. Embryonic neurons of the developing optic chiasm express L1 and CD44, cell surface molecules with opposing effects on retinal axon growth. *Neuron.* 1994;12:957–975.
43. Flurkey K, Stadecker M, Miller RA. Memory T lymphocyte hyporesponsiveness to noncognate stimuli: a key factor in age-related immunodeficiency. *Eur J Immunol.* 1992;2:931–935.
44. Hirano F, Hirano H, Hino E, et al. CD44 isoform expression in periodontal tissues: cell-type specific regulation of alternative splicing. *J Periodontal Res.* 1997;32:634–645.
45. Naot D, Sionov RV, Ish-Shalom D. CD44: structure, function, and association with the malignant process. *Adv Cancer Res.* 1997; 71:241–319.
46. Liu N, Xu XM, Chen J, et al. Hyaluronan-binding peptide can inhibit tumor growth by interacting with Bcl-2. *Int J Cancer.* 2004;109:49–57.
47. Knepper PA, Koga T, Nolan M, Yue BYJT, Sheppard A, Clark A. Multidrug resistance proteins and trabecular meshwork. ARVO annual meeting; 2007
48. Knepper PA, Goossens W, Mayanil CSK. CD44 localization in primary open-angle glaucoma. *Invest Ophthalmol Vis Sci.* 1998;39: 673–680.
49. Camp RL, Krauss TA, Pure E. Variations in the cytoskeletal interaction and posttranslational modifications of the CD44 homing receptor in macrophages. *J Cell Biol.* 1991;115:1283–1292.
50. Lesley J, English N, Perschl A, et al. Variant cell lines selected for alterations in the function of the hyaluronan receptor CD44 show differences in glycosylation. *J Exp Med.* 1995;182:431–437.
51. Thankamony SP, Knudson W. Acylation of CD44 and its association with lipid rafts are required for receptor and hyaluronan endocytosis. *J Biol Chem.* 2006;281:34601–34609.
52. Seiki M. The cell surface: the stage for matrix metalloproteinase regulation of migration. *Curr Opin Cell Biol.* 2002;14:624–632.
53. Stoeck A, Keller S, Riedle S, et al. A role for exosomes in the constitutive and stimulus-induced ectodomain cleavage of L1 and CD44. *Biochem J.* 2006;393:609–618.
54. Yang P, Baker KA, Hagg T. The ADAMs family: coordinators of nervous system development, plasticity and repair. *Prog Neurobiol.* 2006;79:73–94.
55. Lammich S, Okochi M, Takeda M, et al. Presenilin-dependent intramembrane proteolysis of CD44 leads to the liberation of its intracellular domain and the secretion of an Abeta-like peptide. *J Biol Chem.* 2002;277:44754–44759.
56. Liu F, Su Y, Li B, et al. Regulation of amyloid precursor protein (APP) phosphorylation and processing by p35/Cdk5 and p25/Cdk5. *FEBS Lett.* 2003;547:193–196.
57. Tamura H, Kawakami H, Kanamoto T, et al. High frequency of open-angle glaucoma in Japanese patients with Alzheimer's disease. *J Neurol Sci.* 2006;246:79–83.
58. Bayer AU, Ferrari F, Erb C. High occurrence rate of glaucoma among patients with Alzheimer's disease. *Eur Neurol.* 2002;47:165–168.
59. Rajendran L, Schneider A, Schlechtingen G, et al. Efficient inhibition of the Alzheimer's disease beta-secretase by membrane targeting. *Science.* 2008;320:520–523.
60. Tesco G, Koh YH, Kang EL, et al. Depletion of GGA3 stabilizes BACE and enhances beta-secretase activity. *Neuron.* 2007;54: 721–737.
61. Werb Z, Yan Y. A cellular striptease act. *Science.* 1998;282: 1279–1280.
62. Lee MC, Alpaugh ML, Nguyen M, et al. Myoepithelial-specific CD44 shedding is mediated by a putative chymotrypsin-like sheddase. *Biochem Biophys Res Commun.* 2000;279:116–123.
63. Li HL, Wang HH, Liu SJ, et al. Phosphorylation of tau antagonizes apoptosis by stabilizing beta-catenin, a mechanism involved in Alzheimer's neurodegeneration. *Proc Nat Acad Sci U S A.* 2007; 104:3591–3596.
64. Knepper PA, Miller AM, Choi J, et al. Hypo-phosphorylation of aqueous humor sCD44 and primary open-angle glaucoma. *Invest Ophthalmol Vis Sci.* 2005;46:2829–2837.
65. Giovingo MC, Nolan MJ, Koga T, et al. Aqueous humor sCD44 concentration in Diabetes and Primary Open-Angle Glaucoma. ARVO annual meeting; 2008
66. Cavin LG, Romieu-Mourez R, Panta GR, et al. Inhibition of CK2 activity by TGF-beta1 promotes IkappaB-alpha protein stabilization and apoptosis of immortalized hepatocytes. *Hepatology.* 2003;38:1540–1551.
67. Tripathi RC, Li J, Chan WF, Tripathi BJ. Aqueous humor in glaucomatous eyes contains an increased level of TGF-beta 2. *Exp Eye Res.* 1994;59:723–727.
68. Wang WH, McNatt LG, Pang IH, et al. Increased expression of the WNT antagonist sFRP-1 in glaucoma elevates intraocular pressure. *J Clin Invest.* 2008;118:1056–1064.
69. Chen HK, Fernandez-Funez P, Acevedo SF, et al. Interaction of Akt-phosphorylated ataxin-1 with 14-3-3 mediates neurodegeneration in spinocerebellar ataxia type 1. *Cell.* 2003;113: 457–468.
70. Cantley LC. The phosphoinositide 3-kinase pathway. *Science.* 2002;296:1655–1657.
71. Wei W, Wang X, Kusiak JW. Signaling events in amyloid beta-peptide-induced neuronal death and insulin-like growth factor I protection. *J Biol Chem.* 2002;277:17649–17656.
72. Sherman LS, Rizvi TA, Karyala S, Ratner N. CD44 enhances neuregulin signaling by Schwann cells. *J Cell Biol.* 2000;150: 1071–1084.
73. Suo Z, Risberg B, Karlsson MG, et al. The expression of EGFR family ligands in breast carcinomas. *Int J Surg Pathol.* 2002; 10:91–99.
74. Alexander JP, Acott TS. Involvement of protein kinase C in TNF alpha regulation of trabecular matrix metalloproteinases and TIMPs. *Invest Ophthalmol Vis Sci.* 2001;42:2831–2838.

75. Limb GA, Daniels JT, Pleass R, et al. Differential expression of matrix metalloproteinases 2 and 9 by glial Muller cells: response to soluble and extracellular matrix-bound tumor necrosis factor-alpha. *Am J Pathol.* 2002;160:1847–1855.
76. Weinreb RN, Lindsey JD. Metalloproteinase gene transcription in human ciliary muscle cells with latanoprost. *Invest Ophthalmol Vis Sci.* 2002;43:716–722.
77. OH J, Takahashi R, Kondo S, et al. The membrane-anchored MMP inhibitor RECK is a key regulator of extracellular matrix integrity and angiogenesis. *Cell.* 2001;107:789–800.
78. Xu XM, Chen Y, Chen J, et al. A peptide with three hyaluronan binding motifs inhibits tumor growth and inducesapoptosis. *Cancer Res.* 2003;63:5685–5690.
79. Sy MS, Guo YJ, Stamenkovic I. Inhibition of tumor growth in vivo with a soluble CD44-immunoglobulin fusion protein. *J Exp Med.* 1992;176:623–637.
80. Mohapatra S, Yang X, Wright JA, Turley EA, Greenberg AH. Soluble hyaluronan receptor RHAMM induces mitotic arrest by suppressing Cdc2 and cyclin B1 expression. *J Exp Med.* 1996;183: 1663–1668.
81. Wisniewski HG, Naime D, Hua JC, Vilcek J, Cronstein BN. TSG-6, a glycoprotein associated with arthritis, and its ligand hyaluronan exert opposite effects in a murine model of inflammation. *Pflugers Arch.* 1996;431(6 Suppl 2):R225–R226.
82. Rubinstein DB, Stortchevoi A, Boosalis M, et al. Receptor for the globular heads of C1q (gC1q-R, p33, hyaluronan-binding protein) is preferentially expressed by adenocarcinoma cells. *Int J Cancer.* 2004;110:741–750.
83. Liu N, Lapcevich RK, Underhill CB, et al. Metastatin: a hyaluronan-binding complex from cartilage that inhibits tumor growth. *Cancer Res.* 2001;61:1022–1028.
84. Yu Q, Toole BP. A new alternatively spliced exon between v9 and v10 provides a molecular basis for synthesis of soluble CD44. *J Biol Chem.* 1996;271:20603–20607.
85. Zeng CX, Toole BP, Kinney SD, Kuo JW, Stamenkovic I. Inhibition of tumor growth in vivo by hyaluronan oligomers. *Int J Cancer.* 1998;77:396–401.
86. Wang N, Chintala SK, Fini ME, Schuman JS. Activation of a tissue-specific stress response in the aqueous outflow pathway of the eye defines the glaucoma disease phenotype. *Nat Med.* 2001; 7:304–309.
87. Fitzgerald KA, Bowie AG, Skeffington BS, O'Neill LA. Ras, protein kinase C zeta, and I kappa B kinases 1 and 2 are downstream effectors of CD44 during the activation of NFkappa B by hyaluronic acid fragments in T-24 carcinoma cells. *J Immunol.* 2000;164: 2053–2063.
88. Miller AM, Nolan MJ, Choi J, et al. Lactate treatment causes NK-κB activation and CD44 shedding in cultured trabecular meshwork cells. *Invest Ophthalmol Vis Sci.* 2007;48:1615–1621.
89. Schwamborn K, Weil R, Courtois G, Whiteside ST, Israel A. Phorbol esters and cytokines regulate the expression of the NEMO-related protein, a molecule involved in a NF-kappa B-independent pathway. *J Biol Chem.* 2000;275:22780–22788.
90. Stern R, Shuster S, Neudecker BA, Formby B. Lactate stimulates fibroblast expression of hyaluronan and CD44: the Warburg effect revisited. *Exp Cell Res.* 2002;276:24–31.
91. Pache M, Flammer J. A sick eye in a sick body? Systemic findings in patients with primary open-angle glaucoma. *Surv Ophthalmol.* 2006;51:179–212.
92. Wang WH, McNatt LG, Pang IH, et al. Increased expression of serum amyloid A in glaucoma and its effect on intraocular pressure. *Invest Ophthalmol Vis Sci.* 2008;49:1916–1923.

# Chapter 84
# Stem Cells and Glaucoma

Shan Lin, Mary Kelley, and John Samples

Patients frequently ask about the applicability of stem cell research and therapy for their glaucoma. Stem cell therapies do offer significant promise in glaucoma. Like other neurodegenerative diseases where stem cells may be of benefit, glaucoma offers logical targets for stem cell therapy. For glaucoma, these are the optic nerve and the trabecular meshwork. In Parkinson's disease, stem cells delivered to the basal ganglia have proven to have significant therapeutic benefit.[1]

Stem cells may be derived from a variety of sources including embryos, nonfetal cell culture lines, and immortalized cell lines. The defining characteristic of fetal stem cells is that they are often pluripotent and able to differentiate into many cell types. Pluripotent stem cells can give rise to every cell type in the body; unipotent or multipotent cells can differentiate into a lesser number of cell types. Most nonfetal stem cells (adult stem cells) are multipotent or unipotent. As an example, mesenchymal cells from bone marrow are multipotent, while trabecular insert cells from the triangular insert region under Schwalbe's line are likely unipotent.

For the optic nerve, it might be possible to eventually regenerate or renew damaged retinal ganglion cells, perhaps in association with the use of roundabout proteins (as described in an important paper in *Nature Medicine*) that have some potential for assisting with site-directed regrowth.[2] A more likely candidate for stem cells helping glaucoma in the optic nerve is the delivery of cells that can differentiate to become supportive glial elements for the optic nerve. As noted elsewhere in the text, it may be that glial elements at certain specific locations dramatically alter support for the retinal ganglion cells (see Chap. 16). Emphasis on glial elements, long popular in neurological cell biology, has increased. In culture systems, they are significantly hardier and more robust than neural cells.

In the trabecular meshwork, it seems logical to seed cells onto the beams.[3] Delivery of cells to the site of resistance, the juxtacanalicular meshwork, as well as Schlemm's canal, may be clinically useful. The cells that are the most important in glaucoma are the relatively deep cells that mediate aqueous outflow resistance. A potential inability to get the cells directly to the deeper meshwork as well as the considerable macrophage-like capability of trabecular cells on beams suggest that more directed or strategic means of delivery of stem cells in the meshwork will be important. Because the intratrabecular spaces are large, cells may find little physical impediment to reaching deeper structures. Experiments with laser trabeculoplasty and organ culture systems suggest that media from explants with its growth factors could potentially propel cells from the insert region to the deeper trabecular meshwork where an effect on outflow is expected.[3] Growth factors, cytokines, and a variety of other peptides have all proven useful in delivering the necessary instructions for undifferentiated cells to become more differentiated. In the case of the trabecular meshwork, it may help to deliver a chemotactic signal. We think that specific cytokines will help trabecular cells to the area, where they may have the most impact on outflow.[4-7] Our experiments in the late 1980s with human recombinant tumor necrosis factor and interleukin-1 injections intravitreally suggest that the direct injection of these molecules is not suitable for the purpose of directing stem cells.[8,9] However, similar molecules located in alternate pathways may be useful. Some ocular cells, such as trabecular cell, are influenced by their basement membrane to differentiate as well as to orient their apical and basement aspects. Positioning of stem cells in the trabecular region, as well as the lamina cribrosa and elsewhere in the optic nerve may require chemotactic signals to correctly position the cells.

What do we expect from the stem cells in terms of their ability to cure or improve glaucoma in patients? Healthier cells are more likely to perform well in terms of biosynthesis and degradation of extracellular matrix materials, including those that presumably regulate outflow. Our long-held belief has been that one of the main obstructions to outflow is one or more of the proteoglycans in the juxtacanalicular meshwork.[10,11] Proteoglycans can be affected by both synthesis and degradation that may be improved by the arrival of new cells on the beams or other locations. Delivering cells that can deliver "healthy molecules," particularly proteoglycans and extracellular matrix constituents to the critical outflow pathways, is the best way to physiologically correct glaucoma and ultimately eliminate the need for both medications and surgery to treat high pressure-related diseases. Similar principles may apply to the delivery of stem cells to the optic nerve, but because of its location, stem cell therapy to the nerve may lag stem cell therapy to the meshwork.

## References

1. Svensen C. Stem cells and Parkinsons disease: toward a treatment not a cure. *Stem Cell*. 2008;2(5):412-413. PubMed ID: 18462691.
2. Jones CA, London NR, Chen H, et al. Robo4 stabilizes the vascular network by inhibiting pathologic angiogenesis and endothelial hyperpermeability. *Nat Med*. 2008;14(4):448–453. PubMed ID: 18345009.
3. Kelley MJ, Rose AY, Keller KE, Hessle H, Samples JR, Acott TS. Stem cells in the trabecular meshwork: present and future promises. *Exp Eye Res*. 2009;88:747–751.
4. Zhang CC, Lodish HF. Cytokines regulating hematopoietic stem cell function. *Curr Opin Hematol*. 2008;14(4):307–311.
5. Loveland KL, Hogarth C, Mendis S, et al. Drivers of germ cell maturation. *Ann N Y Acad Sci*. 2005;1061:173–182. Review.
6. Heng BC, Cao T, Lee EH. Directing stem cell differentiation into the chondrogenic lineage in vitro. *Stem Cells*. 2004;22(7):1152–1167. Review.
7. Sachinidis A, Fleischmann BK, Kolossov E, Wartenberg M, Sauer H, Hescheler J. Cardiac specific differentiation of mouse embryonic stem cells. *Cardiovasc Res*. 2003;58(2):278–291. Review.
8. Rosenbaum JT, Howes EL, Rubin RM, Samples JR. Ocular inflammatory effects of intravitreally-injected tumor necrosis factor. *Am J Pathol*. 1998;133:47–53.
9. Rosenbaum JT, Samples JR, Hefeneider SH, Howes EL Jr. Ocular inflammatory effects of intravitreal interleukin-1. *Arch Ophthalmol*. 1987;105:1117–1120.
10. Acott TS, Kingsley PD, Samples JR, Van Buskirk EM. Human trabecular meshwork organ culture: morphology and glycosaminoglycan synthesis. *Invest Ophthalmol Vis Sci*. 1988;29:90–100.
11. Fuchshofer R, Welge-Lussen U, Lütjen-Drecoll E. The effect of TGF-beta2 on human trabecular meshwork extracellular proteolytic system. *Exp Eye Res*. 2003;77:757–765.

# Chapter 85
# Cytoskeletal Active Agents for Glaucoma Therapy

Jennifer A. Faralli, Marie K. Schwinn, Donna M. Peters, and Paul L. Kaufman

The conventional outflow pathway, also known as the trabecular meshwork-Schlemm's canal (TM-SC) pathway, consists of three layers.[1,2] The most proximal layer to the anterior chamber consists of collagen beams wrapped with trabecular meshwork (TM) cells. The middle layer is called the juxtacanalicular region (JCT). It is composed of trabecular cells embedded in a thick matrix containing fibronectin, collagen, and laminin. This region is often regarded as the major site of aqueous humor outflow resistance due to its narrow intercellular spaces.[3] The last layer is the inner wall of Schlemm's canal and is made up of a monolayer of specialized endothelial cells situated on a basal lamina that is directly connected to the extracellular matrix of the JCT. The inner wall of Schlemm's canal has a high density of pores across its surface and is thought to contribute perhaps 10% of the total resistance to aqueous humor outflow through the TM.[4]

Recent studies utilizing cultured anterior segments in which the ciliary muscle has been removed suggest that the TM-SC pathway can participate in regulating outflow and, hence, may be a potential target for lowering intraocular pressure (IOP). The TM tissue is a smooth muscle-like, suspended multilayer tissue with contractile properties.[5-7] TM cells express α-smooth muscle actin and myosin[8,9] as well as G-protein coupled receptors and ion channels[10,11] involved in contractility. Numerous studies have recently demonstrated that the contractile properties of the TM-SC pathway can play an important role in the regulation of aqueous humor outflow[10,12-14] and may be one way to target outflow through the conventional pathway.

The contractile properties of smooth muscle tissue are regulated by the phosphorylation state of the 20-kDa myosin regulatory light chain (MLC) of smooth and nonmuscle myosin II in the presence of $Ca^{2+}$ and calmodulin. Phosphorylation of MLC facilitates an interaction between myosin and actin filaments, thereby providing a contractile network that modulates cell shape, the formation of actin stress fibers, cell–matrix contacts, and cell–cell junctions. Likewise when MLC is dephosphorylated, there are fewer actin stress fibers, and a decrease in cell–cell and cell–matrix contacts is observed. It is any, or all, of these changes that can lead to relaxation of a tissue.

In nonskeletal mammalian muscle cells, MLC is phosphorylated by a kinase called myosin light chain kinase (MLCK) and dephosphorylated by a phosphatase called myosin light chain phosphatase (MLCP). MLCK has been shown to modulate a variety of contractile processes, including smooth muscle contraction, cell adhesion, migration, and proliferation and dysregulation of these processes has been shown to contribute to the vascular pathologies that occur during atherosclerosis, restenosis, and hypertension. The activation of MLCK and concomitant inhibition of MLCP is regulated by members of the Rho GTPase family, in particular RhoA (Fig. 85.1). When RhoA is active, it stimulates Rho kinase (also known as ROCK), which in turn promotes MLCK activity and inactivates MLCP by phosphorylating it. This simultaneous activation of MLCK and inhibition of MLCP increases the phosphorylation state of MLC, thereby allowing it to interact with actin filaments to form the contractile actomyosin network.

In the TM, the actomyosin network may act as a regulatory complex to counteract such forces as stretch, shear stress, and other physical factors. For instance, increased IOP that could induce stretching of the TM may be countered by the TM actomyosin network with decreased cellular contraction. Another factor that may affect outflow through the TM is the contractile state of the scleral spur. The elastic fibers in the scleral spur are continuous with the elastic fibers in the TM, and scleral spur cells have been shown to have contractile properties.[15] In addition, scleral spur cells are closely associated with varicose axons,[16] suggesting that nervous signals may alter the tone of the scleral spur. Thus, changes in the contractile state of scleral spur cells may alter the architecture of the TM, thereby modulating outflow of aqueous humor through the TM.

A decrease in contractility of the actomyosin network in the TM can dramatically affect aqueous humor outflow by causing a "relaxation" of the TM and an increase in intercellular spaces leading to an increase in aqueous humor outflow.

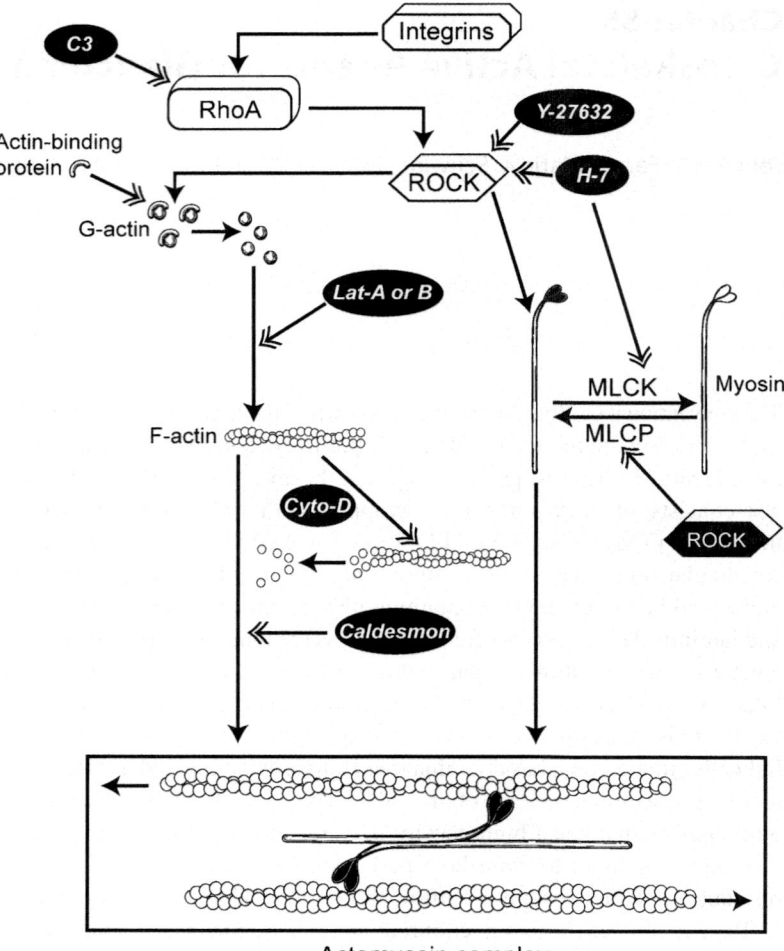

**Fig. 85.1** Schematic of Rho signaling pathway involved in the formation of actomyosin complex. Inhibitors of the pathway are indicated in *black* with *double arrow heads*. G-actin is represented by *circles*. F-actin is the assembled actin filament that consists of two chains of actin monomers. The *half circles* on G-actin are actin-binding proteins that bind G-actin, thus preventing it from being assembled into a filament. ROCK triggers the removal of these actin-binding proteins off G-actin and promotes the assembly of actin filaments. Cytochalasin, (cyto-D) promotes the disassembly of F-actin. Caldesmon binds F-actin and prevents it from being assembled into the actomyosin complex with myosin (shown in box). Unphosphorylated myosin is indicated in *purple*. Its light chain (*oval*) is phosphorylated by myosin light chain kinase (MLCK) and dephosphorylated by myosin light chain phosphatase (MLCP). The rod in myosin represents the helical portion of myosin. The actomyosin complex is indicated in the *box*. It contains two molecules of phosphorylated myosin and two molecules of actin filaments. *Arrows* in the *box* indicate the direction of the contractile force.

Indeed, treating enucleated calf and human eyes or the eyes of living monkeys and humans with actin-disrupting agents such as cytochalasins B and D or the latrunculins (Lat)-A and -B causes an increase in aqueous humor outflow facility.[17-26] These agents work by disassembling actin filaments. Cytochalasins are fungal metabolites that cap the barbed ends of actin filaments, thereby preventing their elongation. The latrunculins are extracted from *Latrunculia magnifica* (nagombata), a sponge that lives in the bottom of the Red Sea, and disrupt the actomyosin network by sequestering monomeric actin (or G-actin), thus preventing assembly of actin filaments.

In living monkey and organ-cultured human eyes treated with cytochalasin B or D, the increase in outflow facility is accompanied by a separation of trabecular cells from their neighboring cells and their surrounding extracellular matrix (ECM) on the beams, in the juxtacanalicular region, and along the inner wall. This leads to distension of the meshwork and ruptures in the inner wall, which can enhance fluid flow and washout of ECM.

Similar changes were seen in eyes and TM cultures treated with Lat-A or Lat-B. In TM cultures, treatment with Lat-A or Lat-B leads to a disruption of both cell–cell and cell–ECM adhesions. In living monkeys and cultured porcine eyes, Lat-A and/or Lat-B increased outflow facility and decreased IOP for up to 24 h. Structurally, Lat-B caused a reorganization of the cytoskeleton, especially in TM cells on the collagen beams, which appeared rounded, and in Schlemm's canal inner wall (IW) cells, which developed numerous giant vacuoles. The sub-canalicular cells developed numerous cytoplasmic processes and there was a massive "ballooning" of the juxtacanalicular (JXT) region creating an expansion of the space between the IW of Schlemm's canal and the trabecular collagen beams. There was also an entrapment of ECM between the altered intercellular spaces created by the cytoplasmic processes (Fig. 85.2). Although these effects were readily seen in the primate eye, they were not always as pronounced in cultured human anterior segments.[27] No detrimental effects on tight junctions, cell–cell, or cell–ECM adhesions were observed. Clinically, latrunculins rather than cytochalasins may be the agent of choice since they appear to be gentler with less adverse side effects. In fact, a derivative of Lat-B (INS117458) is currently in Phase 1 clinical testing. Cytochalasins often caused breaks in the inner wall of Schlemm's canal and the appearance of platelet aggregates at the site of ruptures along the inner wall.

Another way to trigger the relaxation of the TM is to use the novel approach of gene therapy for glaucoma and over-express cytoskeleton-relaxing proteins such as caldesmon in the TM. In smooth muscle cells, caldesmon regulates the activity of myosin II by blocking its interaction with actin.[28-30] In cultured cells, over-expression of caldesmon led to the suppression of cell contractility, manifested by a reduced capacity to develop traction forces applied to the underlying extracellular matrix. Anterior segments transduced with an adenoviral vector that expressed caldesmon for 5 days showed some disruption of trabecular beams, and the TM cells appeared to be rounded up. Schlemm's canal seemed to be intact. The magnitude of the outflow facility increase resulting from caldesmon over-expression in monkey organ-cultured anterior segments in the current study is nearly identical to that found with 300 μM H-7 treatment in this system and to 100 μM H-7[26] or 0.5 μM latrunculin-A[22] in monkey eyes in vivo. More detailed morphological analyses are needed to determine whether structural effects such as cell relaxation, expansion of the juxtacanalicular region, dilation of Schlemm's canal, and luminal protrusion of the inner wall similar to those induced by to H-7 or latrunculin-A or -B are produced.

In addition to actin-disrupting agents, microtubule disrupting agents can also be used to increase outflow facility and decrease IOP. One such drug is ethacrynic acid (ECA), which inhibits microtubule assembly and blocks signaling pathways that normally regulate the formation of cell contacts with the ECM. ECA reduces outflow resistance in enucleated calf and human eyes and in living monkey eyes, and concomitantly reduces IOP in live rabbit, monkey, and human eyes. In enucleated human eyes, low ECA doses that increase outflow do not produce morphologic changes in the TM, whereas higher doses induce separations between TM and inner wall cells.

Diverse protein kinase inhibitors such as staurosporine, H-7, chelerythrine, and ML-7 and the protein kinase C (PKC) activator phorbol ester can also be used to alter the contractile properties of the TM and increase outflow facility. Despite targeting different kinases, all these inhibitors have one thing in common: They perturb the cytoskeleton of cultured TM cells. H-7 in particular has proven to be very effective in regulating outflow facility. H-7 is a serine–threonine kinase inhibitor that inhibits actomyosin-driven contractility and induces general cellular relaxation by preventing the phosphorylation of MLCK. This leads to the eventual deterioration of the actin filaments and the disruption of cell–matrix attachments in human TM and other cultured cells. In living monkeys and enucleated porcine eyes, H-7 increases outflow facility and decreases IOP in a dose- and time-dependent fashion. Ultrastructural studies indicate that the effect of H-7 is similar to that observed with the actin-disrupting agents and leads to the expansion of the juxtacanalicular intercellular spaces, accompanied by removal of extracellular deposits. The inner wall cells also become highly extended, but cell–cell contacts are maintained. H-7 appears to decrease outflow resistance by relaxing and expanding the TM and Schlemm's canal, without significantly changing intercellular adhesion. The effect of H-7 is reversible, indicating that it is not toxic and that the effects are due to targeting cell contractility. Interestingly, the cornea is not affected at the concentrations used to affect the TM, indicating the feasibility of administering this compound as an eye drop.

Finally, targeting Rho kinase itself is a very effective way to increase outflow facility and decrease IOP. This can be accomplished by using a specific ROCK inhibitor (e.g., Y-27632), a dominant negative Rho kinase, or the bacterial protein toxin exoenzyme C3 transferase (C3) from *Clostridium botulinum* to inhibit Rho activity. C3-transferase specifically inactivates RhoA by ADP-ribosylation. Treatment with these inhibitors increased outflow facility in organ cultured porcine and human eyes and in rabbit and monkey eyes in vivo. In vitro treatment of TM cultures showed a reduction in assembled actin filaments and cell rounding. Structural studies on the light microscopic level revealed that expression of C3-transferase in cultured anterior segments triggered a reduction in cellularity and a disorganization of beams. In the majority of cultured anterior segments, Schlemm's canal appeared intact. Derivatives of these compounds (i.e., INS117458) that target Rho kinase, MLCK, and actin filaments are currently in Phase 1 clinical testing.

These studies suggest that disruption of cell–cell or cell–matrix contacts in the TM leads to a change in TM architecture, thereby increasing outflow of aqueous humor. Additional evidence supporting this comes from a recombinant integrin/syndecan binding domain from fibronectin called the Heparin II (Hep II) domain. In human and monkey anterior segment organ cultures, the Hep II domain significantly increased aqueous humor outflow by 25%,[31] suggesting that signaling events mediated by cell–matrix interactions also play an important role in the TM.

The overwhelming success of these compounds in increasing outflow and lowering IOP in experimental models suggests that the Rho-mediated signaling pathway may be part of the natural regulatory mechanisms within the TM that control outflow facility. Lending credence to this idea is the fact that TM cells contain the necessary contractile apparatus including α-smooth muscle actin and smooth muscle myosin. They also contain members of the integrin family of receptors, which regulate Rho-mediated contractility and can act as

**Fig. 85.2** (**a**) Schematic diagram of the layers in the trabecular meshwork. There are three layers. First the beams, which have endothelial-like cells wrapped around them. Second layer is the JCT, which consists of smooth-muscle-like cells embedded in an extracellular matrix of collagen fibrils, amorphous patches of fibronectin, and proteoglycans. Third layer, a monolayer of Schlemm's canal (SC) cells on top of a discontinuous basement membrane. Many cells are flat and elongated, but some are very round. All are connected. Some of the cells have formed giant vacuoles, which is a distended cell protruding into the canal. (**b**) Schematic diagram showing how actin disrupting agents affect the organization of the trabecular meshwork. Diagram adapted from Tripathi and Tripathi[32].

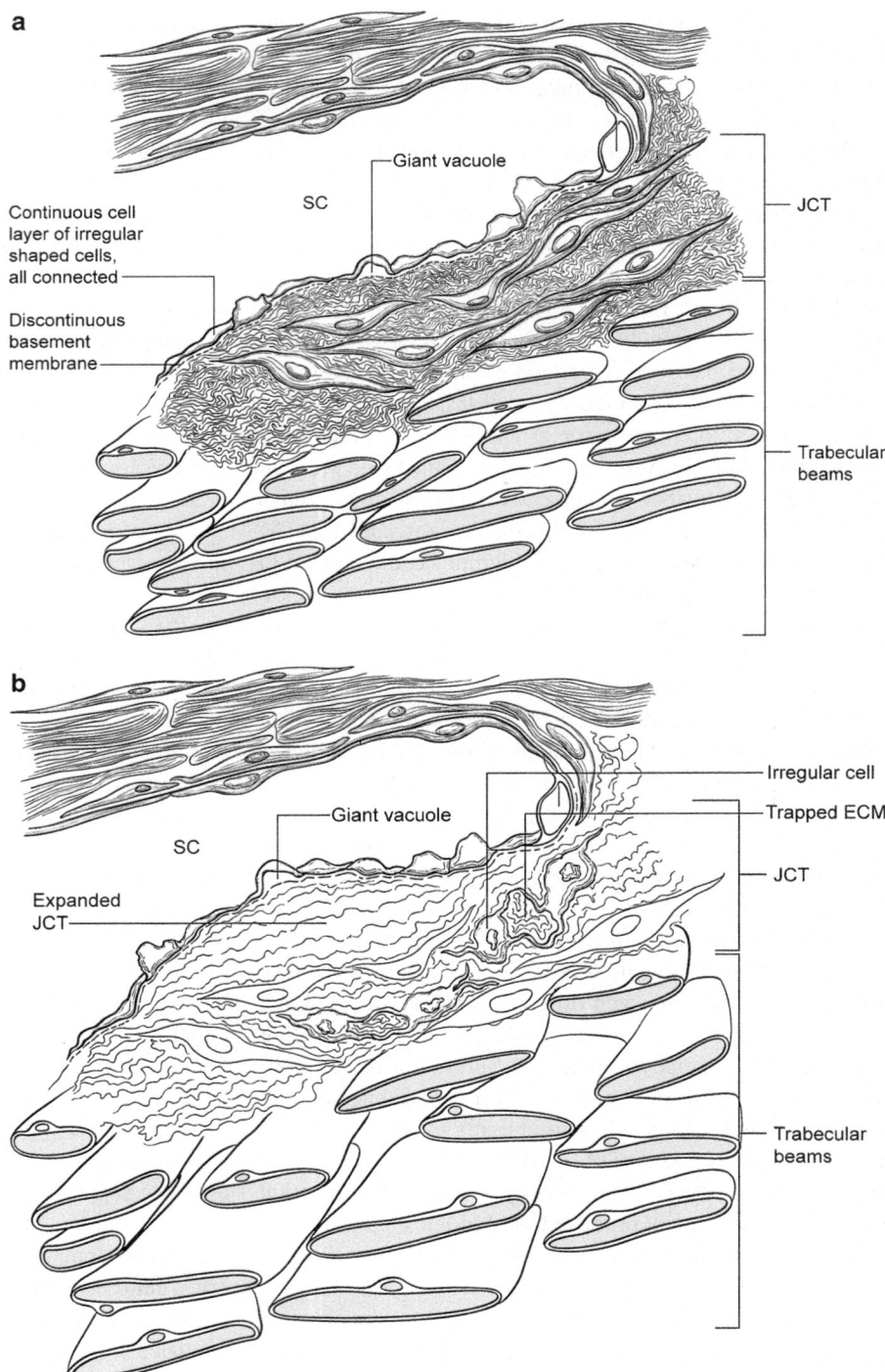

transducers of mechanochemical signals. Integrins form an important physical link between the extracellular and intracellular environment by binding both the extracellular matrix and the actomyosin network. In other systems, in particular the cardiovascular system, integrins transmit signals in response to physical stimuli such as stretch, pressure, and shear force. In summary, these data define a molecular mechanism by which the TM could be an active regulator of outflow facility in response to changes in IOP.

# References

1. Gong H, Tripathi RC, Tripathi BJ. Morphology of the aqueous outflow pathway. *Microsc Res Tech*. 1996;33:336–367.
2. Llobet A, Gasull X, Gual A. Understanding trabecular meshwork physiology: a key to the control of intraocular pressure? *News Physiol Sci*. 2003;18:205–209.
3. Johnson DH, Johnson M. How does nonpenetrating glaucoma surgery work? Aqueous outflow resistance and glaucoma surgery [comment]. *J Glaucoma*. 2001;10:55–67.

4. Bill A. Editorial: the drainage of aqueous humor. *Invest Ophthalmol.* 1975;14:1–3.
5. Barany EH. The mode of action of pilocarpine on outflow resistance in the eye of a primate (Cercopithecus ethiops). *Invest Ophthalmol.* 1962;1:712–727.
6. Wiederholt M, Thieme H, Stumpff F. The regulation of trabecular meshwork and ciliary muscle contractility. *Prog Retin Eye Res.* 2000;19:271–295.
7. Lepple-Wienhues A, Stahl F, Wiederholt M. Differential smooth muscle-like contractile properties of trabecular meshwork and ciliary muscle. *Exp Eye Res.* 1991;53:33–38.
8. de Kater AW, Shahsafaei A, Epstein DL. Localization of smooth muscle and nonmuscle actin isoforms in the human aqueous outflow pathway. *Invest Ophthalmol Vis Sci.* 1992;33:424–429.
9. de Kater AW, Spurr-Michaud SJ, Gipson IK. Localization of smooth muscle myosin-containing cells in the aqueous outflow pathway. *Invest Ophthalmol Vis Sci.* 1990;31:347–353.
10. Rao PV, Deng P, Sasaki Y, Epstein DL. Regulation of myosin light chain phosphorylation in the trabecular meshwork: role in aqueous humor outflow facility. *Exp Eye Res.* 2005;80:197–206.
11. Mitchell CH, Fleischhauer JC, Stamer WD, Peterson-Yantorno K, Civan MM. Human trabecular meshwork cell volume regulation. *Am J Physiol Cell Physiol.* 2002;283:C315–C326.
12. Stumpff F, Wiederholt M. Regulation of trabecular meshwork contractility. *Ophthalmology.* 2000;214:33–53.
13. Thieme H, Stumpff F, Ottlecz A, Percicot CL, Lambrou GN, Wiederholt M. Mechanisms of action of unoprostone on trabecular meshwork contractility. *Invest Ophthalmol Vis Sci.* 2001;42:3193–3201.
14. Tian B, Geiger B, Epstein DL, Kaufman PL. Cytoskeletal involvement in the regulation of aqueous humor outflow. *Invest Ophthalmol Vis Sci.* 2000;41:619–623.
15. Tamm E, Flugel C, Stefani FH, Rohen JW. Contractile cells in the human scleral spur. *Exp Eye Res.* 1992;54:531–543.
16. Tamm ER, Koch TA, Mayer B, Stefani FH, Lutjen-Drecoll E. Innervation of myofibroblast-like scleral spur cells in human money eyes. *Invest Ophthalmol Vis Sci.* 1995;36:1633–1644.
17. Epstein DL, Rowlette LL, Roberts BC. Acto-myosin drug effects and aqueous outflow function. *Invest Ophthalmol Vis Sci.* 1999;40:74–81.
18. Johnson DH. The effect of cytochalasin D on outflow facility and the trabecular meshwork of the human eye in perfusion organ culture. *Invest Ophthalmol Vis Sci.* 1997;38:2790–2799.
19. Kaufman PL. Pharmacologic trabeculocanalotomy. Facilitating aqueous outflow by assaulting the meshwork cytoskeleton, junctional complexes, and extracellular matrix [comment]. *Arch Ophthalmol.* 1992;110:34–36.
20. Kaufman PL, Barany EH. Cytochalasin B reversibly increases outflow facility in the eye of the cynomolgus monkey. *Invest Ophthalmol Vis Sci.* 1977;16:47–53.
21. Kaufman PL, Bill A, Barany EH. Effect of cytochalasin B on conventional drainage of aqueous humor in the cynomolgus monkey. *Exp Eye Res.* 1977;25:411–414.
22. Peterson JA, Tian B, Bershadsky AD, et al. Latrunculin-A increases outflow facility in the monkey. *Invest Ophthalmol Vis Sci.* 1999;40:931–941.
23. Peterson JA, Tian B, Geiger B, Kaufman PL. Effect of latrunculin-B on outflow facility in monkeys. *Exp Eye Res.* 2000;70:307–313.
24. Rao PV, Deng PF, Kumar J, Epstein DL. Modulation of aqueous humor outflow facility by the Rho kinase-specific inhibitor Y-27632. *Invest Ophthalmol Vis Sci.* 2001;42:1029–1037 [erratum appears in Invest Ophthalmol Vis Sci 2001;42(8):1690].
25. Sabanay I, Gabelt BT, Tian B, Kaufman PL, Geiger B. H-7 effects on structure and fluid conductance of monkey trabecular meshwork. *Arch Ophthalmol.* 2000;118:955–962.
26. Tian B, Kaufman PL, Volberg T, Gabelt BT, Geiger B. H-7 disrupts the actin cytoskeleton and increases outflow facility. *Arch Ophthalmol.* 1998;116:633–643.
27. Ethier CR, Read AT, Chan DW. Effects of latrunculin-B on outflow facility and trabecular meshwork structure in human eyes. *Invest Ophthalmol Vis Sci.* 2006;47:1991–1998.
28. Huber PA. Caldesmon. *Int J Biochem Cell Biol.* 1997;29:1047–1051.
29. Chalovich JM, Sen A, Resetar A, et al. Caldesmon: binding to actin and myosin and effects on elementary steps in the ATPase cycle. *Acta Physiol Scand.* 1998;164:427–435.
30. Marston S, Burton D, Copeland O, et al. Structural interactions between actin, tropomyosin, caldesmon and calcium binding protein and the regulation of smooth muscle thin filaments. *Acta Physiol Scand.* 1998;164:401–414.
31. Santas AJ, Bahler C, Peterson JA, et al. Effect of heparin II domain of fibronectin on aqueous outflow in cultured anterior segments of human eyes. *Invest Ophthalmol Vis Sci.* 2003;44:4796–4804.
32. Tripathi BJ, Tripathi PC. Embryology of the Anterior Segement of the Human Eye. Chapter pp 3–40. The Glaucomas, ed. R. Ritch, M. Bruce Shields, and T. Krupin. C.V. Mosby, St Lousis. 1989.

# Chapter 86
# The Drug Discovery Process: How Do New Glaucoma Medications Come to Market?

Michael Bergamini

In the United States of America, no drugs have been approved to treat glaucoma in the past 25 years. The vast majority of drugs in the glaucoma specialist's armamentarium are indicated for the reduction (or treatment) of elevated intraocular pressure (IOP) in patients with open-angle glaucoma or ocular hypertension – or words to that effect. Internationally, the situation is quite different, but this review will focus primarily on how drugs (and more specifically, glaucoma drugs) are discovered and developed for the US market.

Over time, the medical community and the end consumer (patient) have come to expect and demand that the medicine prescribed will be safe and effective. The regulatory controls placed on the pharmaceutical industry can be viewed as a response by society to the decisions made by a few senior managers which were not in the best interest of their customers. Note that these regulatory controls assure the relative safety and efficacy (based on risk/benefit assessment) of new medications for only the indicated patient population. Because of pharmacogenetic variation in patients' responses to drugs, the safety or efficacy of a drug in a specific, individual patient is never assured.

A little regulatory history: The US Pure Food and Drug Act of 1906 (passed in response to the public outcry over adulterated products; e.g., *The Jungle* by Upton Sinclair) addressed only quality (e.g., a drug had to be pure). The Food, Drug, and Cosmetic Act of 1938 (passed following the deaths of about 100 children from diethylene glycol poisoning due to its use as a solvent in an elixir of sulfanilamide) added the requirement that the product be safe.

Enforcement was entrusted to the Food and Drug Administration (FDA) and toxicity studies were expected, although not required. Drug products had to be submitted to the FDA, and if the FDA did not object within 90 days, the product could be distributed and promoted. Formal approval was not included as part of the legislation, no proof of efficacy was required, and the risk-to-benefit ratio was seldom mentioned. The Harris–Kefauver Amendments to the Food, Drug, and Cosmetic Act in 1962 (passed in response to the outbreak of the birth defect of phocomelia induced by thalidomide, a hypnotic with no obvious advantage over other drugs in its class) required formal testing in human beings and approval of a New Drug Application (NDA) before marketing. Prior to testing in humans, investigators are required to submit an application for an Investigational New Drug (IND) exemption. Since 1962, proof of clinical efficacy has been required for all new drugs, as is documentation of relative safety in terms of the risk-to-benefit ratio for the disease entity to be treated. Finally, the legislation held senior management of the sponsor (which is usually the manufacturer) criminally liable for any infractions by their subordinates. The provisions of the Harris–Kefauver amendments have greatly increased the time and the cost required to market a new drug.

More recently, the Food and Drug Administration Modernization Act of 1997 (FDAMA) was enacted by Congress as part of the redesigning of the US Government. Some of the features of the Act include less burdensome requirements for sponsors of device applications, streamlining of clinical research, revisions to the regulations concerning advertising and promotion, and pediatric exclusivity to mention a few. Additionally, as part of FDAMA, the Prescription Drug User Fee Act (PDUFA) was reenacted. Sponsors of human drug applications are required to pay a fee upon filing a New Drug Application (NDA), and the fees collected are utilized by FDA to fund additional reviewers. The PDUFA also encouraged review time lines based upon the NDA filing date. The FDA committed to try to review the majority of priority applications within 6 months and the majority of standard applications within 10 months' time.

FDA Amendments Act (FDAAA) of 2007 extended key user-fee programs, including the Prescription Drug User Fee Act (PDUFA) and the Medical Device User Fee Act (MDUFMA), to reauthorize the Best Pharmaceuticals for Children Act and the Pediatric Research Equity Act. In addition, it provides FDA with additional requirements, authorities, and resources with regard to both pre- and postmarketing drug safety. The statute contains important new authorities to require postmarketing studies and clinical trials, safety labeling changes, and Risk Evaluation and

Mitigation Strategies (REMS). The act requires increased activities for active post market risk identification and analysis and requires an expanded clinical trials database to ensure that clinical trials information is provided to the National Institutes of Health (NIH) ClinicalTrials.gov.

The International Conference on Harmonization (ICH) Common Technical Document (CTD) was enacted in July of 2001 and was intended to allow a sponsor to prepare one common technical submission that can be submitted to all three ICH regions: the U.S., Europe and Japan. In practice, there is still much duplication. The ICH also has issued many guidelines that cover essentially all aspects of drug product development in excruciating detail. Those guidelines with perhaps the greatest impact on the glaucoma specialist are the ones covering the composition, purity, and stability of the marketed drug product and its clinical exposure.

Pharmaceutical stability testing (from ICH QA1(R2) guideline) of the drug product should be conducted for a minimum of 12 months at the time of submission on at least three primary batches of the same formulation and packaged in the same container closure system (including, as appropriate, any secondary packaging and container label) meeting the same specification as that intended for marketing. The long-term testing should be continued for a period of time sufficient to cover the proposed shelf life. These results assure the glaucoma specialist that what is in the bottle is what is on the label.

The ICH guidelines (from ICH E1A) for clinical exposure for drugs intended for chronic use suggest that at least 1,500 patients be exposed, with 300–600 patients exposed for 6 months or more, and 100–200 patients exposed for 1 year or more. This was consistent with FDA's past recommendations for having at least 300 patients in adequate and well-controlled clinical studies for at least 3 months and 100 patients followed for at least a year that the new IOP-lowering drugs have met as a minimum.

The preceding brief foray into regulatory history and guidelines may serve as an explanation for the following: Discovering and developing new drugs is expensive! The research-based (i.e., not the generic) pharmaceutical and biotechnology industry invested $65.2 billion in research and development in 2008 (which was more than double the entire National Institutes of Health's budget for FY2008/9). More specifically, the National Eye Institute (NEI) 2008 budget of $667 million is less than that invested by pharmaceutical companies in ophthalmic research and development (R&D). While it is not possible to determine from publicly available documents what each of the companies spends solely on ophthalmic R&D, Alcon Laboratories, Inc., which describes itself as the world's largest eye care company, invested a total of $619 million in R&D in 2008.

## 86.1 The Drug Discovery and Development Process: An Overview

### 86.1.1 Pre-clinical Testing

Laboratory (in vitro) and animal (in situ or in vivo) studies are conducted to show the pharmacological activity (efficacy) of the compound against the targeted disease and to determine the compound's toxicological activity (safety). See Stages I–III of Fig. 86.1.

### 86.1.2 Investigational New Drug Application

After completing sufficient preclinical testing, a company files an IND (known in Europe as the CTA (Clinical Trial Application) and in Japan as the CTN (Clinical Trial Notification)) with the FDA to begin to test the drug in humans. In the US, the IND becomes effective if FDA does not place a clinical hold on it within 30 days after submission. The IND is actually an "exemption" to the law that requires any drug shipped across a state border to have an approved NDA.

The IND usually includes: (1) the results of previous experiments; (2) how, where, and by whom the new clinical studies will be conducted, including the final protocol; (3) the chemical structure of the compound; (4) how it is thought to work in the body; (5) any toxic effects found in the animal or previous human studies; and (6) how the compound is manufactured and its quality is assured.

All clinical trials must be reviewed and approved by the Institutional Review Board (IRB) or Independent Ethics Committee (IEC) covering the sites where the trials will be conducted. Progress reports on clinical trials must be submitted at least annually to the FDA and the IRB/IEC. All patients must give their "informed consent" to the risks (and benefits) prior to their participation.

#### 86.1.2.1 Clinical Trials, Phase 1

These tests usually involve about 20–80 normal, healthy volunteers. The tests usually involve exaggerated doses in order to study a drug's safety profile and the safe dosage range, although microdosing is becoming popular. The studies also determine how a drug is absorbed, distributed, metabolized, and excreted (ADME) as well as the duration of its action. See Stage IV of Fig. 86.1.

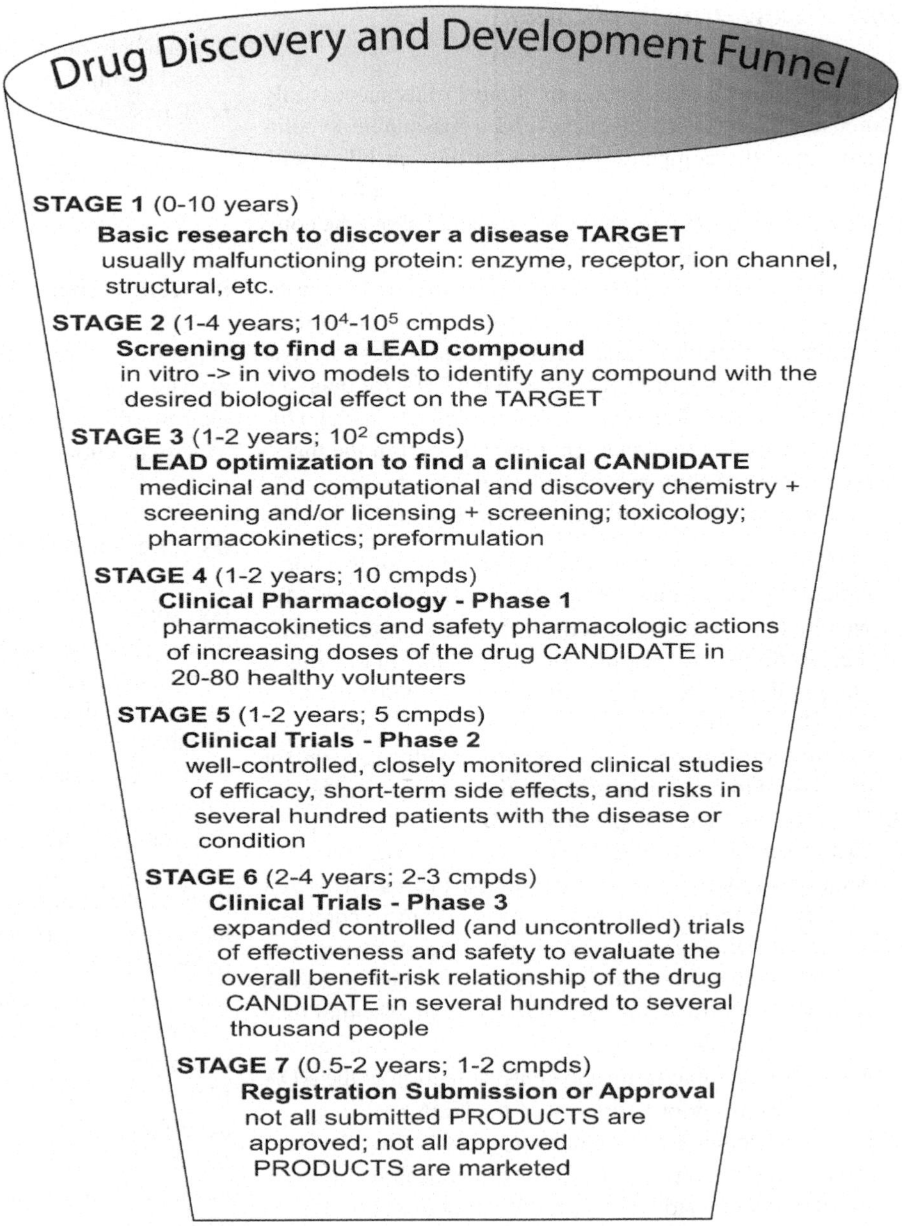

**Fig. 86.1** The stages of drug discovery and development

**Drug Discovery and Development Funnel**

**STAGE 1** (0-10 years)
**Basic research to discover a disease TARGET**
usually malfunctioning protein: enzyme, receptor, ion channel, structural, etc.

**STAGE 2** (1-4 years; $10^4$-$10^5$ cmpds)
**Screening to find a LEAD compound**
in vitro -> in vivo models to identify any compound with the desired biological effect on the TARGET

**STAGE 3** (1-2 years; $10^2$ cmpds)
**LEAD optimization to find a clinical CANDIDATE**
medicinal and computational and discovery chemistry + screening and/or licensing + screening; toxicology; pharmacokinetics; preformulation

**STAGE 4** (1-2 years; 10 cmpds)
**Clinical Pharmacology - Phase 1**
pharmacokinetics and safety pharmacologic actions of increasing doses of the drug CANDIDATE in 20-80 healthy volunteers

**STAGE 5** (1-2 years; 5 cmpds)
**Clinical Trials - Phase 2**
well-controlled, closely monitored clinical studies of efficacy, short-term side effects, and risks in several hundred patients with the disease or condition

**STAGE 6** (2-4 years; 2-3 cmpds)
**Clinical Trials - Phase 3**
expanded controlled (and uncontrolled) trials of effectiveness and safety to evaluate the overall benefit-risk relationship of the drug CANDIDATE in several hundred to several thousand people

**STAGE 7** (0.5-2 years; 1-2 cmpds)
**Registration Submission or Approval**
not all submitted PRODUCTS are approved; not all approved PRODUCTS are marketed

### 86.1.2.2 Clinical Trials, Phase 2

These are controlled trials of approximately 100–300 volunteer patients (people with the disease) to assess a drug's safety and effectiveness. They provide the basis for the posology (amount and frequency of administration) of the drug during the Phase 3 trials. In addition, Phase 2 may include clinical mechanism of action studies. See Stage V of Fig. 86.1.

### 86.1.2.3 Clinical Trials, Phase 3

A total of approximately 500–3,000 volunteer patients in clinics and hospitals closely monitored in placebo or active controlled clinical trials to establish efficacy and identify adverse events (AEs). These studies are used to create dosage statements for each indication. See Stage VI of Fig. 86.1.

### 86.1.3 New Drug Application

If the data from all three phases of clinical trials successfully demonstrate safety, effectiveness, and a reasonable benefit-to-risk ratio, the company (or sponsor) files an NDA with FDA. The NDA contains all of the scientific information (both + and −) that the company has gathered about the compound. See Stage VII of Fig. 86.1.

NDAs typically run 100,000 pages or more and the average review time for new molecular entities, while down from the previous multiple years, remains at more than a year. Though medical practitioners criticize the FDA for delaying the approval of new drugs, some consumer groups demand the recall of drugs that may play an important part in the therapeutic regimen of appropriately selected patients.

In response to these conflicting demands:

1. FDA initiated new "treatment" IND regulations that allow patients with serious or life-threatening diseases, for which there is no satisfactory alternative treatment to receive drugs for therapy prior to general marketing if there is limited evidence of drug efficacy without unreasonable toxicity.
2. FDA established a priority system to expedite reviews for drugs used to treat serious or life-threatening diseases.
3. Congress enacted the previously discussed Prescription Drug User Fee Act (PDUFA) to help fund hiring the FDA personnel required to speed the review process. This Act also sets performance standards for the FDA to complete reviews in a timely manner (6 months for a priority review and 10 months for a standard review) and also obligates companies not to submit an NDA until all essential data are complete. The act does allow a sponsor to submit the chemistry manufacturing and controls section of the NDA up to 120 days prior to the rest of the NDA.
4. FDA has become involved more actively in drug development to facilitate the approval of drugs designed to treat life-threatening and severely debilitating diseases. By the interactive design of well-planned, focused clinical studies using validated surrogate markers or clinical endpoints other than survival or irreversible morbidity, sufficient data are then available earlier in the development process to allow a risk-benefit analysis and a possible decision for approval. In rare cases, this system has reduced or obviated the need for Phase 3 testing prior to approval. Fast Track status can be designated for new drugs intended to treat a serious or life-threatening condition, and if there is an unmet medical need. Fast Track status allows for more frequent meetings with FDA, submission of a "rolling NDA" wherein individual sections of the NDA can be submitted when they are completed.
5. Coupled with this expedited development process is the requirement, when appropriate, for restricted distribution to certain specialists or facilities and for postmarketing studies to answer the remaining issues of risks, benefits, and optimal uses of the drug.
6. If postmarketing studies are inadequate or demonstrate lack of safety or clinical benefit, approval for the new drug may be withdrawn.

#### 86.1.3.1 Approval

Once FDA approves an NDA, the new medicine becomes available for physicians to prescribe. The company must continue to submit periodic reports to FDA, including any cases of adverse reactions and appropriate quality-control records.

#### 86.1.3.2 Clinical Trials, Phase 4

For some medicines, FDA may require additional trials (Phase 4) as postapproval commitments to evaluate long-term safety and efficacy.

Before a drug can be marketed, a package insert for use by physicians must be prepared. The insert usually contains basic pharmacological information, as well as essential clinical information in regard to approved indications, contraindications, precautions, warnings, adverse reactions, usual dosage, and available preparations. Promotional materials used by the company cannot deviate from information contained in the insert; however, dissemination of peer-reviewed published information may be allowed if it is requested by the receiving physician.

Since the FDA only regulates interstate commerce, a seemingly contradictory situation can occur because the FDA does not regulate the practice of medicine. Thus, once the efficacy of a new agent has been proven in the context of acceptable toxicity for a well-defined use, the drug can be marketed. The physician is then allowed to determine its most appropriate use regardless of whether or not the drug was ever intended (or even studied!) for such a use.

## 86.2 Discovery

Paul Ehrlich, credited with initiating the concept of the "magic bullet," is said to have stated that all who are about to embark on developing a new drug must bring to the task four essentials: brains, persistence (balanced between "stick-to-itivity" and perseveration), capital (the $1.25 billion, on average, required to research and develop a new chemical entity (NCE); although, so far, new IOP-lowering drugs have cost less than a quarter of that), and luck (combining serendipity and outright good fortune).

## 86.2.1 Disease Target Discovery

In current pharmaceutical idiom, "Research" and "Discovery" are interchangeable. Disease Target discovery is basic disease research utilizing all available tools (genomics, proteomics, molecular biology, cell biology, biochemistry, pharmacology, etc.) to find an association between the Target, which is usually a malfunctioning subcellular or extracellular component (enzyme, receptor, ion channel, structural, etc.), and a clinical sign of a disease. This is the opening at the top of the Drug Discovery & Development Funnel (see Stage I of Fig. 86.1.) and is at the start of the Drug Discovery and Development Cycle (see Fig. 86.2).

The Target is studied by screening compounds that either inhibit or stimulate the component as it carries out its normal cellular function. This inhibition/stimulation of the Target is then extrapolated to humans in the sense of assuming – or hoping – that the chemical would affect some similar human system. An important point is that until there is a compound that shows clinical efficacy in humans, the Target is not really "validated."

Even when the Target is known to be valid, the pathway to identification of the Lead may still be a long one. Maren[1] originally published the activity of the carbonic anhydrase inhibitor (CAI), acetazolamide, in 1954, and Becker[2] demonstrated its oral IOP-lowering efficacy in glaucoma patients the same year. But the first topical CAI, dorzolamide, was not approved until late in 1994 and followed the synthesis and testing of the approximately 750 compounds by Merck and the clinical evaluation of several.[3]

## 86.2.2 Lead Identification

Using subcellular component (enzyme, receptor, etc.) removed from a living system and studied in vitro, the screen is an assay or series of assays that identifies chemicals that either inhibit or stimulate the component as it carries out its normal cellular function (see Stage II of Fig. 86.1.)

The compounds to be screened can either be chemically synthesized or isolated as "natural product." If synthesized, the structure of the Target and molecular modeling are used to "drug design" the compounds. If a compound with activity at the Target already exists, then new compounds can be designed based on the structure-activity results from the previously tested compounds. Alternatively, pharmaceutical companies may have or lease large libraries of compounds to test in a "high throughput screen" to identify a Lead compound, which has some activity on the Target.

Another source of compounds is that from natural products, for example, soil samples from all over the world. There are other sources as well: from the oceans, from plants, from algae, etc. However, natural products are usually complex mixtures of compounds and the challenge is to determine which compound (or combination of compounds) is the active one.

It should be noted that for both synthesized and natural products, the size of the sample screened is usually in the nanogram to milligram range.

In the end, the initial Lead is any compound with the desired biological effect on the Target.

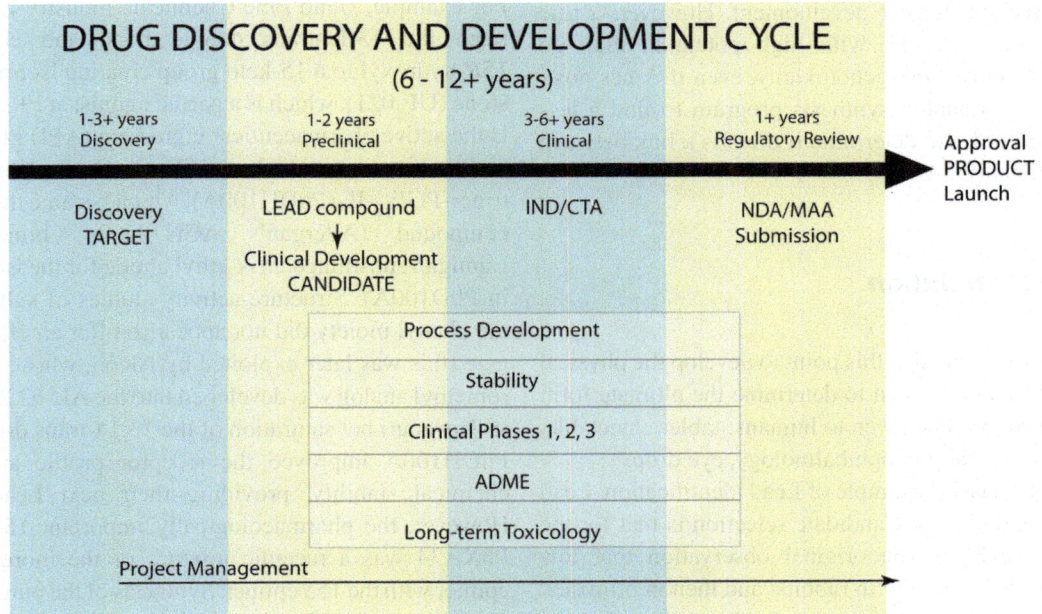

**Fig. 86.2** The drug discovery and development cycle. *ADME* absorbed, distributed, metabolized, and excreted; *IND* Investigational New Drug; *CTA* Clinical Trial Application; *NDA* New Drug Application; *MAA* Marketing "Authorisation" Application

### 86.2.3 Lead Optimization

Since the Lead invariably is not the ideal compound because of some negative characteristic(s) – e.g., solubility, an unfavorable patent position, etc. – more often than not the chemists will start making analogs (chemical modifications) of the Lead and continue to do so until the optimal characteristics are produced. Indeed, in order to create a broad intellectual property (e.g., patents, etc.), the chemists are often called upon to provide unconventional structural analogs with the same biological activity.

Once such issues have been resolved and the Lead is acceptable, it is possible to move on to the next level of profiling in vivo pharmacology.

This entails testing the Lead in animal(s) for efficacy and ADME (absorption, distribution, metabolism, excretion), assuming that there is a clinically validated animal model for the disease under investigation. When the Target is a novel therapeutic approach or an unmet medical need, there is, by definition, no clinically validated animal model. Therein lies the real challenge for preclinical pharmacologists (see Stage III of Fig. 86.1.)

### 86.2.4 Safety Assessment

Preliminary toxicity potential of the Lead is usually assessed by the Ames test to determine the mutagenic potential of the Lead. For most pharmaceutical companies, a positive Ames test or other genetic toxicity predictor is usually of sufficient concern to preclude further development. However, a true breakthrough product, one with high potential, may go through significantly more genotoxicity, even if Ames positive, as well as an analog synthesis program to find a less suspect Lead in order to determine if there is a link between efficacy and toxicity.

### 86.2.5 Preformulation

Studies are often initiated at this point to develop the physical chemical information needed to determine the ultimate form in which the drug will be given to humans: tablet, injectable, patch, or, most typically in ophthalmology, eye drop.

The current "classic" example of Lead identification, Lead optimization, and clinical Candidate selection is that for the prostaglandin analogs. The original observation that low doses of $PGF_{2\alpha}$ lowered IOP in rabbits[4] and then in primates[5] was followed by personal experience that it produced foreign body sensation.[6] Clinically, 200 µg of $PGF_{2\alpha}$ tromethamine salt in 40 µl of sterile water lowered IOP unilaterally in 18 nonglaucomatous normal volunteers (12 females and 6 males) for up to 24 h. It did not produce any change in pupillary diameter or signs of intraocular inflammation visible by anterior segment biomicroscopy or iris fluorescein angiography. However, conjunctival hyperemia was constant and many of the volunteers complained of ocular smarting and headache.[7] This demonstrated that a prostaglandin, in this case $PGF_{2\alpha}$, had the desired IOP-lowering clinical efficacy.

Lead optimization began in 1983 with the involvement of Pharmacia.[8] Initial efforts to improve bioavailability focused on forming esters of the acid moiety of $PGF_{2\alpha}$. The isopropyl ester of $PGF_{2\alpha}$ ($PGF_{2\alpha}$-IE) produced IOP-lowering in normal males with doses as low as 0.5 µg twice daily or 1 µg once daily with 10 µg daily providing 24 h IOP reduction.[9] However, even though the isopropyl ester was several orders of magnitude more potent than $PGF_{2\alpha}$, the maximum IOP-lowering efficacy, duration of action, and, most importantly, side effects of irritation and hyperemia remained essentially the same. The pharmacology of prostanoid receptors was not well defined in the 1980s, and then it was not at all clear that what is now known as the FP prostanoid receptor was responsible for the ocular hypotensive activity of $PGF_{2\alpha}$, its prodrugs, or its analogs. Indeed, much of the confusion may have been because of the higher affinity of $PGF_{2\alpha}$ for the EP3 receptor than for the FP receptor, which was not known at the time.[10,11] That said, under the leadership of Johan Stjernschantz with the collaboration of Lazlo Bito, Pharmacia pushed ahead with preclinical and clinical mechanism of action studies to clarify the exceptional IOP-lowering efficacy of $PGF_{2\alpha}$.[8] A series of modifications of $PGF_{2\alpha}$ were synthesized and screened by Pharmacia and also by their competitors. For example, Ueno Fine Chemicals Industry in Japan saturated the 13,14-trans double bond and converted the 15R-hydroxyl to a 15-keto group creating isopropyl unoprostone (UF-021), which is a partial agonist at FP receptors and is the active pharmaceutical ingredient (API) in Rescula.

Pharmacia persisted and identified 17-phenyl-18,19,20-trinor-$PGF_{2\alpha}$-IE (PhDH100A), which became their next Lead compound (Allergan's AGN192024, bimatoprost, in Lumigan substituted an N-ethyl amide for the isopropyl ester in PhD100A). Structure-activity studies of substitutions on the phenyl moiety did not appear to offer an efficacy advantage (this was later exploited by Alcon, whose meta-trifluoromethyl analog was developed into the AL-6221, travoprost, in Travatan) but saturation of the 13,14-trans double bond of PhDH100A improved the receptor profile and enhanced chemical stability, providing their next Lead, PhXA34. However, the pharmacologically important 15-hydroxyl in PhXA34 was a racemic mixture of the more potent 15R epimer with the 15S epimer. Synthesis of the pure 15R-epimer provided the final Lead, latanoprost, the API in Xalatan.

It is worth noting that each of these Leads became clinical Candidates and that the backup compounds were developed in staggered parallel until the final candidate proved itself. It is also worth noting that Pharmacia and its competitors synthesized more than a thousand compounds in total as they narrowed down the development funnel to their products.

## 86.2.6 Clinical Candidate Selection

If the findings regarding the new compound have been sufficiently favorable so that the decision is to persist, the Lead now becomes a clinical Candidate (a.k.a., Development Candidate or Safety Assessment Candidate). However, in order to reach the market – to pass over the regulatory hurdles summarized previously – a compound has to run a gauntlet of toxicology studies ranging from acute studies lasting for a day to a week up through lifetime carcinogenicity studies (about 24 months) in the mouse and rat. Up to a year before the actual passing into the development stage, some companies create a predevelopment team with members from research, development, and project management. If this team agrees that the Lead is worthwhile pursuing, a preclinical package will be put together for presentation to senior management (see Stage III of Fig. 86.1.)

This package presents:

1. Background of the field and the candidate drug.
2. In vitro assay results with emphasis on biochemical, pharmacological, and physiological assays including activity of drug on human biochemical targets and emphasis on biochemistry and biology results from the same animal species.
3. Whole animal assays results – in vivo or *ex vivo* experiments related to design of projected clinical studies. Blood levels of drug required for activity are presented, as is the bioavailability of the drug in the animals used for tests. The relation of the species used for in vitro and in vivo assays is compared and contrasted.
4. Chemistry – description of synthesis (or isolation) for both preparative and pharmaceutical purposes; also, a description of important related analogs as well as potential back-ups to the Candidate are usually included.
5. Process Chemistry includes the cost and feasibility of the scaled-up process.
6. Pharmaceutical Chemistry describes the stability, physical/chemical characteristics, salt or free acid, stereoisomerism, potential issues for formulation, etc.
7. The Patent and Intellectual Property assessment is a written legal opinion of patentability and freedom to practice.
8. The outline of the Clinical Plan including parallel and nonparallel experimental designs to get to the initial Go/NoGo clinical feasibility decision point.
9. The Regulatory Affairs' commentary on whether the preclinical data might present any unique or substantial regulatory issues that could affect clinical plans. These are linked to the potential problems found in safety, metabolism, formulation, etc. data that may be predictive of issues arising in Development.
10. Competition – these are current and future competitive drugs within this target and other targets in this therapeutic field. This assessment is linked with future research plans to expand upon the projected success of the Candidate or with back-up plans in case the initial development is not successful.
11. Safety results to date, including Ames and Cytochrome P450 induction, mouse lymphoma forward mutation, and mouse micronucleus assay results and interpretation and the acute toxicity studies. And, finally,
12. The Recommendation – a reasoned rationale of why the product candidate should be proposed for development including those potential attributes that could be found in a package insert indicating superiority over the current marketed drugs in the relevant therapeutic area.

## 86.3 Development

Once senior management approves moving forward, the Candidate transitions from Discovery to Development. For conventional systemic pharmaceuticals, a series of studies begin. For example, Chemical Process Development now starts preparing the drug for the initial sub-chronic toxicity studies. These 90-day studies in two species are key to the drug going into humans. Each study takes about 9 months, with about 3 months for the treatment phase, 4 months to prepare and analyze the many histology slides, and about 2 months to write a final report. While the 90-day studies are underway, formulation development will have commenced, as will have metabolism studies. And Clinical Pharmacology will begin to consider how the first studies in humans should be conducted.

For ophthalmic pharmaceuticals, the path is usually somewhat different. With rare exceptions (as noted previously for the topical CAIs and PG analogs), the active pharmaceutical ingredient (API) in all the topical ophthalmic anti-infectives, anti-inflammatories, and antiallergics were initially developed for other systemic indication(s). The same is true for the older generations of IOP-lowering agents. For example, the nonselective beta-adrenoceptor antagonist timolol maleate, in Timoptic 0.5 and 0.25%, came from the Merck Blocadren systemic antihypertensive program (even though Timoptic was launched first in the US). As a result, it is often possible to shorten the timeline for ophthalmic development by referring to the systemic toxicology, safety pharmacology,

ADME, etc. already developed for the Candidate. In addition, the total systemic dose administered from an eyedrop is very small compared with those used systemically. For example, a 33 µl drop of a 1% formulation contains only 330 µg of drug.

Also, the FDA now supports the employment of an Exploratory IND. The exploratory IND focuses on a circumscribed study or group of studies and articulates the rationale for selecting a compound (or compounds) and for studying them in a single trial or related trials, as this represents all that is known about the overall development plan at this stage. Repeat dose clinical studies can be designed with pharmacologic or pharmacodynamic endpoints. In exploratory IND studies, the duration of dosing should be limited (e.g., 7 days). For escalating dose studies done under an exploratory IND, dosing should be designed to investigate a pharmacodynamic endpoint, not to determine the limits of tolerability. Although in each phase of a clinical investigational program sufficient chemistry, manufacturing, and control (CMC) information should be submitted to ensure the proper identification, strength, quality, purity, and potency of the investigational candidate, the amount of information that will provide that assurance will vary with the phase of the investigation, the proposed duration of the investigation, the dosage form, and the amount of information already available. Thus, the CMC section of an Exploratory IND is often less exhaustive than that of a conventional IND. Likewise, the toxicology and safety pharmacology studies are less comprehensive. For clinical trials designed to evaluate higher or repeated doses, each candidate product to be tested should be evaluated for safety pharmacology in the central nervous and respiratory systems, which can be performed as part of the rodent toxicology studies; while safety pharmacology for the cardiovascular system can be assessed in the nonrodent species, generally the dog, and can be conducted as part of the confirmatory or dose-escalation study.

Repeat dose clinical trials lasting up to 7 days can be supported by a 2-week repeat dose toxicology study in a sensitive species accompanied by toxicokinetic evaluations. The goal of such a study would be to select safe starting and maximum doses for the clinical trial. The rat is the usual species chosen for this purpose. The confirmatory study could be a dedicated study involving repeat administrations of a single dose level approximating the rat No-observed-adverse-effect level (NOAEL) calculated on the basis of body surface area. Alternatively, the test in the second species could be incorporated as part of an exploratory, dose-escalating study culminating in repeated doses equivalent to the rat NOAEL. The number of repeat administrations at the rat NOAEL, at a minimum, should be equal to the number of administrations, given with the same schedule, intended clinically. The genetic toxicology tests should include a bacterial mutation assay using all five tester strains with and without metabolic activation as well as a test for chromosomal damage either in vitro (cytogenetics assay or mouse lymphoma thymidine kinase gene mutation assay) or in vivo. The in vivo test can be a micronucleus assay performed in conjunction with the repeated dose toxicity study in the rodent species. The high dose in this case should be a maximally tolerated or limit dose.

The results from the preclinical program can be used to select starting and maximum doses for the clinical trials. The starting dose is anticipated to be no greater than 1/50 of the NOAEL from the 2-week toxicology study in the sensitive species on an mg/m² basis. The maximum clinical dose would be the lowest of the following:

- ¼ of the 2-week rodent NOAEL on a mg/m² basis.
- Up to ½ of the AUC at the NOAEL in the 2-week rodent study, or the AUC in the dog at the rat NOAEL, whichever is lower.
- The dose that produces a pharmacologic and/or pharmacodynamic response, or at which Target modulation is observed in the clinical trial.

### 86.3.1 Observation of an Adverse Clinical Response

Escalation from the proposed maximal clinical dose should only be performed after consultation with and concurrence of the FDA.

Because most IOP-lowering agents have shown efficacy following initial dosing, with rare exception, 7 days of dosing should be sufficient to determine if the drug has IOP-lowering activity. Once efficacy is demonstrated, the full dose–response and duration of action would need to be established once a traditional IND is filed.

It is worth noting that the information for an Exploratory IND is very similar to that usually generated in the preclinical package presented to senior management. Use of the Exploratory IND can thus save the approximately 1 year of time usually spent in 90-day safety assessments, preparation, and submission of the traditional IND/CTA.

### 86.3.2 Clinical Pharmacology (Safety, Dose–Response, Duration of Action, Posology Selection)

By now, a project team has been formed, which consists of representatives of all the various disciplines and divisions throughout the company who will carry the drug through all stages of development to NDA filing, launch, and market support. As mentioned previously, the traditional IND (in Europe, CTA, or in Japan, CTN) provides extensive and detailed information both on the API (in FDA parlance, the drug substance) and on the finished dosage form or formulation to be tested (in FDA parlance "the drug product"). It also provides the pharmacologic rationale as well as sufficient safety (toxicology, pharmacology, ADME) information to support testing in humans. Finally, it provides a detailed summary of all information on the drug (known as the Investigator's Brochure), the qualifications of the investigators who will conduct the clinical trial as well as those who will monitor the investigators, and a detailed step-by-step description of the clinical study and how it is to be conducted (known as the Clinical Protocol) (see Stages IV–V of Fig. 86.1 and the middle of Fig. 86.2).

Because most pharmaceutical companies conduct clinical studies with appropriate investigators at sites around the world, most tend to prepare clinical supplies in at least two locations: one in the United States, one overseas. This is because of US laws limiting shipment of drugs in interstate commerce without an NDA (IND provides an exemption). The FDA also requires that certain documentation requirements, such a informed consent, curricula vitae, signed Form 1572s, financial disclosure, etc. be strictly adhered to under an IND; and many foreign investigators will not agree to these rules.

Up to this point, the developmental process has proceeded in basically a sequential manner. At the time of filing the IND/CTA/CTN (or after initial clinical trials have shown the drug to be tolerated safely at multiples of the expected therapeutic dose), the developmental process branches into five major parallel developmental pathways. These are the chemical process development; formulation development and stability; clinical phase 1, 2, & 3; ADME; and toxicology (see Fig. 86.1.). The actual "network" of pathways is much more complicated and intertwined. Project Management is the function that provides the sequence and interrelationship of the individual studies and experiments (called "work breakdown structures (WBS)") that make up these pathways. Depending on the granularity of management focus, there can be as many as several thousand of these WBS (subpathways).

Once the IND/CTA/CTN is approved (in the US, this is automatically 30 days after submission unless the FDA provides feedback), the first Phase 1 study can begin. Although Phase 1 studies are usually conducted in normal volunteers (there is always the question about how "normal" is a person who volunteers) for whom, by definition, there is no benefit, for IOP-lowering drugs regulatory agencies have allowed relatively healthy patients (e.g., those with ocular hypertension (OHT) or early open-angle glaucoma (OAG)) to be exposed, so that the IOP values will provide useful pharmacodynamic information. As mentioned previously, the Exploratory IND allows for limited duration efficacy to be determined. However, the primary focus of Phase 1 is safety and side effects. In order to evaluate these results in a realistic way, it is necessary to know the safety/side effect profile of the competition. There is no point in developing a drug with an inferior safety profile unless the efficacy/activity of the drug is significantly superior.

Because only one in five drugs (one in ten according to the FDA: page 3 of Guidance for Industry, Investigators, and Reviewers, Exploratory IND Studies, U.S. Department of Health and Human Services Food and Drug Administration, Center for Drug Evaluation and Research (CDER), January 2006, Pharmacology/Toxicology) that begins clinical evaluation successfully completes that evaluation, it is considered good management to have a back-up compound available in order to continue testing the clinical therapeutic hypothesis. Because costs escalate dramatically during the development process (by roughly an order of magnitude at each clinical phase), it is also considered good management to have the back-up (and its back-up) following in a staggered (or echelon) sequence in time so that the project can "fail its way to success." How far the back-up(s) lag behind the Lead or Candidate depends on the resources available, the importance of the project, and the risk tolerance of R&D management.

If the initial Phase 1 results show no unreasonable untoward effects and also some efficacy (if from an Exploratory IND), the work then proceeds to Phase 2. This stage involves dose-ranging in patients to determine the dose–response relationship and the frequency of administration in order to identify the optimal therapeutic benefit. Patients are carefully monitored for all side effects (adverse events (AEs)) in order to gain an initial assessment of the benefit-to-risk ratio. These trials are also generally performed with a placebo as well as a comparator drug known to be active in the targeted disease if such is available. For glaucoma, the current standard for comparison is a prostaglandin analog dosed once daily. Mechanism of action studies are considered to be part of Phase 2. It is important to design the studies in such a way as to obtain information that facilitates decision making.

It should be noted that additional Phase 1 studies will be conducted in parallel with the Phase 2 and 3 studies to determine the clinical ADME profile of the drug and its interactions with other drugs as well as in special patient populations, such as specific age groups, both sexes, patients with renal/hepatic impairment, etc.

The duration and scope of the Phase 2 studies depend upon whether the hypothesized mechanism of action of the drug is similar to a known one or is something unexampled. If the latter, then the Phase 2 program will proceed in a more sequential sequence than if the drug is from a well-known class.

As an aside, combination products usually employ the registered concentrations of the individual APIs and the dosing regimen of the least frequently dosed entity. Considering the formulation compromises usually required, the potential impact of one API on the ocular ADME of the other, and the likely difference in their durations of action, this approach to combination products may explain why none of the

IOP-lowering combination products has been shown to produce efficacy superior to concomitant dosing of the individual products administered at their approved dosing frequency. For example, the IOP-lowering effect of Cosopt b.i.d. was approximately 1 mmHg less than that of concomitant therapy with 2.0% dorzolamide t.i.d. and 0.5% timolol b.i.d. (from the US label approved 10/22/2008) and the IOP-lowering of Combigan b.i.d. was less (approximately 1–2 mmHg) than that seen with the concomitant administration of 0.5% timolol b.i.d. and 0.2% brimonidine tartrate t.i.d. (from the US label dated 2008).

Interestingly, the FDA regulations state, "Two or more drugs may be combined in a single dosage form when each component makes a contribution to the claimed effects and the dosage of each component (amount, frequency, duration) is such that the combination is safe and effective for a significant patient population requiring such concurrent therapy as defined in the labeling for the drug." Contribution to the claimed effects is defined as being a clinically significant effect, which can be based on the efficacy (informally, more than 2 mmHg IOP-lowering superiority of the combination dosed at its proposed regimen compared to each of the individual components dosed at their indicated regimens) or the safety of the combination. Consequently, a number of IOP-lowering combination products available to glaucoma patients outside the US are not approved by the FDA. The prostaglandin analog combinations (Xalacom (latanoprost 0.005% + timolol 0.5%), DuoTrav (travoprost 0.004% + timolol 0.5%), and Ganfort (bimatoprost 0.03% + timolol 0.5%)) have all demonstrated statistically significant IOP-lowering superiority to their individual components of ≥1 mmHg and offer reduced exposure to the preservative, benzalkonium chloride, and enhanced convenience compared with concomitant dosing. The combination of brinzolamide 1% and timolol 0.5% (Azarga) dosed b.i.d. was noninferior to Cosopt b.i.d. across all time points at all visits for 1 year; demonstrated IOP-lowering of 7–9 mmHg that was statistically superior to both brinzolamide 1% b.i.d. (note, US labeling is t.i.d.) and timolol 0.5% b.i.d. at all time points and visits throughout a separate 6-month study; and, in three controlled clinical trials, produced significantly lower ocular discomfort upon instillation than Cosopt (EMEA Summary of Product Characteristics 10/2008). Since a number of trials have shown at least a 10% decrease in glaucoma progression per 1 mmHg IOP-lowering,[12-14] the impact over time that the absence of these IOP-lowering combination products has on the US glaucoma population is a subject for contemplation that is beyond the scope of this chapter.

In parallel with Phase 2 and 3 clinical studies, activities in the Process Development area include: making bulk compound(s) to produce the supplies needed to carry out the developmental work; process evolution and improvement to solve long-term economic and proprietary considerations regarding the manufacture of the compound and the final formulation; generation of the CMC (Chemistry, Manufacturing, and Control) section for registration; and transfer of technology and experience to manufacturing. The description of the validated process that reliably produces the compound is called the Drug Master File (DMF).

Since the initial formulation selected for Phase 1 is rarely the final marketed formulation, dosage form development normally progresses from preformulation to formulation through preliminary stability. This stage can involve a number of decision loops until a formulation demonstrating acceptable stability, bioavailability, and tolerability is developed. When such a formulation is in hand, package selection and the formal stability study can commence. These must be manufactured using "current" Good Manufacturing Procedures (cGMP). Throughout this process, supplies must be manufactured and packaged (also to cGMP standards) for clinical and other studies. To simulate manufacturing conditions, increasingly larger batches are produced. Toward the end of this phase, technology must be transferred to the selected manufacturing site(s) that will be used once the drug is approved for marketing.

Also conducted in an echeloned or staggered parallel fashion with the clinical evaluation are the toxicological studies, with animal exposure always leading human exposure by several months and, usually, at a substantial multiple of the human dose. These studies include:

1. Acute Studies – single or short-term multiple dosing via different routes of administration;
2. Range Finding Studies to determine doses for subacute and chronic studies;
3. Subacute Studies – 28 days and 3 months;
4. Genetic Toxicity – in vitro gene mutation in bacteria and mammalian cells (with and without activation), in vitro chromosomal aberrations in mammalian cells, and an in vivo assay for chromosome damage in rodent bone marrow (usually, mouse micronucleus assay);
5. Segment I Reproductive Toxicity – fertility and reproductive function in male and female;
6. Segment II Reproductive Toxicity – developmental toxicology and teratology;
7. Segment III Reproductive Toxicity – perinatal and postnatal toxicity, three generation back crosses;
8. Chronic Toxicity – 6 months, 1 year;
9. Carcinogenicity Studies (lifetime feeding – usually 2-year dosing) in two species; and
10. Special Target Organ Studies for known classes or specific dosing routes. See Fig. 86.2.

Because of the extensive resources required to conduct all these studies under the Good Laboratory Practices (GLP) regulations, many companies contract out all or part of them to contract research organizations (CROs). However, the sponsoring company remains responsible for the quality of all the data.

### 86.3.3 Clinical Trial Initiation

The FDA IND guidelines strongly encourage sponsors to meet with the FDA at the completion of Phase 2 to review safety and the adequacy of the study design for the Phase 3 program. While the sponsor usually takes advantage of the end of Phase 2 meeting, it should be noted that additional requirements may be added to the sponsor's development plan at that meeting, thereby possibly generating other decision points (see Stages V–VI of Fig. 86.1).

The end of the main Phase 2 clinical studies marks a decision point that can be characterized as the most critical in the drug development process. For most companies, this milestone brings together all available data for a decision to proceed or not to proceed – to persist or not persist – with the project. The Critical Factors that should be reviewed at this time are:

1. Does the drug present an adequate safety profile
2. Has a dose/regimen been identified that demonstrates a reasonable therapeutic benefit
3. Importance of the drug to the medical armamentarium
4. The proposed indications – those desired by marketing versus what realistically appears to be achievable
5. The market potential, including dollar size and growth, competition and estimated market share
6. Scientific criteria and published manuscripts required
7. Results of end of Phase 2 conference with FDA
8. Updated clinical objectives
9. Required manufacturing investment and feasibility
10. Estimate of dosage range and cost of goods of final dosage form
11. Recommended primary packages
12. Estimated time and cost of completion
13. Priority ranking in relation to other projects

Assuming that the review of the Critical Factors is positive, then it is possible to move to the next activities, which revolve around and stem from the major clinical trial program known as Phase 3. Phase 3 consists of several "well controlled" and uncontrolled trials conducted to determine additional safety and efficacy data to establish a benefit-to-risk assessment and a basis for labeling. This phase may incorporate from several hundred to several thousand subjects. There are many interrelated activities and decisions that must take place while conducting each of these trials. They are summarized as follows: (1) protocol definition, (2) prepare financial agreement(s), (3) generate randomization scheme, (4) investigator approvals, (5) IRB approvals (company and site institutions), (6) order and obtain drug, (7) prepare drug and code for centers, (8) design and print case report forms (CRFs) and other forms, (9) obtain each investigator's and sub-investigator's curriculum vitae (CV) and file documentation in IND or IND amendment, (10) initiation visit, (11) patient recruitment and informed consent, (12) obtain lab normal values, (13) monitor trial and acquire data in-house, (14) medical team process data, (15) data with statisticians, (16) statistical analysis, (17) medical report available, (18) investigator approval of report, (19) final reports, and (20) quality assurance of all reports.

Usually, the FDA has interpreted the requirement for adequate and well-controlled studies to mean that at least two Phase 3 trials must be conducted. As mentioned previously, for IOP-lowering drugs, the minimum requirements for an NCE have been exposing 300 patients for 3 months and 100 patients for a year (the latter with endothelial cell counts). A 3-month study with IOP measurements made at the peak and trough times of efficacy throughout the day and on at least three different days that span the length of the efficacy portion of the study appears to be the minimum duration to be considered "adequate" from an efficacy perspective; an additional 3 months often are appended as a safety extension to reach the 6-month exposure time to satisfy European regulators. If a second study is conducted that uses the same times and days as the initial study and then continues on to provide 100 patients on the final formulation for a year, then the results can be combined to meet the minimum totals. However, the requirements for a European Marketing "Authorisation" Application (MAA) may be more extensive; and for a Japanese JNDA, the drug must be studied in Japanese patients. This adds to the complexity of conducting global clinical trials.

However, the clinical trials are just a part of the activities that occur during the Phase 3 Development Program. Figure 86.2 diagrams some of the major activities that occur during this stage. A list of the important components of the Phase 3 program are:

1. Clinical efficacy – the Phase 3 trials provide the major clinical support (the pivotal trials) for the potential therapeutic claim.
2. Clinical safety – since these are the longer-term trials, they provide very important safety data on the compound.
3. Toxicology completion – during the course of Phase 3 trials, several toxicology studies are being completed. These include the 24-month rat and mouse carcinogenicity studies, the 12-month chronic rat study, and the 12-month chronic dog study. Associated with these studies are previously mentioned evaluations of absorption, distribution, metabolism, excretion, and kinetics (ADME).
4. Pharmacology completion – during Phase 3 trials, it is not unusual for additional pharmacological studies to be carried out. These generally fit into the category of generation of data suitable for publication in accordance with a defined publication strategy.
5. Prescribing information – key clinical data that will be incorporated into the package insert emerges from the

Phase 3 program. As Phase 3 progresses, commercial considerations become more heavily involved in the decision-making process, such as Registration/Pricing.

6. Registration/pricing – it is at this time that a worldwide registration strategy (initially developed in late Phase 2) is usually finalized. Decisions must be made in relation to the countries in which the drug will be registered – including which indication for which countries. Pricing, a complex and highly competitive area of consideration, is based upon many interrelated international factors;
7. Sales formulation – during Phase 1 trials a clinical formulation was prepared that could be a modification of the dosage form used in toxicology studies. Later in the course of the Phase 1 studies and on into Phase 2, efforts were directed at formulating and developing the commercial (sales) dosage form. Usually during Phase 3, the final stability studies on the sales dosage form manufactured by cGMP are undertaken at the site(s) intended for commercial manufacture.
8. Manufacture – when the final decision has been made on the sales dosage form, the next step is large-scale production of the drug.
9. Marketing plan – by this time there are an increasing number of commercial issues to take into consideration, the most important of which is the marketing plan. This plan must be reviewed in light of changes that may have taken place during the development process. For example, the competition may have introduced a compound of the same type during the clinical trials, thereby changing the marketing forecast. Or, a newer therapeutic approach may have been introduced that could have a bearing on the marketing decision. During this period, it is also time to rethink the whole commercial lifetime of the drug in light of a host of external considerations.

In what may seem to be ancient history, the development of dipivefrin 0.1% (Propine) occurred in parallel with that of Timoptic but, for a variety of reasons, its approval in May 1980 came nearly 2 years after the approval of Timoptic in August 1978. As their respective labels indicate, the clinical results were clear: "Therapeutic response to Propine ophthalmic solution twice daily is somewhat less than 2% epinephrine twice daily" while "Timoptic 0.25 or 0.5% administered twice a day produced a greater reduction in intraocular pressure than ... 2% epinephrine hydrochloride solution administered twice a day."

Propine is an optimized prodrug of epinephrine, which was a staple of IOP-lowering therapy at the time; however, with a pH around 4.5, it is uncomfortable. While its label still states, "The precise mechanism of the ocular hypotensive action of Timoptic is not clearly established at this time," it is an exceptionally comfortable formulation. Timoptic went on to become the first $100 million dollar drug in ophthalmology and has remained as a mainstay of IOP-lowering therapy globally into the twenty-first century. For Propine, the marketing environment had changed completely and the results speak for themselves.

10. Market support – such trials would provide data for new indications or indication amplification, as well as suggesting the potential for future development of the new compound. Health Economic/Formulary Justification/CMS Reimbursement studies need to have been incorporated in the Phase 3 development plan.

## 86.4 Registration

Assuming that the Phase 3 program has successfully demonstrated not only the safety and efficacy of the drug but also sufficient superiority to current or likely future competitive products, a whole series of decisions now revolve around the filing of New Drug Applications. In the US, this is the NDA (for biologicals, it is the Biological License Application or BLA). In other countries, it is generally referred to as the Marketing "Authorisation" Application (MAA); and in Japan, it is the JNDA (see Stage VII. of Fig. 86.1 and the right side of Fig. 86.2.)

As mentioned previously, the ICH guidelines apply to the format (but not the content) of the Common Technical Document (CTD), which allows companies to write the modules of documents once (sort of) rather than multiple times and provides harmonized presentation of the core technical information. This allows for "top-down" review by Japan and EU and "bottom-up" review by the FDA. These submissions are large. For new systemic drugs, it is not unusual to submit 300 volumes consisting of more than 100,000 pages. New ophthalmic applications are usually a little smaller.

It is a key and critical issue to conduct the Drug Development Process such that the worldwide filing is done as nearly as possible simultaneously so as to maximize the benefit from the intellectual property and the marketing synergy from the presentations of the data on the product at international scientific and medical conferences. In practice, the JNDA usually trails by more than a year.

The FDA suggests that sponsors conduct a Pre-NDA meeting at least 6 months prior to filing the NDA. In the EU, the sponsor must commit to a specific date for the MAA submission. The actual filing is followed by a "fileability" decision from FDA, which means that the FDA and other regulatory agencies have determined the applications are sufficiently complete to warrant a substantial review. The FDA has up to 60 days to do this; in other countries, this period is variable. In the US, extensive interactions with FDA occur during the NDA review period. Such interactions could include:(1) explanations of any data submitted; (2) request for modification or retabulation of data; (3) inspection/audit by FDA of manufacturing and clinical trial sites; (4) Advisory Committee Reviews (which will include recommendations made to FDA); and (5) labeling negotiations (this is an important decision point since labeling can be accepted or rejected).

In the EU, there is a fixed timeline following official receipt (procedural start, Day 0); review, reply to the sponsor with a consolidated list of questions (Day 120) and, once the sponsor responds to those questions, procedural restart (Day 121); joint assessment report (Day 150); Opinion (Day 180); if positive Opinion, then finalize the Summary of Product Characteristics (SPC), Patient Information Leaflet (PIL) and labeling (Day 181–210 ); adoption of the Committee for Medicinal Products for Human Use (CHMP) opinion and CHMP assessment report (Day 210); SPC, PIL and labeling in all languages (Day 215); draft European Commission (EC) decision (Day 260–290); and finalize the European Public Assessment Report (EPAR) by Day 300. As does the Summary Review from the FDA (see the Approval History, Letters, Reviews, and Related Documents link for a specific product at Drugs@FDA: http://www.accessdata.fda.gov/Scripts/cder/DrugsatFDA/), the EPAR (http://www.emea.europa.eu/htms/human/epar) provides a summary of the grounds for the CHMP opinion in favor of granting a marketing authorization for a specific medicinal product. It results from the committee's review of the documentation submitted by the applicant, and from subsequent discussions held during CHMP meetings. The EPAR is updated throughout the authorization period as changes to the original terms and conditions of the authorization (i.e., variations, pharmacovigilance issues, specific obligations) are made.

After completing the monumental task of NDA/MAA preparation(s), a new series of commercially oriented activities begin in preparation for launch and marketing of the Product. These plans must take into account such factors as: (1) the market, (2) the competition, (3) the product profile, (4) the market support trials, (5) the potential for future development, (6) the target audience, (7) promotional methods, (8) promotional costs, (9) trademark, (10) pricing, (11) new formulations, and (12) forecast. A number of process development problems must now be resolved, including purchase of the tooling needed for the filling machines, the punches for tablets; and the bulk drug substance (active pharmaceutical ingredient) required. Long before the NDA/MAA is filed, package development must consider: (1) types of packages, (2) specifications for package, (3) labels (and glue), (4) stability in package, (5) artwork, (6) samples, and (7) the package insert. Items 1–4 must be addressed before Phase 3. Quality Assurance (QA) issues are also very important, and they include such factors as: (1) assay validation, (2) release for bulk drug to be used, (3) release of raw materials, (4) release of samples, (5) release of commercial product for distribution, and (6) any other quality control issues. All the engineering, purchasing, and documentation aspects of a product must be carefully considered so that production will proceed smoothly. Significant issues to be addressed at this point may include: (1) buildings, (2) tooling, (3) parts, (4) package components, (5) blenders and filling machines, (6) bulk drug (API), (7) campaign plans, (8) sample packages, (9) packages, and (10) shipping. It is also important to establish projections on such practical matters as bulk drug substance (API) needs for worldwide sale as well as drug Product needs (in millions) over the forecast period. This also entails making an assessment of current available capacity, capital requirements for stocks, plant costs and operating margins.

Once the Product is approved, the process of obtaining federal, state, or managed care formulary approval (in the US) and price and reimbursement approval (in Europe) begins. During this stage, those pharmacoeconomic aspects of the product that differentiate it from its therapeutic competitors are highlighted to the various health care companies and agencies (in the US, the Centers for Medicare & Medicaid Services (CMS) is the federal agency responsible for administering the Medicare, Medicaid, SCHIP (State Children's Health Insurance), etc.) in order to make the best case for inclusion in their lists of reimbursed products. The data to support this differentiation must have been collected during Phase 3 (or earlier), and, therefore, the pharmacoeconomic/health economic plan must be integrated into the overall development plan at an early stage. The construction of the price in those countries where it is established by governmental agencies is a delicate process, and transfer prices used for customs purposes when samples are shipped internationally during development can have disastrous commercial consequences for the price assigned to the product.

## 86.5 Marketing/Product Launch

The drug is now ready for public announcement. This is usually a major advertising and public relations effort designed to launch the product into the marketplace with maximum thrust and exposure. This is also regulated by the FDA and requires prior approval before use.

Invariably, once a product is approved, Marketing wants more, better, or at least different claims for it. This is why Fig. 86.2 is titled the "Drug Discovery & Development Cycle." In the US, any claim for a new indication or indications requires a new supplemental NDA that entails a longer review process. An example for a systemic medication would be a claim that a product not only is effective for the approved indication, for example hypertension, but can also serve as an antiangina agent. Each additional claim would require its own clinical development plan. For this reason, few products in the glaucoma specialists' armamentarium have received additional indications.

### 86.5.1 Phase 4 Program and Postmarketing Surveillance

Phase 4 was previously market oriented since, periodically, new marketing facts or studies would be needed for continued growth and to attain a competitive edge. This phase was designed to expand upon an already approved claim. However, new regulatory concerns have acted to combine Phase 4 with Postmarketing Surveillance of safety. Phase 4 is conducted under the original IND but may be mandated by the approving regulatory agency(ies). Currently, Phase 4 and Postmarketing Surveillance involve tracking adverse drug experiences, and have become an increasingly important and complex feature of drug development.

Adverse drug experience reporting falls into three categories: regulatory, promotional (to introduce physicians to the Product), and independent (involving university/research institutions). There is also IND/NDA reporting of adverse experiences occurring during ongoing clinical trials for products with approved NDAs. After a drug has received FDA approval for marketing, clinical trials are usually still being conducted under the IND for both new and approved indications; there is also the international requirement for safety reporting for each marketed product on a yearly basis. The timing of these reports is in the process of being standardized internationally as is the dictionary used to describe the medical nature of the events.

## 86.6 Conclusion

What has been described so far speaks to a multidisciplinary, complicated process that entails the interaction and demands the cooperation of many people with different expertise and perspectives. Many things must occur at the same time (or in a specific order) and be brought to completion to make smooth progress possible. Managing this kind of procedure is difficult, and success is dependent on correct decision making at each step. Most companies use a project team approach, which, under a project leader or manager with assistance from a centralized project management group, plans, executes, and monitors every step of the drug development process. See Fig. 86.2 for an overview of the activities and timelines.

How is this accomplished? This approach must be based on an overall or master research and development project operational plan that facilitates the development process. This is one of the key concepts in any R&D organization. The master project operational plan itself may be defined as a living document that takes the strategy from the Strategic Plan and implements it to develop the compounds that flow from the Disease Target Discovery Programs and that are identified by the Program Review as Leads and, eventually, Development Candidates. Ideally, this project plan is composed of three parts and is prepared at various stages in the development of a compound.

The first part of the research and development master project plan covers the development from the beginning of the research project through early Phase 1 clinical studies. This stage of the master operational plan includes the process for selecting or nominating a compound for project status, and a brief outline of planned preclinical, toxicological and clinical studies. Although perhaps obvious, a knowledgeable individual who can summarize the strategy and intended activities to be accomplished, and then obtain written approval from the appropriate management elements should prepare this document.

The second stage covers the period from IND/CTA filing to the end of Phase 2. This must be a more detailed plan aimed at determining whether or not the compound is likely to become a drug Product. The areas covered include toxicology, metabolism, preliminary registration plans for countries other than the United States, and a clinical plan to confirm indications, side effects, and competitive advantages. This part of the plan also covers: formulations to be developed, supply sourcing and scale-up considerations, what the projected product profile will be, and the target dates for the end of Phase 2 meetings.

This third and final stage (from mid Phase 2 to Registration Filings) covers the draft of the intended package insert, manufacturing locations, and such matters as dosage forms, indications, pivotal studies, control and manufacturing section issues, registration plans, required clinical studies by country, specialized studies, comparative studies, and the expert opinions that will be required.

That said, within the past few years, Design Control of the Product Development Process is beginning to be instituted for pharmaceutical products. Brought to drugs from medical devices, Design Control provides a documented sequence of events that control the Planning (establishing project documents), Verification (preclinical testing and review), Validation (clinical studies and review), Launch (regulatory submission and approval), and Post Production (product surveillance and change control) of the product. Employing an entirely different language from conventional pharmaceutical development, it is an approach that is likely to change the way of life in the pharmaceutical industry in the next few years.

The preceding has been a "classic comic" version of the Drug Discovery & Development process. For greater detail, the reader is referred to Bert Spilker's *Multinational Pharmaceutical Companies: Principles and Practices*, 2nd Ed.[15]; or, for lighter and more up to date views, Rick Ng's *Drugs from Discovery to Approval*[16] or John Campbell's *Understanding Pharma – a primer on how pharmaceutical companies really work*.[17]

# References

1. Maren TH, Mayer E, Wadsworth BC. Carbonic anhydrase inhibition. I. The pharmacology of Diamox, 2-acetylamino-1,3,4,-thiadizole 5-sulfonamide. *Bull Johns Hopkins Hosp*. 1954;95:199–243.
2. Becker B. Diamox and the therapy of glaucoma. *Am J Ophthalmol*. 1954;38:16-17.
3. Ponticello GS, Sugrue MF, Plazonnet B, et al. Dorzolamide, a 40-year wait: from an oral to a topical carbonic anhydrase inhibitor for the treatment of glaucoma. In: Borchardt RT, Freidinger RM, Sawyer TK, Smith PL, eds. *Integration of Pharmaceutical Discovery and Development*. New York, NY: Plenum; 1998:555–574.
4. Camras CB, Bito LZ, Eakins KE. Reduction of intraocular pressure by prostaglandins applied topically to the rabbit eye. *Invest Ophthalmol Vis Sci*. 1977;16:1125–1134.
5. Camras CB, Bito LZ. Reduction of intraocular pressure in normal and glaucomatous primate (Aotus trivirgatus) eyes by topically applied PGF2a. *Curr Eye Res*. 1981;1:205–209.
6. Bito LZ. A new approach to the medical management of glaucoma, from the bench to the clinic and beyond. *Invest Ophthalmol Vis Sci*. 2001;42:1126–1133.
7. Giuffrè G. The effects of prostaglandin F2a in the human eye. *Graefes Arch Clin Exp Ophthalmol*. 1985;222:139–141.
8. Stjernschantz JW. From $PGF_{2a}$-isopropyl-ester to latanoprost: a review of the development of Xalatan. *Invest Ophthalmol Vis Sci*. 2001;42:1134–1145.
9. Villumsen J, Alm A, Söderström M. Prostaglandin F2 alpha-isopropylester eye drops: effect on intraocular pressure in open-angle glaucoma. *Br J Ophthalmol*. 1989;73(12):975–979.
10. Hellberg MR, Sallee VL, McLaughlin MA, et al. Preclinical efficacy of travoprost, a potent and selective FP prostaglandin receptor agonist. *J Ocul Pharmacol Ther*. 2001;17:421–432.
11. Hellberg MR, McLaughlin MA, Sharif NA, et al. Identification and characterization of the ocular hypotensive efficacy of travoprost, a potent and selective FP prostaglandin receptor agonist, and AL-6598, a DP prostaglandin receptor agonist. *Surv Ophthalmol*. 2002;47(Suppl 1):S13–S33.
12. Gordon MO, Beiser JA, Brandt JD, et al. The Ocular Hypertension Treatment Study: baseline factors that predict the onset of primary open-angle glaucoma. *Arch Ophthalmol*. 2002;120:714–720.
13. Leske MC, Heijl A, Hussein M, et al. Factors for glaucoma progression and the effect of treatment: the Early Manifest Glaucoma Trial. *Arch Ophthalmol*. 2003;121:48–56.
14. Chauhan BC, Mikelberg FS, Balaszi AG. Canadian Glaucoma Study 2. Risk factors for the progression of open-angle glaucoma. *Arch Ophthalmol*. 2008;126(8):1030–1036.
15. Spilker B. *Multinational Pharmaceutical Companies: Principles and Practices*. 2nd ed. New York, NY: Raven; 1994.
16. Ng R. *Drugs from Discovery to Approval*. Hoboken, NJ: John; 2004.
17. Campbell JJ. *Understanding Pharma – A Primer on How Pharmaceutical Companies Really Work*. Raleigh, NC: Pharmaceutical Institute; 2005.

# Chapter 87
# Glaucoma Clinical Research in the Community Setting

Harvey DuBiner, Helen DuBiner, and Paul N. Schacknow

While medical scientists at both universities and pharmaceutical companies may discover and develop suitable drug candidates to treat glaucoma, the US Federal Drug Administration (FDA) requires that such medications be tested on human patients during structured clinical trials before the drugs may be "approved" and prescribed by physicians. The clinical research that leads to the approval of the medications we use daily to treat our glaucoma patients takes place not only in industry-sponsored laboratories but also in academic centers and community-based office practices. Indeed, community-based ophthalmology practices provide a large proportion of the patients who enroll in clinical trials, especially at later stages of development. This chapter will describe how such clinical trials are incorporated into a busy ophthalmology practice in the United States. Here, we will limit our discussion to medical glaucoma research trials. The approval process is structured differently for research into surgical devices such as glaucoma shunts.

## 87.1 Clinical Research Trials

Clinical research trials are conducted in several "phases." At each stage of the process, different types of information are desired and obtained. The pharmaceutical company sponsoring the research files an Investigational New Drug application and conducts laboratory experiments in vitro, as well as in vivo in suitable animal models, with the drug candidate they have developed to treat the disease process. For example, they may have developed a new prostaglandin analogue that reduces intraocular pressure, is dosed one drop per day, and appears to have few local side effects. After successful preliminary pilot studies and filing a New Drug Application with the FDA, the company is ready to begin formal human trials with the new compound.

In Phase I trials, the goal is to test a new drug in a small group (10–50) of healthy individuals, with the goals of determining safety, tolerability, a range of feasible doses/concentrations, and to look for serious adverse and minor side effects. Sometimes, these trials are performed in an in-patient setting. These trials usually are not performed in a community-based eye practice. Occasionally, placebo treatments are used in Phase I studies.

In Phase II trials, the drug is now tried on more subjects, say 100–300, with efficacy and safety as primary goals. Dosing, concentration, and side effects are evaluated. Many physiological and ocular parameters are monitored with an eye toward patient safety. The subjects may or may not have the disease condition being studied. Given the intensity of the entire ancillary (safety) testing requirements, only community-based practices with extensive experience in drug trials are offered such studies by industry sponsors. Comparisons between test drug, related drugs, and placebos may be undertaken.

In Phase III trials, the new medication is tested on large groups of subjects; 1,000–3,000 subjects are used, often in two or more separate studies. Generally, the research is performed as randomized, double-masked, multicenter clinical trials on subjects with glaucoma or ocular hypertension as stipulated by the protocol. The duration of the studies is several weeks to more than 1 year. Here, the FDA is interested in confirming that the drug reaches the stated therapeutic goal (e.g., significant intraocular pressure reduction), often comparing efficacy to an existing approved medication (e.g., the new drug compared to timolol). Adverse events are carefully monitored in the large number of subjects who participate in the study. For this phase, participants are almost always subjects who have the disease under study (e.g., glaucoma) and in whom it is determined to be safe to stop their current treatments (wash out period), and likely to be safe on the experimental treatment for the duration of the study. In glaucoma Phase III medication studies, few, if any, subjects are enrolled with placebo treatments as controls. The new drug is usually compared for efficacy against an existing medication as opposed to vehicle (placebo). These Phase III trials are combined into one large regulatory submission and are often termed the "registration trials" that, if successful, lead to the premarket approval of the drug by the FDA.

In Phase IV trials, postmarketing studies are designed to provide additional clinical information about the drug once it has been in use in the "real world." These studies yield new data about the drug's side effects, possible dosing changes, advantages, and compliance. Although Phase IV trials provide much useful data to the physician, sometimes they are designed by marketing departments of pharmaceutical companies, which seek to demonstrate some competitive advantage of their drug compared to another product designed to have the same therapeutic benefit. While these may be constructed as well-designed, randomized clinical trials, the FDA regulations are much looser with respect to such design issues. Many open label trials, without adequate controls, are performed as Phase IV clinical trials. Nonetheless, the great majority of Phase IV trials provide the practicing clinician with additional information about the drug in real world use, beyond what is contained in the package insert.

Phase II through III studies are highly structured protocols designed by the pharmaceutical company that is sponsoring the drug. Clinicians who become principal investigators in these projects are basically performing contract research, to enhance their practice income, typically with little creative input on their part regarding the experimental design. They do, however, offer feedback to the sponsor based upon their clinical assessments made during the study visits and at completion. In addition, they are participating in cutting-edge science, will become immersed in the latest literature on the topic, and they also will enjoy the intellectual stimulation of interacting with their peers at investigators' meetings. Some of the contracting physicians may be invited to submit articles to peer-reviewed journals describing the outcome of these projects.

Often, Phase IV studies are designed by clinical physicians who propose them to the pharmaceutical company that sells the drug. These studies allow academic and community-based ophthalmologists to explore research ideas of interest to them, some of which may be germinated by their experiences using the approved drug with their patients. Some of these clinician-generated Phase IV studies are small pilot studies, which may lead to large-scale multicenter projects.

## 87.2 Participants

Clinical trials that may lead to drug approval by the FDA are very expensive undertakings. The sponsors are pharmaceutical companies that usually have extensive in-house research departments that identify drug candidates and write the clinical trial protocol. (Occasionally, a larger pharmaceutical firm will buy the rights to a product being developed by a smaller company.) Some pharmaceutical companies contract with clinical research organizations (CROs) to manage the protocols for them because they do not have their own personnel who can make site visits on a regular basis, or they find it is to their economic advantage to use regional monitors. The CROs are independent organizations whose business is the monitoring of clinical trials. The CROs or sponsor monitors make sure that all aspects of the protocol are being followed and that FDA regulations are being observed. The monitor ensures there is proper source documentation, accuracy of case report forms (data collection documents), ethical treatment of human subjects, and the timely reporting of adverse events – both serious and nonserious, both drug-related and non-drug-related.

Clinical trials themselves are conducted at the practices of both academic and community-based ophthalmologists. At each selected site, the principal investigators (PIs) are practicing physicians (MD, DO, OD) who are responsible for all aspects of the research. They must read and understand the *investigator brochure*, the *research protocol*, and all other documents that are part of the clinical trial. In coordination with the sponsor and their own practice's administrators, they agree upon a suitable budget for the trial. This budget should be sufficient to cover practice overhead (staff and material), pay subject participants a stipend for their time, and provide additional funds for the investigators and the practice. Sponsors usually offer reasonable budgets based on the time and resources to be committed and on years of experience conducting clinical trials.

The principal investigators are helped with the day-to-day aspects of the project by an in-house clinical research coordinator (CRC), or study coordinator (SC). The study coordinator may be a PhD member of a university faculty or in the community setting is more likely to be a certified ophthalmic technician, registered nurse, or pharmacist with considerable experience in conducting human clinical drug trials. In many ways, the SC is the most important member of the research team, even more so than the principal investigators. Without an excellently trained, highly conscientious SC, it is impossible for a practice to coordinate all aspects of a clinical trial; the principal investigator cannot do it alone. The SC is the "go to" person for all aspects of the clinical trial. The SC may be accredited after suitable training and examinations by the Association of Clinical Research Professionals (ACRP) (www.acrpnet.org). The ACRP provides extensive educational opportunities for study coordinators. The SC schedules patients and may participate in aspects of the clinical examination during each study visit by the patient. The study coordinator helps maintain the integrity of the clinical records and protocol-related paperwork that may be audited by the sponsor, CRO, or FDA, both during and after the research trial.

The research protocol proposed by the sponsor must also be accepted, sometimes with modifications, by an Institutional Review Board (IRB) that functions to guard the human rights of the participants in the study. IRBs have been required for all research involving human participants since passage of the US National Research Act of 1974. Academic centers may have their own IRB. Community-based practices usually submit the clinical trial protocol to a regional, "public" IRB (e.g., Schulman and Associates – www.sairb.com; Western

IRB – www.wirb.com; Quorum IRB – www.quorumreview.com) that may have been selected by the sponsor and is familiar with most aspects of the protocol. Sometimes, the site is asked to select a local IRB that they may choose on their own. Additionally, organizations such as the US Office for Human Research Protections (OHRP) (www.hhs.gov/ohrp/) ensure that drug industry sponsored trials protect "the rights, welfare, and well-being of subjects involved in research" conducted under FDA-approved trials (www.hhs.gov/ohrp/about/ohrpfactsheet.htm – September 2005). Clinical trials should be conducted under generally accepted guidelines called Good Clinical Practices (GCP), required of all FDA sponsored research (www.fda.gov/oc/gcp/default.htm) and set up by the International Conference on Harmonisation of Technical Requirements for Registration of Pharmaceuticals for Human Use (ICH) (www.ich.org) that coordinates the pharmaceutical regulating bodies of the USA, Japan, and Europe.

IRBs are beginning to require proof of training regarding protections for human subjects in clinical research for investigators and study coordinators. In addition to the subject matters in the previous paragraph, some other topics that PIs and SCs should be educated about include:

1. The Health Insurance Portability and Accountability Act of 1996 (HIPAA Privacy Rule). http://www.hipaa.org/
2. The Belmont Report, which is subtitled Ethical Principles and Guidelines for the protection of human subjects of research. http://ohsr.od.nih.gov/guidelines/belmont.html
3. FDA regulations (Title 21 CFR, Title 45 CFR, among others). http://www.access.gpo.gov/nara/cfr/waisidx_99/45cfr100_99.html)

Formal training in conducting clinical research and human subject protection can be obtained at in-person seminars or online. Seminars that offer coordinator training, GCP training, and other topics, such as preparing for an FDA audit, may be offered by such organizations as the ACRP, Barnett International, Research Dynamics, Drug Information Association (DIA), and Public Responsibility in Medicine and Research (PRIM&R). Some online sites that provide courses and information are:

1. Collaborative IRB Training Initiative (CITI) – www.citiprogram.org
2. National Institutes of Health (NIH)
   (a) http://phrp.nihtraining.com/users/login.php
   (b) http://ohrp-ed.od.nih.gov/CBTs/Assurance/login.asp

More can be found viewing the "investigator" tab on IRB Web sites such as Sterling IRB, Schulman Associates IRB, or Western IRB.

The sponsor and the principal investigators at each site must develop a written *informed consent* for potential participants. It must provide a description of the trial in terms that any subject can understand, describe potential benefits of the proposed treatment, and describe known side effects of the experimental medication. It should contain emergency contact information in case of worrisome adverse events. Serious adverse events threatening life or sight or requiring hospitalization must be promptly reported to the sponsor and the IRB. The stipend (if any) paid to the study subject should be part of the informed consent. This informed consent document must be approved by the IRB along with the entire clinical trial protocol before enrolling patients in the study.

Patients who become participants in a clinical trial do so for many reasons. Some genuinely want to participate in research that may lead to drugs that will help themselves or other persons. Other patients have difficult economic circumstances and clinical trial participation will provide them with free care during the study, free study medication, and, in some cases, a stipend for doing the research. Some patients like the increased attention, "VIP status," and increased interaction with their doctor and staff that comes from clinical trial participation. The principal investigators and study coordinator must offer trial participation to patients who not only meet the inclusion criteria of the study but who also would appear to receive benefit and no harm from participation. The principle of *primum non nocere* ("first do no harm") must trump the investigators' desire to meet enrollment goals when conducting a clinical trial.

## 87.3 Finding and Obtaining Clinical Research Trials

Clinical trials can nicely supplement the day-to-day patient-related income of a medical practice. You can get an excellent overview of the kinds of major clinical trials currently under way by visiting: clinicaltrials.gov. Before searching for the first clinical trial, the partners in an ophthalmology practice and staff physicians must make the philosophical determination to go down this road. Clinical research is demanding of both physician and staff time and practice resources. A suitable study coordinator must be trained from within the practice or hired. Clinical protocols require that participants be seen at highly structured time intervals with little toleration for deviation. Schedules may have to be altered to allow these VIP patients to be seen promptly. Personal vacation time of the investigators or study coordinator may have to yield to participant visit requirements of the protocol. Some protocols require serial measurements of intraocular pressure from 8 A.M. in the morning until 8 P.M. at night, requiring that the office stay open with various personnel after normal business hours. Someone must be available on call to respond to any adverse events experienced by study participants. The sponsor or CRO will make site visits and need to meet with the principal investigators and study coordinator. Investigator meetings may require the attendance of the investigators and study coordinators at locations around the country for a 1- or 2-day session. Some trials conduct initiation meetings in the investigator's site. Realize that overhead staffing considerations must be flexible enough to accommodate periods with multiple versus few studies simultaneously in progress. If the practice is committed to research and doing all of these listed things, then the hunt for a project can begin.

Drug companies are always on the lookout for large ophthalmology practices with whom they may contract to conduct clinical research trials. It may be difficult to find your first research project. Finding your first study is like finding your first job. Most of the jobs you want provide opportunities to build valuable experience for your resume, but most sponsors, like most employers, are looking for someone with relevant experience and a proven track record. The pharmaceutical companies want to know that if they choose your site to participate in their study, you will be able to follow the protocol, quickly find patients who meet their inclusion/exclusion criteria, enabling you to meet the protocol timelines. They will assess your physical plant and equipment, interview some of your staff – especially your study coordinator – and get a feel for your office flow to see if you are likely to meet the demands of the research protocol. They will see how you maintain patient records; determine if you have a secure area to store data, drugs, and supplies; and assess the practice's ability to perform certain tests in the protocol (e.g., blood draws, specular microscopy, or get a LOGMAR visual acuity).

How do you find out about potential studies? The drug companies' sales representatives are a possible source of such information. Tell them you are interested in doing research and ask them to pass your name and interest along to the proper people. These representatives probably know well many aspects of your practice and are in a good position to informally evaluate your site when they pass along your interest to the research department at the home office. Alternatively, ask them to get you the names of the pharmaceutical study managers who conduct Phase III and IV trials at their company and try a cold call. When new at research, you are more likely to do well if you get your feet wet with a simpler Phase IV study.

Another source for finding clinical studies is regional and national ophthalmology meetings. Go up to representatives at the exhibit booths and ask them who at the meeting might be available to chat with you about research opportunities. Very often, high-level members of research and development departments of the pharmaceutical companies attend these national meetings. You may be able to visit with one of them over coffee and better present yourself and your interest than over just a cold phone call.

You may also call local and regional CROs to determine if they have received any ophthalmology-related drug contracts and if they are recruiting clinical sites. Organizations such as PharmaNet (www.pharmanet.com/) and ClinAssure (www.clinassure.com) conduct many drug trials and are good sources for leads to participation in clinical trials.

Perhaps, the best source for getting a clinical trial for your practice is the recommendation of a colleague who is participating in a trial. Many clinical research trials are conducted simultaneously at dozens of centers throughout the world. Call ophthalmologist friends who have conducted trials or chat with them at scientific meetings. The drug companies are very receptive to recommendations for additional sites from current investigators who understand the demands of conducting a clinical trial.

Possible participation in a clinical trial begins, after initial interest on the part of the drug company, with signing confidentiality agreements. This is followed with phone call discussions about protocol requirements and the site's facilities and equipment and patient base requirements that will be needed for the study. If both the potential principal investigator and sponsor still wish to proceed, a formal copy of the protocol and investigator's brochure are sent to the site. After reading these and further phone conversations (including budget negotiations), a site visit by a sponsor's research staff member or a CRO representative is arranged. If this visit proves suitable, the project is approved. Informed consent documents and the protocol must be approved by the IRB and then more paperwork (including FDA documents) ensues. Once all of this paperwork is complete, shipments of study drugs and supplies are arranged, and patients may be recruited. Unfortunately, most physicians are a bit optimistic about their ability to recruit participants. Strict protocol inclusion and exclusion criteria, along with patient's lack of interest ("I don't have time for all the visits," "I am going on vacation soon," "I don't want to be a guinea pig," "I can't come in for the evening visits") may limit enrollment possibilities. An excellent physician/patient relationship, established during the regular care of the patients, can make all the difference in the patient's willingness to join the trial.

To best ensure that you can reach target enrollment goals, chart review of potential subjects should begin early (after initial contractual agreement has been reached) – often in advance of formal approval by the IRB and before scheduled screening examinations. Recruitment bonuses may give incentive to your staff to more efficiently enroll subjects. Failure to enroll the agreed upon number of subjects in the study tends to lessen your site's chance of having the sponsor invite you for a future project. Also, note that many studies have a competitive enrollment for the total number of subjects. As stated earlier, get your feet wet with a smaller, less ambitious Phase IV study, establish a good track record, and then ask for a more complex Phase III project. Make sure the patients who participate in these trials are indeed treated as VIPs. These folks may then be pleased to make themselves available again for another study.

Sponsored research can be very rewarding to the principal investigator, both economically and intellectually. A participant learns about the latest developments in medical glaucoma therapy, interacts at investigators' meetings with the best minds in the field, earns enhanced prestige among patients and colleagues, and will be financially rewarded at the same time. But realize that conducting clinical research trials is a major undertaking for any practice, even a large, well-run one. Make sure everyone in a decision-making capacity is on board; have low tolerance for errors in conducting the protocol; and see your subjects promptly and respond personally to any concerns they may have about medication side effects. Participating in clinical research trials can remove the day-to-day humdrum of clinical practice and add a worthwhile new dimension to coming to work.

# Chapter 88
# Future Glaucoma Medical Therapies: What's in the Pipeline?

Abbot F. Clark

## 88.1 Challenges with Current Glaucoma Therapy

There are a number of limitations with our current glaucoma therapies. All available current therapies are directed at lowering intraocular pressure (IOP), an important risk factor for the development and progression of glaucoma. However, IOP lowering only treats a symptom of glaucoma and does not address the underlying pathogenic pathways. Current agents lower IOP by suppressing aqueous humor formation or by enhancing aqueous humor outflow, without modifying the disease process(es) responsible for glaucomatous damage to the outflow facility. Clinical efforts to lower IOP only indirectly protect the retina, optic nerve head, and optic nerve. There are currently no approved therapies that directly neuroprotect these tissues. Some glaucoma patients continue to progress despite receiving IOP-lowering therapy, suggesting that factors other than IOP may be involved. In addition, in many patients, there is a progressive loss of therapeutic efficacy, which often leads to patients being on multiple medications. Another challenge is adherence to therapy, as the majority of patients do not take all their prescribed medications at all times.

Disease-modifying therapies need to be developed that treat all of the tissues involved in glaucoma pathogenesis. Agents that address the progressive glaucomatous damage to the trabecular meshwork (TM) and outflow pathway need to be discovered and developed. This also includes glaucomatous retinopathy (apoptosing retinal ganglion cells), axonopathy (damage to the optic nerve head and optic nerve), and glialopathy (that occurs in the retina, optic nerve head, and optic nerve). Glial cells are essential supporting elements for neurons and may be an attractive therapeutic target.

We also need to do a better job in diagnosing glaucoma and following disease progression. Current advances in molecular genetics and biomarker discovery should be applied to glaucoma so that important risk alleles can be identified and quantitative molecular markers of disease can be followed. The potential for biomarkers is addressed elsewhere in this text (see Chap. 82).

## 88.2 Aqueous Outflow as a Therapeutic Target

IOP is still the most important causative risk factor for the development and progression of glaucoma. New classes of agents are being explored as potential future IOP-lowering therapies.[1] The cytoskeleton of the TM endothelial cells lining Schlemm's canal is an attractive therapeutic target. Agents that disrupt actin microfilaments, such as cytochalasin and latrunculin, enhance aqueous outflow and lower IOP in perfusion cultured anterior segments and in nonhuman primates.[2-4] Ethacrynic acid and several ECA analogs disrupt microtubules, inhibit microtubule assembly, and lower IOP in perfused anterior segments as well as in vivo.[5,6] There are a number of regulators of actomyosin contraction, including a number of kinases. Broad-spectrum kinase inhibitors, such as H-7, increase aqueous outflow and lower IOP[7] as do more specific inhibitors of rho kinase (ROCK inhibitors).[8-10] ROCK inhibitors are also associated with the undesired side effect of conjunctival hyperemia. An inhibitor of myosin II ATPase also appears to increase aqueous outflow.[11] However, there still are several outstanding issues related to targeting the cytoskeleton as a glaucoma therapeutic. All cells contain an actin and tubulin cytoskeleton, so this therapeutic approach would be expected to target more than just the outflow pathway. Because of their potential for intraocular toxicity, such agents need to be carefully selected and site directed so as not to harm the corneal endothelium and other intraocular cells. In addition, the TM actin cytoskeleton is reorganized in glaucomatous eyes[12-13] and glaucomatous TM cells,[14] and it is unclear whether many of these cytoskeletal agents tested in normal eyes will be equally effective in glaucomatous eyes.

In addition to providing mechanical support to the TM, the extracellular matrix (ECM) of the aqueous outflow pathway also regulates outflow resistance. The ECM in the outflow pathway is dynamic, and homeostasis is regulated through a balance of ECM synthesis and ECM degradation. Extracellular proteinases, such as matrix metalloproteinases and plasminogen activators, regulate ECM turnover. MMPs can increase aqueous humor outflow, while MMP inhibitors reduce outflow.[15] The physiologic behavior of this enzyme class is determined by the ratio of the enzymes and their constitutively secreted inhibitors. Matrix metalloproteinases are secreted in a proform and require activation in the ECM. A better understanding of MMP activation in the TM[16] led to the discovery of a small molecule that activated MMP-3 expression and increased aqueous outflow in perfusion cultured anterior segments.[17] One of the proposed mechanisms for prostaglandin analogs' outflow enhancing activity is increased expression of MMPs in the ciliary body and TM. All of the prostaglandin analogs appear to increase the expression of MMPs at both sites.

Recently, there have been a number of new studies directed at identifying pathogenic pathways involved in glaucomatous damage to the outflow pathway. One approach is to evaluate differences in mRNA and protein expression between normal and glaucomatous cells and tissues. Levels of the growth factor TGFβ2 (TGF-β2) are elevated in the aqueous humor and in the TM of POAG patients. TGFβ2 alters ECM metabolism and promotes ECM deposition in the TM. TGFβ2 also directly elevates IOP in perfusion cultured anterior segments. Two groups have independently demonstrated that another class of growth factors, BMPs, can block the ECM enhancing effects of TGFβ2 on the TM,[18,19] suggesting a potential new disease altering therapeutic pathway. Interestingly, glaucomatous TM cells have elevated expression of the BMP inhibitor gremlin, which reverses the protective effect of BMPs on TGFβ2, leading to further ECM production in the TM.[19] Soluble CD44 has also been reported to be elevated in the aqueous humor of POAG patients, which correlates with the degree of visual field loss,[20] and sCD44 can be toxic to TM cells[21] (see Chap. 83). Recent studies have shown that overexpression of CD44 in the mouse eye causes elevated IOP,[22] suggesting a cause and effect relationship. It will be interesting to determine whether the sCD44-induced ocular hypertension leads to glaucomatous damage to the retina and optic nerve. If so, this may become an attractive animal model that mimics human POAG.

The Wnt signaling pathway has also been implicated in regulation of aqueous outflow. The expression of the Wnt antagonist sFRP1 is elevated in glaucomatous TM cells, and increased expression of sFRP1 elevated IOP in perfusion cultured anterior segment and in mouse eyes. Topical ocular administration of a GSK3 inhibitor, which restores Wnt signaling, lowered the sFRP1 induced ocular hypertension in mice.[23] The expression of serum amyloid A2 (SAA2) mRNA and protein was elevated in glaucomatous TM cells and tissues, and perfusion with SAA2 elevated IOP in perfusion cultured anterior segments,[24] suggesting another potential pathogenic pathway to therapeutically attack.

## 88.3 Targeting Glaucomatous Retinopathy and Optic Neuropathy

A number of groups are working to identify the molecular pathogenic pathways involved in glaucomatous damage to the retina, optic nerve, and optic nerve head. A better understanding of these pathways will ultimately lead to disease intervening therapeutic agents. Excitotoxic amino acids such as glutamate are elevated in ischemic damage to the retina and can kill retinal ganglion cells (RGCs). The NMDA receptor antagonist memantine protects RGCs in a number of preclinical models of RGC damage,[25] and memantine has been in clinical trials for the treatment of glaucoma. However, this therapeutic approach did not meet the primary efficacy endpoints.[26] Extensive data analysis of subgroups remains ongoing and may yet suggest some benefit. It is important to realize that transsynaptic glutamate and extracellular glutamate may be quite different and have different implications for the RGCs.

Growth factors and cytokines can play both pathologic and neuroprotective roles in glaucomatous damage to the retina and optic nerve. Neurotrophins and neurotrophic factors appear to protect RGCs from a variety of insults. Transduction of RGCs with viral expression vectors for BDNF[27] or CNTF[28] partially protected RGCs in a rat model of glaucoma. However, the receptors for some of these neuroprotective factors are also downregulated with retinal injury, which would appear to limit their overall neuroprotective efficacy.[29] TNFα (TNF-alpha) is upregulated in the glaucomatous retina, and TNFα can kill RGCs. The relationship of TNFα and optineurin, the glaucoma gene associated with the locus GLC1E, is discussed in Chap. 9. Blocking TNFα with neutralizing antibodies or deleting the TNFα receptor protected RGCs in a mouse model of ocular hypertension-induced glaucoma.[30] The profibrotic growth factor TGFβ2 (TGF-beta 2) is elevated in the glaucomatous optic nerve head,[31,32] and this may be responsible for the remodeling to the optic nerve head that occurs in glaucoma. TGFβ2 drives ECM synthesis and deposition in cells of the optic nerve head,[32–34] which can be blocked by BMP4[33] or by inhibition of CTGF.[34]

Although glaucomatous insults damage RGCs, which can result in cellular apoptosis, the process of apoptosis is more complex than originally identified. Administration of a caspase inhibitor, XIAP, partially protected RGCs in a rat model of glaucoma. Likewise, administration of FK506, which among other things is a calcineurin inhibitor, also protected RGCs in a rat glaucoma model.[35] Bax is a major player in apoptosis, and RGCs were protected from glaucomatous damage in Bax deficient mice.[36] Interestingly, although the RGC somas were protected, the optic nerves of these mice developed glaucomatous damage, showing that apoptosis can be compartmentalized within a single cell.

## 88.4 Glaucoma Genetics and Pharmacogenomics

The identification of glaucoma genes and glaucoma-associated genes will help us better understand the molecular pathogenesis of glaucoma as well as help identify those individuals at greater risk for developing glaucoma. There have been a number of glaucoma loci mapped and several glaucoma genes identified. MYOC was the first glaucoma gene identified,[37] and there is a relatively good genotype/phenotype correlation for certain MYOC mutations. Glaucomatous MYOC mutations cause a gain of function phenotype, and there have been a number of hypotheses on the molecular cause(s) of MYOC glaucoma. A genome-wide scan using SNP (single nucleotide polymorphism) chip arrays identified alleles in LOXL1 that are associated with increased risk of developing exfoliation glaucoma.[38] (See also Chaps. 9 and 39.) Most of the glaucomas are complex, multigenic diseases, so the SNP genotyping approach will undoubtedly allow the identification of other DNA markers that are associated with increased risk of disease.

Individual responses to drug therapy are quite heterogeneous and due to a number of factors. Many of these factors are genetically determined, including genetic differences in the drug target as well as differences in drug metabolism and elimination. For example, differences in IOP-lowering responses to beta-blockers in glaucoma patients appear to be associated with a polymorphism in the beta adrenergic receptor gene (ADBR2).[39] A number of clinical trials are now including genetic profiling of patients' DNA for pharmacogenetic markers so that markers can be linked to drug efficacy as well as potential drug side effects.[40] In the future, it may be possible to tailor specific therapies for individual patients.

## 88.5 New Target Identification

Recent scientific advances have led to a better understanding of glaucoma pathogenesis and the discovery of new pathogenic pathways. Both genomics and proteomics techniques have identified differences in gene and protein expression between normal and glaucoma specimens. The identity and quality of samples is absolutely essential for finding relevant differences. It is also important to show that the discovered difference(s) actually cause a glaucoma-like phenotype. For example, if increased expression of a gene/protein or a specific gene mutation is found in the glaucomatous TM, it is essential to demonstrate that this change results in elevated intraocular pressure. Similarly, a discovered change in the glaucomatous retina, optic nerve head, or optic nerve should cause glaucomatous retinopathy or optic neuropathy in an animal model. Although there have been quite a few studies reporting differences in gene and protein expression in glaucoma models and in samples from glaucoma patients, only some of these studies have demonstrated a cause and effect relationship (Table 88.1).

The discovery of pathogenic pathways can also lead to the discovery of new therapeutic agents. Although levels of sFRP1 are elevated in the glaucomatous TM,[23] sFRP1 is currently a very difficult therapeutic target. However, realizing that sFRP1 is an inhibitor of Wnt signaling and that Wnt signaling plays a role in regulating normal IOP led to the evaluation of another member of the Wnt signaling pathway that was more amenable to therapeutic intervention. Glycogen synthase kinase-3 (GSK3) is a kinase that controls the levels of β-catenin (beta-catenin), a key mediator of Wnt signaling. GSK3 inhibition blocks β-catenin degradation, thus restoring Wnt signaling. Topical application of a GSK3 inhibitor lowers sFRP1-mediated ocular hypertension in mice,[23] justifying this approach to new therapeutic target identification.

## 88.6 Gene Therapy

Gene therapy can target the replacement of defective genes or overexpress a gene that regulates or interferes with a specific pathogenic process. The use of AAV2. RPE65 gene replacement therapy for some patients with Leber congenital amaurosis (LCA) is a great example of the potential use of gene therapy in ophthalmology.[41] However, not all genetically determined diseases are amenable to this therapeutic approach. For example, MYOC glaucoma is not due to haploinsufficiency (i.e., the lack of a functional protein), but instead is due to gain-of-function mutations. A novel approach to the treatment of MYOC glaucoma would be to use viral vectors to deliver RNA interference that would selectively knockdown myocilin expression in the TM. Viral delivery of RNAi has been successfully utilized in a rodent model of retinal degeneration.[42] RNA silencing therapy is a

**Table 88.1** Discovery of new glaucoma pathogenic pathways involved in regulating IOP

| Molecule | Pathway | Phenotype |
|---|---|---|
| TGFβ2 | TGFβ2 | Elevates IOP in perfused anterior segments and in mice |
| Gremlin | BMP signaling | Elevates IOP in perfused anterior segments |
| sFRP1 | Wnt signaling | Elevates IOP in perfused anterior segments and in mice |
| SAA2 | ? | Elevates IOP in perfused anterior segments |
| sCD44 | ? | Elevates IOP in mice |

popular concept in which small RNAs are used to activate a cellular process, leading to a highly specific RNA degradation. The RNA pathway consists of the presentation of a triggering dsRNA, which is processed into small interfering RNAs (siRNA) 21–25 base pairs in length by a specific enzyme. The challenge remains to efficiently and effectively deliver siRNA molecules to specific target tissues in vivo.

Neuroprotective trophic factors also can be selectively delivered to RGCs. Intravitreal administration of AAV2 expression vectors can transduce up to 70% of RGCs in the rat retina.[27] AAV2 delivery of BDNF or CNTF partially protected the retina from glaucomatous damage in rats (see previous), and similar approaches might be used to deliver other biological neuroprotective agents.

Several viral vectors have been used to successfully deliver transgenes to the TM. Administration of adenovirus 5 (Ad5) transduces the TM of ex vivo perfusion cultured anterior segments[43] and of monkey[44] and mouse[45] eyes to deliver a variety of transgenes including GFP, myocilin, sFRP1, and CD44. However, Ad5 mediated transgene expression is associated with some ocular inflammation and diminished transgene expression over time. FIV lentiviruses also efficiently transduce the TM and lead to prolonged GFP expression in cat and monkey eyes for over 1 year.[46,47] Attempts to deliver therapeutic transgenes to the TM include C3[48] and the dominant negative Rho-binding domain,[49] and each enhanced aqueous outflow in perfused anterior segments.

## 88.7 Drug Delivery Methods

This chapter would not be complete without mentioning that numerous methods of drug delivery may make possible the therapeutic exploitation of many of the pathways noted. Punctal plugs, subconjunctival reservoirs, sub-Tenon's reservoirs, and scleral reservoirs are all under investigation as potential means of delivering antiglaucoma therapy. Some of these approaches may work with larger molecules. Not only do they have the potential to deliver the conventional drugs delivered elsewhere, but they make therapeutic intervention with small peptides and human recombinant polypeptides possible.

## 88.8 Conclusion

New therapeutic agents are being explored for lowering IOP, one of the most important risk factors for the development and progression of glaucoma. New studies are uncovering the molecular pathways involved in glaucomatous damage to the aqueous outflow pathway, which have opened up new disease modifying therapeutic strategies for lowering IOP. We also are developing a better understanding of the pathways involved in glaucomatous damage to the retina, optic nerve head, and optic nerve, which will be used to develop new neuroprotective agents. Molecular genetics is being used to identify genes associated with the development of glaucoma and will be used in the near future to predict an individual's response (both efficacy and side effects) to a specific drug treatment.

## References

1. Pang I-H, Clark AF. IOP as a target – inflow and outflow pathways. In: Yorio T, Clark AF, Wax MB, eds. *Ocular Therapeutics: Eye on Discovery*. Amsterdam: Elsevier/Academic Press; 2008:45–67.
2. Robinson JC, Kaufman PL. Cytochalasin B potentiates epinephrine's outflow facility-increasing effect. *Invest Ophthalmol Vis Sci*. 1991;32(5):1614–1618.
3. Fan H, Rao SK, Zhou YS, Lam DS. Effect of latrunculin B on intraocular pressure in the monkey eye. *Arch Ophthalmol*. 2005;123(10):1456–1457. author reply 1457.
4. Ethier CR, Read AT, Chan DW. Effects of latrunculin-B on outflow facility and trabecular meshwork structure in human eyes. *Invest Ophthalmol Vis Sci*. 2006;47(5):1991–1998.
5. Melamed S, Kotas-Neumann R, Barak A, Epstein DL. The effect of intracamerally injected ethacrynic acid on intraocular pressure in patients with glaucoma. *Am J Ophthalmol*. 1992;113(5):508–512.
6. Shimazaki A, Ichikawa M, Rao PV, et al. Effects of the new ethacrynic acid derivative SA9000 on intraocular pressure in cats and monkeys. *Biol Pharm Bull*. 2004;27(7):1019–1024.
7. Tian B, Wang RF, Podos SM, Kaufman PL. Effects of topical H-7 on outflow facility, intraocular pressure, and corneal thickness in monkeys. *Arch Ophthalmol*. 2004;122(8):1171–1177.
8. Honjo M, Inatani M, Kido N, et al. A myosin light chain kinase inhibitor, ML-9, lowers the intraocular pressure in rabbit eyes. *Exp Eye Res*. 2002;75(2):135–142.
9. Tian B, Kaufman PL. Effects of the Rho kinase inhibitor Y-27632 and the phosphatase inhibitor calyculin A on outflow facility in monkeys. *Exp Eye Res*. 2005;80(2):215–225.
10. Tokushige H, Inatani M, Nemoto S, et al. Effects of topical administration of y-39983, a selective rho-associated protein kinase inhibitor, on ocular tissues in rabbits and monkeys. *Invest Ophthalmol Vis Sci*. 2007;48(7):3216–3222.
11. Zhang M, Rao PV. Blebbistatin, a novel inhibitor of myosin II ATPase activity, increases aqueous humor outflow facility in perfused enucleated porcine eyes. *Invest Ophthalmol Vis Sci*. 2005;46(11):4130–4138.
12. Read AT, Chan DW, Ethier CR. Actin structure in the outflow tract of normal and glaucomatous eyes. *Exp Eye Res*. 2007;84(1):214–226.
13. Hoare MJ, Grierson I, Brotchie D, Pollock N, Cracknell K, Clark AF. Cross-linked actin networks (CLANs) in the trabecular meshwork of the normal and glaucomatous human eye in situ. *Invest Ophthalmol Vis Sci*. 2009;50(3):1255–1263.
14. Clark AF, Miggans ST, Wilson K, Browder S, McCartney MD. Cytoskeletal changes in cultured human glaucoma trabecular meshwork cells. *J Glaucoma*. 1995;4:183–188.
15. Bradley JM, Vranka J, Colvis CM, et al. Effect of matrix metalloproteinases activity on outflow in perfused human organ culture. *Invest Ophthalmol Vis Sci*. 1998;39(13):2649–2658.

16. Fleenor DL, Pang IH, Clark AF. Involvement of AP-1 in interleukin-1alpha-stimulated MMP-3 expression in human trabecular meshwork cells. *Invest Ophthalmol Vis Sci.* 2003;44(8):3494-3501.
17. Pang IH, Fleenor DL, Hellberg PE, Stropki K, McCartney MD, Clark AF. Aqueous outflow-enhancing effect of tert-butylhydroquinone: involvement of AP-1 activation and MMP-3 expression. *Invest Ophthalmol Vis Sci.* 2003;44(8):3502-3510.
18. Fuchshofer R, Yu AH, Welge-Lussen U, Tamm ER. Bone morphogenetic protein-7 is an antagonist of transforming growth factor-beta2 in human trabecular meshwork cells. *Invest Ophthalmol Vis Sci.* 2007;48(2):715-726.
19. Wordinger RJ, Fleenor DL, Hellberg PE, et al. Effects of TGF-beta2, BMP-4, and gremlin in the trabecular meshwork: implications for glaucoma. *Invest Ophthalmol Vis Sci.* 2007;48(3):1191-1200.
20. Nolan MJ, Giovingo MC, Miller AM, et al. Aqueous humor sCD44 concentration and visual field loss in primary open-angle glaucoma. *J Glaucoma.* 2007;16(5):419-429.
21. Choi J, Miller AM, Nolan MJ, et al. Soluble CD44 is cytotoxic to trabecular meshwork and retinal ganglion cells in vitro. *Invest Ophthalmol Vis Sci.* 2005;46(1):214-222.
22. Shepard AR, Nolan MJ, Millar JC, et al. *CD44 overexpression causes ocular hypertension in the mouse.* Ft. Lauderdale, FL: ARVO; 2008. Abstract #2880.
23. Wang WH, McNatt LG, Pang IH, et al. Increased expression of the WNT antagonist sFRP-1 in glaucoma elevates intraocular pressure. *J Clin Invest.* 2008;118(3):1056-1064.
24. Wang WH, McNatt LG, Pang IH, et al. Increased expression of serum amyloid A in glaucoma and its effect on intraocular pressure. *Invest Ophthalmol Vis Sci.* 2008;49(5):1916-1923.
25. Hare W, WoldeMussie E, Lai R, et al. Efficacy and safety of memantine, an NMDA-type open-channel blocker, for reduction of retinal injury associated with experimental glaucoma in rat and monkey. *Surv Ophthalmol.* 2001;45(suppl 3):S284-S289. discussion S295-6.
26. Osborne NN. Recent clinical findings with memantine should not mean that the idea of neuroprotection in glaucoma is abandoned. *Acta Ophthalmol.* 2009;87:450-454.
27. Martin KR, Quigley HA, Zack DJ, et al. Gene therapy with brain-derived neurotrophic factor as a protection: retinal ganglion cells in a rat glaucoma model. *Invest Ophthalmol Vis Sci.* 2003;44(10):4357-4365.
28. Pease ME, Zack DJ, Berlinicke C, et al. Effect of CNTF on retinal ganglion cell survival in experimentalglaucoma. *Invest Ophthalmol Vis Sci.* 2009;50:2194-2200.
29. Cheng L, Sapieha P, Kittlerova P, Hauswirth WW, Di Polo A. TrkB gene transfer protects retinal ganglion cells from axotomy-induced death in vivo. *J Neurosci.* 2002;22(10):3977-3986.
30. Nakazawa T, Nakazawa C, Matsubara A, et al. Tumor necrosis factor-alpha mediates oligodendrocyte death and delayed retinal ganglion cell loss in a mouse model of glaucoma. *J Neurosci.* 2006;26(49):12633-12641.
31. Pena JD, Taylor AW, Ricard CS, Vidal I, Hernandez MR. Transforming growth factor beta isoforms in human optic nerve heads. *Br J Ophthalmol.* 1999;83(2):209-218.
32. Zode GS, Sethi A, Brun-Zinkernagel AM, Chang IF, Clark AF, Wordinger RJ. Transforming growth factor-b2 increases extracellular matrix proteins in optic nerve head cells via activation of the Smad signaling pathway. *Submitted for Publication.* April 13, 2010.
33. Zode GS, Clark AF, Wordinger RJ. Bone morphogenetic protein 4 inhibits TGF-beta2 stimulation of extracellular matrix proteins in optic nerve head cells: role of gremlin in ECM modulation. *Glia.* 2008;57(7):755-766.
34. Fuchshofer R, Birke M, Welge-Lussen U, Kook D, Lutjen-Drecoll E. Transforming growth factor-beta 2 modulated extracellular matrix component expression in cultured human optic nerve head astrocytes. *Invest Ophthalmol Vis Sci.* 2005;46(2):568-578.
35. Huang W, Fileta JB, Dobberfuhl A, et al. Calcineurin cleavage is triggered by elevated intraocular pressure, and calcineurin inhibition blocks retinal ganglion cell death in experimental glaucoma. *Proc Natl Acad Sci U S A.* 2005;102(34):12242-12247.
36. Libby RT, Li Y, Savinova OV, et al. Susceptibility to neurodegeneration in a glaucoma is modified by Bax gene dosage. *PLoS Genet.* 2005;1(1):17-26.
37. Stone EM, Fingert JH, Alward WL, et al. Identification of a gene that causes primary open angle glaucoma. *Science.* 1997;275(5300):668-670.
38. Thorleifsson G, Magnusson KP, Sulem P, et al. Common sequence variants in the LOXL1 gene confer susceptibility to exfoliation glaucoma. *Science.* 2007;317(5843):1397-1400.
39. McCarty CA, Burmester JK, Mukesh BN, Patchett RB, Wilke RA. Intraocular pressure response to topical beta-blockers associated with an ADRB2 single-nucleotide polymorphism. *Arch Ophthalmol.* 2008;126(7):959-963.
40. Katz DA, Bhathena A. Overview of pharmacogenetics. *Curr Protoc Hum Genet.* 2009;Chap. 9:Unit 9.19.
41. Cideciyan AV, Aleman TS, Boye SL, et al. Human gene therapy for RPE65 isomerase deficiency activates the retinoid cycle of vision but with slow rod kinetics. *Proc Natl Acad Sci U S A.* 2008;105(39):15112-15117.
42. Tam LC, Kiang AS, Kennan A, et al. Therapeutic benefit derived from RNAi-mediated ablation of IMPDH1 transcripts in a murine model of autosomal dominant retinitis pigmentosa (RP10). *Hum Mol Genet.* 2008;17(14):2084-2100.
43. Ethier CR, Wada S, Chan D, Stamer WD. Experimental and numerical studies of adenovirus delivery to outflow tissues of perfused human anterior segments. *Invest Ophthalmol Vis Sci.* 2004;45(6):1863-1870.
44. Borras T, Gabelt BT, Klintworth GK, Peterson JC, Kaufman PL. Non-invasive observation of repeated adenoviral GFP gene delivery to the anterior segment of the monkey eye in vivo. *J Gene Med.* 2001;3(5):437-449.
45. Millar JC, Pang IH, Wang WH, Wang Y, Clark AF. Effect of immunomodulation with anti-CD40L antibody on adenoviral-mediated transgene expression in mouse anterior segment. *Mol Vis.* 2008;14:10-19.
46. Khare PD, Loewen N, Teo W, et al. Durable, safe, multi-gene lentiviral vector expression in feline trabecular meshwork. *Mol Ther.* 2008;16(1):97-106.
47. Barraza RA, Rasmussen C, Loewen N, et al. Prolonged transgene expression with lentiviral vectors in the aqueoushumor outflow pathway of non-human primates. *Hum Gene Ther.* 2009;30:191-100.
48. Liu X, Hu Y, Filla MS, et al. The effect of C3 transgene expression on actin and cellular adhesions in cultured human trabecular meshwork cells and on outflow facility in organ cultured monkey eyes. *Mol Vis.* 2005;11:1112-1121.
49. Rao PV, Deng P, Maddala R, Epstein DL, Li CY, Shimokawa H. Expression of dominant negative Rho-binding domain of Rho-kinase in organ cultured human eye anterior segments increases aqueous humor outflow. *Mol Vis.* 2005;11:288-297.

## Chapter 89
## Anecortave Acetate: A New Approach for the Medical Treatment of Glaucoma

Amy Lewis Hennessy and Alan L. Robin

The medical management of glaucoma is often compromised by patients' nonadherence with prescribed topical therapy – both the ability to execute eye drop administration[1-9] and persistency of medication use.[10-14] This can be made more complex in patients who are taking multiple systemic medications[16,17] and multiple medications to lower IOP.[12-18] The consequence of inadequate treatment arising from patient nonadherence is disease progression, with permanent and irreversible loss of visual function. The Early Manifest Glaucoma Treatment Study (EMGTS)[19] found that among individuals treated and closely monitored for their glaucoma, 57% progressed in a 5-year period. In 2008, Urquhart[20] described noncompliance, nonabsorption, and nonresponse as possibilities for disease progression despite use of prescribed medications. It may be that part of the reason for progression in glaucoma is poor adherence to prescribed therapy.[5,6]

There are numerous reports[21,22] of patients self-reporting trouble with manual dexterity, getting drops into the eye, dislike of drops, and inadequate vision as problems with administering glaucoma medications. Glaucoma patients also frequently cite the complexity of a multi-drug regimen as one explanation for their lack of compliance. This is confirmed in the literature, with 40% of ocular hypertension patients requiring multiple medications to achieve a 20% reduction in intraocular pressure (IOP) after 5 years, and with 75% of those with actual glaucoma requiring multiple pharmacotherapies. Topical beta-adrenergic blockers are commonly used as an adjunctive therapy to first-line prostaglandins, though, despite the advantage of being a once-daily dosage and having complementary mechanisms of action, there is minimal additive effect of a beta-blocker with a prostaglandin.[23-25] When considering the addition of a topical carbonic anhydrase inhibitor or alpha-agonist, practitioners must weigh the fact that these medications are labeled as dosed three times daily, but not much more than 2 mmHg of IOP lowering is achieved with these extra applications of drops.

Adding additional eye drops increases costs for the patient and increases the risk of side effects, preservative-related ocular surface disease, and medication errors.[26] The majority of glaucoma patients are already using other medications for systemic comorbidities, thus adding to the complexity of the overall medication load. There is a need for an antiglaucoma agent that is safe, highly effective, and has a long duration of action that reduces or eliminates patient involvement – and puts control in doctors' hands.

Development of new glaucoma medications peaked in the mid-1990s with the introduction of three new classes of topical IOP-lowering medications: topical carbonic anhydrase inhibitors, alpha-adrenergic agonists, and prostaglandins (Fig. 89.1). Since then, several drugs and combinations of existing drugs have been introduced but no new drug class for IOP lowering has emerged in over a decade. In other chronic ophthalmic conditions such as cytomegalovirus retinitis, chronic uveitis, and diabetic macular edema, slow-release, sustained-delivery devices can be inserted into the eye; IOP-lowering therapy is not currently on this same level.

Anecortave acetate (AL-3789) (Alcon Laboratories, Inc.) represents a potential innovation in both drug class and drug delivery route for glaucoma management and represents an alternative therapy for long-term IOP reduction. It is a cortisene – an angiostatic steroid and a derivative of cortisol that has been established in multiple experimental models of angiogenesis and has been evaluated as a therapy for neovascular age-related macular degeneration in humans.[27-30] Anecortave is formulated by replacing the hydroxyl group at carbon 9 of the cortisol molecule with a double bond between carbons 9 and 11 and the addition of an acetate group at carbon 21 (Fig. 89.2).

These very specific and irreversible chemical modifications to the cortisol structure have been shown to possess angiostatic activity via inhibition of proteases that degrade the extracellular matrix, thus blocking migration of vascular endothelial cells.[28] This has resulted in the potent inhibition of blood vessel growth, and there has been no evidence, clinical or non-clinical, of glucocorticoid receptor-mediated biological activity.[31] There have been three in vivo studies and one in vitro study all demonstrating that anecortave acetate lacks glucocorticoid anti-inflammatory activity.* Unlike corticosteroids such as

---

*Clark AF, Personal communication, Dec 2007.

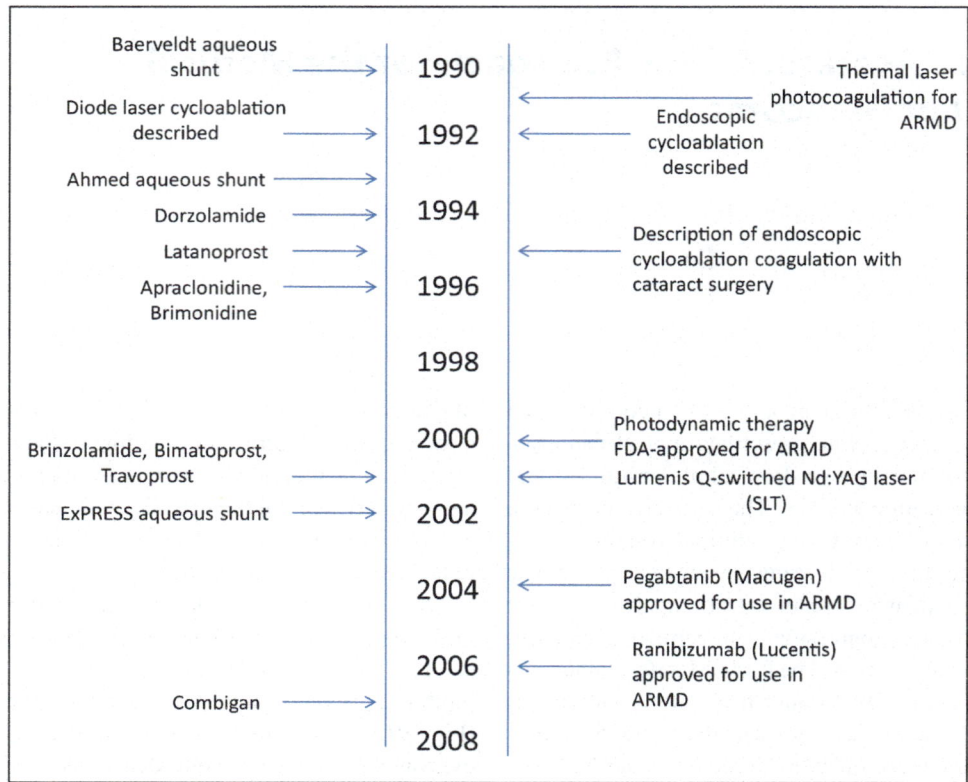

**Fig. 89.1** Timeline showing introduction of various glaucoma treatments from 1990 to 2008

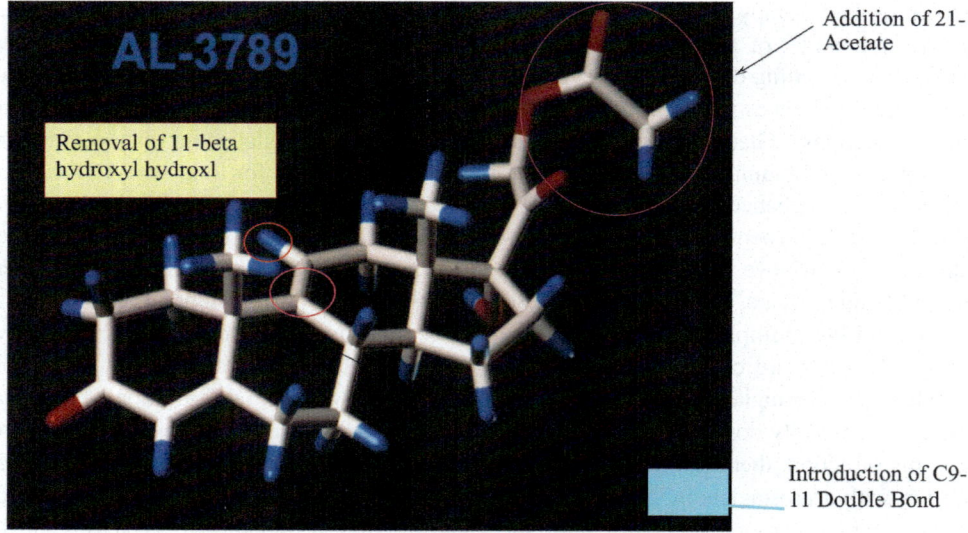

**Fig. 89.2** Comparison of anecortave acetate (AL-3789) and tetrahydrocortisol. Anecortave is formulated by replacing the hydroxyl group at carbon 9 of the cortisol molecule with a double bond between carbons 9 and 11, and the addition of an acetate group at carbon 21

prednisone, dexamethasone, or triamcinolone, anecortave acetate does not reduce inflammation, elevate IOP, or cause cataracts.

Anecortave acetate, given by posterior juxtascleral depot injection, has also been studied as a possible treatment for neovascular age-related macular degeneration (ARMD).[28,29] Problems with this technique include reflux through the injection site, anteriorization along the injection tract, and decreased efficacy due to inability to penetrate the macula from the injection site. Such issues have presented insurmountable problems to the study of this medication for ARMD. Anecortave is relatively insoluble and its action is limited to the area just beneath where it is located. During the retinal administration, just above the macula, there appeared to be no effect on IOP.

Problems with patient self-administration and compliance with glaucoma medications have led investigators to search for other methods of administering IOP-lowering medication. Anecortave acetate is an insoluble compound, that, when injected by an anterior juxtascleral depot (AJD), exerts its effect locally, migrating through sclera over approximately 270°, and acting at the level of the trabecular meshwork and ciliary body, for a prolonged period. It does not block aqueous production; nor does it enter Schlemm's canal. It is thought to slowly diffuse and enhance outflow. Changes to the trabecular meshwork cells following exposure to corticosteroids include increase in cell size,[32] reduction in phagocytic activity,[33] cross-linking of actin molecules,[31,32] and upregulation of myocilin production. Because the injection is not intravitreal, it carries an extremely low-risk of endophthalmitis. If properly administered, the injection procedure is relatively safe and well-tolerated by patients. An AJD injection obviates the need for patient adherence and places the burden of adherence primarily in the doctors' hands. Advantages include the avoidance of an intravitreal injection, relatively infrequent intervals of treatment, and an excellent safety and tolerability profile. Several small uncontrolled studies have evaluated its use in treating various forms of glaucoma and have suggested satisfactory IOP lowering from anecortave.

Robin et al[34] described a novel approach with AJD injection of anecortave in open-angle glaucoma. This involves the use of a 30-gauge needle, modified topical anesthesia, and delivery of medication in the sub-Tenon's space, creating a circumferential deposition surrounding the limbus. Robin and coworkers presented a case series of seven eyes of six patients with primary open-angle glaucoma that was uncontrolled with at least a prostaglandin analogue who were treated with anecortave acetate delivered using an AJD and followed closely for up to 2 years. IOP was lowered by 40–50% at 4 weeks in eyes with baseline IOP ranging from 23 to 52 mmHg on a prostaglandin analogue. In six out of seven eyes, anecortave acetate produced a rapid and substantial reduction in IOP, dropping by 9.5 mmHg after 1 week and by 12.7 mmHg at 4 weeks. This IOP lowering from a single injection lasted for at least 3 months and up to 19 months.

Prata et al described the use of anterior juxtascleral anecortave in 25 eyes of 25 patients with uncontrolled primary open-angle, steroid-induced or uveitic glaucoma.[35] Mean pretreatment IOP was 30.9 mmHg, and at least 30% IOP reduction was demonstrated for at least 3 months after a single injection of anecortave.

Callanan et al studied the use of anecortave to control elevation in IOP following insertion of Retisert implant for noninfectious posterior uveitis in 11 eyes of 10 patients.[36] It is known that one of the major complications of the Retisert implant is IOP elevation in 60%, with glaucoma filtering surgery required in 30% at 2 years, so the anecortave injections for this study were done to prevent this IOP elevation. Doses of 12 mg, 24 mg, or 30 mg were given every 4 months, and no patient required filtering surgery to control IOP.

Landry et al studied the use of anecortave 12 mg or 24 mg in eight pseudophakic patients that were status-post laser trabeculoplasty and at least one additional intraocular procedure.[37] Three of the eight patients had an IOP reduction of more than 30% from baseline and reduced medications. Although anecortave offers an option for IOP lowering in patients with more complex glaucomas, the optimal dosing of the AJD has yet to be determined.

Anecortave acetate delivered by AJD injection has also been reported to lower IOP rapidly and substantially in eyes with steroid-induced ocular hypertension. A prospective placebo-controlled study by Robin et al[38] examined the safety and efficacy of anecortave acetate for this condition. This was a study of eight eyes that had undergone one or more injections of triamcinolone acetate, and received a 24-mg dose of anecortave acetate via AJD if IOP was uncontrolled on current medications. A rapid and sustained reduction in IOP was demonstrated by 1 week in all patients, and no adverse events were noted. By 1 month, seven of eight had IOP that remained reduced by over 30%.

The possibility of use in steroid-induced ocular hypertension is significant given the attractiveness of intravitreal steroid injections for macular edema, vein occlusion, or choroidal neovascular membrane. In fact, up to 40% of eyes receiving approximately 20 mg doses of intravitreal triamcinolone acetate (IVTA) will have a transient elevation of IOP.[39] This elevation can occur within 1 week and may take up to 9 months to return to baseline.[40] Jonas has looked at the 25 mg dose of IVTA for exudative ARMD, diabetic macular edema, central retinal vein occlusion (CRVO), adjunct in proliferative diabetic retinopathy, proliferative vitreoretinopathy, and prephthisical hypotony; his groups noticed that early on some patients experienced IOP elevation after this therapeutic triamcinolone injection. In a meta-analysis of all previously reported data, Jonas et al[40] found that following approximately 20 mg dose of IVTA, 163 of 272 patients experienced IOP greater than 21 mmHg. Most of these were controlled with medications; however, 1% required filtering surgery to adequately lower IOP and prevent optic nerve damage and visual field loss. Challa et al have studied the 4 mg dose of IVTA for exudative ARMD, and found that 3% (1/26) had IOP elevation that required IOP-lowering medications for 6 weeks.[41]

This evidence presents the clinician with a dilemma: steroid-induced IOP elevation is a self-limited condition, and IOP may return to normal in most cases. However, what if the patient is in that small population that experiences an IOP elevation that requires filtering surgery to reduce IOP? Filtering surgery is not without complications, which include wound leak, blebitis, and endophthalmitis.[42-48] Many practitioners may not be willing to weigh a patient's loss of vision due to glaucomatous optic nerve damage against loss of vision due to a surgical complication. Utilization of anecortave to lower IOP in this situation may alleviate this dilemma.

The mechanism for anecortave acetate's IOP lowering is not fully understood at present. Glucocorticoids and transforming growth factor-beta 2 (TGFβ2) have both demonstrated elevation of IOP in humans, animals, and in the laboratory,[31,49] and have been implicated in the pathogenesis of glaucoma. TGFβ2 can cause elevated IOP in perfusion cultured anterior segments,[50,51] as well as in mice transduced with a TGFβ2 expression vector.[52,53] Dexamethasone and TGFβ2 and their effects on cultured human trabecular meshwork (TM) cells are being studied in order to better understand how these insults alter TM cell gene expression. Glucocorticoids and TGFβ2 act to increase the mRNA and protein expression of plasminogen activator inhibitor-1 (PAI-1) in TM cells.[54] PAI-1 directly inhibits the activation of plasminogen and indirectly inhibits the activation of promatrix metalloproteinases (pro-MMPs), playing a major part in extracellular matrix (ECM) metabolism. This activity in turn increases deposition of ECM in the TM; this is a feature of both glucocorticoid-induced and TGFβ2-induced ocular hypertension as well as primary open-angle glaucoma. Increased expression of PAI-1 in the anterior segment can be pathogenic for ocular hypertension and glaucoma.[†] Elevated PAI-1 that has been induced in cultured TM cells can be inhibited by simultaneous addition of anecortave desacetate in the culture medium. This suggests the mechanism for this agent's ability to lower IOP in patients with glaucoma and steroid-induced ocular hypertensive patients.[‡]

## 89.1 Conclusion

The use of an anterior of anecortave acetate by juxtascleral administration may have the potential not only to delay the progression of this chronic disease process, but also have a significant positive impact on the socioeconomic burden of glaucoma.[55] If not yet in the end-stages of glaucoma, the level of visual impairment may involve participation in daily activities, increased rates of falls, car accidents, and mortality. If patients are reaching end-stage glaucoma or blindness, the benefits, healthcare, and reduced tax revenues cost an estimated $1.5 billion per year. Currently, though the mechanism by which anecortave acetate lowers IOP is unclear, the magnitude, rapidity, and duration of IOP reduction following a single AJD injection are noteworthy.

Compliance in glaucoma may come in several forms – not only must the patients accept that they have a disease and must use medications, but they must remember to take the eyedrop as directed, and they also have to get it into the eye. Patients have demonstrated difficulties with all of these issues. In the environment of glaucoma where patient compliance and persistence is a significant obstacle, a treatment administered by the practitioner, which acts locally at the level of the trabecular meshwork, and lasts more than 1 day, and in some cases up to 6 months, would potentially eliminate all need for patient involvement.

## References

1. Norell SE. Improving medication compliance: a randomised clinical trial. Br Med J. 1979;2:1031–1033.
2. Norell S. Medication behaviour. A study of outpatients treated with pilocarpine eye drops for primary open-angle glaucoma. Acta Ophthalmol Suppl (Copenh). 1980;143:1–28.
3. Norell SE, Granstrom PA. Self-medication with pilocarpine among outpatients in a glaucoma clinic. Br J Ophthalmol. 1980;64:134–141.
4. Norell SE, Granstrom PA, Wassen R. A medication monitor and fluorescein technique designed to study medication behaviour. Acta Ophthalmol (Copenh). 1980;58:459–467.
5. Kass MA, Gordon M, Meltzer DW. Can ophthalmologists correctly identify patients defaulting from pilocarpine therapy? Am J Ophthalmol. 1986;101:524–530.
6. Kass MA, Meltzer DW, Gordon M, Cooper D, Goldberg J. Compliance with topical pilocarpine treatment. Am J Ophthalmol. 1986;101:515–523.
7. Winfield AJ, Jessiman D, Williams A, Esakowitz L. A study of the causes of non-compliance by patients prescribed eyedrops. Br J Ophthalmol. 1990;74:477–480.
8. Kholdebarin R, Campbell RJ, Jin Y, Buys YM. Multicenter study of compliance and drop administration in glaucoma. Can J Ophthalmol. 2008;43:454–461.
9. Brown M, Brown G, Spaeth G. Improper topical self-administration of ocular medication among patients with glaucoma. Can J Ophthalmol. 1984;19(1):2–5.
10. Friedman DS, Quigley HA, Gelb L, et al. Using pharmacy claims data to study adherence to glaucoma medications: methodology and findings of the Glaucoma Adherence and Persistency Study (GAPS). Invest Ophthalmol Vis Sci. 2007;48(11):5052–5057.
11. Schwartz GF, Platt R, Reardon G, Mychaskiw MA. Accounting for restart rates in evaluating persistence with ocular hypotensives. Ophthalmology. 2007;114:648–652.
12. Robin AL, Novack GD, Covert DW, Crockett S, Marcic T. Adherence in glaucoma: objective measurements of once-daily and adjunctive medication use. Am J Ophthalmol. 2007;144:533–540.
13. Robin AL, Stone JL, Sleath B, Covert DW, Cagle GD. An Objective Evaluation in Glaucoma Patients of Eye-Drop Instillation Using Video Observations and Patient Surveys. Abstract presented at

---

[†]Pang I, unpublished observation.
[‡]Clark AF, unpublished observation.

*American Glaucoma Society Annual meeting*, Washington DC, March 2008.
14. Tsai JC, McClure CA, Ramos SE, Schlundt DG, Pichert JW. Compliance barriers in glaucoma: a systematic classification. *J Glaucoma*. 2003;12:393–398.
15. Nordstrom BL, Friedman DS, Mozafarri E, Quigley HA, Walker AM. Persistence and adherence with topical glaucoma therapy. *Am J Ophthalmol*. 2005;140:598–606.
16. Covert D, Robin AL, Novack GD. Letter to the editor. Systemic medications and glaucoma patients. *Ophthalmology*. 2005;112(10): 1849–1850.
17. Covert D, Robin AL. Adjunctive glaucoma therapy use associated with travoprost, bimatoprost, and latanoprost. *Curr Med Res Opin*. 2006;22(5):971–976.
18. Robin AL, Covert D. Does adjunctive glaucoma therapy affect adherence to the initial primary therapy? *Ophthalmology*. 2005; 112:863–868.
19. Patel SC, Spaeth G. Compliance in patients prescribed eyedrops for glaucoma. *Ophthalmic Surg*. 2005;26(3):233–236.
20. Leske MC, Heijl A, Hyman L, et al. Predictors of long-term progression in the early manifest glaucoma trial. *Ophthalmology*. 2007;114:1965–1972.
21. Urquhart J. The drugs not taken. *Science*. 2008;321(5890):769.
22. Sleath B, Robin AL, Covert D, Byrd JE, Tudor G, Svarstad B. Patient-reported behavior and problems in using glaucoma medications. *Ophthalmology*. 2006;113:431–436.
23. Tsai T, Robin AL, Smith JP. An evaluation of how glaucoma patients use topical medications: a pilot study. *Trans Am Ophthalmol Soc*. 2007;105:29–35.
24. O'Connor DJ, Martone JF, Mead A. Additive intraocular pressure lowering effect of various medications with latanoprost. *Am J Ophthalmol*. 2002;133:836–837.
25. Higginbotham EJ, Feldman R, Stiles M, Dubiner H. Latanoprost and timolol combination therapy vs monotherapy: one-year randomized trial. *Arch Ophthalmol*. 2002;120:915–922.
26. Pfeiffer N. A comparison of the fixed combination of latanoprost and timolol with its individual components. *Graefes Arch Clin Exp Ophthalmol*. 2002;240:893–899.
27. Young TL, Higginbotham EJ, Zou XL, Farber MD. Effects of topical glaucoma drugs on fistulized rabbit conjunctiva. *Ophthalmology*. 1990;97:1423–1427.
28. Augustin AJ, D'Amico DJ, Mieler WF, Schneebaum C, Beasley C. Safety of posterior juxtascleral depot administration of the angiostatic cortisene anecortave acetate for treatment of subfoveal choroidal neovascularization in patients with age-related macular degeneration. *Graefes Arch Clin Exp Ophthalmol*. 2005;243(1):9–12.
29. Augustin A. Anecortave acetate in the treatment of age-related macular degeneration. *Clin Interv Aging*. 2006;1(3):237–246.
30. Russell SR, Hudson HL, Jerdan JA, Anecortave Acetate Clinical Study Group. Anecortave acetate for the treatment of exudative age-related macular degeneration – a review of clinical outcomes. *Surv Ophthalmol*. 2007;52(suppl 1):S79–S90.
31. Clark AF, Wilson K, deKater AW, Allingham RR, McCartney MD. Dexamethasone-induced ocular hypertension in perfusion-cultured human eyes. *Invest Ophthalmol Vis Sci*. 1995;36:478–489.
32. Wilson K, McCartney MD, Miggans ST, Clark AF. Dexamethasone induced ultrastructural changes in cultured human trabecular meshwork cells. *Curr Eye Res*. 1993;12(9):783–793.
33. Zhang X, Ognibene CM, Clark AF, Yorio T. Dexamethasone inhibition of trabecular meshwork cell phagocytosis and its modulation by glucocorticoid receptor beta. *Exp Eye Res*. 2007;84(2): 275–284.
34. Robin AL, Clark AF, Covert D, et al. Anterior juxtascleral delivery of anecortave acetate in eyes with primary open-angle glaucoma: a pilot investigation. *Am J Ophthalmol*. 2009;147:45–50.
35. Prata TS, Tavares IM, Mello PAA, Tamura CY, Belfort R Jr. Anterior juxtascleral depot of anecortave acetate: intraocular pressure reduction in different types of glaucoma. *Association for Research in Vision and Ophthalmology (ARVO)*; abstract 2008 E-1205, poster A47.
36. Callanan D, Fuller C, Landry TA, Dickerson JE, Bergamini MVW. Prophylactic anecortave acetate in patients with a retisert implant. *Association for Research in Vision and Ophthalmology (ARVO)* 2008; abstract 2008 E-5630.
37. Landry TA, Dickerson J, Merriam JC. The use of anecortave acetate for refractory, complex glaucoma. *Association for Research in Vision and Ophthalmology (ARVO) 2008*; abstract 1206/A48.
38. Robin AL, Suan EP, Sjaarda RN, Callanan DG, DeFaller J. Anecortave acetate lowers intraocular pressure in eyes with steroid injection-related glaucoma. *Arch Ophthalmol*. 2009;127:173–178.
39. Jonas JB, Kreissig I, Degenring R. Intraocular pressure after intravitreal injection of triamcinolone acetonide. *Br J Ophthalmol*. 2003;87:24–27.
40. Jonas JB, Degenring RF, Kreissig I, Akkoyun I, Kamppeter BA. Intraocular pressure elevation after intravitreal triamcinolone acetonide injection. *Ophthalmology*. 2005;112:593–598.
41. Challa JK, Gillies MC, Penfold PL, Gyory JF, Hunyor AB, Billson FA. Exudative macular degeneration and intravitreal triamcinolone: 18 month follow up. *Aust N Z J Ophthalmol*. 1998;26(4):277–281.
42. Wolner B, Liebmann JM, Sassani JW, Ritch R, Speaker M, Marmor M. Late bleb-related endophthalmitis after trabeculectomy with adjunctive 5-fluorouracil. *Ophthalmology*. 1991;98(7):1053–1060.
43. Higginbotham EJ, Stevens RK, Musch DC, et al. Bleb-related endophthalmitis after trabeculectomy with mitomycin C. *Ophthalmology*. 1996;103(4):650–656.
44. Solomon A, Ticho U, Frucht-Pery J. Late-onset, bleb-associated endophthalmitis following glaucoma filtering surgery with or without antifibrotic agents. *J Ocul Pharmacol Ther*. 1999;15(4):283-293.
45. DeBry PW, Perkins TW, Heatley G, Kaufman P, Brumback LC. Incidence of late-onset bleb-related complications following trabeculectomy with mitomycin. *Arch Ophthalmol*. 2002;120(3):297–300.
46. Ashkenazi I, Melamed S, Avni I, Bartov E, Blumenthal M. Risk factors associated with late infection of filtering blebs and endophthalmitis. *Ophthalmic Surg*. 1991;22(10):570–574.
47. Phillips WB 2nd, Wong TP, Bergren RL, Friedberg MA, Benson WE. Late onset endophthalmitis associated with filtering blebs. *Ophthalmic Surg*. 1994;25(2):88–91.
48. Poulsen EJ, Allingham RR. Characteristics and risk factors of infections after glaucoma filtering surgery. *J Glaucoma*. 2000;9(6):438–443.
49. Clark AF. Steroids, ocular hypertension, and glaucoma. *J Glaucoma*. 1995;4:354–369.
50. Gottanka J, Chan D, Eichhorn M, Lutjen-Drecoll E, Ethier CR. Effects of TGF-beta2 in persued human eyes. *Invest Ophthalmol Vis Sci*. 2004;45:153–158.
51. Fleenor DL, Shepard AR, Hellberg PE, Jacobson N, Pang IH, Clark AF. TGFbeta2-induced changes in the human trabecular meshwork: implications for glaucoma. *Invest Ophthalmol Vis Sci*. 2006;47:226–234.
52. Clark AF, Millar C, Pang I-H, Jacobson N, Shepard AR. Adenoviral gene transfer of active human transforming growth factor-b2 induces elevated intraocular pressure in rats. *2006 Annual Meeting Association for Research in Vision and Ophthalmology*. Abstract 4771.
53. Shepard AR, Millar JC, Pang IH, Jacobson N, Clark AF. Adenoviral gene transfer of active human transforming factor-b2 elevates intraocular pressure and reduces outflow facility in rodent eyes. In press.
54. Fleenor DL, Pang I-H, Clark AF. Regulation of PAI-1 protein in human trabecular meshwork cells. *2008 Annual Meeting Association for Research in Vision and Ophthalmology (ARVO)*, Abstract 1631.
55. Distelhorst JS, Hughes GM. Open-angle glaucoma. *Am Fam Physician*. 2003;67(9):1937–1944.

# Chapter 90
# Future Glaucoma Instrumentation: Diagnostic and Therapeutic

Kelly A. Townsend, Gadi Wollstein, and Joel S. Schuman

## 90.1 Why Improve Glaucoma Technology?

Glaucoma is a complex set of diseases that are based on a clinical diagnosis. There is no blood test that can provide a definitive diagnosis of glaucoma, and it is rare that a single diagnostic test can reveal the presence of glaucoma. More often a variety of information is necessary for glaucoma diagnosis. Fortunately, a wide array of data that can be obtained about this disease and medical technology and instrumentation continue to play important roles in the assessment of the glaucomatous disease state and its treatment. The current state of ocular imaging, functional assessment, and surgical treatment has been discussed in previous chapters. This chapter aims to go beyond that, to assess what needs still exist and how technologies could realistically help meet them.

Much of the future of glaucoma diagnostics focuses on obtaining precise reproducible quantitative objective measurements of glaucoma severity and progression, because current assessment is still highly subjective. Diagnostic instruments may never replace a trained glaucoma specialist, but might be able to provide consistent, clear objective information enabling the identification and treatment of the disease at the very early stages of glaucoma, and preventing the disease from progressing to the point of affecting the patient's vision.

As device development technology is able to produce smaller, more complex devices, the possibility of surgical treatment for glaucoma using micron-scale devices is expanding. Stent and shunt technology is developing rapidly far beyond initial uses in areas such as cardiology to uses in ophthalmology to improve aqueous outflow. Moreover, the development of surgical tools is enabling the incorporation of novel procedures. The pharmacokinetics of drug delivery is becoming better understood, leading to the possibility of extended, well-controlled release delivery systems for the eye. It may be possible that future devices are able to safely and reproducibly lower intraocular pressure, without the side effects and compliance problems inherent in medical treatments today.

The management of glaucoma will change as instrumentation designed to diagnose and treat it changes. In the ideal future, we would be able to detect and cure the disease before it causes any effects whatsoever, perhaps through genetic testing or other methods of diagnosis and gene therapy to repair or replace aberrant genetic code. It is understood that earlier treatments are more effective, and pose less risk of progression, with less intensive treatments necessary. This is becoming increasingly possible with new instruments and techniques, which can detect changes in the structure of the eye before functional loss occurs, such as imaging devices. As implants for treatment become available, and are smaller and easier to implement in patients, these techniques may help glaucoma patients move away from frequent tedious eye drops, which might be affected by adherence. The future of technology for glaucoma treatment and diagnosis will depend greatly on future research discovering the root causes and fundamental cures of the complex of diseases that is glaucoma.

## 90.2 How Can Current Techniques Be Improved, and What Shows Promise for the Future?

Measurement of intraocular pressure (IOP) is a valuable component of a standard ophthalmic examination, because IOP is a major causal risk factor for glaucoma and is the only proven treatable aspect of glaucoma. Unfortunately, the types of tonometry instruments most commonly used currently all have some inherent limitations that leave room for improvement in the future. Applanation tonometry requires corneal anesthesia, is difficult for use with uncooperative children, and is not suitable for patients with corneal irregularities due to the corneal contact necessary for this method. Pneumatonometry, which is essentially applanation tonometry as well, can be used in children – where it may provide a more accurate measurement than Goldmann tonometry – and in patients with irregular corneas. Applanation tonometry is significantly affected by corneal biomechanical properties including corneal thickness, stiffness, and elasticity. Air-puff tonometry is noncontact, but its accuracy is lower than the contact methods, and it is also affected by corneal stiffness. Transpalpebral tonometry does not require corneal contact, but it can be difficult to obtain a precise reproducible result with this technique. Schiotz tonometry, though rarely performed, is extremely portable, lightweight, and simple, but is highly susceptible to confounding by factors such as scleral rigidity and intraocular gas.

Electronic indentation tonometry, rebound tonometry, dynamic contour tonometry, and the Ocular Response Analyzer are newer techniques that are currently available, and they attempt to address some of the problems with other methods. Electronic indentation tonometry (Tono-Pen; Reichert, Inc., Depew, New York) is a form of applanation tonometry, using a strain gauge to electronically acquire IOP measurements, and is actually not new at all. The McKay–Marg tonometer of over 50 years ago was such a device, but is no longer available, and has been shrunken down to a small, portable handheld device in the form of the Tono-Pen. The advantage of the electronic indentation tonometry Tono-Pen device is that it can be used in a variety of positions on the subject because it is compact and lightweight. However, it is still subject to the same corneal property effects as other types of applanation tonometry, and accuracy and reproducibility are marginal. Rebound tonometry (iCare Tonometer; Tiolat Oy, Helsinki, Finland) also involves contact with the cornea, but rather than several seconds of applanation, an ultra-light probe touches the cornea gently for just a fraction of a second, so a more comfortable measurement can be taken, without the need for a topical anesthetic. Also, the device is portable, like the Tono-Pen and the tips are disposable, providing a sterile measurement easily in each patient. The small size of the contact area (this technique was originally designed for use on rats and mice) is another advantage, allowing for pressure measurement on a localized unaffected area of the cornea in the case of patients with corneal damage. The portability and ability to use it without anesthesia makes it more feasible for out-of-clinic monitoring of IOP. Rebound tonometry is also affected by corneal biomechanical properties, although possibly to a lesser degree than applanation tonometers.

Dynamic contour tonometry (DCT, Pascal; Ziemer Ophthalmic Systems AG, Port, Switzerland) attempts to minimize the effects of corneal confounding. DCT looks similar to Goldmann applanation tonometry, but rather than applying variable force, it applies a constant force. The contour of the device tip is concave with a radius of 10.5 mm and approximates the shape of the cornea. The pressure change on the sensor inside the tip is calculated as a change in the electrical resistance, and this corresponds to IOP. Once the tip is matched with the surface of the cornea, the device takes 800 measurements over 8 s to define an averaged IOP. By matching the tip to the cornea, this technique can reduce the effects of an individual's corneal properties. This is reflected by the fact that the "LASIK effect," where an individual's IOP is measured to be significantly lower post refractive surgery because of the change in corneal structure, is not present when DCT is used to measure IOP in contrast to the findings with Goldmann applanation tonometry[1]; however, other confounders do still exist that affect the accuracy of DCT's IOP measurements.

The Ocular Response Analyzer (ORA, Reichert, Inc., Depew, New York) calculates variables that describe corneal biomechanical properties in addition to calculating a cornea-compensated IOP. The ORA uses a pulse of air to depress the cornea inward to a slightly concave shape, and monitors the changing shape as the cornea flattens, then bounces back. The two pressures at which the cornea is applanated (flat) – as it moves inward, then back outward – are calculated, and the difference is used to define the corneal hysteresis. Figure 90.1 contains a graphical representation for this. The corneal hysteresis is defined by the viscoelastic properties of the cornea, which are believed to be a major factor affecting IOP measurement.[2] Using this information, the ORA provides a cornea-compensated IOP. This device also has the advantage of being noncontact with the cornea, since the corneal deformation is done by air.

One of the main problems of IOP monitoring clinically is that it consists of just a single measurement, often taken only once every three to 6 months. Because IOP can vary substantially throughout the day, these single measurements might not truly gauge how effectively a patient's glaucoma is managed. The ultimate IOP measuring device would be one that is not confounded by corneal properties, does not require corneal contact, and allows for continuous measurements.

### 90.2.1 Summary for the Clinician

- There are a wide variety of methods for measuring IOP, but many have the problem of being confounded by corneal biomechanical properties, and most rely on several seconds of corneal contact, which can be uncomfortable or difficult to perform in certain situations.
- Some methods (electronic indentation tonometry and rebound tonometry) are portable devices, which improves their flexibility.
- Dynamic Contour Tonometry and the Ocular Response Analyzer both attempt to adjust for certain corneal biomechanical properties, aiming to calculate IOP that is not confounded by the cornea.
- Rebound tonometry and the Ocular Response Analyzer minimize corneal contact, resulting in no need for anesthetic, while providing a more accurate measurement than conventional air-puff tonometry.

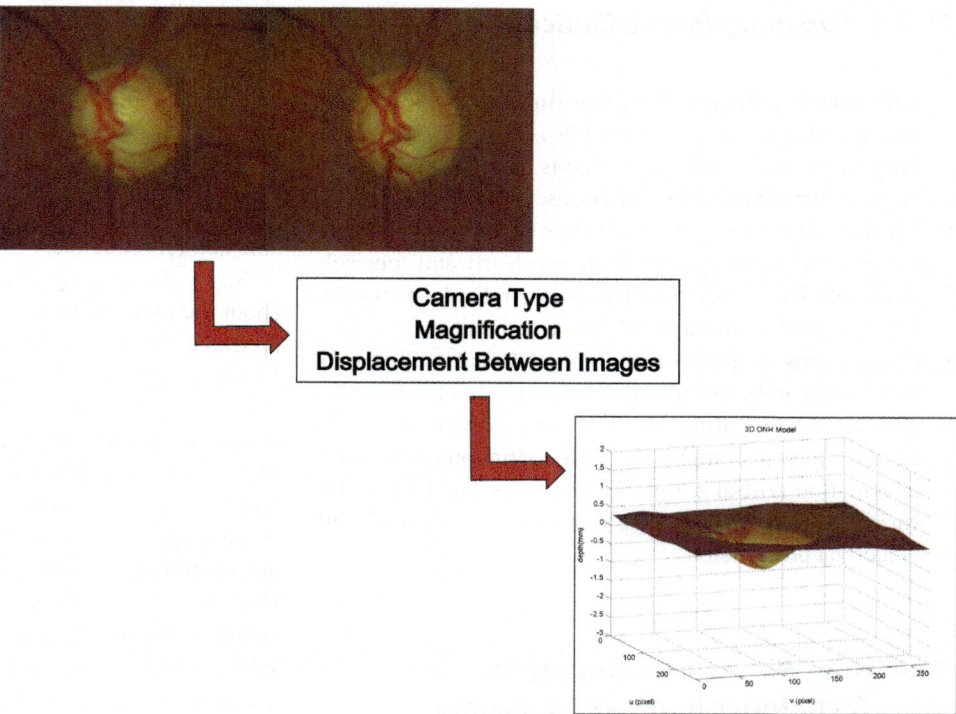

**Fig. 90.1** Three-dimensional rendering from stereo disc photographs. Using camera type, magnification, and distance between images as input information, the stereo photographs can be mathematically rendered to provide a 3D model of the optic nerve head, which can then be measured objectively

## 90.3 Is Continuous Management of IOP Possible Through Telemedicine?

The future of glaucoma IOP management would be an accurate, portable, easy-to-use device that could be purchased by glaucoma patients, or lent to them by their eye care professional, so that patients could self-monitor their IOP, similar to home monitoring for systemic hypertension. By recording frequent IOP measurements such technologies could provide much more detailed and useful information about IOP throughout the day and over time.

At this point, one such device has been developed and is clinically available, the Proview tonometer (Bausch and Lomb; Rochester, New York). It uses a unique approach of having a device that the person presses on their eyelid until they see a phosphene caused by the pressure of the device transpalpebrally and transsclerally mechanically stimulating the retina, and then the patient can read and record the pressure from the device. Its accuracy is substantially poorer than typical clinical measurement methods.[3] It is not the first or only home tonometer, but is one that is generally commercially available.

A unique approach to this problem of frequent IOP monitoring would be the use of a device incorporated into a contact lens or an implantable device that could transmit IOP data electronically to a detector, which could then record the information for the ophthalmologist. This would require less action by the patient and minimize the amount of human error in the measurements. One potential problem with patient self-monitoring is failure to comply fully with their treatment protocol if they are finding their IOP to be "normal." If measurements are recorded electronically for submission to the physician directly, patients might be less likely to have their compliance affected by their continuously monitored IOP. Also, tonometers can be difficult for many patients to use on their own correctly, so a method with minimal input needed from the patient would be of benefit.

The approach of incorporating IOP measurement into a contact lens has been tested to measure changes in corneal curvature with an imbedded micro strain gauge. A contact lens would be less invasive than an implant, which could be integrated into an intraocular lens placed during cataract surgery. However, the internally placed device would be less subject to corneal property changes, and could be more accurate because of measuring pressure directly, rather than the indirect method of measuring corneal curvature change. Initial development has been done with both techniques, but much more research is needed to make this technology safe, affordable, accurate, reproducible and comfortable in order for the device to be clinically feasible.[4]

These constant IOP monitoring devices will be very relevant for the future of glaucoma and of telemedicine in this field. Developing systems to get continuous IOP data cleanly and efficiently to physicians will be as difficult and important as developing the tonometer itself. With the large amounts of data that would be generated by a system like a continuous IOP monitor, it is vital for the information to be summarized clearly, whether graphically or otherwise, so physicians are not overwhelmed by lists of numbers and noisy data.

### 90.3.1 Summary for the Clinician

- IOP varies substantially over time so that a single measurement once every 6 months is not sufficient.
- The future will enable continuous IOP monitoring for more accurate assessment of disease and treatment.
- Telemedicine will provide a better way to provide continuous IOP monitoring information clearly and concisely to the clinician once an easy-to-use, reliable method is developed for continuous IOP measurement.
- Contact lens or intraocular implant based methods for monitoring and recording IOP information electronically will provide continuous IOP measures without the need for patient compliance. This continuous monitoring information will allow physicians to assess diurnal IOP variation and better manage risk factors associated with glaucoma progression.

## 90.4 How Will New Photographic Techniques Improve Glaucoma Diagnosis?

The most recent substantial changes in glaucoma instrumentation have come in the form of ocular imaging, and this continues to be a major area of research focus in the glaucoma field. This includes technologies ranging from stereoscopic disc photography, to scanning systems such as confocal scanning laser ophthalmoscopy, scanning laser polarimetry, and optical coherence tomography (OCT) in its various forms. Improvements are still being made in both the way these devices acquire images, and the way the data can be processed to gain more information.

Disc photographs were the earliest method available for objectively capturing an image of the optic nerve head as seen during clinical examination. While systems for capturing these images have become fairly standardized, there continues to be a need for a standard method of analyzing and quantifying the structures seen in these images. At this point assessment is subjective and variable, even when the disc photographs are read by expert observers.

The two main types of parameters that would be useful to quantify for glaucoma are retinal nerve fiber layer (RNFL) measurements and optic disc parameter measurements. Semi-quantitative scales have been developed to assess the amount of retinal nerve fiber defect in a disc photograph, but this is done manually by a trained physician examining the photograph, and is prone to inter-observer variability.[5-7] A method of quantitatively analyzing the amount of RNFL defect automatically has been proposed by Lee and associates using image processing techniques to locate the optic disc and plot the intensity of pixels around the disc.[8] The area of defect is then determined by comparing the intensity plot of the RNFL and the first derivative of the intensity plot. For clinical use, this and other methods of locating and quantifying the extent of RNFL defects must be established as reliable and reproducible.

Stereo disc photographs also hold substantial information about the optic nerve head, though automatic quantification is scarce due to the complexity of disc margin detection. Moreover, the variety of cameras used clinically, with a variety of displacements between the two images and changes in magnification further complicate disc parameter calculations. Much initial research has been done by Xu and Abramoff, among others, into modeling of the 3D disc structure, as well as peripapillary disc features such as blood vessels.[9,10] A demonstration of this process can be seen in Fig. 90.2. However, these methods still need improvement and stabilization, especially in the case of poorer quality images and subtle abnormalities, where current quantitative methods may not be sensitive enough to detect glaucomatous damage.

An important reason for developing a quantitative method for evaluating stereo disc photos is the large amount of legacy data available. Photography is the oldest and the most common technology for imaging the eye, so there is the potential of developing the most extensive longitudinal data with this modality. This gives researchers the largest data set to look at glaucomatous progression, and gives clinicians the most history for many of their patients. If a consistent, accurate method of quantifying this data can be applied, significant knowledge about the progression of the disease can be obtained.

### 90.4.1 Summary for the Clinician

- Optic disc photographs are the oldest objective method of recording the optic disc appearance, but clinical interpretation of them is primarily subjective.
- Quantification of nerve fiber layer defects objectively through image processing techniques holds potential for clinical use.
- Three-dimensional digital representation of the optic disc based on stereo-photographs could provide objective quantitative optic disc information.
- The use of photography with objective methods of analysis could provide the most extensive longitudinal information, because of photography's clinical use for a longer period of time than any other imaging technique.

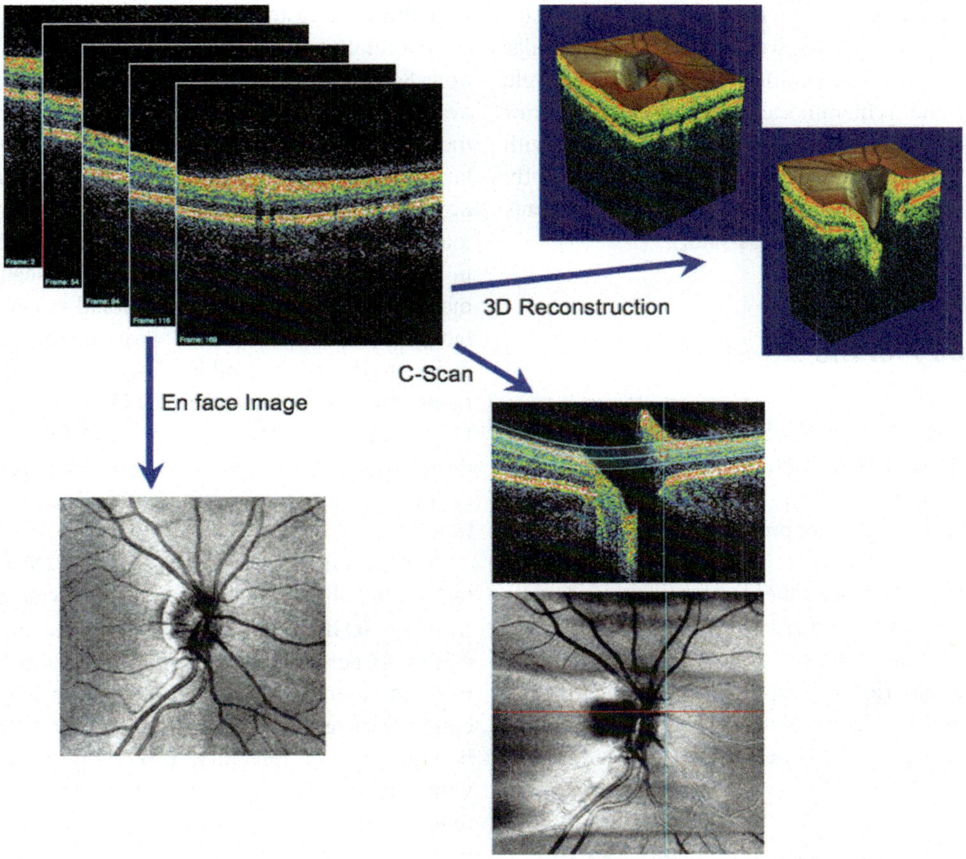

**Fig. 90.2** Three-dimensional optical coherence tomography data. The *upper left corner* represents five selected B-scans from a raster set consisting of 200 B-scans. These can be represented in a 3D reconstruction that can be sliced along any plane (*upper right* shows entire 3D reconstruction and reconstruction sliced through optic nerve head). Summing the intensities along each A-scan creates the en face image in the *lower left*. The 3D data set can also be used to show just a certain thickness along a chosen contour to isolate specific layers like the retinal nerve fiber layer (*lower right*). C-scan includes only data taken within the light blue region of the B-scan above it. The location of the B-scan within the 3D data set is the red line. The light blue line is currently identifying the *right side* of the disc margin at that B-scan

## 90.5 How Will Optical Coherence Tomography Provide New Anterior Segment Information?

Optical coherence tomography is an ocular imaging technique that has shown promise for a variety of important purposes in glaucoma and other eye diseases. In addition to the now common clinical use of time-domain OCT, spectral-domain OCT (SD-OCT) has quickly gained clinical popularity. OCT is being applied to the anterior eye, in addition to the more common retinal imaging use.

OCT has been used in the anterior eye since 1994,[11] but only recently has it been gaining common use clinically for evaluation of the cornea and anterior chamber, and for angle assessment in glaucoma cases. It has the advantage of being much more comfortable than ultrasound biomicroscopy (UBM) because it is noncontact, uses near-infrared light (which is invisible to the patient), able to acquire scans with the patient in a sitting position, and is able to provide a much higher resolution scan, though with lower penetration beyond the iris. This prevents imaging of the ciliary body, an important target tissue in many cases of glaucoma evaluation. However, the noncontact aspect of the OCT makes it more appropriate for imaging of filtering blebs or angle imaging just after surgery than UBM. It could also be of great benefit for use in children or other patients who might not be willing to undergo UBM.[12]

The primary clinical anterior segment specific OCT device currently available is the Visante OCT (Carl Zeiss Meditec, Dublin, California), a time domain system specifically for anterior eye imaging, with a longer wavelength light allowing for more penetration into the sclera and iris than would be available at the wavelengths typically used to image the retina. The future of anterior segment OCT is to move toward spectral domain devices for scanning, which would allow for faster scans with higher resolution. This would allow a near cellular level view of the cornea and detailed information on angle structures such as the Schlemm's canal. Currently, anterior segment spectral domain OCT is only possible clinically with add-on systems to retinal-based devices and are presently limited by the shorter wavelengths used by these instruments (~850 nm) compared to Visante (~1,310 nm).

### 90.5.1 Summary for the Clinician

- Anterior segment OCT is noncontact, and is therefore more comfortable and more suitable for patients just after surgery or for children.
- Anterior segment OCT also provides higher resolution than UBM.
- Anterior segment OCT lacks the depth of tissue penetration of UBM, making visualization of structures behind the iris difficult or impossible.
- Current clinical anterior segment OCT systems are time domain OCT, but the future is anterior segment spectral domain OCT, with improved speed and resolution.

## 90.6 How Does SD-OCT Improve Our Ability to Visualize Ocular Disease?

The primary advantage of using SD-OCT in either the anterior or posterior segment of the eye is the ability to acquire images with higher resolution (up to ~3.5 μm in the eye commercially available) and faster scanning speed (up to 55,000 A-scans/s commercially available) than the time domain OCT (resolution; 8–10 μm, scanning speed: 400 A-scan/s commercially available). This enables the development of new scanning modes such as 3D imaging that can be used to visualize ocular structures. However, because this iteration of the technology is new, software to fully utilize the data acquired by the machine, such as 3D visualization and segmentation, is still in its infancy. Inspecting individual B-scans is a sufficient method to look at the cross-sectional structure of the tissue, but visualization of specific tissue layers en face is difficult due to their contours and motion artifacts. Methods for alignment and registration of the 3D OCT scans may prove helpful in being able to sample the 3D OCT in any desirable direction and to view en-face or C-mode images. Visualization of the various forms of 3D OCT data can be seen in Fig. 90.3.

While producing images from the 3D OCT data is valuable, OCT holds the unique potential to provide quantifiable data from the 3D data set. For example, in the anterior segment, if a 3D scan across the entire anterior chamber is gathered, the relevant parameters regarding the angle 360° around the eye could be measured and summarized. This information could be displayed graphically, providing glaucoma specialists with quantifiable angle measurements that could be easily interpreted and used to identify optimal surgical sites, for example. Three-dimensional data sets of the retina provide a multitude of possibilities for segmentation leading to automated quantifiable information regarding the thickness of retinal layers, or other retinal landmarks, such as quantifying drusen in the macular degeneration, quantifying the intraretinal vasculature in the various retinal layers, or determining the geometry of the optic nerve head as it relates to glaucoma.

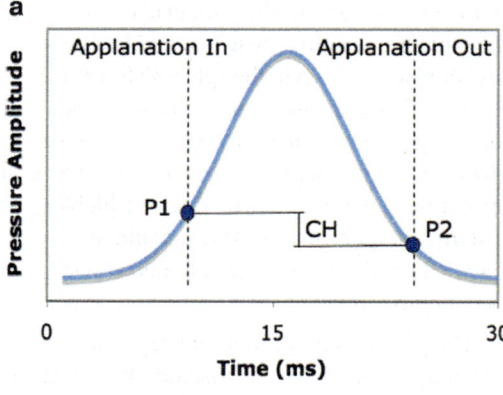
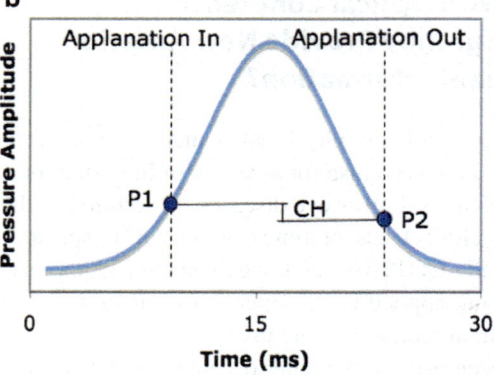

**Fig. 90.3** Corneal hysteresis measurement with the Ocular Response Analyzer. These graphs demonstrate how corneal hysteresis, a measurement of corneal viscoelastic properties, is calculated. Pressure is increased on the cornea smoothly by a pulse of air that indents the central cornea from convex to concave, followed by the cornea rebounding to convex. The two points where the cornea is applanated (*flat*) are found optically, and the pressure difference between them defines corneal hysteresis. (**a**) A graph of a typical healthy cornea. (**b**) A graph of a cornea post-LASIK surgery, where corneal hysteresis is reduced due to weakening of the cornea from flap creation during surgery, making it less capable of absorbing the energy of the air pulse. This weakening affects tonometry results. P1 = Pressure on cornea during applanation from convex to concave, P2 = Pressure on cornea during applanation from concave to convex, CH = corneal hysteresis

Currently, the segmentation and analysis of 3D SD-OCT data sets is a very important area of research in OCT. As segmentation algorithms improve, SD-OCT will provide clear thickness maps for the retinal layers corresponding to glaucoma damage. Another potential advantage of the 3D OCT dataset is the possibility to align one set of scans to another. This would enable highly reproducible measurement at exactly the same location between visits, thus improving the ability to detect even minute structural changes over time.

### 90.6.1 Summary for the Clinician

- SD-OCT is able to quickly create 3D data sets composed of hundreds of B-mode images, rather than just simple B-mode scans acquired with time-domain OCT.
- Software for visualization and interpretation of these 3D data sets is rapidly being developed.
- Segmentation and quantification methods will provide more accurate and reproducible clinically relevant information, enabling early diagnosis and detection of disease progression.

## 90.7 What Other OCT Techniques Have Been Developed for Research Use That May Become Clinically Relevant?

In addition to processing OCT data in new ways, there are several methods of acquiring OCT data in new ways that may have potential for future use in glaucoma. New optical techniques have been applied to SD-OCT, including swept-source imaging, adaptive optics, and the calculation of functional data such as blood flow and changes in reflectance of retinal layers due to light exposure. All of these may have future implications for glaucoma imaging. Swept-source OCT (SS-OCT), is a frequency-domain OCT method with some similarities to SD-OCT.[13] SD-OCT uses a broadband light source to acquire reflections across a variety of light wavelengths, where SS-OCT uses a single tunable light source that emits a single frequency at a time, which can be rapidly swept across a wide range of wavelengths. This method provides a much faster acquisition rate, more than 200,000 A-scans/s, as opposed to SD-OCT's rate of 55,000 A-scans/s. This allows for a much faster scan time and reduced motion artifacts. Because of the high sampling rate of SS-OCT, much more information can be acquired in a given amount of time. An OCT "snapshot" is feasible, or signal averaging can be performed in which multiple scans can be averaged to reduce the noise level and improve the signal. Currently, these systems are expensive and limited to axial resolution of around 10 μm because of technological limitations of the tunable laser and laser–tissue interactions. However, as tunable laser technology improves, the price and resolution will improve, and these devices may become clinically relevant.

SD-OCT is valuable clinically because of the large improvement in scanning speed it provides compared to time-domain OCT. However, transverse resolution in traditional SD-OCT systems is still limited, because of the natural aberrations in the cornea and lens affecting the reflections from the retina. The addition of adaptive optics to SD-OCT systems could help improve OCT transverse resolution in the future. Adaptive optics is the use of a wavefront sensor to identify these aberrations and then correct for them using deformable mirrors, similar to the technique used to image distant objects in astronomy. Adaptive optics has been used with OCT[14] as well as confocal scanning laser ophthalmoscopy[15] and fundus imaging,[16] and can provide sufficient transverse resolution to image photoreceptors in vivo.[17] There is hope that adaptive optics can provide sufficient resolution to visualize ganglion cell bodies, which are typically too small and transparent to see without adaptive optics. This could provide a method for more accurately assessing retinal neuron death because of glaucoma, by measuring actual cell body characteristics and loss rather than simply quantifying the degree of glaucoma damage based on the thinning of the RNFL. One caveat of adaptive optics is that only a small area can be scanned at a given time (e.g., 300 × 300 μm).

OCT and perhaps other imaging techniques will also provide the opportunity for monitoring functional aspects of the eye with glaucoma, including blood flow, aqueous outflow and retinal function. As discussed in previous chapters, retinal blood flow is believed to be relevant to many eye diseases including glaucoma. Doppler OCT is in the beginning stages of being established for clinically measuring ocular blood flow in real time and in vivo. As a better understanding of the parameters measured by Doppler OCT can be developed, it may become a valuable tool for measuring the rate and volume of blood flow in the eye at baseline and following interventions that affect blood flow. Aqueous outflow measurement is important for glaucoma, although Doppler measurement of the aqueous outflow system is much more complicated than measuring contained, primarily laminar flow in blood vessels. With further development of this technology, Doppler OCT assessment of flow may become clinically useful for glaucoma.

Initial research has been begun using the spectroscopic information gained by SD-OCT to examine the oxygenation of the retinal blood supply.[18] The red to infrared broadband light source allows the determination of the ratio of oxygenated to deoxygenated blood in the vessels, comparing reflectance at different wavelengths, using oximetric techniques.

The oxygenation of the blood in the retina may be relevant to glaucoma and other retinal diseases.

Another area of interest is functional OCT – gaining information about the function of the neural retina.[19] The reflectance of the retina increases when exposed to light. The reflectance changes in a predictable pattern, with the first responses occurring in the photoreceptor outer segments. This technology is in the very early stages, but it may be possible to map function across the retina in patients affected by glaucoma and other diseases affecting the retina. It should be noted that the change in signal is *very small* (10–15% of baseline amplitude) and it will need to be amplified into a more robust signal if this is to be clinically relevant, but the advantages of an objective, repeatable functional test would be significant.

### 90.7.1 Summary for the Clinician

- Swept source OCT is a technique that is similar to SD-OCT, but is able to acquire data substantially faster. SS-OCT axial resolution is limited by tunable laser technology and laser–tissue interactions to 10 μm.
- The incorporation of adaptive optics into SD-OCT systems can greatly improve transverse resolution by removing the effect of optical aberration in the lens and cornea, but limits the field of view.
- Doppler OCT can be used for measurement of retinal blood flow and aqueous outflow.
- Spectroscopic information from various wavelengths within the broad spectrum of SD-OCT can be used for oximetry.
- Changes in reflectance of the neural retina when exposed to light may be valuable in the clinical development of functional OCT.

## 90.8 Will Objective Measurements of Visual Field Be Possible?

Currently, the most common techniques for visual field assessment are not objective, but rather, use patient responses to map out the space in which they can see. Perimetry suffers from substantial inter-visit variability for each patient, resulting in significant difficulty in tracking or defining progression in a slowly developing disease like glaucoma. Changes to visual field protocols, such as decreasing the time of test taking, can decrease some of the variability, but the future calls for more objective methods.

Attempts to objectively measure the electrical signals of the functioning retina include multifocal electroretinography (ERG) and multifocal visual evoked potential (VEP). These tests provide an indication of the functional properties of the eye without the need of subjective input. ERG is gathered with electrodes on the cornea and around the eye, and the signal is processed to determine the responses corresponding to certain areas of the visual field. VEP maps the visual field based on the visually related cortical signals from electrodes placed on the scalp. Electrical noise due to poor electrode contacts, poor grounding, or ambient electrical sources can often affect the ERG output. The technician can minimize the first two during the examination, but the third issue means the ERG must be acquired in a room shielded from sources of 50/60 Hz electrical interference. Eye movement can also cause substantial errors, with inconsistent fixation causing smearing of the response between loci. VEP suffers from similar effects, with other complications inherent in the electroencephalogram process.

Smaller test targets and improvement in recording threshold level would allow the detection of localized damage and thus further improve the utility of these devices for glaucoma assessment. Using eye-tracking methods may alleviate some of the artifacts appearing because of the eye movement and allow for changing fixation, so the electrical signals can be processed with their dependence on the location of the subjects' fixation.

Imaging techniques may also provide potential for objective functional assessment of the eye. Besides the functional OCT optophysiology measurements discussed previously, a Retina Function Imager has been developed based on traditional fundus imaging technology, which uses the changes in the optical properties caused by the metabolic state of each specific area of the retina. Other optical methods have also been proposed for monitoring retinal changes, such as reflectance changes of photoreceptors during adaptive optics scanning laser ophthalmology.[20] Imaging methods may be more comfortable for the patient than the electrodes of ERG and VEP, and may provide better resolution, so this remains an important area of research for clinical glaucoma.

### 90.8.1 Summary for the Clinician

- Current visual field techniques are subjective and have substantial patient inter-visit variability.
- ERG and VEP provide an assessment of visual function. These methods are subject to several artifacts, such as electrical interference, movement, and poor electrode placement.
- Functional imaging techniques may someday be valuable for determining localized retinal function.

## 90.9 How Can All of the Diagnostic Data Be Combined into an Automated Diagnosis?

A primary purpose for recent advances in glaucoma diagnostic instrumentation is to provide a variety of valuable information to ophthalmologists who incorporate these results into a diagnosis. In order to differentiate between apparently conflicting results from different devices, ophthalmologists require substantial training and experience. The amount of information now available helps ophthalmologists make more educated decisions about a patient's glaucoma without as much subjective judgment as it required in the past, but there is not yet a cohesive method of knowing how to combine all the data available. Working toward systems for automated diagnosis will help solve this. A calculator that predicts the risk of developing glaucoma was introduced recently using demographic as well as clinical examination information. However, this method does not take into consideration the important information obtained by imaging devices that might substantially improve the performance of these calculators.

Automated diagnosis information based on comparison to a prior normative data set is already available individually for many glaucoma instruments. For example, Heidelberg Retina Tomography III (Heidelberg Engineering; Heidelberg, Germany) provides a Glaucoma Probability Score ranging from 0 to 1 based on a machine classifier algorithm, as well as Moorfields Regression Analysis and several Linear Discriminant Analysis parameters that are used to classify subjects as healthy or glaucomatous using multiple parameters. An example of the clinical representation of each these parameters can be seen in Fig. 90.4. OCT and visual field devices provide comparison to an age-matched normative database that can classify the subject as inside or outside normal limits.

The automated diagnosis given by each individual machine may provide results that contradict one another, and the physician must rely on experience to determine what the true situation is for their patient. It would be beneficial if a system were developed that could take the information from various devices (clinical and demographic information, visual fields and imaging results) and process the data to produce an estimation of the risk of glaucoma or its progression,

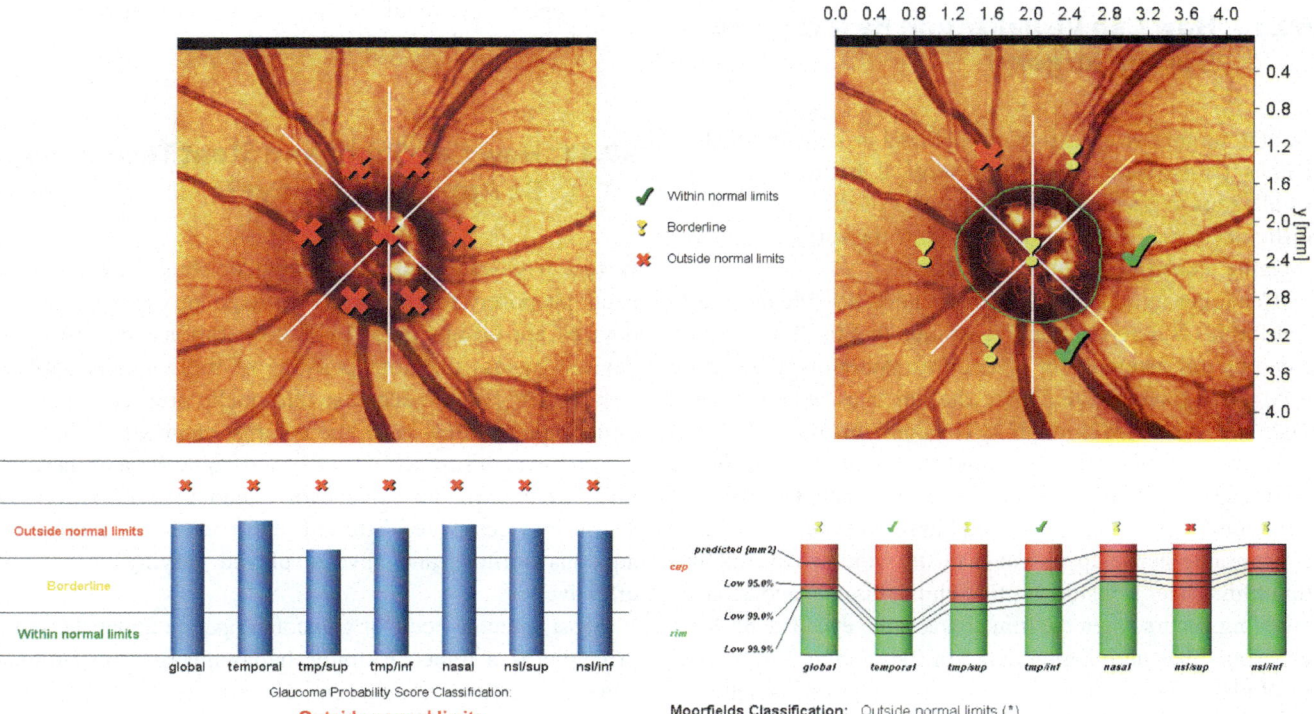

**Fig. 90.4** Single device automated diagnosis based on comparison to normative database. Heidelberg Retinal Tomography III software provides two primary methods for providing a diagnosis of inside normal limits, outside normal limits, or borderline. A glaucomatous patient's results are presented. Glaucoma Probability Score (GPS; *left*) is based on an automatically fit disc shape model independent of disc margin tracing. This patient is classified as outside normal limits overall and in all sectors, with a GPS value of 0.86 overall, indicating an 86% chance of this patient having glaucoma. (GPS value not shown.) The Moorfields Classification (*right*) is based on the operator-traced disc margin, and this patient shows a mixture of all three classifications overall and sectorally, with the final classification of outside normal limits

taking all information into account simultaneously. There is much more that must be learned about how different devices analyze data from the same person to know how a risk calculator should use and weigh information gained by each device. This system would have the advantage of standardizing diagnosis at an expert level.

### 90.9.1 Summary for the Clinician

- Automated diagnosis is already possible for individual diagnostic devices, through comparison to normative databases or discriminatory models based on experimental testing.
- Diagnostic devices may produce contradictory results, making interpretation by the clinician difficult without significant experience with each instrument.
- Future development of systems to integrate information from different devices into a unified multimodal glaucoma diagnostic analysis would be very beneficial.

## 90.10 How Can Visualization Be Improved During Surgery?

Ocular surgery is an extremely delicate process, with challenges far beyond many other surgical fields, due to the small, sensitive nature of the structures of the eye. It can be difficult for the surgeon to clearly view the surgical site, and imaging techniques may aid in this.

Canaloplasty (iScience Interventional; Menlo Park, California) is a new surgical technique that has been greatly aided by the development of an ultrasound probe that can be used during surgery to image the angle as an illuminated microcatheter is fed through it. The combination of the visualization using the ultrasound and the illuminated tip of the microcatheter enables identification and catheterization of Schlemm's canal. The ultrasound biomicroscopic device uses a disposable sterile tip with an acoustic window covered by a thin film. Water is inside this tip behind this cap, and acoustic coupling occurs when the film contacts the eye. The 85 MHz ultrasound has an imaging depth of 2–4 mm at 25-μm axial resolution. There is a tradeoff between depth of penetration and image resolution. The development of a handheld probe using other imaging technology, such as endoscopic imaging or OCT, would be beneficial for higher resolution imaging, either intraocularly though a small endoscope, or ab externo. Some progress has been made in the use of video endoscopy for imaging during goniotomy or cyclophotocoagulation, vitreoretinal surgery, or even intraorbital surgery.

In addition to imaging of the structure of the aqueous outflow system, the ability to image the aqueous flow and quantify it would be of benefit pre-, post-, and intra-operatively. This could give the surgeon information that could lead to surgical modification while the procedure is conducted, such as collector channel location and Schlemm's canal function. Doppler ultrasound and OCT may hold potential for feedback to surgeons with visualization of flow. Currently, Doppler ultrasound and OCT has been used on ocular blood vessels,[21] which are simpler to assess because of their larger size and velocity, but it may be possible to measure flow along Schlemm's canal as technology improves.

### 90.10.1 Summary for the Clinician

- An ocular ultrasound system has been developed for use during surgery, without use of a water bath for acoustic coupling as in traditional UBM.
- Endoscopic imaging or development of a handheld OCT probe could also aid visualization during surgery in the future.
- Imaging of the aqueous outflow system during surgery or perioperatively could help in assessing surgical sites, technique, and outcome.

## 90.11 How Can Shunt and Stent Technology Be Applied to the Eye?

In recent years, a variety of stent or shunt devices have been proposed for aqueous drainage procedures. These devices are designed for bypass operations, but different devices bypass different portions of the aqueous outflow system. They aim to decrease intraocular pressure by facilitating aqueous flow from the anterior chamber to the sub-conjunctival or suprachoroidal space; some devices increase flow directly to the eye's own aqueous outflow system. These devices take different approaches to increasing aqueous outflow, and have displayed varying degrees of effectiveness.

Most shunt devices for glaucoma operate under the same principle as a trabeculectomy, bypassing the conventional aqueous outflow system entirely (trabecular meshwork, Schlemm's canal, and the collector channels), diverting fluid from the anterior chamber into the sub-conjunctival space to form a filtration bleb. For example, the Ex-PRESS Miniature Glaucoma Device (Optonol Ltd., Neve Ilan, Israel) is a stainless steel, less than 3-mm-long, 400-μm-diameter (27 gauge) tube, which acts as a shunt. The implant is placed under a scleral flap, with the tip penetrating into the anterior chamber.

The structure of the device and its ocular placement can be seen in Fig. 90.5a. It has been found to have similar IOP-lowering effects to trabeculectomy.[22] There is potential for tube erosion resulting in the need for device removal, and complications are more common in advanced, complicated glaucoma cases. Other shunts include the Ahmed Glaucoma Valve (New World Medical, Inc., Rancho Cucamonga, California), which attempts to use a valve system to control outflow, the Baerveldt Glaucoma Drainage Device (Pfizer, Inc., New York, New York), the Molteno Implant (Molteno Ophthalmic Ltd, Dunedin, New Zealand) and others are also continually undergoing improvement to provide sufficient IOP lowering with minimal hypotony and other complications.

The SOLX Gold Shunt (SOLX, Inc., Waltham, Massachusetts) bypasses the trabecular meshwork, Schlemm's canal, collector channels and aqueous veins, and uses an approach designed to bring aqueous from the anterior chamber to the suprachoroidal space. It is a flat plate-shaped device made of gold, with multiple micro-tubular channels and perforations. The device and its placement can be seen in Fig. 90.5b. The natural pressure differential between these two areas maintains the flow across the device. As one of the newest glaucoma devices, its efficacy is not yet established in published literature.

The iStent (Glaukos Corp, Laguna Hills, California) trabecular bypass stent uses a different approach to reduce resistance to aqueous outflow by providing a direct conduit between the anterior chamber and Schlemm's canal, avoiding the resistance of the trabecular meshwork and inner wall of Schlemm's canal. The device and its placement can be seen in Fig. 90.5c. This device must be placed carefully to avoid dislocation, and there is little literature to date regarding the utility of the device, but initial results seem promising.[23]

All of these devices have the approach of structurally altering the aqueous outflow pathway in order to reduce IOP. One of the aims of using a glaucoma implant device per se is to effect a more consistent surgical procedure with less variability in outcome between surgeons and fewer postoperative complications and side effects. One specific stent or shunt may not work as effectively in all patients. The future of these surgical implants may be that they will be adjustable allowing for tailoring the device for each patient's needs, such as changing the diameter of the channels or tube. Adjustable stents and shunts are becoming more common in cardiology.

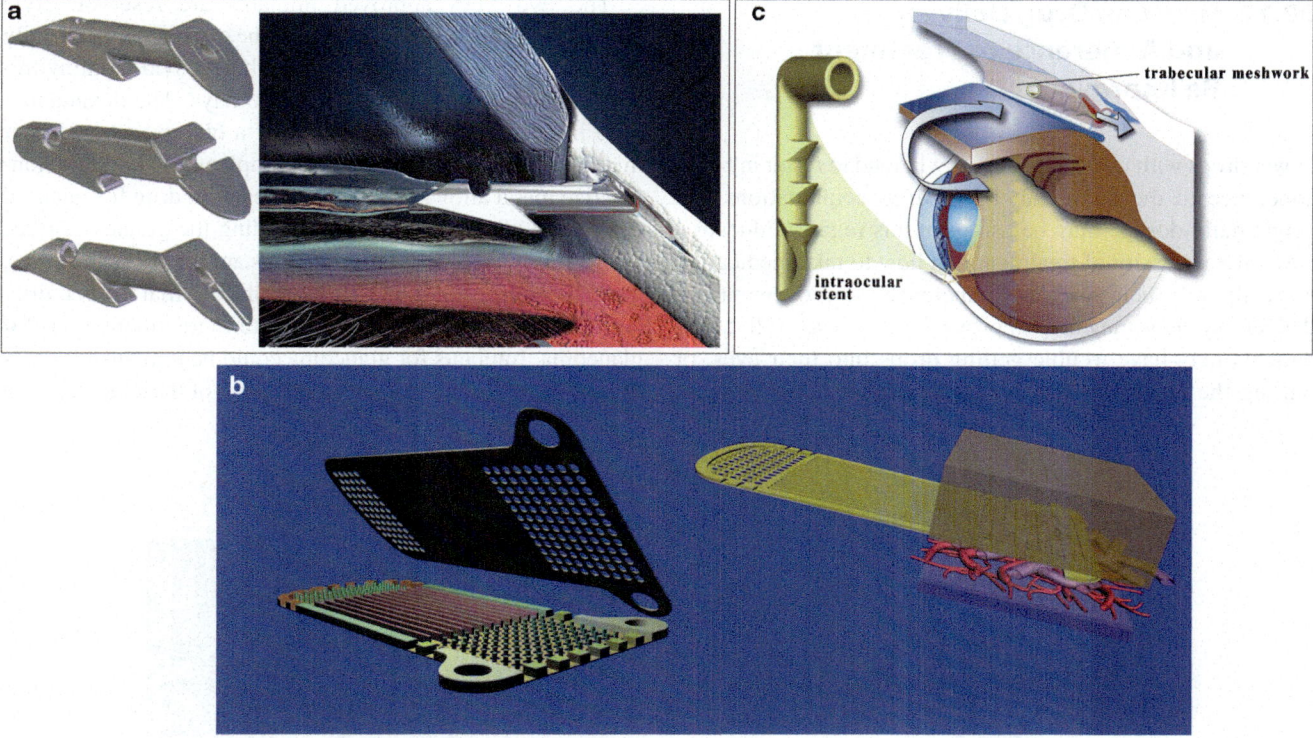

**Fig. 90.5** Glaucoma Stents and Shunts. (**a**) The Ex-PRESS Miniature Glaucoma Implant allows flow from the anterior chamber to the suprachoroidal space. Three slightly different versions are available, depending on the surgical needs. (Optonol Ltd, Neve Ilan, Israel.) (**b**) The SOLX Gold Shunt, which bridges the anterior chamber and suprachoroidal space with microchannels. (SOLX, Inc., Waltham, Massachusetts.) (**c**) The iStent allows flow to bypass the resistance of the trabecular meshwork by creating a direct connection between the anterior chamber and Schlemm's Canal. (Glaukos Corporation, Laguna Hills, California)

Drug eluting stents are an example of tools in another field of medicine that might be relevant to glaucoma technology development. Many of the drug-eluting stents designed for use in coronary arteries are treated with a drug that prevents cell growth and scarring, which can reocclude the vessel. Wound healing is a major issue in glaucoma surgery and this technology could be relevant for the eye.

An ultimate drainage device will be small and simple and would require minimal surgical skills. It would have no complications, including hypotony and infection. The device should be tunable so it can be adjusted to the needs of each patient and the desired level of intraocular pressure.

### 90.11.1 Summary for the Clinician

- A variety of stent and shunt devices are becoming available for clinical trials to help improve glaucoma surgical outcomes by allowing more controlled aqueous outflow.
- Adjustable and drug eluting stent technology that is currently available in cardiac and vascular surgery medicine may someday be applicable to ocular shunt or stent devices.

## 90.12 How Can Drug Delivery and Adherence to Treatment Be Improved?

Fewer drops with fewer side effects will tend to result in better adherence to the treatment. Fixed drug combinations and single daily dosage may be useful in this regard. Education about the necessity of treatment and how to take medication correctly can help increase adherence. Improvements in delivery systems may help improve adherence as well. Many patients may have trouble getting drops into their eyes, or putting the correct number of drops in their eyes. A more accurate method of dispensing eye drops, such as a spray or change in the shape of the dispenser, may aid in this. Electronic monitoring devices attached to the bottle may also help increase adherence to treatment with timely reminders for the patient and tracking of drug use.

Sustained drug delivery implants may serve as a method for getting glaucoma medications directly into the eye with improved treatment adherence and efficiency as compared to daily self-medication with drops. Intravitreal controlled release devices have been developed and FDA approved for cytomegalovirus retinitis and uveitis (Vitrasert and Retisert; Bausch & Lomb, Rochester, New York), and other devices are being developed for intravitreal placement, including a bioerodable dexamethasone implant for persistent macular edema (Allergan; Irvine, California) and a helical coil containing triamcinolone for diabetic macular edema (SurModics: Eden Prarie, Minnesota). Figure 90.6 contains images of the Retisert device as well as the approximate scale of it. Similar devices for sustained release delivery of IOP lowering medications such as prostaglandin analogs, beta-adrenergic receptor antagonists, or Alpha2-adrenergic agonists, or potentially neuroprotective or ocular blood flow stimulating agents could be beneficial in glaucoma. Ocular stents could also act as a platform for controlled-release drug delivery that would improve patient adherence.

The two FDA approved implants are reservoir style implants, which are possible due to the extremely small daily drug doses needed to be effective when provided intravitreally, allowing for use for up to 1,000 days. The dexamethasone implant is made up entirely of a bioerodable polymer mixed with drug. The helical coil implant is made of a nonreactive metal alloy that can be coated with drug for released delivery, with the helical coil providing the greatest surface area for drug coating. These implants are for retinal diseases, not glaucoma, but raise the possibility that direct drug delivery could be possible as a long-term treatment mode for glaucoma. Implants for glaucoma could be implanted intravitreally or in the anterior segment. Some of these devices can

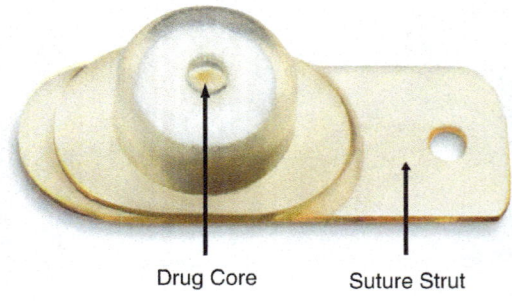
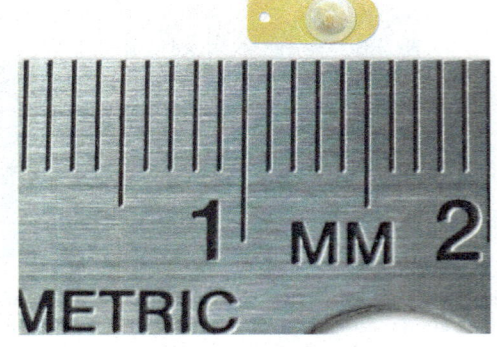

**Fig. 90.6** Bausch & Lomb Retisert. This drug-delivery implant is used to treat chronic non-infectious uveitis affecting the posterior segment of the eye. A scale is provided to identify the size of the device. (Bausch & Lomb, Rochester, New York)

be inserted into the eye fairly simply through a paracentesis. This could lead to simpler treatments compared with complex eye drop routines, with fewer complications compared to more invasive surgeries.

Patients with chronic, slowly progressing diseases like glaucoma may have poor adherence to medical treatment because they have a frequently asymptomatic disease and are being asked to take medication that causes symptoms. Patients tend to underestimate the severity of their disease until it has substantially progressed, and in a disease such as glaucoma where the damage is irreversible which poses a significant treatment challenge.

### 90.12.1 Summary for the Clinician

- There are several devices that could help improve adherence with medical treatment, including devices to improve drop delivery and electronic monitors to track compliance.
- Ocular sustained release implants have been developed and are available for certain diseases, and this technology may be helpful for glaucoma drug delivery as well.
- Sustained release devices could improve patient adherence by replacing or decreasing the need for eye drops.

## 90.13 How are New Surgical Tools Enabling New Surgical Techniques?

Recently new surgical tools have been developed that allow for surgical procedures previously impossible with conventional ophthalmic surgical devices. These new tools allow for site-specific interventions in the anterior chamber of the eye to provide greater aqueous outflow, by using micron-scale operating instruments.

The iTrack Microcatheter (iScience Interventional, Menlo Park, California) mentioned previously combines an optical fiber with a polymer tube, strengthened by a support wire, to create a catheter with a tip illuminated for transscleral visualization, and can be used to deliver ophthalmic substances through the lumen. The tip and shaft are designed specifically to prevent tissue damage or trauma in the eye, and its flexibility allows the catheter to be fed 360° around Schlemm's canal during the canaloplasty. Initial clinical study of this new technique has so far been promising as a safe and effective procedure.[24]

The Trabectome (NeoMedix Inc., Tustin, California) is another device that has enabled a new type of surgery for open-angle glaucoma. It is used to perform an ab interno trabeculectomy, with removal of a section of the trabecular meshwork and inner wall of Schlemm's canal using electrocautery. Through its microtip, which incorporates the electrode, irrigation, and aspiration systems together, it is able to coagulate and clear tissue minimally invasively. The device and its positioning during use can be seen in Fig. 90.7. A curved protective footplate that prevents damage to surrounding tissues, as well as guiding the tip along Schlemm's canal, protects the outer wall. Use of this technique has been shown to produce a patent opening into Schlemm's canal with removal of the trabecular meshwork unlike goniotomy.[25] This has translated clinically into subjects with moderate IOP reduction and a reduction in the need for medication postoperatively. Many of the complications seen with trabeculectomy have not been seen with this technique, and the use of this technique does not preclude trabeculectomy if the initial ab interno trabeculectomy procedure is not successful in lowering the IOP sufficiently.[26]

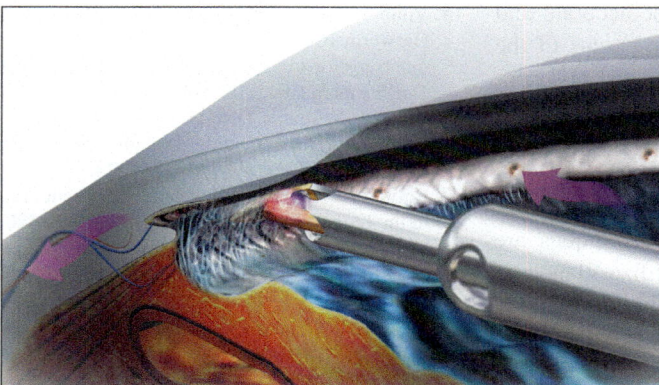
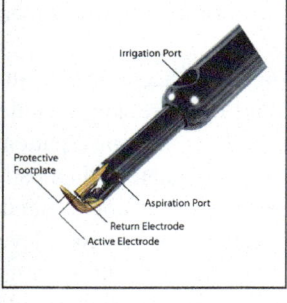

**Fig. 90.7** Trabectome. This glaucoma surgical device uses electrocauterization of the trabecular meshwork and inner wall of Schlemm's canal to increase aqueous outflow facility and decrease IOP. The structure of the tip (*right*) also incorporates irrigation and aspirations ports to clear away the cauterized area. The protective footplate is fed along Schlemm's canal to prevent damage to the outer wall of the canal itself while the current between the electrodes ablates trabecular and inner wall tissue (*left*). (NeoMedix Inc. Tustin, California)

Both of these new surgical instruments demonstrate the potential for newly developed devices to provide novel surgical techniques. The primary progression toward the future of glaucoma surgical devices will probably not be devices to aid in current common surgical techniques such as trabeculectomy, but rather to develop new devices that can provide new surgical options. Developing new, safer, more effective ways of decreasing IOP and protecting the optic nerve is an important task for the future, and as micro-manufacturing processes improve, we can expect a trend toward even less invasive and more controlled and precise surgical procedures.

### 90.13.1 Summary for the Clinician

- Standard surgical procedures typically have standard tools that are not being actively modified for the future.
- The future of the development of new surgical tools is to allow new surgical procedures that are otherwise not possible without these devices.

## 90.14 Conclusion

- Technological devices for the diagnosis and treatment of glaucoma are being developed and improved upon continuously.
- Intraocular pressure measurement techniques are needed that are less invasive, more accurate, less dependent on corneal thickness and ocular biomechanical properties, and available to the patient for home monitoring. Ideally, IOP measurement devices would provide measurements over 24 h, like a Holter monitor for the eye.
- The future of ocular imaging is to provide accurate and reproducible objective quantitative measurements of the structure and function of both the anterior and posterior segments of the eye.
- Objective methods for accurately evaluating a patient's visual field would be extremely beneficial for assessing ocular function and for tracking a patient's progression.
- Telemedicine and automated diagnostic techniques are computerized systems that could standardize glaucoma diagnosis and treatment at an expert level in the future.
- Development of implants for improving aqueous outflow and drug delivery may advance glaucoma surgical techniques.
- New surgical instruments are enabling surgical techniques that were previously difficult or impossible.

## References

1. Kaufmann C, Bachmann LM, Thiel MA. Intraocular pressure measurements using dynamic contour tonometry after laser in situ keratomileusis. *Invest Ophthalmol Vis Sci.* 2003;44:3790–3794.
2. Broman AT, Congdon NG, Bandeen-Roche K, Quigley HA. Influence of corneal structure, corneal responsiveness, and other ocular parameters on tonometric measurement of intraocular pressure. *J Glaucoma.* 2007;16:581–588.
3. Alvarez TL, Gollance SA, Thomas GA, et al. The Proview phosphene tonometer fails to measure ocular pressure accurately in clinical practice. *Ophthalmology.* 2004;111:1077–1085.
4. Detry-Morel M. Update in tonometry. Phosphene and rebound tonometries, self-tonometry and technologies for the future. *Bull Soc Belge Ophtalmol.* 2007;303:87–95.
5. Niessen AG, van den Berg TJ. Evaluation of a reference set based grading system for retinal nerve fiber layer photographs in 1941 eyes. *Acta Ophthalmol Scand.* 1998;76:278–282.
6. Niessen AG, van den Berg TJ, Langerhorst CT, Bossuyt PM. Grading of retinal nerve fiber layer with a photographic reference set. *Am J Ophthalmol.* 1995;120:577–586.
7. Sommer A, Quigley HA, Robin AL, Miller NR, Katz J, Arkell S. Evaluation of nerve fiber layer assessment. *Arch Ophthalmol.* 1984;102:1766–1771.
8. Lee SY, Kim KK, Seo JM, et al. Automated quantification of retinal nerve fiber layer atrophy in fundus photograph. *Conf Proc IEEE Eng Med Biol Soc.* 2004;2:1241–1243.
9. Abramoff MD, Alward WL, Greenlee EC, et al. Automated segmentation of the optic disc from stereo color photographs using physiologically plausible features. *Invest Ophthalmol Vis Sci.* 2007;48:1665–1673.
10. Xu J, Chutatape O, Sung E, Zheng C, Chew Tec Kuan P. Optic disk feature extraction via modified deformable model technique for glaucoma analysis. *Pattern Recognit.* 2007;40:2063–2076.
11. Izatt JA, Hee MR, Swanson EA, et al. Micrometer-scale resolution imaging of the anterior eye in vivo with optical coherence tomography. *Arch Ophthalmol.* 1994;112:1584–1589.
12. Ishikawa H. Anterior segment imaging for glaucoma: OCT or UBM? *Br J Ophthalmol.* 2007;91:1420–1421.
13. Choma MA, Hsu K, Izatt JA. Swept source optical coherence tomography using an all-fiber 1300-nm ring laser source. *J Biomed Opt.* 2005;10:44009.
14. Hermann B, Fernandez EJ, Unterhuber A, et al. Adaptive-optics ultrahigh-resolution optical coherence tomography. *Opt Lett.* 2004;29:2142–2144.
15. Vilupuru AS, Rangaswamy NV, Frishman LJ, Smith EL 3rd, Harwerth RS, Roorda A. Adaptive optics scanning laser ophthalmoscopy for in vivo imaging of lamina cribrosa. *J Opt Soc Am A Opt Image Sci Vis.* 2007;24:1417–1425.
16. Liang J, Williams DR, Miller DT. Supernormal vision and high-resolution retinal imaging through adaptive optics. *J Opt Soc Am A Opt Image Sci Vis.* 1997;14:2884–2892.
17. Roorda A, Williams DR. The arrangement of the three cone classes in the living human eye. *Nature.* 1999;397:520–522.
18. Kagemann L, Wollstein G, Wojtkowski M, et al. Spectral oximetry assessed with high-speed ultra-high-resolution optical coherence tomography. *J Biomed Opt.* 2007;12:041212.
19. Srinivasan VJ, Wojtkowski M, Fujimoto JG, Duker JS. In vivo measurement of retinal physiology with high-speed ultrahigh-resolution optical coherence tomography. *Opt Lett.* 2006;31:2308–2310.
20. Grieve K, Roorda A. Intrinsic signals from human cone photoreceptors. *Invest Ophthalmol Vis Sci.* 2008;49:713–719.
21. Bower BA, Zhao M, Zawadzki RJ, Izatt JA. Real-time spectral domain Doppler optical coherence tomography and investigation

of human retinal vessel autoregulation. *J Biomed Opt.* 2007;12: 041214.
22. Maris PJ Jr, Ishida K, Netland PA. Comparison of trabeculectomy with Ex-PRESS miniature glaucoma device implanted under scleral flap. *J Glaucoma.* 2007;16:14–19.
23. Spiegel D, Wetzel W, Haffner DS, Hill RA. Initial clinical experience with the trabecular micro-bypass stent in patients with glaucoma. *Adv Ther.* 2007;24:161–170.
24. Lewis RA, von Wolff K, Tetz M, et al. Canaloplasty: circumferential viscodilation and tensioning of Schlemm's canal using a flexible microcatheter for the treatment of open-angle glaucoma in adults: interim clinical study analysis. *J Cataract Refract Surg.* 2007;33: 1217–1226.
25. Francis BA, See RF, Rao NA, Minckler DS, Baerveldt G. Ab interno trabeculectomy: development of a novel device (Trabectome) and surgery for open-angle glaucoma. *J Glaucoma.* 2006;15: 68–73.
26. Minckler DS, Baerveldt G, Alfaro MR, Francis BA. Clinical results with the Trabectome for treatment of open-angle glaucoma. *Ophthalmology.* 2005;112:962–967.

# Chapter 91
# What Really Causes Glaucoma?

John R. Samples

Glaucoma can be defined in many different ways, as evidenced in this text. The most common definition is based on anatomy and pressure, with open angle glaucoma being most common among Caucasians in North America, low or normal tension glaucoma being most common among the Japanese, and angle closure being most common among other Asians. (Such clear delineations are not currently recognized in other ethnic groups.) Certain regions of the world give rise to the special circumstances of exfoliation. In the U.S., I am continually surprised with the discovery of new geographic foci of exfoliation. Regionally, it has been recognized for decades that exfoliation has a higher than normal prevalence in the greater Minneapolis area and around Minnesota – it is likely that this is due to the large number of individuals of Scandinavian descent. A week before writing this, I found out that exfoliation was also very common in the Salt Lake City area, where again northern European heritage is considered the causal factor. The genetics of exfoliation may eventually be studied more extensively in the geographic areas that are most highly affected. Ultimately, what really causes glaucoma is likely to be defined in genetic terms, just as exfoliation (but not necessarily exfoliative glaucoma) has been. Risk factors and "environmental factors," as enumerated in the first chapters of this text, will always be important and have an impact upon the susceptible eye.

The following list represents 16 hypotheses of high pressure primary open angle glaucoma. It is in no way "the definitive list"; I am continually changing it, adding to it, and subtracting from it. It is presented as a starting place for clinicians to begin to delve into the cell biology of glaucoma. Interestingly, as one reads through this list, one discovers that most of them are not mutually exclusive. To the contrary, most of the ideas come together and achieve a certain amount of confluence.

## 91.1 16 Hypotheses of High Pressure Open Angle Glaucoma

1. *Trabecular cells age poorly.* Drs. Alvarado[1,2] and Grierson[3,4] put forth the hypotheses that trabecular cell numbers decrease in open angle glaucoma; that the trabecular meshwork has about 200,000–300,000 cells, and cell death occurs with aging and is increased with glaucoma. It may well be that "stem cells" or the cells responsible for replacing dead or lost trabecular cells are less able to move into the juxtacanalicular meshwork with age, and hence there is a decrease in the number of cells. Trabecular cells are capable of mitosis, and it is likely that replacement takes place in the aging eye. Trabeculoplasty, reviewed in this text by Gaasterland in Chap. 61, stimulates trabecular mitosis.
2. *Oxidation and "Senescence" of trabecular cells.* Dr. Dave Epstein[5,6] has called attention to the potential oxidation of trabecular cells and proposed that glaucoma be treated with a reducing agent: Ethacrynic acid. More recently, he has put emphasis on the notion of senescence of trabecular cells.
3. *Myocilin GLC1A.*[7] The story of the discovery of the first glaucoma gene and the phenotypic variability of its various mutations has been an exciting one (see Chap. 9). There are numerous interesting hypotheses for how myocilin is involved in glaucoma; it remains a mystery that it is steroid-induced, but steroids do not really seem directly related to the abnormal gene product.
4. *Optineurin GLC1E.* The GLC1E story, which appeared in *Science* in 2002, is the second gene that was identified for open angle glaucoma[8] (see Chap. 9). As of this writing, there are still widely varying estimates about its frequency in the population, none of which are published. Much remains to be learned about frequency and the actual number of mutations.
5. *Other glaucoma genes.* For the open-angle loci, genes remain to be found. The table in the genetics chapter (Chap. 9, Table 9.1 *Selected Genes and Their Loci*) is likely to become antiquated very quickly. The clinical relevance of single nucleotide polymorphisms and other gene associations with glaucoma are still not worked out. It is likely that susceptibility gene studies will provide us with a new understanding of the disease. Studies with transcription factor chips, soon to be available, may profoundly change our understanding of glaucoma.

6. *Cell stress.* In one sense, open angle glaucoma is about stress for both the optic nerve and the trabecular meshwork. Drs. Joel Schuman[9] and Paul Knepper[10] have both pointed this out. A cellular stress model of glaucoma is important in a biological sense because it can lead to a different perspective on treatment. Perhaps nutritional therapy can alleviate cellular stress (see Chaps. 56 and 60). Personally, I recommend fish oil, zinc, and ascorbic acid (except prior to surgery) to each of my patients. Occasionally, I also recommend resveratrol to patients, though I regard this as an area deserving further investigation.[11] Each of us has to look at the literature and which recommendations we are comfortable with and which seem to be rational. It is unlikely that an expensive multicenter trial will ever be funded to evaluate nutritional therapies for glaucoma. Such clinical trials would be prohibitively expensive.
7. *Ferritin abnormalities.*[12] Quantitatively, H and L chains of ferritin appear to be the types of messenger RNA that are most elevated as a result of cellular injury or stimulation in the meshwork. This may be a non-specific injury response of the eye; further investigation is merited to fully understand the causality and implications.
8. *CD44 toxic to trabecular cells.* The finding that sCD44 is elevated in open angle glaucoma and is cytotoxic to both trabecular cells and retinal ganglion cells is reviewed in Chap. 83 by Dr. Paul Knepper, who has devoted many years to this finding.[13] This story is appealing because of the complete connection it provides between a protein that is elevated in glaucoma and its potential direct connection to causal mechanisms in glaucoma.
9. *Interleukin-1 (IL1) autocrine loop disruption.* IL1 receptors are found in the trabecular meshwork; they appear to be an important cell signal in the eye.[14] Early work injecting IL1 into the eye as a human recombinant protein suggested that it would not be a useful therapeutic agent.[15] Later, we found that it was one of the several signals produced by laser trabeculoplasty and that it seemed to antagonize some of the effects of corticosteroids on the delicate balance of matrix metalloproteinases and their inhibitor.[16,17] IL1 was also implicated in a glaucoma story by Shuman.[9,18]
10. *Stretch theory.* Dr. Acott has pointed out that stretch mechanisms exist on trabecular cells and that they are absolutely essential for cellular function.[19,20] Specifically, he believes that IOP homeostasis is achieved by extracellular matrix turnover, which is modulated by stretch. Changes in IOP are perceived by juxtacanalicular trabecular meshwork cells as mechanical stretch and distortion of their extracellular matrix (ECM). The effects of stretch in the meshwork have been demonstrated to alter ECM turnover, both biosynthesis and degradation. As pointed out in Chap. 34 Sidebar 34.2, the proteoglycan versican is a prime target for the outflow resistance and may be a therapeutic target.
11. *Tubules in Schlemm's canal.* Dr. Johnstone has written about the tubules in Schlemm's canal since the early 1970s, and how their dysfunction may lead to elevated pressure at the level of the juxtacanalicular meshwork.[21-23] Dr. Johnstone was among the first to establish that the meshwork deforms with intraocular pressure and then rebounds.
12. *Trabecular cells size and volume.* Drs. O'Donnell and Stamer, among others, have evaluated the aquaporin receptor on trabecular cells, which appears to be important in regulating cell volume.[24] A patent is pending for the manipulation of RNA producing aquaporin 4 in order to lower intraocular pressure.[25]
13. *Loss of oscillations.* Dr. Stamer (Chap. 4, Sidebar 4.1) and Acott (Chap. 34, Sidebar 34.2) point out that the subtle action of systole and diastole are important in allowing cells to maintain them.
14. *Abnormal proteins.* Dr. Fautsch at the Mayo Clinic has provided useful studies on proteins in the anterior chamber and made the many proteins a seemingly conquerable universe, enabling further studies and it may become possible to associate specific proteins with specific phenotypes of some types of glaucoma.[26,27]
15. *Herniations into the collector channels.* The ostia of the collector channels may play a major role in regulation of outflow into the venous system. Drs. Gong and Freddo have pointed this out and suggested it as a potential mechanism for glaucoma.[28] Certainly, it would explain the finding that direct cannulation of Schlemm's canal lowers IOP about 25%, suggesting that there is a site of resistance between Schlemm's canal and the venous system.
16. *Versican.* Dr. Acott has pointed out that this proteoglycan is a major candidate for outflow obstruction.[19] It is important to understand that proteoglycans in the juxtacanalicular meshwork are regulated by a combination of biosynthesis and degradation (see Chap. 34, Sidebar 34.2).

Collectively, these hypotheses suggest that the meshwork is not a static structure – it is constantly moving. It is segmental, with perhaps only 1 or 2 clock hours working at any given time in terms of outflow. Glaucoma both at the meshwork and in the nerve must ultimately be considered a matter of cellular stress. At present, we alleviate cellular stress by lowering intraocular pressure. We can prevent cellular stress with new drug ideas (and there are many) and nutritional supports to the astrocytes and the supporting glial elements in the nerve and the meshwork. Reversing cellular stress in the future may be possible with the adjunctive use of stem cells as discussed by Dr. Lin in Chap. 84 with growth factors and with other important cellular proteins such as the roundabout proteins.

At the time this chapter is being written, there are at least 14 identified loci for open angle glaucoma loci, and elucidation of more is pending. The currently known loci appear monogenic, but most glaucoma and susceptibility to glaucoma is likely to be polygenic. Three of the genetic loci for open angle glaucoma were found initially in my practice in Portland, Oregon. These were found by old-fashioned detective work and investing time with patients – and asking patients over and over about their family history. Full and accurate patient history is more difficult to elicit than most ophthalmologists recognize, and requires more time than this era of managed appointments easily allows.

In 23 years of my academic experience, I have observed many residents obtain a "full" patient history only to become crestfallen when I found something entirely different upon entering the room. Such is the norm; information elicited at the first patient encounter is rarely accurate or sufficient; that a patient volunteering additional history or reversing himself or herself is normal. Only by educating the patient about his or her disease we can begin to actually elicit all the appropriate information.

There have been a lot of difficulties in providing a genetic test for the known autosomal dominant glaucomas due in large part to intellectual property concerns. Hopefully, these will resolve soon. The US Genetic Privacy Act of 2008 will protect patients from the disclosure of their "genetic glaucoma" to insurance companies, but once these tests finally become available, there will still be issues of interpretation and implementation. The potential for misuse is high; it will be easy for clinicians to misinterpret glaucoma genetics data by attaching more significance to it than it actually has. Many of our patients are desperate for information and may want us to be soothsayers. The list of monogenic glaucomas, susceptibility genes to glaucoma, and polygenic glaucomas will grow. They vary in terms of phenotypic characteristics such as the appearance of the optic nerve, corneal thickness, response to medication, response to laser, and response to surgery. Evidence for this is subtle and is found in various papers reporting loci. It is an area where much more work is needed and will be forthcoming.

Lastly, a fundamental question for clinicians is what makes an optic nerve susceptible to damage from elevated intraocular pressure? As alluded to in the genetics chapter, we may be able to understand this in completely different terms very soon, as transcription factors altered by environmental factors. It is also highly probable that new risk factors will be discovered based on the work outlined by Dr. Harris (see Chap. 11), coupled with the potential importance of oscillations as determined by Dr. Stamer (see Chap. 4, Sidebar 4.1). What causes high pressure open angle glaucoma? It may ultimately be the cellular fragility of the juxtacanalicular meshwork as well as the lining of Schlemm's canal, and the ostia of the collector channels. If one looks at all the evidence, some of which has been presented previously as well as in this text, one concludes that the outflow environment is fragile and complex and that there are numerous ways that it can become dysfunctional.

## References

1. Alvarado J, Murohy C, Polansky J, Juster R. Age-related changes in trabecular meshwork cellularity. *Invest Ophthalmol Vis Sci.* 1981;21:714–727.
2. Alvarado JA, Wood I, Polansky JR. Human trabecular cells – II. Growth pattern and ultrastructural characteristics. *Invest Ophthalmol Vis Sci.* 1982;23:464–478.
3. Grierson I, Lee WR. Pressure-induced changes in the ultrastructure of the endothelium lining of Schlemm's canal. *Am J Ophthalmol.* 1975;80(5):863–884.
4. Grierson I, Lee WR. The fine structure of the trabecular meshwork at graded levels of intraocular pressure. (1) Pressure effects within the near-physiological range (8–30 mmHg). *Exp Eye Res.* 1975;20(6):505–521.
5. Montserrat C, Liton PB, Clahha P, Epstein DL, Gonzalez P. Effects fo donor age on proteasome activity and senescence in trabecular meshwork cells. *Biochem Biophys Res Commun.* 2004;323(22):1048–1054.
6. Epstein DL, Freddo TF, Bassett-Chu S, Chung M, Karageuzian L. Influence of ethacrynic acid on outflow facility in the monkey and coif eye. *Invest Ophthalmol Vis Sci.* 1987;28(12):2067–2075.
7. Stone M, Fingert JH, Alward WL, et al. Identification of a gene that causes primary open angle glaucoma. *Science.* 1997;275:668–670.
8. Rezaie T, Child A, Hitchings R, et al. Adult-onset primary open-angle glaucoma caused by mutations in optineurin. *Science.* 2002;295:1077–1079.
9. Wang N, Chitala SK, Fini ME, Schuman JS. Activation of tissue-specific stress response in the aqueous outfly pathway of the eye defines the glaucoma disease phenotype. *Nat Med.* 2001;7:304–309.
10. Nolan MJ, Giovingo MC, Miller AM, et al. Aqueous humor sCD44 concentration and visual field loss in primary open-angle glaucoma. *J Glaucoma.* 2007;16(5):419–429.
11. Luna C, Li G, Liton PB, et al. Resveratrol prevents the expression of glaucoma markers induced by chronic oxidative stress in trabecular meshwork cells. *Food Chem Toxicol.* 2009;47(1):198–204.
12. Wirtz MK, Samples JR, Hong X, Severson T, Acott TS. Expression profile and genome location of CDNA clones from an infant human trabecular meshwork cell library. *Invest Ophthalmol Vis Sci.* 2002;43:3698–3704.
13. Knepper AP, Miller AM, Choi J, et al. Hyperphosphorylation of aqueous humor sCD44 anad primary open-angle glaucoma. *Invest Ophthalmol Vis Sci.* 2005;46:2829–2837.
14. Samples JR, Alexander PA, Acott TS. Regulation of human trabecular meshwork metalloproteinase and inhibitors by interlukin-1 and dexamethasone. *Invest Ophthalmol Vis Sci.* 1993;34(12):3386–3395.
15. Rosenbaum JT, Samples JR, Hefender SH, Howes EL. Ocular inflammatory effects of intravitreal interleukin-1. *Arch Ophthalmol.* 1986;105:1117–1120.
16. Parshley DE, Bradley JM, Fisk A, et al. Laser trabeculoplasty induces stromelysin expression by trabecular juxtacanalicular cells. *Invest Ophthalmol Vis Sci.* 1996;37:795–804.
17. Bradley JMB, Anderssohn AM, Colvis CM, et al. Mediation of laser trabeculoplasty-induced matrix metalloproteinase expression by IL-1b and TNFa. *Invest Ophthalmol Vis Sci.* 2000;41:422–430.
18. Wang N, Chintala SK, Fini ME, Shuman JS. Ultrasound activates the TM ELAM-1/IL-1/NF-kB response: a potential mechanism for intraocular pressure reduction after phacoemulsification. *Invest Ophthalmol Vis Sci.* 2003;44:1977–1981.

19. Acott TS, Kelley MJ. Extracellular matrix in the trabecular meshwork. *Exp Eye Res*. 2008;86(4):543–561.
20. Keller KE, Aga M, Bradeley JM, Kelley MJ, Acott TS. Extracellular matrix turnover and outflow resisitance. *Exp Eye Res*. 2009;88(4):676–682.
21. Johnstone MA, Grant WM. Pressure-dependent changes in structure of the aqueous outflow system in human and monkey eyes. *Am J Ophthalmol*. 1973;75:365–383.
22. Johnstone MA. A New Model Describes an Aqueous Outflow Pump and Causes of Pump Failure in Glaucoma. In: Grehn F, Weinreb RN, eds. *Essentials in Ophthalmology: Glaucoma*. Berlin: Springer; 2006.
23. Johnstone MA. Aqueous outflow: the case for a new model – moving fluid out of the eye may be the work of a biomechanical pump. *Rev Ophthalmo!*. 2007;14.
24. Stamer WD, Peppel K, O'Donnell MS, Roberts BC, Wu F, Epstein DL. Expression of aquaporin-1 in human trabecular meshwork cells: role in resting cell volume. *Invest Ophthalmol Vis Sci*. 2001;42:1803–1811.
25. Chatterton JE, Patil RV, Sharif N, Clark AF, Wax MB. (Agent, Alcon) RNAi-mediated inhibition of aquaporin 4 for treatment of iop-related conditions. USA Patent Pending, application #20080214486. Applied for in 2008.
26. Fautsch MP, Johnson DH, and the Second ARVO/Pfizer Research Institute Working. Aqueous humor outflow: what do we know? Where will it lead us? *Invest Ophthalmol Vis Sci*. 2006;47:4181–4187.
27. Fautsch MP, Bahler CK, Vrabel AM, et al. Perfusion of his-tagged eukaryotic myocilin increases outflow resistance in human anterior segments in the presence of aqueous humor. *Invest Ophthalmol Vis Sci*. 2006;47:213–221.
28. Battista SA, Lu Z, Hofmann S, Freddo TF, Overby D, Gong H. Acute IOP elevation reduces the available area for aqueous humor outflow and induces herniations into the collector channels of bovine eyes. *Invest Ophthalmol Vis Sci*. 2008;49:5346–5352.

# Chapter 92
# The Glaucoma Book: What Do We Know Now, What Do We Need to Know About Glaucoma?

Paul N. Schacknow

What do we know about glaucoma as we approach the end of the first decade of the twenty-first century? What more do we need to know about glaucoma to advance the diagnosis and treatment of our patients? *The Glaucoma Book* describes the state of the art as practiced by glaucoma subspecialists. In this chapter, I reflect upon the knowledge provided by our contributors and also speculate about what new discoveries loom on the horizon. As glaucoma management is an imperfect science, I would like to indulge my editor's privilege to offer some educated guesses and opinions about the art of taking care of our patients along with occasional whimsical references.

## 92.1 Why Does a Person Develop Glaucoma?

The definition of glaucomatous optic neuropathy has been in flux over the past two decades. The relationships of the components of the classic clinical triad of glaucoma observations, "characteristic optic nerve head changes, elevated intraocular pressures, and certain patterns of visual field defects" that were learned by many of us as gospel during residency training is constantly evolving. Statistically high intraocular pressure (IOP) is no longer the *sine qua non* for diagnosing the disease. Most ophthalmologists *know* (dare I say *grok*?[1])[1] that IOP is somehow integrally related to disk damage over time. Yet, because the continuum of damaging IOPs ranges from "low" (normal tension glaucoma – NTG) to "high" (classical primary open angle glaucoma – POAG), we cannot describe a simple (linear), deterministic role for IOP and glaucomatous damage. Some patients with elevated pressures remain only suspects for glaucoma throughout their lives. Furthermore, the finding of many undetected glaucoma patients with IOPs under 21 mmHg, in population-based projects such as the Baltimore Eye Survey,[2] has also contributed to the paradigm shift that has changed the role of IOP from causation to correlation. Intraocular pressure has changed from an etiology to a risk factor. The *true* cause(s) underlying structural glaucomatous disc damage and functional glaucomatous visual loss are still debated (e.g., dysregulation of vascular perfusion, mechanical damage at the lamina cribrosa related to IOP, secondarily causing axonal damage). As clinicians, our more important obligation is to learn which risk factors are potentially subject to modification. We need to know *what* we can safely treat to slow down or halt the loss of vision from glaucoma, even if we do not fully understand *why* our treatments work or how they may modify the underlying disease mechanisms (e.g., laser trabeculoplasty.[3–6]) We need to take a pragmatic, engineering approach to treating glaucoma, as well as study the science that explains the engineering principles.

Researchers have determined many of the patient risk factors that greatly influence both the likelihood of developing glaucoma as well as the prognosis for disease progression. Intraocular pressure is an important risk factor easily measured during routine examination. It is also the risk factor that has proved easiest to treat with current medical and surgical therapies. Critics such as Eddy[7] and Billings[8] have challenged us to practice evidence-based medicine rather than rely upon "generally accepted" tradition-based training from our professors (Chap. 2).

Beginning in the 1990s, (Chap. 3) many well-designed and well-executed multicenter, randomized clinical studies have been conducted that show that, in almost all situations, reducing intraocular pressure slows or halts the progression of glaucomatous disk damage, *regardless of the level of pressure* at which the disease was first diagnosed or detected. This suggests that while the *diagnosis* of glaucoma may occur at a wide range of IOPs, the *treatment* of glaucoma to prevent progression involves lowering of IOP regardless of how high it was when the glaucomatous optic nerve head changes were discovered by the clinician. The current zeitgeist may not include intraocular pressure in the definition of

---

[1] To *grok* is to comprehend something so well that it is totally absorbed into one's own being. In Robert A. Heinlein's classic science fiction book *Stranger in a Strange Land*, the word is Martian and literally means "to drink," and may be interpreted to mean "to understand fully," or to "be at one with."

glaucoma, but therapeutic benefit follows from "lowering the intraocular pressure (IOP) at early and late stages of the disease."[9]

The role of daily, intervisit, and longer-term fluctuations of IOP in glaucomatous progression is hotly debated (Chap. 4). As with the term "glaucoma," definitions of "fluctuation" are not easily agreed upon. Some studies (not without critics) purport to show that fluctuations in IOP are harmful to the glaucoma patient, while other studies interpret their findings to show no influence of daily or intervisit IOP variability on glaucoma progression.[10–14] Implantable or wearable devices to continuously monitor IOP, similar in concept to cardiac Holter monitors, are under development (Chap. 6). Nonetheless, because homeostasis and autoregulation are general features of many healthy biological systems, it seems prudent that therapies directed at lowering IOP (medical, laser, and incisional surgery) should be studied (and used) with respect to their abilities to minimize intraday, intravisit, and long-term IOP changes as well as being efficacious in lowering IOP.

Nonemergent glaucoma care occurs during the physician's regularly scheduled office hours, usually during the daytime. But glaucoma affects the patient around the clock. We know that the highest levels of IOP often occur outside the diurnal time period.[15–17] Nocturnal IOP elevation, and subsequent glaucoma damage, may truly be "the sneak thief of vision" because it takes place silently, unobserved by the clinician, while the patient is sleeping. Circadian (24-h) control of IOP and the importance of IOP in the recumbent position have only recently begun to have rigorous study in a few places around the world[18–23] (Chap. 5). I predict that regulatory agencies such as the United States Federal Drug Administration will eventually require that medication registration protocols include a subset of patients who were observed over several 24-h time periods. It seems reasonable to use therapies that control IOP both diurnally and nocturnally, even if we cannot conveniently examine our patients in the wee hours of the morning.

During this decade, the accuracy of measuring IOP in the clinic has been reexplored, following the publication of the Ocular Hypertension Treatment Study (OHTS) in 2002.[24] While the physical principles underlying the design of the Goldmann applanation tonometer[25] have been known from the time of its invention in 1955, only since OHTS has it become routine to measure central corneal thickness in newly examined patients (Chap. 8). However, simple pachymetry may not be the best technique for evaluating the role of corneal factors (e.g., elasticity) on IOP determination. Other instruments are coming into use in the clinic that may eventually surpass the Goldmann device for the standard of care.

Although other risk factors for glaucoma may not be as amenable to modification as IOP, their association with glaucoma and their determination for a given patient may influence the severity of the disease and its prognosis. For example, while one cannot choose one's parents, the genetic gifts we receive from them play a strong role in the development of some glaucomas (Chap. 9). This may be expressed and observed phenotypically as gender or race (ethnicity?) (Chap. 10) or may be *sub rosa* in its effects involving no distinguishing macroscopic appearance characteristics but rather subtler alterations in one or more gene loci. There could be many genotypic variations in what we have lumped together phenotypically as the "open-angle glaucomas." Also, there is a strong genetic component to some secondary glaucomas such as exfoliation and pigmentary dispersion syndromes. Angle closure varieties of glaucoma (Chap. 36) are more prevalent in certain Asian ethnic groups, while normal pressure glaucoma is highly prevalent in Americans of Japanese heritage living in California.[26] Genetic testing for glaucoma-related alleles is in its infancy, but it may play a bigger role for early detection and treatment as more specific and less costly testing is developed. Ethical considerations and medical insurance coverage may influence the widespread use of tests that "predict" future disease.[27–30]

Advancing age is a strong risk factor in the development of glaucoma. Spaeth (Chap. 14) reminds us that each patient is an individual human being and not a disease entity. He and colleagues have argued persuasively in various forums that treatment for glaucoma must be customized to the life-stage of the patient, the level of disc damage, and his or her daily living activities.[31,32] Hippocrates' *primum non nocere* should be the guiding principle in glaucoma management as in all fields of medicine.[33] When I was a resident, I wanted to offer all my glaucoma patients maximum therapy. I considered using all medical, laser, and incisional surgical procedures to attempt to halt glaucoma progression in each and every patient; this seemed like the "American way" of treating everyone equally and using all resources possible without regard to cost or convenience. Fortunately, I quickly grew to understand that the effect of glaucoma on each patient would impact his or her life in different, unique ways, for them and their families. Many glaucoma suspects need only psychological support and lifelong monitoring without early or late medical/surgical intervention. Some patients first diagnosed at advanced age, with mild to moderate glaucomatous disc and field changes, may require no or minimal treatment to maintain visual functioning to allow them to engage in their usual activities for the remainder of their lives. Occasionally, elderly patients with mild glaucoma are very frightened of blindness and no amount of discussion will convince them that they are unlikely to suffer functional blindness in their lifetimes. For these patients, it may be reasonable to initiate medical monotherapy as much for psychological as for medical reasons. Economic issues will continue to play a major role in the frequency of offering testing procedure, clinical examinations, and the differential availability for each patient of chronic glaucoma medications based on medical insurance and their personal financial circumstances.[34]

My coeditor John Samples has an excellent essay (Chap. 91) that describes 16 possible "causes" for the development of glaucoma, ranging from genetic mutations to chemical messengers that signal trabecular meshwork functionality. His chapter discusses both risk factors and etiologies, with an eye to future research that should yield abundant areas for diagnosis and therapy.

## 92.2 When Does a Person Develop Glaucoma?

Because glaucoma is a disease involving dysfunction or death of retinal ganglion cells (RGC), it seems obvious to me that structural changes must occur before functional changes in the patient's visual abilities. In the twentieth century, the classic papers by Quiqley et al showed that between 40% and 50% of RGCs could be lost without noticeable Goldmann visual field defects.[35-37] In this population, major structural changes took place before visual functional loss could be detected. The situation may nowadays be reversed, with functional loss *detected* before structural loss can be observed. Glaucomatous structural alterations may first occur intracellularly, biochemically, at a micro- or nanoscopic level that we cannot detect with either ophthalmoscopy, stereo-disc photography, or the current technological capabilities of digital image analyzers. In some cases, functional loss found with modern-day visual fields, electrophysiological or brain-based measurement systems may be manifest before we are able to detect the underlying early structural pathologies. For example, the sensitivities of the newer visual field technologies (e.g., frequency doubling threshold perimetry, short wavelength perimetry) and analytical software (Zeiss-Humphrey "Glaucoma Progression Analysis") may detect functional changes much earlier than the Goldmann perimeter (as per the Quigley et al studies referenced previously). Cell death and retinal nerve fiber layer thinning must occur after the cells are sick for some time, not as the first manifestation of disease. So, while we may see functional loss demonstrable before structural loss because of limitations in our current technologies, it is likely that physical pathologies in retinal ganglion cells are the precursors of the functional damage that we can observe.

Open-angle glaucoma does not develop in a "quantum leap" fashion, fully formed at one moment and not present the moment before. RGCs may be stressed by mechanical, vascular, and biochemical factors. Over time, some cells of the optic nerve and supporting structures (e.g., astrocytes, glial cells) become dysfunctional; then, some of them may die. As more and more of the cells of the retinal nerve fiber layer (RNFL) become compromised, the clinical manifestations of the disease become apparent. Visual field analyzers show Bjerrum scotomas. Digital image analyzers and red-free photography show loss of the RNFL. Optic nerve head cupping, asymmetrical changes between the two disks, flame-shaped disk hemorrhages, and baring of the circumlinear vessel may be observed. Presumed early structural changes, unnoticed and unnoticeable with current technologies, are the precursors of what becomes clinical glaucoma, or "almost" glaucoma when a patient is declared a suspect for the disease. This continuum of glaucoma pathology has been described as having three stages: undetectable disease, asymptomatic disease, and functional impairment.[38] As technologies improve and risk factors are more fully elucidated, it becomes incumbent upon the clinician to decide in whom careful and regular observation is appropriate and in whom (and when) treatment should be initiated. Does very early intervention prevent ultimate significant functional impairment? Does the benefit of starting treatment for barely detectable disease in a younger person outweigh the social, personal, and economic costs associated with ten or twenty more years of additional therapy compared to waiting to see if frank glaucoma declares itself in time? Is it better to treat early certain patients with many risk factors for glaucoma, or just burdensome to do so for the patient and society, if there is to be little long-term benefit to the patient's visual functioning? As the tools for diagnosis continue to improve and the treatments evolve, the decision-making process for caring for the patient becomes more rather than less complicated for the physician.

## 92.3 What Does the Future Hold for Our Ability to Detect the Structural and Functional Changes in Glaucoma?

Until recently, glaucoma management was entirely a contact sport between the patients and their caregivers. The physician or technician performed manual Goldmann perimetry. The doctor observed the optic nerve by direct ophthalmoscopy or with high diopter lenses. Gonioscopy of the anterior chamber angle required coupling gels and examiner skill. Stereoscopic disk photos and red-free retinal nerve fiber layer photos were evaluated for serial change by the ophthalmologist. Glaucoma education was provided one-on-one without the Internet or color DVDs. Glaucoma subspecialists were considered more expert in both performing and interpreting these diagnostic tasks than comprehensive ophthalmologists and optometrists. The newer automated technologies have brought advanced diagnostic capabilities to all eye care doctors. This may seem to have blunted these distinctions among practitioners based on experience and skill.

The analysis software accompanying these technologies may misleadingly yield simple "yes" or "no" conclusions regarding diagnosis and progression of disease. The need for "contact" and some forms of direct observation between the patient and practitioner appear to be less important with the advent of these new machines. However, believing solely in these machines and relying on their interpretations of clinical data is akin to praying to false gods for guidance and acting on their declarations of truth for glaucoma management. Yes, it is true that some eye doctors cannot themselves "read" Zeiss-Humphrey visual fields, that they only look at the grayscale pattern rather than interpret the clinical relationship among pattern standard deviation, mean deviation, reliability parameters, and other numerical parameters. Having advanced technologies to evaluate their patients can help when their personal interpretive skill sets are not sufficient. Unfortunately, I see patients daily in consultation who have had clinical decisions made by their referring physicians, who have initiated or increased medical and surgical therapies only as a result of a computerized visual field or digital image analysis reported as abnormal or progressing by software analysis.

Glaucoma risk calculators[39-43] have been developed that incorporate knowledge obtained from controlled clinical studies (see Chap. 34). These devices allow nonsubspecialty practitioners to incorporate evidence-based risk factors into their decision making. Unfortunately, they remove the physician from the reasoning process behind the diagnosis. The assumptions behind the calculations may be unknown to many physicians. The patient's clinical situation may not meet all the criteria for using the calculator.

Technologies (hardware and software) used appropriately may allow us to learn things we cannot easily see by direct observation. For example, anterior chamber angle anatomy can be viewed in great detail by ultrasound and optical coherence imaging devices (Chap. 27). This technology may someday filter down to the community-based eye doctor who is not extremely skilled or comfortable manipulating gonioprisms (Chap. 26). Instruments that incorporate databases based on thousands of patient observations may have more (artificial) "experience" to rely upon when comparing the current patient to "normal" or "abnormal" exemplars, than does the doctor who has only been in practice a few years. Of course, even the most brilliant and experienced clinician, like all other humans, has a less perfect memory and computative ability than a computer. Conversely, technology available in the foreseeable future cannot substitute for the clinical observation and knowledge and experience of the physician actively engaged in direct patient care. The magical "black box" qualities and "answers" provided by risk calculators, digital image analyzers, and visual field machines are seductive, but deceptive in their lack of applicability to all patients under all circumstances. The algorithms used for decision analysis are constantly being updated as new knowledge becomes available. Perhaps in the more distant future, *Star Trek*-like machines will be able to scan a patient, take a blood sample, and ask him or her a few questions before rendering a definitive glaucoma diagnosis and prescribing a therapeutic plan. For now, the physician who is aware of the glaucoma evidence base and has the experience of dealing with thousands of real world patients will undoubtedly deliver better care than the newbie doctor who relies mostly on instrumentation and lacks clinical experience.

## 92.4 What Are Current Recommendations for Treating Open-Angle Glaucoma?

Current therapy for slowing or halting glaucoma progression is primarily directed to lowering IOP and perhaps to minimizing IOP fluctuations and providing both diurnal and nocturnal control. At present, therapies for direct neuroprotection of RGCs are not proven. In the United States, first-line treatment for primary open-angle glaucoma is usually medical therapy. Hypotensive lipids (HLs) as initial monotherapy lower IOP greater than other drugs, have low IOP fluctuation, and are effective both day and night (Chap. 51). Adjunctive medical therapies (Chap. 52) currently favor topical carbonic anhydrase inhibitors (TCAIs) and alpha agonists for efficacy when added to HLs, although TCAIs may have slight advantages with respect to flat IOP curves and night-time control compared to alpha agonists. Combination products have some advantages over concomitant therapy from separate bottles due to cost, lower preservative loads, and perhaps better compliance. Cosopt was introduced in 1998. Combination products have become more popular recently with several new products introduced in the USA and throughout the world (Combigan, DuoTrav, Ganfort and Xalacom).

Complex dosing regimens and faulty memories in elderly patients result in poor adherence with therapeutic plans. Medications that might be administered only several times each year are undergoing multicenter clinical trials (Chap. 89). In the USA, informal surveys I have taken at scientific meetings suggest that most physicians treating glaucoma patients feel that two bottles (perhaps one with a combination of products), dosed no more frequently than every 12 h, are reasonable maximal medical therapy (see Chap. 51). If target IOP is not reached or maintained, some form of laser trabeculoplasty (LTP) is the next step in treatment escalation. During the twentieth century, this was most commonly employing argon energy (ALTP), while at the start of the twenty-first century, "selective laser trabeculoplasty (SLTP)" is preferred by many because it is less destructive to the trabecular meshwork and thus offers more potential repeatability than ALT (Chap. 61). In some studies, exfoliation and pigmentary glaucomas are even more likely to respond to LTP than POAG.[44-51]

Newer lasers with different spectral wavelengths and new systems for energy delivery are explored in Chaps. 61 through 64. The family of angle closure glaucomas may respond to laser peripheral iridotomy or laser iridoplasty. Longevity of IOP reduction, ease of performing the technique, and the repeatability of treatment without complications or loss of effectiveness are some of the criteria by which newer laser modalities will be judged as replacements for ALTP and SLTP.

In the USA, incisional glaucoma surgeries in their various forms are generally reserved for patients who have failed medical therapy and perhaps LTP. In Europe and Asia, primary incisional glaucoma surgery for both OAGs and chronic angle closure glaucomas is not uncommon.[52]

Incisional glaucoma surgeries advanced in the twentieth century from full-thickness filtering procedures to guarded procedures, with Cairns' trabeculectomy[53] (with modifications) becoming the gold standard surgery that still is the most common glaucoma operation today (Chap. 65). The most important modification of trabeculectomy was the introduction of antifibrotic agents (e.g., mitomycin-C[54] and 5-flourouracil[55-62]) that permitted a degree of modulation of the wound healing process. Tube shunts, both unvalved and valved, continue to be introduced (Chaps. 68 and 69). Although they are generally used for secondary, and not primary glaucoma surgeries, that may be changing.[63-66] Canaloplasty,[67-69] viscocanalostomy,[70-78] and similar techniques require more surgical finesse than trabeculectomy but offer fewer short- and long-term complications (Chap. 67). Unfortunately, current "canal surgery" methods cannot lower pressure to the degree that trabeculectomy or tube shunts can. At this time, their place in the surgical armamentarium is reserved for patients with modest requirements for IOP reduction but insufficient response to medication or laser therapies. Older procedures such as trabeculotomy are being revisited with application to adult glaucoma surgery[79] (Chap. 66).

The most successful glaucoma surgeons are not only excellent at their technical tasks intraoperatively, but they are distinguished by their ability to manage the inevitable complications of the procedures they perform (Chaps. 70, 72–74). Interestingly, incisional surgeries have declined in the USA since the introduction of more effective glaucoma medications beginning in the mid-1990s.[80] More effective future medical or possibly genetic therapies may ultimately render surgery safe but rare.

## 92.5 What Does the Future Hold for Glaucoma Patients?

The evidence base that is the cornerstone of scientific diagnosis and treatment of glaucoma comes from laboratory and clinical research. Both academic centers and private offices conduct government and industry sponsored projects (Chaps. 86–88). These efforts result in discoveries that provided a basic understanding of the glaucoma disease process. From this research, new instruments to determine structural and functional pathologies, new medications, and surgical interventions have proliferated. In this century, we are likely to see blood tests[81] for diagnosing glaucoma, reliable automated instrument systems to stage glaucoma and document its progression,[82] extended duration of action (months to years) medical therapies,[83] and simpler surgical procedures[84,85] with fewer complications. Stem cell research (Chap. 84) offers hope of restoration of visual function in glaucoma patients, while immunological initiatives (Chap. 81) portend vaccines that could prevent glaucoma in high-risk patients.

Today, we can slow the course of glaucoma for many patients, and for some of them, halt the disease. In the future, we may be able to restore visual function and possibly cure some forms of the disease.

## References

1. Heinlein RA. *Stranger in a Strange Land*. New York: Putnam; 1961.
2. Sommer A. Glaucoma risk factors observed in the Baltimore Eye Survey. *Curr Opin Ophthalmol*. 1996;7(2):93–98.
3. Cioffi GA, Latina MA, Schwartz GF. Argon versus selective laser trabeculoplasty. *J Glaucoma*. 2004;13(2):174–177.
4. Latina MA, Tumbocon JA. Selective laser trabeculoplasty: a new treatment option for open angle glaucoma. *Curr Opin Ophthalmol*. 2002;13(2):94–96.
5. Wise JB. Ten year results of laser trabeculoplasty. Does the laser avoid glaucoma surgery or merely defer it? *Eye*. 1987;1(Pt 1): 45–50.
6. Wise JB. Technical considerations in laser trabeculoplasty. *Trans New Orleans Acad Ophthalmol*. 1985;33:210–214.
7. Eddy DM, Billings J. The quality of medical evidence: implications for quality of care. *Health Aff (Millwood)*. 1988;7(1):19–32.
8. Billings J, Eddy D. Physician decision making limited by medical evidence. *Bus Health*. 1987;5(1):23. 26–28.
9. Weinreb RN, Khaw PT. Primary open-angle glaucoma. *Lancet*. 2004;363(9422):1711–1720.
10. Caprioli J, Coleman AL. Intraocular pressure fluctuation a risk factor for visual field progression at low intraocular pressures in the advanced glaucoma intervention study. *Ophthalmology*. 2008;115(7):1123–1129. e1123.
11. Asrani S, Zeimer R, Wilensky J, Gieser D, Vitale S, Lindenmuth K. Large diurnal fluctuations in intraocular pressure are an independent risk factor in patients with glaucoma. *J Glaucoma*. 2000;9(2):134–142.

12. Bengtsson B, Leske MC, Hyman L, Heijl A. Fluctuation of intraocular pressure and glaucoma progression in the early manifest glaucoma trial. *Ophthalmology.* 2007;114(2):205–209.
13. Medeiros FA, Weinreb RN, Zangwill LM, et al. Long-term intraocular pressure fluctuations and risk of conversion from ocular hypertension to glaucoma. *Ophthalmology.* 2008;115(6):934–940.
14. Shuba LM, Doan AP, Maley MK, et al. Diurnal fluctuation and concordance of intraocular pressure in glaucoma suspects and normal tension glaucoma patients. *J Glaucoma.* 2007;16(3):307–312.
15. Nakakura S, Nomura Y, Ataka S, Shiraki K. Relation between office intraocular pressure and 24-hour intraocular pressure in patients with primary open-angle glaucoma treated with a combination of topical antiglaucoma eye drops. *J Glaucoma.* 2007;16(2):201–204.
16. Mosaed S, Liu JH, Weinreb RN. Correlation between office and peak nocturnal intraocular pressures in healthy subjects and glaucoma patients. *Am J Ophthalmol.* 2005;139(2):320–324.
17. Hughes E, Spry P, Diamond J. 24-hour monitoring of intraocular pressure in glaucoma management: a retrospective review. *J Glaucoma.* 2003;12(3):232–236.
18. Dubiner HB, Sircy MD, Landry T, et al. Comparison of the diurnal ocular hypotensive efficacy of travoprost and latanoprost over a 44-hour period in patients with elevated intraocular pressure. *Clin Ther.* 2004;26(1):84–91.
19. Gross RL, Peace JH, Smith SE, et al. Duration of IOP reduction with travoprost BAK-free solution. *J Glaucoma.* 2008;17(3):217–222.
20. Walters TR, DuBiner HB, Carpenter SP, Khan B, VanDenburgh AM. 24-hour IOP control with once-daily bimatoprost, timolol gel-forming solution, or latanoprost: a 1-month, randomized, comparative clinical trial. *Surv Ophthalmol.* 2004;49(Suppl 1):S26–S35.
21. Liu JH, Gokhale PA, Loving RT, Kripke DF, Weinreb RN. Laboratory assessment of diurnal and nocturnal ocular perfusion pressures in humans. *J Ocul Pharmacol Ther.* 2003;19(4):291–297.
22. Liu JH, Kripke DF, Hoffman RE, et al. Nocturnal elevation of intraocular pressure in young adults. *Invest Ophthalmol Vis Sci.* 1998;39(13):2707–2712.
23. Liu JH, Kripke DF, Weinreb RN. Comparison of the nocturnal effects of once-daily timolol and latanoprost on intraocular pressure. *Am J Ophthalmol.* 2004;138(3):389–395.
24. Kass MA, Heuer DK, Higginbotham EJ, et al. The Ocular Hypertension Treatment Study: a randomized trial determines that topical ocular hypotensive medication delays or prevents the onset of primary open-angle glaucoma. *Arch Ophthalmol.* 2002;120(6):701–713. discussion 829–830.
25. Goldmann H. Un neuveau tonometre. *Bull Soc Ophtalmol Fr.* 1955;5:281–292.
26. Pekmezci M, Vo B, Lim AK, et al. The characteristics of glaucoma in Japanese Americans. *Arch Ophthalmol.* 2009;127(2):167–171.
27. Schmidt C. Regulators weigh risks of consumer genetic tests. *Nat Biotechnol.* 2008;26(2):145–146.
28. Collins FS, McKusick VA. Implications of the Human Genome Project for medical science. *JAMA.* 2001;285(5):540–544.
29. Gerard S, Hayes M, Rothstein MA. On the edge of tomorrow: fitting genomics into public health policy. *J Law Med Ethics.* 2002;30 (3 Suppl):173–176.
30. Rothenberg KH, Terry SF. Human genetics. Before it's too late – addressing fear of genetic information. *Science.* 2002;297(5579):196–197.
31. Henderer JD. Disc damage likelihood scale. *Br J Ophthalmol.* 2006;90(4):395–396.
32. Spaeth GL, Henderer J, Liu C, et al. The disc damage likelihood scale: reproducibility of a new method of estimating the amount of optic nerve damage caused by glaucoma. *Trans Am Ophthalmol Soc.* 2002;100:181-185. discussion 185–186.
33. Smith CM. Origin and uses of primum non nocere – above all, do no harm! *J Clin Pharmacol.* 2005;45(4):371–377.
34. Rein DB, Wittenborn JS, Lee PP, et al. The cost-effectiveness of routine office-based identification and subsequent medical treatment of primary open-angle glaucoma in the United States. *Ophthalmology.* 2009;116(5):823–832.
35. Quigley HA, Addicks EM, Green WR. Optic nerve damage in human glaucoma. III. Quantitative correlation of nerve fiber loss and visual field defect in glaucoma, ischemic neuropathy, papilledema, and toxic neuropathy. *Arch Ophthalmol.* 1982;100(1):135–146.
36. Quigley HA, Addicks EM, Green WR, Maumenee AE. Optic nerve damage in human glaucoma. II. The site of injury and susceptibility to damage. *Arch Ophthalmol.* 1981;99(4):635–649.
37. Quigley HA, Green WR. The histology of human glaucoma cupping and optic nerve damage: clinicopathologic correlation in 21 eyes. *Ophthalmology.* 1979;86(10):1803–1830.
38. Weinreb RN, Friedman DS, Fechtner RD, et al. Risk assessment in the management of patients with ocular hypertension. *Am J Ophthalmol.* 2004;138(3):458–467.
39. Boland MV, Quigley HA, Lehmann HP. The impact of risk calculation on treatment recommendations made by glaucoma specialists in cases of ocular hypertension. *J Glaucoma.* 2008;17(8):631–638.
40. Mansberger SL, Medeiros FA, Gordon M. Diagnostic tools for calculation of glaucoma risk. *Surv Ophthalmol.* 2008;53(Suppl 1):S11–S16.
41. Gordon MO, Torri V, Miglior S, et al. Validated prediction model for the development of primary open-angle glaucoma in individuals with ocular hypertension. *Ophthalmology.* 2007;114(1):10–19.
42. Mansberger SL, Cioffi GA. The probability of glaucoma from ocular hypertension determined by ophthalmologists in comparison to a risk calculator. *J Glaucoma.* 2006;15(5):426–431.
43. Mansberger SL. A risk calculator to determine the probability of glaucoma. *J Glaucoma.* 2004;13(4):345–347.
44. Higginbotham EJ, Richardson TM. Response of exfoliation glaucoma to laser trabeculoplasty. *Br J Ophthalmol.* 1986;70(11):837–839.
45. Sherwood MB, Svedbergh B. Argon laser trabeculoplasty in exfoliation syndrome. *Br J Ophthalmol.* 1985;69(12):886–890.
46. Ritch R, Podos S. Laser trabeculoplasty in the exfoliation syndrome. *Bull N Y Acad Med.* 1983;59(4):339–344.
47. Logan P, Burke E, Joyce PD, Eustace P. Laser trabeculoplasty in the pseudo-exfoliation syndrome. *Trans Ophthalmol Soc U K.* 1983;103(Pt 6):586–587.
48. Ritch R, Liebmann J, Robin A, et al. Argon laser trabeculoplasty in pigmentary glaucoma. *Ophthalmology.* 1993;100(6):909–913.
49. Lehto I. Long-term follow up of argon laser trabeculoplasty in pigmentary glaucoma. *Ophthalmic Surg.* 1992;23(9):614–617.
50. Lunde MW. Argon laser trabeculoplasty in pigmentary dispersion syndrome with glaucoma. *Am J Ophthalmol.* 1983;96(6):721–725.
51. Robin AL, Pollack IP. Argon laser trabeculoplasty in secondary forms of open-angle glaucoma. *Arch Ophthalmol.* 1983;101(3):382–384.
52. Sherwood MB, Migdal CS, Hitchings RA, Sharir M, Zimmerman TJ, Schultz JS. Initial treatment of glaucoma: surgery or medications. *Surv Ophthalmol.* 1993;37(4):293–305.
53. Cairns JE. Trabeculectomy. Preliminary report of a new method. *Am J Ophthalmol.* 1968;66(4):673–679.
54. Wilkins M, Indar A, Wormald R. Intra-operative mitomycin C for glaucoma surgery. *Cochrane Database Syst Rev.* 2005;(4):CD002897.
55. Rothman RF, Liebmann JM, Ritch R. Low-dose 5-fluorouracil trabeculectomy as initial surgery in uncomplicated glaucoma: long-term followup. *Ophthalmology.* 2000;107(6):1184–1190.
56. Hefetz L, Keren T, Naveh N. Early and late postoperative application of 5-fluorouracil following trabeculectomy in refractory glaucoma. *Ophthalmic Surg.* 1994;25(10):715–719.
57. Stilma JS. Trabeculectomy with 5-fluorouracil in complicated glaucoma. *Klin Oczna.* 1993;95(2):81–83.

58. Smith MF, Sherwood MB, Doyle JW, Khaw PT. Results of intraoperative 5-fluorouracil supplementation on trabeculectomy for open-angle glaucoma. *Am J Ophthalmol*. 1992;114(6):737–741.
59. Wilson RP, Steinmann WC. Use of trabeculectomy with postoperative 5-fluorouracil in patients requiring extremely low intraocular pressure levels to limit further glaucoma progression. *Ophthalmology*. 1991;98(7):1047–1052.
60. Liebmann JM, Ritch R, Marmor M, Nunez J, Wolner B. Initial 5-fluorouracil trabeculectomy in uncomplicated glaucoma. *Ophthalmology*. 1991;98(7):1036–1041.
61. Taniguchi T, Kitazawa Y, Shimizu U. Long-term results of 5-fluorouracil trabeculectomy for primary open-angle glaucoma. *Int Ophthalmol*. 1989;13(1–2):145–149.
62. Kitazawa Y, Taniguchi T, Nakano Y, Shirato S, Yamamoto T. 5-Fluorouracil for trabeculectomy in glaucoma. *Graefes Arch Clin Exp Ophthalmol*. 1987;225(6):403–405.
63. Rauscher FM, Gedde SJ, Schiffman JC, Feuer WJ, Barton K, Lee RK. Motility disturbances in the tube versus trabeculectomy study during the first year of follow-up. *Am J Ophthalmol*. 2009;147(3):458–466.
64. Gedde SJ, Schiffman JC, Feuer WJ, Herndon LW, Brandt JD, Budenz DL. Treatment outcomes in the tube versus trabeculectomy study after one year of follow-up. *Am J Ophthalmol*. 2007;143(1):9–22.
65. Gedde SJ, Herndon LW, Brandt JD, Budenz DL, Feuer WJ, Schiffman JC. Surgical complications in the Tube Versus Trabeculectomy Study during the first year of follow-up. *Am J Ophthalmol*. 2007;143(1):23–31.
66. Gedde SJ, Schiffman JC, Feuer WJ, Parrish RK 2nd, Heuer DK, Brandt JD. The tube versus trabeculectomy study: design and baseline characteristics of study patients. *Am J Ophthalmol*. 2005;140(2):275–287.
67. Lewis RA, von Wolff K, Tetz M, et al. Canaloplasty: circumferential viscodilation and tensioning of Schlemm canal using a flexible microcatheter for the treatment of open-angle glaucoma in adults: two-year interim clinical study results. *J Cataract Refract Surg*. 2009;35(5):814–824.
68. Grieshaber MC, Pienaar A, Olivier J, Stegmann R. Channelography: imaging of the aqueous outflow pathway with flexible microcatheter and fluorescein in canaloplasty. *Klin Monatsbl Augenheilkd*. 2009;226(4):245–248.
69. Shingleton B, Tetz M, Korber N. Circumferential viscodilation and tensioning of Schlemm canal (canaloplasty) with temporal clear corneal phacoemulsification cataract surgery for open-angle glaucoma and visually significant cataract: one-year results. *J Cataract Refract Surg*. 2008;34(3):433–440.
70. Kobayashi H, Kobayashi K, Okinami S. A comparison of the intraocular pressure-lowering effect and safety of viscocanalostomy and trabeculectomy with mitomycin C in bilateral open-angle glaucoma. *Graefes Arch Clin Exp Ophthalmol*. 2003;241(5):359–366.
71. Shaarawy T, Nguyen C, Schnyder C, Mermoud A. Five year results of viscocanalostomy. *Br J Ophthalmol*. 2003;87(4):441–445.
72. O'Brart DP, Rowlands E, Islam N, Noury AM. A randomised, prospective study comparing trabeculectomy augmented with antimetabolites with a viscocanalostomy technique for the management of open angle glaucoma uncontrolled by medical therapy. *Br J Ophthalmol*. 2002;86(7):748–754.
73. Ahmed II, Crandall AS. Viscocanalostomy vs trabeculetomy. *Ophthalmology*. 2002;109(3):411–412.
74. Jonescu-Cuypers C, Jacobi P, Konen W, Krieglstein G. Primary viscocanalostomy versus trabeculectomy in white patients with open-angle glaucoma: a randomized clinical trial. *Ophthalmology*. 2001;108(2):254–258.
75. Crandall AS. Nonpenetrating filtering procedures: viscocanalostomy and collagen wick. *Semin Ophthalmol*. 1999;14(3):189–195.
76. Bylsma S. Nonpenetrating deep sclerectomy: collagen implant and viscocanalostomy procedures. *Int Ophthalmol Clin*. 1999;39(3):103–119.
77. Stegmann R, Pienaar A, Miller D. Viscocanalostomy for open-angle glaucoma in black African patients. *J Cataract Refract Surg*. 1999;25(3):316–322.
78. Carassa RG, Bettin P, Brancato R. Viscocanalostomy: a pilot study. *Acta Ophthalmol Scand Suppl*. 1998;227:51–52.
79. Godfrey DG, Fellman RL, Neelakantan A. Canal surgery in adult glaucomas. *Curr Opin Ophthalmol*. 2009;20(2):116–121.
80. Strutton DR, Walt JG. Trends in glaucoma surgery before and after the introduction of new topical glaucoma pharmacotherapies. *J Glaucoma*. 2004;13(3):221–226.
81. Wang N, Chintala SK, Fini ME, Schuman JS. Activation of a tissue-specific stress response in the aqueous outflow pathway of the eye defines the glaucoma disease phenotype. *Nat Med*. 2001;7(3):304–309.
82. Diaz-Aleman VT, Anton A, de la Rosa MG, Johnson ZK, McLeod S, Azuara-Blanco A. Detection of visual-field deterioration by Glaucoma Progression Analysis and Threshold Noiseless Trend programs. *Br J Ophthalmol*. 2009;93(3):322–328.
83. Robin AL, Clark AF, Covert DW, et al. Anterior juxtascleral delivery of anecortave acetate in eyes with primary open-angle glaucoma: a pilot investigation. *Am J Ophthalmol*. 2009;147(1):45–50.
84. Minckler D, Baerveldt G, Ramirez MA, et al. Clinical results with the Trabectome, a novel surgical device for treatment of open-angle glaucoma. *Trans Am Ophthalmol Soc*. 2006;104:40–50.
85. Minckler DS, Baerveldt G, Alfaro MR, Francis BA. Clinical results with the Trabectome for treatment of open-angle glaucoma. *Ophthalmology*. 2005;112(6):962–967.

# Index

## A

ABC transporters, 97
Ab externo Schlemm's canal outflow devices
    deep dissection, 801
    laser goniopuncture, 804
    microcatheter, 802
    prolene suture and knots, 803
    scleral flap, 800–801
    trabeculodescemet window (TDW), 801–802
Ab interno Schlemm's canal outflow devices
    trabectome handpiece
        advantage, 807
        complications and outcome, 806
        design, 805–806
    trabecular micro-bypass, 805
Absolute risk reduction (ARR), 30
acetazolamide, 44, 452, 483, 494, 514, 572, 577, 605–608, 612, 634, 681–683, 742, 908, 965
ACG. *See* Angle closure glaucoma
Adherence
    coverage and dosing errors, 651
    economic impact, 654–655
    evaluation and medication, 651
    eye drop administration instillation, 652
    nonadherence, IOP control relationship, 655
    *vs.* outcomes, 651
    provider–patient relationship
        inadequate communication, 653
        inadequate provider monitoring, 654
        rapport issues, 653–654
Adjunctive therapy
    advantages, 637–638
    alpha-adrenergic agonists, 630–631
    beta-blockers, 631
        *vs.* brimonidine, 632–633
        *vs.* topical CAIs, 632
    brimonidine-P, 638
    combination agents, 615–616
    combination medical therapy, 634–636
    diastolic ocular perfusion pressure, 637
    fixed combination agents, 634
    limitations, 937
    medical management, 638
    *vs.* medical therapy, 631–632
    medications classes, 629
    monotherapy
        benzalkonium chloride (BAK), 629
        IOP reduction, 629–630
        PAG therapy, 630
        selection process, 630
    oral CAIs, 634
    PGAs, 629
    pilocarpine, 633
    topical carbonic anhydrase inhibitors, 631
Advanced Glaucoma Intervention Study (AGIS)
    intraocular pressure (IOP), 37
    risk factors, 51
Ahmed valved implants, 813, 816
Alphagan, 609
Alphagan-P, 592, 609, 610
Alpha-lipoic acid, 657
Alpha-tocopherol, 658
ALT. *See* Argon laser trabeculoplasty
Alzheimer's disease (AD)
    optic nerve cupping, 276
    sCD44 and POAG, 941–943
Amniotic membrane transplantation (AMT)
    bleb leak, 863
    conjunctival tube repairing devices, 864
    intraoperative conjunctival buttonholes, 862
    shunt tube covering devices, 864
    trabeculectomy, 861–862
Analysis of variance (ANOVA), 150
Anecortave acetate
    anterior juxtascleral depot (AJD), 991
    intraocular pressure (IOP), 989
    intravitreal triamcinolone acetate (IVTA), 991–992
    *vs.* tetrahydrocortisol, 989, 990
    treatment timeline, 989, 990
Angiotensin converting enzyme (ACE), 115
Angle closure glaucoma (ACG)
    anterior segment imaging, 467–468
    chronic angle-closure, 470
    classification, ISGEO
        PAC, 461
        PACG, 462
        PACS, 461
    combined mechanism, 470
    definitions, 461
    drug-induced secondary, 482–484
    epithelial and fibrous downgrowth, 480
    genetics, 97
    gonioscopy
        compression, 465
        concentric rings, 466
        Goldmann three-mirror lens, 464, 465
        Keoppe lens, 464
        Posner lens, 465–466
        Sussman lens, 466
        synechiae charted, 466
        Zeiss lens, 465

Angle closure glaucoma (ACG) (Con't)
   inflammation, 480–481
   iridocorneal endothelial (ICE) syndrome, 479–480
   mechanistic (pathophysiologic) Classification, 462–463
   methods, 461, 462
   nanophthalmos, 484–485
   neovascular glaucoma, 479
   PAC
      acute and sub-acute, 471–475
      risk factors, 470–471
   pathogenesis and pathophysiology
      iris bombe, 469
      mechanisms, 463, 468
      pupillary block mechanism, 468–469
   plateau iris syndrome, 463
   primary vs. secondary, 464
   progressive iris atrophy, 479
   retinal disorders and posterior segment disorders, 481
   secondary without pupillary block, 478–479
   secondary with pupillary block
      homocystinuria, 476, 478
      laser iridotomy, 478
      marfan syndrome, 476
      penetrating trauma and phacomorphic glaucoma, 475, 476
      Weill–Marchesani syndrome, 475–476
   ultrasound biomicroscope (UBM), 295–298
Angle recession, 563, 565
ANOVA. See Analysis of variance
Anterior chamber angle
   ciliary body band (CBB), 314–315
   Schwalbe's line, 315–316
   scleral spur (SS), 315
   trabecular meshwork (TM), 315
Anterior chamber intraocular lens (ACIOL) optic implantation, 895
Anterior chamber paracentesis, 774
Anterior juxtascleral depot (AJD), 991
Anterior scleral buckling method, 874–875
Anterior segment digital imaging
   angle closure, 295–298
   clinical performance, 298
   normal angle, 294–295
   OCT, 294
   plateau iris, 295
   posterior iris, 298
   pupillary block, 295
   ultrasound biomicroscope (UBM), 293–294
Anterior uveitis, 533–534
Apnea–hypopnea index (AHI), 135, 702
apraclonidine, 494, 514, 595, 608, 609, 683, 716, 720, 725
AQP1, 558
Aqueous humor production, 35–36
Aqueous misdirection. See Malignant glaucoma
Aqueous veins
   aqueous outflow, 72
   distribution, 66
   episcleral vein, 66–67
   episcleral vein pressure and posture
      collapsible veins, 75
      Starling resistor, 75–76
   importance
      direct observation, 65
      gonioscopy, 73
      peripheral iridectomy, 65
   intrascleral mixing of, 66
   mixing veins, 66–67
   origin, 66, 69

   pulsatile aqueous flow
      cardiac source, 68, 71
      causes, 71–72
      driving force, 68
      glaucoma abnormalities, 72–73
      increased stroke volume, 72
      medications, 74–75
      origination, 69
      physiologic pressure effect, 68
      Schlemm's canal (SC), 70
      systole and diastole changes, 71
      systolic stroke volume determinates, 69
      TM tissue abnormalities, 73–74
      trabecular meshwork (TM), 70–71
   recognition method, 67
   stoke volume, 72
   theories validation methods
      collapsible tubes, 70
      enucleated eyes, 69–70
      in vivo tissue load, 70
      TM movement and outflow resistance, 70
   visiblity, 66
Argon laser trabeculoplasty (ALT), 450–451, 513–514, 755, 873
Association of Clinical Research Professionals (ACRP), 978
Axenfeld-Rieger syndrome, 97
Axon screamometer, 15
Azarga, 607, 971
Azopt, 607

**B**
Baerveldt implants, 816
Bailey–Lovie near reading card, 355
Beehler three-point pupil dilator, 899
Benzalkonium chloride (BAK), 591–593
Betagan, 599
Beta-adrenergic antagonists
   brands, 599
   brimonidine, 573, 632–633
   preservatives, 599
   systemic side effects
      cardiovascular medicine, 678
      ophthalmic efficacy, 677
      pharmacology and physiology, 677–678
   topical type, 600
   vs. topical CAIs, 632
Beta-blockers. See Beta-adrenergic antagonists
Betimol, 599, 600
Betoptic-S, 599, 600
bimatoprost, 27–30, 307, 415, 513, 548, 573, 593, 599–605, 615, 616, 629–635, 685, 897, 966, 970
Binocular Esterman testing, 339–340
Binomial scale distributions, 152
Biomarkers
   cytokine molecules, POAG, 935–936
   extracellular matrix (ECM) components, 933–934
   stress and agings, POAG, 936
Biomechanics, 70
Black-and-white photography, 223
Bland–Altman analysis, 153
Bleb leak, AMT, 863
Bleb needling revision, 386
Bradycardia, 679
brimonidine, 74, 75, 277, 463, 494, 502, 504, 513, 573, 577, 585, 591, 592, 595, 608–611, 616, 631–638, 648, 674, 683, 684, 716, 720, 725, 744, 772, 970
brinzolamide, 494, 607, 610, 631–633, 638, 681, 970

Bupivicaine, 675
Busacca nodules, 530, 539

## C

Calcium channel blockers and optic nerve blood flow
  brovincamine, 453
  CCBs caution and OAG development, 453–454
  memantine and excitotoxicity, 454
  nifedipine, 452–453
  nilvadipine and nimodipine, 453
Canaloplasty
  aqueous humor
    pathways, 796
      Schlemm's canal outflow, 796–797
      subconjunctival filtration, 796
      suprachoroidal outflow, 797–798
  emerging devices, 795
  Schlemm's canal devices, 800–807
  subconjunctival filtration device, 798–800
  suprachoroidal gold microshunt device, 807–811
Canon laser Doppler flowmeter (CLBF), 124
Carbonic anhydrase inhibitors (CAI)
  acetazolamide, 605–606
  dorzolamide, 607
  methazolamide, 606
  oral type, 605–606
  systemic side effects
    physiology and pharmacology, 681
    systemic reactions, 682–683
  topical type, 607
  use, 608
Cardiovascular disease
  antihypertensive medications, 691–693
  atherosclerosis, 689
  factors, 689
  glaucomatous optic neuropathy, 690
  hypertension and cardiovascular risk
    blood pressure classification, 690
    definition, 690
    diagnosis, 690
    JNC-VI and VII report, 690
    patterns, 690
    prognostic significance, blood pressure, 690–691
  IOP, 689
  posterior ciliary artery (PCA), 689
  vascular autoregulatory capacity, 689
Carnitine, 658
carteolol HCL, 599
Cataract extraction
  adjunctive procedures
    endocyclophotocoagulation, 910
    filtration procedures, 910–911
    goniosynechialysis, 909–910
    limited pars plana vitrectomy (LPPV), 910
  indications
    acute and chronic angle closure, 906
    adjunctive procedures, 906–907
  lens, angle closure, 905
  technique
    capsulorhexis and iris, 909
    incisions, 908
    phacoemulsification, 909
    postoperative management, 909
    preoperative considerations, 908
Cataract surgery, 512
  cataract extraction with IOL implantation alone, 895
  clear-corneal phacoemulsification, 897
  evidence-based medicine, 889
  preoperative considerations
    implications, 890–893
    slit-lamp examination, 889, 890
  prostaglandin analogs and pseudophakic cystoid macular edema, 902
  selective laser trabeculoplasty (SLT), 897
  sequential surgery vs. combined surgery, 896–897
  surgical techniques
    combined surgery, 900–901
    filtering bleb, 901
    pupil management, 898–900
  topical medications, 897
Catechins, 662
CD44
  cell growth and survival, 945–947
    casein kinase II inhibitors, 946
    CD44 transmembrane receptor, 945
    human TM cells, 946, 947
    phospho-specific western blot analysis, 946
    RGC-5 cells, 946, 947
  cell signalling, 945
  functions, 939
  interactions
    ATP-binding cassette transporter, 941
    signal transduction pathways, 940
  localization, 941
  NF-κB and lactate stress, 948
  trabecular cells, 1012
Center for Medicare and Medicaid Services (CMS), 377–378
Central corneal thickness (CCT)
  case presentation
    IOP mesurement, 79
    racial differences, 79
  corneal hysteresis, 87–88
  correction factors, 87
  differences
    age-related, 80
    corneal refractive surgery, 80–83
    diabetes, 83
    diurnal variations, 83
    lamina cribrosa, 83
    racial, 80
  drug effects, 87
  measuring methods
    anterior segment optical coherence tomography (AS-OCT), 84
    optical pachymetry, 83
    orbscan system, 84
    ultrasonic pachymetry, 83
  ophthalmic assistant role, 305
  practical aspects, 88
Central retinal vein occlusion (CRVO)
  elevated IOP, 518
  neovascular glaucoma risk, 521
  ocular hypotension, 518
  retinal disorders and treatments, 481
Certified Low Vision Therapists (CLVT), 377
Certified Orientation and Mobility Specialists (COMS), 377
Certified Vision Rehabilitation Therapist (CVRT), 377
Chandler's syndrome, 553
Cholinergic agents, 610
Ciliary body
  band (CBB), 314–315
  endoscopic photocoagulation treatment, 731–732
  indications and contraindication

Ciliary body (*Con't*)
    endoscopic photocoagulation (ECP), 730
    transscleral cyclophotocoagulation (TSCPC), 730
    intraoperative and postoperative complications, 732
    IOP reduction, 732–733
    preparation, 731
    surgery and postoperative care, 731
    TSCPC treatment, 731
Circadian IOP variation, 644
Citicoline
    brain pharmacotherapy, 658–659
    phospholipids biosynthesis, 659
    retinal ganglion cells (RGCs), 659
Clinical research organizations (CROs), 978
Clinical research trials
    new drug application, 977
    participants
        association of clinical research professionals (ACRP), 978
        clinical research organizations (CROs), 978
        finding and obtaining of, 979–981
        primum non nocere principle, 979
    phases, 977–978
    real world, 977–978
    registration trials, 977
Clonidine, 609, 683
CNTGS. *See* Collaborative Normal Tension Glaucoma Study
Coding and billing reconciliation, 388
Coenzyme Q10, 659
Cogan-Reese syndrome, 553, 554
Collaborative Initial Glaucoma Treatment Study (CIGTS), IOP, 37
Collaborative Normal Tension Glaucoma Study (CNTGS)
    lowering treatment, 449
    randomized clinical trials, 36–37
Collagen VIII gene, 558
Color Doppler ultrasound imaging, 121–122
Combigan, 610, 616, 634, 635, 970, 1018
Community setting. *See* Clinical research trials
Compliance. *See* Adherence
Computerized optic nerve analysis
    computerized scanning imaging, 219–220
    cup-to-disc ratio, 219
    white-on-white automated perimetry, 219
Confocal scanning laser Doppler flowmeter (CSLDF), 125–126
Confocal scanning laser ophthalmoscopy (CSLO), 209–210, 214–215, 220
Confounding, 151
Congenital glaucoma, genetics, 96
Continuous wave laser systems
    postoperative care, 716
    tissue temperature interpretation, 717
    treatment and settings, 716
Contralateral eye management, 496
Corneal hysteresis, 87–88
Corticosteroid-induced ocular hypertension management, 532–533, 535
Cosopt, 607, 610, 616, 634, 635, 970, 1018
CRVO. *See* Central retinal vein occlusion
Cupping
    nonglaucomatous optic neuropathy
        arteritic AION, 271
        nonarteritic AION, 270–271
        optic nerve photographs, 272
    ONH biomechanics
        laminar deformation, 188
        prelaminar thinning, 188
        tissue types, 185
    optic nerve head, 185

Curcumin
    beneficial effect, 659
    diabetic cataract, 659–660
    neuroprotective, 659
Current Procedural Terminology (CPT) codes, 384
Cyclodestruction, 576
Cyclodialysis (CDC)
    anatomy and pathogenesis, 871
    cleft closure, 564
    diagnosis, 871–872
    sentinel cleft, 873
    signs and symptoms, 871
    treatment
        anterior scleral buckling method, 874–875
        cycloplegia and Argon laser methods, 873
        direct cycloplexy, 874–875
        McCannel suture technique, 874
        surgical methods, 872–874
Cyclophotocoagulation (CPC) technique
    cautions, 531
    endoscopic cyclophotocoagulation, 750–751
    laser therapy, inflow, 760
    techniques/features, 750
Cycloplegia medical treatment, 872
Cystoid macular edema (CME), 551
Cytokine molecules, POAG, 935–936
Cytoskeletal active agents
    actomyosin complex, 955, 956
    latrunculia magnifica, 956
    myosin light chain phosphatase (MLCP), 955
    trabecular meshwork, 958

**D**

Dan shen *(Salvia miltiorrhiza)*, 660
Daranide, 606
Darkroom infrared gonioscopy (DIG), 467–468
Definition, 3
Depression, 679–680
Descemet's membrane (DM), 557
Descemet's stripping endothelial keratoplasty (DSEK)
    incidence, 885–886
    intraocular pressure (IOP), 886
    surgical management
        glaucoma drainage devices, 886–887
        posterior corneal lamellar surgery, 886
Diabetes
    Baltimore eye survey, 697
    cardiovascular diseases, 697
    diagnosis, 696–697
    diet, exercise and life style, 698–700
    Los Angeles Latino Eye Study (LALES), 697
    metabolic abnormalities, 696
    risk factor, 696
Diamox, 606
Diastolic ocular perfusion pressure, 637
dichlorphenamide, 606
Diffuse neuroretinal rim loss, 204
Diffuse RNFL loss, 204
DIG. *See* Darkroom infrared gonioscopy
Digital fundus photography, 225–226
Direct cycloplexy, 874–875
Discam digital camera, 226
Disc damage likelihood scale (DDLS), 160
Disc hemorrhages (DH)
    consequences, 196–197
    definition, 195

local and systemic factors, 197
morphologic relationships, 196
ocular blood flow, 195
pressure reduction, 197–198
prevalence, 195–196
Diurnal IOP, 55
Diurnal–nocturnal variation and fluctuation, 422–423
Docosahexaenoic acid (DHA), 657
dorzolamide, 25, 29, 38, 56, 87, 494, 513, 607, 610, 616, 631, 632, 634–638, 692, 965, 970
Drainage devices
  categories, 813
  clinical outcomes
    keratoplasty, 822–823
    ocular surface disease, 823
    pediatric, uveitic and neovascular glaucoma, 821
    retinal detachment, 823
  complications
    elevated intraocular pressure, 824
    hypotony, 823
  design features, 816
  glaucoma tube insertion technique, 575–576
  indications, 816
  nonvalved implants, Baerveldt and Molteno types, 816
  surgical techniques
    basic methods, 817–819
    flow restriction devices, 819
    Pars plana tube insertion devices, 820
  valved implants
    Ahmed type, 813, 816
    Eagle Vision type, 816
  valve failure, 817–818
Driving activity
  Advance Glaucoma Intervention Study (AGIS)-scoring system, 340
  Binocular Esterman testing, 339–340
  crash rates, 339
  functional abilities, 340
  motor vehicle accidents (MVAs), 339
  vision-threatening diseases, 339
Drug management process
  development
    adverse clinical response observation, 968
    clinical pharmacology, 968–970
    clinical trial initiation, 971–972
    no-observed-adverse-effect level (NOAEL), 968
  discovery
    clinical candidate selection, 967
    disease target discovery, 965
    lead identification, 965
    lead optimization, 966
    preformulation, 966–967
    safety assessment, 966
  efficacy assessment, 645–646
  marketing
    drug discovery and development cycle, 965, 973
    phase 4 program and postmarketing surveillance, 974
  pre-clinical testing
    investigational new drug application, 962–963
    new drug application, 964
  registration
    factors, 973
    fileability, 972
    safety and efficacy, 972
    stages, 963, 972
DuoTrav, 616, 634, 635, 970, 1018
Dynamic Contour Tonometry (DCT)
  corneal confounding effect, 996
  corneal refractive surgery, 80–83
  intraocular pressure (IOP) measurement, 40
Dysrhythmia, 679

E
Eagle Vision valved implants, 816
Early manifest glaucoma trial (EMGT), IOP
  randomized clinical trials, 38
  risk factors, 51
Eccentric fixation training, 372
Electronic health record (EHR) systems
  initial task force, 343
  legal aspects
    available information, 347–348
    confidentiality issues, 348
    documentation and installation time, 346
    policies and resources, 348
    printed format, 347
    recordkeeping changes, 346
    system downtime, 348
    training time, 346–347
  selection
    internet searches, 343–344
    record-keeping methods, 344–345
    records and format, 345
    upgrades and implementation, 345
    vendors, 344
Electronic magnifiers
  inline closed-circuit television (CCTV), 362
  portable lightweight handheld, 363
  swing-arm, 363
Electronic prescribing, 389
Electroretinography
  flash (ERG), 265
  multifocal (mfERG), 266
  pattern (PERG), 265–266
  visual evoked potential, 266
Encapsulated filtering blebs, 814–816
Endoscopic cyclophotocoagulation
  advantage and disadvantage, 760–761
  limbal approach and a pars plana entry, 761
  phacoemulsification surgery, 762
Endoscopic cyclophotocoagulation (ECP), 750–751
Endothelins, ocular blood flow, 114
Epigallocatechin gallate (EGCG), 662
epinephrine, 26, 74, 531, 594, 595, 608, 609, 635, 674, 683, 684, 731, 818, 851, 891, 972
Episcleral venous identification, 67
Episcleral venous pressure (EVP), 797
Epithelial downgrowth
  diagnosis
    aqueous humor aspiration, 879
    differential diagnosis, 879–880
    iris surface, 880
    specular microscopy and fluorophotometry, 879
  etiology and pathogenesis, 877–878
  *vs.* fibrous ingrowth, 880
  glaucoma mechanisms, 879
  incidence, 877
  pathology, 880
  signs and symptoms
    anterior chamber angle, 879
    retrocorneal membrane, 878
    scalloped edge, 878
  *vs.* transplant rejection, 879

Epithelial downgrowth (Con't)
　treatment
　　glaucoma drainage methods, 881
　　surgical methods, 880–881
Esterman visual field test (EVFT), 15
Evaluation and Management (EM) codes, 385
Evidence-based medicine (EBM)
　definition, 23
　evidence cart, 28
　evolution, 24–25
　glaucoma care evolution
　　golden age and polypharmacy era, 26
　　individualized medicine era, 27
　　postgonioscope and postophthalmoscope era, 26
　　randomized clinical trial era, 26–27
　meta-analysis, 27
　process
　　application, 29–30
　　basic calculus, 30–31
　　clinical problem formulation, 27–28
　　evidence cart assemble, 28
　　evidence quality evaluation, 28–29
　　suprachoroidal hemorrhages, 31–32
　usage reasons
　　learning, principle and sense of control, 25
　　risk calculators, 25
Excimer laser trabeculostomy (ELT), 755
Exfoliative glaucoma (XFG)
　appearance
　　biomicroscope, 509
　　classic slit-lamp, 508
　　electron microscope, 508
　　light microscope, 508
　　ultrastructure, 509
　argon laser trabeculoplasty (ALT), 513–514
　clinical diagnosis
　　dense deposition, 510, 511
　　typical gonioscopic appearance, 510, 511
　definition, terminology and prevalance, 507
　differential diagnosis
　　cataract surgery, 512
　　IOP characteristics, 511
　evolution, XFS, 510
　genetics, 96
　medical therapy
　　IOP characteristics, 512
　　POAG, 512–513
　surgery, 514–515
EX-PRESS shunt devices
　gonioscopic view, 800
　sapphire blade, 799
　schematic diagram, 798
　vs. trabeculectomy, 800
Extensive conjunctival scarring, 816
Eye codes, 385

F
Ferritin abnormalities, 1012
Filtering blebs, surgery complications
　early failure, 854–855
　encapsulated type, 855–856
　late failure, 855
　ocular infection, 856–857
　symptomatic type, 856
Flash (ERG) electroretinogram, 265
Flow restriction techniques, 819
Flow-restrictive drainage devices. See Valved implants
5-Fluorouracil (5-FU), 777
Focal ischemic disc, 199
Folic acid
　exfoliation syndrome (XFS), 660
　homocysteine, 660
Fornix-based flap technique
　advantages and disadvantages, 772
　creation steps, 772
　postoperative complications, 768
Fresnel prisms, 367–368
Fuchs' endothelial dystrophy (FED)
　angle closure glaucoma
　　anterior chamber, 557
　　bilateral endothelial dystrophy, 557
　AQP1, 558
　collagen VIII gene, 558
　oxidative stress and apoptosis, 558
　primary open angle glaucoma, 557
Fuchs' uveitis syndrome (FUS)
　etiology and pathogenesis, 541
　history and clinical features
　　cataracts, 540–541
　　iris changes, 539
　　subtle heterochromia, 539
　　vitreous debris, 540
　management
　　medical and surgical therapy, 542
　　prognosis, 541
FUS. See Fuchs' uveitis syndrome

G
Ganfort, 616, 631, 634, 635, 970, 1018
GDx, 215–216
Gene therapy, 985–986
Genetics
　angle closure glaucoma, 97
　congenital glaucoma, 96
　definitions and nomenclature
　　gene and exons, 91–93
　　inheritance, 91–92
　　mutations and diseases, 92–93
　　polymorphism, 94
　　single nucleotide polymorphisms (SNPs), 94
　　transcription factors, 93–94
　early observations, 94
　exfoliation glaucoma, 96
　genes and loci associated, 92
　gene therapy, 97
　genetic testing, 97–98
　mesodermal dysgenesis syndromes, 97
　open angle glaucoma (OAG), types
　　genetic loci, 95
　　gene variants, 95–96
　pharmacogenetics, 98, 985
　potential phenotypic differences, OAG, 93
Gentle digital pressure, 67
Ghost cell glaucoma, 314, 563–564
　anterior chamber aspirate, 556
　cataract surgeries, 555
　definition, 555
　diagnosis, 555
　IOP reduction, 555
Ginkgo biloba extract (GBE)
　bioactive compound, 660
　diabetic retinopathy, 661

neuroprotective, 660–661
  protective effects, 660
Ginseng RB1/RG3, 661
Glaucoma drainage implants, PK-glaucoma, 883–884
L-Glutathione, 661
Glycerin, 613
Goldmann applanation tonometry (GAT), 39, 55
Goldmann equation, 35
Goldmann perimetry. *See* Kinetic perimetry
Goldmann-style 3 mirror lens, 404, 405
Goldmann visual field testing (III-4e target), 340
Gold microshunt suprachoroidal outflow device
  fornix-based conjunctival peritomy
    complications and medication usage, 810
    non-toothed forceps, 808–809
    nylon sutures, 809–810
    postoperative goniophotograph, 809
    scleral cutdown, 808
    toothed forceps, 808
  implantation, 807
  interior view, 808
  models, 807
  schematic diagram, 808
Gonioscopy
  anterior chamber angle
    ciliary body band (CBB), 314–315
    Schwalbe's line, 315–316
    scleral spur (SS), 315
    trabecular meshwork (TM), 315
  comparison, 283–285
  compression, 465
  concentric rings, 466
  direct and indirect method, 283–285
  four-mirror lenses, 288
  FUS, 539–540
  Goldmann lens technique, 288
  Goldmann three-mirror lens, 464, 465
  grading systems
    Scheie system, 289
    Shaffer system, 289
    Spaeth system, 289–291
  guidelines, 285–287
  indentation, 288–289
  Keoppe lens, 462
  lenses, 404
  Posner lens, 463–464
  Posner style goniolens, 314–315
  Sussman lens, 464
  synechiae charted, 466
  view, 287–288
  Zeiss lens, 465
Goniotomy
  indications, 573
  results, 574
  technique, 573–574
Grape seed proanthocyanidins, 661

# H
Handheld magnifiers, 361
Handheld scanner/reader, 364–365
Heidelberg retina tomographs (HRT), 209–210, 214–215
Herpes simplex virus (HSV)
  management
    anti glaucoma medications, 547, 548
    anti-inflammatory agents, 547
    oral acyclovir and eye medications, 547

  ocular area
    conjunctival and stroma disease, 545
    dendritic/amoeboid ulcer, 545
    epithelial/stromal keratiti, 545–546
    intraocular pressure (IOP), 545
    keratouveitis, 545
  pathogenesis
    enucleated eyes, 546
    keratouveitic glaucoma, 546
    trabecular meshwork cells, 546
  types, 545
Herpes zoster ophthalmicus (HZO)
  management, 549–551
  varicella–zoster virus (VZV), 549
High pressure open angle glaucoma, 1011–1013
Hill of vision
  Humphrey field analyzer, 230
  procedure, 229
  schematic representation, 230
  sensitivity profile, 230
  testing
    lens induced artifacts, 233
    rim defects, 234–235
  visual field defects, 231
Home tonometers, 61
Humphrey field analyzer (HFA)
  multiple field analysis, 257
  single field analysis
    deficit features, 257
    gaze tracking, 255
    information interpretion, 255–257
    retinal ganglion cell arrangements, 257–258
    total and pattern deviation probability plots, 254
  test frequency, 253–254
Humphrey visual field, 81
Hyaluronic acid receptor CD44 (sCD44)
  Alzheimer's disease
    ectodomain shedding of CD44 and B-amyloid, 941, 942
    metalloproteinase inhibitors, 942
    protein kinase C activators, 943
    putative phosphorylation and influence, 943
  antagonists, 947
  aqueous humor concentration, 943–944
  cell growth and survival
    casein kinase II inhibitors, 946
    CD44 transmembrane receptor, 945
    human TM cells, 946, 947
    phospho-specific western blot analysis, 946
    RGC-5 cells, 946, 947
  cell signaling, 945
  disease process, 944–945
  ectodomain shedding, 941
  internalization, 947–948
  NF-κB and lactate stress, 948
Hyperosmotic agents
  intravenous (IV) mannitol, 612–613
  oral glycerin, 613
  side effects, 613–614
Hyphema, 563, 565
Hypopyon, 314
Hypotensive lipids (HLs)
  bimatoprost, 27–30, 307, 415, 513, 548, 573, 593, 599–605, 615, 616, 629–635, 685, 897, 966, 970
  chemical structure, 601
  cystoid macular edema (CME), 604
  first-line agents, 600–601

Hypotensive lipids (HLs) (Con't)
   functional activity, 602–603
   lash changes, bimatoprost, 604–605
   latanoprost, 27–30, 51, 56, 75, 414, 513, 548, 573, 585, 591, 593, 599–604, 615, 616, 629–635, 637, 638, 644, 674, 685, 686, 897, 966, 970
   Lumigan, 304, 600, 638, 966
   ocular-related side effects, 604
   prostaglandin FP receptors, 601–603
   Rescula, 600, 966
   systemic side-effects, 603–604
   Travatan, 304, 414, 592, 600, 966
   Travatan Z, 592, 600
   travoprost, 27–29, 56, 87, 415, 513, 573, 591, 593, 599–604, 615, 616, 629–635, 685, 966
   unoprostone, 600, 601, 685
   Xalatan, 60, 304, 600, 966
Hypothyroidism
   ICD-9 diagnosis, 695
   mucopolysaccharide deposition, 695
   open-angle glaucoma, 695–696
   relationship, 696
Hypotony
   glaucoma drainage devices, 823
   maculopathy (HM)
      disc edema and chorioretinal folds, 845–846
      occurence and diagnosis, 847
      scleral flap suture, 846
   serous choroidal effusions, 867
   surgery complications
      choroidal effusions, 842
      corneal edema and Descemet's folds, 842
      flat anterior chamber, 842–844
      management, 841
      treatment, 845–847

# I

Immunology
   glaucoma vs. immune responses, factors, 929
   neurodegenerative disease
      abnormal accumulation, 926–927
      apoptotic signals, 927
      excessive glutamate, increased calcium levels, and excitotoxicity, 926
      intraocular pressure (IOP), 925
      neurotrophins and growth factors, 926
      oxidative stress and free radicals, 926
   pharmacological neuroprotection, 927
   potential glaucoma therapy, 928–929
   retinal ganglion cells (RGCs)
      anti-self T cells, 928
      immune system, 927
      protective autoimmunity, 928
Implantable pressure transducer, 61–63
Improved techniques
   adherence, sustained drug delivery implants, 1006
   anterior segment, optical coherence tomography, 999, 1000
   aqueous outflow, 1004
   automated diagnosis, 1003–1004
   diagnosis
      optical disc photographs, 998
      three-dimensional optical coherence tomography, 998, 999
   Doppler OCT, 1001
   Dynamic Contour Tonometry (DCT), 996
   intraocular pressure (IOP) measurement, 995
   iTrack Microcatheter, 1007
   ocular disease, (SD-OCT), 1000, 1001
   ocular response analyzer (ORA), 996
   stent and shunt devices, 1004–1006
   surgery, ocular ultrasound system, 1004
   swept source OCT, 1001
   telemedicine, 997
   Trabectome, 1007
   visual field, 1002
Incisional therapies
   canaloplasty
      aqueous humor, 796–798
      emerging devices, 795
      Schlemm's canal devices, 800–807
      subconjunctival filtration device, 798–800
      suprachoroidal gold microshunt device, 807–811
   fibrin glue, 851–852
   glaucoma drainage devices
      categories, 813
      clinical outcomes, 820–823
      complications, 823–824
      design features, 816
      elevated pressure, 827–828
      indications, 816–817
      nonvalved implants, 816
      surgical techniques, 817–820
      valved implants, 813, 816
   iStent
      development, 831–832
      goniophotograph, 832–833
      surgical techniques, 832–837
   physiologic function restoration, surgery, 831
   surgery complications
      bleb-related ocular infection, 856–857
      early bleb leak, 851
      filtering bleb failure, 854–855
      hyphema, 848–849
      hypotony and overfiltration, 841
      late bleb leak, 853–854
      malignant glaucoma, 849–850
      postoperative suprachoroidal hemorrhage, 842–844
      releasable sutures, 848
      symptomatic blebs, 856
      types, 841
      wipe-out phenomenon, 850–851
   trabeculectomy surgery
      adults, 789–794
      alternative filtration routes, 765
      anesthesia, 765–766
      anterior chamber paracentesis, 774
      anticoagulants, 769–770
      antimetabolites, 777–780
      conjunctival closure, 781–782
      conjunctival incision, 768, 771
      corneoscleral flap, 766
      eye exposure, 766, 768
      flap suturing techniques, 776–777
      guarded filtration procedure, 765
      intraocular pressure (IOP), 767–768
      peripheral iridectomy (PI), 781
      postoperative follow-up, 782–786
      scleral flap, 774–776
      traction suture, 768
   tube shunt surgery
      hypertensive phase (HP), 824–826
      Tube Versus Trabeculectomy Study (TVT), 814–815
Infantile, childhood, and juvenile glaucomas

clinical examination
    angle appearance, 571–572
    examination-under-anesthesia (EUA), 572
    infantile glaucoma, 571
    iris and pupil, 571
    medical and family history, 571
    optic nerve head, 572
    tonometry, 571
clinical features
    PCG diagnoses, 570
    signs and symptoms, 570
epidemiology and genetics
    anterior segment dysgenesis, 569
    chromosome locus, 569
    evaluation, 569–570
nomenclature
    developmental glaucoma, 567
    genetic basis, 567
    primary and secondary pediatric glaucomas, 568
pathophysiology
    angle histopathology, 569
    PCG, 568
    Schlemm's canal and trabecular meshwork, 569
treatment
    beta-adrenergic agonist, 573
    beta-adrenergic antagonists, 573
    cyclodestruction, 576
    glaucoma drainage devices, 575–576
    goniotomy, 573–574
    oral carbonic anhydrase inhibitors, 572
    prostaglandin analogues, 573
    trabeculectomy, 574–575
    trabeculotomy, 574

Inflammatory disease, elevated IOP
  mechanisms
    affects, 527
    clinical classification, 527–530
  uveitis patients
    principles, 530–531
    therapeutic armamentarium, 531–532
    treatment, 532–535

Inflammatory ocular hypertension syndromes (IOHS) management, 532
Inline closed-circuit television (CCTV), 362
Insurance coding
  office services
    diagnosis, 386–387
    office procedures, 385–386
    patient past visits, 384
    service level, 385
    special tests and exam modifiers, 385
  postoperative period, 387–388
  surgical procedures, 387

Interleukin-1 (IL1) autocrine loop disruption, 1012
Intermediate uveitis, 534
Intraocular pressure (IOP)
  Advanced Glaucoma Intervention Study (AGIS), 51
  aqueous humor production and outflow
    ciliary body, 36
    Goldmann equation, 35
  clinical import, 56–57
  continuous monitoring method
    current methods and limitations, 59–60
    home tonometers, 61
    implantable pressure transducer, 61–63
    necessity, 60–61
  cyclic oscillations, 54
  distribution, 41
  diurnal role, 54
  exfoliative glaucoma (XFG), 507
  early manifest glaucoma trial (EMGT), 51
  history, glaucoma link, 35
  influencing factors
    cardiac pulse wave, 42
    circadian and seasonal variation, 41–42
    fluid intake, 42–43
    nutrition and recreational substances, 43
    physical exercise and postural changes, 42
    respiration and valsalva maneuver, 42
  intravitreal triamcinolone (IVTA) effects
    delayed, 672
    early, 671–672
    immediate, 672
  long-term IOP fluctuation, 51
  measurement
    Dynamic Contour Tonometry (DCT), 40
    Goldmann applanation tonometry (GAT), 39
    noncontact air puff and tono-pen tonometry, 40
    phasing, 12
    pneumatonometer, 40
    Schiotz tonometry, 41
    telemetry and water-drinking test, 12
    transpalpebral scleral palpation, 40
  medication efficacy analysis
    aqueous suppressants, 56
    nocturnal measurements, 56
  medications influence
    corticosteroids, 43
    drug-induced intraocular hypertension, 43
    general anesthetics, 44
    pupillary block, 43–44
  nocturnal and diurnal IOP, 55
  ocular hypertensive patients, 53
  randomized clinical trials
    Advanced Glaucoma Intervention Study (AGIS), 37
    Collaborative Initial Glaucoma Treatment Study (CIGTS), 37
    Collaborative Normal Tension Glaucoma Study (CNTGS), 36–37
    Early Manifest Glaucoma Trial (EMGT), 38
    Ocular Hypertension Treatment Study (OHTS), 37–38
  rapid oscillations, 52
  risk factor, glaucoma development, 38
  target IOP, 44
  tonometry measurements, 54

Intraoperative considerations, 913–914
Intravitreal colchicine, 220
Intravitreal gas, 918–919
Intravitreal triamcinolone (IVTA)
  indications, 671
  intraocular pressure (IOP) elevation
    delayed, 672
    early, 671–672
    immediate, 671
  pharmacokinetics, 671
Intravitreal triamcinolone acetate, 991–992
Iopidine, 609, 716, 725
Iridocorneal endothelial (ICE) syndrome
  clinical variations, 553
  Cogan-Reese syndrome, 554
  corneal endothelium, 553
  glaucoma prevalence and surgical intervention, 553
Iridoplasty
  history, 727
  surgery and postoperative care, 727–728

Iridotomy
    complications, 727
    history, 725
    postoperative care, 726–727
    preparation, 725
    treatment and laser system settings, 725–726
Iris bombe, 528, 529
Iris heterochromia, 530
Iris hooks, 899
Irradiance, 753, 754
Ismotic, 612, 613
Isosorbide, 44, 472, 494, 612, 613
Istalol, 599, 600
iStent
    development, 831–832
    goniophotograph, 832–833
    implantation
        applicator tubing, 834
        sequence, 835
        with and without cataract surgery, 836
    surgical techniques
        implantation, 834–837
        trabectome trabecular excision, 836–838
iTrack Microcatheter, 1007

## K
Keoppe lens, 464
Keratouveitis, 546, 550
Kestenbaum's vision rule, 359
Kinetic perimetry
    binocular testing, 237–238
    grayscale and sensitivity, 237
    polar and Cartesian coordinate systems, 237
    suprathreshold static type, 237
Koeppe nodules, 539
Krukenberg spindle, 499, 500
Kurzweil-National Federation of the Blind Reader, 364–365

## L
Laser assisted in situ keratomileusis (LASIK) effects, 424–425
Laser Doppler flowmeter (LDF), 124–125
Laser iridoplasty technique
    acute angle closure, 742–743
    clinical assessment
        ancillary testing, 744
        examination, 743–744
        history, 743
    crystalline lens, 741
    lens extraction, 743
    malignant or ciliary block, 743
    pupillary block, 741
    pathophysiology and mechanism
        anatomic levels, 741
        angle closure, 741–742
        plateau iris, 741
        pupil block, 741
    phacomorphic glaucoma, 743
    plateau iris syndrome, 742
    primary angle closure (PAC) management, 742
    quantitative imaging techniques, 746
    technique
        coherence tomography image, 745
        complications, 746
        contraction burns and laser setup, 745
        pilocarpine, 744
        posttreatment, 746
    risks, 744–745
    Urrets-Zavalia syndrome, 746
Laser therapy
    angle closure mechanism
        iridoplasty, 727–728
        iridotomy, 725–727
        pupilloplasty and pupillary sphincterotomy, 728–729
    bleeders coagulation, 735
    ciliary body
        complications, 732
        endoscopic photocoagulation treatment, 731–732
        history, 730–731
        indications and contraindication, 730
        IOP reduction, 732–733
        preparation, 731
        surgery and postoperative care, 731
        TSCPC treatment, 731
    cyclophotocoagulation
        endoscopic, 750–751
        techniques/features, 750
    indications, 749
    inflow
        cyclophotocoagulation, 760
        endoscopic cyclophotocoagulation, 760–762
    iris
        corneal edema and angle closure, 723–724
        indications and contraindications, 723
    light properties and parameters
        absorption path length, 753
        irradiance, 753
        principles, 753
        tissue interaction, 753
    micropulse diode laser trabeculoplasty (MDLT), 757–758
    Nd:YAG laser, 749
    neovascular glaucoma, 735
    nonpenetrating deep sclerectomy (NPDS), 759
    occluded inner ostium, 734–735
    outflow
        argon laser trabeculoplasty (ALT), 755
        excimer laser trabeculostomy, 755
    peripheral iridotomy, 531
    process, 713
    sealing hypotonous cyclodialysis clefts, 734
    suture lysis, 733–734
    technique and treatment pararmeters comparison, 736
    titanium, sapphire laser trabeculoplasty (SLT), 757
    trabecular meshwork
        history, 714–716
        indications and contraindications, 714
        methods, 717–723
Laser trabeculoplasty, 531, 675
LASIK effects. See Laser assisted in situ keratomileusis effects
latanoprost, 27–30, 51, 56, 75, 414, 513, 548, 573, 585, 591, 593,
    599–604, 615, 616, 629–635, 637, 638, 644, 674, 685,
    686, 897, 966, 970
Latisse, 604
Latrunculia magnifica, 956
Lebensohn's vision rule, 360
Leber's hereditary optic neuropathy (LHON), 276
levobunolol, 599, 600, 629, 631
Limbal-based flap technique
    advantages and disadvantages, 773
    creation steps, 773
    postoperative complications, 768
Lumigan, 304, 600, 638, 966
Limited pars plana vitrecomy (LPPV), 910

Localized neuroretinal rim loss, 205
Localized RNFL loss, 205–206
Low vision
    blindness networking systems
        organizations, 378–379
        primary service providers, 376–377
        reimbursement sources, 377–378
    contact lenses
        complications, 359
        fitting characteristics, 357–358
        uses, 358–359
    examination sequence
        health history, 353
        observation, 353
        ocular history, 353–354
        social history, 354
    field enhancement devices
        amorphic lens, 369
        electronic type, 369–370
        field expanders, 365–366
        Fresnel prisms, 367–368
        glare control, 370–372
        inwave channel lenses, 368
        minus lenses, 366
        reverse telescopes, 368–369
        scanning, 365
    glare, 352
    lighting, 372
    magnification
        computer screen programs and reader, 363–364
        electronic magnifiers, 362–363
        handheld magnifiers, 361
        handheld scanner/reader, 364–365
        Kestenbaum's rule, 359
        Lebensohn's rule, 360
        microscopes, 360
        stand magnifiers, 361–362
    non-optical devices
        adaptive and talking devices, 374–375
        embossed paper and large-print checks, 374
        labeling systems, 375–376
        plasticized and bold line marker, 373–374
        signature guides, 373
        tactile dots, 373
        talking books, 376
        typoscopes, 372–373
    PRL and eccentric fixation training, 372
    vision rehabilitation, 352–353
    visual acuity
        blindness standard, 352
        measurement, 354–357
    visual field loss, 351–352
Lutein, 662

## M

Malignant glaucoma
    anterior chamber, 495
    argon laser treatment, 495
    classic, 489, 490
    clinical manifestations, 489, 490
    clinical picture consistent, 490, 491
    contralateral eye management, 496
    differential diagnosis
        choroidal effusion, 493
        overfiltration and wound leakage, 494
        pupillary block, 493
        suprachoroidal hemorrhage, 493–494
        ultrasound biomicroscopy (UBM), 494
    medical and surgical management, 494–495
    non-phakic, 490–491
    pathogenesis
        aqueous misdirection or posterior aqueous diversion, 490, 491
        ciliary block, 491
        vitreous cavity, 491, 492
        vitreous mechanisms, 492
    surgery complications
        management, 849–850
        prevention, 850
    surgical therapy, 495–496
Malyugin ring, 900
mannitol, 472, 483, 484, 494, 612–615, 908
McCannel suture technique, 874
Medical insurance
    coding
        office services, 384–387
        postoperative period, 387–388
        surgical procedures, 387
    infrastructure
        billing department, 383–384
        imperative items, 384
    reconciliation, 388
    resources and suggestions, 388
Medical legal considerations, glaucoma care
    clinical practice guidelines, 394
    compliance
        drug side effects, 392–393
        physician instructions, 392
    patient expectations
        complaints, 394
        postsurgical recovery, 393–394
    prognosis and diagnosis errors, 391
    standard therapy, 395
    triage, 392
Medical therapies
    aqueous outflow, 983–984
    beta-adrenergic antagonists, 598–600
    carbonic anhydrase inhibitors (CAI), 605–608
    challenges, 983
    drug delivery methods, 986
    drug selection characteristics, 596–597
    gene therapy, 985–986
    genetics and pharmacogenomics, 985
    hyperosmotics, 612–615
    hypotensive lipids (HLs), 600–605
    intraocular pressure-lowering effects, 600
    new glaucoma pathogenic pathways, 985
    parasympathomimetic agents, 610–611
    sympathomimetic agonists, 608–610
    targeting glaucomatous retinopathy and optic neuropathy, 984
    treatment options and timeline, 598
Mesodermal dysgenesis syndromes, 97
methazolamide, 494, 565, 572, 605, 606, 608, 634, 681
Methylcobalamin, 662
metipranolol, 599, 629, 631
Micropulsed diode laser trabeculoplasty
    anterior chamber angle, 718
    laser energy, 715
    postoperative care, 718
    tissue temperature interpretation, 717
    treatment and settings, 717–718
Micropulse diode laser trabeculoplasty (MDLT), 757–758
Migraine, ocular blood flow, 119–120

Miotic agents. *See* Parasympathomimetic agents
Miotics, systemic side effects
    pharmacology and physiology
        cholinomimetics classes, 684
        neural pathways, 684–685
    systemic toxicity, 685
Mitomycin C (MMC), 777, 820, 861–862
Molteno implants, 816
Monocular photography, 224
Monocular therapeutic drug trial, IOP reduction
    circadian rhythm, 644
    clinical utility, 643
    contralateral crossover, 644
    drug efficacy assessment, 645–646
    lowering medication, 644
    medical therapy, 643
    patient use, 644–645
    retrospective evaluation, 645
    spontaneous variation, 643–644
Moorfields regression analysis (MRA), 214
Morcher pupil dilating ring, 900
Multifocal (mfERG) electroretinogram
    advanced instrumentation, 1002
    diagnosis, 266
Multifocal visual evoked potential (VEP), 1002
Multiple sphincterotomies, 898
Myocillin
    locus, 96
    optineurin, 96
    prevalance, 95
    TIGR sequence homology, 95
Myocillin GLC1A, 1010
Myopic disc, 199
Myosin light chain phosphatase (MLCP), 955

## N
*N*-Acetyl-L-cysteine, 662
Nasolacrimal occlusion digital massage technique, 594
Natural compound treatments
    alpha-lipoic acid, 657
    alpha-tocopherol and tocotrienol, 658
    carnitine, 658
    citicoline
        brain pharmacotherapy, 658–659
        phospholipids biosynthesis, 659
        retinal ganglion cells (RGCs), 659
    coenzyme Q10, 659
    curcumin
        beneficial effect, 659
        diabetic cataract, 659–660
        neuroprotective, 659
    Dan shen *(Salvia miltiorrhiza),* 658
    fish oil and omega-3 fatty acids
        age-related macular degeneration (ARMD), 658
        oxidative damage, 657–658
        retina protection, 658
        types, 657
    folic acid
        exfoliation syndrome (XFS), 660
        homocysteine, 660
    *Ginkgo biloba* extract (GBE)
        bioactive compound, 660
        diabetic retinopathy, 661
        neuroprotective, 660–661
        protective effects, 660
    Ginseng RB1/RG3, 661
    grape seed extract, 661
    green tea catechins, 662
    hemorheologic abnormalities, 657
    L-glutathione, 661
    lutein and zeaxanthine, 662
    methylcobalamin, 662
    *N*-acetyl-L-cysteine, 662
    neuroprotection, 657
    optic nerve head perfusion, 657
    pycnogenol
        angiotensin-converting enzyme (ACE), 663
        composition, 663
        cytotoxicity, 663
        oral administration, 662
        vascular endothelial cells, 663
    quercetin, 663
    resveratrol, 663
    taurine, 663–664
Neovascular glaucoma (NVG), 733
    clinical presentations, 518–520
    diabetes, 520–522
    differential diagnosis, 517–518
    pathophysiology, 517
    treatment
        anti-VEGF, 523
        aqueous shunts, 523–524
        cyclophotocoagulation, 524
        medical therapy, 523
        pan-retinal photocoagulation (PRP), 522
        trabeculectomy, 523
Neptazane, 606
Neuroprotection, retinal ganglion cells
    causes
        excitotoxicity and antioxidants
        gene therapy
        immune system
        natural compounds
        neurotrophins
        technique
Nitric oxide synthase, 648
*N*-methyl-d-aspartate (NMDA) antagonists, 647
Nocturnal hypotension, ocular blood flow, 116
Nocturnal IOP
    24H IOP curves, 55
    pneumatonometry measurement, 55
Nominal scale distributions, 152
Nonarteritic anterior ischemic optic neuropathy (NAION), 270–271
Noncontact air puff tonometry, IOP, 40
Nonglaucomatous optic neuropathy
    *vs.* glaucoma
        afferent pupillary defects (APD), 272
        Alzheimer's disease, 276
        clinical features, 270
        compressive lesions, 275
        cupping, 270–272
        intermittent IOP elevation, 276–277
        nasal step, 272
        optic nerve excavation, hereditary, 276
        optociliary shunt vessels (OCSV), 274–275
        peripapillary nerve fiber hemorrhage, 274
        prevalence, 270
        shock, 275–276
        temporal visual field defects, 272–274
        traumatic, 276
    neuro-imaging, 279
    neuroprotection, 277

prophylactic IOP lowering, 277
vascular events mimicking, 278–279
Nonpenetrating deep sclerectomy (NPDS), 759
Nonselective beta-blockers, 599
Nonvalved implants, Baerveldt and Molteno type, 816
Norepinephrine, 594
Normal pressure glaucoma. *See* Normal tension glaucoma (NTG)
Normal tension glaucoma (NTG)
   argon laser trabeculoplasty (ALT), 450–451
   definition, 421
   differential diagnosis, 448
   epidemiology
      clinical studies, 422
      population studies, 421–422
   filtering surgery, 451–452
   IOP-lowering treatment
      Collaborative Normal Tension Glaucoma Study (CNTGS), 448–450
      compliance issues, 450
      differential diagnostic possibilities, 449
      elements of the medical and ocular exam, 449–450
      medications, 450
   non-IOP-lowering therapy, 452–454
   *vs.* primary open angle glaucoma (POAG), 270
   risk factors
      IOP-related, 422–425
      optic-nerve related, 425–434
   sleep apnea syndrome (SAS), 135
   systemic factors
      migraine headache and Raynaud's phenomenon, 445–447
         obstructive sleep apnea syndrome, 448
   visual field defects
      age, gender and refractive error, 444–445
      patterns of loss, 433–436
      progression characteristics, 436–445
Neurotrophic keratitis, 550

## O

Obstructive sleep apnea (OSA)
   apnea/hypopnea index (AHI), 135
   diagnosis, 702
   glaucoma prevalence
      normal-tension glaucoma (NTG), 136
      polysomnography result, 135
      prevalence, 701–702
      relationship, glaucoma, 703
      retinal nerve fiber layer (RNFL), 136
      sleep disordered breathing (SDB), 135
   treatment, 136
Occluded inner ostium, 734–735
OCT. *See* Optical coherence tomography
Ocular blood flow
   anatomy
      central retinal artery, 112–113
      ophthalmic artery, 112
      uveal system, 113
   ischemia and optic neuropathy
      retinal ganglion cells, 111
      vascular role, 112
   measuring methods
      canon laser Doppler flowmeter (CLBF), 124
      color Doppler ultrasound imaging, 121–122
      confocal scanning laser Doppler flowmeter (CSLDF), 125–126
      laser Doppler flowmeter (LDF), 124–125
      pulsatile ocular blood flow, 126–128
      retinal oximetry, 128–129
      retina vessel analyzer (RVA), 128
      scanning laser ophthalmoscope (SLO), 122–124
   open angle glaucoma (OAG), 115–119
   optic nerve vascular anatomy
      lamina cribrosa and the retrolaminar region, 113–114
      prelaminar region, 113
      superficial nerve fiber layer, 113–114
   prospective studies, glaucoma patients, 120
   regulation
      angiotensinconverting enzyme (ACE), 115
      autonomic nervous system, 114
      endothelins, 115
      extrinsic and intrinsic controls, 114
      soluble vasoactive molecules, 114–115
      superoxide anions, 115
   signs and conditions
      diabetes, 120
      disc hemorrhages, 119
      migraines, 119–120
   vascular risk factors, OAG
      nocturnal hypotension, 116
      ocular perfusion pressure, 116–119
      systemic hypertension and hypotension, 115–116
   visual function and structure
      neuroretinal rim blood flow, 129
      ocular perfusion pressure (OPP), 129
      retrobulbar blood flow, 129
Ocular Hypertension Treatment Study (OHTS)
   central corneal thickness (CCT), 79, 105–106
   randomized clinical trials, IOP, 37–38
Ocular perfusion pressure (OPP), 195, 411–413
Ocular trauma
   diagnosis, 561
   early onset glaucoma
      chemical injuries, 563
      hyphema, 563
      intraocular inflammation, 561–562
      trabecular meshwork injury, 563
   epidemiology and pathogenesis, 561
   late onset glaucoma
      angle recession, 563
      cyclodialysis cleft closure, 564
      epithelial downgrowth, 564
      ghost cell glaucoma, 563–564
      lens injury, 564
      retained intraocular foreign body, 564
      rhegmatogenous retinal detachment, 564
      secondary angle closure, 564
   treatment
      angle recession and ghost cell glaucoma, 565
      hyphema, 565
      medical and surgical management principles, 564–565
Ocupress, 599, 600
Omega-3 fatty acids
   age-related macular degeneration (ARMD), 658
   oxidative damage, 657–658
   retina protection, 658
   types, 657
Open angle glaucoma
   clinical information, 200
   findings, 201
   fluorescein angiography, 199
   glaucoma populations, 201–202
   optic nerves, 199
   principal component analysis, 201
   stereo optic disc photographs, 199
Open tube drainage devices. *See* Nonvalved implants

Ophthalmic assistant–patient interview
   chart review, 303
   Glaucoma Consultation Report, 327–334
   information recording
      central corneal thickness (CCT), 305
      current eyeglasses, 305
      demographic, 304
      pupillary responses to light, 306
      tonometry, 306–307
      visual acuity, 304–305
      visual fields, 305–306
   language translation, 303
   open-ended and directed questions, 304
Ophthalmic literature evaluation
   Bland–Altman analysis, 153
   citations, 142
   discussion section, 141–142
   distributions
      density function, 146
      mean, median and mode, 146
      measures of variability, 146–147
      null hypothesis, 145
      statistical power, 145
   figures, tables, and graphs, 142
   measurement scales, data types
      ordinal and interval data, 144
      ratio, nominal and timeline data, 144
      robust test, 145
      student's t-test, 145
   methods, 153
   publishing criteria, 140
   randomization
      double-masked experimental treatments, 143
      key elements, 143
      post hoc analysis, 144
   results section, 141
   reviewing process, 152–153
   statistical testing
      clinically significance, 149
      inference, 147
      level of statistical significance, 147
      sample size, 148
      study power, 148
   statistic essentials, box of truth, 142–143
   tests and errors
      analysis of variance (ANOVA), 150
      confounding, 151
      nominal and binomial scale distributions, 152
      nonparametric test, 151–152
      parametric tests, 149–150
      parametric *vs.* non-parametric statistical tests, 149
      Poisson test, 152
Optical coherence tomography (OCT), 79, 210, 215, 220, 467
   drawback and advantage, 294
   iris, pigment dispersion, 299
   narrow angle, plateau component., 297
   normal angle, 295
   pupillary block angle closure, 296
   time domain, 294
Optic nerves
   anatomy
      intralaminar, 169
      normal optic disc, 170
      optic disc, 169
      retinal nerve fiber layer (RNFL), 169
      retrobulbar, 170
   cameras
      Canon CR-1, 226
      Nidek AFC-230-210, 225, 226
      Topcon TRC-50DX, 227
   comparisons, 425, 433
   differential diagnosis
      anterior ischemic optic neuropathy (AION), 178–181
      compressive optic neuropathy, 182–183
      congenital optic disc pits, 182
      morning glory syndrome, 181–182
      optic disc drusen (ODD), 181
      optic neuritis, 181
   digital imaging devices
      comparison, 210
      confocal scanning laser ophthalmoscopy (CSLO), 209–210, 214–215
      detecting ability, 210
      GDx, 215–216
      optical coherence tomography (OCT), 210, 215
      progression assessing ability, 216
      scanning laser polarimetry (SLP), 210
   examining methods
      direct ophthalmoscope, 170
      indirect ophthalmoscopy, 171
      optic disc photography, 171
      retinal nerve fiber layer examination, 171
      RNFL and optic disc analyzers, 172
   focal ischemic discs, 430, 431
   generalized optic cup enlargement, 431
   head (ONH)
      biomechanics, 185–188
      clinical implications, 188–191
      cupping, 185, 188
      IOP-related stress and strain, 186
      lamina cribrosa, 185
   myopic glaucomatous discs, 431
   neuroretinal rim loss, 431
   optic disc evaluation
      classification systems, 172
      disc asymmetry, 175
      disc damage likelihood scale (DDLS) determination, 173–174
      disc drawing, 172
      hemorrhages, 176
      neuroretinal rim size, shape and pallor, 175
      peripapillary atrophy (PPA), 176
      size, 174–175
   optic disc hemorrhages (ODHs), 431–432
   optic disc size, 425
   patterns of, 426–430
   peripapillary atrophy (PPA), 432–434
   photography
      black and white, 223
      digital fundus, 225–226
      monocular, 224
      Polaroid, 227
      retinal nerve fiber layer (RNFL), 223–224
      stereo color, 224–225
   progressive damage evaluation
      disc hemorrhages, 206
      neuroretinal rim loss, 204–205
      optic disc photographs, 203
      quality evaluation, 203–204
      retinal nerve fiber layer (RNFL) loss, 204–206
   senile sclerotic discs, 431
   stereo image viewing frequency, 227–228
   structural changes, 176–178

OptiPranolol, 599
Optineurin, 96
Optineurin GLC1E, 1011
Oral carbonic anhydrase inhibitors, 572, 605–606
Osmitrol, 612, 613
Osmoglyn, 612, 613
Overfiltration and wound leakage, 494

# P

PAC. *See* Primary angle closure
PACG. *See* Primary angle-closure glaucoma
Pachymetry
    advantages and disadvantages, 85
    anterior segment optical coherence tomography (AS-OCT), 84
    central corneal thickness CCT measurement, 84–86
    consistency, 85
    Goldmann applanation tonometry (GAT), 85
    partial coherence interferometry, 85
    ultrasound, 84
PACS. *See* Primary angle-closure suspect
Panretinal photocoagulation (PRP), 522
Parasympathomimetic agents
    classes, 610
    local and systemic side effects, 611
Pars plana tube insertion devices, 820
Pars plana vitrectomy, 919
Partial radial sphincterotomy, 898
Pathogenesis
    malignant glaucoma
        aqueous misdirection or posterior aqueous diversion, 490, 491
        ciliary block, 491
        vitreous cavity, 491, 492
        vitreous mechanisms, 492
    POAG
        aqueous humor, 411
        ocular perfusion pressure (OPP), 411–413
        population studies, OPP, 411
        proteoglycan biosynthesis and degradation, 411–413
Patient examination
    consultation reports and dictations, 320
    digital image analysis, 319
    dilation, 316
    gonioscopy
        anterior chamber angle, 314–316
        Posner style goniolens, 314–315
    indigent patients, 319
    intake process
        consent for dilation, 303, 325
        consent for medical photography, 303, 326
        Medical History Questionnaire (MHQ), 302, 321–322
        ophthalmic assistant role, 303–307
        physician role, 307
        welcome letter, 302–303, 323–324
    ophthalmic assistant role
        chart review
        glaucoma consultation report, 327–330
        information recording, 4–7
        language translation
        open-ended and directed questions
    physician role, 307
    refill requests, 319–320
    slit-lamp
        anterior chamber (AC), 313–314
        conjunctiva, 308–309
        cornea, 309–313
        extraocular muscles and lids, 307

        iris, 308
        lens, 316
        optic nerve and retinal nerve fiber layer, 317
        pupils, 307–308
        retina, 317–319
    telephone appointment booking process
        medical records, 301
        visual field print-out, 302
        Zeiss-Humphrey visual field examination (HVF), 302
Pattern (PERG) electroretinogram, 265–266
Penetrating keratoplasty (PK)-glaucoma
    incidence and medical therapy, 883
    mechanisms, 883
    surgical management
        cyclophotocoagulation (CPC), 884
        glaucoma drainage implants, 883–884
        trabeculectomy with mitomycin C, 883
Peng Khaw's adjustable suture technique, 777
Peripapillary atrophy (PPA), 195
Peripheral anterior synechia (PAS), 519
Peripheral iridectomy (PI), 781
Peripheral iris, 499, 501
Phacoemulsification surgery, 762
Phacotrabeculotomy, 794
Pharmacokinetics, Intravitreal triamcinolone (IVTA), 671
Phospholine, 611, 684, 685, 767
Photodisruption, 753
Photorefractive keratectomy (PRK) effects, 424–425
Photovaporization, 753
Physician Quality Reporting Initiative (PQRI), 389
Pigmentary dispersion syndrome (PDS)
    asymmetric or unilateral, 502
    differential diagnosis, 502
    examination, 501–502
    inheritance, 502–503
    pathophysiology
        iris transillumination defects, 499, 500
        Krukenberg spindle, 499, 500
        mechanisms, 499
        peripheral iris, 499, 501
        pupillary block, 499
        trabecular meshwork, 499, 500
    presentation, 500–501
    temporal evolution, 503
    treatment, 503–504
pilocarpine, 26, 73, 75, 149, 304, 359, 414, 451, 472, 475, 476, 484, 503, 504, 531, 573, 586, 595, 598, 600, 608, 611, 633–635, 652, 657, 684, 685, 725, 744, 746, 767, 803, 844, 892, 909
Plateau iris
    anterior segment imaging, 468
    configuration and syndrome, 463
Pneumatonometer, IOP, 40
Polaroid photography, 227
Portable lightweight handheld electronic magnifiers, 363
Posner lens, 465–466
Posner–Schlossman syndrome (PSS), 537
Posner style goniolens, 314–315
Posterior aqueous diversion syndrome. *See* Malignant glaucoma
Posterior corneal lamellar surgery, DSEK, 886
Posterior uveitis, 534–535
Post-herpetic neuralgia (PHN), 549, 550
Postoperative bleb evaluation
    anatomical sites, 783–784
    bleb leakage, 785
    flat blebs, 785–786
    iris tissue, 786

Postoperative considerations, 913–914
Preferred retinal locus (PRL), 372
Pregnancy
    glaucoma therapy
        β-blockers, 674
        concentration and frequency, 674–675
        medications' effects, 673–674
        miotics, 674
        prostaglandin analogs, 674
    intraocular pressure (IOP), 673
    laser trabeculoplasty, 675
Preoperative considerations, 913
Primary angle closure (PAC)
    acute and sub-acute
        laser and surgical treatment, 472–473
        medical treatment, 472
        narrow or occludable anterior chamber angle, 473–475
        signs, 471–472
        symptoms, 471
    management, 742
    risk factors
        age, race and gender, 470
        biometrics, 470–471
        genetic predisposition, 470
        iris cross-sectional area, 471
Primary angle-closure glaucoma (PACG), 462
Primary angle-closure suspect (PACS), 461
Primary congenital glaucoma (PCG)
    angle histopathology, 569
    diagnoses, 570
    epidemiology and genetics, 569–570
    infantile, 567
    trabecular meshwork, 569
Primary open angle glaucoma (POAG)
    CD44
        cell growth and survival, 945–947
        cell signalling, 945
        functions, 939
        interactions, 939–940
        localization, 941
        NF-κB and lactate stress, 948
    clinical assessment
        generalized enlargement, 406
        glaucoma suspect situation, 409–410
        Goldmann-style 3 mirror lens, 404, 405
        gonioscopy lenses, 404
        nerve fiber layer hemorrhage, 408
        preferred practice pattern (PPP), 405
        superior nerve fiber layer hemorrhage, 408
        thin rim inferiorly with nerve fiber layer, 408
        vertical elongation, 434–436
        Zeiss-style 4 mirror lens, 404
    cost, 414
    definition, 400
    genetics, 400–401
    Gonio lens
        narrow angle, 401
        open angle, 400
    pathogenesis
        aqueous humor, 411
        population studies, OPP, 411
        proteoglycan biosynthesis and degradation, 411–413
    patient unawareness, 399, 400
    risk factors
        early manifest glaucoma trial (EMGT), 401, 402
        intraocular pressure (IOP), 401
        ocular hypertensives (OHTS), 401
        types, 403
    risk of monocular or binocular blindness, 399, 400
    sCD44
        Alzheimer's disease, 941–943
        antagonists, 947
        aqueous humor concentration, 943–944
        cell growth and survival, 945–947
        cell signaling, 945
        disease process, 944–945
        ectodomain shedding, 941
        internalization of, 947–948
        NF-κB and lactate stress, 948
    treatment and compliance, 414–415
    Zeiss-style 4 mirror lens, 400
Primary open-angle glaucoma (POAG), 104
PRK effects. *See* Photorefractive keratectomy effects
Prognosis
    future treatment, 1019
    intraocular pressure (IOP), 1015
    open-angle glaucoma treatment, 1018–1019
    risk calculations, 1018
    risk factors, 1016–1017
    structural and functional changes, 1017–1018
    technologies, 1018
Progression characteristics, normal pressure glaucoma
    age, gender and refractive error, 444–445
    risk factors, 442, 443
    VF damage
        color disc, 436, 439, 442
        dense paracentral VFD, 439–442
        SITA standard, 442–447
    VF test, 436–442
    measurement
        axon screamometer, 15
        functional and structural tests, 13
        provisos, 12
        visual loss effects, 13–15
Progressive iris atrophy, 553
Propine, 591, 609, 972
Prostaglandin analogs
    bimatoprost, 27–30, 307, 415, 513, 548, 573, 593, 599–605, 615, 616, 629–635, 685, 897, 966, 970
    latanoprost, 27–30, 51, 56, 75, 414, 513, 548, 573, 585, 591, 593, 599–604, 615, 616, 629–635, 637, 638, 644, 674, 685, 686, 897, 966, 970
    Lumigan, 304, 600, 638, 966
    pseudophakic cystoid macular edema, 902
    Rescula, 600, 966
    systemic side effects
        pharmacology and physiology, 685
        systemic reactions and clinical recommendations, 685–686
    Travatan, 304, 414, 592, 600, 966
    Travatan Z, 592, 600
    travoprost, 27–29, 56, 87, 415, 513, 573, 591, 593, 599–604, 615, 616, 629–635, 685, 966
    unoprostone, 600, 601, 685
    Xalatan, 60, 304, 600, 966
Pseudo neovascularization, NVG
    clinical presentations
        anterior segment NV, 518
        contraction, 520
        IOP rate, 520
        iris angiogram, 519
        massive end-stage fibrosis, 519
        peripheral anterior synechia (PAS), 519

smooth muscle antigen (SMA), 519
  VEGF influence, 519
 differential diagnosis, 515–518
Pupillary block, 467–468
Pupil management, 898–900
Pupil-stretching technique, 899
Purite, 591, 609, 631, 638
Pycnogenol
 angiotensin-converting enzyme (ACE), 663
 composition, 662
 cytotoxicity, 663
 oral administration, 662
 vascular endothelial cells, 663

## Q
Q-switched laser, 713
Quality of life (QOL) measurement
 familiarity and application, 18
 human resources utilization, 18–19
 instruments, 18
 questionnaire, 19
Quercetin, 663

## R
Radial sphincterotomy, 898
Rectangular scleral flap technique, 774–775
Refractive surgery
 intraoperative considerations, 913–914
 preoperative considerations, 913
Relative risk reduction (RRR), 30
Rescula, 600, 966
Resveratrol, 663
Retinal ganglion cells (RGCs)
 anti-self T cells, 928
 cell death mechanisms
  apoptosis, 647
  excitotoxicity, 647
  genes control, 647
  metabolic substrates, 647
  neurotrophin, 647
  nitric oxide synthase, 648
  optic nerve, 648
 Citicoline, 659
 histologic studies, 647
 immune system, 927
 neuroprotection
  causes, 648–649
  excitotoxicity and antioxidants, 648
  gene therapy, 648
  immune system, 648
  natural compounds, 649
  technique, 649
 protective autoimmunity, 928
Retinal nerve fiber layer (RNFL)
    photography, 223–224
Retinal oximetry, 128–129
Retinal surgery
 intravitreal gas, 918–919
 panretinal photocoagulation, 918
 pars plana vitrectomy, 918
 scleral buckle, 917
 silicone oil, 919–920
Retina vessel analyzer (RVA), 128
Retinopathy of prematurity (ROP), 517
RGC nerve fiber layer, electroretinography, 265
Rhegmatogenous retinal detachment, 564

Risk factors
 central corneal thickness (CCT)
  case presentation, 79
  corneal hysteresis, 87–88
  correction factors, 87
  differences, 80–83
  drug effect, 87
  measuring methods, 83–87
  practical aspects, 88
 genetics
  angle closure glaucoma, 97
  congenital glaucoma, 96
  definitions and nomenclature, 91–94
  early observations, 94
  exfoliation glaucoma, 96
  genes and loci associated, 92
  gene therapy, 97
  genetic testing, 97–98
  mesodermal dysgenesis syndromes, 97
  pharmacogenetics, 98
  potential phenotypic differences, OAG, 93
  types of glaucoma, 94–96
 intraocular pressure (IOP), 509, 545, 673
  Advanced Glaucoma Intervention Study (AGIS), 51
  aqueous humor production and outflow, 35–36
  clinical import, 56–57
  continuous monitoring method, 59–63
  cyclic oscillations, 54
  distribution, 41
  diurnal role, 54
  early manifest glaucoma trial (EMGT), 51
  history, glaucoma link, 35
  influencing factors, 41–43
  intravitreal triamcinolone (IVTA) effects, 671–672
  long-term IOP fluctuation, 51
  measurement, 39–41
  medication efficacy analysis, 56
  medications influence, 43–44
  nocturnal and diurnal IOP, 55
  ocular hypertensive patients, 53
  randomized clinical trials, EMGT, 38
  rapid oscillations, 52
  risk factor, glaucoma development, 38
  target IOP, 44
  tonometry measurements, 54
 obstructive sleep apnea syndrome (OSA)
  apnea/hypopnea index (AHI), 135
  normal-tension glaucoma (NTG), 136
  retinal nerve fiber layer (RNFL), 136
  sleep disordered breathing (SDB), 135
  treatment, 136
 ocular blood flow
  anatomy, 112–113
  ischemia and optic neuropathy, 111–112
  measuring methods, 120–129
  open angle glaucoma (OAG), 115–119
  optic nerve vascular anatomy, 113–114
  prospective studies, glaucoma patients, 120
  regulation, 114–115
  vascular risk factors, OAG, 115–119
  visual function and structure, 129–130
 signs and conditions
 race/ethnicity
  age, 104–105
  incidence, 104
  Latinos, 102–103

Risk factors (Con't)
  non-ocular risk factors, 107
  ocular risk factors, 105–106
  prevalence, 101
  primary open-angle glaucoma (POAG), 104
  variability, 103–104

## S
Sapphire laser trabeculoplasty (SLT), 757
Sara document reader, 364
Scanning laser ophthalmoscope (SLO)
  fluorescein angiography, 122–123
  indocyanine green angiography, 123–124
Scanning laser polarimetry (SLP), 210, 220
Scanning peripheral anterior chamber depth analyzer (SPAC), 467
sCD44. See Hyaluronic acid receptor CD44 (sCD44)
Schiotz tonometry, IOP, 41
Schlemm's canal outflow
  ab externo devices
    deep dissection, 801
    iScience microcatheter, 802
    laser goniopuncture, 804
    prolene suture and knots, 803
    scleral flap, 800–801
    trabeculodescemet window (TDW), 801–802
  ab interno devices
    trabectome handpiece, 805–807
    trabecular micro-bypass iStent, 805
  distal system, 797
  proximal system, 796–797
  scleral flap
    exposing technique, 790–792
    location, 790
    opening technique, 792–794
  vs. trabecular meshwork, 797
  tubules, 1012
Schwalbe's line, 315–316
Scleral buckle, 917
Scleral spur (SS), 315
Sealing hypotonous cyclodialysis clefts, 734
Selective alpha agonists, systemic side effects
  pharmacology and physiology, 683
  systemic reactions, 683–684
Selective laser trabeculoplasty (SLT)
  anterior chamber angle, 718
  postoperative care, 716
  treatment and settings, 716
Senile sclerotic disc, 199
Sequential stereoscopic optic disc photography
  Allen stereo separator, 224
  manual shift technique, 224
Serologic evaluation, nonglaucomatous optic atrophy, 280
Serous choroidal effusions
  conservative management, 868
  diagnosis and symptomatology, 867
  filtering bleb and sclerostomy, 868
  vs. hemorrhagic choroidals, 867
  reform methods, 869
Silicone oil, 919–920
Simultaneous stereoscopic optic disc photography, 224–225
Sleep disordered breathing (SDB), 135
Slit-lamp examination
  anterior chamber (AC), 313–314
  conjunctiva, 308–309
  cornea, 309–313
  extraocular muscles and lids, 307
  iris, 308
  lens, 316–317
  optic nerve and retinal nerve fiber layer, 317
  pupils, 307–308
  retina, 317–318
Smooth muscle antigen (SMA), 520
Snuff syndrome, 850–851
SPAC. See Scanning peripheral anterior chamber depth analyzer
Stand magnifiers, 361–362
Statins
  HMG-CoA inhibitors, 703
  immune activity and LDL lowering potential, 703
  medications, 704–705
  optic nerve injury, 704
Stem cells, 953–954
Stereo color photography
  sequential, 224
  simultaneous, 224–225
Sterile neurotrophic ulcer, 550
Stress and agings, POAG, 936
Stretch theory, 1012
Stromal keratitis, 549, 550
Student's t-test, 145
Subconjunctival filtration
  anterior and posterior types, 796
  Ex-PRESS shunt devices
    gonioscopic view, 800
    sapphire blade, 799
    schematic diagram, 798
    vs. trabeculectomy, 800
Suprachoroidal outflow
  ab interno cyclodialysis, 797–798
  gold microshunt device
    fornix-based conjunctival peritomy, 807–811
    implantation, 807
    models, 807
Surgical techniques
  combined surgery, 900–901
  filtering bleb, 901
  pupil management, 898–900
Sussman lens, 466
Swing-arm electronic magnifiers, 363
Sympathomimetic agonists
  brimonidine, 609–610
  epinephrine, 608–609
  iopidine, 609
  systemic side effects
    nonselective agonists, 684
    pharmacology and physiology, 684
    systemic reactions, 684
  types, 608
Systemic side effects
  beta-adrenergic blockers
    cardiovascular medicine, 678
    pharmacology and physiology, 677–678
  carbonic anhydrase inhibitors
    physiology and pharmacology, 681
    systemic reactions, 605–606, 681–683
  hypotensive lipids (HLs), 603–604
  miotics
    pharmacology and physiology, 684–685
    systemic reactions, 685
  parasympathomimetic medications, 611
  prostaglandin analogs

pharmacology and physiology, 685
systemic reactions and clinical recommendations, 685–686
selective alpha agonists
pharmacology and physiology, 683
systemic reactions, 683–684
sympathomimetics
nonselective agonists, 684
pharmacology and physiology, 684
systemic reactions, 684
sympathomimetic agonists, 608–610
systemic reactions and clinical recommendations
advantage and disadvantage, 680–681
asthma and obstructive lung disease, 679
bradycardia and dysrhythmia, 679
depression, 679–680
lipoprotein inhibition, 680
topical beta-blockers, 600

## T

Targeting glaucomatous retinopathy and optic neuropathy, 986
Taurine, 663–664
T cut exposing technique, 789–792
Teachers of children with visual impairment (TCVI), 377
Telemetry, 12
Tenon's cyst, 779
Therapeutic armamentarium
laser procedures, 531
POAG, 531
surgery
aqueous drainage devices, 532
trabeculectomy, 531
Therapy and indications
adjunctive therapy and combination agents, 615–616
aqueous humor outflow, 588–590
colored glaucoma graph
activities of daily living (ADL), 158
cup/disc ratio system, 159
disc damage likelihood scale (DDLS), 160
treatment justification factors, 161
corneal penetration
drug penetration anatomy, 591
preservatives, 592–593
disease stage
definite damage, 162
purposes, 162
uncertain damage, 161–162
drug activity
parasympathetic nerve system, 595
sympathetic nerve system, 594–595
duration, 163
effectiveness and safety, 163–164
eye drops, 590–591
goals and approaches, 583
history taking primacy, 156
individualizing indications
change predicting speculations, 156
reasons, 156
intraocular pressure (IOP) control
circadian variation, aqueous humor dynamics, 584–586
multicenter, randomized clinical trials, 587–588
maximum tolerated medical therapy (MTMT), 584
medications
beta-adrenergic antagonists, 598–600
carbonic anhydrase inhibitors (CAI), 605–608
drug selection characteristics, 596–597
hyperosmotics, 612–615
hypotensive lipids (HLs), 600–605
intraocular pressure-lowering effects, 599
parasympathomimetic agents, 610–611
sympathomimetic agonists, 608–610
treatment options and timeline, 598
pragmatic considerations, 616–617
predictors of
intraocular pressure (IOP), 157
standard risk factors, 157–158
visual field, 158
prostaglandins vs. prostamides
bimatoprost, 593
nasolacrimal occlusion digital massage technique, 594
socioeconomic factors, 164
treatment purposes, 155–156
Timolol GFS, 599, 600
timolol hemihydrate, 599
timolol maleate, 599, 674, 967
Timoptic, 304, 592, 599, 600, 967, 972
Timoptic Ocudose, 592, 599
Timoptic XE, 599, 600
Tocotrienol, 658
Tolerable treatment
lasers, 16
medications, 16
surgical techniques, 16–17
Tonometry, 306–307
Tono-pen tonometry, IOP, 40
Topical beta-blockers, 600
Topical carbonic anhydrase inhibitors, 607
Topical steroids, 549, 550
Trabectome surgery
IOP reduction, medications, 837–838
scanning electron micrograph, 836
Trabecular bypass surgical gonioscope, 833
Trabecular cells
age, 1011
CD44 toxic, 1012
oxidation and senescence, 1011
size and volume, 1012
Trabecular iStent
applicator tubing, 834
development, 831–832
gonioscopes, 833
Trabecular meshwork (TM)
Fuchs' Endothelial Dystrophy, 557
gonioscopy, 317
injury, 563
schematic diagram, 958
Trabeculectomy
alternative filtration routes, 765
AMT, 861–862
anesthesia, 765–766
anterior chamber paracentesis, 774
anticoagulants, 769–770
antimetabolites
avascular cystic bleb, 778
complications, 780
encapsulated bleb, 779
conjunctival closure, 781–782
conjunctival incision
limbal-base vs. fornix-base techniques, 768, 772–773
Tenon's capsule, 771
wet field cautery, 771

Trabeculectomy (Con't)
   corneoscleral flap, 766
   external approach, Schlemm's canal
      location, 790
         opening technique, 792–794
         T cut exposing technique, 789–792
   eye exposure, 766, 768
   failure and complications, 575
   flap suturing techniques, 776–777
   5-fluorouracil and mitomycin C, 452–453
   guarded filtration procedure, 765
   intraocular pressure (IOP), 767–768
   peripheral iridectomy (PI), 781
   PK-glaucoma, 883
   postoperative follow-up
      bleb evaluation, 783–786
      complications, 783
   potential candidates, 790
   procedure, 574–575
   scleral flap
      corneal tunnel and surgical limbus, 775
      rectangular technique, 774–775
      triangular technique, 774–776
   technique, 575
   traction suture, 768
Trabeculoplasty
   history
      continuous wave laser system, 714–715
      micropulsed diode laser trabeculoplasty (MDLT), 715–716
      spot size, 716
   indications and contraindications
      beneficial response, 714
      IOP reduction, 714
   methods
      complications, 718
      continuous wave laser system, 716
      inflammation, 718
      infrared laser energy application, 722–723
      instruments comparison, 719–721
      IOP response, 718–719
      micropulsed diode laser trabeculoplasty, 717–718
      preparation, 716
      pressure spikes, 718
      selective laser trabeculoplasty, 716
Trabeculotomy
   indication, 574
   results, 574
   technique, 574
Transpalpebral scleral palpation, IOP, 40
Travatan, 304, 414, 592, 600, 966
Travatan Z, 592, 600
travoprost, 27–29, 56, 87, 415, 513, 573, 591, 593, 599–604, 615, 616, 629–635, 685, 966
Trial frame refractions
   Halberg clips, 357
   Oculus universal, 356
Triangular scleral flap technique, 774–776
Trusopt, 607
Tube shunt surgery
   hypertensive phase (HP)
      etiology, 824–825
      treatment techniques, 825–826
   TVT, 814–815
Tube Versus Trabeculectomy Study (TVT), 814–815

**U**

Ultrasound biomicroscope (UBM)
   anterior segment imaging, 467–468
   axial resolutions, 293
   ciliary body cleft, 300
   ciliary sulcus posterior, iris, 300
   cyst, 298
   higher frequency, 293
   iris, pigment dispersion, 299
   narrow angle, plateau component., 297
   normal angle, 294
   occludable angle, 296
   peripheral anterior synechiae, 298
   pupillary block angle closure, 296
Uveitic angle closure management, 532
Uveitis-related elevation, IOP
   acute uveitic angle closure
      Iris bombe, 528, 529
      non-pupillary block, 529
      pupillary block, 528–529
   chronic, mixed-mechanism ocular hypertension, 530
   corticosteroid-induced ocular hypertension, 529
   IOHS
      herpes zoster keratouveitis, 528, 529
      Posner Schlossman syndrome, 528

**V**

Valved implants
   Ahmed type, 813, 816
   Eagle Vision type, 816
Varicella–zoster virus (VZV), 549
Vascular risk factors
   hypertension, blood flow, and glaucoma risk
      blood pressure, 694
      intraocular pressure, 695
      optic nerve, 964
   systolic blood pressure, 693nocturnal hypotension, 116
   ocular perfusion pressure, 116–119
   systemic hypertension and hypotension, 115–116
Vision distance test chart, 354–355
Visual acuity
   blindness standard, 352
   measurement
      Bailey–Lovie near reading card, 355
      trial frame refractions, 356–357
      vision distance test chart, 354–355
      visual field assessment, 355
Visual evoked potential (VEP) electroretinogram, 266
Visual field assessment, 355
Visual field defects
   age, gender and refractive error, 444–445
   patterns of loss, 433–436
   progression characteristics, 436–445
      age, gender and refractive error, 444–445
      risk factors, 442, 443
      VF damage, 436–448
      VF test, 436–442
Visual function
   automated visual fields
      Humphrey *vs.* Goldmann, 251
      nonspecific defects, 252
   hill of vision
      Humphrey field analyzer, 230
      procedure, 229
      schematic representation, 230

testing, 230, 233
visual field defects, 231
Humphrey field analyzer
multiple field analysis, 257
single field analysis, 254–257
test frequency, 253–254
screening methods
effectiveness, 239
flicker perimetry, 244, 245
frequency doubling technology perimetry, 240, 242
high pass resolution perimetry (HPRP), 244, 246
kinetic *vs.* static perimetry, 236–238
motion perimetry, 240, 243
multifocal electroretinograms, 246–247
multifocal visual evoked potentials, 247, 248
rarebit perimetry, 244, 246
short wavelength automated perimetry (SWAP), 239–241
structural *vs.* functional methods, 229–236
testing strategies
threshold evaluation, 247
visual field screening, 247–248
Vitamin E. *See* Alpha-tocopherol

**W**
Water-drinking test (WDT), 12
WDR36, 96
Weill–Marchesani syndrome, 475–476
Wet field cautery, 771

**X**
Xalacom, 616, 631, 634, 635, 970, 1018
Xalatan, 60, 304, 600, 966

**Y**
YAG iridotomy, 895

**Z**
Zeaxanthine, 662
Zeiss lens, 465
Zeiss-style 4 mirror lens, 404
ZoomText magnifier, 364